D0535195

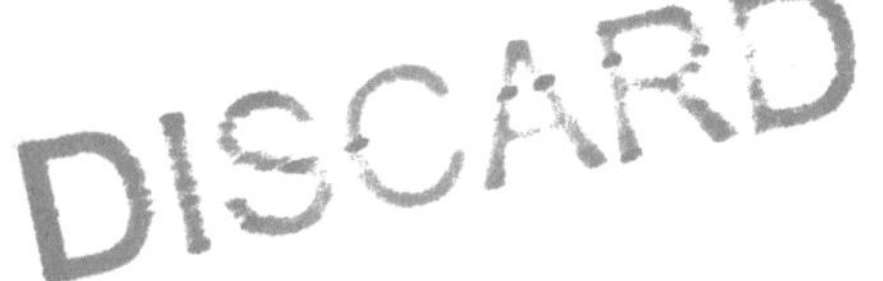
For Reference
Not to be taken from this room

Clinical Management of POISONING AND DRUG OVERDOSE

Clinical Management of POISONING AND DRUG OVERDOSE

LESTER M. HADDAD, MD
Attending Emergency Physician and Active Staff
Bon Secours St. Francis Xavier Hospital
Clinical Professor in Family Medicine
Medical University of South Carolina
Charleston, South Carolina
Active Staff, St. Joseph's Hospital
Consultant Staff, Memorial Medical Center
Savannah, Georgia

MICHAEL W. SHANNON, MD, MPH
Associate Chief of Emergency Services
Pediatric Emergency Medicine
Director, Lead and Toxicology Clinic
The Children's Hospital
Associate Professor of Pediatrics
Harvard Medical School
Staff Toxicologist
Massachusetts Poison Control System
Boston, Massachusetts

JAMES F. WINCHESTER, MD
Professor of Medicine
Division of Nephrology
Department of Medicine
Georgetown University Medical Center
Washington, DC

3rd edition

W.B. SAUNDERS COMPANY
A Division of Harcourt Brace & Company
Philadelphia London Toronto Montreal Sydney Tokyo

W.B. SAUNDERS COMPANY
A Division of Harcourt Brace & Company

The Curtis Center
Independence Square West
Philadelphia, Pennsylvania 19106

Library of Congress Cataloging-in-Publication Data

Clinical management of poisoning and drug overdose / [edited by] Lester M. Haddad, Michael W. Shannon, James F. Winchester—3rd ed.

p. cm.

Includes bibliographical references and index.

ISBN 0–7216–6409–1

1. Poisoning. 2. Medication abuse. 3. Drugs—Overdosage. I. Haddad, Lester M. II. Shannon, Michael W. III. Winchester, James F. [DNLM: 1. Poisoning—therapy. 2. Overdose—therapy. QV 600 C639 1998]

RA1211.C584 1998 615.9′08—dc20

DNLM/DLC 96–43968

CLINICAL MANAGEMENT OF POISONING AND DRUG OVERDOSE, 3rd Edition ISBN 0–7216–6409–1

Printed in the United States of America.

Last digit is the print number: 9 8 7 6 5 4 3 2 1

To all the pioneers of toxicology.

James F. Winchester, MD

To my beloved family, Elaine, Evan, and Lila,
whose patience made this possible,
and to my parents for their inspiration.

Michael W. Shannon, MD

To my wonderful friend and colleague of 20 years, Jim Winchester,
always thoughtful and generous,
and to Michael Shannon,
for putting his heart and energy into our creation.

Lester M. Haddad, MD

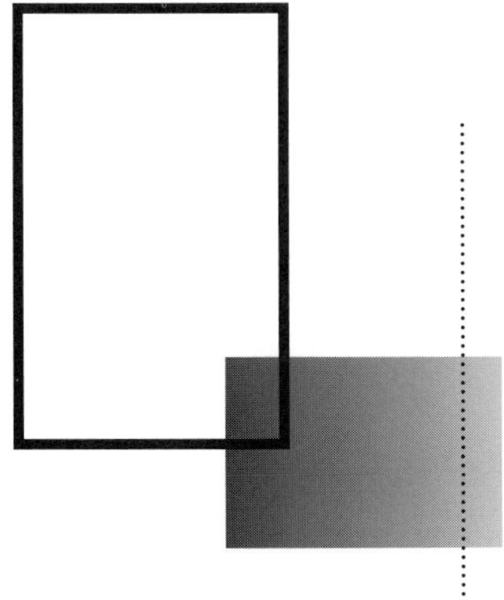

Contributors

Jawaid Akhtar, MD
Medical Toxicology Fellow, Pennsylvania State University College of Medicine, Hershey, Pennsylvania
Clinical Neurotoxicology

Timothy E. Albertson, MD, PhD
Professor of Medicine and Pharmacology and Toxicology, Medical Director, University of California, Davis, Medical Center, Regional Poison Control Center; Chief, Division of Pulmonary and Critical Care Medicine, University of California, Davis, School of Medicine, Sacramento, California
Cocaine; Amphetamines

Alfred Aleguas, Jr., RPh, PharmD
Adjunct Clinical Professor, University of Rhode Island, Kingston; Certified Specialist in Poison Information, Rhode Island Poison Control Center, Rhode Island Hospital, Providence, Rhode Island
Petroleum Distillates and Turpentine

Roblee P. Allen, MD
Associate Professor of Clinical Internal Medicine, Division of Pulmonary and Critical Care Medicine, University of California, Davis, School of Medicine, Davis, California
Amphetamines

John Ambre, MD, PhD
Formerly Associate Professor, Department of Medicine, Northwestern University Medical School; Attending Physician, Northwestern Memorial Hospital; American Medical Association, Chicago, Illinois
Principles of Pharmacology for the Clinician

Angela C. Anderson, MD
Assistant Professor, Brown University School of Medicine; Attending Physician, Hasbro Children's Hospital, Department of Pediatric Emergency Medicine; Medical Consultant, Rhode Island Poison Control Center, Rhode Island Hospital, Providence, Rhode Island
Toxic Injury to the Eye

Robert Bartlett, MD
Vice Chair, Emergency Medicine, Richland Memorial Hospital, University of South Carolina School of Medicine, Columbia; Associate Professor of Pharmacy, University of South Carolina, Columbia; Director, Hyperbaric Medicine, Richland Memorial Hospital, University of South Carolina School of Medicine, Columbia, South Carolina; Diving Medical Officer, National Oceanic and Atmospheric Administration, Washington, DC
Carbon Monoxide Poisoning; Phenol and Related Agents

Brian A. Bates, MD
Clinical Assistant Professor of Pediatrics, University of Texas Health Science Center at San Antonio; Director, Children's Emergency Center, Methodist Women's and Children's Hospital, San Antonio, Texas
Mercury

Neal L. Benowitz, MD
Professor of Medicine and Chief, Division of Clinical Pharmacology and Toxicology, University of California San Francisco; Staff Physician, San Francisco General Hospital; Consultant, Northern California Bay Area Poison Control Center, San Francisco, California
Cardiac Disturbances

Michelle Blanda, MD
Assistant Professor of Emergency Medicine, Northeastern Ohio Universities College of Medicine, Rootstown; Research Director, Attending Physician, Department of Emergency Medicine, Summa Health System, Akron, Ohio
Freon and Other Inhalants

Jeffrey L. Blumer, PhD, MD
Professor of Pediatrics and Pharmacology, Case Western Reserve University School of Medicine; Chief, Division of Pediatric Pharmacology and Critical Care, Medical Director, Greater Cleveland Poison Control Center, Rainbow Babies and Childrens Hospital, Cleveland, Ohio
Drug-Drug Interactions

Jonathan Borak, MD
Associate Clinical Professor of Medicine, Yale University; Consulting Physician, Department of Emergency Medicine, St Raphael's Hospital; Member, Yale Occupational and Environmental Medicine Program, Yale–New Haven Hospital, New Haven, Connecticut
Chlorine

George Braitberg, MB, BS
Senior Associate, Department of Medicine, Faculty of Medicine and Dentistry, University of Melbourne, Parkville; Director of Emergency Medicine, Consultant Medical Toxicologist, Austin and Repatriation Medical Centre, Heidelberg, Victoria, Australia
Poisonous Plants

Mary H. Branton, MD
Assistant Professor, George Washington University School of Medicine; Dialysis Director, Veterans Affairs Medical Center, Washington, DC
Chemotherapeutic Agents and Transplant Agents—Transplant Agents

Jeffrey Brent, MD, PhD
Associate Clinical Professor of Medicine, Surgery, and Pediatrics, University of Colorado Health Sciences Center, Denver, Colorado
Mushrooms; Monoamine Oxidase Inhibitors and the Serotonin Syndrome

Keith K. Burkhart, MD
Associate Professor of Medicine and Pharmacology, Pennsylvania State University College of Medicine; Medical Director, Central Pennsylvania Poison Center, The Milton S. Hershey Medical Center, Hershey, Pennsylvania
Clinical Neurotoxicology

Michael J. Burns, MD
Instructor of Medicine, Harvard Medical School; Associate of Medicine, Section of Toxicology, Division of Emergency Medicine, Beth Israel Deaconess Medical Center, Boston, Massachusetts
The Antipsychotic Drugs

Louis Cannon, MD
Assistant Professor, Departments of Emergency Medicine and Cardiology, Michigan State University School of Medicine; Chairman, Department of Internal Medicine, The Heart Group, Saginaw, Michigan
Ammonia, Nitrogen, Nitrogen Oxides, and Related Compounds

Thomas R. Caraccio, PharmD
Assistant Professor of Toxicology/Pharmacology, New York College of Osteopathic Medicine, Old Westbury; Clinical Manager, Long Island Regional Poison Control Center, Winthrop University Hospital, Mineola, New York
Volatile Substance Abuse

Frederick B. Carlton, Jr., MD
Associate Professor of Emergency Medicine, University of Mississippi Medical Center; Associate Professor of Emergency Medicine, University Hospitals and Clinics, Jackson, Mississippi
The Organophosphates and Other Insecticides

Michael W. Carlton, MD
Fellow, Department of Medical Toxicology, Good Samaritan Regional Medical Center; Medical Director, META Center, Phoenix, Arizona
Hematologic Consequences of Poisoning; Hydrofluoric Acid; Ergot

Marcel Casavant, MD
Assistant Professor of Emergency Medicine and Pediatrics, The Ohio State University; Consulting Toxicologist, Central Ohio Poison Center, Columbus, Ohio
Lidocaine

William K. Chiang, MD
Clinical Assistant Professor of Surgery/Emergency Medicine, New York University School of Medicine; Attending Physician, Emergency Department, Bellevue Hospital Center, New York, New York; Medical Director, Hudson Valley Poison Center, North Tarrytown, New York
Radiation Poisoning

James Cisek, MD
Clinical Assistant Professor of Emergency Medicine, Wayne State University School of Medicine, Detroit; Program Director, Emergency Medicine, William Beaumont Hospital, Royal Oak, Michigan
Disaster Management of Massive Toxic Exposure

David J. Cohen, MD, PhD
Assistant Professor of Medicine, George Washington University School of Medicine; Assistant Chief, Renal Section, Medical Service, Veterans Affairs Medical Center, Washington, DC
Chemotherapeutic Agents and Transplant Agents—Transplant Agents

Steven C. Curry, MD
Associate Professor of Clinical Medicine, University of Arizona College of Medicine; Director, Department of Medical Toxicology, Associate Director, Samaritan Regional Poison Center, Good

Samaritan Regional Medical Center, Phoenix, Arizona
Hematologic Consequences of Poisoning

William E. Davis, MD
Assistant Professor, Department of Emergency Medicine, Emory University School of Medicine, Atlanta, Georgia
Thrombolytic Agents and Anticoagulants

Sheila Dawling, PhD
Associate Professor of Pathology, Vanderbilt University School of Medicine; Director, Analytical Toxicology Laboratories, Vanderbilt University Medical Center, Nashville, Tennessee
Sedatives

Kathleen A. Delaney, MD
Assistant Professor of Surgery, Division of Emergency Medicine, University of Texas Southwestern Medical School; Staff Physician, Parkland Memorial Hospital, Dallas, Texas
Ethanol

Andrew R. Donato, MD
Clinical Associate Professor of Surgery, University of South Carolina School of Medicine, Columbia; Attending Emergency Physician, Lexington Medical Center, Columbia, South Carolina
Cyanoacrylates

J. Ward Donovan, MD
Associate Professor of Medicine, Pennsylvania State University College of Medicine; Director, Central Pennsylvania Poison Center, The Milton S. Hershey Medical Center, Pennsylvania State University, Hershey, Pennsylvania
Nonsteroidal Anti-Inflammatory Drugs and Colchicine

Constance J. Doyle, MD
Clinical Instructor, Section of Emergency Medicine, Department of Surgery, University of Michigan Medical School; Core Faculty University of Michigan/St. Joseph Emergency Medicine Residency; Staff Attending Physician, St. Joseph Mercy Hospital, Ann Arbor, Michigan
Disaster Management of Massive Toxic Exposure

Milou-Daniel Drici, MD, PhD
Merck Fellow in Clinical Pharmacology, Division of Clinical Pharmacology, Georgetown University Medical Center, Washington, DC; Maître de Conférences des Universités de Pharmacologie Clinique, Université de Nice–Sophia Antipolis, Nice, France
Nitroprusside, ACE Inhibitors, and Selected Antihypertensive Agents

Garabed Eknoyan, MD
Professor of Medicine, Baylor College of Medicine, Houston, Texas
Renal Toxicity—Acute Renal Toxicity

Timothy B. Erickson, MD
Associate Professor, Emergency Medicine, Director, Division of Toxicology, Residency Director, University of Illinois at Chicago Department of Emergency Medicine, University of Illinois College of Medicine, Chicago, Illinois
Management Principles of Overdose in Pregnancy

Susan E. Farrell, MD
Assistant Professor, Department of Emergency Medicine, Division of Toxicology, Allegheny University of the Health Sciences, Medical College of Pennsylvania, Philadelphia, Pennsylvania
Benzodiazepines

Donald A. Feinfeld, MD
Professor of Clinical Medicine, State University of New York, Health Sciences Center at Stony Brook, Stony Brook; Associate Director of Nephrology, Nassau County Medical Center, East Meadow, New York
Volatile Substance Abuse

Richard Feldman, MD
Associate Professor of Clinical Emergency Medicine, University of Illinois at Chicago; Chairman, Department of Emergency Medicine, Illinois Masonic Medical Center, Chicago, Illinois
The Volatile Oils

Miguel C. Fernández, MD
Medical Director, South Texas Poison Center, University of Texas Health Science Center at San Antonio, San Antonio, Texas
North American Venomous Snakebite

David A. Flockhart, MD, PhD
Assistant Professor of Medicine and Pharmacology, Division of Clinical Pharmacology, Georgetown University Medical Center, Washington, DC
Nitroprusside, ACE Inhibitors, and Selected Antihypertensive Agents

Marsha Ford, MD
Clinical Associate Professor of Emergency Medicine, Department of Emergency Medicine, University of North Carolina, Chapel Hill; Director, Division of Toxicology, Assistant Chairman, Department of Emergency Medicine, Medical Director, Carolinas Poison Center, Carolinas Medical Center, Charlotte, North Carolina
Acids and Antacids

R. Brent Furbee, MD
Assistant Clinical Professor of Emergency Medicine, Indiana University; Medical Director, Indiana Poison Center, Methodist Hospital, Indianapolis, Indiana
Class IA Antiarrhythmics: Quinidine, Procainamide, and Disopyramide

Nora Goldschlager, MD
Professor of Clinical Medicine, University of California School of Medicine; Director, Coronary Care Unit, Cardiac Clinic and Pacemaker Clinic, and ECG Laboratory, San Francisco General Hospital, San Francisco, California
Cardiac Disturbances

Lloyd S. Goodman, MD
Clinical Professor, Department of Medicine, School of Medicine, Medical College of Georgia, Augusta; Associate Professor of Internal Medicine (Cardiology), Mercer University, School of Medicine, Macon; Medical Director, Department of Adult Cardiology, Memorial Medical Center, Savannah, Georgia
Digitalis

Andis Graudins, MBBS
Staff Specialist in Emergency Medicine and Medical Toxicology, Westmead Hospital, Westmead, New South Wales, Australia
Tear Gas and Riot Control Agents

Lester M. Haddad, MD
Attending Emergency Physician and Active Staff, Bon Secours St. Francis Xavier Hospital; Clinical Professor in Family Medicine, Medical University of South Carolina, Charleston, South Carolina; Active Staff, St. Joseph's Hospital; Consultant Staff, Memorial Medical Center, Savannah, Georgia
The Emergency Management of Poisoning; North American Venomous Snakebite; Toxic Marine Life; Tricyclic Antidepressants and Selective Serotonin Reuptake Inhibitors; Barbiturates; Antibiotics and Anthelminthics—Antibiotics; The Organophosphates and Other Insecticides; Phenol and Related Agents; LSD, Natural Hallucinogens, and Miscellany

Alan H. Hall, MD
Clinical Assistant Professor of Preventive Medicine and Biometrics, University of Colorado Health Sciences Center, Denver; Editor-in-Chief, TOMES and TOMES Plus Information Systems, Micromedex, Inc, Englewood; Senior Consultant, Rocky Mountain Poison and Drug Center, Denver, Colorado
Arsenic and Arsine; Cyanide and Related Compounds

Darell E. Heiselman, DO
Professor, Internal Medicine, Northeastern Ohio Universities College of Medicine, Rootstown; Chief, Critical Care Medicine, Akron General Medical Center, Akron, Ohio
Benzene and the Aromatic Hydrocarbons

Grady H. Hendrix, MD
Professor of Medicine, Division of Cardiology, Medical University of South Carolina, Charleston, South Carolina
The New Cardiac Antiarrhythmic Agents

Fred M. Henretig, MD
Associate Professor of Pediatrics, University of Pennsylvania School of Medicine; Director, Section of Clinical Toxicology, Children's Hospital of Philadelphia; Medical Director, The Poison Control Center, Philadelphia, Pennsylvania
The Vitamins

Stephen M. Herman, MD
Private Practice, Department of Internal Medicine, St. Joseph Hospital, Savannah, Georgia
Antibiotics and Anthelminthics—Antibiotics

Thomas S. Herman, PhD
Technical Director, LabCorp, Tampa Division, Tampa, Florida
Appendix: Chemical Conversions of Toxicologic Laboratory Values

Thomas J. Hetrick, MD
Assistant Professor of Emergency Medicine, Northeastern Ohio Universities College of Medicine, Rootstown; Emergency Medicine Attending Staff Physician, Akron General Medical Center, Akron, Ohio
Ammonia, Nitrogen, Nitrogen Oxides, and Related Compounds

Walter J. Hunter, PharmD
Clinical Assistant Professor, University of South Carolina, College of Pharmacy; Clinical Pharmacist, Internal Medicine, Richland Memorial Hospital, Columbia, South Carolina
Principles of Pharmacology for the Clinician

Ian D. Jones, MD
Resident Physician, Department of Emergency Medicine, Vanderbilt University Medical Center, Nashville, Tennessee
Botulism and Food Poisoning

Jeffrey Jones, MD
Associate Professor, Department of Internal Medicine, Michigan State University College of Human Medicine, East Lansing; Research Director, Emergency Medicine Residency Program, Butterworth Hospital, Grand Rapids, Michigan
Industrial Toxicology

Katherine Jones, PharmD
Manager of Pharmacy Clinical Services, Memorial Medical Center, Savannah, Georgia
Pharmaceutical Excipients

Michael T. Kelley, MD
Associate Professor, Emergency Medicine and Pediatrics, Ohio State University; Medical Director, Central Ohio Poison Center, Children's Hospital, Columbus, Ohio
Sympathomimetics

Fergus Kerr, MB, BS, MPH
Medical Toxicology Fellow/Instructor, University of Pittsburgh; Medical Toxicology Fellow, University of Pittsburgh Medical Center, Pittsburgh, Pennsylvania
Salicylate Toxicity

Christopher Keyes, MD, MPH
Chief, Section of Toxicology, Division of Emergency Medicine, University of Texas Southwestern Medical Center; Medical Director, North Texas Poison Center, Dallas, Texas
Antibiotics and Anthelminthics—Anthelminthics

Daniel E. Keyler, PharmD
Associate Professor, College of Pharmacy, University of Minnesota; Co-Director, Toxicology Research, Department of Medicine, Hennepin County Medical Center, Minneapolis Medical Research Foundation, Minneapolis, Minnesota
Tricyclic Antidepressants and Selective Serotonin Reuptake Inhibitors

Mark A. Kirk, MD
Assistant Clinical Professor, Indiana University School of Medicine; Medical Toxicology Fellowship Director, Associate Medical Director, Indiana Poison Center, Methodist Hospital, Indianapolis, Indiana
Anticholinergics and Antihistamines

Kurt C. Kleinschmidt, MD
Assistant Professor of Surgery, Division of Emergency Medicine, University of Texas Southwestern Medical School; Staff Physician, Parkland Memorial Hospital, Dallas, Texas
Ethanol

Edward P. Krenzelok, PharmD
Professor of Pharmacy and Pediatrics, University of Pittsburgh Schools of Pharmacy and Medicine; Director, Pittsburgh Poison Center, Children's Hospital of Pittsburgh, Pittsburgh, Pennsylvania
Salicylate Toxicity

Kenneth Kulig, MD
Associate Clinical Professor, University of Colorado Health Sciences Center; Chairman, Department of Medicine, Director, Porter Regional Toxicology Center, Porter Care Hospital, Denver, Colorado
Mushrooms; Chlorophenoxy Herbicides and Dioxin Contaminants; Other Herbicides and Fungicides

Donald B. Kunkel, MD
Associate in Pharmacology and Toxicology, University of Arizona, Tucson; Medical Director, Samaritan Regional Poison Center, Good Samaritan Regional Medical Center, Phoenix, Arizona
Poisonous Arthropods—Scorpions; Poisonous Plants; Ergot

Paul W. Ladenson, MD
Professor of Medicine, Johns Hopkins University School of Medicine; Director, Division of Endocrinology and Metabolism, Johns Hopkins Hospital, Baltimore, Maryland
Thyroid

Christopher P. Langford, MD
Attending Emergency Physician, Lexington Medical Center, Columbia, South Carolina
Phenol and Related Agents

Richard F. Lee, PhD
Professor of Oceanography, Skidaway Institute of Oceanography, University of Georgia System, Savannah, Georgia
Toxic Marine Life

William J. Lewander, MD
Associate Professor of Pediatrics, Brown University School of Medicine; Director, Pediatric Emergency Medicine, Hasbro Children's Hospital; Medical Director, Rhode Island Poison Control Center, Rhode Island Hospital, Providence, Rhode Island
Petroleum Distillates and Turpentine

Erica L. Liebelt, MD
Director, Pediatric Emergency Services, Geisinger Medical Center, Danville; Medical Toxicology Consultant, Central Pennsylvania Poison Center, The Milton S. Hershey Medical Center, Hershey, Pennsylvania
Iron

James G. Linakis, PhD, MD
Associate Professor of Pediatrics, Brown University School of Medicine; Associate Director, Pediatric Emergency Medicine, Hasbro Children's Hospital/Rhode Island Hospital, Providence, Rhode Island
Toxic Emergencies in the Neonate

Christopher H. Linden, MD
Associate Professor, University of Massachusetts Medical School, Worcester, Massachusetts
Smoke Inhalation

Toby Litovitz, MD
Director, National Capital Poison Center; Professor, Emergency Medicine, Georgetown University Medical Center; Clinical Professor, Emergency Medicine, The George Washington University Medical Center, Washington, DC
Alkali Injury—The Miniature Battery Hazard

Frederick H. Lovejoy, Jr., MD
William Berenberg Professor of Pediatrics, Harvard Medical School; Associate Physician-in-Chief, The Children's Hospital, Boston, Massachusetts
Prevention of Childhood Poisonings

Judith K. Lucas, MD
Assistant Professor of Clinical Pediatrics, University of Arizona; Associate Director, Pediatric Emergency Medicine, Maricopa Medical Center, Phoenix, Arizona
Cosmetics and Toilet Articles

Timothy Mader, MD
Assistant Clinical Professor of Emergency Medicine, Tufts University School of Medicine, Boston; Associate Director of Emergency Medicine Research, Baystate Medical Center, Springfield, Massachusetts
Introduction to Geriatric Toxicology

Gregory P. Marelich, MD
Assistant Professor of Clinical Internal Medicine, Division of Pulmonary and Critical Care Medicine, University of California, Davis, School of Medicine, Davis, California
Cocaine

John L. Marshall, MD
Assistant Professor, The Vincent Lombardi Cancer Center, Georgetown University Medical Center, Washington, DC
Chemotherapeutic Agents and Transplant Agents—Chemotherapeutic Agents

Billy Martin, PhD
Louis and Ruth Harris Professor, Virginia Commonwealth University, Richmond, Virginia
Marijuana

Thomas Mason, MD
Emergency Physician, Mecklenburg Emergency Medical Associates, Department of Emergency Medicine, Presbyterian Hospital, Charlotte, North Carolina
Acids and Antacids

James F. McAnally, MD
Clinical Associate Professor of Medicine, Seton Hall University Graduate School of Medicine; Chief of Nephrology, St. Elizabeth's Hospital; Director of Nephrology, Alexian Brothers Hospital, Elizabeth, New Jersey
Acid-Base, Fluid, and Electrolyte Balance in Adults

Michael A. McGuigan, MD, MBA
Associate Professor of Pediatrics, Pharmacology, and Health Administration, University of Toronto; Medical Director, Ontario Regional Poison Control Centre (Toronto), Hospital for Sick Children, Toronto, Ontario, Canada
Alkali Injury—Caustics; Bleach, Soaps, Detergents, and Other Corrosives

Charles A. McKay, Jr., MD
Assistant Professor of Surgery, Division of Emergency Medicine, University of Connecticut School of Medicine, Farmington; Director, Division of Medical Toxicology, Department of Emergency Medicine, Hartford Hospital, Hartford, Connecticut
Chlorine

Thomas W. McKee, MD
Director, Pediatric Intensive Care Unit, Memorial Medical Center, Savannah, Georgia
Pediatric Resuscitation and Fluid Management; Pharmaceutical Excipients

Patrick E. McKinney, MD
Assistant Professor, Department of Emergency Medicine, School of Pharmacy; Medical Director, New Mexico Poison Center, University of New Mexico Health Sciences Center, Albuquerque, New Mexico
Designer Drugs

Mary Jo McMullen, MD
Assistant Professor Clinical Emergency Medicine, Northeastern Ohio Universities College of Medicine, Rootstown; Senior Attending Staff Physician, Department of Emergency Medicine, Akron General Medical Center, Akron, Ohio
Industrial Toxicology; Ammonia, Nitrogen, Nitrogen Oxides, and Related Compounds

Timothy J. Meredith, MD
Professor of Medicine and Pathology, Vanderbilt University School of Medicine; Director, Center for Clinical Toxicology, Vanderbilt University Medical Center, Nashville, Tennessee
Sedatives

Brooks C. Metts, Jr., PharmD
Associate Professor, Clinical Pharmacy; Director, Palmetto State Poison Center, College of Pharmacy, University of South Carolina, Columbia, South Carolina
Principles of Pharmacology for the Clinician; Rodenticides

Mary Beth Miller, DO
Department of Emergency Medicine, Michigan Capital Medical Center, Lansing, Michigan
Poisonous Arthropods—Scorpions

Howard C. Mofenson, MD
Professor of Pediatrics and Emergency Medicine, Medical School of State University of New York at Stony Brook, Stony Brook; Medical Director, Long Island Regional Poison Control Center, Winthrop University Hospital, Mineola, New York
Volatile Substance Abuse

Darlena M. Monet, MD
Emergency Physician, DeKalb Medical Center, Atlanta, Georgia
Thrombolytic Agents and Anticoagulants

Lindsay Murray, MB, BS
Conjoint Lecturer, Department of Medicine, Prince Henry/Prince of Wales Hospital Clinical School; Faculty of Medicine, University of New South Wales, Sydney; Staff Specialist, Emergency

Department, The Prince of Wales Hospital, Randwick, New South Wales, Australia
Oral Hypoglycemic Agents

Donella Nazzaro, RPh
Clinical Pharmacist, Georgetown Infusion Services, Rockville, Maryland
Chemotherapeutic Agents and Transplant Agents—Chemotherapeutic Agents

Valerie D. Neylan, MD
Assistant Professor, Education Director, University of Illinois, Department of Emergency Medicine, University of Illinois Hospital, Chicago, Illinois
Management Principles of Overdose in Pregnancy

K. Patrick Ober, MD
Professor of Internal Medicine (Endocrinology and Metabolism), Bowman Gray School of Medicine, Wake Forest University, Winston-Salem, North Carolina
Endocrine Agent Toxicity

Boon S. Ooi, MD
Professor of Medicine, George Washington University School of Medicine; Chief, Renal Section, Veterans Affairs Medical Center, Washington, DC
Chemotherapeutic Agents and Transplant Agents—Transplant Agents

John D. Osterloh, MD
Professor of Clinical Laboratory Medicine and Medicine, University of California, San Francisco; Associate Chief of Biochemistry/Toxicology, Clinical Laboratories, San Francisco General Hospital, San Francisco, California
Laboratory Diagnoses and Drug Screening

Mark S. Paller, MD
Professor of Medicine, University of Minnesota, Minneapolis, Minnesota
Renal Toxicity—Chronic Renal Toxicity

Paul D. Pearigen, MD
Residency Program Director, Department of Emergency Medicine, Naval Medical Center, San Diego; Clinical Assistant Professor of Military and Emergency Medicine, The Uniformed Services University for Health Sciences, Bethesda, Maryland; Assistant Clinical Professor of Medicine, University of California at San Diego Medical Center, San Diego, California
Calcium Channel Blocker Poisoning

Kimberley C. Pearson, MD, MPH
Instructor in Medicine, Harvard Medical School, Boston; Associate Medical Director, Occupational Health Service, Morton Hospital and Medical Center, Taunton, Massachusetts
Chlorinated Hydrocarbons

Paul R. Pentel, MD
Professor of Medicine and Pharmacology, University of Minnesota; Chief, Clinical Pharmacology and Toxicology, Hennepin County Medical Center, Minneapolis, Minnesota
Tricyclic Antidepressants and Selective Serotonin Reuptake Inhibitors

Holly Perry, MD
Instructor in Pediatrics, Harvard Medical School; Assistant in Medicine, The Children's Hospital, Boston, Massachusetts
Acetaminophen

Scott D. Phillips, MD
Toxicology Associates, Denver, Colorado
Environmental Toxicology

Heidi Pinkert, MD
Assistant Professor of Clinical Pediatrics, Columbia University College of Physicians and Surgeons; Assistant Director, Pediatric Emergency Services, St. Luke's–Roosevelt Hospital Center, New York, New York
Baby Powder, Borates, and Camphor

Susan M. Pond, MBBS, MD
Professor of Medicine, The University of Queensland; Director of Clinical Pharmacology, Princess Alexandra Hospital, Brisbane, Queensland, Australia
Methyl Bromide and Related Compounds

A. T. Proudfoot, BSc
Director, Scottish Poisons Information Bureau, The Royal Infirmary, Edinburgh, Scotland
Salicylate Toxicity

James Raymond, MD
Associate Dean, University of South Carolina School of Medicine; Senior Vice President for Education and Research, Richland Memorial Hospital, Columbia, South Carolina
Introduction to Geriatric Toxicology

Michael D. Reed, PharmD
Professor of Pediatrics, Case Western Reserve University School of Medicine; Director, Pediatric Clinical Pharmacology/Toxicology, Director, Greater Cleveland Poison Control Center, Rainbow Babies and Childrens Hospital, Cleveland, Ohio
Drug-Drug Interactions

T. J. Rittenberry, MD
Associate Professor of Clinical Emergency Medicine, University of Illinois at Chicago; Director, Emergency Medicine Education, Illinois Masonic Medical Center, Chicago, Illinois
The Volatile Oils

James R. Roberts, MD
Professor, Emergency Medicine, Director, Division of Toxicology, Allegheny University of the Health

Sciences/Medical College of Pennsylvania/Hahnemann University; Chairman, Department of Emergency Medicine, Mercy Health Systems, Philadelphia, Pennsylvania
Benzodiazepines

Barry H. Rumack, MD
Clinical Professor of Pediatrics, University of Colorado Health Sciences Center, Denver, Colorado
Cyanide and Related Compounds

Daniel T. Schelble, MD
Professor of Clinical Emergency Medicine, Northeastern Ohio Universities College of Medicine, Rootstown; Chairman, Department of Emergency Medicine, Akron General Medical Center, Akron, Ohio
Phosgene and Phosphine

Michael Schwartz, MD
Clinical Instructor in Medicine, Harvard Medical School, Boston; Attending Physician, Emergency Department, Mount Auburn Hospital, Cambridge, Massachusetts
Opiates and Narcotics

Donna L. Seger, MD
Assistant Professor of Medicine, Fellowship Director, Center for Clinical Toxicology, Department of Medicine, Medical Director, Middle Tennessee Poison Center, Vanderbilt University Medical Center, Nashville, Tennessee
Anticonvulsants

K. M. Mohamed Shakir, MD
Associate Professor of Medicine, Uniformed Services University of the Health Sciences; Director, Division of Endocrinology and Metabolism, Department of Medicine, National Naval Medical Center, Bethesda, Maryland
Thyroid

Michael W. Shannon, MD, MPH
Associate Chief of Emergency Services, Pediatric Emergency Medicine; Director, Lead and Toxicology Clinic, The Children's Hospital; Associate Professor of Pediatrics, Harvard Medical School; Staff Toxicologist, Massachusetts Poison Control System, Boston, Massachusetts
The Emergency Management of Poisoning; Acetaminophen; Antibiotics and Anthelminthics—Antibiotic Toxicity; Isoniazid; Lead; The Toxicology of Other Heavy Metals; Bromine and Iodine Compounds; Theophylline and Caffeine; Herbal, Traditional, and Alternative Medicine; Muscle Relaxants

Mahesh Shrestha, MD
Adjunct Professor of Medicine and Surgery, University of Texas Southwestern Medical School, Dallas, Texas; Emergency Department Physician, Crozer-Chester Medical Center, Upland, Pennsylvania
Antibiotics and Anthelminthics—Anthelminthics

William M. Simpson, Jr., MD
Professor of Family Medicine and Associate Medical Director, Occupational and Environmental Medicine, Agromedicine Program, Medical University of South Carolina; Medical University of South Carolina Hospital, Charleston, South Carolina
The Organophosphates and Other Insecticides

Corey M. Slovis, MD
Professor of Emergency Medicine and Medicine, Chairman, Department of Emergency Medicine, Vanderbilt University School of Medicine; Director, Emergency Services, Vanderbilt University Medical Center Hospital, Nashville, Tennessee
Botulism and Food Poisoning

N. John Stewart, Jr., MD
Adjunct Instructor, College of Pharmacy, University of South Carolina; Director of Education and Professional Services, Department of Emergency Medicine, Richland Memorial Hospital; Medical Director, Palmetto State Poison Center, University of South Carolina, Columbia, South Carolina
Rodenticides

Williamson B. Strum, MD
Staff Physician, Department of Gastroenterology, Scripps Clinic and Research Foundation, La Jolla, California
Gastrointestinal Effects of Poisoning

Young-Jin Sue, MD
Assistant Clinical Professor of Pediatrics, Albert Einstein College of Medicine; Attending Physician, Pediatric Emergency Services, Montefiore Medical Center, Bronx, New York
Baby Powder, Borates, and Camphor

Stephen Szara, MD, DSc
Former Chief, Biomedical Branch, National Institute on Drug Abuse, Rockville, Maryland
Marijuana

Angelo M. Taveira da Silva, MD, PhD
Associate Professor of Medicine and Pharmacology, Georgetown University School of Medicine; Director, Medical Intensive Care Unit, Georgetown University Hospital, Washington, DC
Management of Respiratory Complications in the Poisoned Patient

Fred Tecklenburg, MD
Associate Professor of Pediatrics, Medical University of South Carolina; Director, Division of Pediatric Critical Care, Medical University of South Carolina, Charleston, South Carolina
Pediatric Resuscitation and Fluid Management

R. Steven Tharratt, MD
Associate Professor of Clinical Internal Medicine, Division of Pulmonary and Critical Care Medicine, University of California, Davis; Associate Medical Director, University of California, Davis, Medical Center, Regional Poison Control Center, University of California, Davis, School of Medicine, Sacramento, California
Cocaine

Christian Tomaszewski, MD
Clinical Assistant Professor of Emergency Medicine, University of North Carolina, Chapel Hill; Medical Director of Hyperbaric Medicine, Department of Emergency Medicine, Carolinas Medical Center, Charlotte, North Carolina
Poisonous Arthropods—Spiders

Francis X. Tunney, MD
Emergency Physician, Medical University of South Carolina, Charleston, South Carolina
Poisonous Arthropods—Stinging Insects

Mark J. Upfal, MD, MPH
Director and Associate Professor, Division of Occupational and Environmental Medicine, Wayne State University, Detroit, Michigan
Disaster Management of Massive Toxic Exposure

Michael V. Vance, MD
Consultant, Good Samaritan Poison Center, Phoenix, Arizona
Hydrofluoric Acid

Brent E. Van Hoozen, MD
Assistant Professor in Residence, Division of Pulmonary and Critical Care Medicine, University of California, Davis, School of Medicine, Davis, California
Amphetamines

Ingrid M. O. Vicas, MD
Clinical Associate Professor, Pharmacology, and Clinical Assistant Professor, Internal Medicine, University of Calgary; Director, Poison and Drug Information Service, Division of Emergency Medicine, Foothills Hospital; Department of Emergency Medicine, Alberta Children's Hospital, Calgary, Alberta, Canada
Hydrogen Sulfide

Philip D. Walson, MD
Professor of Pediatrics, Pharmacology, and Pharmacy, The Ohio State University; Division/Section Head, Clinical Pharmacology/Toxicology, Medical Director, Toxicology Lab, Children's Hospital, Columbus, Ohio
Lidocaine

Frank G. Walter, MD
Associate Professor of Clinical Surgery, Division of Emergency Medicine, Department of Surgery, Chief, Section of Medical Toxicology, Director, Medical Toxicology Fellowship, Director of Clinical Toxicology, The University of Arizona College of Medicine, University Medical Center, Tucson, Arizona
North American Venomous Snakebite

Richard Y. Wang, DO
Assistant Professor, Department of Medicine, Brown University School of Medicine; Director, Division of Medical Toxicology, Department of Emergency Medicine, Rhode Island Hospital, Providence, Rhode Island
Radiation Poisoning

John V. Weigand, MD
Associate Professor of Clinical Emergency Medicine, Northeastern Ohio Universities College of Medicine, Rootstown; Attending Physician, Department of Emergency Medicine, Summa Health System, Akron, Ohio
Freon and Other Inhalants

James F. Wiley II, MD
Associate Professor of Pediatrics, Head, Division of Emergency Medicine, Department of Pediatrics, The School of Medicine at the University of Connecticut Health Center; Consultant and Medical Advisory Board Member, Connecticut Regional Poison Control Center, Farmington, Connecticut
Clonidine and Related Imidazoline Derivatives

James F. Winchester, MD
Professor of Medicine, Division of Nephrology, Department of Medicine, Georgetown University Medical Center, Washington, DC
Acid-Base, Fluid, and Electrolyte Balance in Adults; Active Methods for Detoxification; Lithium; Methanol, Isopropyl Alcohol, Higher Alcohols, Ethylene Glycol, Cellosolves, Acetone, and Oxalate; Barbiturates; Paraquat and the Bipyridyl Herbicides

Jane K. Witman, MD
Clinical Staff Physician, St. Vincent's Hospital and St. Mary's Hospital, Green Bay, Wisconsin
Class IA Antiarrhythmics: Quinidine, Procainamide, and Disopyramide

Leslie Rae Wolf, MD
Assistant Professor/Toxicology Coordinator, Departments of Emergency Medicine and Pharmacology/Toxicology, Wright State University School of Medicine, Dayton, Ohio
β-Adrenergic Blocker Toxicity

Alan D. Woolf, MD, MPH
Associate Professor of Pediatrics, Harvard Medical School; Director, Program in Clinical Pharmacology and Toxicology, Director, Massachusetts Poison Control System, The Children's Hospital, Boston, Massachusetts
Prevention of Childhood Poisonings; Phencyclidine

Robert O. Wright, MD
Clinical Fellow in Pediatrics, Program in Pharmacology/Toxicology, Harvard Medical School; Clinical Fellow, The Children's Hospital, Boston, Massachusetts
Phencyclidine

Joseph J. Zealberg, MD
Associate Professor of Psychiatry, Director, Emergency Psychiatry Service/Mobile Crisis Program, Medical University of South Carolina; Charleston, South Carolina
Psychiatric Evaluation of the Suicidal Patient

Hyman J. Zimmerman, MD
Distinguished Scientist, Armed Forces Institute of Pathology; Professor of Medicine, Emeritus, George Washington University School of Medicine; Clinical Professor of Medicine, Uniformed Services University of Health Sciences; Consultant, Veterans Affairs Medical Center, Clinical Center, NIH, US Naval Medical Center, Bethesda, Maryland; Walter Reed Medical Center, Washington, DC
Chemical Hepatic Injury

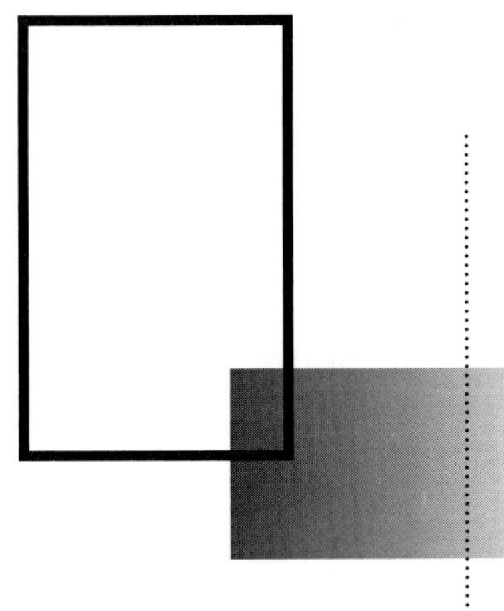

Preface

The third edition of *Clinical Management of Poisoning and Drug Overdose* finds toxicology an essential subject for practicing emergency physicians; primary care physicians in family medicine, internal medicine, and pediatrics; and physicians in public health.

The dramatic advances in the care of the toxicology patient, such as new and specific antidotal therapy, improved standards in the specialty of emergency medicine, and the organization of regional poison centers over the past 25 years are most gratifying to those of us dedicated to the field. Especially heartwarming is the creation of toxicology fellowships to train interested physicians, enabling us to continue our specialty. None of us in emergency medicine and primary care could ever have predicted that toxicology would become such an important subject as we head for the third millennium.

Toxicology has become intertwined with the very fabric of our society and, unfortunately, has begun to reflect the spiritual and moral crisis prevalent in our culture. The foundation of Western civilization is the Biblical ethic, as noted, for example, in our Declaration of Independence, which speaks of God our Creator and the natural law. The weakening of family and traditional values has spawned rampant teenage drug abuse and other social horrors. For the first time in American history, a major antidepressant, Prozac, is one of the top-selling prescription drugs. A chemical dimension has been added to man's inhumanity to man with the first massive terrorist attack in the Tokyo subway on March 20, 1995, involving the organophosphate sarin, and the Oklahoma City bombing on April 19, 1995, involving an explosive made from store-bought fertilizer.

Physicians deal with these toxicology and social issues on an individual and daily basis. In addition to becoming even more sophisticated in our knowledge base, physicians more than ever must practice the art of medicine and serve as sources of light and hope to the growing number of drug-dependent and troubled souls in our modern times.

Dr. James F. Winchester and I express deep gratitude for the tremendous effort that our new editor Dr. Michael W. Shannon has given this third edition, which has been almost completely rewritten, and represents the same effort as the first edition. The textbook includes ten new chapters to reflect new developments in medicine and toxicology, such as chapters on Pediatric Resuscitation and Fluid Management; Thrombolytic Agents and Anticoagulants; and Herbal, Traditional, and Alternative Medicine.

The three of us thank our outstanding group of contributors, both our experienced authors who continue to be innovative, and our new authors, the majority, who are now productive in the field of toxicology. We thank our many colleagues who have supported our effort by being generous with the schedule at our respective hospitals and have made helpful suggestions. We wish to thank our secretarial staff, especially Geri LaVia at the Medical University of South Carolina, our library staff, especially Marilyn Seymour at Memorial Medical Center, and all who helped us complete this textbook. Thanks to Charlene and Elizabeth Anne Haddad for their help with the Toxic Marine Life chapter, and to Matthew, Joseph, Jeanne, Daniel, and Madeleine Haddad for proofreading and commentary. We appreciate the efforts of Melissa Messersmith, our developmental editor, Carolyn Naylor, Les Hoeltzel, Judy Fletcher, Denise LeMelledo, Deborah Thorp, Ellen Zanolle, Bob Keller, Mary Finuoli, and the W.B. Saunders staff who helped bring our textbook to fruition.

Finally, we extend to our readers the hope that this text will benefit them in their pursuit of knowledge and in their clinical practice of medicine.

Lester M. Haddad, MD
Michael W. Shannon, MD, MPH
James F. Winchester, MD

DRUG NOTICE

Toxicology is an ever-changing field. Standard safety precautions must be followed, but as new research and clinical experience broaden our knowledge, changes in treatment and drug therapy become necessary or appropriate. Readers are advised to check the product information currently provided by the manufacturer of each drug to be administered to verify the recommended dose, the method and duration of administration, and contraindications. It is the responsibility of the treating physician relying on experience and knowledge of the patient to determine dosages and the best treatment for the patient. Neither the Publisher nor the editor assumes any responsibility for any injury and/or damage to persons or property.

THE PUBLISHER

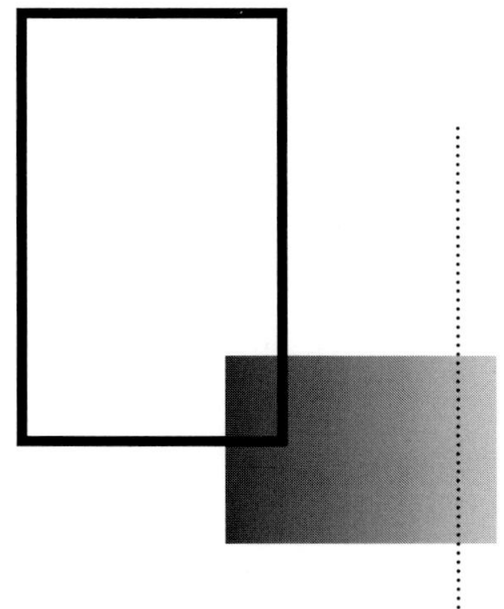

Contents

Color figures follow p. xxiv

I

General Information

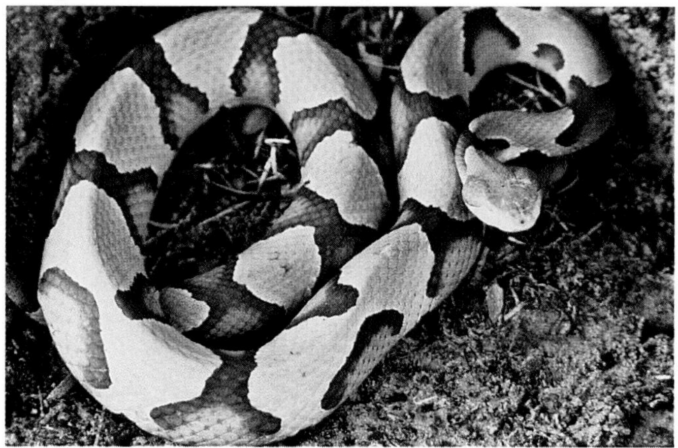

Color Figure 23–1. The copperhead, *Agkistrodon contortrix.* (Courtesy of the Savannah Science Museum, Savannah, GA.)

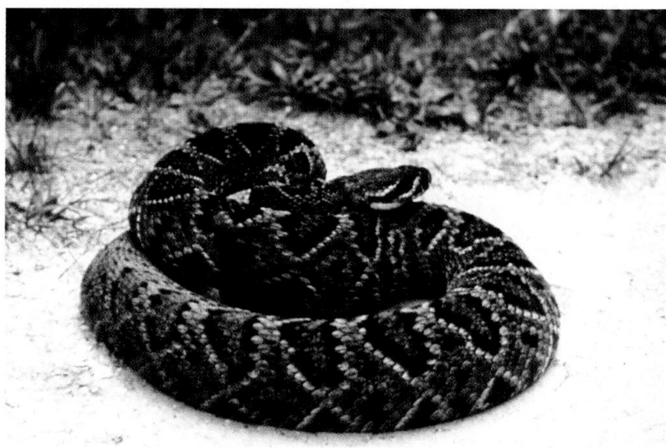

Color Figure 23–2. The eastern diamondback rattlesnake, *Crotalus adamanteus.* (Courtesy of Savannah Science Museum, Savannah, GA.)

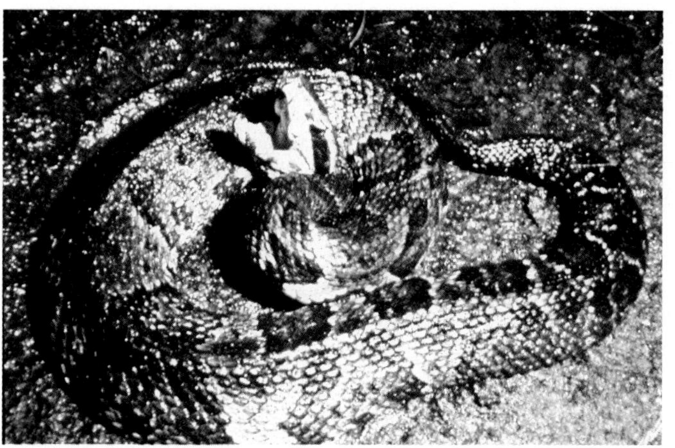

Color Figure 23–3. The water moccasin, or cottonmouth, *Agkistrodon piscivorus,* named for the cotton-white interior of its mouth. (Courtesy of Winchester Seyle, herpetologist, and the Savannah Science Museum, Savannah, GA.)

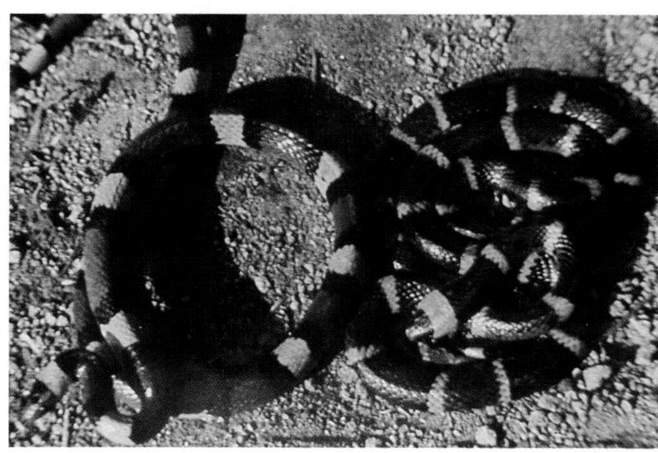

Color Figure 23–4. The eastern coral snake (*right*), *Micrurus fulvius,* highly lethal, but rarely seen ("red next to yellow, kill a fellow"), next to the harmless scarlet king snake (*left*), *Lampropeltis triangulum elapsoides* ("red next to black, venom lack"). (Courtesy of Michael D. Ellis of Galveston, TX, and the Texas Parks and Wildlife.)

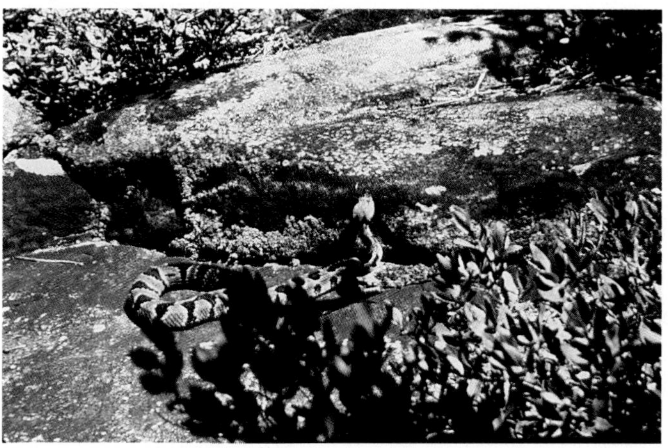

Color Figure 23–5. The timber rattlesnake, *Crotalus horridus.* (Courtesy of Adam Safer and the Savannah Science Museum, Savannah, GA.)

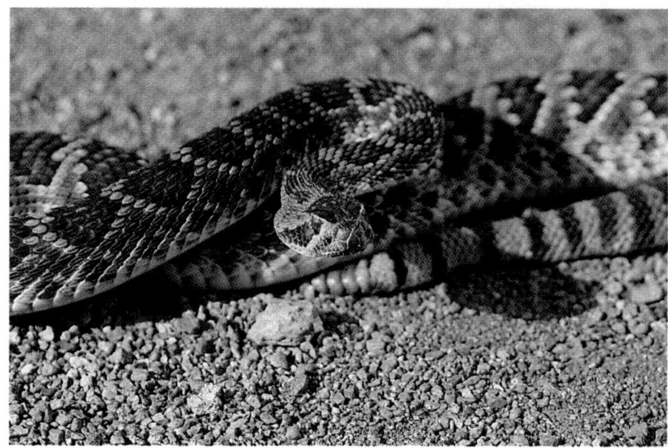

Color Figure 23–6. The Mojave rattlesnake, *Crotalus scutulatus scutulatus.* (Courtesy of Donald Kunkel, M.D., and the Good Samaritan Poison Center, Tucson, AZ.)

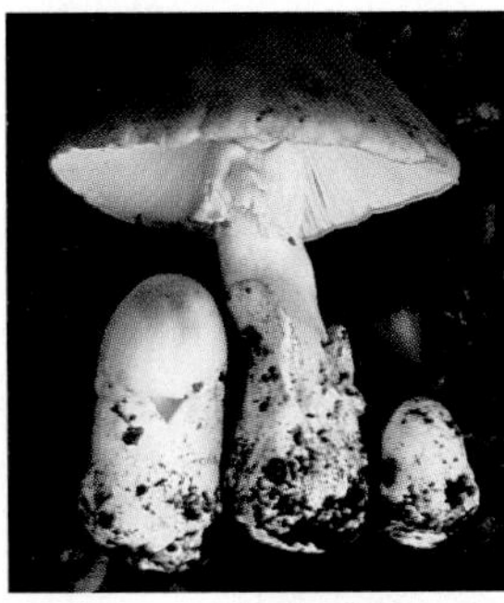

Color Figure 25–1. The death cap, *Amanita phalloides* (cyclopeptide). (Courtesy of Marilyn Shaw, Denver.)

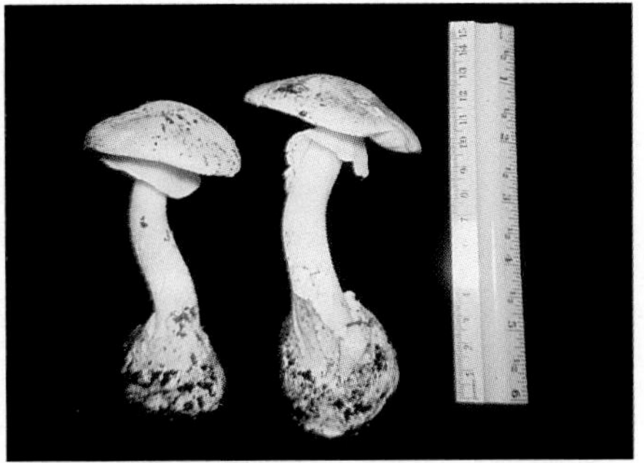

Color Figure 25–2. The destroying angel, *Amanita virosa* (cyclopeptide). (Courtesy of D. H. Mitchel and the Denver Botanic Gardens—Herbarium of Denver.)

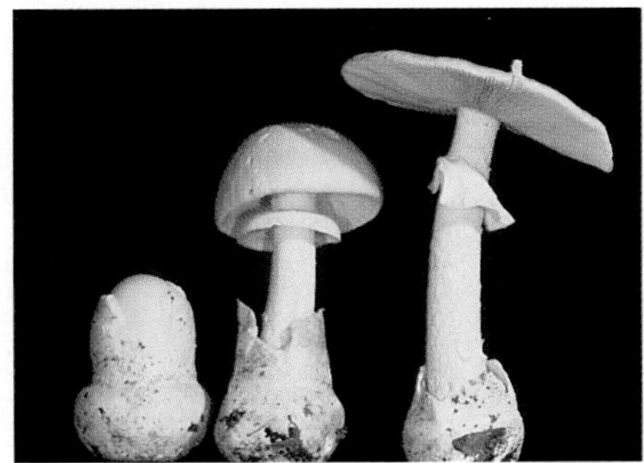

Color Figure 25–3. Fool's mushroom, *Amanita verna* (cyclopeptide). (Courtesy of Donald Simon, Wilmington, DE.)

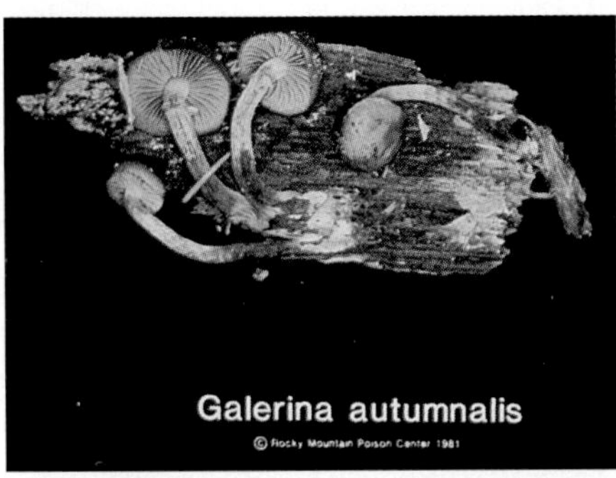

Color Figure 25–4. *Galerina autumnalis* (cyclopeptide). (Courtesy of Linnea Gilman, Denver.)

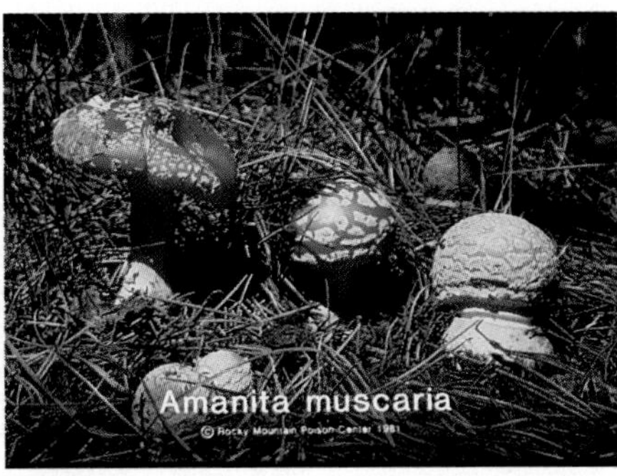

Color Figure 25–5. The fly agaric, *Amanita muscaria* (muscimol, ibotenic acid). (Courtesy of Linnea Gilman, Denver.)

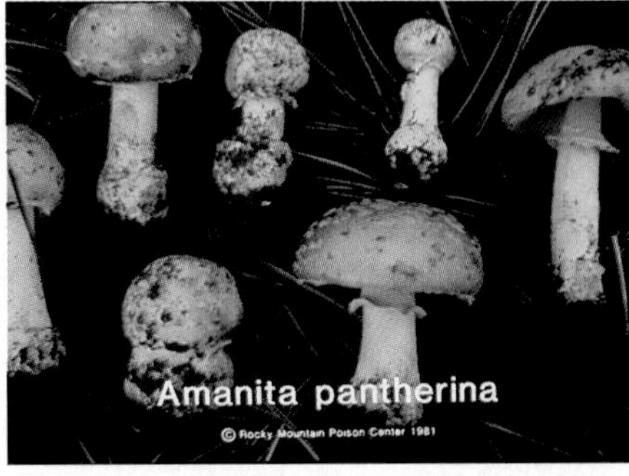

Color Figure 25–6. *Amanita pantherina* (muscimol, ibotenic acid). (Courtesy of Linnea Gilman, Denver.)

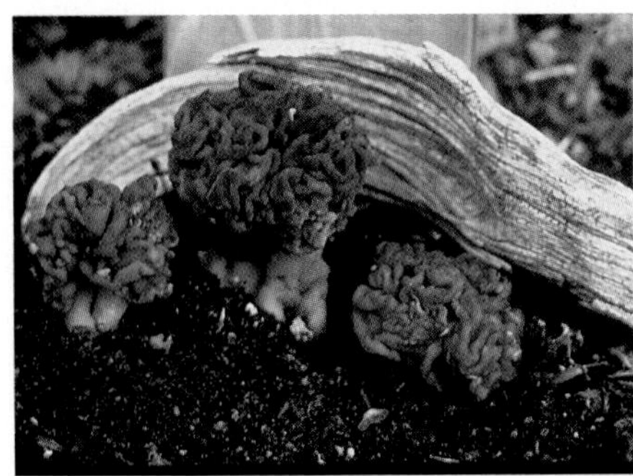

Color Figure 25–7. *Gyromitra esculenta* (monomethylhydrazine). (Courtesy of Joy Spurr, Issaquah, WA.)

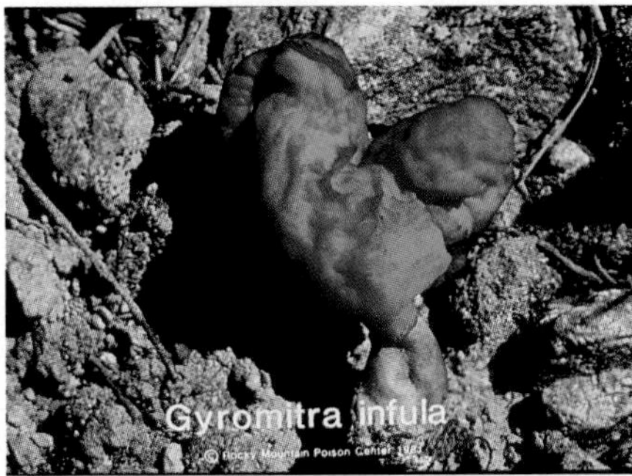

Color Figure 25–8. *Gyromitra infula* (monomethylhydrazine). (Courtesy of the late George Grimes.)

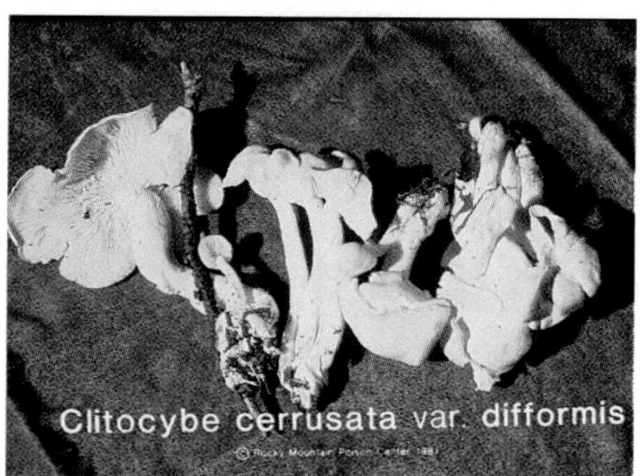

Color Figure 25–9. *Clitocybe cerrusata* (muscarine). (Courtesy of Linnea Gilman, Denver.)

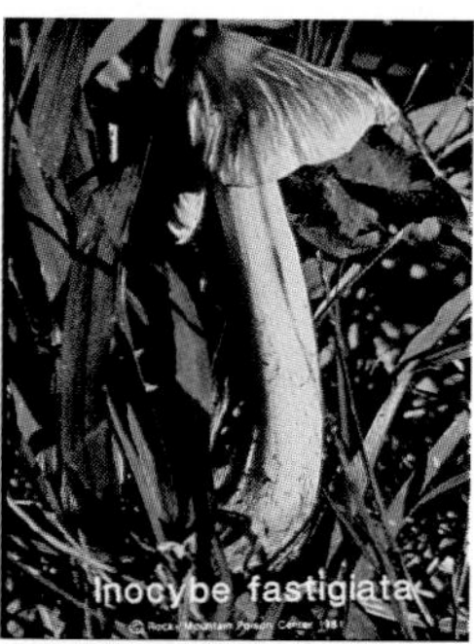

Color Figure 25–10. *Inocybe fastigiata* (muscarine). (Courtesy of the late George Grimes.)

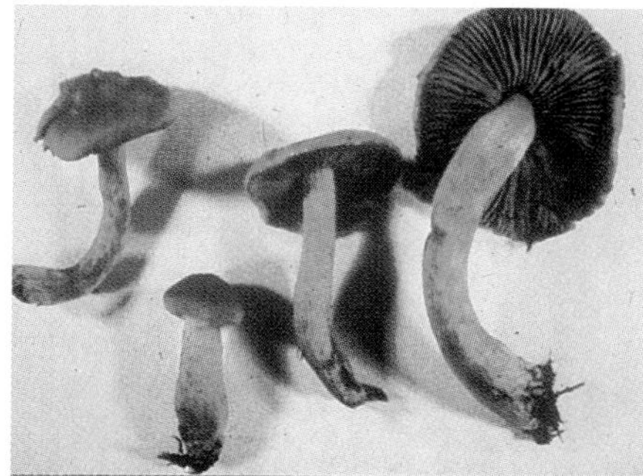

Color Figure 25–11. *Cortinarius speciosissimus* (orellanine). (Reprinted with permission from Lampe KF (ed): AMA Handbook of Poisonous and Injurious Plants. Chicago, American Medical Association, 1985.)

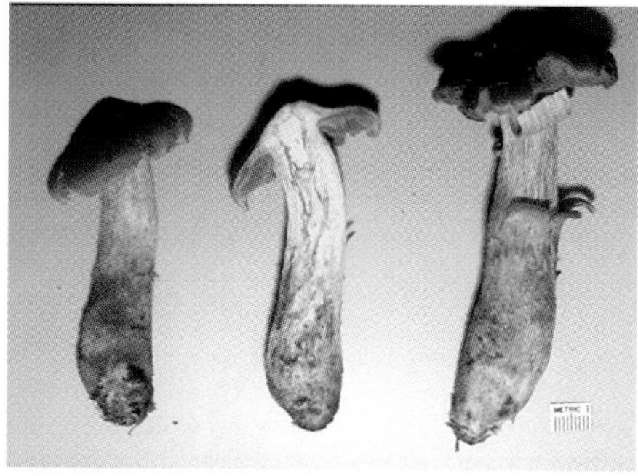

Color Figure 25–12. *Cortinarius orellanoides* (orellanine). (Courtesy of Joseph Ammirati, Ph.D., University of Washington, Seattle.)

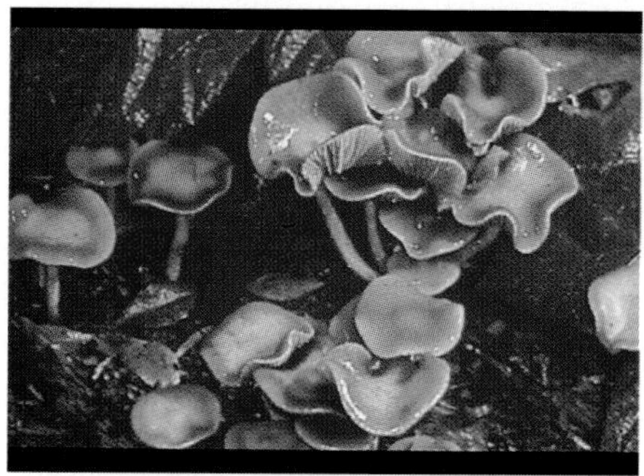

Color Figure 25–13. *Psilocybe cyanescens* (indole). (Courtesy of Kit Scates, Post Falls, ID.)

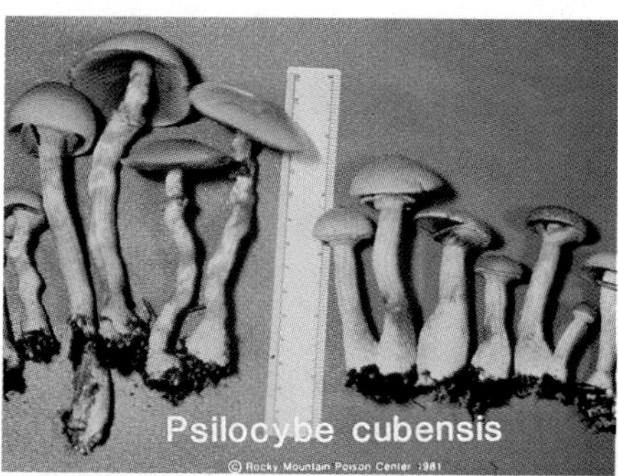

Color Figure 25–14. *Psilocybe cubensis* (indole). (Courtesy of the Rocky Mountain Poison Center, Denver.)

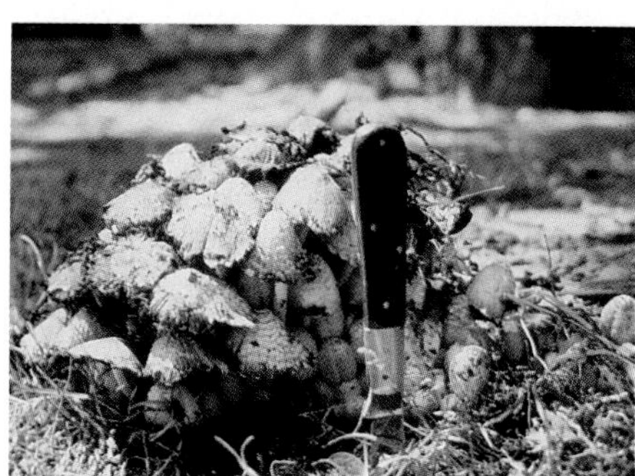

Color Figure 25–15. *Coprinus atramentarius* (coprine). (Courtesy of Joe H. Restivo, Savannah, GA.)

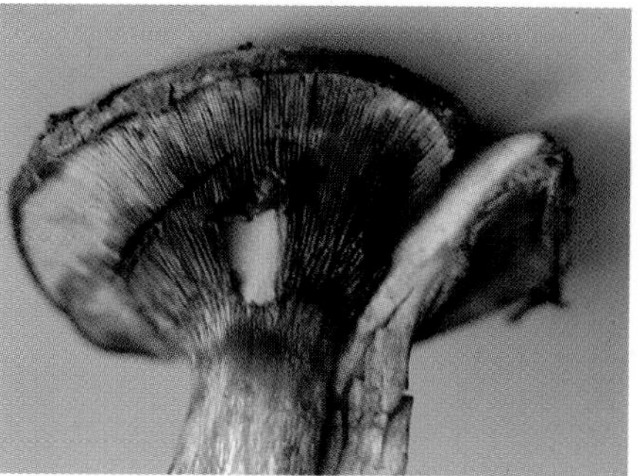

Color Figure 25–16. *Paxillus involutus* (hypersensitivity). (Courtesy of Marilyn Shaw, Denver.)

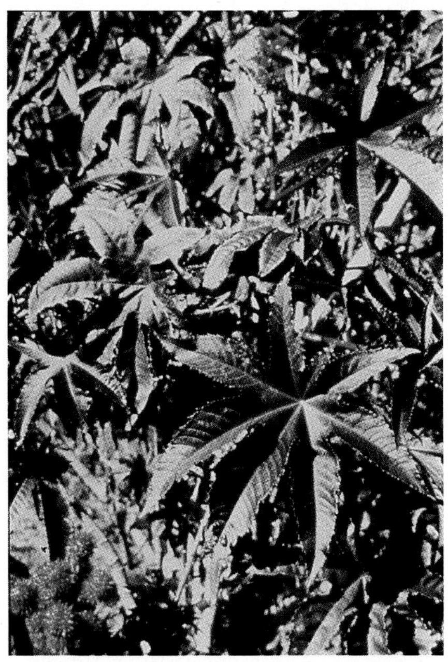

Color Figure 26–1. Castor bean bush.

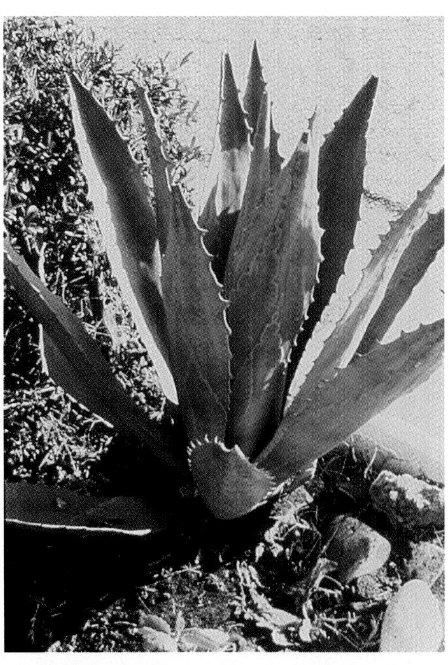

Color Figure 26–2. Century plant.

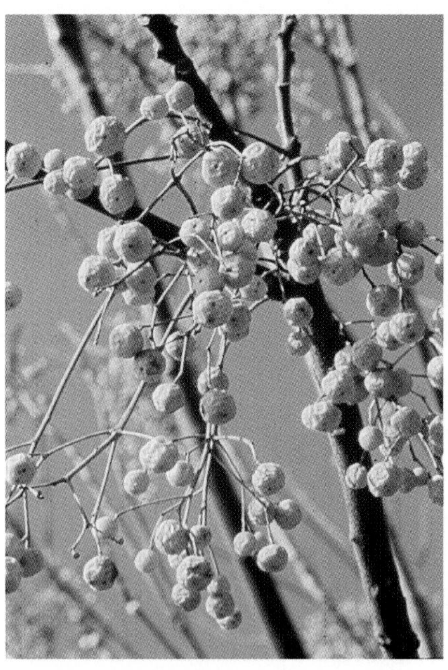

Color Figure 26–3. Chinaberry (drying fruit).

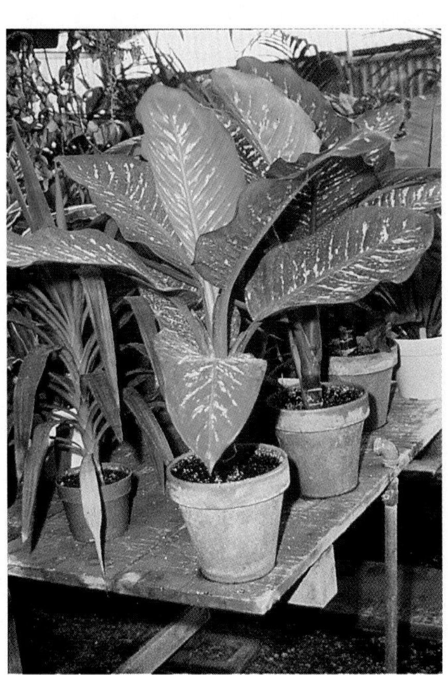

Color Figure 26–4. Dieffenbachia.

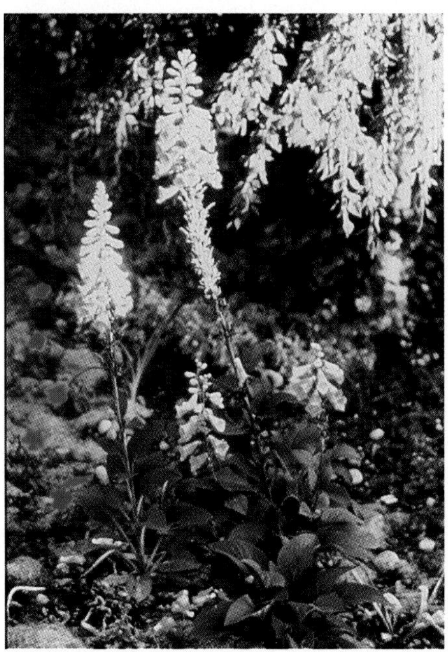

Color Figure 26–5. Foxglove (*Digitalis purpurea*).

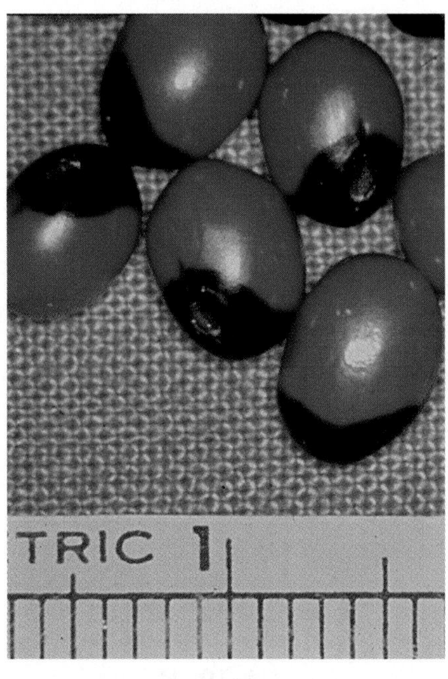

Color Figure 26–6. Jequirity beans, or "rosary peas."

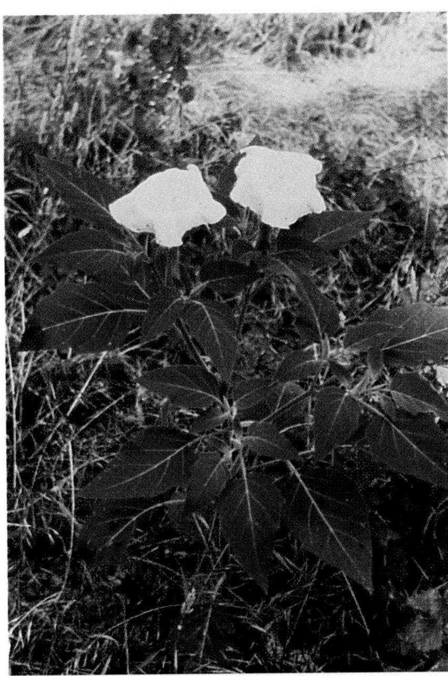

Color Figure 26–7. Jimson weed.

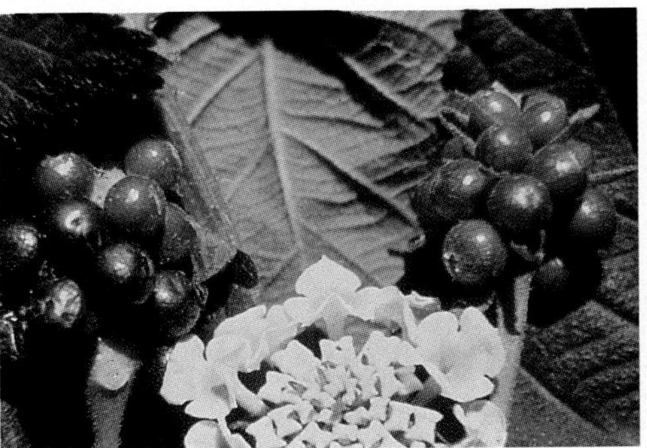

Color Figure 26–8. Lantana.

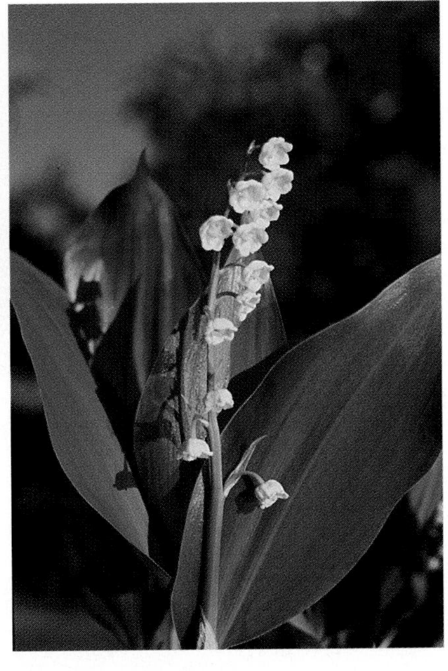

Color Figure 26–9. Lily of the Valley.

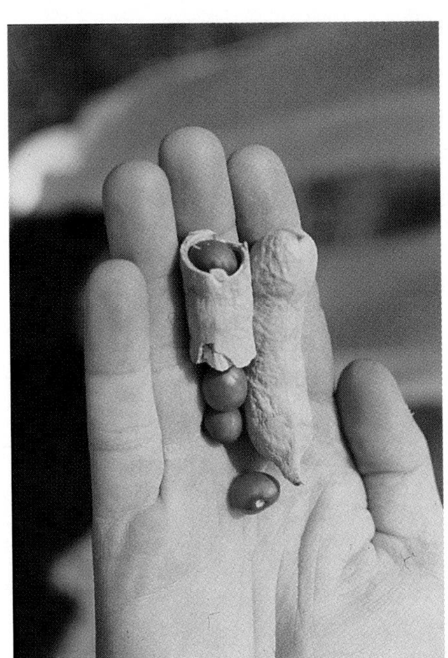

Color Figure 26–10. Mescal beans.

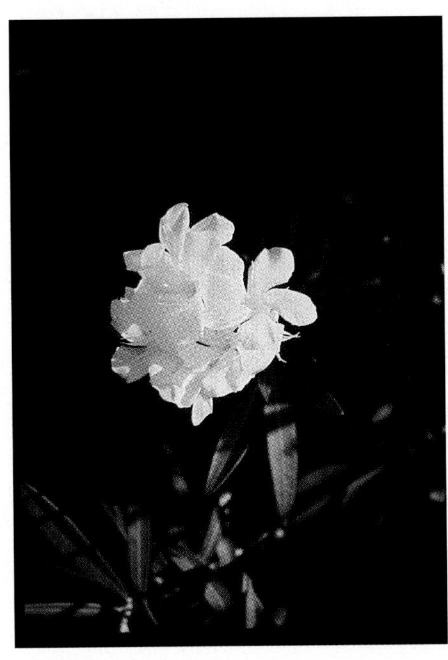

Color Figure 26–11. Oleander.

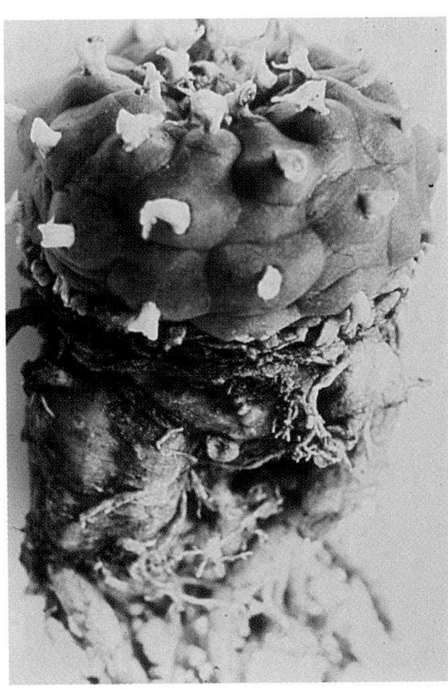

Color Figure 26–12. Peyote.

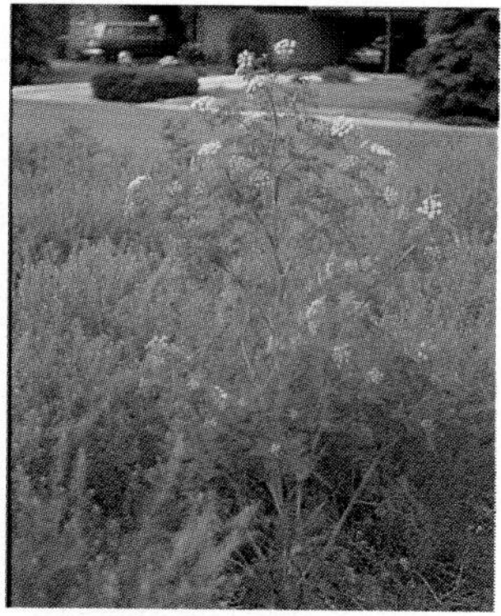

Color Figure 26–13. Poison hemlock.

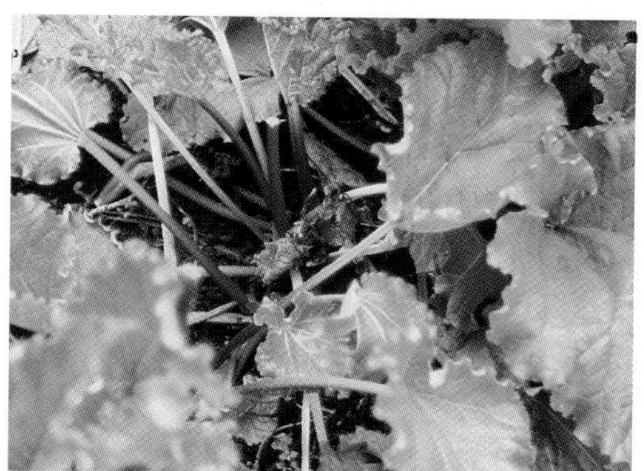

Color Figure 26–14. Rhubarb.

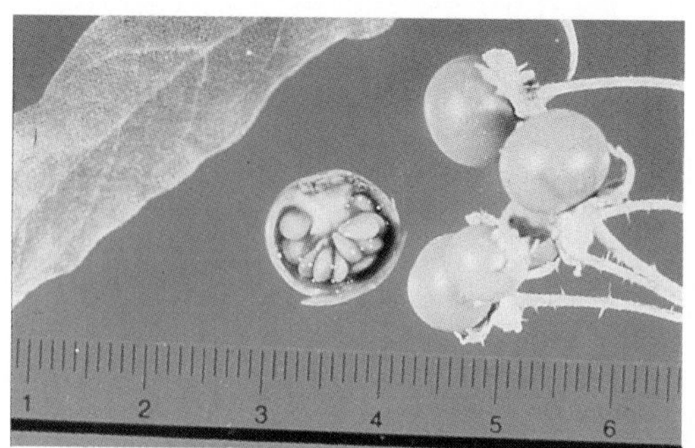

Color Figure 26–15. Silverleaf nightshade.

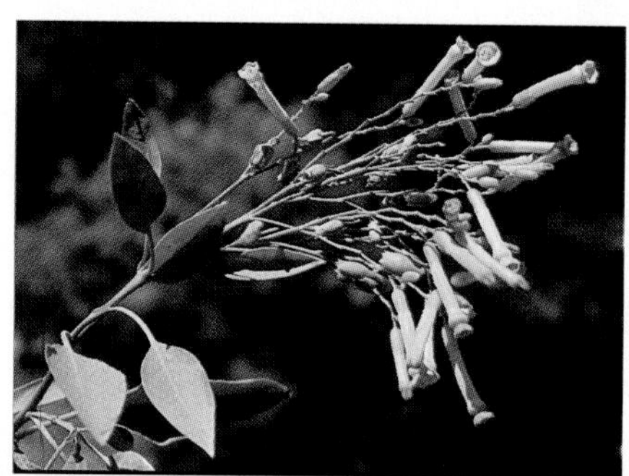

Color Figure 26–16. Tree tobacco.

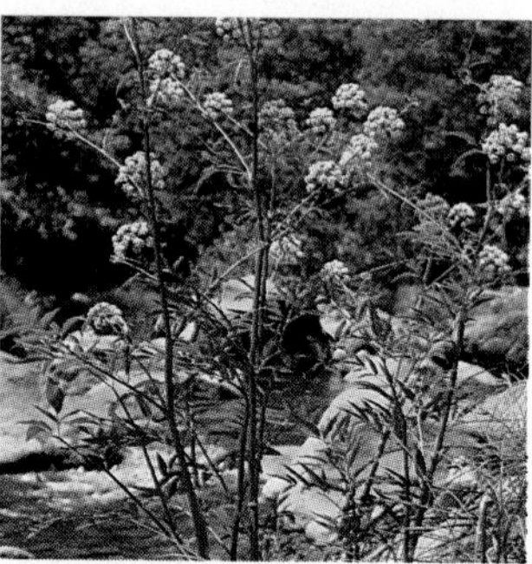

Color Figure 26–17. Water hemlock.

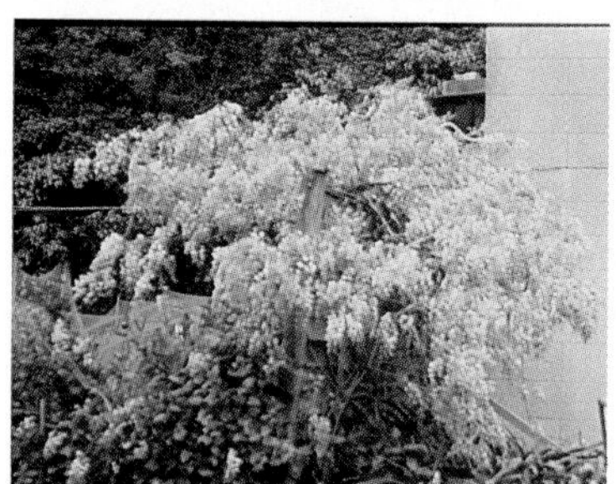

Color Figure 26–18. Wisteria.

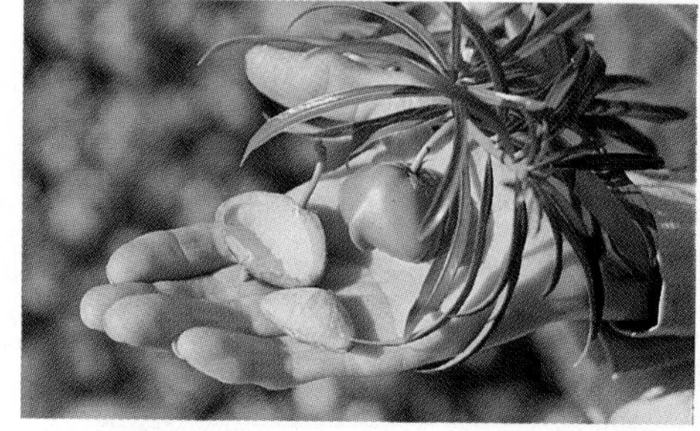

Color Figure 26–19. Yellow oleander, fruit with "lucky nut."

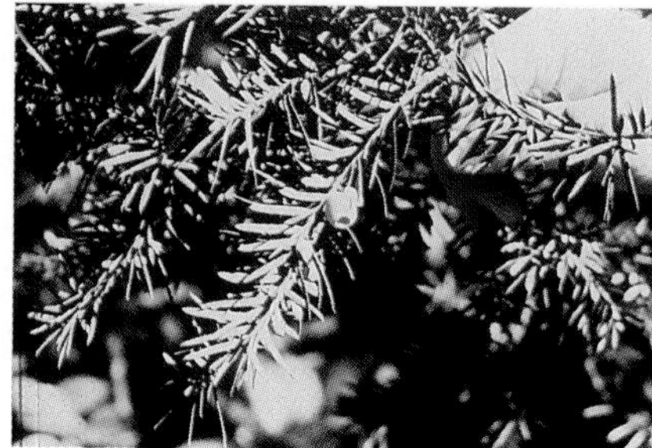

Color Figure 26–20. Yew.

Color figures 26–1 to 26–20 courtesy of Donald B. Kunkel, MD.

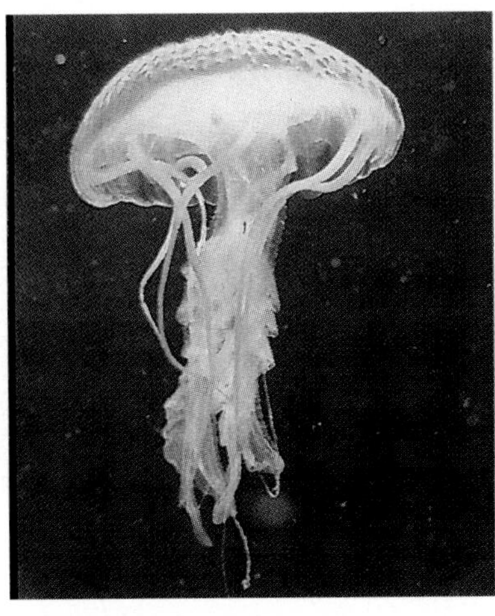

Color Figure 27–1. The purple stinger jellyfish, *Pelagia noctiluca.* (With permission from Humann P: Reef Creature Identification. Jacksonville, FL, New World Publications, 1992.)

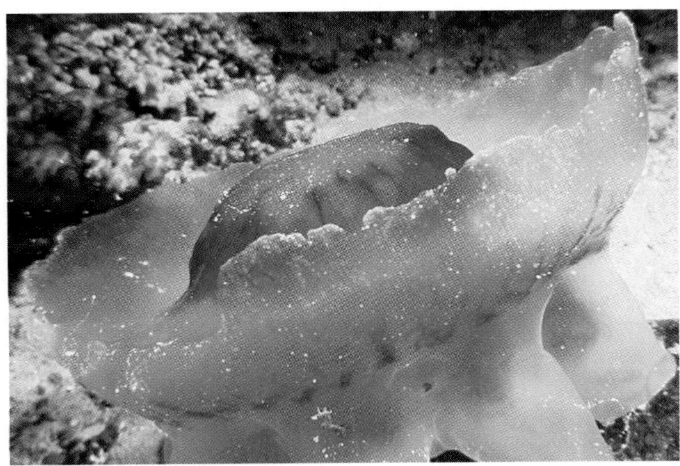

Color Figure 27–2. Jellyfish "with no name," photographed off the Fiji islands. (Courtesy of Leonard S. Wojnowich, MD, Savannah, GA.)

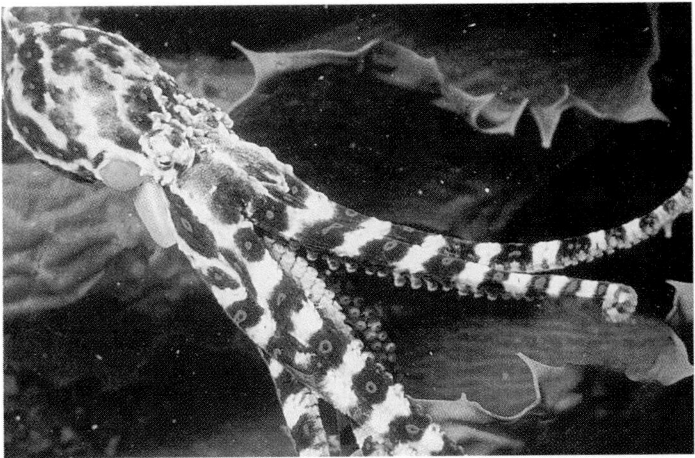

Color Figure 27–3. The Australian blue-ringed octopus, *Octopus maculosa.* (Copyright David Parer and E. Parer Cook, Auscape International, in VanDenbeld J; Nature of Australia: A Portrait of the Island Continent. New York, Facts on File (in cooperation with the Australian Broadcasting Corporation), 1988.)

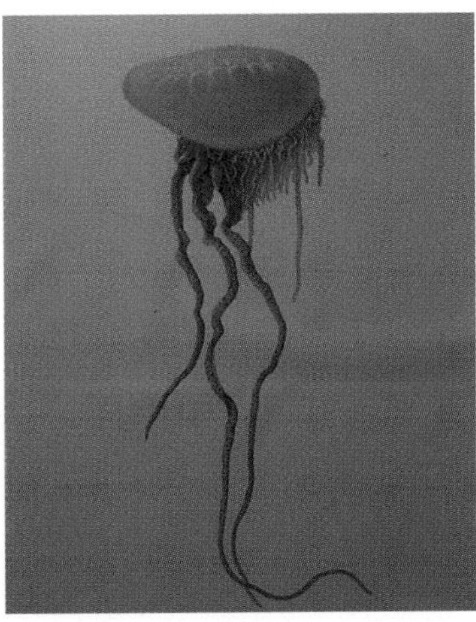

Color Figure 27–4. Portuguese man-of-war, *Physalia physalis.* (Courtesy of Bruce W. Halstead and the World Life Research Institute, Colton, CA.)

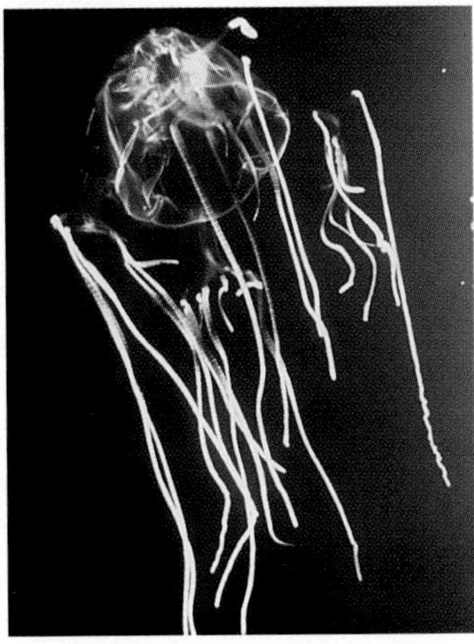

Color Figure 27–5. The sea wasp, *Chironex fleckeri.* (Courtesy of Bruce W. Halstead and the World Life Research Institute, Colton, CA.)

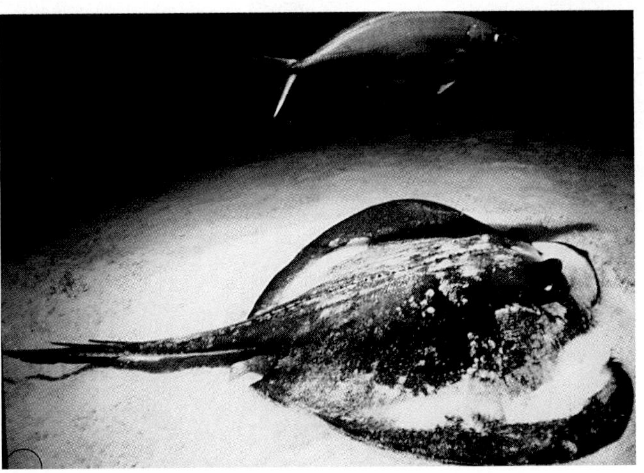

Color Figure 27–6. The blunt-nosed stingray, *Dasyatis sayi.* (Courtesy of Bruce W. Halstead and the World Life Research Institute, Colton, CA.)

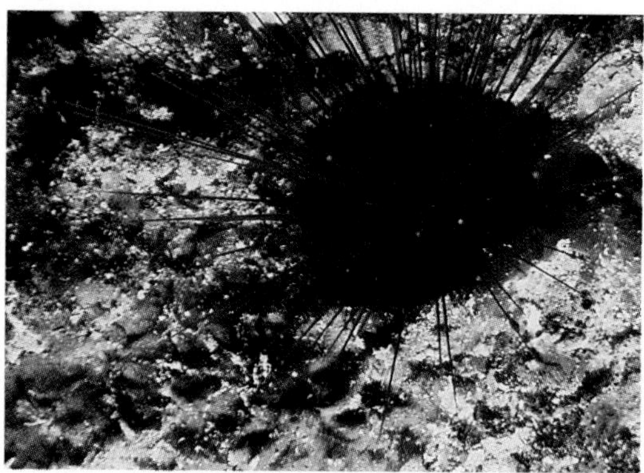

Color Figure 27–7. The sea urchin, *Diadema setosum*, from the Pacific Ocean near the Fiji islands. (Courtesy of Leonard S. Wojnowich, MD, Savannah, GA.)

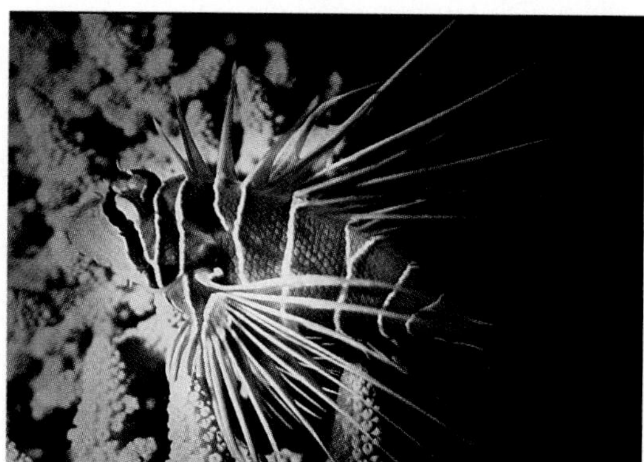

Color Figure 27–8. The zebrafish, *Dendrochirus zebra.* (Courtesy of Sea World, Orlando, FL.)

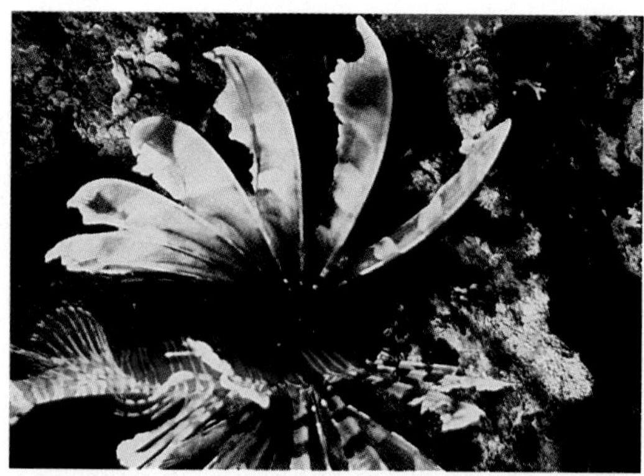

Color Figure 27–9. The lionfish, *Pterois volitans*, near the Fiji islands. (Courtesy of Leonard S. Wojnowich, MD, Savannah, GA.)

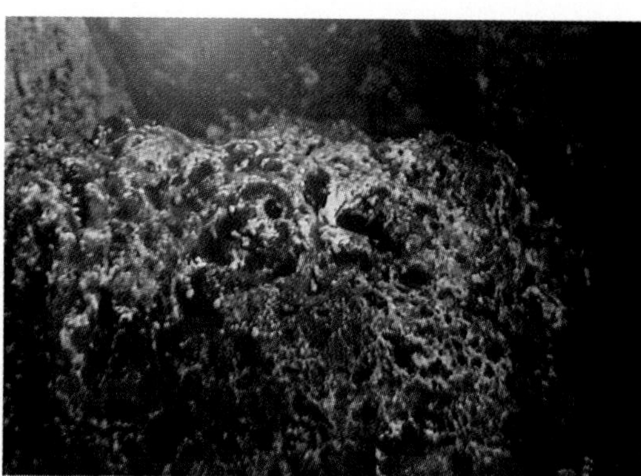

Color Figure 27–10. The stonefish, *Synenjeca verrucosa.* (Courtesy of Sea World, Orlando, FL.)

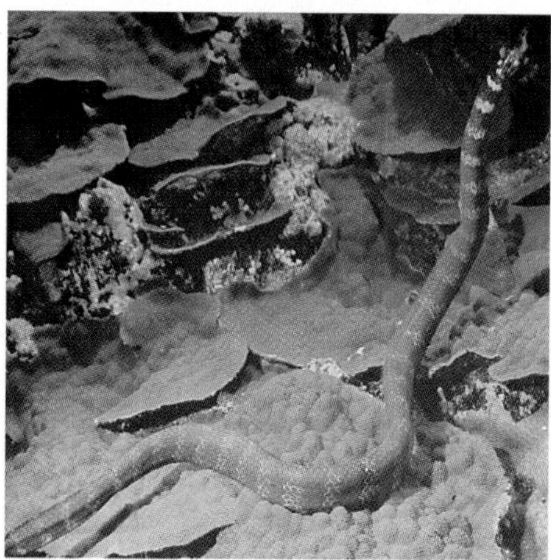

Color Figure 27–11. The sea snake, *Enhydrina schistosa.* (Courtesy of S. Keiser, the Sea Library, and Time-Life, Alexandria, VA.)

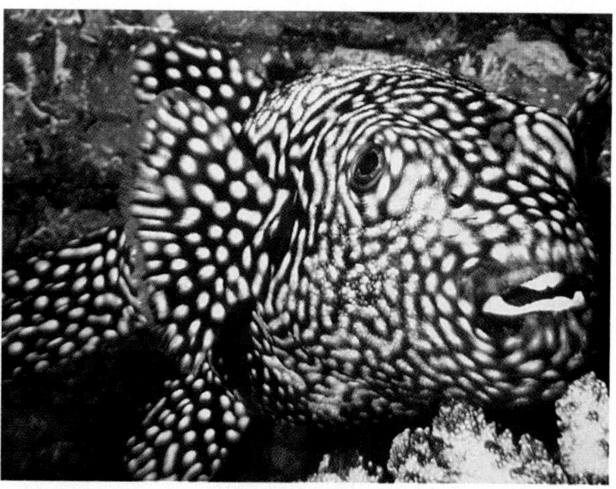

Color Figure 27–12. The puffer fish, *Arophron meleagris.* (Courtesy of Sea World, Orlando, FL.)

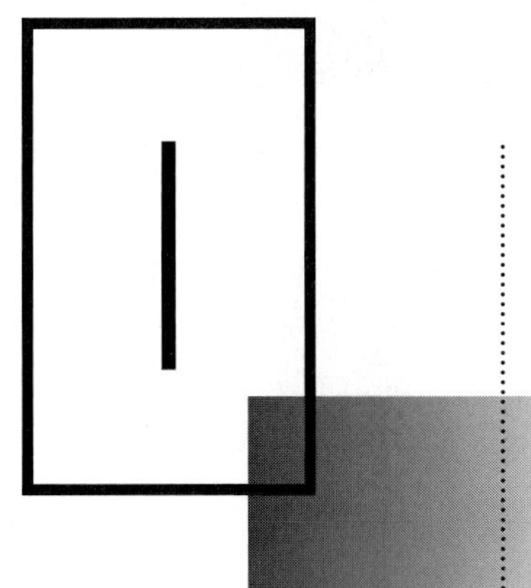

General Information

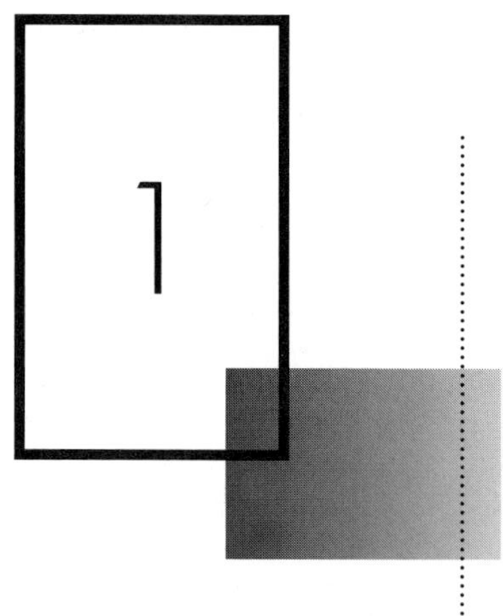

1 The Emergency Management of Poisoning

MICHAEL W. SHANNON, MD, MPH
LESTER M. HADDAD, MD

Clinical toxicology is one of the most dynamic fields in medicine today, as the practicing physician is continually faced with the management of poisoning and drug overdose. The alarming increase in illicit drug use in the United States reflects a worldwide trend. There has been a phenomenal growth in the prescription and subsequent overdose of mood-altering medications, as our society becomes ever more confining and less tolerant of the individual and of the natural ebb and flow of his or her emotions.

Defining the extent of human poisoning is not easy because the three major sources of data reflect different viewpoints and because the information that they contain overlaps. Ninety-nine per cent of all patients with significant poisoning present directly to a hospital emergency department.[1] The National Institute of Drug Abuse surveys emergency department visits through the *Drug Abuse Warning Network (DAWN),* and in 1993 reported that a total of 8541 deaths resulted from drug abuse, with cocaine being the most commonly implicated agent.[2] The *Toxic Exposure Surveillance System (TESS)* of the American Association of Poison Control Centers tabulates phone information referrals, and in 1994 it recorded 1,926,438 exposures with 766 deaths, with cyclic antidepressants being the most common cause.[3] The *National Center for Health Statistics* reviews primarily medical examiner death certificates; yearly, it reports carbon monoxide poisoning as the leading cause of death.

Data from all three of these sources still do not reflect the extent of human poisoning. For example, reports of intoxicated patients who die from trauma, drowning, and fires are not consistently included, nor are those of patients with medical complications from therapy, such as chemotherapy, anesthesia, and adverse drug reactions. Morbidity resulting from chronic abuse (e.g., heart disease from cocaine or nicotine use and cirrhosis from alcohol abuse) or industrial exposures, or the long-term effects of environmental hazards are not included and are probably impossible to quantify.

The most common causes of poisoning-related death in the United States have been carbon monoxide poisoning, cocaine use, and tricyclic antidepressant overdose. Poisoning with analgesics, aspirin and acetaminophen, remains a leading cause. Calcium channel blocker overdose has surpassed digitalis overdose as the most common cause of cardiovascular drug–related death.

DEFINITION

To poison means to injure or kill with poison, a chemical substance that usually kills, injures, or impairs an organism. Thus, the term *poisoning* connotes clinical symptomatology. It also implies that the toxic exposure is *accidental* (e.g., in the case of an elderly patient who misreads a drug label) or *unintentional* (e.g., in the case of an inquisitive toddler or a child who gives drugs to another child when "playing doctor"), or that the patient is *unaware* of the toxic exposure (e.g., he or she is the victim of an intended homicide).

In contrast, the term *overdose* implies *intentional* toxic exposure, either in the form of a suicide attempt or as inadvertent exposure secondary to intentional drug abuse.

The terms *poisoning* and *drug overdose* often are used interchangeably, especially when prescription drugs are the agents, even though by definition a drug overdose does not produce poisoning unless it causes clinical symptoms.

Poisoning most commonly occurs in children who are 1 to 5 years of age and in the elderly. Overdose, whether motivated by suicidal intent or secondary gain or whether the result of abuse, is recognized through adulthood. Toxic exposure in those between the ages of 6 to 12 years is uncommon and difficult to determine, and in each case the patient must be assessed individually to ensure that psychiatric follow-up is provided when indicated.

HISTORY

The history of poisons and poisoning dates to antiquity; their use originally fell within the province of ancient magicians and priests. It was once believed that poisons were mystical substances that were lethal to the guilty while remaining harmless to the innocent.

The first recognition of poisons comes to us from the Bible,[4] in which Moses provides sound advice concerning the consumption of toxic marine life:

"These you shall eat of all that are in the waters which have fins and scales; and whatsoever hath not fins and scales you may not eat, for it is unclean."

DEUTERONOMY 14:9–10

In the first century before Christ, in his quest for the universal antidote, Mithridates, King of Pontus, was the first person to develop antidotes.

The earliest recognized poisons were plant and animal substances used for murder or official executions. Plato reported the death of Socrates by poisoning with hemlock *(Conium maculatum)*.[5]

In the 13th-century work *De Venenis*, Peter of Abanos reviewed literary collections of Arabic thought and divided all poisons into the three Arabic categories of animal, vegetable, and mineral.[6]

Paracelsus, in the 16th century, was the first to relate poisoning to the dosage of the toxic substance. To him is attributed the historic comment, "All substances are poisons; there is none which is not a poison. The right dose differentiates a poison from a remedy."

MODERN ERA

Modern clinical approaches to the field of toxicology were initiated primarily in the specialty of pediatrics. In 1952, the American Academy of Pediatrics established an Accident Prevention Committee. The Committee's survey of the membership produced the surprising finding that 50% of the reported accidents involved some type of poisoning. Flavored children's aspirin, which had been introduced in the mid-1940s at a dosage of 2.5 grains (150 mg) and available in bottles containing 100 or more tablets, was responsible for 25% of poisonings in children younger than 5 years of age and for approximately 400 deaths annually. Dr. Jay M. Arena, a pediatrician at Duke University, worked with the Plough Company, maker of St. Joseph's Aspirin for children, to develop the safety closure cap for drug containers.[7] Use of the safety closure cap, which was introduced in 1959, was mandated by federal law in 1972, the same year that Arena served as president of the American Academy of Pediatrics. Over the years, the use of safety caps has eliminated aspirin as a major cause in childhood poisoning and since 1980 has reduced the overall incidence of mortality from childhood poisoning to fewer than 100 deaths per year.

On October 21, 1958, the first meeting of the American Association of Poison Control Centers (AAPCC) was held in Chicago. The AAPCC has been a leader in the poison control movement and has been especially active in developing standards for the proper rendering of poison information by regional poison centers.[8]

Death by drug overdose became almost commonplace in the late 1950s and early 1960s, typified by the tragic death of Marilyn Monroe at age 36 years on August 4, 1962 from an overdose of barbiturates. The use of dialysis for removal of drugs was introduced and became accepted as a therapeutic regimen primarily because of the work of nephrologist George Schreiner at Georgetown University.[9]

The nationwide growth of hospital emergency departments and the proliferation of lysergic acid diethylamide (LSD), methaqualone (Quaaludes), and other street drugs in the late 1960s necessitated rapid involvement of emergency physicians in toxicology. In 1978, the American College of Emergency Physicians established its Committee on Toxicology, and it has been active in improving standards of care in poison treatment. Emergency department care of poisoning has improved considerably with the advent of the burgeoning specialty of emergency medicine. Emergency medicine was established as the 22nd primary medical specialty by the American Board of Medical Specialties on September 21, 1989 (which, ironically, is the same day Hurricane Hugo struck Charleston, South Carolina). The first subspecialty examination in toxicology was administered by the American Board of Emergency Medicine in November of 1994 and has been available to emergency physicians, pediatricians, internists, and other physicians dedicated to toxicology. The future should bring further refinement of this exciting and dynamic new field.

THE GENERAL APPROACH TO POISONING

The general approach to the toxicologic patient can be divided into seven phases: (1) emergency manage-

Table 1–1. Common Emergency Antidotes

Poison	Antidote	Adult Dosage*	Comments
Acetaminophen	*N*-Acetylcysteine	140 mg/kg initial oral dose, followed by 70 mg/kg q4h × 17 doses	Most effective within 16 hours; may be useful up to 24 hours; IV *N*-acetylcysteine protocols available
Atropine	Physostigmine	Initial dose 0.5–2 mg (IV); children: 0.02 mg/kg	Can produce convulsions, bradycardia
Benzodiazepines	Flumazenil	0.2 mg (2 mL) (IV) over 15 seconds; repeat 0.2 mg (IV) every minute as necessary; initial dose not to exceed 1 mg	Recommended *only* for reversal of pure benzodiazepine sedation; competitive γ-aminobutyric acid antagonist
β-Blockers	Glucagon	1-mg/mL ampule; 5–10 mg (IV) initially	Stimulates cyclic adenosine monophosphate synthesis, increasing myocardial contractility
Calcium channel blockers	Calcium	Calcium chloride 10% 1 g (10 mL) (IV) over 5 minutes as initial dose; repeat as necessary in critical patients	Each syringe contains 1 gram or 10 mL of 10% calcium chloride; each milliliter contains 100 mg of calcium chloride or 1.4 mEq of Ca^{2+}
Carbon monoxide	Oxygen		Hyperbaric oxygen may be indicated
Cyanide	Amyl nitrate, *then* sodium nitrite	Pearls every 2 minutes; 10 mL of 3% solution over 3 minutes (IV); 0.33 mL (10 mg of 3% solution)/kg initially for children	Methemoglobin cyanide complex; causes hypotension; dosage assumes normal hemoglobin
	Sodium thiosulfate	25% solution 50 mL (IV) over 10 minutes; 1.65 mL/kg for children	Forms harmless sodium thiocyanate
Digitalis	Digibind, digoxin immune Fab (ovine)	IV dose of digoxin immune Fab in critical patients with unknown ingestion = 800 mg (20 vials); dosage if serum digoxin and patient's weight (in kilograms) are known: the number of vials to administer = (concentration [in ng/mL] × 5.6 × kg)/600	IV dose of digoxin immune Fab should be equimolar to total-body load of digoxin; one vial of digoxin immune Fab (Digibind) contains 40 mg of Fab, which neutralizes 0.6 mg digoxin; the number of milligrams of digoxin ingested divided by 0.6 is the number of vials required; indicated for life-threatening cardiac arrhythmias and hyperkalemia, and if serum digoxin level > 10 ng/mL in adults, or 4 ng/mL in children
Hydrofluoric acid	Calcium	Calcium gluconate gel or calcium carbonate paste; 10% calcium gluconate 10 mL in 40 mL D_5W via intra-arterial infusion over 4 hours may be indicated for significant digital hydrofluoric acid burns	A single intra-arterial infusion of 10% calcium gluconate provides 84 mg (4.7 mEq) of elemental calcium to bind fluoride ion, preventing cellular injury and tissue necrosis
Iron	Deferoxamine mesylate	Initial dose: 40–90 mg/kg (IM), not to exceed 1 gram; 15 mg/kg per hour (IV)	Deferoxamine mesylate forms excretable ferrioxamine complex
Lead	DMSA (succimer), 2,3-dimercaptosuccinic acid	5-Day course of 30 mg/kg per day in 3 divided doses; then 14-day course of 20 mg/kg per day divided in 2 doses	Succimer 100-mg capsule; oral congener of chelator dimercaprol, indicated for blood lead levels > 45 μg/dL
Mercury (arsenic, gold)	British antilewisite (BAL)	5 mg/kg (IM) as soon as possible	Each milliliter of BAL in oil has dimercaprol, 100 mg, in 210 mg (21%) benzyl benzoate and 680 mg peanut oil; forms stable, nontoxic, excretable cyclic compound
Methyl alcohol (ethylene glycol)	Ethyl alcohol in conjunction with dialysis	1 mL/kg of 100% ethanol initially in glucose solution; dilute ethanol to 10%; maintain blood level of 100 mg/dL; maintenance dose 0.15 mL/kg per hour (double during dialysis)	Competes for alcohol dehydrogenase; prevents formation of formic acid, oxalates
Nitrites	Methylene blue	0.2 mL/kg of 1% solution (IV) over 5 minutes	Often, exchange transfusion is needed for severe methemoglobinemia
Opiates, Darvon, Lomotil	Naloxone	2.0 mg (IV); 0.1 mg/kg (IV) for children; repeat as needed	No respiratory depression (0.4 mg per 1-mL ampule)
Organophosphates	Atropine	Initial dose: 0.5–2 mg (IV); 0.05 mg/kg (IV) initially for children	Physiologic: blocks acetylcholine; cardiac monitoring and proper oxygenation are indicated
	Pralidoxime (2-PAM chloride) (Protopam chloride)	Initial dose: 1 gram (IV); children: 25–50 mg/kg (IV)	Specific: breaks alkyl phosphate–cholinesterase bond; up to 500 mg every hour may be necessary in the critical adult patient
Tricyclic antidepressants	Sodium bicarbonate	Sodium bicarbonate 1–2 ampules (IV); (1 mEq/kg) IV bolus for initial dose; IV drip to maintain arterial pH of 7.5	One ampule of 50-mL sodium bicarbonate contains 50 mEq of $NaHCO_3$ in 50 mL or 1M sodium bicarbonate; IV bolus for life-threatening cardiac arrhythmias

* Dosages listed may require modification according to specific clinical conditions; see each specific chapter for details.

Updated and adapted from Haddad LM: Acute Poisoning. *In* Bennett JC, Plum F (eds): Cecil Textbook of Medicine. 20th ed. Philadelphia, W.B. Saunders Co., p 504, 1996; and the American College of Emergency Physicians Poster on Poisoning, Dallas, 1980.

IV, intravenous; IM, intramuscular; Fab, antigen-binding fragments.

ment, which may include administration of an antidote; (2) clinical evaluation; (3) elimination of poison from the gastrointestinal tract, skin, and eyes, or removal from the site of exposure in inhalation poisoning; (4) administration of an antidote; (5) elimination of absorbed substance; (6) supportive therapy; and (7) observation and disposition.

Emergency Management

Because overdose patients often present in moribund states, resuscitation with establishment of the airway, adequate support of ventilation and perfusion, and maintenance of all vital signs (including temperature) must be accomplished first. Continuous cardiac and pulse oximetry monitoring is essential. Rapid-sequence intubation may be indicated. Naloxone, 2 mg intravenously (IV); thiamine, 100 mg IV; and 50% dextrose, 50 mL IV (if patients are shown on Dextrostix testing to be hypoglycemic) are generally given to all adults in coma after the insertion of an intravenous line and the performance of appropriate blood studies. Maintenance of blood pressure and tissue perfusion may require adequate volume replacement, correction of acid-base disturbance, antidotal therapy (e.g., IV calcium chloride for calcium channel blocker overdose, or sodium bicarbonate for tricyclic antidepressant overdose), and administration of pressor agents. Table 1–1 lists the common emergency antidotes.[10] Cardiac arrhythmias and seizures should be appropriately treated, if possible.

Advanced Airway Management

In addition to basic airway management, many victims of poisoning require advanced management that includes endotracheal intubation. Clinical situations in which endotracheal intubation may be necessary in poisoned patients are numerous (Table 1–2). Intubation offers the advantages of complete airway control, protecting the patient from aspiration of gastric contents, providing a route for suctioning of secretions, and optimizing both oxygenation and ventilation. However, the process of intubating an awake patient is difficult and produces a number of adverse effects, including coughing, gagging, vomiting, tachycardia, hypertension, hypoxia, and increased intracranial pressure. Moreover, emergency intubation can be complicated by vocal cords that are obscured by secretions, by unusual airway anatomy, by a full stomach, or by active vomiting. Therefore, this task requires a thorough understanding of advanced airway management principles and of their application in a manner that prevents worsening of the clinical situation. Rapid-sequence intubation (RSI) is a method of rapidly obtaining airway control with minimal physiologic disturbance. The process of RSI involves a patterned sequence of preparation, drug administration, intubation, and postintubation management.[11]

In the emergency department, RSI has historically had its greatest role in the patient with severe head trauma in whom intubation could exacerbate already increased intracranial pressure. However, because it is designed to blunt or prevent all adverse responses associated with endotracheal intubation, RSI is the ideal method of intubation in the poisoned patient. With the use of drugs having a short duration of action, RSI also is advantageous because it is a temporary measure that permits temporary airway control for the patient with mildly compromised airway reflexes who requires gastrointestinal decontamination (lavage followed by activated charcoal administration) but who does not require prolonged intubation.

Table 1–2. Clinical Conditions in the Poisoned Patient That May Require Endotracheal Intubation

Acute Upper Airway Obstruction
Corrosive ingestion (sodium hydroxide, sulfuric acid)
Corrosive inhalation (ammonia, chlorine)
Envenomation
Anaphylaxis
Excess Bronchial Secretions
Pulmonary edema (opioids)
Bronchorrhea (organophosphates)
Loss of Airway Reflexes
Severe CNS depression (ethanol, opioids, barbiturates)
Cerebrovascular accident (cocaine)
Seizures (isoniazid, theophylline)
Respiratory Failure
Aspiration (hydrocarbons)
Hypoxia (drug-induced adult respiratory distress syndrome or pulmonary edema [cardiogenic or noncardiogenic])
Hypercarbia (CNS depressants, muscle relaxants [barium, organophosphates, botulism])

CNS, central nervous system.

RSI requires several essential steps that include the use of pharmacologic agents (Table 1–3). To be performed safely, RSI must occur in the following sequence.

Evaluation. The clinician must first evaluate the patient's airway to determine the necessary equipment and the best technique for safe intubation. Particular attention should be paid to abnormalities in the cervical spine and temporomandibular joint. If there is any question about the stability of the cervical spine, immobilization must be maintained. The oral cavity should be closely examined for the presence of foreign bodies.

Preparation. Before intubation, all necessary equipment must be present so that serious delays or unforeseen complications can be avoided. An IV line should be established and the patient connected to a cardiac monitor and pulse oximeter. The equipment necessary for endotracheal intubation is outlined in Table 1–4. The proper function of all equipment should be ensured before it is used. Appropriate endotracheal tube size also should be determined (Table 1–5).

Preoxygenation. Oxygen should be administered

Table 1–3. Pharmacotherapy Used in Rapid Sequence Intubation

Agent	Dose*	
Pretreatment Agents		
Atropine	0.01–0.02 mg/kg (minimum, 0.1 mg; maximum, 0.5 mg)	
Lidocaine	1–2 mg/kg	
Sedatives and Anesthetics		
Benzodiazepines		
Midazolam	0.1 mg/kg	
Opioids		
Fentanyl	5–7 μg/kg	
Barbiturates		
Sodium thiopental	3–5 mg/kg	
Methohexital	1 mg/kg	
Ketamine	1–4 mg/kg	
Skeletal Muscle Relaxants		
Depolarizing		
Succinylcholine	1–2 mg/kg	
Nondepolarizing	Defasciculating Dose	Full Dose
Pancuronium	0.01–0.05 mg/kg	0.1 mg/kg
Vecuronium	0.01–0.05 mg/kg	0.1–0.2 mg/kg
Atracurium		0.5 mg/kg
Rocuronium		0.5–1.0 mg/kg

* Doses listed are for intravenous administration.

for 4 to 5 minutes before intubation; this produces a washout of nitrogen from the lungs, replacing this gas with an oxygen reservoir. The oxygen reservoir allows several minutes of apnea during which intubation can be performed without the risk of producing hypoxia. Assisted ventilation should only be provided if the patient's own respiratory efforts are inadequate because it risks inflation of the stomach, which increases the likelihood of vomiting. Patients who are breathing spontaneously should be given 100% oxygen by face mask for several minutes before intubation.

Pretreatment. Pretreatment involves the administration of pharmacologic agents that prevent adverse physiologic changes that may occur during intubation. Agents included in this category are lidocaine and atropine.

Table 1–4. Equipment Needed for Endotracheal Intubation

- 100% Oxygen
- Face mask
- Bag-valve apparatus
- Suction equipment
  - Catheter
  - Yankauer suction tube
- Stylet
- Magill forceps
- Oral airway
- Nasopharyngeal airway ("trumpet")
- Laryngoscope handle and blades
- Endotracheal tubes
- Tongue depressors
- Syringe for endotracheal cuff inflation
- Tape
- Tincture of benzoin

Table 1–5. Age-Specific Endotracheal Tube Sizes

Age	Internal Diameter (mm)
Infant	
Premature	2.5
Term	3.0
1–6 mo	3.5
6–12 mo	4.0
Child	
2 y	4.5
4 y	5.0
6 y	5.5
8 y	6.5
10 y	7.0
Adolescent and Adult	
12 y	7.5
≥14 y	8.0–9.0

Accompanying principles:
1. Small sizes are necessary for nasotracheal intubation.
2. Endotracheal tubes two sizes smaller than age-appropriate should be immediately available.
3. Pediatric endotracheal tubes are uncuffed to reduce the risk of injury and because of "physiologic cuffing" of the pediatric airway.

IV administration of the anesthetic lidocaine appears to blunt the increase in intracranial pressure that accompanies intubation. Although scientific proof of lidocaine's efficacy is somewhat lacking, it is appropriate—particularly in the patient with suspected intracranial hypertension—to administer lidocaine, 1.0 to 2.0 mg/kg IV, 3 to 4 minutes before intubation.

Bradycardia can accompany RSI in two circumstances. In young children, both posterior pharyngeal stimulation and administration of succinylcholine can result in severe bradycardia. Therefore, in children younger than 5 years of age, atropine should be administered before induction. The dose of atropine is 0.01 to 0.02 mg/kg (maximum, 0.5 mg). No less than 0.1 mg of atropine should be administered because smaller doses can produce paradoxical bradycardia.

Severe bradycardia can also occur in patients of any age who have been exposed to medications or toxins with negative chronotropic actions. For example, in patients who have ingested β-antagonists (e.g., propranolol, calcium channel blockers, and digoxin), RSI can produce an abrupt decrease in heart rate or frank cardiac arrest. Therefore, in patients who are undergoing RSI after exposure to these agents, atropine should either be administered prophylactically or kept immediately available should emergency administration become necessary.

Induction. Induction consists of two components: administration of a sedative/anesthetic agent to produce unconsciousness, and the subsequent administration of an agent that produces complete skeletal muscle relaxation (paralysis); both actions facilitate intubation. Because administration of these drugs leads to apnea and paralysis, it is essential that induction proceed quickly and efficiently; this underscores the importance of having all intubation equipment immediately available and in working order.

A number of medications of different pharmacologic classes are used to produce sedation before skeletal muscle relaxation (see Table 1–3). These drugs include benzodiazepines, opioids, barbiturates, and ketamine. Among the benzodiazepines, midazolam, when given in a dose of 0.1 mg/kg IV (up to a range of 5 to 6 mg in an adult), is ideal because its effects are rapid in onset and short in duration. The drug also offers the advantage of producing muscle relaxation and amnesia. Opioids are another class of drugs that can be used; however, many opioids, such as morphine, may prompt histamine release, with resultant hemodynamic changes. Fentanyl in a dose of 5 μg/kg is highly effective at producing rapid sedation and relaxation with minimal cardiovascular change. Several barbiturates can produce rapid sedation and relaxation. The most popular of these is sodium thiopental (dose, 3 to 5 mg/kg). Equally effective but with a shorter duration of action is methohexital (dose, 1 mg/kg). Finally, ketamine is a dissociative anesthetic that can produce rapid onset of a state in which the patient is insensitive to pain but maintains an awake appearance and continues to have protective airway reflexes. The typical IV dose of ketamine is 1 to 2 mg/kg. Unlike other sedatives/anesthetics, ketamine can produce significant elevations in pulse, blood pressure, intracranial pressure, and myocardial oxygen consumption, and such an increase in any of these could worsen the patient's clinical condition. Because ketamine has a potent bronchodilating effect, it retains its important role as an induction agent in the patient with severe bronchospasm.

After administration of a sedative/anesthetic, skeletal muscle relaxation is performed. Skeletal muscle relaxants, all of which interrupt acetylcholine function at the myoneural junction, are typically divided into depolarizing and nondepolarizing categories. *Depolarizing agents,* of which succinylcholine is the model drug, produce muscle depolarization before paralysis; this results in initial generalized muscle fasciculation. *Nondepolarizing relaxants* produce paralysis without initial depolarization. The nondepolarizing skeletal muscle relaxants include pancuronium, vecuronium, atracurium, and rocuronium.

Succinylcholine is the most popular muscle relaxant because it has several desirable properties, including a rapid onset of action (less than 1 minute) and an extremely short duration of action. Customary paralyzing doses of succinylcholine are 1 to 2 mg/kg IV.

Despite its efficacy and popularity, succinylcholine can produce several adverse effects. These include hyperkalemia, prolonged paralysis, malignant hyperthermia, and hemodynamic changes. Hyperkalemia, which can be severe, has been most commonly associated with administration of succinylcholine to those with burns, crush injuries, select neuropathies (e.g., Guillain-Barré syndrome), and myopathies (e.g., childhood muscular dystrophies). Prolonged paralysis can occur in those who have a genetic deficiency in serum cholinesterase, the enzyme which inactivates the drug. Prolonged paralysis may also occur in patients with liver disease, the elderly, and those who have ingested anticholinesterase insecticides (carbamates or organophosphates). *Malignant hyperthermia* is a syndrome characterized by muscle rigidity, hyperthermia, autonomic disturbances, acidosis, rhabdomyolysis, myoglobinuria, renal failure, and coagulopathy. Occurring in genetically predisposed individuals, malignant hyperthermia may appear without warning in those who are given inhalation anesthetics or succinylcholine. The mortality rate associated with this syndrome is approximately 5% to 10%. Finally, succinylcholine-induced muscle depolarization can lead to transient increases in intracranial and intra-abdominal pressure, with accompanying changes in cardiac output. Because of these potential adverse effects, nondepolarizing muscle relaxants are often recommended as adjuncts to or substitutes for succinylcholine use. As adjuncts, nondepolarizing agents, when given before succinylcholine, can prevent muscle fasciculation and its attendant physiologic effects. The so-called "defasciculating dose" of a nondepolarizing agent is approximately one-tenth the full dose of that agent. For example, pancuronium can be given in a dose of 0.01 mg/kg IV before the administration of succinylcholine to prevent fasciculation. Nondepolarizing agents can also be used solely for skeletal muscle relaxation. However, they generally have a much slower onset of action (as long as 3-5 minutes) and produce a longer duration of paralysis. Also, many nondepolarizing agents stimulate histamine release, producing significant hemodynamic changes. Therefore, they are not ideal agents for RSI. A new nondepolarizing relaxant, rocuronium, appears to have the most rapid onset of all nondepolarizing agents, approaching that of succinylcholine with regard to time to complete muscle relaxation.[12]

Intubation. Suction must be immediately available when intubation is performed. The patient undergoing emergency intubation often has a full stomach; the risk of vomiting and aspiration is therefore significant. This risk is minimized both by the RSI technique and by the direct application of pressure upon the cricoid cartilage (Sellick's maneuver), which occludes the esophagus. Preoxygenation and limiting the duration of the intubation attempt to less than 20 to 30 seconds should prevent significant hypoxia.

The differences between the airway of the child and that of the adult have important implications for endotracheal intubation.

1. The child has a relatively large tongue; this makes direct visualization of the larynx difficult.
2. The child has larger tonsils, which also obscure visualization.
3. The infant's larynx is located more cephalad than that of the adult. As a result, the angle between the tongue and the glottis is more acute and visualization of the larynx is impaired.

4. The subglottic area of the infant is the narrowest part of the larynx and may impede the passage of an endotracheal tube passed through the vocal cords.

Post-Intubation Management. Immediately after successful endotracheal intubation, placement of the endotracheal tube must be confirmed by detection of the combination of bilateral equal breath sounds on chest auscultation, end-tidal carbon dioxide monitoring, or chest radiography. After confirmation, the tube should be secured either with a strap or with benzoin and adhesive tape. Inflation of the endotracheal tube cuff should be performed to minimize aspiration of gastric contents (although aspiration of activated charcoal around cuffed endotracheal tubes is a frequent occurrence). Because the airway of the young child has an area of narrowing ("physiologic cuffing"), cuffed endotracheal tubes are not used in the pediatric patient. If long-term intubation is necessary, sedatives/anesthetics and nondepolarizing muscle relaxants should continue to be administered.

In unskilled or unprepared hands, emergency endotracheal intubation can have disastrous consequences. Even when performed by the most experienced hands, this complex procedure can have complications that should be anticipated so that they can be quickly recognized and treated. These complications include:

- dental or oral cavity trauma
- gagging and vomiting
- hypoxia
- hypercarbia
- bradycardia
- tachycardia
- hypertension
- hypotension
- increased intracranial pressure
- pneumomediastinum
- pneumothorax
- cardiac arrhythmias
- myocardial ischemia or infarction
- aspiration
- laryngospasm
- esophageal intubation
- tracheal injury

Circulatory Support

The poisoned patient often presents to the emergency department with hypotension or frank shock. The provision of circulatory support through interventions that may include volume expansion, antidote administration, correction of electrolyte and acid-base disturbances, and vasopressor therapy is essential in initial management.

Many medications and toxins produce hypotension (Table 1–6). Depending on the ingested substance, the low blood pressure may have a number of causes. For example, blood pressure depressions may occur from direct depression of myocardial contractility (e.g., quinidine), disturbances of central nervous system cardiorespiratory centers (e.g., clonidine), severe gastrointestinal fluid losses (e.g., acetaminophen, iron, arsenic, ricin, mushrooms), peripheral vasodilatation (e.g., angiotensin-converting enzyme inhibitors), or a combination of these effects (e.g., theophylline, calcium channel blockers, tricyclic antidepressants). Hypotension also can result from the secondary effects of toxins (e.g., cocaine-induced myocardial infarction). Finally, blood pressure disturbances in the poisoned patient may represent accompanying trauma (e.g., severe spinal cord injury or internal hemorrhage). With the multitude of possible causes, the clinician, on the basis of the known pathophysiology of a particular drug and after having performed a thorough physical assessment, should determine, if at all possible, the probable cause of hypotension if he or she is to provide a specific intervention.

Table 1–6. Intoxications Commonly Associated with Hypotension

Arsenic
Calcium-channel blockers
Clonidine
Iron
Theophylline
Tricyclic antidepressants
Phenothiazines
Quinidine
Digoxin
β-Blockers
Angiotensin-converting enzyme (ACE) inhibitors
α-Antagonists
Monoamine oxidase inhibitors
Barbiturates
Opioids
Envenomations
Marine
Reptile
Hymenoptera

Volume Expansion

Appropriate cardiac output relies on the adequacy of intravascular volume. After poisoning, intravascular volume may decrease abruptly. This decrease can be *absolute,* occurring as a result of a direct loss of intravascular volume (e.g., pulmonary edema, gastrointestinal pooling), or *relative,* resulting from severe peripheral vasodilatation (e.g., angiotensin-converting enzyme inhibitor or α-antagonist ingestion). In either case, hypotension should first be treated with the administration of volume-expanding agents.

Fluids that are acceptable for volume expansion are numerous. However, normal saline and lactated Ringer's solution are generally the most readily available isotonic agents. Adults should receive up to 500- to 1000-mL boluses of isotonic fluid while blood pressure is monitored (children should be given 10 to 40 mL/kg). After the administration of each bolus, the patient should be reassessed for improvements in cardiac output.

Alternative fluids that can be used for volume

expansion in the poisoned patient include albumin, Plasmanate (plasma protein fraction 5%), and whole blood. Each of these fluids has a role that is best determined by the pathophysiologic mechanism responsible for the hypotension. Being colloid rather than crystalloid in nature, these fluids in theory maintain intravascular volume better than saline solutions do. In clinical situations in which a "leaky capillary syndrome" is mechanistically the source of intravascular volume loss, the use of colloid solutions may be preferred. Whole blood is most valuable in situations in which there is frank blood loss. With severe hemolysis (e.g., after arsine or stibine exposure), exchange transfusion with whole blood may be necessary.

Usually, the adequacy of volume expansion is determined clinically by an increase in blood pressure. Other clinical signs of improved cardiac output include resolution of cyanosis and normalization of capillary refill time. Central venous pressure and Swan-Ganz catheter monitoring, although invasive, provide the best evidence of appropriate intravascular volume.

Fluid overload is a potential complication of volume expansion. This is most likely to occur in patients who receive excess fluids over a short period of time. Also, after overdoses of myocardial depressants such as tricyclic antidepressants, a fluid bolus that could be tolerated by a healthy individual can produce pulmonary edema in the overdose patient. Therefore, administration of modest boluses of fluid is generally recommended; if cardiac output remains inadequate after fluids have been given, vasopressor therapy should be initiated.

Vasopressor Therapy

In the patient with severe hypotension, vasopressor therapy is necessary if blood pressure is not satisfactorily improved after volume expansion. In the poisoned patient who is also a trauma victim, definitive treatment of hypotension may include operative intervention.

Vasopressors are drugs that are administered to maintain cardiac output. These agents have specific effects on the heart or blood vessels, augmenting myocardial function or increasing vasomotor tone, or both. With rare exception, vasopressors used in the acute management of hypotension are short-acting drugs that are given by continuous IV infusion. Vasopressors generally act at adrenergic (α and β), D (dopamine), or glucagon receptors (Table 1–7). The adrenergic system has been further defined with the recognition of two major α-adrenergic receptor subtypes (α_1 and α_2) and three β-adrenergic receptor subtypes (β_1, β_2, and β_3). Coupled with intracellular G proteins, these membrane-bound receptors effect an intracellular chain of events that includes changes in the activity of adenylate cyclase. This action goes on to modulate the level of intracellular cyclic adenosine monophosphate (cAMP), which in turn alters phospholipase activity or opens gated calcium channels. Although the cellular mechanisms of this system have become much better defined, the general principles of vasopressor action remain unchanged. For example, α-adrenergic receptor agonists produce vascular smooth muscle contraction. β_1-Adrenergic receptor agonists produce increased heart rate and contractility, whereas β_2-adrenergic receptor agonists promote generalized smooth muscle relaxation (including bronchial and vascular). Vasopressor therapy is designed to improve cardiac output through manipulation of the specific receptor most appropriate for the clinical situation.

A number of vasopressors can be used to provide blood pressure support (see Table 1–7). The indications for the use of these drugs may vary slightly, depending on the clinical circumstance.

Epinephrine. Epinephrine elevates low blood pressure primarily through its α-adrenergic stim-

Table 1–7. Common Vasopressors by Dose Range and Mechanism of Action

	Receptor Type			
Agent	*α-Adrenergic*	*β_1-Adrenergic*	*β_2-Adrenergic*	*Dopaminergic*
Epinephrine (0.1–0.5 μg/kg per min)				
Low-dose		+ +	+ + +	
Moderate-dose	+	+ + +	+ + +	
High-dose	+ + +	+ + +	+ + +	
Norepinephrine (0.1–0.5 μg/kg per min)	+ + +	+ +		
Dopamine (2–20 μg/kg per min)				
Low-dose				+ + +
Moderate-dose		+ + +		
High-dose	+ + +			
Dobutamine (2–20 μg/kg per min)	+	+ + +	+	
Phenylephrine (0.1–0.5 μg/kg per min)	+ + +			
Metaraminol (5–10 μg/kg)	+ + +		+ +	
Nonadrenergic agents				
Amrinone (5–15 μg/kg per min)				
Glucagon (50–150 μg/kg per h)				
Calcium chloride				

+, Mild effect; + +, Moderate effect; + + +, Major effect.

ulating properties. This effect also is valuable in improving myocardial and cerebral blood flow. Because it also has prominent β-adrenergic agonist effects, epinephrine is variably effective at producing marked increases in blood pressure. Epinephrine therapy is initiated at a dose of 0.1 to 0.5 μg/kg per minute. Epinephrine is particularly effective in intoxications associated with hypotension and bronchospasm (e.g., Hymenoptera envenomation and anaphylactic reactions).

Norepinephrine. Norepinephrine stimulates both α- and β-adrenergic receptors, with slightly greater stimulation of α-adrenergic receptors. The effect is improved vasomotor tone in conjunction with increased myocardial chronotropy and inotropy. Norepinephrine infusions are initiated in a dose of 0.1 to 0.5 μg/kg per minute.

Dopamine. Dopamine is a precursor to norepinephrine. The most popular of vasopressors, dopamine appears to have at least three mechanisms of action: (1) promotion of norepinephrine synthesis, (2) a tyramine-like effect that stimulates release of preformed norepinephrine, and (3) direct stimulation of vascular dopamine receptors.

The cardiovascular effects of dopamine are variable, depending on the infusion rate. At relatively low doses (1 to 2 μg/kg per minute), it dilates renal and mesenteric vessels without marked increases in heart rate or blood pressure. At doses of 2 to 10 μg/kg per minute, β-adrenergic receptor stimulation predominates, producing significant increases in cardiac output. Finally, at doses greater than 10 μg/kg per minute, α-adrenergic receptor stimulation is the primary action, resulting in marked peripheral vasoconstriction. The general dose range for dopamine infusion is 2 to 20 μg/kg per minute.

Dopamine is safe and effective for any type of drug-induced hypotension. In the past, there have been theoretic concerns that dopamine's β-adrenergic effect in the face of phenothiazine or tricyclic antidepressant intoxication would increase the peripheral vasodilatation associated with overdose, exacerbating hypotension. However, experimental data and clinical experience have failed to confirm this adverse effect from dopamine use. Also, with hypotension after monoamine oxidase inhibitor overdose, dopamine's effects are somewhat unpredictable; it may be relatively ineffective (owing to the lack of preformed norepinephrine), or it can produce an exaggerated response (because of its tyramine-like action).

Dobutamine. Dobutamine is a synthetic catecholamine with almost exclusive β-adrenergic receptor–stimulating effects. Its primary mechanism of blood pressure improvement is direct myocardial inotropy; thus, reflex peripheral vasodilatation may occur with its use. Unlike dopamine, dobutamine does not release preformed norepinephrine. The usual dosage range for dobutamine is 2 to 20 μg/kg per minute, although doses as high as 40 μg/kg per minute have been used. High-dose infusions often increase myocardial oxygen demands which, if unmet, can result in myocardial ischemia. Nonetheless, dobutamine is extremely effective in congestive heart failure.

Phenylephrine. Phenylephrine has both α- and β-adrenergic receptor–stimulating properties, although its α-adrenergic receptor actions predominate. Phenylephrine is a potent stimulator of vasomotor tone; it is therefore very effective in patients in hypotensive states resulting from severe peripheral vasodilatation (e.g., following overdose with an α-adrenergic antagonist, such as prazocin). Phenylephrine infusions are given in a typical dose range of 0.1 to 0.5 μg/kg per minute.

Metaraminol (Aramine). Metaraminol is a synthetic amine vasopressor with both α- and β-adrenergic effects. β-Adrenergic effects are specifically β_1, but not β_2. Metaraminol also stimulates the release of norepinephrine from its storage sites; thus, its main effects are cardiac stimulation and peripheral vasoconstriction. Because of its potential ability to produce arrhythmias in those with myocardial irritability, metaraminol can produce rhythm disturbances, including ventricular tachycardia, ventricular premature beats, and atrioventricular dissociation. Cardiac arrhythmias are more likely to occur in patients who have myocardial ischemia or infarction. Bradycardia occasionally occurs as a complication, resulting from a reflex response to an increase in blood pressure. This reflex bradycardia is blocked by the administration of atropine. Monoamine oxidase inhibitors and inhibitors of catecholamine uptake (e.g., tricyclic antidepressants) may potentiate the effects of metaraminol, precipitating a hypertensive crisis. Because it has a prolonged duration of action (20 to 60 minutes), metaraminol usually is given in single dose (approximately 10 μg/kg IV) rather than as a continuous infusion; this makes the drug difficult to titrate. As with other drugs that stimulate the release of preformed norepinephrine, long-term use of metaraminol may deplete endogenous catecholamine stores, resulting in tachyphylaxis. Unlike other vasopressors, metaraminol is relatively stable in bicarbonate-containing solutions; because it is subject to oxidation, it should be protected from light.

Amrinone. Amrinone is a novel, nonadrenergic cardiac stimulant that improves myocardial contractility while inducing vasodilatation. Its mechanism of action appears to be direct inhibition of phosphodiesterase; the result of this is increased intracellular cAMP activity, an action that increases transmembrane calcium flux, potentiating cardiac chronotropy and inotropy. Amrinone's effects have been compared with those of dobutamine and nitroprusside combination therapy. Amrinone can be used to treat syndromes of left ventricular failure but should not be administered in the presence of myocardial ischemia; like dobutamine, it may increase myocardial demands, resulting in infarction. Because of its potent vasodilating action, amrinone may cause a hypotensive response in those with low intravascular volume. The usual dosage range for this agent is 5 to 15 μg/kg per minute; the total daily dose should not exceed 10 mg/kg per day.

Glucagon. Glucagon is a single-chain pancreatic polypeptide that is an effective inotropic and chronotropic agent. Its mechanism of action is direct stimulation of myocardial glucagon receptors; these receptors, when stimulated, increase the formation of myocardial cAMP. The resultant effect is positive inotropy and, to a lesser degree, positive chronotropy. Glucagon is theoretically most effective after β-blocker overdose, in which decreased β-adrenergic receptor activation leads to diminished cAMP production. Glucagon is given in an initial dose of 1 to 10 mg (50 to 150 μg/kg in children). If effective in augmenting blood pressure, it can be given as a continuous infusion of 5 to 10 mg/h (100 μg/kg per hour in children). The diluent, which is provided with lyophilized glucagon, contains 0.2% phenol. Therefore, although single doses can be given after standard reconstitution, glucagon for continuous infusion should be reconstituted with saline to prevent phenol toxicity. Adverse effects from glucagon include hyperglycemia, nausea, vomiting, and ileus.

Calcium. Calcium plays a key role in regulating cardiac inotropy through its binding to troponin C, an action that permits interaction between actin and myosin. Although most of the calcium that produces this change resides in an intracellular calcium pool, extracellular calcium does diffuse into cells and contributes to increased contractility. Although diffusion of calcium into the myocardium is "gated"—that is, it is tightly controlled—high concentrations of extracellular calcium, particularly in the face of channel blockade (e.g., after overdose of calcium-channel blockers), sometimes improve contractility. Administration of IV calcium chloride is indicated in the management of hypotension resulting from calcium channel blocker overdose (see Table 1–1), hyperkalemia, and hypocalcemia.

Clinical Evaluation

A thorough history-taking and physical examination are essential to the diagnosis of the toxic patient. *Poisoning should be suspected in any patient who presents with multisystemic involvement until proved otherwise.* Although the initial manifestations of poisoning are myriad, a patient with acute poisoning often presents with coma, cardiac arrhythmia, seizures, metabolic acidosis, or gastrointestinal disturbance, either together as symptom complexes or as isolated events. Symptom complexes, or *toxidromes* (Table 1–8), may give clues to an unknown poisoning. For example, a patient with a history of depression who presents with coma, seizures, a widened QRS complex or evidence of dysrhythmia on electrocardiography, and dilated pupils suggests tricyclic antidepressant overdose. Hepatic, renal, respiratory, and hematologic disturbances are generally delayed manifestations of poisoning.

The clinical evaluation, in addition to the history-taking and physical examination, includes an assessment of major signs of toxicity presented by the patient and evaluation of the laboratory data.

History

The primary goal is identification of the toxic agent when one suspects poisoning or drug overdose. Sometimes, diagnosis is easy, as in the case of the toddler who ingests iron tablets in the mother's presence. Sometimes it is difficult, as in the case of the patient who is hiding a history of drug abuse and passes out at work or who has an unexpected seizure.

Prior medical or psychiatric history, current medications, and allergies should be obtained from family or friends if the patient is unable to relate the information. These individuals should be asked the following questions:

What other medicines are in the house?
What was the patient doing that day?
Was he working on the car in the garage, spraying the roses, working on the farm, cleaning out the bilge of a ship with chemicals, or driving a forklift inside a poorly ventilated warehouse?
Does the patient live alone, did he or she just lose a job, or is he or she suffering the end of a meaningful relationship?
Is the patient on a special diet or eating some exotic new health food?
Has the patient inadvertently taken too much medication with an adverse effect (e.g., acetaminophen overdose in an alcoholic, or two medications from two different physicians)?
Is the substance nontoxic (see Table 1–9)?

A young patient who presents with chest pain and cardiac arrhythmia may be abusing cocaine. A patient who has abused a street drug may be completely unaware of the actual substance taken.

Children who are afebrile and have unexplained lethargy, neurologic symptoms, bizarre behavior, and other puzzling presentations must be evaluated for poisoning.

A patient may have two simultaneous disorders. For example, the patient may have had an accident because he or she had been abusing drugs, or an intoxicated patient may have fallen down a flight of stairs. Alternatively, a patient with an overdose may exacerbate an underlying condition, such as diabetic ketoacidosis. The emergency medical service paramedics can be a valuable source of information regarding the history and surrounding events of a particular case. The presence of an empty bottle of medication next to a collapsed patient is a valuable clue.

Physical Examination

The physical examination can help in determining the extent of poisoning and may reveal the presence of a toxic syndrome, of any underlying disease, or of any concomitant trauma. *Repeated assessment, espe-*

Table 1–8. Examples of Symptom Complexes, or Toxidromes

Toxidrome or Complex	Consciousness	Respirations	Pupils	Other	Possible Toxic Agent/ Mechanism
Cholinergic	Coma	↑ ↓	Pinpoint	Fasciculations Incontinence Salivation, wheezing Lacrimation Bradycardia	Organophosphate insecticides, carbamates, nicotine
Anticholinergic	Agitation, hallucinations	↑	Dilated	Fever, flushing Dry skin and mucous membranes Urinary retention	Anticholinergics (Atropine, Jimson weed) (Antihistamines)
Opioid	Coma	↓	Pinpoint	Tracks Hypothermia Hypotension	Opiates, Lomotil (diphenoxylate hydrochloride; atropine sulfate), pentazocine, Darvon (propoxyphene hydrochloride)
Extrapyramidal	Wakefulness	↑	—	Torsion of head/neck	Phenothiazines, haloperidol
Phenothiazine	Coma	↓	Pinpoint	Cardiac arrhythmia Orthostatic hypotension, anticholinergic findings	Phenothiazines
Tricyclic antidepressant	Coma (initially, agitation)	↓	Dilated	Cardiac arrhythmia Convulsions Hypotension QT interval prolongation Cardiac conduction defect Myoclonus, hyperreflexia	Tricyclic antidepressants
Uremia	Coma	↑	—	Uremic frost Detectable shunt Hyperkalemia Acidosis	(Uremia)
Sedative/hypnotic	Coma	↓	Dilated	Hypothermia Decreased reflexes Hypotension	Sedatives, barbiturates
Salicylates	Semicoma, agitation	↑	—	Diaphoresis Tinnitus Agitation Alkalosis (early) Acidosis (late) Fever	Salicylates Oil of wintergreen
Sympathomimetic	Agitation, hallucinations	↑	Dilated	Seizures Tachycardia Hypertension Diaphoresis Metabolic acidosis Tremor Hyperreflexia	Cocaine Theophylline Amphetamines Caffeine

cially of vital signs and of cardiac, pulmonary, and neurologic status is critical to proper management of the toxicologic patient. The physical examination also can provide valuable clues as to the particular toxin involved (Table 1–10).

Vital Signs. As part of the initial evaluation, complete determination of vital signs, including measurement of body temperature initially and throughout the emergency department assessment, is mandatory. Obtaining a core body temperature measurement may be necessary. *Hyperthermia* can occur with a number of ingestions and in infectious illness, but it is characteristic of poisoning with salicylates, anticholinergics, monoamine oxidase inhibitors, and dinitrophenols, and it occasionally is seen in intoxication with phencyclidine, LSD, and cocaine, especially following seizures. Life-threatening malignant hyperthermia following drug overdose may occur. *Hypothermia* is common and often occurs because of exposure to cold, hypoglycemia, or overdose of a number of sedatives, especially barbiturates, ethanol, carbamazepine, narcotics, and phenothiazines. *Bradycardia* can be seen with overdose of digitalis, cholinergic agents, β-blockers, and calcium channel blockers (especially verapamil), but it also may be seen with hypothermia or spinal cord trauma. *Hypertension* is characteristic of intoxication with cocaine, amphetamines, phencyclidine, and sympathomimetics. An overdose of almost any drug may result in *hypotension* or *tachycardia*.

Skin. The skin should be examined for needle tracks, burns, bruises, or lacerations. Needle tracks may be confined to the groin or other areas that are not readily visible. A *"boiled lobster" appearance*

Table 1–9. Nontoxic Ingestions

abrasives	Elmer's glue	petroleum jelly (Vaseline)
adhesives	Etch-A-Sketch	Play-Doh
antacids	fabric softeners	Polaroid picture coating fluid
antibiotics	fish bowl additives	porous-tip marking pens
baby product cosmetics	glues and pastes	Prussian blue (ferricyanide)
ballpoint pen inks	hand lotions and creams	putty (less than 2 oz)
bath oil (castor oil and perfume)	3% hydrogen peroxide, medicinal	rubber cement
bathtub floating toys	incense	sachets (essential oils, powder)
birth control pills	indelible markers	shampoos (liquid)
bleach (< 5% sodium hypochlorite)	ink (black, blue)	shaving creams and lotions
body conditioners	iodophil disinfectant	soap and soap products
bubble bath soaps (detergents)	laxatives	spackles
calamine lotion	lipstick	suntan preparations
candles (beeswax or paraffin)	lubricant	sweetening agents (saccharin)
chalk (calcium carbonate)	Magic Markers	teething rings (water sterility)
cigarettes or cigars (nicotine)	makeup (eye, liquid, facial)	thermometers (mercury)
colognes	matches	toothpaste with or without fluoride
cosmetics	mineral oil	toy pistol caps (potassium chlorate)
crayons marked AP, CP	modeling clay	vitamins with or without fluoride
dehumidifying packets (silica or charcoal)	newspaper	watercolors
deodorants	pencil (graphite lead, coloring)	zinc oxide
deodorizers, spray and refrigerator	perfumes	zirconium oxide

Adapted from Mofenson HC, Greensher J: The non-toxic ingestion. Pediatr Clin North Am *17*:583, 1970.

suggests borate poisoning, particularly in a child who may have ingested roach powder insecticide. *Flushing* suggests an allergic reaction, niacin overdose, anticholinergic poisoning, fever, scombroid fish poisoning (histamine reaction), the toxic shock syndrome, or an alcohol-disulfiram reaction.

Diaphoresis suggests hypoglycemia, salicylate or organophosphate poisoning, hyperthyroidism, drug or alcohol withdrawal, or shock from cardiac or other etiology. *Jaundice* or hepatic coma usually is seen 2 to 5 days after the acute poisoning incident and may follow acetaminophen overdose, aspirin ingestion (Reye's syndrome), iron poisoning, carbon tetrachloride, mushroom, copper, or phosphorus ingestion. *Petechiae* and *ecchymosis* suggest a coagulopathy, coumadin or aspirin overdose, or meningococcemia. *Bullae* may be secondary to skin hypoxia or prolonged pressure and are seen with most sedative-hypnotic overdoses (especially barbiturate overdose), carbon monoxide poisoning, and thermal burns. Bullae often are seen following rattlesnake envenomation. Bullous lesions or soft tissue swelling should prompt evaluation for rhabdomyolysis, an occasional finding in patients following prolonged coma or malignant hyperthermia, such as in cocaine abuse.

Table 1–10. Important Clues on Physical Examination

Clinical Finding	Diagnostic Example
Needle tracks	Intravenous drug abuse
Characteristic odor of breath	Gasoline
Destruction of nasal mucosa/cartilage	Cocaine abuse
New significant heart murmur	Infective endocarditis
Pulmonary edema	Heroin abuse
Boardlike abdomen	Black widow spider bite
Salivation and lacrimation	Organophosphates
"Boiled lobster" skin	Boric acid poisoning

Breath. It is important to smell the patient's breath. Alcohol is the most common odor detected on the breath of an intoxicated patient in the emergency department. The accurate identification of other odors varies greatly among physicians. A fruity odor may be detectable in the patient with diabetic ketoacidosis, but ketosis also is seen with isopropyl alcohol ingestion. Cyanide poisoning can produce the smell of silver polish. A smell of cleaning fluid suggests carbon tetrachloride poisoning. Gasoline, camphor, hydrogen sulfide, ether, turpentine, methyl salicylate, paraldehyde, phenol, and organophosphate insecticides all have a characteristic odor. Arsenic intoxication is associated with the odor of garlic.

Ear, Nose, and Throat. An ear, nose, and throat examination may disclose hidden needle marks (ears), and a nasal examination may reveal chronic insufflation of cocaine. An edematous, often elongated uvula may be seen with marijuana abuse as well as in other conditions.

Lungs. Auscultation of the lungs may provide diagnostic clues. In narcotic or tricyclic antidepressant overdose, pulmonary edema may be a complication. In all overdose patients, *aspiration pneumonitis* is a possibility. Inhalation of toxic gases may produce wheezing and pulmonary compromise. *Pneumothorax* may be detected in patients with underlying trauma. *Mediastinal emphysema* from marijuana or crack cocaine smoking also may be detected by auscultation.

Heart. Examination of the heart may reveal a new *murmur*, which in an intravenous drug abuser suggests endocarditis. A slow rhythm, which on electrocardiography indicates complete heart block in a young patient, suggests calcium channel blocker overdose (especially verapamil), just as a ventricular arrhythmia on electrocardiography in a young patient suggests cocaine toxicity. An irregularly irregular heartbeat that is new in a patient on an alcoholic binge suggests atrial fibrillation—the so-called "holiday heart" syndrome.

Abdomen. A *boardlike abdomen* in a patient with a history of spider bite is characteristic of black widow envenomation. Examination of the abdomen in an overdose patient often reveals an *adynamic ileus*. In patients with abdominal pain, a surgical abdomen must be ruled out. *Hepatomegaly* suggests a cause for coma other than poisoning, such as Reye's syndrome.

Neurologic Assessment. All patients should undergo a careful neurologic examination. Issues of major concern are concomitant head trauma and spinal cord trauma in comatose patients. Serial neurologic examinations are key to proper assessment (see discussion of coma).

Extremities. The extremities should be evaluated to detect thrombophlebitis, fracture or dislocation, or vascular insufficiency. *Rhabdomyolysis* and the *compartment syndrome* are definite concerns in overdose patients, especially in those with prolonged coma or underlying trauma.

Assessment of Major Signs of Toxicity

The toxicologic patient presenting in the acute setting often exhibits the following, either alone or in combination: coma, cardiac arrhythmia, metabolic acidosis, gastrointestinal disturbance, and seizures.

Coma

One of the most common manifestations of acute poisoning is coma. The principles of coma management are relatively straightforward. Patients in coma must be stabilized initially by establishment of an airway, proper oxygenation with continuous pulse oximetry, insertion of an IV line with normal saline, and resuscitation, if necessary (see discussion of emergency management). The clinical evaluation of the comatose patient is invaluable not only in determining the depth of coma and assessing for trauma, but also in providing a baseline for repeated clinical assessment.

Level of Consciousness. *Consciousness* is defined as an awareness of self and the environment.[13] *Coma* is unarousable unresponsiveness. *Wakefulness* implies the ability to be aroused. These three functional states are mediated by the ascending reticular activating system, a tract that courses through the diencephalon, midbrain, and pons (the brain stem). Diseases produce coma either by diffusely affecting the brain or by encroaching upon the brain stem.[13] Coma may be effected by (1) a supratentorial mass lesion, such as a subdural hematoma; (2) a brain stem lesion (uncommon); or (3) metabolic disorders that widely depress or interrupt brain function.

The major causes of coma in patients seen in the emergency department include poisoning (e.g., carbon monoxide poisoning), drug overdose, head trauma, cerebrovascular accident, anoxia, infection (e.g., meningitis), and diabetes and other systemic disorders such as renal failure, hepatic coma, and cardiac arrhythmia. The physician must rule out each condition before establishing the diagnosis of poisoning.

Supratentorial structural lesions are suggested by a rapid progression of signs, including changes in respiratory pattern, disconjugate gaze, lateralizing signs, loss of doll's eyes movements, and other signs of trauma in the patient.

A metabolic cause of coma may be indicated by the persistence of the pupillary light reflex; a depression of respiration and consciousness more pronounced than other neurologic signs; preceding altered mental states; asterixis or fasciculations, or both; the presence of a ciliospinal reflex; and extracranial signs, such as jaundice or uremic frost.

Repeated assessment of the comatose patient is critical to proper management of poisoning.

Pupils. Evaluation of the patient's pupils is most helpful. *Midpoint fixed pupils* or a unilateral dilated pupil suggests a structural lesion. *Pinpoint pupils* suggest overdose of opiates, clonidine, organophosphate insecticides, chloral hydrate, phenothiazine, or nicotine; the use of pilocarpine-containing eye drops; or a structural pontine lesion. Dilated pupils are nonspecific.

Respirations. It is important to review the pattern of breathing. *Posthyperventilation apnea, Cheyne-Stokes respirations,* and *apneustic and ataxic breathing* strongly suggest that a structural lesion is the cause of the patient's coma. Whereas central neurogenic hyperventilation is a classic presentation of brain stem injury, the differential diagnosis of rapid, deep breathing is a challenge in inself. Salicylate poisoning, dinitrophenol insecticide poisoning, Kussmaul's breathing in the diabetic, pulmonary embolus, carbon monoxide poisoning, or hypoxia from any cause can produce a similar pattern. *Compensatory hyperventilation* may accompany methanol or ethylene glycol poisoning or other toxin-producing metabolic acidosis. *Respiratory arrest* is a common presentation in the overdose patient and may lead to multisystemic dysfunction resulting from severe hypoxic injury.

Ocular Movements. A disturbance of ocular movements (e.g., loss of doll's eyes movements) suggests a structural lesion. *Nystagmus* suggests intoxication with phenytoin, phencyclidine, carbamazeine, and, occasionally, ethanol.

Motor Function. *Decorticate and decerebrate posturing* suggests a structural lesion. It is important to realize that patients with poisoning or drug overdose may appear brain dead, have fixed, dilated pupils, be in an unresponsive coma, and lack the cold caloric response, yet they recover fully in time (see Chapter 8).

Cardiac Arrhythmia

A 12-lead electrocardiography and cardiac monitoring are essential for any patient with significant

Table 1–11. Common Toxic Causes of Cardiac Arrhythmia

Tricyclic antidepressants	Digitalis
Arsenic	Dinitrophenol
β-Blockers	Fluoroacetate
Calcium channel blockers	Phenol
Carbon monoxide	Phenothiazine
Chloroquine	Phosphorus
Chloral hydrate	Physostigmine
Clonidine	Quinine
Cocaine	Succinylcholine
Cyanide	

poisoning. Evidence of an arrhythmia or other important diagnostic clues may be present on electrocardiography, such as a widened QRS complex in cyclic antidepressant overdose, or a prolonged QT interval in phenothiazine overdose. Table 1–11 lists common toxic causes of cardiac arrhythmia.

The patient with life-threatening cardiac arrhythmia or cardiac arrest should be managed on the basis of the general principles of resuscitation and the American Heart Association's Advanced Cardiac Life Support (ACLS) guidelines. If cyclic antidepressant overdose is suspected, administration of IV sodium bicarbonate is indicated for correction of ventricular arrhythmia or conduction disturbances. Administration of IV calcium chloride is the primary therapeutic measure for calcium channel blocker overdose.[14, 15] Use of digoxin antibody fragments (Digibind) is indicated for digitalis poisoning,[16] and glucagon[17, 18] and isoproterenol (Isuprel) for β-blocker overdose (see Table 1–1). In referred patients who have already been hospitalized elsewhere, ventricular arrhythmia may be due to hyperkalemia because renal failure may have ensued; in such patients, IV sodium bicarbonate, glucose/insulin, and, if necessary, calcium chloride administration may be warranted. In all intoxicated patients, correction of hypoxia, metabolic acidosis, and fluid and electrolyte disturbance serves to reduce the incidence of cardiac arrhythmias (see Chapter 6).

Metabolic Acidosis

Causes of a *high–anion gap metabolic acidosis* are listed in Table 1–12. The assessment of metabolic acidosis includes not only arterial blood gas analysis, but also studies of serum sodium, potassium, chloride, carbon dioxide, blood urea nitrogen, creatinine, glucose, acetone, serum osmolality, and urine pH, as well as urinalysis. Determination of the anion gap[19] is helpful in the diagnosis and management of poisoning.

Table 1–12. Causes of a High–Anion Gap Metabolic Acidosis

Methanol	Ethylene glycol poisoning
Uremia	Salicylates
Diabetic ketoacidosis	Cyanide
Paraldehyde	Iron
Isoniazid	Nondiabetic alcoholic ketoacidosis
Lactic acidosis	

The clinician can measure serum osmolality either directly by determining the freezing point (osmometry) or by calculation. The formula for calculating osmolality is

$$\text{Serum osmolality} = 2 \times \text{Na}^+ \text{ (mEq/L)} + \frac{\text{BUN (mg/dL)}}{2.8} + \frac{\text{Glucose (mg/dL)}}{18},$$

where BUN is the blood urea nitrogen level.

The normal serum osmolality is 280 to 295 mOsm/L. An osmometer measurement indicating a serum osmolality that is more than 10 mOsm/L greater than the calculated osmolality is termed an *osmolal gap,* and this suggests the presence of an osmotically active substance that is not accounted for by the calculated osmolality. Substances such as ethanol, methanol, isopropyl alcohol, ethylene glycol, glycerol, and mannitol produce an increase in the measured osmolality over the calculated osmolality—the most common is, of course, ethanol. A substance contributes to osmolality only if it achieves relatively high blood levels and has a low molecular weight. Most drugs or intoxicants cannot be detected with use of the osmolal gap (see Chapter 5).

Gastrointestinal Disturbance

The causes of toxic gastrointestinal disturbance are many. The patient with iron poisoning has severe, repeated episodes of vomiting and may develop gastrointestinal hemorrhage. Theophylline overdose also causes persistent retching. Acute lithium and arsenic poisoning characteristically produce massive diarrhea. Patients with acute mercury poisoning have a mucous-type diarrhea, with the subsequent development of hemorrhagic colitis. One of the most striking presentations is caused by phosphorus poisoning, which produces luminescent vomitus and flatus. The early presentation of organophosphate poisoning is similar to that of acute gastroenteritis and is characterized by abdominal cramps, vomiting, and diarrhea, with subsequent development of neurologic signs. Poisoning from mushrooms (Chapter 25), toxic marine life (Chapter 27), botulism, and food (Chapter 28) should be included in the differential diagnosis. Chemotherapeutic agents (Chapters 10 and 54) are well-known causes of toxic gastroenteritis.

The management of gastrointestinal disturbance in the toxic patient includes following the general principles of blood, fluid, and electrolyte resuscitation, when indicated; judicious use of parenteral antiemetics to control persistent vomiting; specific measures such as antidotal therapy (e.g., in iron or organophosphate poisoning), or interventional therapy, such as charcoal hemoperfusion (in theophylline overdose) or hemodialysis (in lithium overdose), when indicated; and supportive care.

Table 1–13. Common Toxic Causes of Seizures

Amoxapine	Lithium
Anticholinergics	Lysergic acid diethylamide (LSD)
Bupropion	Oral hypoglycemics
Camphor	Parathion
Carbon monoxide	Phencyclidine
Cocaine	Phenothiazines
Ergotamine	Physostigmine
Insulin	Propoxyphene
Isoniazid	Strychnine
Lead	Theophylline
Lindane	Tricyclic antidepressants

Seizures

Common agents that cause seizures are listed in Table 1–13. Almost any drug or toxin is capable of producing a seizure. Delayed seizures occurring during a recovery period may be a sign of drug or alcohol withdrawal.

Seizures should be managed first with establishment of an airway and oxygenation. Patients with simple isolated seizures may require only observation and supportive care, whereas repetitive seizures or status epilepticus can be life-threatening and must be managed aggressively. Some seizures are particularly difficult to control, such as those seen with theophylline or amoxapine[19] overdose.

The standard regimen for seizure control in overdose of an unknown agent is use of the full therapeutic dosages of benzodiazepines (e.g., diazepam or lorazepam), followed by administration of phenytoin or a barbiturate (e.g., phenobarbital or pentobarbital), or both. In patients with status epilepticus, RSI may be necessary and the use of thiopental is indicated, with electroencephalographic monitoring to ensure control of electrical seizure activity; the use of additional paralytics, such as pancuronium bromide, may be warranted.[20]

Specific measures to control seizures may be indicated, such as administration of pyridoxine for isoniazid-induced seizures, naloxone for propoxyphene-induced seizures, or glucose for hypoglycemia.

Laboratory Evaluation

Table 1–14 lists specific blood studies whose results may be used to direct therapy of the overdose patient. In every significant poisoning, routine studies include a complete blood count; determination of serum electrolytes, glucose, blood urea nitrogen, creatinine, and calcium; urinalysis; prothrombin time; pulse oximetry; and 12-lead electrocardiography. Arterial blood gas analysis is necessary for evaluating respiratory status and acid-base abnormalities, especially in the comatose or seizure patient. A measurement of salicylate and acetaminophen levels is generally added in the case of the patient with overdose of an unknown substance, as these agents are often coingestants or are contained in combination drugs. Measurements of hepatic enzymes often are obtained for evaluation of acetaminophen toxicity. The advantage of a toxicologic drug screen is equivocal, as its effect on outcome is rarely beneficial. Table 1–15 gives a partial list of drugs and toxins not commonly detected with routine drug screening. Further laboratory blood studies are tailored to assess the individual diagnostic and therapeutic needs of the patient.

It is extremely important to remember to "treat the patient, not the lab." One should *never* withhold therapy while waiting for a confirmatory drug level in a critical patient, such as a patient with tricyclic antidepressant overdose who is exhibiting a widened QRS complex. In contrast, performing hemodialysis on a completely asymptomatic patient with lithium overdose on the basis of one test result indicating an elevated level of serum lithium would be equally unwise.

Serial blood level determinations are often helpful in guiding therapy in patients undergoing hemodialysis; in patients in whom concretions have formed, such as those with barbiturate, glutethimide, iron, salicylates, or meprobamate intoxication; or in patients receiving antidotal therapy (e.g., serial measurement of serum calcium levels is useful in patients on IV calcium chloride for management of calcium channel blocker overdose).

Urinalysis is necessary. Performing urine or serum pregnancy testing is wise in all women of child-bearing age. Urine pH monitoring is helpful in the management of salicylate overdose. Urine is the best specimen to use for "screening" purposes.

The intravenous drug abuser requires special blood testing, such as evaluation for HIV, a hepatitis profile, blood culture for septicemia, and evaluation for rhabdomyolysis and myoglobinuria.

Chest radiography is an aid for diagnosing aspiration pneumonia or pulmonary edema. Table 1–16 lists agents that are radiopaque on plain film radiography of the abdomen. Computed tomography may be useful if underlying trauma is suspected. Finally,

Table 1–14. Toxicologic Blood Studies That May Direct Therapy

Acetaminophen	Lithium
Carboxyhemoglobin	Methanol
Digoxin	Salicylate
Ethylene glycol	Theophylline
Iron	

Table 1–15. A Partial List of Drugs and Toxins Not Commonly Detected with Routine Drug Screening

Antiarrhythmics	Iron
Antihypertensives	Isoniazid
Carbon monoxide	Lithium
Cyanide	LSD
Digitalis	Mushrooms
Ethylene glycol	Organophosphates
Heavy metals	Paraquat
Hydrocarbons	Venom
Hypoglycemics	

Table 1–16. Radiopaque Toxins

Calcium carbonate
Chloral hydrate
Crack vials
Drug packets
Iron
Potassium chloride
Sustained-release products

lumbar puncture may be indicated for ruling out meningitis in a patient with fever and coma.

Elimination of Poison from the Eyes, Skin, and Gastrointestinal Tract

Ocular Decontamination

Ocular exposures account for 6.2% of all poisonings reported annually to the AAPCC. These cases almost invariably represent unintentional splashes of liquid into the eye or exposure to corrosive gases such as chlorine, bromine, and ammonia. Nonetheless, in the absence of a prompt, rational approach to management, ocular toxins can produce permanent injury, including blindness. Toxins can also be absorbed from the eye and thus can produce systemic effects.

The structures most vulnerable to injury after chemical exposure are the conjunctivae and cornea. The cornea is composed of layers of transparent epithelium. Beneath the cornea is the anterior chamber of the eye, which contains the ciliary apparatus, including the iris. Posterior to this is the posterior chamber, which contains the vitreous humor.

The cornea is richly innervated; as a result, even minor epithelial loss can produce substantial pain. In addition to de-epithelialization, ocular toxins can produce corneal clouding or perforation, either of which can result in permanent visual impairment.

Solvents

Solvents are a class of substances that are commonly sprayed or splashed into the eyes. These substances include hydrocarbons, alcohols, and detergents. All solvents are capable of dissolving lipids in the corneal epithelium, producing intense pain and tearing. Fortunately, corneal injury is superficial and generally heals without sequelae.

Corrosive Agents

Both acid and alkaline corrosives can produce tissue destruction that results in blindness. As with corrosive ingestions, the type of eye injury produced by the agent is pH specific: with acid corrosives, coagulation necrosis is produced; with alkaline corrosives, liquefaction necrosis occurs. Acid corrosives do not penetrate conjunctival or epithelial barriers because hydrogen ions precipitate surface ocular proteins, impeding further acid spread. Therefore, as a general rule, most acid burns produce only superficial damage. Except with extremely low (less than 2.5)–pH solutions, acid injuries to the eye are generally associated with a good prognosis (with the exception of injury with hydrofluoric acid).[21] In contrast, alkaline corrosives, because of their properties of saponification and lipid emulsification, can rapidly penetrate all layers of the conjunctiva and corneal epithelium. The most serious ocular injuries are associated with exposure to agents having a pH of greater than 11.5. The alkaline corrosives are associated with the greatest likelihood of corneal perforation or permanent clouding.

The severity of eye injury often is made evident by the presenting clinical features. With eye injuries caused by mildly corrosive agents, conjunctival injection occurs. Fluorescein examination may reveal scattered filling defects. Moderate ocular injuries are often associated with periorbital skin burns. Instead of being hyperemic, the conjunctivae are pale and chemotic. The pallor represents local ischemia; limbal blanching is correlated with later corneal ischemia and ulceration. Fluorescein examination, in addition to revealing large areas of corneal injury, demonstrates corneal edema (which may result in a cloudy cornea that obscures visualization of the iris). In patients with severe corrosive injuries, there is prominent conjunctival chemosis, complete loss of corneal epithelium on fluorescein examination, and corneal clouding. These features may be associated with marked increases in intraocular pressure. Such injuries may ultimately result in cataract, glaucoma, and blindness. Corrosive injuries are generally confined to the anterior chamber and are characterized by little to no involvement of the posterior chamber.[21]

Management. Toxic injuries of the eye, particularly chemical burns, are ophthalmologic emergencies and require immediate decontamination.[22] General principles of initial management must be followed in the treatment of ocular exposure to toxins. First, as soon as an exposure is recognized, the eye should receive immediate and effective irrigation with water, lactated Ringer's solution, or isotonic saline for 30 minutes. As long as irrigation is effective, several liters of fluid should be instilled before transfer of the patient to a health care facility. Upon arrival to the health care facility, copious irrigation should continue. Solutions such as Balanced Saline Solution and lactated Ringer's solution with bicarbonate may be better tolerated than normal saline; however, saline is more readily available and should be the initial agent used. Because patients often complain of discomfort, there may be some benefit to topical anesthesia before continuation of irrigation.[22] However, topical anesthesia should not be performed unless it is certain that no rupture of the globe has occurred. *Irrigation should be performed for a minimum of 30 minutes.* With corrosive injuries to the eye, the pH of the ocular fluid should be tested. If the pH is not approximately neutral (pH ≅7.0), the eye should be irrigated further.

In cases of persistent pain, particularly after an alkaline corrosive exposure, patients should be referred on an emergent basis to an ophthalmologist for further care.

Dermal Decontamination

Being the largest and most superficial organ in the body, the skin is often subject to exposure to toxins and is affected in 7.9% of reported cases. At least 50% of occupational illnesses involve the skin. The effects of these exposures can be local or systemic (Table 1–17).

The skin provides many barriers to the absorption of toxins. The stratum corneum forms an important first barrier and is highly effective when it is completely intact. However, when skin wounds are present, when the wounds are wet, and when exposure is to certain highly lipophilic substances (e.g., organophosphate insecticides), significant absorption of toxin through the skin can occur. The skin of infants is notable for being more permeable than that of adults to substances of all classes.

The range of dermal toxins is broad. Most of these substances are corrosive agents capable of producing burns that may become full-thickness (i.e., third degree). Other types of agents are irritants, sensitizers (including photosensitizers), allergens, vesicants, and exfoliants.

Management. As with ocular exposures, the general principles of management after exposure to dermal toxins are many. As soon as a toxic dermal exposure is recognized, decontamination efforts should begin. If the victim is immersed in a toxic fluid, the first step in management is his or her extrication without injury to the assistant. The victim should disrobe him- or herself at the scene. If assistance is needed because the victim is unable, undressing should be done as safely as possible. Protective gear should be donned before assistance with decontamination is rendered. Unless the agent is highly reactive (e.g., elemental sodium), it is appropriate to wash the victim thoroughly with water, preferably in a nearby decontamination shower. *Water should not be used to decontaminate skin in exposures to sodium, phosphorus, calcium oxide, chlorosulphonic acid, and titanium tetrachloride.* When emergency medical personnel arrive to the scene, they should continue skin decontamination. Again, if the agent is known to have significant dermal absorption, emergency medical personnel should provide themselves every available level of self-protection. Certain toxins such as organophosphates can contaminate the air within the ambulance and produce ill effects among personnel if prehospital decontamination efforts are inadequate.

Table 1–17. Toxins Associated with Systemic Toxicity After Dermal Absorption

Organophosphate insecticide	Aniline dyes
Hydrofluoric acid	Nitrates
Lindane (γ-benzene hydrochloride)	Phenol
Hexachlorophene	Acrylamide
Nitrobenzene	Dinitrophenol
Organic mercury	Thallium
Lidocaine	Camphor

Table 1–18. Specific Interventions for Toxic Dermal Exposure

Toxin	Therapeutic Intervention
Hydrofluoric acid	Calcium gluconate
Instant-bonding adhesive ("Super glue")	Polyoxyethylene sorbitan (Neosporin)
Elemental sodium	Mineral oil
Organophosphate insecticide	Protected decontamination

Upon arrival at a health care facility, the victim may require quarantine, depending on the nature of the agent. Skin decontamination in a decontamination shower should continue. Particular caution should be exercised in the decontamination of victims of organophosphate insecticide or organophosphate-based nerve gas exposure; health care personnel have been overcome secondarily by contaminants on victims when they assisted in their care without donning proper protective gear.

Water is the most commonly used skin decontaminant and is highly effective for most dermal exposures. In select cases, specific agents should be used to assist in management (Table 1–18).

Without exception, toxin-induced skin burns should be treated according to existing burn management guidelines. These include wound débridement and dressing, monitoring for infection, fluid management, and surgical consultation when appropriate.

Gastrointestinal Decontamination

After the ingestion of a toxic substance, with the exception of agents that have a direct toxic effect on the gastrointestinal tract (e.g., iron or corrosives), that substance must be systemically absorbed and circulated before it reaches a target organ and exerts clinical toxicity. *Preventing the absorption of toxin is therefore the foundation of treatment after ingestion of a toxin has occurred.* The term *gastrointestinal decontamination (GID)* has been coined to describe those interventions that are useful in preventing toxin absorption. With the exception of rare interventions such as gastroscopy, GID is considered to have only three components: (1) gastric evacuation, (2) administration of adsorbent, and (3) catharsis.

Each of the components of GID has a long history. For example, it is said that the principle of gastric emptying after ingestion of toxic substances was first established when man discovered his finger (i.e., that vomiting could be induced by gagging).[23] It was later that chemical agents and mechanical instruments were invented as means of gastric evacuation. The discovery of adsorbents, particularly activated charcoal, was chronicled by Hippocrates. Finally, cathartics also have ancient origins, historically being used to "cleanse" the gut.

Gastric Emptying

It is logical that shortly after a toxic substance has been ingested, the most effective intervention is likely to be gastric evacuation. The length of time food or any other substance remains in the stomach before it passes beyond the pylorus into the small intestine is highly variable, depending on many factors that include lipophilicity, dispersion characteristics, the presence of other substances in the stomach, and the pharmacologic characteristics of the agent (e.g., its ability to slow gastrointestinal motility). Nonetheless, unless there is a complete absence of gut motility or mechanical obstruction, every agent leaves the stomach eventually, making any gastric evacuation efforts futile. Therefore, the principle of gastric emptying has always focused on the ability to perform it promptly, through either the induction of emesis or the mechanical evacuation of the stomach.

Emesis. The vomiting reflex is a normal physiologic response to irritating substances. This response, much like sneezing and coughing, is one of many host reflexes designed to facilitate the removal of substances that produce a noxious stimulus. The vomiting "circuit" has three components: an afferent arc, a control center, and an efferent arc. The *afferent arc* for vomiting includes parasympathetic nerves that innervate the full length of the gastrointestinal tract. Impulses from these nerves are directed to the vomiting center, a cluster of neurons located in the reticulum of the medulla oblongata. Direct stimulation of the vomiting center initiates efferent impulses to the gastrointestinal tract that result in vomiting. Distinct but closely related to the vomiting center is the *chemoreceptor trigger zone (CTZ),* located on the floor of the fourth ventricle.[24] Additional input reaching the CTZ comes from olfactory, lingual, and ocular afferents, and the CTZ activates the vomiting center. The neurons in both the CTZ and vomiting center use dopamine and acetylcholine as their primary neurotransmitters. This forms the basis for the use of antidopaminergic agents, such as phenothiazines and anticholinergic agents (e.g., dimenhydrinate [Dramamine]) for the treatment of vomiting. Output from the CTZ and vomiting center is directed to both skeletal and visceral muscles of the gastrointestinal tract. These efferent nerves produce a coordinated action of pylorospasm, relaxation of the gastroesophageal sphincter, abdominal wall contraction, and forced contraction of the stomach.[24] Chemical emetics were created to produce prompt vomiting after toxic ingestion.

A number of emetics have been created and used for the treatment of poisoning. These have included oral medicinal agents, such as ipecac, copper sulfate, mustard water, zinc sulfate, and tartar emetics; parenteral agents, such as apomorphine; and homemade agents, such as salt or soapy water.[23, 25] With the exception of ipecac syrup, the use of all of these agents has been abandoned because of their toxicity.[26] For example, apomorphine enjoyed several years of popularity because of its efficacy as a rapidly-acting emetic.[27] However, it had to be administered parenterally, and it produced significant central nervous system depression; these characteristics led to its abandonment.[28] Copper sulfate also was used briefly as a chemical emetic before it was recognized as an extremely toxic agent.[23, 25, 26] Emetics that could be made in the home, including salt water, were once widely used (and are still occasionally used as an emergency measure when no other emetic is available) but can be very toxic. Smith and Palevsky reported the case of a 2-year-old child who was given salt water by a baby sitter after an ingestion of a substance that was thought to be toxic. The child rapidly developed severe hypernatremia and died.[29]

Ipecac was discovered in Latin America and introduced into Europe in 1648.[30] According to legend, ipecac gained public prominence in France when it was used by J.A. Helvetius in 1686 to treat Dauphine, the daughter-in-law of Louis XIV, for amebic dysentery.[30] Ipecac remained popular as a treatment for dysentery until the beginning of the 1900s, when both its effectiveness as a treatment for poisoning and the toxicity associated with its chronic use were appreciated.

Ipecac is prepared from the dried roots (rhizomes) of the plants *Cephaelis ipecacuanha* or *C. acuminata*.[30, 31] It contains two alkaloids: emetine and cephaline. A 30-mL (1-oz) bottle of ipecac contains approximately 11.4 mg of emetine and 23.4 mg of cephaline.[32] A small amount of emetine is absorbed into the systemic circulation[32]; emetine's potent emetic effects are thought to be due to both local and central nervous system actions.[30, 33] Emetine has a very long elimination half-life; thus, cumulative toxicity can result from repeated use; after 35 days, as much as 35% of the emetine administered is still retained in the body.[33] Chronic emetine exposure is particularly toxic to the heart, producing T wave disturbances and both atrial and ventricular arrhythmias.[31, 33, 34] Death from ipecac syrup toxicity may occur after total emetine ingestion of greater than 1.25 g.[31] Cephaline is twice as potent as emetine in producing vomiting, and primarily is a direct gastrointestinal irritant.[33]

Ipecac was originally available in three forms: a powder, a fluid extract, and a syrup.[31] However, because the fluid extract was 14 times more concentrated than the syrup, its inadvertent administration led to serious toxicity and fatalities. Now, only syrup of ipecac is available for public use.[30, 33, 35] Spurred by ipecac's safety and apparent efficacy as an emetic, the American Academy of Pediatrics lobbied to make syrup of ipecac available without a prescription; ipecac gained nonprescription status from the Food and Drug Administration in 1965. At that time, administration of ipecac syrup was considered one of the most important measures in reducing the morbidity and mortality resulting from childhood ingestions.[23]

Pediatricians and toxicologists campaigned to place syrup of ipecac in every home that a child might enter so that, if indicated, it could be administered as soon as an ingestion was recognized.

Syrup of ipecac is extremely effective as an emetic. Its efficacy is not reduced by concomitant administration of activated charcoal. Its alkaloids remain effective for long periods: syrup of ipecac is effective up to 4 years after the expiration date on the label.[36]

Dosing guidelines for syrup of ipecac are given in Table 1–19. General indications are the ingestion of a toxic substance in an awake, alert patient with an intact gag reflex. The youngest age at which ipecac can be used safely has been variously published as 6 months, 9 months, and 12 months. Under present general poison center protocols, ipecac can be given to any child older than 6 months of age. For infants aged 6 to 12 months of age, 10 mL is given; this dose *cannot* be re-administered if the patient does not vomit.[37] For those 1 to 12 years of age, 15 mL is administered; this dose can be repeated in 20 minutes if vomiting has not occurred. For those 12 years of age through adulthood, 30 mL is administered; a repeat dose can be administered in 20 minutes if no vomiting has occurred. Ipecac should *never* be given repeatedly because of the risk of emetine cardiotoxicity. Large amounts of fluid should be given after ipecac to promote vomiting.[37] Vomiting after ipecac administration generally occurs within 20 minutes and persists for 30 to 120 minutes.[32]

Contraindications to ipecac use are many. It should not be given after ingestion of corrosive agents. Although ipecac use has been contraindicated after the ingestion of hydrocarbons because of the risk of aspiration, this recommendation is not entirely supported by the literature. Other contraindications to ipecac use are the presence of seizures, coma, loss of protective airway reflexes, or ingestion of an agent that can induce coma or seizures. Since the mid-1980s, the last category has served to narrow the accepted uses for ipecac.

Adverse effects from routine ipecac use have been extremely rare, and this fact serves to document the safety of this agent. Reported complications from its use include fatal gastric rupture,[38] Mallory-Weiss tear,[39] intracranial hemorrhage, hemorrhagic gastritis, and pneumomediastinum.[40] Most adverse effects, including death, have been seen almost exclusively in those who abuse ipecac (e.g., those with bulimia nervosa).[41, 42]

Table 1–19. Dosing Guidelines for Ipecac Use

Indications:	Toxic ingestion in an awake, alert patient with an intact gag reflex
Contraindications:	Nontoxic substance Nontoxic amount Ingestion of corrosive agents Presence of seizures or coma Ingestion of any agent that can produce coma or seizures Loss of protective airway reflexes
Dose by age:	
0–6 months	No ipecac
6–12 months	10 mL; dose cannot be repeated.
12 mo–12 y	15 mL; can be repeated in 20 min.
Older than 12 y	30 mL; can be repeated in 20 min.

Historically, ipecac's ease of administration and apparent efficacy resulted in its widespread use in emergency departments. Administration of ipecac upon arrival to the emergency department became protocol; in many areas of the country, administration of ipecac by emergency medical technicians and paramedics was included in prehospital protocols. However, the efficacy of ipecac has been closely reexamined in recent years. A number of studies have set out to determine whether use of a substance that has nearly 100% effectiveness in producing emesis is a beneficial intervention.

Early studies by Abdallah and Tye, Corby and coworkers, and Arnold and associates suggested that ipecac was highly effective in removing ingested toxins from the stomach and was generally more effective than gastric lavage.[43–45] However, their studies suffered from significant methodologic flaws, including use of an animal model and the performing of gastric lavage with small tubes. Subsequently, ipecac's effectiveness was studied in humans in both natural and experimental settings. In experimental models, ipecac's ability to prevent absorption of toxins, measured either by diminution in the area under the curve of the ingested drug, reduction in the urinary excretion of the drug, or direct measurement of the toxin in vomitus, has been mixed. At 1 hour postingestion, toxin recovery ranges from 0% to 78%, with a mean of 30%.[23] A delay to ipecac administration of 90 minutes renders it virtually ineffective. This finding has important clinical consequences in an emergency department when one recognizes that the usual time to emergency department presentation after a poisoning is 1 hour for children and more than 4 hours for adults.

Gastric Lavage. Gastric lavage (historically referred to as "pumping the stomach") is the process of gastric intubation whose purpose is the evacuation of stomach contents. Its first use as a treatment for poisoning is attributed to Physick, who used a hollow tube to lavage two infants with a laudanum (tincture of opium) overdose in 1812.[46, 47] The procedure, like induced emesis, is performed so that toxic agents are removed before they leave the stomach and pass into the small intestine, where they are systemically absorbed.

The process of gastric lavage is optimally performed according to a specific protocol: first, a thorough clinical evaluation must be made for the purpose of assessing the patient's airway. If the patient demonstrates depressed consciousness, active convulsions, or any other condition that may compromise airway reflexes, then he or she should undergo endotracheal intubation in order to secure the airway. In the awake patient, prior intubation is unnecessary. The patient is placed in the left lateral decubitus position in 15-degree Trendelenburg.[46] This position decreases movement of gastric contents into the duodenum and reduces the likelihood of aspiration. A large, single-lumen tube with multiple distal ports is necessary. The Ewald tube, which has a single distal aperture, may be less effective than lavage tubes with numerous lateral holes. Tube size should be 32 to 40 French for adults and 24 to 32 French for children. Proper positioning is confirmed by the spontaneous return of gastric contents or by detection of insufflation of air into the stomach with a stethoscope. After the position has been confirmed, the stomach is emptied. This is followed by the administration of aliquots of tap water or saline; saline is preferred in children because of the risk of excessive free water absorption.[46] The volume of each aliquot should be 100 to 150 mL for adults and 10 to 15 mL/kg for children. Return of toxin may be facilitated by gastric massage, a maneuver advocated by Bartecchi.[48, 49] After the fluid has been instilled it is removed either by gravity drainage or syringe suction. Double-lumen ("sump") tubes should never be used to perform lavage unless the ingested toxin is a liquid; pill fragments cannot be removed from these tubes. Along similar lines, orogastric intubation is always preferred to nasogastric intubation because the latter necessitates use of a smaller tube. In the extremely uncooperative patient, nasogastric intubation may be the only option.

Gastric lavage is technically difficult to perform. First, it is labor intensive; typically, at least two providers are needed to restrain the patient and assist in its performance. Lavage is time consuming; with ingestions occurring after a large meal, several liters of water must be instilled before the return is clear. In a study of gastric lavage after tricyclic antidepressant overdose, Watson and colleagues reported a mean 1.3-hour duration to perform "aggressive" gastric lavage (instilling 12.8 L of fluid).[50] Finally, in studies examining the efficacy of gastric lavage, the general finding has been that average toxin recovery is 30% when lavage is performed immediately after an ingestion; however, one study found that less than 10% of a tricyclic antidepressant dose was removed after gastric lavage.[50]

Because of the risk of vomiting and aspiration, gastric lavage should not be performed in patients who have compromised airway (gag) reflexes (e.g., those with obtundation or coma). In these patients, airway protection with endotracheal intubation should be performed before gastric lavage is initiated. Contraindications to lavage include corrosive ingestion and history of esophageal or gastric surgery. Gastric lavage is relatively contraindicated in the elderly because it has been associated with significant cardiorespiratory disturbances when performed in this population. Thompson and colleagues, investigating cardiorespiratory function during lavage, found that mean pulse rate increased and mean Po_2 decreased during the procedure. These changes were more significant in smokers, and they were marked in smokers aged 45 years or older. Electrocardiographic changes were noted in 41% of patients, including potentially serious disturbances in 2 patients.[51]

Complications reported after gastric lavage have been numerous. These include inadvertent intubation of the trachea and esophageal perforation.[46, 47] Large amounts of fluid can potentially produce hypothermia in young children unless the lavage fluid is slightly warmed.[46] Epistaxis may occur if the lavage tube is introduced by a nasogastric route.[46] Some studies have shown that gastric lavage can be counterproductive in that it can facilitate the propulsion of drug into the small intestine. Harstad and coworkers, in a study of gastric lavage in acutely poisoned patients, reported that 25% of lavage fluid passed into the small intestine.[52]

The comparative efficacy of ipecac-induced emesis and gastric lavage has been examined in a number of studies. Initial studies in animal models found ipecac syrup to be superior to lavage.[43, 44] However, later studies suggested that gastric lavage was superior. In a volunteer study, Tandberg and associates found that the mean recovery of an ingested tracer was 28% for ipecac versus 45% for gastric lavage.[53] In a study of poisoned patients, lavage recovered a larger amount of tracer than did ipecac (90% versus 50%).[54] In a study of poisoned patients who underwent endoscopy after gastric emptying, 38.5% of patients who received ipecac had retained gastric contents compared with 88.2% of patients who underwent gastric lavage; this result indicates a significant benefit from ipecac-induced emesis.[55] Collectively, these studies suggest that these two methods of gastric emptying have comparable efficacy.

Administration of Adsorbent

Any agent that is capable of binding to a toxic substance in the gastrointestinal tract is considered an *adsorbent*. Several adsorbents have been proved effective after toxic ingestion (Table 1–20). With the possible exception of sodium polystyrene sulfonate (Kayexalate), all of these substances act by means of noncovalent attachment to the substance. Once the adsorbent has bound toxin, the toxin-adsorbent complex is expelled in the feces.

Among adsorbents used in clinical toxicology, *activated charcoal* has been the best characterized. His-

Table 1–20. Adsorbents Used in the Management of Toxic Ingestions

Adsorbent	Toxin
Activated charcoal	Pharmaceuticals, organic agents
Fuller's earth, bentonite	Paraquat
Sodium polystyrene sulfonate (Kayexalate)	Lithium, potassium
Cholestyramine	Organochlorines (chlordecone, lindane)
Starch	Iodine
Potassium ferricyanate (Prussian blue)	Thallium
Sodium silicate gel	Pharmaceuticals, organic agents

torically, charcoal-based substances have been used since the age of Hippocrates to "bind" toxic agents. This was in part the origin of the "universal antidote" of burnt toast and tea formerly promoted as a treatment for poisoning.

"Activated" charcoal is created by subjecting carbonaceous materials (e.g., wood, coal, rye starch, or coconut shells) to steam (at 600 to 900°C) and acid.[56, 57] This produces a substance with innumerable interstices capable of trapping organic chemicals.[58, 59] The efficacy of activated charcoal was made famous in 1831 by Touery when, before the French Academy of Medicine, he drank a lethal dose of strychnine combined with activated charcoal and sustained no ill effects![56]

Most activated charcoals in current use have a surface binding area of 900 to 1500 m^2/g (compared with 2 to 4 m^2/g for "unactivated" carbonaceous materials).[57] Therefore, one 50-g dose of charcoal has the surface area of 10 football fields. Recently, there has been clinical use of "superactivated" charcoals, which have surface areas that are threefold greater than that of standard activated charcoals.[60]

Commercially available activated charcoal preparations are dispensed in many forms. Tablets and capsules of activated charcoal are available, but these are generally impractical because of the large doses of activated charcoal that must be given after toxic ingestions. Charcoal powder is available for reconstitution in whatever liquid medium is desired. However, the powder is extremely messy and its use has become unpopular. The preparation most commonly available is charcoal that is already suspended in a liquid medium. The liquid medium may be a sweetened water suspension (for increased palatability) or a cathartic. Wax and co-workers found that 47% of surveyed hospitals stocked a charcoal-sorbitol mixture; in 16% of hospitals, premixed activated charcoal-sorbitol was the only activated charcoal preparation available.[61]

Charcoal is capable of strongly binding organic substances ranging from pharmaceuticals to biologic toxins to hormones (e.g., thyroid hormone). The maximal amount of adsorption to charcoal by chemicals is an estimated to be 500 to 1000 mg/g.[57] However, all substances are not adsorbed equally. For example, many substances have minimal adsorption to activated charcoal; administration of charcoal is therefore not recommended after ingestion of these substances (Table 1–21). *In vitro* studies that have examined activated charcoal's binding to alcohols, minerals, and hydrocarbons have variously shown that up to 15% of the substance is adsorbed—a clinically insignificant amount. However, it is occasionally recommended that activated charcoal be provided after ingestions of poorly adsorbed agents because the likelihood of the agents' being severely toxic is high, and thus all efforts to reduce this toxicity are justified.

Table 1–21. Substances Not Well Adsorbed to Activated Charcoal

Alcohols (ethanol, methanol, isopropyl alcohol, glycols, acetone)
Hydrocarbons (petroleum distillates and plant hydrocarbons [e.g., pine oil])
Metals and inorganic minerals (e.g., sodium, iron, lead, arsenic, iodine, fluorine, boric acid)
Corrosives

Despite the fact that charcoal binding is noncovalent, desorption of substances from activated charcoal appears to be minimal. Another important feature of charcoal is that it traverses the length of the gastrointestinal tract, making it superior to gastric emptying techniques, whose efficacy ends at the pylorus. Being inert, activated charcoal is nonirritating to mucous membranes. Even when aspirated, charcoal appears to be nontoxic; charcoal-associated aspiration pneumonias are thought to result from either the aspiration of gastric acid or of irritative substances in the liquid medium.

Dosing of activated charcoal is based on scientific data that define the charcoal-to-drug ratio necessary for a protective degree of binding. This has led to the "10:1 gram-for-gram maxim," which states that the dose of activated charcoal administered should be at least 10-fold greater than the dose of ingested toxin.[62] Theoretically, higher ratios (e.g., 25:1) would lead to an even greater degree of drug binding and even greater clinical protection. In a study in which the activated charcoal dose was fixed (50 g) and increasing doses of para-aminosalicylic acid were given, Olkkola demonstrated that with a charcoal-to-drug ratio of 50:1, less than 5% of para-aminosalicylic acid was absorbed from the gastrointestinal tract. This rate compared with absorption rates of 25% and 37% with charcoal-to-drug ratios of 5:1 and 2.5:1, respectively.[63] In clinical practice, the recommended charcoal dose is 1 g/kg for children. In adults, published recommended charcoal doses have included 1 g/kg with no maximum dose (e.g., a 100-kg man would receive a single 100-g dose of activated charcoal), 100-g, 60-g, and 50-g maximum single doses. This wide range of published recommendations illustrates the lack of clear scientific data establishing an optimal dose. Based on existing data, a maximum single adult dose of 50 to 60 g should be sufficient for all toxic ingestions. Superactivated charcoals have a greater binding surface area and are more effective than standard charcoal preparations[64, 65]; theoretically, this permits the administration of doses that are smaller but equally effective.

Efficacy studies have proved charcoal to be highly effective at both reducing absorption of ingested toxin and improving clinical course. Even when administered more than 1 hour postingestion, activated charcoal diminishes the absorption of ingested drug by as much as 60%. Also, in studies that have examined the use of activated charcoal alone in comparison with other components of GID, charcoal has been shown to be superior to the other interventions.

Generally, activated charcoal is successfully administered to adults as a slurry in a liquid medium.

If the slurry does not already contain a cathartic, one can be added. In children, activated charcoal administration is more problematic. Generally, a young child will not drink the black, gritty suspension, despite the addition of a sweet liquid. This problem has been investigated by adding charcoal to mixtures including ice cream, chocolate, and fruit flavors. These studies have found that the efficacy of charcoal is reduced by the addition of many such excipients; however, the extent of reduction may not be clinically important.[66] Therefore, the addition of flavor enhancers remains an option. The alternative is placement of a nasogastric tube for charcoal administration.[67] If gastric lavage has been performed before charcoal administration, the charcoal can be instilled through the same tube. Otherwise, a tube must be inserted for the sole purpose of charcoal administration. Studies have shown that with present protocols, 20% to 60% of children younger than 5 years of age require gastric intubation for administration of charcoal. Using standard placement techniques, a 12- to 14-French nasogastric tube should be introduced into the stomach.[67] Charcoal should be suspended in enough liquid to permit its administration through a small-bore tube. After administration of the charcoal, the nasogastric tube can be removed.

Because it is inert and completely nonabsorbed from the gastrointestinal tract, activated charcoal is extremely safe to use. Bronchiolitis obliterans, empyemas, and aspiration pneumonia have been reported after charcoal aspiration.[68] However, these outcomes are more likely the result of aspiration of sorbitol or gastric acid. Charcoal administration is associated with a 10% rate of spontaneous emesis, which possibly is the result of the vehicle.

Catharsis

After a toxic ingestion, a third measure that may be useful in reducing systemic toxicity is facilitating the expulsion of the toxin.[69] This measure has led to the principle of *catharsis* after toxic ingestion. When cathartics are added to activated charcoal, the toxin-charcoal complex can be rapidly eliminated from the body, further reducing the opportunity for absorption. *Cathartics,* also known as *purgatives* or *laxatives*, are therefore the third component of GID after a toxic ingestion. A list of commonly used cathartics and their recommended doses is found in Table 1–22.

All cathartics act by disturbing the balance between intestinal absorption and secretion of fluid.[69] The cathartics used in clinical toxicology can generally be placed in the broad category of osmotic cathartics. This category can be subdivided into the saccharides (e.g., sorbitol, mannitol, lactulose) and salines (e.g., magnesium citrate, magnesium sulfate). Stimulant cathartics (e.g., phenolphthalein, senna, castor oil) are rarely used in the treatment of toxic ingestions. The mechanism of action of cathartics is variable. For example, saccharide cathartics hygroscopically attract water into the gastrointestinal lumen from the splanchnic circulation.[69] Saline cathartics also act by exerting an osmotic effect; however,

Table 1–22. Commonly Used Cathartics

	Dose	
Cathartic	*Pediatric*	*Adult*
Saccharides		
Sorbitol	1–2 g/kg	1–2 g/kg
Mannitol	1–2 g/kg	1–2 g/kg
Salines		
6% Magnesium citrate	4 mL (225 mg)/kg	300 mL (17.5 g)
Magnesium sulfate	200–300 mg/kg	15–20 g
Sodium sulfate	200–300 mg/kg	15–20 g

there is evidence that they have other actions, including stimulation of gastrointestinal hormones (e.g., vasoactive intestinal peptide), which increase gastrointestinal motility.[69, 70] Saline cathartics may also act on the myenteric plexus and other gastrointestinal nerves to enhance gastrointestinal motility.

The cathartics have varying degrees of effectiveness at producing stooling. For example, in a study of the use of activated charcoal with or without cathartic, activated charcoal in water had a mean transit time of 23.5 hours. This transit time was reduced to 9.3 hours with the addition of magnesium sulfate, to 4.2 hours with the addition of magnesium citrate, and 0.9 hours with the addition of sorbitol.[71] Thus, sorbitol is the most effective cathartic. In a study of cathartic efficacy in children, Sue and associates reported that giving 4 mL/kg of magnesium citrate (with charcoal) produced stool significantly faster than did administration of activated charcoal in water (13 versus 19.5 hours, respectively).[72]

Like induced emesis, however, a distinction must be made between the intervention's ability to produce the desired action and the evidence that this action in turn reduces or prevents clinical toxicity after a toxic ingestion. Thus, although cathartics are capable of producing stool in a relatively brief period of time, studies examining their clinical efficacy after a toxic ingestion have revealed a disappointing degree of effectiveness. The view that cathartics confer little added benefit to activated charcoal therapy after a toxic ingestion is growing. *Therefore the use of cathartics is best considered an option in clinical management, secondary to the administration of activated charcoal.*

Contraindications to the use of cathartics are few. Cathartics should not be used in patients with absent bowel sounds because of the risk of abdominal distention and reflex vomiting. Similarly, because hypotension can be associated with marked reductions in gut motility, cathartics should be used cautiously, if at all, in patients with cardiovascular instability.[69] Saline cathartics such as magnesium citrate should not be administered in patients with renal disease, profound electrolyte imbalance, and bowel obstruction.[56]

Although the use of cathartics is generally safe, adverse effects have been associated with their administration. Fluid and electrolyte disturbances are the most common of these. Fecal fluid has a significant concentration of electrolytes, containing approximately 32 mmol/L of sodium, 75 mmol/L of potassium, 16 mmol/L of chloride, and 40 mmol/L of bicarbonate. And, whereas typical fecal fluid volume is approximately 100 mL daily, fluid losses with the use of cathartics can be as great as 6 L (average, 2.7 L).[69] Cathartics, particularly sorbitol, are also associated with a significant rate of spontaneous emesis (with sorbitol, up to 57%, depending on the dose) likely owing to their extremely sweet, syrupy taste. Administration of cathartic (especially sorbitol) to young children has been associated with excessive pooling of fluid in the gastrointestinal lumen, which leads to intravascular depletion, hypernatremia, and cardiovascular collapse.[73, 74] Similar excess fluid losses have been reported in adults who receive repetitive doses of cathartic. In the case of magnesium cathartics, single doses have not produced significant toxicity because gastrointestinal systemic absorption of magnesium ion is minimal (although Weber and Santiago have reported a patient who developed a serum magnesium level of 10.3 mg/dL after receiving a single dose of magnesium citrate[75]). However, multiple doses of cathartic have been associated with the development of hypermagnesemia manifested by hypotonia, areflexia, generalized muscle weakness (to the point that ventilatory support is required), and coma.[76–79] In a study of single-versus multiple-dose magnesium sulfate therapy, Smilkstein and associates found that the incidence of hypermagnesemia was 20% in the single-dose group versus 64% in those receiving multiple-dose therapy.[78] The threat of adverse effects from repetitive administration of a cathartic has been compounded by the increasing use of premixed charcoal-cathartic mixtures. One case report described a 55-year-old woman who died secondary to cathartic-induced bowel perforation after she had received both magnesium sulfate and an activated charcoal-sorbitol mixture.[80]

Whole-Bowel Irrigation. Historically, the importance of having a fully evacuated gastrointestinal tract before gastrointestinal surgery led to the creation of the "bowel-prep," consisting of administration of cathartics. Because of the risk of fluid and electrolyte disturbances from the use of cathartics, Hewitt and co-workers introduced the concept of *whole-bowel irrigation (WBI)* in 1973.[81] This technique led to the development of electrolyte-balanced, inert solutions that could mechanically flush the gut of material.[82] WBI crossed over to the realm of poison management in the early 1980s. In the poisoned patients, large volumes of solution are administered to flush toxic substances out of the body before they can be absorbed. In principle, WBI can be used as the sole method of gastrointestinal decontamination, obviating the need for gastric emptying and activated charcoal administration. Clinical studies in both children and adults have shown that WBI is highly effective in expelling toxic substances and in reducing clinical toxicity. WBI's peculiar mechanism of action has found its greatest value in the management of toxins that are poorly adsorbed by activated charcoal, such as arsenic and lithium.[83] WBI has also become a valuable intervention for the management of patients who have ingested drug packets (so-called "body stuffers" or "body packers"), as well as of those with overdoses of sustained-release capsules, such as ones containing calcium channel blockers.

The WBI solution consists of a mixture of polyethylene glycol and salts and is designed to produce minimal fluid shifts and no electrolyte disturbances. The solution is either drunk by the subject or administered by nasogastric tube. The WBI solution is administered until the rectal effluent is clear. For this goal, the required volume varies from 5 to 50 L. In one case report, 44 L of WBI solution was administered to a young child, with no adverse effects being observed.[84] The recommended rate of fluid administration is 1 to 2 L/h for adults, 500 mL/h for children over 1 to 6 years of age, and 1 L/h for children 6 to 12 years of age.

WBI is made problematic by the copious amounts of liquid stool it produces. In actual practice, the patient must either lie in the bed, in which case frequent linen changes are required because of recurrent soiling, or receive this therapy while sitting on a commode. If the patient is receiving intensive monitoring, placement on a toilet or the frequent need to get him or her in and out of a bed may compromise supportive care. "Cholera beds," once used for those with massive diarrhea, are ideal for successfully performing WBI.

Theoretically, WBI is an effective intervention for any type of toxic ingestion. However, its efficacy has been explored primarily in situations in which activated charcoal use may not be adequate as a means of GID. Therefore, ingestions of metals and minerals, such as iron, lithium, and lead, and sustained-release pharmaceuticals have been closely examined.[85] In these cases, WBI has been proved to be highly effective, even when used as the sole measure. Tenenbein showed that WBI, when performed 1 hour after ingestion, could produce a 67% decrease in drug absorption.[86] After administration of a mean 7.7 L of polyethylene glycol solution, Tenenbein's subjects experienced no adverse effects. Smith and colleagues demonstrated an identical degree of reduction in the absorption of lithium.[85]

WBI is generally a decontamination procedure that is performed in isolation—that is, without prior gastric emptying or administration of activated charcoal. In fact, administration of ipecac syrup impairs the ability to perform WBI. However, because there are circumstances in which adjunctive therapy with activated charcoal is recommended (e.g., in the ingestion of drug packets), it has been questioned whether WBI solutions reduce the efficacy of activated charcoal. A study by Kirshenbaum and co-workers demonstrated minimal adsorption of polyethylene glycol solution to activated charcoal.[87] However, Hoffman and associates and Makosiej and colleagues found a significant reduction in activated charcoal's effectiveness.[88, 89]

An Integrated Approach to Gastrointestinal Decontamination After Toxic Ingestion

Gastrointestinal decontamination after a toxic ingestion is ideally performed immediately after the ingestion. It is this ideal that led to the movement to place syrup of ipecac in every location where there are children, including day care centers, churches, baby sitters' homes, and the homes of any relatives. These settings now seem to be the only appropriate places for ipecac to be readily available. For example, Kirk and co-workers showed that in young children with ingestions of acetaminophen, ipecac administration within 1 hour of ingestion resulted in lower acetaminophen concentrations than in those who received activated charcoal in emergency departments.[90] However, because of the data demonstrating its relative lack of efficacy, coupled with the typical time delay to activated charcoal administration, there is an active (and appropriate) movement to end ipecac use, both in the emergency department and in the prehospital medical setting (ambulance).

With four general options in acute poison management after a toxic ingestion—gastric evacuation, administration of adsorbent, addition of cathartic, and WBI—*developing one approach that adequately treats all poisoned patients is impossible.* Given the multiplicity of important clinical factors that must be considered after an ingestion, such as the substance ingested, the amount ingested, the time postingestion, the patient's age, the presence or absence of coingestants, past medical history, and whether intervention was carried out at home by the family or by emergency medical personnel, *multiple options enhance the ability of the clinician to customize intervention in a particular situation.*

The comparative efficacy of specific decontamination measures, used singly or in combination, have been evaluated in a number of studies. As early as 1983, Neuvonen and associates compared the efficacy of ipecac with that of activated charcoal alone and found activated charcoal to be far superior.[91] In a later study comparing orogastric lavage, ipecac-induced emesis, and activated charcoal alone, instituted 1 hour after ampicillin ingestion, reduction in the absorption of ampicillin was greatest for activated charcoal alone (57%), followed by lavage (32%) and ipecac (38%).[92]

In a study of poisoned patients randomized to receive ipecac followed by activated charcoal or activated charcoal alone, Albertson and colleagues[93] showed that patients who received ipecac remained in the emergency department longer before their discharge and that they had a higher complication rate when compared with patients who received activated charcoal alone (5.4% versus 0.9%, respectively). In a pediatric study, Kornberg and Dolgin[94] randomized children to receive activated charcoal alone or activated charcoal following administration of syrup of ipecac. In this study, they found that those who received ipecac spent significantly more time in the emergency department compared with those who received only activated charcoal.

Several large, prospective studies have evaluated the benefit conferred by gastric emptying. In a landmark study, Kulig and co-workers[95] conducted a prospective evaluation of 592 patients with drug overdose, randomizing patients into three groups: (1) those receiving ipecac followed by activated charcoal, (2) those receiving gastric lavage followed by activated charcoal, and (3) those receiving activated charcoal alone. Use of syrup of ipecac did not significantly improve the clinical outcome of patients under any circumstances. Gastric lavage before activated charcoal administration provided benefit when it was instituted within 1 hour of ingestion. This study signaled a turning point in the practice of emergency medicine, as it showed that the standard of care for gastrointestinal decontamination need not necessarily include a gastric emptying procedure before the administration of activated charcoal.

Merigian and associates[96] studied 808 poisoned patients who on odd days underwent insertion of a nasogastric tube if they were obtunded, followed first by aspiration of stomach contents (without lavage) and then by administration of activated charcoal. On even days, a gastric emptying procedure (ipecac-induced emesis or gastric lavage until the lavage effluent was clear) was followed by administration of activated charcoal. Although the authors concluded that in symptomatic patients gastric emptying combined with activated charcoal therapy offered no benefit when compared with the use of activated charcoal alone, it is important to note that the group receiving the activated charcoal only *did* have aspiration of gastric contents.

In a study of 876 patients presenting to an emergency department after poisoning, Pond and colleagues[97] could not identify any benefit to performing gastric emptying prior to administration of activated charcoal. They also showed that the incidence of aspiration pneumonitis was related to airway intubation rather than to gastric lavage because the percentage of patients intubated in the study and the complication rates were similar in both the group with gastric emptying and in that receiving charcoal alone. No comment was made concerning prehospital (emergency medical service) administration of charcoal.

Bosse and co-workers[98] carefully examined the management of tricyclic antidepressant overdose, comparing three methods of gut decontamination in 51 patients: group 1 received activated charcoal alone, group 2 received gastric lavage with saline followed by activated charcoal, and group 3 received activated charcoal, followed first by saline lavage and then by activated charcoal. The average hospital stay among admitted patients was 93.3 hours in group 1, 107.2 hours in group 2, and only 66.7 hours in group 3. Of those patients admitted to an intensive care unit, the average time spent in the unit was 66.9 hours in group 1, 54.1 hours in group 2, and 34.4 hours in group 3. Of those requiring mechanical ventilation, the average ventilator time was 43.4 hours in group 1, 24.1 hours in group 2, and 17.8 hours in group 3. Although the authors concluded, recognizing the limits of sample size, that the three methods produced similar outcomes, the data suggest a trend toward a decrease in the length of hospital stay, intensive care unit time, and mechanical ventilation time in the charcoal-lavage-charcoal group.

Collectively, these studies indicate that the single most important intervention that can be provided to an overdose patient is *administration of activated charcoal*. Furthermore, they indicate that use of ipecac before administration of activated charcoal should be completely abandoned. Kulig and co-workers found that gastric lavage provided benefit within the first hour of ingestion,[95] and at least aspiration of gastric contents before use of activated charcoal was performed in one of these studies. Indeed, the practice in emergency medicine of EMS' giving charcoal at the scene, followed by emergency department aspiration of gastric contents with *prudent* (i.e., limited to 1 to 4 aliquots of saline) lavage to remove pill fragments within the first hour of ingestion, and then followed by activated charcoal administration appears to be supported by the study of Bosse and co-workers[98] and not disproved by the other studies. The ritual of overaggressive gastric lavage with many liters of lavage fluid until the lavage effluent is clear is clearly a thing of the past.

The combined efficacy of WBI and activated charcoal therapy has also been investigated. In an experimental study, Burkhart and associates found that WBI conferred no benefit to activated charcoal therapy.[99] This study and those that have suggested that there is an important interaction between activated charcoal and polyethylene glycol (GoLYTELY)[88, 89] prompt the clinician to take a flexible approach, depending on treatment priorities. If WBI is the most important intervention, activated charcoal therapy may provide an added benefit and its use should be considered in customary doses. If, on the other hand, activated charcoal administration is the primary intervention, the evidence for its reduced efficacy with polyethylene glycol suggests that either activated charcoal should precede WBI by some interval or that larger doses of activated charcoal should be administered.

The combination of activated charcoal with a cathartic is another potential intervention.[100] An experimental study that investigated the value of activated charcoal combined with sorbitol and that of activated charcoal alone demonstrated that the addition of sorbitol reduced salicylate absorption by 28% compared with the use of activated charcoal alone.[101] However, others have found that the addition of sorbitol to activated charcoal conferred no added benefit in a simulated acetaminophen overdose.[102] Easom and associates observed that the addition of magnesium citrate did not enhance the efficacy of activated charcoal in inhibiting aspirin absorption.[103] In the absence of clear demonstration of its efficacy and in view of the evidence that charcoal binding to toxin is so avid that desorption is minimal, use of a cathartic should be considered optional and not essential to poison management.

The need for all three interventions should also be dictated by the severity of the poisoning. *In cases in which life-threatening ingestion is suspected, the modest benefit derived from gastric emptying and catharsis may be important.* Therefore, in serious ingestions, all three components of GID should be considered. For patients in whom mild to moderate toxicity is expected, there appears to be little need for application of all of the components of GID; the only intervention necessary is administration of activated charcoal, with or without a cathartic.

The role of WBI in the management of toxic ingestions requires further clarification. WBI is the treatment of choice after ingestions of iron, lithium, drug packets, and, possibly, sustained-release pharmaceutical agents. For other toxic ingestions, administration of activated charcoal remains the most effective and practical therapy.

Multiple-Dose Activated Charcoal

The desire to prevent gastrointestinal absorption and enhance the elimination of already absorbed toxin has resulted in the creation of the concept of *multiple-dose oral activated charcoal (MDAC)*.[59]

There are two major goals in the use of MDAC: (1) preabsorptive and (2) postabsorptive elimination enhancement (Table 1–23).[56, 104]

Preabsorptive Elimination Enhancement. It is well recognized that many drugs, prior to their absorption from the gut, may, because of their physical characteristics, remain in the gastrointestinal tract for extended periods of time. Such agents include (1) anticholinergic agents, which slow gastrointestinal motility; (2) sustained-release agents, which dissolve slowly; and (3) drugs whose absorption is typically poor or erratic (e.g., phenytoin, which, when taken in overdose, may not be completely absorbed for as long as 5 days after ingestion).[59] In poisoning with each of these agents, theoretically benefit is

Table 1–23. Rationale for Multiple-Dose Activated Charcoal Therapy

Preabsorptive Elimination Enhancement
Anticholinergics
Sustained-release agents
Poorly absorbed pharmaceuticals (e.g., phenytoin)
Postabsorptive Elimination Enhancement
Gastrointestinal Dialysis
Theophylline
Phenobarbital
Phenytoin
Salicylates
Interruption of Enterohepatic Circulation
Cyclic antidepressants
"Classic" benzodiazepines (e.g., diazepam, chlordiazepoxide)
Carbamazepine
Phenothiazines
Thyroid hormones

Table 1–24. Pharmacokinetic Features of Drugs Reportedly Eliminated by Gastrointestinal Dialysis

Drug	Volume of Distribution (L/kg)	Protein Binding (%)
Theophylline	0.50	50–60
Phenobarbital	0.54	50–60
Aspirin	0.17	70–90
Phenytoin	0.64	80–90
Atenolol	0.90	<5

derived from giving more than a single dose of activated charcoal.

Postabsorptive Elimination Enhancement. In the 1970s, a theory emerged that multiple oral doses of charcoal could also be used to enhance the elimination of drugs that had already been absorbed from the gut or given intravenously. This concept of *postabsorptive elimination enhancement* was proved in a seminal article by Berg and colleagues who examined the ability of MDAC to enhance the elimination of intravenously administered phenobarbital. Using a crossover experimental design, they showed that repeated charcoal administration reduced the elimination time of phenobarbital from a mean of 110 hours to a mean of 45 hours.[105] In an accompanying editorial, Levy coined the term "gastrointestinal dialysis" to describe this phenomenon.[106] Levy suggested that certain drugs are capable of diffusing across the mucous membrane of the gastrointestinal tract, with the mucosa taking on the characteristics of a hemodialysis membrane, adsorbing to charcoal and then being eliminated in the stool. This phenomenon has also been referred to as "enterocapillary exsorption."[107] The fact that drug was administered intravenously has made this theory more credible. Intravenously administered theophylline and phenytoin have been shown to have an identical profile of rapid elimination with MDAC.[108] Finally, case reports have suggested that other substances, including salicylates, atenolol, and valproate, can be eliminated more rapidly with administration of MDAC[109] (although there is considerable controversy about enhanced salicylate excretion after MDAC use[110]). It is notable that, with the exception of phenytoin, all of these drugs have in common a small volume of distribution (less than 1 L/kg) and low protein binding (less than 70% to 80% [Table 1–24]). These characteristics are thought to be prerequisite for MDAC to act via gastrointestinal dialysis.[104, 107]

Another theory suggests that the elimination of absorbed drugs is enhanced by the interruption of their enterohepatic recirculation.[104] The normal pharmacokinetics of many drugs, particularly lipophilic drugs, includes hepatic uptake followed by either phase I biotransformation or phase II conjugation. In the case of phase I biotransformation (e.g., the demethylation of tricyclic antidepressants, propoxyphene, diazepam, meperidine, carbamazepine, and other agents), pharmacologically active metabolites are produced. With phase II reactions (e.g., the glucuronidation of morphine), the resultant metabolite is pharmacologically inactive. Both types of metabolites are secreted into the bile acid pool.[56] When bile is secreted into the gastrointestinal lumen, these metabolites are also present. In the gut, bacterial flora can remove the conjugate from phase II metabolites, releasing the active parent drug.[56] In the distal ileum, the active parent drug and pharmacologically active metabolite are reabsorbed along with bile acids. From here, they repeat the cycle of hepatic uptake, excretion, and ileal reabsorption, creating an enterohepatic cycle. With such drugs, MDAC is thought to adsorb the drug or metabolite when it reaches the gut, preventing reabsorption and interrupting the enterohepatic cycle.[56]

The effectiveness of MDAC in producing important increases in drug elimination is highly dependent on the drug (Table 1–25). With many drugs, clearance rates can approach those seen with hemodialysis. For example, with theophylline ingestion, MDAC produces clearance rates that approximate those of hemodialysis.[111]

Although MDAC therapy is being recommended for an enlarging list of drugs, in many cases this recommendation has been based on isolated case reports or, in some cases, no data whatsoever. A critical reanalysis of the role of MDAC has suggested that the range of toxic ingestions for which it is clearly beneficial is very narrow. For drugs with delayed gastrointestinal absorption, such as anticholinergics and sustained-release drugs, no firm scientific data demonstrate the efficacy of MDAC. In the case of the gastrointestinal dialysis model, studies have suggested that although drug elimination can be enhanced by the administration of MDAC, this enhancement cannot always be correlated with improvement in clinical outcome. For example, in patients with phenobarbital overdose, Pond and colleagues demonstrated that, despite the dramatic reduction in serum phenobarbital concentration effected by MDAC, the time to extu-

Table 1–25. Efficacy of Multiple-Dose Activated Charcoal in Enhancing Drug Elimination

Efficacy	Drug
Effective	Phenobarbital
	Theophylline
	Carbamazepine
	Salicylates
	Quinine
	Digitoxin
	Phenytoin
	Dapsone
Questionably effective	Sustained-release pharmaceuticals
	Thyroid hormone
	Valproate
	Anticholinergic/antihistaminic agents
Unlikely to be effective	Tricyclic antidepressants
	Phenothiazines
	Propoxyphene
	Aminoglycoside antibiotics
	Calcium channel blockers

bation and the duration of intensive care unit length of stay was comparable with those of patients who received a single dose of activated charcoal.[113] Finally, with respect to drugs with enterohepatic circulation, few studies show benefit from MDAC. In light of this critical examination, the list of drugs for which MDAC should be recommended for poisoning management is extremely small (see Table 1–25).

The diminishing role of MDAC is further supported by the important adverse effects it can produce.[112] The most common of adverse effects have been inspissation of charcoal in the gut, which produces charcoal concretions with resultant mechanical obstruction; bowel infarction; and perforation.[113–115] In particular, bowel catastrophes have been associated with MDAC use for drugs known to slow gastrointestinal motility, such as tricyclic antidepressants and phenobarbital. MDAC has also been associated with instances of charcoal aspiration that have resulted in bronchiolitis obliterans or death.[59, 116–118] Finally, due to the popularity of the activated charcoal–cathartic slurry, MDAC therapy has led to multiple-dose cathartic use, which results in fluid and electrolyte disturbances. Collectively, these cases demonstrate the potential toxicity of MDAC therapy.

A number of treatment regimens have been proposed for MDAC, when appropriate. The most common is administration of 1 g/kg every 4 hours. If the patient is unable to swallow, charcoal can be administered by continuous infusion. An alternative regimen of 20 g every 2 hours is as effective as 1 g/kg every 4 hours for theophylline intoxication.[119] Repeat doses of charcoal are sufficiently safe for use in those at extremes of age, including neonates.[120] Cathartics should be administered with every two to three doses of activated charcoal in order to prevent its inspissation.[59] The endpoint of MDAC therapy is a reduction in serum drug level to a nontoxic range or significant clinical improvement, or both. MDAC therapy should not be continued for longer than 24 hours because after this point the potential risks may exceed the benefits.

Antidotes

With the development of sophisticated new antidotes and the changing spectrum of clinical poisoning, the use of emergency antidotes is becoming the primary treatment method in clinical toxicology. Table 1–1 lists the common emergency antidotes. In poisoning with a known substance, early antidote use is indicated for emergency stabilization, often within the first hour. Other antidotes are available, such as pyridoxine (the initial adult dosage is 5 mg IV for significant isoniazid overdose) and snakebite antivenin. A promising new antidote for cyanide poisoning presently under investigation is hydroxycobalamin.

Hyperbaric oxygenation can provide oxygen at pressures greater than normal atmospheric pressure, which is given as 1 atm (atmosphere) or 760 mm Hg. Three atmospheres is the maximal pressure humans can tolerate over a reasonable period of time; hyperbaric medicine units generally do not exceed 2.5 to 2.8 atm. The use of hyperbaric oxygenation is becoming standard therapy for patients with significant carbon monoxide poisoning, and it is becoming more available (see Chapter 70) for carbon tetrachloride poisoning, and, possibly, for cyanide and hydrogen sulfide poisoning.

Admission to an intensive care unit following antidotal therapy for further management and observation is generally indicated. Further discussion of each antidote and its use is provided in the chapter on each specific poison.

Elimination of Absorbed Substance

Table 1–26 outlines treatment methods and indications for elimination of absorbed substances, such as charcoal hemoperfusion and hemodialysis. Hemodialysis also is indicated for any drug overdose patient who has severe intractable metabolic acidosis, electrolyte abnormalities, or renal failure. Dialysis is not indicated in a patient who has ingested a substance that is markedly protein-bound, such as tricyclic antidepressants; in a drug overdose that is rarely, if ever, lethal (e.g., benzodiazepine overdose); when the plasma concentration of the drug is not significant enough to ensure drug removal (as with digitalis); when the action of the agent is irreversible (as with cyanide); when the patient is in shock; or when the dangers of hemodialysis outweigh the benefits. Further discussion of elimination of a substance that has already been absorbed is provided in Chapter 10.

Observation and Supportive Care

Observation and supportive care are the mainstay of therapy for the poisoned patient. *Indiscriminate use of gastric lavage, antidotes, and drugs should be avoided.* All too often, the toxic agent is unknown, multiple drugs have been taken, or the patient is too unstable to undergo an aggressive therapy such as hemodialysis. Monitoring of vital signs, cardiac telemetry, and oxygen saturation is mandatory.

Table 1–26. Additional Treatment Methods for Elimination of Absorbed Substance

Treatment	Drug
Alkalization of urine	Phenobarbital Salicylates
Hemodialysis	Lithium Ethylene glycol Methanol Salicylate Theophylline
Hemoperfusion	Theophylline Barbiturates

Hospitalization in an intensive care unit is generally indicated for the patient with serious poisoning. Multisystem monitoring with blood studies and assessment of other parameters is indicated, and upon detection of any specific system disturbance, appropriate subspecialty consultation is warranted.

Some agents such as iron, mercury, acetaminophen, paraquat, carbon tetrachloride, and *Amanita phalloides* toxin have a latent phase, in which the patient appears to recover from the initial insult, only to decompensate 24 to 72 hours postingestion. Patients with overdose of sustained-release capsules, such as calcium channel blocker or theophylline preparations, also may have delayed manifestation of poisoning. Rarely, the tricyclic antidepressants have been known to cause fatal arrhythmia up to 3 days following ingestion. Some effects are not seen until later, such as hypertension following phencyclidine ingestion, hemorrhagic colitis following mercury ingestion, and disseminated intravascular coagulation following snakebite. One must also watch for the delayed pulmonary (Chapter 7), hepatic (Chapter 9), renal (Chapter 11), and hematologic (Chapter 13) manifestations of poisoning.

Patients may require observation because of an underlying disease that may be exacerbated because of the overdose, such as diabetic ketoacidosis. Observation may be necessary to evaluate or treat complications, such as in a patient with an overdose who fell and sustained trauma or in a patient who develops aspiration pneumonitis or interstitial pulmonary edema.

The IV use of illicit drugs is associated with multiple complications; observation is especially indicated for patients experiencing these complications, which include bacterial endocarditis, rhabdomyolysis, and neurologic sequelae.

Disposition

The disposition of the patient with intoxication may involve medical and psychiatric care as well as social follow-up. All patients admitted to the hospital with intentional overdose warrant close observation and the institution of suicide precautions. These patients may need appropriate restraint or observation if further injury or additional overdose attempts are to be prevented. Overt or subtle attempts or gestures indicate the need for psychiatric evaluation. Often, outpatient follow-up is necessary; for example, a child with kerosene ingestion may require further examination and chest radiography, and a child who has ingested anticoagulant rat poison may require serial outpatient monitoring of prothrombin times. The issue of child abuse or neglect may need consideration whenever a pediatric patient is treated. Finally, long-term follow-up may be indicated; for example, hepatitis and HIV testing may be needed in the IV drug abuser.

References

1. Haddad LM: Emergency physicians and poison treatment. N Engl J Med *300*:1223, 1979.
2. DAWN (Drug Abuse Warning Network): 1993 Annual Medical Examiner Data. Publication 95-3019. Rockville, MD, Department of Health and Human Services, 1995.
3. Litovitz T: 1994 Toxic Exposure Surveillance System (TESS) of the American Association of Poison Control Centers. Am J Emerg Med *13*:551–597, 1995.
4. The New American Bible, *St. Joseph's Edition*. New York, The Catholic Publishing Company, 1992; or *The Authorized King James Version of the Holy Bible*. Gordonsville, TN, The Mid-America Bible Society, 1993; or *The Holy Scripture*. Philadelphia, The Jewish Publication Society, 1993.
5. Plato: The Republic and Phaedo. New York, P. F. Collier and Sons, 1909.
6. Halstead BW: Poisonous and Venomous Marine Animals of the World. Revised ed. Princeton, NJ, Darwin Press, Inc., 1978.
7. Arena JM: Safety closure caps. JAMA *169*:1187, 1959.
8. Lovejoy FH Jr, Caplan DL, Rowland T, Fazen L: A statewide plan for care of the poisoned patient: the Massachusetts Poison Control System. N Engl J Med *300*:1223, 1979.
9. Schreiner GE: The role of hemodialysis (artificial kidney) in acute poisoning. Arch Intern Med *102*:896, 1958.
10. Haddad LM: Acute poisoning. *In* Bennett JC, Plum F (eds): Cecil Textbook of Medicine. 20th ed. Philadelphia, W. B. Saunders Co., 1996.
11. Walls RM: Rapid sequence intubation. Ann Emerg Med *22*:1008–1013, 1993.
12. Wright PMC, Caldwell JE, Miller RD: Onset and duration of rocuronium and succinylcholine at the adductor pollicis and laryngeal adductor muscles in anesthetized humans. Anesthesiology *81*:1110–1115, 1994.
13. Plum F, Posner JB: Diagnosis of Stupor and Coma. 3rd ed. Philadelphia, F. A. Davis Co., 1980.
14. Lipman J, Jardine I, Roos C, Dreosti L: Intravenous calcium chloride as an antidote to verapamil-induced hypotension. Intensive Care Med *8*:55, 1982.
15. Haddad LM: Case Report: Resuscitation of nifedipine (Procardia) overdose exclusively with intravenous calcium chloride. Am J Emerg Med *14*:602–603, 1996.
16. Smith TW, Haber E, Yeatman L, Butler VP: Reversal of advanced digoxin intoxication with Fab fragments of digoxin-specific antibodies. N Engl J Med *294*:797, 1976.
17. Parmley WW: The role of glucagon in cardiac therapy. N Engl J Med *285*:801, 1971.
18. Kozinski EJ, Stein N, Malindzak GS, Boone E: Glucagon and propranolol (Inderal) toxicity. N Engl J Med *285*:1325, 1971.
19. Litovitz TL, Troutman WH: Amoxapine overdose: Seizures and fatalities. JAMA *250*:1069, 1983.
20. Kulig K: Initial management of ingestions of toxic substances. N Engl J Med *326*:1677–1681, 1992.
21. Safran MJ: Chemical ocular injuries. Hosp Physician 53–58, January 1989.
22. Herr RD, White GL, Bernhisel K, et al: Clinical comparison of ocular irrigation fluids following chemical injury. Am J Emerg Med *9*:228–231, 1991.
23. Decker WJ: In quest of emesis: Fact, fable and fancy. Clin Toxicol *4*:383–387, 1971.
24. DiGregorio GJ, Fruncillo RJ: Antiemetics. Am Fam Physician *26*:200–202, 1982.
25. Karlsson B, Noren L: Ipecacuanha and copper sulphate as emetics in intoxications in children. Acta Paediatr Scand *54*:331–335, 1965.
26. Stein RS, Jenkins D, Korns ME: Death after use of cupric sulfate as emetic. JAMA *235*:801, 1976.
27. Hanson TA: Apomorphine in the management of accidental ingestion of poisons. South Med J *60*:603–605, 1967.
28. MacLean WC: A comparison of ipecac syrup and apomorphine in the immediate treatment of ingestion of poisons. J Pediatr *82*:121–124, 1973.
29. Smith EJ, Palevsky S: Salt poisoning in a two-year-old child. Am J Emerg Med *8*:571–572, 1990.

30. Smith RP, Smith D: Acute ipecac poisoning: Report of a fatal case and review of the literature. N Engl J Med *265*:523–525, 1963.
31. MacLeod J: Ipecac intoxication: Use of a cardiac pacemaker in management. N Engl J Med *268*:146–147, 1963.
32. Moran DM, Crouch DJ, Findle BS: Absorption of ipecac alkaloids in emergency patients. Ann Emerg Med *13*:1100–1102, 1984.
33. Manno BR, Manno JE: Toxicology of ipecac: A review. Clin Toxicol *10*:221–242, 1977.
34. Klatskin G, Friedman H: Emetine toxicity in man: Studies on the nature of early toxic manifestations, their relation to dose level, and their significance in determining safe dosage. Ann Intern Med *28*:892–915, 1948.
35. Miser JS, Robertson WO: Ipecac poisoning. West J Med *128*:440–443, 1978.
36. Grbcich P, Lacouture PG, Kresel JJ, et al: Expired ipecac syrup efficacy. Pediatrics *78*:1085–1089, 1986.
37. King WD: Syrup of ipecac: A drug review. Clin Toxicol *17*:353–358, 1980.
38. Knight KM, Doucet HJ: Gastric rupture and death caused by ipecac syrup. South Med J *80*:786–787, 1987.
39. Tandberg D, Liechty EJ, Fishbein D: Mallory-Weiss syndrome: An unusual complication of ipecac-induced emesis. Ann Emerg Med *10*:521–523, 1981.
40. Wolowodiuk OJ, McMicken DB, O'Brien P: Pneumomediastinum and retropneumoperitoneum: An unusual complication of syrup-of-ipecac-induced emesis. Ann Emerg Med *13*:1148–1151, 1984.
41. Adler AG, Walinsky P, Krall RA, Cho SY: Death resulting from ipecac syrup poisoning. JAMA *243*:1927–1928, 1980.
42. Pope HG, Hudson JI, Nixon RA, Herridge PL: The epidemiology of ipecac abuse. N Engl J Med *314*:245–246, 1986.
43. Abdallah AH, Tye A: A comparison of the efficacy of emetic drugs and stomach lavage. Am J Dis Child *113*:571–575, 1967.
44. Arnold FJ, Hodges JB, Barta RA, et al: Evaluation of the efficacy of lavage and induced emesis in treatment of salicylate poisoning. Pediatrics *23*:286–301, 1959.
45. Corby DG, Lisciandro RC, Lehman R, Decker WJ: The efficiency of methods used to evacuate the stomach after acute ingestions. Pediatrics *40*:871–874, 1967.
46. Lanphear WF: Gastric lavage. J Emerg Med *4*:43–47, 1986.
47. Kulig K: Gastric lavage and acute poisoning. J Emerg Med *7*:403–404, 1989.
48. Bartecchi CD: A modification of gastric lavage technique. J Am Coll Emerg Physicians *3*:304–305, 1974.
49. Bartecchi CD: Removal of gastric drug masses. N Engl J Med *296*:282–283, 1977.
50. Watson WA, Leighton J, Guy J, et al: Recovery of cyclic antidepressants with gastric lavage. J Emerg Med *7*:373–377, 1989.
51. Thompson AM, Robins JB, Prescott LF: Changes in cardiorespiratory function during gastric lavage for drug overdose. Hum Toxicol *6*:215–218, 1987.
52. Harstad E, Moller KO, Simesen MH: The value of gastric lavage in the treatment of acute poisoning. Acta Med Scand *112*:478–484, 1942.
53. Tandberg D, Diven BG, McLeod JW: Ipecac-induced emesis versus gastric lavage: A controlled study in normal adults. Am J Emerg Med *4*:205–209, 1986.
54. Auerbach PS, Osterloh J, Braun O, et al: Efficacy of gastric emptying: Gastric lavage versus emesis induced with ipecac. Ann Emerg Med *15*:692–698, 1986.
55. Saetta JP, Quinton DN: Residual gastric content after gastric lavage and ipecacuanha-induced emesis in self-poisoned patients: An endoscopic study. J R Soc Med *84*:35–38, 1991.
56. Derlet RW, Albertson TE: Activated charcoal: Past, present and future. West J Med *145*:493–496, 1986.
57. Park GD, Spector R, Goldberg MJ, Johnson GF: Expanded role of charcoal therapy in the poisoned and overdosed patient. Arch Intern Med *146*:969–973, 1986.
58. Greensher J, Mofenson HC, Caraccio TR: Ascendency of the black bottle (activated charcoal). Pediatrics *80*:949–951, 1987.
59. Jones J, McMullen MJ, Dougherty J, Cannon L: Repetitive doses of activated charcoal in the treatment of poisoning. Am J Emerg Med *5*:305–310, 1987.
60. Cooney DO: A "superactive" charcoal for antidotal use in poisonings. Clin Toxicol *11*:387–390, 1977.
61. Wax PM, Wang RY, Hoffman RS, et al: Prevalence of sorbitol in multiple-dose activated charcoal regimens in emergency departments. Ann Emerg Med *22*:1807–1812, 1993.
62. Chin L, Piccioni AL, Bourn WM, et al: Optimal antidotal dose of activated charcoal. Toxicol Appl Pharmacol *26*:103–108, 1973.
63. Olkkola KT: Effect of charcoal-drug ratio on antidotal efficacy of oral activated charcoal in man. Br J Clin Pharmacol *19*:767–773, 1985.
64. Krenzelok EP, Heller MB: Effectiveness of commercially available aqueous activated charcoal products. Ann Emerg Med *16*:1340–1343, 1987.
65. Dillon EC, Wilton JH, Barlow JC, Watson WA: Large surface area activated charcoal and the inhibition of aspirin absorption. Ann Emerg Med *18*:547–552, 1989.
66. Eisen TF, Grbcich PA, Lacouture PG, et al: The adsorption of salicylates by a milk chocolate–charcoal mixture. Ann Emerg Med *20*:143–146, 1991.
67. Schneider SM, Michelson EA: Enhanced activated charcoal delivery through small-bore tubing. Vet Hum Toxicol *35*:503–505, 1993.
68. Elliott CG, Colby TV, Hicks HG: Charcoal lung: Bronchiolitis obliterans after aspiration of activated charcoal. Chest *96*:672–674, 1989.
69. Shannon M, Fish SS, Lovejoy FH: Cathartics and laxatives: Do they still have a place in management of the poisoned patient? Med Toxicol *1*:247–252, 1986.
70. Donowitz M: Magnesium-induced diarrhea and new insights into the pathobiology of diarrhea. N Engl J Med *324*:1059–1060, 1991.
71. Krenzelok EP, Keller R, Stewart RD: Gastrointestinal transit times of cathartics combined with charcoal. Ann Emerg Med *14*:1152–1155, 1985.
72. Sue Y-J, Woolf A, Shannon M: Efficacy of magnesium citrate cathartic in pediatric toxic ingestions. Ann Emerg Med *24*:709–712, 1994.
73. Farley TA: Severe hypernatremic dehydration after use of an activated charcoal-sorbitol suspension. J Pediatr *109*:719–722, 1986.
74. McCord MM, Okun AL: Toxicity of sorbitol-charcoal suspension. J Pediatr *111*:307–308, 1987.
75. Weber CA, Santiago RM: Hypermagnesemia: A potential complication during treatment of theophylline intoxication with oral activated charcoal and magnesium-containing cathartics. Chest *95*:56–59, 1989.
76. Garrelts JC, Watson WA, Holloway KD, Sweet DE: Magnesium toxicity secondary to catharsis during management of theophylline poisoning. Am J Emerg Med *7*:34–37, 1989.
77. Jenkins J, Shannon M, Lacouture P, Woolf A: Serum magnesium concentrations after repetitive magnesium cathartic administration. Am J Emerg Med *8*:297–300, 1990.
78. Smilkstein MJ, Steedle D, Kulig KW, et al: Magnesium levels after magnesium-containing cathartics. Clin Toxicol *26*:51–65, 1988.
79. Gren J, Woolf A: Hypermagnesemia associated with catharsis in a salicylate-intoxicated patient with anorexia nervosa. Ann Emerg Med *8*:200–203, 1989.
80. Brent J, Kulig K, Rumack BH: Iatrogenic death from sorbitol and magnesium sulfate during treatment for salicylism. Vet Hum Toxicol *31*:334, 1989.
81. Hewitt J, Reeve J, Rigby J, Cox AG: Whole-gut irrigation in preparation for large-bowel surgery. Lancet *2*:337–340, 1973.
82. Michael KA, Kipiro JT, Bowden TA, Tedesco F: Whole-bowel irrigation for mechanical colon cleansing. Clin Pharmacol *4*:414–424, 1985.
83. Lee DC, Roberts J, Kelly J, Fishman SM: Whole-bowel irrigation as an adjunct in the treatment of radiopaque arsenic. Letter. Am J Emerg Med *13*:244–245, 1995.
84. Kaczorowski J, Waax P: Whole-bowel irrigation with 44 liters of polyethylene glycol in a pediatric iron overdose. Abstract. Vet Hum Toxicol *36*:340, 1994.

85. Smith SW, Ling LJ, Halstenson CE: Whole-bowel irrigation as a treatment for acute lithium overdose. Ann Emerg Med *20*:536–539, 1991.
86. Tenenbein M: Whole-bowel irrigation in iron poisoning. J Pediatr *111*:142–145, 1987.
87. Kirshenbaum LA, Sitar DS, Tenenbein M: Interaction between whole-bowel irrigation solution and activated charcoal: Implications for the treatment of toxic ingestions. Ann Emerg Med *19*:1129–1132, 1990.
88. Hoffman RS, Chiang WK, Howland MA, et al: Theophylline desorption from activated charcoal caused by whole-bowel irrigation solution. J Toxicol Clin Toxicol *29*:191–201, 1991.
89. Makosiej FJ, Hoffman RS, Howland MA, Goldfrank LR: An *in vitro* evaluation of cocaine hydrochloride adsorption by activated charcoal and desorption upon addition of polyethylene glycol electrolyte lavage solution. J Toxicol Clin Toxicol *31*:381–395, 1993.
90. Kirk MA, Peterson J, Kulig K, et al: Acetaminophen overdose in children: A comparison of ipecac versus activated charcoal versus no gastrointestinal decontamination. Abstract. Ann Emerg Med *20*:472–473, 1991.
91. Neuvonen PJ, Vartiainen M, Tokola O: Comparison of activated charcoal and ipecac syrup in prevention of drug absorption. Eur J Clin Pharmacol *24*:557–562, 1983.
92. Tenenbein M, Cohen S, Sitar DS: Efficacy of ipecac-induced emesis, orogastric lavage, and activated charcoal for acute drug overdose. Ann Emerg Med *16*:838–841, 1987.
93. Albertson TE, Derlet RW, Foulke GE, et al: Superiority of activated charcoal alone compared with ipecac and activated charcoal in the treatment of acute toxic ingestions. Ann Emerg Med *18*:56–59, 1989.
94. Kornberg AE, Dolgin J: Pediatric ingestions: Charcoal alone versus ipecac and charcoal. Ann Emerg Med *20*:648–651, 1991.
95. Kulig K, Bar-Or D, Cantrill SV, et al: Management of acutely poisoned patients without gastric emptying. Ann Emerg Med *14*:562–567, 1985.
96. Merigian KS, Woodard M, Hedges JR, et al: Prospective evaluation of gastric emptying in the self-poisoned patient. Am J Emerg Med *8*:479–483, 1990.
97. Pond SM, Lewis-Driver DJ, Williams G, et al: Gastric emptying in acute overdose: A prospective randomised controlled trial. Med J Aust *163*:345–349, 1995.
98. Bosse GM, Barefoot JA, Pfeifer MP, Rodgers GC: Comparison of three methods of gut decontamination in tricyclic antidepressant overdose. J Emerg Med *13*:203–209, 1995.
99. Burkhart KK, Wuerz RL, Donovan JW: Whole-bowel irrigation as adjunctive treatment for sustained-release theophylline overdose. Ann Emerg Med *21*:1316–1320, 1992.
100. Burton BT, Bayer MJ, Barron L, Aitchison JP: Comparison of activated charcoal and gastric lavage in the prevention of aspirin absorption. J Emerg Med *1*:411–416, 1984.
101. Keller RE, Schwab RA, Krenzelok EP: Contribution of sorbitol combined with activated charcoal in prevention of salicylate absorption. Ann Emerg Med *19*:654–656, 1990.
102. McNamara RM, Aaron CK, Gemborys M, Davidheiser S: Sorbitol catharsis does not enhance efficacy of charcoal in a simulated acetaminophen overdose. Ann Emerg Med *17*:243–246, 1988.
103. Easom JM, Caraccio TR, Lovejoy FH: Evaluation of activated charcoal and magnesium citrate in the prevention of aspirin absorption in humans. Clin Pharmacol *1*:154–156, 1982.
104. Pond SM: Role of repeated oral doses of activated charcoal in clinical toxicology. Med Toxicol *1*:3–11, 1986.
105. Berg MJ, Berlinger WG, Goldberg MJ, et al: Acceleration of the body clearance of phenobarbital by oral activated charcoal. N Engl J Med *307*:642–644, 1982.
106. Levy G: Gastrointestinal clearance of drugs with activated charcoal. N Engl J Med *307*:676–678, 1982.
107. Chyka PA: Multiple-dose activated charcoal and enhancement of systemic drug clearance: Summary of studies in animals and human volunteers. Clin Toxicol *33*:399–405, 1995.
108. Kulig KW, Bar-Or D, Rumack BH: Intravenous theophylline poisoning and multiple-dose charcoal in an animal model. Ann Emerg Med *16*:842–846, 1987.
109. Mofenson HC, Caraccio TR, Greensher J, et al: Gastrointestinal dialysis with activated charcoal and cathartic in the treatment of adolescent intoxications. Clin Pediatr *24*:678–684, 1985.
110. Kirshenbaum LA, Matthews SC, Sitar DS, Tenenbein M: Does multiple-dose charcoal therapy enhance salicylate excretion? Arch Intern Med *150*:1281–1283, 1990.
111. Heath A, Knudsen K: Role of extracorporeal drug removal in acute theophylline poisoning: A review. Med Toxicol *2*:294–308, 1987.
112. Tenenbein M: Multiple doses of activated charcoal: Time for reappraisal? Ann Emerg Med *20*:529–531, 1991.
113. Pond SM, Olson KR, Osterloh JD, Tong TG: Randomized study of the treatment of phenobarbital overdose with repeated doses of activated charcoal. JAMA *251*:3104–3108, 1984.
114. Ray MJ, Padin R, Condie JD, Halls JM: Charcoal bezoar: Small-bowel obstruction secondary to amitriptyline overdose therapy. Dig Dis Sci *33*:106–107, 1988.
115. Watson WA, Cremer KF, Chapman JA: Gastrointestinal obstruction associated with multiple-dose activated charcoal. J Emerg Med *4*:401–407, 1986.
116. Benson B, VanAntwerp M, Hergott T: A fatality resulting from multiple-dose activated charcoal therapy. Abstract. Vet Hum Toxicol *31*:335, 1989.
117. Harsch HH: Aspiration of activated charcoal. Letter. N Engl J Med *314*:318, 1986.
118. Menzies DG, Busuttil A, Prescott LF: Fatal pulmonary aspiration of oral activated charcoal. BMJ *297*:459–460, 1988.
119. Park GD, Spector R, Goldberg MJ, et al: Effect of the surface area of activated charcoal on theophylline clearance. J Clin Pharmacol *24*:289–292, 1984.
120. Shannon M, Amitai Y, Lovejoy FH Jr: Multiple-dose activated charcoal for theophylline poisoning in young infants. Pediatrics *80*:368–370, 1987.

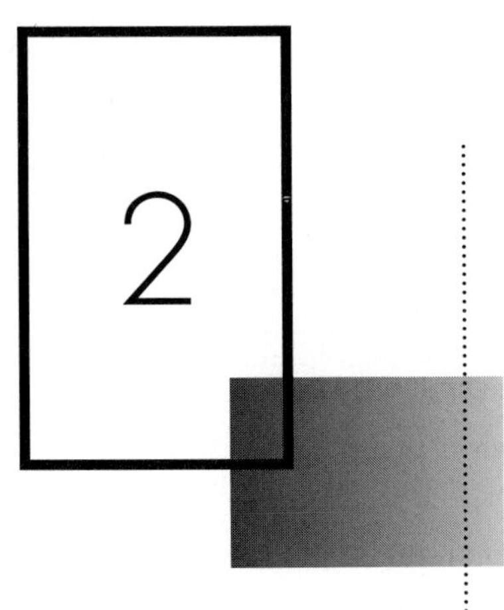

Pediatric Resuscitation and Fluid Management

FRED TECKLENBURG, MD
THOMAS W. McKEE, MD

When confronted with a critically ill child, the physician must rapidly provide cardiopulmonary support on the basis of the patient's physiologic status regardless of the underlying cause. Resuscitation of the pediatric patient proceeds with the sequential assessment and stabilization of the *airway, breathing,* and *circulation (ABC's).* This chapter reviews the ABC's of resuscitation and subsequently presents the management of fluids and electrolytes in the pediatric patient.

RESUSCITATION PHYSIOLOGY

Oxygen Delivery

The primary physiologic objective of resuscitation is optimization of oxygen (O_2) delivery to the body (measured in milliliters of O_2 per minute). *Oxygen delivery* is the product of the O_2 content of the blood (in milliliters of O_2 per deciliter) and cardiac output (in liters per minute) multiplied by 10 (deciliters per liter) (Fig. 2–1). The O_2 content equation demonstrates the importance of ensuring a high arterial hemoglobin saturation (i.e., greater than 90%) and an adequate hemoglobin concentration. The most common reason for low O_2 content in a critically ill child is low arterial hemoglobin saturation due to the hypoxemia caused by pulmonary ventilation-perfusion mismatch. Anemia is the second most common cause of inadequate O_2 content. Both of these problems can usually be corrected rapidly.

Normal hemoglobin is nearly completely saturated with O_2 when the arterial partial pressure of O_2 ($Pa{O_2}$) is 70 mm Hg or greater (Fig. 2–2). The sigmoid shape of the oxyhemoglobin dissociation curve allows rapid unloading of O_2 at the lower O_2 partial pressures of peripheral tissues. Carboxyhemoglobin and methemoglobinemia obviously have a deleterious impact on this important aspect of O_2. Analysis of the equation also reflects the minimal contribution that dissolved O_2 (0.003 mL O_2/dL per mm Hg $\times$ $Pa{O_2}$) makes to the total O_2 content. On the other hand, hyperbaric conditions can significantly increase the $Pa{O_2}$, and, in turn, the amount of O_2 dissolved in the plasma, which impacts directly on carbon monoxide poisoning.

The other major factor in O_2 delivery is the *cardiac output,* which is the product of the heart rate and stroke volume. The venous return and end-diastolic myocardial fiber length (preload), myocardial contractility, and resistance to ventricular emptying (afterload) determine the stroke volume. The cardiac

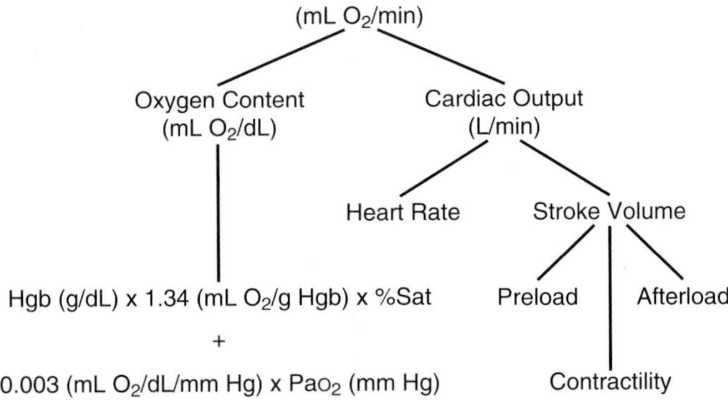

Figure 2–1. Oxygen delivery to the body. Hgb, hemoglobin; %Sat, per cent saturation; $Pa{O_2}$, partial pressure of arterial oxygen.

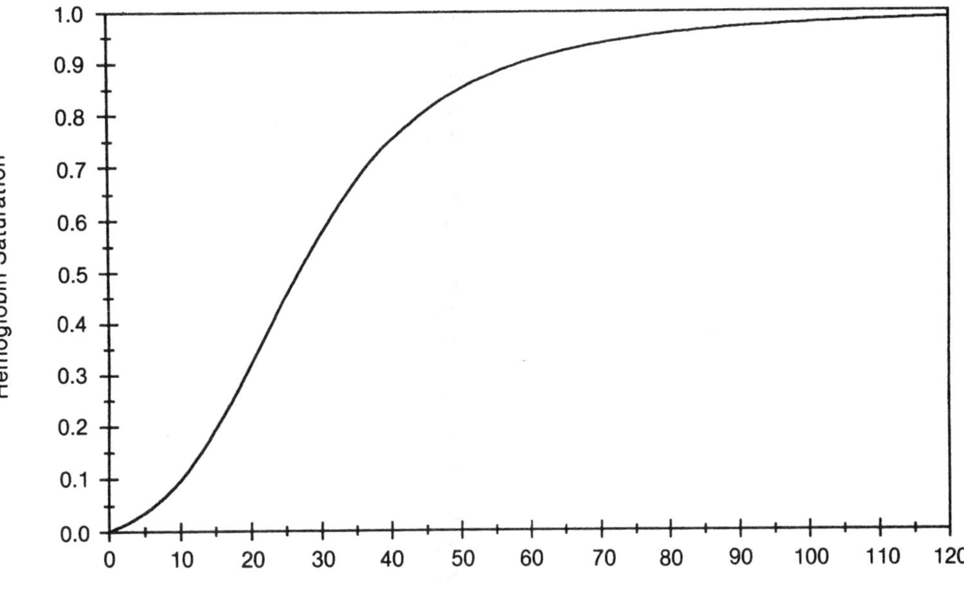

Figure 2–2. Standard oxyhemoglobin dissociation curve. (From Dantzker DR: Cardiopulmonary Critical Care. 2nd ed. Philadelphia, W.B. Saunders Co., p 201, 1991.)

output of the stressed infant is very dependent on heart rate because of the relatively small inotropic response to an increase in sympathetic tone. Seriously ill infants do not tolerate bradycardia. Also, it is important to appreciate that most pediatric patients in shock—especially those in shock attributable to toxins—have a reduction in preload due to hypovolemia or relative hypovolemia created by an increase in venous capacitance and arteriolar vasodilatation. All factors that relate to O_2 delivery should be assessed and corrected in the practical application of cardiopulmonary resuscitation.

Oxygen Utilization

Although the immediate physiologic priority is improvement of systemic O_2 delivery, resuscitation efforts should continue to address factors that influence overall O_2 utilization (Fig. 2–3). Microcirculatory abnormalities and the attendant end-organ perfusion abnormalities may be improved by infusion of vasoactive agents. Metabolic acidosis should not be overzealously treated because the oxyhemoglobin dissociation curve shifts to the left in the setting of alkalosis; this increases hemoglobin affinity for O_2 and decreases O_2 unloading in the peripheral tissues. Evidence of cellular hypoxia and poor extraction (e.g., narrow arterial–mixed venous O_2 content difference) in the setting of a normal arterial O_2 content suggests the presence of a toxin that is creating a cellular metabolic block. For example, cyanide can inhibit oxidative phosphorylation by binding cytochrome oxidase, in effect dismantling aerobic metabolism. In the patient with massive cocaine overdose, a hypermetabolic storm that negates the resuscitative effects of O_2 delivery may require aggressive cooling and neuromuscular blockade. Simply stated, a toxin is capable of harmfully impacting every factor that contributes to O_2 delivery and utilization. Resuscitation based on physiologic principles is necessary for achieving the best possible clinical outcome.

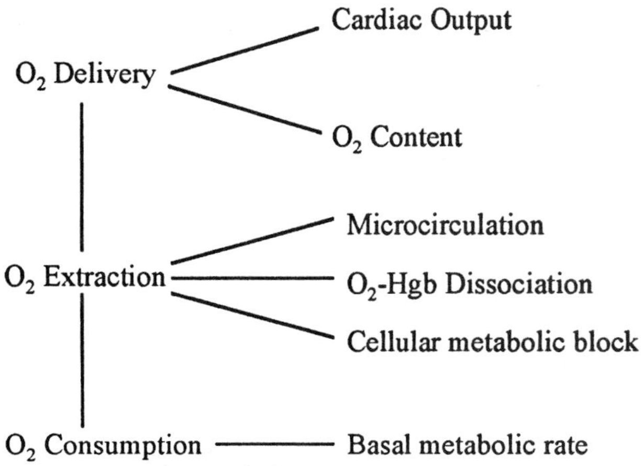

O_2 Delivery — Cardiac Output
O_2 Delivery — O_2 Content
O_2 Extraction — Microcirculation
O_2 Extraction — O_2-Hgb Dissociation
O_2 Extraction — Cellular metabolic block
O_2 Consumption — Basal metabolic rate

Figure 2–3. Oxygen utilization.

CARDIOPULMONARY ASSESSMENT

Case Report

A previously healthy 2-year-old toddler was found unresponsive. On presentation to the emergency department, she was pale and obtunded with agonal respirations, a central pulse rate of 180 bpm, and a systolic blood pressure of 65 mm Hg.

Rapid assessment of ventilation, oxygenation, and perfusion generally place a patient into one of the following categories: stable, potential, or probable respiratory failure; compensated or decompensated shock; or cardiopulmonary collapse.[1]

Airway and Breathing Assessment

The evaluation of an ill-appearing child typically starts from the doorway of a hospital room. From this distance, the experienced clinician subconsciously registers the patient's facial color and global mental status while visually assessing the airway and breathing. When the clinician approaches the child, signs that characterize airway patency, work of breathing, and respiratory rate usually are obvious. Assessment of chest expansion and auscultation of the chest reflect the adequacy of air exchange. A low-pitched, biphasic (inspiratory greater than expiratory) stridor associated with suprasternal retractions is typical of hypopharyngeal obstruction due to posterior displacement of the tongue block—a common reason for upper airway obstruction in an obtunded patient. Tachypnea greater than 80 respirations per minute (rpm) in an infant, 60 rpm in a toddler or preschooler, and 40 rpm in a school-age child or adolescent usually signifies severe pulmonary disease or, less frequently, cardiac disease, the latter lacking the intensity of retractions and work of breathing ("quiet" tachypnea). Hyperpnea and mild tachypnea may indicate respiratory compensation for a metabolic acidosis.

The work of breathing is demonstrated by the intensity of retractions, nasal flaring, and accessory muscle use. *Head bobbing* associated with respiratory effort is typically a sign of maximal effort and probable respiratory failure. Similarly, grunting on expiration is a sign of significant respiratory dysfunction. A striking pallor and altered mental status are typical of significant hypoxemia or decreased cardiac output, whereas frank cyanosis and coma often are markers of imminent cardiopulmonary arrest. A low, irregular respiratory rate (less than 10 breaths per minute) in an ill-appearing, lethargic child represents overt respiratory failure due to either central nervous system depression or an advanced cardiopulmonary process.

Circulation Assessment

A rapid cardiovascular examination starts with assessment of the amplitude and rate of peripheral and central pulses—usually, at the basilic and femoral arteries in a young child. The heart rate of infants and toddlers may normally vary from approximately 90 to 200 beats per minute, depending on their level of activity; in older children, it varies from 60 to 140 beats per minute. The lower norm for systolic blood pressure in children may be approximated by use of the following formula: $70 + (2 \times \text{age in years})$. An infant generally should have a systolic blood pressure of at least 70 mm Hg.

Peripheral perfusion is assessed on the basis of the differential skin temperature and color of the extremities and trunk, the presence or absence of mottling or flushing, and the capillary refill time. One determines the capillary refill time by firmly pressing the patient's palm or sole and measuring the time required for the blanching to disappear. A refill time longer than 2 seconds suggests circulatory insufficiency but may also indicate mild vasospasm associated with cool ambient temperatures or elevated body temperature. Abnormal central nervous system signs also may reflect inadequate circulatory perfusion. The child's mental status, motor response to voice or pain, and muscle tone should be noted. (Even a young infant's mental status may be assessed on the basis of his or her visual fixation and environmental interaction.)

Shock is a clinical state of inadequate organ perfusion due to hypovolemia, maldistribution of vascular volume and tone ("distributive" shock), or cardiac dysfunction, or any combination of these. Early shock may be difficult to recognize in children because homeostatic mechanisms (e.g., tachycardia and increases in systemic vascular resistance) may very effectively maintain a normal blood pressure. Typically, children in *compensated shock* have tachycardia; are mildly tachypneic, oliguric, confused, or lethargic; and demonstrate subtle signs of poor peripheral perfusion such as a delayed capillary refill time, coolness of the extremities, and rapid, low-amplitude peripheral pulses. *Decompensated shock* is distinguished by hypotension and more profound circulatory dysfunction that may progress to cardiopulmonary collapse and death in the absence of treatment. Clinically, the signs in the patient in this type of shock may progress from a constellation of hypotension, tachycardia, tachypnea, mottled appearance, coldness of the extremities, and obtundation to absence of pulse and unresponsiveness with agonal respirations.

The cardiopulmonary constellation of signs, especially the heart rate, may be altered in the setting of toxic ingestion because of inhibition or stimulation of the autonomic nervous system. In evaluating symptoms and signs, it is also useful to consider that the vast majority of poisoning fatalities in children are due to a relatively small number of substances: iron, antidepressants, cardiovascular drugs, alcohols and glycols, hydrocarbons, pesticides, and salicylates.[2]

Although not part of the rapid physical examination, pulse oximetry and continuous electrocardiography should be automatically performed on all seriously ill children on presentation to the emergency department.

CARDIOPULMONARY STABILIZATION

Case History

(Continuation) Unresponsive 2-year-old with agonal respirations; heart rate, 180 beats per minute; systolic blood pressure, 65 mm Hg.

Rapid assessment: respiratory failure. Airway and breathing were controlled by bag-valve-mask ventilation as intravenous access was established. Intubation with a 4.5 mm endotracheal tube, taped at 14 cm; breath sounds bilaterally equal. Pallor, tachycardia, and hypotension persisted despite ventilation and oxygenation. Electrocardiography revealed sinus tachycardia with increased QRS complex (0.15 second).

Reassessment: Decompensated shock.

Resuscitation of the seriously ill child proceeds simultaneously with the rapid cardiopulmonary assessment of the airway, breathing, and circulation. Recognition of a physiologic state and the appropriate stabilization must be constantly modified on the basis of serial assessments and anticipation of deterioration.

Airway and Breathing Resuscitation

Protection of the airway in the critically ill child is first approached with proper positioning of the head and the administration of supplemental O_2 during maintenance of cervical neutrality if there is any possibility of head injury. Excessive hyperextension should be avoided because it can displace the anterior glottis of the young child further anteriorly and out of the direct line of air flow. A "sniffing" position and a jaw thrust usually optimize airway patency and resolve any hypopharyngeal tongue obstruction. Airway adjuncts such as oropharyngeal and nasopharyngeal airways occasionally are useful. In the context of toxic ingestion with altered mental status, signs of airway obstruction (even if relieved by the above maneuvers) or a decreased gag reflex are indications for endotracheal intubation.

The child with overt respiratory failure or cardiopulmonary collapse must first be supported with bag-valve-mask ventilation with good airway positioning and mask seal. If sufficient personnel are available, a two-person method may improve the assisted ventilation. One rescuer uses both hands to perform a jaw thrust and mask seal, while the other rescuer compresses the self-inflating bag with one hand and exerts gentle cricoid pressure with the other. The cricoid pressure (Sellick's maneuver) occludes the cervical esophagus, preventing gastric insufflation and regurgitation.

Airway and ventilation support should be followed by intubation in an organized fashion, with all equipment of appropriate size for the patient's age ready at hand (Table 2–1). Several caveats regarding pediatric intubation are important. Most pediatric authorities prefer to use straight blades in infants and toddlers because of the relatively anterior position of their glottis. For the same reason, use of the "sniffing" position and cricoid pressure may be necessary for adequate visualization on direct laryngoscopy. The glottis is also anatomically more cephalad in the young child than it is in the adult; this explains the tendency of an inexperienced laryngoscopist to view the esophagus rather than the glottis. The anatomic position precludes blind nasotracheal intubation in young children. The clinician can generally calculate the correct endotracheal tube size by using the following formula:

Table 2–1. Pediatric Emergency Equipment

Age	Body Weight (kg)	Endotracheal Tube Size (mm)	Laryngoscope Blade Size
Newborn	3.5	3.0, 3.5	0, 1
6 mo	7.0	3.5	1
1 y	10	4.0	1
2–3 y	12–14	4.5	1.5, 2
4–5 y	16–20	5.0	2
6–8 y	22–27	5.5, 6.0	2
10–12 y	30–40	6.0, 7.0	2, 3
16 y	>50	7.0, 8.0	3

$$\text{Internal diameter} = (\text{age [y]} + 16) \div 4$$

It not uncommon for the selected endotracheal tube to be too large or too small; therefore, a larger tube and a smaller tube should always be available at the bedside. Generally, uncuffed endotracheal tubes are used in patients up to 8 years of age because the conical shape of the pediatric subglottic space forms a physiologic cuff. It should be noted that pediatric endotracheal tube usually has 1 to 3 black rings, or vocal cord markers, at its distal end; these rings assist in placement of the tube to the correct depth. After intubation of the trachea, the centimeter mark at the lip is noted, breath sounds are checked bilaterally, and, ideally, end-tidal CO_2 confirmed. Although drugs for rapid-sequence induction are covered elsewhere in this textbook, one should be aware that succinylcholine has potential vagotonic properties in the young child, and its use should generally be preceded by administration of a dose of atropine for the prevention of bradycardia.

Whether a ventilation bag or mechanical ventilator is used, air exchange should be clinically demonstrated by adequate chest rise, appropriate breath sounds, and improved oxygenation. Generally, the neonatal self-inflating bag (250 mL) should remain in the nursery. The pediatric size (450 mL) is more appropriate for bag-mask ventilation of infants and children up to 25 kg in weight. Mechanical ventilation is usually performed in a synchronous intermittent mandatory ventilation mode, with the rate initially being set at physiologic respiratory norms (in breaths per minute): infant, 30; toddler, 24; school age, 16 to 18; and adolescent, 12. In the critically ill, the fraction of inspired O_2 should be 1.0, and weaning should be undertaken as dictated by the clinical course. Positive end-expiratory pressure is generally set at a pressure of 2 to 3 cm H_2O but is increased in increments of 2 to 3 cm H_2O to achieve adequate oxygenation in clinical conditions associated with diffuse bilateral alveolar disease or pulmonary edema, or both. On a volume-cycled ventilator, a tidal volume setting of approximately 10 mL/kg is appropriate, with the flow adjusted to provide a normal inspiratory time. Time-cycled pressure-limited ventilators are sometimes used in young infants in whom an initial pressure limit of 20 to 25 cm H_2O and an inspiratory time of 0.5 to 0.8 seconds generally suffice. In patients with poor pulmonary compliance, even higher pressures are necessary for achieving adequate air exchange.

The respiratory management discussed so far has pertained to the child with evident respiratory failure or cardiopulmonary collapse. Many more seriously ill children present with significant respiratory signs but at least temporary preservation of airway patency, ventilation, and oxygenation. These patients should be considered to be in potential respiratory failure until further observation and laboratory assessment prove otherwise. They should be nil per os and allowed to maintain a position of respiratory comfort with continuous pulse oximetry, repeated assessments, and blood gas determination. Progressive clinical deterioration should signal the need for more aggressive airway and ventilatory support before a life-threatening physiologic state occurs.

Circulation Resuscitation

Shock states and cardiopulmonary collapse with or without dysrhythmias demand immediate circulatory support. Vascular access should be established with a protocol-defined escalation of invasiveness to minimize elapsed time in patients with circulatory collapse or decompensated shock.[3, 4] In general, intraosseous access should be obtained in moribund pediatric patients who are younger than 6 years of age after 90 seconds of failed attempts to establish intravenous access.

Volume infusion in the form of aliquots of isotonic crystalloid solution (20 mL/kg) is the mainstay of initial circulatory support in hypovolemic and distributive shock. (The 20-mL/kg fluid bolus is derived from the knowledge that hemodynamic compromise occurs with an acute loss of 25% of intravascular volume and that the child's blood volume is approximately 80 mL/kg.) The bolus of normal saline or lactated Ringer's solution should be administered as fast as it can be infused in the patient in decompensated shock because every minute of hypotension translates into additional end-organ injury. Note that 5% dextrose is not given in the fluid resuscitation of shock because each 20-mL/kg bolus contains 1 g/kg of glucose, the infusion of which would create a severe iatrogenic hyperglycemia. After the first bolus has been administered, the cardiovascular status is reassessed, and if signs of shock are persistent, an additional bolus is infused. This sequence is repeated as necessary, with the cardiovascular response increasingly evaluated on the basis of additional parameters such as urinary output, chest radiography, blood gas analysis, and, in recalcitrant cases, central venous pressure monitoring. Patients with hemorrhagic hypovolemic shock who fail to demonstrate improvement with 2 or 3 rapidly administered boluses should receive blood. Similarly, blood component therapy may be necessary in the patient in a shock state associated with a coagulopathy. A patient with significant intravascular depletion in severe hypovolemic or distributive shock may require up to 5 or 6 boluses of fluid in the first hour.

Pharmocologic vasoactive support is indicated in the patient in distributive shock if poor perfusion is unresponsive to fluid administration. Cardiogenic shock is less common in pediatric patients but also requires catecholamine support (Table 2–2). The choice of catecholamine drip may be influenced by the patient's cardiovascular status. For example, a toxic overdose that causes vasodilatation and shock via α-adrenergic inhibition may be better treated with norepinephrine, an α-adrenergic agent. On the other hand, an epinephrine drip may be a better agent in severe distributive shock states of sepsis or anaphylaxis, in which both β- and α-adrenergic support is needed. In less severe cases, many clinicians use dopamine because it can be titrated from predominantly β-adrenergic doses of 5 μg/kg per minute to increasingly α-adrenergic doses of 20 to 25 μg/kg per minute. Regardless of which agent is used, vigilant monitoring and titration to clinical effect is necessary. (It is not unusual for dosages higher than the given ranges to be required in severe distributive shock.)

In pulseless arrest, the cardiac rhythms encountered are asystole, electromechanical dissociation, ventricular fibrillation, or pulseless ventricular tachycardia (Table 2–3). The most important drug to administer to patients with these "collapse" rhythms is epinephrine, dosing of which should be repeated every 3 to 5 minutes during cardiopulmonary resuscitation (Table 2–4). The recommendation for second and subsequent doses of epinephrine in pulseless arrest is 10-fold the initial 0.01 mg/kg.[4] As in the adult population, ventricular fibrillation or pulseless ventricular tachycardia is treated with defibrillation, but at an energy level of 2 J/kg; this level is doubled if no effect is observed. Infant defibrillator paddles are used for infants weighing less than 10 kg. In the setting of cardiotoxin poisoning (e.g., with tricyclic antidepressants or class IA and IC antiarrhythmics), other therapeutic modalities such as overdrive pacing and administration of sodium bicarbonate or

Table 2–2. Emergency Infusions*

Drug	Dose (μg/kg per min)	Dilution
Dobutamine	5–20	6 × weight (kg) = mg/100 mL of D_5W, then 1 mL/h (1 μg/kg per min)
Dopamine	3–20	
Lidocaine	20–50	
Nitroprusside	1–10	
Epinephrine	0.1–1.0	0.6 × weight (kg) = mg/100 mL of D_5W, then 1 mL/h (0.1 μg/kg per min)
Isoproterenol	0.1–1.5	
Norepinephrine	0.1–1.0	

* Route: intravenous or intraosseous.

Table 2–3. Pediatric Arrhythmias

Type	Cause	Treatment
Slow	Sinus bradycardia or heart block	If HR < 60 and unstable: CPR; epinephrine; atropine; consider pacing
Fast	Supraventricular tachycardia	Adenosine, synchronized cardioversion
	Ventricular tachycardia	Lidocaine, synchronized cardioversion
Collapse		CPR plus:
	Electromechanical dissociation	Epinephrine
	Asystole	Epinephrine
	Ventricular fibrillation or pulseless ventricular tachycardia	Defibrillate × 3; epinephrine, defibrillate; lidocaine, defibrillate; consider bretylium

HR, heart rate; CPR, cardiopulmonary resuscitation.

magnesium sulfate may be considered. Unfortunately, the most common rhythm disturbance in pediatric arrest is asystole or a pulseless, idioventricular rhythm, which portends a poor outcome in the vast majority of cases.

The emergency treatment of symptomatic bradyarrhythmias with decompensated shock involves chest compressions and administration of epinephrine if ventilatory support does not immediately improve heart rate. (The most common reason for bradycardia in the pediatric age group is hypoxia.) Subsequent doses of epinephrine for sustained, symptomatic bradycardia are not increased beyond the 0.01-mg/kg dosage. In the unusual circumstance of atrioventricular block, atropine may be an appropriate first-line medication. In addition, isoproterenol infusion and pacing may be utilized for persistent bradycardia.

The "fast" rhythms of ventricular tachycardia and supraventricular tachycardia in the pediatric patient deserve comment. It must be appreciated that infants may have heart rates of up to 220 or 230 beats per minute with sinus tachycardia associated with fever, hypovolemia, or pain; these should *not* be confused with supraventricular tachycardia. Ventricular tachycardia in a pediatric patient should prompt investigation of a possible cardiotoxin ingestion or metabolic abnormality, such as hyperkalemia.

Table 2–4. Emergency Drugs and Interventions

Drug or Intervention	Dose
Epinephrine (1:10,000)	0.01 mg (0.1 mL)/kg IV
(1:1000)	0.1 mg (0.1 mL)/kg ET
(1:1000)	0.1 mg (0.1 mL)/kg IV every 3–5 min for subsequent doses in pulseless patient
Atropine	0.02 mg/kg IV, ET, or IM (maximum, 1 mg)
Dextrose ($D_{25}W$)	0.5 g (2mL)/kg
Lidocaine (2%)	1 mg/kg IV, ET
Sodium bicarbonate (8.4%)	1 mEq/kg IV
Cardioversion	0.5–1 J/kg
Defibrillation	2 J/kg, then 4 J/kg
Fluid bolus (crystalloid)	20 mL/kg
Fluid bolus (colloid)	10 mL/kg
Adenosine	0.1–0.2 mg/kg (maximum, 12 mg)
Naloxone	0.1 mg/kg (maximum, 2 mg, repeat as needed)

IV, intravenously; ET, via endotracheal tube; IM, intramuscularly.

After the ABC's

The resuscitation of the pediatric patient obviously extends beyond stabilization of the airway, breathing, and circulation. The prioritization may continue with "D" for *disability*, *distention*, *dextrose*, and other *drugs*, and in the case of poisonings, *decontamination* (Table 2–5). By the completion of the initial cardiopulmonary evaluation, the patient's motor response has generally been observed; however, at this juncture assessment of the pupillary reflex and a cursory check for focal findings are important. Similarly, a nasogastric tube if not already inserted, should be placed in all critically ill children because gastric distention is common, especially after bag-mask ventilation, and can limit diaphragmatic excursion in young children. A bedside glucose check should be performed in all patients with altered mental status; if not, then an empirical dose of dextrose should be delivered. Young children in particular have low glycogen stores and may become hypoglycemic with serious illnesses. Likewise, the use of other drugs such as naloxone may be indicated, depending on the clinical situation. Relevant to this text, decontamination may be a priority at this point.

Finally, "E" may stand for *exposure* of the patient as well as the search for an *etiology* of the presentation. It must be remembered, however, that infants and young children quickly become hypothermic with severe illness and may require environmental sup-

Table 2–5. ABC(D and E)'s of Resuscitation

Airway
Breathing
Circulation
Disability
  Distention
  Dextrose and other drugs
  Decontamination
Exposure
  Etiology
serial assessments

port for maintenance of body temperature. The search for a cause usually involves emergency laboratory testing, radiography, cultures, drug screening, and more extensive history-taking.

In concluding this section, the importance of serial assessments of the ABC(D and E)'s cannot be overemphasized.

Case History

(Conclusion). Intubated, unresponsive 2-year-old child; heart rate, 180 bpm; systolic blood pressure, 65 mm Hg; 100% hemoglobin saturation by pulse oximetry. Electrocardiography showed sinus tachycardia and QRS interval of 0.15 second. Normal saline, 20 mL/kg was given three times over 30 minutes, with progressive systolic blood pressure response to 85 mm Hg. Norepinephrine drip was prepared and available at bedside. Sodium bicarbonate, 1 mEq/kg was given empirically, with subsequent narrowing of QRS complex; an additional 1 mEq/kg was administered over 1 hour. Defibrillator pads were placed prophylactically. A 6-French sheath in the femoral vein and a central venous pressure catheter were placed. A transvenous, balloon-tipped pacing catheter and a programmable stimulator capable of delivering impulses at high energy levels were available at bedside. A nasogastric tube was inserted; bedside glucose measurements were normal; gastrointestinal lavage was followed by administration of charcoal, 1 g/kg, via nasogastric tube. Further history-taking revealed evidence of tricyclic antidepressant bottle tampering. The patient recovered intact.

PEDIATRIC FLUIDS AND ELECTROLYTES

The composition of pediatric body fluids and the principles of the use of maintenance fluids and electrolytes are reviewed in the remainder of this chapter. The evaluation and treatment of dehydration and other common pediatric electrolyte disorders also are discussed.

Body Fluid Composition

In the neonate, almost 80% of body weight is composed of water. This ratio decreases to approximately 70% by 6 months of age and to 60% by the age of 1 year. Fluid requirements of pediatric patients are proportionately much greater than those of adults. The relative daily turnover of fluids as a percentage of total-body water is much greater in infants than in older children and adults; this places infant patients at greater risk for illnesses and conditions that cause derangements in fluid status.

Total-body water comprises the *extracellular fluid (ECF)* and the *intracellular fluid (ICF)*. At birth, the ECF is approximately 40% of body weight. This value decreases to 30% by the age of 1 year and to 25% by adolescence (Fig. 2–4). The ECF consists of blood plasma and interstitial fluid. The ICF increases from approximately 35% of body weight at birth to 45% by late childhood and adolescence. The remaining body water (approximately 2%) is *transcellular water,* which is the body fluid not directly connected with either ICF or ECF, such as fluid within the gastrointestinal tract and cerebrospinal fluid.

The chemical composition of the intracellular and extracellular spaces in children is similar to that of those in adults. In the ECF, sodium is the predominant cation, and chloride and bicarbonate account for most of the anions. In the ICF, however, potassium is the major cation, and negative charges are supplied mostly by phosphates, sulfates, and proteins. Under physiologic conditions, electrical neutrality is maintained within each space. The large concentration gradient of sodium and potassium between the intra- and extracellular spaces is maintained by the so-called "sodium pump." This is an active process dependent on sodium/potassium–adenosine triphosphatase (Na^+,K^+-ATPase) found in cell membranes.

Maintenance Requirements

Maintenance fluid and electrolyte requirements vary with the metabolic rate, which is expressed as caloric expenditure in kilocalories per 24 hours. When insensible fluid loss, obligatory renal and stool water losses, and the gain of water from endogenous metabolism are considered, maintenance water requirements are found to equal approximately 100 mL/100 kcal. The clinician can estimate caloric requirements, using the formulas outlined in Table 2–6. This method assumes that a child has normal metabolic activity and no excess requirements.

Sodium, potassium, and chloride are electrolytes necessary for the short-term administration of maintenance fluids. Daily sodium requirements are approximately 3 mEq/100 kcal. Requirements for chloride are similar to those for sodium. These electrolytes are generally provided together as sodium chloride. Maintenance potassium requirements are approximately 2 mEq/100 kcal. For short-term therapy, potassium also is usually administered in combination with chloride. A parenteral solution containing 30 mEq/L of sodium chloride and 20 mEq/L of potassium chloride delivered at a maintenance rate provides average daily requirements of sodium,

Table 2–6. Caloric Requirements

Body Weight (kg)	Caloric Expenditure (per d)
≤10	100 kcal/kg
11–20	1000 kcal + 50 kcal/kg for each kg above 10 kg
>20	1500 kcal + 20 kcal/kg for each kg above 20 kg

From Holliday MA, Segar WE: The maintenance need for water in parenteral fluid therapy. Pediatrics *19*:824, 1957.

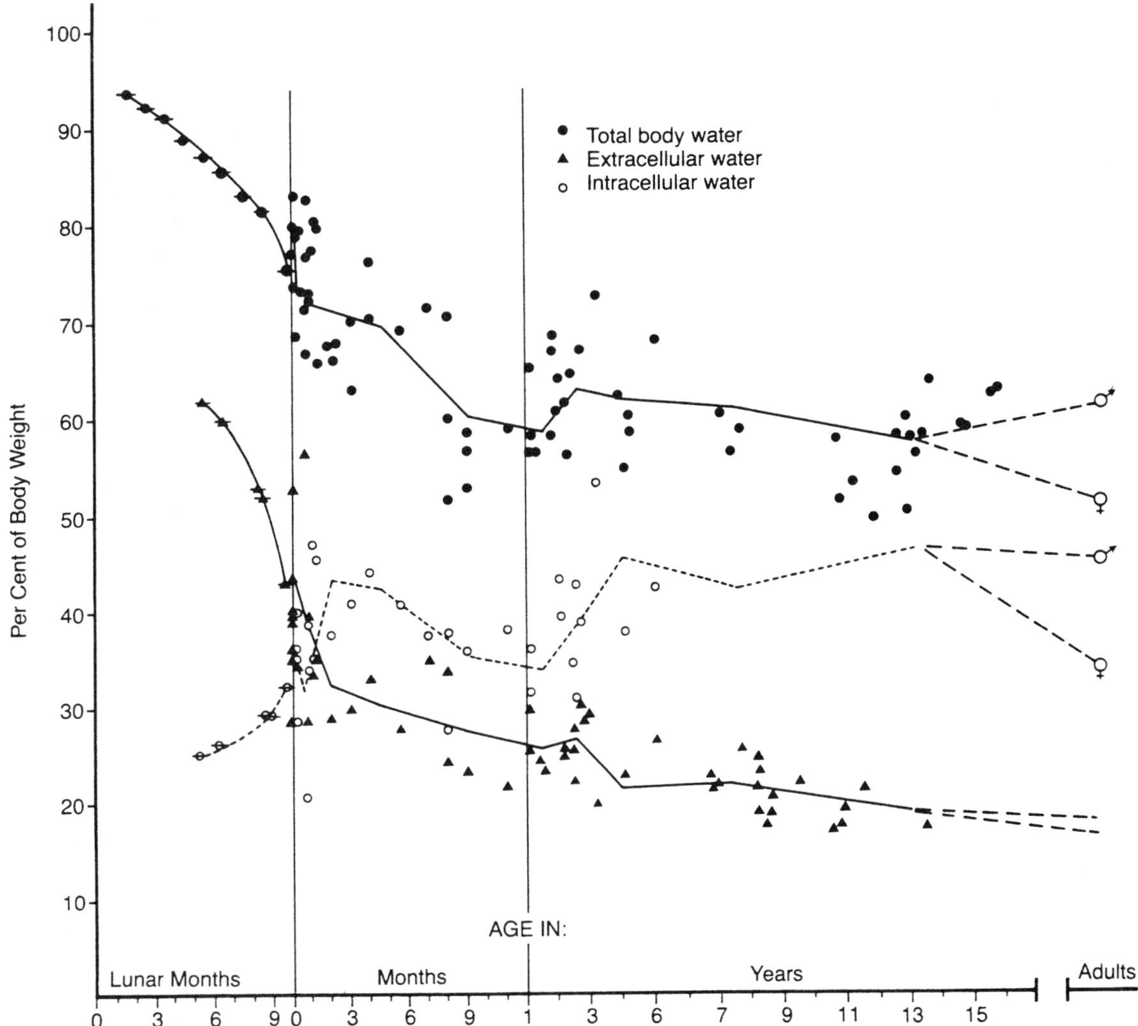

Figure 2–4. Body water compartments. (From Friis Hansen B: Body water compartments in children. Pediatrics *28*:171, 1961. Copyright American Academy of Pediatrics 1961.)

potassium, and chloride. As in adults, parenteral fluids are usually administered as a solution containing 5% dextrose so that endogenous protein breakdown is minimized.

Of course, daily fluid and electrolyte requirements must be individualized. Maintenance requirements are decreased in many disease states. In anuric renal insufficiency, fluids should be reduced to insensible losses only (approximately 40 mL/100 kcal per day); administration of electrolytes, particularly potassium, should be reduced accordingly. Patients with the syndrome of inappropriate antidiuretic hormone have an abnormally low urine output and benefit from fluid restriction. Small children in highly humidified environments (e.g., mist tents) have a reduced insensible water loss. Daily fluid and electrolyte requirements may also be reduced in hypometabolic states such as drug-induced coma.

The acutely ill child often has abnormal fluid and electrolyte losses and thus requires an increase in maintenance requirements. In the patient with fever, metabolic rate (and thus the requirement for maintenance fluids) increases by 12% for each 1°C increase in body temperature. A hypermetabolic state is produced in certain intoxications, such as salicylate poisoning. Vomiting and diarrhea frequently accompany childhood poisonings and can significantly increase fluid and electrolyte losses. The hypochloremic alkalosis resulting from gastric fluid loss is associated with renal potassium loss. Supplemental potassium chloride should be added to replacement fluids to prevent the development of hypokalemia in this situation. Whereas enteric and renal losses can be estimated or quantified by direct measurements, "third space" losses are more difficult to evaluate.

Occasionally, it is necessary to administer maintenance fluids at an accelerated rate so that adequate urinary output is ensured or the renal excretion of certain toxins enhanced. Most children with healthy cardiovascular systems tolerate up to twice their normal maintenance fluid rate without experiencing problems. However, compensatory mechanisms may be limited in the acutely ill or poisoned child. In such a child, close monitoring is essential if volume overload, cerebral edema, and iatrogenic electrolyte derangements are to be prevented.

Fluid and Electrolyte Deficits

Adequacy of hydration in pediatric patients is generally described as a per cent change in body weight. Any acute gain or loss of body weight of greater than 1% is assumed to be the result of fluid gain or loss. For example, a child with gastroenteritis who has lost 10% of body weight is said to be 10% dehydrated. Of course, accurate pre- and postillness weights usually are not available, so estimates must be made on clinical grounds. Such judgments are rough estimates only because the severity of signs and symptoms vary not only with the degree of dehydration, but also with the rate of fluid loss and the underlying tonicity of the plasma.

Deficits of less than 5% are difficult to detect clinically. A child who has mild (5%) dehydration may have diminished skin turgor and thickened oral secretions. In small infants, the anterior fontanelle is somewhat depressed. Other than presence of mild tachycardia, however, vital signs are stable. A child with moderate (10%) dehydration appears acutely ill, with sunken eyes and, in infancy, a sunken fontanelle. Skin turgor is diminished, and mucous membranes are dry. Tachycardia is evident, but peripheral perfusion and blood pressure are maintained. A child with severe (15%) dehydration often presents in shock. The extremities may be cool and poorly perfused, with peripheral pulses being thready or nonpalpable. Skin turgor is poor, and mucous membranes are dry. Such patients are often lethargic and respond poorly to stimulation. In these children, hemodynamic compensatory mechanisms are maximally stressed, and cardiovascular collapse may follow.

Dehydration is further classified according to the osmolality or tonicity of the plasma. Sodium is the most prevalent osmotically active particle in the extracellular fluid, and dehydration can be classified as hypotonic, isotonic, or hypertonic on the basis of the measured serum sodium concentration. In *isotonic dehydration,* sodium and water have been lost from the ECF in approximately equal amounts. The resultant serum sodium levels range from 130 to 150 mEq/L. The clinical changes seen with isotonic dehydration are those outlined earlier.

In *hypotonic dehydration,* a net loss of sodium in excess of water from the ECF has occurred, and the measured sodium level is less than 130 mEq/L. Such a situation may occur in a child with isotonic dehydration whose deficits are partially replaced with a non–electrolyte-containing solution. Clinical signs of hypotonic dehydration may be more severe than a similar degree of isotonic dehydration because water moves from the ECF to the ICF to maintain osmotic equilibrium, and this transfer further depletes the circulatory volume.

In *hypertonic dehydration,* the serum sodium concentration is greater than 150 mEq/L. This condition results from loss of water in excess of sodium, which is seen in some diarrheal states; from excessive insensible water loss; and from diabetes insipidus. Hypernatremic dehydration also has been reported in infants and young children given repeated doses of charcoal and sorbitol, the latter inducing an osmotic diarrhea.[5] The ECF is hypertonic compared with the ICF; thus, fluid moves from the ICF to the ECF. As a result, classic physical findings of dehydration are less pronounced than in isotonic or hypotonic dehydration. The cellular dehydration that occurs with this condition often gives the skin what is described as a "doughy" consistency. Central nervous system signs and symptoms are often seen in hypernatremic states. Lethargy, irritability, and seizures are common.

Treatment of Dehydration

Fluid therapy must provide for maintenance requirements and ongoing losses in addition to the replacement of deficits. It is now well recognized that the oral route, when available, is preferred for fluid and electrolyte maintenance therapy and the replacement of moderate deficits. Solutions containing from 50 to 90 mEq/L of sodium, 20 mEq/L of potassium, and 20 g/L of glucose have been shown to be effective in treating most infants with mild or moderate dehydration secondary to enteric illness. For purposes of this chapter, however, discussion is limited to parenteral fluid therapy.

Of critical importance is the rapid restoration of adequate circulatory volume in patients who present with severe volume depletion and cardiovascular instability. As discussed in the section on resuscitation, the emergency phase of treatment should be accomplished with the rapid infusion of isotonic fluid, 20 mL/kg, for restoration of circulatory volume. If improvement in peripheral perfusion and blood pressure is not evident after infusion of the initial bolus, then the dose should be repeated.

In isotonic dehydration, estimated fluid deficits are usually replaced over 24 to 36 hours. Many clinicians advocate replacing one half of the deficit within the first several hours; however, in less critically ill patients, fluid deficits may be evenly replaced over 24 to 36 hours. Sodium and water losses are proportional in isotonic dehydration. Part of the sodium lost from the ECF moves to the ICF to compensate for intracellular potassium losses. Actual losses of sodium from the total-body water are approximately 80 to 100 mEq/L of fluid lost, or 8 to 10 mEq/kg in the small child with moderately severe dehydration. Daily maintenance sodium requirements and ongoing losses should be added to replacement solutions. Most children with isotonic dehydration can be successfully treated with a parenteral solution of approximately 75 mEq of sodium chloride per liter, or 0.5% normal saline.

Fluid management of the child with hypotonic dehydration is similar to that of the child with isotonic dehydration. Estimated deficits and maintenance requirements are administered over 24 to 36 hours once hemodynamic stability has been achieved. The sodium deficit in the child with hypotonic dehydration, however, is greater than that of a child with a similar degree of isotonic dehydration. For replacement purposes, this extra sodium deficit can be calculated from the following formula:

$$Na^+ \text{ deficit} = (\text{Desired } Na^+ - \text{Measured } Na^+ \text{ [mEq/L]}) \times 0.6 \times \text{Body weight (kg)}$$

(Six tenths of lean body weight approximates total-body water, the fluid space in which sodium exerts an osmotic effect. Even though sodium is an extracellular cation, the concentration of sodium in the ECF affects the water content in the ICF.) Initial therapy in hypotonic dehydration should begin with administration of normal saline. Once serum sodium levels are greater than 130 mEq/L, replacement may continue with 0.5% normal saline. Sodium deficits need not be corrected rapidly unless the patient exhibits neurologic symptoms associated with hyponatremia. Such symptoms rarely occur unless the serum sodium concentration is less than 120 mEq/L. The amount of sodium needed to increase the serum level to 120 mEq/L can be calculated from the formula and can be given as an infusion of 3% saline (approximately 0.5 mEq of sodium per milliliter) over several hours, if necessary. If the patient is experiencing seizures, then more rapid administration is indicated.

Although most children with isotonic or hypotonic dehydration recover if given adequate fluid and sodium chloride, children with hypertonic dehydration (i.e., sodium level is greater than 150 mEq/L) present a difficult challenge. Children usually develop hypernatremic dehydration over a period of days, and osmotic equilibrium between the ECF and ICF is maintained by intracellular water loss and possibly by the formation of "audiogenic osmoles" in central nervous system cells. The estimated fluid deficit is predominantly intracellular and should be replaced slowly over 48 hours or more. Rapid administration of fluid can create an osmotic gradient between the ECF and ICF, precipitating cerebral edema and convulsions. Sodium deficits are smaller than in isotonic dehydration and are usually replaced with 0.2% saline. Once urine output is established, potassium chloride (30 to 40 mEq/L) is added to correct intracellular potassium deficits and to increase the osmolality of the replacement fluid. The choice of fluid, however, is less important than the rate at which it is administered. The rate of lowering the serum sodium should not exceed 10 mEq per 24 hours. Frequent monitoring of serum sodium levels is necessary.

It should be stressed that these suggestions for parenteral fluid therapy are general guidelines only and are based on gross estimations of body fluid deficits. The most complex calculations are no substitute for frequent clinical evaluation and close monitoring of the course of treatment.

Other Sodium Disorders

Abnormalities of serum sodium status also may be seen in the normovolemic or hypervolemic patient. Several of the more common disorders are reviewed in this section.

The *syndrome of inappropriate antidiuretic hormone (SIADH)* is the result of inappropriate secretion of the hormone vasopressin in the normovolemic patient, which results in free water retention and hyponatremia. The diagnosis is based on the demonstration of an inappropriately concentrated urine in the presence of a dilute serum in the normovolemic patient. Symptoms rarely occur unless the serum sodium concentration is less than 120 mEq/L, and most patients are readily managed with fluid restriction. More rapid correction of serum sodium level usually can be accomplished with the use of loop diuretics, such as furosemide, and by means of volume replacement with sodium-containing solutions. SIADH is seen most often in pediatric patients with meningitis or other central nervous system disease, although a number of other causes, including drug toxicity, have been described (Table 2–7).

Dilutional hyponatremia may occur as the result of the ingestion or administration of excessive free water in infants and small children. The infant's ability to excrete a large volume of free water is reduced compared with that of an adult. Hyponatremia and seizures may be seen in infants younger than 6 months of age who are fed dilute formulas and excessive amounts of water. Hyponatremia may also be seen with inappropriate administration of hypotonic parenteral fluids. In the euvolemic patient, simple fluid restriction and provision of adequate sodium chloride suffice. The hypervolemic patient with hyponatremia usually is edematous and may also require diuresis in addition to sodium chloride replacement for correction.

Table 2–7. Disorders Associated with Excessive Antidiuretic Hormone Effect

Central nervous system: Infection, tumor, injury, vascular accidents, Guillain-Barré syndrome		
Drug-related:	acetaminophen (Tylenol)	morphine
	barbiturates	thiothixene (Navane)
	carbamazepine (Tegretol)	nicotine
	chlorpropamide	phenformin
	clofibrate	polymyxin B
	cyclophosphamide	thiazides
	amitriptyline (Elavil)	tolbutamide
	indomethacin	vincristine
	isoproterenol	
Endocrine: Myxedema, cortisol deficiency, pituitary stalk section		
Heart: Congestive heart failure, left atrial stretching, constrictive pericarditis		
Infections: Acute childhood infectious disorders, especially viral		
Liver: Cirrhosis, hepatic failure, portal hypertension		
Metabolic: Acute intermittent porphyria		
Pulmonary: Asthma, infections, emphysema, fibrosis, tumors, ventilation (continuous positive airway pressure)		
Renal: Changes in sodium handling by the kidney related to volume contraction and/or diuretic; hypoalbuminemia		
Surgery-related: Anesthesia or premedication, peritoneal reflexes, intracranial manipulation, postoperative pain		
Tumors: Duodenum, pancreas, salivary gland, thymus		

From Gruskin AB, Baluarte HJ, Prebis MS, et al: Serum sodium abnormalities in children. Pediatr Clin North Am *29*:924, 1982.

Pseudohyponatremia occurs as the result of the presence of high concentrations of nonaqueous solids like lipids and proteins in the serum. These solids displace water and cause the serum to appear falsely diluted, even though the physiologic concentration of sodium may be normal. A similar situation occurs with hyperglycemic states, in which serum sodium concentration is lowered 1.6 mEq/L for every 100 mg/dL increase in glucose level.

Hypernatremia and Salt Poisoning

Hypernatremic states in the absence of dehydration are uncommon in children and usually result from the inappropriate administration or ingestion of excessive sodium. This may be observed after the ingestion of table salt or the excessive administration of sodium bicarbonate—for example, following cardiac resuscitation. Free water deficits in hypernatremic states can be estimated from the following formula:

$$\text{Free water deficit (L)} = (0.6 \times \text{body wt [kg]} \times [1 - \text{measured Na}^{+} \text{ \{mEq/L\}}]) \div 140$$

The hypernatremic state should be gradually corrected with the use of hypotonic fluid in a fashion similar to that described for the treatment of hypertonic dehydration, such that serum sodium level is lowered by no more than 10 mEq/L per day. Rapid correction may be associated with circulatory overload or may create an osmotic gradient between the ICF and the ECF and thus precipitate cerebral edema.

Fatal salt poisoning has occurred in children following the inadvertent substitution of table salt for sugar in infant formulas and the administration of salt as an emetic. Symptoms are generally seen within hours of oral ingestion and include seizures, obtundation, coma, and cardiorespiratory arrest. Serum sodium levels may be greater than 180 mEq/L. Such high levels of sodium create a large osmotic gradient between the ECF and ICF, leading to extreme cellular dehydration and brain injury. Autopsy studies of children dying from salt poisoning have shown capillary and venous congestion of the central nervous system, subarachnoid and parenchymal hemorrhage, and dural sinus occlusion. In acute salt poisoning with serum sodium levels greater than 180 mEq/L, removal of excess sodium chloride by means of dialysis improves the outcome. Hemodialysis or peritoneal dialysis with a 4.25% glucose solution can effectively lower sodium levels and limit the severity of symptoms.

Disorders of Potassium

Because potassium is predominantly an intracellular cation, the measured serum potassium level reflects only a small portion of total-body stores. However, relatively small changes in serum potassium level can have profound physiologic effects.

Hypokalemia (serum potassium level of less than 2.5 mEq/L) can cause muscle weakness, renal tubular dysfunction, and electrocardiographic changes. T wave depression, U waves, and ST depression are seen with progressive hypokalemia. Low-potassium states are seen with inadequate dietary intake or result from excessive gastrointestinal or renal losses. Hypochloremic states resulting from gastric losses or diuretic therapy enhance renal potassium excretion. Potassium chloride can be given safely in concentrations of up to 40 mEq/L in parenteral fluids. Higher concentrations should be given only when clearly indicated, in a monitored setting, to reduce the risk of hyperkalemia. In extreme circumstances, an infusion of 0.5 mEq/kg of potassium chloride over 30 to 60 minutes may be given to pediatric patients for the correction of severe potassium deficits. Such infusions should be administered only in an intensive care unit setting and with constant electrocardiographic monitoring.

Falsely elevated serum potassium levels are often seen as the result of hemolysis of red blood cells associated with blood collection in pediatric patients. *True hyperkalemia* (serum potassium level greater than 5.5 mEq/L) may be precipitated by acidosis, excessive administration of potassium, adrenal insufficiency, massive cellular destruction, or renal failure. Signs and symptoms of hyperkalemia are predominantly cardiac. Electrophysiologic changes that occur with increasing potassium levels include peaked T waves, first-degree atrioventricular block, loss of P waves, a widened QRS complex, sine wave formation, ventricular tachycardia or fibrillation, and asystole. If serum potassium levels are greater than 5.5 mEq/L, all supplemental administration of potassium should be discontinued. If levels are greater than 6.5 mEq/L or if electrocardiographic changes are present, immediate treatment directed at lowering serum levels should be started (Table 2–8). Calcium given by slow intravenous push temporarily counteracts the electrophysiologic effects of hyperkalemia. This measure may cause bradycardia and thus should be used only in a monitored setting. Sodium bicarbonate given parenterally raises the blood pH and causes potassium to move into cells temporarily. Similarly, the use of glucose and insulin causes a shift of potassium from the extracellular to the intracellular space. Lowering the body's potassium load can be accomplished by the oral or rectal administration of an exchange resin such as sodium polystyrene sulfonate (Kayexalate). Potassium is most effectively removed by dialysis.

CONCLUSION AND EXAMPLE: SALICYLATE POISONING

A wide spectrum of fluid and electrolyte derangements occur in childhood poisonings. The patient's

Table 2–8. Therapy for Hyperkalemia

Drug	Dose and Route	Onset (Duration)	Mode of Action	Comments
1. Calcium gluconate, 10% (100 mg/mL)	20 mg/kg IV over 5 min. May repeat × 2	Immediate (30–60 min)	Counteracts electrophysiologic effects of hyperkalemia	Monitor electrocardiogram for bradycardia. Stop infusion if heart rate <100
2. Sodium bicarbonate, 7.5% (1 mEq/mL)	1–2 mEq/kg IV bolus or infusion over 20 min	20 min (1–4 h)	Causes movement of potassium into cells	Assure adequate ventilation. Do not administer simultaneously with calcium gluconate: will precipitate
Glucose plus	1–2 g/kg (5–10 mL of 20% dextrose)	15–30 min (3–6 h)	Same	
Insulin	0.3 unit/g of glucose; administer by infusion together over 2 h	15–30 min (3–6 h)	Same	Monitor blood glucose level
3. Sodium polystyrene sulfonate) (Kayexalate)	1 g/kg PO in 70% sorbitol or PR in 30% sorbitol every 6 h		Removal of potassium from body	Removes 1 mEq of potassium per g resin: 1 g resin = 4.1 mEq of sodium. Watch for volume overload due to sodium. Do not administer with magnesium- or aluminum-containing antacids, since it may cause obstipation
4. Dialysis				Do not ignore Steps 1, 2, and 3 while preparing for Step 4

PO, perorally; PR, per rectum.
From Maxwell LG, Firush BA, McLean RH: Renal failure. *In* Rogers MC (ed): Textbook of Pediatric Intensive Care. Baltimore, Williams & Wilkins, p 1025, 1987.

age and underlying state of health, the specific toxin and amount of exposure, and the magnitude and duration of resultant symptoms all affect fluid and electrolyte status. A prime example of the importance of early recognition and aggressive management of fluid and electrolyte disorders is the case of salicylate poisoning.

Salicylate intoxication (see also Chapter 50) is a complex poisoning that produces fever, central nervous system symptoms (e.g., lethargy, seizures, or coma), disorders of glucose metabolism, acid-base derangements, dehydration, and electrolyte abnormalities. Dehydration results from fever, increased metabolic demands, hyperventilation, vomiting, decreased oral intake, and obligatory renal water losses. Fluid deficits may be severe. Hypernatremia can be seen after the marked increase in insensible water loss. Hypokalemia frequently results from obligatory urine losses and is further aggravated by iatrogenically induced metabolic alkalosis.

Parenteral fluid therapy in salicylate poisoning is directed toward replacement of deficits and enhancement of renal salicylate excretion. Fluid deficits should be estimated on the basis of clinical presentation. Patients with severe dehydration should receive isotonic fluid as a bolus of 20 mL/kg for restoration of circulatory volume and urine output. Acidosis favors the intracellular movement of salicylate and should be treated with sodium bicarbonate administration. In addition, the renal elimination of salicylate is greatly enhanced by alkalization of the urine. This may be accomplished with the administration of sodium bicarbonate in intermittent boluses (1 mEq/kg over several minutes) and with its addition to rehydrating fluids. Generally, 0.5% normal saline with 1 ampule (44 mEq) of sodium bicarbonate added per liter suffices. The amount of sodium bicarbonate needed and the fluid infusion rate should be adjusted to achieve a urine pH of 7.5 and a urinary output of 3 to 6 mL/kg per hour. It should be remembered that the addition of sodium bicarbonate can significantly increase the sodium load to the patient, producing or worsening hypernatremia. As in other hypernatremic states, serum sodium excess should be corrected gradually. Once urinary output is established, supplemental potassium chloride, 20 to 40 mEq/L, should be added for the correction of potassium deficits. Overly vigorous hydration can cause volume overload, cerebral edema, hypo- or hypernatremia, hypokalemia, hypocalcemia, or severe alkalosis. As with all critically ill patients, frequent clinical assessment and close monitoring of appropriate laboratory parameters are essential to providing optimal care.

References

1. American Heart Association/American Academy of Pediatrics: Textbook of Pediatric Advanced Life Support. Chameides L, Hazinski MF (eds). Dallas, American Heart Association, 1994.
2. Litovitz T, Manoguerra A: Comparison of pediatric poisoning hazards: An analysis of 3.8 million exposure incidents. Pediatrics *89*:999, 1992.
3. Kanter RK, Zimmerman JJ, Strauss RH, et al: Pediatric emergency intravenous access. Am J Dis Child *140*:132, 1986.
4. American Heart Association: Pediatric Advanced Life Support. JAMA *268*:2262, 1992.
5. Farley TA. Severe hypernatremic dehydration after use of an activated charcoal-sorbitol suspension. J Pediatr *109*:719, 1986.

Further Reading

Berkowitz ID, Banner W, Rogers MC: Poisoning and the critically ill child. *In* Rogers MC (ed): Textbook of Pediatric Intensive Care. 2nd ed. Baltimore, Williams & Wilkins, pp 1290–1354, 1992.

Finberg L, Kiley J, Luttrell CN: Mass accidental salt poisoning in infancy: A study of a hospital disaster. JAMA *184*:187, 1963.

Finberg L, Kravath RE, Fleishman AR: Water and Electrolytes in Pediatrics. Philadelphia, W.B. Saunders Co., 1982.

Gruskin AB, Baluarte HJ, Prebis MS, et al: Serum sodium abnormalities in children. Pediatr Clin North Am *29*:294, 1982.

Khilnani P: Electrolyte abnormalities in critically ill children. Crit Care Med *20*:241, 1992.

Robson AM: Parenteral fluid therapy. *In* Behrman RE, Vaughan VC (eds): Nelson Textbook of Pediatrics. 12th ed. Philadelphia, W.B. Saunders Co., pp 228–249, 1983.

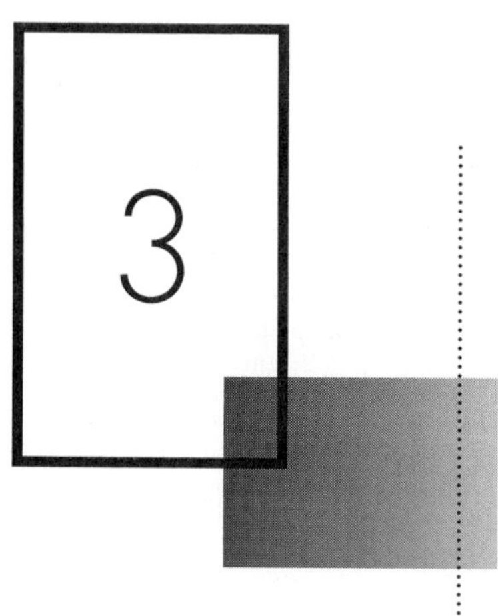

Laboratory Diagnoses and Drug Screening

JOHN D. OSTERLOH, MD

Clinical laboratory tests that indicate the effects or presence of drugs can be useful in the emergency evaluation of the patient with overdose. However, the majority of toxicologic diagnoses and therapeutic decisions are made on the basis of clinical findings, even though advances in technology have provided the potential ability to measure many toxins. Numerous reviews extol the technologic virtues of toxicologic measurement techniques,[1] but the application of these laboratory techniques is limited by practical considerations. The time required for analysis is often longer than the critical time course of an overdose case. Also, laboratories cannot support the cost of performing the variety of procedures, maintaining the instruments, and providing the training and specialized labor needed for analyzing every toxin.

Most important, the interpretation of laboratory toxicologic measurements requires that the relationship between the presence or the concentration of a toxin and its pharmacologic or toxicologic effects be known. For most toxins, our knowledge of such relationships is limited or unstudied, precluding the meaningful use of advanced technologic measures in direct clinical evaluations. Even when well studied, no clear relationship may exist. For example, a toxin at an effector site may not be in rapid equilibrium with the sampled fluid (e.g., lithium in the serum is not representative of lithium in the brain during acute overdose), or the measured toxin may be metabolized to an unknown, unmeasured and active metabolite (e.g., as in organophosphate toxicity). Occasionally, limited information about pharmacologic relationships for common drug toxins has been derived from the monitoring of low-dose drug therapy. However, predictions based on pharmacokinetics or pharmacodynamics of drugs administered in the therapeutic range do not always extrapolate to overdose (e.g., theophylline elimination is first order at therapeutic doses and zero order in overdose).

Although the utility of many toxicologic measurements may be limited, the proper use of certain laboratory tests (both drug tests and biochemistry tests) in the emergency setting can be applied to common clinical toxicologic presentations. This chapter reviews and evaluates the circumstances and types of toxicologic testing, as well as the utility, reliability, and application of these tests in the emergency evaluation of the intoxicated patient. Throughout this chapter, it should be remembered that the best guide to the diagnosis, therapy, and appropriate use of these tests is the clinical presentation of the patient.

USING MEDICAL AND TOXICOLOGIC TESTS

Medical tests can be categorized as belonging to one of three types: monitoring, diagnostic testing, and screening. In each setting, there is a different prior probability that the test condition exists (Table 3–1). This prior probability dramatically affects the reliability of a test for each of these situations (see discussion of reliability later in this chapter). In the *monitoring* of a patient, the change in a highly prevalent test condition—such as blood pressure, body temperature, or therapeutic drug concentrations—is being followed. The most important requisite for this type of test is precision or the ability to detect change. Thus, therapeutic drug monitoring and quantitative toxicologic tests that follow drug concentrations over time (e.g., those for lithium) must be precise. *Diagnostic tests* are applied in situations in which the presence of one of several test conditions is highly likely or suspected. Because these suspected test conditions are moderately prevalent (prior probability), sensitivity is less important than specificity (i.e., no misidentification of a test condition). Diagnostic tests aid in making choices from a limited set of alternatives in narrowly defined populations of patients. For example, a patient with chest pain may have a myocardial infarction, esophagitis, or musculoskeletal injury. Electrocardiography findings and CK-MB testing can be applied to the selection of myocardial infarction from among these alternative conditions. Toxicologic panel testing or "screening" (e.g., comprehensive drug screen or coma panel) can be considered a diagnostic test when overdose is considered in the differential diagnosis and when the initial medical evaluation does not provide a clear picture of what is causing the signs or symptoms. Such testing may help answer the question, Is the patient's condition due to drugs or a disease? and secondarily, Which drug(s)? Screening tests must have good sensitivity if they are to detect the test condition in a low-prevalence situation. An example of this is screening for phenylketonuria in newborns. In the application of this test, there is no prior suspicion or preselection, and all persons are tested. Nonspecificity arising from the screening tests can be corrected with subsequent, more specific testing, if it is not costly.

The prevalence of test condition (e.g., drugs present) or the prior probability strongly influences the reliability (i.e., predictive value of a positive or negative test result, posterior probabilities) at any given sensitivity and specificity. In employee drug screening (low prior probability of drugs being present), toxicologic methods are adapted in order to improve sensitivity for finding low concentrations of drugs, or for detecting only a few drugs in unselected populations.[2, 3] Without such adaptations, the ratio of false-positive results to true-positive results would be high in this low-prevalence setting. In emergency toxicologic testing, procedures are designed to detect a larger number of drugs at a high concentration in populations clinically suspected of overdose (i.e., high prior probability, diagnostic situations). Thus, with regard to these definitions, the term *toxicologic screen* is a misnomer.

This raises the issue of what types of laboratories perform these tests. The development and use of toxicologic methods have evolved from a number of varied situations. Medical examiners investigating cause of death have other forensic evidence that often

Table 3–1. Types of Medical and Toxicologic Test Situations

Type of Medical Setting	Purpose	Preselection of Population	Prior Probability or Prevalence of Test Condition in Population Tested	Primary Attribute Required of Test	Clinical Example	Toxicologic Example
Monitoring	Measure change	Yes	85–100%	Precision	BP, T	TDM
Diagnostic	Sort, categorize	Yes	30–85%	Specificity	CK-MB	Toxicologic screen
Screening	Find	No	0–30%	Sensitivity	PKU	Employee drug testing

BP, blood pressure; T, temperature; CK-MB, MB fraction of creatine kinase; PKU, phenylketonuria; TDM, therapeutic drug monitoring.

suggests a drug-related cause (raising the prior probability or prevalence that the test condition exists in those forensic specimens). The concentrations of drugs or toxins are frequently very high, so sensitivity is often not an issue; however, the type of tissue examined may frequently alter the ability of the analytic technique to detect a toxin. In surveillance (employee) drug screening, low concentrations of drugs are expected to be detected for a small group of selected drugs of abuse, but these tests are applied to populations in which the prevalence of persons abusing drugs is low. Methadone drug testing programs also test individuals for drug use. However, the prevalence of drug use in this selected population is much greater, as are the concentrations of the few drugs monitored. Therefore, the number of procedures applied might be reduced to enable the clinician to have adequate confidence in the result. In each of these situations, the toxicologic methods are tailored to specific needs.

The laboratory performing emergency toxicologic testing[4–6] must consider the prevalence and the types of drugs that must be tested and should adapt methods to the sensitivity, specificity, accuracy, and precision required in their locale (see Toxicologic Screens, later in this chapter). Also, before any test is applied, it must be (1) analytically *valid* (i.e., defined and tested for detection limits, the calibration-response relationship, precision, referenced accuracy, dynamic range, interferents), (2) *reliable* (i.e., have appropriate clinical sensitivity, specificity, and predictive value), and demonstrate *utility* (i.e., the test result will assist the clinician in making a diagnosis or in effecting a change in the course of therapy or disposition of the patient).

DRUG TESTING TECHNIQUES

The techniques for detecting the presence of drugs include a variety of chromatographic methods, immunoassays, chemical tests, and spectrometric techniques. Each of these general techniques can be developed or adapted so that they detect a large number of drugs and chemicals, or it can be focused specifically to detect and quantitate only certain drugs. The analysis of drugs, chemicals, or toxins is predicated on the matching of the properties or behavior (e.g., chemical, chromatographic, or light absorption) of a substance with that of a valid reference compound—that is, the analysis is comparative. For a laboratory to be able test for a particular drug, it must possess that drug for the comparative process. Because the biologic sample matrix may contain components that can interfere in the detection of a drug, isolation of the drug from the biologic matrix is often necessary before characterization procedures are applied. A comparison of the attributes of common toxicologic methods is given in Table 3–2. With regard to usefulness, immunoassays and gas chromatographic techniques have the widest applications for discrete and broad screens, respectively, or for quantitation. Ferrara and co-workers have compared all of the major techniques for their sensitivity and specificity to commonly screened illicit drugs.[7] Most broad screening methods are limited by the range of drugs detectable at one time or sensitivity. In addition, methods can vary considerably with respect to individual drugs. For example, without application of derivation techniques, ease of detection for morphine would be ranked as follows: immunoassay > thin-layer chromatography > gas chromatography. In contrast, in the detection of trazodone, the order may be reversed.

Chemical spot tests are often used as initial quick screening tests for certain drugs. They rely on the chemical reactivity of the drug in the presence of specific reagents. These tests are usually not applied in settings in which a high degree of sensitivity or specificity is required (e.g., *not* in employee drug testing), but they do demonstrate utility, offer ease of application, and have a quick turnaround time when they are applied in emergency settings in which high drug concentrations are present (e.g., urine testing).[8, 9]

Spectrometric assays may require a chemical reaction that converts the target drug into a light-absorbing species. Fifteen years ago, these assays were still very commonly used for the routine determination of barbiturates, acetaminophen, salicylates,

Table 3–2. Comparison of Generic Toxicologic Methods for Drug Determination

Method	Specificity*	Sensitivity*	Multidrug Detection Possible	Quantitative Ability	Turnaround Time (h)	Labor Intensivity	Technical Expertise	Initial Capital Costs ($)
Chemical-spot	+	+	No	No	<0.5	+	0	500
Spectrometric†	+	+	No	Yes‡	<2–4	+ +	+ +	10,000
IA†	+ +	+ +	Some	Some	<1	+	+	15,000
TLC	+ +	+	Yes	No	2–4	+ + +	+ +	1500
GC	+ +	+ +	Yes	Yes‡	<4	+ +	+ +	15,000
HPLC	+ +	+ +	Yes	Yes‡	<4	+ +	+ +	20,000
GC-MS	+ + +	+ + +	Yes	Yes‡	<6	+ + +	+ + + +	60,000

IA, immunoassays; TLC, thin-layer chromatography; GC, gas chromatography; HPLC, high-performance liquid chromatography; GC-MS, gas chromatography–mass spectrometry.

* Relative comparison for a specific analyte.

† Can be performed on analyzers widely used in the clinical laboratory.

‡ Adaptable.

quinidine, methaqualone, and chlordiazepoxide. Still used today for less frequently encountered toxins are the spectrometric assays for carboxyhemoglobin, methemoglobin, cyanide, salicylates, borate, and acetaminophen. In uncomplicated cases, these methods have adequate accuracy for quantifying spectrometric chemicals in overdose situations. However, these methods are very prone to interference. Sulfhemoglobin and the antidote for methemoglobin, methylene blue, cause false elevation of methemoglobin levels with the co-oximetry method. Ketoacidosis, phenylketonuria, phenothiazines, diflunisal, salicylamide, and renal failure can cause false elevations with the salicylate colorimetric method.[10] Salicylate, salicylamide, high bilirubin levels, and the presence of renal failure interfere with the colorimetric nitrosation reaction for acetaminophen determination.[11] Many of these assays have been replaced by enzymatic or immunologic assays that can be performed on automated analyzers, which also can perform a variety of other laboratory tests.

Immunoassays are available for rapid identification of about 10 individual classes or specific drugs in urine and for quantitation of about a dozen drugs in serum. Use of immunoassays has increased dramatically since the mid-1980s because of their ease of automation and applications to screening. Any immunoassay relies on the ability of a drug-specific antibody to bind to either labeled drug (which may be bound to a fluorescent molecule or to an enzyme, or attached to a solid matrix) or to free drug in a sample. Immunoassay techniques are available with a variety of endpoints based on aggregation-light transmission, enzyme product formation, fluorescent polarization, and other principles. Each specific drug assay is commercially available as a kit, but kits are available for only a limited number of drugs. All such assays have analytic sensitivity in excess of that needed for the detection of overdose concentrations. These tests are also rapid and easy to automate, and they have been used as presumptive tests in emergency department settings. Disposable, prepackaged manual devices are now available for bedside diagnosis. Immunoassays are often used as initial screens; their results are then confirmed by a second method, particularly in employee drug testing circumstances. The most common immunoassay in use is the *enzyme immunoassay (EIA)* (EMIT7, Syva Co.; see Fig. 3–1). *Fluorescent polarization inhibition assays* (TDX, Abbott) and *immunoaggregation assays* (KIMS, Roche) also are used in many laboratories.

Chromatographic assays are widely used in emergency toxicology because a large number of drugs can be detected on a single chromatogram. Sensitivity is adequate for detecting the presence of many common pharmaceuticals at concentrations seen in overdose. For most chromatographic procedures, drugs first must be extracted from serum, gastric material, or urine. In many cases, further chemical derivation is necessary for making the drug or drugs compatible with the chromatographic phase or detection system. For example, in the detection of morphine by gas

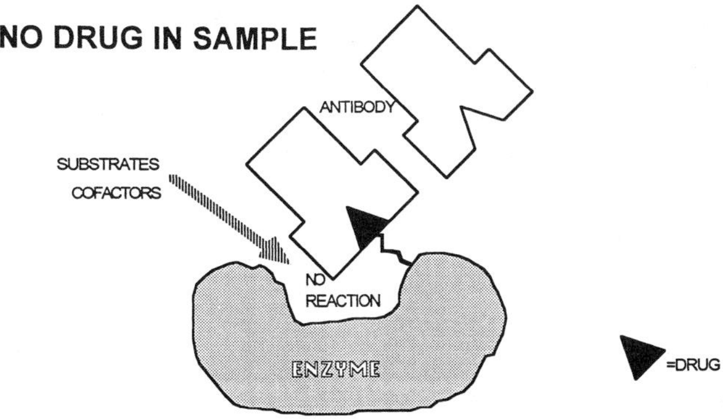

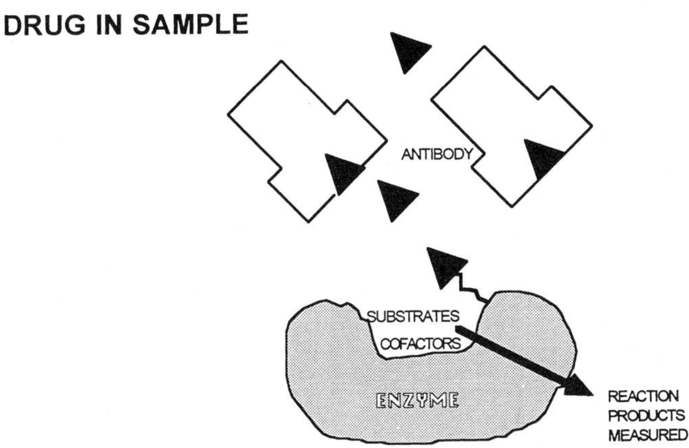

Figure 3–1. Principle of an enzyme immunoassay. A drug-specific antibody inhibits an enzymatic reaction because of a drug label on the enzyme. The greater the amount of free drug in the sample, the less the inhibition by the antibody and the faster the reaction of the enzyme system.

chromatography, the extracted morphine may be *N*-acetylated to decrease its polarity, increase its volatility, and enhance its detectability. Once prepared for chromatography, the partially isolated drug (extract) is separated from other solutes during its interaction with the chromatographic stationary phase. There are three general types of chromatography used in toxicologic analyses: thin-layer chromatography, gas chromatography, and high-performance liquid chromatography.

In *thin-layer chromatography (TLC),* extracted drugs are dried onto silica gel–coated plates. During the migration of a solvent up the plate, separation of the components and drugs in the extract is achieved by their differential interaction with the silica gel and solvent (Fig. 3–2). Chemical reactants sprayed on the plate localize (detect) the drugs, and the drugs' locations are compared with the locations of comigrated drugs on reference plates. Usually, a series of different chemical reactions are used in this process. The "staining" sequence and the ability to specify the migration distance of each drug endow TLC with the specificity that often is unachievable with the use of more elaborate procedures. However, with TLC, the analytical sensitivity for most drugs is limited to about 1.0 mg/L or greater, and it varies with the being drug tested, the detection method, and the

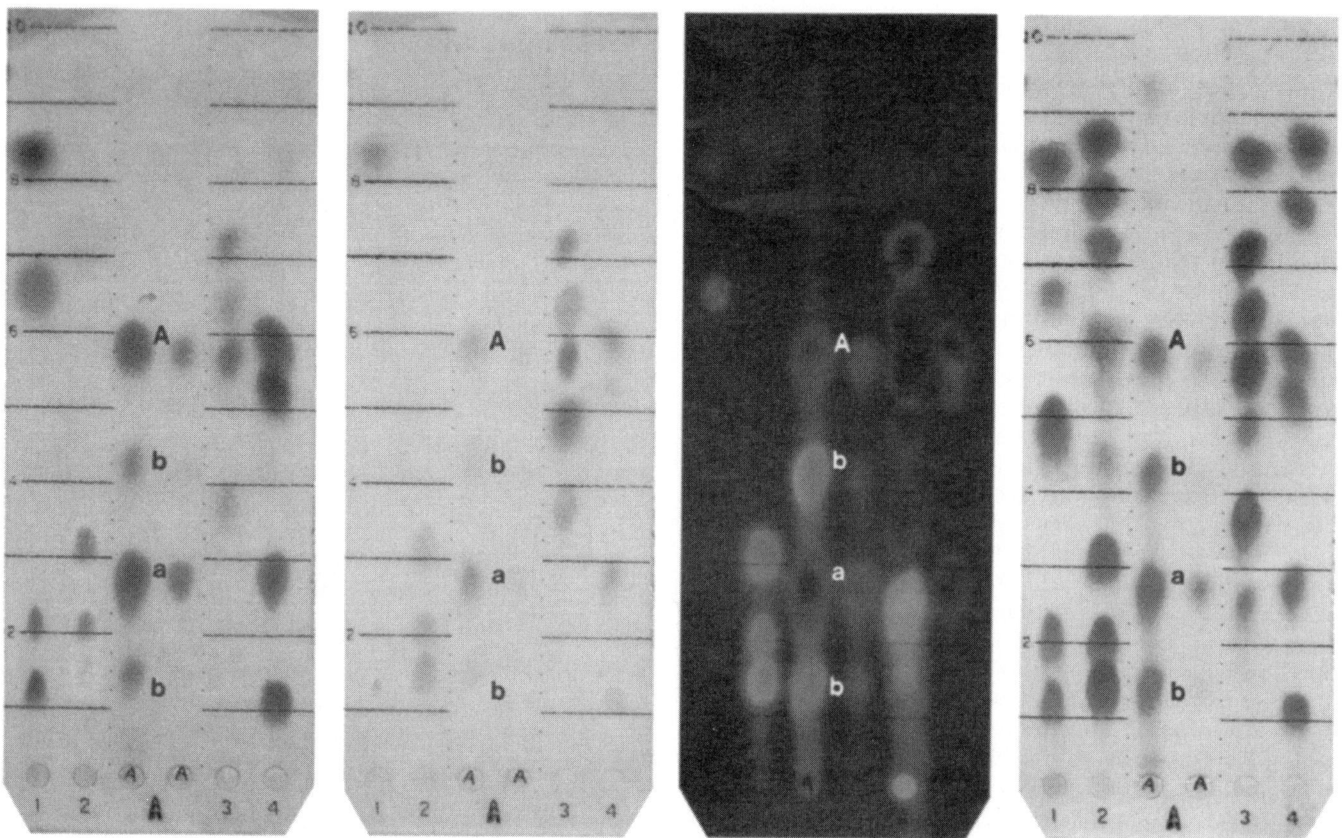

Figure 3–2. Diagram of a standardized thin-layer chromatography system for identification of a wide spectrum of drugs (Toxilab, Ansys Inc.). Drugs from urine were extracted and plated in the middle lanes A and chromatographed. Lanes 1 to 4 are standard drugs comigrated with lane A. Sequential staining with chemical reagents (phases I through IV) and migration distance aid in the identification of the unknown drug in lane A. Amitriptyline (A) and its metabolite nortriptyline (a) are detected. Other metabolites (b) are also detected. (Courtesy of ToxiLab, Ansys, Inc., Irvine, CA.)

amount of starting sample material. Many potent drugs—and often new drugs—may not be detectable with this technique (e.g., digoxin, lysergic acid diethylamide [LSD]).[12] Most current modifications of TLC-based drug screening have been adapted from the earlier procedures of Davidow and associates.[13] TLC for drug detection in emergency situations has become standardized owing to the availability of commercially prepared TLC systems (e.g., Toxilab, Ansys, Inc.). This has allowed expertise in the TLC identification of drugs to be less technologist dependent and results to be similar from laboratory to laboratory (see Fig. 3–2). Comigration of 30 or more standard drugs can be carried out on a single plate, allowing the identification of a large number of other drugs with the use of comigrated standards and information in a reference compendium. TLC will probably remain a common technique in testing for a broad range of unknown drugs.

High-performance liquid chromatography (HPLC) is similar in many respects to TLC. Drugs are separated within tightly packed columns; high pressure is applied to the columns to elute the drugs. Column material for HPLC may be silica gel, as with TLC, or nonpolar phases (alkyl groups) bonded to small particles. With the former, drug is eluted with organic solvents, and with the latter solvents miscible in aqueous buffers are used. Often, drugs eluting from the end of the column are detected on the basis of their absorption of ultraviolet light. Other detection techniques are based on refractometry, conductivity, and electrochemical (redox) reactions. Drugs are identified only by the time that it for takes each to be eluted from the column and to pass the detector (retention time) in a highly standardized procedure. HPLC systems have not been widely used in broad drug screening partly because of the narrow range of drug polarity that can be chromatographed in one run. However, systems that change the composition of eluting solvent during a single run (gradient systems) or those that use multiple-column processing can perform this task. Because of this high selectivity (resolution or separation of similar drugs), much HPLC work is directed toward screening for classes of similar compounds, confirming the presence of selected agents or quantitating specified drugs. Quantitation involves the measurement of the sizes of peaks relative to those of a standard compound added in a fixed quantity to all samples (internal standard). With extraction and preconcentration of the extract, detection limits of 0.01 to 1.0 mg/L often are achieved with HPLC. Certain automated instruments have been shown to be useful in screening for a wide variety of drugs of overdose[14]; however, application in practice has been limited.

Gas chromatography (GC) requires that the extracted drug be volatile at the temperatures inside the GC column (80 to 300° C). Drugs and toxins can be chemically modified to make them more volatile. During injection onto the beginning of the column, the drugs are heated. Drugs in the gas phase are separated from each other by interaction with the "liquid" stationary phase (at high temperatures) on the column. Drugs eluting from the column can be detected on the basis of their thermal conductivity, combustibility, ability to donate electrons, ability to capture β-particle beams, ionization, and other characteristics. The range of selective detectors for GC is quite broad. One mode of detection that merits discussion is *gas chromatography/mass spectrometry (GC/MS)*. A portion of the effluent gases from GC are ionized by bombardment in an electron beam or other methods. The molecular fragments that result are characteristic of the eluting drug. GC/MS is very specific. When unique fragments are monitored, the sensitivity can extend into the nanogram-per-liter range.

Whether GC or GC/MS is used, the range of drugs that can be chromatographed on a single column is wide, but it is also limited by volatility and polarity. Most current GC applications for screening of the many drugs seen in overdose cases are similar to those developed years ago by Forester and colleagues.[15] With the introduction of capillary columns, many similar drug molecules can be screened with good resolution (specificity). An example of a chromatogram of standards used in emergency urine screening is shown in Figure 3–3. After extraction, evaporation of solvent, and reconstitution, the mixture is injected and volatilized into the gas stream of the column. Detection in this case is with a nitrogen-phosphorus–type alkali detector. As with other similar systems, about 0.1 to 0.5 mg/L of a large number of drugs is detectable. Another common GC application is the determination of volatile alcohols. Ethanol, methanol, isopropanol, and other volatile solvents can be identified specifically and quantitated quickly in simple GC systems.

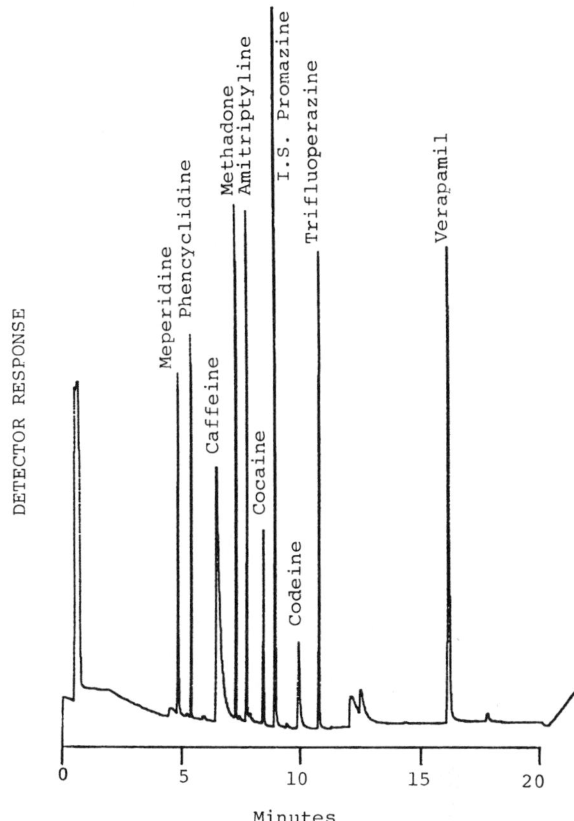

Figure 3–3. Chromatogram of a quality control urine sample containing 10 drugs after extraction from urine and detection by capillary gas chromatography with nitrogen-phosphorus detection. The concentration of caffeine and verapamil is 2.0 mg/L; that of each other drug is 0.5 mg/L. The limit of detection is about 0.1 mg/L.

SERUM QUANTITATION OF OVERDOSED DRUGS

Rationale and Uses

Drug and toxin quantitations in overdose are used for monitoring the course of the patient and for determining whether toxicity is occurring but not yet clinically apparent or whether it will occur after a delay. In the emergency setting, there are relatively few drugs for which quantitative measurements meet these goals. These drugs include acetaminophen, salicylates, theophylline, methanol, ethylene glycol, iron, carbon monoxide, and lithium. Quantitation also is useful in circumstances in which the presence of a hazardous therapy is being considered or in the evaluation of the efficacy of that therapy (see later).

Two criteria must be satisfied for quantitation to be useful. First, good clinical indicators that would otherwise reveal the status or condition of the patient must be absent. If the suspected toxin is known or its presence highly probable and if toxicity is apparent (i.e., clinical effects are observed), knowledge of drug concentration is of limited utility except in the patient who has overdose of the drugs listed in the previous paragraph. For most patients with drug intoxication, the clinical indicators of toxicity are better than measurements of drug concentration. For example, the clinical manifestations in the patient with overdose of a tricyclic antidepressant indicate the course and severity of the ingestion better than do measurements of drug concentrations. Initially, norepinephrine reuptake blockade and anticholinergic effects caused by a tricyclic drug result in sinus or supraventricular tachycardia. Later, after tissue concentrations have increased, blockade of sodium channel conductance widens the QRS complex on the electrocardiogram and, thus, leads to ventricular arrhythmias. Subsequently, as tissue concentrations increase, α-adrenergic blockade together with cardiac pump failure leads to cardiovascular collapse. Status in most cases of overdose can be monitored on the basis of clinical signs.

The second criterion that must be satisfied for measurements of drug concentrations to be useful is confirmation of the existence of a concentration-effect relationship. Unfortunately, only a few drugs have known relationships, and many more remain unstudied. In therapeutic drug monitoring, these relationships are well described for the endpoints of efficacy or toxicity. These therapeutic relationships cannot simply be extrapolated to the overdose setting. For instance, carbamazepine is an anticonvulsant at therapeutic concentrations of 5 to 10 mg/L, but it may cause seizures when taken in overdose. Similarly, a therapeutic dose of theophylline would be completely eliminated in a single day; in contrast, in the patient with an overdose of theophylline, several days may be required for complete elimination of the drug.

Prescott had considered the most important task of the toxicology laboratory to be the quantitation of drug concentrations for the evaluation of dangerous or expensive therapeutic procedures.[16] Quantitation on this basis is applied when any drug that may require hemoperfusion (e.g., theophylline, phenobarbital, ethchlorvynol) or hemodialysis (e.g., salicylates, methanol, lithium) is used so that toxic life-threatening concentrations may be avoided, the coma time associated with drugs with long residence times shortened, and the efficacy of the extracorporeal elimination techniques evaluated. Quantitation of drug concentrations is required for similar reasons when a clinician is deciding whether to treat a patient with digoxin overdose with digoxin immune antigen-binding fragments (Digibind) and when determining the appropriate use of metal chelators in metal poisoning. Certainly, other clinical data may alter how the balance of clinical management is carried out. For example, it is well known that hypomagnesemia, hypokalemia, and underlying atherosclerotic heart disease are factors in the manifestation of digoxin toxicity.

Availability and Reliability

If real change in the concentration of a substance in a given patient is to be discerned, measurements should be available immediately on a 24-hour basis and they should be precise (i.e., not semiquantitative). In the mid-1980s, only a small proportion of hospital laboratories had quantitative capabilities. Because of the increasing use of quantitative immunoassays performed on rapid chemistry analyzers, most large hospital laboratories are now able to perform therapeutic drug monitoring assays. However, of all hospitals capable of performing routine chemistry tests, only 63% performed assays for iron, 38% for lithium, 79% for theophylline, 51% for salicylate, and 51% for acetaminophen.[17]

Not only must serum quantitation techniques be adequately *precise* to recognize a change occurring from one time point to another, but they should also be *accurate* (reference to a true value) so that management decisions may be made correctly (relative to predetermined decision values). The accuracy and interlaboratory variability of the quantitation of concentrations may be assessed on the basis of results from proficiency testing programs.[17] In general, accuracy (i.e., nearness to target concentrations) and agreement of results obtained by different laboratories are most apparent for drugs measured commonly and by uniform techniques (e.g., antiepileptic drugs). For drugs that are measured infrequently and by more diverse methods, the results obtained are more diverse. Today, interlaboratory coefficients of variation less than 8% and biases less than 15% have been demonstrated for the quantitation of most therapeutic drug monitoring–type drugs.[17]

Altered Pharmacokinetic and Pharmacodynamic Relationships in Overdosage

Serum drug quantitations must be evaluated with respect to each patient's clinical condition. The variation in the metabolism of pharmaceuticals from person to person (Fig. 3–4), the interactions of disease processes and medications, the altered pharmacologic properties of drugs taken in overdose, and the potential for interference in assays may affect how a measured drug concentration is interpreted.[18] For example, when taken in overdose, salicylates are more toxic than the linear extrapolation of effects of therapeutic concentrations would predict. This discrepancy is the result of the elevation of free (unbound) concentrations with increasing serum concentrations, an increase in central nervous system penetration at acidotic blood pH, and the saturation of metabolic pathways in the presence of the higher concentrations. Interpretation of drug levels may be altered by the consideration of several factors together. For instance, a renal failure patient receiving normal doses of digoxin may have no digoxin-related symptoms even though the patient has a serum digoxin level of 4 ng/mL. Falsely measured digoxin-like substances in renal failure may raise the patient's measured "digoxin" level by 1 ng/mL. In addition, cross-reaction of accumulated metabolites due to poor renal clearance may falsely elevate the measured level an additional 2 ng/mL. In contrast, a different patient with a measured digoxin level of 2 ng/mL may exhibit digoxin-related toxicity that is due to exacerbation from hypokalemia. Therefore, measured drug concentrations must be interpreted relative to the condition of the patient, and therapeutic ranges should be used only as a guide.

TOXICOLOGIC "SCREENS"

Components of a Toxicologic "Screen"

A *toxicologic screen* is a combination of laboratory procedures that is aimed at identifying the drugs

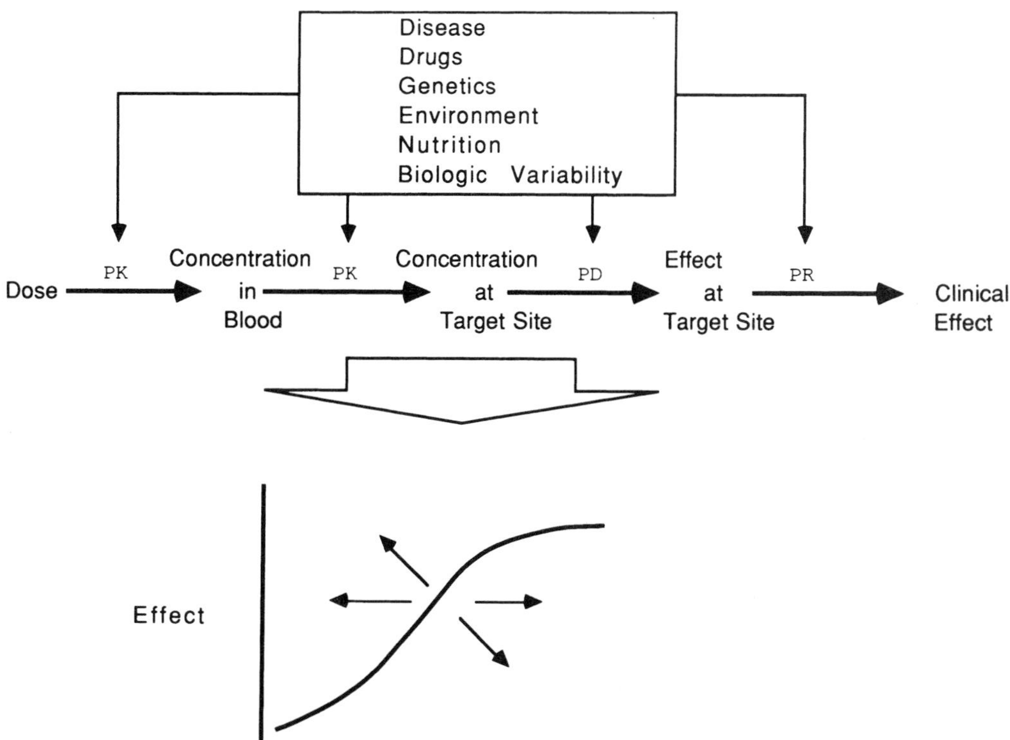

Figure 3–4. Factors producing altered pharmacologic relationships. PK, pharmacokinetics; PD, pharmacodynamics; PR, physiologic response to pharmacologic effect.

most commonly encountered in emergency toxicology. Screens may include as many procedures as are necessary for the identification of target drugs; alternatively, to shorten turnaround time, screens can be focused or abbreviated so that they test for only a few common, critical, or difficult-to-recognize drugs. The numbers and types of drugs on the screen can be adapted somewhat to reflect regional differences in drug prevalence.[19] Ultimately, in the cost-contained environment, availability of inexpensive commercial methods is often the greater determinant.

Comprehensive screening that includes spot tests, immunoassays, TLC, and GC procedures may require 3 to 4 hours of intensive labor. During the application of multiple procedures, the presence of a detected drug may be confirmed by any two of the procedures. Presently, most laboratories do not report a drug identification unless the agent has been detected on two procedures or unless the single method is known to be highly specific for a highly prevalent intoxicant (e.g., GC for ethanol). Initial identification of a drug (e.g., codeine/morphine on immunoassay) would be considered only presumptive. Subsequent confirmation (e.g., by TLC or GC/MS) would make the result reportable. Lack of confirmation or the absence of initial identification would be reported as not detected. Confirmation is not always a requirement in clinical testing, depending on the prevalence of the drug being tested, the specificity of the single test used, and the implications of a positive test result. In a case of illicit drug use, results should always be confirmed because the ramifications of such use (subsequent to the results' being reported in the medical chart) may extend beyond the patient's care. The detection of some highly prevalent drugs, such as benzodiazepines, may not require confirmation or individual identification because these drugs often are present in hospital and drug-using populations (i.e., high prior probability) and because they contribute little to the clinical picture. The sequence and choice of tests can vary, depending on the information provided to the laboratory. In this regard, communication between the laboratory and the treating physician is encouraged; exchange of information may raise the prior probability that a given class of drugs is present and thus reduces the likelihood of false-positives or false-negative results, speeds analysis, and helps the laboratory make the best use of its resources.

At the San Francisco General Hospital's (SFGH's) clinical laboratories, the following procedures are performed on urine specimens with requests for comprehensive toxicology screens: two spot tests (for salicylates and phenothiazines); eight IAs (for codeine/morphine, benzodiazepine metabolites, amphetamine-methamphetamine, methadone, phencyclidine, ethanol, cocaine metabolite, and barbiturates); TLC for 30 to 60 drugs; two-column GC using nitrogen-phosphorus and flame ionization detectors for about 60 to 80 drugs. The drugs screened by this combination of methods are listed in Table 3–3. Toxins not usually detectable in comprehensive toxicologic screens are listed in Table 3–4. Many of these unscreened drugs are either not very prevalent or not very toxic, but many important intoxicants are not detected in screening procedures (e.g., ethylene

Table 3–3. Common Drugs Included on Most Toxicologic Screens

Drug Type	Examples
Alcohols	Ethanol, methanol, isopropanol, acetone
Barbiturates/ sedatives	Amobarbital, secobarbital, pentobarbital, butalbital, butabarbital, phenobarbital, glutethimide, ethychlorvynol, methaqualone
Antiepileptics	Phenytoin, carbamazepine, primadone, phenobarbital
Benzodiazepines	Chlordiazepoxide, diazepam, alprazolam, temazepam
Antihistamines	Diphenhydramine, chlorpheniramine, brompheniramine, tripennelamine, trihexyphenidyl, doxylamine, pyrilamine, methyprylene
Antidepressants	Amitriptyline, nortriptyline, doxepin, imipramine, desipramine, trazodone, amoxapine, maprotiline, fluoxetine
Antipsychotics	Trifluoperazine, perphenazine, prochlorperazine, chlorpromazine
Stimulants	Amphetamine, methamphetamine, phenylpropanolamine, ephedrine, MDA and MDMA (other phenylethylamines), cocaine, phencyclidine
Narcotics, analgesics	Heroin, morphine, codeine, oxycodone, hydrocodone, hydromorphone, meperidine, pentazocine, propoxyphene
Other analgesics	Salicylates, acetaminophen
Cardiovascular drugs	Lidocaine, propranolol, metoprolol, quinidine, procainamide, verapamil
Others	Theophylline, caffeine, nicotine, oral hypoglycemics, strychnine

glycol, isoniazid, and cyanide). Assays for drugs not included in the toxicologic screen can often be requested separately, or specimens can be sent to other institutions for testing. Clinicians can prevent the reporting of clinical false-negative results (which can occur when a test not capable of finding the test condition in question is ordered) by knowing which drugs and toxins are not included on the screens at their hospitals. *Also, the earlier the urine is collected, the greater the chance that a drug will be found, because the duration of detectability for many drugs is short (see Table 3–5 for detection intervals of commonly found illicit drugs).*

Table 3–4. Toxins Not Detectable by Emergency Toxicologic Screens Classified by Area of Difficulty

Difficulty	Drugs/Toxins
Too polar	Antibiotics, diuretics, isoniazid, ethylene glycol, lithium, lead, iron
Too nonpolar	Steroids, THC, digoxin
Too nonvolatile	Plant and fungal alkaloids, some phenothiazines
Too volatile	Aromatic and halogenated hydrocarbon solvents, anesthetic gases, noxious gases (hydrogen sulfide, nitrogen dioxide, carbon monoxide)
Concentration too low	Potent drugs or drugs with large volume of distribution (e.g., clonidine, fentanyl, colchicine, ergot alkaloids, LSD, dioxin, digoxin, THC)
Toxic anions (too polar)	Thiocyanate, cyanide, fluoride, bromide, borate, nitrite
New drugs	Buspirone

THC, tetrahydrocannabinol; LSD, lysergic acid diethylamide.

A smaller screen for illicit drugs also is commonly offered. At SFGH, the "drugs of abuse screen" comprises the aforementioned eight immunoassays, with confirmation procedures performed as needed. (Refer to Table 3–6 for comparison of the drugs of abuse screen and the comprehensive drug screen.) This screen has most frequently been used by the emergency and psychiatric services (refer to Table 3–7 for utilization data) and accounts for 79.1% of all screening requests. Although many hospitals test for marijuana, the laboratory at SFGH does not screen for marijuana metabolite (wide commercial availability) in emergency situations because (1) it is present in many overdoses within the drug-using population, (2) it is rarely considered responsible for serious toxicologic effects, and (3) it is excreted in urine for long periods of time after use and thus temporally may not be related to the acute clinical picture.

The composition of toxicologic screens vary quite widely from laboratory to laboratory. Some laboratories advocate limited application of spot tests only, or combinations of spot tests and rapid immunoassays for specific drugs. Comprehensive screens composed of multiple complementary methods are the norm.[8, 20, 21*] Hepler and colleagues have emphasized a comprehensive approach to screening and indicated that 98.8% of all drugs found in patients with positive test results can be detected with the use of urine and IA, TLC, spot tests, GC, and HPLC techniques.[8] Yet, today only 6% of hospital or clinic laboratories are enrolled in proficiency testing for comprehensive screening; this fact suggests that the capability to perform such comprehensive testing is not widespread.[17]

Rationale and Use of Toxicologic "Screens"

In the emergency setting, urine, blood, and aspirates of gastric contents should be obtained as soon as a toxicologic diagnosis is considered in the differential diagnosis. It is unlikely that comprehensive screening will produce results that affect emergency management (see Clinical Utility of Toxicologic "Screens," later in this chapter), but the subsequent results of findings may assist the ward physicians in evaluating a patient if the diagnosis remains unclear. In the emergency department, if the diagnosis is not intoxication or the clinical picture indicates a manageable toxicologic syndrome, specimens may be retained in the emergency department or stored frozen in the laboratory.

Techniques that use urine specimens identify the greatest number of drugs in easily detectable quantities. When compared with assays using serum or

*See also references 7, 10, 72, and 100 cited in reference 1 of this chapter.

Table 3–5. Approximate Duration of Detectability of Selected Drugs in Urine

Drug	Approximate Duration of Detectability*	Method	Limits of Sensitivity of Analytic Techniques	Interferences
Amphetamines	<2 d	IA	1000 ng/mL†	Newer generation assays react with MDA, MDMA, STP, and I-amphetamine; older assays cross-react with adrenergic amines as phenylpropanolamine
Barbiturates				
Short-Acting				
Pentobarbital	~1 d	IA	500 ng/mL	NSAIDs, adulterants, other barbiturates
Secobarbital	~1 d			
Butalbital	~2–3 d			
Long-Acting				
Phenobarbital	~7 d	IA	500 ng/mL	
Benzodiazepines	3 d‡	IA	300 ng/mL	NSAIDs, other less used benzodiazepines
Cannabinoids (Tetrahydrocannabinol Metabolites)	3 d§ 5 d‖ 7–10 d¶ <30 d**	IA	50 ng/mL† (ER drug screen) 20 ng/mL (confirmatory test)	Adulterants
Cocaine (Metabolite: Benzoylecgonine)	2 d	IA	300 ng/mL†	Adulterants Teas made from coca leaf
Ethanol	<1 d (social) <2 d (toxic)	GC (serum)		
Opiates				
Methadone	<5 d	IA	300 ng/mL†	Opiates, antihistamines, poppy seed morphine, adulterants, rifampin
Codeine	<2 d			
Morphine	<2 d			
Phencyclidine	~8 d	IA	25 ng/mL†	PCP analogues

IA, immunoassay; GC, gas chromatography; NSAIDs, nonsteroidal anti-inflammatory drugs; PCP, phencyclidine hydrochloride; MDA, 3,4-methylenedioxyamphetamine; MDMA, 3,4-methylenedioxymethamphetamine; STP, "serenity, tranquility, and peace" (4-methyl 2,5-dimethoxyamphetamine).

* Durations are given for single recreational use or therapeutic dosages, unless otherwise specified; drug overdose or chronic abuse will generally give longer durations of detectability. Factors such as drug metabolism, half-life, patient's physical condition, fluid balance and state of hydration, and route and frequency of ingestion may also affect duration of detectability.

† Recommended screening cut-off concentrations by the Substance Abuse and Mental Health Services Administration.

‡ Therapeutic dosage.

§ Single use.

‖ Moderate smoker (4 times per wk).

¶ Heavy smoker (Daily use).

** Chronic heavy smoker.

gastric aspirates, urinalysis yields the highest rate of positive findings.[1, 8, 20] Drawing a blood sample in addition to a urine specimen produces a slightly greater overall yield of positive results. These added positive results obtained on serum testing may be due to the application of specific methods for drugs commonly measured in serum (e.g., a group of therapeutic drug monitoring tests), but they also may be owing to early sample acquisition. No true serum or blood screen capable of identifying as many drugs as urinalysis is currently available. The analytic limitations of serum screening are that lower concentrations of drugs are found in serum and blood, the size of available samples is small, and the use of serum samples is incompatible with some testing methodologies. In some cases, however, drugs may not have reached the urine in detectable quantities soon after ingestion, but they may be present in the plasma. Also, some drugs are highly metabolized, and thus little of the parent drug may be detectable in the urine. Furthermore, gastric samples often contain high concentrations of the parent drugs, and thus their collection facilitates identification. In one study, patients who had undergone gastric lavage for initial management demonstrated the following percentage of the positive results for the presence of drugs on analyses of their specimens: urine, 93%; serum, 54% (samples screened for sedative-hypnotics only); and gastric aspirate or lavage effluent, 38%.[22]

Toxicologic screens should be applied as diagnostic tests—that is, they should be used by the clinician considering several possible diagnoses. When used after a working diagnosis has been made, toxicologic screens serve to document or to confirm what was considered highly likely. However, toxicologic screens often have utility in clinical situations other than acute overdose (see Clinical Utility of Toxicologic "Screens," later in this chapter). When ordering a toxicologic screen, the clinician should write suspected drugs or drug classes and either the key symptoms or the working diagnosis on the requisition. This facilitates both the screening process and the

Table 3–6. Comparison of Drugs of Abuse Screen (DAU) and Comprehensive Drug Screen (CDS)

	DAU	CDS
Availability	All days, all shifts	6 d/wk, day shift
Sample	30 mL of urine	30 mL of urine
Methods used	8 IA	8 IA, 2 spots, 2 TLC, 2 GC
Time to negative results	45 min (stat); 2 h (routine)	6–30 h
Time to positive results	45 min for cocaine, ethanol, and benzodiazepines; 2–8 h for others	6–30 h
Total number of drugs/group screened	8 illicit	50 illicit plus pharmaceuticals

IA, immunoassays; GC, gas chromatography; TLC, thin-layer chromatography.

communication of results back to the ordering physician. For instance, if a toxicologic screen is ordered and clonidine is specified as the drug suspected of causing pinpoint pupils and respiratory depression, the laboratory can call the physician and inform him or her that the screening methods would be unlikely to detect clonidine but that they could rule out the possibility that other narcotics are causing the pinpoint pupils and respiratory depression. In another case, a physician may order only a test for amphetamines in urine because his or her patient is "acting bizarrely." In the psychiatric emergency service at SFGH, patients with antihistamine abuse (in conjunction with narcotics and cocaine abuse) commonly present to medical attention. Antihistamines are able to produce anticholinergic delirium that is somewhat similar to that occurring in both functional and amphetamine-related psychoses. In this case, a toxicologic screen or a limited screen may be recommended. Fligner and colleagues[23] indicated that the best method of communication is the use of a requisition form containing adequate prompts and sufficient space for written comments. In a survey addressing the use of these forms, only 48% had space for the listing of suspected drugs.[23]

Drug Overdose and the Drugs Found

One and one-half million cases of accidental (86.3%) or intentional (10.9%) chemical exposures are reported annually.[24] The estimated number of deaths occurring in the United States as a result of toxin exposure is about 12,000. This low incidence of fatality reflects the low toxicity of exposure in the majority of cases and the outcome of medical treatment; however, drug ingestions (i.e., not other toxins) accounted for 91% of the deaths. The drug categories responsible for the deaths reported by poison control centers were analgesics (narcotic and non-narcotic), antidepressants, stimulants (including amphetamines, cocaine, and phencyclidine), sedative-hypnotics, cardiovascular drugs, and alcohol.[24] All of these drugs are detectable on comprehensive toxicologic screening. A sample of screening results at SFGH in 1995 is representative of other past compilations (see Table 3–7).[1] These data confirm older studies of emergency settings showing that toxicologic screening yields positive results in 50% to 80% of patients in whom testing is requested and that the top five drug classes account for 70% to 90% of all drugs found. The top five drugs found in various screening situations are listed in Table 3–8. From the 1970s through the 1980s, the incidence of detection of barbiturates and ethanol has decreased while that of benzodiaze-

Table 3–7. Toxicologic Screen Results from SFGH (6 Months, 1995)

	DAU	CDS
Percent of Requests	79.1	20.9
Requisition Source		
General medicine wards	14.5	22.4
Psychiatric wards	13.3	16.1
Emergency and psychiatric emergency departments	48.1	21.1
Other in/outpatient settings	24.1	40.4
*Results**		
n	1949	406
Per cent negative for all drugs†	27.2	19.9
Per cent positive in any drug group‡	72.8	80.1
Per cent positive for amphetamine/methamphetamine	11.9	10.8
Per cent positive for barbiturates	3.6	5.4
Per cent positive for benzodiazepine metabolites	13.8	20.0
Per cent positive for cocaine metabolite	25.9	32.7
Per cent positive for ethanol	9.7	9.4
Per cent positive for methadone	5.1	15.5
Per cent positive for morphine/codeine	15.2	31.0 (15.2% morphine as alone)
Per cent positive for phenyclidine	0.4	0.7
Positive for drugs other than the above DAU groups§	N/A	23.9%

N/A, not applicable.

Per cent other drugs found on CDS: diphenhydramine, 11.1; acetaminophen, 7.9; salicylate, 6.9; trimethoprim, 6.4; phenytoin, 3.2; chlorpheniramine, 2.5; phenothiazines, 2.5; carbamazepine, 2.2; and nortriptyline/amitriptyline, 1.5. Drugs <1% are quinidine/quinine, benztropine, caffeine (overdose), desipramine, dextromethorphan, doxylamine, meperidine, doxepin, ephedrine/pseudoephedrine, tripennelamine, brompheniramine, and trihexiphenidyl.

* Results for all drugs/groups confirmed with second method except those of ethanol and benzodiazepines.

† For DAU, the results for the eight drug groups listed (immunoassays) were all negative. For CDS, the results for the eight drug groups listed were negative, and the results on the chromatographic screens were negative.

‡ For DAU, the results for any of the eight drug groups listed could be positive. For CDS, the results for any of the drug groups listed or the results on chromatographic screens could be positive.

§ Positive results for drugs other than those found on the initial eight-drug group immunoassays (i.e., DAU).

Table 3–8. Top Five Drugs Found on Toxicologic Screens and Death Reports

Rank	Poison Control Death Reports (AAPCC 1993)	Forensic Deaths (1982, 1985)[27, 28]	Hospital Toxicologic Screens (1985)[8]	Hospital Toxicologic Screens (SFGH 1989)	Hospital Toxicologic Screens (SFGH 1995)
1	Analgesics* (0.103)§	Carbon monoxide	Benzodiazepines	Stimulants‡	Stimulants‡
2	Antidepressants (0.372)	Ethanol	Ethanol	Opiates	Opiates
3	Stimulants‡ (0.395)	Sedatives	Acetaminophen	Benzodiazepines	Benzodiazepines
4	Sedatives/antipsychotics (0.147)	Opiates	Tricyclics	Analgesics†	Analgesics†
5	Cardiovascular agents (0.285)	Tricyclics	Barbiturates	Ethanol	Antihistamines

SFGH, San Francisco General Hospital.
* Includes opiates.
† Does not include opiates.
‡ Includes cocaine and amphetamines.
§ Per cent mortality of that drug category.

pines, tricyclic antidepressants, sympathomimetic amines, and most recently, cocaine has increased. Bailey reported that the incidence of toxicologic screens' yielding positive results for cocaine had risen from 1% in 1978 to 10% in 1986.[25] Currently, test results for cocaine are positive in over 25% of all screens ordered at the SFGH laboratory.

In contrast to toxicologic screening results and poison control center reports (see Table 3–8), the reports of medical examiners show a slightly different spectrum of toxic exposures, listing carbon monoxide (along with exposure to fire), ethanol, sedatives, opiates, tricyclic antidepressants, and propoxyphene as the more common causes of toxin-related deaths.[26, 27] In pediatric overdose, suicide and drug abuse are less likely circumstances. Drugs are responsible for only a minority of all exposures in children (40%), but they account for a large portion of intoxications, hospital admissions, and deaths, particularly among teenagers.[24, 28–30] Also, drug exposures in pediatric patients younger than 6 years of age usually involve single agents, whereas in adults 27% to 66% of all cases are characterized by the ingestion of multiple drugs.* The most common second drug group reported to be detected is benzodiazepines regardless of the primary drug abused.[31]

The drugs found on toxicologic screens vary by report because of regional differences, ordering patterns, and the composition of the screens. For instance, the incidence of detection of ethanol on urinary toxicologic screens is relatively low. The reverse is true for serum samples submitted for quantitation of ethanol because the use of serum samples for ethanol quantitation is indicative of a greater suspicion of the presence of ethanol. The source of these samples may also reflect a high prevalence, as in trauma cases.

Analytic Accuracy of Toxicologic "Screens"

Screening performed for workplace drug testing programs has become very accurate because of the time allowed for analysis, the definitive techniques that need to be applied (GC-MS), and the small number of drugs that are targeted.[32] During the 1970s, the strategies and methods of workplace drug testing were similar to those for emergency toxicologic screening, methadone testing, and medical examiners' cause-of-death determinations. Usually, TLC and GC were used, with IA and radioimmunoassay methods finding applications in the mid- to late 1970s. In reports of proficiency testing surveys from the late 1970s, detection limits for drugs were quite high when compared with current limits or cutoffs. Incidences of false-negative results as high as 40% for common drugs were the major problem.* In the early 1980s, surveys of drug screening accuracy focused on methadone testing laboratories. These surveys demonstrated that false-positive and false-negative reporting rates were high, indicating that little improvement in testing had occurred from the 1970s to 1980s.

Currently, testing in emergency hospital laboratories can be assessed by hospital laboratories' participation in proficiency testing programs administered by the American Association of Clinical Chemists and the College of American Pathologists. The incidence of false-negative results on testing for a rare drug such as carisoprodol can be as high as 60%, compared with about 10% for a common drug such as codeine. The occurrence of false-positive results is low in part because of high drug concentrations seen in cases of overdose and because of confirmatory techniques.

A more difficult challenge than the routine proficiency samples was presented to 26 specialty toxicology laboratories in the West.[33] A case history was presented along with a urine sample containing four drugs. Only two of the laboratories were able to identify all of the four drugs present. Sixty-five per cent of the laboratories identified dihydrocodeine, 54% identified MDEA (methylene dioxyethyl amphetamine), 23% identified naloxone, and 23% identified

*See Table 3–11 found in reference 1 of this chapter.

*See reference 1 at the end of this chapter for other studies.

aminoflunitrazepam (a metabolite of flunitrazepam [Rohypnol]). For the average laboratory, false-negative results occur at a rate of 10% to 30%, and false-positive results at a rate of 0% to 10%. It should be noted that many false-positive and some false-negative results are due to misidentification within a drug class (i.e., pentobarbital for amobarbital). Thus, the impact of this error on clinical diagnosis would be small.

As stated earlier in the section on methods, drugs usually must be identified by two methods before a positive result can be reported. The choice and sequence of screening and confirmatory procedures is affected by costs, the labor intensiveness of the procedures, and the number of positive results. No matter what test is used first or second, each has its own fallibility; however, the complementary use of two testing methods with different analytic principles of detection usually precludes most false identifications.[7] Even GC-MS techniques, when improperly applied, resulted in the misidentification of drugs. False-negative identification due to interference from adulterants is unlikely in emergency toxicologic screening. Common adulterations include dilution (by ingestion or direct addition of water), substitution (with purchased urine or the urine of a second person or animal), ingestion of weak acids or bases (e.g., vinegar or bicarbonate, respectively) to influence the excretion of acidic or basic drugs, the use of interfering substances to alter test results (e.g., benzalkonium chloride), and the addition of strong chemicals (e.g., soap, bleach, or glutaraldehyde) to impair biologically based immunoassays.[12]

Accuracy of the Clinical Diagnosis

In Norway, Rygnestad and Berg[34] showed in 265 overdoses due to self-poisoning that the correct drug or class of drug could be identified in 85% of the cases through the use of data in the patient history, the findings on physical examination, and the results of basic laboratory tests, including quantitations of acetaminophen, salicylates, barbiturates, and lithium. Diagnoses were wrong or unknown in 14% of cases when initial findings were compared with data collected during extensive follow-up and other toxicologic testing. Toxicologic screening was needed to identify drugs in only 5% of cases, being most useful in identifying ethanol and benzodiazepines. Nice and co-workers[21] assessed the use of "toxidromes" for the identification of drug-intoxicated patients and showed that nurses, physicians, and clinical pharmacists identified the drug or drug class causing intoxication in over 80% of cases. In contrast, Bury and Mashford[35] indicated that information on drug intake was unreliable or unavailable in 75% of 167 drug overdose cases, confirming earlier suspicions of Teitelbaum and associates.[36] The rate of complete concordance of clinical predictions with toxicologic testing results is estimated to be only 20% to 32%, in that other additional drugs often are found (20% to 48% of the time). The clinically predicted drug is not found in 9% to 25% of cases when a number of surveys are reviewed.[1]

Clinical Reliability of Toxicologic "Screens"

Overall clinical reliability depends on (1) analytic sensitivity and specificity, (2) whether a laboratory tests for the drugs that are expected in the screen, and (3) the prevalence of drug-positive cases and intoxications in a given clinical setting. The prevalence of positive results on drug screens in past surveys of overdoses is about 50% to 80%.* In other words, of the suspected cases where tox screens were submitted, results were positive in 50–80%. Prevalence of positive screens will vary from situation to situation and by region.

If it is assumed that the prior probability of drugs being present in a patient who appears to have an overdose is 50% and if the toxicologic screen has a sensitivity of 70% to 90% (based on proficiency testing data given earlier), the predictive value of a negative test result is 63% to 83%. If the specificity is from 90% to 100%, then the predictive value of a positive test result is 83% to 100%. Thus, the "rule-in" value of the toxicologic screen is better than its "rule-out" value (Fig. 3–5). Kellerman and associates[37] indicated that most physicians tend to use toxicologic screens to "rule-out" drug toxicity as a diagnosis and are less likely to use these screens for "rule-in" purposes. This finding is disconcerting if the positive predictive value of toxicologic screens is higher than their negative predictive value in high prevalence settings. On the other hand, when diagnostic choices are few and the running diagnosis is less likely to be drug intoxication, rule-out testing makes some sense (see Fig. 3–5). For example, if a patient were strongly considered to have a metabolic coma, the prior probability of the involvement of detectable drugs might be considered very low (e.g., 5%) in light of other data indicating metabolic causes (e.g., liver failure). With this prior probability and the same specificity and sensitivity of the toxicologic screen, the predictive value of a negative test result is from 76% to 90%, and the predictive value of a positive test result is 33%—hence, the rule-out value is better (see discussion in the following section).

Clinical Utility of Toxicologic "Screens"

Toxicologic screens are reliable for limited clinical use, but do their results establish a diagnosis or effect a change in a plan of management? Toxicologic screens would be suspected to have limited utility for the following reasons:

---

*See references 5, 44, 46, 76, 88, 90, and 99 cited in reference 1 of this chapter.

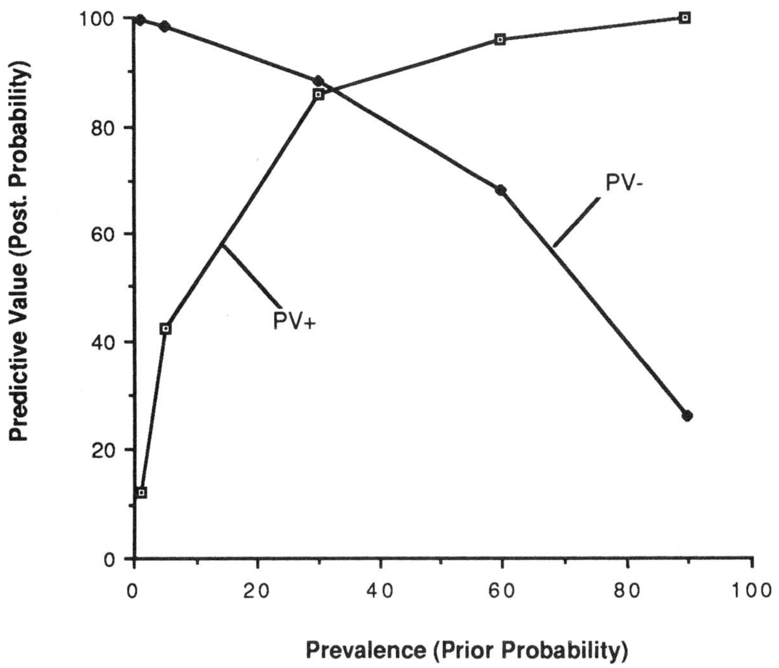

Figure 3–5. Posterior probability of finding any common drug in the toxicologic screen at various prevalences (prior probabilities) given a screen that is 70% sensitive (on average to any of the drugs detectable) and a specificity of 95%. PV+, posterior probability of a positive test result; PV−, posterior probability of a negative test result.

1. Diagnostic and management decisions are made before results are returned.
2. Benign and diagnostic intervention may preclude the need for these tests (e.g., response to naloxone in opiate intoxication).
3. There are only a few specific interventions or antidotes in toxicologic management that could possibly hinge on toxicologic test outcomes.[38]
4. The incidence of morbidity is low (<1%[24, 43]), in part owing to the nature of the drugs but also to effective standardized decontamination procedures and supportive therapy.
5. Toxicity is very often apparent on presentation.

Clinical features not only allow identification of a toxic syndrome but also are prognostic for outcome. Brett and colleagues[38] have studied 209 overdose patients and have shown that they can be categorized as being at low risk or high risk with respect to the development of complications or the need to undergo intensive care interventions as determined by initial clinical, blood gas, or electrocardiographic findings. Alternatively, the drugs that cause most of the deaths (see discussion earlier in this chapter) are detectable by screening, and screening can detect many drugs unsuspected by the physician. In studies assessing the utility of toxicologic screens, endpoints have included retrospective chart review to find alteration in management or diagnosis and prospective assessment with the completion of questionnaires by physicians receiving drug test results. Most recent studies in Table 3–9 indicate that the impact of screening on clinical diagnosis and management is low (<15%).[39–42] Kellerman and associates[37] have examined the subject of the utility of toxicologic screens most carefully. In prospective evaluations of diagnostic certainty, both before and after the return of toxicologic screen results, they showed that diagnostic certainty only increased by a mean value of 16.5% (the prior probability of drug toxicity was 75.5% and increased to a posterior probability or post-test probability of 92.0%) and that these changes in diagnostic

Table 3–9. Impact of Toxicologic Screening on Clinical Diagnosis and Management

Reference (Year)	No. of Patients Studied	Per cent of Cases in Which Diagnosis or Management Altered Due to Toxicologic Screen Results	Study Methods	Type of Patient
Wiltbank et al (1974)[40]	148	<7	R, chart review	ED
Helliwell et al (1979)[42]	108	15	P, verbal, chart review	ED coma
Bury and Mashford (1981)[35]	167	66	R, chart review	OD*
Mahoney et al (1985)[41]	176	8	R, ?	OD
Kellermann et al (1987)[37]	183	4.4 (66.3)†	P, questionnaire before/after	ED-OD
Brett (1988)[39]	198	1.5	R, records review	Intentional OD

P, prospective; R, retrospective; ED, emergency department patients suspected to have drug toxicity; OD, overdose patients.
* Self-poisoning excluded.
† 4.4% altered management; 66.3% slightly improved diagnostic certainty.

certainty occurred in 66% of the 183 cases evaluated. The authors concluded that other clinical information received by physicians may have inflated the estimated utility of toxicologic screens in the diagnostic process. Such estimates of utility validate the impressions of most toxicologists. However, many of the studies presented in Table 3–9 have focused only on positive toxicologic screen results. The impact of a negative test result is difficult to assess. No intervention as a result of a negative test result may also be considered contributory to the diagnostic and treatment process. In the duo-diagnosis of drug-induced or functional psychosis, the negative toxicologic screen result is considered by some as a predictor of the need for greater psychiatric care; however, thorough study of this hypothesis is still needed.[44]

TESTING FOR OTHER NONDRUG TOXINS

Testing for nondrug toxins is an area of great deficiency with respect to clinical utility. Few tests in this area have been developed or studied or have any commercial potential. Toxins from plants, animals, microorganisms, and chemical sources are numerous but are ingested with a much lower frequency than are drugs. Although potent and deadly toxins in these categories are many, most exposures tend to result in little, short-lived, or benign toxicity. Certain plant toxins such as nicotine, strychnine, and atropine can be recognized on comprehensive toxicologic screens. Specific tests for digoxin (and oleander) and cyanide (from cyanogenic glycoside–containing plants, fire exposure, or ingestion), and carboxyhemoglobin can be ordered from the laboratories of larger hospitals. Few specific plant and fungal toxins can be measured, and the clinician must use the data obtained during the history-taking and physical examination to guide diagnosis and management. However, most regional poison centers have contacts with a wide variety of agencies that can help in identifying materials from plants, mushrooms, and chemicals used in agriculture.

Guidelines for interpreting concentrations in chemical exposures (e.g., to metals or hydrocarbons) are usually based on timed or chronic exposure. These guidelines and cutoffs are often used for discerning excessive (but not necessarily toxic, as in monitoring) exposure rather than for identifying amounts associated with effects (i.e., for diagnosis). Although not the topic of this chapter, guidelines and laboratory methods for determining a narrow selection of commonly encountered inorganic substances (e.g., lead, mercury, cadmium, arsenic trichloroethylene, benzene, toluene, hexane, and polychlorinated biphenyls) are available. The reader is directed to other reference texts on these topics.[45, 46]

SUMMARY

Emergency physicians who use toxicologic testing should learn the capabilities of their institutions' laboratories: What is detectable? What is not detectable? What are the expected turnaround times? Do pharmacologic relationships exist? With regard to requests for testing, the laboratory should allow the physician to order limited test combinations; similarly, the physician can assist the laboratory in the search for unknowns by indicating the running diagnosis and what drugs are suspected. Only a few drugs require serum quantitation if results are to be useful for the making of therapeutic decisions (Table 3–10). Urine drug screening is useful in documenting drug-related intoxications and frequently detects the presence of more or different drugs than were clinically suspected. The impact of findings from emergency drug screening on diagnosis and therapy appears to be minimal. Although the positive predictive ("rule-in") value of comprehensive drug screening in the emergency setting is greater than its negative ("rule-out") predictive value, toxicologic screening may be useful as a rule-out test in other diagnostic applications of lower prior probability.

Future directions in the laboratory diagnosis of the intoxicated patient are likely to include growth in the direct application of new immunoassays, particularly in the emergency department. Also, with improvements in technology, screening of drugs in serum will become more common, as will the identification of more quantitative relationships between serum concentration and toxic effects.

Table 3–10. Summary: Situations in Which Toxicologic Testing Is Useful

1. Overdoses requiring serum drug concentration to diagnose severity or monitor course:
   - Acetaminophen
   - Salicylate
   - Theophylline
   - Iron
   - Methanol
   - Ethylene glycol
2. Overdoses requiring serum drug concentrations as criteria for therapy or to assess effectiveness of therapy:
   - All drugs in 1.
   - Lithium
   - Digoxin
   - Long-acting sedatives and benzodiazepines
   - Carbon monoxide
   - Lead, mercury, arsenic
   - Organophosphates (cholinesterases)
3. Situations in which toxicologic screens have utility:
   - When the differential diagnosis is sufficiently narrowed to a drug cause versus a disease cause (e.g., psychosis: functional versus amphetamines).
   - When drugs are an unlikely cause ("rule-out" value).
   - When there is documentation that the working diagnosis was correct (post factum).

References

1. Osterloh JD: Utility and reliability of emergency toxicologic testing. Emerg Med Clin North Am *8*:693–723, 1990.
2. Griner PF, Glaser RJ: Misuse of laboratory tests and diagnostic procedures. N Engl J Med *307*:1336–1339, 1982.

3. Spiehler VR, O'Donnell CM, Gokhale DV: Confirmation and certainty in toxicologic screening. Clin Chem *34*:1535–1539, 1988.
4. Ellenhorn MJ, Barceloux DG: Medical Toxicology: Diagnosis and Treatment of Human Poisoning. New York, Elsevier Science Publishing Co., 1988.
5. Olson KR: Comprehensive Evaluation and Treatment of Poisoning and Overdose. *In* Olson KR et al (eds): Poisoning and Drug Overdose. 2nd ed. Norwalk, CT, Appleton & Lange, 1994, pp 1–58.
6. Kulig K: Utilization of emergency toxicology screens. Am J Emerg Med *6*:573–574, 1985.
7. Ferrara SD, Tedeschi L, Frison G, et al: Drugs-of-abuse testing in urine: Statistical approach and experimental comparison of immunochemical and chromatographic techniques. J Anal Toxicol *18*:278–291, 1994.
8. Hepler BR, Sutheimer CA, Sunshine I: The role of the toxicology laboratory in emergency medicine. II. Study of an integrated approach. Clin Toxicol *22*:503–528, 1984–5.
9. Higgins G: Screening tests for common drugs. *In* Clark EGC (ed): Isolation and Identification of Drugs in Pharmaceuticals, Body Fluids and Post-Mortem Material. Vol. 1. London, The Pharmaceutical Press, 1974.
10. Dalrymple RW, Sterns FM, Diflunisal interferes with determination of salicylate by Trinder, Abbott TDx, and Du Pont aca methods. Clin Chem *32*:230, 1986.
11. Osterloh J: Limitations of acetaminophen assays. J Clin Toxicol *20*:19–22, 1983.
12. Mikkelsen SL, Ash KO: Adulterants causing false negatives in illicit drug testing. Clin Chem *34*:2333–2336, 1988.
13. Davidow B, Petri NL, Quarne B: A thin-layer chromatographic screening procedure for detecting drug abuse. Am J Clin Pathol *50*:714–719, 1968.
14. Binder SR, Regalia M, Biaggi-McEachern, Mazhar M: Automated liquid chromatographic analysis of drugs in urine by on-line cleanup and isocratic multi-column separation. J Chromatogr *473*:325–341, 1989.
15. Forester EH, Hatchett D, Garriott JC: A rapid, comprehensive screening procedure for basic drugs in blood or tissues by gas chromatography. J Anal Toxicol *2*:50–55, 1978.
16. Prescott LF: Limitations of hemodialysis and forced diuresis. *In* Curry AS (ed): Symposium on the Poisoned Patient—Role of the Laboratory. CIBA Foundation Symposium. New York, Elsevier Science Publishing Co., 1974.
17. College of American Pathologist Surveys: Urine Toxicology Survey 1995 Set UT-B; Therapeutic Drug Monitoring Survey 1995 Set Z-B; and Chemistry Survey 1995 Set C4-B. Chicago, IL, College of American Pathologists, 1995.
18. Rosenberg J, Benowitz NL, Pond S: Pharmacokinetics of drug overdose. Clin Pharmacokinet *6*:161–192, 1981.
19. Lasky FD, Wesley JF, Marx AJ: Changes in the pattern of drugs detected in a toxicology screen in an upstate New York hospital. Pathol Annu *20*:161–187, 1985.
20. Kellerman AL, Fihn SD, Logerfro JP, et al: Utilization and yield of drug screening in the emergency department. Am J Emerg Med *6*:14–20, 1988.
21. Nice A, Leikin JB, Maturen A, et al: Toxidrome recognition to improve efficiency of emergency urine drug screens. Ann Emerg Med *17*:676–680, 1988.
22. Auerbach PS, Osterloh J, Braun O, et al: Efficacy of gastric emptying: Gastric lavage vs. emesis induced with ipecac. Ann Emerg Med *15*:692–698, 1986.
23. Fligner CL, Robertson WO: Request and report forms in toxicology screening. Abstract. *In* Proceedings of the American Association of Poison Control Centers (AACT/AAPCC/ABMT/CAPCC) Annual Scientific Meeting, Kansas City, KS, August 4–9, 1985.
24. Litovitz TL, Clark LR, Soloway RA: 1993 Annual Report of the American Association of Poison Control Centers National Data Collection System. Am J Emerg Med *12*:546–584, 1994.
25. Bailey DN: Changing trends in drug abuse. Abstract. California Association of Toxicologists—Newsletter, Winter 1990, p 20.
26. Caplan YH, Ottinger WE, Park J, et al: Drug and chemical related deaths: Incidence in the state of Maryland—1975 to 1980. J Forensic Sci *30*:1012–1021, 1985.
27. Norton LE, Garriott JC, Di Maio VJM: Drug detection at autopsy: A prospective study of 247 cases. J Forensic Sci *27*:61–71, 1982.
28. Fazen LE, Lovejoy FH, Crone RK, et al: Acute poisoning in a children's hospital: A 2-year experience. Pediatrics *77*:144–151, 1986.
29. Jacobsen D, Halvorsen K, Marstrander J, et al: Acute poisonings of children in Oslo. Acta Paediatr Scand *72*:553–557, 1983.
30. Trinkoff AM, Baker SP: Poisoning hospitalizations and deaths from solids and liquids among children and teenagers. Am J Public Health *76*:657–660, 1986.
31. Schwartz JG, Stuckey JH, Prihoda TJ, et al: Hospital-based toxicology: Patterns of use and abuse. Tex Med *86*:44–51, 1990.
32. Frings CS, Battaglia DJ, White RM: Status of drug-of-abuse testing in urine under blind conditions: An AACC study. Clin Chem *35*:891–894, 1989.
33. Quality Assurance Committee Report. Proceedings of the California Association of Toxicologists Meeting, Napa, CA, August, pp 13–16, 1995.
34. Rygnestad T, Berg KJ: Evaluation of benefits of drug analysis in the routine clinical management of acute self-poisoning. Clin Toxicol *22*:51–61, 1984.
35. Bury RW, Mashford ML: Use of a drug-screening service in an inner-city teaching hospital. Med J Aust *1*:132–133, 1981.
36. Teitelbaum DT, Morgan J, Gray G: Nonconcordance between clinical impression and laboratory findings in clinical toxicology. Clin Toxicol *10*:417–422, 1977.
37. Kellermann AL, Fihn SD, Logerfro JP, et al: Impact of drug screening in suspected overdose. Ann Emerg Med *16*:1206–1216, 1987.
38. Brett AS, Rothschild N, Gray R, et al: Predicting the clinical course in intentional drug overdose: Implications for use of the intensive care unit. Arch Intern Med *147*:133–137, 1987.
39. Brett AS: Implications of discordance between clinical impression and toxicology analysis in drug overdose. Arch Intern Med *148*:437–441, 1988.
40. Wiltbank TB, Sine HE, Brody BB: Are emergency toxicology measurements really used? Clin Chem *20*:116–118, 1974.
41. Mahoney JD, Gross PL, Stern TA: The use of the toxic screen in the management of overdosed patients. Abstract. *In* Proceedings of the AACT/AAPCC/ABMT/CAPCC Annual Scientific Meeting. Vancouver, BC, p 29, September 27 to October 2, 1987.
42. Helliwell M, Hampel G, Sinclair E: Value of emergency toxicological investigations in differential diagnosis of coma. BMJ *2*:819–821, 1979.
43. Jacobsen D, Fredericksen PS, Knutsen KM, et al: A prospective study of 1212 cases of acute poisoning: General epidemiology. Hum Toxicol *3*:93–106, 1984.
44. Sanguineti VR, Samuel SE: Comorbid substance abuse and recovery from acute psychiatric relapse. Hosp Community Psych *44*:1073–1076, 1993.
45. Tarcher AB: Principles and Practice of Environmental Medicine. New York, Plenum Publishing Corp., 1992.
46. Kneip TJ, Crable JV: Methods for Biologic Monitoring. A Manual for Assessing Human Exposure to Hazardous Substances. Washington, DC, American Public Health Association, 1988.

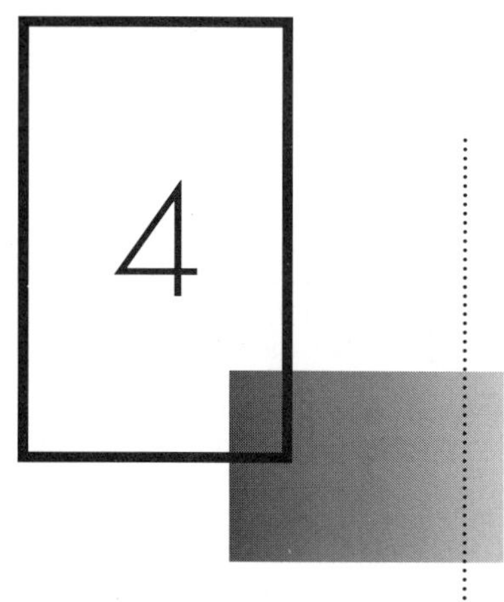

Principles of Pharmacology for the Clinician

BROOKS C. METTS, JR., PHARMD
WALTER J. HUNTER, PHARMD
JOHN AMBRE, MD, PHD

Knowledge of basic pharmacologic principles is key to a rational approach in solving clinical problems. This chapter reviews fundamental concepts in pharmacology and kinetics, with specific examples illustrating how these concepts relate to the diagnosis and treatment of drug overdose and poisoning.

DISPOSITION OF DRUGS AND TOXINS

Exposure to toxins can result from environmental contamination or from accidental or intentional administration of a toxin. Intoxication or poisoning is the result of the presence of a substance in a critical concentration at the site of the toxic action in the body. Factors that have a role in determining the concentration in the body include the amount of the toxin and the rates of its *absorption, distribution, metabolism,* and *excretion.*[1]

All of these disposition processes involve passage across cell membranes. Drugs and other substances pass through cell membranes by diffusing through aqueous pores in the membrane, or they pass directly through the lipoprotein membrane by dissolving in it and diffusing out the other side.

Diffusion and dissolution are passive processes (i.e., they do not require chemical energy), and they occur in response to and in the direction of a concentration difference (gradient). Dissolution in the lipoprotein membrane structure requires that the substance have some degree of lipid solubility. Movement across the membrane occurs from the side of higher concentration toward the side of lower concentration until the concentrations on both sides are the same. Filtration through cell membrane pores involves the flow of water in response to a hydrostatic or osmotic gradient. Water-soluble substances are transported with the water if they are small enough to pass through the pores.

The primary mode of passage of substances across capillaries, with the exception of the capillaries in the central nervous system, is by flow through intercellular spaces. For example, this is the process involved in filtration across glomerular capillaries. The absence of such spaces between endothelial cells in capillaries of the central nervous system constitutes the anatomic basis for the blood-brain barrier.

Specialized transport mechanisms are available for some substances. *Active transport processes* move substances against a concentration gradient. In active transport, there is relative selectivity for certain chemical structures, saturability, a requirement for metabolic energy, and susceptibility to inhibition. *Facilitated diffusion processes* are similar to active transport in that they have selectivity, saturability, and susceptibility to inhibition, but they do not require energy and do not work against a concentration gradient. High-molecular-weight substances, such as venoms, often enter cells through *pinocytosis.*

ABSORPTION

Absorption generally means movement of a substance into the blood. Of the various sites where absorption occurs, the gastrointestinal tract is the most important because the majority of acute poisonings involve ingestion. Several factors influence absorption from the stomach and intestines. Gastrointestinal absorption involves diffusion across lipid cell membranes of the lining epithelium because movement between lining cells is limited by tight intercellular junctions.

Nonionized, lipid-soluble substances are most readily absorbed in the gastrointestinal tract. Lipid-soluble, nonelectrolyte substances such as alcohols and glycols are rapidly absorbed, and absorption is limited only by factors that reduce their contact with the membrane, such as the presence of food.

For drugs and chemicals that are weak electrolytes, the pH at the absorption site may influence the degree of ionization and thus influence absorption, since membrane passage is easiest for the nonionized form. The extent of ionization at a particular pH depends on the ionization constant (p*K*) of the weak acid or base. The p*K* is the pH at which 50% of an electrolyte exists in the ionized form, and 50% in the nonionized form (Fig. 4–1). Absorption is best from the medium in which the substance is ionized the least. As shown in Figure 4–2, the nonionized form moves in response to its concentration gradient until concentrations are equal on each side of the membrane. Because the degree of ionization changes as the substance moves to the plasma compartment, the total concentration of the acidic substance becomes greater in the plasma. Similarly, for a basic substance, concentration in the plasma is favored by an alkaline-absorbing medium. The pH of the gastrointestinal tract can be influenced by disease (e.g., achlorhydria) or by administration of substances (e.g., antacids); these factors, in turn, can influence absorption from these sites.

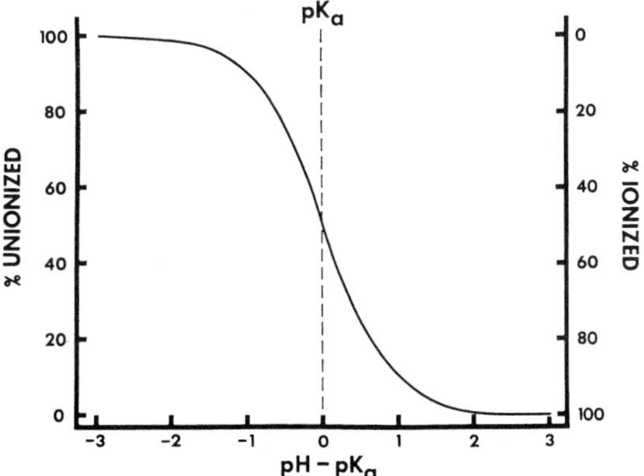

Figure 4–1. The effect of pH on the ionization of a weak acid. The acid is 50% ionized at a pH equal to pK_a. At higher pH values, it becomes increasingly more ionized; at lower pH values, it becomes increasingly more nonionized. The rate of change of ionization is greatest at pH values near the pK_a. (From LaDu BN, Mandel HG, Way EL: Fundamentals of Drug Metabolism and Disposition. Baltimore, Williams & Wilkins, p 5, 1971.)

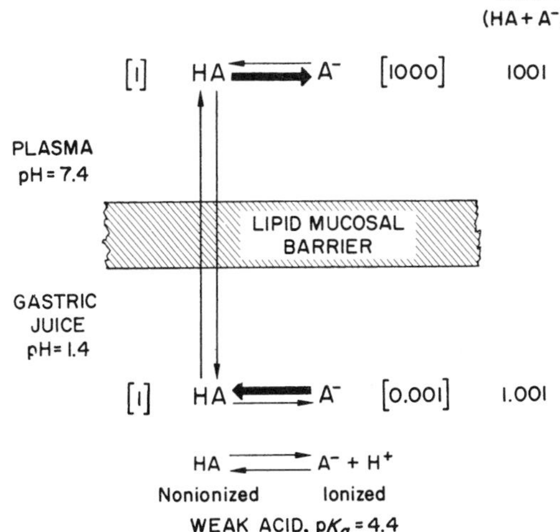

Figure 4–2. Influence of pH on the distribution of a weak acid between plasma and gastric juice, separated by a lipid barrier. (From Mayer SE, Melmon KL, Gilman AG: Introduction: The dynamics of drug absorption, distribution, and elimination. In Gilman AG, Goodman, LS, Gilman A (eds): The Pharmacological Basis of Therapeutics. New York, Macmillan Publishing Co., p 4, 1980.)

Strong electrolytes are absorbed to a limited extent. They are not influenced by pH because they are essentially completely ionized at any pH in the physiologic range. They diffuse slowly or depend on specialized mechanisms for absorption.

A few substances can be absorbed by specialized active transport processes, apparently because their chemical structures closely resembles those of natural substances that are normally transported by the system. The antitumor drug 5-fluorouracil is actively carried across intestinal mucosa by a process that transports the natural pyrimidine bases uracil and thymine.

In general, substances in solution are better absorbed than those in solid form. A certain degree of aqueous solubility also is required for efficient absorption. Some highly lipid-soluble materials are poorly absorbed for that reason. Finely divided, small particulate substances are better absorbed than are large particles.

Other factors modifying absorption that apply to gastrointestinal absorption are the concentration of the drug at the absorption site, the presence of food or binding agents, the total area of the absorbing surface, the rate of gastric emptying, the blood flow to the site, and intestinal motility.

A high concentration of a substance at the absorption site maximizes the concentration gradient into blood. The presence of food or other binding substances essentially reduces the concentration of absorbable material. The large absorbing surface of the small intestine makes it the primary site of gastrointestinal absorption for most substances—in fact, the absorbing area is so great that other factors such as pH may become relatively insignificant. The effect of rate of gastric emptying on absorption is probably the result of the hastening or the retarding of delivery of gastric contents to the large absorptive surface of the intestine. Blood flow to the stomach and intestines via the splanchnic vessels ordinarily is not rate limiting for absorption but presumably could be in the shock state. An increase in intestinal motility might reduce absorption by shortening intestinal transit time and reducing contact time with the absorbing surface. In the intoxicated patient, decreased motility might reduce absorption by allowing the formation of tablet masses, or it might increase absorption by prolonging transit time.

The value of thinking about these various influences on absorption is in knowing that the therapist can alter some of them. The drug or poison may affect these factors in such a way that intoxication is more severe or prolonged than it need be. The physician can facilitate recovery by recognizing and reversing effects that are detrimental or by influencing these factors in the patient's favor. For example, in a patient with tricyclic antidepressant overdose, the anticholinergic effects on the gastrointestinal tract might include delayed gastric emptying and decreased intestinal motility. Retention of some drug in the stomach may allow removal by lavage. Decreased intestinal motility may reduce absorption from a tablet mass but may also prevent expulsion of unabsorbed tablets. Administration of activated charcoal may bind a drug or toxin and reduce the absorbable drug concentration, but the charcoal may also form a stagnant mass in the intestine that eventually takes on the consistency of concrete. Administration of an osmotic cathartic should aid in rectal passage of undissolved tablets or material and charcoal-bound substance.

Skin Absorption

The skin, to a great extent, is an effective barrier to toxic chemical absorption. The intact skin behaves qualitatively like cellular membranes. Thus, substances penetrate the skin at rates determined by their lipid solubility. Lipid-soluble organophosphate insecticides are readily absorbed from skin and thus represent a hazard to medical personnel who handle the exposed patient. Organic solvents, such as carbon tetrachloride, methanol, and others that are present as vehicles for some industrial toxins, may enhance skin absorption. Dimethyl sulfoxide, a common commercial solvent, is particularly efficient as a carrier in skin absorption. Inflammation, rubbing, and other causes of increased skin blood flow may increase absorption, whereas the application of tourniquets or the local application of ice may retard absorption.

Absorption from the Respiratory Tract

Some toxic fumes, particulate matter, and gases may be absorbed via the lungs. Particle size is an important factor in lung retention of a particulate substance, because only particles smaller than 1 μm in diameter can penetrate to the lower airways. Generally, the only means of reducing lung absorption is removal of the patient from the toxic atmosphere.

DISTRIBUTION

After absorption, which involves movement into the blood and the mechanical displacement of the blood to the various body organs by the pumping action of the heart, the substance moves into organ tissues. This is the process of *distribution.*

Volume of Distribution

As a rule, the amount of drug or poison at the specific site of its toxic action is a very small part of the total amount of that substance in the body. Each substance is distributed to the tissues of the body in a definite pattern. This pattern is established when the concentrations of that substance in the various tissues are in equilibrium. Equilibrium does not mean that all tissue concentrations are equal; rather, it means that there is no net transfer of substance from one tissue to another. Usually, it is not possible or practical to measure concentrations in each tissue at the substance's site of action. Actually, even in the target tissue, most of the substance present is associated with tissue membranes or molecules having nothing to do with the substance's action; that is, only a fraction of the drug is bound to specific receptors. Because plasma is the tissue in which drugs' and other substances' concentrations are most easily measured, and since plasma is the medium of distribution, drug and toxin distribution usually are related to plasma concentrations.

The *volume of distribution* is the apparent volume in which the substance is distributed. It is the volume that the drug would occupy if it were present elsewhere at the same concentration found in plasma. The volume of distribution is clinically useful because it tends to be characteristic of the substance and is constant over a wide range of doses. It allows prediction of the plasma concentrations that will be produced by a given amount of the substance.

Factors Influencing Distribution

The rate and extent to which a substance reaches the tissues of each organ is determined by the blood flow through the organ, the substance's ability to cross capillary and cell membranes, and the substance's relative partitioning between blood and tissue.

Blood Flow

The early phase of distribution is primarily a reflection of the rate of blood flow to various organs.

Distribution into highly perfused tissues, such as the brain, liver, and kidney, is faster than distribution into adipose tissue and muscle. This feature is dramatically illustrated by the time course of blood and tissue concentrations after an intravenous dose of thiopental (Fig. 4–3).

Capillary Membrane Passage

Movement from blood into the extracellular or interstitial space of tissues (except for brain) occurs readily because most drugs and toxins are smaller than albumin and are able to pass through the intercellular channels of the capillary endothelial membrane. Lipid-soluble substances may also move directly across capillary endothelial cells to reach the interstitial space. Lipid-insoluble substances are not able to pass cell membranes (see discussion later in this chapter) and therefore may be limited to the extracellular tissue spaces.

The term *blood-brain barrier* refers to the brain capillary membranes' lack of intercellular channels or pores; movement directly across cell membranes is the only means of access to brain extracellular fluid. The blood-brain barrier is therefore essentially a lipid barrier, and in general, lipid-insoluble substances have limited access to—and thus little effect on—the central nervous system.

Cell Membrane Passage

The ability of a drug to cross cell membranes is a function of its lipid solubility and the degree of protein binding. The same factors influencing membrane passage that were considered under the section on absorption also apply here. Lipid-soluble nonelectrolytes pass readily into cells, whereas strong electrolytes pass poorly. Passage by weak electrolytes depends on their ionization state and the relative lipid solubility of their un-ionized form.

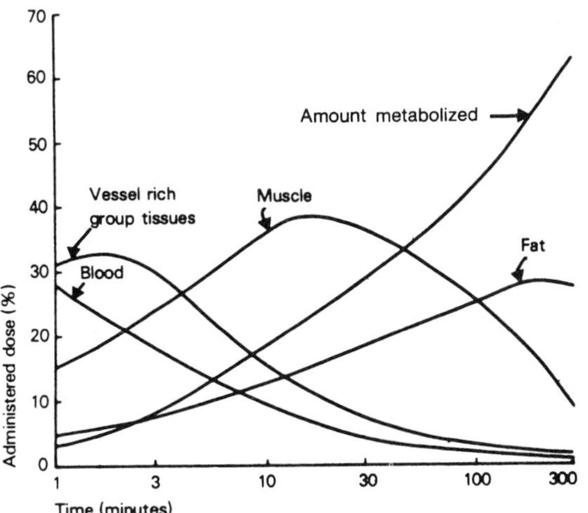

Figure 4–3. Distribution of thiopental after an intravenous injection. The time course of distribution is a reflection of tissue blood flow. The drug moves quickly into highly perfused tissues, such as brain, liver, and kidney, and more slowly into muscle and fat tissue. (From Ghoneim MM, Korttila K: Pharmacokinetics of intravenous anaesthetics: Implications for clinical use. Clin Pharmacokinet 2:344, 1977.)

EFFECT OF pH

It is generally assumed that only the non-ionized forms of organic acids and bases are sufficiently lipid soluble to pass through cell membranes. The ionized form is too polar to penetrate the membrane. Because many drugs and other substances are weak organic acids or bases, the relative pH of blood and tissue fluids influences the proportion of ionized to non-ionized species in these fluids and, therefore, the amount in the form capable of penetrating cell membranes. Therefore, normal pH differences between body fluids and tissues influence the normal distribution of these substances. The influence of changes in pH on distribution is seen only with substances whose p*K* is in a range in which ionization state changes substantially with pH changes that fall within the physiologic range. The p*K* of a weak acid or base is the pH at which 50% exists in the ionized and 50% in the non-ionized form. As pH decreases, weak bases become more ionized; in contrast, as pH increases, weak acids become more ionized. The distribution of these substances is altered if they move into a tissue fluid in which the pH—and, consequently, their ionization state—is different.

The practical application of this phenomenon can be seen in the effect systemic pH changes have on the anesthesia produced by the weak acid phenobarbital. When phenobarbital is administered and blood pH is lowered, there is a drop in plasma drug level, an increase in brain levels, and a deepening of anesthesia. Blood alkalosis produces the opposite effects.[2] This phenomenon must be considered when the physician is deciding what method to use to alkalinize the urine in order to hasten phenobarbital excretion.

PROTEIN BINDING

Many drugs and poisons are bound to some extent to plasma proteins, particularly albumin. The binding involves reversible weak electrostatic, hydrophobic, or van der Waals forces but, in some cases, may involve the formation of covalent bonds. The extent of binding varies greatly. Some lipophilic organic acids are more than 90% bound, whereas small, neutral hydrophilic organic bases may also bind to plasma proteins. However, albumin tends to bind acids more strongly and extensively than bases. Some basic substances are bound to other plasma components, such as the acute-phase reactant α_1-acid glycoprotein.

Binding in the plasma limits movement of substances through capillaries and into the tissues. Only the unbound substance crosses cell membranes because the large molecular size of substance-protein complexes limits such movement. Equilibrium is established between the unbound substance in plasma and the tissue water. Because a drug or poison ordinarily must pass some membranes to reach its site of action, only the unbound portion represents the active substance. Binding may influence the processes of liver uptake and renal excretion (discussed later).

In the case of drug overdose, distribution may be altered by increasing drug concentrations if plasma protein binding sites become saturated. Then, as the concentrations increase, the fraction of unbound drug rises, and the volume of distribution increases. More drug would move into tissues and penetrate to the site of toxic action. This concentration-dependent decrease in protein binding could be responsible for the poor correlation between total (free plus bound) plasma concentrations and the clinical status of the patient.

The converse of the above process is the basis for treating a drug toxicity. Hybridoma techniques may allow production of large quantities of substance-specific antibodies. The high affinity-specific antibodies (or their Fab fragments) can be administered to bind a substance in an inactive complex that is excreted. This is demonstrated by the digoxin-specific Fab fragments (Fig. 4–4).[3]

Free digoxin in the serum is bound immediately, and digoxin in the tissues is redistributed back to the vascular system, where it, in turn, also is bound. Signs of toxicity dissipate. Total serum digoxin level, consisting almost entirely of bound inactive drug, increases 10-fold, reflecting the influx of digoxin from tissue; the level then begins to decline at a rate determined by the excretion of the Fab-drug complex.

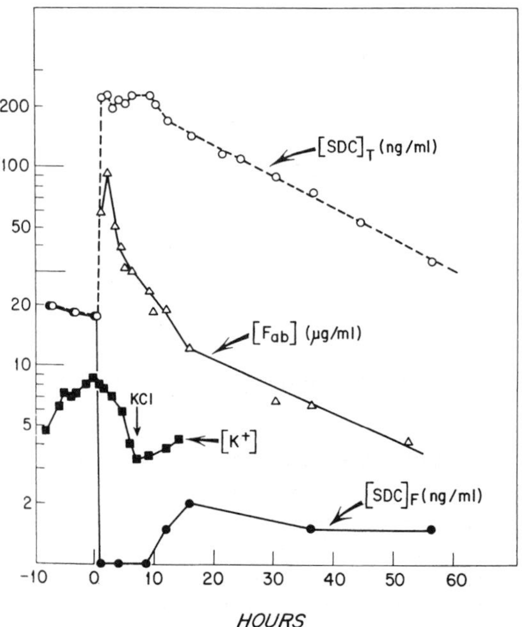

Figure 4–4. Fab therapy of digoxin toxicity. (From Smith TW, Haber E, Yeatman L, Butler VP: Reversal of advanced digoxin toxicity with Fab fragments of digoxin-specific antibodies. N Engl J Med *294:*797–800, 1976. Reprinted, by permission, from the *New England Journal of Medicine.*)

REDISTRIBUTION

In some cases, movement of substances into more slowly penetrated tissues, rather than metabolism and excretion of the substance, may be responsible for the termination of effects. An example is the redistribution of lipid-soluble thiopental from its site of action in the brain to the more slowly perfused muscle and fat tissues. After single intravenous doses, redistribution to these tissues is primarily responsible for the termination of its anesthetic effect, as initially high levels in rapidly perfused brain tissue continue to equilibrate with decreasing blood levels (see Fig. 4–3). In circumstances in which repeated administration or continuous infusion is used, levels in these more slowly perfused muscle and fat tissues equilibrate and the lipophilic drug accumulates. When infusion is stopped, the anesthetic effect disappears at the slower rate, being dependent on metabolism rather than on redistribution.

TISSUE RESERVOIRS

For lipophilic drugs, slowly perfused muscle and fat tissues may serve as a reservoir for storage. For other drugs, slowly mobilized intracellular drug present in many tissues may function as a reservoir. In toxicology, the *reservoir effect* is most evident in situations in which drug removal from plasma is augmented by artificial means, such as with hemodialysis or hemoperfusion.

The drug lithium, after a single dose, initially is distributed to extracellular fluid and then more slowly moves inside cells. With repeated dosing, it eventually has a distribution volume similar to that of total body water and has fairly uniform concentration in all body tissue.[4] Plasma concentrations are lowered very efficiently by hemodialysis. When dialysis is discontinued, however, plasma levels may rise again, owing to the movement of lithium out of cellular stores (Fig. 4–5).

BIOTRANSFORMATION PATHWAYS (METABOLISM)

Most foreign chemicals introduced into the body undergo a chemical transformation before excretion. This process has been called *metabolism* to draw a parallel between it and the chemical transformations undergone by normal or endogenous body chemicals. The term *biotransformation* is now more widely used to describe the process; however, the products of this process are generally called *metabolites*. Transformation of drugs and chemicals can result in compounds that are more active or toxic than the original compound, or in those that are less active or toxic. In general, biotransformation can be characterized as processes that produce more water-soluble or polar compounds. Metabolites are, therefore, chemical

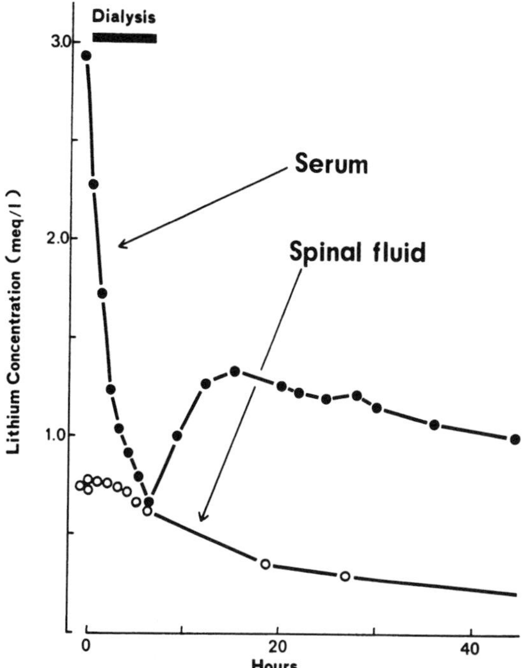

Figure 4–5. Serum and spinal fluid lithium levels in a 48-year-old lithium-intoxicated man who was anuric. Serum levels decline rapidly with dialysis and rise again as lithium redistributes from tissues. Spinal fluid levels respond slowly to changes in serum level. (From Amdisen A, Skjoldborg H: Haemodialysis for lithium poisoning. Lancet *2*:213, 1969.)

forms that are less able to move through biomembranes; more restricted in their distribution to tissues; less readily reabsorbed from renal tubules, bile duct or intestine; and ultimately more easily excreted.

Biotransformation may occur in any tissue, including the blood. However, it is generally most active or quantitatively most important in the liver. The metabolizing enzymes are present in various parts of the liver cell. Their location is conventionally indicated by the *in vitro* fraction of the homogenized liver tissue in which the enzymatic activity is present, rather than by the subcellular structure with which the enzyme is associated *in vivo.* Drug-metabolizing enzymes are therefore referred to as *soluble, mitochondrial,* or *microsomal* enzymes.

Drugs and other foreign chemicals may undergo three general types of biotransformation: *oxidation/reduction, hydrolysis,* and *conjugation.*[5] Drug-metabolizing enzymes subserving oxidation reactions are primarily found in the microsome (Table 4–1), whereas hydrolytic and conjugating enzymes may be found in the cytosol or extracellularly in the plasma. Substances that chemically resemble endogenous substances may be metabolized by the same enzymes as these normal body constituents.

Most of the reactions involved in metabolism may be considered chemical oxidations. A hemoprotein involved in many of the microsomal reactions as an electron transport function is *cytochrome P-450.* An outline of the electron transport chain involving P-450 and the oxidation of substances by the hepatic endoplasmic reticulum is shown in Figure 4–6. NADPH is oxidized by the flavoprotein cytochrome P-450 reductase, and an electron is transported to the oxidized form of cytochrome P-450, which has formed a complex with the compound. The reduced form of the P-450 chemical complex binds oxygen, and another electron is introduced to generate oxidized chemical, oxidized P-450, and water (see Chapter 21 on drug-drug interactions).

The cytochrome P-450 system was originally thought to consist of a few hemoproteins with broad substrate activity. It is now known that there are several classes or families of P-450 isoenzymes with varying substrate specificity. Different inducers of drug metabolism, such as phenobarbital and other chemicals (mentioned in a following section), may promote the formation of specific isoenzymes. Different P-450 isoenzymes may also be preferentially involved in production of different metabolites from a particular substance.

Other routes of chemical metabolism involve chemical reduction, hydrolysis, and glucuronide conjugation. Figure 4–7 illustrates specific examples of the major pathways of drug metabolism.

Many drugs undergo sequential reactions; a common example is hydroxylation followed by conjugation with glucuronic acid or activated sulfate (or both) on the hydroxyl group. This process is so common that drug metabolism is often described as taking place in two phases.[6] *Phase one* reactions include an oxidation, reduction, or hydrolysis step that introduces or unmasks a functionality such as hydroxyl (—OH), sulfhydryl (—SH), amine (—NH_2, or carboxyl

Table 4–1. Sites of Drug Metabolism

Metabolic Pathways	Location of Enzymes*
Oxidations	
Hydroxylation	M
Dealkylation	M
Epoxidation	M
S- and *N*-Oxidation	M
Desulfuration	M
Dehalogenation	M
Deamination	M, mitochondria
Alcohol oxidation	M, S
Aldehyde oxidation	S
Reductions	
Aldehyde reduction	S
Azoreduction	M
Nitroreduction	M, S
Hydrolyses	
De-esterification	M, S, plasma
Deamination	M, S
Conjugations	
Glucuronidation	M
Sulfation	S
Glutathione conjugation	S
Methylation	S
Acylation	S

*M, microsomes (endoplastic reticulum); S, soluble fraction (cytosol).

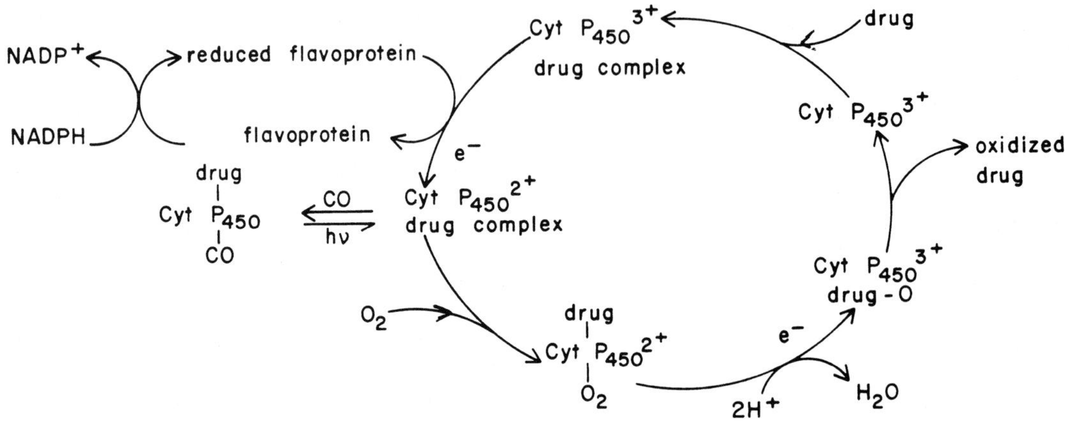

Figure 4–6. Electron flow pathway in microsomal drug metabolizing system. NADPH is oxidized by the flavoprotein cytochrome P-450 reductase (cyt P-450), and an electron is transferred to the oxidized form of cytochrome P-450 that has formed a complex with the drug. The reduced form of cytochrome P-450 drug complex binds oxygen and another electron and is introduced to generate oxidized drug, oxidized P-450, and water. The oxidized cytochrome P-450 is then available to bind another drug molecule and continue the cycle. (Adapted from Goldstein A, Aronow L, Kalman S: Principles of Drug Action. 2nd ed. New York, John Wiley & Sons, 243, 1974.)

(—COOH) group on the chemical structure. These are primarily microsomal (endoplastic reticulum) enzymatic reactions. *Phase two* reactions consist of a synthetic or conjugation reaction in which the substance or a phase one metabolite is linked through the functional group to an endogenous compound such as glucuronic acid or sulfate to form a conjugate. These are primarily cytosol or soluble-phase enzymes. The conjugate is not only more water soluble and ionizable but may also be handled by the acid transport mechanism of the excretory systems.

As indicated previously, important conjugation reactions and some oxidative and hydrolytic enzyme systems are available for metabolism at nonmicro-

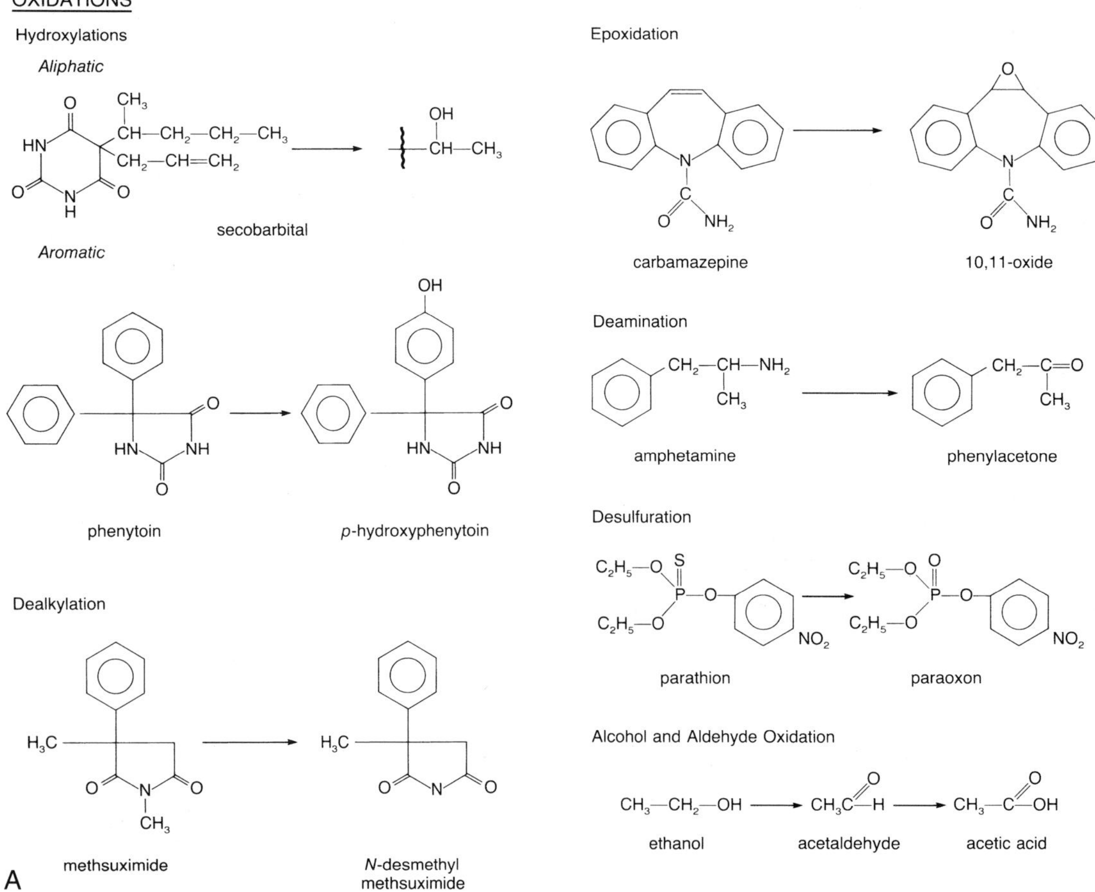

Figure 4–7. Typical metabolic reactions. *A,* Oxidations.

somal sites in liver, in other tissues, and in plasma (see Table 4–1).

Microsomal substance–metabolizing enzymes are subject to induction. Some common drugs, such as phenobarbital and various chemicals, are capable of inducing the rate of metabolism of many other substances processed by microsomal enzymes. Phenobarbital and glutethimide, which induce the metabolism of other substances, also induce their own rate of metabolism with repeated administration. Unfortunately, induction of the rate of metabolism is not useful in the treatment of acute intoxication because the process requires synthesis of new enzyme and takes place over a period of days. A compound that "activates" enzymes already present in the liver might be useful in this manner, but such a compound is not available.

Metabolizing enzymes also are subject to inhibition of their activity on one substance (substrate) by competition from alternate substances (substrates). Inhibition may also be noncompetitive, resulting from inactivation of metabolizing enzymes by highly reactive substances. Inhibition is a phenomenon that can take place acutely. Significant competitive inhibition is likely when the substance has saturated its metabolizing enzyme system. Few drugs or toxins saturate the system, even when they are taken in overdose. Exceptions are salicylates, methanol, ethanol, theophylline, acetaminophen, and phenytoin. Ethyl alcohol can induce microsomal drug metabolism chronically and inhibit it acutely. For example, when alcoholic subjects are sober, they have a faster-than-normal rate of phenobarbital metabolism, which slows when alcohol also is present in their blood. Inhibition of metabolism has a definite but limited place in the treatment of acute intoxication. The best example involving inhibition of metabolism is the treatment of acute methanol metabolism to formate by administration of ethanol and, more recently, by the administration of 4-methylpyrazole.[7]

The phenomenon of induction and inhibition of microsomal drug metabolism is superimposed on a normal interindividual variation in rates of metabolism of approximately 3- to 20-fold.[8]

It is widely believed, as a result of Vesell's[8] studies in identical and fraternal twins, that the major cause

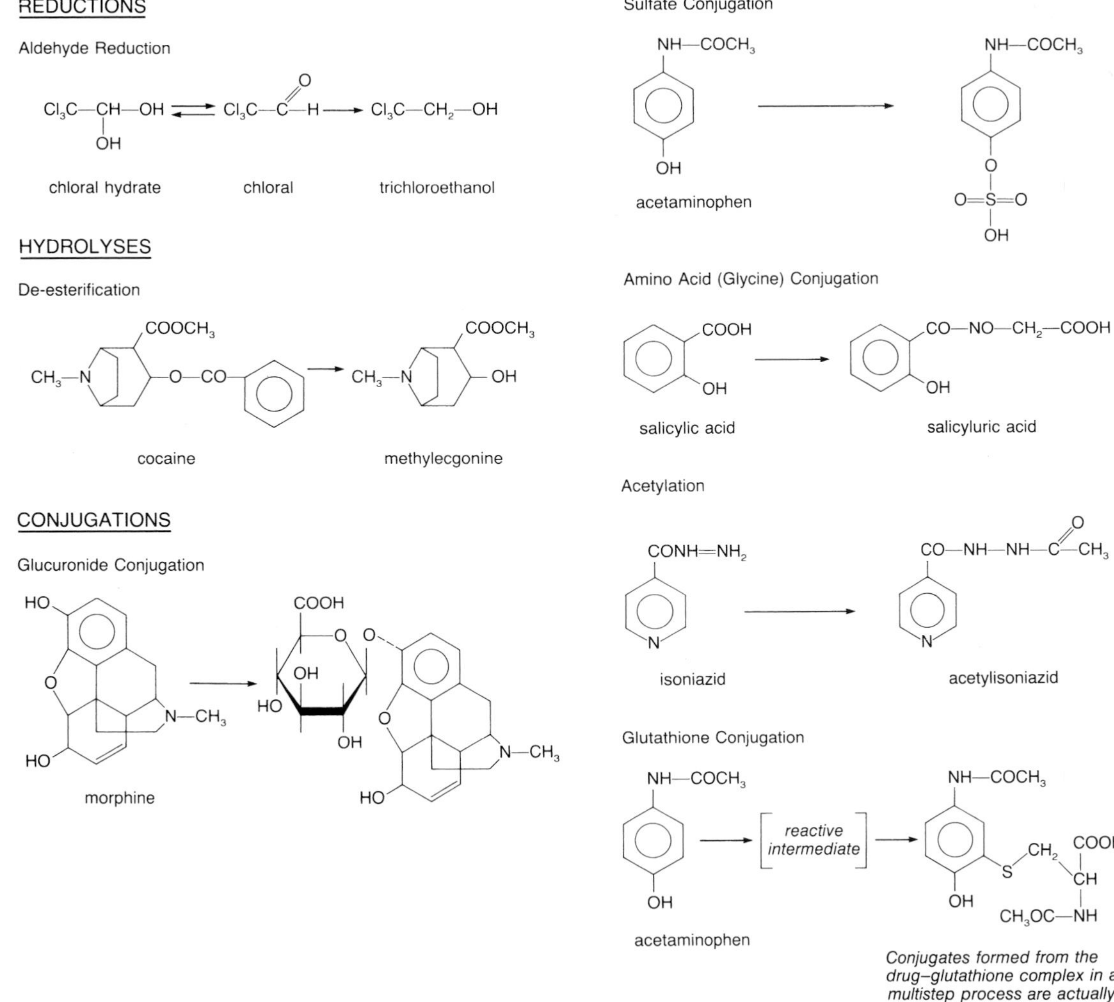

Figure 4–7 *Continued B,* Reductions and other reactions.

of the large interindividual differences in rates of metabolism is genetic. Environmental factors seemed to play a minor roll. Individuals with the slowest rates of metabolism were subject to the greatest degree of induction when treated with phenobarbital, an inducer of microsomal drug metabolism. The extent to which variation in rates of metabolism makes different individuals more or less susceptible to drug toxicity has not been fully explored.[9]

Nonmicrosomal enzyme systems exhibit similar interindividual variations in rates, and some, such as the cholinesterase system in plasma, exhibit genetic polymorphism. However, they are generally not subject to enzyme induction.

Some compounds may be metabolized nonenzymatically (chemical decomposition) within the body. Benzoylecgonine, a major metabolite of cocaine, probably arises from cocaine by spontaneous hydrolysis.[10]

ACTIVE METABOLITES

In some cases, toxicity is directly related to the products of drug metabolism (Tables 4–2 and 4–3).[11] Although drug metabolism is designed to render agents more water soluble and less toxic, there are occasions when the metabolite possesses greater toxicity than the parent compound.

The products may be major metabolites that accumulate in the systemic circulation, or they may be quantitatively minor, acting locally in the cell where they are formed. Toxicity due to accumulation of an active metabolite characteristically exhibits a latency that is due to the time required for accumulation.[12–14] Clinically, the patient exhibits increasing toxic effects rather than improvement in the hours after hospital admission. Such *drug toxification* occurs in methanol, ethylene glycol, and acetaminophen poisoning.

Table 4–2. Active Metabolites of Therapeutic Agents

Acetohexamide	Hydroxyhexamide
Allopurinol	Oxypurinol
Amitriptyline	Nortriptyline 10-Hydroxynortriptyline
Carbamazepine	Carbamazepine epoxide
Chlordiazepoxide	*n*-Desmethychlordiazepoxide Demoxepam
Diazepam	*n*-Desmethyldiazepam Oxazepam
Disopyramide	*n*-Desalkyldisopyramide
Flurazepam	*n*-Desalkylflurazepam
Glutethamide	4-Hydroxyglutethamide
Imipramine	Desipramine
Lidocaine	Monoethylglycinexylidide, glycinexylidide
Meperidine	Normeperidine
Phenylbutazone	Oxyphenbutazone
Procainamide	*n*-Acetylprocainamide
Propranolol	4-Hydroxypropranolol
Sulindac	Sulfide metabolite
Tolbutamide	Hydroxytolbutamide
Verapamil	Norverapamil

Adapted from Wilkinson GR, Rawlings MD (eds): Drug Metabolism and Disposition: Considerations in Clinical Pharmacology. Boston, MTP Press, 1985.

Table 4–3. Toxic Agents with Active Metabolic Intermediates

Agent	Active Product
Acetaminophen	*n*-Hydroxylated intermediate
Acetylhydrazine	*n*-Hydroxylated intermediate and rearrangement
Aflatoxin B_1	Epoxide
Benzene	Epoxide
Benzo[α]pyrene	Epoxide
Carbon tetrachloride	Free radical
Chloroform	Phosgene
Cyclophosphamide	Hydroxylation and rearrangement
Halothane	Free radical
Parathion	Paraoxon
Vinyl chloride	Epoxide

Methanol is an example of a substance whose toxicity is enhanced by metabolism. The active metabolite in this case is formic acid. Formate is responsible for the ocular toxicity of methanol and may account for the metabolic acidosis in humans.[14] The time required for metabolite accumulation is responsible for the usual 10- to 20-hour latent period between methanol ingestion and the development of clinical signs and symptoms. As already mentioned, it is possible to inhibit the metabolism of methanol to formate by administration of ethanol, which has much greater affinity for the alcohol-oxidizing enzyme system. More recently, the use of 4-methylpyrazole, a potent inhibitor of alcohol dehydrogenase, has been proposed as a treatment for preventing the formation of toxic metabolites in methanol and ethylene glycol exposures.[7]

The clinical course following ingestion of a single large overdose of the anticonvulsant methsuximide (Celontin) is strikingly biphasic. The initially stuporous patient appears to recover and then lapses into deep coma several hours later. The prolonged second phase of coma is apparently due to accumulation of the active metabolite *N*-desmethylmethsuximide.[15]

Other active, toxic metabolites are not quantitatively prominent and do not accumulate systemically but act locally as the proximate toxin. These metabolites are reactive intermediates that are ordinarily inactivated by protective mechanisms in the cell. Two examples of reactive metabolites formed by microsomal oxidation are epoxides and quinones (Fig. 4–8). The sulfhydryl compound glutathione results in formation of an inactive conjugate. When a large overdose of acetaminophen is taken, the limited glutathione stores of the cell are depleted by excessive formation of the reactive metabolites, and the conjugation process is overwhelmed. The intermediate then reacts with vital cell components, and cell damage occurs. Induction of the microsomal oxidation pathway producing the reactive product may lead to glutathione depletion and tissue damage in circumstances in which excessive therapeutic amounts of the drug are taken.

The finding that the availability of glutathione in

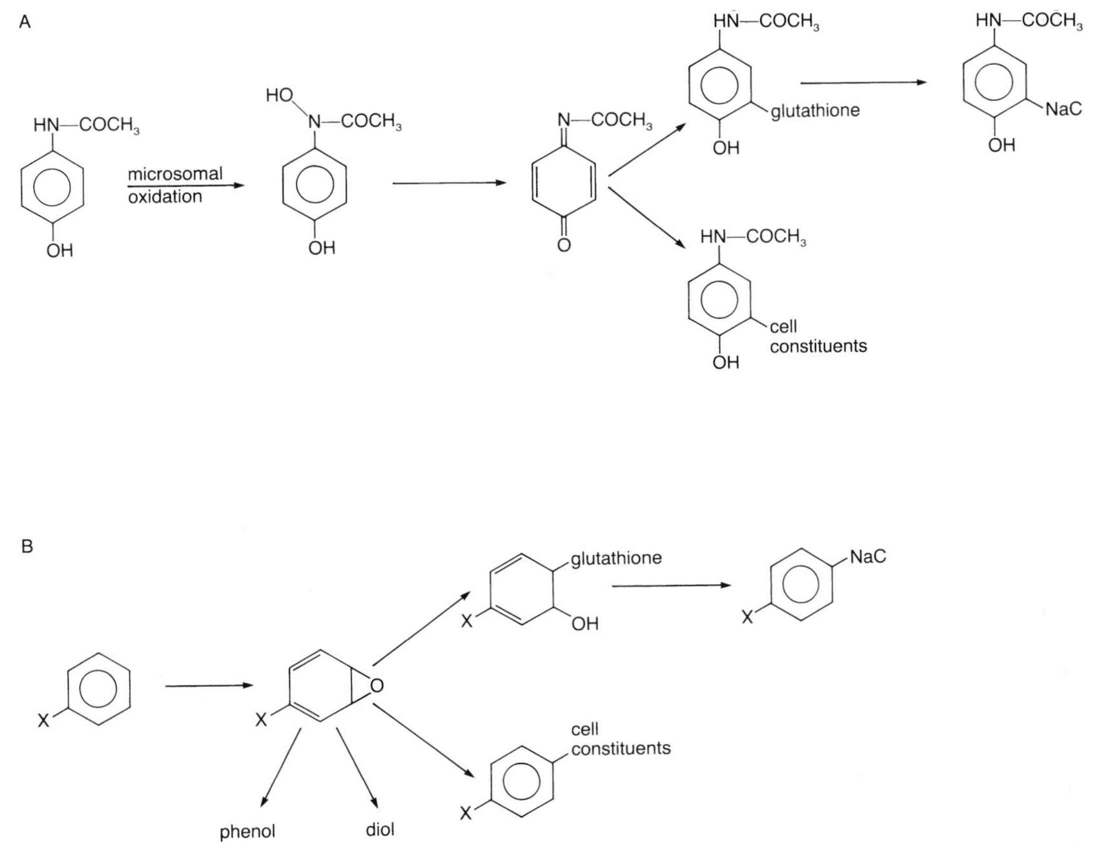

Figure 4–8. *A,* Acetaminophen may react with tissue components by formation of a quinone intermediate. Normally, the quinone form reacts with liver cell glutathione and is excreted as the mercapturic conjugate. *B,* An aromatic compound such as monohalogenated benzene may be metabolized to an epoxide. This reactive intermediate is converted spontaneously to the phenol or by further oxidation to the dihydroxy compound (diol). It may also react with glutathione and eventually be excreted as a mercapturic conjugate. If glutathione is not available, the epoxide may react with tissue components.

liver cells correlates inversely with the extent of liver necrosis induced by acetaminophen was an important step in the understanding of this mechanism of toxicity.[16] Since exogenous glutathione cannot enter the liver cell, the search for an acetaminophen antidote involved trials of various other sulfhydryl compounds that might substitute for glutathione. *N*-Acetylcysteine was found to be effective and well tolerated.

Polycyclic aromatic hydrocarbons, naphthalene, monohalogenated benzene, aflatoxins, and presumably benzene are metabolized to epoxides. Halogenated benzenes are hepatotoxins that produce liver damage in a manner analogous to that of acetaminophen. Polycyclic aromatic hydrocarbons and aflatoxins are carcinogenic substances that apparently interact with DNA by means of the reactive epoxide intermediates to initiate the neoplastic transformation of cells. Possibly, individual susceptibility to the carcinogenic effects of these chemicals is related to the level of activity of the cellular oxidative enzyme producing the toxic metabolite.[17, 18]

EXCRETION

Excretion or the process of drug/toxin/metabolite elimination plays a significant role in the practice of toxicology. In the acute setting, the clinician has two therapeutic options for excretion that often are drug/toxin specific. The first therapeutic option involves allowing the drug or toxin to be normally eliminated from the body while at the same time supportive care and hemodynamic monitoring are provided to prevent adverse consequences.[1] The best example of this type of approach involves phenytoin overdoses in which the drug is believed to be already in the systemic circulation. Phenytoin can be bound and inactivated by activated charcoal if it is not already in the blood stream. There is no antidote or reversal agent for phenytoin; hemodialysis and hemofiltration also are ineffective. Therefore, the only option is to allow the medication to be excreted normally and to provide monitoring and supportive care in order to prevent adverse cardiovascular and neurologic consequences.[19]

The other therapeutic option involves enhancing elimination of the drug/toxin/metabolite to prevent or decrease the contact time with organ systems and tissues of the body. The rationale is that decreasing this contact time will prevent irreversible damage and enhance the potential for full recovery. A prototypical example of enhanced excretion can be seen with potassium supplement overdoses.[1] Potassium often is given orally and parenterally to replace or maintain serum potassium concentrations for patients receiving diuretics, aminoglycosides, or amphotericin B. These agents are known to renally waste endogenous potassium. Potassium oversupplementation may cause induction of cardiac arrhythmias. Potassium can be driven from the extracellular fluid into intracellular fluid by administration of glucose and insulin. This measure is generally temporary, and enhancement of excretion by administration of sodium polystyrene sulfonate (Kayexalate) or fluid and diuretics generally is required. Most often, both methods (normal excretion with supportive care plus enhanced excretion) are instituted if plausible, and data to support such endeavors have been published. Drug/toxin/metabolite elimination can be attained via a number of organ systems. Renal elimination is the most viable and important system in toxicology. Biliary and pulmonary elimination has a minor role in the excretion process.[20]

Renal Elimination

Drugs/toxins/metabolites are processed by the kidneys in the same fashion as are endogenous substances (catecholamines, neurotransmitters). Most substances are filtered at the glomerulus. The larger the molecule, the less likely it will be filtered at the glomerulus; thus, plasma protein binding can inhibit glomerular filtration. Once the drugs/toxins/metabolites are in the tubule, they may remain and be eliminated. The lipophilicity of the substance is a major determinant. The more polar (hydrophilic) the substance, the more likely it will remain in the tubule and be excreted. The more nonpolar (lipophilic) the compound, the greater the chance that tubular reabsorption will occur. Tubular reabsorption occurs by means of passive diffusion across the tubule wall into the blood stream. As with enterohepatic recirculation, the goal is to eliminate the drug/toxin/metabolite and prevent reabsorption. Urinary divergence can be accomplished by a process known as *ion trapping*.[21] This process is highly dependent on the pH of the urine and p*K* of the substance. The p*K* of a weak acid (salicylates and phenobarbital) or a weak base (quinidine and amphetamines) is the pH at which it is half ionized. When the pH is increased, weak acids become more ionized; when the pH is decreased, weak bases become more ionized. Once in the ionized form, the drug/toxin/metabolite is unable to pass through the tubule membrane and becomes trapped and is excreted—hence, the term *ion trapping*. Only the un-ionized form has the ability to cross membranes and return to the blood stream to potentially cause further toxicity. Therefore, the excretion of toxic weak acids may be enhanced through alkalization of the urine. The use of sodium bicarbonate is the preferred method. Enhancement of the excretion of weak bases, such as phencyclidine and amphetamine, can be accomplished by urinary acidification through the use of ascorbic acid, hydrochloric acid, or ammonium chloride; this method is now discouraged because of the associated risk of metabolic acidosis and myoglobinuria. The final step in the renal process is tubular secretion. *Secretion* can occur in the proximal tubule by one of two processes. One process handles acids and the second one handles bases. In tubular secretion, drug/toxin/metabolites are secreted back into the tubule for excretion. This is obviously advantageous, but control or enhancement of the process is not possible. Tubular secretion is an active transport process that requires energy. It also is competitive and saturable, and this limits its true advantage.

Diuresis

Enhancement of urine flow is a beneficial means of drug/toxin/metabolite excretion, but it is substance specific. Drugs known to be highly dependent on glomerular filtration may be excreted in proportion to the glomerular filtration rate (see Chapter 5).

Biliary/Enteric Excretion

Drugs/toxin metabolites excreted or eliminated in this manner enter the intestine for fecal excretion. They can enter from the biliary system or diffuse into the intestine from the general circulation along a concentration gradient. The biliary/enteric route of elimination can be a beneficial and useful tool to the clinician. Many drugs/toxin/metabolites can be bound up and inactivated by certain agents. Activated charcoal and cholestyramine have been shown to be effective in binding, inactivating, or adsorbing drugs/toxins/metabolites and allowing them to be harmlessly eliminated in the feces (see Chapter 1).

Pulmonary Excretion

The body has the ability to excrete volatile anesthetics by the lungs. Paraldehyde also is partially eliminated by the lungs. Toxic gases such as carbon monoxide and hydrogen sulfide also are excreted by the pulmonary route. Determining factors that can affect pulmonary excretion include minute ventilation, ventilation-perfusion status, drug solubility, and tidal volume.

PHARMACOKINETICS

Clinical pharmacokinetics is the mathematic study or description of a drug/toxin/metabolite concentration following entry into the body. Simply stated, it is what the body "does" to the substance. It involves absorption, distribution, metabolism, and finally, elimination. Conversely, *pharmacodynamics* relates an agent's concentration to effect. Simply stated, pharmacodynamics is what the substance "does" to

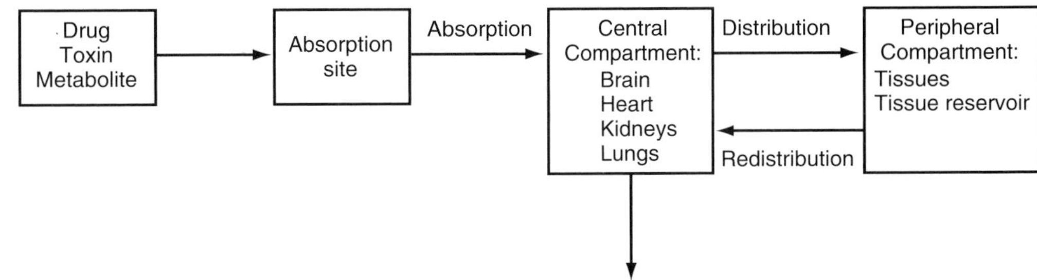

Figure 4–9. Example of a two-compartment model.

the body. Effects can be the desired outcome or undesired adverse consequences.

Most drugs/toxins/metabolites that are predominantly renally excreted follow two-compartment model changes in concentrations[22] (Fig. 4–9). Following absorption, the drug/toxin/metabolite can be found in the central compartment.

Once in the central compartment, the substance can be eliminated or distributed into the peripheral compartment. The central compartment includes the highly perfused organs and tissues of the heart, brain, lungs, and kidneys. The peripheral compartment includes poorly perfused organs and tissues, as well as tissue storage reservoirs. A prototypical two-compartment model medication is digoxin.

From a single dose of an agent, a concentration-versus-time curve can be plotted or predicted. Figure 4–10 depicts an absorption phase, a distribution α phase, and finally an elimination β phase. Serum concentration (Cs) can be determined with the following equation:

$$\mathrm{Cs} = \frac{\mathrm{Dose}}{\mathrm{Vd}}$$

where Vd is the volume of distribution. In the acute intoxication presentation, the actual dosage is generally unknown or can only be estimated. Therefore, this equation is of academic interest only. However, as is discussed later in this chapter, the measured Cs can be useful to the clinician.

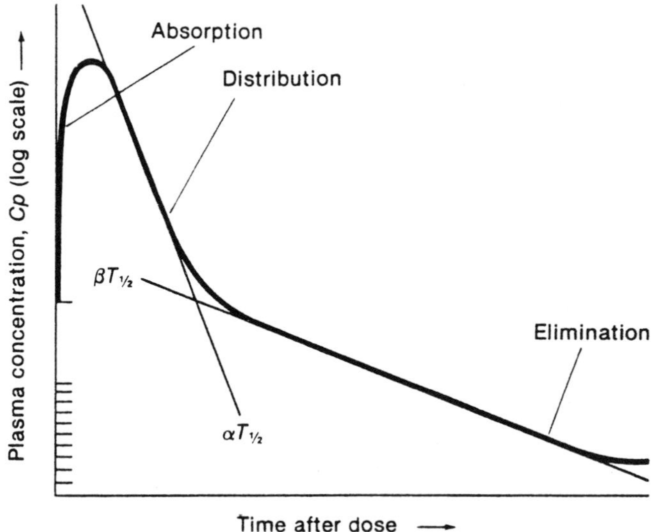

Figure 4–10. Phases of drug movement in a two-compartment model.

Other terms related to pharmacokinetics include first order, zero order, and Michaelis-Menten pharmacokinetics. Most medications follow *first-order pharmacokinetics.*[22] This is a process of elimination in which the rate of drug elimination is directly proportional to drug concentration.[22] More simply stated, a constant *fraction* of drug is handled per unit of time. Other medications (most notably, phenytoin) or conditions follow *zero-order pharmacokinetics.* This involves a process of elimination that is not proportional to drug concentration; in other words, a constant *amount* is handled per unit of time.[22] This indicates that small increases in chronic drug treatments can cause large increases in drug concentration. The rate limiting factor for zero-order pharmacokinetics involves capacity-limited metabolism from the saturation of metabolizing enzymes.[22]

Phenytoin is a medication used chronically for numerous seizure disorders. Many patients with seizures exhibit a prodromal phase before a seizure and therefore can judiciously medicate themselves with their phenytoin. Saturation occurs, and large increases in drug concentration and toxicities are realized.[22] *Michaelis-Menten pharmacokinetics* is a mathematic description of certain zero-order processes that involve saturation enzymatic pharmacokinetics.[22]

Pharmacokinetic information is useful to clinicians when drugs concentrations can be obtained, assayed, and reported timely for evaluation. Pharmacokinetic parameters that provide useful information to the clinician include the Vd, the elimination rate constant (ke), clearance (Cl), and half-life ($t_{1/2}$).5 Half-life can be further defined as either distribution (α) half-life ($\alpha t_{1/2}$) and elimination (β) half-life ($\beta t_{1/2}$).5 The $\alpha t_{1/2}$ is not usually determined because it has generally elapsed between the time of exposure and presentation.[23]

Once a patient presents, plotting toxic serum concentrations graphically allows for the calculation of these useful parameters.[22]

$$\mathrm{ke} = \frac{\ln C_2 \div C_1}{\mathrm{Time}}$$

where C_1 is the first concentration, C_2 is the second concentration, and time is the time between the measurement of the two concentrations. For this equation to be valid, the two concentrations need to be at least one $\beta t_{1/2}$ apart.[23] The population $\beta t_{1/2}$ for most drugs and toxins for which concentration measurements are important are generally available in drug information resources commonly found in clinical or acute areas (e.g., *Physician's Desk Reference*). These values are derived from population estimates and pharmacokinetic literature. Often, a range is provided. For example, digoxin has a $\beta t_{1/2}$ of 36 to 48 hours. Therefore, in the clinical setting of digoxin toxicity, levels should be measured at intervals no less than 36 hours. Levels determined too early invalidate the true slope (ke) of the serum concentration line. Many clinicians do not wait the desired time for determining the true slope, favoring either the measurement of levels early for interpretation and treatment or the use of reversal agents (e.g., digoxin Fab) when available. Concerns about observing the proper time to sample are valid in the face of overt toxicity, but clinicians must be aware of the principle just discussed and of the potential for misinterpretation.

Once the ke is known and the slope of the serum concentration curve has been determined, the $\beta t_{1/2}$ can be predicted with the use of the following equation:

$$\beta t_{1/2} = \frac{\ln 2}{ke} \text{ or } \frac{0.693}{ke}$$

This information provides the clinician with the patient-specific $\beta t_{1/2}$, which is more useful than ranges from population studies and estimates found in the literature.[4] The ke and $\beta t_{1/2}$ now can be used to predict when serum drug/toxin/metabolite concentrations will decrease into an acceptable range for reimplementation of a chronic medication or total elimination from the body. For example, a patient on theophylline presents with nausea, vomiting, palpitations, and tachycardia. Because these are known concentration-dependent adverse effects of theophylline, levels are obtained and supportive treatment is initiated:

Toxic theophylline concentration = 37 mg/L
Second concentration measured 6 h later = 24 mg/L
Clinically desired level for chronic obstructive pulmonary disease = 15 mg/L
Calculated and plotted ke = $.072\ h^{-1}$
$t_{1/2} = 9.6$ h

If first-order pharmacokinetics are assumed for theophylline, then in one $\beta t_{1/2}$ (6 hours), the theophylline level would approach 15 to 18 mg/L if no additional theophylline is given. The equation predicts:

$$Cp = (CpT)\ e^{(-ke)(t_{1/2})}$$

where Cp is the concentration predicted from ke and $\beta t_{1/2}$, CpT is the toxic theophylline concentration, and ke is the elimination rate constant.

$$Cp = (37 \text{ mg/L})\ e^{(.072)(10)}$$

$$Cp = 18.01 \text{ mg/L}$$

The level decreased from 37 mg/L to 18.01 mg/L in 10 hours.

The goal for this patient is reinstitution of the theophylline at an adjusted dose and dosing interval. The same principles and calculations can be utilized in situations in which the goal is complete removal of a drug/toxin/metabolite or its removal until an acceptable, less toxic concentration is reached at which monitoring and support can be safely discontinued.

For example, a patient is admitted with an imipramine overdose. A toxic concentration of 400 μg/L is obtained. The estimated $\beta t_{1/2}$ from the literature or in a reference is 15 hours. The clinician provides supportive treatment and monitoring for cardiac conduction disturbances and other anticholinergic side effects. A second imipramine level is obtained in 18 hours (a time greater than the expected $\beta t_{1/2}$) and is reported as 300 μg/L. The actual ke is calculated as follows:

$$ke = \frac{\ln 400\ \mu g/L \div 300\ \mu g/L}{18 \text{ hours}}$$

$$ke = 0.016 h^{-1}$$

and

$$\beta t_{1/2} = \frac{0.693}{0.016\ h^{-1}}$$

$$\beta t_{1/2} = 43.4 \text{ h}$$

Therefore, the concentration will decrease by approximately one half every $\beta t_{1/2}$. The therapeutic range for imipramine is 180 to 350 μg/L. Supportive treatment could be discontinued once the level decreases below this range. One or two $\beta t_{1/2}$'s would be sufficient to attain this value. In five to six $\beta t_{1/2}$'s, the drug would essentially be gone. One $\beta t_{1/2}$ is calculated as 148 μg/L, as follows:

$$Cp = (300\ \mu g/L)(e^{(-0.016)(4\ h)}$$

$$Cp = 148\ \mu g/L$$

Two other parameters have yet to be determined. The Vd following a single dose is calculated as follows:

$$Vd = (dose)(Cpeak)$$

Cpeak must follow the absorption and distribution ($\alpha t_{1/2}$) phases. Often, this is difficult to predict because of the length of elapsed time between exposure and presentation. In such cases, population estimates are again utilized to predict Vd, if needed. Most medications have an estimated range for Vd that is determined in a similar fashion as $\beta t_{1/2}$ (e.g., theophylline, 0.5 to 0.7 L/kg). Knowledge of the Vd pertains mainly to subsequent doses of drugs that may be required for chronic treatment. In cases of toxic exposures to harmful chemicals or toxins, the Vd is not a significant parameter. The goal is complete elimination and prevention of further exposures. The last parameter of interest is clearance. Clearance can be calculated from the following equation:

$$Cl = (ke)(Vd)$$

Therefore, knowing ke (slope) and assuming that Vd is within the population estimated range, clearance can be determined from the previous equation. Clearance can also be calculated with multiple dosing of chronic medications if the dosage, drug preparation/formulation, and a single concentration are known.

The following equation can be used to calculate true drug clearance:

$$Cl = \frac{(S)(F)(Dose)}{C_1}$$

where S is the salt factor (procainamide, quinidine), F is the bioavailability (amount absorbed), dose is the dose in appropriate time, and C_1 is the level. For example, in a patient with quinidine-induced torsades de pointes after receiving two 324-mg doses of quinidine gluconate every 8 hours:

Trough serum concentration obtained at 9 h = 4.3 mg/L
Quinidine information is available or can be found in available resources.
S = 0.62
F = 0.73
Dose = 324 mg 2 PO q8h, or 81 mg/h
Vd = 2.7 L/kg of ideal body weight (IBW)
IBW = 70 kg (patient specific)
C_1 = 4.3 mg/L
Therapeutic range: 1 to 4 mg/L
Desired concentration: 2.0 mg/L

$$Cl = \frac{(S)(F)(Dose)}{C_1}$$

$$Cl = \frac{(0.62)(0.73)(81 \text{ mg/h})}{4.3 \text{ mg/L}}$$

$$Cl = 8.5 \text{ L/h}$$

$$ke = \frac{Cl}{Vd}$$

$$ke = \frac{8.5 \text{ L/h}}{(2.7 \text{ L/kg})(70 \text{ kg})}$$

$$ke = 0.045 \text{ h}^{-1}$$

$$t_{1/2} = \frac{0.693}{ke}$$

$$t_{1/2} = \frac{0.693}{0.045\text{h}^{-1}}$$

$$t_{1/2} = 15 \text{ h}$$

Therefore, the level may decrease by half if first-order pharmacokinetics is assumed.

$$Cp = (4.3 \text{ mg/L})(e^{-(0.045)(15)})$$

$$Cp = 2.23 \text{ mg/L}$$

Therefore, all quinidine should be withheld for 15 hours and restarted at a lower dose if toxicity is resolved. The dose can be determined by use of the following equation:

$$MD = \frac{(Css\ des)(Cl)(T)}{(S)(F)}$$

where MD is the maintenance dose, Css des is the concentration desired at steady state (2.0 mg/L), Cl is 8.5 L/h (new clearance), T is the dosing interval (24 h; must be greater than calculated $t_{1/2}$ [15 h]), S is the salt factor (0.62), and F is the bioavailability (0.73).

$$MD = \frac{(2.0 \text{ mg/L})(8.5 \text{ L/h})(24 \text{ h})}{(0.62)(0.73)}$$

MD = 901 mg/24 h or given as 3 tablets (324 mg) PO daily

Pharmacokinetics can be a beneficial tool for practicing toxicologists in the acute intoxication setting. Simple equations and readily available population parameters can be employed to assist in the decision and treatment processes.

References

1. Franz SW, Beatty PW, English JC, et al: The use of pharmacokinetics as an interpretative and predictive tool in the chemical testing and risk assessment: A position paper on the appropriate use of pharmacokinetics in chemical toxicology. Regul Toxicol Pharmacol *19*:317–337, 1994.
2. Waddell WJ, Butler TC: The distribution and excretion of phenobarbital. J Clin Invest *36*:1217, 1957.
3. Smith TW, Haber E, Yeatman L, Butler VP: Reversal of advanced digoxin intoxication with Fab fragments of digoxin-specific antibodies. N Engl J Med *294*:797–800, 1976.
4. Amdisen A: Serum level monitoring and clinical pharmacokinetics of lithium. Clin Pharmacokinet *2*:73, 1977.
5. Hardman JC, Limbird LE, Molinoff PB, et al (eds): Goodman

and Gilman's The Pharmacologic Basis of Therapeutics. 9th ed. New York, Macmillan, 1996.
6. Testa B, Jenner P: Drug metabolism: Chemical and Biochemical Aspects. New York, Marcel Dekker, 1976.
7. Baud FJ, Galliot M, Astier A, et al: Treatment of ethylene glycol poisoning with intravenous 4-methylpyrazole. N Engl J Med *319*:97–100, 1988.
8. Vesell E: Polygenic factors controlling drug response. Med Clin North Am *58*:951, 1974.
9. Newbert DW, Jensen NM: The Ah locus: Genetic regulation of the metabolism of carcinogens, drugs and other environmental chemicals by cytochrome P-450–mediated mono-oxygenases. CRC Crit Rev Biochem *6*:401, 1979.
10. Stewart DJ, Inaba T, Tank BK, Kalow W: Hydrolysis of cocaine in human plasma by cholinesterase. Life Sci *20*:1557, 1977.
11. Suftin TA, Jusko WJ: Compendium of active drug metabolites. *In* Wilkinson GR, Rawlings DM (eds): Drug Metabolism and Disposition: Considerations in Clinical Pharmacology. Hingham, MA, MTP Press Ltd., 1985.
12. Forrest JAH, Clements JA, Prescott LF: Clinical Pharmacokinetics of Paracetamol. Clin Pharmacokinet *7*:93, 1982.
13. Sangster B, Prenen JAC, DeGroot G: Ethylene Glycol Poisoning. N Engl J Med *302*:465, 1980.
14. McMartin KE, Ambre JJ, Trephly TR: Methanol poisoning in human subjects: Role for formic acid accumulation in the metabolic acidosis. Am J Med *68*:414, 1980.
15. Karch SB: Methsuximide overdose: Delayed onset of profound coma. JAMA *233*:1463, 1973.
16. Mitchell JR, Thorgeirsson J, Potter WZ, et al: Acetaminophen-induced hepatic injury: Protective role of glutathione in man and rationale for therapy. Clin Pharmacol Ther *16*:676, 1974.
17. Ambre JJ, Bures F, Haupt D, et al: Antipyrene metabolism in patients with lung cancer. J Med *8*:57, 1977.
18. Ayesh R, Idle J, Ritchie JC, et al: Metabolic oxidation phenotypes as markers for susceptibility to lung cancer. Nature *312*:169–170, 1971.
19. Troupin AS: Phenytoin therapy and toxicities. Ann Intern Med *101*:568, 1984.
20. Levy G: Gastrointestinal clearance of drugs with activated charcoal. N Engl J Med *307*:676, 1982.
21. Done AK: Ion trapping in the pathogenesis and treatment of poisoning. Vet Hum Toxicol *22* (Suppl):2–9, 1980.
22. Allen L, Kimura K, MacKickin J, Ritschel WA: Manual of symbols, equations, and definitions in pharmacokinetics. J Clin Pharmacol 22(Suppl):3S–23S, 1982.
23. Gibaldi M, Levy G: Pharmacokinetics in clinical practice. JAMA *235*:1864–1867, 1976.

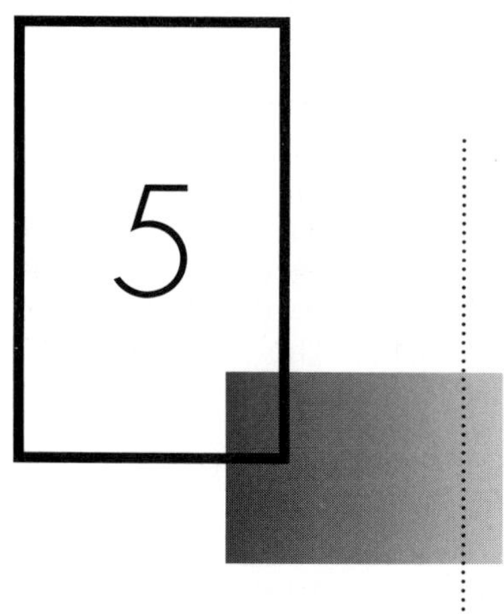

5 Acid-Base, Fluid, and Electrolyte Balance in Adults

JAMES F. WINCHESTER, MD
JAMES F. McANALLY, MD

The poisoned patient commonly presents with acid-base disturbances and with disturbances of volume and electrolyte control. The purpose of this chapter is to discuss the basic principles of acid-base disorders, regulation of body fluid volumes, intracellular and extracellular fluid, and electrolyte composition in the adult.

ACID-BASE DISORDERS

Acid-base homeostasis may be affected by a toxic substance itself, by a metabolite, or by dysfunction or failure of various organ systems. In addition, disorders may arise because of administration or withdrawal of a substance (e.g., gastric lavage leading to metabolic alkalosis, or the use of cathartics leading to hyperchloremic metabolic acidosis) or as a consequence of hemodialysis, which alters the partial pressures of oxygen and carbon dioxide (Po_2 and Pco_2, respectively), as well as bicarbonate level. In the unconscious or otherwise uncommunicative patient, physical findings and laboratory data may suggest an alteration in acid-base homeostasis and may be accompanied by changes in arterial blood gases, electrolytes, anion gap and osmolal gap.

Fundamental Concepts of Acid-Base Homeostasis

The pH of body fluids is regulated within a narrow range because of the participation and interplay of several regulatory systems. The most important are the lungs and the respiratory control center in the central nervous system (CNS), the kidney, and the body's buffer systems. The most important buffer system is the *bicarbonate-carbonic acid system,* which regulates extracellular bicarbonate level and partial pressure of carbon dioxide (Pco_2) independently, whereas Pco_2 represents the respiratory component regulated by the respiratory center and pulmonary mechanisms. Endogenous production of carbon dioxide leads to an increase in its concentration and combination with water to form carbonic acid; carbonic acid itself readily dissociates to hydrogen ion and bicarbonate:

$$CO_2 + H_2O \rightarrow H_2CO \rightarrow H^+ + HCO3^-$$

From this equation, the Henderson-Hasselbalch derivation is made, which states that

$$pH = pK_a + \log \frac{(HCO_3)}{(Pco_2)}$$

where pH is the negative logarithm of hydrogen ion concentration, which reflects plasma acidity and represents the balance between serum bicarbonate level (the metabolic component) and Pco_2 (the respiratory component). The normal serum bicarbonate level is 24 to 28 mEq/L, and the normal Pco_2 is 36 to 44 mm Hg.

Definitions

Acidemia Versus Alkalemia

When pH—the degree of plasma acidity—is less than 7.36, it defines acidemia, and when greater than 7.44, it defines alkalemia. The pH itself indicates neither the origin of the disorder nor whether there is physiologic compensation in response to the initial disorder. In contrast, acidosis and alkalosis are disease states that, if left unopposed, can alter plasma acidity and change the plasma pH. If the initial change in bicarbonate level or Pco_2 is severe enough to over-ride the body's buffer and defense mechanisms, then acidemia or alkalemia ensues. Acidosis or alkalosis can be present without concomitant acidemia and alkalemia, particularly if there is secondary compensation (e.g., as occurs in respiratory alkalosis accompanying a severe lactic metabolic acidosis secondary to septicemia, such that the pH is normal or even alkalemic despite the presence of metabolic acidosis).

Metabolic Versus Respiratory

The *metabolic acid-base disorder* is a disturbance caused by a change in serum bicarbonate level. *Metabolic acidosis* is defined as a decrease in serum bicarbonate level to less than 24 mEq/L, whereas *metabolic alkalosis* is defined as an increase in the serum bicarbonate level to greater than 28 mEq/L. In contrast, a *respiratory acid-base disorder* refers to a disorder caused by a change in the Pco_2. *Respiratory acidosis* is defined as a Pco_2 greater than 44 mm Hg, and *respiratory alkalosis* as a decrease in Pco_2 to less than 36 mm Hg. Secondary defense or compensatory mechanisms are set at force to minimize an ensueing change in pH. Metabolic acidosis leads to hyperventilation and a decrease in Pco_2, whereas metabolic alkalosis leads to secondary hypoventilation and an increase in Pco_2. Respiratory acidosis leads to increased renal reabsorption of bicarbonate and net acid excretion, which increases the serum bicarbonate level, whereas respiratory alkalosis leads to an increase in the renal excretion of bicarbonate accompanied by a decrease in the serum bicarbonate level. These defense mechanisms possess the quality of appropriateness in that they are physiologic responses proportional to the magnitude of the initial disorder and tend to return pH toward normal—but never completely to normal.

Simple/Mixed Acid-Base Disorders

A *simple acid-base disorder* is defined as a single acid-base disorder with an appropriate accompanying secondary physiologic response. A response that is greater in magnitude than the appropriate response—for instance, marked respiratory acidosis accompanied by only a mild increase in serum bicarbonate level implies the coexistence of another primary disorder and therefore is a *mixed acid-base disorder.* Mixed acid-base disorders are particularly common in critically ill poisoned patients, such as those with salicylate poisoning leading to both metabolic acidosis and respiratory alkalosis and those with ethanol poisoning leading to lactic acidosis and metabolic acidosis, with respiratory acidosis occurring secondary to a CNS-depressing effect.

METABOLIC ACIDOSIS

Metabolic acidosis, characterized by a serum bicarbonate level of less than 24 mEq/L is usually, but not always, accompanied by a decrease in bicarbonate level to give a pH of less than 7.36, and thus results in acidemia. Four mechanisms produce metabolic acidosis: (1) a loss of extracellular bicarbonate greater than extracellular chloride (e.g., with diarrhea and renal tubular acidosis; (2) gain of hydrogen ions exogenously or endogenously, with subsequent metabolic consumption of extracellular bicarbonate (e.g., as with methanol ingestion and lactic acidosis); (3) failure to excrete the daily acid load (e.g., as in renal failure); (4) dilution of extracellular bicarbonate. With the initial decrease in serum bicarbonate level and subsequent acidemia, secondary mechanisms initiate the return of pH toward normal. These mechanisms include extracellular buffering, intracellular buffering, the renal excretion of the acid load, and the respiratory compensatory response. Following an acid load, bicarbonate, the most important extracellular buffer, is called into action to buffer acid loss, milliequivalent for milliequivalent. After several hours, intracellular buffers also participate and buffer approximately 55% to 60% of the acid load. Excess extracellular hydrogen ions then enter the cell in exchange for sodium and potassium ions. In general, metabolic disorders tend to cause a greater shift of intracellular potassium to the extracellular space than do respiratory disorders. Bicarbonate itself can cause shifts of potassium ions without changes in pH. In organic acidosis, the organic acid ions—that is, keto acids or lactic acid—can enter cells with the excess hydrogen ions, whereas chloride cannot. Therefore, organic acidosis does not cause significant potassium redistribution when compared with mineral acidosis. Although the described mechanisms act in concert to minimize drastic changes in pH, the kidney alone possesses the ability to generate new bicarbonate by excreting the excess hydrogen ions. This process begins early but takes several days and occurs due to an increase in both ammonium excretion and titratable acidity.

An initial decrease in pH stimulates the ventilatory response mediated both by peripheral chemoreceptors and the medullary receptors in the CNS, which respond to changes in cerebral interstitial pH. A characteristic of the ventilatory response is an increase in tidal volume more so than in respiratory rate. Although occurring within minutes to hours, the maximum ventilatory response to metabolic acidosis may take 12 to 24 hours and probably reflects slow movement of hydrogen ions across the relatively impermeable blood-brain barrier. The ventilatory protective effect lasts only several days, probably because P_{CO_2} lowers renal bicarbonate reabsorption and results in an appropriate bicarbonate loss. Secondary hyperventilation is a physiologic response to an initial aberration in homeostasis and should be proportional to the initial decrease in serum bicarbonate level. Mathematically, the appropriate P_{CO_2} response is determined by the following equation:

$$P_{CO_2} = 1.5(HCO_3) + 8$$

which defines a predictable relationship between P_{CO_2} and bicarbonate for any degree of metabolic acidosis. Any P_{CO_2} responses outside the predicted range would imply the presence of a secondary primary disturbance, that is, a mixed acid-base disturbance. For example, in severe metabolic acidosis, the serum bicarbonate of 10 mEq/L would have an expected P_{CO_2} response of approximately 23 mm Hg; a P_{CO_2} greater than this would suggest concomitant respiratory acidosis along with metabolic acidosis. Conversely, if P_{CO_2} were less than 23 mm Hg, respiratory alkalosis with concomitant metabolic acidosis would occur. Metabolic acidosis is described as either high or normal anion-gap acidosis. The anion-gap equals the serum sodium level minus the sum of the serum chloride and serum bicarbonate levels, and it represents other unmeasured anions not accounted for by chloride and bicarbonate, such as plasma proteins and albumin, needed to maintain electric neutrality. The normal anion gap is 12 ± 2 (range, 8 to 16 mEq/L). If serum albumin is less than 4 g/dL, a corrective addition of 3 for each gram of albumin below 4 must be added.

Elevated Anion-Gap Metabolic Acidosis

Metabolic acidosis with a high anion-gap results from an accumulation of organic and inorganic acids and a subsequent decrease in extracellular bicarbonate level. The causes are listed in Table 5–1. Patients with elevated anion-gap acidosis frequently have multiple severe electrolyte disorders, a greater frequency of admission to intensive care units, and a greater mortality rate compared with those with a normal anion gap. Most often, elevated anion-gap acidosis is accompanied by identifiable increases in organic acids levels (e.g., as in salicylate, ethylene glycol, and methanol ingestions, and in lactic acidosis). Solvent ingestion and salicylate ingestions are associated with anion gaps in the range of 15 to

Table 5–1. Causes of Elevated Anion-Gap Metabolic Acidosis

- Renal failure
- Lactic acidosis
- Ketoacidosis
  - Diabetic ketoacidosis
  - Alcohol ketoacidosis
  - Starvation
- Isopropanol*
- Salicylate intoxication
- Methanol intoxication
- Ethylene glycol intoxication
- Paraldehyde
- Toluene
- Miscellaneous causes
  - Formaldehyde
  - Ibuprofen
  - Rhabdomyolysis
  - Inborn errors of metabolism

*With co-ingestion of ethanol or the induction of lactic acidosis.

20 mEq/L, whereas ethylene glycol and methanol ingestions and lactic acidosis are associated with anion gaps greater than 30 mEq/L. Although an anion gap is most commonly associated with metabolic acidosis, it may also be present in metabolic alkalosis. This can be explained on the basis of coexisting elevated anion gap acidosis and metabolic alkalosis (the mixed metabolic disorder), an alkalemia-induced increase in lactic acid production, and an increase in the negative charges on plasma proteins. Other causes are dehydration and therapy with sodium salts, strong acids, and certain antibiotics. Occasionally, organic acidosis (e.g., ketoacidosis) may be associated with a normal anion-gap metabolic acidosis if the organic acid excretion in catabolism equals the rate of organic acid production. Because excess organic acids are buffered milliequivalent for milliequivalent by extracellular bicarbonate, any elevation in anion gap is accompanied by a proportional decrease in serum bicarbonate level. Therefore, examination of both the decrease in serum bicarbonate level and the increase in the anion gap may suggest a mixed metabolic disorder. For instance, if the decrease in serum bicarbonate concentration is greater than the increment in the anion gap, another mechanism other than the elevated anion-gap acidosis is causing a decrease in serum bicarbonate (i.e., hyperchloremic metabolic acidosis), which therefore constitutes the mixed elevated-normal anion gap acidosis. On the other hand, an increase in the anion gap exceeding the decrement in serum bicarbonate level suggests that another mechanism is responsible for an increase in serum bicarbonate level (i.e., metabolic alkalosis), which now constitutes a mixed elevated anion-gap metabolic acidosis/metabolic alkalosis. In lactic acidosis, the ratio of change in the anion gap to the change in serum bicarbonate is approximately 1.6 to 1.24 owing to buffering of much of the acidosis in the intracellular space.

The osmolal gap may also be helpful in establishing the diagnosis of an elevated anion-gap acidosis. The osmolal gap is the difference between the measured and the calculated plasma osmolality and is given by the following formula:

$$\text{Serum osmolality} = 1.8 \times Na^{+} + \frac{\text{Blood glucose (mg/dL)}}{18} + \frac{\text{BUN (mg/dL)}}{2.8}$$

If the measured osmolality exceeds the calculated osmolality by 10 mOsm/kg or more, then other osmotically active substances such as ethanol, methanol, ethylene glycol, isopropanol, mannitol, ethyl ether, acetone, paraldehyde, and trichloroethane, or lactic acidosis, ketoacidosis, and chronic renal failure may be the cause. (See Chapter 35 for discussion of the alcohols.)

Renal Failure

Acute renal failure and chronic renal failure are common causes of elevated anion-gap acidosis. The metabolic acidosis of renal failure is the result of the inability to excrete the acid load. The anions contributing to the elevated anion gap are predominantly sulfate, phosphate, and other unmeasured ions. In chronic renal failure, the anion gap usually is normal until the glomerular filtration rate decreases to below 30 mL/min and is accompanied by an anion-gap increase to 17 to 23 mEq/L. The drug-induced causes of acute renal failure are discussed in Chapter 11.

Lactic Acidosis

Conversion of lactic acid back to pyruvate and in turn to glucose (via the Cori cycle) or to carbon dioxide (via the Krebs cycle) is the metabolic fate of lactic acid. However, conversion of lactic acid to pyruvate would release extracellular bicarbonate initially consumed during the generation of lactic acidosis. The normal serum lactic acid level is 1 mEq/L (range, 0.5 to 1.5 mEq/L). In most cases of lactic acidosis, there are components of increased production and decreased catabolism of lactic acid. Most often as a result of anaerobic metabolism, the cellular delivery of oxygen or its utilization is impaired, and anaerobic glycolysis with production of lactic acid results. Lactic acidosis is a common feature of severely poisoned patients and may be seen alone or superimposed on other forms of acidosis, such as alcoholic ketoacidosis, methanol intoxication, and salicylate poisoning. Table 5–2 lists the causes of lactic acidosis in the poi-

Table 5–2. Drug or Chemical Causes of Lactic Acidosis

Drug or Chemical	Mechanism
Acetaminophen	Acute liver failure
Ethanol	Acetate-induced increase in NADH/NAD, inhibition or conversion of lactate to glucose, thiamine deficiency, liver disease, seizures
Methanol	Acidemia, decreased lactate utilization, formic acid, hypotension
Ethylene glycol	Seizures, acute renal failure, ethanol, cardiovascular collapse
Salicylates	Uncoupled oxidative phosphorylation
Biguanides	Decreased utilization and increased production of lactate
Isoniazid	Seizures
Carbon monoxide, epinephrine, norepinephrine	Tissue hypoxia
Fructose	Conversion (30%) to lactic acid
Cyanide	Anaerobic glycolysis
Sodium nitroprusside	Anaerobic glycolysis
Cocaine	Seizures, vasoconstriction
Papaverine, nalidixic acid, iron, streptozotocin, strychnine, chloramphenicol, sorbitol, xylitol	Unknown

soned patient. Lactic acidosis is associated with a profound illness that includes weakness, anorexia, impaired mentation, hypotension, tachycardia, and hyperventilation. Blood lactate levels are uniformly elevated, and the higher they are, the worse the prognosis. In the absence of renal failure, lactic acidosis is accompanied by a phosphate-to-creatinine ratio in blood greater than 3 and may be associated with hyperuricemia because lactate and urate compete for the same secretory pathways in the renal tubule. As mentioned above, potassium shifts from intracellular to extracellular compartments do not occur, and any associated hyperkalemia is due to another cause. Drug-induced causes of lactic acidosis are shown in Table 5–2 along with the proposed mechanisms responsible for the lactic acid production.

In the treatment of lactic acidosis, attention should be directed toward the underlying cause. In addition, cardiovascular function and ventilation must be improved, and hypovolemia and hypoxemia corrected. Although intravenous sodium bicarbonate has been standard therapy, controversy exists regarding its use in the treatment of lactic acidosis. Dichloroacetate, which stimulates pyruvate dehydrogenase, the catalyst for oxidation of lactate to pyruvate, may be helpful in its treatment, especially if volume overload or renal failure is present.

Ketoacidosis

Alcohol ketoacidosis is a common clinical entity and must be considered in the differential diagnosis of elevated anion-gap metabolic acidosis in the alcoholic. Depleted glycogen storage, poor caloric intake, and the direct effect of alcohol in suppressing gluconeogenesis can lead to hypoglycemia. Hypoglycemia along with volume depletion suppresses insulin release and stimulates the release of glucagon, which predisposes to ketosis. In addition, alcohol can stimulate lipolysis to produce acetaldehyde and, ultimately, acetate, which allows for increased keto production. Alcohol increases the NADH/NAD ratio in its metabolism; this, in turn, favors the conversion of acetoacetate to β-hydroxybutyrate, and an increase in the β-hydroxybutyrate-to-acetoacetate ratio is a characteristic feature of alcoholic ketoacidosis. Lactic acidosis also may accompany the ketoacidosis as a result of hypotension, sepsis, or gastrointestinal bleeding or as a consequence of ethanol intoxication. Blood glucose level is usually normal; however, if it is in the hyperglycemic range, this should suggest the presence of diabetes mellitus. The treatment is volume resuscitation with glucose-containing solutions; this treatment usually effects reversal of ketosis within hours. Any accompanying electrolyte abnormalities should also be corrected; also, the administration of bicarbonate is required, as is the use of insulin.

Isopropanol

This aliphatic alcohol with a characteristic odor is often found in combination with methanol, ethylene glycol, or ethanol. Approximately 80% is metabolized to acetone by hepatic alcohol dehydrogenase; in turn the acetone is excreted by the kidney. The remaining 20% is excreted unchanged in the urine. Isopropanol ingestion leads to acetonemia and acetonuria without hyperglycemia. Any elevation in the anion gap often reflects lactic acidosis secondary to the ingestion of either ethanol or to hypotension and tissue hypoxia. This topic is discussed more fully in another chapter. Treatment is largely supportive, and dialysis should be considered in the presence of hypotension, coma, and serum isopropanol levels greater than 400 mg/dL.

Salicylate Intoxication

The metabolic acid-base disturbances concomitant with salicylate intoxication are most commonly profound metabolic acidosis accompanied by compensatory respiratory alkalosis. They are seen most commonly in adults, unless the adults have ingested an agent that depresses the respiratory drive; the commonest acid-base disturbance seen in this setting is simple metabolic acidosis. In children, simple metabolic acidosis is found in 100% of cases of salicylate ingestion. The anion gap is usually less than 20 mEq/L (range, 10 to 34 mEq/L), probably because of uncoupled oxidative metabolism and salicylate stimulation of production of lactic acid, keto acids, and other organic acids. Ketone products may be found in 25% of cases, and lactate production is stimulated by the respiratory alkalosis. This, in turn, may promote an elevation of the anion gap, either via the lactic acid itself or directly by salicylic acid. A blood salicylate level of 100 mg/dL increases the anion gap by approximately 7.3 mEq/L. The importance of recognizing complex acid-base disorders and salicylate intoxication cannot be overemphasized. The mixed elevated anion-gap metabolic acidosis/respiratory alkalosis occurs in 57% of patients; 30% of patients have a simple respiratory alkalosis, and 10% have a pure elevated anion-gap metabolic acidosis (this is seen in adults). The diagnosis of salicylate intoxication can be made on the basis of the results of a urine ferric chloride test, or by obtaining a plasma salicylate level. Treatment is largely supportive and includes maintenance of vital signs and ensuring adequate ventilation and hydration as well as other measures such as dialysis (outlined in Chapter 10).

Methanol

Methanol intoxication is accompanied by the production of formaldehyde and formic acid; production of the latter leads to a significantly elevated anion gap (greater than 35 mEq/L, and occasionally greater than 50 mEq/L), which usually develops 12 to 18 hours after ingestion. Although controversial, formic acid seems to be the earliest cause of anion-gap elevation, although the lactic and other organic acids may contribute to this; accompanying multiple-organ failure, which results in decreased hepatic lactate utilization, is also implicated. The treating physician must be cautious, however, in that pretreatment with ethanol—which is preferentially metabolized by hepatic ethanol dehydrogenase—may reverse the anion-gap acidosis by preventing formic acid accumulation; thus, an associated anion-gap acidosis may not be present. In untreated patients, the early high osmolal gap and normal or slightly elevated anion gap, which later changes to a decrease in the osmolal gap and an increase in the anion gap, should suggest methanol intoxication because the methanol is metabolized. Treatment largely includes correction of the profound acidemia, ethanol administration to inhibit the metabolism of methanol, folic acid to enhance formate oxidation, and bicarbonate hemodialysis to correct the profound acidemia and remove the toxic compounds. Mortality is approximately 20% and is related to the duration and severity of the metabolic acidosis, and prognosis correlates poorly with the initial methanol concentration in blood.

Ethylene Glycol

Ethylene glycol intoxication leads to serious life-threatening elevated anion-gap acidosis, with anion gaps ranging from 11 to 58 mEq/L (in the majority of cases, anion gap is greater than 35 mEq/L). The decrease in serum bicarbonate level is due to buffering of excess glycolic acid, which contributes mostly to the elevation of the anion gap. However, small increases in lactic acid and β-hydroxybutyrate levels also are observed. Lactic acidosis usually occurs in the later stages of ethylene glycol intoxication and appears to be the result of hypotension, seizures, concurrent consumption or administration of ethanol, and multiple-organ failure rather than a direct consequence of ethylene glycol ingestion. Hyperchloremic metabolic acidosis may occur also from diarrhea, proximal renal tubular dysfunction, bromide intoxication, which give a spuriously decreased anion gap in the presence of ethylene glycol. If there has been significant vomiting, the clinician should be alert to the presence of metabolic acidosis and mixed anion-gap alkalosis. As with methanol, ethylene glycol is associated with an increased osmolal gap, and like methanol, the metabolism of ethylene glycol causes a reciprocal in the osmolal gap as the anion gap becomes elevated. The common accompaniments of ethylene glycol poisoning include hypocalcemia, profound calcium oxalate, crystalluria, and other renal manifestations. Treatment is the same as that for methanol intoxication: correction of the acidosis, administration of ethanol for preferential metabolism by hepatic ethanol dehydrogenase, or the administration of 4-methylpyrazole, as outlined in Chapter 35. Dialysis also removes ethylene glycol and its breakdown products and corrects the acidosis.

Paraldehyde

Paraldehyde is a pungent, colorless liquid used for the treatment of seizures and for sedation; it has been supplanted by safer and more effective agents. It is metabolized predominantly to acetaldehyde and acetic acid and ultimately to carbon dioxide and water. It produces an elevated anion-gap metabolic acidosis by ill-defined mechanisms, possibly through the increased NADH/NAD ratio, which favors the conversion of acetoacetate to β-hydroxybutyrate which is responsible for the elevation of the anion gap. Large quantities of paraldehyde may cause an elevated osmolal gap. Paraldehyde also causes a false-positive ketone reaction because it reacts with nitroprusside directly to give the positive reaction.

Toluene

Toluene is metabolized to benzoic acid and hippuric acid, which accumulate to yield an elevated anion-gap metabolic acidosis accompanied by hepatic and renal failure. Long-term toluene exposure can lead to type 1 distal tubular acidosis and type 2 proximal tubular acidosis associated with Fanconi's syndrome.

Miscellaneous Causes of Elevated Anion-Gap Metabolic Acidosis

The miscellaneous causes of elevated anion-gap metabolic acidosis are formaldehyde, ibuprofen overdose, rhabdomyolysis (from cocaine, theophylline, or phencyclidine, or prolonged coma from any cause) and inborn errors of metabolism such as type 1 glycogen storage disease, maple syrup urine disease, isovaleric acidemia, propionic acidemia, and methylmalonic acidemia.

Metabolic Acidosis with a Normal Anion Gap (Hyperchloremic Metabolic Acidosis)

Metabolic acidosis with normal anion gap results from a loss of fluid with a bicarbonate concentration greater than chloride concentration, the addition of acids with chloride as their associated anion, or the transient dilution of extracellular bicarbonate with nonbicarbonate solutions. To maintain electroneutrality, the decrease in serum bicarbonate is associated with a proportionate increase in the serum chloride level. For example, in diarrhea, bicarbonate loss is greater than chloride loss, and thus hyperchloremia develops. Accompanying this is extracellular volume contraction, which stimulates renal retention of sodium with chloride, rather than of bicarbonate, because of the increased availability of chloride. This, in turn, leads to the development of hyperchloremic metabolic acidosis. Normal anion-gap metabolic acidosis can be divided into hypochloremic and hyperchloremic forms. Table 5–3 lists the causes of normal anion-gap metabolic acidosis.

In the poisoning situation, diarrhea may be seen with colchicine, alcohol, antibiotics, and cholestyramine. Drug-induced renal tubular acidosis (Table 5–4) may be seen with the use of amphotericin, lithium, toluene, vitamin D, analgesics, and cyclamate

Table 5–3. Causes of Normal Anion-Gap Metabolic Acidosis

Diarrhea
Ureterosigmoidostomy/obstructed ileal conduit
Small bowel/pancreatic drainage
Anion exchange resins
Renal tubular acidosis
Primary hyperparathyroidism
Parenteral alimentation
Post hypocapnia
Recovery phase of diabetic ketoacidosis
Dilution acidosis
Miscellaneous ingestions
Sulfur
Chlorine
Hydrochloric acid
Ammonium chloride
Calcium chloride
Magnesium chloride
Lysine hydrochloride
Arginine hydrochloride

(all of which produce type I renal tubular acidosis). In contrast, type II renal tubular acidosis may be caused by tetracycline, carbonic anhydrase inhibitors, cadmium, mercury, lead, uranium, toluene, mafenide acetate, 6-mercaptopurine, methyl-5-chrome, and streptozotocin. Type II renal tubular acidosis is usually accompanied by a greater than 15% fractional excretion of bicarbonate, aminoaciduria, phosphaturia, glycosuria, and uricosuria (Fanconi's syndrome). Type IV renal tubular acidosis may be induced by tubular interstitial disease caused by drugs or β-blockers, and or ingestion of amiloride, spironolactone, triamterene, lithium, nonsteroidal anti-inflammatory drugs (NSAIDs), angiotensin-converting enzyme inhibitors, and cyclosporine. Type IV renal tubular acidosis is hyporeninemic, hypoaldosteronism, and is most commonly seen in diabetes mellitus. A normal anion-gap metabolic acidosis may also be seen in ingestions of elemental sulfur and of sulfur-containing amino acids, methionine, cystine, and cysteine. Similarly, chlorine gas inhalation and intoxication with hydrochloric acid, ammonium chloride, lysine hydrochloride, arginine hydrochloride, calcium chloride, and magnesium chloride—all of which contribute to generation of chloride ions—lead to normal anion-gap acidosis.

Table 5–4. Causes of Drug-Related Renal Tubular Acidosis

Type I
Amphotericin
Lithium
Toluene
Vitamin D
Analgesics
Cyclamates
Type II
Outdated tetracycline
Carbonic anhydrase inhibitors
Cadmium
Mercury
Lead
Uranium
Toluene
Mafenide acetate
6-Mercaptopurine
Methyl-5-chrome
Streptozotocin
Type IV
Amiloride
Spironolactone
Lithium
Triamterene
Nonsteroidal anti-inflammatory agents
Angiotensin-converting enzyme inhibitors
Cyclosporine
β-Blockers

Clinical Features, Consequences, and Treatment of Metabolic Acidosis

Metabolic acidosis and acidemia produce several cardiovascular effects. Acidemia directly impairs myocardial contractility; it also has some indirect positive inotropic action in that it stimulates catecholamine release. As pH decreases to less than 7.2, the negative inotropic effects predominate, and heart rate increases; however, as pH decreases to less than 7.1, the heart rate also may fall. Acidemia also predisposes to life-threatening ventricular arrhythmias and to arterial vasodilatation and venoconstriction, which increase central blood volume. In combination with the negative inotropic effects, acidemia leads to pulmonary edema. The hemodynamic consequences of acidemia lead to a vicious cycle of decreased myocardial contractility that produces tissue hypoxia and lactic acidosis, which in turn increase acidemia, further impairing myocardial contractility. All of these factors produce shock.

Acidemia induces an increase in tidal volume and in the rate of respiration and, because of the Bohr effect, a shift to the right of the oxyhemoglobin dissociation curve. In the CNS, acidemia induces a spectrum of consciousness—from confusion to coma—probably as a result of changes in cerebrospinal fluid pH. Respiratory acidosis tends to have a greater effect than metabolic acidosis. Other factors in the development of neurologic symptoms include changes in osmolality.

Gastrointestinal effects include abdominal pain, nausea, and vomiting, especially in the setting of ketoacidosis. Changes in serum potassium levels depend on the form of the acidosis (metabolic or respiratory) and the specific types of metabolic acidosis (mineral or organic), as well as other factors, including changes in serum osmolality and changes in plasma insulin, aldosterone, and catecholamine levels. Acidemia displaces bone calcium, leading to an increase in ionized calcium concentration.

The principle treatment is directed at the underlying cause of the metabolic acidosis. Factors to be considered are the magnitude of the metabolic acidosis and the rate at which it develops. The management of rapidly developing severe metabolic acidosis secondary to ethylene glycol poisoning with cardiovascular collapse is far more important than the treatment of a patient with a mildly elevated anion-gap metabolic acidosis after a seizure. Controversy surrounds the use of sodium bicarbonate in the treatment of metabolic acidosis. Proponents recommend the use of bicarbonate sufficient to maintain a blood pH greater than 7.20 because a systemic pH less than 7.20 is associated with adverse hemodynamic effects, including reduced cardiac output, cardiac contractility, venoconstriction, arterial vasodilatation, and arrhythmias. Conversely, critics argue that this is not helpful and might be detrimental because, in models of lactic acidosis alkali might increase lactic acid production. Therefore, it would seem prudent to use sodium bicarbonate judiciously in the treatment of metabolic acidosis, particularly if the pH is less than 7.2 and the bicarbonate level is less than 10 to 12 mEq/L. Several formulae have been suggested to express the bicarbonate deficit. They are based on body weight and volume distribution of bicarbonate. However, these formulae should only be used as guides, especially because acidemia increases the volume of distribution of bicarbonate (e.g., at a pH of 7.1, the volume of distribution of bicarbonate is approximately 80% of total body weight). Because rapid-bolus administration of bicarbonate is dangerous, it is recommended that large amounts be infused slowly over 30 to 60 minutes. "Overshoot alkalosis" may be seen in lactic acidosis and in ketoacidosis when the lactic acid and ketoacids are oxidized to bicarbonate under severe reductive conditions in response to exogenous bicarbonate. Bicarbonate administration may also cause hypokalemia and hypocalcemia, which present their own risks. Similarly, volume overload from sodium bicarbonate may be seen, and when the presence of volume overload precludes the use of sodium bicarbonate, then dialysis in its various forms should be considered.

METABOLIC ALKALOSIS

Metabolic alkalosis is defined as an increase in the serum bicarbonate level to greater than 28 mEq/L. Usually, but not always, this is accompanied by an increase in pH to greater than 7.40. Metabolic alkalosis is quite common in hospitalized patients and is associated with significant morbidity and mortality. It develops from (1) a net gain of extracellular bicarbonate or of one of its precursors, (2) a net loss of hydrogen ions from the extracellular space, or (3) a loss of fluid containing more chloride than bicarbonate from the extracellular space. Metabolic alkalosis is maintained by a decrease in the glomerular filtration rate, a decrease in the real or effective extracellular volume, hypokalemia, hypochloremia, and hypercapnia, and an increase in mineralocorticoid effects. The initial increase in serum bicarbonate level produces alkalemia, which initiates secondary mechanisms to prevent drastic changes in pH. These include extracellular and intracellular buffering, increased renal excretion of excess alkali, and a respiratory compensatory response. Excess extracellular bicarbonate is derived from phosphate and proteins and from an increase in lactic acid production. The initial increase in pH depresses central and peripheral chemoreceptors and leads to hypoventilation and hypercapnia, which minimize the initial increase in pH. However, the respiratory response is not as predictable as it is in metabolic acidosis and is limited by the development of hypoxemia, which occurs as a result of hypoventilation. Any decrease in Po_2 to below 70 to 80 mm Hg stimulates ventilation, which counterbalances the effects of metabolic alkalosis—hence, the respiratory response to metabolic alkalosis is more variable. Rarely does Pco_2 increase to greater than 55 to 60 mm Hg as a response to simple metabolic alkalosis. Hypoxemia is a result of hypoventilation and, therefore, the alveolar-arterial oxygen gradient is normal. Pco_2 increases by 0.5 to 0.7 mm Hg for each milliequivalent per liter increase in serum bicarbonate level. A Pco_2 that is less than predicted suggests the presence of respiratory alkalosis along with metabolic alkalosis, whereas a Pco_2 that is greater than predicted suggests respiratory acidosis along with the metabolic alkalosis.

Causes of Metabolic Alkalosis

Metabolic alkalosis is divided into three categories: (1) sodium chloride–responsive metabolic alkalosis, (2) sodium chloride–resistant metabolic alkalosis, and (3) miscellaneous. In sodium chloride–responsive metabolic alkalosis, there is a decrease in real or effective extracellular volume and hypochloremia accompanied by avid renal reabsorption of sodium chloride and a urine chloride concentration of less than 10 mEq/L (however, in diuretic-induced metabolic alkalosis, urine chloride level may be greater than 10 mEq/L) due to an increase in mineralocorticoid activity. Characteristically, there is an increase in the distal reabsorption of sodium and an increase in potassium and hydrogen ion excretion with urinary chloride levels greater than 20 mEq/L. Hypovolemia is not responsible, and administration of sodium chloride does not correct the alkalosis; rather, treatment is directed at inhibiting excess mineralocorticoid activity. Table 5–5 summarizes the causes of metabolic alkalosis that do not fall into the categories already discussed.

Metabolic Alkalosis in Poisoning and Drug Overdose

Metabolic alkalosis is a fairly uncommon acid-base disorder in the poison patient, but it may occur in bulimics, diuretic abusers, and those with drug-induced Bartter's syndrome. The latter may be caused by administration of capreomycin, viomycin, and gentamicin. Chewing tobacco and imported licorice con-

Table 5–5. Causes of Metabolic Alkalosis

Sodium Chloride–Responsive
Vomiting
Villous adenoma
Congenital chloride diarrhea
Diuretics
Posthypercapnia
Cystic fibrosis
Sodium Chloride–Resistant
Cushing's syndrome
Primary aldosteronism
Bartter's syndrome
Adrenogenital syndrome
Liddle's syndrome
Renal artery stenosis
Licorice ingestion
Chewing tobacco
Carbenoxolone
Capreomycin
Gentamicin
Severe potassium depletion
Miscellaneous
Bicarbonate administration
Overshoot alkalosis
Bicarbonate precursor administration
Antacid–sodium polystyrene in renal failure
Milk-alkali syndrome
Penicillin, carbenicillin, ticarcillin
Nonparathyroid hypercalcemia
Poststarvation refeeding
Hypomagnesemia

taining glycyrrhizic acid have potent mineralocorticoid activity, as does carbenoxolone, and use of these products leads to metabolic alkalosis. Ingestion of excess bicarbonate may lead to metabolic alkalosis only if the kidney is unable to excrete the excess alkali or if renal failure is present. Overshoot alkalosis may occur in response to the correction of organic acidosis by excess bicarbonate.

Clinical Features of Metabolic Alkalosis

The features of metabolic alkalosis are in large part related to the specific cause; however, alkalemia *per se* may produce neuromuscular irritability along with seizures, tetany, delirium, and hyperreflexia. Cardiac arrhythmias may occur in the digitalized patient secondary to increased sensitivity to digitalis. Oxygen delivery to tissues is reduced because metabolic alkalosis shifts the oxyhemoglobin dissociation curve. Concomitant with the alkalosis, there may be hypokalemia, hypocalcemia, decreased ionized calcium, hypomagnesemia, hypophosphatemia, and hypoxemia, and this can further complicate the clinical picture.

Treatment

The primary treatment is to identify and manage the underline cause. Sodium chloride is administered for sodium chloride–responsive metabolic alkalosis, and volume expansion will correct it. Sodium–resistant metabolic acidosis may respond to measures to increase the glomerular filtration rate and to correction of mineralocorticoid activity. In patients with metabolic alkalosis who are volume overloaded, such as in those with congestive heart failure, acetazolamide—a carbonic anhydrase inhibitor—may be helpful and can lead to increased renal bicarbonate excretion. In the patient undergoing continuous nasogastric suction or with protracted vomiting, the histamine$_2$ blockers reduce hydrochloric acid secretion and can be used as therapy. In the renal failure patient with significant metabolic alkalosis, dialysate with a low bicarbonate or low acetate concentration and a low chloride concentration may be used in correcting the metabolic alkalosis.

RESPIRATORY ACIDOSIS

Respiratory acidosis is defined as an increase in the P_{CO_2} to greater than 44 mm Hg in the patient with compromised pulmonary function. The increase in P_{CO_2} and subsequent acidemia initiate changes aimed at the prevention of drastic changes in pH. Intracellular buffering via red cell hemoglobin, phosphate, and protein exchange intracellular sodium and potassium for the excess extracellular hydrogen ions. Hypercapnia leads to increased renal hydrogen ion secretion and net acid excretion, as well as to an increase in reabsorption of bicarbonate. Although beginning early, the maximum effect takes several days. For each 10-mm Hg increase in P_{CO_2}, serum bicarbonate level increases by 1 to 2 mEq/L: in chronic respiratory acidosis, for every 10-mm Hg in P_{CO_2}, the bicarbonate level increases 3 to 4 mEq/L. Any changes in P_{CO_2} outside those predicted indicate coexisting metabolic alkalosis as well as respiratory acidosis; likewise, bicarbonate levels less than those predicted imply the existence of metabolic acidosis as well as respiratory acidosis. Respiratory acidosis is one of the most common acid-base disturbances in the poisoned patient and may result from the drugs in Table 5–6, particularly if coma leads to aspiration pneumonia or laryngeal edema.

Features and Treatment of Respiratory Acidosis

Altered states of consciousness are common in respiratory acidosis, as are abnormal ventilatory patterns, tachycardia, arrhythmias, diaphoresis, visual disturbances, headache, delirium, and coma. Many of the CNS effects are related to increased cerebral blood flow secondary to hypercapnia and subsequently increased cerebrospinal fluid pressure. The acidemia itself can have significant adverse hemodynamic effects. Treatment is directed to improving ventilation.

Table 5–6. Causes of Respiratory Acidosis

Central Causes
Drugs
Opiates
Ethanol
Barbiturates
Anesthetics
Sedatives
Methanol
Ethylene glycol
Central Nervous System Lesions
Trauma
Tumor
Infection
Vascular accidents
Neuromuscular Causes
Guillain-Barré syndrome
Botulism
Myasthenia gravis
Hypokalemia
Aminoglycoside toxicity
Pickwickian syndrome
Primary hypoventilation
Thoracic/Pulmonary Causes
Pneumonia
Smoke inhalation
Pulmonary embolism
Pneumothorax
Pulmonary edema
Chronic obstructive lung disease
Aspiration pneumonia
Airway Obstruction
Foreign body
Epiglottal/laryngeal edema (e.g., phencyclidine poisoning)
Bronchoconstriction

RESPIRATORY ALKALOSIS

Respiratory alkalosis is defined as an acid-base disturbance characterized by a P_{CO_2} less than 36 mm Hg; secondary change is brought about to prevent drastic changes in pH. Intracellular hydrogen ions are exchanged for sodium and potassium to neutralize the excess bicarbonate and, thus, minimize the increased P_{CO_2}. The kidney decreases net acid excretion and bicarbonate reabsorption, and thus tends to return pH toward normal. Although this process begins early, maximal response does not occur for several days. Serum bicarbonate level decreases by 1 to 3 mEq/L for each 10-mm Hg decrease in P_{CO_2}, whereas in chronic respiratory alkalosis, bicarbonate level decreases by 3 to 5 mEq/L for every 10-mm Hg decrease in P_{CO_2}. Values outside this prediction indicate a concomitant metabolic alkalosis as well as respiratory alkalosis (when serum bicarbonate level is greater than predicted) and metabolic acidosis as well as respiratory alkalosis (when the serum bicarbonate is less than predicted). Rarely does serum bicarbonate decrease to less than 14 to 16 mEq/L in compensation. Respiratory alkalosis is the most common acid-base disorder encountered in intensive care, and the greater the degree of hypocapnia and alkalemia, the worse is the prognosis. Table 5–7 lists the causes of respiratory alkalosis, of which salicylate ingestion is the most common.

Features and Treatment of Respiratory Alkalosis

The main features are related to neuromuscular irritability, with certain oral and digital paresthesias, carpopedal spasm, tetany, seizures, and altered consciousness. Significant hypocapnia leads to a decrease in cerebral blood flow and is linked to the symptoms. The small increase in anion gap may be observed secondary to an increase in lactic acid production due to an increase in tissue anaerobic glycolysis brought on by alkalemia. Treatment is directed at the primary disorder; raising the P_{CO_2} by administering enriched inhaled carbon dioxide or by rebreathing mask may hasten the recovery from this disorder.

MIXED ACID-BASE DISORDERS

Drug intoxication may result in mixed acid-base disorders (i.e., the presence of two or more primary acid-base disorders). These are common in the overdose situation, either as a result of the primary ingestant or as a result of the therapeutic interventions used to correct the poisoning.

REGULATION OF BODY FLUID VOLUMES AND TONICITY

The body fluid, or *whole-body water,* in an average 70-kg man consists of about 42 L of water. The fluid

Table 5–7. Causes of Respiratory Alkalosis

General
Anxiety
Salicylates
Brain stem lesions
Encephalitis and meningitis
Metabolic encephalopathy
Pregnancy
Tumors
Pain
Fever
Thyrotoxicosis
Peripheral
Hypotension
Hypoxemia
Pneumonia
Congestive heart failure
Interstitial lung disease
Pulmonary embolism
Miscellaneous
Mechanical ventilation
Sepsis
Cirrhosis

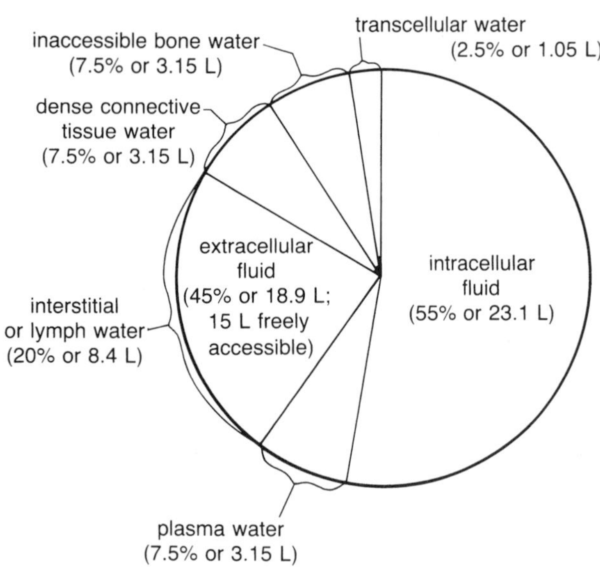

Figure 5–1. Distribution of whole-body water in a 70-kg human adult. Men = 42 L; women = 35 L. Most values shown are for men.

is divided into two distinct subgroups: the intracellular fluid, and the extracellular fluid (Fig. 5–1).

Except for bone, tissues that do not contain fat (the lean body mass) are 60% to 85% water; muscle and the gray matter of brain are the "wettest" tissues of the body, being 70% to 85% water. Connective tissue and erythrocytes are the driest nonadipose tissues (60% water). Fatty tissue, in contrast, is 20% water; therefore, an obese person contains proportionately less water by weight than a thin person. In obese individuals, whole-body water decreases to closer to 40%. In general, women contain more fat than men, thus the water content of women is relatively less than that of men (see Fig. 2–4).

The water content of the body is relatively high in infancy, decreases to adult levels in late childhood, and thereafter decreases slowly but progressively with age. The sex difference in body water content develops at puberty and continues throughout life.

Intracellular water constitutes some 55% to 60% of whole-body water. Excluding the relatively inaccessible bone water, total extracellular fluid water (plasma, as well as interstitial and transcellular water) makes up the difference. For an average man, total extracellular fluid water is 15 L (or approximately 20% to 25% of the body weight). The extravascular or interstitial fluid space accounts for 12 L of the extracellular fluid, whereas 3 L are present as plasma within the circulation. In an average young man, total blood volume is 6% to 8% of body weight (70 mL/kg); this gives absolute values for blood and plasma volumes of 5 L and 3 L, respectively.

Intracellular and extracellular fluid compartments are separated by cell membranes that selectively control passage of ions and nutrients but are freely permeable to water; although ionic gradients may exist across cell membranes, movement of water establishes an osmotic equilibrium, and any osmotic gradients are rapidly corrected.

INTRACELLULAR FLUID COMPOSITION

The ionic composition of body fluids can be discussed in terms of chemical equivalents. Concentrations of all ionic constituents are expressed as the sum of concentrations of the positive ions (cations) and negative ions (anions). Ionic balance is obligatory in order to maintain the electrical neutrality of the body fluids. The principal cations in extracellular fluid are sodium, potassium, calcium, and magnesium, whereas the principal cations in intracellular fluid are potassium and magnesium. Conversely, the principal anions in extracellular fluid are chloride and bicarbonate, whereas the principal anions in intracellular fluid are phosphate, sulfate, and proteins.

Electrical neutrality is maintained in all body fluids by a balance of cations and anions; however, in clinical practice, usually only plasma or serum sodium, potassium, chloride, and bicarbonate are measured, and it is assumed that levels of the rest of the cations and anions are balanced.

The high intracellular–low extracellular concentration of potassium and the reverse for sodium favor the movement of potassium out of and that of sodium into cells. Such ionic gradients are maintained by the presence of sodium-potassium pumps in the cell membrane and are critical in protecting cell volume. High concentrations of osmotically active anionic protein within cells, relative to the interstitial fluid, establish a Donnan equilibrium that increases the osmotic activity within the cell. Any movement of water into cells is prevented by the act of extrusion of sodium, whereas interference with the potassium-sodium pump mechanism results in cellular accumulation of sodium and chloride, with loss of potassium and resultant cellular edema.

Transcellular fluids are predominantly products of cell secretion. The composition of the fluids varies according to their cellular origin. Under physiologic conditions, secreted fluids tend to be recirculated or reabsorbed, but under pathologic (or treatment) conditions, failure to reabsorb continuously secreted fluids may lead to significant losses of volume and electrolytes, as seen with diarrhea, vomiting, and nasogastric suction. Drainage of intestinal fluids may result in considerable losses of chloride and bicarbonate (e.g., in the presence of small intestinal fistulae or with extreme diarrhea, such as that seen in cholera). Similarly, drainage of gastric and salivary juices may result in loss of considerable quantities of hydrogen ions as well as chloride. Diarrhea produced by cholera also results in massive sodium and water loss, which produces not only hypovolemia but also hyponatremia. *Third space fluid loss* refers to sequestration of fluids within cavities (e.g., pleural, pericardial, and intraperitoneal).

MOVEMENT OF WATER BETWEEN INTRACELLULAR AND EXTRACELLULAR FLUID SPACES: OSMOLARITY AND OSMOLALITY

Water moves freely across cell membranes, and an osmotic disequilibrium cannot be sustained. Thus, distribution of total-body water depends on the number of active particles in the intracellular and extracellular spaces. The osmotically driven "shifts" of body water adjust intracellular and extracellular osmolality to maintain osmotic neutrality. One osmole is the mass of a solute (or mixture of a solute) that, when dissolved in 1 L, gives a solution that has an osmotic pressure of 22.4 atm at 0°C. Osmolar concentrations are generally determined indirectly by measuring changes of the physical function of solutions, such as depression of the freezing point below that of water. Osmolality determined in this fashion (or osmoles per 100 g of plasma water) is obtained. The term "osmolality" is preferred to the commonly misused term "osmolarity" (osmoles per liter of whole plasma) and is more appropriate in considering physiologic relationships.

In practice, plasma osmolality mainly reflects plasma sodium concentration, and it must be remembered that water added to or removed from any fluid compartment behaves as though it were added to or removed from whole-body water. Second, sodium added to or removed from extracellular fluid alters sodium concentration, as though it had been added to or removed from whole-body water. Third, sodium concentration in plasma does not necessarily reflect changes in extracellular fluid volume because hypernatremia may exist with low, normal, or increased extracellular fluid. The same remarks apply to hyponatremia or normal serum sodium concentrations. Fourth, changes in the volume of intracellular fluid and extracellular fluid usually are proportional (and in the same direction) with a gain or loss of water, with intracellular and extracellular fluid volumes changing in opposite directions with gains or losses of restricted solutes, such as sodium and potassium. Other important solutes that contribute to plasma osmolality are glucose and blood urea nitrogen.

CELLULAR RESPONSES TO REDISTRIBUTION OF FLUID

Changes in extracellular osmolality can bring about major swelling or contraction of cells, but the primary effects are seen in the brain. Hyponatremia induced in animals causes brain swelling initially, with diminishing changes occurring within several hours. Correction of brain swelling is essentially complete at 24 hours, with the brain responding to extracellular hypotonicity by losing potassium and chloride. In hypernatremia in experimental animals, brain water is initially lost, with gains of sodium, potassium, and chloride being achieved by brain cells. Between 4 hours and several days, brain water content returns to normal, and an increased osmotic activity is sustained through the generation and accumulation of organic solutes such as amino acids. Hypoglycemia can also cause an acute loss of brain water, with a return to normal levels within a few hours, principally because of changes in the concentration of ions and organic solutes. Similarly, urea, mannitol, and glycerol remove water from brain but do not result in the generation of new intracellular organic molecules (idiogenic osmoles). For this reason, use of these compounds is not associated with effective adaptive changes in the regulation of intracellular volume of the brain, and consequently, brain volume decreases.

REGULATION OF BODY FLUID VOLUMES AND DAILY FLUID BALANCE (Table 5–8)

Because sodium is the dominant cation of extracellular fluid, it is the critical determinant of extracellu-

Table 5–8. Daily Basal Fluid, Electrolyte, and Caloric Requirements

Water/Electrolyte Requirements	*Basal Requirements*	*Metabolic Requirements*
Water	1.5–2.0 L*	100 mL/100 cal
Sodium	75 mEq	2–3 mEq/100 cal
Potassium	60 mEq	2–3 mEq/100 cal
Magnesium	8 mEq	—
Chloride	—	4–6 mEq/100 cal
Caloric Requirements		
0–10 kg	100 cal/kg	
11–20 kg	1000 cal plus 50 cal/kg over 10 kg	
>20 kg	1500 cal plus 20 cal/kg over 20 kg	

*Insensible losses (approximately 700 mL) plus volume equivalent to urine volume.

lar fluid volume by virtue of its osmotic activity, and by virtue of its effect on renal sodium chloride reabsorption. It is the major determinant of renal water reabsorption. It is through the reabsorption of sodium and water that the kidney regulates extracellular fluid volume. The reabsorption of sodium by the kidney is an intensely and finely regulated process for the conservation of sodium and water, and also for its secondary effects on hydrogen ion excretion through bicarbonate reabsorption (also linked to potassium secretion). A detailed discussion of sodium reabsorption by the kidney is beyond the scope of this text, but two major mechanisms in sodium homeostasis are worth discussing in relationship to the diagnosis and management of intoxicated patients.

Sodium is freely filtered at the glomerulus and is reabsorbed isotonically at the proximal convoluted tubule, with 60% to 70% of filtered sodium being proximally reabsorbed. Consequently, the glomerular filtrate volume is reduced by 60% to 70% in the proximal tubule; this provides substantial control of fluid balance. In the descending limb of the loop of Henle, the tubule is less permeable to sodium and urea but more permeable to water; consequently, the glomerular filtrate passing through the loop of Henle increases in sodium concentration, with consequent increases in osmolality. The thin ascending limb of the loop of Henle is permeable to sodium and urea but relatively impermeable to water, whereas in the thick ascending limb of the loop of Henle there is active transport of chloride, which also facilitates sodium reabsorption. Subsequently, the ascending limb of the loop of Henle accounts for 20% to 25% of sodium reabsorption. In the distal nephron (the distal convoluted tubule and collecting duct), 5% to 10% of sodium is reabsorbed, facilitating potassium secretion, and in part responsive to aldosterone.

Because the renal excretion of sodium is variable and, under physiologic conditions, is equal to sodium intake, the kidney must vary its excretion of sodium in the wide range encountered in humans (i.e., one to several hundred milliequivalents every 24 hours). It follows that regulatory mechanisms govern sodium excretion. Glomerular filtration; physical factors, such as postglomerular protein oncotic pressure, aldosterone, and antidiuretic hormone; and, finally, a natriuretic substance are all coordinated to maintain the balance of the extracellular fluid volume. It is well known that infusion of saline increases glomerular filtration rate and reduces renin excretion, thereby reducing aldosterone secretion; such physical forces favor natriuresis and release of a natriuretic substance, both of which increase urinary sodium excretion. The reverse occurs when volume contraction is present and sodium is retained by the kidney. Compensatory mechanisms, principally mediated by antidiuretic hormone secretion, are initiated to conserve water, whereas a reduction in renal blood flow probably leads to conservation of sodium.

Antidiuretic hormone (ADH) is an octapeptide produced in the supraoptic and paraventricular nuclei of the hypothalamus. It is transported in the nerves from the hypothalamus in the posterior hypophysis and median eminence, where it is stored. In response to a variety of stimuli, ADH is released and alters the permeability of the late distal tubule and collecting duct to water; the renal tubular cell contains receptors for ADH. A resultant increase in the water permeability of the distal tubule and collecting duct occurs, and, if there is hypertonicity of the medullary interstitium (brought about by the countercurrent concentration mechanism in the loop of Henle), then water reabsorption occurs. The prime factor in producing ADH secretion is the plasma osmolality. It has been known since the late 1940s and early 1950s that a 1% change in osmolality produces ADH secretion, and that a 1% to 2% change in osmolality initiates drinking. In contrast, a 6% change in the extracellular fluid volume is required to produce the same effect on ADH.

Dehydration and hypernatremia lead to reduced renal perfusion and increased ADH secretion. The result is the excretion of small amounts of urine that is low in sodium and highly concentrated. Replacement of free water corrects the problem in patients with pure insensible water loss. In the syndrome of diabetes insipidus, the problem of water loss arises either because of a central defect in ADH production or release, or because of renal insensitivity to ADH (nephrogenic diabetes insipidus), in which water is lost via the kidney. Because of the action of ADH on the most distal sites of the nephron, it is possible for the patient to retain sodium maximally but still excrete volumes of water equal to 10% to 50% of the glomerular filtration rate. The loss of water in diabetes insipidus results in 10 to 15 L of dilute

Table 5–9. Drug-Induced Alterations in Antidiuretic Hormone (ADH) Release and Activity

Central Reduction in ADH Secretion	*Peripheral Reduction in ADH Activity*
Ethanol	Lithium
Phenytoin/diphenylhydantoin	Demeclocycline
Glucocorticoids	Acetohexamide
Chlorpromazine	Tolazamide*
Reserpine	Glyburide*
Morphine†	Propoxyphene*
Central Stimulation of ADH Release	Amphotericin
Clofibrate	Methoxyflurane
Chlorpropamide	Colchicine
Nicotine	Vinblastine
Vincristine	Norepinephrine
Cyclophosphamide	*Peripheral Enhancement of ADH Activity*
Tolbutamide	Chlorpropamide
Carbamazepine	Acetaminophen
Acetylcholine	Indomethacin
Carbachol	
Methacholine	
Barbiturates	
Meperidine	
Prostaglandin E_1	
Isoproterenol	

*Mechanism not fully eludicated; not due to reduction in ADH secretion.
†Mechanism not fully elucidated; raises threshold for osmotically induced ADH secretion.

urine with a low total sodium excretion. The result is concentration of plasma and stimulation of the thirst mechanism, which leads to the ingestion of large quantities of water for replacement of water losses. Clinically, there is polyuria and polydipsia, the latter also being induced by psychogenic polydipsia—a syndrome that is difficult to distinguish from central or nephrogenic diabetes insipidus unless ADH concentrations in plasma are known. Drugs known to have an effect on ADH status are shown in Table 5–9.

Detailed discussion of the factors involved in the production of hypernatremia and hyponatremia, and of hyperkalemia and hypokalemia, is beyond the scope of this text. However, the principal disorders associated with abnormalities of these cations in poisoned patients are shown in Table 5–10. The management of derangements of both sodium and potassium also is outlined in Table 5–10.

ASSESSMENT AND MANAGEMENT OF FLUID AND ELECTROLYTE IMBALANCE

The most useful clinical guides in the assessment of fluid balance are volume overload and volume of contraction. *Volume overload* is manifested by the

Table 5–10. Principal Disorders of Sodium and Potassium in Intoxicated Patients

		Disorder and Examples	Treatment
Hypernatremia	Normal body Na^+	Drug-induced diabetes insipidus Sweating (salicylates, organophosphates)	Diuretics and water replacement
	High body Na^+	Steroids Hypertonic saline, NaCl, $NaHCO_3$ Saline emetics	Water replacement
	Low body Na^+	Osmotic diuretics (mannitol) Sweating (salicylates) Diarrhea (organophosphates, antibiotics)	Hypotonic saline
Hyponatremia	↓ ECF volume	Diuretics (tubular and osmotic) Rhabdomyolysis Steroid deficiencies Vomiting/diarrhea/pancreatitis	Isotonic saline
	↑ ECF volume (nonedematous)	Steroid deficiency Hypothyroidism Beer-drinker's hyponatremia Drugs (see Table 5–4)	Water restriction
	↑ ↑ ECF volume (edematous)	Drug-induced Hepatic, renal, cardiac failure ACE inhibitors	Water restriction
Hyperkalemia	↑ True K^+	Acidosis Arginine hydrochloride Digitalis intoxication Geophagia K^+-sparing diuretics Steroid deficiency NSAIDs Hemolysis Rhabdomyolysis Salt substitutes Penicillin-K^+ β-Blockers Heparin	Correct Stop drug Glucose/insulin Ion exchange resins Dialysis
Hypokalemia	Without K^+ deficit	Respiratory alkalosis (salicylate or respirator induced)	Adequate K^+ replacement
	With K^+ deficit	Nasogastric suction, vomiting Alcoholism Inadequate K^+ replacement Laxative abuse Drug-induced diarrhea Excessive steroids Licorice abuse Osmotic diuretics (mannitol, glucose) Diuretics Carbenicillin/penicillin/ aminoglycosides	Adequate K^+ replacement

ECF, extracellular fluid; ACE, angiotensin-converting enzyme.

presence of peripheral edema or ascites, or both, or by the existence of pleural effusions. In this respect, a useful reminder is that a 4% increase in whole-body water is required to produce a trace of peripheral edema. Other signs of volume overload are distended neck veins, normal skin turgor, and axillary sweating, as well as the signs of congestive heart failure. On the other hand, *volume contraction* is manifested by the absence of peripheral edema, collapsed neck veins, diminished skin turgor, and the absence of axillary sweat. Also important, resting or orthostatic tachycardia and hypotension may be seen with volume contraction.

With an increased extracellular fluid volume, such as occurs in cirrhosis, nephrosis, or congestive heart failure, urinary sodium concentrations are low while urinary osmolality is high (or isotonic), and blood urea nitrogen level is normal or high. Treatment in this setting requires sodium and water restriction. In conditions of decreased extracellular fluid, as in nonrenal loss of sodium with gastrointestinal or skin losses, urinary sodium is low and urinary osmolality is high (or isotonic), whereas the blood urea nitrogen level is normal or high. When renal loss of sodium is common, as with diuretics, renal disease, or Addison's disease, urinary sodium concentration is high, urinary osmolality is isotonic, and the blood urea nitrogen level is normal or high. Treatment of renal disease and Addison's disease requires judicious use of isotonic saline.

In normal extracellular fluid volume, as in the syndrome of inappropriate ADH (SIADH) secretion, urine sodium concentration is high, urine osmolality is high, and the blood urea nitrogen level is low; the condition is best treated with water restriction.

In intoxicated patients, especially those requiring ventilation and intravenous fluids, it is imperative that body weight be measured daily and that fluid intake and output be recorded accurately. Using these measurements, the clinician can determine daily changes in fluid and electrolyte balance. It is stressed that in the absence of peripheral edema, certain drugs may produce pulmonary edema (see Chapter 7) or cerebral edema.

Day-to-day management of fluid electrolyte and caloric requirements depends on the probable duration of coma; the total-body deficits or excesses prior to institution of intravenous fluid therapy; the likely therapeutic maneuvers to be used, such as forced diuresis and dialysis; and the intoxicating agents. In the absence of complicating factors, it is reasonable to assume a normal fluid electrolyte and caloric requirements for a 70-kg man, which are defined as "basal" requirements, as outlined in Table 5–8. For each increase of 0.1 unit in plasma pH, there is a reciprocal decrease in plasma potassium of 0.6 mEq/L; the reverse effects a reduction in serum pH. Such shifts are due to the transfer of plasma potassium into and out of cells because of changes in pH. The daily basal fluid, electrolyte, and caloric requirements outlined in Table 5–6 do not take into account the potassium and bicarbonate requirements necessary for forced diuresis; these are outlined in Chapter 10.)

MANAGEMENT OF RELATIVE HYPOVOLEMIA IN POISONING

In acute poisoning due to barbiturate, opiate, and other sedative drugs, it is well recognized that an increase in the venous capacitance occurs, with a relative deficit of plasma volume. This often responds to augmentation of plasma volume by volume expansion and, in some instances, the use of vasopressor drugs, with a consequent increase in cardiac output and mean blood pressure and a decrease in total peripheral vascular resistance. However, changes in central venous pressure may not be significant, even with copious administration of fluids. The relative hypovolemia due to increased venous capacitance may also be compounded by decreased venous return and extravascular fluid loss. In these circumstances, it is recommended that a flow-directed pulmonary arterial catheter (Swan-Ganz) be used to assess both central venous pressure and pulmonary capillary wedge pressure, which serve as guides to accurate fluid replacement.

In such circumstances, volume expansion with the use of crystalloid solutions may be disadvantageous because these solutions may reduce the osmotic hydrostatic gradient, thereby increasing pulmonary capillary water. This occurrence has been implicated in the development of shock lung in severely hypotensive patients (see Chapter 7). In view of the adverse effects of crystalloid solutions, colloid solutions such as albumin and plasma protein fractions (Plasmanate) are best chosen for the treatment of relatively hypovolemic shock in those patients who might develop pulmonary edema. Plasma protein fractions or dextrans are suitable colloidal agents, whereas human protein solutions are available in various concentrations, ranging from 5% to 25%; human albumin solutions contain between 130 and 160 mEq/L of sodium chloride.

Other colloidal expanders, such as dextran or hetastarch, also are available. Dextran solutions have the advantages of lowering blood viscosity and preventing red blood cell aggregation within the microcirculation in low blood flow states, but volume replacement with large quantities of dextran may impair blood coagulation. In patients with poor cardiac function, it may result in transfer of extracellular fluid to the intravascular compartment and cause pulmonary edema by virtue of its powerful oncotic properties.

Persistent hypotension, despite adequate volume replacement, and elevated pulmonary capillary wedge pressure suggest myocardial dysfunction. In this situation, drugs capable of improving myocardial performance, such as dopamine, dobutamine, and isoproterenol, must be used.

CALCULATION OF WATER EXCESS AND DEFICIT

Water Excess

Whole-body water (Actual weight [in kg] $\times$ 0.6) $\times$ serum Na^+ (in mEq/L) = Desired body water (in L) $\times$ Desired serum Na^+ (in mEq/L)

Example:

$$80 \times 0.6 \text{ (i.e., 48 L)} \times 125 = \text{Desired body water} \times 140$$

$$\text{Desired body water} = 42.8 \text{ L}$$

$$\text{Excess water: } 48 - 42.8 = 5.2 \text{ L}$$

Water Deficit

Desired whole-body water (in L) = Actual whole-body water (Actual weight [in kg] $\times$ 0.6) $\times$

$$\frac{\text{Actual serum Na}^+ \text{ (in mEq/L)}}{\text{Desired serum Na}^+ \text{ (in mEq/L)}}$$

Example:

$$\frac{42 \times 150}{140} = 45 \text{ L}$$

Thus, 3 L (45 − 42) are needed to correct serum sodium level.

Note: Serum sodium level in hyponatremic states probably should not be corrected more quickly than 1 mEq/h because of the risk of central pontine myelinolysis.

Further Reading

Ayus JC, Krothapalli RK, Arieff Al: Treatment of symptomatic hyponatremia and its relation to brain damage. N Engl J Med *317*:1190, 1987.

Buerkert J: The pathophysiologic bases for alterations in water balance. *In* Kiahr S (ed): The Kidney and Body Fluids in Health and Disease. New York, Plenum Medical Book Co., p 149, 1984.

Campbell EJM, Dickinson CJ, Slater JDH: Clinical Physiology. Oxford, Blackwell Scientific Publications, 1969.

Jacobson HR, Striker GE, Klahr S (eds) Principles and Practice of Nephrology. St. Louis, C. V. Mosby Co., 1995.

Leaf A, Cotran RS: Renal Pathophysiology. 2nd ed. New York, Oxford University Press, 1980.

Levi M, Bichet DG, Berl T: Treatment of hypoosmolar and hyperosmolar states. *In* Suki WN, Massry SG (eds): Therapy of Renal Diseases and Related Disorders. Dordrecht, Martinus Nijhoff Publishing, p 1, 1984.

Massry SG, Glassock RJ (eds): Textbook of Nephrology. Baltimore, Williams & Wilkins, 1995.

Narins RG, Emmett M: Simple and mixed acid base disorders: A practical approach. Medicine *59:* 161,1980.

Pitts RP. Physiology of the Kidney and Body Fluids. 2nd ed. Chicago, Year Book Medical Publishers, 1968.

Schrier RW (ed): Renal and Electrolyte Disorders. 3rd ed. Boston, Little, Brown & Co., 1986.

Thier SO: The kidney. *In* Smith LH, Thier SO (eds): Pathophysiology: The Biological Principles of Disease. Philadelphia, W.B. Saunders Co., p 799, 1981.

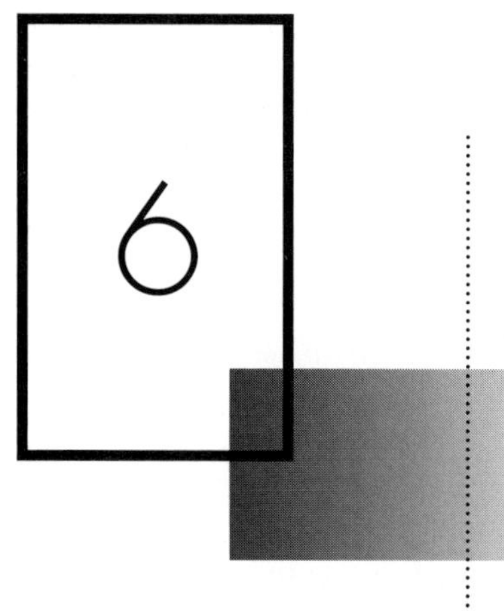

Cardiac Disturbances

NEAL L. BENOWITZ, MD
NORA GOLDSCHLAGER, MD

Cardiovascular complications account for a substantial proportion of the morbidity and mortality of drug overdose. Drug- or toxin-induced cardiovascular syndromes include hypotension and circulatory shock, hypertension, arrhythmias, and pulmonary edema. This chapter focuses on disturbances of cardiac function, particularly circulatory failure, and arrhythmias. Pathophysiology, recognition of specific types of overdose, and principles of management are discussed.

HYPOTENSION AND CIRCULATORY SHOCK

Mechanisms

Hypotension occurs after overdosage with many different types of drugs. The mechanisms of hypotension are diverse, and hemodynamic patterns vary with different drugs in different stages of overdose and according to the presence and nature of underlying medical illness. Cardiac output may be reduced as a result of drug-induced myocardial depression, relative hypovolemia resulting from venous pooling, or true hypovolemia resulting from vascular injury and fluid loss from the vascular space. Peripheral vascular resistance may be reduced because of drug-induced vascular relaxation, adrenergic receptor blockade, or depression of central vasomotor tone. Myocardial and vascular dysfunction resulting from hypoxia, acidosis, and hypotension may complicate the picture.

The major importance of hypotension is that it warns the physician of possible circulatory insufficiency; blood pressure is also one of several indicators of response to treatment. The diagnosis of circulatory shock depends on evidence of tissue hypoperfusion. In previously healthy individuals, urine output is usually the most sensitive indicator of hypoperfusion. Lactic acidosis is biochemical evidence that a substantial amount of tissue is hypoperfused. In patients with underlying coronary artery or cerebrovascular disease, cardiac or cerebral dysfunction may limit the tolerable extent of hypotension.

Management

Hypotensive patients should be placed in an intensive care unit where vital signs, fluid intake and output, body weight, and other parameters of circulatory function can be monitored continuously. Because indirect measurements of arterial blood pressure are difficult to obtain and often do not reflect true intra-arterial pressure in hypotensive states, direct measurement of intra-arterial blood pressure is preferred.

If a patient has hypotension without signs of tissue hypoperfusion, fluids should be administered at sufficient rates to maintain urine output and to compensate for insensible losses. Fluids should be of appropriate composition to provide electrolyte needs. In many patients with signs of hypoperfusion of tissues, correction of acid-base and electrolyte disturbances and modest fluid therapy are sufficient to increase perfusion to adequate levels. However, increased pulmonary vascular permeability complicates many cases of drug overdose, and fluid therapy may cause pulmonary edema. For this reason, fluids must be administered cautiously. A reasonably safe way to administer fluids is by short infusions of small volumes (100 to 200 mL) of normal saline solution. If the clinical response is inadequate and if the patient has no evidence of pulmonary edema, the short infusions should be repeated but should not exceed a total of 1000 to 2000 mL over 1 to 2 hours. Evidence of pulmonary edema includes worsening hypoxia, decreasing lung compliance (manifested by increasing pressure necessary to ventilate a patient with a given tidal volume), and development of pulmonary rales.

If shock persists despite fluid challenge, catheterization of the pulmonary artery and measurement of pulmonary capillary wedge pressure, cardiac output, or venous oxygen saturation are recommended to monitor subsequent fluid therapy and to optimize drug therapy. The goal of fluid therapy is to re-establish adequate tissue perfusion with as little effect as possible on the pulmonary capillary wedge pressure. As long as the pulmonary capillary wedge pressure remains low, further fluid can be administered. Although no data have been published in this regard, an endpoint of a mean pulmonary capillary wedge pressure of 8 to 12 mm Hg in a person with previously normal cardiac function appears to be reasonable in light of the possibility of increased pulmonary vascular permeability. This is in contrast to treatment of hemorrhagic or cardiogenic shock, in which a pulmonary capillary wedge pressure of 15 to 18 mm Hg is often the endpoint. If evidence of tissue hypoperfusion persists when pulmonary capillary wedge pressures have been restored to normal or pulmonary edema is evident, pressor or inotropic agents should be administered to restore adequate perfusion. It should be noted that in persons with chronic cardiac failure, higher pressures (up to 20 mm Hg) may be necessary to maintain an adequate cardiac output, and fluid therapy must be managed more on the basis of clinical assessment of pulmonary edema than on filling pressures per se.

Hemodynamic monitoring aids in the selection of pressor or inotropic drugs. For example, if circulatory failure is associated with low or low-normal peripheral vascular resistance, pressor drugs with substantial direct vasoconstricting activity, such as norepinephrine and dopamine, should be selected. Normalization of vascular resistance is a useful endpoint for titration of infusion rate.

If vascular resistance is normal or high and depressed cardiac output is the determining factor in circulatory failure, drugs or interventions that increase cardiac output should be selected. Isoproterenol is particularly useful when myocardial depression is associated with bradyarrhythmias, although it may be arrhythmogenic; dobutamine, a dopamine analogue with relatively selective inotropic activity and less arrhythmogenic potential, is useful when heart rate is already adequate. In some patients, the addition of the phosphodiesterase inhibitor amrinone to dobutamine or dopamine has resulted in hemodynamic improvement. Amrinone is both an inotropic and a vasodilating agent and should not be used when peripheral vascular resistance is low. In patients with both myocardial depression and low vascular resistance, epinephrine or combinations of norepinephrine or dopamine and isoproterenol may be useful.

Primarily because of its renal vasodilating effect, dopamine has now become the pressor agent of choice in most cases of drug overdose, with the exception of overdose with drugs that have α-adrenergic receptor-blocking effects, such as phenothiazines or tricyclic antidepressants, in which more selective α-adrenergic agonists, such as norepinephrine or phenylephrine, may be required.

Pressor therapy has potential risks: Pressor-induced venoconstriction can increase venous return and worsen pulmonary edema, and arteriolar constriction can further reduce tissue perfusion. However, in studies of the effects of infusion of norepinephrine in patients who overdosed with sedative drugs, the positive effects of norepinephrine on cardiac output outweighed the vasoconstrictor effects, and blood pressure increased without an increase in vascular resistance.[1]

ARRHYTHMIAS

General Mechanisms

Three basic mechanisms are involved in the production and maintenance of arrhythmias: (1) abnormal impulse formation, (2) abnormal impulse conduction, and (3) triggered automaticity.[2]

Abnormal Impulse Formation

The intrinsic firing rate of automatic tissues (those that can develop spontaneous diastolic depolarization) depends on certain characteristics of their action potentials: the slope of diastolic depolarization (phase 4), the duration, the refractory period, and the resting membrane and threshold potentials.

Conditions or agents that increase the slope of phase 4, lower the threshold potential toward the resting potential, or raise the resting membrane potential so that it approaches the threshold potential result in an increase in the spontaneous firing rate of automatic tissue. Conversely, conditions or agents that decrease the rate of diastolic depolarization, raise the threshold potential toward 0, or lower the resting membrane potential so that it takes longer to reach threshold potential result in a decrease in the spontaneous firing rate.

Abnormal Impulse Conduction

Delays in conduction or block of conduction of electric impulses, together with differential refractoriness of myocardial tissues, may lead to re-entry tachyarrhythmias. Such arrhythmias are initiated by early impulses that encounter refractory tissue or anatomic obstacles (e.g., scar) through which they cannot propagate because of their prematurity; thus, they travel down alternate slowly conducting pathways. If the impulses return to the area originally refractory but now excitable, the tissue is able to conduct them. This particular set of electrophysiologic circumstances (unilateral conduction delay and slow impulse transmission in alternate pathways) can lead to paroxysmal or sustained arrhythmias (Fig. 6–1).

Triggered Rhythms

Certain arrhythmias may arise from cells and fibers that are normally quiescent but, when stimulated, develop early or delayed afterdepolarizations that can then depolarize them for short periods.[3] Afterdepolarizations reflect current fluxes that persist after an action potential. If they reach threshold, they result in re-excitation of the cell or fiber. Affected fibers do not normally develop spontaneous phase 4 diastolic depolarization, nor is impulse conduction within them impaired, but when stimulated or triggered, the fibers may become rhythmically active. In an experimental setting, triggered rhythms arise in the presence of stretch, hypoxia, digitalis, high concentrations of calcium, and low concentrations of potassium and during catecholamine stimulation. β-Blocking agents may antagonize triggered rhythms that are catecholamine dependent, and calcium channel blocking agents such as verapamil may abolish those resulting from increased afterpotential amplitude. Although triggered rhythms have not been incontrovertably proved to be responsible for arrhythmias in patients, many rhythm disturbances, particularly if digitalis induced, pause dependent, bradycardia dependent or occurring in association with a prolonged QTU interval, behave as though this was their underlying mechanism.

Arrhythmogenesis in Poisoned Patients

In the setting of drug overdose, cardiac arrhythmias can be caused by direct or indirect sympathomimetic effects, anticholinergic effects, the effects of altered central nervous system (CNS) regulation of peripheral autonomic activity, and direct effects on myocardial membranes. Contributing factors to arrhythmogenesis during the course of drug overdose include hypotension, hypoxia, and disturbances in acid-base and electrolyte balance.

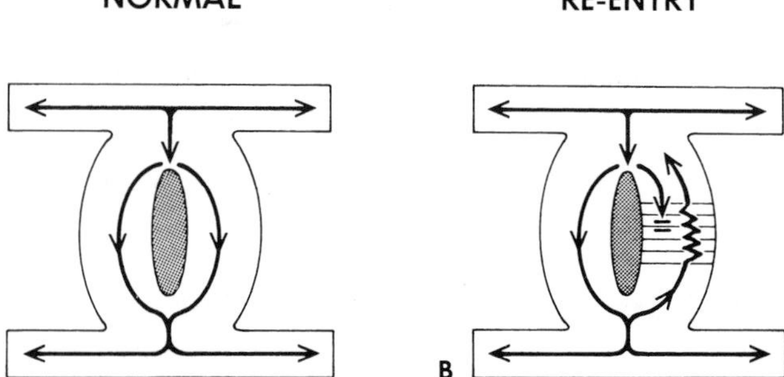

Figure 6–1. Drug-induced re-entry: Schema of Purkinje's tissue or ventricular muscle through which impulse transmission occurs. *A*, Normal depolarization of a muscle segment. Impulses spread simultaneously down various conduction pathways to depolarize distal areas. Depolarization and repolarization proceed homogeneously. *B*, Re-entry. The hatched area represents a local area with depressed conduction, which might be produced by a membrane-depressant drug. An impulse traveling anterogradely in an area of depressed conduction is blocked (*dark horizontal lines*); impulses traveling in adjacent pathways, however, can pass through the area of conduction delay in retrograde fashion. If tissue proximal to the depressed area is already repolarized and is now excitable, restimulation (re-entry) will occur.

Sympathetic Influences

Because the action of many drugs involves the autonomic nervous system, it is useful to understand the effects of sympathetic and parasympathetic activity on cardiac electrophysiology. β-Adrenergic stimulation accelerates spontaneous diastolic depolarization, thereby increasing the sinus rate; enhancement of automaticity in other pacemaker tissues (atrial, atrioventricular [AV] junctional, Purkinje's) may result in accelerated ectopic rhythms. β-Adrenergic stimulation also increases conduction velocity in slow (calcium-dependent) channel fibers, thus leading to more rapid sinoatrial and AV nodal conduction of impulses. The effect of catecholamines on fast channel fibers such as normal Purkinje's fibers is to accelerate repolarization and shorten the action potential duration and refractory period, although effects on conduction velocity are relatively negligible. Finally, β-adrenergic stimulation enhances afterdepolarization magnitude, thereby increasing the potential for triggered tachyarrhythmias.

Parasympathetic Influences

Parasympathetic stimulation slows the rate of spontaneous diastolic depolarization, resulting in slowing of the firing rates of pacemaker tissues. Slowing of the sinus rate may result in the emergence of an escape rhythm originating in supraventricular or ventricular tissue. Delay in impulse transmission through the AV node as a result of parasympathetic stimulation may produce AV block; this "vagotonic block" usually occurs in the presence of sinus slowing and can take the form of progressive delay in impulse conduction through the AV node (Figs. 6–2 and 6–3). The effects of cholinergic stimulation on ventricular conduction tissue include the raised electric threshold necessary for induction of ventricular fibrillation, particularly in the presence of high sympathetic activity.

An interesting arrhythmia resulting from increased parasympathetic tone has been recognized. It is characterized by supraventricular tachyarrhythmias occurring during periods of high vagal tone, such as sleep, and is not found during exercise or stress. Drugs such as digitalis or β-adrenergic blocking agents tend to precipitate or worsen these arrhythmias. This arrhythmia can be effectively treated (suppressed) by cardiac pacing to eliminate the pause or bradycardia dependence. The underlying mechanism of production of this arrhythmia may be acetylcholine-mediated shortening and dispersion of atrial refractory periods, resulting in inhomogeneous atrial repolarization and depolarization sequences. Because this arrhythmia does not connote

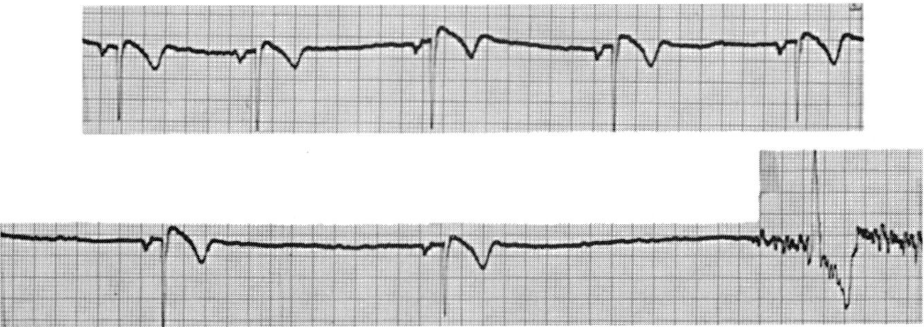

Figure 6–2. MCL_1 tracing recorded during ipecac-induced emesis in a patient with alleged barbiturate overdose. During the Valsalva maneuver of vomiting, marked slowing of sinus rate with prolongation of the PR interval occurs, resulting in a prolonged pause in rhythm terminated by a ventricular escape beat. Sinus slowing with or without concomitant atrioventricular block, such as depicted here, is due to hypervagotonia, and the arrhythmia is known as *vagotonic block*. This has no prognostic significance for underlying heart disease. The arrhythmia is usually transient and requires no specific treatment.

underlying heart disease, its recognition is important. Anticholinergic effects may also predispose to AV nodal re-entrant tachyarrhythmias via differential effects on nodal conduction velocity and refractoriness of re-entrant pathways.

Membrane Depression

In a drug-overdosed patient, a direct effect on myocardial membranes is another important mechanism contributing to arrhythmogenesis. Depressant effects on membrane responsiveness are exemplified by quinidine, which inhibits the fast sodium current, so that, for a given resting membrane potential, depolarization is associated with a reduced rate of voltage change and a reduced maximum achieved voltage. As a result, impulse conduction is slowed. In addition, membrane depressants shift the threshold potential toward 0, thus requiring stimuli of greater intensity to initiate the action potential. Additional effects of quinidine include prolongation of the action potential duration and refractory period, which prolong repolarization time. These electrophysiologic effects result in slowed repolarization and depolarization times, especially in His-Purkinje tissue. These events are reflected in the surface electrocardiogram (ECG) as a prolongation of the QT interval and, in toxic doses, of the QRS duration. With severe intoxication, intraventricular block and asystole supervene, with inability to generate a response for any stimulus strength; this is manifested clinically by failure to respond to cardiac pacing at high-pacing stimulus voltage.

The basis for the arrhythmogenic effect of quinidine lies in part in its ability to produce disparate depolarization and repolarization times in His-Purkinje tissue and to delay impulse transmission. The production of unidirectional conduction block and the delay in impulse propagation in other areas enable re-entry tachycardias to occur. Quinidine and quinidine-like agents can also cause polymorphous ventricular tachycardia, termed *torsades de pointes* (Fig. 6–4), probably due to triggered rhythms, as discussed previously.

The arrhythmogenic effects of most drugs during overdose are best understood as the combination of autonomic influences, membrane-depressant effects, and triggered rhythms. Our analysis attempts to categorize them in this way.

Management of Arrhythmias

Hypotension, hypoxia, and acid-base and electrolyte disturbances occurring during the course of drug

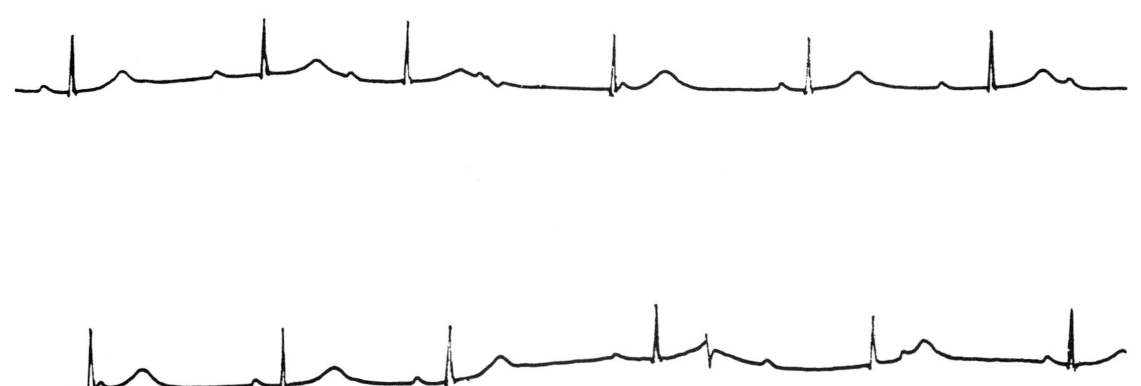

Figure 6–3. A 13-year-old girl ingested 325 mg of phenylpropanolamine and presented with a headache and blood pressure of 130/100 mm Hg. The electrocardiogram showed sinus arrhythmia with Wenckebach-type atrioventricular block, reflecting surges of vagal tone. The vagal discharge is a reflex response to phenylpropanolamine-induced vasoconstriction and hypertension.

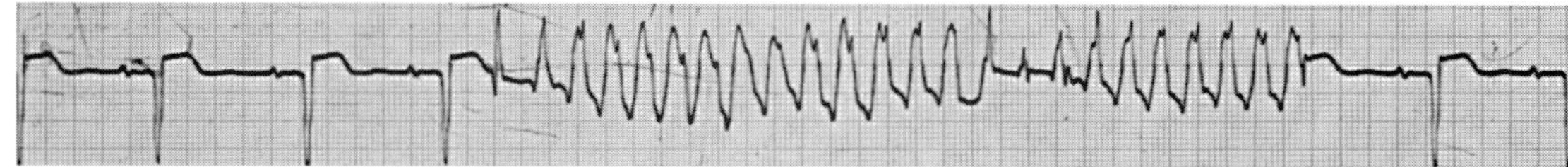

Figure 6–4. V_1 rhythm strip showing polymorphous ventricular tachycardia occurring abruptly and without warning. This particular arrhythmia is often referred to as *torsades de pointes*, reflecting a twisting of the QRS complexes around the electrocardiographic baseline. It occurs in association with prolongation of the QT interval due to any cause (including idiopathic) and may also be seen in acute ischemic heart disease. In this tracing, the QT interval, measured from other leads, was 0.56 second.

overdose may contribute to arrhythmia production and should be corrected (Table 6–1).

Supraventricular Arrhythmias

Sinus tachycardia and other supraventricular arrhythmias usually respond to supportive therapy and subside as the offending drug is excreted, but if they are associated with hemodynamic compromise, especially in patients with pre-existing coronary or cerebrovascular disease, specific therapy is warranted. β-Blockers (esmolol or propranolol) and physostigmine may be indicated for sympathomimetic and anticholinergic drug ingestions, respectively. However, with concomitant evidence of cardiac membrane depression, as occurs with overdose of tricyclic antidepressants, such an approach may itself be hazardous, as discussed later. Administration of digitalis, propranolol, esmolol, sotalol, verapamil, diltiazem, or amiodarone may be useful in slowing a rapid ventricular response to atrial fibrillation or flutter, although these arrhythmias may be only transient. Electric conversion is an acceptable alternative when arrhythmias are life threatening and fail to respond to pharmacologic treatment.

Ventricular Arrhythmias

Pharmacologic therapy for drug-induced ventricular irritability is similar to that used in the setting of acute myocardial ischemia. An important exception exists in cases of overdose of membrane-depressant drugs such as quinidine or tricyclic antidepressants; in these instances, similar agents such as procainamide and disopyramide are contraindicated, and lidocaine or mexiletine is the drug of choice. Selection of secondary drugs depends on the particular overdose; thus, a β-blocker might be indicated for sympathomimetic drug overdose, magnesium or digitalis antibodies for digitalis overdose, and magnesium and isoproterenol for polymorphous ventricular tachycardia with a long QT interval caused by quinidine-like drugs.[4] Administration of bretylium tosylate may be useful in the treatment of intractable ventricular arrhythmias occurring in the setting of acute ischemic heart disease, especially fibrillation unresponsive to defibrillation, and might be tried for similar arrhythmias occurring during drug overdose. Its use has a potential disadvantage of causing or worsening hypotension. Sustained ventricular tachycardia and fibrillation require electric conversion or intravenous administration of amiodarone.

Wide Complex Tachycardia of Uncertain Origin

The ECG occasionally shows a regular wide complex QRS rhythm without readily discernible atrial activity; the origin of the QRS rhythm may thus be uncertain. Rate alone is not a particularly useful criterion in distinguishing ventricular tachycardia from supraventricular tachycardia with intraventricular aberration, especially in a patient suffering from an overdose. QRS morphology, on the other hand, can be helpful. Ventricular tachycardia is suggested by very bizarre QRS complexes; superior deviation of the mean frontal plane QRS axis; qR, RR′, or R waves in leads aVr and V_1; rS or QS in leads aVL and V_6; or concordance (similarity) of QRS morphology in the precordial leads.[5] Supraventricular tachycardia with intraventricular aberration is suggested by QRS morphology that closely resembles typical bundle branch block patterns. Past ECGs with which to compare current ones may be helpful if they have shown a previously present bundle branch block pattern or ventricular premature complexes that resemble the present rhythm (Fig. 6–5).

The relationship of ventricular to atrial activity may afford another clue to the origin of the QRS rhythm. Establishing this relationship when atrial activity is not easily seen on the surface ECG often

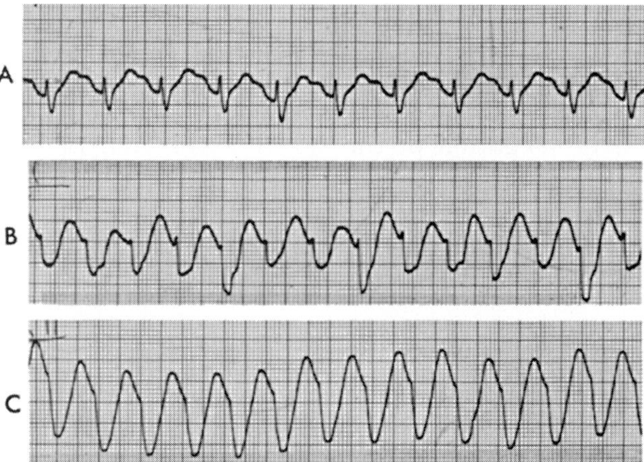

Figure 6–5. These lead I rhythm strips were obtained from a 40-year-old woman who ingested 6 g of amitriptyline (Elavil). In *A*, the rhythm is sinus with a long PR interval. In strips *B* and *C*, recorded within a 20-minute period, no P waves are seen and the QRS complexes are broad and bizarre. Close scrutiny reveals that the QRS complexes in strips *B* and *C* resemble those in strip *A* except that they are more aberrant. The value of previously recorded tracings when evaluating a wide complex tachycardia, as in strip *C*, is illustrated by these electrocardiograms.

Table 6–1. Arrhythmias and Their Management

Type	Comment	Treatment
Tachyarrhythmias		
All		Correct hypotension and acid-base and electrolyte disturbances
Sinus tachycardia	Usually can be made to vary with respiration, exercise, carotid sinus massage	No specific treatment indicated. If hemodynamic compromise, β-blockade
Ectopic atrial tachycardia	If 2:1 AV conduction ratio, suspect digitalis toxicity	If hemodynamic compromise, β-blockade, sotalol, amiodarone, or calcium channel blockade. If digitalis toxic, withdraw digitalis
Atrial flutter	Adenosine produces sufficient AV block to discern atrial activity. If QRS rhythm is regular and slow (<100), suspect AV block, which might be due to digitalis toxicity and/or β- and calcium entry blocker overdosage	Direct current cardioversion (low energy levels usually suffice); pace termination; IV verapamil, esmolol, or metoprolol will slow ventricular rate; digitalis and quinidine or procainamide IV ibutilide for pharmacologic conversion
Atrial fibrillation	May appear to be regular at more rapid rates. Distinguish from multifocal atrial tachycardia by lack of defined atrial activity	Intravenous digitalis, verapamil, esmolol, and/or metoprolol or amiodarone to slow ventricular response (if necessary). Direct current cardioversion if an accessory pathway is known or suspected and ventricular response is rapid.
Junctional tachycardia	No variation in rate with respiration, exercise. Distinguish from sinus tachycardia with long PR interval or ventricular tachycardia (if QRS complex is wide). May be due to digitalis toxicity	If rate is rapid, β-blockade, physostigmine,* pace termination; direct current cardioversion
Ventricular ectopy (couplets, triplets, multiform complexes, sustained tachycardia, fibrillation)	If due to membrane-depressant drugs, other drugs in this class are to be avoided. If due to bradycardia, increase basic rate	IV lidocaine, β-blockade, isoproterenol, magnesium, and/or cardiac pacing if due to bradycardia or associated with long QT. Direct current cardioversion or defibrillation. Procainamide IV if sustained in ischemic setting. IV amiodarone if hemodynamically destabilizing rapid ventricular tachycardia
Bradyarrhythmias		
Sinus bradycardia, including sinus arrest, sinoatrial block, and vagotonic bradycardia		No specific therapy. If hemodynamic decompensation, IV atropine, isoproterenol, cardiac pacing
Vagotonic AV block	AV block with varying PR intervals is associated with slowing of sinus rates. Seen in states with high vagal tone, including sleep and specific situations such as suctioning or endoscopy	No specific therapy. Atropine, theophylline, transdermal scopolamine, if sustained. Note: Atropine should not be administered if vagotonic rhythm is a reflex response to drug-induced hypertension, because it will aggravate the hypertension
AV block type I (Wenckebach)		If hemodynamic compromise, atropine, IV isoproterenol, cardiac pacing
Type II (Mobitz II) high-degree or complete block	If atrial rate is increased by atropine or isoproterenol, increase in degree of AV block may occur	Cardiac pacing

AV, atrioventricular; IV, intravenous.
*May be hazardous if associated with membrane-depressant drug overdose.

requires placing an electrode catheter in the esophagus or right atrium to register atrial electric signals. The simultaneous recording of a surface ECG lead and intracardiac or intraesophageal electrogram permits recognition of atrial activity. If this activity is occurring independently of (is dissociated from) the regular ventricular rhythm, the QRS rhythm is almost certainly ventricular tachycardia. If atrial activity is occurring irregularly at rates faster than the regular ventricular rhythm, the rhythm is ectopic atrial tachycardia or atrial fibrillation, depending on its rate, and is dissociated from the regular ventricular rhythm, which may then be junctional or ventricular in origin. If atrial activity is occurring at a rate that is a multiple of the QRS rate, atrial flutter is suggested. If a 1:1 relationship between atrial and ventricular activity is demonstrated, the direction of impulse transmission (AV or ventriculoatrial) is not known; only by changing the conduction ratios may the correct diagnosis be made. For example, if carotid sinus massage is applied in a patient with regular wide complex tachycardia and 1:1 AV relationship, and ventricular asystole occurs despite persistence of atrial activity, the rhythm was supraventricular in origin (Fig. 6–6). Some patients with hyperkalemia have a wide QRS complex rhythm without discernible P waves, in which the QRS complexes are nevertheless stimulated by the sinus node. This rhythm is termed *sinoventricular conduction*. The absence of P waves is due to hyperkalemia-related atrial arrest, and treatment of the hyperkalemia results in restoration of atrial muscle depolarization and appearance of P waves.

Management of hemodynamically significant wide complex tachycardia while the diagnosis is being established should include carotid sinus massage as a readily applied initial maneuver but should be directed toward the potentially most life-threatening arrhythmia. Thus, intravenous lidocaine should be used for presumed ventricular tachycardia as the agent of first choice. When the nature of the overdose is unknown, however, direct current cardioversion may be the procedure of choice to avoid compounding the problem of arrhythmia and hemodynamic instability, provided there is reasonable certainty that the rhythm is not sinus in origin. It is emphasized that failure to convert a wide complex tachycardia to another rhythm after direct current cardioversion should suggest that sinus tachycardia may indeed be present. It should also be recognized that certain antiarrhythmic agents, notably flecainide, can cause monomorphic ventricular tachycardia refractory to cardioversion attempts.

Bradyarrhythmias

Bradyarrhythmias, particularly AV block, may occur unpredictably and may require temporary transvenous cardiac pacing. Before pacemaker insertion, transcutaneous pacing and pharmacologic therapy may be necessary in an attempt to maintain heart rate, blood pressure, and cardiac output. Intravenous administration of atropine should be tried to treat sinus or junctional bradycardia; intravenous administration of isoproterenol may be used for unresponsive sinus or junctional or ventricular bradycardias. These agents should be used with caution, however, because both may cause significant sinus or junctional tachycardia, and isoproterenol may cause ventricular extrasystolic activity, including ventricular tachycardia. Low doses of atropine (<0.5 mg) may cause paradoxical ventricular bradycardia by increasing the number of atrial impulses that enter the AV node and render it refractory.

Cardiac Pacing in Drug Overdose

Pacemaker-related difficulties encountered in drug-overdosed patients may be related to inability to sense a suboptimal intracardiac signal or to capture the atria or ventricles. To be sensed properly by a pacemaker generator, an intracardiac signal must have certain characteristics: adequate amplitude, rapid rate of change of voltage, and optimal signal duration. In patients overdosed with agents that alter impulse conduction or cause or contribute to myocardial ischemia or failure, the intracardiac signal is often of too poor a quality to be sensed, leading to improper demand pacemaker function. The resulting earlier-than-expected pacing stimulus that follows unsensed spontaneous beats may cause repetitive atrial or ventricular rhythms, including ventricular tachycardia and fibrillation.

Another problem encountered in drug-overdosed patients is failure of the pacing stimulus to depolarize sufficient amounts of myocardial tissue to cause ventricular activation, resulting in failure to pace.[6] This can come about as a result of myocardial intercellular or intracellular edema or as a result of fail-

Surface lead V_1

Intracardiac electrogram

Intracardiac electrogram during carotid sinus massage

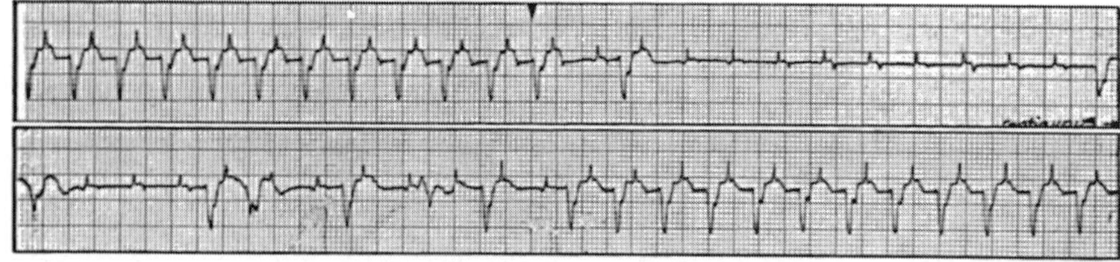

Figure 6–6. The patient is a 67-year-old man with chronic obstructive pulmonary disease. He developed tachycardia during treatment with aminophylline. The surface electrocardiographic V_1 lead *(top strip)* shows a QRS duration of 0.12 second and no clearly discerned atrial activity. Intracardiac electrography *(second strip)* reveals a 1:1 relationship between ventricular (the broad, large deflections) and atrial (the sharp, small deflections) activity. The direction of impulse transmission is not known. Carotid sinus massage *(lower two continuous strips)* shows no change in atrial activity, whereas ventricular response is blocked, probably at the atrioventricular node. The change in the atrioventricular conduction ratio produced by carotid massage allows the diagnosis of atrial tachycardia to be made.

ure of pacing stimulus propagation throughout the muscle due to hyperkalemia, hypoxia, acidosis, or membrane-depressant agents. The failure to pace may be total, with all pacing stimuli failing to depolarize the ventricles, or various degrees of pacemaker exit block may be exhibited, including Wenckebach-type conduction (Fig. 6–7).

Because transcutaneous pacing is not effective over time, it should not be used except in emergencies and should be followed by transvenous pacing to ensure stable heart rate support.

Some patients in whom failure to pace is life threatening may require cardiopulmonary bypass or intra-aortic balloon (triggering off the pacing stimulus) support to maintain circulatory function.

PULMONARY EDEMA

Pulmonary edema frequently complicates overdose with drugs such as narcotics, sedative-hypnotic drugs, salicylates, and sympathomimetic drugs. The pathophysiology of drug-induced pulmonary edema involves increased pulmonary capillary permeability, as evidenced by normal or low pulmonary capillary wedge pressures and pulmonary edema fluid with a protein concentration similar to that of plasma. In a series of 24 patients with pulmonary edema, those with drug-induced and other noncardiogenic pulmonary edema had pulmonary capillary wedge pressures of less than 20 mm Hg and ratios of edema fluid protein concentration to plasma protein concentration exceeding 0.6.[7] Patients with hydrostatic or cardiogenic pulmonary edema had pulmonary capillary wedge pressures greater than 20 mm Hg and ratios of edema fluid protein concentration to plasma protein concentration of less than 0.56.

The mechanisms by which sedative-hypnotic drugs produce capillary endothelial damage are not fully understood. Depression of respiration may lead to hypoxemia, precapillary pulmonary hypertension, increased vascular permeability, and finally extravasation of fluid. An analogy has been made to cases of pulmonary edema at high altitude, in which hypoxia produces a similar picture, which is rapidly reversed by oxygen therapy. Ethchlorvynol, when injected intravenously, is an example of a drug that directly injures the alveolocapillary membrane. Infused salicylate, possibly by effects on prostaglandin synthesis, increases microvascular permeability. Pulsatile lymphatic activity is reduced and lymphatic drainage is retarded during barbiturate anesthesia. This might also contribute to the net accumulation of fluid in the lungs after drug overdose.

Neurogenic pulmonary edema, possibly mediated by massive sympathetic discharge, has been well described after brain injury and has been suggested to occur after overdoses of drugs such as narcotics and salicylates. Sympathomimetic drugs can cause pulmonary edema owing to severe hypertension and diastolic noncompliance. This is most common after intravenous administration. By the time such a patient is evaluated by a physician, blood pressure may be normal or even low, with evidence of hypovolemia due to sequestration of fluid into the lungs and other extravascular sites. Direct depression of myocardial function by drugs may aggravate pulmonary edema caused by pulmonary capillary damage or, in the context of fluid therapy for hypotension, may result in cardiogenic pulmonary edema in the absence of pulmonary capillary damage.

Drug-induced pulmonary edema can be present on admission or may develop subsequently during the

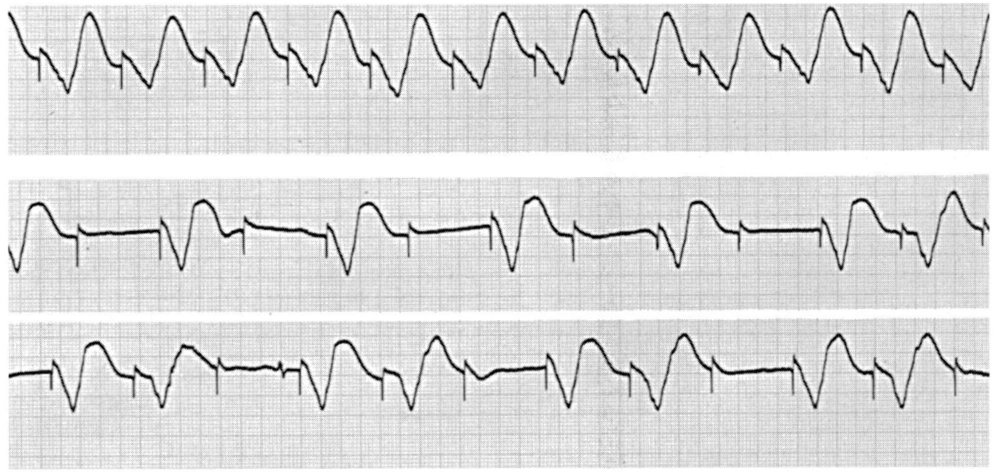

Figure 6–7. The patient was a 76-year-old man who had chronic congestive heart failure, recurrent ventricular tachycardia for which he was being treated with procainamide, paroxysmal atrioventricular block for which a transvenous pacing system had been implanted, and renal failure. He was admitted to the hospital with acute pulmonary edema. His serum potassium level was 5.0 mEq/L, and his serum procainamide level was 19 ng/mL. The top MCL_1 rhythm strip shows a paced QRS rhythm with extremely wide QRS complexes; atrial activity is not discerned. The bottom two continuous MCL_1 rhythm strips, recorded shortly after the top strip, show episodic failure of ventricular capture by the pacing stimuli, with a pattern suggesting Wenckebach's block of the pacing stimuli. Because there was no evidence of pacemaker generator malfunction, the failure to capture in this clinical setting was considered to result from myocardial stimulation threshold elevation and failure of impulse conduction owing to the membrane-depressant effects of the procainamide. Treatment with low-dose isoproterenol and intravenous steroids was without effect, and the patient died.

clinical course; in either case, it complicates management of shock states. Fluid filtration into the lungs depends in part on pulmonary capillary pressure and, therefore, on left atrial pressure. A difficult clinical situation may arise in which intracardiac filling pressures adequate to maintain cardiac output may result in pulmonary transudation. Suggestions about fluid therapy and the use of pulmonary capillary wedge pressures have been discussed. Diuretics are not useful for drug-induced pulmonary edema because filling pressures are already normal or low, and further diuresis can potentiate hypotension. Infusions of albumin have been proposed to increase plasma oncotic pressure and to draw fluid from the lungs. This is not rational because the protein content of the edema fluid is of similar composition to that of plasma, and this indicates that albumin passes through vascular endothelium as freely as water.

The use of mechanical ventilation with positive end-expiratory pressure is an important tool in the management of drug-induced pulmonary edema. Positive end-expiratory pressure increases functional residual capacity, reduces intrapulmonary shunting, and increases pulmonary compliance. Supplemental oxygen is usually necessary to maintain arterial oxygen tension at 60 to 70 mm Hg.

RECOGNITION AND MANAGEMENT OF CARDIAC DISTURBANCES CAUSED BY SPECIFIC DRUGS

Sedative-Hypnotic Drugs

Pathophysiology

Sedative-hypnotic drugs are involved in many or even the majority of cases of drug overdose. Although cardiac complications per se are uncommon, it is important to understand how this class of drugs might influence cardiovascular disturbances caused by coingested drugs. The major action of sedative-hypnotic drugs is on the CNS and results in reduced sympathetic and increased parasympathetic peripheral autonomic tone. Barbiturates have been shown to depress myocardial function in animals, but severe myocardial depression is uncommon in humans.[1] Cardiac output is commonly reduced because of relative hypovolemia caused by increased venous capacitance and absolute hypovolemia due to fluid loss into tissues, the latter a consequence of increased vascular permeability.[8] Cardiac output and heart rate may be lower than normal as a result of hypothermia and reduced metabolic demands. As a consequence of inhibition of sympathetic function, heart rate is frequently less than expected for the degree of hypotension.

An important complication of sedative-hypnotic drug overdose is pulmonary edema, which results from increased pulmonary vascular permeability, as just discussed. As a consequence, hypoxia and metabolic acidosis develop, and they may worsen myocardial performance and potentiate arrhythmias.

General Management

The management of hypotension and shock due to sedative-hypnotic overdose includes judicious use of fluids and pressor drugs. Because venous pooling contributes to reduced cardiac output, the head-down legs-up (Trendelenburg's) position may substantially increase venous return, cardiac output, and blood pressure. Infusion of modest amounts of colloid or crystalloid fluids is sufficient to correct hypovolemia and to increase cardiac output and tissue perfusion to adequate levels in many patients. Failure to achieve adequate tissue perfusion despite increased cardiac filling pressure or evidence of pulmonary edema is an indication for the use of pressor drugs, as discussed.

Sympathomimetic Drugs

General Considerations

As shown in Table 6–2, many drugs and toxins (as well as sedative-drug abstinence syndromes) can cause sympathetic overactivity. This typically results in sinus or atrial tachycardia (Fig. 6–8), hypertension, seizures, and, after massive ingestions, cardiovascular collapse and respiratory arrest. Occasionally, ventricular irritability and, rarely, ventricular fibrillation with death are observed. Sympathomimetic drug-induced hypertension may result in pul-

Table 6–2. Cardiac Disturbances due to Sympathomimetic Drugs and Toxins

Drugs	
Amphetamines	Δ-9-tetrahydrocannabinol
Cocaine	Lysergic acid diethylamide and other hallucinogens
Phencyclidine	Chloral hydrate*
Monoamine oxidase inhibitors	Ethanol
Phenylpropanolamine and other over-the-counter sympathomimetics	Hydrocarbon solvents* (such as toluene)
Theophylline	Freon* (and other fluorocarbon aerosols)
Caffeine	Sedative drug abstinence
Cardiovascular Disturbances	
Sinus tachycardia	Ventricular tachycardia
Atrial tachycardia	Ventricular fibrillation
Sinus bradycardia†	Hypertension
Ventricular premature beats	Hypotension‡
Other Common Manifestations	
Dilated pupils§	Tremor
Diaphoresis	Seizures
Fever	Hypokalemia
Excitement, anxiety, psychosis (often paranoid)‖	Metabolic acidosis

*Sensitizes myocardium to catecholamines.
†Reflex response to vasoconstrictors such as phenylpropanolamine.
‡Late manifestation, usually severe overdose.
§Excepting phencyclidine and alcohols.
‖Phencyclidine, alcohols, and solvents may cause ataxia, lethargy, or coma.

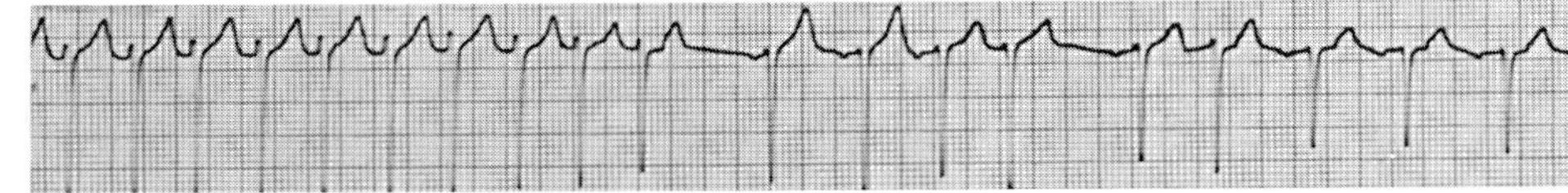

Figure 6–8. The patient, a 27-year-old cocaine user, was admitted to the coronary care unit for electrocardiographic monitoring after having had two syncopal spells. The MCL_1 rhythm strip shows bursts of atrial tachycardia, which terminate spontaneously, and atrial premature beats, some of which are not conducted.

monary edema (although blood pressure may be normal or even low at the time of medical evaluation) or may be complicated by intracerebral hemorrhage.[9] Many sympathomimetic drugs, particularly amphetamine-like drugs and phencyclidine, produce muscular hyperactivity (fasciculations, myoclonus, convulsions) and hyperpyrexia, sometimes associated with rhabdomyolysis, acute renal failure, and disseminated intravascular coagulation.[10] Of note are studies of amphetamine and cocaine toxicity in conscious dogs that indicate that hyperpyrexia contributes significantly to death.[11] Pretreatment with pancuronium, which paralyzes the muscles that are the source of heat generation; diazepam, which prevents convulsions; and chlorpromazine, which sedates the animal, lessened the severity of the seizures and possibly also facilitated heat dissipation via peripheral α-adrenergic blockade. Environmental cooling substantially improved survival. In contrast, propranolol, which effectively blocked cardiovascular responses to amphetamines, or bicarbonate infusion, which reversed metabolic acidosis, did not improve survival.

Amphetamine-Like Drugs and Cocaine

Many amphetamine-like drugs are available as anorectic agents. Along with these, illicitly manufactured amphetamines and their derivatives and cocaine are widely abused, primarily for their euphoric effects.[12] The euphoria is associated with CNS and adrenomedullary sympathetic activation, which produces typical sympathomimetic syndromes. Tolerance to CNS effects develops rapidly, however, and thus the duration of euphoria is much shorter than the presence of the drug in the body. Repeated doses may result in accumulation of drug and cardiovascular toxicity at a time when the user is no longer euphoric.

Amphetamines displace and release catecholamines stored in neurons, directly stimulate postsynaptic adrenergic receptors, and may inhibit monoamine oxidase (MAO), the enzyme responsible for intraneuronal degradation of catecholamines. Cocaine in particular is a potent inhibitor of neuronal catecholamine uptake, which is a major route of detoxification for norepinephrine released from nerve endings or the adrenal medulla or administered exogenously. Continual administration of amphetamines and cocaine has also been reported to result in myocarditis and cardiomyopathy.[13]

Cocaine intoxication has been associated with a number of additional cardiovascular complications, including acute myocardial infarction, myocardial necrosis, and dissecting aortic aneurysm and shock.[14, 15] Myocardial infarction occurs as a consequence of increased myocardial work in the presence of fixed coronary artery disease, coronary vasospasm, or coronary thrombosis. Patchy myocardial necrosis with contraction band necrosis has been described after acute cocaine intoxication, and it is believed to be a result of intense catecholamine stimulation of the heart.[16] Fibrosis and chronic cardiomyopathy may ensue. In high doses, cocaine depresses myocardial function and ventricular depolarization (widening the QRS), effects due to a local anesthetic-type blockade of the fast sodium channel.

The management of amphetamine and cocaine drug toxicity depends on the specific manifestations (Table 6–3). Hypertension and tachycardia can be managed by α- and β-adrenergic blocking agents or vasodilators such as sodium nitroprusside or rate-sparing calcium channel blockers or both. Because arrhythmias result primarily from β-adrenergic stimulation, a β-blocking agent is the drug of choice. Theoretically, a relatively specific β1-blocker such as metoprolol or esmolol would be preferred to avoid antagonizing the β2-mediated arteriolar dilation that may be opposing α-mediated constriction. Thus, β2-blockade could result in unopposed α effects and could worsen hypertension.

Table 6–3. Treatment of Cardiovascular Complications of Sympathomimetic Drug Poisoning

Manifestations	Treatment
Tachyarrhythmias	Reduce environmental stimulation*
Sinus or atrial	None, metoprolol, esmolol, verapamil
Ventricular	Metoprolol, lidocaine, cardioversion
Hypertension	Reduce environmental stimulation*
	Phentolamine
	Nitroprusside
	β-Blocker (β_1-specific if possible) if associated with tachycardia
Convulsions	Diazepam, phenytoin, phenobarbital
Hyperthermia	Stop seizures
	Pancuronium if seizures uncontrollable
	External cooling
	Chlorpromazine or haloperidol
	High inspired oxygen
Myocardial ischemia/ infarction	Nitrates, calcium channel blockers, thrombolysis-esmolol/metoprolol
Cardiovascular collapse	Fluids (may require massive amounts in presence of hyperthermia)
	Pressors (unpredictable sensitivity)

*Especially phencyclidine and hydrocarbons.

Hyperpyrexia is potentially life threatening.[17] Chlorpromazine or haloperidol may reverse hyperthermia by CNS or peripheral vascular actions, as discussed. Although these drugs are known to lower the seizure threshold in some experimental seizure models, chlorpromazine seems to lessen the severity of seizures caused by sympathomimetic drugs. Seizures should be treated as rapidly and effectively as possible. Intravenous administration of lorazepam or diazepam is usually effective in terminating seizures, but loading with phenobarbital should then be accomplished.

If hyperthermia or severe metabolic acidosis complicates seizures or other evidence of muscular hyperactivity, external cooling and paralysis with pancuronium or curare are indicated. Even when muscular hyperactivity is prevented by paralysis, persistent seizure activity may cause brain injury. Therefore, electroencephalograms should be used to monitor paralyzed patients, and their seizures should be controlled with anticonvulsant drugs or general anesthesia, if necessary. Ventilation with high oxygen concentrations is indicated for all hyperthermic patients to meet the extreme metabolic demands of muscular hyperactivity and the effects of hyperthermia on metabolism in other body organs. Acute renal failure may result from hypovolemia, hypotension, and rhabdomyolysis with myoglobinuria and may be prevented by vigorous fluid replacement and use of mannitol and diuretics to increase urine flow and bicarbonate to alkalize the urine.

Phencyclidine

The cardiovascular effects of phencyclidine resemble those of the amphetamines. In most cases, hypertension and tachycardia are present.[18] Seizures are common, are often difficult to treat, and may be fatal. However, unlike patients who have ingested amphetamines, phencyclidine-intoxicated patients usually appear ataxic, sedated, or even comatose. Blood pressure and heart rate are often quite labile and increase with environmental stimulation. With severe overdose, hypotension and respiratory depression occur.

The mechanism of action of phencyclidine includes increased CNS-mediated sympathetic activity, potentiation of endogenous catecholamine actions, and direct vasoconstrictor effects, all of which are reversed by α-adrenergic blocking agents. Neuronal uptake of norepinephrine may be inhibited, as it is with cocaine. The labile cardiovascular responses may be explained by increased sensitivity to endogenously released catecholamines.

Therapy of cardiovascular complications of phencyclidine consists of the use of α- and β-adrenergic blocking drugs and vasodilators, as discussed for amphetamines. Both nitroprusside and diazoxide have been used to treat phencyclidine-induced hypertension. Because phencyclidine enhances sensitivity to catecholamines, increased sensitivity to pressor drugs may be observed when these are used to treat hypotensive patients. Reducing environmental stimulation is helpful in minimizing toxicity. Diazepam is often given for sedation and haloperidol for extreme agitation.

Monoamine Oxidase Inhibitors

Clinical manifestations of MAO inhibitor toxicity resemble those of other sympathomimetic drugs: restlessness, hyperactivity, confusion or stupor, neuromuscular irritability, hypertension, seizures, and hyperpyrexia.[19–21] Hypertension, which most often occurs after ingestion of tyramine-containing foods or beverages or after taking other sympathomimetic drugs but can also occur after an overdose, may be severe, often is associated with severe headache, and has been associated with intracerebral hemorrhage. Hypotension can also occur after overdose.

Understanding the pathophysiology of MAO inhibitor reactions requires understanding of the role of MAO in the body. MAO is located within adrenergic neurons, where it metabolizes catecholamines and related monoamines, and in the gastrointestinal mucosa and liver, where it metabolizes dietary monoamines, such as tyramine. Inhibition of MAO within the adrenergic neuron results in accumulation of both active and relatively inactive (such as octopamine) monoamines. Octopamine and other relatively inactive monoamines act as false neurotransmitters in that they are released by neuronal stimulation into nerve endings, where they do not effectively activate vascular receptors. As a consequence, MAO inhibitors, when taken continually, may lower blood pressure. However, MAO inhibitors, by slowing metabolism, may also increase pressor responses to catecholamines released by other drugs. Most important in causing hypertension is that MAO inhibitors in the gut and liver increase the bioavailability of tyramine, which in turn releases catecholamines stored in adrenergic neurons. Ingestion of foods rich in tyramine can lead to massive catecholamine release and hypertensive crisis. Tranylcypromine is a MAO inhibitor that itself causes catecholamine release and, among the MAO inhibitor class of drugs, has been most commonly implicated in cardiovascular toxicity. It is important also to recognize the potential interaction between meperidine and MAO inhibitors. The combination has resulted in severe hypertension, hyperthermia, and seizures. The mechanism is unknown. Therapy for MAO toxicity is similar to that of other sympathomimetic drugs.

Serotonin reuptake inhibitors such as fluoxetine do not cause direct cardiovascular toxicity but do interact with monamine inhibitors to produce the so-called serotonin syndrome.[22] This syndrome is associated with confusion, fever, diaphoresis, and myoclonus.

Phenylpropanolamine and Other Over-the-Counter Sympathomimetic Drugs

Phenylpropanolamine, ephedrine, and many other over-the-counter decongestants and appetite-suppressant drugs have both direct and indirect (catecholamine-releasing) sympathomimetic effects. In most cases of overdose with cold or decongestant preparations, mild hypertension is observed and requires no specific therapy. After ingestion of predominantly vasoconstrictor drugs such as phenylpropanolamine, heart rate may be slow owing to reflex slowing or rapid owing to coingested caffeine or anticholinergic antihistamines. After overdose and occasionally after therapeutic doses, severe hypertension occurs, sometimes associated with stroke, ventricular arrhythmias, or ST-T changes on the ECG and abnormally elevated myocardial creatine phosphokinase concentrations suggesting myocardial injury.[23, 24] Unusual responsiveness to catecholamines may explain some of the exaggerated blood pressure response in some patients. In one such patient, pressor hypersensitivity to infused norepinephrine was documented and was related to a previously unrecognized autonomic insufficiency state.[25]

Enhanced pressor sensitivity to sympathomimetic drugs is expected in persons taking tricyclic antidepressants, which block uptake of released catecholamines.[26] Antihistamines found in common cold preparations may contribute to sympathomimetic-induced hypertension by inhibiting vagally mediated cardiac deceleration, which normally serves to compensate for vasoconstrictor-mediated hypertension.

Amphetamine "look-alikes," containing phenylpropanolamine, ephedrine, or caffeine, are available without prescription. Sudden deaths, presumably due to arrhythmias, in the context of overdosage have occurred.

Management of overdose with phenylpropanolamine and related drugs includes careful monitoring of blood pressure and ECGs. Management of hypertension, tachycardia, and arrhythmias is as discussed for amphetamines.

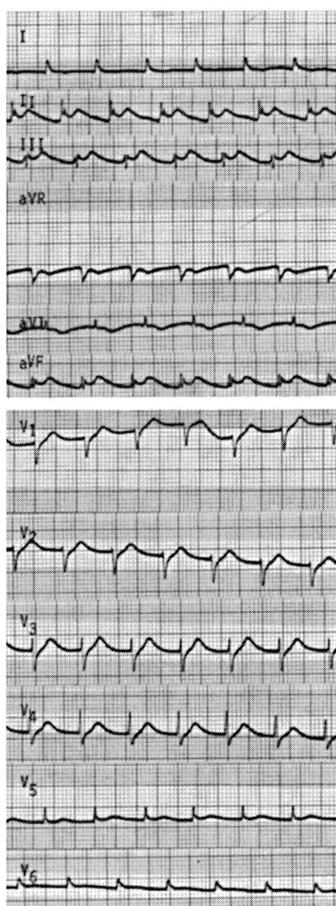

Figure 6–9. This 12-lead electrocardiogram was recorded from a 60-year-old man with chronic obstructive pulmonary disease. He had ingested aminophylline and terbutaline in a suicide attempt. His peak theophylline concentration was 152 μg/mL. A narrow QRS tachycardia is present without discernible atrial activity, suggesting a junctional origin. J point and ST segment elevation are present in the inferolateral leads (II, III, aV_F, V_5, and V_6). Serial enzyme determination failed to confirm myocardial infarction. The patient died 2 days later with refractory cardiovascular collapse.

Theophylline and Caffeine

Cardiac toxicity of theophylline occurs in a different context from that of stimulant drugs. The most common circumstance is overdosage during therapy for obstructive airway disease, often as a result of hepatic dysfunction, which reduces the rate of theophylline metabolism. Accidental or suicidal overdose often occurs in persons with underlying medical illnesses. The nature and severity of these medical conditions have a strong impact on the course and severity of cardiac toxicity.

The typical cardiovascular manifestations of theophylline overdose result from β-adrenergic stimulation and include tachycardia and arrhythmias[27, 28] (Fig. 6–9). Hypotension (rather than hypertension, as occurs with most other sympathomimetic drugs) is encountered in severe intoxications. Like amphetamines, theophylline causes systemic and local vascular catecholamine release but, in addition, at high concentrations, such as those occurring in severe poisonings, may inhibit phosphodiesterase, an enzyme that degrades cyclic adenosine monophosphate, which, in turn mediates β-adrenergic actions. Theophylline also directly relaxes vascular smooth muscle. Convulsions typically occur with an overdose, and cardiac and respiratory arrest are causes of death. Management of cardiac toxicity due to theophylline ingestion in persons with chronic lung disease may be difficult. β-Adrenergic blocking agents are logical and effective treatment for supraventricular and ventricular arrhythmias, but they also may worsen airway obstruction. Relatively cardiospecific β-blockers, such as esmolol or metoprolol, might be tried and the antiarrhythmic effects closely titrated against evidence of worsening airway obstruction.

Hypotension due to theophylline use usually results from peripheral vasodilation, at least early in the course of overdose. However, with prolonged β-sympathetic stimulation, myocarditis with reduced ventricular function may occur late in the course of theophylline overdose. In addition, many older patients with chronic lung disease have ischemic heart disease. Tachycardia and hypotension may reduce myocardial perfusion, resulting in impaired myocardial function. Hypoxia caused by underlying lung disease, hypokalemia caused by sustained β-adrenergic stimulation, and acidosis due to lung disease or convulsions may also contribute to hypotension.

Management of theophylline-induced hypotension includes correction of metabolic disturbances and arrhythmias and administration of fluids and pressor agents. If pressor drugs are to be used, it is useful to know the cardiac output and to be able to compute the systemic vascular resistance. If cardiac output is high and systemic vascular resistance is low, as in many cases of theophylline overdose, administration of vasoconstrictors such as norepinephrine and nonselective β-adrenergic antagonists is indicated. If cardiac output is low despite adequate cardiac filling pressures and systemic vascular resistance is normal or high as sometimes occurs late in the case of theophylline overdose and in persons with pre-existing myocardial disease, inotropic agents such as dobutamine might be selected.

In the presence of severe toxicity, particularly in a patient with serious underlying medical disease, the persistence of theophylline in the body and the time course of toxicity may be prolonged, and acceleration of drug removal by hemoperfusion should be undertaken.[28]

Caffeine is widely consumed in beverages such as coffee and colas, in over-the-counter stimulants, and in various other combination analgesic and cold medications. Caffeine has pharmacologic actions similar to those of theophylline. Caffeine potentiates the effects of sympathomimetic drugs and might contribute to adverse cardiac events, including sudden death due to amphetamine look-alikes, as discussed earlier. Caffeine alone is thought to cause severe cardiac toxicity rarely, although cases of supraventricular tachycardias are reported. Severe caffeine intoxication with tachyarrhythmias followed by cardiovascular collapse and death has occurred in children. We treated an adult who had ingested a massive amount of caffeine (NōDōz) and who had sinus tachycardia with a rate of 190 beats per minute, hypokalemia, hyperglycemia, metabolic acidosis, and rhabdomyolysis (Fig. 6–10).

Δ^9-Tetrahydrocannabinol and Hallucinogens

The usual cardiovascular effects of Δ^9-tetrahydrocannabinol (THC), the principal psychoactive component in marijuana and other cannabis products, are tachycardia, a slight increase in recumbent blood pressure, and, with large doses or in susceptible persons, orthostatic hypotension. The effects of THC on heart rate result from CNS-mediated sympathetic activation and reduced parasympathetic activity and from systemic release of catecholamines. Orthostatic hypotension results from impaired sympathetic reflex responses and, in particular, deficient venoconstriction.

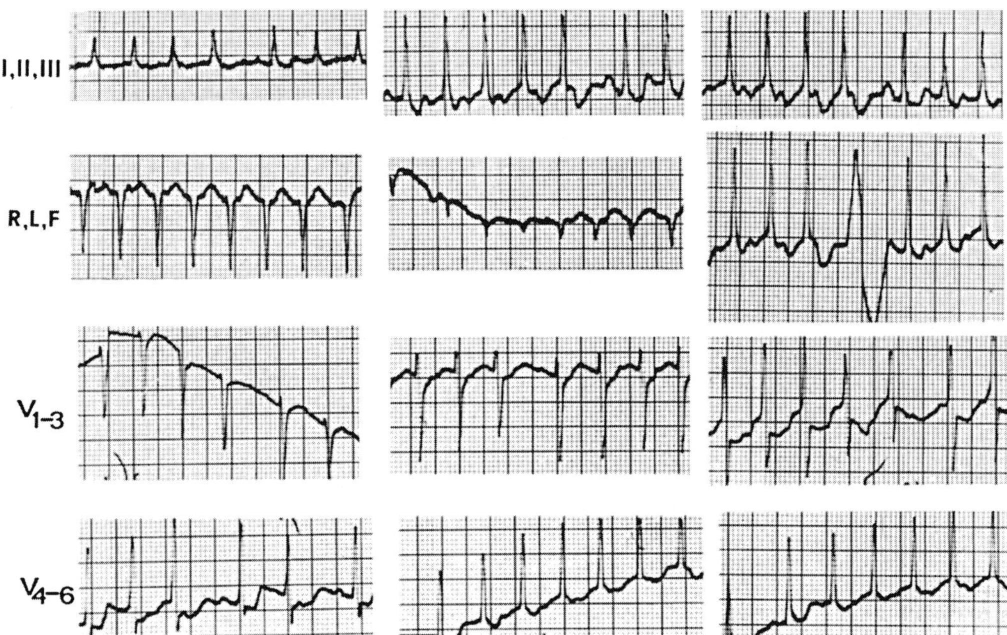

Figure 6–10. The patient is a 30-year-old schizophrenic woman who allegedly ingested the contents of four bottles of the over-the-counter preparation NōDōz, each containing 60 100-mg caffeine tablets. She was brought to the emergency room awake but mute and apparently hallucinating. Blood pressure was 112/74 mm Hg; heart rate, 180 to 200 beats per minute; serum potassium level, 2.2 mEq/L; and serum caffeine level, 200 μg/mL.

This admission electrocardiogram shows a supraventricular tachycardia at a rate of about 180 to 190/min. The tachycardia is probably sinus in origin, judging from the P wave configurations. Atrioventricular nodal Wenckebach's block is present and is probably the result of the tachycardia rate (and the inability of the atrioventricular node to respond) rather than to the pharmacologic effects of caffeine. Ventricular ectopic complexes are also present.

The patient was treated with potassium and fluids, with prompt initial slowing of the sinus rate to 150/min, then with gradual return to normal during the next 48 hours.

Sinus tachycardia can reach rates of 140 to 150 beats per minute or higher and, manifested as palpitations, can contribute to the anxiety reaction occasionally reported by novice users or those consuming marijuana containing unusually large amounts of THC. In otherwise healthy persons, no specific treatment other than reassurance is necessary. Patients with ischemic heart disease are at greater risk from the effects of THC (as they are from those of all sympathomimetic drugs). The combination of (1) increased myocardial oxygen demand due to the tachycardia and increased myocardial contractility and (2) decreased myocardial oxygen delivery due to effects of carbon monoxide derived from marijuana smoke may aggravate the ischemia. For example, persons with angina pectoris are not able to exercise as long after smoking marijuana as they can after smoking tobacco or not smoking at all. Ischemia combined with systemic release of catecholamines also might result in potentially severe arrhythmias.

Orthostatic dizziness is occasionally reported by recreational users of cannabis, particularly after eating larger than usual quantities of THC in cookies or brownies. Patients receiving THC as an adjunct to cancer chemotherapy may also exhibit orthostatic hypotension, particularly when they are dehydrated because of their disease. Hypotension responds well to placing the patient into the horizontal or Trendelenburg posture and administering fluids; administration of pressors is rarely necessary.

Lysergic acid diethylamide, psilocybin, and other hallucinogens commonly result in tachycardia and mild hypertension as part of a general sympathetic arousal syndrome. Cardiovascular disturbances are rarely serious and require only supportive care.

Chloral Hydrate and Ethanol

Chloral hydrate overdose has been associated with supraventricular (mainly junctional) tachycardia, ventricular tachycardia (often polymorphous), and ventricular fibrillation.[29] Chloral hydrate is metabolized to trichloroethanol, which is believed to produce the arrhythmias. Trichloroethanol as well as other alcohols releases catecholamines. Trichloroethanol also is believed to sensitize the myocardium to the effects of circulating catecholamines, an effect similar to that of hydrocarbon anesthetics, to be discussed.

Chronically alcoholic patients with toxicologic problems frequently are seen in emergency rooms. Chronic or acute cardiovascular disorders may appear as primary problems or may complicate other overdoses.[30] Chronic alcoholism is well known to be associated with congestive cardiomyopathy and, less commonly, beriberi heart disease. Congestive cardiomyopathy with low cardiac output, pulmonary congestion, diverse arrhythmias, or sudden death may result from the chronic toxic effects of ethanol.[31] Alcoholic cardiomyopathy is treated like other types of congestive failure.

Beriberi heart disease results from thiamine deficiency. Patients present with high cardiac output manifested by tachycardia and wide pulse pressure, as well as peripheral neuritis. The heart may be enlarged, and dyspnea caused by pulmonary congestion, as well as neck vein engorgement and peripheral edema, may be present. Prolonged QT interval, low QRS voltage, and T wave abnormalities may be present on the ECG. Decreased peripheral vascular resistance is responsible for the high cardiac output. Initial doses of thiamine occasionally result in pulmonary edema because of a sudden increase in vascular resistance combined with mobilization of edema fluid.

Heavy binge drinkers may present with a sudden onset of arrhythmias, particularly atrial fibrillation or flutter with rapid ventricular response but also atrial or junctional tachycardia and ventricular arrhythmias (this syndrome has been termed "holiday heart") (Fig. 6–11). The arrhythmias may be due to preclinical cardiomyopathy, electrolyte abnormalities (including deficiency of potassium, phosphate, or magnesium), or early stages of alcohol withdrawal.

Abstinence from ethanol (and other sedative drugs) may be associated with intense sympathetic hyperactivity, hypertension, and many types of tachyarrhythmias, usually supraventricular but also ventricular arrhythmias, and sudden, unpredictable death.

Lidocaine, β-adrenergic antagonists, and phenytoin have been used to treat arrhythmias caused by chloral hydrate and other alcohols. β-Blockers, verapamil, or diltiazem may be necessary to control the ventricular response rate in cases of alcohol-induced atrial fibrillation or flutter. Metabolic disturbances, particularly hypokalemia, hypophosphatemia, and hypomagnesemia, common in alcoholic persons, may contribute to arrhythmias and should be corrected.

Hydrocarbon Solvents and Fluorocarbon Aerosols

An epidemic of sudden deaths was associated with widespread abuse of solvents by inhalation in the late 1960s.[32] Witnesses reported that victims collapsed after sniffing glue, cleaning fluids, paint, or aerosol propellants (hair sprays, deodorant sprays, and frying pan lubricants) from plastic bags, becoming excited or panicky and then exercising. The presumed cause of death was ventricular fibrillation. Sudden death and atrial fibrillation have been reported after occupational exposure to solvents.[33, 34] Animal studies have shown that many solvents, including toluene, benzene, chloroform, trichloroethane, trichloroethylene, trichlorofluoroethane, and other fluoroalkenes (freons), potentiate arrhythmias due to infused epinephrine. Thus, doses of epinephrine that usually produce no arrhythmias may cause ventricular tachycardia or fibrillation after solvent or fluorocarbon exposure. Arrhythmias are also more easily produced in the presence of hypoxemia, which might also be expected when breathing gases from a plastic bag.

Solvent inhalation, even when normal oxygenation

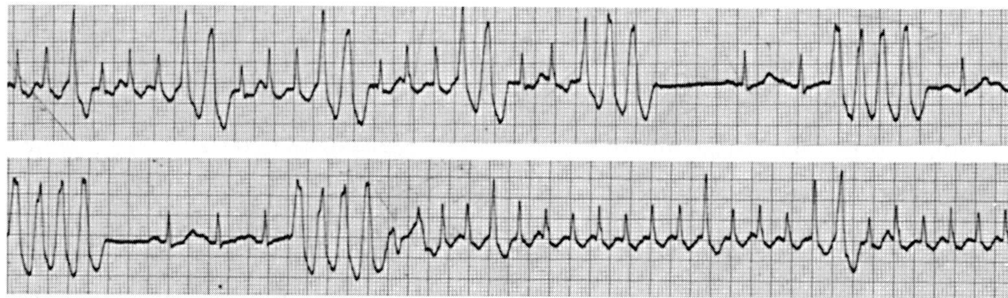

Figure 6–11. These two continuous lead II rhythm strips were recorded in a 48-year-old alcoholic man admitted to the hospital after a syncopal spell preceded by palpitations. Sinus rhythm is interrupted by atrial tachycardia. Frequent premature ventricular complexes are also present, as well as bursts of ventricular tachycardia, which occasionally interrupt the atrial tachyarrhythmia. The rhythm was treated with intravenous lidocaine, which abolished the bursts of ventricular tachycardia but had no effect on the atrial arrhythmia. All arrhythmias resolved within 12 hours of admission. Work-up for organic heart disease was nondiagnostic, and 24-hour ambulatory electrocardiographic monitoring before hospital discharge failed to reveal any rhythm abnormalities.

is maintained, may cause sinoatrial slowing followed by escape junctional or ventricular rhythms and subsequently asystole or ventricular fibrillation. The combination of depressed sinoatrial automaticity and myocardial sensitization to catecholamines, released by exercise or emotional stimuli, possibly accounts for the fatal ventricular arrhythmias. Toluene sniffing in particular causes renal tubular dysfunction, as well as severe hypokalemia, hypophosphatemia, and metabolic acidosis, which might aggravate arrhythmias. Ingestion of hydrocarbons is typically associated with pneumonitis and CNS depression; however, arrhythmias with ECG and enzyme changes, suggesting acute myocardial injury, have been reported. Seizures and ventricular tachycardia occurred in a 2-year-old child after accidental exposure to nonfluorinated hydrocarbon aerosol propellants (isobutane and *n*-butane) used in a deodorant spray can.[35]

Obviously, little can be done to treat victims of "sudden sniffing death." However, in persons who are intoxicated with solvents or fluorocarbons, steps can be taken to lessen the risk of arrhythmias, at least according to our current hypothesis of pathogenesis. Before evaluation at the hospital, patients should be advised to avoid strenuous exercise. In the hospital, patients can be placed in a quiet, nonthreatening environment and sedated if necessary. If they are hypoxic, oxygen should be administered and metabolic abnormalities corrected. Sympathomimetic drugs should be avoided. Ventricular arrhythmias are best treated with β-blocking agents.

Sympathetic-Inhibiting Drugs

Cardiac disturbances caused by sympathetic-inhibiting drugs are listed in Table 6–4.

β-Adrenergic Receptor Blockers

Cardiac disturbances caused by β-adrenergic receptor blockers result from both receptor blockade, which all drugs in this class demonstrate, and other actions such as membrane-depressant or sympathomimetic effects, which differ among drugs within the class. β-Adrenergic blockade itself is associated with sinus bradycardia, AV block (usually first degree) and the emergence of ectopic escape pacemakers in healthy hearts. In persons with underlying cardiac conduction disease, advanced AV block with slow ventricular rates can occur. Occasionally, in the presence of severe underlying myocardial disease in which contractility depends on sympathetic activity, acute β-adrenergic receptor blockade can result in hypotension or cardiac failure, including shock or acute pulmonary edema and death. With gradual dose escalation, however, many patients with severe cardiac failure are able to tolerate β-blockers with beneficial effects on mortality.

In previously healthy persons, drugs such as propranolol, with membrane-depressant effects, can in large doses directly depress myocardial function and result in hypotension caused by reduced cardiac output. Drugs such as pindolol, with intrinsic sympathomimetic activity, can cause tachycardia and hypertension despite concurrent β-blockade after an overdose.

Therapy is summarized in Table 6–5. Sinus brady-

Table 6–4. Cardiac Disturbances Caused by Sympathetic-Inhibiting Drugs

Drugs	
Propranolol and other β-blockers	Resperine
Methyldopa	Guanethidine
Clonidine	Prazosin and other α-blockers
Cardiovascular Disturbances	
Sinus bradycardia	Hypotension
Atrioventricular block	Cardiac failure*
Other Common Manifestations	
Sedation†	Seizures§
Small pupils‡	Hyperkalemia
Diarrhea	Bronchoconstriction‖

*Usually in patients with underlying myocardial disease.
†Except guanethidine and prazosin.
‡Particularly clonidine and prazosin.
§Propranolol and other membrane-depressant β-blockers; rarely clonidine.
‖Usually in patients with previous asthma.

Table 6–5. Treatment of Cardiovascular Complications of Sympathetic-Inhibiting Drug Poisoning

Manifestation	Treatment
Bradyarrhythmias	
Sinus or atrial	None, atropine, isoproterenol, glucagon,* pacing
Junctional and ventricular	Isoproterenol, pacing, glucagon*
Ventricular tachyarrhythmias	Lidocaine, overdrive pacing Cardioversion
Hypotension	Trendelenburg's position Treat bradyarrhythmias if present Fluids (hemodynamic monitoring advised with pre-existing cardiac disease) Glucagon, dobutamine* (if normal or high systemic vascular resistance) Dopamine, norepinephrine (if low systemic vascular resistance)
Hypertension†	Phentolamine, tolazoline Nitroprusside

*Particularly when related to β-blocker overdose.
†Clonidine, methyldopa, guanethidine; note hypertension is often *transient* and is followed by hypotension.

cardia is usually well tolerated and requires no specific therapy. If sinus bradycardia results in hemodynamic compromise, atropine, isoproterenol, glucagon, or intracardiac pacing should be considered. Because of the competitive nature of drug-induced β-blockade, extraordinary doses of isoproterenol may be required to increase heart rate. The dose may be limited by peripheral vasodilation and decline in blood pressure. AV block resulting in hemodynamic compromise is an indication for dual-chamber intracardiac pacing.

Hypotension can usually be managed with fluids and correction of bradyarrhythmias. In the presence of myocardial depression, glucagon, which activates adenylate cyclase by a nonadrenergic mechanism, may enhance myocardial contractility and increase cardiac output. Epinephrine, dobutamine, amrinone, and milrinone are potentially useful inotropic agents, although the doses may need to be higher than usual because of β-blockade. Calcium chloride has been reported to increase blood pressure after severe propranolol overdose that is unresponsive to other medications.[36]

Sympatholytic Antihypertensive Drugs

Most patients who have ingested excessive doses of sympatholytic antihypertensive drugs have sinus bradycardia and hypotension when first seen. Drugs such as methyldopa, clonidine, and reserpine, which are active in the CNS, commonly cause sedation or coma. After an overdose of clonidine, miosis and respiratory depression resembling narcotic overdose can also ensue. However, after clonidine poisoning, hypotension and bradycardia are more prominent than respiratory depression. The reverse is true for narcotics. Clonidine, by direct α-adrenergic receptor agonist activity, and methyldopa, reserpine, and guanethidine, through systemic release of catecholamines, also have been associated with transient and sometimes severe hypertension.

In most cases, hypotension due to antihypertensive drug overdose is not severe and can be managed by the legs-up head-down position and intravenous fluids. When hypotension is severe in the presence of bradycardia, use of atropine, isoproterenol, or cardiac pacing increases heart rate and cardiac output and may increase blood pressure. Although not often necessary, modest doses of dopamine and norepinephrine are usually effective. Hypertension resulting from use of clonidine or other sympatholytic drugs is best treated with the short-acting α-adrenergic receptor antagonist phentolamine and, if necessary, vasodilators such as nitroprusside. Use of oral nifedipine also has been effective. It should be recognized that the hypertensive phase after clonidine overdose is relatively brief, and its treatment should be tapered before the subsequent hypotensive effects become manifested.

Because clonidine exerts its hypotensive and sedating effects by actions on α-adrenergic receptors in the brain, the use of centrally active α-blockers such as tolazoline has been recommended for clonidine overdose. Although tolazoline can reverse the effects of therapeutic doses of clonidine, no benefit has been proved for its use in overdose. Because most clonidine-intoxicated patients fare well with supportive care, we do not use tolazoline. Clonidine has been shown to reduce symptoms of narcotic withdrawal and thus is used as an adjunct in this therapy. (This explains clonidine overdose in heroin addicts.) In animals, high doses of naloxone reverse the hypotension and bradycardia due to clonidine and might be expected to be of benefit in overdose cases in humans. However, the response to naloxone in individuals poisoned with clonidine is variable and should not be relied on as the primary therapy for cardiovascular toxicity from this drug.

Anticholinergic Drugs and Toxins

Cardiac disturbances caused by anticholinergic drugs and toxins are listed in Table 6–6.

The various anticholinergic drugs or toxins that may be ingested are too numerous to list each drug separately. In most cases, they cause sinus or atrial tachycardia with mild hypertension. Serious arrhythmias resulting from purely anticholinergic compounds are uncommon unless a patient has underlying ischemic heart disease. Thus, by increasing myocardial oxygen demand owing to tachycardia, atropine has caused ventricular tachycardia and fibrillation in patients after myocardial infarction. Many patients with anticholinergic signs have ingested antihistamine-sympathomimetic combinations or drugs

Table 6–6. Cardiac Disturbances Caused by Anticholinergic Drugs and Toxins

Drugs	
Atropine, belladonna, scopolamine	Tricyclic antidepressants
Antihistamines (including most over-the-counter hypnotics)	Plants (such as jimsonweed)
Propantheline	Mushrooms (such as *Amanita muscaria**)
Cardiac Disturbances	
Sinus tachycardia	Ventricular premature beats
Atrial tachycardia	Hypertension
Other Common Manifestations	
Sedation	Dry mucous membranes
Delirium, coma	No sweating
Fever	Hypoactive or absent bowel sounds
Dry, flushed skin	Urinary retention
Dilated pupils	

*May have muscarinic as well as anticholinergic activity.

such as tricyclic antidepressants or neuroleptics with both anticholinergic and membrane-depressant effects that result in more serious cardiovascular disturbances.

If treatment is necessary because of hypotension, organ ischemia, or severe hypertension due to use of anticholinergic drugs, the most specific therapy is administration of cholinesterase inhibitors. Physostigmine is most commonly used because it enters the brain and antagonizes the CNS and peripheral autonomic effects. Alternatively, because anticholinergic drugs result in an imbalance between sympathetic and parasympathetic activity with a predominance of the former, β-blockers also may be effective in treating supraventricular tachyarrhythmias. Both physostigmine and β-blockers may be hazardous when given to persons with depressed AV conduction[37] (Fig. 6–12).

Cholinomimetic Toxins and Drugs

Cardiac disturbances and other common manifestations of poisoning by cholinomimetic drugs and toxins are listed in Table 6–7. The most common type of cholinomimetic poisoning is that due to ingestion of organophosphate or carbamate insecticides resulting in excess cholinesterase inhibition.[38, 39] The cardiovascular effects of organophosphates are unpredictable and often change over the time course of the poisoning. Early in the course, acetylcholine stimulates nicotinic receptors at sympathetic ganglia and causes tachycardia and mild hypertension. Later it stimulates muscarinic receptors or blocks ganglionic transmission by hyperpolarization, and bradycardia and hypotension result. The most common cardiac finding in organophosphate poisoning is sinus tachycardia. In severe poisonings, however, advanced AV block, bradyarrhythmias with hypotension, and asystole may occur.

Delayed ventricular tachycardia of the torsades de pointes type may occur as late as 5 days after acute intoxication with organophosphates.[40] The mechanism is believed to be a persistent imbalance between sympathetic and parasympathetic influences on the heart. The result is nonhomogeneous repolarization (associated with a long QT interval) and a predisposition to ventricular arrhythmias. In patients with severe cardiac depression resulting from tricyclic antidepressant drugs, the use of physostigmine has caused loss of atrial activity, worsening of AV block, severe sinus or ventricular bradycardia, and asystole (see Fig. 6–12).[37]

Bradyarrhythmias, if hemodynamically significant, can usually be effectively treated by administration of atropine or glycopyrrolate.[41] Atropine or glycopyrrolate must compete with excess acetylcholine at the receptor site, and thus extremely large doses may be required. Doses should be increased until cholinergic signs such as salivation, diaphoresis, and bronchorrhea are reversed. When anticholinergic drugs are not effective, cardiac pacing is indicated. Sinus or atrial tachycardia causing hemodynamic compromise is a greater problem to treat because drugs such as propranolol that might slow the rate might also worsen bronchoconstriction or aggravate conduction disturbances later in the course of the overdose. Patients with clinical signs of cholinesterase inhibition or an abnormal ECG (including QT interval prolongation) should have continuous cardiac monitoring for the possibility of developing ventricular tachycardia. The ECG findings may remain abnormal for several days.[40] Treatment of ventricular tachycardia is similar to that previously described for torsades de pointes, except that anticholinergic drugs also may be used to normalize autonomic influences on the heart. Pulmonary secretions (sometimes presenting as apparent acute pulmonary edema) or respiratory

Table 6–7. Cardiac Disturbances Due to Cholinomimetic Drugs and Toxins

Drugs	
Organophosphates	Pilocarpine
Carbamates	Neostigmine, pyridostigmine
Physostigmine	Nicotine
Bethanecol	
Cardiac Disturbances	
Sinus bradycardia	Ventricular tachycardia associated with QT interval prolongation†
Atrial or junctional or ventricular bradycardia	Hypotension
Atrioventricular block	Hypertension*
Sinus tachycardia*	Asystole
Other Common Manifestations	
Pulmonary secretions and/or edema	Abdominal cramps
Small pupils	Diarrhea
Diaphoresis	Fasciculations
Lacrimation	Convulsions
Salivation	Muscle weakness and paralysis
Urinary frequency and/or incontinence	Respiratory failure

*May be seen in the early stages of cholinesterase inhibition and nicotine poisoning due to ganglionic stimulation.
†May be delayed up to several days after initial intoxication.

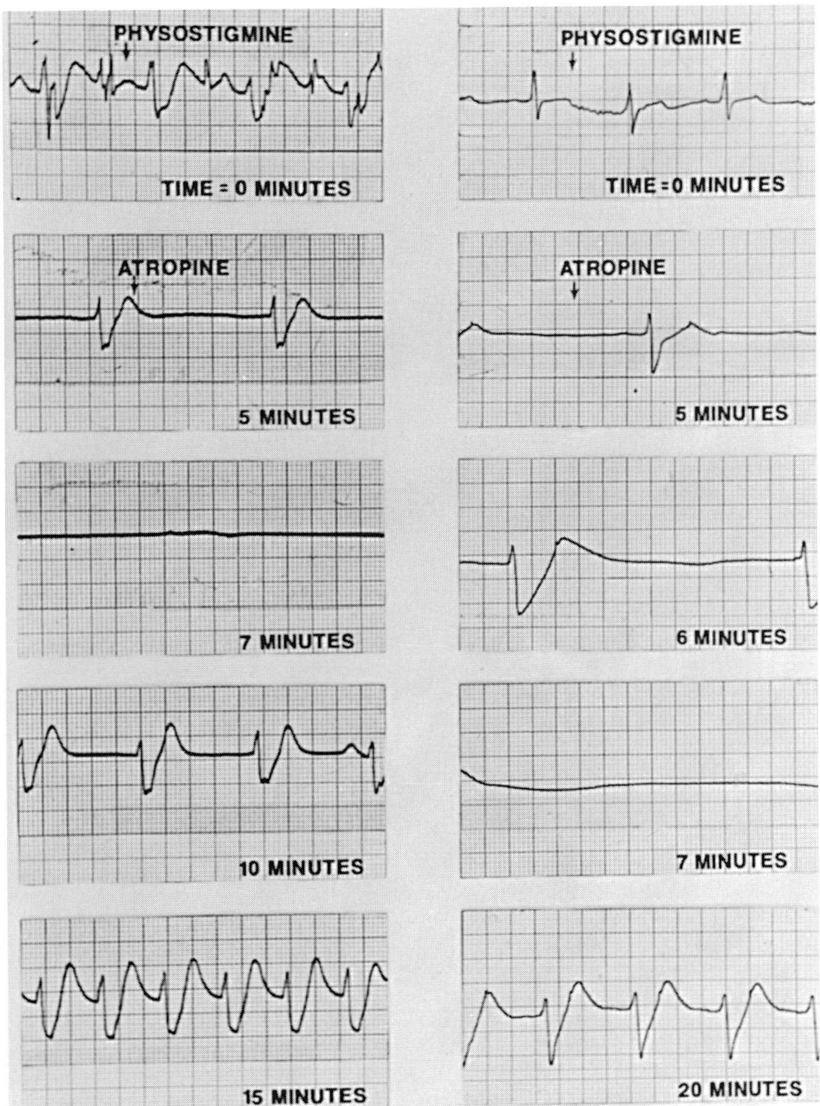

Figure 6–12. The strips in the *left panel* are from a 32-year-old man who had ingested 2300 mg of amitriptyline and who received physostigmine, 2 mg intravenously, for treatment of status epilepticus. Subsequently, junctional bradycardia developed and was unresponsive to atropine, and asystole occurred. Junctional rhythm was restored after treatment with epinephrine and bicarbonate. Sinus rhythm returned, the QRS narrowed during the next 12 hours, and the patient recovered fully.

The strips in the *right panel* are from a 25-year-old man who ingested 5000 mg of imipramine and 150 mg of propranolol. He received two doses of physostigmine, 2 mg intravenously, for recurrent motor seizures. After the second dose, sinus bradycardia developed and was unresponsive to atropine, and asystole occurred. After 10 minutes of closed chest cardiac massage and treatment with epinephrine and bicarbonate, sinus rhythm returned, although severe hypotension persisted. This patient's electrocardiogram results and blood pressure eventually became normal, but he died as a result of irreversible brain damage.

failure also may result in hypoxia and acidosis, which aggravate arrhythmias and hypotension; anticholinergic drugs are the treatment of choice for bronchorrhea. Pralidoxime is often effective in reversing the neuromuscular-blocking effects of organophosphates but has little effect on cardiovascular toxicity.

Membrane-Depressant Drugs and Toxins

Type I Antiarrhythmic Drugs

Type IA, B, and C antiarrhythmic agents affect phase 0 (upstroke velocity of the action potential) and action potential durations to various degrees in different portions of the conduction system and in ventricular and atrial muscle. These differences are reflected in varying effects on the ECG (Table 6–8).

The cardiac disturbances caused by membrane-depressant drugs and toxins are listed in Table 6–9.

Quinidine is the prototypical membrane-depressant drug. Quinidine and other type IA antiarrhythmic drugs (including procainamide and disopyramide) impede the fast sodium current across cardiac cell membranes and slow conduction, particularly in the His-Purkinje system.[42] In toxic doses, slowed conduction is demonstrated by progressively marked QT prolongation, QRS widening, or AV block, with loss of atrial activity and slow ventricular rhythm (Fig. 6–13). Ventricular tachycardia and fibrillation may occur after therapeutic doses ("quinidine syncope"),

Table 6–8. Electrophysiologic Differences Among Antiarrhythmic Agents

Class	Class Name	Examples	Depress Phase 0 Sodium Channel Blockade	Prolong Action Potential Duration	Symphatholytic Effect	Depress Slow Response Calcium Entry Blockade	Depress Phase 4 Depolarization	Prolongation of Surface ECG Intervals			
								PR	*QRS*	*QTc*	*JTc*
IA	Membrane anesthetics	Quinidine Procainamide Disopyramide	2+	1+	0/+	0	1+	0/+	0/+	2+	2+
IB	Same	Lidocaine Tocainide Mexiletine	2+	—	0	0	—	0	0	0	0
IC	Same	Flecainide Encainide Propafenone	2+	0/−	0/+	0/+	1+	2+	2+	1+	0
II	β-Blockers	Propranolol Metoprolol Esmolol	0/+	0/−	2+	0	1+	0/+	0	0	0
III	—	Amiodarone Sotalol Ibutilide	1+	2+	1+	0	1+	1+	0	2+	2+
IV	Calcium blockers	Verapamil Diltiazem	0	1+	1+	2+	1+	0/+	0	0	0/+

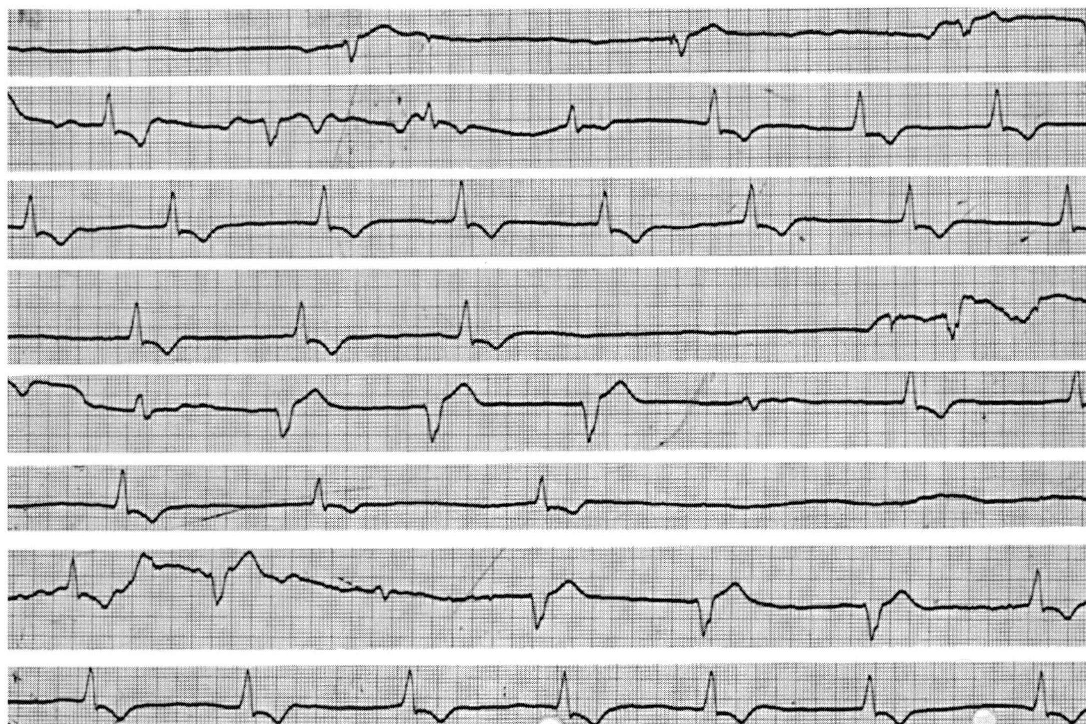

Figure 6–13. These strips are from a 76-year-old woman who was admitted to the coronary care unit with syncopal spells. She had been taking digoxin and quinidine for congestive heart failure and ventricular arrhythmias. Serum levels of both these agents were in the toxic range (serum digoxin level was 3.4 ng/mL, and quinidine 10 mg/mL). This continuously recorded V_1 rhythm strip demonstrates absence of atrial activity and prolonged pauses in QRS rhythm, which are terminated by different ventricular escape foci at different rates. Despite aggressive medical management, the patient died within 48 hours with electromechanical dissociation.

as well as after overdose. Ventricular tachycardia in the presence of a long QT interval is usually of the polymorphous (torsades de pointes) type, characterized by undulation of the QRS polarity about an isoelectric point (Fig. 6–14; see also Fig. 6–8).

In addition to its electrophysiologic effects, quinidine in large doses depresses myocardial contractility and relaxes blood vessels, resulting in hypotension. In cases of massive overdose, this may produce shock. Disopyramide, and quinidine to a lesser extent, also has anticholinergic effects that may result in sinus tachycardia after a mild overdose. Similarly, overdoses of type IC antiarrhythmic drugs, such as flecainide and propafenone, may result in bradyarrhythmias, conduction delays, and depressed cardiac contractility with shock. These drugs may have a significant arrhythmic action, causing ventricular tachycardia, even at therapeutic doses.[42, 43]

Therapeutic options for ventricular tachycardia due to quinidine or quinidine-like drugs include use of magnesium, overdrive pacing, lidocaine, phenytoin, isoproterenol, bretylium, and possibly amiodarone[44] (Table 6–10). Isoproterenol increases the heart rate and shortens the QT interval and is recommended by some as the drug of choice, although the prospect of treating ventricular tachycardia with catecholamines is believed too hazardous by other clinicians. Treatment of conduction disturbances and hypotension is discussed in the section on tricyclic antidepressant toxicity.

Calcium Entry Blockers

The primary electrophysiologic action of verapamil is to impede the calcium current responsible for depolarization of slow-response cardiac cells. Nifedipine and other dihydropyridines act preferentially on vascular smooth muscle, resulting in vasodilation. Diltiazem is similar to verapamil but produces less cardiac depression at therapeutic doses.

Serious toxicity can occur after therapeutic doses of calcium entry blockers in persons with predisposing cardiac disease, and similar effects are observed in healthy people after an overdose.[45] Verapamil- and diltiazem-induced depression of slow-response cardiac cells can result in sinus bradycardia or arrest and AV block, particularly in persons with underlying cardiac conduction disease. Inhibition of calcium entrance into the cell, which is necessary for muscle contraction, results in depression of myocardial contractility. This may cause worsening of cardiac failure or hypotension or both, particularly in persons with underlying myocardial disease. In overdose, heart block, bradyarrhythmias, and hypotension may be expected. Overdose with nifedipine and other dihydropyridines usually results in hypotension without depressed cardiac conduction or contractility, although cardiac depression has occasionally been observed. Cardiac conduction and contractility are maintained because reflex sympathetic stimulation counterbalances the intrinsic myocardial depressant action.

Table 6–9. Cardiac Disturbances Caused by Membrane-Depressant Drugs and Toxins

Drugs	
Quinidine	Phenothiazines and related neuroleptics
Procainamide	Propranolol (and other membrane-depressant β-blockers)*
Disopyramide	
Encainide	
Flecainide	
Tricyclic antidepressants	
Cardiac Effects and Disturbances	
QT interval prolongation†	Ventricular tachycardia (often polymorphous)‡
Intraventricular conduction delay (QRS interval prolongation)	Ventricular fibrillation‡
Atrioventricular block	Asystole
Junctional or ventricular bradycardia	Hypotension
Other Common Manifestations	
No syndromes about which one can generalize, although many agents in this group have anticholinergic effects	

*Membrane depression seen with massive overdose; this is *not* a manifestation of β-blockade.
†Among β-blockers, only sotalol is reported to increase the QT interval. Flecainide and encainide usually do not increase the QT interval.
‡In the case of β-blockers, usually occurs in association with bradyarrhythmia.

Table 6–10. Treatment of Cardiovascular Complications of Membrane-Depressant Drug Poisoning

Manifestation	Treatment
Arrhythmias	
Sinus tachycardia	None, esmolol or propranolol
Atrial tachycardia or fibrillation	Same as above plus verapamil, cardioversion
Ventricular premature beats and tachycardia	Magnesium, lidocaine, phenytoin, isoproterenol (with long QT only), bretylium
	Overdrive pacing
Bradyarrhythmias	Atropine
	Isoproterenol
	Pacemaker*
Hypotension	Fluids (hemodynamic monitoring advised in evidence of cardiac failure or myocardial depression)
	Treat bradyarrhythmias
	Dopamine, norepinephrine (low systemic vascular resistance)
	Dobutamine, isoproterenol (low cardiac output)
	Intra-aortic balloon pump or cardiopulmonary bypass (if intractable cardiogenic shock)

*May require higher than usual pacemaker voltage.

In addition to supportive care, the use of calcium chloride or calcium gluconate is recommended, particularly for treatment of hypotension. It is noteworthy that calcium completely reverses the negative inotropic effects of calcium entry blockers and may partially reverse the electrophysiologic toxicity but appears to have no effect in reversing vasodilation.[46] Glucagon has also been used with success in some cases of calcium blocker poisoning.[47]

Tricyclic Antidepressants and Antipsychotic Drugs

Tricyclic antidepressants account for more cardiac morbidity and mortality than any other class of drugs. Their mechanisms include a strong anticholinergic effect, inhibition of neuronal uptake of catecholamines, membrane depression, peripheral α-adrenergic blockade, and CNS-mediated inhibition of sympathetic reflexes.[48]

In mild and moderate cases of tricyclic antidepressant overdose, anticholinergic effects and increased circulating catecholamines result in supraventricular tachycardia, increased cardiac output, and normal or increased blood pressure. In severe cases, impaired intracardiac conduction and depressed myocardial contractility predominate, and hypotension is observed. Prolongation of the QRS duration is present in most cases of serious tricyclic antidepressant toxicity. The finding of a rightward terminal 40-millisecond frontal plane QRS vector (130 to 270 degrees) is

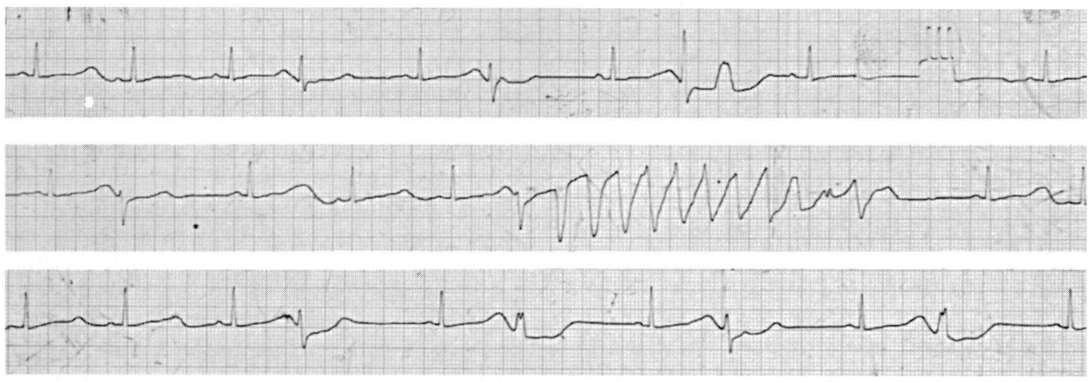

Figure 6–14. The patient is a 64-year-old woman who was begun on oral quinidine therapy for frequent premature ventricular beats associated with palpitations. These continuous lead II rhythm strips were recorded after the third 200-mg dose and show a markedly prolonged QT interval, frequent multiform ventricular ectopic beats, and a self-terminating burst of polymorphous ventricular tachycardia. The serum level of quinidine obtained after the recording of these tracings was 3.6 mg/mL. Quinidine was withdrawn, and oral procainamide substituted without further complications.

reported to be more sensitive than QRS widening in detecting tricyclic poisoning in adults but not in children (who may normally have a rightward axis).[49, 50] The finding of an ECG lead aV_R greater than 3 mm was seen to be another predictor of the development of seizure or arrhythmias.[51] Bundle branch block, AV block, and slow ventricular rhythm and asystole may occur in the most severe poisonings (Fig. 6–15; see also Figs. 6–5 and 6–12). Responsiveness to electric stimulation is decreased so that pacing thresholds are often higher than normal; in extreme cases, the heart does not respond at all to pacing. Hypotension usually results from depressed cardiac output. Cardiac output may be reduced as a result of venous pooling with inadequate cardiac filling (associated with low pulmonary capillary wedge pressure) or, in more severe poisoning, as a result of myocardial depression (associated with normal or high wedge pressure).

Therapy for tricyclic antidepressant overdoses should be tailored to the particular cardiovascular disturbance. Sinus tachycardia and supraventricular arrhythmias, if associated with hemodynamic disturbances (either excessive hypertension or hypotension), can be controlled with physostigmine or propranolol. As noted, these drugs can depress cardiac conduction. They should be avoided, if possible, when membrane-depressant effects, manifested by the presence of a wide QRS interval, AV block, or the presence of a bradyarrhythmia, are present unless a temporary cardiac pacemaker is in place. Severe bradyarrhythmias and asystole have occurred after treatment with physostigmine[37] (see Fig. 6–12). Atropine also should be readily available to counteract the cholinergic effects of physostigmine.

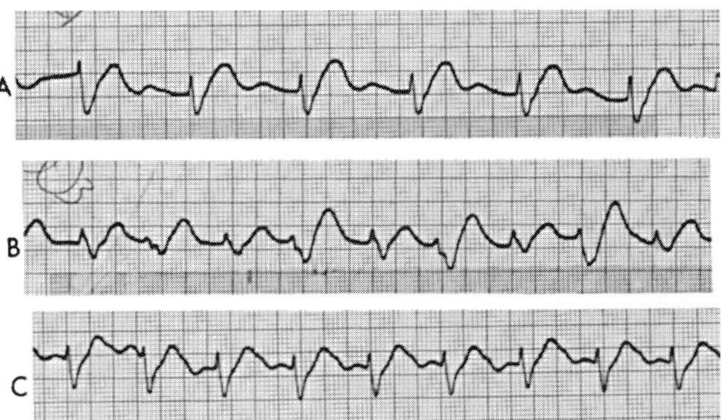

Figure 6–15. Lead II electrocardiograms recorded in a 40-year-old woman who ingested 6 g of amitriptyline (Elavil). The top strip (*A*), recorded on admission, shows a wide QRS rhythm and markedly prolonged QTU interval; atrial activity is not clearly discernible. Strips *B* and *C* were recorded 30 and 60 minutes, respectively, after intravenous administration of 44 mEq of $NaHCO_3$. In *B*, the QRS rate has increased and alternation of QRS complexes is present. The QT interval remains prolonged, but the U wave is less prominent, and the QRS duration of alternate complexes has narrowed. Atrial activity is still not readily seen. In *C*, P waves precede each QRS complex and QRS duration remains prolonged but the QT interval has shortened. This series of tracings suggests a supraventricular origin of the rhythm in strips *A* and *B*.

Administration of either sodium bicarbonate or lactate or hyperventilation to correct acidemia and induce alkalemia reduces arrhythmias in animals and in humans[48] (Fig. 6–15). The use of bicarbonate may be safer than hyperventilation because the hypocapnia due to the latter may lower the seizure threshold, and seizures are a common and serious complication of tricyclic antidepressant overdose. The mechanism of beneficial effects of alkali therapy is not proved, but it most likely works by increasing extracellular sodium concentration, increasing extracellular pH, or decreasing extracellular potassium concentration, all of which may improve membrane responsiveness and increase conduction velocity in fast-response (His-Purkinje) cells.

After sodium bicarbonate, administration of lidocaine is the treatment of choice for ventricular arrhythmias. Type IA or IC antiarrhythmic drugs (quinidine, procainamide, disopyramide, flecainide), which have additive membrane-depressant effects, should be avoided. Overdrive pacing has been successfully used to treat ventricular tachycardia caused by quinidine or long QT syndrome and would be expected to be useful in treating tricyclic antidepressant overdose as well. Bretylium should be considered for refractory ventricular tachycardia or fibrillation, although it also might worsen the hypotension.

Because both tachycardia and intraventricular conduction delay are characteristic and ventricular tachycardia is not uncommon, the diagnostic problem of a wide complex tachycardia of uncertain origin is common. Diagnosis and treatment of this arrhythmia were discussed in detail in an earlier section of this chapter.

Intracardiac pacing is indicated in patients with high-grade AV block. If intraventricular conduction is worsening (i.e., if the QRS complex is widening) early in the clinical course, when the extent of ultimate myocardial depression is not yet known, prophylactic insertion of a transvenous pacemaker is advised because of the chance of sudden deterioration. The presence of sinus or ventricular bradycardia rather than the usual supraventricular tachycardia indicates severe toxicity and warrants pacing as well. Bradyarrhythmias associated with reduced cardiac output and hypotension can be treated with isoproterenol until intracardiac pacing can be instituted.

Hypotension is common after a tricyclic antidepressant overdose. In many patients, hypotension can be managed successfully with fluids. If pressors are required, α-adrenergic agonists such as norepinephrine or dopamine are preferred. In the presence of selective α-blockade due to tricyclic antidepressants, the predominant effects of mixed α- and β-adrenergic agonists such as epinephrine may be β-mediated vasodilation and worsening of hypotension. Dobutamine may prove to be useful in managing myocardial depression with normal or increased vascular resistance. Profound cardiogenic shock resulting from tricyclic antidepressant overdose is often unresponsive to medical treatment and has a poor prognosis. In these cases, extracorporeal circulatory aids such as cardiopulmonary bypass or intra-aortic balloon pumping may be the only means of sustaining life until the body can eliminate the drug. Intra-aortic balloon pumping for drug intoxication associated with intractable shock has been successful.

Phenothiazines and other antipsychotic drugs have pharmacologic properties similar to those of tricyclic antidepressants, but arrhythmias are generally not as difficult to control, and cardiogenic shock is uncommon. Hypotension caused by chlorpromazine is more likely due to peripheral α-adrenergic blockade and usually responds well to posture and intravenous fluids. Differences between tricyclic antidepressants and antipsychotic drugs probably reflect dissimilar potencies with respect to membrane actions and different concentrations in cardiac tissue. The tricyclic antidepressants and their potentially toxic demethylated and hydroxylated metabolites are concentrated in the myocardium to a much greater extent than are the phenothiazines.

Miscellaneous Drugs and Toxins

Cardiovascular disturbances due to miscellaneous drugs and toxins are listed in Table 6–11.

Digitalis

Mortality and major morbidity due to digitalis overdose result from arrhythmias, heart block, and hyperkalemia. Digitalis inhibits the sodium-potassium adenosine triphosphatase–dependent pump located on the cell membrane. In the therapeutic situation, this results in greater calcium movement into the cell, which is believed to account for increased myocardial contractility. After an overdose, disruption of sodium and potassium movement across membranes results in depressed conduction velocity, as described for membrane-depressant drugs. In addition, automaticity of previously nonautomatic tissue is enhanced due to increased rate of diastolic depolarization and possibly to spontaneous afterdepolarizations ("triggered" rhythms). Digitalis also may increase sympathetic and parasympathetic neural activity. Sympathetic stimulation enhances automaticity and excitability, whereas parasympathetic stimulation further decreases conduction velocity. Thus, an overdose with digitalis is characterized by arrhythmias demonstrating both increased automaticity and depressed intracardiac conduction.

Tachyarrhythmias due to digitalis intoxication typically include ectopic atrial tachycardia with AV block, AV junctional tachycardia, and ventricular tachycardia or fibrillation (Figs. 6–16 and 6–17). Ventricular arrhythmias are reported to occur more commonly in persons with underlying heart disease. Bradyarrhythmias include sinus bradycardia, sinoatrial block, second-degree and complete AV block, atrial fibrillation with slow ventricular response, idioventricular rhythm, and asystole (Fig. 6–18). Severe hyperkalemia due to inhibition of sodium-potassium exchange in skeletal muscle can contribute to AV block and depressed myocardial excitability (Fig. 6–19).

Therapy for digitalis-induced arrhythmias is directed at the specific arrhythmia and normalization of serum potassium level. Supraventricular arrhyth-

Table 6–11. Cardiovascular Disturbances—Miscellaneous Drugs and Toxins

Drug/Toxin	Mechanisms of Action	Cardiovascular Disturbances	Other Common Manifestations
Digitalis (including foxglove, oleander, lily of the valley, and toad venom [bufotoxin])	Inhibits Na^+-K^+ ATPase-dependent pump, increases automaticity, afterdepolarizations, decreases atrioventricular conduction velocity, increases vagal and ? sympathetic activity	Atrial tachycardia with atrioventricular block Junctional tachycardia Ventricular ectopy, tachycardia, fibrillation Sinus bradycardia Sinoatrial block High-grade atrioventricular block Slow ventricular response to atrial fibrillation or flutter Asystole	Nausea, vomiting Hypokalemia (with diuretic use) Hyperkalemia (severe intoxication)
Opiates	Central nervous system –mediated increase in parasympathetic and decrease in sympathetic tone	Bradycardia Atrial fibrillation Hypotension	Miosis Respiratory depression Coma Pulmonary edema
Lithium	Disturbed cardiac potassium metabolism	Sinus bradycardia ST-T abnormalities Ventricular ectopy	Tremor, ataxia Confusion, stupor, coma Neuromuscular irritability, convulsions Azotemia
Ergot derivatives	Constriction of vascular smooth muscle	Cardiac ischemia (angina, coronary spasm with possible myocardial infarction) Peripheral vasospasm Gangrene	Headache (reason for excessive use of ergots)

Table 6–11. Cardiovascular Disturbances—Miscellaneous Drugs and Toxins *(Continued)*

Drug/Toxin	Mechanisms of Action	Cardiovascular Disturbances	Other Common Manifestations
Carbon monoxide, hydrogen sulfide	Binds to hemoglobin, preferentially to oxygen, causing chemical asphyxia	Cardiac ischemia (electrocardiographic abnormalities, myocardial infarction) Hypotension	Headache Coma Metabolic acidosis (with normal oxygen tension) Pulmonary edema
Cyanide	Binds to cytochrome oxidase, causing chemical asphyxia	Hypotension	
Arsenic	Interferes with cellular respiration	Cardiac ischemia Myocarditis ST-T abnormalities QT prolongation Polymorphous ventricular tachycardia Hypotension	Abdominal pain Vomiting, diarrhea Hepatitis Skin rash Renal failure Peripheral neuropathy (late) Chills, fever
Arsine	Hemolysis, anemia	Cardiac ischemia Peaked T waves Pulmonary edema	Hyperkalemia Hemoglobinuria Renal failure
Phosphorus	"Protoplasmic poison"	ST-T abnormalities QT prolongation Ventricular tachycardia/ fibrillation Asystole Hypotension	Corrosive burns of skin and gastrointestinal tract Severe gastroenteritis "Smoking" luminescent vomitus and stool
Iron	Cellular membrane injury	ST-T wave abnormalities Hypovolemia Myocardial necrosis Hypotension	Nausea, vomiting, diarrhea Gastrointestinal bleeding Hyperglycemia Leukocytosis Metabolic acidosis Hepatic necrosis
Fluoride	Hypocalcemia Hyperkalemia	QT interval prolongation Peaked T waves Ventricular fibrillation Sudden death	Nausea, vomiting, diarrhea Tetany, hyperreflexia Respiratory depression
Organic mercury (chronic)		ST-T abnormalities QT prolongation	Sore mouth, metallic taste, vomiting, diarrhea, tremor, dysarthria, ataxia
Lead		Chest pain Cardiac failure ST-T abnormalities Hypertension	Anorexia Abdominal pain, constipation Anemia Peripheral neuropathy Encephalopathy
Scorpion and spider venom	? Massive catecholamine release; myocarditis	Hypertension Tachycardia ST-T abnormalities QT prolongation Atrial and ventricular arrhythmias Pulmonary edema Hypotension	Pain at site of envenomation Anxiety Diaphoresis, fasciculations and/ or muscle spasm Abdominal pain and rigidity† Paresthesias, convulsions‡
Ciguatera fish poisoning	Increased membrane sodium permeability	Bradycardia Hypotension	Paresthesias Abdominal pain, nausea, vomiting, diarrhea Respiratory depression
Emetine (syrup of ipecac)	Inhibition of protein synthesis Disrupts oxidative phosphorylation	ST wave abnormalities QT interval prolongation Cardiomyopathy (biventricular cardiac failure) Ventricular arrhythmias	Recurrent vomiting Cachexia Skeletal myopathy
Colchicine	Cellular microtubular toxin	Myocardial injury ST segment abnormalities Hypovolemia Hypotension Pulmonary edema Sudden death	Nausea, vomiting, abdominal pain Respiratory failure Pancytopenia, leukopenia Coagulopathy Myopathy Polyneuropathy
γ-Hydroxybutyrate (GHB)	Unclear	Bradycardia Hypotension	Coma Seizures
Aconite (Chinese herbs—fuzi, chuanwu, cauwu)	Aconitive and shock-related alkaloids block sodium channel	Bradycardia Ventricular tachycardia (may be monomorphic or polymorphic)	Paresthesias Ataxia

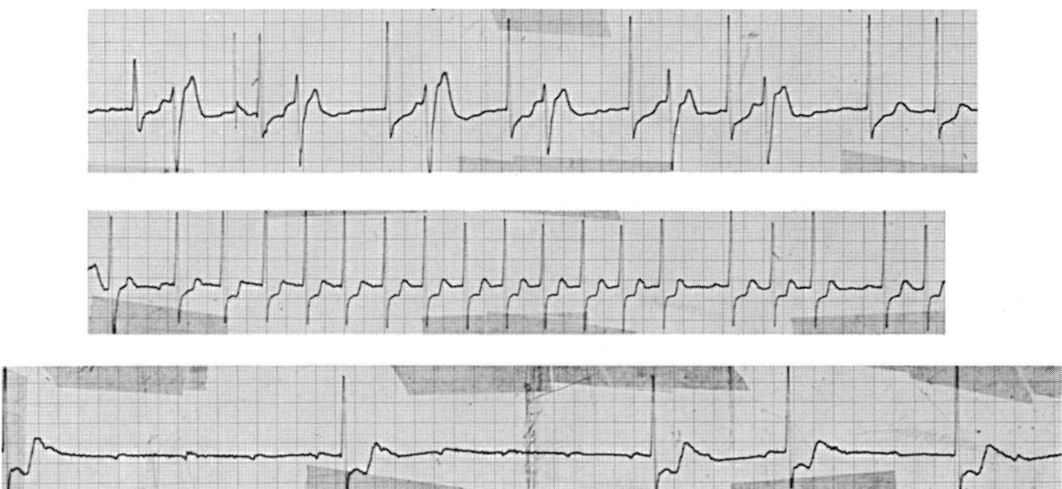

Figure 6–16. Three lead II rhythm strips were recorded during a period of several hours in a 30-year-old patient who intentionally ingested 24.8 mg of digoxin. The *top strip* shows atrial fibrillation and R-on-T ventricular bigeminy. The *middle strip* shows a run of atrial tachycardia that terminates spontaneously to sinus rhythm and resumes immediately. The *bottom strip* illustrates high-degree atrioventricular block that, because of the morphology of the QRS complexes, is considered to be originating in the atrioventricular node or the His bundle. Because all these rhythms occurred and recurred within short periods, treatment was difficult and consisted of only transvenous cardiac pacing for bradyarrhythmias. All bradyarrhythmias disappeared by 22 hours, and all arrhythmias by 1 week.

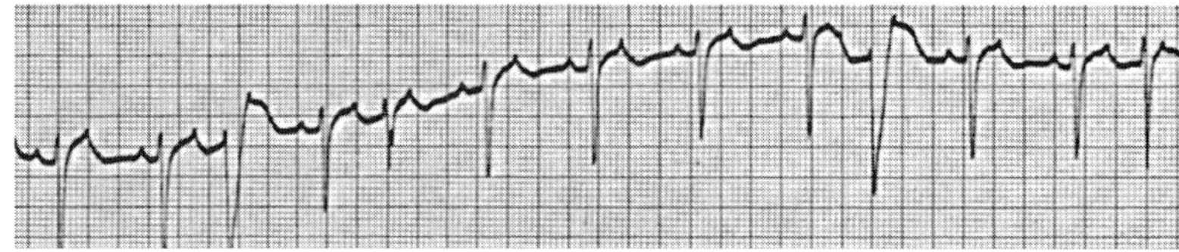

Figure 6–17. The patient is a 69-year-old man who was admitted to the hospital with acute congestive heart failure 7 weeks after having suffered an anterior wall myocardial infarction. This MCL_1 rhythm strip was recorded after administration of 1.5 mg of intravenous digoxin during an 18-hour period. The atrial rate is somewhat irregular at about 150/min. Periods of atrioventricular nodal Wenckebach's block are present, with the second QRS complex of the period conducted aberrantly. Episodes of 2:1 atrioventricular block are also present. The serum digoxin level at this time was 4 ng/mL. The rhythm was restored to sinus after withdrawal of digoxin.

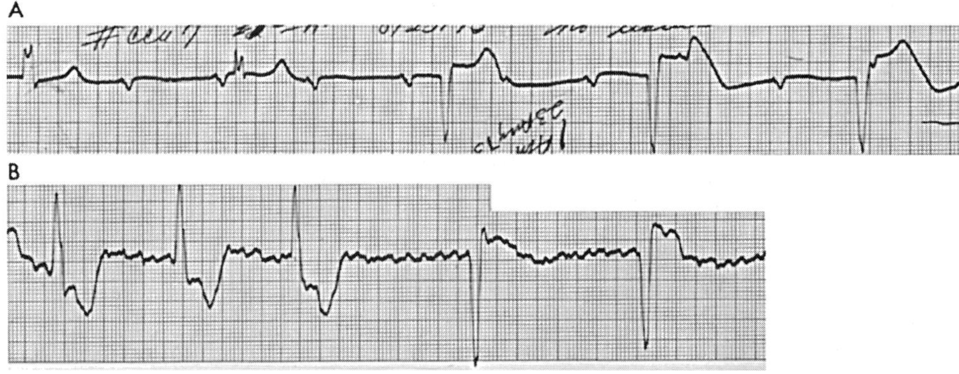

Figure 6–18. These two MCL_1 rhythm strips depict examples of atrioventricular block in the setting of digitalis toxicity. In *A*, sinus rhythm and complete atrioventricular block are present. The QRS complexes are of two types: The first two have a right bundle branch block pattern, and the last three have a left bundle branch block pattern; they occur at two different rates. The long duration of the QRS complexes as well as their very slow rate suggests that the origin of these escape beats is in the distal His-Purkinje system. In this situation, atropine may not result in improved atrioventricular conduction, and temporary cardiac pacing is often required.

In *B*, the atrial rhythm is fibrillation. High-grade atrioventricular block is present, as evidenced by the slow ventricular response. The QRS complexes have two morphologies: right and left bundle branch block patterns. The first three complexes occur at a nearly regular rate, suggesting a ventricular escape focus. The last two complexes occur at a slower escape interval and rate, suggesting instability of the origin of the first three complexes and emergence of a yet more distal pacemaker. Again, atropine may not be of benefit in this situation, and cardiac pacing may be required.

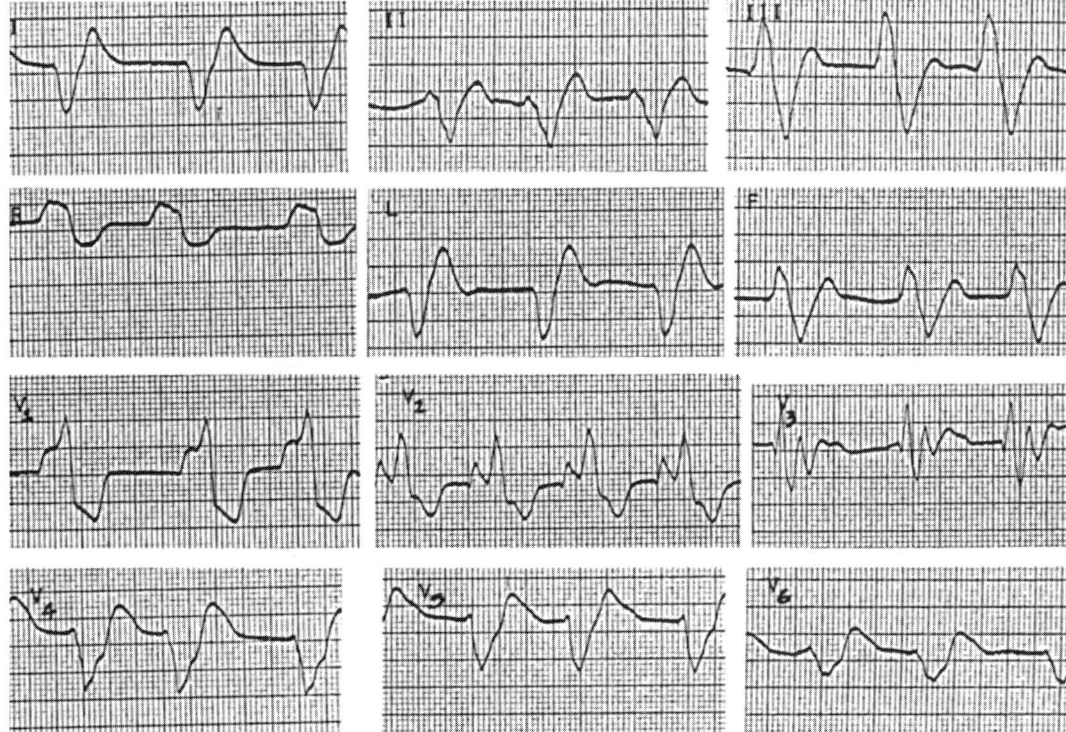

Figure 6–19. The patient was a 68-year-old man who was admitted to the hospital in moribund condition. He had long-standing congestive heart failure and was being treated with oral digoxin and diuretics. His serum potassium level on admission was 10.0 mEq/L, and his serum digoxin level was 5.2 ng/mL. He died shortly after this 12-lead electrocardiogram was obtained, with electromechanical dissociation. The electrocardiogram shows absence of discernible atrial activity and an irregular, wide, complex QRS rhythm having a right bundle branch block configuration. The markedly increased QRS duration suggests hyperkalemia, which in this patient may have been due in part to digitalis toxicity.

mias often do not require specific treatment because the ventricular response is reasonably slow. If necessary, β-blockers may be used to treat atrial tachycardia. Patients who have been continually taking diuretics may be depleted of potassium and magnesium, and supraventricular tachyarrhythmias may respond to potassium or magnesium supplementation. However, use of potassium may depress AV conduction, and as described earlier, life-threatening hyperkalemia may ensue.

The definitive treatment for life-threatening ventricular arrhythmia or hyperkalemia is administration of digoxin-specific antibodies.[52, 53] The antibodies bind free digoxin and may completely reverse digitalis toxicity within 15 to 30 minutes. Quinidine-like membrane-depressant drugs should be avoided. Phenytoin has been reported to be effective in treating arrhythmias, because it may enhance AV conduction while depressing automaticity, but its effect is inconsistent and unpredictable. Lidocaine, propranolol, and esmolol also have been used to treat ventricular arrhythmias; the β-blockers may also worsen conduction disturbances.

Sinus bradycardia and AV conduction block, in light of the vagal actions of digitalis, may respond to administration of atropine. Isoproterenol is usually effective in treating bradyarrhythmias refractory to atropine but can result in increased ventricular excitability. Cardiac pacing is indicated in patients with complete AV block or second-degree heart block or when bradyarrhythmias result in hemodynamic compromise. Correction of hyperkalemia may in itself reverse AV block.

Of note is that ingestion of oleander leaves or tea or toad venom (bufatoxin) can also cause digitalis-like poisoning.[54] Toad venom is currently sold as an aphrodisiac (“Love Stone,” “Rock Hard”) and in Chinese herbal medications (Chan Su). Anecdotal reports suggest that these poisonings may respond to digoxin antibody.

Opiates

Although toxicity from acute opiate overdose is primarily related to respiratory depression, opiates may have significant cardiac and vascular effects. They generally have little effect on the myocardium, although norpropoxyphene, a major metabolite of propoxyphene, may be cardiotoxic. CNS effects of narcotics result in increased vagal activity. Narcotics dilate peripheral veins and arterioles, presumably through a CNS-mediated effect on sympathetic tone. Consequently, hypotension and relative bradycardia are common. Arrhythmias occur occasionally, most commonly atrial fibrillation. Quinidine and procaine, as well as other local anesthetics, commonly adulterate heroin sold on the street and may themselves contribute to myocardial depression or even cardiac arrest.

Pulmonary edema is a common and serious complication of narcotic overdose and is noncardiogenic in origin. Although pulmonary edema usually occurs after injection of narcotics, it may not become evident until naloxone has been administered. It is most likely that sudden reversal of narcotic-induced venodilation and venous pooling combined with pulmonary capillary injury to the extent that fluid enters the lungs at relatively low cardiac filling pressures accounts for naloxone-induced pulmonary edema.

Therapy for opiate overdose in general includes administration of naloxone. No specific therapy for arrhythmias usually is necessary. Naloxone may convert coarse atrial fibrillation to fine atrial fibrillation with a faster ventricular response rate rather than to normal sinus rhythm. If atrial fibrillation with rapid ventricular response rate persists, use of digitalis, verapamil, or propranolol is indicated to slow the rate. The use of intermittent positive expiratory pressure is beneficial in the treatment of pulmonary edema, as discussed previously.

Lithium

Cardiac toxicity of lithium overdose has not been prominent, and no deaths due primarily to cardiovascular complications have been reported. Administration of lithium in usual therapeutic doses produces flattening or inversion of the T wave in nearly all patients. Sinus node disturbances, manifested by sinus bradycardia or sinoatrial block sometimes associated with ventricular ectopy, and junctional or ventricular escape rhythms have been reported in patients with lithium intoxication and during long-term therapy. Ventricular tachyarrhythmias in association with lithium therapy have been reported but are uncommon. Hypotension may complicate lithium overdose, but this appears to be related to dehydration or pulmonary complications in the course of prolonged coma rather than caused by direct cardiovascular toxicity. A mechanism for the cardiac effects of lithium has been suggested by animal studies. Lithium enters myocardial cells and displaces intracellular cations, predominantly potassium. Lithium then leaves the cell more slowly than does potassium and thereby disturbs the usual transmembrane ionic currents.

Treatment is directed toward the specific arrhythmia, as described in Table 6–1, and toward acceleration of lithium elimination, as discussed in Chapter 33.

Ergot Derivatives

Ergotamine and other ergot derivatives are widely used in the treatment of migraine headache and have resulted in significant cardiac and vascular toxicity. The basic action of ergot drugs is constriction of vascular smooth muscle (both α-adrenergic agonist and nonadrenergic effects), although many of the drugs also have α-adrenergic receptor-blocking activity. Intense constriction of peripheral arteries, with resultant coolness, pallor, or cyanosis of the extremity, sometimes progressing to gangrene, is a typical manifestation of ergotism. Intermittent claudication occurs initially, and ischemic rest pain develops with progression of vasospasm. Hypertension is uncommon. In addition, ergot derivatives have been reported to worsen angina or cause myocardial infarction, presumably owing to coronary vasoconstriction in persons with underlying heart disease. Intravenous administration of ergonovine has been used diagnostically during cardiac catheterization to provoke coronary vasospasm. We treated a patient who took excessive quantities of ergotamine tablets for severe migraine headaches; the patient had chest pain and diffuse ST segment elevation suggesting coronary vasospasm (Fig. 6–20).

Amphetamine-like drugs also can produce vascular spasm similar to that produced by ergot derivatives. In particular, 4-bromo-2,5-dimethoxyamphetamine injection has produced severe vascular insufficiency and in one case led to a bilateral lower extremity amputation.

Therapy for ergot-induced vasospasm includes anticoagulation with heparin, the use of direct vasodilators such as sodium nitroprusside for peripheral vasospasm, nitroglycerin for coronary vasospasm, and α-adrenergic blockers. Rapid dilation of vessels in an intensely vasoconstricted patient results in relative hypovolemia and hypotension, and thus fluid replacement must be anticipated. If a specific vessel is affected, vasoconstrictors should be infused intra-arterially into that vessel to allow maximal local vasodilation to be achieved without effecting excessive systemic hypotension. Nifedipine or other calcium channel blockers may also prove useful in treating ergot-induced coronary vasospasm. Other treatments with varying results have included anticoagulants, epidural anesthesia, low-molecular-weight dextran, hyperbaric oxygen, and surgical sympathectomy.

Chemical Asphyxiants

Carbon monoxide, hydrogen sulfide, and cyanide inhibit oxygen transport to tissues or use of oxygen within tissues, resulting in tissue hypoxia. The usual presentation in severe cases of poisoning is coma or metabolic acidosis or both. Tachypnea (with evidence of respiratory alkalosis), tachycardia, and hypotension are common, although carbon monoxide poisoning in particular can be associated with hypertension. ECG changes, including T wave flattening or inversion, ST segment depression or elevation, and conduction disturbances, are frequently observed, and myocardial necrosis or infarction may occur. Premature ventricular contractions and atrial fibrillation are occasionally noted. Pulmonary edema may complicate acute carbon monoxide poisoning, and noncardiogenic versus cardiogenic edema resulting from myocardial damage must be differentiated.

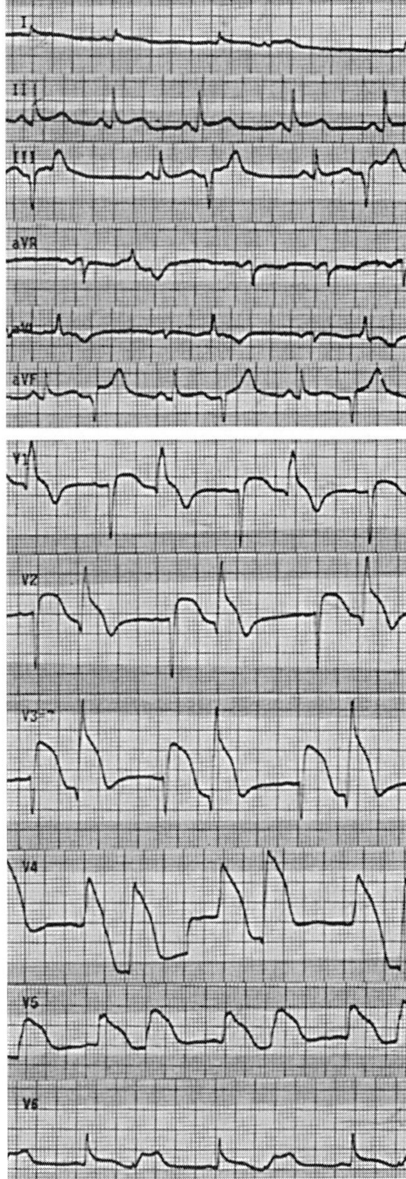

Figure 6–20. The patient is a 50-year-old man who was taking ergotamine for cluster headaches. When the headaches worsened, he ingested up to 10 mg/h, developed severe substernal chest pain, and had an episode of syncope. This 12-lead electrocardiogram was recorded on admission to the coronary care unit. The rhythm is sinus with ventricular bigeminy; diffuse ST segment elevation is present, consistent with coronary artery spasm. After large oral and intravenous doses of nitrates, chest pain and ST segment elevation resolved, but recurrent episodes of pain were associated with return of ST elevation, ventricular ectopy, and bursts of ventricular tachycardia. Myocardial infarction was not documented. Selective coronary arteriography documented coronary spasm during a spontaneous attack of chest pain. Pain and ST segment elevation resolved over 2 weeks coincidentally with oral nifedipine therapy.

Even mild exposure to carbon monoxide can have significant effects in persons with underlying vascular disease. With carboxyhemoglobin concentrations as low as 3%, the duration of exercise to the onset of chest pain in persons with angina pectoris, or leg pain in persons with intermittent claudication, is significantly reduced. Therapy is directed toward improving tissue oxygenation, as described in Chapter 70. Of note is that ECG abnormalities after carbon monoxide poisoning may persist for days or even weeks after treatment, possibly as a result of focal myocardial injury. Mitral valve prolapse related to papillary muscle necrosis due to carbon monoxide exposure has been suggested on the basis of an unexpectedly higher incidence of prolapse found by echocardiography in one small series.[55]

Arsenic and Other Metals

Acute arsenic poisoning, by interfering with cellular respiration, may produce an ECG picture of myocardial ischemia and may be associated with focal myocardial hemorrhage, although patients who recover have no cardiac symptoms. Acute and chronic arsenic poisoning can be associated with T wave changes and QT prolongation and with ventricular tachycardia and fibrillation. Arsenic-induced torsades de pointes type of polymorphous ventricular tachycardia has been reported.

Arsine gas, by causing massive hemolysis and severe anemia, also results in ECG abnormalities, most commonly peaked T waves (possibly related to hyperkalemia), but myocardial ischemia (due to severe anemia and possibly myocardial effects of arsine) is also evident. Death due to arsine exposure in patients who reach the hospital is often secondary to cardiac failure; pathology shows myocardial degeneration. Treatment should include correction of hyperkalemia, transfusion, and therapy of cardiac failure.

Elemental phosphorus and organic mercury poisonings have been associated with ST-T wave abnormalities, QT prolongation, and various arrhythmias (including ventricular tachycardia). After elemental phosphorus ingestion, shock resulting from depressed myocardial contractility and abnormally low systemic vascular resistance occurs and is often difficult to treat. Death in the early phase of phosphorus poisoning is due to shock, ventricular fibrillation, or asystole.

Although uncommon, chronic lead poisoning may be associated with myocarditis characterized by chest pain (angina pectoris saturnina), tachycardia, ventricular gallop, pulmonary congestion, hypertension, ST-T abnormalities, and premature ventricular contractions on the ECG. Autopsy of children dying of lead encephalopathy may show chronic myocarditis. Clinical features usually subside after treatment with the chelating agent ethylenediaminetetraacetic acid.

Acute severe iron (and other heavy metal) poisoning causes shock owing to vasodilation and hypovolemia, the latter resulting from vascular damage and fluid loss. Myocardial injury and dysfunction may also contribute. ECG abnormalities, including T wave inversion, may be present.

Scorpions, Spiders, and Hymenoptera

Patients with poisonous scorpion stings typically show anxiety, profuse diaphoresis, and hypertension.

Myocarditis, characterized by tachycardia, conduction abnormalities, and ST-T abnormalities, including tall peaked T waves, QT prolongation, and atrial and ventricular arrhythmias, may be evident.[56] In severe poisoning, pulmonary edema, hypotension, and ECG changes suggesting myocardial infarction occur. Death is due to congestive heart failure or shock or both; sudden deaths presumably due to arrhythmias are also reported. The clinical and myocardial histologic manifestations of scorpion sting resemble those of massive catecholamine infusion, and urinary catecholamine excretion has been noted to be increased in scorpion sting victims. Although there is little published experience in this regard, the use of α- and β-adrenergic blocking drugs for treatment of hypertension and arrhythmias would be logical. Treatment of cardiac failure and shock is supportive.

Labile blood pressure, atrial arrhythmias, and cardiovascular collapse are occasionally observed in patients after black widow spider bites.[57] Increased urinary catecholamine metabolite excretion also has suggested a role of excess catecholamines in this syndrome, and adrenergic blockers may be useful in management.

Hymenoptera (bees and wasps) stings are well known to cause anaphylaxis, manifested by hypotension, cyanosis, bronchospasm, and collapse in allergic patients. Chest pain and myocardial infarction, probably resulting from profound hypotension, occasionally occur as well.[58]

Some Other Natural Products

Many natural products have cardiovascular effects, and a comprehensive review of these is beyond the scope of this chapter. Three toxins have become of particular interest to poison centers and are mentioned briefly.

γ-Hydroxybutyrate is a suspected human neurotransmitter that is sold illicitly as a muscle builder (purportedly releasing growth hormone). γ-Hydroxybutyrate overdose is associated with coma, sinus or junctional bradycardia, and mild hypotension.[59] The bradycardia is thought to be vagally mediated and should be responsive to atropine.

Ciguatera fish poisoning, caused by ingestion of fish contaminated with ciguatera toxins, produces cardiovascular toxicity as well as gastrointestinal and neurologic symptoms. Patients often experience bradycardia and hypotension, which may be quite severe. Detailed autonomic studies of one such patient revealed that the bradycardia and hypotension were due to both excessive vagal tone and depression of sympathetic nervous responses.[60] Hypotension usually responds to volume expansion and anticholinergic drug therapy.

Aconite poisoning can occur after ingestion of Chinese herbs or teas that contain *Aconitum carmichaelii* or *Aconitum kusnezoffii*. The herbal preparations that contain these herbs include fuzi, chuanwu, and cauwu. If these herbs are not boiled for an adequate time, the alkaloids aconitine, mesaconitine, and others, which are extremely potent toxins, may be ingested. Cardiovascular manifestations include shock with bradycardia or ventricular tachycardia (either monomorphic or polymorphic) or ventricular fibrillation.[61] Several fatalities have been reported. Amiodarone and flecanide have been suggested as first-line antiarrhythmic agents for ventricular tachycardia due to aconite poisoning.

References

1. Shubin H, Weil MH: The mechanism of shock following suicidal doses of barbiturate, narcotics and tranquilizing drugs, with observations on the effects of treatment. Am J Med *38*:853, 1965.
2. Janse MJ: Mechanisms of Arrhythmias. New York, Futura Publishing Co., 1993.
3. Antzelevitch C, Sicouri S: Clinical relevance of cardiac arrhythmias generated by afterdepolarizations. J Am Coll Cardiol *23*:259, 1994.
4. Faber TS, Zehender M, Just H: Drug-induced torsade de pointes. Drug Saf *11*:463, 1994.
5. Brugada P, Brugada J, Mont L, et al: A new approach to the differential diagnosis of a regular tachycardia with a wide QRS complex. Circulation *83*:1649, 1991.
6. Gay RJ, Brown DF: Pacemaker failure due to procainamide toxicity. Am J Cardiol *34*:728, 1974.
7. Fein A, Grossman RF, Jones JG, et al: The value of edema fluid protein measurement in patients with pulmonary edema. Am J Med *67*:32, 1979.
8. Shubin H, Weil MH: Shock associated with barbiturate intoxication. JAMA *215*:263, 1971.
9. Levine SR, Brust JCM, Futrell N, et al: Cerebrovascular complications of the use of "crack" form of alkaloidal cocaine. N Engl J Med *323*:699, 1990.
10. Roth D, Alarcéon MD, Fernandez MD, et al: Acute rhabdomyolysis associated with cocaine intoxication. N Engl J Med *319*:673, 1988.
11. Catravas JD, Waters IW: Acute cocaine intoxication in the conscious dog: Studies on the mechanism of lethality. J Pharmacol Exp Ther *217*:350, 1981.
12. Buchanan JF, Brown CR: "Designer drugs." A problem in clinical toxicology. Med Toxicol *3*:1, 1988.
13. Wiener RS, Lockhart JT, Schwartz RG: Dilated cardiomyopathy and cocaine abuse. Report of two cases. Am J Med *81*:699, 1986.
14. Isner JM, Chokshi SK: Cardiac complications of cocaine abuse. Annu Rev Med *42*:133, 1991.
15. Hollander JE: The Management of cocaine associated myocardial ischemia. Curr Concepts Nutr *333*:1267, 1995.
16. Karch SB, Billingham ME: The pathology and etiology of cocaine-induced heart disease. Arch Pathol Lab Med *112*:225, 1988.
17. Rosenberg J, Pentel P, Pond S, et al: Hyperthermia associated with drug intoxication. Crit Care Med *14*:964, 1986.
18. Burn RS, Lerner SE, Corrado R, et al: Phencyclidine of acute intoxication and fatalities. West J Med *123*:345, 1975.
19. Linden CH, Rumack BH, Strehike C: Monoamine oxidase inhibitor overdose. Ann Emerg Med *13*:1137–1144, 1984.
20. Wells DG, Bjorksten A: Monoamine oxidase inhibitors revisited. Can J Anaesth *69*:64, 1989.
21. Lippman SB, Nash K: Monoamine oxidase inhibitor update. Drug Saf *5*:1990.
22. Sporer KA: The serotonin syndrome. Drug Saf *13*:94, 1994.
23. Pentel P: Toxicity of over-the-counter stimulants. JAMA *252*:1898, 1984.
24. Lake CR, Gallant S, Masson E, et al. Adverse drug effects attributed to phenylpropanolamine: A review of 142 case reports. Am J Med *89*:195, 1990.
25. Pentel P, Mikell F: Reaction of phenylpropanolamine/

chlorpheniramine/belladonna compound on a woman with unrecognized autonomic dysfunction. Lancet *2*:274, 1984.
26. Boakes AJ, Laurence DR, Teoh PC, et al: Interactions between sympathomimetic amines and antidepressant agents in man. BMJ *1*:311, 1973.
27. Olson KR, Benowitz NL, Woo OF, Pond SM: Theophylline overdose: Acute single ingestion versus chronic repeated overmedication. Am J Emerg Med *3*:386, 1985.
28. Benowitz NL, Toffelmire EB: The use of hemodialysis and hemoperfusion in the treatment of theophylline intoxification. Semin Dial *6*:243, 1993.
29. Graham SR, Day RO, Lee R, et al: Overdose with chloral hydrate: A pharmacological and therapeutic review. Med J Aust *149*:686, 1988.
30. Regan TJ: Alcohol and the cardiovascular system. JAMA *264*:377, 1990.
31. Vikhert AM, Tsiplenkova VG, Cherpachenko NM: Alcoholic cardiomyopathy and sudden cardiac death. J Am Coll Cardiol *8*:3A, 1986.
32. Bass M: Sudden sniffing death. JAMA *212*:2075, 1970.
33. Kaufman JD, Silversterin MA, Moure-Eraso R: Atrial fibrillation and sudden death related to occupational solvent exposure. Am J Ind Med *25*:731, 1994.
34. Ford ES, Rhodes S, McDiarmid M, et al: Deaths from acute exposure to Trichloroethylene. J Occup Environ Med *37*:749, 1995.
35. Wason S, Gibler WB, Hassan M: Ventricular tachycardia associated with non-freon aerosol propellants. JAMA *256*:78, 1986.
36. Brimacombe JR, Scully M, Swainston R: Propranolol overdose—a dramatic response to calcium chloride. Med J Aust *155*:267, 1991.
37. Pentel P, Peterson CD: Asystole complicating physostigmine treatment due to organophosphate of tricyclic antidepressant overdose. Ann Emerg Med *9*:11, 1980.
38. Minton NA, Murray VSG: A Review of organophosphate poisoning. Med Toxicol *3*:350, 1988.
39. Bardin PG, Van Eeden SF, Joubert JR: Intensive care management of acute organophosphate poisoning. S Afr Med J *72*:593, 1987.
40. Ludomirsky A, Klein HO, Sarelli P, et al: Q-T prolongation and polymorphous ("torsades de pointes") ventricular arrhythmias associated with organophosphorus insecticide poisoning. Am J Cardiol *49*:1654, 1982.
41. Bardin PG, Van Eeden SF: Organophosphate poisoning: Grading the severity and comparing treatment between atropine and glycopyrrolate. Crit Care Med *18*:956, 1990.
42. Kim SY, Benowitz NL: Poisoning due to class IA antiarrhythmic drugs. Drug Saf *5*:393, 1990.
43. Stanton MS, Prystowsky EN, Fineberg NS, et al: Arrhythmogenic effects of antiarrhythmic drugs: A study of 406 patients treated for ventricular tachycardia or fibrillation. J Am Coll Cardiol *14*:209, 1989.
44. Tan HL, Hou CJY, Lauer MR, et al: Electrophysiologic mechanisms of the long QT interval syndromes and torsades de pointes. Ann Intern Med *122*:701, 1995.
45. Pearigen PD, Benowitz NL: Poisoning due to calcium antagonists. Drug Saf *6*:408, 1991.
46. Hariman RJ, Mangiardi LM, McAllister RG Jr, et al: Reversal of the cardiovascular effects of verapamil by calcium and sodium: Differences between electrophysiologic and hemodynamic responses. Circulation *59*:797, 1979.
47. Walter FG, Frye G, Mullen JT, et al: Amelioration of nifedipine poisoning associated with glucagon therapy. Ann Emerg Med *22*:1234, 1993.
48. Pentel PR, Benowitz NL: Tricyclic antidepressant poisoning. Management of arrhythmias. Med Toxicol *1*:101, 1986.
49. Berkovitch M, Matsui D, Fogelman, R, et al: Assessment of the terminal 40-millisecond QRS vector in children with a history of tricyclic antidepressant ingestion. Pediatr Emerg Care *11*:75, 1995.
50. Niemann JT, Bessen HA, Rothstein RJ, et al: Electrocardiographic criteria for tricyclic antidepressant cardiotoxicity. Am J Cardiol *57*:1154, 1986.
51. Liebelt EL, Francis PD, Woolf AD: ECG lead aVR versus QRS interval in predicting seizures and arrhythmias in acute tricyclic antidepressant toxicity. Ann Emerg Med *26*:195, 1995.
52. Wenger TL, Butler VP Jr, Haber E, Smith TW: Treatment of 63 severely digitalis-toxic patients with digoxin-specific antibody fragments. J Am Coll Cardiol *5*:118A, 1985.
53. Woolf AD, Wenger T, Smith, TW, et al: The use of digoxin-specific Fab fragments for severe digitalis intoxication in children. N Engl J Med *326*:1739, 1992.
54. Brubacher J, Hoffman RS: Digoxinlike toxicity and death from a purported aphrodisiac. JAMA *275*:988, 1996.
55. Corya BC, Black MJ, McHenry PL: Echocardiographic findings after acute carbon monoxide poisoning. Br Heart J *38*:712, 1976.
56. Gueron M, Yaron R: Cardiovascular manifestations of severe scorpion sting: Clinicopathologic correlations. Chest *57*:156, 1970.
57. Weitzmen S, Margulis G, Lehmann E: Uncommon cardiovascular manifestations and high catecholamine levels due to "black widow" bite. Am Heart J *93*:89, 1977.
58. Levine HD: Acute myocardial infarction following wasp sting: Report of two cases and critical survey of the literature. Am Heart J *91*:365, 1976.
59. Chin MY, Kreutzer RA, Dyer JE: Acute poisoning from gamma-hydroxybutyrate in california. West J Med *156*:380, 1992.
60. Geller RJ, Benowitz NL: Orthostatic hypotension in ciguatera fish poisoning. Arch Intern Med *152*:2131, 1992.
61. Tai YT, But PP, Young K, et al: Cardiotoxicity after accidental herb-induced aconite poisoning. Lancet *340*:1254, 1992.

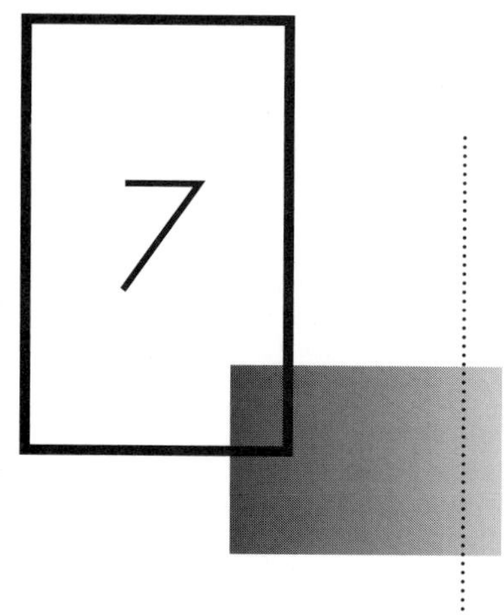

Management of Respiratory Complications in the Poisoned Patient

ANGELO M. TAVEIRA DA SILVA, MD, PhD

Poisoning or overdose with many commonly used drugs depresses respiration and causes apnea. Not infrequently, treatment with mechanical ventilation is required. Acidosis and hypoxia develop as a result of respiratory failure and together with an altered state of consciousness impair lung defense mechanisms against infectious agents.[1] Aspiration of oral secretions or gastric contents is also likely. Cardiovascular collapse, excessive fluid administration, or direct lung injury caused by drugs leads to acute respiratory distress syndrome (ARDS).

Respiratory care of the patient with drug overdose is essential to provide supportive care, prevent complications, and gain time for natural drug elimination mechanisms to operate and therapeutic measures to be implemented to enhance elimination of drugs.

In this chapter are discussed the effects of the most common intoxications that affect the respiratory system; the pathophysiology of respiratory failure and ARDS associated with drug intoxication; and a systematic approach to the management of poisoning and drug overdose, including airway care in the patient with altered mental status and treatment of ARDS and other pulmonary complications.

RESPIRATORY EFFECTS OF POISONS AND DRUGS

Of drugs that directly affect the respiratory system (Table 7–1), two main categories must be considered. Alcohol, opioids, and hypnotic and sedative drugs produce coma and depress respiration, resulting in impairment of lung defense mechanisms, hypoventilation, respiratory acidosis, and respiratory arrest. Salicylates, radiographic contrast media, and nitrofurantoin produce diffuse lung damage and cause severe respiratory failure.

The remainder of intoxicating drugs compromise respiratory function because they alter mental state, making aspiration of oral secretions and gastric contents more likely, or cause renal, hepatic, or cardiac failure, leading to fluid balance abnormalities and pulmonary edema.

Narcotics

Opioids depress respiration. Tidal volume, respiratory rate, and the ventilatory response to carbon dioxide (CO_2) and hypoxia are depressed.[2, 3] Opioids also cause a fulminant but rapidly reversible form of pulmonary edema.[4] Pulmonary edema is frequently observed at autopsy in victims of opioid overdose. Further, in narcotic addicts and abusers a variety of pulmonary pathologic findings can develop, including pneumonias, septic pulmonary emboli, pulmonary granulomatosis, fibrosis, and arteritis, which may lead to pulmonary hypertension.[5–7] Pulmonary function in narcotic addicts is frequently abnormal. Abnormal lung scans and carbon monoxide (CO) diffusing capacity of the lungs (DLCO) have been reported in such patients.[8, 9] The DLCO is most frequently abnormal but usually returns to normal after discontinuation of the drug.[9]

Pulmonary edema due to heroin usually has rapid

Table 7–1. Respiratory Effects of Poisons and Drugs

Class of Drug	Agent	Respiratory Depression or Apnea	Pulmonary Edema (ARDS)	Other Effects
Narcotics	Heroin	Yes	Yes	Chronic use results in pulmonary function abnormalities
	Morphine	Yes	Yes	
	Codeine	Yes	Yes	
	Methadone	Yes	Yes	
	Pentazocine	Yes	?	
	Diphenoxylate	Yes	?	
Hypnotics and sedatives	Barbiturates	Yes	Yes	
	Glutethimide	Yes	Yes	
	Methaqualone	Yes	Yes	
	Ethanol	Yes	Yes	
	Ethchlorvynol	Yes	Yes	
	Chloral hydrate	Yes	Not reported	
	Methyprylon	Yes	Not reported	
	Nitrazepam	Yes	Not reported	Sleep apnea
	Chlordiazepoxide	Yes	Yes	
	Diazepam	Yes	Not reported	Sleep apnea
	Meprobamate	Yes	Yes	
	Midazolam	Yes	Not reported	
Anesthetics	Halothane	Yes	Yes	
	Cocaine	Yes	Yes	Myocardial infarction, cerebrovascular accident, pneumothorax
	Ketamine	Yes	No	
Neuromuscular blockers	D-Tubocurarine	Yes	No	
	Pancuronium bromide	Yes	No	
	Succinylcholine	Yes	No	
	Gallamine	Yes	No	
Antipsychotics	Isocarboxazid	Yes	Yes	Severe cardiovascular toxicity may play a role in the pathophysiology of pulmonary edema
	Phenelzine	Yes	Yes	
	Amitriptyline	Yes	Yes	
	Nortriptyline	Yes	Yes	
	Imipramine	Yes	Yes	
	Doxepin	Yes	Yes	
	Phenothiazines	No	No	
Cholinergic agonists and cytotoxins	Mushroom poisoning	Yes	No	Severe bronchospasm may occur
Anticholinesterases	Parathion, malathion	Yes	No	Severe bronchospasm may occur
Antimuscarinics	Atropine, belladonna alkaloids	Yes	No	
Sympathicomimetics	Epinephrine, amphetamines	Yes	Yes	
Psychedelics	LSD	No	No	
	Phencyclidine	Yes	No	
Analgesics	Propoxyphene	Yes	Yes	
	Salicylates	No	Yes	
Intravenous contrast media	Methylglucamine iothalamate	No	Yes	
	Sodium iothalamate	No	Yes	
	Meglumine diatrizoate	No	Yes	
	Ethiodized oil	No	Yes	
Miscellaneous	Nitrofurantoin	No	Yes	
	Colchicine	No	Yes	
	Disopyramide	No	Yes	
	Hydrochlorothiazide	No	Yes	
	Insulin	Yes (hypoglycemic coma)	Yes	
Herbicides	Paraquat	No	Yes	Causes rapidly progressing pulmonary fibrosis
Smoke inhalation	Carbon monoxide	Yes		
Hydrocarbons	Aliphatic	No	Yes	
	Gasoline	No	Yes	
	Kerosene	No	Yes	

ARDS, acute respiratory distress syndrome; LSD, D-lysergic acid diethylamide.

onset, sometimes occurring hours after respiratory depression has already subsided. Improvement is also rapid, within 24 to 48 hours, although roentgenologic abnormalities may take longer to resolve.[10] The prevalence of pulmonary edema in patients with heroin overdose is about 90%, and because patients may be found unconscious in various positions, the pulmonary edema may be unilateral or may be noted in an unusual site.[11] In chronic narcotic users the prevalence of episodes of pulmonary edema is lower, probably no more than 5 to 20%.[12] In a review of 149 cases of heroin overdose, 71 patients (48%) had pulmonary edema.[13] Mean arterial blood gas concentrations in 39 of the 71 patients were Pa_{O_2} 50 mm Hg and Pa_{CO_2} 53 mm Hg, with pH 7.22. All 13 patients who died had evidence of pulmonary edema. Hemodynamic measurements showed a high cardiac index of 4.1 L/m_2, slight elevation of pulmonary artery pressure (32/12 mm Hg), and normal pulmonary capillary wedge pressure (PCWP) of 8 mm Hg. Cardiac output in heroin-induced pulmonary edema has been reported as either depressed or elevated.[10, 13] No substantially elevated PCWP has been reported.

Pulmonary function abnormalities were reported in 16 patients with heroin-induced pulmonary edema[14]: mean Pa_{O_2} 37 mm Hg and Pa_{CO_2} 56 mm Hg, with pH 7.15. Chest roentgenograms showed bilateral alveolar infiltrates (Fig. 7–1). Vital capacity (VC) was decreased to 46% of predicted normal, and DLCO to 53%. The alveolar-arterial oxygen gradient $(A\text{-}a)_{O_2}$ was increased, and dynamic compliance (Cdyn) was decreased. Hypoxemia was also present in those patients without overt pulmonary edema. Return of VC and Cdyn to normal was slow, and impairment of DLCO persisted for many weeks. Pulmonary edema has been reported also with morphine, methadone, codeine, and pentazocine.

The pathophysiology of narcotic-induced pulmonary edema is obscure. The edema fluid is rich in protein, and its composition approaches that of plasma. Katz et al.[15] reported that in opioid-induced pulmonary edema the fluid protein content was within 98.3 ± 10% of the plasma proteins, whereas in cardiogenic pulmonary edema it was only 40 ± 9%. These observations indicate that this form of pulmonary edema is due to capillary leak syndrome, leading to increased permeability of the lung vessels, interstitial edema, and alveolar flooding. That this form of pulmonary edema can resolve rapidly indicates the capillary damage is not severe.

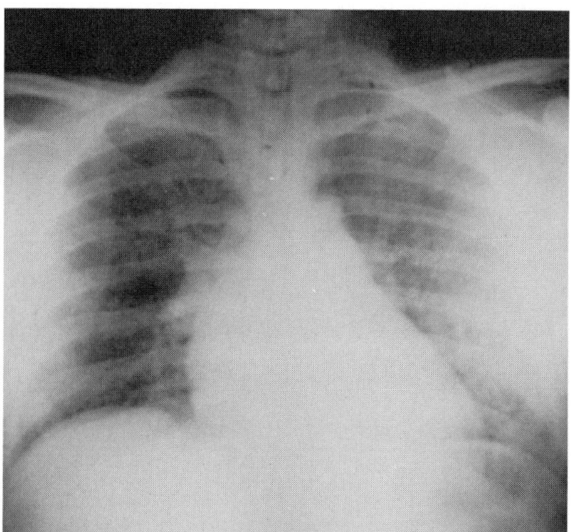

Figure 7–1. Heroin-induced pulmonary edema in a 30-year-old man. Note the predominance of infiltrates in the left lung.

Hypoxemia could be important in the pathogenesis of opioid-induced pulmonary edema. As in the case of high-altitude pulmonary edema, acute hypoxemia may induce severe pulmonary, arterial, capillary, or venous constriction, thus increasing pulmonary vascular pressure.[16] In addition, sudden release of catecholamines or other mediators such as histamine, bradykinin, and cytokines may increase both vascular pressure and permeability of the pulmonary vessels, leading to pulmonary edema.[17]

Hypnotics and Sedatives

Hypnotic and sedative drugs cause circulatory shock, respiratory depression, and noncardiogenic pulmonary edema. Cardiac output is usually depressed, and plasma volume is reduced, probably because of increased capillary permeability and redistribution of extracellular fluid.[18] Systemic vascular resistance is normal or increased.[18] This state of shock itself may cause ARDS. Administration of intravenous fluids as part of the treatment of circulatory shock and as a means of enhancing renal elimination of the toxic drug is at least in part responsible for the frequent occurrence of pulmonary edema. Probably some damage to the alveolocapillary membrane also occurs.

Pulmonary infection is the major cause of morbidity and mortality in patients with barbiturate overdose[19] (Fig. 7–2). Pneumonias are usually due to aspiration of oral or gastric secretions or both. Aspiration is common because in comatose patients clearance of tracheal bronchial secretions is abnormal and macrophage and leukocyte functions are impaired by hypercapnia, acidosis, hypoxia, and effects of associated alcohol intake.[1] Pneumonia is particularly frequent in patients requiring endotracheal intubation (35% to 96%). Fluid overload and pulmonary edema are the next most serious complications.[19] Close monitoring of central venous pressure or PCWP is recommended.

Benzodiazepines are a group of drugs widely used as anxiolytics, hypnotics, and anticonvulsants and preoperatively in patients undergoing invasive diagnostic and therapeutic procedures. These drugs have a wide margin of safety; in patients with cardiorespiratory disorders, however, hypotension, cardiorespiratory depression, and apnea may occur.[20, 21] Apnea is more likely to occur if narcotics or alcohol is taken concurrently. Apnea may occur in as many as 20% of all patients receiving the new short-acting benzodiazepine midazolam by the intravenous route.[20] Diaze-

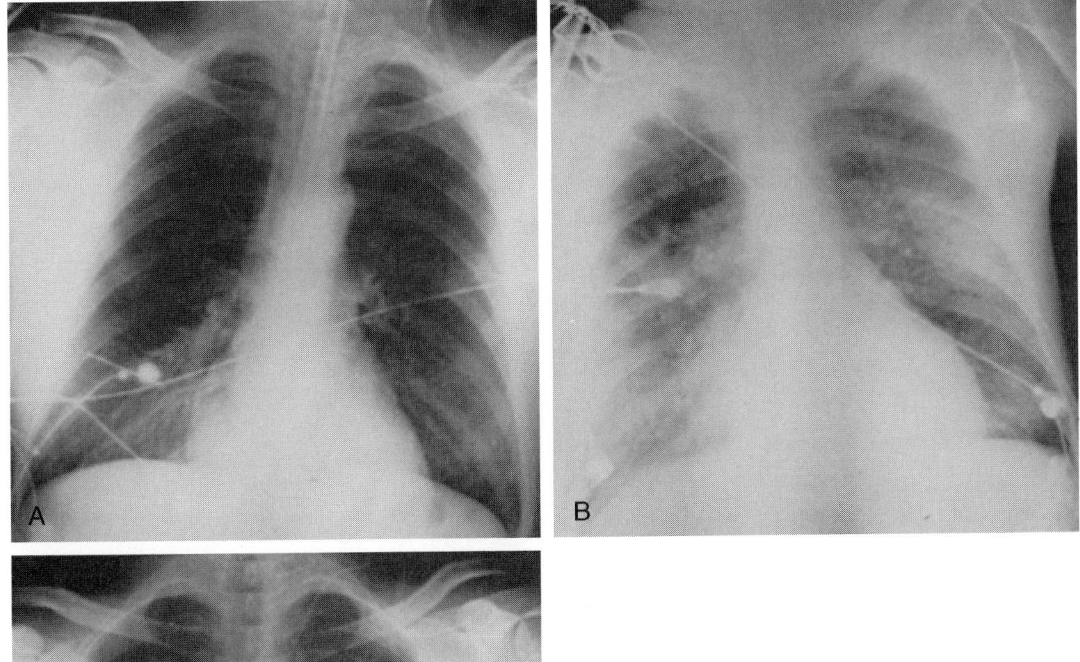

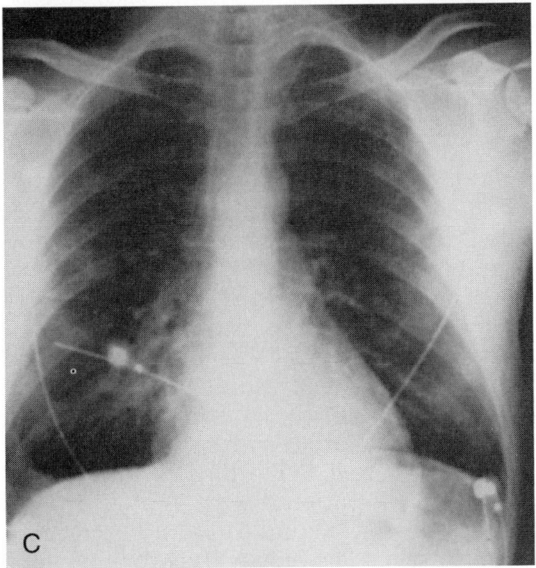

Figure 7–2. Barbiturate overdose in a 52-year-old man. *A,* An endotracheal tube, nasogastric tube, and CVP catheter have been inserted. The lung fields are clear. *B,* Fluid replacement and alkaline diuresis resulted in acute pulmonary edema and severe respiratory failure ($Pa{O_2}$ = 100 mm Hg on 50% $Fi{O_2}$). *C,* Two days later: the bilateral infiltrates have cleared and extubation was successful.

pam decreases alveolar ventilation, increases $Pa{CO_2}$, and impairs the ventilatory response to CO_2.[22] Midazolam has similar effects, decreasing the ventilatory response to CO_2 and other indices of central respiratory activity.[23] These effects are more pronounced in patients with chronic obstructive pulmonary disease, and recovery may take longer. Benzodiazepines increase the number and severity of obstructive episodes in patients with obstructive sleep apnea, because they have an inhibitory effect on genioglossus muscle activity.[24]

The cardiorespiratory depressant effects of benzodiazepines are exerted centrally.[25] The specific benzodiazepine antagonist flumazenil reverses the cardiorespiratory depressant effects of benzodiazepines. Indeed, administration of flumazenil may avert the necessity for endotracheal intubation.[26] The prevalence of seizures after administration of flumazenil is low, even in patients who abuse benzodiazepines or ethanol.[26, 27]

Ethchlorvynol overdose is uncommon but particularly dangerous because of the duration of coma and the potential for severe acute pulmonary edema, which may be fatal.[28]

Intoxication with meprobamate is now rare. The pharmacologic effects are similar to those of barbiturates and are characterized by shock and coma, usually of short duration.[29] Pulmonary edema has been reported.[30] Rapid drug removal by continuous arteriovenous hemoperfusion may be life-saving in patients with severe shock.[31]

Anesthetics and Curare

Accidental or suicidal administration of anesthetics and curarizing agents may be fatal. Epinephrine, which may be administered along with a local anesthetic, may cause severe pulmonary edema.[32] Accidental intravenous administration of halothane also may cause fatal acute pulmonary edema.[33] Halothane may be abused by hospital personnel, and its inhalation has been reported to cause pulmonary edema, cardiac arrhythmias, and death.[34]

Analgesics

Salicylates cause mixed metabolic acidosis and respiratory alkalosis in adults, metabolic acidosis in children, and pulmonary edema[35–38] (Fig. 7–3). Ingestion of salicylates to treat toothache caused severe respiratory failure in a young woman, who required mechanical ventilation.[39]

Studies of the pathophysiology of salicylate-induced pulmonary edema[37, 38] demonstrated normal cardiac output and normal or low PCWP. Severe hypovolemia caused by pulmonary loss of protein-rich fluid has been reported.[38] Urinary losses of protein may be also substantial. Available data indicate this form of pulmonary edema is due to a direct toxic effect on the alveolocapillary membrane.[37] In an experimental sheep model of salicylate intoxication, salicylates increased lung lymph flow, transvascular flux of protein, and lung water.[37] Direct damage to capillaries, mediated by vasoactive substances, is probably responsible for analgesic-induced pulmonary edema.[37]

Propoxyphene, a narcotic analgesic structurally related to methadone, causes respiratory depression and pulmonary edema.[40] Three cases of acute pulmonary edema, two fatal, were reported after ingestion of doses between 1.6 and 3.5 g.[40] However, pulmonary edema has occurred after ingestion of lower doses. Pulmonary edema is probably due to increased capillary permeability, not cardiac failure.

Tricyclic Antidepressants and Antipsychotic Drugs

Tricyclic antidepressants (TCAs) are extremely toxic drugs that cause severe cardiovascular toxicity, shock, and death.[29] TCAs are the most common cause of death from prescribed drugs.[41] Pulmonary edema and respiratory failure have been reported in patients with TCA overdose.[42, 43] Pulmonary edema may be the result of excessive fluid administration, which may be required to treat hypotension and shock.[43] Myocardial depression caused by the drug itself may cause cardiogenic pulmonary edema.[42, 43] Less frequently, TCAs may cause noncardiogenic pulmonary edema and acute respiratory distress syndrome[42, 44–46] (Figs. 7–4 and 7–5). Roy et al.[42] reported that 66 (80%) of 82 patients with TCA overdose had abnormal oxygenation and 61 (76.8%) required mechanical ventilation. The mean duration of ventilation was 46.2 hours. ARDS developed in 9 patients.

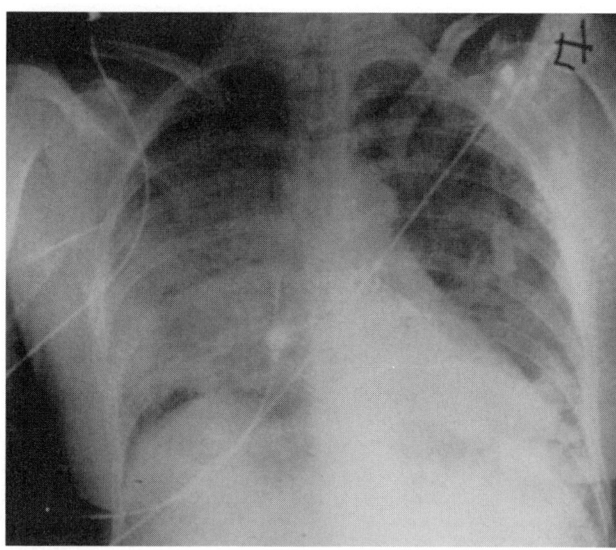

Figure 7–4. Tricyclic antidepressant overdose in a 37-year-old woman. Bilateral pulmonary edema and a right pneumothorax secondary to subclavian vein puncture for insertion of a central venous pressure line are seen.

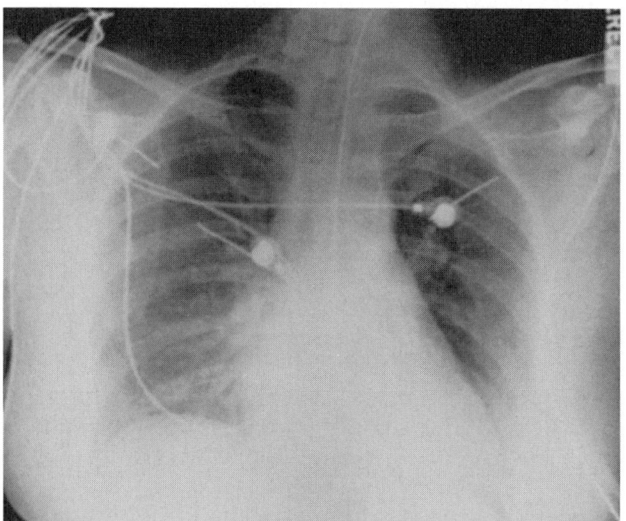

Figure 7–3. Acetaminophen overdose and pulmonary edema (ARDS) in a 40-year-old woman.

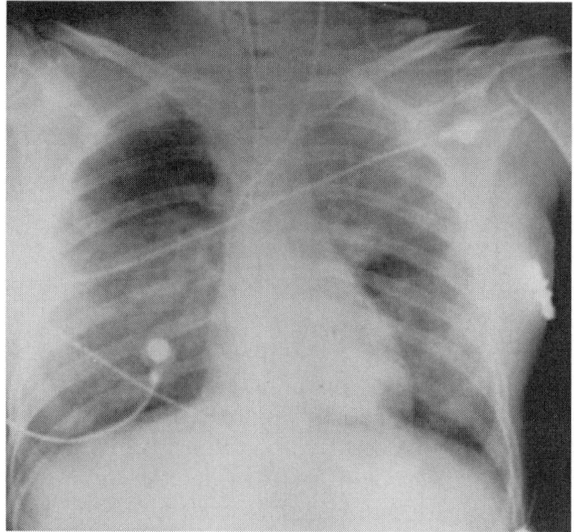

Figure 7–5. Tricyclic antidepressant overdose and severe ARDS in a 22-year-old woman. With 50% FiO_2, PEEP 12 cm H_2O, and PaO_2 84 mm Hg, the cardiac output was 5.7 L/min, and PCWP was 12 mm Hg.

Cocaine and Other Central Nervous System Stimulant Drugs

This group of drugs includes cocaine, amphetamine and its derivatives, phencyclidine (PCP), lysergic acid diethylamide (LSD), and methylphenidate. Most of these drugs have significant cardiovascular effects owing to their sympathomimetic actions. Tachycardia, hypertension, arrhythmias, shock, and respiratory arrest occur with severe overdose. The recreational use of cocaine has been associated with an increasing number of reports of respiratory and cardiovascular toxicity. Acute myocardial infarction, cardiac arrhythmias, rupture of the aorta, and cerebrovascular accidents all have been reported.[47, 48] Intravenous injection of freebase (cocaine), as well as its inhalation, can precipitate acute pulmonary edema and shock.[49] Other respiratory manifestations include lung hemorrhage, asthma, pulmonary edema, bronchiolitis obliterans, and hypersensitivity pneumonitis.[50–52]

We have seen a fatal case in a young woman who had shock complicated by pulmonary edema and severe cardiorespiratory failure. Cardiac output was 8 L/min, and PCWP was normal, ruling out the presence of cardiogenic shock. Therefore, it appears that cocaine may cause not only acute myocardial infarction and cardiogenic pulmonary edema but also noncardiogenic pulmonary edema (ARDS).[50–52] Inhalation of freebase causes diffuse alveolar damage, which can manifest with fever, hypoxemia, hemoptysis, diffuse alveolar infiltrates, and respiratory failure.[52] Lung tissue specimens obtained at biopsy showed diffuse alveolar damage, alveolar hemorrhage, and eosinophil-rich interstitial infiltrates. Immunoglobulin E deposits were identified in lymphocytes and macrophages.[52] Other complications of cocaine abuse are pneumothorax and pneumomediastinum,[53] believed to result from the deep inspirations followed by Valsalva maneuvers performed by the victims during smoking or inhalation of freebase vapors. Repeated inhalation of freebase results in lung function abnormalities, particularly decreased DLCO.[51, 54] Bronchiolitis obliterans in a patient known to be a cocaine user was reported by Patel et al.[55] Good response to treatment with corticosteroids was observed. Cocaine also causes seizures and respiratory arrest, particularly when it is injected intravenously or inhaled as freebase.[50, 51]

Cocaine-related respiratory toxicity is discussed further in Chapter 39.

Roentgenographic Intravenous Contrast Media

Noncardiogenic pulmonary edema may develop after intravenous administration of radiographic contrast products, usually in the context of an anaphylactoid reaction. Several cases of pulmonary edema after injection of methylglucamine iothalamate and meglumine diatrizoate have been reported. Severe respiratory failure may occur, and mechanical ventilation and positive end-expiratory pressure (PEEP) may be required.[56] Hemodynamic measurements show hypotension, high cardiac output, and low systemic vascular resistance. Pulmonary edema fluid has been reported to be rich in protein. Marked hemoconcentration occurs as a result of massive leakage of plasma into the lungs.

Herbicides and Insecticides

Among these compounds, paraquat is most likely to cause severe respiratory failure and death.[57, 58] Ingestion of 10 to 20 mL of a 20% solution of paraquat is usually lethal (Fig. 7–6). Transcutaneous absorption has been documented, especially if skin is damaged (e.g., in the presence of skin ulceration).[58] Absorption of small amounts is compatible with survival, but continuous skin absorption due to improper use of sprays may cause death.[59] The clinical findings are acute pulmonary edema followed by rapidly progressive lung fibrosis, severe hypoxemia, and death. Pneumothoraces, pneumomediastinum, pneumopericardium, and subcutaneous emphysema also may develop.[60] The radiographic changes initially include diffuse consolidation, pneumomediastinum, and cardiomegaly. Interstitial disease develops at the end of the first week, and honeycombing at 4 weeks.[61] Paraquat concentrations in the lung may reach a level 50 times that in the blood. Depending on the amount of paraquat accumulated in the lungs, either a fulminant form of pulmonary edema or rapidly progressive pulmonary fibrosis will develop. Intra-alveolar fibrosis with small airway involvement, medial hypertrophy of the pulmonary arterioles, and fibrosis and destruction of these vessels have been

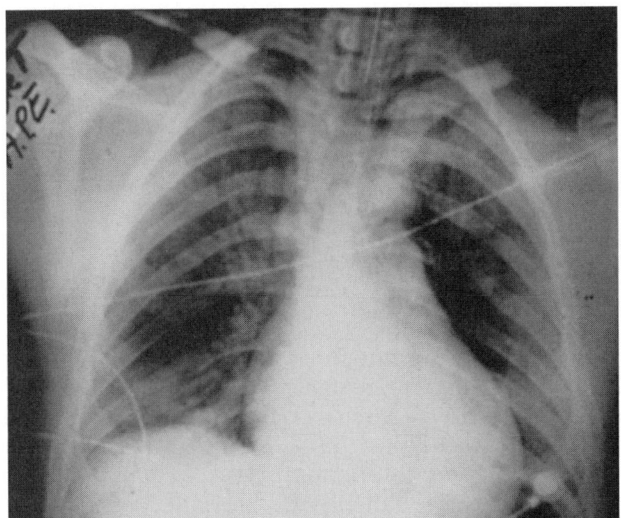

Figure 7–6. Paraquat overdose in a 21-year-old man. Bilateral pulmonary infiltrates are evident. While the patient was breathing room air, PaO_2 was 75 mm Hg. The patient died of intractable respiratory failure.

described. Evidence of endothelial cell damage is suggested by increased serum angiotensin-converting enzyme levels after exposure to paraquat.[62]

Paraquat interferes with the ability of the lung to inactivate superoxide radicals and therefore enhances oxygen toxicity.[63] Conversely, after paraquat poisoning, oxygen may cause and contribute to further lung damage. Serial pulmonary function studies in patients with paraquat poisoning have shown that lung volumes are decreased, but initially arterial oxygen tension may be normal. An increased (A-a)O_2 gradient and an abnormal DLCO measurement are constant findings. Increased shunting caused by development of very low ventilation-perfusion ratio units occurs terminally, making oxygenation of the lungs virtually impossible even with 100% oxygen. Treatment with antioxidants such as desferoxamine and acetylcysteine may be useful.[64]

Paraquat toxicity is discussed further in Chapter 66.

Organophosphate compounds include parathion and malathion, and nerve gases (e.g., sarin) used in chemical warfare. These agents inhibit acetylcholinesterases.[65] Exposure to these substances causes muscarinic symptoms including conjunctival congestion, rhinorrhea, bronchoconstriction, bronchorrhea, nausea, vomiting, and diarrhea.[65] Severe intoxication, manifested by coma, seizures, respiratory failure, and respiratory paralysis, may result in death. ARDS has been reported.[66] Tsao et al.[67] reported that 43 (40.2%) of 107 patients with acute organophosphate and carbamate poisoning required mechanical ventilation, and 22 (51.2%) of these died.[67] Sixty-four patients in whom respiratory failure did not develop survived. In 28 patients, pneumonia developed.

Central respiratory depression is a major cause of the respiratory toxicity produced by organophosphate compounds. Acute central nervous system (CNS) toxicity caused by these compounds may be due to a loss of central respiratory drive, resulting from disruptions of normal patterned activity in respiratory-related unit discharge.[68] The intermediate area of the ventral surface of the medulla oblongata appears to be the most sensitive site for CNS responses elicited by cholinesterase inhibition.[69] The respiratory effects observed after application of cholinesterase inhibitors to this area consist of an initial stimulatory response characterized by increased tidal volume, followed by apnea. These respiratory depressant effects are counteracted by atropine. Poisoning with organophosphates has also been reported to cause fatal ARDS.[70]

Treatment of organophosphate poisoning consists of administering large doses of specific antagonists (atropine and pralidoxime) while supporting the patient with mechanical ventilation. However, treatment with atropine and pralidoxine may not avert the need for mechanical ventilation, which is required in approximately 40% to 60% of patients.[67, 71]

Aspiration or intravenous administration of hydrocarbon insecticides causes severe pneumonitis and a severe form of noncardiogenic pulmonary edema.[72, 73]

Carbon Monoxide

Carbon monoxide (CO) poisoning accounts annually for more than 2000 accidental or suicidal deaths. The affinity of carbon monoxide for hemoglobin (Hb) is about 200 times greater than for oxygen. Indeed, at concentrations of 0.1% CO, hemoglobin becomes 70% saturated, and victims become comatose. Generalized convulsions, shock, and death may follow. Usually no symptoms are observed at COHb concentrations of 5% to 10%. Headache, dyspnea, a feeling of drunkenness, nausea, and vomiting are seen with COHb levels of 10% to 40%.[74] Respiratory failure and coma are seen at COHb levels above 50%.[74, 75] The most common source of carbon monoxide is incomplete combustion of materials in confined spaces (e.g., fires). Carbon monoxide poisoning, however, has been reported in open spaces and in subjects standing near smoldering fires or riding in the back of trucks. Besides decreasing the oxygen-carrying capacity of hemoglobin, carbon monoxide shifts the hemoglobin dissociation curve to the left, resulting in increased affinity of hemoglobin for oxygen. It also inhibits oxidative metabolism by interfering with cytochrome systems throughout the body.

The diagnosis of carbon monoxide poisoning is established by measurement of COHb or oxyhemoglobin concentrations. The arterial oxygen tension and oxygen saturation by pulse oximetry are normal. Treatment of carbon monoxide poisoning consists of speeding the elimination of this gas by the administration of 100% oxygen, which decreases the half-life of COHb by a factor of 4. When COHb levels are above 40% or there is neurologic or cardiovascular impairment, treatment with hyperbaric oxygen is recommended.[74] If this is not available, endotracheal intubation and mechanical ventilation with 100% oxygen should be considered. This treatment should be continued until COHb is reduced to less than 5% and symptoms resolve.

Miscellaneous Drugs

Nitrofurantoin may cause various types of pulmonary toxicity, including pulmonary edema and progressive pulmonary fibrosis.[76] Idiosyncratic reactions to hydrochlorothiazide were responsible for two cases of pulmonary edema.[77] Colchicine, a drug used to treat acute gout, can cause ARDS.[78] Disopyramide, an antiarrhythmic drug, was reported to cause fatal pulmonary edema in three patients without previous cardiac disease.[79] Hypoglycemia secondary to insulin administration or ethanol intoxication also may cause pulmonary edema.[80] The list of drugs potentially capable of causing lung damage is large, and among these is the ever increasing number of chemotherapeutic agents used to treat malignant disease.[81] Inhalation of cadmium and mercury fumes can cause severe respiratory failure.[82, 83] Overdose with iron tablets also may cause ARDS.[84]

TREATMENT OF ADULT RESPIRATORY DISTRESS SYNDROME, RESPIRATORY INSUFFICIENCY, AND RESPIRATORY ARREST

Airway Care in the Intoxicated Patient

If a poisoned patient is comatose or has a depressed sensorium, the upper airway must be protected.

Indications for endotracheal intubation include the following:

- Respiratory arrest
- Coma
- Mechanical ventilation
- Seizures
- Gastric lavage in an unresponsive, unconscious patient
- Severe hypoxemia, acute respiratory acidosis, or both
- Emergency bronchoscopy
- Severe metabolic acidosis

In adult patients, oral intubation with an endotracheal tube having an inside diameter of at least 8 mm is recommended. Tubes this size or larger will permit passage of a fiberoptic bronchoscope, which may be required to (1) remove foreign bodies and food particles (aspiration), (2) assess the upper airway (fire victims, inhalation of toxic gases), (3) remove secretions (atelectasis), or (4) collect specimens of tracheobronchial secretions and perform bronchoalveolar lavage. Nasotracheal intubation in general is contraindicated because it requires a spontaneously breathing cooperative patient and may trigger vomiting and aspiration of gastric contents. Airway protection by means of an endotracheal tube with administration of a humidified gas mixture containing a concentration of oxygen that will ensure Po_2 70 mm Hg or more is recommended. If the patient has had a respiratory arrest or has respiratory failure, mechanical ventilation is added. Respiratory failure is another indication for endotracheal intubation. Patients with seizures or those who are severely agitated may also need endotracheal intubation, particularly if they require chemical sedation (which may itself cause respiratory depression). In these circumstances *rapid-sequence intubation* is recommended. After oxygenating the lungs with 100% oxygen for 5 minutes, we prefer the use of rapid administration of fentanyl (25 μg at a time), midazolam (0.5 mg at a time), and succinylcholine (1 to 2 mg/kg). Thiopental (1 to 4 mg/kg), diazepam (2.5 mg increments), and ketamine (1 to 2 mg/kg) may be used instead.[85, 86] Succinylcholine is contraindicated in patients with hyperkalemia, and ketamine may be the drug of choice in patients with bronchospasm (organophosphate poisoning). After these drugs have been administered, an assistant applies pressure against the cricoid cartilage, occluding the esophagus (Sellick maneuver). After the muscle relaxant takes effect, laryngoscopy and intubation are performed, and ventilation is begun. Appropriate positioning of the endotracheal tube can be ascertained by auscultation at the midaxillary lines or monitoring of the end-tidal CO_2 by capnography.[85, 86] Oxygen saturation should also be monitored throughout the entire procedure.

Another indication for endotracheal intubation is gastric lavage, particularly if lavage is to be undertaken in a patient who is lethargic or unconscious. In these instances, because the risk of aspiration is great the airway must be protected. Finally, severe metabolic abnormalities such as metabolic acidosis (methanol poisoning) are an indication for intubation. Figure 7–7 gives an algorithm helpful in decision-making for airway management in the poisoned patient.

Among some of the immediate complications of endotracheal intubation are bleeding, traumatic avulsion of a tooth, intubation of the esophagus, and intubation of the right main stem bronchus. Laryngeal and tracheal damage may result from traumatic intubation. Once the proper position of the tube has been ascertained, tidal volume and minute ventilation can be measured and the presence of hypoventilation can be detected. Preferably, arterial blood gas concentrations should be determined, and oxygen should be given to maintain Pao_2 above 70 mm Hg. If blood gas measurements cannot be obtained immediately, 100% oxygen administration is recommended. If the patient is apneic or has a slow, shallow respiratory pattern, mechanical ventilation should be initiated.

General Principles of Mechanical Ventilation in the Intoxicated Patient

When the victim of drug intoxication has bradypnea and low tidal volume or when arterial blood gas measurements show an elevated $Paco_2$ level, hypoventilation is present. In these circumstances, intravenous naloxone should be administered; intravenous flumazepam may be indicated in pure benodiazepine overdose. A prompt response should occur, consisting of arousal and increased rate and depth of breathing. Treatment with these drug(s) may have to be repeated. The indications for mechanical ventilation after drug overdose are as follows:

- Respiratory arrest
- Severe hypoxemia
- Severe metabolic acidosis
- Alveolar hypoventilation and respiratory acidosis
- Seizures requiring the use of diazepam or barbiturates
- Administration of curarizing agents
- Aspiration of gastric contents causing ARDS

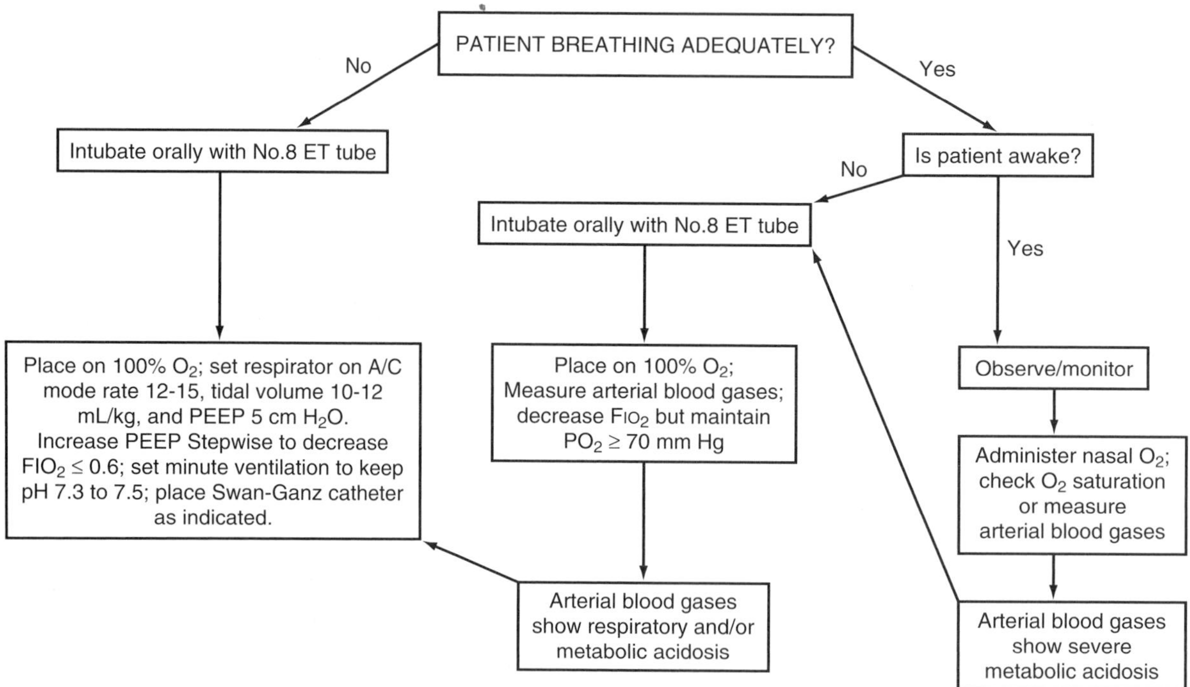

Figure 7–7. Algorithm for airway care and mechanical ventilation in the poisoned patient. ET, endotracheal tube.

- Severe shock
- Pa_{O_2} <70 mm Hg with Fi_{O_2} >50%
- $(A\text{-}a)_{O_2}$ with 100% Fi_{O_2} >350 mm Hg

The objective of mechanical ventilation is to achieve Pa_{O_2} 70 mm Hg or more at an Fi_{O_2} below 50% and to maintain normal pH (7.36 to 7.45), unless otherwise indicated. In a patient with chronic obstructive pulmonary lung disease and chronic hypercapnia, this may entail keeping Pa_{CO_2} around 50 mm Hg by either decreasing the rate or the tidal volume. With severe metabolic acidosis, it may be necessary to hyperventilate the lungs to a Pa_{CO_2} of 20 or 30 mm Hg to obtain normal pH, until the acidosis is corrected. In a patient with tricyclic antidepressant overdose, an alkaline pH is desirable, and thus the patient should be hyperventilated.

In patients who are agitated, are having seizures, or have tachypnea secondary to severe respiratory distress, adequate mechanical ventilation may be difficult to achieve. In these instances, the use of sedatives and muscle relaxant drugs may be required. We commonly use midazolam (0.03 mg/kg), lorazepam (0.044 mg/kg), fentanyl (1 to 2 μg/kg per hour), and pancuronium bromide. Pancuronium is given first as a test dose of 0.01 mg/kg. If no arrhythmias occur, an intravenous loading dose of 0.06 to 0.08 mg/kg is given. Doses of 0.02 to 0.03 mg/kg are then repeated hourly as required. Intravenous haloperidol (2 to 10 mg every 2 to 4 hours) may also be used in the severely agitated patient.[87, 88]

Acute Respiratory Distress Syndrome

ARDS is characterized by impaired oxygenation (ratio between Pa_{O_2} and Fi_{O_2} less than 200 mm Hg), bilateral pulmonary infiltrates, and PCWP less than 18 mm Hg.[89] There is acute injury to the alveolocapillary unit, leading to disruption of the endothelial barrier, increased vascular permeability, and pulmonary edema.[89, 90] This syndrome is associated with shock (particularly septic shock), fat embolism, aspiration of toxic gases or liquids (including gastric contents), toxic inhalation, and drug overdose.[89, 90]

Drug overdose may cause severe respiratory failure. This form of ARDS is generally rapidly reversible because it is due to a self-limited form of capillary leak syndrome. An excess of extravascular lung water is observed, but progression to a fibrotic state does not occur. An exception is intoxication with paraquat, in which progression to fibrosis is the rule. Other drugs such as amphetamines, PCP, and tricyclic antidepressants have the potential to cause serious cardiac dysfunction. In these cases, pulmonary edema may be due to left ventricular failure. Some drugs such as opioids and salicylates have the potential to cause massive fluid loss and lead to hypovolemic shock. The edema fluid has a protein content similar to that of plasma.

The equation defining the forces that regulate fluid exchange in the lungs states that

$$QF = K(Pmv - Ppmv) - \rho(\pi mv - \eta mv)$$

where Qf is the average capillary filtration or lymph flow, K is the capillary filtration coefficient, Pmv and Ppmv are, respectively, the microvascular and perimicrovascular (tissue) hydrostatic pressures, ρ is a term for defining the permeability of pulmonary vessels for proteins, and πmv and ηpmv are the microvascular and perimicrovascular (tissue) osmotic pressures.[91] Anything that changes the hydrostatic pressure gradient (Pmv − Ppmv), osmotic pressure (ηmv − πpmv), or the filtration coefficient K causes pulmonary edema. Increase in fluid filtration secondary to an increase in the Pmv − Ppmv gradient is the cause of the so-called cardiogenic pulmonary edema due to cardiac failure.[92] Increased permeability to fluid and protein through lung capillaries or veins is the cause of ARDS in patients with drug overdose. Fluid overload, heart failure, and shock may play additional roles.

The lungs of patients with ARDS due to drug overdose contain an excessive amount of water, and alveoli are either flooded or unstable, with a tendency to collapse. The lungs are heavy and stiff and have decreased compliance and resting lung volume. Breathing at these low lung volumes requires large inspiratory pressure; thus the work of breathing is increased. Lack of ventilation of flooded or collapsed alveoli results in a low ventilation-perfusion ($\dot{V}$/Q) ratio, venous admixture, and hypoxemia (shuntlike effect).

Treatment of Adult Respiratory Distress Syndrome in Patients with Drug Overdose

The treatment of ARDS in the setting of drug intoxication can be summarized as follows. Mechanical ventilation is indicated for treatment of hypoxemia requiring more than 50% Fio_2, respiratory acidosis, and an alveolar to arterial oxygen gradient $(A\text{-}a)o_2$ on 100% oxygen above 350 mm Hg,[93] particularly in the patient with altered mental status. The $(A\text{-}a)o_2$ can be calculated by subtracting the arterial oxygen tension (Pao_2) from the alveolar oxygen tension (PAo_2). The alveolar oxygen tension (PAo_2) can be derived from the simplified alveolar air equation for 100% oxygen breathing: $PAo_2 = (PB - 47 \text{ mm Hg}) - Paco_2$ where PB is the barometric pressure in millimeters of mercury and 47 mm Hg is the water vapor pressure at 37°C, and $Paco_2$ is the arterial CO_2 tension noted on arterial blood gases.

In general, these patients have high respiratory rates (>30) with low VC (less than 10 mL/kg).

Mechanical ventilation is begun at a frequency of 10 to 12 per minute, a net tidal volume of 10 to 12 mL/kg, and 100% Fio_2. Arterial blood gases are measured 15 to 20 minutes later, and the severity of impairment of oxygen exchange is assessed by calculating again the $(A\text{-}a)o_2$ gradient. As a general rule, for each 20 mm Hg of gradient there is a 1% shunt (normal is 5%). Frequently it is observed that gas exchange improves somewhat with use of the respirator; however, high oxygen concentrations may still be required. In this case PEEP should be started, usually beginning at 5 cm H_2O. PEEP increases functional residual capacity (FRC) and Pao_2 and decreases the $(A\text{-}a)o_2$ gradient and shunt. In addition, perfusion to areas of low V/Q ratio is decreased by PEEP, thus improving Pao_2.[94] The objectives of using PEEP are to (1) recruit unstable and collapsed alveoli and therefore increase FRC, (2) decrease venous admixture (shunt) and improve Pao_2, (3) allow a decrease in Fio_2 to nontoxic levels, and (4) prevent further alveolar collapse and closure. If the arterial blood gas measurements show acidosis or alkalosis, the minute ventilation (tidal volume times frequency) should be adjusted to correct the pH. The minute ventilation should be increased if the pH is decreased, and decreased if the pH is alkaline. For various reasons (e.g., antidiuretic hormone release), patients receiving positive-pressure ventilation have a tendency to retain fluids.[95] Fluid intake should be restricted, but urinary output should be kept at 1 ml/kg per hour. Frequently patients with drug intoxication are in shock or require forced diuresis for the purpose of drug elimination. This is usually translated into administration of as much as 500 mL of fluids per hour. Volume status is further complicated because mechanical ventilation and PEEP may compromise cardiovascular function.[96, 97] This occurs through several mechanisms, the most important of which are a decrease in venous return caused by increased intrathoracic pressure and increased pulmonary vascular resistance caused by overdistention and compression of alveolar vessels.

Regardless of the mechanism, a drop in cardiac output with PEEP, though accompanied by an increase in Pao_2, may result in the availability of less oxygen for cellular metabolism. Oxygen delivery (Do_2) is given by the product of cardiac output (CO) in liters times arterial oxygen content (Cao_2) in milliliters per deciliter of blood:

$$Do_2 = CO \times 10 \times Cao_2$$

where Cao_2 = hemoglobin × 1.34 × oxygen saturation. Oxygen delivery should be monitored as PEEP is increased. If no blood pressure and urinary output changes are observed with PEEP 5 to 8 cm H_2o, Pao_2 increases substantially, and Fio_2 can be decreased to 50% or less, nothing needs to be added.

In cases in which severe ARDS has developed and the lungs are stiff and inspiratory pressure is more than 40 cm H_2O, pressure-controlled (PC) ventilation may be used.[98] This mode of ventilation is recommended in pediatric patients. To improve oxygen tension and decrease Fio_2, inverse ratio ventilation (IRV) may be added to pressure-controlled ventilation (PC-IRV).

Pressure-controlled ventilation may limit peak inspiratory pressures, thus decreasing the prevalence of barotrauma while simultaneously improving oxygenation and CO_2 elimination.[98]

If blood pressure or urinary output drops, adequate Pao_2 at low Fio_2 is not achieved, the patient is in shock, or large volumes of fluids are being administered, a Swan-Ganz catheter should be inserted to monitor PCWP and cardiac output. With this information it is possible to assess the effect of PEEP on cardiac output. In addition, measurement of PCWP will give information about the patient's fluid status.

What should be the approach in the patient who has low cardiac output initially or in whom cardiac output drops with the use of PEEP? In patients with drug overdose, normal compensatory mechanisms to positive-pressure breathing may be impaired. In addition, some types of drugs produce hypovolemia as a result of massive volume loss into the lungs. Fluids should be given in a patient with low PCWP in a shock state undergoing mechanical ventilation with PEEP. Because most of these forms of ARDS associated with drug overdose are self-limited, an increase in PEEP to very high values is not recommended, even if that means FiO_2 is above 50% for 12 to 24 hours.

If blood pressure and cardiac output remain low, vasopressors such as dopamine, norepinephrine, and dobutamine may be used.

Once the objectives are achieved and the patient's lungs are well oxygenated at FiO_2 less than 50% and vital signs are otherwise stable, attention must be directed to weaning the patient from the ventilator. Meanwhile, acidosis and alkalosis should be corrected by improving perfusion and oxygenation or by adjusting minute ventilation. Intermittent mandatory ventilation with pressure support may be used as soon as the patient has spontaneous respirations, and the ventilation rate should be slowly decreased while arterial blood gas levels are monitored. Once the vital capacity is 10 mL/kg or more and the negative inspiratory force is less than 25 cm H_2O, the patient should be able to breathe spontaneously.

PEEP is then discontinued. It is our practice to ascend by increments of 2 to 3 cm H_2O and descend by the same amount, while monitoring the patient and observing respiratory parameters and blood gas levels. A sudden drop in PEEP may cause an abrupt drop in PaO_2.

After the patient has been weaned from the respirator and PEEP, extubation should follow, provided the patient is alert, has an effective cough, and is capable of swallowing.

Besides the cardiovascular complications of mechanical ventilation and PEEP, an increase in the incidence of barotrauma (pneumomediastinum, subcutaneous emphysema, and pneumothorax) has been noted in these patients.[99] A pneumothorax in a patient on receiving mechanical ventilation and PEEP necessitates immediate placement of a chest tube.

Only occasionally does a patient with drug overdose require a tracheostomy. Frequently, the endotracheal tube is needed for only a few days. It is safer to keep it in place for 2 weeks or longer than to proceed with a tracheostomy. The complications of prolonged endotracheal intubation are multiple and vary from oral pressure ulcers to laryngeal damage and subglottic or tracheal stenosis. The latter are the most serious. By keeping the endotracheal tube cuff pressure below 25 mm Hg, ensuring the tube is properly anchored, using swivel adaptors, and keeping the patient calm by means of sedatives, these risks can be minimized.

Aspiration Pneumonia

Aspiration pneumonia (Fig. 7–8) is another serious complication of drug overdose. Because of altered mental status and impairment of lung defense mechanisms, patients with overdose are at risk for aspiration with subsequent pulmonary infection. The cause of these pneumonias depends on the nature of the patient's mouth flora. Commonly, the oropharynx is colonized with aerobic organisms such as *Streptococcus pneumoniae* and *Staphylococcus aureus*. Aspiration of oral secretions outside the hospital or nursing home environment produces anaerobic (*Bacteroides, Fusobacterium,* and *Peptostreptococcus* spp.) or gram-positive pneumonia; therefore, penicillin, a second- or third-generation cephalosporin, erythromycin, and clindamycin (anaerobes) are the antibiotics of choice.[100] In hospitalized or institutionalized patients, changes develop in their mouth flora that result in a significant overgrowth of gram-negative organisms (*Klebsiella, Escherichia,* and *Enterobacteriaceae* spp.) in the oropharynx; thus, treatment must include antibiotics effective against these organisms.[101]

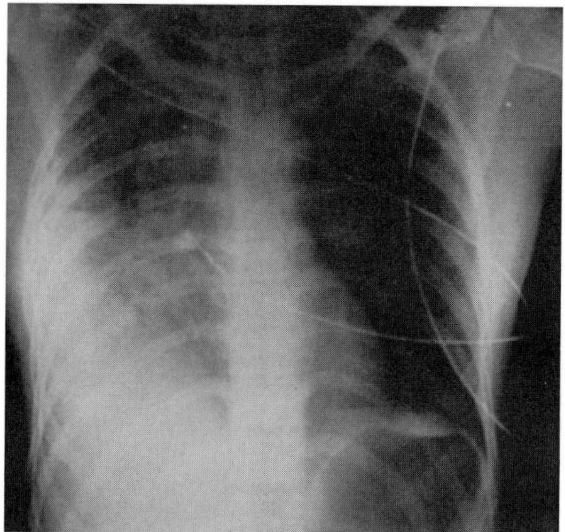

Figure 7–8. Barbiturate overdose and aspiration pneumonia involving the right lower lobe in a 15-year-old boy.

Aspirated bacteria, aerobic or anaerobic, may also cause lung abscesses and empyemas. Acute bronchial obstruction may be produced by solid particles in the tracheobronchial tree that cause atelectasis and infection. Finally, aspiration of gastric contents produces a chemical pneumonitis and respiratory failure with severe hypoxemia, requiring mechanical ventilation and PEEP. This form of aspiration pneumonia is common in the drug-intoxicated patient. It may occur spontaneously or during cardiopulmonary resuscitation resulting from gastric distention, emesis induction, attempts to pass a nasogastric tube, or endotracheal intubation. The pathologic findings of this condition are similar to those of ARDS except that bronchiolar damage is more severe and bronchiolitis obliterans often results.[102] Decreased lung compliance and hypoxemia ensue as a result of edema, alveolar instability, and alveolar collapse. Tachycardia, hypotension, wheezing, and severe respiratory failure also may develop.

Aspiration of food particles without acid causes a

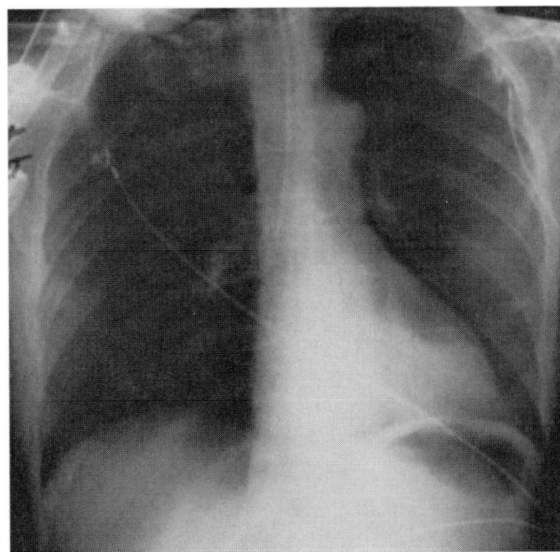

Figure 7–9. Multiple drug overdose in a 52-year-old man. The endotracheal tube tip is in the right main stem bronchus.

hemorrhagic pneumonia and a granulomatous reaction in the lung. Hypercapnia is seen more commonly with this condition than with aspiration of acid. Once the lung is damaged, it probably becomes more susceptible to infections. Unlike the situation of aspiration of oral secretions in nonhospitalized patients, in whom gram-positive organisms and anaerobes predominate, the aspiration of gastric contents produces a chemical pneumonitis. Infection commonly occurs late and may be caused by gram-negative organisms.

The treatment of aspiration pneumonia consists of administration of antibiotics, oxygen, and mechanical ventilation. For aspiration that occurs outside the hospital, the drugs of choice are a second-generation cephalosporin, clindamycin, and erythromycin, if *Legionella* infection is suspected. In those patients in whom colonization with gram-negative organisms is likely, options are a third-generation cephalosporin and an aminoglycoside, *or* a semisynthetic penicillin such as ticarcillin and an aminoglycoside. Once the organism is identified, antibiotic coverage can be changed to the most effective, least toxic, and least expensive drug.

In cases of aspiration of gastric contents, endotracheal suction may be helpful in removing secretions and aspirated material. When feasible, a size 8 endotracheal tube should be placed immediately. Bronchoscopy should be performed if there is a question of aspiration of large particulate matter.

Prophylactic antibiotics are frequently administered immediately after aspiration. In a review of 50 cases of gastric content aspiration, Bynum and Pierce[102] could not demonstrate any benefit from use of prophylactic antibiotics. Nosocomial pneumonia with gram-negative organisms usually occurred when improvement from the initial chemical pneumonitis was already evident. This was interpreted as representing infection; therefore, only after appropriate cultures have been obtained should presumptive antibiotic therapy be initiated. Antibiotics can be discontinued if cultures are negative.

The cornerstone of the treatment of gastric content aspiration is ventilatory support. Mechanical ventilation and PEEP not only keep the patient alive but do it without use of excessive concentrations of oxygen. Close monitoring of fluid balance, cardiac output, and PCWP is necessary, particularly if the patient requires high levels of PEEP. Even with optimal therapy, mortality from aspiration pneumonia ranges from 28% to 60%.

Other Complications

Besides pneumonia, other respiratory complications common in patients with drug overdose, particularly those with severe intoxication requiring endotracheal intubation and mechanical ventilation, include atelectasis, pneumothorax, pulmonary edema caused by fluid overload, and traumatic intubation causing vocal cord damage or tracheal stenosis.

Jay et al.[103] reviewed the respiratory complications

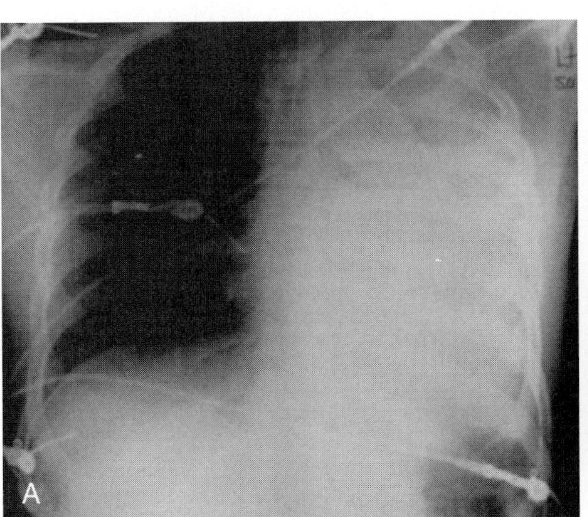

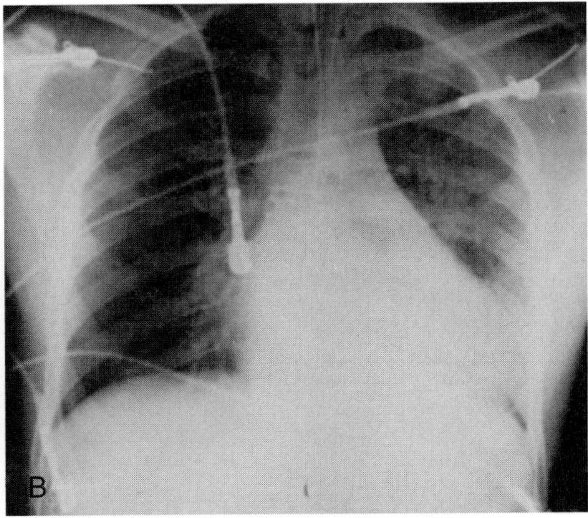

Figure 7–10. *A,* Complete atelectasis of the left lung secondary to intubation of the right main stem bronchus in a patient with barbiturate overdose. *B,* The endotracheal tube has been pulled up, and the left lung is now re-expanded.

in 195 patients with drug overdose admitted to a medical intensive care unit, in whom an endotracheal tube was placed in 77% (a high percentage). Traumatic intubation and right main stem bronchus intubation (Figs. 7–9 and 7–10) were documented in 10.7% of the patients. Aspiration was reported in 10.8%, and aspiration of gastric contents (24%) was observed only in patients with endotracheal tubes. Dislodgement or obstruction of the tube, post-extubation upper airways obstruction, and subglottic stenosis occurred in about 10% of all patients with endotracheal tubes. Three cases of pneumothorax were described. Nine patients died, eight of progressive respiratory insufficiency.

Of 131 patients with drug overdose admitted to our intensive care unit over a 3-year period (1977 to 1980), 33 (25%) required endotracheal intubation, and only 20 (15%) required mechanical ventilation. Of the 33 who required intubation, four had pulmonary edema. Six patients had pneumonia, seven had atelectasis, one had pneumothorax, two had intubation of the right main stem bronchus, and one had severe subglottic edema due to traumatic intubation. None had tracheal stenosis. Only four patients died: of paraquat, tricyclic antidepressant, cocaine, and salicylate overdose, respectively. As more progress is made in the respiratory care of patients with poisoning and drug overdose, it is anticipated the complications of intubation and mechanical ventilation will become less common than previously reported and have less effect on patient survival. Indeed, Henderson et al.[104] reported that although almost 80% of 732 patients with acute overdose admitted to an intensive care unit required mechanical ventilation, only 2% died.

References

1. Reynolds HY: Host defense impairments that may lead to respiratory infections. Clin Chest Med *8:*339, 1987.
2. Dripps RD, Comroe J: The immediate effect of morphine administered intravenously and intramuscularly upon the respiration of normal man. Anesthesiology *6:*462, 1945.
3. Weil JV, McCullough RE, Kline JS, et al: Diminished response to hypoxia and hypercapnia after morphine in normal man. N Engl J Med *292:*1103, 1975.
4. Silber R, Clerkin EP: Pulmonary edema in acute heroin poisoning. Am J Med *27:*187, 1959.
5. Louria DB, Hensle T, Rose J: The major medical complications of heroin addiction. Ann Intern Med *67:*1, 1967.
6. Sapira JD: The narcotic addict as a medical patient. Am J Med *45:*555, 1968.
7. Cherubin CE, Shapira JD: The medical complications of drug addiction and the medical assessment of the intravenous drug user: 25 years later. Ann Intern Med *119:*1017, 1993.
8. Spiritus EM, Wilson AF, Berke RA: Lung scans in asymptomatic heroin addicts. Am Rev Respir Dis *108:*994, 1973.
9. Overland ES, Nolan AJ, Hopewell PC: Alteration of pulmonary function in intravenous drug abusers. Am J Med *68:* 231, 1980.
10. Steinberg AD, Karliner J: The clinical spectrum of heroin pulmonary edema. Arch Intern Med *122:*122, 1968.
11. Morrison WJ, Wetherill S, Zyroff J: The acute pulmonary edema of heroin intoxication. Radiology *97:*347, 1970.
12. Joseph WL, Fletcher HS, Giordano JM, et al: Pulmonary and cardiovascular implications of drug addiction. Ann Thorac Surg *15:*263, 1973.
13. Duberstein JL, Kaufman DM: A clinical study of an epidemic of heroin-induced pulmonary edema. Am J Med *51:*704, 1971.
14. Fran UI, Shim CS, Williams MH: Heroin-induced pulmonary edema. Ann Intern Med *77:*29, 1972.
15. Katz S, Aberman A, Frand UI, et al: Heroin pulmonary edema: Evidence for increased capillary permeability. Am Rev Respir Dis *106:*472, 1972.
16. Jerome EH, Sveringhaus JW: High altitude pulmonary edema. N Engl J Med *334:*662, 1996.
17. Van der Zee H, Malik AB, Lee BC, et al: Lung fluid and protein exchange during intracranial hypertension and role of sympathetic mechanisms. J Appl Physiol *49:*73, 1980.
18. Shubin H, Weil MH: The mechanism of shock following suicidal doses of barbiturates, narcotics and tranquilizer drugs with observations on the effect of treatment. Am J Med *38:*853, 1965.
19. Goodman JM, Bischel MD, Wagers PW, et al: Barbiturate intoxication: Morbidity and mortality. West J Med *124:*179, 1976.
20. Reves JG, Fragen RJ, Vinik HR, et al: Midazolam: Pharmacology and uses. Anesthesiology *62:*310, 1985.
21. Model DG: Nitrazepam-induced respiratory depression in chronic obstructive lung disease. Br J Dis Chest *67:*128, 1973.
22. Catchlove RFH, Kafer ER: The effect of diazepam on the ventilatory response to carbon dioxide and on steady state gas exchange. Anesthesiology *39:*9, 1971.
23. Forster A, Gardaz JP, Suter PM, et al: Respiratory depression by midazolam and diazepam. Anesthesiology *53:*494, 1980.
24. Leiter JC, Knuth SL, Krol RC, et al: The effect of diazepam on genioglossal muscle activity in normal subjects. Am Rev Respir Dis *132:*136, 1985.
25. Gillis RA, Namath IJ, Easington C, et al: Drug interaction with gamma-aminobutyric acid/benzodiazepine receptors at the ventral surface of the medulla results in pronounced changes in cardiorespiratory activity. J Pharmacol Exp Ther *248:*863, 1989.
26. Hajer J, Baehrendtz S, Matell G, et al: Diagnostic utility of flumazenil in coma with suspected poisoning: A double blind, randomized controlled study. BMJ *301:*1308, 1990.
27. Spivey WH, Roberts JR, Derlet RW: A clinical trial of escalating doses of flumazenil for reversal of suspected benzodiazepine overdose in the emergency department. Ann Emerg Med *22:*1813, 1993.
28. Glauser FL, Smith WR, Caldwell A, et al: Ethchlorvynol (placidyl)–induced pulmonary edema. Ann Intern Med *84:* 46, 1976.
29. Benowitz NL, Rosenberg J, Becker CE: Cardiopulmonary catastrophes in drug-overdosed patients. Med Clin North Am *63:*267, 1979.
30. Axelson JP, Hagaman JF: Meprobamate poisoning and pulmonary edema. N Engl J Med *296:*1481, 1977.
31. Lin JL, Lim PS, Lai BC, et al: Continuous arteriovenous hemoperfusion in meprobamate poisoning. J Toxicol Clin Toxicol *31:*645, 1993.
32. Woldorf NM, Pastore PN: Extreme epinephrine sensitivity with a general anesthesia. Arch Otolaryngol *96:*272, 1972.
33. Franks CR, Hudson PM, Rees AJ, et al: Accidental intravenous halothane. Guy Hosp Rep *123:*89, 1974.
34. Spencer JD, Raasch FO, Trefny FA: Halothane abuse in hospital personnel. JAMA *235:*1034, 1976.
35. Granville-Grossman KL, Sergeant HGS: Pulmonary edema due to salicylate intoxication. Lancet *1:*575, 1960.
36. Hill JB: Salicylate intoxication. N Engl J Med *288:*1110, 1973.
37. Bowers RE, Brigham KL, Owen PJ: Salicylate pulmonary edema: The mechanism in sheep and review of the clinical literature. Am Rev Respir Dis *115:*261, 1977.
38. Hormaechea E, Carlson RW, Rogove H, et al: Hypovolemia, pulmonary edema and protein changes in severe salicylate poisoning. Am J Med *66:*1046, 1979.
39. Hernicek G, Skelton J, Miller WC: Pulmonary edema and salicylate overdose. JAMA *230:*866, 1974.

40. Bogartz LJ, Miller WC: Pulmonary edema associated with propoxyphene intoxication. JAMA *215*:259, 1971.
41. Haddad LM: Managing tricyclic antidepressant overdose. Am Fam Physician *46*:153, 1992.
42. Roy TM, Ossorio MA, Cipolla LM, et al: Pulmonary complications after tricyclic antidepressant overdose. Chest *96*:852, 1989.
43. Shannon M, Lovejoy FH: Pulmonary consequences of severe tricyclic antidepressant ingestion. Clin Toxicol *25*:443, 1987.
44. Marshall A, Moore K: Pulmonary disease after amitriptyline overdose. BMJ *1*:176, 1973.
45. Lindstrom FD, Floodmark O, Gustafsson B: Respiratory distress syndrome and thrombotic, non-bacterial endocarditis after amitriptyline overdose. Acta Med Scand *202*:203, 1977.
46. Flaherty JJ, Ceva D, Graff J: ARDS associated with massive imipramine overdose. Am J Emerg Med *202*:203, 1977.
47. Isner JM, Estes M, Thompson PD, et al: Acute cardiac events temporally related to cocaine abuse. N Engl J Med *315*:1438, 1986.
48. Wojak JC, Flamm ES: Intracranial hemorrhage and cocaine use. Stroke *18*:712, 1987.
49. Allred RJ, Ewer S: Fatal pulmonary edema following intravenous "freebase" cocaine use. Ann Emerg Med *10*:441, 1981.
50. Ettinger NA, Albin RJ: A review of respiratory effects of smoking cocaine. Am J Med *87*:664, 1989.
51. Albertson TE, Walby WF, Derlet RW: Stimulant-induced pulmonary toxicity. Chest *108*:1140, 1995.
52. Forrester JM, Steele AW, Waldron JA, et al: Crack lung: An acute pulmonary syndrome with a spectrum of clinical and histopathologic findings. Am Rev Respir Dis *142*:462, 1990.
53. Wiener MD, Putnam CE: Pain in the chest in a user of cocaine. JAMA *258*:2087, 1987.
54. Glassroth J, Adams GD, Schnoll S: The impact of substance abuse on the respiratory system. Chest *91*:596, 1987.
55. Patel RC, Dutta D, Schonfeld SA: Free-base cocaine use associated with bronchiolitis obliterans organizing pneumonia. Ann Intern Med *107*:186, 1987.
56. Chamberlin WH, Stockman GD, Wray NP: Shock and noncardiogenic pulmonary edema following meglumine diatrizoate for intravenous pyelography. Am J Med *67*:684, 1979.
57. Smith P, Heath D: Paraquat lung: A reappraisal. Thorax *29*:643, 1974.
58. Levin PH, Kaff LJ, Rose AG, et al: Pulmonary effects of contact exposure to paraquat: A clinical and experimental study. Thorax *34*:150, 1979.
59. Papiris SA, Maniati MA, Kyriakidis V, et al: Pulmonary damage due to paraquat poisoning through skin absorption. Respiration *62*:103, 1995.
60. Chen KW, Wu MH, Huang JJ, et al: Bilateral spontaneous pneumothoraces and subcutaneous emphysema: A rare presentation of paraquat intoxication. Ann Emerg Med *23*:1132, 1994.
61. Im JF, Lee KS, Han MC, et al: Paraquat poisoning: Findings in chest radiography and CT in 42 patients. AJR *157*:697, 1991.
62. Hollinger MA, Patwell SW, Zuckerman JE, et al: Effect of paraquat on serum angiotensin–converting enzyme. Am Rev Respir Dis *121*:795, 1980.
63. Fisher HK, Clements JA, Wright RR: Enhancement of oxygen toxicity by the herbicide paraquat. Am Rev Respir Dis *107*:246, 1973.
64. Lheureux P, Ledric D, Vanbinst R, et al: Survival in a case of massive paraquat ingestion. Chest *107*:285, 1995.
65. Wyckoff DW, Davies JE, Barquet A, et al: Diagnostic and therapeutic problems of parathion poisonings. Ann Intern Med *68*:875, 1968.
66. Kass R, Kochar G, Lippman M: Adult respiratory distress syndrome from organophosphate poisoning. Am J Emerg Med *9*:32, 1991.
67. Tsao TC, Juang YC, Lan RS, et al: Respiratory failure of acute organophosphate and carbamate poisoning. Chest *98*:631, 1990.
68. Ricket DL: Differentiation of peripheral and central actions of soman-produced respiratory arrest. Research News Letter of the US Army Medical Research and Development Command, April 1983, p 7.
69. Gillis RA, Walton DP, Quest JA, et al: Cardiorespiratory effects produced by activation of cholinergic muscarinic receptors on the ventral surface of the medulla. J Pharmacol Exp Ther *247*:765, 1988.
70. Kass R, Kochar G, Lippman M: Adult respiratory distress syndrome from organophosphate poisoning. Am J Emerg Med *9*:32, 1991.
71. Goswamy R, Chandhuri A, Mahashur AA: Study of respiratory failure in organophosphate and carbonate poisoning. Heart Lung *23*:466, 1994.
72. Eade NR, Taussig LM, Marks MI: Hydrocarbon pneumonitis. Pediatrics *54*:351, 1974.
73. Neeld EM, Limacher MC: Chemical pneumonitis after intravenous injection of hydrocarbon. Radiology *129*:36, 1978.
74. Llano AL, Raffin TA: Management of carbon monoxide poisoning. Chest *97*:165, 1990.
75. Wald PH, Balmes JR: Respiratory effects of short term high-intensity toxic inhalations: Smoke, gases and fumes. J Intensive Care Med *2*:260, 1987.
76. Murray MJ, Kronenberg R: Pulmonary reactions simulating cardiac pulmonary edema caused by nitrofurantoin. N Engl J Med *273*:1185, 1965.
77. Steinberg AD: Pulmonary edema following ingestion of hydrochlorothiazide. JAMA *204*:167, 1968.
78. Hill RN, Spragg RC, Wedel MK, et al: Adult respiratory distress syndrome associated with colchicine intoxication. Ann Intern Med *83*:523, 1975.
79. Hayler AM, Holt DW, Volans GN: Fatal overdosage with disopyramide. Lancet *1*:968, 1978.
80. Baruh S, Sherman L: Hypoglycemia, a cause of pulmonary edema. J Natl Med Assoc *67*:200, 1975.
81. Rosenow EC III, Myers JL, Swensen SY, et al: Drug-induced pulmonary diseases. Chest *102*:239, 1992.
82. Seidal K, Jorgensen N, Elinder CG, et al: Fatal cadmium-induced pneumonitis. Scand J Work Environ Health *19*:429, 1993.
83. Moromisato DY, Anas NG, Goodman G: Mercury inhalation poisoning and acute lung injury in a child: Use of high-frequency oscillatory ventilation. Chest *105*:613, 1994.
84. Cheny K, Gumbiner C, Benson B, et al: Survival after severe iron poisoning treated with intermittent infusions of desferoxamine. J Toxicol Clin Toxicol *33*:61, 1995.
85. Hee MKJ, Plevak DJ, Peters SJ: Intubation of critically ill patients. Mayo Clin Proc *67*:669, 1992.
86. Einarsson O, Rochester CL, Rosenbaum S: Airway management in respiratory emergencies. Clin Chest Med *15*:13, 1996.
87. Shapiro BA, Warren J, Egol AB, et al: Practice parameters for intravenous analgesia for adult patients in the intensive care unit: An executive summary. Crit Care Med *23*:1596, 1995.
88. Shapiro BA, Warren J, Egol AB, et al: Practice parameters for sustained neuromuscular blockade in the adult critically ill patient: An executive summary. Crit Care Med *23*:1601, 1995.
89. Bernard GR, Artigas A, Brigham KL, et al: The American-European Consensus Conference on ARDS: Definitions, mechanisms, relevant outcomes, and clinical trial coordination. Am J Respir Crit Care Med *149*:818, 1994.
90. Kolleff MH, Shuster DP: The acute respiratory distress syndrome. N Engl J Med *332*:27, 1995.
91. Taylor AE, Parker JC: Pulmonary interstitial spaces and lymphatics. *In* Fishman AP (ed): Handbook of Physiology: The Respiratory System. Bethesda, MD, Am Physiological Society, 1985, pp 167–230.
92. Staub NC: Pulmonary edema: Physiological approaches to management. Chest *74*:559, 1978.
93. Pontoppidan H, Wilson RS, Rie MA, et al: Respiratory intensive care. Anesthesiology *47*:96, 1977.
94. Dantzker DR, Brook CJ, Dehart P, et al: Ventilation-perfusion distributions in the adult respiratory distress syndrome. Am Rev Respir Dis *120*:1039, 1979.
95. Sladen A, Laver MB, Pontoppidan H: Pulmonary complications and water retention in prolonged mechanical ventilation. N Engl J Med *279*:448, 1968.

96. Falke KJ, Pontoppidan H, Kumar A, et al: Ventilation with end-expiratory pressure in acute lung disease. J Clin Invest *51:*2315, 1972.
97. Broaddus VC, Berthiaume Y, Biondi JW, et al: Hemodynamic management of the adult respiratory distress syndrome. J Intensive Care Med *2:*190, 1987.
98. Tharratt RS, Allen RP, Albertson TE: Pressure controlled inverse ratio ventilation in severe adult respiratory distress syndrome. Chest *94:*755, 1988.
99. Cullen DJ, Caldera DL: The incidence of ventilator-induced pulmonary barotrauma in critically ill patients. Anesthesiology *50:*185, 1979.
100. Finegold SM: Aspiration pneumonia. Rev Infect Dis *13:* S737, 1991.
101. LaForce FM: Hospital-acquired gram-negative rod pneumonias: An overview. Am J Med *70:*664, 1981.
102. Bynum LJ, Pierce AK: Pulmonary aspiration of gastric contents. Am Rev Respir Dis *114:*1129, 1976.
103. Jay SJ, Johanson WG, Pierce AK: Respiratory complications of overdose with sedative drugs. Am Rev Respir Dis *112:*591, 1975.
104. Henderson A, Wright M, Pon SM: Experience with 732 acute overdose patients admitted to an intensive care unit over years. Med J Aust *158:*28, 1993.

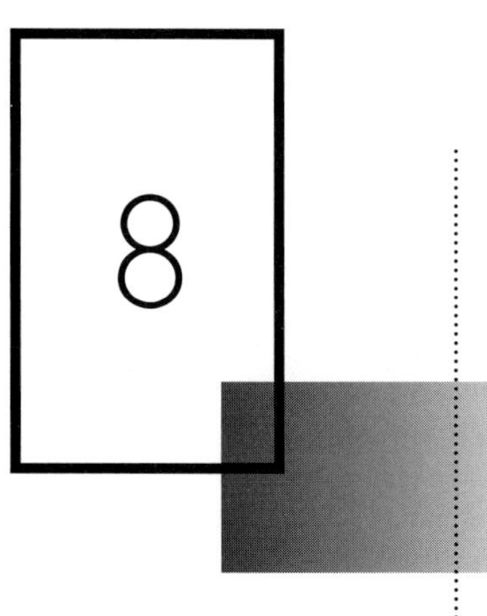

Clinical Neurotoxicology

KEITH K. BURKHART, MD
JAWAID AKHTAR, MD

A wide variety of neurologic syndromes result from toxic exposures. Some neurotoxins produce specific and characteristic syndromes, whereas others may produce conditions that are insidious or diagnosed as other common illnesses. Many toxins share common mechanisms and therefore manifest similar toxicities. This chapter provides a general review of neurotoxicology based on the physiologic actions of drugs and neurotoxins. It begins with a brief review of synaptic neurotransmission because many toxins disrupt steps in this multifaceted process (Table 8–1). Each neurotransmitter system is then individually reviewed, and the toxins that disrupt its action and the syndromes that result are highlighted. Finally, a review of toxin-induced neuropathies is presented.

SYNAPTIC NEUROTRANSMISSION

Neurons are specialized cells involved with communication and information processing[1] (Fig. 8–1). The main structural features of nerve terminals are synaptic vesicles, mitochondria, elements of the smooth endoplasmic reticulum, cytoskeletal structures, and the plasma membrane that surrounds the axon and is separated from the plasma membrane of the postsynaptic neuron by a thin cleft. Neuronal communication occurs through the exocytotic release of neurotransmitters, for which specific receptors exist on neighboring neurons (Table 8–2).

Neurotransmitters are stored in synaptic vesicles. Synaptic vesicles tend to cluster at discrete regions underneath the presynaptic plasma membrane, and each cluster behaves as an anatomic and functional unit composed of equivalent elements of neurotransmitters. Presynaptic plasma membrane shows areas of structural specialization at areas of synaptic clustering, and it is at these "active zones" that exocytosis of classic neurotransmitters occur. The neurotransmitter, on release into the synaptic cleft, recognizes and binds to postsynaptic receptors. Synaptic vesicles, after exocytosis, are recycled and used in subsequent secretory cycles (see Table 8–2).

Calcium ions are necessary for transmission at synaptic junctions and have a dual role in neuronal secretion. Calcium influx following the action poten-

Table 8–1. Cellular Targets and Potentially Neurotoxic Agents

Adrenergic receptors	Clonidine and imidazolines, sympathomimetics, sympatholytics, ergot alkaloids, antipsychotic agents (chlorpromazine, haloperidol), yohimbine
Cannabinoid receptor	Cannabinoid (marijuana, hashish)
Cholinesterase	Organophosphates, carbamates, nerve gas agents, physostigmine
Dopamine receptors	Apomorphine, bromocriptine, antipsychotic drugs
GABA receptors	Benzodiazepine, cyclopyrrolones (zopiclone), imidazopyridines (zolpidem), barbiturates, ethanol, penicillin, muscimol (*Amanita muscaria*), bicuculline, neuroactive steroids (alphaxalone), flumazenil, baclofen
Glycine receptors	Strychnine, brucine
Histamine receptors	Antihistamines, TCAs
Membrane lipid	General anesthetic drugs, e.g., halothane
MAO	MAO inhibitors (iproniazid, phenelzine, isocarboxazid)
Muscarinic receptors	Curare, *A. muscaria, Atropa belladonna*
Nicotinic receptors	Nicotine, neuromuscular blocking drugs, α-bungarotoxin
NMDA receptor	Arylcyclohexylamine (phenycyclidine, ketamine), ethanol, domoic acid
Norepinephrine reuptake	TCAs, reserpine, amphetamine, cocaine
Opioid receptors	Opioid agonists (heroin, morphine, opium, meperidine, methadone) and antagonists (naloxone, naltrexone)
Potassium channel	Barium, 4-aminopyridine, tetraethylammonium ion, cesium, polypeptide toxins from scorpion (charybdotoxin), bee (apamin), snake (dendrotoxin)
Purine receptors	Adenosine, caffeine, theophylline
Serotonin receptor	Atypical neuroleptics, buspirone, ondansetron, granisetron, LSD, mescaline, psilocybin, cyproheptadine, methysergide
Serotonin reuptake	TCAs, selective serotonin reuptake inhibitors, nefazodone, venlafaxine
Sodium channel	Local anesthetics, TCAs, tetrodotoxin (puffer fish), saxitoxin (paralytic shellfish), frog-skin poison (batrachotoxin), aconitine, veratridine, scorpion and anemone toxins

GABA, γ-aminobutyric acid; MAO, monoamine oxidase; TCA, tricyclic antidepressants; NDMA, *N*-methyl-D-aspartate; LSD, lysergic acid diethylamide.

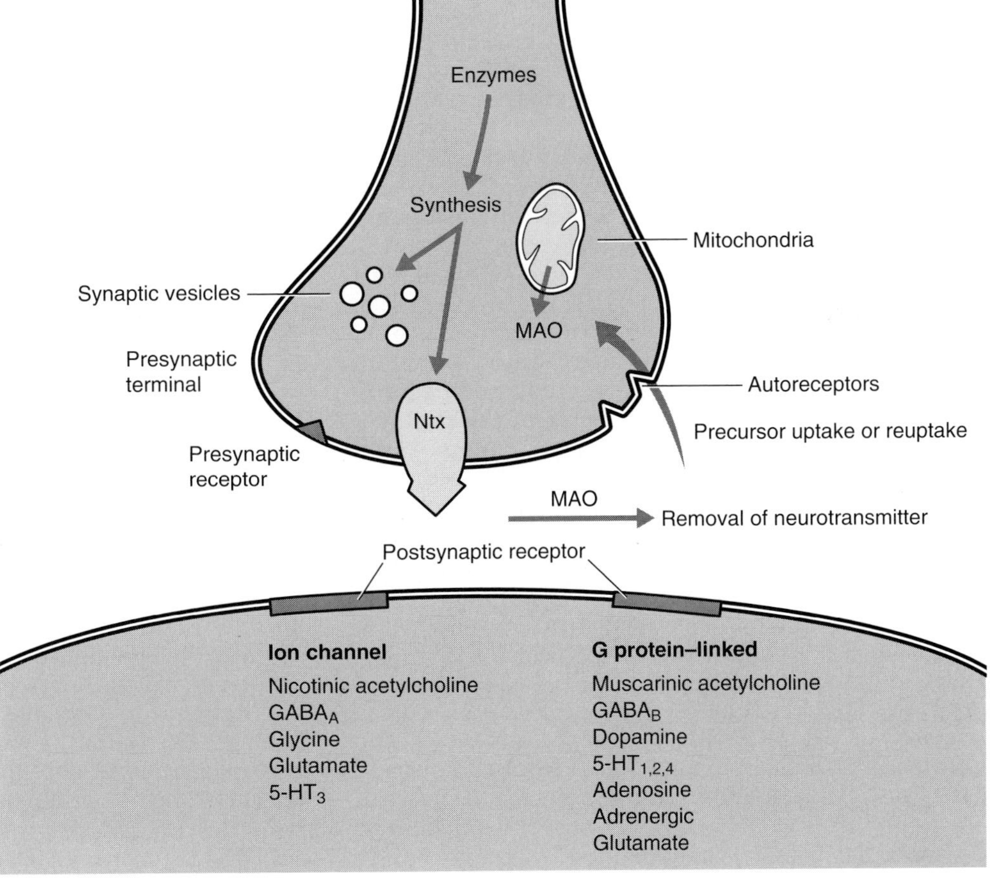

Figure 8–1. A schematic representation of a synapse showing the principal structures and sites of drug action. This synapse is a hybrid for the purpose of visualization; as outlined in the text, a neuron is typically highly specialized for a specific neurotransmitter system. MAO, monoamine oxidase; Ntx, neurotransmitter; GABA, γ-aminobutyric acid; 5-HT, 5-hydroxytryptamine.

Table 8–2. Synaptic Neurotransmitters

Biogenic Amines	*Amino Acids*
Catecholamines	Excitatory
Epinephrine	Glutamate
Norepinephrine	Aspartate
Dopamine	
Indolamines	Inhibitory
Serotonin	γ-Aminobutyric acid
Histamine	Glycine
Ester	*Peptides*
Acetylcholine	Enkephalins
Purines	
Adenosine	

tial triggers synaptic vesicle exocytosis and regulates the amount of vesicles released. The action potential, caused by a depolarizing stimulus, begins with a transient, voltage-gated opening of sodium channels that allows sodium to enter the fiber and depolarize the membrane fully. This is followed by a transient voltage-gated opening of potassium channels that allows potassium to leave and repolarize the membrane.

Receptors are structures that have the ability to recognize a drug, hormone, or neurotransmitter. The activity of these substances is mediated through interaction with these receptors. The receptors include ligand-gated ion channels that are coupled to ion flow, G protein–coupled receptors, growth factors with tyrosine kinase activity that cause tyrosine phosphorylation, and steroid receptors that transport steroids into the nucleus.

Ligand-gated ion channels mediate fast excitatory and inhibitory synaptic neurotransmission in the central nervous system (CNS). The family of ligand-gated ion channels now comprises nicotinic acetylcholine receptors, γ-aminobutyric acid (GABA) type A receptors, glycine receptors, the serotonin 5-HT_3 receptors, and the structurally distinct glutamate receptor channels. Activation of ligand-gated ion channels results in a conformational change and opening of a pore (ionopore) in the membrane of the postsynaptic cells. This allows the passage of ions, to which the membrane was previously impermeable. The prototypic member of this receptor family is the nicotinic cholinergic receptor. Ionopores for other ions such as chloride ions are associated with inhibitory transmission in the CNS.

The G protein family of receptors (so named because it binds guanosine triphosphate [GTP]) are not linked to ionopores but to enzymes that are located within the membrane of the postsynaptic cell.[2] These enzymes act as transducers for the action of the neurotransmitter (first messenger) from the outside of the cell to the inside and produce second messengers. G protein receptors are able to regulate the rate of second messenger production and degradation via control of the activity of a number of effector enzymes. These include isoenzymes of adenylate cyclase, phospholipase C, and cyclic guanosine monophosphate (cGMP) phosphodiesterase families. G protein–linked receptors also regulate ionic flux through ion channels by either direct G protein regulation or via second messenger–mediated phosphorylation events.

Binding of GTP to a G protein changes the activity of adenylate cyclase. Increased formation of cyclic adenosine monophosphate (cAMP) activates specific protein kinases by phosphorylation, and these in turn phosphorylate other proteins. At some receptors, however, stimulation of the receptors causes inhibition of adenylate cyclase and a decrease in intracellular cAMP. Some receptors are linked to the enzyme guanylate cyclase, which converts guanosine triphosphate to cGMP, which in turn acts as a second messenger in a manner analogous to that of cAMP. Phosphorylation of the membrane proteins cAMP and cGMP results in changes in membrane permeability to specific ions and in others to activation of further enzyme systems, which then mediate the biologic response. Termination of the signal involves hydrolysis of cAMP and cGMP by phosphodiesterase enzymes. Response of the postsynaptic cell can thus be influenced by drugs acting on the enzymes involved (i.e., adenylate cyclase, guanylate cyclase, and phosphodiesterase). Phosphatidylinositol breakdown stimulated by phospholipase C, located in cell membranes, represents another type of second messenger system. The breakdown of phosphatidylinositol 4,5-biphosphate leads to the release of inositol triphosphate and diacylglycerol. Diacylglycerol is an activator of kinase C, whereas inositol triphosphate in turn stimulates other intracellular messengers such as calcium or calmodulin. Lithium exerts its therapeutic actions by damping or altering the cellular responses to those neurotransmitters whose actions are mediated by phosphatidylinositol turnover.

THE NEUROTRANSMITTER SYSTEM AND NEUROTOXICITY

The neurotransmitter system has many components, and toxins may interact with, augment, or disrupt any step in neurotransmission. A toxin can thus disrupt ionic channels, block or stimulate a postsynaptic receptor, block or be taken up by a presynaptic reuptake system, or block degradation enzyme systems. Many of these substances are used as pharmaceutical agents in clinical practice, and some are naturally occurring biologic toxins or man-made chemicals. The details of the processes involved in synaptic transmission vary from one transmitter to another and are discussed as the individual neurotransmitter system is reviewed.

A drug that produces a response and mimics the effect of an endogenous regulatory compound is known as an *agonist*. *Antagonists* bind to the receptor site with *zero* intrinsic regulatory activity to initiate a response and therefore cause inhibition of the agonist. Some antagonists do not display an intrinsic activity *of zero* and in certain situations display inverse agonism, a phenomenon also described as *negative efficacy* or *negative intrinsic activity.*

The Purinergic System

Adenosine and adenosine triphosphate (ATP) are purines that are released from neurons and other cells and produce widespread effects on many organ systems by binding to cell-surface purinergic receptors. ATP also is released from non-neuronal sources including platelets, mast cells, and possibly endothelial cells. Receptors for both ATP and adenosine are widely distributed in the nervous system and in other tissues such as the heart, intestine, and bladder. Receptors that bind adenosine or ATP are designated P_1 and P_2 purinergic receptors, respectively.[3] Adenosine and some adenosine analogues activate adenosine receptors but not ATP receptors, and some ATP analogues activate ATP receptors but not adenosine receptors.

A_1 adenosine receptors are widely distributed in the CNS. Central A_1 receptor activity includes sedation, analgesia, neuroprotection, and anticonvulsant activity. Adenosine potentiates the antinociceptive action of norepinephrine in the spinal cord. Many of the central effects of adenosine are attributed to the modulation of neurotransmitter release in the CNS. Opiates have been shown to induce the release of adenosine, and some effects of opiates are blocked by adenosine receptor antagonists. In the periphery, adenosine A_1 receptors are found in the heart, where they produce negative inotropic, chronotropic, and dromotropic responses. In adipose tissue, they inhibit lipolysis and enhance insulin-stimulated glucose transport. In the kidneys, they reduce glomerular filtration pressure and produce antidiuresis. A_1 receptors produce their effect by inhibiting adenylate cyclase, by increasing potassium channel and decreasing calcium channel conductance, and by increasing or decreasing phospholipase activity. The A_2 receptors are further classified into A_{2a} and A_{2b} subtypes, depending on their affinity for adenosine. A_2 receptors present on sensory nerves in the carotid body, aortic body, and pulmonary circulation, and elsewhere produce excitatory sensory input. A_{2a} receptor activation in the vascular bed is classically associated with vasodilation and hypotension. These effects are mediated in part by the elevation of intracellular cAMP and by activation of ATP-dependent potassium channels. Activation of the A_{2a} receptor on platelet membranes elevates intracellular cAMP levels, resulting in inhibition of platelet aggregation. The A_3 receptors are found throughout the brain and are heavily expressed in the pineal body, lungs, and spleen. It is not known what central effects are mediated by A_3 receptors.

Adenosine decreases neurotransmitter release from terminals (presynaptic effect) and binds to adenosine receptors. It is an effective antiepileptic agent in experimental animals. Carbamazepine interacts with the adenosine system, causing enhanced inhibition and reducing epileptogenesis.[4] Caffeine, theophylline, and theobromine are three important alkaloids derived from xanthine. Methylxanthines selectively block adenosine and act as competitive antagonists at adenosine receptors. These agents interfere with the uptake and storage of calcium by the sarcoplasmic reticulum in striated muscle and increase cAMP levels by inhibiting phosphodiesterase. Methylxanthines may cause seizures, and patients with chronic intoxication are more prone to seizures than those with an acute overdose. Seizures may occur without other evidence of toxicity and have a reported mortality of up to 50%. The reason for this high mortality results from A_1 antagonism and consequent inability of self-termination of seizure activity.[5] $GABA_A$ receptor agonism, especially by barbiturates, is most effective in preventing and stopping methylxanthine-induced seizures. Intravenous adenosine may attenuate theophylline-induced seizures by receptor antagonism or from nonspecific adenosine actions.[6] Phenytoin remains ineffective in treating theophylline-induced seizures and may increase mortality.[7]

ATP receptors have a wide tissue distribution. In the autonomic nervous system, ATP is released as a cotransmitter from both sympathetic and parasympathetic neurons. ATP that is released is rapidly broken down by widely distributed 5′-nucleotidases; this results in the formation of adenosine. ATP has a biphasic or inhibitory effect due to its breakdown to adenosine. The physiologic and pharmacologic actions of ATP are mediated through activation of P_2 purinergic receptors, of which at least five subtypes (P_{2u}, P_{2t}, P_{2x}, P_{2y}, and P_{2z} purinergic receptors) have been identified. The receptors are classified largely on the basis of the relative agonist potencies of ATP and a number of structural analogues. The role of these receptors in neurotoxicity is yet to be defined.

The Catecholaminergic System

Three distinct catecholamines—dopamine, norepinephrine, and epinephrine—are involved in neurotransmission. *Norepinephrine* is the predominant catecholamine in peripheral tissue and sympathetic nerves. *Epinephrine*, formed by *N*-methylation of norepinephrine, is released from the adrenal glands and stimulates catecholamine receptors in various organs. Small amounts of epinephrine are also found in the CNS, particularly in the brain stem.[8] A few sympathetic fibers release acetylcholine. *Dopamine*, the precursor of norepinephrine, also has biologic activity in the periphery, especially in the kidneys.

The amino acid L-tyrosine is hyroxylated to dihydroxy-L-phenylalanine (L-dopa) by tyrosine hydroxylase, a mixed-function oxidase located in the cytoplasm and on cell membranes. Tyrosine hydroxylase also hydroxylates phenylalanine to form tyrosine, which is then converted to L-dopa. Dopa decarboxylase, a pyridoxine-dependent enzyme, catalyzes the removal of the carboxyl group from dopa to form dopamine. In neurons that synthesize epinephrine or norepinephrine, dopamine diffuses into synaptic vesicles, where the enzyme dopamine-β-hydroxylase hydroxylates dopamine, forming norepinephrine. In chromaffin cells that synthesize epinephrine, the final step in the pathway is catalyzed by the enzyme phenylethanolamine *N*-methyltransferase. Catecholamines are concentrated in the synaptic vesicles and are also found free in the cytoplasmic fluid. The action of catecholamines released at the synapse is terminated by reuptake. The excess catecholamine is repackaged in storage vesicles or degraded by mitochondrial monoamine oxidase (MAO). These isoenzymes are integral flavoproteins on outer mitochondrial membranes. The MAO enzymes exist in two forms, A and B. MAO-A preferentially deaminates norepinephrine and serotonin and is selectively inhibited by clorgyline or moclobemide, whereas MAO-B acts on dopamine and is selectively inhibited by deprenyl. Catechol-*O*-methytransferase acts on extraneuronal catecholamine and is responsible for inactivation of catecholamine that is not effectively removed from the synaptic cleft.

The effects of catecholamines are mediated by cell-surface receptors.[9] Adrenergic neurons belong to the large family of G protein–coupled receptors. These adrenergic receptors are subdivided into α and β subunits. α-*Adrenergic receptors* have the following order of potency: epinephrine ≥ norepinephrine >> isoproterenol. β-*Adrenergic receptors* have the following order of potency: isoproterenol > epinephrine ≥norepinephrine. The α-adrenergic receptors are responsible for the excitatory actions of norepinephrine and mediate the contraction of some smooth muscles, particularly vascular smooth muscles, resulting in vasoconstriction, while relaxing other smooth muscle cells (e.g., intestine). β-Adrenergic receptors mediate the action of norepinephrine in stimulating contractions of heart muscles and relaxing smooth muscles in the bronchioles and the uterus, as well as cause vasodilation. In addition to postsynaptic adrenergic receptors, presynaptic α-adrenergic and β-adrenergic receptors called α_2 and β_2 are also present. The presynaptic α_2-adrenergic receptors control the rate of norepinephrine release; α_2-adrenergic stimulation decreases norepinephrine release.

Five subtypes of the dopamine receptor have been identified. The D_1 and D_5 receptors are coupled to stimulation of adenylate cyclase. D_2 receptors have an opposing effect on adenylate cyclase. Biochemical second messengers have not yet been identified for the D_3 and D_4 receptors. In the brain, the principal functions mediated by dopamine are the control of movements of behavior, including motivation, cognitive function, and emotion. In the pituitary gland, dopamine controls the release of prolactin and α-melanocyte–stimulating hormone. In the cardiovascular system, it is important in the regulation of blood pressure. Dopamine receptors have therefore been identified functionally in tissues related to these effects (e.g., pituitary gland and certain blood vessels). The largest concentrations of dopamine receptors, however, are in the basal ganglia and the limbic system.

Tyrosine analogues such as metyrosine (α-methyl-*p*-tyrosine) impair the synthesis of dopamine and norepinephrine by blocking the enzyme tyrosine hydroxylase. Reserpine and tetrabenazine inhibit the uptake of dopamine and other catecholamines into vesicles, causing depletion of endogenous neuronal catecholamines. α-Methyldopa causes dopamine depletion by replacement of dopamine with a relatively inactive false transmitter, α-methyldopamine; this causes hypotension and sedation. Other false neurotransmitters include metaraminol and octopamine. Peripheral presynaptic antiadrenergic drugs such as guanethidine and bretylium inhibit norepinephrine release from the presynaptic terminal by depleting the nerve endings of noradrenaline. The neurotoxin 6-hydroxydopamine is taken up by an active uptake mechanism and accumulates in catecholamine-containing neurons, destroying them through the auto-oxidative liberation of hydrogen peroxide or from formation of a quinone. Indirect-acting agents do not bind to adrenergic receptors but cause norepinephrine release from presynaptic terminals. These drugs enter the presynaptic terminals and displace stores of norepinephrine from storage vesicles (e.g., amphetamine and tyramine) or inhibit reuptake of catecholamine already released (e.g., cocaine and tricyclic antidepressants) (Table 8–3). Indirect agents exhibit tachyphylaxis—that is, their effects diminish on repeated administration as the catecholamine pools become depleted. Tricyclic antidepressants affect the catecholamines and serotonin, as well as dopamine reuptake to a lesser degree. Amphetamine also can inhibit reuptake, whereas lithium facilitates reuptake. The MAO inhibitors block metabolism of biogenic amines (norepinephrine, serotonin, dopamine), increasing the synaptic concentration of these neurotransmitters.

Direct sympathetic agonists such as norepinephrine, epinephrine, and isoproterenol bind to α- or β-adrenergic receptors to stimulate them. Phenylpropanolamine acts mostly on the α-adrenergic receptors, and its toxicity is characterized by hypertension and a reflex bradycardia. Ingestion of α_2-adrenergic agonists such as clonidine or other imidazolines may produce a mixed picture; stimulation of central α_2-adrenergic receptors in the brain decreases central sympathetic out-

Table 8–3. Sympathomimetics

Direct Acting	Indirect Acting
Norepinephrine	Amphetamine
Epinephrine	Ephedrine
Isoproterenol	Phenylpropanolamine
Dopamine	
Phenylephrine	
Methoxamine	
Metaraminol	
Albuterol	
Terbutaline	
Dobutamine	

flow, whereas stimulation of peripheral α_1-adrenergic receptors results in vasoconstriction and transient hypertension. Peripheral postsynaptic α-adrenergic antagonists such as phenoxybenzamine and phentolamine compete with endogenous catecholamines for binding to α_1- and α_2-adrenergic receptors. The α-adrenergic receptors are also blocked by tricyclic antidepressants and by antipsychotic agents such as chlorpromazine and haloperidol. β-Blockers antagonize the effects of catecholamines at β-adrenergic receptors. β-Blocking drugs occupy β-adrenergic receptors and competitively block receptor occupancy by catecholamines and other β-adrenergic agonists. Most β-blocking drugs are pure antagonists; however, a few are partial agonists and cause partial activation of the receptors. They also have varying affinity for the β_1- and β_2-adrenergic receptors, causing intrinsic sympathomimetic activity.

Sympathomimetic toxicity often leads to CNS and cardiovascular complications. Cocaine is an active constituent of the leaves of the South American plant Erythroxylum coca. Its primary actions are local anesthetic effects, CNS stimulation, and inhibition of neuronal uptake of norepinephrine, dopamine, serotonin, and acetylcholine, with a toxicity profile similar to that of amphetamine. In the presence of ethanol, cocaine is transesterified to cocaethylene, which has similar pharmacologic effects and a longer half-life than cocaine. Amphetamine toxicity includes euphoria, restlessness, excessive speech and motor activity, tremor, and insomnia. Intracerebral and subarachnoid hemorrhage may occur owing to hypertension or amphetamine-induced cerebral vasculitis. The actions of pemoline and methylphenidate are similar to those of amphetamine. *Many of the phenylamphetamines and amphetamines may produce hallucinations.* 3,4-Methylenedioxyamphetamine (MDMA, "ecstasy") causes the release of serotonin and blocks its reuptake. It is like a more specific amphetamine targeted to the 5-hydroxytryptamine (5-HT, serotonin) system. 5-Methoxy-3,4-methylenedioxyamphetamine (MMDA) can be formed *in vivo* from myristicin, present in the dried seeds of the nutmeg tree *(Myristica fragrans)* and can produce psychomimetic effects when consumed in large amounts. Mescaline is an alkaloid component of the peyote cactus and produces psychotomimetic activity by its amphetamine-like actions. *Cathinone*, *cathine*, and *methcathinone*, related natural alkaloids found in the leaves and stems of *Catha edulis*, or khat, produces effects indistinguishable from those of amphetamines. *Ephedrine is both an α- and a β-adrenergic agonist*; in addition, it enhances release of norepinephrine from sympathetic neurons. It is a naturally occurring drug found in various species of the plant *Ephedra* (mahuang), indigenous to China.

Blockade of the nigrostriatal dopamine receptors produces extrapyramidal symptoms such as parkinsonism, akathisia, and dystonia. Cholinergic input to the caudate and putamen appears to be unaffected, with resultant cholinergic excess. Neuroleptics and drugs such as metoclopramide cause parkinsonism through such a mechanism. Chronic manganese poisoning damages the globus pallidus, leading to permanent neurologic damage.[10] "Manganese madness" is characterized by emotional lability, hallucinations, irritability, and aggressiveness. Carbon disulfide, a volatile, lipid-soluble industrial solvent, and carbon monoxide inhalation produce parkinsonian features owing to damage to the globus pallidus. Although acute carbon monoxide poisoning has a high mortality, a delayed extrapyramidal syndrome can develop in those who recover from the acute effects. Carbon monoxide produces symmetric necrosis of the globus pallidus with demyelination of the subcortical white matter.[11] Methanol poisoning produces optic atrophy and low-density lesions on computed tomography in the region of the putamen, and putaminal necrosis has been confirmed histologically.[12] A plant and fungal neurotoxin, 3-nitropropionic acid, found in mildewed sugar cane is a succinate dehydrogenase inhibitor that produces basal ganglion injury.[13] In 1983, some intravenous drug abusers injected 1-methyl-4-phenyl-1,2,3,6-tetrahydropyridine (MPTP), a compound produced during illicit synthesis of a narcotic related to meperidine.[14] MPTP selectively destroys dopaminergic neurons in the substantia nigra, producing a condition indistinguishable from idiopathic Parkinson's disease. Treatment of these side effects attempts to re-establish the dopamine/acetylcholine balance required for smooth motor movements.

A central hyperexcitation syndrome with fever, delirium, and hypertension occurs when MAO inhibitors such as phenelzine, isocarboxazid, or tranylcypromine are coadministered with phenothiazines, tricyclic antidepressants, serotonergic reuptake inhibitors, and sympathomimetic amines (amphetamine, methamphetamine, ephedrine, phenylpropanolamine). Sympathomimetic amines are commonly found in some nasal sprays, nose drops, and over-the-counter cold preparations. MAO in the gastrointestinal tract and liver prevents access to the general circulation of ingested, indirectly acting agents such as tyramine and phenylethylamine, contained in foods such as aged cheese, yeast, chicken liver, and pickled herring. However, individuals taking MAO inhibitors do not have this protection and can suffer severe hypertensive crises after eating a large amount of tyramine-containing food. An exaggerated response to the usual dose of meperidine has also been observed.

Neuroleptic malignant syndrome (NMS) is an uncommon but life-threatening disorder that occurs in those who are sensitive to the extrapyramidal effects of antipsychotics. However, it is important to consider the diagnosis of NMS in any patient who has recently received medications that affect CNS dopaminergic pathways. Lithium, carbamazepine, cocaine, and droperidol are some of the drugs implicated in the etiology of NMS. The syndrome may begin from a few days to a few weeks after initiation or alteration of neuroleptic drug therapy. NMS is thought to be mediated by a reduction in dopaminergic activity in the CNS, affecting both the basal ganglia and the hypothalamus.[15] Rigidity, catatonia, and fluctuating consciousness associated with autonomic hyperactivity, including hyperpyrexia, and elevated serum creatinine kinase concentrations are typical features of NMS. Treatment consists of discontinuation of the antipsychotic drug with supportive therapy, possibly including the administration of dantrolene, bromocriptine, or a benzodiazepine. The mortality in untreated cases can be as high as 20%.

The Serotonergic System

5-HT is an indolealkylamine present in many neurons in the CNS. 5-HT does not cross the blood-brain barrier, and thus neurons must synthesize their own transmitters. L-Tryptophan readily crosses the blood-brain barrier and is taken up into serotonergic nerve terminals via an active transport process. Hydroxylation to 5-hydroxytryptophan (5-HTP) occurs by the enzyme tryptophan hydroxylase and the cofactor tetrahydrobiopterin. This is the rate-limiting step, because the enzyme tryptophan hydroxylase is not saturated under normal conditions. Diets high in L-tryptophan can result in increased synthesis of 5-HT in the CNS. The 5-HTP is decarboxylated by the nonspecific aromatic L-amino acid 5-HTP decarboxylase to 5-HT. The mechanisms of sequestration of 5-HT in storage granules is similar to that of catecholamines. 5-HT is then packaged into storage vesicles that protect them from cytosolic degradation by MAO. It is released by an exocytotic mechanism and acts on both presynaptic and postsynaptic receptors. Serotonergic transmission is terminated primarily by reuptake of the amine by a specific 5-HT transporter. After reuptake, the free indolamine is either repackaged or metabolized by MAO and aldehyde dehydrogenase to 5-hydroxyindoleacetic acid.

The serotonin receptors are divided into three major subtypes (i.e., 5-HT_1, 5-HT_2, and 5-HT_3). A 5-HT_4 receptor has also been described. All 5-HT receptors interact with G proteins, with the exception of the 5-HT_3 receptors, which are transmitter-gated ion channels. The 5-HT_1 receptor family contains receptors that are negatively coupled to adenylate cyclase. The 5-HT_2 receptors include the 5-HT_{2A}, 5-HT_{2B}, and 5-HT_{2C} receptors that stimulate phospholipase C. The adenylate cyclase stimulatory receptors are a heterogenous group that includes the 5-HT_4 receptor.

Serotonin is involved in feeding, control of sleep and wakefulness, sexual behavior, mood and emotion, thermoregulation, circadian rhythmicity, drug-induced hallucinatory states, and neuroendocrine function in the CNS. It also serves as a precursor for the pineal hormone melatonin. Inhibition of 5-HT uptake has both an antidepressant and anxiolytic effect. Buspirone represents a new class of antianxiety agent whose anxiolytic action is related to interaction with the 5-HT_{1A} receptor in the brain. Atypical neuroleptics such as risperidone and clozapine, in contrast to conventional agents, strongly block serotonin 5-HT_2 receptors in the frontal cortex and striatal system while also blocking adrenergic and dopamine receptors. In neurochemical terms, atypicality may relate to the ratio of 5-HT_2 to D_2 blockade, and drugs with 5-HT_2 to D_2 ratios of 10 or greater are usually atypical. Lysergic acid diethylamide (LSD) and related psychedelic drugs have been found to have an inhibitory action on the firing of 5-HT–containing neurons in the raphe nucleus. They act relatively selectively at the 5-HT_2 receptor. The antiemetic effects of ondansetron and granisetron are mediated through the 5-HT_3 receptors, and agonists at 5-HT_{1D} receptors such as sumatriptan are effective in treating migraine headaches.

Tryptophan hydroxylase can be blocked by *p*-chlorophenylalanine, decreasing the concentration of 5-HT. Drugs such as reserpine that disrupt the storage of catecholamines also impair the storage of 5-HT. Serotonin reuptake is blocked by some of the tricyclic antidepressants; however, the selective serotonin reuptake inhibitors (SSRIs) such as sertraline, fluoxetine, and venlafaxine are more potent inhibitors of serotonin uptake than of norepinephrine and increase serotonin concentration in the presynaptic cleft. MAO inhibitors increase 5-HT concentration by preventing its breakdown. *LSD is the diethylamide derivative of lysergic acid. It alters serotonin turnover and has agonistic activity of 5-HT_{1A} and 5-HT_{1C} receptors*. Lysergic acid is produced by the fungus *Claviceps purpurea*, which grows on grain and is also found in the seeds of several species of the morning glory family (*Rivea corymbosa, Ipomoea violacea*). The hallucinogenic mushrooms of the *Psilocybe* genus contain the thermostable indole-alkylamine psilocybin and its dephosphorylated congener, psilocin. These substances are structurally related to serotonin and are about 100 times less potent than LSD. Bufotenin is the hallucinogenic indole derivative similar to serotonin found in cohoba snuff and in the skin and parotid glands of the toad *Bufo marinus*.

Concurrent use of two or more serotonergic drugs may result in a marked increase of serotonin in the synapses and may produce the "serotonin syndrome."[16] The syndrome is often unrecognized because of the varied and nonspecific nature of its symptoms. This syndrome includes hyperthermia, muscle rigidity, myoclonus, and mental status changes. This important pharmacodynamic interaction has been commonly reported when fluoxetine or one of the SSRIs is used in the presence of an MAO inhibitor. Moreover, a number of other combinations seem just as capable of producing this syndrome. The SSRIs have been implicated in combination with tryptophan, dextromethorphan, and lithium.

Opioids

The term *opiate* was originally used to designate narcotic drugs derived from opium—that is, morphine and codeine and their many semi-synthetic derivatives prepared from the seed capsules of the poppy *Papaver somniferum*. Later, the term *opioid* was coined to refer in a generic sense to all drugs, natural and synthetic, that have morphine-related actions, as well as to the endogenous peptides later discovered to have such actions. Opioid receptors differ in their regional distribution in the CNS.[17] The opioids induce their biologic effects by interacting with three major classes of receptors, the δ, κ, and μ receptors. σ Opioid receptors are also present in the CNS. Naloxone does not reverse σ receptor–mediated actions. Also, there is an overlap between σ sites and binding sites for phencyclidine, a nonopiate drug of abuse. Morphine and β-endorphin are potent μ receptor agonists, whereas the enkephalins are less potent. μ Receptors mediate supraspinal analgesia, respiratory depression, miosis, euphoria, and physical dependence. Most of the clinically used opiates such as morphine, methadone, and codeine selectively interact with the μ opioid receptor. Naloxone and naltrexone are more potent antagonists at μ receptors than at δ or κ receptors. The κ receptor mediates spinal analgesia and sedation but not respiratory depression. Agonists at the κ receptor are less addictive and do not produce as severe respiratory depression as do μ agonists. Tramadol is a centrally acting opioid-type analgesic that is structurally similar to morphine. It also inhibits the uptake of norepinephrine and 5 = HT; this suggests that its antinociceptive property is mediated by both opioid and nonopioid mechanisms.

The opioid receptors work by activation of G protein, and each opioid receptor type can be linked to either the potassium channel or the calcium channel. Binding to the μ and δ receptors leads to opening of the potassium channel, whereas binding to κ sites results in closing of calcium channels. Opioid receptors function primarily by exerting inhibitory modulation of synaptic transmission in both the CNS and the myenteric plexus. They are often found on presynaptic nerve terminals, where their action results in decreased release of excitatory neurotransmitters. All three major receptor sites are involved in pain modulation. δ Receptors have been implicated in cardiovascular effects, whereas κ receptors seem to have a role in salt and water balance. A given opioid drug may interact to a variable extent with all three types of receptors and can act as an agonist, a partial agonist, or an antagonist at each.

Opiates and opioids in overdose cause sedation and respiratory depression. Death is usually due to respiratory failure, usually as a result of apnea or pulmonary aspiration. The respiratory depression is complicated by bradycardia and hypotension. Pinpoint pupils are usually considered to be the classic sign of narcotic poisoning. Normeperidine, the metabolite of meperidine, a synthetic opioid structurally different from morphine, is known to produce seizures on multiple dosing.[18] The neurotoxicity of normeperidine is manifested by signs of CNS stimulation that include tremors, twitching, myoclonus, and seizures. Treatment consists of giving benzodiazepines to reduce CNS excitation. The use of naloxone is contraindicated because it may increase the incidence of seizures. Propoxyphene causes delusions, hallucinations, and seizures, often with naloxone-resistant cardiodepression.

Opioid-associated depression of respiration and mental status can be reversed by administration of opioid antagonists. The half-life of naloxone is shorter than that of most opioids, and patients may again manifest signs of toxicity after the effect of naloxone wears off. Nalmefene is a new injectable methylene analogue of naltrexone with a half-life of about 11 hours, which is much longer than naloxone's half-life of 1 to 2 hours. Opioid reversal in opioid-dependent patients also poses a risk of precipitating withdrawal symptoms.

The Cholinergic System

Acetylcholine is released from the presynaptic nerve terminal in both the sympathetic and parasympathetic ganglia. It was the first compound to be identified pharmacologically as a transmitter in the CNS, and its action closely mimics the response of parasympathetic nerve stimulation.

The enzyme choline acetyltransferase catalyzes the acetylation of choline by acetyl coenzyme A to form acetylcholine in the motor nerve terminals. Acetylcholine is sequestered in synaptic vesicles and is released when extracellular calcium enters the neuron after depolarization. The released acetylcholine diffuses through the synaptic cleft to interact with the cholinergic receptor. The action of acetylcholine is terminated by hydrolysis by acetylcholinesterase, which is present in high concentrations in the synapse. Metabolism produces acetate and choline, and the breakdown products are used for resynthesis of acetylcholine. The enzyme acetylcholinesterase is widely distributed throughout the body in both neuronal and non-neuronal tissues. It is known as *true* or *specific cholinesterase*, unlike pseudocholinesterase, which is made primarily in the liver and appears in plasma. It has a lower affinity for acetylcholine and metabolizes some drugs, including cocaine and succinylcholine.

Nicotinic and muscarinic receptors are the two major receptors, and both exhibit distinct subtypes. Both nicotinic and muscarinic receptors are present in the brain, and their properties are similar to those of peripheral receptors. Many drugs with actions at peripheral cholinergic receptors are without central effects because they do not cross the blood-brain barrier. Nicotinic receptors are found in the peripheral ganglion and skeletal muscles.[19] Ganglion receptors are found in postsynaptic neurons in both the parasympathetic and sympathetic ganglia and in the adrenal ganglia. Muscarinic receptors are responsible for postganglionic parasympathetic neurotransmission; however, some sympathetic responses such as piloerection also are mediated through muscarinic receptors. Muscarinic receptors also are found in the visceral smooth muscle, in cardiac muscle, in secretory glands, and in the endothelial cells of the vasculature. The muscarinic receptors belong to the family of cell-surface receptors, which transduce their signals across membranes by interacting with GTP-binding protein. Nicotinic receptors are part of the ligand-gated channel, and neuronal receptors show ligand specificity distinct from receptors in the neuromuscular junction.

The cholinergic agonists and the cholinesterase inhibitors comprise a large group of drugs that mimic the effects of acetylcholine. Direct cholinergic agents are divided into esters of choline (acetylcholine) and alkaloids (muscarine and nicotine). Most cholinergic agonists bind to both muscarinic and nicotinic receptors, but a few are highly selective. Their spectrum of action depends on the receptor type stimulated—that is, muscarinic or nicotinic. The immediate clinical effects of excessive muscarinic stimulation include salivation, vomiting, diarrhea, sweating, cutaneous vasodilation, miosis, and bronchial vasoconstriction, whereas excessive nicotinic stimulation leads to muscle fasciculation, weakness, paralysis, hypertension, and tachycardia. Muscarinic antagonists block the actions of acetylcholine at muscarinic sites and block responses evoked by stimulation of parasympathetic nerves. At therapeutic doses, muscarinic antagonists do not bind to nicotinic receptors and neuromuscular blockers do not bind to muscarinic receptors. Ganglion blockers such as hexamethonium, mecamylamine, and trimethaphan block the action of acetylcholine and similar agonists at the nicotinic receptors of both parasympathetic and sympathetic ganglia. They are seldom used clinically.

Jimson weed (*Datura stramonium*) and the deadly nightshade (*Atropa belladonna*) contain the alkaloids atropine, hyoscyamine, and hyoscine. *These alkaloids also are found in other plants belonging to the Solanaceae family* and in toxic amounts produce the anticholinergic syndrome characterized by hot dry skin, hyperthermia, hyperactivity, confusion, delirium and hallucinations, and eventually coma, respiratory depression and cardiovascular collapse. Mushrooms of the family *Amanita muscaria* and *A. pantherina* contain ibotenic acid, muscazon, and muscimol, which are anticholinergics. Neuroleptics, tricyclic antidepressants, and certain antihistamines also have antimuscarinic activity, and overdoses may mimic atropine poisoning. Physostigmine is used as an antidote in anticholinergic poisoning. It is a quaternary compound that crosses the blood-brain barrier and acts as a reversible inhibitor of acetylcholinesterase.

Direct-acting muscarinic agents such as pilocarpine and choline esters produce predictable signs of muscarinic excess when given in overdose. *A. muscaria* contains clinically insignificant amounts of muscarine, a cholinergic agonist, but mushrooms of the genera *Inocybe*, *Clitocybe*, and *Omphalotus* contain muscarine and are usually responsible if cholinergic symptoms dominate. This is clinically manifested as the "SLUDGE" phenomenon of *s*alivation, *l*acrimation, *u*rination, *d*efecation, *g*astrointestinal cramping, and *e*mesis. All the effects are blocked by atropine and its congeners. Cholinesterase inhibitors are used as insecticides and nerve gas poisons. Nerve agents are organophosphorus compounds that are similar to but much more potent than organophosphorus insecticides. They lead to accumulation of acetylcholine, with hyperactivity at both muscarinic and nicotinic receptors and stimulation of the CNS. Atropine blocks the action of excess acetylcholine primarily at muscarinic sites, decreasing secretions, bronchoconstriction, and intestinal motility. Oximes such as pralidoxime work by reactivating phosphorylated cholinesterase enzyme and protecting the enzyme from further inhibition. They act primarily at nicotinic sites with reversal of skeletal muscle weakness and should be used in conjunction with atropine. Pralidoxime's action on muscarinic symptoms is less pronounced than that of atropine. An "intermediate syndrome" has been described 1 to 4 days after the acute phase of organophosphate toxicity, presenting with sudden respiratory paralysis, cranial nerve palsy, and weakness of neck flexors and proximal limb muscles, but this may be related to inadequate pralidoxime therapy.[19a, 19b] In addition, some organophosphates such as tri-orthocresylphosphate cause a peripheral neuropathy associated with axonal demyelination that usually appears 2 to 3 weeks after exposure. *Preceding cholinergic symptoms may be mild or even absent*. These axonal effects are independent of cholinesterase inhibition and are due to inhibition of a second enzyme known as neuropathy target esterase.

Acetylcholine is also the neurotransmitter involved in the neuromuscular junction. A number of biologic toxins produce effects at the neuromuscular junction. Cessation of toxic exposure usually results in complete recovery. A number of toxins disrupt neuromuscular transmission by altering the release of acetylcholine or by producing receptor blockade. The heat-labile neurotoxin botulin produced by the anaerobic bacterium *Clostridium botulinum* produces muscle paralysis by preventing the release of acetylcholine from nerve terminals. Venoms of snakes, such as the Mojave rattlesnake, impair neuromuscular transmission by postsynaptic receptor blockade, which may be irreversible or partially reversible, in addition to inhibiting acetylcholine release.[20] The black widow spider (*Latrodectus mactans*) and some species of tarantula produce a venom, α-latrotoxin, that causes presynaptic release and depletion of acetylcholine from presynaptic vesicles.[21] Other arachnids that produce neurotoxins include ticks, funnel-web spiders, and scorpions. The funnel-web spider toxin, atraxotoxin, contains calcium channel inhibitors, which can produce neuromuscular blockade. A toxin found in the salivary glands of pregnant North American ticks (*Dermacentor andersoni* and *D. variabilis*) causes presynaptic block of acetylcholine release but can also affect conduction in small-diameter motor and sensory axons.[22] Removal of the tick is often curative, leading to complete clinical recovery. Drugs called *hemicholiniums* can block transmission at the neuromuscular junction by blocking the uptake of choline. Cholinesterase inhibitors such as the organophosphate compounds and carbamates inactivate acetylcholinesterase by phosphorylation, preventing acetylcholine degradation to produce a syndrome of cholinergic excess.

The sodium channel of cholinergic neurons is the target of several potent poisons. Venoms of the *Centruroides* genus of scorpions of Arizona and Mexico and *Leiurus quinquestriatus* are neurotoxic. They affect sodium channels with resultant prolongation of action potentials as well a spontaneous depolarization of nerves of both the adrenergic and parasympathetic nervous systems. Tetrodotoxin found in the puffer fish species, suborder Tetraodontoidea, selectively blocks fast sodium channels in nerves and muscle membranes. It is found in fish (Echinodermata), the California newt *(Taricha)*, blue-ringed octopus *(Hapalochlaena maculosa)*, frogs *(Atelopus)*, and marine bacteria. Tetrodotoxin relaxes vascular smooth muscle and blocks preganglionic cholinergic motor, sensory, and sympathetic neurotransmission. Saxitoxin, produced by the dinoflagellate *Protogonyaulax catenella* and by some bacteria, is found in plankton-eating shellfish (clams, oysters, mussels, scallops) and has an action similar to that of tetrodotoxin. Ciguatoxin, a toxin elaborated by the dinoflagellate *Gambierdiscus toxicus*, enhances quantal acetylcholine release at the neuromuscular junction by prolonging the duration of sodium channel opening. Batrachotoxin, found in the skin of a South American frog *(Phyllobates aurotaenia)*, and the plant alkaloids aconitine and veratridine prevent closure or inactivation of voltage-dependent sodium channels. A second important class of sodium channel blockers includes local anesthetics such as lidocaine and related antiarrhythmic agents. This quinidine-like membrane-stabilizing effect is shared with the tricyclic antidepressants and is responsible for the cardiotoxicity. Potassium channel blockers such as 4-aminopyridine are convulsants, and polypeptide toxins from scorpion (charybdotoxin), bee (apamin), or snake (dendrotoxin) venoms also affect the potassium channels.

The Histaminergic System

The histaminergic system functions in the regulation of arousal, body temperature, locomotor activity, analgesia, regulation of biologic rhythms, feeding, drinking, and vascular dynamics.[23] Many of the psychotropic drugs interact with histamine receptors.

Histamine in the brain is formed from L-histidine by decarboxylation by histidine and L-amino acid decarboxylase. Unlike the monoamines and amino acid transmitters, there does not appear to be an active reuptake process for histamine after its release. Histamine is metabolically inactivated by histamine methyltransferase.

Most of the histamine receptors are located in the ventral posterior hypothalamus and give rise to long ascending and descending tracts to the entire CNS. Three subtypes of histamine receptors have been described. *H_1 receptors,* the most prominent, may be located on glia and vessels as well as on neurons and are associated with increased formation of cAMP and cGMP. *H_2 receptors* are directly linked to adenylate cyclase through a G protein. *H_3 receptors* coupled to G protein are predominantly located in the basal ganglia and are most sensitive to histamine. The H_1 receptor is blocked by antihistamines (e.g., pyrilamine). Cimetidine and ranitidine block H_2 receptors, and the H_3 receptor is selectively antagonized by thioperamide.

Antihistamines are structurally related to histamine and antagonize the effects of histamine on H_1 receptor sites. They also possess anticholinergic effects, and the major signs of acute overdose are similar to those caused by classic antimuscarinic agents and are treated accordingly. They may also stimulate or depress the CNS, and some agents such as diphenhydramine possess local anesthetic and membrane-depressant effects when they are taken in large doses.

The Glutaminergic System

Amino acids found in the brain can function as neurotransmitters and can be either excitatory or inhibitory. Glutamic acid and aspartic acid are excitatory, whereas the main inhibitory transmitters are GABA and glycine.

Glutamates are present in high concentration in the CNS. They do not cross the blood-brain barrier and are synthesized from glucose and other precursors. The synthesis of glutamate is mediated by the enzyme glutamate dehydrogenase. Glutamate released from nerve terminals is inactivated by reuptake into the tissues. Glutamate, taken up into glial cells, is oxidized through the Krebs cycle or converted to glutamine by the enzyme glutamine synthetase. Glutamine is recycled back into the nerve terminal to be converted to glutamate.

Receptors for glutamate have a wide distribution in the CNS and are present on neurons that receive input from other neurotransmitter systems.[24] Glutamate receptors convey most of the fast excitatory transmission in the CNS. The ionotropic glutamate receptor is named after the agonists kainate, α-amino-3-hydroxy-5-methyl-4-isoxazolepropionate (AMPA), and *N*-methyl-D-aspartate (NMDA). AMPA also activates G protein–coupled metabotropic glutamate receptors. The metabotropic glutamate receptors do not act on ion channels but rather on intracellular enzymes. The AMPA and the kainate receptor are collectively known as the *non-NMDA* receptor.[25]

At least five distinct sites of pharmacologic or regulatory significance have been identified on the NMDA receptor.[26] There are two different agonist recognition sites for glutamate and glycine: a polyamine regulatory site that promotes receptor activation, and separate recognition sites for magnesium and zinc that act to inhibit flux through agonist-bound receptors. The NMDA receptor requires simultaneous binding of glutamate and glycine for activation.[27] They are known as coagonists because neither glycine nor glutamate alone can open the channel. The glycine site on the NMDA receptor is pharmacologically distinct from the classic spinal inhibitory glycine receptor in that it is not blocked by strychnine. Polyamines such a spermine and spermidine increase the ability of glutamate and glycine to open ion channels by binding on their modulatory sites.[28] Thus, glutamate, glycine, and certain polyamines act in concert to open NMDA ion channels. Zinc and magnesium are endogenous blockers of the NMDA receptor and bind to different receptor sites. Magnesium, unlike zinc, exerts a voltage-dependent block on the open ion channel. Other voltage-dependent blockers of the NMDA receptor channels include dizocilpine (MK-801), phencyclidine, and ketamine. Ethanol acts as an allosteric inhibitor at the NMDA receptor, and it is suggested that the behavioral disinhibition produced by ethanol is mediated by an action on the NMDA receptor and that the ataxia, somnolence, and CNS depression are mediated through other receptors.[29] Acute alcohol withdrawal is accompanied by excessive NMDA activity and is thought to explain some of the characteristic agitation, hallucinations, and convulsions.[30]

AMPA receptors are widely distributed in the CNS, and in the absence of other excitatory activity, AMPA receptors may mediate fast depolarizing responses at most excitatory synapses in the CNS. Kainate receptors activate neuronal membrane channels that are distinguishable from those associated with NMDA and AMPA receptors on the basis of their conductance and desensitization properties. Distinct kainate receptors are involved in some neuropathologic events mediated by excitatory amino acids in the CNS.

Glutamate receptors are thought to have a role in acute neuronal death in response to various insults to the nervous system, including anoxia, hypoglycemia, seizures, and mechanical trauma. The non-NMDA receptors too may be involved in pathologic processes. Glutamate receptor activation can cause seizures, and excitatory amino acid receptor antagonists may be of primary value for the treatment of epilepsy. Postischemic neuronal damage is attributed in part to overactivity of the excitatory amino acid neurotransmitter systems. Elevated extracellular glutamate levels result in glutamate receptor–mediated increase in postsynaptic intracellular calcium levels. Excitotoxicity, the "excitation to death" of neurons, results mainly from the intracellular calcium increase subsequent to overexcitation of neurons. This translocation of calcium leads to a cascade of events with formation of free radicals, activation of nitric oxide synthetase, and cell death. Nitric oxide is produced after stimulation of the enzyme nitric oxide synthetase. Nitric oxide is a novel neuronal messenger that acts with surrounding neurons, not by synaptic transmission but by diffusion between cells. In excess, nitric oxide is toxic to neurons. This toxicity is mediated largely by an interaction with the superoxide anion, presumably through the generation of the oxidant peroxynitrite. This cascade can be halted by administration of NMDA receptor antagonists.[31] Studies show that NMDA antagonists are more effective in reducing penumbral damage after cerebral arterial occlusion. Chronic neurodegenerative disorders such as olivopontocerebellar atrophy and Huntington's chorea are associated with disorders of excitatory amino acid transmission, as is amyotrophic lateral sclerosis. Much is yet to be learned about the role of NMDA receptors in ischemic and nonischemic neurotoxicity.

Domoic acid was identified as the toxin in a major outbreak of food poisoning in Canada in 1987.[32] An alga *Nitzschia pungens* was found to be the source of the toxin, which contaminated blue mussels. Domoic acid is a glutamate analogue and produces neurotoxicity by overstimulation of the glutaminergic system. Dietary consumption of the chickling (*not* chick) pea *Lathyrus sativus* or other potentially neurotoxic *Lathyrus* species is associated with lathyrism characterized by spastic paraparesis. The offending agent in the pea is thought to be β-*N*-oxaloamino-L-alanine (BOAA). The cycad *Cycas circinalis* has a BOAA-like constituent, β-*N*-methylamino-L-alanine (BMAA), and may be the cause of the motor neuron disease that occurs in Guam. Phencyclidine and ketamine are known as *dissociative anesthetics* because they produce a feeling of being apart from one's environment. They are antagonists at the *N*-methyl-D-aspartate subtype of the glutamate receptor and act by blocking the ion. The primary antiepileptic action of felbamate is believed to be at the strychnine-insensitive glycine binding site at the *N*-methyl-D-aspartate receptor. It is also shown to weakly potentiate GABA receptor binding. Lamotrigine, another antiepileptic drug, is thought to act by inhibiting the release of glutamate.

The GABAergic System

The amino acids GABA and glycine both are inhibitory neurotransmitters that mediate fast postsynaptic inhibition in the nervous system. Their action is to bind specifically to GABA and glycine receptors, respectively. The GABA and glycine receptors belong to the family of ligand-gated ion channels.

Glucose is the principal precursor for GABA production, although pyruvate and other amino acids can also act as precursors. Glutamic acid is formed from the transamination of α-ketoglutarate, formed from glucose metabolism in the Krebs cycle by GABA α-oxoglutarate transaminase. Glutamic acid decarboxylase catalyzes the decarboxylation of glutamic acid to form GABA. The cofactor is pyridoxal phosphate. Pyridoxal phosphate is synthesized from pyridoxine (vitamin B_6) by the enzyme pyridoxine kinase. The action of GABA released into the synaptic cleft is inactivated by a high-affinity uptake process. Enzymatic breakdown entails transamination to succinic semialdehyde by GABA transaminase. The next step is oxidation to succinic acid by succinic semialdehyde dehydrogenase, with the succinic acid then entering the Krebs cycle.

GABA receptors predominate in the brain, where they have a widespread distribution.[33] Two types of receptors for GABA have been proposed: *$GABA_A$ receptors* open chloride channels, causing hyperpolarization of the recipient neuronal cell. Muscimol is a naturally occurring GABA analogue isolated from the hallucinogenic mushroom *A. muscaria* and acts as a potent agonist.[34] Bicuculline and picrotoxin are competitive antagonists. The binding of GABA is enhanced by benzodiazepines, barbiturates, and certain steroids. At the *$GABA_B$ sites,* the antispastic drug baclofen is an agonist, and GABA has a relatively low potency that is unaffected by benzodiazepines. $GABA_B$ receptors are indirectly coupled to potassium channels, decrease calcium conductance, and inhibit cAMP production by binding to G proteins.

$GABA_A$ receptors are multimembered, with five subunits assembled into a functional complex. The five major binding sites are for GABA, benzodiazepines, barbiturates, picrotoxin, and the anesthetic steroid. These binding domains serve to modulate the receptors to GABA stimulation. A number of agonists bind to the binding site and elicit GABA-like responses. Benzodiazepines enhance GABAergic transmission, and a wide variety of nonbenzodiazepines, such as β-carbolines, cyclopyrrolones (zopiclone), and imidazopyridines (zolpidem), also bind to the benzodiazepine site.[35] Barbiturates facilitate GABA-mediated synaptic transmission by increasing chloride influx and at pharmacologic concentrations are known to allosterically increase binding of benzodiazepine and GABA to their binding sites. Bicuculline, a plant alkaloid, is a competitive GABA antagonist and is selective for the $GABA_A$ receptor that controls chloride permeability. Penicillin is a chloride channel blocker with a net negative charge that occludes the chloride channel by interacting with the positively charged amino acid residues within the channel pore. The allosteric regulation of $GABA_A$ receptor function by neuroactive steroids is well known, and the steroid recognition site provides a potentially important target in the development of new therapeutic agents.[36] General anesthetics, including barbiturates, volatile gases, steroids, and alcohols, enhance GABA-mediated chloride conductance.[37]

Pyridoxal phosphate antagonists such as isoniazid and other hydrazines, such as monomethylhydrazine in the mushroom *Gyromitra (Helvella) esculenta,* produce seizures by impairing GABA synthesis.[38] Intravenous pyridoxine is used to combat the toxicity. Cyanide inhibits glutamic acid decarboxylase, thereby decreasing GABA, and may partly account for seizures occurring in cyanide toxicity.[39] GABA is the major inhibitory neurotransmitter in the CNS, and impairment of GABAergic transmission is involved in the pathogenesis of epilepsy. Drugs such as penicillin and bicuculline impair inhibitory transmission mediated by GABA and therefore produce seizures. Picrotoxin found in the berries of the shrub *Anamirta cocculus* is a $GABA_A$ receptor channel blocker. The active principle picrotoxinin works on the gating process of the channel. The chlorinated hydrocarbons inhibit the action of GABA by binding to the picrotoxin site on the $GABA_A$ receptor to produce seizures.[40] Gabapentin, an amino acid structurally related to GABA, is currently being used in the treatment of epilepsy. Gabapentin appears to have GABA-mimetic properties, but its precise mechanism of action remains unclear. An effect on central serotonin metabolism has been postulated by some investigators. The anticonvulsant valproic acid works by inhibiting GABA transaminase and succinic semialdehyde dehydrogenase, enzymes that degrade GABA. γ-Vinyl-GABA is an irreversible inhibitor of GABA transaminase and increases GABA concentration. Alcohol is known to augment GABA-mediated chloride flux, and ethanol may exert some of its effect by enhancing the function of the GABA receptor.[41] Baclofen is an orally active GABA-mimetic agent and acts as a $GABA_B$ agonist.[42] It causes hyperpolarization by increasing potassium conductance and has presynaptic inhibitory functions. Baclofen in an overdose produces drowsiness, coma, seizures, respiratory depression, and arrhythmias. Pure benzodiazepine overdoses are usually not fatal. However, the newer, short-acting agents may greatly increase the frequency of complication, especially when benzodiazepines are combined with other CNS depressant drugs and alcohol. The benzodiazepine antagonist flumazenil is one of several 1,4-benzodiazepine derivatives with high affinity for the benzodiazepine receptor that acts as a competitive antagonist. Caution in flumazenil administration is warranted in mixed overdoses, when benzodiazepine may provide a neuroprotective or cardioprotective action.

Glycine is another inhibitory neurotransmitter that mediates fast postsynaptic inhibition in the nervous system. Like GABA, it inhibits neuronal firing by chloride channel gating but with a different pharmacology.[43] The glycine receptors are predominantly found in the spinal cord and the brain stem. Glycine is also the most likely inhibitory transmitter in the reticular formation. The pharmacology of the glycine receptor is less extensively known than that of the GABA receptors. They are defined by the antagonism by the convulsive alkaloid strychnine, in contrast to the strychnine-insensitive glycine-binding site that is associated with the excitatory NMDA subclass of the glutamate receptor. This explains strychnine's effect to be localized to the spinal cord and the medulla only.

Strychnine, an alkaloid found in the seeds of the tree *Strychnos nux-vomica,* increases the level of neuronal excitability by a selective antagonist action at glycine receptors. The result is generalized seizure such as contraction of skeletal muscles, rhabdomyolysis, myoglobinuria, and in some cases acute renal failure. It is used primarily as a rodenticide and is sometimes found as an adulterant in illicit drugs such as cocaine or heroin. Barbiturates and diazepam are effective antagonists of strychnine. *Calycanthus* species (Carolina allspice) contain the strychnine-like toxin calycanthine, which may produce convulsions.

TOXICITY SPECIFIC TO THE PERIPHERAL NERVOUS SYSTEM

Neurotoxins almost invariably produce polyneuropathy and are rarely implicated in focal neuropathy. Neurologic dysfunction usually occurs as part of a systemic toxicity.[44] The neurotoxicity may occur in isolation, however, and then need to be differentiated from other nontoxic causes of neuropathies. The development of a neuropathy is directly related to continued exposure to a particular toxin. The neuropathy often improves when the exposure is discontinued. If the neuropathy progresses after removal of a suspected toxin, then other causes should be considered (Table 8–4).

Diseases of the peripheral nervous system can be classified in two ways. The first categorization depends on the distribution: focal, multifocal, diffuse, proximal, distal, symmetric, or segmental. The second system depends on the anatomic location of the pathologic process: muscle, neuromuscular junction, or peripheral nerve. Further differentiation is based on involvement of the neuron, axon, or myelin.

Symmetric Generalized Neuropathies

The most common form of drug- or toxin-induced neuropathy is a symmetric distal axonopathy. The neuropathy reflects failure of axonal transport and begins distally, where the axons are most vulnerable, and predominantly affects long and large-diameter axons, progressing proximally. Axonopathies usually have a subacute onset with gradual progression and are clinically reflected by a symmetric, distal, diffuse, stocking and glove–type sensorimotor loss. Sensory signs and symptoms initially predominate over motor deficits. Complete recovery is subject to withdrawal of the toxic insult and is often prolonged and slow. Axonal regeneration occurs at a rate of 2 mm/d, with recovery in an order reverse to that of the initial loss (i.e., proximal before distal).

Demyelinating neuropathy is characterized by lesions that occur in the myelin sheath or Schwann's cells. The axons usually are spared. The onset usually is subacute, and the involvement in myelinopathy, unlike in axonopathy, is predominantly distal and motor because the heavily myelinated large motor fibers are more severely affected than the small-diameter myelinated and unmyelinated sensory fibers. The demyelination may be patchy, however, with early proximal involvement. Areflexia is characteristic, and sensory symptoms are minimal. Recovery from a myelinopathy is usually rapid, early, and complete, when compared with that from an axonopathy. The buckthorn toxin, found in high concentrations in the endocarp of the fruit of *Karwinskia huboldtiana*, and perhexiline are the few toxins causing a peripheral myelinopathy.

Toxic injury to the cell body directly is termed a *neuropathy.* The dorsal root ganglions are especially involved. This vulnerability is because of a poorly formed nerve-blood barrier and the fenestrated blood vessels with increased vascular perfusion. Neuronopathies are rarely the cause of toxic insults. Neuronopathies are characterized by the rapid or subacute onset of motor or sensory deficits. The neurologic defect mirrors the nerve root involved and can occur anywhere. Recovery is variable and often incomplete because of incomplete neuronal recovery. Toxic neuronopathies can be caused by mercury, pyridoxine, and doxorubicin.

Acute and chronic heavy metal exposure may produce neuropathies. Metal compounds tend to be stored in bones, from where they may be gradually released into the circulation, subsequently delaying recovery time. Other systems (i.e., hematopoietic, renal, and gastrointestinal) dysfunctions usually accompany the neuropathy. Arsenic produces a generalized axonal peripheral neuropathy with predominant sensory involvement. Symptoms of toxicity usually appear 5 to 10 days after ingestion, with painful dysesthesias and numbness in the feet and hands. Arsenic reacts with the sulfhydryl groups on various enzymes necessary for cellular metabolism. Both inorganic and organic lead are neurotoxic. Lead intoxication produces a demyelinating neuropathy with predominantly motor involvement. Lead intoxication in children, unlike that in adults, may produce an encephalopathy rather than a peripheral neuropathy. Mercury exposure causes a subacute, diffuse, predominantly motor neuropathy. Thallium compounds have been used as rodenticides, and toxicity produces an axonal neuropathy with prominent systemic features that include alopecia and autonomic dysfunction. Aluminum has been implicated in the causation of dialysis encephalopathy, a progressive acute syndrome found in patients undergoing dialysis.

A number of organic compounds also produce neuropathies. The rodenticide Vacor causes a severe, rapid-onset distal axonopathy with associated autonomic dysfunction and diabetes mellitus due to necrosis of pancreatic β cells.[45] The neuropathy can be prevented by nicotinamide, and Vacor may inhibit nicotinamide dinucleotide–dependent enzyme with disruption of an axonal-dependent process. Peripheral neurotoxic organic solvents include *n*-hexane and methyl-*N*-butyl ketone, carbon disulfide, and trichlorethylene.[46] *n*-Hexane and methyl-*N*-butyl ke-

Table 8–4. Characteristic Features of Toxic Neuropathy

Consistent pattern of neurologic dysfunction
Reproducible pathophysiologic or pathologic findings
Temporal relationship between exposure and onset of the clinical finding
Nonfocal disorder
Neurotoxicity improves with cessation of exposure

Table 8–5. Selected Neurotoxins That Produce Neuropathy

Toxins	Exposure Risk	Pathologic Finding	Clinical Features
Arsenic	Metallurgy, pesticides, wood preservatives, pigments, ant stakes, weed killers	Axonopathy (S>M)	GI distress, psychosis, hyperkeratosis, hyperpigmentation, Mees' lines, anemia
Lead	Lead production, solders, batteries, pigment, insecticides, auto radiators, moonshine, construction workers, folk medicine (*azarcon* and *greta*)	Axonopathy (M>S)	GI distress, microcytic anemia, basophilic stippling, encephalopathy, acute tubular dysfunction, gout, hyperuricemia
Mercury	Gold and silver extraction, dental amalgams, fungicides, environmental contamination, thermometers	Axonopathy (M>S)	GI distress, tremor, ataxia, gingivostomatitis, neuropsychiatric disturbances
Thallium	Manufacture of optical lenses, photoelectric cells, and costume jewelry; rodenticide	Axonopathy (M>S)	GI distress, delirium, seizures, coma, alopecia, choreoathetosis, ataxia, tremor, Mees' lines
Carbon disulfide	Insecticides, rayon fiber production	Axonopathy (MS)	Encephalopathy, parkinsonian syndromes, nystagmus, psychosis
Acrylamide	Production of acrylamide resins	Axonopathy (MS)	Irritant, contact dermatitis, ataxia
Allyl chloride	Epoxy resin and glycerin production	Axonopathy (S>M)	Irritant, pulmonary edema
Ethylene oxide	Sterilizing agent, solvent, plasticizer, chemical intermediate	Axonopathy (MS)	Convulsions, arrhythmias, leukemia
Hexacarbons, e.g., hexane	Solvents	Axonopathy (SM)	GI dysfunction, hyperhidrosis, autonomic dysfunction
Methyl bromide	Insecticidal fumigant, fire extinguisher ingredient	Axonopathy (MS)	Irritant, dermatitis, tremor, seizure, coma, dementia, psychosis, extrapyramidal symptoms
Trichloroethylene	Typewriter correction fluid, insecticides, spot removers, paint removers	Myelinopathy	Extrapyramidal dysfunction, degreaser's flush
Polychlorinated biphenyls (PCBs)	High-temperature insulators, transformers, carbonless copy papers	Myelinopathy	Chloracne, hepatic transaminitis, porphyria
Organophosphates	Pesticides	Axonopathy (M>S)	Cholinergic symptoms, agitation, seizures, coma
Vacor (PNU)	Rodenticides	Axonopathy (M>S)	Nausea, vomiting, autonomic dysfunction, insulin-dependent diabetes mellitus

M, motor; S, sensory; GI, gastrointestinal; PCB, polychlorinated biphenyl.

tone are metabolized to 2,5-hexanedione, the active agent that damages the peripheral nerves. Methyl ethyl ketone enhances the neurotoxic effects of *n*-hexane and methyl-*N*-butyl ketone without itself being neurotoxic. Trichloroethylene may cause trigeminal neuropathy through its breakdown product, dichloroacetylene. Allyl chloride, used in the manufacture of epoxy resin, produces a characteristic distal axonopathy with sensory loss and loss of ankle jerks. Acrylamide monomer, unlike its polymer, is neurotoxic and produces a distal axonopathy involving large myelinated fibers. Ethylene oxide, commonly used as a sterilizing agent, produces a distal sensorimotor axonopathy with numbness, weakness, and areflexia. Residual ethylene oxide in dialysis tubing after the sterilization process may contribute to peripheral neuropathy in patients undergoing long-term hemodialysis.[47] Methyl bromide exposure causes a distal symmetric axonopathy with involvement of the pyramidal tracts and cerebellum. Polychlorinated biphenyls have been associated with outbreaks of neuropathy when cooking oil has been contaminated with tetrachlorobiphenyl[48] (Table 8–5).

An exciting future lies ahead in neurotoxicology. The knowledge of normal brain physiology and its response to insult has grown tremendously. The number of new antidepressants has greatly increased. Clinical trials of drugs that treat ischemic and traumatic brain injury are under way. The results of these studies will further expand the understanding of neurotoxicity and lead to the development of better therapies.

References

1. Kandel ER, Schwartz JH, Jessel TM (eds): Principles of Neural Science, 3rd ed. New York, Elsevier Science Publishing Co., 1991.
2. Bourne HR, Sanders DA, McCormick F: The GTPase superfamily: Conserved structure and molecular mechanism. Nature *349*:117–129, 1991.
3. Palmer TM, Stiles GL: Adenosine receptor. Neuropharmacology *34*:683–694, 1995.
4. Clark M, Post RM: Carbamazepine, but not caffeine, is highly selective for adenosine A1 binding sites. Eur J Pharmacol *164*:399–401, 1989.
5. Eldridge FL, Paydarfar D, Scott C, et al: Role of endogenous

adenosine in recurrent generalized seizures. Exp Neurol *103*:179–185, 1989.
6. Shannon MW, Maher TJ: Anticonvulsant effects of intracerebro-ventricular adenosine in theophylline-induced seizures. Vet Hum Toxicol *36*:350, 1994.
7. Blake KV, Massey KL, Hendes L, et al: Relative efficacy of phenytoin and phenobarbital for the prevention of theophylline-induced seizures in mice. Ann Emerg Med *17*:1024–1028, 1988.
8. Molinoff PB, Axelrod J: Biochemistry of catecholamines. Annu Rev Biochem *40*:465–500, 1971.
9. Caron MG, Lefkowitz RJ: Catecholamines receptors: Structure, function, and regulation. Recent Prog Horm Res *48*:277, 1993.
10. Mena I: Manganese poisoning. *In* Vinken PJ, Bruyn GW (eds): Handbook of Clinical Neurology. Vol. 21. New York, Elsevier Science Publishing Co., pp 821–823, 1977.
11. Ginsberg MD: Carbon monoxide. *In* Spencer PS, Schaumburg HH (eds): Experimental and Clinical Neurotoxicology. Baltimore, William & Wilkins, pp 374–394, 1980.
12. Aquilonius SM, Asmark H, Enoksson P, et al: Computerised tomography in severe methanol intoxication. BMJ *2*:929, 1978.
13. He FS: Extrapyramidal lesions induced by mildewed cane poisoning (with report of three cases). Chung Hua I Hsueh Tsa Chih *67*:395–396, 1987.
14. Tanner CM, Langston JW: Do environmental toxins cause Parkinson's disease? A critical review. Neurology *322*:1781–1787, 1990.
15. Granner MA, Wooten GF: Neuroleptic malignant syndrome or parkinsonism hyperpyrexia syndrome. Semin Neurol *11*:228–335, 1991.
16. Mill KC: Serotonin syndrome. Am Fam Med *52*:1475–1482, 1995.
17. Reisine T: Opiate receptors. Neuropharmacology *34*:463–472, 1995.
18. Kaiko RF, Foley KM, Grabinski PY, et al: Central nervous system excitatory effects of meperidine in cancer patients. Ann Neurol *13*:180–185, 1983.
19. Galzi JL, Changeux JP: Molecular organization and regulations. Neuropharmacology *34*:563–582, 1995.
19a. Benson BJ, Tolo D, McIntire M: Is the intermediate syndrome in organophosphate poisoning the result of insufficient oxime therapy? J Toxicol Clin Toxicol *30*:347–349, 1992.
19b. Haddad LM. Organophosphate poisoning: Intermediate syndrome? J Toxicol Clin Toxicol *30*:331–332, 1992.
20. Kitchens CS, Van Mierop LH: Envenomation by the eastern coral snake *(Micrurus fulvius)*. JAMA *258*:1615–1618, 1987.
21. Rauber A: Black widow spider bites. J Toxicol Clin Toxicol *21*:473, 1983–84.
22. Kincaid JC: Tick bite paralysis. Semin Neurol *10*:32–34, 1990.
23. Hough LB: Cellular localization and possible functions for brain histamine: Recent progress. Prof Neurobiol *30*:469–505, 1987.
24. Pin JP, Duvoisin R: The metabotrophic glutamate receptors: Structure and functions. Neuropharmacology *34*:1219–1237, 1995.
25. Bettler B, Mulle C: AMPA and kainate receptors. Neuropharmacology *34*:123–139, 1995.
26. Mori H, Mishina M: Structure and function of the NMDA receptor channel. Neuropharmacology *34*:1219–1237, 1995.
27. Kleckner NW, Dingledine R: Requirements for glycine in activation of NMDA receptors expressed in *Xenopus* oocyte. Science *241*:835–837, 1988.
28. Williams K, Romano C, Dichter MA, et al: Modulation of the NMDA receptor by polyamines. Life Sci *48*:469–498, 1991.
29. Weight FF, Lovinger DM, White G, et al: Alcohol and anaesthetic actions on excitatory amino acid–activated ion channels. Ann N Y Acad Sci *625*:97–107, 1990.
30. Hoffman PL, Grant KA, Snell LD, et al: NMDA receptors: Role in ethanol withdrawal seizures. Ann N Y Acad Sci *654*:52–60, 1992.
31. Olney JW: Excitatory amino acids and neuropsychiatric disorders. Annu Rev Pharmacol Toxicol *30*:47–71, 1990.
32. Perl TM, Bedard L, Kosatsky T, et al: An outbreak of toxic encephalopathy caused by eating mussels contaminated with domoic acid. N Engl J Med *322*:1775–1780, 1990.
33. Luddens H, Korpi ER, Seeburg PH: $GABA_A$/benzodiazepine receptor heterogeneity: Neurophysiological implications. Neuropharmacology *34*:245–254, 1995.
34. Krogsgaard-Larsen P, Brehm L, Schaumburg K: Muscimol, a psychoactive constituent of Amanita muscaria, as a medicinal chemical model structure. Acta Chem Scand [B] *35*:311–324, 1981.
35. Mohler H, Okada T: Benzodiazepine receptor: Demonstration in the central nervous system. Science *198*:849–851, 1977.
36. Majewska MD, Harrison NL, Schwartz RD, et al: Steroid hormone metabolites are barbiturate-like modulators of the GABA receptor. Science *232*:1004–1007, 1986.
37. Allan AM, Harris RA: Anesthetic and convulsant barbiturates alter γ-aminobutyric acid–stimulated chloride flux across brain membranes. J Pharmacol Exp Ther *238*:763–768, 1986.
38. William HL, Killah MS, Jenny EH, et al: Convulsant effects of isoniazid. JAMA *152*:1317–1321, 1951.
39. Gosselin RE, Smith RP, Hodge HC: Clinical Toxicology of Commercial Products. 5th ed. Baltimore, William & Wilkins, 1984.
40. Lummis SCR, Buckinham SD, Rauh JJ, et al: Blocking actions of heptachlor at an insect central nervous system GABA receptor. Proc R Soc Lond Biol Sci *240*:97–106, 1990.
41. Suzdak PD, Schwartz RD, Skolnick P, et al: Ethanol stimulates γ-aminobutyric acid receptor–mediated chloride transport in rat brain synaptoneurosomes. Proc Natl Acad Sci U S A *83*:4071–4075, 1986.
42. Ogata N: Pharmacology and physiology of $GABA_B$ receptors. Gen Pharmacol *21*:395–402, 1990.
43. Langosch D, Becker CM, Betz H: The inhibitory glycine receptor: A ligand-gated chloride channel of the central nervous system. Eur J Biochem *194*:1–8, 1990.
44. Schaumberg HH, Spencer PS, Thomas PK (eds): Disorder of Peripheral Nerves. Philadelphia, F.A. Davis Co., 1983.
45. LeWitt P: The neurotoxicity of the rat poison vacor. N Engl J Med *302*:73–77, 1980.
46. Spencer PS, Schaumberg HH, Sabri M, et al: The enlarging view of hexacarbon neurotoxicity. Crit Rev Toxicol *7*:279–356, 1980.
47. Windebank AJ, Blexrud MD: Residual ethylene oxide in hollow fiber hemodialysis units is neurotoxic in vitro. Ann Neurol *26*:63–68, 1989.
48. Murai Y, Kuroiwa Y: Peripheral neuropathy in chlorobiphenyl poisoning. Neurology *21*:1173–1176, 1971.

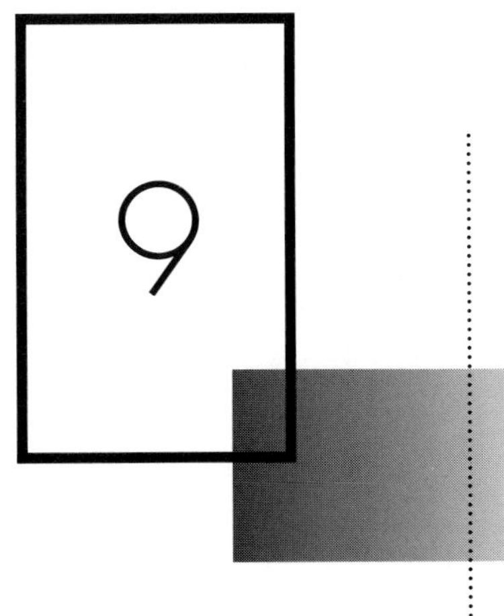

Chemical Hepatic Injury

HYMAN J. ZIMMERMAN, MD

Poisonous doses of any of a huge number of chemical and biologic agents can lead to hepatic injury.[1–3] Some hepatotoxins are plant or fungal products. Some are minerals. Many are industrial products, byproducts, or wastes (Table 9–1).

Hepatotoxic agents may be encountered at home or at work (Table 9–2). Toxic exposure to some agents has occurred only in industry (e.g., trinitrotoluene [TNT]); to others only in the home (e.g., poisonous mushrooms); and to some in both settings (e.g., carbon tetrachloride [CCl_4]). Occupational exposure to hepatotoxic agents has long been a worrisome cause of hepatic injury. Indeed, various agents with experimentally proven hepatotoxic potential (Table 9–3) have been used in numerous industries (Table 9–4). Improved industrial hygiene in recent years, however, apparently has led to a reduced incidence of acute toxic liver damage.[1] The risk of chronic hepatic disease should be monitored and evaluated.

Table 9–1. Hepatotoxin Agents

Types of Agents	Examples
Organic	
Natural	Tannic acid
Plant products	
Mycotoxins	
Macro	Mushroom toxins
Micro	Aflatoxins
Bacterial	Diphtheria toxin
Animal	Hornet venom
Synthetic	
Nonmedicinal	Tetrachloroethane
Medicinal	Acetaminophen
Inorganic	
Metals	Ferrous salts, copper salts
Metalloids	Inorganic arsenicals
Hydrazine derivatives	Methylhydrazine
Iodides	

Household poisonings are today, by far, the more frequent cause of acute hepatic injury.[3] Poisoning may result from accidental or suicidal intake of a known toxin (CCl_4, acetaminophen); from inhalation of a hepatotoxic solvent as a result of careless use, accident, or solvent sniffing; or from ingestion of natural toxins or synthetic chemicals that are contaminants of food or drink.

HEPATOTOXIC AGENTS

All agents that can produce hepatic injury might be defined as hepatotoxins. It is essential, however, to distinguish agents that are true toxins from those whose hepatotoxic effects are idiosyncrasy dependent.[1] Those that can produce dose-dependent hepatic injury in humans and in experimental animals are considered to be true (intrinsic, predictable) hepatotoxins, whereas agents that produce hepatic injury in only unusually susceptible humans, seemingly not dose dependent, are designated idiosyncrasy dependent (nonpredictable) hepatotoxins.[1] This

Table 9–2. Circumstances of Exposure of Chemical Hepatic Injury

Toxicologic
Occupational
Domestic
Accidental or suicidal
Ingestion of food or contaminant
Drug abuse
Solvent or glue sniffing
Ingestion or injection of illicit drugs
Alcoholism
Pharmaceutical
Iatrogenic
Self-medication

Table 9–3. Partial List of Agents Likely to Be Encountered Occupationally, with Indication of Hepatotoxic Effects in Experimental Animals and Humans*

	Experimental† Animals	Humans†	Lesion*
Organic, non-halogenated			
Alcohols and glycols			
Allyl alcohol	+	?	Necrosis, zone 1
Dioxane	+	+	Necrosis, zone 3
Ethyl alcohol	+	+	See Chapter 34
Ethylene glycol	±	±	
Methyl alcohol	±	±	
Iospropyl alcohol	0	0	
Aldehydes, acetyls, acetates, esters	0	0	
Amines, aliphatic			
Ethanolamine	+	?	Degeneration
Ethylenediamine	±	?	Degeneration
Amines aromatic			
4,4′-Diaminodiphenylmethane (methylene dianiline)	+	+	Cholestasis
4-Dimethylaminobenzene	+	?	Degeneration, CA‡
Cyanides and nitriles			
Acetonitrile	±	?	Degeneration
Acrylonitrile	±	?	Degeneration
Hydrogen cyanide	0	0	
Hydrocarbons, aliphatic			
Alicyclic	±	0	
Cyclopropane	±	0	
Cyclohexane	±	0	
Gasoline (C8-C10)	±	0	
n-Heptane	±	0	
Hexane	±	0	
Turpentine	±	0	
Hydrocarbons, aromatic			
Benzene	±	±	Trivial steatosis
Diphenyl	+	+	Necrosis
Naphthalene	0	0	
p-Terbutyl toluene	±	0	
Styrene	+	0	Degeneration, steatosis
Tetraline	+	0	Steatosis, necrosis
Toluene	±	±	Trivlial steatosis
Xylene	±	±	Steatosis, necrosis in fatal poisoning after ingestion
Nitroaliphatic compounds			
Nitroethane	+	+	Necrosis
Nitromethane	+	+	Necrosis
2-Nitropropane	+	+	Necrosis
1-Nitropropane	+	+	Steatosis, necrosis
Nitroaromatic compounds			
Dinitrobenzene	+	+	Necrosis
Dinitrophenol	±	±	?Cholestasis
2,6-Dinitrotoluene	+	+	Necrosis, CA‡
Nitrobenzene	+	±	Degeneration
Nitrodiphenyl	±	±	
Picric acid (2,4,6-trinitrophenol)	+	+	Necrosis
Tetryl	+	+	Necrosis
Trinitrotoluene (TNT)	+	+	Necrosis
Organic, Halogenated			
Haloaliphatic compounds			
Bromoform	+	+	Necrosis, zone 3
Bromoethene (vinyl bromide)	+	?	Degeneration, CA‡
Carbon tetrachloride	+	+	Necrosis, zone 3, fat, CA‡
Carbon tetrabromide	+	+	Necrosis, zone 3
Chloroform	+	+	Necrosis, zone 3, fat
Chloroethane (vinyl chloride)	+	+	Degeneration, CA‡, angiosarcoma hepatoportal sclerosis
Chloroprene	±	?	Degeneration
1,2-Dibromoethane	+	+	Necrosis, zone 3, CA‡
1,2-Dichloroethane	+	+	Necrosis, CA‡

Table 9–3. Partial List of Agents Likely to Be Encountered Occupationally, with Indication of Hepatotoxic Effects in Experimental Animals and Humans *(Continued)*

	Experimental† Animals	Humans†	Lesion*
Haloaliphatic compounds *(Continued)*			
Fluoroethane	?	?	
Halothane	+	+	Necrosis, zone 3
Methyl chloride	±	±	Degeneration
Methylene chloride	±	±	Degeneration
Propylene chloride	+	+	Necrosis
Tetrachloroethane	+	+	Necrosis
Tetrachloroethylene	+	±	Steatosis, degeneration, necrosis only with severe exposure
1,1,2-Trichloromethane	+	+	Necrosis, steatosis
1,1,1-Trichloromethane	+	±	Steatosis, degeneration, necrosis only with severe exposure
Haloaromatic compounds			
2-Acetylaminofluorine	+	+	Degeneration, CA‡
Benzyl chloride	±	±	
Brominated biphenyls†	+	±	Steatosis, necrosis in animals
Brominated benzenes	+	+	Necrosis, zone 3
Chlordecone	+	±	Steatosis, CA‡
Chlorinated biphenyls†	+	±	Steatosis, necrosis in animals Steatosis in man
3,3′-Dichlorobenzidine	+	?	Degeneration, CA‡
4,4′-Methylenebis (2-chloroaniline)	+	?	Necrosis, CA‡
0-Dichlorobenzene	+	?	Necrosis, zone 3§
p-Dichlorobenzene	+	?	Degeneration, CA‡
Chlorinated benzenes	+	+	Necrosis, zone 3
Chlorinated naphthalanes	+	+	Necrosis
Pentachlorophenol	+	±	Degeneration, CA‡
Nitrochloroaliphatics	+	+	Necrosis
Nitrochloroaromatics	+	+	Necrosis, CA‡
Organic miscellaneous			
β-Propiolactone	+	?	Necrosis
Carbon disulfide	±	?	Steatosis
Decalin	+	0	Steatosis, necrosis
Dimethyl sulfate	0	0	
Dimethylacetamide	+	+	Degeneration
Dimethylformamide	+	+	Steatosis, necrosis
Diphenyl oxide	+	+	Necrosis
Ethyleneimime	+	?	CA‡
Furans	±	±	
Hydrazine	+	+	Steatosis, necrosis
Mercaptans	–	0	
N-Nitrosodimethylamine (dimethylnitrosamine)	+	+	Necrosis, CA‡
Pyridine	+	+	Necrosis
Bipyridyls			
Paraquat	+	+	Necrosis early, bile duct injury and cholestasis later
Diquat	+	+	Necrosis
Inorganic			
Arsenic	+	+	Steatosis, necrosis angiosarcoma, CA‡
Arsine	0	0	
Beryllium	+	+	Granuloma in humans
Boron hydrides	+	+	Zone 2 necrosis in exposed animals Granulomas, hepatoportal
Bordeaux mixture (copper salts and lime as spray)	?	+	Steatosis Sclerosis, cirrhosis, angiosarcoma
Cadmium	+	?	Necrosis, cirrhosis
Chromium	+	±	Degeneration
See Table 9–6			

*Ability to cause injury on ingestion or injection, not in ordinary occupational exposure.
†0, No known injury; ±, trivial injury, i.e. minor degeneration or steatosis; +, definite hepatic injury.
‡Hepatocarcinogenic in experimental animals.
§2-Chloro-2-bromo, 1,1,1, trifluoroethane. Injury is due to idiosyncrasy.

Table 9–4. Some Occupations That Entail Exposure to Hepatotoxic Chemicals

Airplane dope makers	Lacquer makers and lacquerers
Airplane pilots (insecticide sprayers)	Leather workers
Airplane hangar employees	Linoleum makers
Artificial pearl makers	Lithographers
Burnishers	Paint remover makers and users
Cement (rubber, plastic) makers	Painters, paint makers
Cementers (rubber)	Paraffin workers
Chemical industry workers	Perfume makers
Chemists	Petroleum refiners
Chlorinated rubber makers	Pharmaceutical workers
Cobblers	Photographic material workers
Color makers	Polish (metal) makers and users
Degreasers	Printers
Dry cleaners	Pyroxylen-plastics workers
Dye makers	Rayon makers
Dyers	Refrigerator workers
Electric transformer and condenser makers	Resins (synthetic) makers
Electroplaters	Rubber workers
Enamel makers and enamelers	Scourers (metal)
Extractors, oil and fats	Shoe factory workers
Fillers (plastics)	Soap makers
Fire extinguisher makers	Spreaders (rubber works)
Galvanizers	Straw hat makers
Garage workers	Tapers (airplanes)
Gardeners (insecticides)	Thermometer makers
Gas (illuminating) workers	Tobacco denicotinizers
Glass (safety) makers	Varnish makers and users
Glue workers	Varnish removers
Ink makers	Waterproofers
Insecticide makers	Wax makers
Insulators (wire)	

From Zimmerman HJ: Hepatotoxicity: Adverse Effects of Drugs and Other Chemicals on the Liver. New York, Appleton-Century-Crofts, 1978, with permission of copyright holder.

chapter is concerned mainly with true hepatotoxins. Indeed, hepatic injury due to a medicinal agent is usually a therapeutic misadventure resulting from individual susceptibility (idiosyncrasy) (see Tables 9–18 to 9–21). Accordingly, most forms of drug-induced liver damage are not included in this discussion. Reference is made to the few drugs that, in overdose, do lead to important hepatic injury.

A large number of chemicals are found in the home as components of household products (Table 9–5) or as pesticides (Table 9–6). In addition, some of the agents encountered in industry (see Table 9–3) may find their way into the home. Chemicals used in industry or in research laboratories may be "borrowed" for use in the household.[3] The presence of these in the home, often in unlabeled containers and in the absence of the discipline of the occupational setting, may set the stage for accidental intoxication.

Household Products

The household products likely to contain hepatotoxic chemicals are those used for cleaning clothes and furniture and for paint removal. Chloroaliphatic solvents are the likely toxic agents (see Table 9–5). The chloroaliphatics used today, however, are less toxic than CCl_4, which was widely used in the past; they include ethylene dichloride, tetrachloroethylene, trichloroethylene, methyl chloroform, and methylene chloride.[3] Polishes for furniture, floors, and shoes are likely to contain nitrobenzene and antimony trichloride.[3] These agents have a potential for producing hepatic injury.[2] Despite the potential toxicity of some household products, the number of reported instances of serious hepatic injury attributable to them seems very low.

Pesticides

Little evidence shows that hepatic injury has occurred as a result of exposure to pesticides being used as such (Table 9–6). Organochlorine insecticides, herbicides,* fungicides, copper salts, or compounds of trivalent arsenic can lead to hepatic injury but only on ingestion. Indeed, ingestion of rodenticides containing phosphorus, by accident or with suicidal intent, has led to numerous instances of severe hepatic injury.[4] Rare instances of liver damage caused by accidental ingestion of rodenticides containing thallium or warfarin also have been recorded.[3] In general, however, acute hepatic injury due to pesticides, even as a result of ingestion, has been very rare.[1]

Rare instances of gross contamination of food or

*The herbicide 2,4,5-T is subject to regular contamination, during manufacture or processing, by the highly toxic chlorinated dibenzodioxins. It seems reasonable to ascribe the hepatotoxic effects of the herbicide to the contaminant.

Table 9–5. Household Products That Might Be Hepatotoxic

Product	Toxic Agent
Antifreeze	Chlorobenzene
Carburetor cleaner	Chlorobenzene
Christman tree lights (bubbling)	Methylene chloride
Dry-cleaning fluids	Chlorinated aliphatic compounds
Drugs hepatotoxic in overdose	Acetaminophen
	Aspirin
	Ethanol
	Ferrous salts
	Phenylbutazone
Furniture polishes and waxes	Antimony (trivalent)
	Nitrobenzene
	Cellosolve
Mothballs	Chlorobenzenes
Paint products	
Brush cleaners	Cresols
Paints	Arsenic (trivalent)
Plasticizers, lacquers, resins	Varied
Removers, paint, wax, etc.	Chlorinated aliphatic compounds
Pesticides	See Table 9–6
Plastic menders, greasers, plasticizers, glues	Ethylenedichloride, phthalates
Shoe cleaners	Aniline
	Nitrobenzene
Spray repellent	Vinyl chloride
Stamping inks	Phenol
Toilet bowl blocks	Paradichlorobenzene

Any unknown product should be considered potentially hepatotoxic, and all halogenated ones should be considered hepatotoxic until otherwise determined.

water[5] by pesticides have been described; however, for the most part, no recognized hepatic injury has resulted. Several reports have attributed chronic hepatic disease to toxic levels of trivalent arsenic in well water, however, presumably derived from use of arsenical insecticides.[5]

Hexachlorobenzene (HCB) in wheat was responsible for an epidemic of severe liver disease in Turkey more than 40 years ago. The hexachlorobenzene had been added as a fungicide to wheat intended for use as seed grain. Diversion of the seed grain to use as food led to ingestion of toxic amounts of hexachlorobenzene and the subsequent epidemic of a syndrome resembling porphyria cutanea tarda, accompanied by severe liver disease and characterized by a mortality rate exceeding 10%.[3]

Accidental contamination of food by industrial chemicals can lead to domestic hepatotoxicity. A prime example is the epidemic of cholestatic jaundice in Epping, England (Epping jaundice), caused by contamination of flour by a leaking container of 4,4′-diaminodiphenylmethane (methylenedianiline).[3] Similar injury by this chemical agent also has been occupationally acquired.[6] Somewhat similar to Epping jaundice but far more disastrous was the epidemic of the toxic oil syndrome in Spain caused by contaminated cooking oil.[7]

Polychlorinated biphenyls (PCBs) also have been implicated as causes of hepatic disease.[8, 9] Before and during World War II, serious subacute hepatic necrosis occurred in patients occupationally exposed to chloronaphthalene–chlorinated biphenyl mixtures. However, these agents, under ordinary circumstance, would not be found in the home except as components of electric appliances and household fixtures and as pollutants of food and water.[1] Although the hazard of hepatotoxicity from the general pollution of the food chain and water by PCBs is entirely speculative, specific contamination of food has been reported to lead to hepatic disease. Indeed, in 1968, hepatic disease developed in 11% of more than 1000 persons in Japan who had ingested food prepared in cooking oil contaminated with PCBs.[9*]

Contamination of animal feed with polybrominated biphenyls in Michigan several years ago was associated with appearance of minor hepatic injury in animals ingesting the feed and in human beings, presumably as a result of ingesting the contaminated meat.

Natural Hepatotoxins

A large number of botanic and microbiologic products are poisonous.[1, 3] Many include hepatic injury in their repertoire of toxic effects (Table 9–7). These are discussed in a subsequent section dealing with foods as hepatotoxins. Relevant to the hepatotoxic role of botanic products are the reports of hepatic injury resulting from herbal preparations taken as folk medicine or nutritional adjuncts[10–24] (Table 9–8).

MODES OF EXPOSURE

Exposure to hepatotoxins in the home may be by inhalation of a volatile agent. It also may be mediated by ingestion of the toxins as a result of ignorance, accident, or suicidal intent, or of food contaminated by toxic agents[1] (Table 9–9). Exposure also may be a byproduct of a form of drug abuse, such as solvent sniffing or even cocaine use (Table 9–10).

*Evidence suggests that the contaminating PCB mixture also contained small amounts of polychlorinated dibenzofurane. These chemicals, rather than the PCBs, may have been responsible for the disease.[1]

Table 9–6. Specific Uses of Various Potentially Hepatotoxic Pesticides

	Halogen Compounds	As	Cu	Dioxins*	P, Th, Warfarin
Fumigants	+	–	–	–	–
Fungicides	+	+	+	–	–
Herbicides	+	–	–	+	–
Insecticides	+	+	+	–	–
Rodenticides	–	+	–	–	+

As, inorganic arsenic derivatives; Cu, copper compounds; P, white allomorph of phosphorus; Th, thallium compounds.

*Dioxins present in herbicides as contaminants.

Table 9–7. Hepatotoxic Agents Found in Nature

	Relevance*		
	Experimental	*Human*	*Veterinary*
Plants			
Albitocin	+	−	+
Cycasin	+	+	−
Hypoglycin A	+	+	−
Icterogenin	+	−	+
Indospicine	+	−	+
Lantana	+	−	+
Mushrooms (amanitins,	+	+	−
phalloidins)	+	−	+
Ngaione	+	±	−
Nutmeg	+	+	+
Pyrrolizidine alkaloids	+	±	−
Safrole	+	+	+
Tannic acid			
Mycotoxins			
Aflatoxins	+	+	+
Cyclochloritine	+	±	+
Ethanol	+	+	−
Griseofulvin	+	±	−
Ipomeamarone	+	−	+
Luteoskyrin	+	±	+
Ochratoxin	+	±	+
Sporidesmin	+	±	+
Sterigmatocystin	+	+	−
Tetracycline	+	−	+

*Considered of human relevance if human hepatic injury has been attributed to the agent on the basis of evidence (+) or suspicion (±). Considered of veterinary relevance if disease in livestock is attributed to the agent.

The number of occupations that permit exposure to hepatotoxic agents is large. The list includes the manufacture of munitions, rubber, rocket fuels, cosmetics and perfumes, processed foods, paints, insecticides, herbicides, pharmaceuticals, and, of course, chemical products (see Table 9–4). The risk, however, is largely hypothetical, and little evidence today supports acute hepatic injury due to ordinary occupational exposure to hepatotoxic agents. Chronic hepatic injury, however, has been attributed to occupational exposure to toxic chemicals.[25] Evaluation of its extent, frequency, and importance awaits appropriate epidemiologic studies.

Careless Use or Accidental Ingestion of Toxic Agents

Many instances of poisoning from exposure to CCl_4 have resulted from the use of this volatile solvent as a dry-cleaning agent in a poorly ventilated room, particularly by alcoholics.[1] Alcohol potentiates the toxicity of CCl_4,[26] and drinkers are often careless with its use. Formerly a solvent with many domestic uses, this toxin is rarely found in the home today; yet its availability as an industrial and laboratory reagent may permit both occupational and household exposure.[1] Inadvertent ingestion of CCl_4 also has led to devastating hepatotoxic events. Alcoholic individuals have mistaken CCl_4 for a potable beverage.

Ingestion of various other toxic substances found in the home can occur. Large doses of chlorinated pesticides and fungicides are hepatotoxic for experimental animals, but hepatotoxic accidents from their ingestion by humans are rare. Nevertheless, instances of serious hepatic injury resulting from ingestion of DDT, chlordane, and paraquat have been reported.[3] Also, children have ingested other pesticides containing white phosphorus, thallium compounds, copper compounds, and warfarin.[3]

Suicide and Homicide by Hepatotoxic Agents

Homicide by poisoning is an ancient practice. History and fiction provide many examples of arsenic

Table 9–8. Herbal Products That Can Lead to Hepatic Injury

Herbal Product	Active Ingredient	Ostensible Effect	Hepatic Injury
Comfrey	PAs	Nutritional supplement	VOD
Gordolobo yerba tea	PAs	Health aid	VOD
Mate tea	PAs	Health aid	VOD
Chinese herb preparations			
Medicinal tea	?PAs*	Medicinal	VOD
Chinese herbs	?Glycerrhyza	Medicinal	Hepatitis
Jin Bu Auan	?Levotetrahydropalmitine	Anodyne hypnotic	Hepatitis, also microvesicular steatosis
Germander		Weight loss	Necrosis, zone 3
Chaparral leaf	Nordihydroguardtic acid	Medicinal	Necrosis, zone 3
Mistletoe (plus other herbs)		Health aid	Chronic hepatitis
Syo-saika-to (Xiau-Chai-Humtang)	?Scuylaria	Medicinal	Necrosis, steatosis
Margosa oil	Pulegone		Microvesicular steatosis
Pennyroyal oil	Pulegone Isopulegone	Abortifacient Also medicinal	Necrosis, microvesicular steatosis

VOD, veno-occlusive disease; PAs, pyrrolizidine alkaloids.
*The composition of this preparation is not clear. The entity is suggested in view of the character of the injury.

Table 9–9. Examples of Hepatotoxic Agents Encountered in the Home

Agents	Exposure	Lesion		
		Necrosis	*Fat*	*Other*
Toxic Chemicals				
Carbon tetrachloride and other haloaliphatics	Careless use Accident/suicide Sniffing	CZ	+	−
Phosphorus	Accident/suicide	PZ	4+	−
4,4′-Methylenedianiline	Food contamination (Epping jaundice)	−	−	Cholestasis
Rapeseed oil—aniline	Toxic oil syndrome	±	−	Cholestasis
Drugs				
Acetaminophen	Suicide/accident Therapeutic misadventure	CZ	−	−
Ferrous sulfate*	Accident	PZ	−	−
Phenylbutazone*	Accident	+	±	−
Drug Abuse	See Table 9–10			
Toxic Foods				
Mushrooms	Food	CZ	+	−
Pyrrolizidine alkaloids	Food	CZ	−	Veno-occlusive disease
Herbal preparations	Purported medicinal	+	+	See Table 9–8
Mycotoxins (aflatoxins)	Food	+	4+	Carcinoma

CZ, Centrizonal (zone 3); PZ, peripheral zone (zone 1).
*Ingestion of overdose by children.
†Ingestion of therapeutic doses leading to toxic effects.

poisoning.[3] Purposeful arsenic poisoning, however, is of more than historical interest; instances of deliberate poisoning still occur.[27] The dramatic clinical features of poisoning by inorganic arsenic, which include dementia, neuropathy, skin changes, myocarditis, and other systemic manifestations,[4] may overshadow the hepatic disease, but the liver damage can be an important part of the toxicity.

A major cause of hepatic injury in the home is attempted suicide. Most agents taken with suicidal intent are not hepatotoxic. Suicide by ingestion of white phosphorus, however, continues to be an important entity in some parts of the world. Indeed, 70% of cases of phosphorus poisoning are a result of deliberate suicidal intent; the remainder are a result of accidental ingestion, usually by children.[3]

Ingestion of large doses of acetaminophen is today a popular means of attempting suicide in Britain and to a lesser degree in other countries.[28–30] This agent, a weak and nontoxic analgesic and antipyretic in single therapeutic doses, becomes a potent hepatotoxin in large overdose.[28, 29] In patients with enhanced susceptibility (e.g., alcoholics), even modest, therapeutically intended doses may lead to hepatic injury.[30]

Table 9–10. Drug Abuse as Cause of Hepatic Injury*

Drug	Exposure	Necrosis	Lesion Fat
Chloroform	Sniffing	CZ	+
Cocaine	Abuse	+	+
Trichloroethylene	Sniffing	CZ	+
Perchloroethylene†	Sniffing	CZ	+
Halothane	Sniffing	CZ	−
Ethanol	Abuse	−	+
Toluene	Sniffing	−	±
MMDA	Abuse	+	−
Phencylidine	Abuse	+	−

CZ, Central zone (zone 3); MMDA, 5-methoxy-3,4 methylenedeoxymethamphetamine (street name "ecstasy").
*Effect of glue sniffing depends on solvents included.
†Potential for injury minor.

Abuse of Euphorogenic Hepatotoxic Agents

It has become increasingly clear that alcohol per se is a hepatotoxin. It is largely responsible for liver disease of alcoholics, perhaps abetted by the usual accompanying malnutrition. Other forms of drug abuse can lead to hepatic injury (see Table 9–9). Hepatic injury occurs in sniffers of trichlorethylene,[31] chloroform,[3] and even halothane.[32] The hepatic injury resembles that of CCl_4 poisoning. The demonstrations that cocaine is hepatotoxic for mice[3] and the report[33, 34] of hepatic disease in humans attributed to cocaine use suggests that cocaine should be added to the list of substances threatening the liver. Also, several hallucinogens including 5-methoxy-3,4-methylenedioxymethamphetamine (MMDA) (street name "ecstasy")[35] and phencyclidine[36] have led to hepatic injury (see Table 9–10).

Foods as Hepatotoxins

Natural Toxins as Food or Contaminants

Hepatotoxic mushrooms may be mistaken for edible ones. Also, poisonous plants of *Senecio, Heliotrop-*

ium, Crotolaria, and related genera may be eaten as contaminants of foods or as medicinal decoctions, because their toxic effects are not appreciated.[1] The unripened fruit of the *Blighia sapida* tree, on ingestion by Jamaican infants, leads to Jamaican vomiting sickness.[3] The fruit of the cycad tree, found on Guam, contains a potent hepatotoxin that also can lead to hepatic injury when eaten.[46] The most important of the natural hepatotoxins appears to be the mycotoxins, of which the aflatoxin group has attracted the greatest attention.[1]

Poisonous mushrooms and the fatalities they cause have been known since the 5th century B.C. Several hundred deaths per year are still attributable to these plants, especially in Europe.[37] Fatal mushroom poisoning is relatively rare in North America. Although there are many genera and thousands of species of mushrooms, the number of poisonous species is relatively small. Most fatal poisonings are due to the ingestion of *Amanita phalloides* or the closely related *A. verna* or *A. virosa*.[37]

Poisonous mushrooms remain a significant cause of hepatotoxicity in the home. The amount ingested need not be great. The content of toxin in *A. phalloides* is so great and the toxic peptides are so potent that a single mushroom has been estimated to contain a fatal dose.[37] The clinical syndrome is described in a later section of this chapter.

Pyrrolizidine alkaloids (PAs) also are important household hepatotoxins in some parts of the world.[38–43] More than 100 alkaloids have been identified in the more than 200 plants that have been studied.[38, 39] The total number of PA-bearing plants is about 10 times as great. The best-known genera are *Crotolaria, Heliotropium*, and *Senecio*. The hepatic injury produced by the PAs consists of centrizonal necrosis and damage to the small branches of the hepatic veins, producing a syndrome called *veno-occlusive disease* (VOD).[39, 40] The picture may be that of relatively acute or subacute hepatic failure, with ascites, slight jaundice, and a mortality rate of approximately 20%; or the syndrome may be one of prolonged chronic insufficiency with severe ascites.[2, 38–43] Although PA toxicity is far more likely to be encountered in the Third World, the toxic plants are found in many other areas.[38, 39] Indeed, cases have occurred in the United States, and it is clear that these hepatotoxins can be bought in some "natural food" stores.[44, 45]

Cycasin, found in the cycad nut, is a potent experimental hepatotoxin and hepatocarcinogen.[3] In chemical structure and in the effects on the liver of its aglycon, cycasin (methylazoxymethanol) resembles dimethylnitrosamine. Despite the known ingestion of cycad nuts by humans,[46] evidence that cycasin causes human liver disease has been scant, perhaps because the populations that eat cycad nuts have learned to process the fruit in a manner that removes the toxin.[3] Nevertheless, a report from Japan described a small epidemic of acute hepatic injury attributable to the ingestion of cycad nuts,[46] and this toxic plant warrants inclusion among the domestic hepatotoxins.

Hypoglycin A, a compound found in the unripened fruit (called *akee*) of the *B. sapida* tree in Jamaica, clearly warrants listing with the domestic hepatotoxins. Ingestion of the unripe fruit, especially if poorly cooked, leads to an acute fatty liver with severe hypoglycemia and a syndrome (Jamaican vomiting sickness) that can be fatal if untreated. This entity resembles Reye's syndrome. It seems particularly likely to occur in winter, when food is scarce.[47]

Tannic acid is a known experimental hepatotoxin, especially when administered parenterally.[1,3] Human toxicity has resulted from its use for the treatment of burns and, in barium sulfate suspensions, for colonic roentgenography.[1] Despite the toxicity of tannic acid when fed to experimental animals or when ingested by grazing livestock,[1] no evidence showed that oral intake of tannic acid had ever led to human disease until a report[3] described a patient whose eccentricity led to the ingestion of a half pound of tea every 3 to 4 days. These large amounts of dried tea were presumed to be responsible for the hepatic injury that she developed.[3]

Other botanic hepatotoxins are sufficiently numerous and potent to warrant the concern that yet unrecognized opportunities for human exposure may exist.[1] Safrole, hydroxysafrole, and isosafrole are hepatotoxic and, in large doses, hepatocarcinogenic for experimental animals.[48] Despite having been barred from use in soft drinks, safrole remains available in substances sold in natural food shops. Indeed, a large variety of herbal products sold in these shops contain botanic agents of diverse and obscure chemical nature, and rare reports describe some as being apparently hepatotoxic.[48]

Mycotoxins include a large number of compounds of diverse chemical nature (see Table 9–7) that are produced as metabolites by a number of different mycotic species.[1, 49] Many are known to cause hepatic injury in experimental animals, and some may possibly cause human liver disease. Instances of acute disease attributed to aflatoxins have been reported from several parts of the world. In Uganda, fatal hepatic necrosis occurred in a 15-year-old boy who was found to have eaten food with a very high content of aflatoxin.[50] Groups in Thailand,[51] New Zealand,[52] Czechoslovakia,[53] and the United States[54] have demonstrated aflatoxin in the livers of patients dying of Reye's syndrome, the lesions of which closely resemble the acute fatty liver produced in monkeys[55] and other animals[56] by aflatoxins. A report of 106 fatal instances of hepatic disease among 397 individuals who became ill after eating maize containing very large amounts of aflatoxin also suggests that acute aflatoxicosis can occur in human beings.[57]

Chronic disease is readily produced in experimental animals given food contaminated by aflatoxins.[1] Although it has been difficult to prove that humans develop chronic liver disease as a result of ingesting aflatoxin-contaminated food, epidemiologic studies have demonstrated a relationship between cirrhosis in humans and aflatoxin exposure and have provided convincing support that these agents are hepatocarcinogenic or cocarcinogenic for human beings.[58, 59] In general, the hazard of aflatoxin contamination of foods has seemed to apply particularly to tropical parts of the world.[3, 59] The aflatoxins are produced in grains, cereals, nuts, and rice under conditions of temperature and moisture provided best by the tropics. Evidence that aflatoxin contamination can occur even in temperate climates, however, is provided by reports of aflatoxin in the liver of a patient with Reye's syndrome in Minnesota[54] and of aflatoxin in corn harvested in Iowa.[3]

Chemical Contaminants of Foods

Toxic chemicals may be found in food as accidental contaminants.[1] Classic examples are the cases of cholestatic jaundice (Epping jaundice) that involved 84 people who had eaten bread baked from flour accidentally and heavily contaminated by *methylenedianiline (4,4'-diaminodiphenylmethane),*[3] the epidemic of Yusho that involved more than 1000 Japanese who had eaten rice prepared in oil contaminated by PCBs,[9] and the devastating epidemic of severe liver disease and toxic porphyria involving more than 3000 Turkish Kurds who had ingested wheat treated with the fungicide hexachlorobenzene.[3]

A dramatic example of the phenomenon is the epidemic toxic oil syndrome due to use of cooking oil containing rapeseed oil contaminated with aniline.[60] The hepatic injury of the toxic oil syndrome includes severe cholestatic disease as well as veno-occlusive injury. Extensive vascular lesions are also found in other organs. The mortality rate has been approximately 20%.

Nitrites and nitrates added to foods as preservatives have posed hypothetical hazards of potential hepatotoxicity and carcinogenicity.[3, 61] The potential toxicity of nitrites in foods was first noted as hepatic necrosis among sheep and mink that had been fed herring meal preserved with nitrite.[3] The hepatic injury was found to be due to dimethylnitrosamine, which had been formed by reaction of the nitrite with secondary amines in the fish. Subsequent studies have shown that nitrites may be present in plant food products as a result of enzymatic reduction of nitrates from the soil and in meat and fish products to which nitrites have been added as preservatives and colorants.[61] These may react with diethylamine and other alkylamines that occur in fish, fish meal, and other fish products; in cereals and tea; and in some drugs. The reaction can occur nonenzymatically at the acid pH of the gastric juice.[61] Formation of dimethylnitrosamine also can occur by reaction of nitrites with diethylamine produced by intestinal bacteria. Furthermore, some foods and alcoholic beverages have been found to contain measurable amounts of nitrosamines.[3] The magnitude of the human hazard of nitrites and nitrosamines in food and drink is unknown. Nevertheless, there is no doubt that dimethylnitrosamine and other nitrosamines are potent experimental hepatotoxins and carcinogens and that feeding nitrites and secondary amines as well as nitrite-preserved feed can produce hepatic injury in experimental animals.

Morphologic Types of Chemical Hepatic Injury

Chemical injury in human beings can lead to acute, subacute, or chronic hepatic disease (Table 9–11). A

Table 9–11. Morphologic Types of Toxic Hepatic Injury

Type of Injury	Agents
Acute	
Parenchymal	
Cytotoxic (cytolytic)	
Necrosis	
Zonal	CCl_4, ACM, MSH
Central (zone 3)	Ngaione, beryllium
Mid (zone 2)	Phosphorus, ferrous salts
Peripheral (zone 1)	Many drugs (see Table 9–20)
Nonzonal	Severe zonal or nonzonal
Massive	Many toxic agents and drugs
Degeneration, ballooning, apoptosis	
Steatosis	
Microvesicular	Aspirin, hypoglycin A, tetracycline
Macrovesicular	Ethanol
Cholestastic	See Tables 9–12 and 9–20.
Vascular (hepatic veins and branches)	
Hepatic venule injury (VOD)	Pyrrolizidine alkaloids
Peliosis hepatitis	Vinyl chloride, anabolic steroids
Subacute	
Subacute necrosis	Trinitrotoluene, tetrachloroethane
Subacute VOD	Pyrrolizidine alkaloids
Chronic	
Parenchymal	
Cirrhosis	
Macronodular	CCl_4
Micronodular	CCl_4, aflatoxin
Congestive (cardiac type)	Pyrrolizidine alkaloids
Biliary	Chlorpromazine and a few other drugs
Steatosis	Ethanol,* methotrexate
Neoplasm	
Carcinoma	
Hepatocellular	Aflatoxins, vinyl chloride, and many other chemicals
Cholangiocellular	Thorotrast
Adenoma	Anabolic and contraceptive steroids
Sarcoma	Dimethylnitrosamine
Angiosarcoma	Vinyl chloride, Thorotrast, inorganic arsenicals
Vascular	
Veno-occlusive	Pyrrolizine alkaloids
Peliosis hepatitis	Anabolic and contraceptive steroids, vinyl chloride†
Hepatic vein thrombosis	Contraceptive steroids
Granulomas	Copper sulfate–lime spray

CCl_4, carbon tetrachloride; ACM, acetaminophen; MSH, mushroom poisoning; VOD, veno-occlusive disease.

*Also leads to degenerative lesion called *alcoholic hyaline* or *Mallory's body.*

†Other agents (e.g., phalloidin) can produce lesions experimentally.

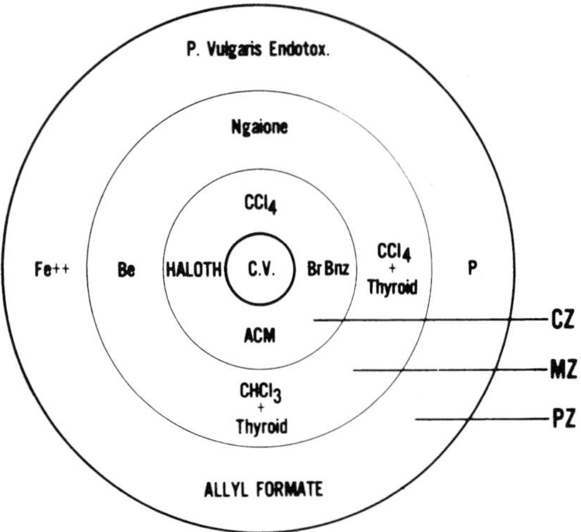

Figure 9–1. Types of zonal necrosis, containing examples of etiologic agents for each. ACM, acetaminophen; Be, beryllium; Br Bnz, bromobenzene; C.V. central vein; Fe^{++}, ferrous ion; HALOTH, halothane; P, white phosphorus; P. Vulgaris Endotox., *Proteus vulgaris* endotoxin; CZ, zone 3; MZ, zone 2; PZ, Zone 1. (From Zimmerman HJ: Hepatotoxicity. Adverse Effects of Drugs and Other Chemicals on the Liver. New York, Appleton-Century Crofts, 1978.)

single, relatively heavy exposure may lead to acute disease, while repeated exposure of lesser intensity may lead to subacute or chronic liver disease.

Acute

Chemical injury may be mainly cytotoxic (cytolytic), involving overt damage to hepatocytes, or mainly cholestatic, involving arrested bile flow (see Table 9–11). Some relationship exists between the type of hepatotoxin and the form of injury. Most true toxins produce mainly cytotoxic injury; only a few produce mainly cholestatic injury. Many of the drugs that produce hepatic damage in humans as an idiosyncratic reaction produce mainly cholestatic injury, others produce cytotoxic injury, and some produce a mixed pattern (see Tables 9–18 to 9–21).

Cytotoxic Injury. This includes degeneration, necrosis, and steatosis of hepatocytes. Necrosis may be zonal or diffuse. That produced by true toxins is often zonal (Fig. 9–1), whereas the necrosis due to idiosyncrasy-dependent hepatic injury in most instances is not zonal. The zonal necrosis produced by some hepatotoxins is in the central zone (zone 3) of the lobule; fewer agents lead to peripheral zone (zone 1) necrosis. Midzonal (zone 2) necrosis is most uncommon. The necrosis produced by CCl_4, acetaminophen, mushroom poisoning, and many other toxins is centrizonal; that produced by phosphorus and ferrous salts is in the peripheral zone.

The zonality appears to be related to the mechanism of injury. The centrizonal necrosis produced by CCl_4 (Fig. 9–2) and acetaminophen, for example, appears to be a consequence of the centrizonal concentration of cytochrome P-450, the enzyme system responsible for conversion of these agents to hepatotoxic metabolites. The necrosis in the peripheral zone produced by allyl formate has been attributed to the location in that zone of the enzyme system that converts the compound to its toxic metabolites.[3] The basis for the peripheral zone necrosis of phosphorus and ferrous salts is not clear.

Steatosis can be produced by a large number of toxic agents. Two main types can occur. Some agents (e.g., tetracycline, hypoglycin A) produce microvesicular steatosis—that is, the droplets are small, there are many in each hepatocyte, and the nucleus remains in the center of the cell. Other substances

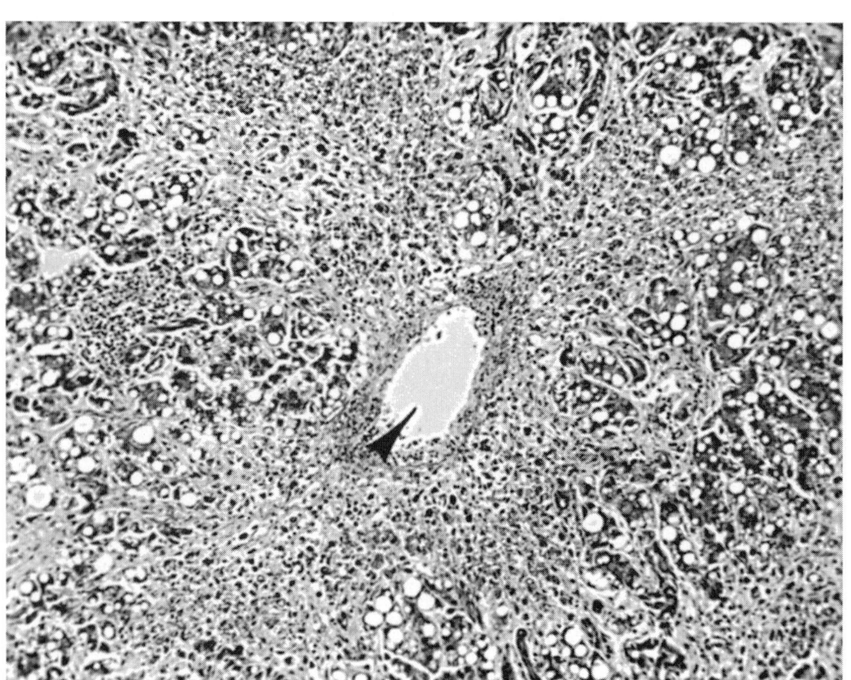

Figure 9–2. Fatal centrizonal necrosis in carbon tetrachloride poisoning. *Arrow* in central vein. (Courtesy of Dr. Kamal G. Ishak, Armed Forces Institute of Pathology.)

(e.g., ethanol, methotrexate) lead to macrovesicular steatosis: Individual large fat droplets within each cell displace the nucleus to the periphery.

Necrosis and *steatosis* constitute the lesion produced by some agents. With some (e.g., CCl_4), the necrosis is more prominent; with others (e.g., toxic mushrooms, phosphorus), the steatosis stands out more.

Cholestatic Injury. Some agents lead to hepatic injury characterized mainly by arrested bile flow with little or no parenchymal damage. This is particularly true of some drugs, but cholestasis-producing chemicals can also be found among natural hepatotoxins, among synthetic industrial compounds, and even among the secondary bile acids (Table 9–12).

Chronic

The forms of chronic hepatic disease attributable to chemical injury are listed in Table 9–11. A few warrant special comment.

Cirrhosis. Chronic or repeated chemical injury can lead to necrosis, fibrosis, nodular regeneration, and the pseudolobule development that produces the distortion of hepatic architecture that is cirrhosis. It may be a consequence of prolonged and repeated parenchymal injury, a result of subacute hepatic necrosis, or, rarely, a sequel to a single episode of necrosis. In general, a single bout of zonal necrosis in experimental animals (e.g., CCl_4 poisoning), even when extensive, is followed by complete histologic restitution in surviving animals, and cirrhosis does not develop. Given repeatedly to experimental animals at intervals too short to permit recovery from each dose, CCl_4 can lead to cirrhosis.[3] Long-term occupational exposure has been incriminated in the causation of cirrhosis.[25]

Some of the toxic agents that can lead to experimental cirrhosis are listed in Table 9–13. Among them are toxins to which there has been human exposure. Nevertheless, relatively few convincing examples of chemical poisoning have led to human cirrhosis. Drug-induced idiosyncratic hepatic injury that apparently can lead to cirrhosis is identified in Tables 9–18 to 9–21, later in this chapter.

Hepatoportal Sclerosis. Hepatoportal sclerosis is a curious portal and periportal fibrosis and deposition of collagen in the space of Disse, with occlusion of branches of the portal veins and consequent portal hypertension.[3] It has been attributed to prolonged exposure to inorganic compounds of arsenic[62] and to vinyl chloride.[3] Also referred to as *noncirrhotic portal hypertension*, it consists of portal and periportal fibrosis, as seen by light microscopy, and of collagen fibrils in the space of Disse, as seen by electron microscopy. This curious deposition of fibrous material is held accountable for the development of portal hypertension. The lesion leads to no clinical manifestations until the varices, collateral venous pattern, and splenomegaly become evident. Other forms of noncirrhotic portal hypertension include fibrosis in zone 3 as a result of the toxic effects of prolonged

Table 9–13. Toxic Agents Known to Cause Cirrhosis in Experimental Animals

Aflatoxins	Manganese
Arsenicals	Mushroom toxins
Azocompounds	Nitrosamines
Bromobenzene	Pyridine
Carbutamide	Pyrrolizidine alkaloids
Cadmium	Safrole
Carbon tetrachloride	Selenium
Chlorinated biphenyls	Stilbamidine
Chloronaphthalene	Tetrachloroethane
DDT	Thioacetamide
Dioxins	Thorotrast
Ethionine	Trinitrotoluene
Galactosamien	Trypan blue
Indospicine	Vinyl chloride

Table 9–12. Agents That Cause Cholestasis

	Cholestatic Effect				
	Experimental	*Grazing Animals*	*Occupational*	*Drug*	**Comments**
Intrinsic hepatotoxin					
Natural					
Bile acids	+	–	–	–	Especially lithocholate
Cytochalasin B	+	–	–	–	
Endotoxins	+	–	–		?Responsible for jaundice in neonates with infection
Icterogenin	+	+	–	–	
Rifampicin	+	–	–	+	Acts at both sites
Sporidesmin	+	+	–	–	In some species
Synthetic					
α-Naphthylisothiocyanate	+	–	–	–	
4,4′-Diaminodiphenylmethane	+	–	+	–	Cause of Epping jaundice
Paraquat	–	–	+	–	
Steroids					
C-17 anabolic	+	–	–	+	
Oral contraceptive	+	–	–	+	
Rapeseed oil and aniline	+	–	–	–	Cause of toxic oil syndrome in Spain

intake of large overdoses of vitamin A[63] and partial nodular transformation of the liver.[64]

Veno-Occlusive Disease. A form of chronic hepatic disease resembling the hepatic change of prolonged right heart failure (cardiac cirrhosis) results from ingestion of PAs. These agents can lead to central necrosis and occlusion of hepatic venules, hence the designation VOD.[38–41] A similar lesion has been produced by reactions to several drugs used in cancer chemotherapy and immunosuppressive treatment and by radiation injury (radiation hepatitis). Thrombosis of the hepatic veins, which leads to a somewhat similar histologic picture, can result from the thrombogenic effect of the estrogenic component of oral contraceptives. This lesion and VOD can lead to the Budd-Chiari syndrome.[1] The syndrome may present as acute disease with abdominal pain, acutely evolving ascites and edema, mild jaundice, and aminotransferase levels sufficiently high to reflect necrosis; or it may present as chronic disease resembling cardiac cirrhosis with severe ascites, edema, and portal hypertension.

Peliosis Hepatis. This curious lesion consists of blood-filled lacunae of various sizes. It appears as a complication of the administration of anabolic and contraceptive steroids[65] and after prolonged occupational exposure to vinyl chloride.[3] It also has been produced in experimental animals by administration of lasiocarpine and phalloidin. The lesion has been ascribed to injury of sinusoidal supporting membranes.[3]

Syndrome of Toxic Hepatic Injury

Acute

Liver disease, often accompanied by renal failure, dominates the syndrome of poisoning caused by some agents (Table 9–14). In the syndrome produced by others, the hepatic injury may be only one facet of systemic injury (Table 9–15). The acute injury produced by most agents is hepatocellular in character.

Acute hepatic failure, usually accompanied by renal failure, is the dominant feature of poisoning due to chlorinated hydrocarbons, white phosphorus, and poisonous mushrooms (see Table 9–14). It is usually preceded by neurologic and gastrointestinal (GI) manifestations. The syndrome of acetaminophen poisoning is similar, but the hepatic failure is not preceded by the neurologic manifestation associated with the other three toxic agents.[1]

Severe hepatic injury results from the intake of toxic doses of iron and copper compounds also. However, the liver damage is usually only one facet, although a serious one, of the total systemic toxicity.

Significant hepatic injury, as part of a syndrome that is dominated by the extrahepatic manifestations of toxicity, is caused by a number of other toxic

Table 9–15. Relative Importance of Hepatic Injury in Several Forms of Acute Toxicity

Toxicity manifested chiefly with or without renal injury
Carbon tetrachloride and other chlorinated hydrocarbons
Phosphorus (white)
Mushroom, mycotoxins, cycasin, others; natural toxins
Acetaminophen
Ferrous and copper salts in high doses
Toxicity manifested by systemic effects with hepatic injury only one facet
Arsenic (inorganic)
Thallium salts
Insecticides
Hypoglycin A
Borates

Table 9–14. Salient Features of Syndromes of Acute Toxic Hepatic Injury*

	Carbon Tetrachloride	Phosphorus	Toxic Mushrooms	Acetaminophen
Phase I (first 24h)				
Diarrhea	+	+†	−	−
Vomiting	±	+†	+	±
Pain	±	+	−	−
Hemorrhage	−	+	−	−
Shock	−	+	±	±
Phase II (24–72h)				
"Asymptomatic" period	−	+	+	+
Jaundice	+	−	−	−
Renal	±	±	+	−
Central nervous system	−	−	+	−
Phase III (48–72h)				
Hepatic failure	+	+	+	+
Jaundice	4+	4+	4+	+
Renal failure	+	+	+	±
Hemorrhagic phenomena	+	+	+	+
Hepatic lesion—fat	+	4+	4+	±
Necrosis	Zone 3	Zone 1	Zone 3	Zone 3
Death	10–20%	30–40%	50%	15%

*Similar syndrome produced by ferrous and copper salts. Copper sulfate toxicity leads to zone 3 (centrizonal) necrosis. Ferrous salts lead to zone 1 (peripheral zone) necrosis.
†Phosphorescent appearance and garlic odor to vomitus and feces.
From Zimmerman HJ: Hepatotoxicity: Adverse Effects of Drugs and Other Chemicals on the Liver. New York, Appleton-Century-Crofts, 1978.

agents. Thallium poisoning, for example, leads to severe hepatic steatosis, but the manifestations of the liver injury are overshadowed by neurologic and systemic features of the poisoning. This is also true of the fatty liver resulting from borate poisoning.[3]

A form of hepatic injury resembling that of Reye's syndrome may be caused by toxic agents.[3] Reye's syndrome is a curious, acute illness of children characterized by microvecular hepatic steatosis and encephalopathy. It is usually considered to be caused by a virus or by the interaction of viral infections and a chemical toxin. Nevertheless, a similar hepatic lesion is produced by some toxic agents—for example, parenteral tetracycline,[1] hypoglycin A,[47] dimethylformamide,[66] and cocaine.[34] Most important is the evidence that aspirin in large doses[67] or even in the therapeutic doses given to children with acute viral illness[68] may precipitate Reye's syndrome.

Acute cholestatic jaundice is a rare manifestation of poisoning (see Table 9–12), although it is a characteristic syndrome resulting from the adverse effects of some medicinal agents (see Table 9–21). The foregoing material has described the production of cholestatic injury by 4,4′-diaminodiphenylmethane (methylenedianiline), as a contaminant of bread[3] or by occupational exposure[6, 7]; by poisonous intake of paraquat, and by the mixture of rapeseed oil and aniline (toxic oil syndrome).[60]

SPECIAL SYNDROME OF HEPATOTOXICITY

Acute Hepatic and Renal Failure

Carbon Tetrachloride Poisoning

Three quarters of a century ago, the usual setting for CCl_4 poisoning was the hepatic injury induced by use of the agent as a vermifuge. Since abandonment of the practice, almost all cases have resulted from industrial or domestic accidents.[25, 69] Exclusion of this solvent from most of its former industrial uses, increased caution in its use, and removal of it from the list of readily available household cleaning agents have minimized opportunities for exposure to this toxin.[69] Nevertheless, instances of toxicity continue to be reported.[69]

Exposure in industry to acute intoxicating doses has occurred by inhalation, as in the cleaning of large vats without proper aeration or as a result of exposure of heavy fumes in other closed settings. In the home, ingestion by mistake and inhalation in a poorly ventilated small room have been the common modes of intoxication.[1, 25, 69]

Most instances of CCl_4 poisoning have occurred in alcoholic individuals, who are more vulnerable than others to the toxic effects of this agent and are likely to be more careless with its use.[25, 26, 69] Alcoholic persons exposed to an atmospheric concentration that led to no apparent hepatic injury in simultaneously exposed nonalcoholic individuals have been severely poisoned. Ingestion of CCl_4, mistaken for a potable beverage, has led to instances of hepatic injury in alcoholic individuals. Persons who are not alcoholic, although less likely to develop CCl_4 hepatotoxicity, are not immune.

Histopathology. Centrizonal (zone 3) hepatic necrosis is characteristic (see Fig. 9–2). Necrosis of renal tubular epithelium is also usual. The lungs usually show edema, an alveolar pseudomembrane, and thickened fibrotic alveolar walls with epithelial cell proliferation, perhaps secondary to renal failure rather than to CCl_4 per se.[3] "Focal pancreatitis" similar to that noted in association with other forms of renal failure also has been observed in fatal CCl_4 poisoning, but true pancreatitis also occurs.[69]

Clinical Features. The syndrome consists of hepatic and renal failure, usually preceded by transitory neurologic and GI symptoms, and in some patients is complicated in the late phases by cardiac failure and pulmonary edema. Immediately after exposure to the agent, dizziness, headache, visual disturbances, and confusion are usual, reflecting the anesthetic properties of haloalkanes.[1, 25, 69] Indeed, a small proportion of deaths due to CCl_4 poisoning are "anesthetic" deaths.[3] Nausea, vomiting, abdominal pain, and diarrhea also occur during the first 24 hours, especially after ingestion of the toxin; to a lesser degree they may also occur after inhalation. Both neurologic and GI symptoms, however, may be mistaken for symptoms of the acute and chronic alcoholism so frequent in victims of CCl_4 poisoning.

Evidence of hepatic disease usually follows the exposure by 2 to 4 days but may be observed as early as 24 hours. Jaundice develops in about half of the cases of poisoning. Severely affected patients develop ascites and hepatic coma, often accompanied by hemorrhagic phenomena. The jaundice is hepatocellular in type and usually rapid in its evolution. The rapidity of increase of the bilirubin levels probably reflects both rapid progression of hepatic injury and loss of excretory function. Increased production of bilirubin by hemolysis and perhaps by destruction of cytochrome P-450 also might contribute to the hyperbilirubinemia.[3] It is probable that the renal injury induced by this toxin also contributes to the rapid intensification of the depth of jaundice by interference with renal excretion of the bilirubin.

Renal failure usually begins a few days after the hepatic damage is manifested and reaches a peak in the second week. It may be heralded by the oliguria that is usually noted between the second and fourth days after exposure, presumably mainly of prerenal origin. Continued oliguria or anuria beyond the early phase and mounting azotemia during the first and second weeks indicate the presence of tubular necrosis. Renal failure has been the cause of death in a majority of fatal cases.[1, 25]

Pulmonary edema is observed in most patients who survive for more than 1 week. Cardiac failure, which occurs in the second week or later, has been ascribed to the administration of excess amounts of fluid in the treatment of azotemia and to the sodium retention incident to the renal failure. Nevertheless, toxic effects of CCl_4 on the myocardium may be inferred from the tendency of early acute poisoning to produce ventricular arrhythmias and might contribute to the heart failure.[3]

Laboratory Features. Anemia is common, and a moderate degree of neutrophilic leukocytosis is usual.[3] The urine usually contains protein, erythrocytes, leukocytes, and epithelial cells, as well as hyaline, epithelial, granular, or rarely even red blood cell casts. The levels of blood urea nitrogen (BUN) and total nonprotein nitrogen (NPN) may be elevated early in the episode as a manifestation of extrarenal azotemia secondary to nausea, vomiting, and dehydration or of early renal tubular necrosis. Toward the end of the first week, frank azotemia secondary to tubular necrosis develops. Although the BUN, NPN, and creatinine levels all are elevated, the severe liver damage may lead to a disproportionately modest degree of elevation of BUN relative to the level of NPN and creatinine.[1]

Biochemical manifestations of hepatic injury include striking elevation of a number of serum enzymes. Serum levels of aspartate aminotransferase (AST) (glutamic-oxaloacetic transaminase [GOT]) may be increased 50- to 500-fold,[1] and an instance of a 700-fold elevation to 27,000 Karmen units has been reported.[70] Values for alanine aminotransferase (ALT) (glutamate pyruvate transaminase [GPT]) and a number of other enzymes also reach very high levels.[1] Values for alkaline phosphatase are elevated to only a modest degree. Evidence of impaired coagulation includes hypoprothrombinemia as well as decreased levels of plasma clotting factors. Evidence suggests increased fibrinolysis in experimental CCl_4 toxicity.[3]

Prognosis. Before the era of hemodialysis, the case fatality rate could be estimated to be approximately 25%.[1] In about one fourth of the fatal cases, patients had died in hepatic failure, usually during the first or early part of the second week of illness, and about three fourths had died in renal failure, usually during the second week or later.[3] The current availability of hemodialysis has improved the outlook for patients with severe renal failure.[68]

Treatment. Management is mainly supportive, as in other forms of acute hepatic failure. Careful attention to fluid and electrolyte balance, attending to dehydration during the first day or two, and judicious replenishment thereafter, with care to avoid overloading with fluids, is important. Repeated small feedings rich in carbohydrate provide a means of maintaining caloric intake. If azotemia is slight or absent, a standard intake of protein (1 g/kg) seems permissible. It is wise to restrict protein, however, in patients with mounting azotemia. An elevated BUN value beyond the fourth day seems a reasonable basis for reduction of protein intake to 0.25 g/kg per 24 hours if hemodialysis is not available. Reduction of protein also is in order, of course, if asterixis or other evidence of hepatic encephalopathy develops. If available, alternate-day hemodialysis should be substituted for the protein restriction unless the latter seems required for the management of hepatic encephalopathy.

Other Haloaliphatic Compounds

A number of other chlorinated, brominated, and iodinated aliphatic hydrocarbons, depending on their structure, can induce similar hepatic injury and the same syndrome after sufficiently heavy, acute exposure[1] (Table 9–16). Trichloroethylene, as a result of accidental industrial exposure[3] or sniffing,[24] can lead to a similar syndrome—usually of lesser severity than that due to CCl_4. Chloroform toxicity, formerly an iatrogenic disease and now a potential laboratory accident or due to deliberate chloroform sniffing, also leads to a similar syndrome on accidental ingestion or inhalation.[1] Carbon tetrabromide has been reported to produce a syndrome similar to that of CCl_4 poisoning as a result of exposure in the laboratory. Tetrachloroethane (TCE), a potent occupational hepatotoxin, in the past has caused subacute hepatic disease in industrially exposed humans. Ingestion or inhalation of high concentration, however, leads to acute disease similar to that induced by CCl_4.[3]

Phosphorus Poisoning

Phosphorus poisoning is relatively rare today.[1] Large groups of cases, however, have been reported from Latin America and elsewhere. Before the use of white phosphorus as a constituent of firecrackers and matches was outlawed in 1942, poisoning was much more common. Cases that have occurred since then have been a result of ingestion of rat or roach poison or firecracker contents, by accident or with suicidal intent.[71, 72] Despite its relative infrequency, phosphorus poisoning remains an important form of intoxication as one of the classic syndromes of hepatotoxicity with a high (>50%) mortality.[1]

Histopathology. The characteristic lesion is steatosis. It may involve the entire lobule but begins or is most prominent in the periportal area (zone 1). Necrosis, which usually accompanies the steatosis, is also most prominent in zone 1. Renal tubular necrosis is regularly noted in fatal cases. Droplets of fat also engorge the renal tubules that have not undergone necrosis and are also found in the myocardium.[1]

Clinical Features. The clinical picture has been

Table 9–16. Relative Estimated Toxicity of Haloaliphatic Compounds

Compound	Toxicity
Tetrachlorethane	4+
Carbon tetrachloride	4+
Chloroform	2+
1,1,2-Trichlorethane	1–2+
1,1,1-Trichlorethane	±
Dichloromethane	±
Methyl chloride	–

4+, Maximum hepatotoxic potential among agents listed; ±, minor hepatic injury.

characterized[73] as consisting of three stages (see Table 9–14). An immediate acute toxic stage that consists of severe GI and neurologic symptoms, often accompanied by vascular collapse, is followed by the second stage (a symptom-free period). The third stage is characterized by hepatic and renal failure and serious neurologic abnormalities.

The *first stage* reflects the immediate, severe, irritative effects of phosphorus on the GI tract. Nausea, vomiting, abdominal pain, and at times diarrhea dominate the picture. Hematemesis occurs in about 30% of patients, a reflection of acute gastric and duodenal ulceration. Thirst is extreme; shock, convulsions, and coma are frequent. The vomitus and feces are characteristically phosphorescent and have a strong odor of garlic, an odor that may also be detected on the breath; the feces may emit a vapor resembling smoke (the "smoking stool syndrome").[73] This acute phase is brief, with a duration of 8 to 24 hours. Approximately one fourth of the patients die during this stage.[73] About one third recover; the remainder go on to the third stage with or without going through the second, "asymptomatic" stage.

The *second stage* classically has been described as a symptom-free or latent period of 1 to 3 days.[4] Some investigators, however, have emphasized the merging of the first with the third stage and have minimized the benign aspects of the asymptomatic stage.[4]

The *third stage* is characterized by hepatic failure, renal insufficiency, and recurrent involvement of the central nervous system. Jaundice occurs in the majority of patients who reach this stage. In most reported cases, the jaundice becomes apparent between 3 and 5 days after poisoning. It is usually preceded by rapidly increasing hepatomegaly. Renal failure may be noted as early as the first or as late as the fourth day after ingestion of the toxin.[3]

Restlessness, delirium, and toxic psychosis occur during the first stage and often progress to coma. Indeed, this is the usual sequence in the 25% of patients who die early in the course. Early coma apparently reflects the neurotoxicity of phosphorus; that which occurs later results from the hepatorenal failure.

Laboratory Features. The jaundice of phosphorus poisoning is hepatocellular in type. The urine contains bilirubin and urobilinogen and has been said to show leucine and tyrosine crystals. The leukocyte level is normal or low, and anemia is not usual.[4]

Serum enzyme levels are only moderately elevated.[1] In experimental poisoning, values for the serum AST (GOT) and ALT (GPT) levels are usually elevated only two- to sixfold.[74] Higher values may be noted, but they are usually far lower than those in severe CCl_4 poisoning. The development of shock presumably accounts for higher levels in some patients. Abnormal coagulation parameters and a hemorrhagic tendency are usual.

Diagnosis. The diagnosis is based on a history of ingestion of roach powder, rat poison, firecracker contents, or other material containing white phosphorus. Phosphorescence of the vomitus and stools and the garlic odor of these and the breath provide diagnostic clues. These clues, in a patient with hepatic and renal failure preceded by violent GI complaints, may lead to the diagnosis when the history has been incomplete.

Prognosis. Large doses of phosphorus, ingestion of the poison in a liquid medium, and late treatment appear to be associated with a high mortality. A mortality of 15% has been recorded for patients who had ingested less than 0.8 g and of more than 90% for those who had taken 1.5 g or more. Ingestion of phosphorus without liquid has been reported to lead to a lower mortality rate (25%) than that associated with ingestion of the agent in water, rum, beer, or wine (50% to 90%). In general, jaundice, azotemia, shock, and convulsions early in the course appear to augur a poor prognosis.[73]

Treatment. The most important aspect of management is early (within 1 hour) gavage; this has appeared to decrease the mortality rate. The use of potassium permanganate to convert the elemental phosphorus to harmless oxidation products has been recommended on theoretic grounds,[71] but there is scant evidence of benefit. Hepatic and renal failure probably should be treated in a manner similar to that recommended for CCl_4 poisoning. Glucocorticoid therapy seems to be of no value.[72] Exchange transfusion has been credited with benefit.[3] Extracorporeal perfusion using a charcoal column, accordingly, might help.

Mushroom Poisoning

The poisonous *A. phalloides* mushroom and related species produce hepatic and renal failure. This form of mushroom poisoning has been called *mycetismus choleriformis* to distinguish it from *mycetismus nervosus*, the muscarine poisoning due to *Amanita muscaria*. The latter produces no hepatic lesions.[29]

Hepatotoxic mushroom poisoning in the United States is usually a result of ingestion of *A. verna* (or *A. virosa*), whereas in Europe it is usually the result of ingestion of *A. phalloides*.[1, 37, 38] The responsible mushroom, which grows in all parts of the country, may be found from early June until the first frost. Young forms, which are the most poisonous, are also most likely to be mistaken for edible mushrooms.[3] The toxicity results from the presence in the mushroom of thermostable toxins (amatoxins and phallotoxins). These substances together produce a syndrome of hepatorenal failure that somewhat resembles that caused by CCl_4 and white phosphorus (see Table 9–14).

Histopathology. The hepatic lesion produced by mushroom poisoning is steatosis and centrizonal (zone 3) necrosis. Degenerative changes of the GI tract, kidneys, heart, and central nervous system also occur.[25, 75] Fatal cases often show severe steatosis and variable degrees of necrosis.[75] The relative degree of hepatic fat and necrosis seems to vary from case to case. Necrosis without steatosis has been found in biopsy specimens from nonfatal cases, and it has been suggested that the necrosis and steatosis are of independent pathogenesis. Indeed, in experimental animals, phallotoxins produce only necrosis and amatoxins cause mainly steatosis. The reasonable hypothesis that balance between necrosis and steatosis, accordingly, might be governed by the relative roles played by the two toxins is belied by the evidence that phalloidin is not absorbed from the GI tract.[3]

Clinical Features. The syndrome consists of extremely severe GI symptoms, neurologic abnormalities, and collapse, usually followed by jaundice and renal failure (see Table 9–14). A latent period of 6 to 20 hours after ingestion of the poisonous mushrooms precedes the first symptoms. Severe spasm and abdominal pain, vomiting (at times blood streaked), and diarrhea, follow thereafter. These symptoms usually are promptly followed by cyanosis and shock. Within 1 or 2 days, hepatocellular jaundice and azotemia are noted. Central nervous system damage, as indicated by confusion, delirium, coma, and convulsions, may occur during the first 3 days after ingestion.[37] Electrocardiographic evidence of myocardial involvement may include bundle branch block and premature ventricular beats.[3]

Laboratory Features. Anemia, presumably hemolytic, may occur, or it may be obscured by the extreme dehydration. The biochemical reflections of the liver damage resemble those of CCl_4 poisoning. Aminotransferase values are strikingly elevated, as much as 500 times normal in some patients,[1, 75] and are only modestly elevated in others. Hyperbilirubinemia is characteristic. The coagulation abnormalities have attracted considerable attention.[75] A reduction of the prothrombin complex to less than 30% has an adverse prognostic significance, but even patients with these values may recover. Levels below 10% usually augur a fatal outcome.[76] The suggestion that disseminated intravascular coagulation is an important part of the syndrome is controversial.

Prognosis. The outlook is poor but not as grim as previous estimates. Thirty to 90% of the patients in the series reported a quarter century ago died.[75] Current figures are 10% to 25%.[37] Death within 4 to 8 days results from hepatic failure, severe dehydration and collapse, or central nervous system complications. Death may occur during the first 48 hours as a result of the choleriform diarrhea.[37] Children younger than 10 years appear to have a higher case fatality than adults.

Treatment. The management is similar to that of other forms of acute hepatorenal failure. During the first 1 to 2 days, adequate diuresis should be maintained (if renal function is normal) and emesis should be induced.[76, 77] Activated charcoal should be given hourly to prevent absorption of ingested toxins undergoing enterohepatic circulation. Also insertion of a duodenal take or even cannulation of the common bile duct to aspirate toxin excreted in the bile may be helpful in severe poisoning.[76, 77] As renal failure evolves, carefully limited fluid and electrolyte replacement and restriction of protein intake are in order. Renal failure may require treatment with hemodialysis or peritioneal dialysis. Impressions of benefit from glucocorticoid therapy are controversial,[3] although experimental lysosomal injury by phalloidin can be blunted by hydrocortisone.[3] Early hemodialysis or hemoperfusion has been suggested as treatment for removal of the circulating toxins (see Chapter 10). However, measurement of levels of toxins in the blood suggests that dialysis would be of little benefit.[78]

A number of studies have reported that administration of cytochrome C, thioctic acid, or an antitoxin principle from milk thistle (silybin, formerly silymarin) after ingestion of mushroom toxins can prevent or ameliorate the hepatotoxic syndrome in animals. These have been recommended for human use, but the claims have not been substantiated.[79] Huge doses of penicillins (40 million units/d) have been reported to be of benefit.[79]

Acetaminophen Toxicity

Acetaminophen poisoning is discussed in Chapter 49. The hepatic injury and the clinical syndrome of acute acetaminophen poisoning resemble somewhat those of CCl_4, phosphorus, and hepatotoxic mushroom poisoning, in that they also have three phases (see Table 9–14). The first consists of the acute GI symptoms of the irritative effects of the large dose of drug. In the second, the symptoms abate. The third is marked by overt hepatic injury.[1]

Most published instances of acetaminophen-induced hepatic injury are a result of a single intake of a large overdose.[28, 29] In 80% of cases, the individual has taken at least 15 g of the drug; in most of the remainder, 6 to 15 g.[80] A number of instances have now been reported, however, in which doses in the therapeutic range (2.5 to 4 g/24 h) have appeared to produce hepatic injury in patients whose susceptibility was enhanced by alcoholism, fasting, or other factors.[30]

Iron Salts

Acute hepatic necrosis can result from ingestion of large amounts of ferrous sulfate.[4] Indeed, accidental intake of ferrous sulfate tablets has been one of the most frequent causes of poisoning in children. The resulting syndrome resembles that described for CCl_4, phosphorus, mushroom, and acetaminophen poisoning, in that three phases are noted. Shortly after ingestion, evidence of severe GI injury is noted, with nausea, vomiting, diarrhea, and, often, melena. Shock is frequent. Usually, if the patient does not die during this phase, symptoms may abate for a short period (phase 2), followed within 1 to 3 days by the third phase in which evidence of hepatic injury, jaundice, elevated aminotransferase levels, and striking hypoprothrombinemia appear.

The necrosis is periportal. Striking degrees of hyperferremia are observed, and a heavy tissue overload of iron would be expected. Accordingly, it is curious that some fatal cases may show little or no iron in the liver by staining.

Treatment consists of efforts to remove iron from the stomach by gavage and from the tissues by intravenous administration of the chelator deferoxamine. In addition, the supportive measures for hepatic failure already described should be followed.

Copper Poisoning

The clinical features of copper poisoning[81, 82] are similar to those of ferrous sulfate overdose. Ingestion of toxic amounts (1 to 10 g) by infants and children is usually accidental; in adults, it may be with suicidal intent. Hepatotoxic effects also have been ascribed to the absorption of copper ion from sites of local application of cupric sulfate as an astringent antiseptic.[83]

Copper salts produce GI erosions, centrizonal hepatic necrosis, and renal tubular necrosis. Jaundice is a result of the hepatic injury, enhanced by the hemolysis produced by high blood copper levels.

The course resembles that of the other forms of acute hepatorenal failure (see Table 9–14). Severe nausea, vomiting, diarrhea, and abdominal pain, accompanied by a metallic taste, characterize the first few hours after ingestion. During this phase, shock may develop. Hepatic injury is manifested by jaundice, high aminotransferase levels, and hepatomegaly by the second or third day after ingestion.

Treatment is directed at removing excess copper and providing support. Penicillamine, the chelator used to treat the copper overload of Wilson's disease, has been credited with benefit in enhancing copper excretion and leading to clinical improvement.[3]

Acute Necrosis Due to Insecticide Poisoning

A number of insecticides are chlorinated hydrocarbons. Some are hepatotoxic for experimental animals and, in large doses, for human beings. Specifically, isolated instances of ingestion of large amounts of DDT (approximately 6 g)[17] and of paraquat (approximately 20 g)[19] have led to zone 3 (centrizonal) hepatic necrosis and a clinical syndrome of hepatic failure resembling CCl_4 poisoning. Paraquat poisoning has been reported to lead to a biphasic type of hepatic injury. The early lesion after intake of paraquat is zone 3 necrosis; the later lesion is selective destruction of bile ducts and cholestasis.[3]

Acute Hepatic Injury as a Feature of Systemic Toxicity

Poisonous doses of a number of agents can lead to serious injury accompanied by liver damage that is a relatively minor facet of the syndrome (see Table 9–15). Large doses of inorganic arsenicals, thallium salts, borates, and several insecticides lead to neurologic, muscular, renal, and GI manifestations that may indeed be responsible for a fatal outcome.[1, 4] Hepatic injury is a regular feature of the intoxication but has only a contributory role in determining the gravity of the syndrome.

Inorganic arsenic, in the trivalent state, is a strong protoplasmic poison with a long tradition of use as a homicidal or suicidal agent.[84] Large doses (> 3 g) can cause death in 1 to 3 days.[84] Hepatic injury is a regular feature but is eclipsed by the GI, neurologic, and vascular effects. Severe nausea, vomiting, diarrhea, depression of the central nervous system, and vascular collapse dominate the clinical picture.[3] Necrosis of capillary walls is apparently responsible for congestion, edema, and hemorrhagic necrosis of gastric and intestinal mucosa.[4] The liver shows severe steatosis and various degrees of necrosis.

Descriptions of the zonality of arsenic-induced necrosis have differed.[83] Von Glahn and associates[85] have emphasized periportal (zone 1) necrosis in experimental animals. Other investigators have emphasized centrizonal (zone 3) predominance of the necrosis, perhaps as a result of shock. Jaundice and other evidence of hepatic failure in arsenic poisoning are rare and can be recognized only among patients who survive for a few days. That the hepatic injury is significant, however, is clear from the histologic findings in acute poisoning and the cirrhogenic effects of prolonged exposure to arsenic.[1, 3]

Acute Cholestatic Hepatic Injury

In humans, almost all forms of acute hepatic injury caused by true toxins involve the hepatic parenchyma and produce hepatocellular jaundice. Interesting exceptions include the cholestasis produced by 4,4′-diaminodiphenylmethane (methylenedianiline), the cause of Epping jaundice,[3] the toxic oil syndrome, and the ductal destruction produced by paraquat poisoning.[86] However, there is no doubt that other experimental toxins (see Table 9–12) can produce a cholestatic type of jaundice[1] by selective injury of the canaliculi or bile ducts or by an effect on the hepatocytes.

Epping jaundice was named for an epidemic of toxic hepatic injury that involved 84 persons in Epping, England. The victims had eaten bread made from flour contaminated with the aromatic amine.[3] Methylenedianiline, used in industry as a hardener for epoxy resin, had spilled from a plastic container on the floor of a van that was also carrying flour. The compound had apparently seeped into the flour. Subsequent to this report, a syndrome similar to that of Epping jaundice was reported to result from occupational exposure to this aromatic amine.[6, 7] The clinical picture consisted of cholestatic jaundice preceded or accompanied by abdominal pain, fever, and chills. Onset in 60% of the cases was abrupt, with severe abdominal pain. In the remainder, the illness was more insidious.

The cholestatic nature of the jaundice has been evident in the prominence of itching, the histologic predominance of bile stasis and portal inflammatory infiltration, accompanied by only slight parenchymal injury in most cases, and by the only moderately elevated aminotransferase values. Alkaline phosphatase values, however, also have been only moderately elevated, and a number of patients showed some hepatocellular injury. The pattern of jaundice, accordingly, appears to have been of a mixed cholestatic-hepatocellular type, as associated with a number of drugs. Indeed, Epping jaundice is a form of hepatic injury very similar to that caused by many drugs. It also is accompanied by clinical (fever, chills, rash) and laboratory (eosinophilia) features considered to be hallmarks of hypersensitivity.[1] Yet, unlike the drugs that are considered to cause hepatic injury as a result of hypersensitivity, 4,4′-diaminodiphenylmethane is a true (intrinsic) toxin. It produces similar hepatic injury in experimental animals.[3]

The cholestatic injury of the toxic oil syndrome resembles that of Epping jaundice. The systemic manifestations, which reflect vascular, pulmonary, and other extrahepatic injury, tend to overshadow the hepatic lesion.

Subacute Hepatic Injury

Several syndromes of subacute hepatic disease may be caused by toxic agents. One form has been the subacute hepatic necrosis seen as a result of prolonged exposure to industrial hepatotoxins (Table 9–17). Another is the VOD caused by ingestion of PAs.[1]

Subacute Hepatic Necrosis

Subacute hepatic necrosis (SHN) is a form of toxic hepatic injury that was a major problem for industrial medicine during World Wars I and II. Most attention was directed to the liver disease caused by prolonged exposure to trinitrotoluene (TNT), TCE, and chloronaphthalene-PCB mixtures.[3] Dinitrobenzene (DNB) and dimethylnitrosamine also have been found to cause SHN. Fortunately, SHN as a form of industrial hepatotoxicity has virtually disappeared. Nevertheless, as a classic syndrome of the past and one that might reappear in another setting, it warrants description. Little difference appeared among the syndromes of hepatic disease caused by TNT, TCE, chloronaphthalene-PCB mixtures (see Table 9–17), and DNB. The two nitro-derivatives, especially TNT, however, were prone to lead to aplastic anemia and methemoglobinemia in addition to hepatic disease.

Table 9–17. Hepatotoxicity of Trinitrotoluene (TNT), Tetrachloroethane (TCE), and Chloronaphthalene-Polychlorinated Biphenyl (CNP-PCB) Mixture

Occupational Injury	TNT*	TCE	CNP-PCB
Acute necrosis	+	+	+
Massive	+	+	+
Zonal (central)	−	+	+
Fat	±	+	+
Subacute necrosis and cirrhosis	+	+	+
Delayed onset	+	+	+
Case fatality rate	25%	16%	50%
Associated features			
Dermatitis	+	+	+
Blood			
Methemoglobinemia	+	−	−
Aplastic anemia	+	−	−
Monocytosis (early)	−	+	−

*Dinitrobenzene toxicity produces a similar syndrome.

The *syndrome* of SHN caused by these agents was a smoldering illness characterized by the delayed onset of jaundice. With the appearance of jaundice, a syndrome of grave prognostic import characterized by ascites and progressive hepatic insufficiency was set in motion. Death occurred in some patients within 1 to 4 months, although others survived this phase and achieved at least clinical recovery. Some were later found or assumed to have developed macronodular cirrhosis.

The liver disease caused by these agents was serious. The estimated case fatality rates ranged from 17% to 50%. In patients with a relatively brief course (1 month or less), the syndrome was that of acute hepatic failure rather than SHN. Indeed, in approximately half of the fatal cases of TNT-induced liver disease, the patients died of acute hepatic failure. Many patients had less severe disease characterized only by jaundice and hepatomegaly with ultimate clinical recovery.

Trinitrotoluene Poisoning. The severe hepatic disease caused by TNT was recorded among workers in munitions factories during World Wars I and II. The incidence among exposed workers was low, estimated to be 5% or less.[3] Susceptibility seemed greater among workers with direct manual contact with the agent, especially those with grease on the skin. Women seemed far more susceptible than men. Individual differences, beyond the differential exposure and caution at work, also appeared to account for apparent striking differences in susceptibility. Indeed, the very low incidence, analogous to that of idiosyncratic reactions to some drugs, suggests that a metabolic aberration permitting conversion to toxic metabolites may have accounted for the uncommon susceptibility.

Clinical features were those of acute or subacute hepatic necrosis. Onset of illness was usually delayed for 1 to 4 months (at times even longer) after initial exposure. Indeed, in some instances, illness did not appear until days or weeks after cessation of exposure to TNT. Early symptoms consisted of fatigue, weakness, anorexia, and nausea. Some patients had had overt methemoglobinemia, as manifested by cyanosis, but many patients developed jaundice without having shown cyanosis. Jaundice usually followed the digestive complaints by several weeks.

Prognosis was grim. Death occurred in about 25%

of the approximately 500 cases that occurred in Great Britain during World War I. In approximately half of the fatal cases, patients developed acute hepatic failure and died in hepatic coma within 5 to 30 days of the appearance of jaundice. The others had a more prolonged (1 to 3 months) downhill course, characterized by persistent jaundice and the development of ascites and portal hypertension. Among surviving patients, some were found to have cirrhosis at a later date. Many, however, seemed to have returned to normal health.

The histologic picture ranged from massive hepatic necrosis, in patients who had survived only a few days, to various degrees of fibrosis and architectural distortion accompanying the necrosis in patients who had survived for weeks or months. The latter lesion has been called *toxic cirrhosis*, *subacute yellow* or *red atrophy*, *subacute necrosis*, or *submassive necrosis*.[3]

Also noted were extrahepatic manifestations of TNT toxicity. Erythematous dermal plaques and methemoglobinemia were common but quite independent of hepatic injury and posed no threat to survival. Methemoglobinemia was far more common than hepatic injury and, of course, reversible. Aplastic anemia, a somewhat more common result of exposure to TNT than was hepatic injury, was usually fatal.[3]

Treatment of TNT-induced injury consisted of prompt withdrawal from exposure on recognition of hepatic injury. Despite the observation that some patients showed progression of liver disease or even its first appearance after withdrawal, many instances of liver damage appeared to have been aborted by cessation of exposure to the agent. Prevention of hazardous exposure is by far the most important approach to this form of injury. Indeed, proper preventive measures have virtually wiped out TNT toxicity.

Tetrachloroethane Toxicity. The syndrome of hepatic injury produced by exposure to this highly toxic chloroalkane resembled that of TNT-induced hepatic disease. A delayed onset of a few to many weeks was also characteristic. Toxic exposure, apparently, was most often by inhalation, although ingestion or percutaneous absorption can also lead to toxicity. Susceptibility appeared to have been enhanced among women and alcoholic persons.

Premonitory symptoms resembled those of TNT toxicity; digestive complaints (anorexia, nausea, vomiting) were common. Neurologic symptoms (dizziness, headache, paresthesias) were also prominent but presumably were evidence of anesthetic effects of TCE vapor rather than of early hepatic damage. Indeed, jaundice was in some instances the first evidence of toxicity; in others, it appeared after weeks of premonitory symptoms. The appearance of jaundice ushered in the syndrome of SHN or of acute hepatic failure.

The prognosis of SHN caused by exposure to TCE was probably almost as grave as from TNT. In one series, a 15% case fatality rate was recorded.[3] However, attention to early cases of jaundice and prompt withdrawal from exposure apparently helped abort hepatic injury at milder levels. Among the clues to early injury, the digestive complaints and a curious hematologic abnormality—increased numbers of circulating large monocytes—appeared to be helpful.[3]

Chloronaphthalene-Polychlorinated Biphenyl Toxicity. Hepatic injury acquired as the result of industrial exposure to these compounds usually has been subacute or chronic, at times acute. During World War II, it was a serious entity with a grave prognosis.

The clinical syndrome of this type of industrial poisoning also resembled that of TNT toxicity. It appeared as early as 7 weeks after beginning exposure or as late as many months. Toxic exposure of cases described during World War II appeared to have resulted from inhalation of toxic fumes released by the melting of the chloroaromatic agent during the soldering of electrical materials.[3]

Initial symptoms among reported cases usually included fatigue, anorexia, and nausea, sometimes accompanied by edema of the face and hands. The complaints were usually followed by jaundice. In some instances, severe abdominal pain occurred, perhaps a manifestation of the acute pancreatitis that can accompany the hepatic injury.[83] The appearance of jaundice often signaled the beginning of a downhill course, either as fulminant disease with death in less than 2 weeks or as SHN with death in 1 to 3 months.

It appears that the SHN attributed to PCBs was the result of a toxic "cocktail" containing mixtures of several PCBs, the toxic chloronaphthalenes, and probably the contaminating tetrachlorodibenzofurans and tetrachlorodibenzodioxins.[8] It appeared to differ from toxicity due to the ingestion of food heavily contaminated by PCBs (Yusho poisoning), mentioned earlier.[9]

Veno-Occlusive Disease

VOD is caused by ingestion of PAs. Ingestion of plants containing PAs had led to a number of epidemics of liver disease among humans in various parts of the world and, in retrospect, can be recognized as having been a scourge of livestock as far back as the 19th and perhaps even the 18th centuries.[39] Epidemic liver disease due to ingestion of PAs has been reported from India[43] and Afghanistan.[44]

Focus on PA poisoning of humans came with Bras and associates' description in the 1950s of a syndrome in children characterized by abdominal distention, hepatomegaly, ascites, and edema.[40, 41] They named the syndrome *veno-occlusive disease* because they were able to attribute the centrilobular hepatic congestion, congestive cirrhosis, and clinical features to the regularly demonstrable occlusion of the hepatic venules.

Cultural practices, economic circumstances, and the plants involved determine the mode of exposure to the PAs.[39–42] Drinking "bush tea," a decoction of *Senecio jacobaea* taken as a folk remedy for acute illness, has been responsible for the VOD of Jamaican children. Cases in South Africa have appeared to be a result of ingestion of *Senecio*-contaminated bread.[39] Those in central Asia appeared to have resulted from ingestion of cereal grain contaminated by seeds of *Heliotropium lasiocarpium*. An epidemic of VOD in central India was due to ingestion of cereal contaminated by seeds of a species of *Crotolaria*,[43] and the epidemic in Afghanistan was attributed to the ingestion of wheat contaminated by a species of *Heliotropium*.

Exposure to PAs has occurred in the United States. Preparations containing the toxic alkaloids can be obtained in some natural food stores.[44, 45] Pharmacies in New Mexico, Arizona, and Texas also sell various preparations containing PAs as home remedies.[44]

VOD can also be produced by drugs used in the treatment of neoplastic diseases.[86] Radiation to the liver can also lead to this change. The curious cholestatic injury of the toxic epidemic syndrome of Spain has in some instances been accompanied by veno-occlusive changes.

Factors predisposing to the development of VOD from intake of PAs have appeared to be malnutrition and childhood. Among the Jamaican patients, the majority have been young children, usually older than 1 year.[40, 41] Relatively few adults have been involved. That susceptibility to toxic effects of the alkaloid is not limited to children, however, is demonstrated by reports of epidemics of subacute and chronic VOD in other parts of the world that have involved various age groups or even been predominantly among the adults.[39, 42, 43] The greater tendency for acute VOD to occur among children in Jamaica is presumably related to the manner in which the toxic agent has been taken—namely, as bush tea.

Nutrition appears relevant in that the incidence of VOD in a given area has been greater among the poor.[39] Whether this relates to the effects of protein deprivation on conversion of PAs to toxic metabolites or to the increased likelihood that the impoverished ingest contaminated foods is unclear. Perhaps both factors play a part. Experimental attempts to clarify the role of nutrition in the toxicity of the alkaloids also have led to inconclusive results.[38, 39, 87] The adverse effects of some alkaloids are enhanced by protein deprivation, and those of others inhibited by it.

Clinical Features.[39, 41, 43] VOD may present as acute, subacute, or chronic illness. All three forms are characterized by hepatomegaly, ascites and edema, and collagenous occlusion of the small branches of hepatic vein. The clinical features result from the interference with hepatic flow and can lead to the Budd-Chiari syndrome.

Acute VOD generally refers to cases with abrupt onset of hepatomegaly and ascites and may be accompanied by modest degrees of jaundice. These cases usually have a relatively short course with fatal outcome or apparent recovery within 2 to 8 weeks. However, almost half the cases undergo transition to subacute or chronic VOD.[40, 41]

Onset of acute VOD is usually marked by gnawing or colicky epigastric pain that usually precedes the first evidence of ascites by a few days. Jaundice occurs in only one fifth of the patients, and vomiting and diarrhea are variably present. The average duration of the acute form in the cases of Stuart and Bras[41] was 4 weeks, but instances with rapid development of hepatic failure and death within 1 week were recorded. A fatal outcome or recovery as late as 4 months after onset also has been observed. Acute VOD has been attributed to a single ingestion of the toxic alkaloids or to their ingestion over a brief period of time.

Subacute VOD consists of a syndrome lasting for many months and manifested mainly by persistent hepatomegaly and various degree of ascites but by few other complaints. The course is punctuated by acute episodes similar to those of acute VOD. Subacute VOD may develop by transition from the acute form or may be a result of the ingestion of small amounts of toxic substances over a prolonged period.

Chronic VOD includes cirrhosis. Similar to subacute VOD, the course of the chronic form can be punctuated by acute injury. Chronic VOD may be either a sequel to the acute form or may be a result of ingestion of the toxic alkaloid for a prolonged period.

Morphologic Features. Histologic changes consist of collagenous, fibrotic partial or total occlusion of the efferent (central and sublobular) veins. In the acute form of the syndrome, centrilobular (zone 3) hepatic necrosis and sinusoidal dilation are noted.[39, 41] The subacute and chronic forms are characterized by central fibrosis and bridging between central veins, leading to a form of cirrhosis similar to cardiac cirrhosis and to the cirrhosis of the classic Budd-Chiari syndrome. This "nonportal" cirrhosis, caused by PA toxicity, apparently accounts for one third of the cirrhosis found in Jamaica.[39] Megalocytosis is a characteristic finding in clinical and experimental PA poisoning and consists of huge hepatocytes, presumed to result from the interference with the multiplication of the hepatocytes by the toxic effect of the alkaloid.[88]

Prognosis and Treatment. The prognosis of VOD has been well studied. The acute form is characterized by a rapidly fatal course in 15% to 20% of patients and by apparently complete recovery in about 25% of patients. Approximately one sixth of the patients with the acute disease undergo transition into the subacute or chronic form and succumb to the illness within 1 to 3 years. In one fourth of the patients whose follow-up has been possible, transition to chronic disease with little progression during the years of follow-up has been noted, as well as the presence of apparently inactive cirrhosis with various evidences of portal hypertension. Transition from acute disease to cirrhosis may occur with extraordinary rapidity in VOD. Indeed, a period as brief as 3 months may intervene between onset of the syndrome and fully established cirrhosis. Death in the acute phase is often due to liver failure. In the chronic phase, it appears to be usually a result of portal hypertension.[40, 41]

Treatment of this condition consists of prevention. Adequate education with regard to the use of folk

Table 9–18. Classification of Hepatotoxic Drugs and Major Characteristics of Each Group

Category of Agents	Incidence	Experimental Reproductivity	Dose Dependent	Mechanism	Histologic Lesion	Examples
Intrinsic toxicity	High	Yes	Yes			
Direct				Direct physicochemical distortion and destruction of hepatocytes	Necrosis (zonal)	CCl_4, $CHCl_3$
Indirect						
Cytotoxic				Interference with specific metabolic pathway leads to structural injury	Steatosis or necrosis	Tetracycline, oncotherapeutic drugs, others
Cholestatic				Interference with hepatic excretory pathways leads to cholestatic	Bilirubin cast	C-17 alkylated steroids
Host idiosyncrasy*	Low	No	No			
Immunologic (hypersensitivity)				Hypersensitivity	Necrosis or cholestasis	Phenytoin, PAS, HALO, CPZ, PBZ
Metabolic				Production of hepatotoxic metabolites (aberrant metabolism of drug)	Necrosis	INH, VPA

PAS, *p*-aminosalicylate; HALO, halothane; CPZ, chlorpromazine; PBZ, phenylbutazone; INH, isoniazid; VPA, valproic acid; $CHCl_3$, chloroform.
*Intrinsic toxicity may participate in injury.

remedies containing these toxic alkaloids and public health measures to ensure minimal chances of contamination of wheat or cereals by the seeds of toxic plants are obviously essential steps. Nevertheless, the combination of famine and availability of plants, the toxicity of which is not appreciated, will lead to epidemics such as those described in India[42] and Afghanistan.[43] It is also clear that education to prevent PA toxicity in the United States is in order.

Chronic Hepatic Injury. A single episode of acute hepatic injury apparently rarely leads to chronic disease. I am aware of no evidence showing that the severe necrosis of white phosphorus or of toxic mushroom poisoning leaves a residue of cirrhosis after recovery from the acute episode. The picture with CCl_4 poisoning, however, is more complex. Although single necrotizing doses given to animals do not usually lead to cirrhosis as a sequel, they have been reported to do so in humans.[83] In poisoning of humans by CCl_4, because alcoholism is a predisposing factor, the presence of cirrhosis in a patient recovered from acute toxicity would not necessarily or even probably be a sequel to the bout of acute injury.

Cirrhosis can result from the syndrome of SHN. Indeed, SHN may be regarded as consisting of continued smoldering necrosis, paralleled by increasing degrees of fibrosis, architectural distortion, and regeneration—that is, cirrhosis. The terms *toxic cirrhosis* and *active postnecrotic cirrhosis* have been applied to this lesion. In cases of recovery from the phase of subacute necrosis, which have followed removal from exposure to the offending agent, a residual macronodular scarring has been described.[3]

Cirrhosis also may develop more slowly as a result of prolonged subtle injury. Examples are provided by cases of cirrhosis in refrigeration engineers, workers in dry-cleaning plants exposed to chlorinated hydrocarbons,[25] and vintners exposed to inorganic arsenicals.[89]

Neoplasms should be included among the delayed results of exposure to toxins. Many toxic synthetic chemicals and some botanic toxins can produce hepatocellular carcinoma in experimental animals, but cancer of the liver in humans has never been proved to be a result of exposure to toxic chemicals other than aflatoxin and thorium dioxide. Aflatoxins, however, have been implicated epidemiologically in hepatic carcinogenesis, and, of course, the virus of virus B hepatitis has been shown to be involved in hepatic carcinogenesis.[90] Exposure to Thorotrast,[91] inorganic arsenic,[91] vinyl chloride,[91] and a spray made of copper sulfate and lime (Bordeaux mixtures)[92] has been incriminated in the etiology of angiosarcoma.

CONCLUDING COMMENTS

Acute, subacute, and chronic hepatic disease may result from domestic and occupational exposure to hepatotoxic agents. The classic syndromes of acute and subacute hepatic injury are today more likely to have resulted from accidental or suicidally motivated exposure to hepatotoxins in the home than from occu-

Table 9–19. Histologic Types of Acute Hepatic Injury and Associated Biochemical and Clinical Aspects

Histologic Lesion	Biochemical Abnormalities of Serum*			Clinical Syndrome	Examples
	Aminotransferases	*Alkaline Phosphatase*	*Cholesterol*		
Cytotoxic					
Necrosis					
Zonal	8–500 ×	1–2 ×	N, ↓	Hepatic and renal failure	CCl_4, ACM, HALO
Diffuse	8–200 ×	1–2 ×	N, ↓	Severe hepatitis	INH, α-Methyldopa
Steatosis					
Microvesicular	5–20 ×	1–2 ×	N, ↓	FLP, RS	Tetra, VPA
Macrovesicular	1–5 ×	1–2 ×	N, ↓	Resembles AFL	MTX
Cholestasis					
Hepatocanalicular	1–8 ×	3–10 ×	↑	Resembles EHOJ	CPZ, EE
Canalicular	1–5 ×	1–3 ×	N, ↑	Resembles EHOJ	Anabolic and contraceptive steroids
Mixed (mixture of cytotoxic and cholestatic)	Variable	Variable	N, ↑	Resembles hepatitis or EHOJ	PBZ, PAS, sulfonamides

AFL, Alcoholic fatty liver; EHOJ, extrahepatic obstructive jaundice; FLP, fatty liver of pregnancy; RS, Reye's syndrome; ACM, Acetaminophen; CPZ, chlorpromazine; EE, erythromycin estolate; HALO, halothane; INH, isoniazid; MTX, methotrexate; PAS, *p*-aminosalicylic acid; PBZ, phenylbutazone; Tetra, tetracycline; VPA, valproic acid.

*Degree of abnormality indicated as fold increase; N indicates normal; ↑ indicates elevated values; ↓ indicates depressed values.

pational exposure. Chronic hepatic disease may result from occupational exposure. Knowledge of the syndromes and circumstances of exposure to the toxic agent permits prevention.

APPENDIX

Drugs as a Cause of Hepatic Injury

A large number of drugs can produce hepatic injury as therapeutic misadventures. Some of these drugs are intrinsic hepatotoxins. Others produce the injury as a result of a special vulnerability of the exposed individual (idiosyncrasy). Several types of intrinsic hepatotoxins and at least two categories of idiosyncrasy have been identified (Table 9–18). The hepatic injury may be acute or chronic. The forms and characteristics of acute injury are summarized in Table 9–19 and of chronic injury in Table 9–20. Table 9–21 contains a list, by pharmaceutical category, of a large number of drugs with an indication of the type of hepatic injury each is likely to produce.

Table 9–20. Chronic Hepatic Lesions Caused by Medicinal Agents

Lesion	Agents	
Chronic necroinflammatory disease (chronic active hepatitis, CAH)	Oxyphenisatin	Sulfonamides
	α-Methyldopa	Perhexiline maleate*
	Isoniazid	Prophylthiouracil
	Nitrofurantoin	Aspirin†
	Dantrolene	Acetaminophen†
Steatosis	Methotrexate, glucocorticoid, L-asparaginase, and various oncotherapeutic drugs	
Phospholipidosis	Coralgil‡, amiodarone, perhexiline	
Vascular lesions		
Peliosis hepatis	Anabolic and contraceptive steroids	
Hepatic vein thrombosis§	Contraceptive steroids	
Veno-occlusive disease§	Thioguanine, urethane	
Granulomas	Allopurinol, halothane, hydralazine, penicillin, phenylbutazone, quinidine, sulfonamides. sulfonylureas, methyldopa, carbamazepine	
Cirrhosis		
Micronodular type	Ethanol, methotrexate, inorganic arsenic	
Macronodular type	Drugs that lead to chronic active hepatitis and subacute hepatic necrosis	
"Primary biliary" type	Chlorpromazine, organic arsenical, tolbutamide, thiobendazole	
Congestive type	Drugs that lead to hepatic vein thrombosis and veno-occlusive disease§	
Noncirrhotic portal hypertension	Vinyl chloride, inorganic arsenic	
Hepatoportal sclerosis	Vitamin A overdoses	
Centrilobular fibrosis	Alcoholic hepatitis	
Neoplasms		
Adenoma and hepatocellular carcinoma	Contraceptive and anabolic steroids	
Cholangiocarcinoma, angiosarcoma	Thorotrast, vinyl chloride, inorganic arsenic	

*Perhexiline leads to lesion with features of both CAH and alcoholic liver disease.
†Causative role in lesion is in doubt.
‡4,4′-Diethylaminoethoxyhexestrol, an amphiphilic compound used to treat coronary disease in Japan.
§Can cause Budd-Chiari syndrome.

Table 9–21. Types of Acute Hepatic Injury Caused by Drugs in Various Therapeutic Categories

Cytotoxic (Hepatocellular) and Mixed*	Cholestatic and Mixed*	Some Cytotoxic and Some Cholestatic†
Anesthetics‡		
Enflurane		
Fluroxene		
Halothane		
Isoflurane§		
Methoxyflurane		
Neuropsychotropics		
Amineptine	Chlorpromazine (and other phenothiazines)	Chlordiazepoxide
Clozapine	Haloperidol	Diazepam
Cocaine	Trimipramine	Mianserin
Famoxitine	Benzodiazepines	Trazodone
Hydrazides (all)		Tricyclics (some)
Maprotiline		
Metopimazine		
Methylphenidate		
Molindone		
Tranylcypromine		
Tricyclics (most)		
Zimelidine		
Anticonvulsants		
Phenytoin		Carbamazepine
Progabide		Phenobarbital
Valproate‖		
Felbamate		
Analgesic, Anti-Inflammatory, Anti–Muscle Spasm, Antigout agents		
Acetaminophen	Benoxaprofen	Allopurinol**
Chlorzoxazone	Diflunisal	Gold compounds
Clomatacine	Penicillamine	Naproxen
Dantrolene	Propoxyphene	Phenylbutazone**
Diclofenac		Piroxicam
Fenclozic acid		Sulindac
Glafenine		
Ibuprofen		
Indomethacin		
Salicylates		
Pirprofen		
Tolmetin		
Zoxazolamine		
Hormonal Derivatives and Drugs Used in Endocrine Disease		
Acetohexamide	Carbimazole	Thiouracil
Carbutamide	Chlorpropamide**	
Cyclofenil	Tolazamide**	
Glipizide	Tolbutamide**	
Metahexamide	Methimazole	
Propylthiouracil**	Methylthiouracil	
Tamoxifen††	Anabolic and contraceptive steroids	
Diethylstilbestrol††	Danazol	
Antimicrobials		
Amodiaquine	Amoxicillin-clavulanate	Cephalosporins
Amphotericin B	Erythromycin‡‡	Chloroamphenicol
Antimonials	Griseofulvin	Clarithromycin
Clindamycin	Thiabendazole	Nitrofurantoin**
Hycanthone	Menelamine	Penicillins§§
Hydroxystilbamidine	Cloxacillin	Sulfamethoxazole-trimethoprim
Didanosine	Zidovudine	Sulfadoxine
Ketoconazole	Dicloxacillin	Pyrimethamine
Mebendazole	Floxacillin	Idoxuridine
Mepacrine		Zidovudine
Metronidazole		Ampicillin
p-Aminosalicylate		Oxacillin
Rifampin		
Sulfonamides**		
Sulfones		
Tetracyclines‖		
Prothionamide		

Table continued on following page

Table 9–21. Types of Acute Hepatic Injury Caused by Drugs in Various Therapeutic Categories *Continued*

Cytotoxic (Hepatocellular) and Mixed*	Cholestatic and Mixed*	Some Cytotoxic and Some Cholestatic†
Cardiovascular Drugs		
Amiodarone‖††‖‖	Ajmaline	Amrinone
Aprindine	Captopril	Disopyramide
Benziodarone	Chlorthalidone	Enalapril
Diltiazem	Coumadin	
Methyldopa	Phenindone	
Mexiletine	Prajmaline	
Hydralazines**	Propafenone	
Nicotinic acid	Thiazides	
Nifedipine††	Verapamil**	
Papaverine		
Perhexiline‖††‖‖		
Procainamide		
Pyridinol carbamate		
Quinidine**		
Suloctidil		
Ticrynafen		
Tocainamide		
Labetalol		
Lisinopril		
*Antineoplastic****		
Asparaginase‖†††	Aminoglutethimide	Azathioprine
cis-Platinum‖	Busulfan	
Cyclophosphamide	Floxuridine	
Dacarbazine		
Diethylstilbestrol††		
Doxorubicin		
Etoposide		
Fluorouracil		
Indicine-*N*-oxide		
Methotrexate†††		
N-methyl-formamide‖		
Mithramycin		
6-Mercaptopurine		
Nitrosoureas		
Tamoxifen		
Thioguanine‡‡		
Vincristine		
Flutamide		
Miscellaneous		
Disulfiram	Propoxyphene	Cimetidine
Iodide ion	Rapeseed oil—aniline‡‡‡	Ranitidine
Oxyphenisatin	Methylene dianiline§§§	Etretinate
Phenazopyridine		
Salizopyridine		
Tannic acid		
Vitamin A		
p-Aminobutyric acid		

*Mixed forms of injury are categorized according to the predominant injury as cytotoxic or cholestatic.
†Refers to agents that are inconsistent in the form of injury produced, with some instances having been cholestatic and others cytotoxic.
‡Hepatic injury produced by volatile anesthetic agents is always cytotoxic.
§Two credible cases reported.
‖Microvesicular steatosis. Valproate injury also includes necrosis in some cases.
**Can cause granulomas.
††Can lead to changes resembling alcoholic liver disease (alcoholic hyaline).
‡‡E-Estolate, E-Ethylsuccinate, E-Proprionate, E-Stearate.
§§Semi-synthetic penicillins and penicillin.
‖‖Also leads to phospholipidosis.
***Some of these agents alone or as combinations lead to veno-occlusive disease.
†††Macrovesicular steatosis.
‡‡‡Responsible for "toxic oil" epidemic in Spain.
§§§Responsible for "Epping jaundice."

References

1. Zimmerman HJ: Hepatotoxicity: The Adverse Effects of Drugs and Other Chemicals on the Liver. New York, Appleton-Century-Crofts, 1978.
2. Klaassen CD: Casarett and Doull's Toxicology. The Basic Science of Poisons. 5th ed. New York, Macmillan Publishing Co., 1995.
3. Zimmerman HJ: Chemical hepatic injury. *In* Haddad LM, Winchester JF (eds): Clinical Management of Poisoning and Drug Overdose. 2nd ed. Philadelphia W.B. Saunders Co., pp 266–296, 1990.
4. Arena JM, Drew RH (eds): Poisoning: Toxicology–Symptoms–Treatment. 5th ed Springfield, IL, Charles C Thomas, Publisher, 1986.
5. Feinglass El: Arsenic intoxication from well water in the United States. N Engl J Med *288*:828, 1973.
6. Bastian PG: Occupational hepatic caused by methylenedianiline. Med J Aust *141*:533, 1984.
7. Posada M, Castro M, Kilbourne EM, et al: Toxic oil syndrome: Case report associated with the Ith oil refinery in Sevilla. Food Chem Toxicol *25*:87, 1987.
8. Kimbrough RD: The toxicity of polychlorinated polycyclic compounds and related chemicals. CRC Crit Rev Toxicol *2*:445, 1974.
9. Kuratsune M, Yoshimura T, Matsuzaka J, Yamaguchi A: Epidemiologic study of oil contaminated with a commercial brand of polychlorinated biphenyls. Environ Health Perspect *1*:119, 1972.
10. Ridker PM, Ohkuma S, McDermott WV, et al: Hepatic veno-occlusive disease associated with the consumption of pyrrolizidine containing dietary supplement. Gastroenterology *88*: 1050, 1985.
11. Stillman AE, Huxtable R, Consroe P, et al: Hepatic veno-occlusive disease due to pyrrolizidine (Senecio) poisoning in Arizona. Gastroenterology *73*:349, 1977.
12. McGee JO'D, Patrick RS, Wood CB, Blumgart LH: A case of veno-occlusive disease of the liver in Britain associated with herbal tea consumption. J Clin Pathol *29*:788, 1976.
13. Kumana CR, Ng M, Lin HJ, et al. Herbal tea induced hepatic veno-occlusive diseases: Quantification of toxic ethanoild exposure in adults. Gut *26*:101, 1985.
14. Davies EG, Pollork J, Steal HM: Chronic herb for eczema. Letter. Lancet *336*:177, 1990.
15. Woolf GM, Petrovic LM, Rojter SE, et al: Acute hepatitis associated with the chinese herbal product Jin Bu Huan. Ann Intern Med *121*:729, 1994.
16. Larrey D, Vial T, Pauwels A, et al: Hepatitis after Germander (*Teucrium chamaedrys*) administration: Another instance of herbal medicine hepatotoxicity. Ann Intern Med *117*:129, 1992.
17. Katz M, Saibil F: Herbal hepatitis: Subacute hepatic necrosis secondary to chaparral leaf. J Clin Gastroenterol *12*:203, 1990.
18. Gordon DW, Rosenthal G, Hart J, et al: Chaparral ingestion. The broadening spectrum of liver injury caused by herbal medications. JAMA *273*:489, 1994.
19. Harvey J, Colin-Jones DG: Mistletoe hepatitis. BMJ *282*:186, 1981.
20. Itoh S, Marutani K, Nishijima T, et al: Liver injuries induced by herbal medicine, syo-saiko-to (xiao-chai-hu-tang). Dig Dis Sci *40*:1845, 1994.
21. Sinniah D, Baskaras BH, Thomas J, et al: Margosa oil as a cause of Reye's syndrome. Lancet *1*:487, 1981.
22. Anderson IB, Mullin WH, Meeker JE, et al: Pennyroyal toxicity. Measurement of toxic metabolite levels in two cases and review of the literature. Ann Intern Med *117*:165, 1992.
23. Larrey D: Liver involvement in the course of phototherapy. Presse Med *16*:691, 1994.
24. Huxtable RJ: The myth of beneficent nature: The risk of herbal preparations. Ann Intern Med *117*:165, 1992.
25. Dossing M, Skinhoj P: Occupational liver injury. Present state of knowledge and future perspectives. Int Arch Occup Environ Health *56*:11, 1985.
26. Zimmerman HJ: Effects of alcohol on other hepatotoxins. Alcohol Clin Exp Res *10*:3, 1986.
27. Poklis A, Saady J: Arsenic poisoning: Acute or chronic. Suicide or murder. Am J Forsenic Med Pathol *11*:226, 1990.
28. Prescott LF: Paracetamol overdosage. Pharmacological considerations and clinical management. Drugs *25*:290, 1983.
29. Rumack BH, Peterson RC, Koch GG, Amara IA: Acetaminophen overdose; 662 cases with evaluation of oral acetylcysteine treatment. Arch Intern Med *141*:380, 1987.
30. Zimmerman HJ, Maddrey WC: Acetaminophen (paracetamol) hepatotoxicity with regular intake of alcohol: Analysis of instances of therapeutic misadventure. Hepatology *22*:767, 1995.
31. Clearfield JR: Hepatoreneal toxicity from sniffing spot remover (metchloroethylene). Am J Dig Dis *15*:851, 1970.
32. Tucker SC, Patteson TE: Hepatitis and halothane sniffing. Ann Intern Med *30*:667, 1974.
33. Perino LE, Warren GH, Levine J: Cocaine-induced hepatotoxicity in humans. Gastroenterology *93*:176, 1987.
34. Wanless IR, Dore S, Gopinath N, et al: Histopathology of cocaine hepatotoxicity. Report of four patients. Gastroenterology *98*:497, 1990.
35. Henry JA, Jeffreys KJ, Dawling S: Toxicity deaths from 3,4 methlenedioxyamphetamine (ecstasy). Lancet *340*:384, 1992.
36. Armen R, Kanel G, Reynolds T: Phencyclidine-induced malignant hyperthermia causing submassive liver necrosis. Am J Med *77*:167, 1984.
37. Spoerke DG, Rumack BH (eds): Handbook of Mushroom Poisoning. Diagnosis and Treatment. Baca Raton, FL, CRC Press, 1994.
38. Bull LB, Culvenor CCJ, Dick AT: The Pyrrolizidine Alkaloids. New York, John Wiley & Sons, p 249, 1968.
39. McLean EK: The toxic actions of pyrrolizidine *(Senecio)* alkaloids. Pharmacol Rev *22*:429, 1970.
40. Bras G, Jelliffe DB, Stuart KL: Veno-occlusive disease of the liver with non-portal type of cirrhosis occurring in Jamaica. Arch Pathol *57*:285, 1954.
41. Stuart KL, Bras G: Veno-occlusive disease of the liver. Q J Med *26*:291, 1957.
42. Mohabbat O, Younos M, Merzad AA, et al: An outbreak of hepatic veno-occlusive disease in northwestern Afghanistan. Lancet *2*:269, 1976.
43. Tandon BN, Tandon RK, Randon HD, et al: An epidemic of veno-occlusive disease of liver in central India. Lancet *2*:271, 1976.
44. Huxtable R: New aspects of the toxicology and pharmacology of pyrrolizidine alkaloids. Gen Pharmacol *10*:159, 1979.
45. Rottman JN: Comfrey and liver damage. Lancet *1*:944, 1990.
46. Fukunishi R: Acute hepatic lesions induced by cycasin. Acta Pathol *23*:639, 1973.
47. Tanaka K, Kean EA, Johnson B: Jamaican vomiting sickness: Biochemical investigation of two cases. N Engl J Med *295*:161, 1976.
48. Segelman AB, Segelman FP, Karline L, Sofi I: Sassafras and herb tea: Potential health hazard. JAMA *263*:477, 1976.
49. Wogan GN: Mycotoxins. Annu Rev Pharmacol Toxicol *15*:437, 1975.
50. Serck-Hansen A: Aflatoxin-induced fatal hepatitis? Arch Environ Health *20*:729, 1970.
51. Shank RC, Bourgeois CH, Neschamaras N, Davimol P: Aflatoxins in autopsy specimens from Thai children with an acute disease of unknown etiology. Food Cosmet Toxicol *9*:501, 1971.
52. Becroft DMO, Webster DR: Aflatoxins and Reye's disease. BMJ *2*:117, 1972.
53. Dvorackova L, Zilkova L, Brodsky F, Cerrnar J: Aflatoxin and liver damage with encephalopathy. Sb Ved Pr Lek Fak Univ Karlovy *15*:521, 1972.
54. Chaves-Carballo E, Ellefson RD, Gomez MR: Aflatoxin in the liver of a patient with Reye-Johnson syndrome. Mayo Clin Proc *51*:47, 1976.
55. Bourgeois CH, Shank RC, Grossman RA, et al: Acute aflatoxin B1 toxicity in the macaque and similarities to Reye's syndrome. Lab Invest *24*:206, 1971.
56. Rogers AE: Toxicity and carcinogenicity of aflatoxins in experimental animals. *In* Pollack JD: Reye's Syndrome. New York, Grune & Stratton, p 135, 1974.
57. Krishnamarchan K, Nagarjan V, Bhat RV, Tilak TBG: Hepati-

tis due to aflatoxicosis. An outbreak in Western India. Lancet *1*:1061, 1975.
58. Wogan GN: Aflatoxins as risk factors for hepatocellular carcinoma in humans. Cancer Res *52*:1145, 1992.
59. Mantisano R, Kirby GM: Chemical carcinogens in humans liver. *In* Brechot C (ed): Primary Liver Cancer. Etiological and Progression Factors. Boca Raton, FL, CRC Press, pp 52–78, 1994.
60. Tabuenca JM: Toxic-allergic syndrome caused by ingestion of rapeseed oil derivatives with aniline. Lancet *2*:567, 1981.
61. Shirley RL: Nutritional and physiological effects of nitrates, nitrites, and nitrosamine. BioScience *25*:790, 1975.
62. Neale G, Azzopardi JG: Chronic arsenical poisoning and noncirrhotic portal hypertension—a case for diagnosis. BMJ *4*:725, 1971.
63. Russell RM, Boyer IL, Baghen SA, Huban Z: Hepatic injury from chronic hypervitaminosis A resulting in portal hypertension and ascites. N Engl J Med *291*:435, 1974.
64. Wanless IJ: Vascular disorders. *In* MacSween RNM, Anthony PP, Scheuer PJ, et al (eds): Pathology of the Liver. 3rd ed. Edinburgh, Churchill Livingstone, pp 535–562, 1994.
65. Bagheri SA, Boyer JL: Peliosis hepatis associated with androgenic-anabolic steroid therapy. A severe form of hepatic injury. Ann Intern Med *81*:610, 1974.
66. Redlich CA, Becket WS, Sparer J, et al: Liver disease associated with occupational exposure to the solvent dimethylformatide. Ann Intern Med *108*:680, 1988.
67. Remington PL, Rowley D, McGee H, et al: Decreasing trends in Reye syndrome and aspirin use in Michigan, 1979 to 1984. Pediatrics *77*:93, 1986.
68. Barrett MJ, Hurwitz ES, Schonberger LB, Rogers MF: Changing epidemiology of Reye syndrome in the United States. Pediatrics *77*:598, 1986.
69. Ruprah M, Mont TGK, Flannagan RJ: Acute carbon tetrachloride poisoning in 19 patients: Implications for diagnosis and treatment. Lancet *1*:107, 1985.
70. Wroblewski F: Clinical significance of alterations in transaminase activities in serum and other body fluids. Adv Clin Chem *1*:313, 1958.
71. Brewer E, Haggerty RJ: Toxic hazards. Rat poisons. II. Phosphorus. N Engl J Med *258*:147, 1958.
72. Rodriguez-Iturbe B: Acute yellow phosphorus poisoning. N Engl J Med *284*:157, 1971.
73. Simon FA, Pickering LK: Acute yellow phosphorus poisoning. Smoking stool syndrome. JAMA *235*:1343, 1976.
74. Ghostal AK, Porta EA, Hartroft WS: The role of lipoperoxidation in the pathogenesis of fatty liver by phosphorus poisoning in rats. Am J Pathol *54*:275, 1969.
75. Herold R, Straub PW: Acute hepatic necrosis of hepatitis and mushroom poisoning. The value of coagulation tests in their differentiation, prognostic assessment and pathogenesis. Helv Med Acta *37*:5, 1978.
76. Hanrahan JP, Gordon MA: Mushroom poisoning. Case reports and a review of therapy. JAMA *251*:1057, 1984.
77. Duffy TJ, Verggeer P: Treatment of mushroom amanitin poisoning. West J Med *145*:521, 1986.
78. Marugg D, Reutter EW: Die Amanita-phalloides-intoxication: Moderne therapeutische Massnahmen und klinischer Verlauf. Schweiz Rundsch Med Prax *74*:972, 1985.
79. Floersheim GL: Treatment of human amatoxin poisoning. Myths and advances in therapy. Med Toxicol *2*:1, 1987.
80. Hamlyn AN, Douglas AP, James O: The spectrum of paracetamol (acetaminophen) overdose: Clinical and epidemiological studies. Postgrad Med J *54*:400, 1978.
81. Goyer RA; Toxic effects of metals. *In* Klaassen CD (ed): Casarett and Doull's Toxicology: The Basic Science of Poisons. 5th ed. New York, Macmillan Publishing Co., p 691–736, 1996.
82. Jantsch W, Kulig K, Rumack BH: Massive copper sulfate ingestion resulting in hepatotoxicity. J Toxicol Clin Toxicol *22*:585, 1984.
83. Klatskin G: Drug-induced hepatic injury. *In* Schaffner F, Sherlock S, Leevy CM (eds): The Liver and Its Diseases. New York, Intercontinental M Book Corporation, p 173, 1974.
84. Moeschlin S: Poisoning, Diagnosis and Treatment. New York, Grune & Statton, 1965.
85. Von Glahn WC, Flinn FB, Keim WF Jr: Effect of certain arsenates on the liver. Arch Pathol *25*:488, 1937.
86. Zimmerman HJ: Hepatotoxic effects of oncotherapeutic agents. Progr Liver Dis *8*:621, 1986.
87. Jago M: Factors affecting the chronic hepatotoxicity of pyrrolizidine alkaloid poisoning. Am J Pathol *105*:1, 1971.
88. Jago MV: The development of the hepatic megalocytosis of chronic pyrrolizidine alkaloid poisoning. Am J Pathol *56*:405, 1969.
89. Luchtrath H: Cirrhosis of the liver in chronic arsenical poisoning. German Med Mon *2*:127, 1972.
90. Miller EC, Miller JA: Hepatocarcinogenesis by chemicals. Prog Liver Dis *5*:699, 1976.
91. Popper H, Thomas LB, Telles NC, et al: Development of hepatic angiosarcoma in man induced by vinyl chloride, Thorotrast, and arsenic: Comparison with cases of unknown etiology. Am J Pathol *92*:349, 1978.
92. Pimental JC, Menezes AP: Liver disease in vineyard sprayers. Gastroenterology *72*:295, 1977.

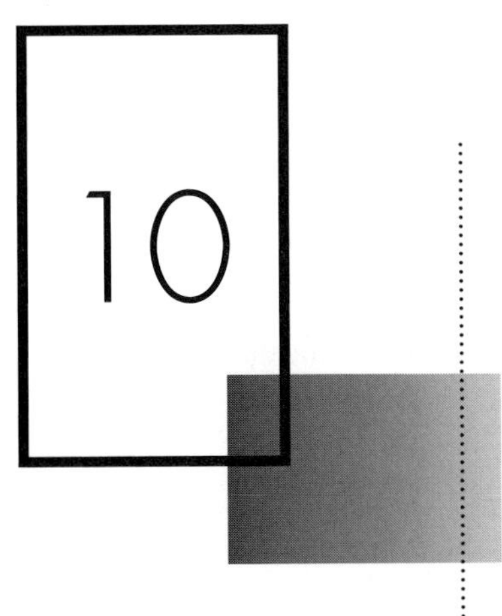

Active Methods for Detoxification

JAMES F. WINCHESTER, MD

This chapter discusses active methods of detoxification, primarily recent advances in *hemodialysis* and *hemoperfusion,* and enumerates specific criteria that should allow clinicians to judge rationally when these techniques should be used in the management of poisoning.[1] Also discussed are other techniques for solute removal, such as alkalization with or without forced diuresis, hemofiltration, continuous arteriovenous hemofiltration (CAVH), plasmapheresis, exchange blood transfusion, and the use of specific antibodies to drugs.

Special attention is given to three types of poisonings: (1) those in which routine measures, such as urinary alkalization in salicylate poisoning or correction of fluid and electrolyte balance in lithium overdose, are ineffective in removing the toxin, and hemodialysis is required; (2) those with drugs for which significant quantities of the intoxicant are metabolized to more noxious substances, such as the conversion of methanol to formaldehyde and ethylene glycol to oxalic acid; and (3) those with agents known to produce delayed toxicity, such as paraquat and related compounds.

Litovitz and colleagues[2] have shown in the 1995 Annual Report of the American Association of Poison Control Centers (AAPCC) that of 2,023,089 human exposure cases, 970,152 poisoned patients were treated by oral charcoal dilution/irrigation, a further 140,359 by single-dose charcoal, and 1690 by whole-bowel irrigation. Enhanced elimination of drugs using alkalization of urine was performed in 7261, hemodialysis in 772, hemoperfusion in 59, and other extracorporeal techniques in 53. An analysis of poisonings for which dialysis or hemoperfusion was used in the 1986 AAPCC report[3] is shown in Table 10–1.

ORAL SORBENTS

Oral sorbents (particularly activated charcoal) are discussed in Chapter 1. Oral charcoal contributes significantly to the management of poisoning by shortening drug half-life through interruption of enterohepatic circulation of specific agents such as phenobarbital.

ALKALIZATION AND FORCED DIURESIS

Most drugs are weak acids or bases and in solutions exist as both non-ionized and ionized species. The non-ionized molecules are usually lipid soluble and diffuse across the cell membrane by the process known as *nonionic diffusion.* The ionized form, in contrast, is usually unable to penetrate lipid membranes.

Excretion of drugs by the kidneys also depends on the ionization state of the specific drug or its metabolites and involves three main processes. The first is glomerular filtration. In the glomeruli, drugs that are not bound to albumin are ultrafiltered, depending on the degree of protein binding, whereas drugs that are strongly bound to albumin are retained by the glomerulus. The second process by which drugs are excreted by the kidneys is tubule secretion at the proximal convoluted tubule. This takes place through transport systems that carry drugs from plasma to urine. There is one transport system for acidic drugs and another for basic drugs. Tubule epithelium can also secrete free drug and drug bound to protein-binding sites. As free drug is

Table 10–1. Poisons for Which Hemoperfusion or Dialysis Was Used in the 1986 AAPCC Report

Poison	Hemoperfusion	Dialysis
Acetaminophen	1	9
Aspirin	1	25
Barbiturate	9	13
Boric acid	0	5
Cardiac glycosides	1	6
Cyclic antidepressants	20	8
Ethanol	4	10
Formaldehyde	0	6
Glycols	0	41
Isopropanol	0	7
Lithium	0	39
Methanol	0	31
Mushrooms	3	5
Phenothiazines	3	5
Theophylline	30	15
Total cases: 297 hemodialysis, 99 charcoal, and 23 resin hemoperfusion.		

Note: Many cases are multiple ingestions.
From Litovitz TL, Martin TG, Schmitz B: 1986 Annual Report of the American Association of Poison Control Centers National Data Collection System. Am J Emerg Med *5*:405, 1987.

removed by the tubule cells, rapid breakdown of the circulating drug-protein complex takes place in the plasma. Examples of drugs that compete for proximal secretion are acidic drugs such as probenecid, which can be used to reduce the elimination of penicillins and to prolong their half-life in the body. Little is known, however, of competitive interplay among basic drugs.

The third process by which drugs are excreted by the kidneys is passive tubule reabsorption. This process involves a bidirectional movement of drugs across the renal tubule epithelium; however, as water and electrolytes are progressively reabsorbed from the tubule fluid (as it passes through the loop of Henle and the collecting system), a favorable concentration gradient is created for net absorption of dissolved materials back into the blood stream. This reabsorption requires little energy and is limited to lipid-soluble drugs and the non-ionized fraction of those drugs that are weak electrolytes and that undergo partial ionization at physiologic pH. Increasing the pH of tubular fluid increases the degree of ionization of weak acids and reduces passive tubule free drug absorption by lowering its non-ionic diffusion, whereas the reverse applies to weak bases. The dissociation of a weak acid or base is determined by its dissociation constant (pK_a) and the pH gradient across the tubule membrane.

The ratio of non-ionized to ionized drug can be calculated from the Henderson-Hasselbalch equation. At a pK_a equal to the pH, the concentrations of non-ionized drug and ionized drug are equal (see Chapter 4). Elimination of weak acids by the kidneys is increased in the range of 3.0 to 7.5, whereas for weak bases elimination is increased in acid urine if their pK_a is 7.5 to 10.5. This is illustrated in Figure 10–1.

For drugs to respond to pH manipulation of the urine, they must first satisfy the following criteria: (1) The drug is predominantly eliminated in the unchanged form via the kidneys, (2) the drug is a weak electrolyte with a pK_a in the appropriate acidic or basic pK_a range (see Fig. 10–1); and (3) the drug is distributed mainly to the extracellular fluid compartment and is minimally protein bound. Table 10–2 contains representative listing of pK_a values for various drugs. It is inappropriate to manipulate pH and attempt forced diuresis when the drug is eliminated from the circulation mainly by hepatic or tissue metabolism, is strongly protein bound, or has a large volume of distribution and is highly lipid soluble.

As can be seen in Figure 10–1, phenobarbital (pK_a 7.2) and thiopental (pK_a 7.6) have similar dissociation constants. However, their lipid solubility is quite different; as measured by the methylene chloride water partition coefficient, phenobarbital has a coefficient of 3, whereas thiopental has a partition coefficient of about 80. This means that although 25% to 50% of a dose of phenobarbital is excreted unmetabolized in the urine—and this can be even higher in a large overdose—the renal excretion of thiopental, unchanged in the urine, is less than 1%. Therefore, it is clear that forced alkaline diuresis is of no value in the treatment of overdosage with thiopental or other highly lipid-soluble drugs. Although no fatalities have been recorded, the use of forced diuresis may be complicated by the development of hyponatremia and water intoxication, pulmonary edema, cerebral edema, hypokalemia, and either alkalemia or acidemia secondary to the use of alkaline or acidic agents, respectively, in promoting the diuresis. For these reasons, any commitment to the use of forced diuresis must be accompanied by close attention to the patient and measurement of urinary pH at least hourly and electrolytes every 1 to 2 hours initially and frequently thereafter.

The advantages of alkalization of urine in salicylate poisoning can be illustrated by the following facts: Salicylic acid has a pK_a of 3.0; therefore, at urinary pH 3.0, the ratio of salicylate (ionized) to salicylic acid (non-ionized) is 1:1. At a urine pH of 7.0, this ratio increases to 10,000:1. When the pH is increased to 7.4, the ratio is increased to about 25,000:1. It is not surprising that the elimination half-time for salicylate is greatly prolonged when the urinary pH is less than 7.4. Blood acidemia also increases the amount of non-ionized and diffusible salicylic acid and enhances its accumulation within the cerebral tissue.[4, 5]

Urinary alkalization by systemic bicarbonate and a saline-glucose fluid-induced diuresis increases the ratio of ionized salicylate to non-ionized salicylic acid in the renal tubule; consequently, "ion trapping" of salicylate occurs in the tubule lumen. Accompanying these changes, potassium shifts into cells as blood pH increases and potassium excretion is enhanced by alkaline diuresis. Consequently, the serum potassium concentration declines. It is therefore essential to replace potassium in such situations. The opposite effect occurs with the induction of acidemia. Every

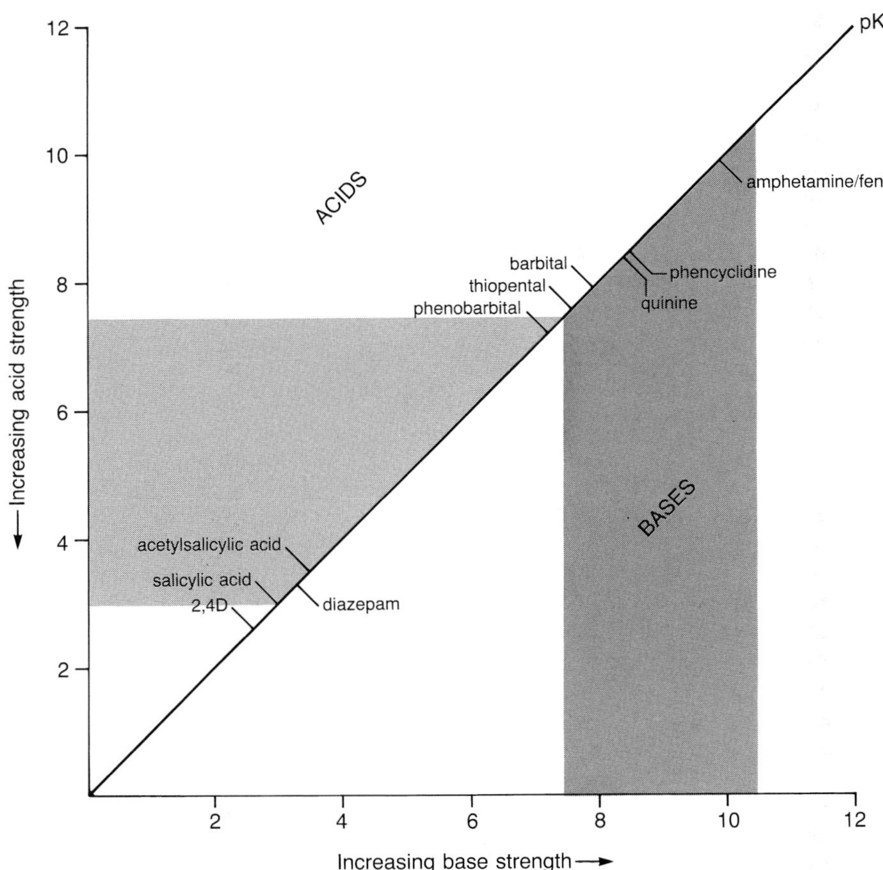

Figure 10–1. Dissociation constants pK_a for several drugs. *Shaded areas* represent urinary pH limits that allow increased excretion of drug.

rise in pH of 0.1 unit in the blood is accompanied by a reduction in plasma potassium level of 0.6 mEq/L, with identical but reciprocal changes occurring with decrements in pH. Therefore, in forced acid diuresis, careful attention must also be paid to the measurement of plasma potassium levels.[6]

It has also been shown that in moderate salicylate poisoning, the same quantity of salicylate was excreted in the urine when identical quantities of sodium bicarbonate were administered with or without forced diuresis.[7, 8] Such a measure avoided the risk of copious fluid administration (6 L) and illustrates the importance of ion trapping alone in moderate salicylate poisoning (32.8 to 46.7 mg/dL plasma concentrations at the start of therapy).

In moderate to severe salicylate poisoning, it may be necessary to resort to dialysis or hemoperfusion when the levels of salicylate exceed 100 mg/dL at 6 hours after ingestion or when acidosis is unresponsive or renal failure develops. When other measures have failed, persistence of the manifestations of salicylate poisoning, with progressive deterioration, are another indication for consideration of dialysis.[4, 9]

For alkaline diuresis, it is wise to measure baseline electrolyte values and arterial and urinary pH as well as drug levels in the blood. It is also preferable to place a bladder catheter in the patient because urine flow rates should be accurately assessed. When appropriate, a flow-directed pulmonary arterial line (Swan-Ganz line) should be used to assess the dangers of fluid overload during intravenous infusion of fluids. The latter is necessary because patients may have impairment of renal or cardiac function. In the presence of hypotension with a high pulmonary capillary wedge pressure, forced diuresis is contraindicated.

The urinary pH should be maintained within the range of 7.5 to 8.5 by adjusting the amount of bicarbonate administered. The diuresis can be initiated by using furosemide or osmotic diuretic agents such as mannitol or urea. The use of mannitol as the diuretic agent may be associated with hyponatremia and hyperosmolality in patients with acute barbiturate or salicylate poisoning. Theoretically, if hemodialysis were subsequently administered to patients in whom diuresis was maintained by high-dose mannitol therapy, the dialysis disequilibrium syndrome might be induced. For this reason, it is recommended that the total dose of mannitol not exceed 300 g. In practice, however, it is rare to use such high doses of mannitol, and the usual clinical case of salicylate poisoning may be treated by doses of between 20 and 100 g of mannitol.

In salicylate poisoning, some degree of dehydration is frequently present before initiation of treatment, so 1 L of 5% dextrose containing 25 mEq/L of bicarbonate and 75 mEq/L of sodium and appropriate levels of potassium judged on the initial serum potassium level should also be given. In the presence of severe acidosis, however, the bicarbonate supple-

Table 10–2. Dissociation Constants (pK_a) for Various Drugs

Acids		Bases	
Drug	*pK_a*	*Drug*	*pK_a*
Acetazolamide	7.2	Allopurinol	9.4
Acetylsalicylic acid	3.49	Amiloride	7.2
Amobarbital	7.7	Amitriptyline	9.4
Barbital	7.91	Amphetamine	9.9
Boric acid	9.24	Atropine	9.8
Chlorpropamide	4.8	Chlorpheniramine	9.2
2,4-Dichlorophenoxyacetic acid	2.6	Chlorpromazine	9.3
Ethosuximide	9.3	Clonidine	8.25
Furosemide	3.8	Codeine	8.2
Hydrochlorothiazide	7.9	Diazepam	3.3
Indomethacin	4.5	Diphenhydramine	8.3
Methotrexate	5.5	Phenytoin	8.3
Pentobarbital	8.2	Ephedrine	9.36
Phenobarbital	7.2	Fenfluramine	9.9
Probenecid	3.4	Haloperidol	8.7
Salicylic acid	3.0	Hydralazine	7.1
Sulfadiazine	6.48	Imipramine	9.5
Theophylline	8.75	Ketamine	7.5
Thiopental	7.6	Lidocaine	7.9
Tolbutamide	5.3	Meperidine	8.7
Valproate sodium	4.8	Methadone	8.6
		Morphine	8.05
		Naloxone	7.94
		Nortriptyline	9.73
		Pentazocine	9.0
		Phencyclidine	8.5
		Procainamide	9.2
		Procaine	8.8
		Quinidine	8.4
		Quinine	8.4
		Reserpine	6.6
		Triamterene	6.2

ments should be increased and adjusted to maintain the urinary pH in the optimal range. Such solutions are best administered for 1 to 2 hours until volume expansion occurs. Thereafter, in an adult, 100 to 200 mL/h of 5% dextrose in half-normal saline containing 20 to 35 mEq of bicarbonate should be given until the salicylate level declines to the therapeutic range (30 to 35 mg/dL).

Alkaline diuresis is suitable for treating overdoses of the following drugs: phenobarbital, when the plasma level exceeds 10 mg/dL; barbital, when the plasma level exceeds 10 mg/dL; and salicylates, when the plasma level exceeds 50 mg/dL (relative to time of ingestion). Forced alkaline diuresis has also been shown to be of benefit in the treatment of 2,4-dichlorophenoxyacetic acid poisoning.[10]

Although forced acid diuresis can increase the excretion of amphetamines, fenfluramine, phencyclidine, and quinine, this intervention has fallen into disfavor because of the possibility of myoglobinuria and the development of acute renal failure. One liter of 5% dextrose in normal saline per hour is given in the first 1 or 2 hours, with added arginine or lysine hydrochloride (10 g given intravenously over 30 minutes). Thereafter, 5% dextrose in normal saline is given every 2 hours. Ammonium chloride, 4 g every 2 hours, should be administered orally, or in a patient who cannot tolerate a nasogastric or duodenal tube, a 1% to 2% solution of ammonium chloride in normal saline should be given intravenously. With either technique, the dose is adjusted to maintain a urinary pH of 5.5 to 6.5. Plasma potassium level should be monitored frequently. Urinary pH should be measured at least hourly. Ascorbic acid (1 g every 6 hours in adults) can also be administered orally to acidify the urine.

It is clear that chloride loading (especially ammonium chloride) increases the excretion of bromides; bromide excretion can be further increased with administration of mannitol or loop diuretics. On the other hand, lithium excretion is not further enhanced by ammonium chloride, water, saline, or loop diuretics (furosemide, ethacrynic acid) administration. Bicarbonate, acetazolamide, urea, and aminophylline may increase lithium excretion in volunteers with normal renal function; however, the data are inconclusive, and no firm evidence shows that forced diuresis (after correction of fluid deficits) is of benefit to lithium-intoxicated patients.

DIALYTIC TECHNIQUES FOR REMOVING POISONS

Many substances can be removed by hemodialysis and peritoneal dialysis, and exhaustive reviews of the state of the art of dialysis in poisoning have been published. Before discussion of dialysis in specific drug poisoning, it is worthwhile to consider the basic principles of dialysis, factors favoring drug removal with dialysis, and the potential problems associated with dialysis in poisoned patients.

Principles of Dialysis

Various forms of dialytic techniques are available in modern therapeutics. *Peritoneal dialysis and hemodialysis* use artificial semi-permeable membranes, with either aqueous dialysate, sorbent-containing dialysate,[11] or, in the past, lipid-containing dialysate (soybean oil). Direct extensions of hemodialysis have used the principle of *ultrafiltration,* in which drug removal accompanies the ultrafiltrate in the process of "solvent drag." Drug removal may also be increased by *CAVH, CAVHD, CVVH, and CVVHD,* modifications of hemodialysis that process continuous (C) arterial (A) or venous (V) blood, hemofiltered/ultrafiltered (H) or ultrafiltered/dialyzed (D) at high rates, through membranes that have a pore structure larger than conventional dialysis membranes[12] rapidly or slowly for a continuous 24-hour period.[13] The different techniques are portrayed in Figure 10–2.

Solute (or drug) removal by dialysis has numerous determinants but involves principally the juxtaposition of a replaceable stream of blood and an appropriate rinsing solution, or dialysate. In peritoneal dialysis, the blood supply is in the capillary bed supplying the peritoneum; in hemodialysis, blood is supplied through the dialysis circuit. Drug removal depends not only on drug characteristics but also on physical factors of the specific dialyzer used.

The factors governing drug removal are the solute (or drug) size, its lipid-water partition coefficient (or lipid solubility), the degree to which it is protein bound, its volume of distribution, and the maintenance of a concentration gradient.[14] Table 10–3 lists drug volumes of distribution and protein binding. The physical factors governing drug removal by the dialyzer itself depend on blood flow rate through the dialyzer, dialysate flow rate, dialyzer surface area, and the characteristics of the specific membrane chosen. To illustrate the effect of dialysis on these important points, it is worthwhile to discuss analysis of two markedly different drugs—lithium and amitriptyline.

Table 10–3. Volume of Distribution and Protein Binding of Some Selected Drugs in a 70-kg Person

Drug	Volume of Distribution		Protein Binding
	L/kg	*Liters*	
Acetaminophen	1.1	77	2–3
Acetylsalicylic acid	0.1–0.2	7–14	50–90
Amitriptyline	15	1050	95
Cyclophosphamide	0.79	55	12
Diazepam	0.95	67	97
Digoxin	6.8	476	2
Digitoxin	0.61	43	93
Phenobarbital	0.7	49	51
Phenytoin	0.54	38	90
Prednisone	1	70	70–95
Theophylline	0.33–0.74	23–52	59

Adapted from Gurland HJ, Samtleben W, Lysaght MJ, Winchester JF: Extracorporeal blood purification techniques: Plasmapheresis and hemoperfusion. In Jacobs C, Kjellstrand CM, Koch KM, Winchester JF (eds): Replacement of Renal Function by Dialysis. 4th ed. Boston, Kluwer Academic Publishers, p 472, 1996.

Lithium, the lightest cation known, is not lipid soluble, is freely distributed in whole-body water, and does not have any degree of plasma protein binding. Its apparent volume of distribution equates to about 0.8 L/kg of body weight. Because it is not present in dialysate, there is a continuous concentration gradient across either the peritoneal membrane or across an artificial semi-permeable membrane. Consequently, lithium is one of the most highly dialyzable drugs; its clearance from blood is proportional to blood flow rate, dialysate flow rate, and dialyzer surface area. Owing to its low molecular weight, its removal rate by different dialyzer membranes does not depend on the pore characteristics, because its clearance by the membrane is proportional to that of sodium. On the other hand, amitriptyline is of larger molecular weight, is somewhat lipid soluble, and is 96.4% bound to serum albumin in plasma. Its apparent volume of distribution is also extremely large (8.3 L/kg of body weight). Although this drug is also not found in dialysate, with a consequent high concentration gradient possible, it is very poorly dialyzable in view of its characteristics just noted.

For drugs that are diffusible across semi-permeable membranes under the usual operating conditions, the solute removal rate for small molecules is predominantly flow limited; in other words, clearance increases with increase in blood flow rate. For larger solutes, the rate of diffusion across the membrane is less, concentration gradients across the membrane remain high, and increasing flow rates have a smaller effect on drug clearance rates. In short, drug removal is limited by the membrane area times the permeability. Clearances reach a plateau above a blood flow rate of 200 to 300 mL/min. For larger drugs, therefore, the removal rate can be increased by increasing the surface area, a situation similar to removal of larger uremic solutes. For this reason, also, in uremic patients treated with various drugs, which are usually greater than 300 daltons, it is to be expected that drug accumulation occurs even in the presence of dialysis, which is more effective for removal of small solutes.

Dialysance, or Clearance

Dialysance (D) is the traditional term used for solute removal by dialysate, which is given by the following formula:

$$D = Q_b \frac{B_i - B_o}{B_i - B_i} = Q_d \frac{D_o - D_i}{B_i - D_i}$$

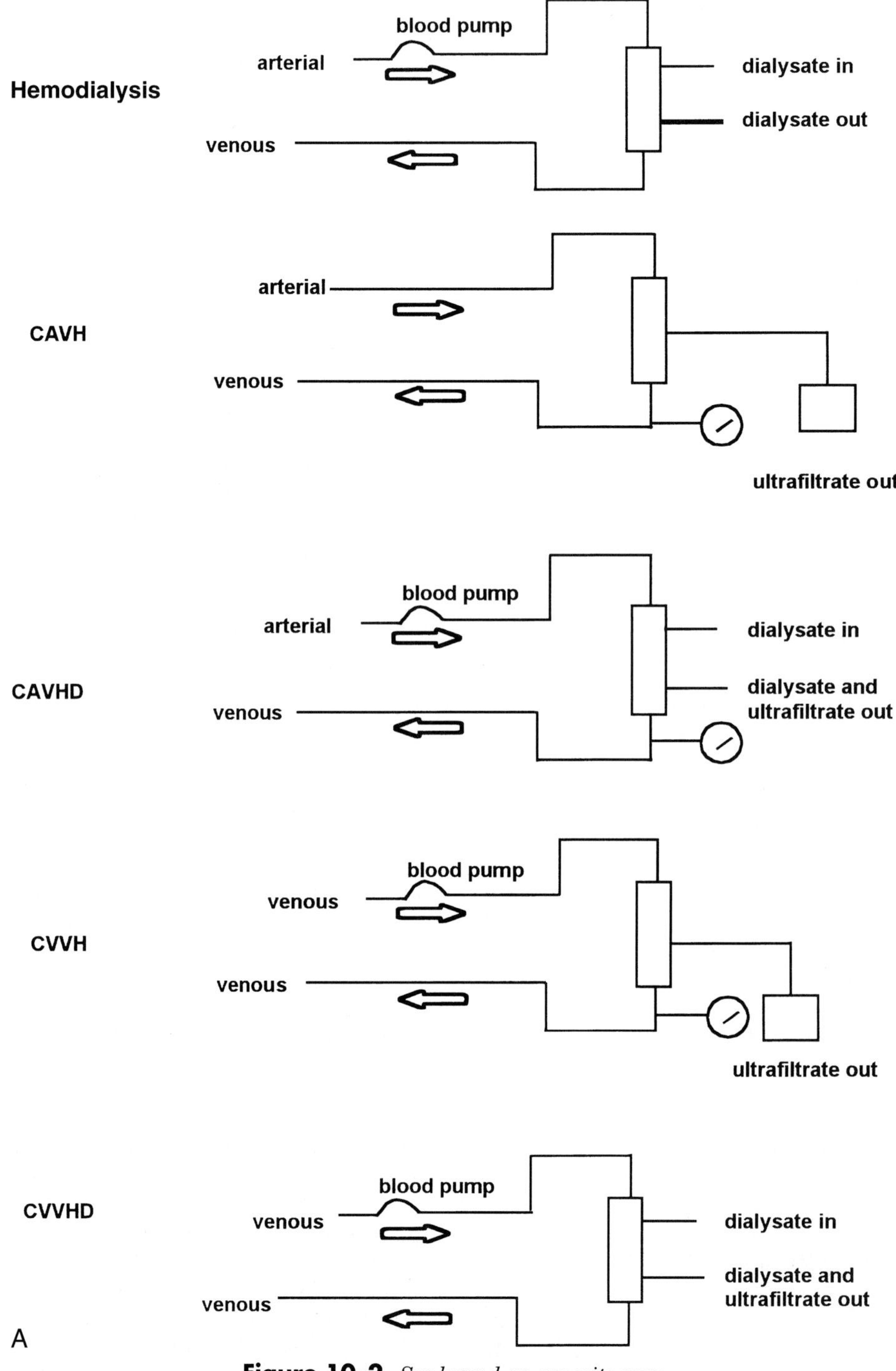

Figure 10–2 *See legend on opposite page*

where Q_b and Q_d are flow rates of blood and dialysate, respectively; B_i and B_o are blood concentrations entering and leaving the dialyzer; and D_i and D_o are the dialysate inlet and outlet concentrations. Dialysance takes into account the concentration of drug in the dialysate. However, when the concentration of drug in dialysate is negligible (i.e., when the dialysate does not come into further contact with the dialyzer in the process known as *single-pass dialysis,* such as used in hollow-fiber and flat-plate modern dialyzers), then such a formula gives the *clearance* of solute from the blood:

$$\text{Clearance} = Q_b \frac{A-V}{A}$$

where A is arterial, or inlet, concentration; V is venous, or outlet, concentration of drug going through the dialyzer; and Q_b is blood flow rate through the dialyzer. The ratio $A-V/A$ also equates to the drug

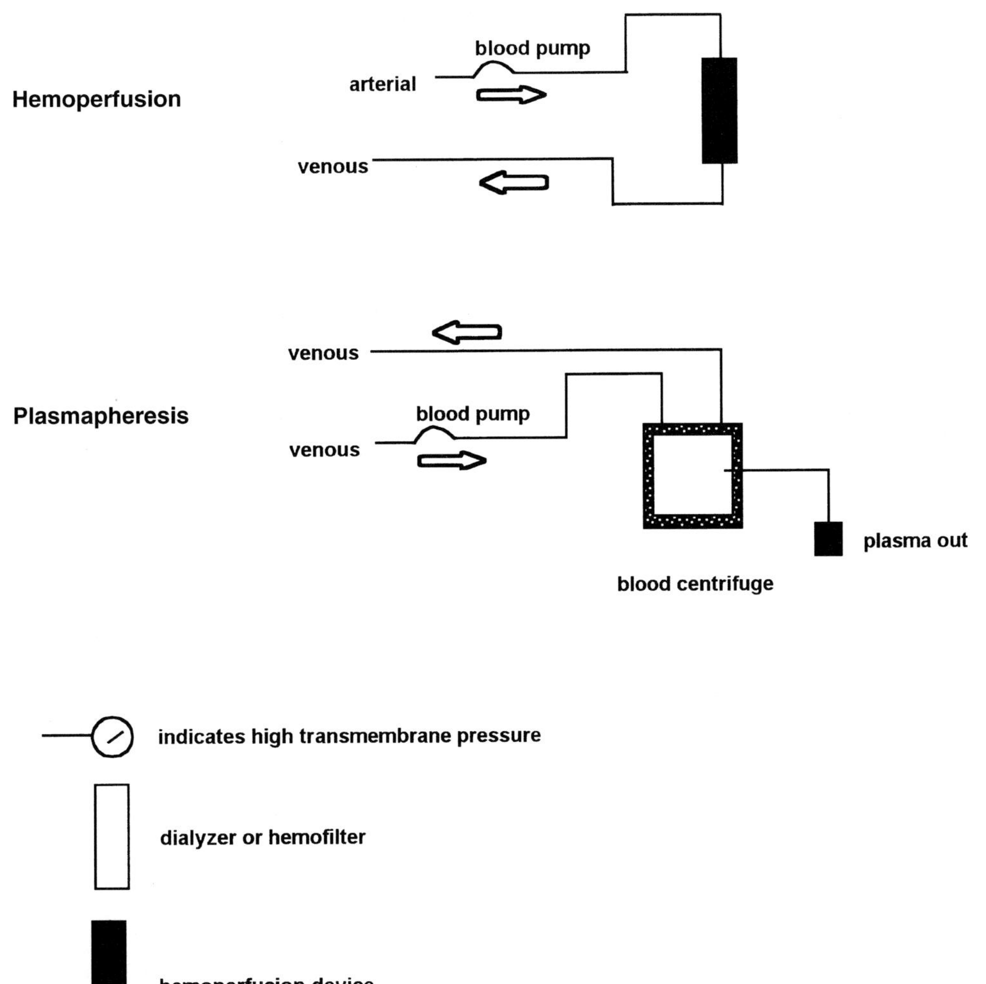

Figure 10–2. *A* and *B*, Extracorporeal circuits for procedures used in drug or chemical removal. CAVH, continuous arteriovenous hemofiltration; CAVHD, continuous arteriovenous hemodialysis; CVVH, continuous venovenous hemofiltration; CVVHD, continuous venovenous hemodialysis.

extraction ratio across the dialyzer, and this is dealt with in some detail in the following section.

Factors Governing Drug Removal with Dialysis

Drug removal rates with dialysis can be calculated from *in vitro* experiments, the accuracy of which is increased if *in vitro* experiments use protein-containing drug or chemical solutions to mimic the clinical situation. It is often assumed that the plasma concentrations are representative of whole blood concentrations, and blood flow rates have been used for calculations of clearances on the assumption that blood represents the volume from which the solute is removed to dialysate. However, drugs are removable from red blood cells, and failure to use the whole blood flow rates through dialyzers (or hemoperfusion devices) can introduce considerable errors into calculation of clearances. Although the volume of distribution of drugs and their lipid solubility are extremely important in relation to drug removal with dialysis, it is also important to consider the intercompartmental transfer of drugs from tissues into plasma and its influence on drug removal rates;[15] the influence of this factor on drug removal for most drug is unknown and is not discussed further.

Although plasma protein binding is an important factor and the degree of protein binding depends on plasma protein concentrations and solute concentrations, it must be pointed out that some solutes do not saturate binding sites at the usual pharmacologic concentrations but others demonstrate an increase in the ultrafilterable fraction at very high drug levels. This is noted with salicylate poisoning and renders salicylate an ideal dialyzable drug.

Lipid solubility of drugs also governs their removal by dialysis. Removal of ethchlorvynol and glutethimide, as examples of highly lipid-soluble drugs, has been shown to be low with aqueous dialysis; this rate is increased by the use of lipid dialysis, which allows partitioning of these drugs in lipid globules within the dialysate. However, with modern dialysis and with large surface area dialyzers, this technique has fallen into disfavor. In addition, lipid-soluble drugs are more readily removed with activated charcoal or resin hemoperfusion; these techniques are discussed later.

Ultrafiltration dialysis is the term used to describe aqueous hemodialysis, with hydrostatic ultrafiltration of water through the semi-permeable membrane. This process is known to increase solvent drag of solute, thereby making its clearance higher than at a degree at which no ultrafiltration occurs. This type of dialysis was tried (unsuccessfully) for treating poisoning with agents such as paraquat,[16] but with conventional hemodialyzer membranes the degree of increase in clearance is rather small. The clearance of solutes by the process of ultrafiltration, however, is greatly enhanced if the membrane has larger pores.[17] Although these large-pore membranes were not specifically introduced for poisoning therapy, it is known that removal of solutes ranging from 64 (urea) up to 1500 (vitamin B_{12}) daltons is identical; therefore, this type of treatment theoretically should allow higher clearance rates for rather high-molecular-weight drugs. CAVH, CAVHD, CVVH, and CVVHD also use large-pore membranes and rely on ultrafiltration for solute and fluid removal (see Fig. 10–2).

It thus can be appreciated that peritoneal dialysis is the least effective method for removing drugs compared with hemodialysis and hemofiltration, in view of the slower dialysate transit times within the abdominal cavity. Peritoneal dialysis should therefore be used for removing dialyzable poisons only if the other methods are unavailable. Drugs such as calcium channel blockers have been shown to slightly increase peritoneal clearances of various solutes by inducing changes in vascular permeability, but this method has not been used in human clinical poisoning.

Peritoneal Dialysis

Peritoneal dialysis uses the instillation of sterile, preheated, commercially available dialysate solutions (2 L) into the abdominal cavity of a poisoned patient, using a semi-rigid peritoneal catheter placed 4 to 5 inches below the umbilicus under local anesthesia. The peritoneal dialysate is changed, usually hourly, with the dialysate "dwelling" within the peritoneal cavity for about 30 minutes, after which it is drained and discarded. As pointed out earlier, this technique is less efficient than hemodialysis, but in certain situations it is of some use. In hypothermic patients, instillation of preheated solutions into the abdominal cavity can rapidly reverse the hypothermia; theoretically, equilibration across the gastrointestinal wall may influence removal of ingested drugs before equilibration with body stores is achieved.

Hemodialysis

Hemodialysis requires the passage of anticoagulated (heparinized) blood through dialyzer lines and dialyzers consisting of semi-permeable membranes through which dialysate is brought into juxtaposition with blood on the other side of the semi-permeable membrane. Dialyzers are available as flat-plate or hollow-fiber models. Blood is usually pumped through the dialyzer lines with a roller pump. Blood is derived from an arteriovenous shunt (for CAVH, when blood flow is not controlled by a pump) or from venous or arterial catheters (single or double lumen) placed in the arm or leg, and blood flows are adjusted according to a patient's blood pressure. Whole blood clotting time or activated clotting time must be maintained within limits by adjusting heparin dosage.

In a hypotensive patient who requires dopamine or dobutamine for blood pressure control, these drugs must be placed distal to the drug-removing device. Requirements of these catecholamines may increase during the procedure, because they are readily removed through the hemodialyzer membrane or sorbent. Lipid hemodialysis requires the addition of quantities of soybean oil to aqueous dialysate to form an emulsion, but as previously noted, the advantages of modern hemodialyzers and hemodialyzer apparatus largely outweigh the benefits of lipid hemodialysis. Single-pass dialysis systems are the most efficient methods for removing drugs (or other solutes) because they maintain a constant concentration gradient, which enhances drug removal.

Dialysate regeneration apparatus in which the dialysate is regenerated using a sorbent system (the REDY system) may be used in the treatment of poisoned patients. However, it must be pointed out that the sorbent system may theoretically become saturated with drug, and removal rates decrease over time for certain drugs.

CRITERIA FOR CONSIDERATION OF HEMODIALYSIS IN POISONING

The decision about whether a patient should undergo active drug removal is not always easily made, and it is certainly not the purpose of this discussion to suggest that every patient suffering from poisoning of an extractable drug undergo hemodialysis. The *prime consideration in the decision is based on the clinical features of poisoning; hemodialysis or hemoperfusion should be considered in general if the patient's condition progressively deteriorates despite intensive supportive therapy.*

The use of active drug-removing techniques has engendered a great deal of controversy. Some clinicians are conservative in their approach; others are more aggressive. Appraisal of each viewpoint, however, reveals little difference and may be explained by patient spectrum and geographic area. Both groups are, however, very close in their use of intervention techniques for specific poisonings as well as for specific clinical indications. Supportive therapy includes appropriate fluid balance, correction of acid-base abnormalities, pressor infusion, and forced diuresis.

Table 10–4. Clinical Considerations for Hemodialysis or Hemoperfusion in Poisoning

- Progressive deterioration despite intensive supportive therapy
- Severe intoxication with depression of midbrain function leading to hypoventilation, hypothermia, and hypotension
- Development of complications of coma, such as pneumonia or septicemia, and underlying conditions predisposing to such complications (e.g., obstructive airway disease)
- Impairment of normal drug excretory function in the presence of hepatic, cardiac, or renal insufficiency
- Intoxication with agents with metabolic and/or delayed effects (e.g., methanol, ethylene glycol, and paraquat)
- Intoxication with an extractable drug or poison that can be removed at a rate exceeding that of endogenous elimination by the liver or kidneys

Suggested clinical criteria are outlined in Table 10–4. These criteria should be used along with the plasma concentrations of common drugs (Table 10–5), above which hemodialysis or hemoperfusion should be considered. Table 10–6 lists the reported dialyzable drugs; note that many of the reports are anecdotal and uncritical, and it is suggested that dialysis be reserved for only those drugs that are not placed in parentheses in Table 10–6. For further discussion of specific agents, see the appropriate chapter and the review by Golper and colleagues.[18]

SORBENT HEMOPERFUSION

Hemoperfusion, by which anticoagulated blood is passed through a column containing sorbent particles, was introduced in the 1940s,[19] refined in 1950 to 1970,[20–22] and adopted for clinical use in poisoning in the 1970s and 1980s.[23–25] Both activated charcoal hemoperfusion and resin hemoperfusion devices are available. In addition, antibody- or antigen-coated charcoal hemoperfusion is available for specific autoimmune states (lupus erythematosus[26] and removal of cytotoxic antibody before renal transplantation[27]).

Table 10–5. Plasma Concentrations of Common Poisons in Excess of Which Hemodialysis or Hemoperfusion Should Be Considered

Drug	Serum Concentration* (μg/mL)	(mmol/L)	Method of Choice
Phenobarbital	100	430	HP>HD
Other barbiturates	50	200	HP
Glutethimide	40	160	HP
Methaqualone	40	160	HP
Salicylates	800	5000	HD
Theophylline	400	2200	HP>HD
Paraquat	0.1	0.5	HP>HD
Methanol	50		HD
Trichloroethanol	50	335	HP>HD
Meprobamate	100	460	HP

HD, hemodialysis; HP, hemoperfusion.

*Suggested concentrations only: Clinical condition may warrant intervention at lower concentrations (e.g., in mixed intoxications).

Table 10–6. Representative Drugs Removed by Dialysis

Alcohols

Ethanol
Ethylene glycol
Isopropanol
Methanol

Analgesics

Acetaminophen
Colchicine
Salicylates

Antibiotics and Chemotherapeutics

Amoxicillin
Clavulanic acid
Penicillin
Ticarcillin
Cefixime
Cefuroxime
Cephalexin
Amikacin
Gentamicin
Kanamycin
Neomycin
Streptomycin
Tobramycin
Metronidazole
Nitrofurantoin
Sulfisoxazole
Sulfonamides
Tetracycline
Imipenem
Ciprofloxacin
Acyclovir
Isoniazid
Ethambutol
Didanosine
Zidovudine
Foscarnet
Ganciclovir
Cyclophosphamide
5-Fluorouracil

Sedatives-Anticonvulsants

Butabarbital
Pentobarbital
Phenobarbital
Carbamazepine
Chloral hydrate
Ethchlorvynol
Glutethimide
Meprobamate
Primidone
(Valproic acid)

Cardiovascular Drugs

Atenolol
Captopril
Enalapril
Metoprolol
Methyldopa
Nadolol
Procainamide
Propranolol
Sotalol
Tocainide

Solvents

Acetone
Camphor
Thiols
Toluene
Trichloroethylene

Miscellaneous

Lithium
Theophylline
Paraquat
Aniline
Boric acid
Chromic acid
Chlorates
Diquat
Thiocyanate

Parentheses indicate not well removed.

Early hemoperfusion devices produced transient side effects such as facial flushing, dyspnea, and burning sensations as well as platelet depletion and reduction of fibrinogen concentrations. Such side effects have been overcome with preparatory techniques including selection of materials, washing, and coating with a polymer solution, which impairs particle generation and platelet aggregation without losing efficiency of adsorption.

Certain resins have been shown to be most effective for removal of lipid-soluble drugs, with drug clearance rates from blood often exceeding those achieved by charcoal hemoperfusion. Although used in Europe, they are no longer available in the United States. The clinically available hemoperfusion devices and the contained sorbents are listed in Table 10–7.

Hemoperfusion relies on the physical process of drug adsorption for its efficiency, and in many instances drug removal in terms of clearance is far better than with hemodialysis, peritoneal dialysis, or forced diuresis. With activated charcoal, drugs are

Table 10–7. Available Hemoperfusion Devices

Manufacturer	Device	Sorbent Type	Amount of Sorbent	Polymer Coating
Bioencapsulation Technology	DiaKart	Petroleum-based charcoal	70 g	Collodion
Clark	Biocompatible system	Charcoal	50, 100, 250 mL	Heparinized polymer
Gambro	Adsorba	Norit	100 or 300 g	Cellulose acetate
Organon-Teknika	Hemopûr 260	Norit extruded charcoal	260 g	Cellulose acetate
Smith and Nephew	Hemocol or Haemocol	Sucliffe Speakman charcoal	100 or 300 g	Acrylic hydrogel
Braun	Haemoresin	XAD-4	350 g	None

often so tightly bound with Van der Waals' forces that they are unextractable from the sorbent. On the other hand, with the resin preparations, the drug is tightly but not irreversibly bound within the resin bead matrix and can be eluted with organic solvents. Water- and lipid-soluble substances with molecular weights ranging from 113 to 40,000 daltons are well adsorbed, although substances at the higher molecular weights are adsorbed less efficiently to charcoal when a coating polymer solution is used.[28]

A typical hemoperfusion circuit for treatment of drug intoxication is shown in Figure 10–2; in general, hemoperfusion is instituted with a column that contains between 100 and 300 g of activated charcoal or 650 g (wet weight) of polystyrene resin. Most devices are flushed with saline before use (because most come already sterilized), and blood is withdrawn through an arteriovenous shunt or venovenous shunt, as in hemodialysis, using a blood pump. Blood flow rates are graduated, depending on the clinical condition of the patient, but the most efficient drug removal is achieved with blood flow rates of approximately 300 mL/min. Pressure devices can detect interior increases in pressure, which serve as an index of thrombosis occurring inside the device. With the resin preparations, greater decrements in platelet counts were observed.

Table 10–8 shows that the plasma-drug extraction ratios for many drugs are greater with hemoperfusion than with hemodialysis. Removal of lipid-soluble drugs, such as glutethimide and methaqualone, is far more efficient with XAD-4 resin hemoperfusion than with activated charcoal.

Table 10–9 lists representative drugs that have been reported to be removed by various types of hemoperfusion; again, it cannot be overstated that many of these reports are anecdotal, but critical review of drug removal rates indicates that those drugs not enclosed in parentheses are most efficiently removed.

Criteria for Consideration of Hemoperfusion in Poisoning

The criteria outlined in Tables 10–4 and 10–5 for hemodialysis also apply to hemoperfusion. However, in certain situations one is preferred over the other, so Table 10–10 is provided as a guide in choosing either hemoperfusion or hemodialysis.

Complications of Hemoperfusion

The principal side effect of hemoperfusion with charcoal or resin preparations is platelet depletion. Most studies of hemoperfusion in humans show an average loss of 30% of platelets with coated or uncoated charcoal or resin preparations. A larger decrement in platelet count can occasionally occur and may give rise to clinical bleeding problems. Other side effects noted are reductions in serum calcium and serum glucose levels and transient reductions in

Table 10–8. Plasma Drug Extraction Ratios with Different Hemodialysis/Hemoperfusion Devices*

	Standard Hemodialysis Charcoal	Coated or Uncoated Hemoperfusion	XAD-2 or XAD-4 Resin Hemoperfusion
Acetaminophen	0.4	0.5	0.7
Amobarbital	0.26	0.3	0.9
Acetylsalicylic acid	0.5	0.5	—
Carbromal	0.31	0.55	1.0
Digoxin	0.2	0.3–0.6	0.4
Ethchlorvynol	0.32	0.7	1.0
Glutethimide	0.16	0.65	0.8
Paraquat	0.5	0.6	0.9†
Phenobarbital	0.27	0.5	0.85
Theophylline	0.5	0.7	0.75
Tricyclics	0.35	0.35	0.8

*Calculated for blood flow rate 200 mL/min.
†Ion exchange resin.

Table 10–9. Drugs and Chemicals Removed with Hemoperfusion

Barbiturates	Amobarbital Butabarbital Hexabarbital Pentobarbital Phenobarbital Quinalbital Secobarbital Thiopental Vinalbital
Nonbarbiturate Hypnotics, Sedatives, and Tranquilizers	Carbromal Chloral hydrate Chlorpromazine (Diazepam) Diphenhydramine Ethchlorvynol Glutethimide Meprobamate Methaqualone Methsuximide Methyprylon Promazine Promethazine (Valproic acid)
Analgesics, Antirheumatics	Acetaminophen Acetylsalicylic acid Colchicine D-Propoxyphene Methylsalicylate Phenylbutazone Salicylic acid
Antimicrobials/Anticancer	(Adriamycin)† Ampicillin Carmustine† Chloramphenicol Chloroquine Clindamycin Dapsone Doxorubicin (5-Fluorouracil) Gentamicin Isoniazid (Methotrexate) Thiabendazole)
Antidepressants	(Amitryptiline) (Imipramine) (Tricyclics)
Plant and Animal Toxins, Herbicides, Insectides	Amanitin Chlordane Demeton sulfoxide Dimethoate Diquat Methylparathion Nitrostigmine (Organophosphates) Parathion Paraquat Phalloidin Polychlorinated biphenyls
Cardiovascular	Digoxin Diltiazem (Disopyramide) Flecainide Metoprolol *N*-acetylprocainamide Procainamide Quinidine
Miscellaneous	Aminophylline Cimetidine (Fluoroacetamide) (Phencyclidine) Phenols (Podophyllin) Theophylline
Solvents, Gases	Carbon tetrachloride Ethylene oxide Trichloroethane Xylene
Metals	(Aluminum)* (Iron)

( ), Not well removed; ( )*, removed with chelating agent; †, well removed in regional hemoperfusion.

white blood cell counts, all of which are usually mild and can be managed clinically. In addition, with the recirculating of blood in the extracorporeal circuit a mild reduction of 1 to 2°F in body temperature occurs, and body temperatures should be frequently measured in deeply comatose patients. Although hypotension as a consequence of circulation of blood in the extracorporeal circuit is an infrequent phenomenon in drug overdosage, pressor agents such as dopamine for hypotensive comatose patients should be administered distal to the sorbent devices, because they are also adsorbed by the sorbent preparations. The observed reductions in platelet concentrations have usually returned to normal limits within 24 to 28 hours after a single hemoperfusion. Such decrements are far outweighed by the clinical benefits to be obtained.

Table 10–10. Choice of Hemodialysis or Hemoperfusion for Certain Drugs

Hemodialysis	Hemoperfusion
Lithium	Lipid-soluble drugs
Bromide	Barbiturates
Ethanol	Nonbarbiturate hypnotics, sedatives, and tranquilizers
Methanol	Digitalis glycosides
Ethylene glycol	Theophylline
Salicylates	

INFLUENCE OF ACTIVE DRUG REMOVAL PROCEDURES ON DRUG ELIMINATION RATE

In barbiturate poisoning, forced diuresis has not been conclusively shown to alter duration of coma or overall mortality; in one large study of forced diuresis in barbiturate poisoning, mortality was reduced from 3.5% to 2.4%, but if deaths in the most severely affected groups were excluded, mortality with diuresis was 2.1% compared with 2.6% without diuresis, results that may not be significantly different. Peritoneal dialysis is not substantially more effective than diuresis, because peritoneal clearance of most drugs is usually less than 10 mL/min. However, as mentioned, pharmacologic agents or albumin added to dialysate may increase drug removal rates, although it has not been confirmed that peritoneal dialysis shortens coma time or substantially increases total clearance of barbiturates.

Maher and Schreiner pointed out that any procedure used in poisoning treatment must be demonstrated to have a greater effect on drug elimination than that which occurs spontaneously.[29] In human beings, the spontaneous half-life of barbiturates in barbiturate poisoning ranges from 37 to 96 hours, and hemodialysis does seem to have some effect on this, with reported rates of drug half-life ranging from 3.6 to 9.7 hours.[30] Hemoperfusion, on the other hand, has been shown in animals to reduce mortality in barbiturate, salicylate, and paraquat poisoning and to reduce the duration of coma in barbiturate-poisoned dogs.[31] In humans, in comparison with standard supportive therapy, hemoperfusion also appears to shorten the duration of coma, but no controlled studies have been undertaken. For further discussion of specific agents, see the appropriate chapter.

Using appropriate pharmacokinetic models, it has been shown that hemoperfusion increases drug elimination rates in animals intoxicated with acetaminophen, amobarbital, ethchlorvynol, doxorubicin (Adriamycin), digoxin, and digitoxin. In all these experiments, as well as in clinical experience, it has been observed that "rebound" of drug concentration occurs after hemoperfusion as drug redistributes from tissues into the plasma after its removal from the plasma compartment. This is consistent with pharmacokinetic handling of drugs after their removal from the central compartment, but clinically it may return the patient to coma—for instance, as occurs after hemoperfusion for glutethimide poisoning.

Intermittent hemoperfusion has two major advantages: reduction in blood concentrations and attenuation of the hematologic side effects of prolonged hemoperfusion. Replacement of saturated devices with fresh devices is not usually necessary but is another positive aspect of short intermittent hemoperfusion. Any rebound in plasma drug concentrations released from tissue can be reduced with further hemoperfusion (e.g., paraquat and glutethimide). Review of pharmacokinetic data not unexpectedly has shown that hemodialysis and hemoperfusion enhance drug elimination for only specific drugs. In humans, in view of the difficulties in conducting controlled prospective clinical trials, reduction in the duration of coma or overall mortality has not conclusively been demonstrated, although it has been suggested by retrospective studies. In severely hypothermic patients, hemoperfusion can be combined with hemodialysis for blood warming.

Hemoperfusion of blood draining a limb or the cerebral circulation may effect significant regional removal of anticancer drugs and reduce systemic exposure and has been used experimentally in human cancers.

PLASMA EXCHANGE AND EXCHANGE BLOOD TRANSFUSION

Both plasma exchange and exchange blood transfusions have been used infrequently in the treatment of poisoning.[32] Plasma exchange, or plasmapheresis, involves removal of a patient's plasma by means of centrifugal or filtration devices, with substitution of fresh plasma. Exchange blood transfusion involves the removal of a quantity of blood and its replacement with an identical quantity of fresh whole blood. Plasma exchange involves a 3- to 4-L exchange of plasma in a 4-hour treatment period; therefore, the total maximal quantity of drug removed is its concentration times the volume of plasma removed. This technique, therefore, is most applicable to strongly protein-bound drugs that are not well removed with hemodialysis. (Examples are chromic acid and chromate poisoning, although it may not be successful in every case.[33]). The effectiveness of plasmapheresis in various poisonings has been reported anecdotally, but at present the role of plasmapheresis is unclear. Exchange blood transfusion has also been used infrequently in the treatment of poisoning, principally when hemolysis and methemoglobinemia have complicated the poisoning (e.g., sodium chlorate poisonings), whereas plasma exchange with subsequent plasma perfusion over sorbents has been used for various poisons.

HEMOPERFUSION AND HEMODIALYSIS WITH CHELATING AGENTS

In dialyzed patients, aluminum and iron intoxication can be treated with deferoxamine in conjunction with dialysis (continuous ambulatory peritoneal dialysis or hemodialysis) or hemoperfusion, for removal of the deferoxamine-aluminum complex. Clinical improvement in the osteomalacia component of renal osteodystrophy, encephalopathy, iron overload, or anemia has been reported.[34, 35]

Heavy metals and their salts are not removed efficiently by dialysis or hemoperfusion alone. During hemodialysis, metal removal may be enhanced with certain chelating agents, such as N-acetylcysteine or cysteine. On the other hand, removal of mercury and thallium by hemoperfusion appears modest at best. Chelating microspheres or chelate-metal groups for adsorption may eventually prove useful clinically for heavy metal removal.[36, 37]

IMMUNOPHARMACOLOGY AS AN ACTIVE TREATMENT METHOD IN POISONING

An antibody is composed of two Fab fragments and an Fac fragment. Fab fragments retain the binding sites of the antibodies and have a molecular weight of about 50,000 daltons. By appropriately binding the drug to a hapten, an antibody response can be mounted, and antibody fractions can be subjected to splitting to obtain Fab fragments. When injected, these Fab fragments combine with specific antigens (drug) with a high degree of specificity to neutralize their toxic effects. In potentially fatal cases of glycoside poisoning, such procedures have resulted in a response far greater than that obtained with conventional therapy. In the presence of renal failure, however, for drugs that depend on renal elimination, the effectiveness of Fab fragment administration may be minimized.

Poisoning treated by immunopharmacology is now limited to digoxin poisoning. In digoxin poisoning, the elimination half-life of digoxin in anephric patients can be substantially reduced with the addition of hemoperfusion. Potentially fatal cases of digoxin poisoning have been successfully treated by Fab antibody fragments, but failures have also been reported, and the cost of treatment averages $1680 (range of $175 to $7000).[38] Immobilized antibody on hemoperfusion devices may offer an alternative.[39] In dialyzed patients (in whom vascular access facilitates interventional therapy), a judgment to use either hemoperfusion or Fab antibody fragments is required. Moreover, recrudescence of digoxin poisoning has been reported 24 to 48 hours after Fab antibodies have been administered to *patients with renal failure.*[40]

References

1. Jacobs C, Kjellstrand CM, Koch KM, Winchester JF: Replacement of Renal Function by Dialysis. 4th ed. Boston, Kluwer Academic Publishers, 1996.
2. Litovitz TL, Felberg L, Soloway RA, et al: 1995 Annual Report of the American Association of Poison Control Centers Toxic Exposure Surveillance System. Am J Emerg Med *14:*487, 1996.
3. Litovitz TL, Martin TG, Schmitz B: 1986 Annual Report of the American Association of Poison Control Centers National Data Collection System. Am J Emerg Med *5:*405, 1987.
4. Winchester JF: Active methods for detoxification. *In* Haddad LM, Winchester JF (eds): Clinical Management of Poisoning and Drug Overdose. 2nd ed. Philadephia, W. B. Saunders Co., 1990.
5. Mayer SE, Melman KL, Gilman AG: Introduction: The dynamics of drug absorption, distribution and elimination. *In* Gilman AG, Goodman LS, Gilman A (eds): The Pharmacological Basis of Therapeutics. 6th ed. New York, Macmillan Publishing Co., p 1, 1981.
6. Gabow PA, Peterson LN: Disorders of potassium metabolism. *In* Schrier RW (ed): Renal and Electrolyte Disorders. 2nd ed. Boston, Little, Brown & Co, p 183, 1980.
7. Prescott LF, Balali-Mood M, Critchley JA, et al: Diuresis or urinary alkalinization in salicylate poisoning? BMJ *285:* 1383, 1982.
8. Done AK: Salicylate intoxication: Significance of measurements of salicylate in blood in cases of acute ingestion. Pediatrics *26:*800, 1960.
9. Schreiner GE: Dialysis of poison and drugs—annual review. Trans Am Soc Artif Intern Organs *16:*544, 1970.
10. Vale JA, Rees AJ, Widdop B, Goulding R: Use of charcoal haemoperfusion in the management of severely poisoned patients. Br Med J 1:5, 1975.
11. Ash SR, Carr DJ, Blake DE, et al. Effect of sorbent-based dialytic therapy with the Biologic-DT on an experimental model of hepatic failure. Trans Am Soc Artif Intern Organs *39:*M675, 1993
12. Henderson LW, Silverstein MAE, Ford CA, Lysaght MJ: Clinical response to maintenance hemodiafiltration. Kidney Int *7:*S52, 1975.
13. Kaplan AA: Continuous arteriovenous hemofiltration and related therapies. *In* Jacobs C, Kjellstrand CM, Koch KM, Winchester JF (eds): Replacement of Renal Function by Dialysis. 4th ed. Boston, Kluwer Academic Publishers, p 390, 1996.
14. Maher JF: Principles of dialysis and dialysis of drugs. Am J Med *62:*475, 1977.
15. Gibson TP, Atkinson AI: Effect of changes in intercompartment rate constants on drug removal during hemoperfusion. J Pharm Sci *67:*1178, 1978.
16. Pond SM, Johnston SC, Schoof DD, et al: Repeated hemoperfusion and continuous arteriovenous hemofiltration in a paraquat poisoned patient. J Toxicol Clin Toxicol *25:*305, 1987.
17. Henderson LW: Biophysics of ultrafiltration and hemofiltration. *In* Jacobs C, Kjellstrand CM, Koch KM, Winchester JF (eds): Replacement of Renal Function by Dialysis. 4th ed. Boston, Kluwer Academic Publishers, p 146, 1996.
18. Golper TA, Marx MA, Shuler C, Bennett WM: Drug dosage in dialysis patients. *In* Jacobs C, Kjellstrand CM, Koch KM, Winchester JF (eds): Replacement of Renal Function by Dialysis. 4th ed. Boston, Kluwer Academic Publishers, p 750, 1996.
19. Muirhead EE, Reid AF: Resin artificial kidney. Lab Clin Med *33:*841, 1948.
20. Schreiner GE: The role of hemodialysis (artificial kidney) in acute poisoning. Arch Intern Med *102:*896, 1958.
21. Yatzidis IT, Voudiclari S, Oreopoulos D, et al: Treatment of severe barbiturate poisoning. Lancet *2:*216, 1965.
22. Chang TMS: Artificial Cells. Springfield, IL, Charles C Thomas, Publisher, 1972.
23. Hampel G, Crome P, Widdop B, Goulding R: Experience with fixed-bed charcoal haemoperfusion in the treatment of severe drug intoxication. Arch Toxicol *45:*133, 1980.
24. Gelfand MC, Winchester JF, Knepshield JH, et al: Charcoal hemoperfusion in severe drug overdosage. Trans Am Soc Artif Intern Organs *23:*599, 1977.
25. Verpooten GA, De Broe ME: Combined hemoperfusion-hemodialysis in severe poisoning: Kinetics of drug extraction. Resuscitation *11:*275, 1984.
26. Terman DS, Buffaloe G, Mattioli C, et al: Extracorporeal immunoabsorption: Initial experience in human systemic lupus erythematosus. Lancet *2:*824, 1979.
27. Hakim, RM, Milford E, Himmelfarb J, et al: Extracorporeal removal of anti-HLA antibodies in transplant candidates. Am J Kidney Dis *16:*423, 1990.
28. Denti E, Luboz MP, Tessore V: Adsorption characteristics of cellulose acetate coated charcoals. J Biomed Mater Res *9:*143, 1975.
29. Maher JF, Schreiner GE: The dialysis of poison and drugs. Trans Am Soc Artif Intern Organ *13:*369, 1967.
30. Hadden J, Johnson K, Smith S, et al: Acute barbiturate intoxication: Concepts in management. JAMA *209:*893, 1969.
31. Winchester JF, Gelfand MC, Tilstone WJ: Hemoperfusion in drug intoxication: Clinical and laboratory aspects. Drug Metab Rev *8:*69, 1978.
32. Gurland HJ, Samtleben W, Lysaght MJ, Winchester JF: Extracorporeal blood purification techniques: Plasmapheresis and hemoperfusion. *In* Jacobs C, Kjellstrand CM, Koch KM, Winchester JF (eds): Replacement of Renal Function by Dialysis. 4th ed. Boston, Kluwer Academic Publishers, p 472, 1996.
33. Meert KL, Ellis J, Aronow R, Perrin E: Acute ammonium dichromate poisoning. Ann Emerg Med *24:*748, 1994.
34. Winchester JF: Management of iron overload. Semin Nephrol *4*(Suppl 1):22, 1986.
35. Chang TMS, Barre P: Effect of desferrioxamine on removal of aluminum and iron by coated charcoal haemoperfusion and haemodialysis. Lancet *2:*1051, 1983.
36. Margel S: A novel approach for heavy metal poisoning treatment, a model. Mercury poisoning by means of chelating microspheres; hemoperfusion and oral administration. J Med Chem *24:*1263, 1981.
37. De Groot G, van Heijst AN, van Kesteren RG, Maes RA: An evaluation of the efficacy of charcoal haemoperfusion in the treatment of three cases of acute thallium poisoning. Arch Toxicol *57:*61, 1985.

38. Martiny SS, Phelps SI, Massey KL: Treatment of severe digitalis intoxication with digoxin-specific antibody fragments: A clinical review. Crit Care Med *16:*629, 1988.
39. Savin H, Marcus L, Margel S, et al: Treatment of adverse digitalis effects by hemoperfusion through columns containing antidigoxin antibodies bound to agarose polyacrolein microsphere beads. Am Heart J *113:*1078, 1987.
40. Ujhelyi MR, Robert S, Cummings DM, et al: Disposition of digoxin immune Fab in patients with kidney failure. Clin Pharmacol Ther *54:*388, 1993.

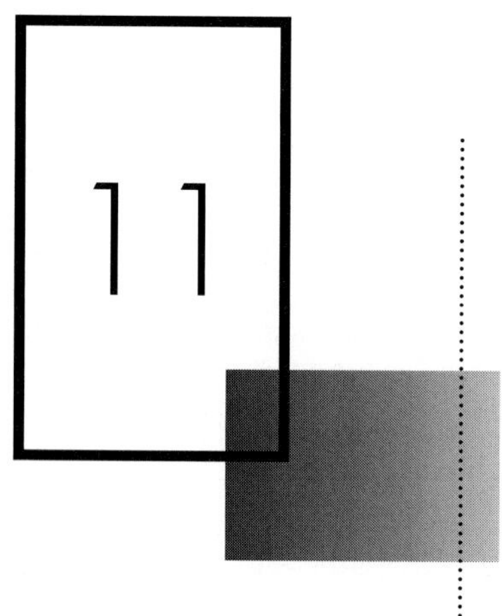

Renal Toxicity

A Acute Renal Failure

GARABED EKNOYAN, MD

A common consequence of the renal injury that results from any poisoning or drug overdose is the entity that has come to be known as *acute renal failure* (ARF). ARF itself is a clinical syndrome of diverse causes (Table 11A–1) in which a sudden deterioration of renal function results in the inability of the kidneys to regulate normal homeostasis. Its importance stems from the acuteness and severity of the clinical manifestations that develop and the potential for reversibility of the condition, particularly if it is recognized early and the appropriate preventive and therapeutic measures are instituted promptly. Despite the fact that it is a self-limited condition and that it is one instance of organ failure that is totally reversible and for which replacement therapy is available, ARF is associated with a high mortality rate, principally because of the seriousness of the underlying conditions that lead to its onset and in turn are aggravated by the loss of renal regulatory functions.[1]

ARF as we have come to understand it occupies a very brief span in the history of medicine. Clearly it must have afflicted humankind from the dawn of history, when the very effort of daily existence exposed individuals to infected wounds, crush injuries, and massive hemorrhage. Yet, the problem initially recognized as acute anuria or cessation of urine and addressed in much of recorded medicine concerns that due to obstruction or associated with dropsy. The clinical description of the entity, as much of the rest of medical knowledge, becomes somewhat clearer in the Age of Enlightenment when suppression of urine or *ischuria renalis,* as it was then termed, came to be attributed to either inflammation or "paralysis of the kidneys" as opposed to that of retention of the urine associated with obstruction that had been previously identified.[2] The name "paralysis of the kidneys" was soon criticized on the grounds that palsy is a term that should be restricted to the loss of muscle power.

The state of affairs by the turn of the century is perhaps best summarized by Osler in his 1909 edition of *The Principles and Practice of Medicine.* He classified ARF under the general heading of acute Bright's disease, a rather broad and vague group of cases of ARF among which he included toxic agents (turpentine, potassium chlorate, carbolic acid), extensive skin burns, and trauma. Shortly afterward, the acute renal lesions that affected crushed or wounded soldiers were described in the German literature during and immediately after the First World War.[3] Sporadic reports of ARF in traumatized civilians began to appear in the literature thereafter and were soon followed by reports of cases of ARF that ensued after

Table 11A–1. Major Causes of Acute Renal Failure

Prerenal Failure
Extracellular circulating fluid volume contraction
Gastrointestinal losses: vomiting, diarrhea
Fluid sequestration: burns, pancreatitis, peritonitis, crush injury, venous ligation
Renal losses: diuretics, diabetic ketoacidosis
Blood loss
Central or cardiac shock: congestive heart failure, myocardial infarction, tachyarrhythmias, central nervous system injury
Septicemia: endotoxic shock
Anoxia (requires salt depletion)
Postrenal Failure
Prostatic hypertrophy, tumors, calculi, blood clots, ureteral edema, retroperitoneal fibrosis, inadvertent ureteral ligation, papillary necrosis
Renal Failure
Primary damage to tubular epithelium
Ischemia
Nephrotoxic
Drugs: aminoglycosides, methoxyflurane, cytolytic agents, phenytoin, cisplatin, bismuth, rifampin
Radiopaque contrast agents
Respiratory pigments: hemoglobin, myoglobin
Poisons: heavy metals, carbon tetrachloride, animal toxins
Intratubular precipitation: uric acid, myeloma proteins, mucoprotein, sulfas, calcium, xanthine, oxalate
Primary damage to glomeruli and small renal vasculature
Acute glomerulonephritis, collagen vascular diaease, malignant hypertension, serum sickness, thrombotic microangiopathy
Primary damage to major renal vessels
Thrombosis, embolization, atheroembolism
Parenchymal necrosis
Cortical, papillary

prolonged, complicated, and infected surgical procedures.[4] However, the picture that emerged remained hazy, the terminology applied to it vague, and its pathophysiology uncertain. This was to change dramatically during the Second World War, when, early in the course of the Battle of Britain, Bywaters and Beall reported on four patients who developed ARF after crush injury sustained during the bombing of London.[5] The detailed studies of ARF that followed and the ongoing concerted war effort at elucidating the mechanism of shock in battle injuries resulted in an exponential rise in the understanding of ARF.[6] This, coupled with the then beginning attempts of Willem J. Kolff at renal replacement therapy, were to lead to an explosion of knowledge that began in the 1950s when hemodialysis became available.[7] The work of pioneers in the area such as Merrill, Schreiner, and Maher soon changed not only the understanding but the outcome of ARF.[7,8] In fact, much of the initial literature published in the 1960s concerned the role of renal replacement therapy in removing drugs and poisons from the bodies of patients whose kidneys had failed because of the acute renal toxicity of these agents.[8]

Since then, the causes of ARF have come to be classified into those due to underperfusion of the kidneys (prerenal), those due to intrinsic parenchymal lesions of the kidneys (renal), and those due to obstruction of the urinary outflow passages (postrenal). These general categories and their relative prevalence as a cause of ARF are shown in Figure 11A–1.

PATHOPHYSIOLOGY

The hallmarks of ARF are the onset of progressive *oliguria* (the ischuria of old) and *azotemia*.[9] *Oliguria* is said to be present if the daily urine volume is lower than the volume necessary to excrete the waste products of the body. The daily urine excretion necessary to maintain homeostasis is about 400 to 500 mL in an individual who is on a *normal diet,* who has *normal renal function,* and who is *concentrating the urine maximally.* To maintain normal homeostasis, the amount of solute to be excreted by an adult is about 600 mOsm, with urea constituting 40% to 50%

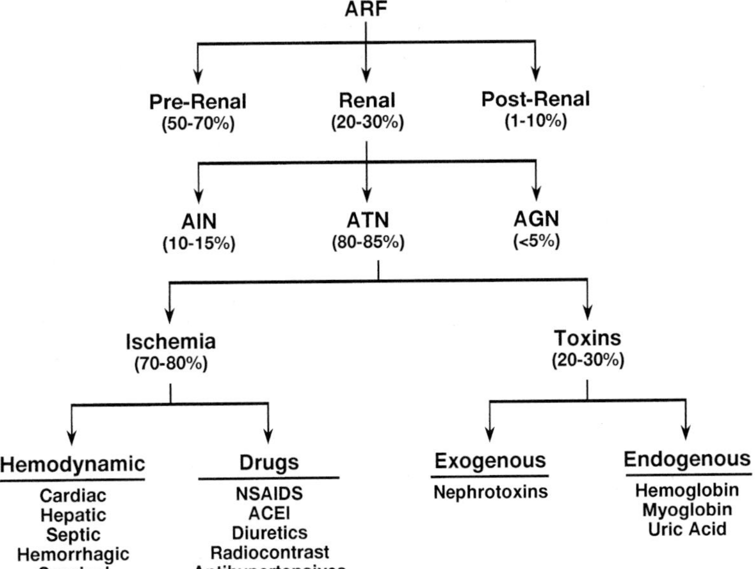

Figure 11A–1. Prevalence and principal forms of acute renal failure. ARF, acute renal failure; AIN, acute interstitial nephritis; ATN, acute tubular necrosis; AGN, acute glomerulonephritis; NSAIDs, nonsteroidal anti-inflammatory drugs; ACEI, angiotensin-converting enzyme inhibitors.

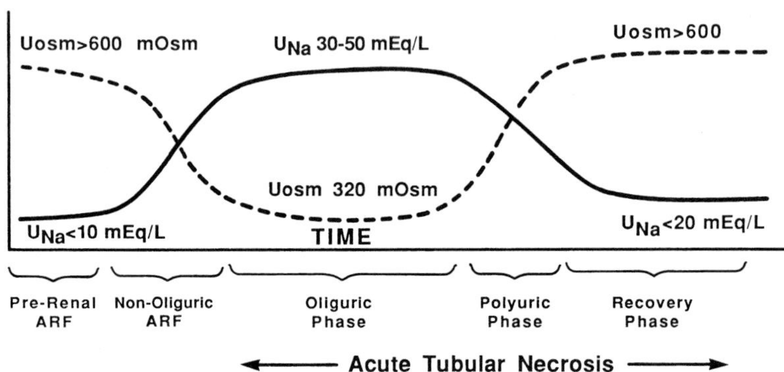

Figure 11A–2. Changes in urine osmolality and sodium concentration during the various phases of acute renal failure.

of the load. Because the normal human kidneys are able to concentrate maximally the urine to 1200 mOsm/kg of water, it follows that the maximally concentrating kidney would be able to excrete the *obligatory solute load* in about 400 to 500 mL of urine, hence the level below which *oliguria* is said to be present. The normal daily urine output of 1000 to 1500 mL reflects the intake of water, which is in excess of the amount necessary to maintain homeostasis. Obviously, this results in the excretion of a less concentrated urine—not an undesirable outcome, because concentrating the urine maximally entails added work and energy consumption by the kidneys and renders them all the more susceptible to injury.[10]

In individuals on a low dietary intake of protein or in a person unable to break down protein to urea (*cirrhosis of the liver*), the amount of urea to be excreted is diminished. Because urea constitutes half of the normal solute load, the urine output to maintain balance in these individuals is more in the range of 300 mL/d, because the amount of water necessary to excrete urea is now considerably reduced. By the same token, in individuals on restricted salt intake or patients whose kidneys are in a sodium retention state (*congestive heart failure, nephrotic syndrome, liver cirrhosis*), the urine output necessary to maintain balance is also reduced to the extent that the load of sodium excreted and, therefore, the amount of water obligated to it are now reduced. Conversely, in a hypercatabolic state (*trauma, burn,* or *sepsis*), when urea production is increased, or in conditions in which *diuretics* are used to inhibit sodium reabsorption, a proportionately larger urine volume would be necessary to clear the solute load.

If the kidneys are injured and unable to absorb and concentrate maximally, a larger volume of water would be needed to excrete the daily load of solutes. Thus, in kidneys able to concentrate urine to 600 mOsm only, 1000 mL of urine would have to be excreted to maintain homeostasis, whereas in kidneys able to concentrate to 300 mOsm only, 2000 mL of urine would have to be excreted. This would be the case of chronically diseased kidneys, but much more important for purposes of this chapter is the situation in the early stages of acute renal injury. One of the first structural consequences of injured tubular cells appears to be a loss of the polar distribution of the sodium-potassium–adenosine triphosphatase (Na-K-ATPase) pump, with consequent impairment of the capacity to absorb filtered sodium and, hence, the subsequent natriuresis and inability to achieve medullary hypertonicity necessary to concentrate the urine maximally.[1, 11] The duration of this otherwise invariable phase of early acute renal injury varies, depending on the magnitude and severity of the insult to the kidneys. This stage when the urine output is high at a time that the glomerular filtration rate (GFR) is declining has been termed *nonoliguric ARF* (Fig. 11A–2). Its early detection, by noting increasing blood urea nitrogen (BUN) and creatinine (Cr) levels, is important because removal of the insult can prevent progression to oliguric ARF, with its graver prognosis.

Under any circumstance, it is evident that an acute reduction in the normal regulatory function of the kidneys can occur in the presence of reduced, normal, or high urine flow rates (Table 11A–2). The clinical jargon of "good urine output" is a misnomer that provides a false sense of security and should be abandoned. By contrast, an increase in the levels of BUN and Cr is progressive in ARF, and it is the changes in BUN and Cr level that should be sought in the early diagnosis of ARF.[12]

Commonly used definitions of ARF include an increase in Cr level of 0.5 mg/dL, BUN increase of 10 to 15 mg/dL, or an increase of more than 50% over the baseline levels of either one. Although these are reasonable values for the diagnosis of ARF, it is prudent clinically to consider any incremental trend of BUN or Cr as an early warning sign of potential renal injury and to initiate a quest for the cause of the changes noted before ARF becomes established.

Table 11A–2. Range of Daily Urine Composition

				Acute Renal Failure	
		Normal	**Prerenal Failure**	*Oliguric*	*Nonoliguric*
Volume	(mL/24h)	300–1500	<400	<400	1500+
Urea	(g/24h)	20	15	5	10
	(mM/24 h)	350	250	85	170
Creatinine	(g/24h)	1–1.5	>1.0	<1.0	<1.0
Sodium	(mEq/24h)	100	5	25	100
Potassium	(mEq/24h)	50–79	10	>50	>50

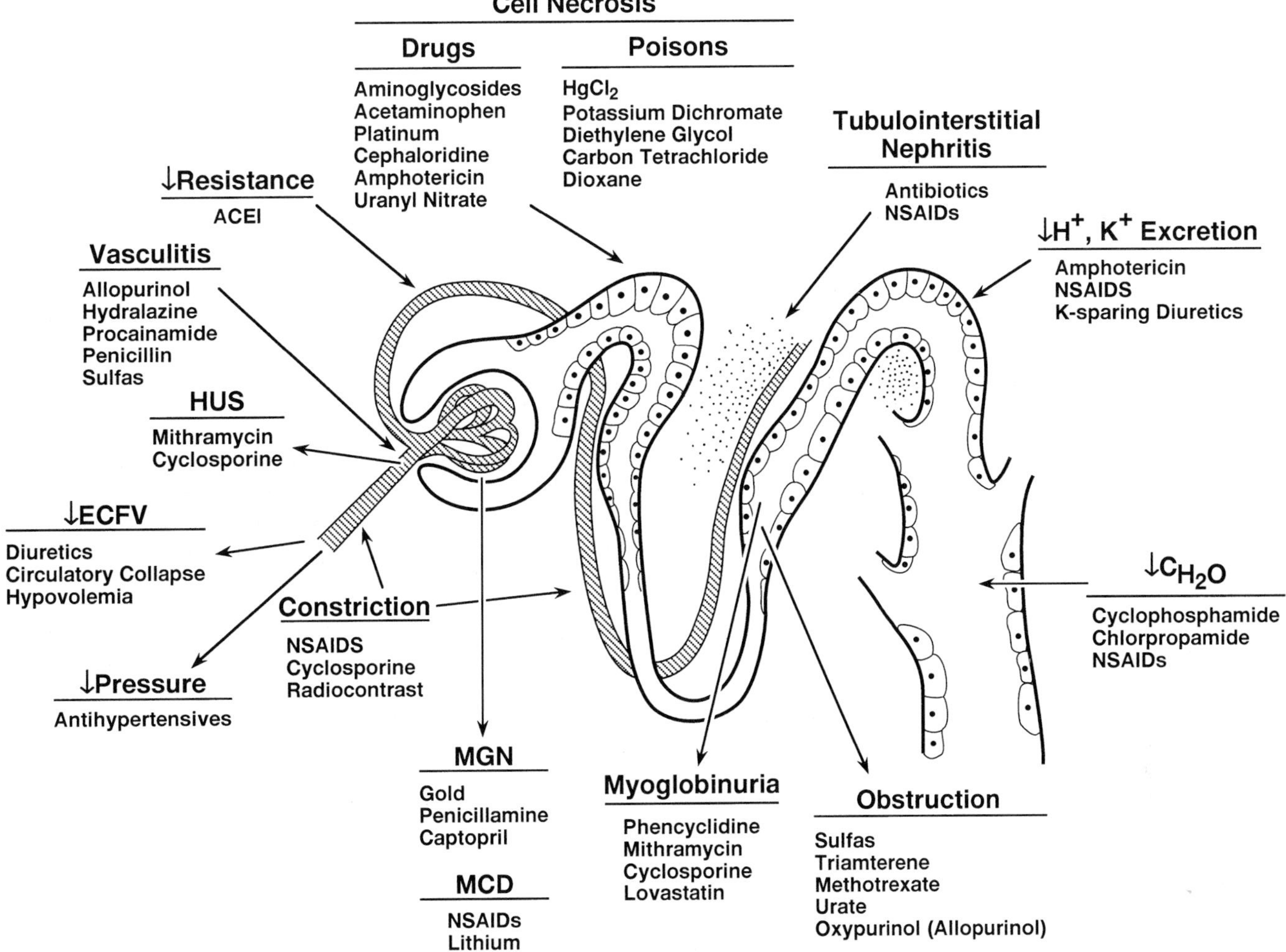

Figure 11A–3. Schematic representation of the mechanisms and sites of injury within the nephron of the major nephrotoxic drugs. HUS, hemolytic-uremic syndrome; ECFV, extracellular fluid volume; CH_2O, free water clearance; MGN, membranous glomerulopathy; MCD, minimal change disease.

TOXIC ACUTE RENAL FAILURE

Strictly defined, toxic ARF is acute tubular cell injury and ultimate acute tubular necrosis (ATN) that is caused by a dose-dependent direct cell damage by a toxic agent, which is usually limited to a specific part of the tubule. More broadly defined, in the general context of ARF, the renal injury may be induced by a host of agents that exert a detrimental effect at various sites within the entire nephron by mechanisms other than direct cell injury and that are not necessarily dose dependent (Fig. 11A–3).

Injury due to exogenous poisons, such as mercuric chloride ($HgCl_2$) formerly the best-characterized form of toxic ATN, is now rare. Much of the ARF currently encountered is due to drugs,[13, 14] whose increased availability and wider use have been associated with a host of undesirable side effects. The kidneys as the principal organs for the excretion of drugs and their metabolites are particularly prone to their side effects. The renal factors that render the kidneys particularly susceptible to injury are listed in Table 11A–3. The nonrenal factors that contribute to increased drug-induced injury are listed in Table 11A–4. Clearly, the physician-related factors noted in Table 11A–4 can be circumvented. By the same token, of the patient-related factors, recognition of reduced renal function to make appropriate adjustments of drug dosage and correction of volume depletion to avert renal underperfusion can prevent renal injury. Volume depletion is extremely important to recognize and correct early, because the associated increase in renal vascular resistance and consequent ischemia is central to much of the nephrotoxicity encountered in clinical practice.[1, 9, 11]

Furthermore, although strictly defined acute renal toxicity is a result of toxic effects on the renal paren-

Table 11A–3. Factors Predisposing the Kidneys to Drug Toxicity

High blood flow
Tubular transport and metabolism of drugs
Tubular fluid concentration in the medulla
Distal tubular fluid acidification

Table 11A–4. Factors Affecting Drug-Related Nephrotoxicity

Patient Related
Kidney disease
↓ Extracellular circulating fluid volume/ ↑ renal vascular resistance
Abuse/dependence
Drug Related
Nephrotoxicity
Immunogenicity
Vasoconstrictive
Hypersensitivity
Physician Related
Dosing
Monitoring
Duration
Mixing

chyma, several toxic agents exert their effect by causing impaired perfusion of the kidneys (prerenal) or their direct renal toxicity (renal) is magnified in the presence of reduced extracellular circulating fluid volume (ECFV). As such, it is essential to fully appreciate the sequence of events that characterize prerenal ARF.

PRERENAL FAILURE

Prerenal failure is usually present in patients with vascular collapse or circulatory insufficiency (see Table 11A–1). In their attempt to preserve ECFV, the kidneys sustain functional changes without demonstrable organic or structural damage (Fig. 11A–4). The most important of these is severe but reversible renal vasoconstriction with a preferential renal cortical underperfusion. The resultant reduction in renal blood flow may be associated with reduced glomerular filtration and thus a decreased filtration of solute. In addition, a greater fraction of this filtrate (urea, water, sodium) is reabsorbed under the influence of volume-stimulated factors. Simultaneous stimulation of antidiuretic hormone secretion usually occurs in response to volume changes. Thus, the oliguria that results is associated with urine that is characteristically highly concentrated and low in sodium content. The azotemia that may be present is the result of increased reabsorption of urea and may develop in the absence of an actual decline in GFR. When renal circulation is restored, these patients respond with a prompt diuresis with correction of the azotemia and oliguria.[15] An important aspect of prerenal ARF is that it represents an earlier and reversible change in renal circulation that, if left uncorrected, may ultimately lead to organic renal damage (see Fig. 11A–2). At the very least, it renders the underperfused kidneys much more susceptible to toxic injury.

Although this category of ARF may be identified by the usual accompanying signs of peripheral circulatory failure and low ECFV, the composition of the urine is the main clue to its diagnosis (see Figs. 11A–2 and 11A–4). The urine is characteristically low in sodium content (<10 mEq/L, fractional sodium excretion <1%) and high in concentration (Uosm >500 mOsm/KgH_2O).

A number of drugs exert their detrimental effects on the kidneys by inducing or aggravating prerenal

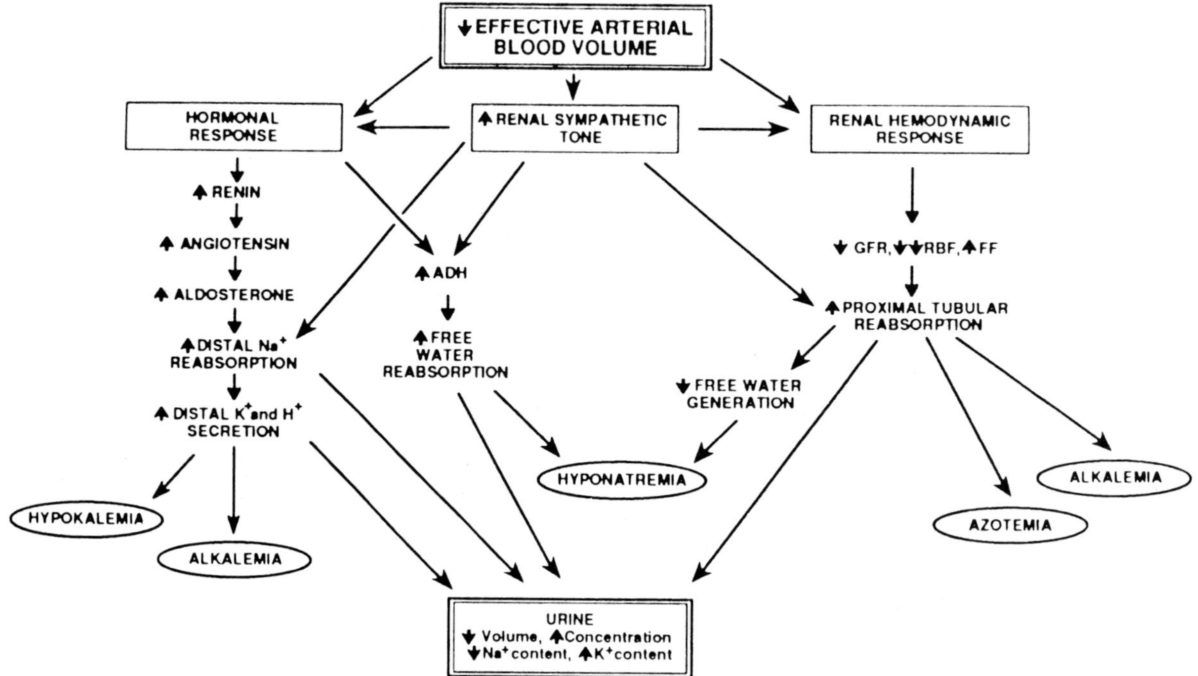

Figure 11A–4. Pathogenetic pathways implicated in prerenal failure. The arrows reflect the directional changes in the parameters depicted. The legends enclosed in the ovals indicate the changes in the blood chemistries that might be expected. GFR, glomerular filtration rate; RBF, renal blood flow; FF, filtration fraction; ADH, antidiuretic hormone.

ARF (see Fig. 11A–3). Most notable among these are *diuretics,* whose injudicious and nondiscriminating use accounts for most cases of ARF in the hospital setting.[15, 16] A second and common cause is *nonsteroidal inflammatory drugs* (NSAIDs).[16, 17] By inhibiting cyclooxygenase, the principal enzyme in prostaglandin synthesis, NSAIDs deprive the kidneys of the protective vasodilatory prostaglandins and thereby aggravate any existing vasoconstriction and initiate a hemodynamically mediated ARF. This is usually a mild and reversible effect but on occasion results in severe oliguric ARF requiring renal replacement therapy.[17] Patients with pre-existing ineffective ECFV and decreased renal perfusion (congestive cardiomyopathy, cirrhosis, sepsis, or diuretic therapy) or those with pre-existing renal disease (nephrotic syndrome, chronic renal failure) are at risk of NSAID-induced ARF. A third group of drugs that inhibit the protective effect of efferent arteriolar vasoconstriction on maintaining GFR in the presence of reduced renal perfusion are the *angiotensin-converting enzyme (ACE) inhibitors.* The vasodilatory effect of these agents on the afferent arteriole is potentially salutary but essentially modest; by contrast, their effect on the post-capillary efferent arterioles is greater and results in a sudden decline in the glomerular intracapillary hydrostatic pressure (P_{GC}) necessary for filtration. Unless blood flow (QA) to the kidneys is increased by the afferent dilatation, the result is a sudden reduction in GFR. As is the case with NSAIDs, the renal effects of ACE inhibition are usually modest and reversible but on occasion result in severe oliguric ATN necessitating renal replacement therapy.[18] The detrimental effect of ACE inhibitors is most evident in patients who have severe congestive cardiomyopathy, renal artery stenosis, or reduced ECFV; they are unable to compensate for the loss of P_{GC} by increasing QA. Given the role of diuretics in causing ECFV depletion, it is not unexpected that most cases of ACE inhibitor–induced ARF observed clinically are in patients who have severe congestive cardiomyopathy and who are diuresed aggressively.

Notable among the causes of prerenal ARF are those due to *antihypertensive agents,* which, even in the absence of decreased ECFV, induce a reduction in renal perfusion pressure that can result in ARF. Not unexpectedly, this is most evident in individuals who have accelerated or malignant hypertension and in whom the endothelial swelling caused by the pre-existing severe hypertension results in a narrowed lumen with a high renal vascular resistance that requires high pressure levels to perfuse the narrowed and constricted renal vasculature.[19] It is in these individuals that the sudden and severe reduction in the mean arterial blood pressure (>25 mm Hg) can result in the onset of progressive ARF often necessitating renal replacement therapy. Hence, gradual titration of the blood pressure downward in slow increments is important in such cases, while monitoring renal function and maintaining adequate ECFV.

RENAL FAILURE

Although in its broad definition renal failure includes among others such diverse entities as acute glomerulonephritis, vasculitis, thrombotic microangiopathy, and papillary necrosis (see Table 11A–1), those forms of ARF that are due to ischemia, nephrotoxic agents, or a combination of both most commonly account for the vast majority of cases encountered clinically (see Fig. 11A–1). The ultimate picture that results is that of ATN, although strictly defined this term may be a misnomer because the apparently necrotic cells that are excreted have been shown to be viable and to grow *in vitro* in cultures of tubular epithelial cells isolated from the urine.[20] Their shedding into the urine is one of the consequences of cell injury, rather than actual necrosis, which in addition to the loss of their polarity sustain a loss of cell-wall integrins and a decomposition of their attachment to the basement membrane and to each other. This accounts for the loss of their anchorage and ultimate shedding into the urine.[1, 9, 21] In addition to microscopic examination of the urine for tubular epithelial cells that are shed, analysis of the urine is extremely valuable in the diagnosis (see Figs. 11A–2 and 11A–4). The urine is characteristically high in sodium (>50 mEq/L, fractional sodium excretion >1%) and literally isosmotic in concentration (320 to 350 mOsm/kg of water).

Should the patient survive, in the absolute majority of cases regeneration of tubular cells sets in and restores renal function. The regenerative and repair process of the injured tubules is an early event that is activated at the very start of injury, culminates during the ensuing days, and results in the ultimate restoration of normal renal structure and function.[22, 23] The clinical course that ATN follows has been divided into four phases that correspond to the various phases of epithelial cell injury, necrosis, and regeneration. They are of variable duration and have considerable overlap.

Initial Phase

The initial phase is the period of ischemia or exposure to the nephrotoxic agent; it continues until oliguria develops (see Fig. 11A–2). The importance of identifying this phase stems from the fact that it represents a potentially reversible stage. Its length varies and depends largely on the causative agent (may last 5 to 7 days). In general, an abnormal sediment (cylindruria), tubular proteinuria (β_2-microglobulins), lysozymuria, and a renal concentrating defect precede by several days any decrease in GFR caused by nephrotoxic agents. Other tubular dysfunctions (renal glycosuria, tubular acidosis, sodium loss) may be detectable and should be sought.

The efficacy of prophylactic measures that on occasion are effective during this phase *(mannitol, loop diuretics, dopamine)* relates to their ability to increase renal blood flow and solute excretion. These measures may also have the capacity to convert oliguric to nonoliguric renal failure (see Fig. 11A–2 and Table 11A–2). As a rule, their efficacy in preventing ARF clinically is questionable.[24] On the other hand, *prostaglandins* have a protective role in the renal autoregulation that is associated with vasoconstricting insults. Inhibitors of prostaglandin synthesis *(NSAIDs)* or inhibitors of efferent constriction (*ACE* inhibitors), used during this phase, can accentuate the ischemia and precipitate oliguria.[16–18]

Oliguric Phase

No single pathogenetic sequence appears to account for all the varieties of ATN and the development of oliguria. The balance of evidence favors the view that excessive *backleak* across the damaged tubular epithelium and *tubular obstruction* by the sloughed cells are important. Changes in *glomerular permeability* and *filtration rate* also appear to be contributing mechanisms.[1, 9] The degree of involvement of any of these potential pathogenetic mechanisms varies and depends on the nature, severity, and duration of the initial nephrotoxic insult.

Oliguria is present in 60% to 70% of cases encountered clinically; another 30% to 40% are diagnosed earlier and are associated with a nonoliguric ARF (see Fig. 11A–2 and Table 11A–2). The average duration of the oliguria is 1 to 2 weeks, and daily urine volume averages 150 mL. *Anuria* (urine output <50 to 75 mL/d) is uncommon. If oliguria continues for longer than 4 weeks, more likely possibilities to rule out are cortical necrosis, acute glomerulonephritis, and vasculitis. The duration of oliguria is of some prognostic significance; longer duration portends a greater chance of complications and undesirable outcomes.

Diuretic Phase

The diuretic phase begins when the 24-hour urine volume exceeds 500 mL/d. Classically, at the onset of this phase, urine volume doubles on successive days until a volume of 2000 to 3000 mL is reached. This phase lasts from 7 to 14 days. With the onset of diuresis, the renal blood flow and GFR gradually increase. The urine is at first isosmotic and literally appears to be pure plasma filtrate. As the regenerating tubular cells recover some ability to reabsorb sodium and concentrate urea, the urine gradually contains less sodium and more urea than plasma. Thus, blood chemistry values do not begin to correct with the onset of the diuretic phase, and days may pass before these values begin to normalize. As diuresis continues, however, the azotemia gradually diminishes. Factors contributing to the diuresis observed in this phase include (1) *osmotic diuresis* resulting from mobilization of the urea accumulated during the oliguric phase, (2) *functional inadequacy* of the regenerating tubular cells to reabsorb the glomerular filtrate and concentrate the urine, and (3) *pushing intravenous fluids,* because overzealous replacement of urine output maintains a patient in a continuous state of volume expansion. Thus, one ends up "chasing" the urine output by infusing gradually larger volumes of fluid.[9, 25]

Although apparently similar to nonoliguric ARF, the diuretic phase of ATN is a totally different entity in that unlike the increasing BUN and Cr of the former, the BUN and Cr levels gradually decline during the diuretic phase. Although the decrement is modest during the first few days, it gradually increases in pace as cellular function matures and the GFR is restored. It is important to remember that many drugs are still poorly excreted during the diuretic phase, and dosage adjustments may be necessary if further drug toxicity is to be avoided.

Convalescent Phase

BUN and Cr levels are usually normal within 5 to 60 days after the onset of the diuretic phase. GFR, however, increases more slowly and may be 70% to 80% of normal within months. The ability to elaborate a maximally concentrated urine will return but may take several months. The principal renal symptoms during this phase are nocturia and polyuria, which gradually subside as the ability to concentrate urine improves. As a rule, there is no convincing evidence of progressive renal disease in recovered patients.

Although urinary tract infection is common during the oliguric phase because of prior urethral catheterization, evidence of persistent chronic infection is rare.

TOXIC ACUTE TUBULAR NECROSIS

The principal agents associated with toxic ATN are listed in Table 11A–5. The exact incidence of nephrotoxicity for any of these agents is not known, but the sequence in which they are listed parallels that with which they are encountered.[13, 14, 16, 19, 26]

Table 11A–5. Agents Associated with Toxic Acute Tubular Necrosis

• Antibiotics:	Aminoglycosides, cephalosporin, amphotericin, vancomycin, pentamidine, sulfas, acyclovir, foscarnet, penicillin, tetracycline
• Antineoplastic agents	
Alkylating agents:	Cisplatin, carboplatin, ifosfamide
Antimetabolites:	Methotrexate, ara-C,5-fluorouracil, 5-azacitidine, 6-thioguanine
• Metals:	Mercury, bismuth, cadmium, chromium, lead, gold, platinum, uranium, lithium
• Organic solvents:	Ethylene glycol, diethylene glycol, carbon tetrachloride
• Miscellaneous:	Radiocontrast agents, heroin, phencyclidine, cocaine, mannitol

Antibiotics

Aminoglycosides are among the most widely prescribed antibiotics. Nephrotoxicity develops in 10% to 15% of persons who use these drugs and depends on the total dose, the duration of treatment, and the frequency of administration. These highly water-soluble agents are freely filtered and absorbed in the proximal tubule. It is their accumulation within the epithelial cells that accounts for their nephrotoxicity. The variations in degree of nephrotoxicity observed remain unexplained but have been attributed to a number of risk factors such as age, gender, reduced renal function, volume depletion, potassium and magnesium depletion, and hepatic failure. As a rule, toxicity results in nonoliguric ARF, with recovery from mild renal failure if the drug is discontinued, but it can lead to oliguric ARF if the insult remains undetected and drug administration is continued. The role of monitoring drug levels to predict nephrotoxicity is equivocal because the antibiotic levels actually increase when nephrotoxicity is already established.[26, 27]

The increased availability of *cephalosporins* has been associated with an increasing incidence of reported cases of ARF, some of which are due to their nephrotoxic effect, particularly evident with use of cephaloridine, whereas others are a result of a hypersensitivity reaction and are due to acute interstitial nephritis.[28]

The vast number of antibiotics used in the treatment of HIV-infected patients renders this group of patients particularly susceptible to toxic ATN.[29, 30] Incriminated agents include *pentamidine, foscarnet, amphotericin, acyclovir,* and *sulfas.* Approximately a third of patients receiving pentamidine and two thirds of those receiving foscarnet have clinical evidence of ARF due to tubular injury. By contrast, the *sulfas* and *acyclovir* exert their detrimental effect by intratubular precipitation, and *amphotericin* exerts its detrimental effect by complexing with the plasma membrane and increasing the cellular aqueous pores (see Fig. 11A–3). The latter accounts for the early polyuria and distal renal tubular acidosis, which with continued therapy result in a dose-dependent toxic ATN.[14, 19, 26]

Antineoplastic Agents

The nephrotoxicity associated with antimetabolites is generally cumulative and chronic, although acute injury can result in the presence of severe volume compromise, excessive dosing, and multiple-drug use.[31] Cancer is the underlying disease in as many as one fifth of cases of ARF in some series, not because of the nephrotoxic effect of antimetabolites alone but rather because of the antimicrobials and analgesics used in their management. Yet another cause of ARF is that of acute massive tumor tissue necrosis, particularly in lymphoproliferative disorders, with resultant acute urate nephropathy—a potentially preventable lesion with adequate hydration, alkalization of the urine, and inhibition of uric acid synthesis with prophylactic allopurinol.[31–33] Thrombotic microangiopathy is a rare cause of ARF that has been associated with *mithramycin, cyclosporine,* and *5-fluorouracil* therapy.[34, 35]

Heavy Metals

Exposure to heavy metals is usually chronic in nature and results in various renal abnormalities that are primarily tubular in nature, ranging from proximal tubular dysfunction to oliguric ARF and chronic tubulointerstitial nephritis. Of the metals listed in Table 11–5, *mercuric chloride* is the one that is most typically associated with toxic ATN, but this cause of toxicity has literally vanished. *Uranium* also gives rise to a toxic ATN that closely resembles that of mercuric chloride nephrotoxicity. A similar picture has been reported after excessive doses of *bismuth* and *chromium.*[8, 14]

Organic Solvents

Cases of accidental ingestion or attempted suicide with the antifreeze solution *ethylene glycol* are not rare. Oxalate, one of the metabolites of ethylene glycol, accounts for much of its nephrotoxicity owing to the intratubular precipitation of oxalate crystals (see Fig. 11A–3). *Diethylene glycol,* an organic chemical solvent, causes tubular necrosis and recently was the cause of an epidemic of toxic ATN in children in Haiti. *Carbon tetrachloride,* another industrial solvent, causes direct, dose-dependent renal and hepatic toxicity, which is much less commonly encountered nowadays.[8, 14]

OTHER FORMS OF PARENCHYMAL ACUTE RENAL FAILURE

Of the renal parenchymal forms of ARF, other than ATN, both acute interstitial nephritis (AIN) and acute glomerulonephritis can be a side effect of a number of drugs (see Fig. 11A–3). By far the more common of these two is that of AIN, which although first identified as due to infection in the preantibiotic era is now most commonly encountered with the very drugs used to treat infections.[28]

The principal drugs that have been associated with AIN are listed in Table 11A–6. Unlike toxic ATN, AIN is not dose dependent, develops in only some individuals, and is usually associated with the classic findings of a hypersensitivity reaction (fever, eosinophilia, elevated IgE levels) that are often transient and on occasion with eosinophiluria. The impairment in renal function begins with discrete abnormalities of tubular function and progresses to ARF. The renal failure is nonoliguric in the early stages of the dis-

Table 11A–6. Principal Agents Associated with Acute Interstitial Nephritis

Antimicrobials
Penicillins, cephalosporins, sulfonamides, rifampin
Nonsteroidal Anti-inflammatory Drugs
Propionic acid derivatives, others
Miscellaneous
Phenindione, phenytoin, thiazide diuretics, allopurinol, cimetidine

ease and is usually accompanied by findings of tubular dysfunction (renal glycosuria, hypouricemia, and β_2-microglobinuria due to their decreased tubular reabsorption). If renal failure is undetected and administration of the incriminated agent continues, oliguric ARF ensues and is severe enough to require renal replacement therapy. Renal failure is more common in the elderly and more severe in those who become oliguric. In most, the renal failure is reversible and its course can be shortened by brief use (2 to 4 weeks) of steroid therapy. In some (10% to 15%) of those with severe renal failure, irreversible renal failure may persist.

Among the agents that produce AIN, that due to *NSAIDs* is unique in that it generally presents with renal failure that is accompanied by the nephrotic syndrome. The onset after initiation of therapy with NSAIDs is usually longer than that observed with other agents and takes longer (months) to subside after discontinuation. In addition, no beneficial effect of steroids has been noted in cases of AIN due to NSAIDs.[17, 28]

Iodinated *radiocontrast agents* are a cause of acute renal toxicity. The injury that results ranges from modest tubular dysfunction, which may remain undetected, to severe ARF, which may require renal replacement therapy. In patients who sustain renal injury, the ARF is generally nonoliguric and develops within 2 to 4 days of the procedure, although a sudden onset of oliguric ARF can ensue on occasion. Although the precise mechanism of ARF remains undetermined, renal ischemia due to intrarenal vasoconstriction, particularly in the presence of volume depletion, appears to be an important factor. The protective effect of calcium channel blockers, demonstrated experimentally and documented clinically, supports the role of intrarenal vasoconstriction as a cause of radiocontrast agent–induced ARF. Of the several predisposing factors incriminated, that of decreased ECFV, reduced renal function (Cr >2 mg/dL), diabetes mellitus, and total dose of radiocontrast agent injected are specially important. Adequate volume expansion with a brisk diuresis initiated before and maintained well after the procedure, coupled with use of calcium channel blockers and limitation of the dose of radiocontrast agents administered, is effective in circumventing the undesirable side effect of these agents.[36, 37]

Rhabdomyolysis consequent to the overuse of *heroin* can result in ARF. Myoglobinuria and hyperuricosuria, due to muscle injury, in a setting of severely compromised ECFV account for the ARF that develops. Prompt recognition, with restoration of intravascular volume and alkalization of urine, can prevent progression to oliguric ARF. A similar picture can occur after overdosage with *cocaine* and *phencyclidine.*[38]

Other less common forms of ARF are due to glomerular lesions that result from a vasculitis that has been reported in association with the use of *allopurinol, hydralazine, procainamide, penicillin,* and *sulfas.* The thrombotic microangiopathy associated with certain antineoplastic agents has been mentioned. Finally, membranous glomerulopathy has been noted with the use of *gold, penicillamine,* and *captopril.*[14, 19, 26]

TREATMENT

Renal replacement therapy has greatly simplified the management of ARF. Nevertheless, certain principles governing fluid and electrolyte management are important to monitor and correct in order to avoid the invasive nature of dialysis, when possible.

Prerenal Failure

Prompt recognition of the manifestations of prerenal ARF is extremely important.[23, 39] Prerenal ARF represents an early and reversible change in renal hemodynamics that if left uncorrected can lead to ATN. It is characterized by symptoms of peripheral circulatory failure (low blood pressure, rapid pulse, orthostatic hypotension, dry mucous membranes); urine that is low in volume, sodium content (<10 to 20 mEq/L), and fractional sodium excretion (<1%) but highly concentrated (Uosm >500 mOsm/kg of water); and rising levels of BUN and Cr (see Figs. 11A–2 and 11A–4).

Apart from discontinuing drugs that aggravate the effects of decreased ECFV discussed previously (*diuretics, antihypertensives, ACE inhibitors, NSAIDs*), the principal effort should be directed at judiciously restoring ECFV. Direct measurement of pulmonary artery wedge pressure is indicated if the diagnosis is in doubt and before volume replacement in the presence of cardiac disease. Volume replacement is with isotonic saline or lactated Ringer's solution in increments of 500 mL until ECFV is restored or the pulmonary artery wedge pressure is 18 mm Hg.[15] If no response to volume replacement is noted, use of low-dose dopamine (2 to 3 μg/kg per minute) can enhance renal perfusion. Administration of mannitol (12.5 to 25 g) or high-dose furosemide (up to 120 mg but never >240 mg), after volume replacement, may induce diuresis. Both furosemide and mannitol can be used alone or in conjunction with dopamine. The salutary effect of these pharmacologic maneuvers is, at best, transient and equivocal, particularly once oliguric ARF is established.[22] In fact, mannitol itself can induce ARF.[40] If no response to their initial administration is observed, their continued use would be contraindicated.

Renal Failure

During the *initial phase* of ARF, efforts to restore intravascular volume outlined for prerenal ARF should be continued. Appropriate antibiotics for coexistent infection or sepsis should be initiated at the full loading dose, but any subsequent dosing should be modified for a GFR of less than 20 mL/min until this usually reversible phase is actually reversed or its progression to oliguric ARF is ruled out. The use of potentially aggravating and nephrotoxic agents (*NSAIDs, ACE inhibitors, antihypertensives, diuretics*) should be avoided and the use of *radiocontrast agents* minimized and restricted to those that are absolutely essential for a definitive diagnosis.

During the *oliguric phase* of ARF, in well-managed cases without serious complications, the BUN level rises 10 to 20 mg/dL per day and Cr level 0.5 to 1 mg/dL per day. In hypercatabolic patients (trauma, rhabdomyolysis), Cr level may increase by more than 2 mg/dL per day. In patients without complications, plasma potassium values can increase by 0.5 mEq/L per day; in catabolic states, it may increase by as much as 1 to 2 mEq/L in hours. Weight losses of 0.2 to 0.5 kg/d are expected because of catabolism; in complicated hypercatabolic states, weight loss may be 1 kg/day. Hypocalcemia (6 to 8 mg/dL) is common, reflecting hypoalbuminemia, hyperphosphatemia, and skeletal resistance to parathyroid hormone.

Water replacement should be restricted to a volume equivalent to urine volume plus extrarenal losses (gastric suction, diarrhea, wound drainage). Insensible losses (800 mL/d) should be restored by 400 to 500 mL of fluid only, because endogenous water production is 300 to 400 mL/d. Water requirements increase in the presence of high ambient temperature, fever, and low relative humidity. Adequate fluid replacement can best be monitored by the following:

1. Daily weight measurement. ARF is a catabolic state, and a daily weight loss of 0.5 kg or 1 lb should be expected. Any weight gain can represent only excess fluid administration.
2. Measuring serum sodium concentration. An increase in serum sodium level (>145 mEq/L) would indicate insufficient water replacement, whereas a decline in serum sodium level (<135 mEq/L) would reflect excess water replacement.

The administration of *sodium chloride* should be restricted once the initial volume replacement during the prerenal ARF or the initial phase of ARF has been accomplished. The guiding principles of sodium chloride replacement are as follows:

1. Body weight losses in excess of 300 g/d in the presence of a normal serum sodium level should be replaced, 1 mL of isotonic saline for each gram of weight loss.
2. Gastrointestinal losses, wound drainage, and estimated sequestered fluid require replacement with isotonic sodium chloride.
3. If acidosis develops, salt losses should be replaced with sodium bicarbonate. Available forms of sodium bicarbonate are concentrated (7.5% $NaHCO_3$) and hypertonic (890 mOsm). They must not be administered as a bolus or added to isotonic saline solution. They should be restored to isotonicity in glucose or half normal saline solution.

Potassium intake must be restricted. Small deficits need not be replaced. Hypokalemia, unless severe (<3mEq/L), should not be corrected. Hyperkalemia, if present, can be best treated with correction of acidosis and with exchange resins (Kayexalate). The exchange resins are most effective when used as retention enemas. Hyperkalemia is always an indication to consider dialysis.

Caloric requirements (30 kcal/kg of body weight per day) must be met to avoid increased catabolism. In the presence of sepsis, surgery, or burns, the usual caloric requirements are increased by as much as 50%. Caloric intake can be given as glucose (20% to 70%) and fat emulsions (10% to 20%). Any protein given should consist of high-biologic-value essential amino acids and should not exceed 0.5 g/kg of body weight per day.

The potential for *upper gastrointestinal bleeding* is high in ARF. H_2-receptor blocking agents should be used. Antacids, if used, represent added loads of aluminum and calcium. The use of magnesium-containing antacids is contraindicated.

Dialysis should be started early and performed daily. Continuous renal replacement seems to have a distinct advantage in the dialysis management of these patients.[41] The dialysis bath should be adjusted to the level of serum potassium and should be bicarbonate based. Convincing evidence for the advantage of biocompatible membranes in ARF has been presented.[42] Dialyzers used should have a biocompatible membrane.

The onset of the *diuretic phase* requires continued vigilance. *Dialysis* must be continued through this phase until predialysis BUN levels begin to diminish well below 100 mg/dL and patients have no problems with elevated potassium levels. The serum sodium level must be monitored by measurements of body weight and sodium concentration as outlined for the oliguric phase. Although urinary losses must be replaced, pushing fluids must be avoided. This can best be accomplished by replacing urine output no more frequently than every 8 to 12 hours, depending on the previous urine volume, in order to avoid the continued overexpansion of ECFV that is present often. It is unusual for patients to have urine volumes greater than 3 to 4 L/d during this phase unless too much fluid is being administered. It is important to remember that renal function remains compromised, and many drugs are still poorly excreted during the diuretic phase. Dosage adjustment should remain in effect if drug toxicity is to be avoided.

References

1. Thadani R, Pascual M, Bonventre JV: Acute renal failure. N Engl J Med *334:*1448, 1996.
2. Dickinson WH: On Renal and Urinary Affections. New York, William Wood & Co., 1885.
3. Minami S: Über Nierenveränderungen nach Verschüttung. Virchows Arch Pathol Anat *245:*247, 1923.
4. Husfeldt E, Bjering T: Renal lesions for traumatic shock. Acta Med Scand *91:*279, 1937.
5. Bywaters EGL, Beall D: Crush injuries and renal function. BMJ *1:*427, 1941.
6. Van Slyke DD: The effects of shock on the kidney. Ann Intern Med *28:*701, 1948.
7. Swann RC, Merrill JP: The clinical course of acute renal failure. Medicine *32:*215, 1953.
8. Schreiner GE, Maher JF: Toxic nephropathy. Am J Med *38:*409, 1965.
9. Paller MS: Pathophysiology of acute renal failure. *In* Greenberg A, Cheung AK, Coffman TM, et al (eds): Primer on Kidney Diseases. San Diego, Academic Press, pp 126–133, 1994.
10. Brezis M, Rosen S: Hypoxia of the renal medulla—its implications for disease. N Engl J Med *332:*647, 1995.
11. Fish EM, Molitoris BA: Alterations in epithelial polarity and the pathogenesis of disease states. N Engl J Med *330:*1580, 1994.
12. Perrone RD, Madras NE, Levey AS: Serum creatinine as an index of renal function: New insights into old concepts. Clin Chem *38:*1933, 1992.
13. Mathew TH: Drug-induced renal disease. Med J Aust *156:*724, 1992.
14. Swan SK, Bennett WM: Nephrotoxic acute renal failure. *In* Lazarus M, Brenner B (eds): Acute Renal Failure. New York, Churchill Livingstone, pp 357–392, 1993.
15. Eknoyan G: Diagnosis of disturbances. *In* Seldin DW, Giebisch G: The Regulation of Sodium and Chloride Balance. New York, Raven Press, pp 237–259, 1990.
16. Davidman M, Olson P, Kohen J, et al: Iatrogenic renal disease. Arch Intern Med *151:*1809, 1991.
17. Palmer BF, Henrich WL: Clinical acute renal failure with nonsteroidal anti-inflammatory drugs. Semin Nephrol *15:*214, 1995.
18. Toto R, Mitchell H, Lee H, et al: Reversible renal insufficiency due to angiotensin converting enzyme inhibitors in hypertensive nephrosclerosis. Ann Intern Med *115:*512, 1991.
19. Garella S: Drug-induced renal disease: A clinical approach to its detection. AKF Nephrol Letter *4:*32, 1990.
20. Racusen LC, Fivush BA, Li Y-L, et al: Dissociation of tubular cell detachment and tubular cell death in clinical and experimental "acute tubular necrosis." Lab Invest *64:*546, 1991.
21. Goligorsky MS, DiBona GF: Pathogenetic role of arg-gly-asp recognizing integrins in acute renal failure. Proc Natl Acad Sci U S A *90:*5700, 1993.
22. Toback FG: Regeneration after acute tubular necrosis. Kidney Int *41:*226, 1992.
23. Humes HD: Recovery phase of acute renal failure: The cellular and molecular biology of regenerative repair. Kidney *24:*1, 1991.
24. Denton MD, Chertow GM, Brady HR: "Renal-dose" dopamine for the treatment of acute renal failure: Scientific rationale, experimental studies and clinical trials. Kidney Int *49:*4, 1996.
25. Hutchinson FN: Management of acute renal failure. *In* Greenberg A, Cheung AK, Coffman TM, et al (eds): Primer on Kidney Diseases. San Diego, Academic Press, pp 157–162, 1994.
26. Cooper K, Bennett WM: Nephrotoxicity of common drugs used in clinical practice. Arch Intern Med *147:*1213, 1987.
27. Tune BM: Renal tubular transport and nephrotoxicity of beta-lactam antibiotics: Structure-activity relationships. Miner Electrolyte Metab *20:*221, 1994.
28. Eknoyan G: Acute tubulointerstitial nephritis. *In* Schrier RW, Gottschalk CW (eds): Diseases of the Kidney. 6th ed. Boston, Little Brown & Co., pp. 1249–1272, 1996.
29. Berns JS, Cohen RM, Stumacher RJ: Renal aspects of therapy for human immunodeficiency virus and associated opportunistic infections. J Am Soc Nephrol *1:*1061, 1991.
30. Rao TK, Friedman EA: Outcome of severe acute renal failure in patients with acquired immunodeficiency syndrome. Am J Kidney Dis *25:*390, 1995.
31. Cobos E, Hall RR: Effects of chemotherapy on the kidney. Semin Nephrol *13:*297, 1993.
32. Simmonds HA, Cameron, JS, Morris GS, Davies PM: Allopurinol in renal failure and the tumor lysis syndrome. Clin Chem Acta *160:*189, 1986.
33. Curry SC, Chang D, Connor D: Drug- and toxin-induced rhabdomyolysis. Ann Emerg Med *18:*1068, 1989.
34. Jackson AM, Rose BD, Graff LG: Thrombotic microangiopathy and renal failure associated with antineoplastic chemotherapy. Ann Intern Med *101:*41, 1984.
35. Poch E, Gonzalez-Clemente JM, Torres A, et al: Silent renal microangiopathy after mitomycin C therapy. Am J Nephrol *10:*514, 1990.
36. Krinloosky FA, Simon N, Santhanam S: Acute renal failure: Association with administration of radiographic contrast material. JAMA *239:*125, 1993.
37. Porter GA: Contrast-associated nephropathy: Presentation, pathophysiology and management. Miner Electrolyte Metab *20:*232, 1994.
38. Roth D, Alarcon FJ, Fernandez JA, et al: Acute rhabdomyolysis associated with cocaine intoxication. N Engl J Med *319:*673, 1988.
39. Better OS, Stein JH: Early management of shock and prophylaxis of acute renal failure in traumatic rhabdomyolysis. N Engl J Med *322:*825, 1990.
40. Dorman HR, Sondheimer JH, Cadnapaphornchai P: Mannitol-induced acute renal failure. Medicine *69:*153, 1990.
41. Mehta RL: Therapeutic alternatives to renal replacement for critically ill patients in acute renal failure. Semin Nephrol *14:*64, 1994.
42. Hakim R, Wingard RL, Parker RA: Effect of dialysis membrane in the treatment of patients with acute renal failure. N Engl J Med *331:*1338, 1994.

B Chronic Renal Toxicity

MARK S. PALLER, MD

Chronic renal toxicity may be defined as a persistent and progressive functional and structural defect in the kidneys produced by a drug or an environmental toxin. This chapter addresses those toxins that cause renal injury over a period of months to years. Nephrotoxins causing acute renal dysfunction are discussed in Chapter 11A. Acute nephrotoxicity is most commonly caused by aminoglycoside antibiotics, amphotericin B, radiographic contrast agents, cyclosporine, cisplatin, and methoxyflurane. The important causes of chronic renal toxicity are listed in Table 11B–1.

CLINICAL PRESENTATION

The diagnosis of chronic renal toxicity is based almost exclusively on the detection of a decrease in renal function. Unlike acute renal toxicity, in which urine output may abruptly decrease in as many as half of all patients, chronic renal toxicity is by nature insidious and clinically difficult to recognize. A decrease in renal function is determined by the measurement of serum creatinine level. Serum creatinine determination is most informative when considered in the context of total body muscle mass and gender. Serum creatinine is derived from the metabolism of creatinine in muscle and therefore reflects total muscle mass. Dietary meat intake also affects serum creatinine but to a lesser extent. Creatinine is eliminated from the body predominantly by glomerular filtration, with a small contribution from renal secretion. Cockcroft and Gault proposed an empirical formula that uses serum creatinine value (in mg/dL) to assess glomerular filtration rate (GFR) (Equation 1).

$$\text{Creatinine clearance} = \frac{(140 - \text{age}) \times \text{Weight in kg}}{72\,(\text{Scr})}$$

Their formula is as accurate a determinant of GFR as is the more cumbersome procedure of 24-hour urine collection for creatinine clearance determination.[1] Note that this equation for predicting GFR also has a term for age (in years). For women, the result is multiplied by 0.85. GFR decreases by approximately 1 mL/min per year after the age of 40 years. However, the serum creatinine value does not increase with age while GFR falls because a fortuitous, almost equivalent decrease occurs in muscle mass. Using the Cockcroft-Gault equation yields a far more accurate estimate of renal function than does serum creatinine determination because laboratories usually use far too wide a range for the normal serum creatinine value. Some form of renal disease should therefore be suspected when the GFR is less than the age-appropriate value.

The differential diagnosis of chronic renal failure is extensive (Table 11B–2). The four most common causes of chronic progressive renal disease are diabetes mellitus, hypertension, glomerulonephritis, and polycystic kidney disease. Therefore, chronic renal disease due to drugs and environmental toxins represents a small subset of the large population of patients with chronic renal disease. Patients with chronic renal toxicity generally have the histologic lesion of chronic interstitial nephritis, a description that is also useful as a disease category. By definition, all patients with chronic renal failure have a decreased GFR (elevated serum creatinine value). Compared with patients having other categories of chronic renal failure, those with chronic interstitial nephritis tend to have low-grade proteinuria (<1.5 g/24 h), urinary sediment with few cells or casts, infrequent or mild hypertension, preserved or increased urine volume with a tendency toward sodium wasting, elevated uric acid level, hyperchloremic metabolic acidosis, and anemia disproportionately severe for the degree of renal failure.

These abnormalities are a consequence of injury to renal epithelial cells throughout the nephron. Proximal tubule epithelial cells reabsorb filtered sodium,

Table 11B–1. Major Causes of Chronic Renal Toxicity

Drugs
Analgesics
Cyclosporine
Lithium
Cisplatin
Nitrosoureas
Environmental and Occupational Toxins
Lead
Cadmium

Table 11B–2. Common Causes of Chronic Renal Failure

Diabetic nephropathy
Chronic glomerulonephritis
Hypertensive nephrosclerosis
Hereditary renal disease
Polycystic kidney disease, Alport's disease
Obstructive nephropathy, reflux nephropathy
Chronic interstitial nephritis
Metabolic (hypercalcemia, hypokalemia, hyperoxaluria)
Drugs and environmental toxins
Hematologic disorders (multiple myeloma)
Radiation
Ischemic nephropathy
Chronic transplant rejection

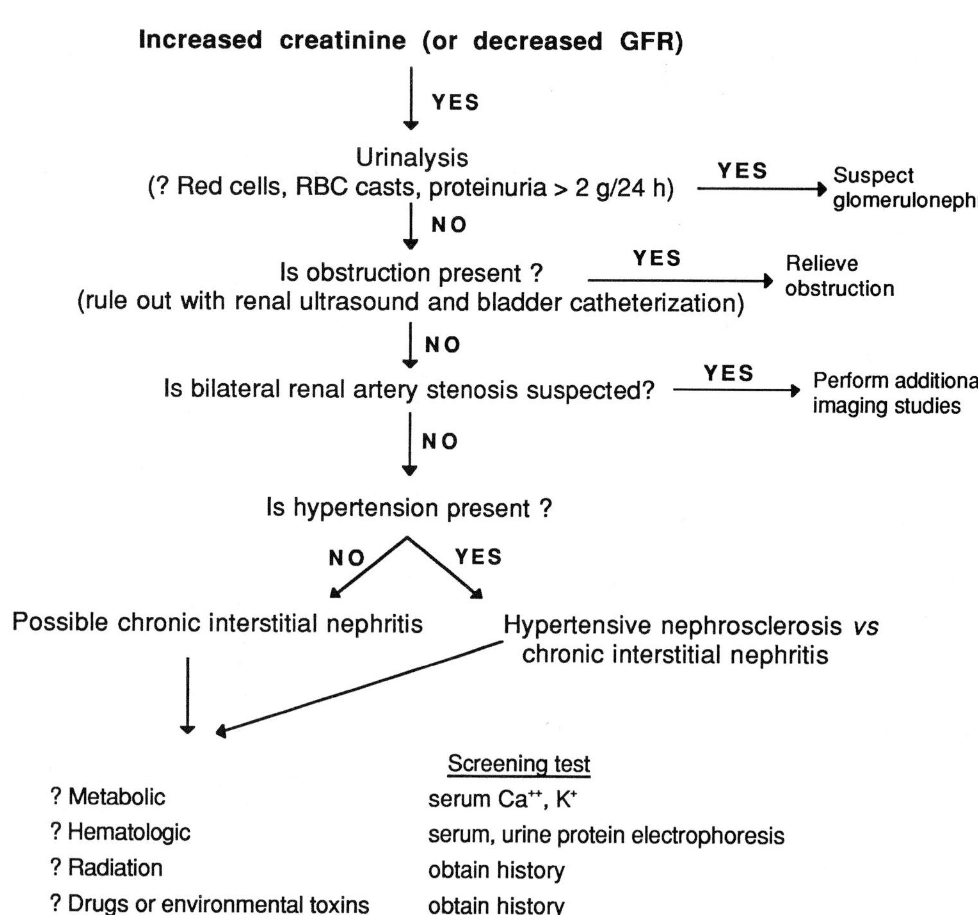

Figure 11B–1. Approach to the patient with chronically decreased renal function. GFR, glomerular filtration rate; RBC, red blood cell.

chloride, bicarbonate, glucose, calcium, phosphate, amino acids, and low-molecular-weight proteins, and they secrete organic anions. Proximal epithelial cell injury results in impaired reabsorption (increased urinary excretion) of these substances. *Fanconi's syndrome* is the clinical term for defective proximal tubule dysfunction resulting in these urinary abnormalities. Distal tubule epithelial cells secrete hydrogen ions and potassium. Injury to these cells results in metabolic acidosis and hyperkalemia. Collecting tubule epithelial cells are responsible for concentrating the urine by water reabsorption. Injury of these cells causes nephrogenic diabetes insipidus, which in minor form may be manifested as increases in urine volume and urinary frequency.

Epithelial cell injury also leads to appearance in the urine of proteins that are normal cellular constituents—mainly, brush border membrane and lysosomal proteins. Alanine aminopeptidase, alkaline phosphatase, γ-glutamyl transpeptidase, *N*-acetylglucosaminidase, and β-galactosidase have been measured and proposed as markers for identifying early or mild renal injury before the occurrence of a detectable reduction in GFR.

CLINICAL APPROACH TO PATIENTS WITH CHRONIC RENAL FAILURE

A useful guideline for the clinical approach to patients with increased serum creatinine level (or a decrease in GFR) is shown in Figure 11B–1. The presence of numerous red blood cells or red blood cell casts leads one to suspect glomerulonephritis. Similarly, urinary protein in excess of 2 g/24 h is more characteristic of glomerular disease than chronic interstitial disease. The possibility that the renal disease is caused by multiple myeloma or another monoclonal gammopathy can be ruled out by serum and urine protein electrophoresis and immunofixation. If a patient has unremarkable urinalysis results, the possibility of obstruction should be ruled out with bladder catheterization and renal ultrasonography. In patients with diffuse atherosclerosis or risk factors for atherosclerosis, the possibility of bilateral renal artery stenosis should be considered. The presence or absence of hypertension does not eliminate the possibility of chronic interstitial nephritis, whereas the absence of hypertension certainly eliminates the possibility of hypertensive nephrosclerosis. When considering the possibility of chronic interstitial nephritis, metabolic factors need to be considered. At a minimum, the serum potassium and calcium levels need to be ascertained. The possibility that other causes of chronic interstitial nephritis are relevant can be considered by the careful taking of the history of drug ingestion (both prescription and over-the-counter drugs; see Table 11B–1), evaluation of the past medical history (particularly a history of tumor and type of therapy), and determination of environmental exposure (including occupational and domestic exposures). In many cases of chronic renal toxicity, it is not possible to establish firmly a causal relationship, although the circumstantial evidence may be very convincing.

No unique pathophysiologic process is responsible for the development of chronic renal toxicity. Therefore, disease-specific descriptions are most informative.

THERAPEUTIC AGENTS

Analgesics

Epidemiology

Analgesics have long been suspected to be a cause of chronic renal disease.[2, 3] The full impact of analgesics on renal function is unknown because it is difficult to measure accurately the total quantity of analgesic drugs consumed over a long period. Most studies have suggested that a cumulative intake of more than 1 to 3 kg of the harmful analgesic is required to produce chronic renal disease. Therefore, clinical disease would not be recognized until a patient had consumed large daily doses of analgesics for 3 or more years. Conservative estimates are that between 1% and 3% of patients with end-stage renal disease in the United States have analgesic nephropathy. In some areas of the country, however, analgesic nephropathy is more common. For example, in northwestern North Carolina, about 10% of cases of end-stage renal disease may be due to analgesic use. Throughout the world, a striking variation is noted in the incidence of analgesic nephropathy, with areas of greater frequency in Belgium, Australia, Scotland, and Switzerland.

Phenacetin was the earliest recognized nephrotoxic analgesic drug. Because of its association with renal disease, it is no longer marketed. Phenacetin was linked not only to the development of renal disease but also to hypertension, cardiovascular disease, and cancer. In a 20-year prospective study of women who were identified as regular users of phenacetin, the relative risk of death due to urologic or renal disease was 16.1.[4] Many case-control studies also supported the relationship between the use of phenacetin and the risk of developing chronic renal disease.

Acetaminophen, the major metabolite of phenacetin, has also been associated with the development of chronic interstitial nephritis and renal failure. In a case-control study of subjects hospitalized with a new diagnosis of chronic renal disease, the odds ratio of end-stage renal disease was 3.21 when daily users of acetaminophen were compared with infrequent user.[5] A more recent case-control study using a similar experimental design found the odds ratio of end-stage renal disease to be 2.1 for subjects who took 366 or more acetaminophen pills for a year, compared with those who consumed fewer than 104 pills per year.[6] This study further estimated that between 8% and 10% of all cases of end-stage renal disease were attributable to acetaminophen use.

The risk of renal disease for patients using nonsteroidal anti-inflammatory drugs (NSAIDs), including aspirin, is less clear. In many cases, patients have used combinations of acetaminophen and NSAIDs, and it has been difficult to determine consumption and the independent contribution of each agent. In one case-control study, a twofold increased risk of chronic renal disease was noted in subjects with previous daily use of NSAIDs.[7] In men older than 65 years of age, the odds ratio for chronic renal disease was 10.0 for daily use of NSAIDs. In another study, an estimated cumulative lifetime dose of 5000 or more pills containing NSAIDs was associated with increased odds of developing end-stage renal disease (odds ratio, 8.8).[6] These case-control studies have been criticized because they are retrospective, rely on recall of drug use for estimation of analgesic exposure, and present difficulties in identifying appropriate control subjects. Nevertheless, it seems likely that phenacetin and acetaminophen are chronic nephrotoxins. NSAIDs may also be toxic to the kidneys when consumed continually and may contribute to the toxicity caused by acetaminophen and phenacetin when these drugs are consumed together (discussed later).

Aspirin has also been questioned as a cause of chronic renal disease. Because of its ability to inhibit renal prostaglandin synthesis, aspirin has the ability to cause acute renal failure through a reduction in renal blood flow. This effect is particularly striking in persons with pre-existing renal disease.[8] On the other hand, long-term aspirin use alone may not be an independent cause of chronic renal disease.[6]

Pathophysiology

Analgesics produce chronic interstitial nephritis and papillary necrosis. The precise mechanism of analgesic nephropathy is unclear but probably includes some combination of injury produced by toxic metabolites of the drug and medullary ischemia. Acetaminophen accumulates in the renal medulla and papilla, where it is further metabolized by conjugation or oxidation.[9, 10] Conjugation is the usual mechanism. Under toxicologic conditions, more oxidation occurs. This oxidation is catalyzed by cytochrome P-450 and results in generation of a toxic free radical intermediate. The eventual oxidation product is *N*-acetyl-*p*-benzoquinone imine. Acetaminophen can also be deacetylated to yield *p*-aminophenol, which is then oxidized by cytochrome P-450 to *p*-benzoquinone imine. Glutathione preferentially reacts with these metabolites to protect intrinsic renal macromolecules. When renal glutathione is depleted, renal injury occurs. This mechanism is similar to that observed in the liver. In animal studies, inhibitors of cytochrome P-450 prevent renal cell injury, as do therapies that enhance glutathione availability.[9]

NSAIDs and aspirin inhibit cyclo-oxygenase, decrease the synthesis of vasodilatory prostaglandins, and predispose to renal ischemia. The medulla and papilla, having a tenuous oxygen supply, are therefore susceptible to ischemic injury and papillary necrosis.[11] Synergism between acetaminophen and NSAIDs can be explained by the accumulation of acetaminophen, which is metabolized to toxic intermediates, in combination with renal vasoconstriction due to ischemic injury caused by renal prostaglandin inhibition.

Clinical Presentation

Analgesic nephropathy occurs more frequently in women than men. The prototypical patient is one who has suffered chronically from headache or low back pain. Some of these patients also have chronic gastrointestinal symptoms caused by chronic use of NSAIDs. The majority of patients have consumed a mixture of analgesic agents rather than drugs of a single category.

Long-term use of analgesics results in interstitial nephritis and papillary necrosis. In addition to renal insufficiency, patients develop impaired renal concentrating ability and have sterile pyuria. During episodes of papillary necrosis, patients can have flank pain, pyuria, and hematuria. Acute ureteral obstruction may result, and necrotic papillary tissue is often passed in the urine. Intravenous pyelography reveals the characteristic ring sign, which is actually contrast agent surrounding the sloughed papilla. Later, only a puddle of contrast medium is seen in the space previously occupied by the papilla. Renal ultrasonography reveals small, irregularly contoured kidneys with irregular thinning of the renal cortex. Previous papillary necrosis produces triangular papillary calcifications.[12] The presence of papillary calcification on computed tomography is probably the most sensitive indicator of analgesic nephropathy (Fig. 11B–2).[13] On renal biopsy, the kidneys have interstitial infiltrates and fibrosis.

Long-term use of analgesics also increases the risk of developing transitional cell carcinoma of the urinary collecting system and bladder.[14, 15] This risk may continue even after cessation of analgesic use. Therefore, hematuria that develops in a patient with a history of chronic analgesic abuse should prompt an exceptionally thorough search for bladder and collecting system tumors.

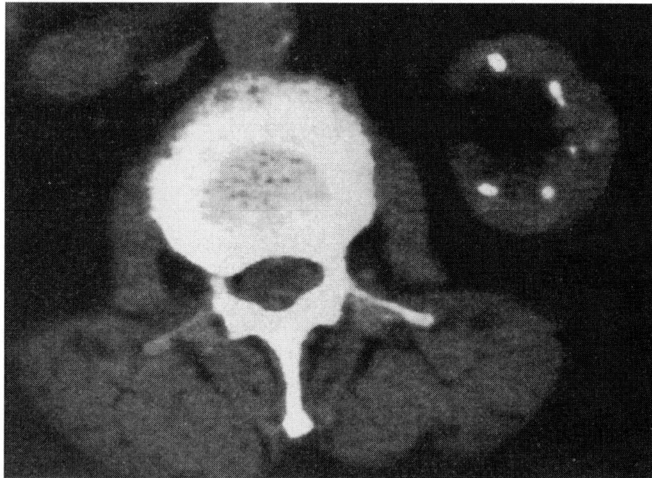

Figure 11B–2. Analgesic nephropathy. This CT scan demonstrates papillary calcification characteristic of analgesic nephropathy. Calcifications appear as triangular, ringlike, or polygonal calcifications on the papillary line. Other CT findings in analgesic nephropathy include a decrease in renal volume and irregular contour. (From Elseviers MM, De Schepper A, Corthouts R, et al: High diagnostic performance of CT scan for analgesic nephropathy in patients with incipient to severe renal failure. Kidney Int *48*:1316, 1995. Reprinted by permission of Blackwell Scientific, Inc.)

Outcome and Treatment

The natural history of the disease in patients who continue to use analgesics is end-stage renal disease. Renal function often stabilizes in patients who are able to discontinue analgesic use or switch to a nontoxic drug, even when they already have substantial renal impairment. Because patients often intentionally or unintentionally underestimate their consumption of analgesics, diagnosis requires a high index of suspicion and a carefully taken history. Once chronic renal insufficiency has developed as a result of analgesic use, even aspirin, which is unlikely to cause chronic interstitial nephritis, may reversibly impair renal function through inhibition of vasodilatory prostaglandins. Therefore, if chronic pain persists and must be treated with medications, carefully supervised use of narcotics may be necessary. However, substantial efforts at alleviating underlying physical and psychologic conditions requiring continued pain medication should first be attempted.

Cyclosporine

Epidemiology

With the widespread use of cyclosporine as an immunosuppressant agent in solid organ transplantation, bone marrow transplantation, and immune-mediated diseases, it has become apparent that chronic renal disease is an unavoidable consequence of long-term cyclosporine use.[16, 17] The incidence and severity of cyclosporine-mediated renal disease are debated and depend in large part on the dose of cyclosporine administered and the presence of other risk factors for impaired renal function. However, even in patients without pre-existing renal disease, long-term use of cyclosporine results in depression of glomerular filtration and renal blood flow and a high incidence of hypertension. In some patients, these renal effects are reversible as soon as use of the drug is discontinued. In other patients, however, structural injury that is not immediately reversible occurs. Of this latter group of patients, some develop progressive renal insufficiency or progressive histopathologic injury but others maintain stable renal function for a number of years.

Pathophysiology

Acute administration of cyclosporine causes renal vasoconstriction in both experimental animals and humans.[18, 19] Renal vasoconstriction causes a decrease in renal blood flow and a consequent decrease in GFR. These effects are immediately reversible and can be demonstrated to occur repeatedly in patients after administration of each dose of cyclosporine. Multiple mediators for renal vasoconstriction have been proposed and include activation of the sympathetic nervous system, with participation of endothelin as a second messenger, alterations in the balance of vasoconstrictor and vasodilator prostaglandins, and activation of the renin-angiotensin system.

The relationship between acute and chronic nephrotoxicity has not been clarified. It is suspected that recurrent or persistent vasoconstriction causes chronic ischemic injury of the kidneys. Chronic cyclosporine-related nephropathy is characterized by the same physiologic alterations of reduced renal plasma flow and GFR as well as by the development of histologic indicators of chronic renal injury. Both preglomerular and glomerular vessels are involved, as is the renal parenchyma. Cyclosporine arteriolopathy is characterized by arterial hyalinosis and, in severe cases, myocyte degeneration and thrombosis of the arteriole (Fig. 11B–3). Glomerular injury is characterized by focal segmental sclerosis. Renal parenchymal disease is characterized by tubular atrophy and interstitial fibrosis, which is often described as patchy or striped in appearance (Fig. 11B–4).[20]

Arteriolopathy and interstitial fibrosis have been reproduced in rodents after administration of cyclosporine for 2 to 4 or more weeks. In rodents, salt depletion markedly enhances the development of these lesions. The earliest vascular change observed was eosinophilic granular transformation of smooth muscle cells in the glomerular afferent arterioles.[21] The renal parenchymal lesion of interstitial fibrosis is preceded by tubular and interstitial cell proliferation and macrophage infiltration.[22] Increased accumulation of type I and type IV collagen eventually results in fibrosis.

Clinical Presentation

Cyclosporine has a number of side effects, including neurotoxicity, hypertrichosis, and gingival hyperplasia, but its most common and severe complication is chronic nephrotoxicity.[23] Renal dysfunction often appears in the absence of other problems and is recognized only by an increase in serum creatinine values. Cyclosporine toxicity has no other specific renal or clinical markers, although 60% to 100% of patients also have hypertension. Chronic cyclosporine toxicity is associated with the use of higher doses of cyclosporine (>5 mg/kg per day) and may be more common in patients who have had episodes of acute nephrotoxicity.[24, 25] Attempts to correlate the development of chronic nephrotoxicity with blood levels of cyclosporine or its metabolites have largely been unsuccessful. The diagnosis of chronic cyclosporine nephrotoxicity is usually made when all other potential contributing factors have been eliminated and

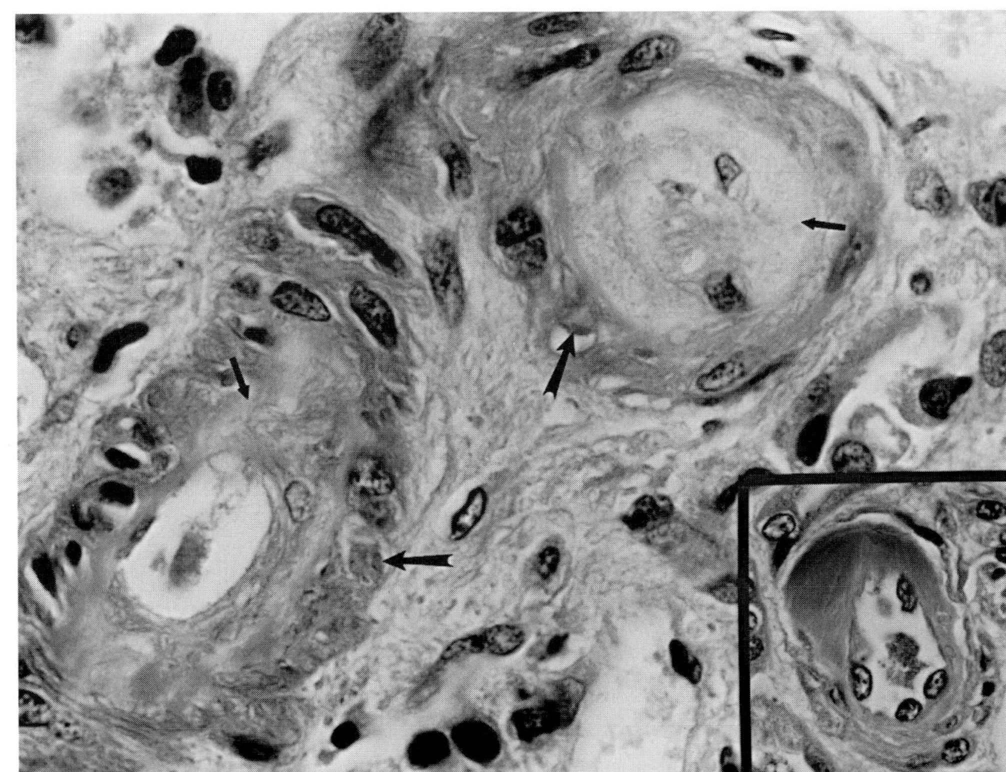

Figure 11B–3. Acute cyclosporine arteriolopathy is characterized by focal smooth muscle degeneration *(large arrows)* and mucoid intimal thickening *(short arrows)*. Note the loss of smooth muscle cells in the lower right quadrant of the vessel on the left. *Inset:* Chronic cyclosporine arteriolopathy. The myocytes are replaced by hyaline deposits that protrude toward the outer aspect of the media. (Courtesy of Dr. J.C. Manivel.)

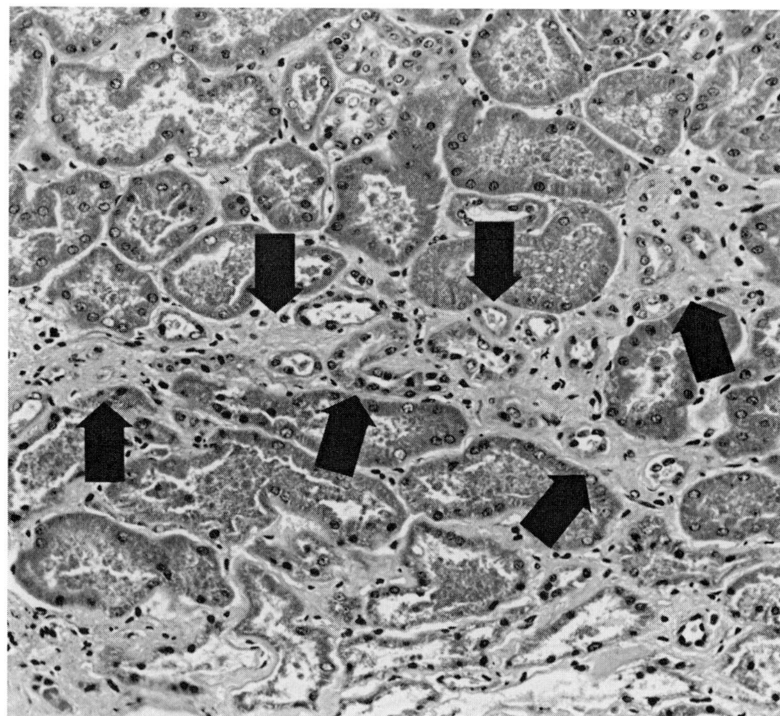

Figure 11B–4. Interstitial fibrosis resulting from cyclosporine toxicity. Bandlike "striped" areas of fibrosis and tubular atrophy are seen between the *arrows*. This interstitial fibrosis is not fundamentally different from that seen with other causes of chronic nephrotoxicity. (Courtesy of Dr. J.C. Manivel.)

renal function remains impaired. Functional and pathologic involvement may be dissociated, and some patients with well-preserved renal function have shown arteriolopathy and interstitial fibrosis on renal biopsy.[26]

Outcome and Treatment

The long-term outcome of chronic cyclosporine nephrotoxicity is unclear. Initial reports of cardiac transplant recipients' receiving high doses of cyclosporine suggested that long-term administration of cyclosporine resulted in the development of end-stage renal disease that necessitated the use of dialysis in a substantial portion of patents.[20, 27] Many other studies, however, have suggested that after the initial decrease in GFR induced by renal vasoconstriction, renal function stabilizes for many years.[28, 29] Some have cautioned that despite stabilization in renal function, progressive glomerulosclerosis and interstitial fibrosis may occur and may ultimately result in further impairment of renal function and possible development of end-stage renal disease.

Most would agree that cessation of cyclosporine use leads to stabilization or improvement in renal function. However, many patients being treated with cyclosporine do not have this option (as do heart or liver transplant recipients). Avoiding high doses of cyclosporine is recommended but must be balanced against the possibility that too low a dose of cyclosporine may result in ineffective immunosuppression with partial loss of therapeutic efficacy. When cyclosporine use can be discontinued in patients with severe nephrotoxicity, eventual improvement may occur. Even severe cyclosporine arteriopathy has been observed to reverse with discontinuation or lowering of the dose of cyclosporine.[30] Various renal vasodilators have been demonstrated to reduce the acute vasoconstriction induced by cyclosporine. Therefore, dopamine, dopamine agonists such as fenoldopam, and calcium channel blockers improve renal blood flow and GFR in patients receiving long-term cyclosporine therapy.[31–33] However, it is not known whether these agents can prevent the development of chronic renal disease in patients exposed to cyclosporine for prolonged periods.

Lithium

Lithium is an effective and frequently prescribed drug for the treatment of bipolar affective disorders. Unfortunately, lithium has a number of important effects on renal function. These include nephrogenic diabetes insipidus, renal tubular acidosis, and chronic interstitial nephritis.[34] Demonstrable defects in the renal concentrating ability occur in more than half of patients taking lithium, but clinically significant polyuria occurs in approximately 20%. An intermediate fraction of patients complain of polydipsia or are noted to have it. Lithium induces nephrogenic diabetes insipidus through several cellular effects. The most important effect of lithium is to impair generation of cyclic adenosine-3′, 5′,-monophospate in the collecting tubule of the distal nephron in response to antidiuretic hormone. This defect results in a failure to reabsorb filtered water adequately, and the result is water wasting, hyperosmolality, and secondary polydipsia. Although this defect usually responds to discontinuation of lithium therapy, some patients clearly have persistent nephrogenic diabetes insipidus for months or even years after cessation. The diuretic amiloride has been shown to improve concentrating ability in patients taking lithium.[35] A major effect of amiloride is to prevent the renal cellular uptake of lithium. Thus, although not yet proved, it is possible that coadministration of amiloride with lithium would prevent lithium-induced nephrogenic diabetes insipidus.

A great concern is that long-term administration of lithium leads to interstitial nephritis and decreased GFR. Surprisingly, this has been a very difficult subject to study. Early data were retrospective and identified selected patients who came to medical attention because of renal functional abnormalities. Renal biopsies of a number of these patients showed tubular atrophy and interstitial fibrosis.[36] However, the attribution of these lesions to lithium was put in doubt because similar renal histologic changes have been observed in psychiatric patients who have never received lithium.[37] At least one prospective study demonstrated no difference in renal interstitial fibrosis between psychiatric patients taking lithium for more than 5 years and those who had never received the drug. Nevertheless, prospective studies have suggested an increased incidence of impaired GFR in lithium-treated patients, and a number of well-documented case reports describe patients who had normal baseline renal function yet progressed to end-stage renal disease after long-term therapy with lithium.[38, 39] The incidence of severely impaired renal function in patients receiving lithium is probably low, and it is reasonable to assume that maintenance of serum lithium levels in the therapeutic range would limit progressive renal damage. Patients who demonstrate progressive renal insufficiency while receiving lithium should be considered for discontinuation if their psychiatric disease permits. Amiloride has not been reported to prevent further deterioration in renal function once interstitial nephritis has developed.

Cisplatin

Cisplatin (*cis*-diamminedichloroplatinum) has activity against various solid tumors and is frequently used in combination chemotherapy. Its toxicities include myelosuppression and renal dysfunction. Cisplatin causes acute renal failure, chronic interstitial nephritis, and Fanconi-type tubular dysfunction that includes renal salt wasting and renal magnesium wasting.[40]

Cisplatin is largely protein bound and is actively taken up by renal cells. Cisplatin remains in the kidneys for weeks after intravenous administration. Both antitumor and nephrotoxic properties are dependent on the stereoisomer, because *trans*-dichlorodiammineplatinum has no toxicity. It is believed that biotransformation of the molecule involving removal of chloride to form the aquated dihydroxydiamminoplatinum contributes to toxicity. Binding of the metal to sulfhydryl groups of cellular macromolecules may also mediate toxicity.[41]

Cisplatin causes focal acute tubular necrosis with tubular dilatation, interstitial edema, and sparing of the glomerulus. Although doses in excess of 100 mg/m^2 have caused acute renal failure, a more typical presentation with cumulative administration is the slow progressive rise in creatinine levels. Magnesium wasting, a consequence of impaired tubular reabsorption, may be severe, resulting in hypomagnesemia as well as hypokalemia and hypocalcemia.[42]

Vigorous hydration is important in reducing acute and probably chronic nephrotoxicity. Carboplatin has similar nephrotoxicity, although nephrotoxicity appears less frequently at equieffective tumoricidal doses.

Nitrosoureas

Streptozocin, lomustine, and carmustine are chemotherapeutic agents causing various degrees of chronic nephrotoxicity. Of these agents, streptozocin is the most nephrotoxic and lomustine the least. Renal dysfunction is usually not apparent until months to years after administration of the drug, although it may be progressive and may lead to end-stage renal disease.[43] As is typical in cases of interstitial nephritis, the kidneys become small and shrunken and renal biopsy reveals tubular atrophy and interstitial fibrosis. Glomerulosclerosis, endarteritis, and cellular atypia have also been identified in patients who had earlier received these drugs. This specific mechanism for development of chronic renal disease by nitrosoureas is not known. No treatment is known to be effective once the disease has developed. However, nephrotoxicity is infrequent with cumulative doses of less than 1200 mg/m^2.

ENVIRONMENTAL AND OCCUPATIONAL TOXINS

Lead

Children who ingest paint chips containing lead-based paints or soil contaminated by exhaust fumes from automobiles using leaded gas are continuously exposed to lead. Adults may be continually exposed to lead by the inhalation route. Exposure may occur in smelting and refining processes, casting of battery plates, welding, or petroleum distillation. Plumbers and miners have a lower risk of exposure. Although now relatively rare, consumption of moonshine made in improper containers or the use of pottery glazed with lead-containing glazes is another source of lead ingestion. Leaded gasoline is still produced and available overseas in many Asiatic countries.

Acute exposure to lead results in proximal tubular dysfunction or Fanconi's syndrome. Long-term exposure leads to hyperuricemia (saturnine gout), hypertension, and chronic renal failure. The pathologic lesion of lead nephropathy is chronic interstitial nephritis.[44] End-stage renal disease may not develop until 20 or 30 years after exposure, and thus it has been difficult to implicate lead in specific cases of renal failure of unknown cause.[45] About 5% of patients undergoing hemodialysis have elevated bone lead concentrations; this findings may be of etiologic importance.[46] In a cross-sectional study in Belgium, an inverse correlation was found between blood lead concentrations and creatinine clearance.[47] However, other studies have failed to find such a relationship.

Diagnosis is best made by determination of whether a patient has excessive body lead stores. This can be determined by parenteral administration of calcium disodiumedetate (EDTA) (2 g) followed by 24-hour urine collections for 1 to 3 days. Patients with a reduced GFR should have a 72-hour urine collection. Normal subjects excrete less than 400 μg/72 h. Subjects with lead nephropathy excrete more than 600 μg of lead chelate.

Chronic lead toxicity can be treated by long-term chelation therapy with EDTA. Improvement in GFR has been reported in patients with minimal reductions in GFR. However, patients with advanced chronic renal failure do not usually demonstrate improvement.

Cadmium

Industrial workers may develop chronic renal disease by inhalation exposure to cadmium. Much like lead, cadmium exposure results in Fanconi's syndrome and chronic interstitial nephritis.[48] Workers with high-level industrial exposure show reductions in GFR and increased urinary excretion of various enzymes such as β_2-microglobulin and *N*-acetyl-β-glucosaminidase.[49, 50] β_2-Microglobulin undergoes glomerular filtration and is then reabsorbed by proximal tubule epithelial cells. Increased excretion suggests impaired proximal tubule function. *N*-Acetyl-β-glucosaminidase is a lysosomal enzyme; increased urinary excretion suggests chronic cellular injury. Treatment of cadmium nephropathy consists of elimination of exposure. As is true of all forms of chronic renal disease, however, if renal function is already moderately impaired, progressive dysfunction may continue even when the initiating factor is withdrawn.

References

1. Cockcroft DW, Gault MH: Prediction of creatinine clearance from serum creatinine. Nephron *16*:31, 1976.
2. Kincaid-Smith P: Analgesic abuse and the kidney. Kidney Int *17*:250, 1980.
3. Murray T, Goldberg M: Chronic interstitial nephritis: Etiologic factors. Ann Intern Med *82*:453, 1975.
4. Dubach UC, Rosner B, Stürmer T: An epidemiologic study of abuse of analgesic drugs. Effects of phenacetin and salicylate on mortality and cardiovascular morbidity. N Engl J Med *324*:155, 1991.
5. Sandler DP, Smith JC, Weinberg CR, et al: Analgesic use and chronic renal disease. N Engl J Med *320*:1238, 1989.
6. Perneger TV, Whelton PK, Klag MJ: Risk of kidney failure associated with the use of acetaminophen, aspirin, and nonsteroidal antiinflammatory drugs. N Engl J Med *331*:1675, 1994.
7. Sandler DP, Burr F, Weinberg CR: Nonsteroidal anti-inflammatory drugs and the risk for chronic renal disease. Ann Intern Med *115*:165, 1991.
8. Kimberly RP, Plotz PH: Aspirin-induced depression of renal function. N Engl J Med *296*:418, 1977.
9. Mitchell JR, McMurtry RJ, Statham CN, et al: Molecular basis for several drug-induced nephropathies. Am J Med *62*:518, 1977.
10. Lash LH: Role of metabolism in chemically induced nephrotoxicity. *In* Goldstein RS (ed): Mechanisms of Injury in Renal Disease and Toxicity. Boca Raton, CRC Press, pp 209–210, 1994.
11. Brezis M, Rosen S, Silva P, et al: Renal ischemia: A new perspective. Kidney Int *26*:375, 1984.
12. Weber M, Braun B, Kohler H: Ultrasonic findings in analgesic nephropathy. Nephron *39*:216, 1985.
13. Elseviers MM, De Schepper A, Corthouts R, et al: High diagnostic performance of CT scan for analgesic nephropathy in patients with incipient to severe renal failure. Kidney Int *48*:1316, 1995.
14. Gonwa TA, Corbett WT, Schey HM, et al: Analgesic-associated nephropathy and transitional cell carcinoma of the urinary tract. Ann Intern Med *93*:249, 1980.
15. McCredie M, Stewart JH, Carter JJ, et al: Phenacetin and papillary necrosis: Independent risk factors for renal pelvic cancer. Kidney Int *30*:81, 1986.
16. Myers BD: Cyclosporine nephrotoxicity. Kidney Int *30*:964, 1986.
17. Remuzzi G, Bertani T: Renal vascular and thrombotic effects of cyclosporine. Am J Kidney Dis *13*:261, 1989.
18. Murry BM, Paller MS, Ferris TF: Effect of cyclosporine administration on renal hemodynamics on conscious rats. Kidney Int *28*:767, 1985.
19. Curtis JJ, Luke RG, Dubovsky E, et al: Cyclosporine in therapeutic doses increases renal allograft vascular resistance. Lancet *2*:477, 1986.
20. Myers BD, Ross J, Newton L, et al: Cyclosporine-associated chronic nephropathy. N Engl J Med *311*:699, 1984.
21. Young BA, Burdmann, EA Johnson RJ, et al: Cyclosporine A induced arteriolopathy in a rat model of chronic cyclosporine nephropathy. Kidney Int 48:431, 1995.
22. Young BA, Burdmann, EA, Johnson RJ, et al: Cellular proliferation and macrophage influx precede interstitial fibrosis in cyclosporine nephrotoxicity. Kidney Int *48*:439, 1995.
23. Kahan BD: Cyclosporine. N Engl J Med *321*:1725, 1989.
24. Feutren G, Mihatsch MJ: Risk factors for cyclosporine-induced nephropathy in patients with autoimmune diseases. N Engl J Med *326*:1654, 1992.
25. Pei Y, Scholey JW, Katz A, et al: Chronic nephrotoxicity in psoriatic patients treated with low-dose cyclosporine. Am J Kidney Dis *23*:528, 1994.
26. Ludwin D, Alexopoulou I, Esdaile JM, et al: Renal biopsy specimens from patients with rheumatoid arthritis and apparently normal renal function after therapy with cyclosporine. Am J Kidney Dis *23*:260, 1994.
27. Bertani T, Ferrazzi P, Schieppati A, et al: Nature and extent of glomerular injury induced by cyclosporine in heart transplant patients. Kidney Int *40*:243, 1991.
28. Bantle JP, Paller MS, Boudreau RJ, et al: Long-term effects of cyclosporine on renal function in organ transplant recipients. J Lab Clin Med *115*:233, 1990.
29. Ruggenenti P, Perico N, Amuchastegui S, et al: Following an initial decline, glomerular filtration rate stabilizes in heart transplant patients on chronic cyclosporine. Am J Kidney Dis *24*:549, 1994.
30. Morozumi K, Thiel G, Albert FW, et al: Studies on morphological outcome of cyclosporine-associated arteriolopathy after discontinuation of cyclosporine in renal allografts. Clin Nephrol *38*:1, 1992.
31. Conte G, Dal Canton A, Sabbatini M, et al: Acute cyclosporine renal dysfunction reversed by dopamine infusion in healthy subjects. Kidney Int *36*:1086, 1989.

32. Jorkasky DK, Audet P, Shusterman N, et al: Fenoldopam reverses cyclosporine-induced renal vasoconstriction in kidney transplant recipients. Am J Kidney Dis *19*:567, 1992.
33. Ruggenenti P, Perico N, Mosconi L, et al: Calcium channel blockers protect transplant patients from cyclosporine-induced daily renal hypoperfusion. Kidney Int *43*:706, 1993.
34. Boton R, Gaviria M, Batlle DC: Prevalence, pathogenesis, and treatment of renal dysfunction associated with chronic lithium therapy. Am J Kidney Dis *10*:329, 1987.
35. Batlle DC, von Riotte AB, Gaviria M, et al: Amelioration of polyuria by amiloride in patients receiving long-term lithium therapy. N Engl J Med *312*:408, 1985.
36. Hestbech J, Hansen HE, Amdisen A, et al: Chronic renal lesions following long-term treatment with lithium. Kidney Int *12*:205, 1977.
37. Walker RG, Bennett WM, Davies BM, et al: Structural and functional effects of long-term lithium therapy. Kidney Int *21*:513, 1982.
38. Jorkasky DK, Amsterdam JD, Oler J, et al: Lithium-induced renal disease: A prospective study. Clin Nephrol *30*:293, 1988.
39. Gitlin MJ: Lithium-induced renal insufficiency. J Clin Psychopharmacol *13*:276, 1993.
40. Madias NE, Harrington JT: Platinum nephrotoxicity. Am J Med *65*:307, 1978.
41. Fillastre JP, Godin M: An overview of drug-induced nephropathies. *In* Goldstein RS (ed): Mechanisms of Injury in Renal Disease and Toxicity. Boca Raton, CRC Press, pp 131–133, 1994.
42. Schilsky RL, Anderson T: Hypomagnesemia and renal magnesium wasting in patients receiving cisplatin. Ann Intern Med *90*:929, 1979.
43. Weiss RB, Posada JG, Kramer RA, et al: Nephrotoxicity of semustine. Cancer Treat Rep *67*:1105, 1983.
44. Emmerson BT: Chronic lead nephropathy. Kidney Int *4*:1, 1973.
45. Batuman V, Landy E, Maesaka JK, et al: Contribution of lead to hypertension with renal failure. N Engl J Med *309*:17, 1983.
46. Van De Vyver FL, D'Haese PC, Visser WJ, et al: Bone lead in dialysis patients. Kidney Int *33*:601, 1988.
47. Staessen JA, Lauwerys RR, Buchet JP, et al: Impairment of renal function with increasing blood lead concentrations in the general population. N Engl J Med 327:151, 1992.
48. Wedeen RP: Environmental renal disease: Lead, cadmium and Balkan endemic nephropathy. Kidney Int *40*:S-4, 1991.
49. Smith TJ, Anderson RJ, Reading JC: Chronic cadmium exposure associated with kidney function effects. Am J Industr Med *1*:319, 1980.
50. Meyer BR, Fischbein A, Rosenman K, et al: Increased urinary enzyme excretion in workers exposed to nephrotoxic chemicals. Am J Med *76*:989, 1984.

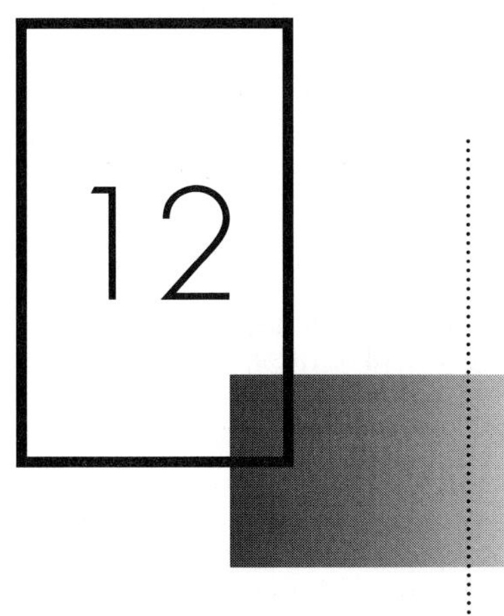

Gastrointestinal Effects of Poisoning

WILLIAMSON B. STRUM, MD

The effect of poisoning on the gastrointestinal (GI) tract is a consequence of the interaction of specific chemical agents (xenobiotics) on a susceptible tissue. In certain ways, the GI tissue is uniquely resistant; in other ways, it is vulnerable to certain poisons. To understand the GI tissue response to poisons, an awareness of certain critical aspects of its epithelial structure, cell renewal characteristics, and specific functions is required. Although the GI tract is lined throughout with an epithelium of entodermal origin, both the structure and function vary considerably from esophagus to colon. This chapter begins with a concise assessment of the essential features of epithelial cell structure, cell kinetics, and function as they occur in human beings and as they relate to poisoning.

GASTROINTESTINAL EPITHELIAL CELL STRUCTURE

Esophagus

The epithelium of the esophagus differs strikingly from the epithelium found elsewhere in the GI tract.[1] The esophagus is lined with stratified squamous cells that are similar to the squamous cell covering of the skin except for the absence of a keratin surface and cells of skin appendages (hair, nails, and sweat glands). Mucus is secreted from small superficial glands, which are identical in appearance to the cardiac glands of the stomach and are located beneath the epithelial surface at the levels of the cricoid cartilage and the esophagogastric junction. The mucus provides a protective and lubricant surface to facilitate the passage of food from the mouth into the stomach. The proliferating zone is the layer of polygonal cells in the basal portion of the epithelium. The squamous epithelial cell lining of the esophagus is a protective coating of cells for the underlying tissue.

Stomach

The stomach has an epithelial cell lining that is 0.5 mm thick. The epithelium is characterized by a uniform surface with shallow pits (foveolae gastricae), below which are gastric glands. The epithelium lining the surface and pits consists of surface mucous cells uniformly distributed throughout the stomach. Differences in the underlying glands permit histologic separation of three distinct gastric regions: the cardia, body (body and fundus), and pyloric antrum.[1]

The cardia is the first 1 to 3 cm of gastric epithelium distal to the esophagogastric junction. The cardia epithelium is composed of columnar mucous cells lining the surface and pits and mucus-secreting cells in the glands, as well as undifferentiated neck cells. As a rule, parietal, chief, and endocrine cells are absent. A characteristic feature is the presence of one or more dilated cystic glands.

The epithelial cell lining of the body and fundus is more complex and accounts for approximately 80% of the remaining stomach. In addition to the surface and pit mucous cells, mucous neck cells, and undifferentiated neck cells, the glands contain parietal (oxyntic) cells, chief (zymogen) cells, mucous cells, and endocrine cells. The parietal cells are located in the mid to upper half of the glands and secrete hydrochloric acid and intrinsic factor. Electron microscopy reveals that the cytoplasm is packed with mitochondria and contains a system of secretory canaliculi with microvillous lining. The chief cells are located in the deepest portion of the glands, and their cytoplasm contains pepsinogen granules, precursors of the proteolytic enzyme pepsin. The mucous cells of the glands also secrete mucus and pepsinogens. The endocrine cell population of this region includes argentaffin and argyrophilic cells that are scattered singly or in small clusters in the midzone of the glands. The argentaffin cells secrete serotonin and histamine. The endocrine cells are thought to have their embryologic origin in the neural crest. The undifferentiated neck cells are thought to be multipotential proliferating cells from which the other cell types are derived.

The epithelium of the pyloric antrum occupies a triangular area in the distal fifth of the stomach. The architecture of the epithelium differs from that of the body, in that the pits are deeper and the glands shorter but more extensively coiled. The cell population differs in that parietal cells are less frequent and chief cells are rarely found at all; gastrin-secreting (G) cells are added to the endocrine cell types. The gastrin-secreting cells are found most frequently in the midportion of the glands; these cells are able to synthesize DNA and to replicate through mitosis.

Small Intestine

The small intestine is composed of the duodenum, jejunum, and ileum. It is about 280 cm in length and 4 cm in internal diameter.[1] However, the surface area is much greater than these measurements suggest, because the surface is extensively folded and contains numerous finger-like projections called *villi*. Villi are visible under the microscope at low power and have been estimated to number 25 million.[2] The length and shape of the villi change in the three portions of the intestine; they are longest and broadest in the duodenum and shortest and most fingerlike in the ileum. The villi project from cryptlike glands. The number of cells that compose the crypts (of Lieberkühn) does not differ in the three regions of the bowel. In fact, the basic structure of the epithelium is the same throughout the small intestine.

The epithelial cell lining is a single layer of columnar cells, 40 to 50 μm in height, which make up the cover of the villi and the crypts. The villous epithelium is composed of absorptive, goblet, and a few endocrine cells. The crypt epithelium is composed of undifferentiated goblet, endocrine, and Paneth's cells. Of particular interest to toxicologists are the undifferentiated proliferating cells of the crypts and the absorptive cells of the villi. Because of the great proliferative activity of the undifferentiating crypt cells, the intestinal epithelium is particularly susceptible to damage by mitotic inhibitors that interfere with normal cell growth. This subject is discussed further in the next section, on epithelial cell proliferation. Because the major function of the small intestine is the digestion and absorption of nutrients and this function also can be poisoned by various agents, the highly specialized role of the absorptive cells is discussed further.

The absorptive cells are distinguished by a surface brush border that is a complex organelle containing hydrolytic enzymes, receptors, and other proteins involved in transport and contraction. The brush border is a membranous sheet, 6.0 nm wide, that has on the luminal side a carbohydrate-rich layer known as the *glycocalyx* (fuzzy coat).[3] Filamentous structures, thought to be actin, are attached to the inner aspect of the brush border membrane. These fibrils extend into the region of the terminal web, where they intertwine and form attachments to each other so that the contractions of the filaments shorten the microvilli. Mitotic figures are never seen in the villous epithe-

Table 12–1. Key Metabolic Steps Involved in the Cell Cycle

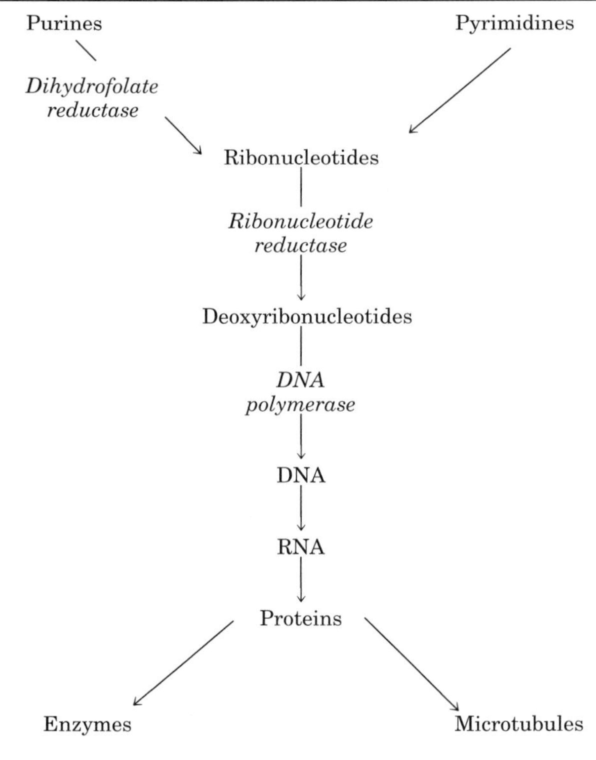

Metabolic poisons interrupt the pathway by enzyme inhibition or substrate alteration, resulting in injury or death to the cell.

lium. All the recognized human brush border enzymes are hydrolases that degrade polymeric substances. These enzymes include disaccharidases, peptidases, phosphatases, and others (Table 12–1). Other nonenzymatic proteins, such as the receptors for intrinsic factor–B_{12} complex, are also found in the brush border.

Colon

The colon is composed of several anatomically distinct regions: cecum, ascending colon, transverse colon, descending colon, sigmoid colon, and rectum. The basic architecture of the epithelial lining is the same throughout.[1] The epithelial lining differs from that of the small bowel in that villi are absent; therefore, the absorptive surface is flat. However, numerous straight tubular crypts, up to 0.7 mm in depth, are present. The crypts are lined with three main cell types: proliferating differentiated cells, mucus-secreting goblet cells, and absorptive cells. The absorptive cells vary from the similar cells of the small intestine, and the microvilli are much less abundant. Paneth's cells are seen occasionally in the proximal colon. Of particular interest to toxicologists are the proliferating cells and the absorptive cells, which are subject to damage by internal and external toxins.

GASTROINTESTINAL EPITHELIAL CELL RENEWAL

A number of agents, including chemotherapeutic drugs used in the treatment of cancer and other diseases of proliferating tissues, are poisonous to the rapidly dividing cells of the GI epithelium. An understanding of how these agents adversely affect the GI epithelium requires a general appreciation of the kinetics of epithelial cell growth. It is beyond the scope of this chapter to review the subject in great detail, and a brief overview with emphasis on the epithelium of the small intestine should suffice. A number of excellent reviews,[4–12] from which these comments are derived, are available for readers who desire more information.

Cell Cycle

The cell cycle in human intestine is the most rapid of all cycles in normal tissue and is the reason for the intestine's exquisite sensitivity to various poisons. The events of cell proliferation are studied by mitotic counting, which identifies the cells in mitosis, and by autoradiography, using tritiated thymidine to label cells entering DNA synthesis. Concomitant estimation of the *mitotic index* (percentage of cells undergoing mitosis) and the DNA *synthesis index* (percentage of cells involved in DNA synthesis) provides a more dynamic picture of the cell cycle than either alone. The phases of the cell cycle are identified by serial examination of the epithelium at intervals after labeling. The cell cycle is the period between the midpoint of mitosis and the midpoint of the subsequent mitosis in one daughter cell, including the cellular and biochemical events that regulate cell growth.[4] Tissues grow primarily through an increase in the number of cells. They occasionally grow by increasing the amount of intracellular substance. In either case, cells also must increase in mass, and all cell components double their mass before mitosis.

Cycling cells pass through various phases. The G_1 (initial growth) phase is the most variable period of the cell cycle, and its duration largely determines the rate of cell proliferation. In general, rapidly growing populations of the intestine consist of cells with G_1 periods shorter than those of slowly growing cells. Some rapidly proliferating cell lines do not even have a G_1 period. The S (synthesis) phase is the period during which DNA replicates and chromosomal proteins are laid down on the newly synthesized DNA. The G_2 phase is the interval between completion of DNA synthesis and mitosis.

Many biochemical events that apply specifically to certain phases of the cell cycle (cell cycle specific) have been described. These events seem to occur only in proliferating cells and are absent or undetectable in nongrowing cells. A number of enzymes that are strictly related to DNA synthesis increase in activity during the S phase. These enzymes include thymidine kinase, DNA polymerase, dihydrofolate reductase, and ribonucleotide reductase. DNA replication occurs during only a discrete and brief period (S phase) of the intestinal cell cycle. The sequence of events and the position of the key enzymatic steps in the sequence are outlined in Table 12–1.

From the standpoint of cell proliferation, the intestinal epithelium contains a mixture of two cell populations: (1) Some cells are continuously dividing (i.e., going from one mitosis to the next in a short time). After mitosis, these cells go through the G_1 phase, the S phase, and the G_2 phase and then back into mitosis. Because they regularly traverse the cell cycle, they are called *cycling cells*. In the intestine, they are represented by rapidly proliferating cells of the crypt epithelium. (2) Other cells leave the cell cycle after a certain number of divisions and differentiate. These cells are destined to die without dividing again. Absorptive cells of the villous epithelium are an example of this class of nondividing, mature cells. Absorptive cells migrate onto the villus after at least two divisions within the crypt and, having lost the ability to incorporate thymidine, undergo further mitosis. Differentiation into a mature columnar cell is accompanied by the appearance of enzymes necessary for the primary function of nutrient digestion. Cell migration is more rapid in the ileum than the jejunum as a result of the decreasing aboral gradient of villus height down the small intestine.

A third class of cells found in most normal tissue leaves the cycle temporarily and remains in a dormant state until environmental conditions stimulate re-entry into the cell cycle. Some stem cells belong to this third group, because they do not cycle until tissue depletion causes them to re-enter the cycle and proliferate in order to replenish the tissue. These cells are G_0 cells.

Normal intestinal epithelial tissue growth depends on (1) the cell cycle time, (2) the growth fraction, and (3) the rate of cell loss. The *cell cycle time* in cycling cells refers to the interval between mitosis—the shorter the interval, the faster cells are produced. The *growth fraction* refers to the fraction of cycling cells; when all the cells participate in the process of cell renewal, the growth fraction equals 1 and the cell cycle time equals the turnover time. The larger the fraction of cycling cells in a population, the faster the increase in cell number. The *rate of cell loss* in the cell population refers to the fraction of cells that dies or migrates to other tissues. The cell cycle time and the growth fraction determine the number of cells produced per unit of time, and the rate of cell loss determines the number of cells lost per unit of time. In an adult's intestine, in which cell proliferation is rapid yet growth has ceased, the number of cells produced per unit of time is equal to the number that die—the tissue is in a steady state. Measurement of DNA exfoliated into the intestinal lumen can be used to determine the rate of cell renewal, because under these steady-state conditions, cell loss from the villus tip is balanced by cell birth at the crypt base.

Cell division in enteric epithelium is restricted to the base of the crypts of Lieberkühn, where cells have high activities of the enzymes of nucleic acid synthesis. The complete cell cycle in human intestine lasts approximately 24 hours. The M phase of actual mitosis occupies only a brief part (about 1 hour). DNA synthesis is confined to a discrete period (S phase) lasting 6 to 11 hours, but RNA and proteins are actively elaborated throughout the S phase and during the premitotic (G_2) and postmitotic (G_1) periods.

The epithelial surface of the GI tract is in a constant state of renewal. As described, the renewal process can be divided into three phases: replication, migration, and differentiation. The epithelium has the fastest rate of turnover for any normal tissue of the body. Enteric epithelium is completely replaced in 3 to 6 days. The constant turnover of the epithelium is maintained by a delicate balance between cell population in the proliferative zones and cell loss from the differentiated regions. This rate of turnover is so rapid that cells do not normally enter the prolonged interphase (G_0) found in other, more slowly renewing tissue. The turnover time, or epithelial cell renewal time, for each organ of the GI tract is shown in Table 12–2.

Table 12–2. Turnover Time of Human Gastrointestinal Epithelial Cells

Site	Method	Turnover Time* (d)	References
Esophagus (rodent)†	Labeling	7–10	
Stomach‡	Labeling	2–6	MacDonald et al[9]; Lipkin et al[10]
Duodenum	Mitotic counting	2	Bertalanffy and Nagy[11]
	Labeling	5–6	MacDonald et al[9]
Jejunum	Labeling	5	Shorter et al[12]
Ileum	Labeling	3	Lipkin et al[42]
Colon	Labeling	4–8	Cole and McKalen[43]

*Turnover time refers to the surface epithelium; Paneth's cells, argentaffin cells, chief cells, and parietal cells renew more slowly, estimated on the order of weeks.

†Comparable data in humans are not available, but human esophageal epithelial renewal is probably much slower, estimated on the order of weeks to months.

‡The glandular portion of the stomach renews itself more slowly than the surface epithelium.

GASTROINTESTINAL EPITHELIAL CELL FUNCTION

The functions of GI epithelium are numerous, and a complete discussion is beyond the scope of this chapter. However, selected functions bear a relationship to poisoning and have been chosen for discussion.

Esophagus

The function of the esophagus is to transport food from the mouth and pharynx to the stomach. The normal process of swallowing is a function of the underlying muscular coats and occurs in a peristaltic manner requiring 5 to 7 seconds. The role of the epithelium is to protect the underlying tissue.

Gastric Acid Secretion

Hydrochloric acid is secreted into the gastric lumen by parietal cells.[13] The process requires energy, which is derived from hydrolysis of adenosine triphosphate (ATP). As mentioned, parietal cells are well endowed with mitochondria that generate the high-energy phosphate bonds of ATP during aerobic metabolism. For each H^+ secreted, a molecule of carbon dioxide derived from arterial blood or epithelial cell metabolism is converted to HCO_3^-, which ultimately enters the interstitial fluid. Parietal cells contain a high concentration of carbonic anhydrase, which catalyzes the conversion (Reaction 1).

$$H_2O \longrightarrow OH^- + H^+ \longrightarrow H^+$$

$$HCO_3^- \longleftarrow HCO_3^- \xleftarrow[\text{anhydrase}]{\text{carbonic}} OH^- + CO_2$$

(Reaction 1)

The H^+ concentration in gastric juice is 3 million times greater than that in blood tissue, and the maximum concentration is between 140 and 160 mM. In addition to H^+, the other principal cations are Na^+ (137 mM) and K^+ (17 mM). There is an inverse relationship between the concentration of H^+ and Na^+; the concentration of K^+ is relatively stable. The principal anion is Cl^- (166 mM). In the fasting state, acid secretion has a circadian rhythm, with a peak at 6 PM to 1 AM and a valley from 5 AM to 11 AM; periods of achlorhydria are not uncommon.

Acid secretion is regulated by three major endogenous chemicals: acetylcholine, gastrin, and histamine.[13] A diagram of the interrelationship of these secretagogues is presented in Reaction 2.

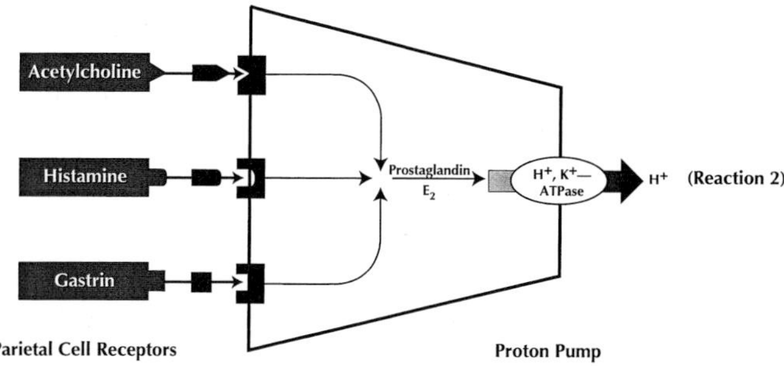

Acetylcholine release at the neuroeffector site of the parietal cell can be initiated by vagal efferent nerves and local nerves. Acetylcholine causes direct stimulation of acid secretion, and the effect is potentiated by histamine. The effect of acetylcholine can be mimicked by cholinomimetic drugs such as carbachol and inhibited by muscarinic antagonists such as atropine at the neuroeffector site.

Gastrin has two major forms—big gastrin, or G34, and little gastrin, or G17—which are distinguished by the number of amino acid residues. On a molar basis, little gastrin is six times more potent than big gastrin. Pharmacologically, the effect can be reproduced with the five-terminal amino acid synthetic peptide, pentagastrin. The highest concentration and total amount of gastrin are in the G cells of antral glands. Appreciable amounts of gastrin are also found normally in the epithelium of the duodenal bulb, where the concentration is about 10% to 20% of that in antral epithelium. Antral gastrin is 90% to 95% little gastrin, and duodenal gastrin is about 50% big gastrin. After meals, the predominant form of gastrin in plasma is big gastrin, which accounts for 60% to 70% of the total gastrin, although little gastrin remains the main stimulant of acid secretion. The predominance of big gastrin in the plasma is accounted for by the slower removal—a half-life of about 50 minutes compared with a half-life of about 6 minutes for little gastrin. Gastrin causes direct stimulation of acid secretion, and the effect is potentiated by histamine.

Histamine is present abundantly in most tissues of the body, and the gastric mucosa is not excepted. Histamine originates from mast cells, which are especially numerous around small blood vessels and basophils. Histidine decarboxylase, present in gastric endocrine cells of rats but not of humans, can convert histidine to histamine. This enzyme has not been found in any human tissue, however, and the mechanism of human biosynthesis of histamine is not known. Nor is it known whether mast cells or basophils are more important to histamine release or how release occurs. Nevertheless, the appearance of histamine H_2 antagonists (cimetidine, ranitidine, famotidine, and nizatidine) confirms that histamine is involved in all or most forms of acid secretion.[13] H_2 antagonists inhibit acid secretion stimulated not only by histamine but also by various other agents including gastrin, caffeine, and insulin-induced hypoglycemia. It is hypothesized that histamine is released constantly and sensitizes the parietal cells to other stimuli. Therefore, when the effect of histamine is blocked by H_2 antagonists, acid secretion in response to other stimuli is inhibited. Proton pump inhibitors are more recent additions to drugs that block stomach acid secretion and include omeprazole and lansoprazole. Proton pump inhibitors are the more potent blockers of acid secretion (Reaction 2).

In reality, the physiology and biochemistry of acid secretion are much more complex than suggested by this brief overview. A general presentation has been provided to give at least the major concepts regarding endogenous stimulation of acid secretion and to provide some background for an appreciation of the effects on the stomach of various chemicals, including drugs, and of strong acids and alkalis.

Digestion and Absorption

Virtually all food enters the GI tract in polymeric form and requires enzymatic digestion to hydrolyze the subunits to monomers that can be absorbed by specific transport systems. These digestive enzymes originate primarily from the stomach chief cells, pancreas, and small intestinal absorptive cells. Absorptive cells of the small intestinal epithelium have a highly specific brush border on which many enzymes reside. All brush border enzymes are hydrolases that degrade substances in the lumen of the intestine.[14] These enzymes include disaccharidases, peptidases, and phosphatases and are listed in Table 12–3. The enzymes hydrolyze their substrates outside the cell, so at least some part of the protein faces the external surface of the membrane. The surface exposure of these enzymes renders them susceptible to damage by poisons within the lumen of the intestinal tract, including drugs, but also by infectious organisms, foreign antigens, and pancreatic proteases. The proteolytic digestion of the surface enzymes leads to a rapid turnover of some of these proteins and reduces the half-life to 4 to 6 hours. Therefore, the maintenance of activity of some brush border enzymes requires several cycles of protein synthesis during the approximately 5-day life span of jejunal cells.[3]

Absorption of dietary nutrients follows their digestion from polymers to monomers. Complex starches are digested to hexoses, proteins to dipeptides and amino acids, and vitamin complexes to free vitamins.[13, 14] These monomers are then absorbed by specific carrier-mediated mechanisms. Sodium-dependent active transport systems have been described for glucose and galactose, amino acids and peptides, pteroylglutamate, vitamin C, biotin, bile salts, riboflavin, thiamine, and other water-soluble organic substrates. It is hypothesized that the sodium gradient across the intestinal absorptive cell membrane is the driving force for active transport. The carrier systems for these nutrients have not been isolated in humans but are thought to be represented by integral proteins situated in the lipid membrane of the brush border. For a membrane protein to have a carrier function, it must be able to orient to the internal and external surfaces of the cell. As with the surface orientation of brush border digestive enzymes, it is the external orientation that is most susceptible to toxic injury from ingested poisons.

Lipids do not appear to require a membrane protein for absorption. After dietary neutral fat (triglycerides) is digested to long-chain fatty acids and monoglycerides by pancreatic lipase, the monomers as well as cholesterol are solubilized in bile salts to form micelles. Micellar formation requires bile salts at a concentration of 2 mM or higher. The concentration of bile salts in the duodenum after gallbladder contraction averages 2 to 10 mM under normal circumstances. Long-chain fatty acids, monoglycerides, and cholesterol are absorbed by diffusion when the molecules by chance collide with the absorptive cell membrane. Fat absorption then is diminished by factors that interrupt the formation of micelles or alter the absorptive membrane.

Colon Function

The functions of the colon mediated by the epithelium include (1) absorption of water and electrolytes and (2) secretion of potassium. The storage and dis-

Table 12–3. Human Brush Border Enzymes

Enzyme	Principal Substrate	Products
Peptidases		
Oligopeptidases	Oligopeptides	Peptides
Dipeptidases	Dipeptides	Amino acids
Folate conjugase	Folate polyglutamate	Folate monoglutamate
Enterokinase	Trypsinogen	Trypsin
Carbohydrases		
Glucoamylase	α-Dextrins, maltose, maltotriose*	Glucose, oligosaccharides
Isomaltase (α-dextrinase)	α-Dextrins	Glucose, oligosaccharides
Lactase	Lactose	Glucose, galactose
Sucrase	Sucrose, maltose, maltotriose	Glucose, fructose
Trehalase	Trehalose	Glucose
Others		
Alkaline phosphatase		
Guanylate cyclase		

*α-Dextrins, maltose, and maltotriose are products of starch digestion that originate in the intestinal lumen from pancreatic amylase hydrolysis.

charge functions of the colon depend on the motor activity and may be altered by poisons affecting the autonomic nervous system. They are not considered here. The fact that colonic epithelium has a much more decisive role than intestinal motility in controlling stool water secretion has been discovered in recent years.[15]

Colonic epithelium is confronted with about 1500 mL of water, 200 mEq of sodium, 5 mEq of potassium, 120 mEq of chloride, and 60 mEq of bicarbonate for absorption per 24 hours. A normal stool contains about 100 to 150 mL of water, 5 mEq of sodium, 9 to 13 mEq of potassium, 2 mEq of chloride, and 3 mEq of bicarbonate, thus indicating the net absorption of water, sodium, chloride, and bicarbonate and the net secretion of potassium. Various agents can alter fluid and electrolyte movement. These agents exert their effect by different mechanisms: (1) decrease in electrolyte absorption, (2) stimulation of active electrolyte secretion, (3) increase in mucosal permeability, (4) increase in mucosal cyclic AMP levels, and (5) alteration of the mucosal morphology. Water and electrolyte movement is affected by pH, osmolality, and ions (bile acids, sulfates, hydroxy fatty acids) but not by glucose, amino acid, or bicarbonate. Mucosal cyclic AMP may affect water and electrolyte movement. A number of hormones clearly affect water and electrolyte movement, including aldosterone, 9α-fluorohydrocortisone, and antidiuretic hormone. Pentagastrin, glucagon, angiotensin, and prostaglandins E_3 and $F_{2\alpha}$ have not altered water and electrolyte movement.

The absorption of bile acids by colonic epithelium is a special situation.[16] In healthy adults, a bile acid pool of 2 to 4 g recycles through the enterohepatic circulation six to eight times per day. Each cycle results in the release of 0.2 to 0.6 g of bile acids into the proximal small intestine after each meal. More than 90% of the bile acids secreted are reabsorbed by ionic, non-ionic, and active transport systems within the small intestine. The remaining 0.4 to 0.8 g of bile acid reaches the colon in 24 hours, where 30% to 40% is absorbed by non-ionic diffusion and 0.3 to 0.6 g is lost in the feces per 24 hours. Dihydroxy bile acids—chenodeoxycholic acid and deoxycholic acid—have cathartic properties. Water and sodium secretion results from perfusion of the colon with a dihydroxy bile acid at a concentration greater than 3 mM. Diarrhea is a serious consequence of bile salt malabsorption due to ileal disease and is a potential side effect of chenodeoxycholic acid therapy when given for the dissolution of cholesterol gallstones. The mechanism may involve cyclic AMP because bile acids activate adenyl cyclase.

INHIBITORS OF CELL GROWTH

Chemotherapeutic agents serve as a model for GI toxicity. These agents exert their poisonous effect on GI epithelium by a number of mechanisms, each of which results in interference with cell proliferation without reducing the normal rate of cell death. Thus, the steady state is interrupted. Chemotherapeutic toxicity is discussed in detail in Chapter 54; therefore, only the specific features of these poisons that affect the GI epithelium are described here. A list of chemotherapeutic agents that are potentially poisonous to the GI epithelium is presented in Table 12–4. The table lists the mechanism of action, cell cycle specificity, metabolic activation requirements, nature of GI toxicity, excretion mechanisms, and treatment alternatives. It is of special interest to use one well-studied example from the list of agents for more detailed review. Methotrexate is a good example for this purpose because intestinal toxicity due to this drug is a major limitation in its use.

Methotrexate, or amethopterin (4-amino-10-methylpteroylglutamic acid), is a folate antagonist that has been effective in the treatment of acute leukemia, choriocarcinoma, lymphomas, Wegener's granulomatosis, certain solid tumors, and severe psoriasis.[17, 18] Results with high-dose methotrexate in the treatment of osteogenic sarcoma and lung and breast cancer have encouraged the hope that improved methotrexate therapy of other solid tumors may be possible. Low-dose therapy has applications including use in ulcerative colitis, Crohn's disease, rheumatoid arthritis, less severe forms of psoriasis, and other disorders.[19–22] Primary physicians need to recognize both acute dose-related damage to rapidly dividing tissue and unpredictable idiosyncratic reactions.

The chemotherapeutic usefulness of methotrexate appears to be referable to two separate effects of the drug at the molecular level: (1) inhibition of intracellular dihydrofolate reductase (the enzyme responsible for the reduction of pteroylglutamate or dihydrofolate to tetrahydrofolate) (Reaction 3), which in turn leads to decreased synthesis of certain metabolites (thymidylate, inosinate, methionine, serine, histidine) that serve as precursors of DNA, RNA, and protein; and (2) inhibition of the transport of 5-methyltetrahydrofolate into cells. The effect of this metabolic block on DNA synthesis is illustrated in Reaction 3. The anti-inflammatory effect may relate to the release of adenosine and a reduction in methylation reactions.[23]

Toxicity toward the nonmalignant proliferating cells of the intestinal epithelium is a major limitation in the therapeutic use of methotrexate. Efforts to circumvent this undesirable side effect have used *reduced* folate derivatives (e.g., 5-formyltetrahydrofolate and 5-methyltetrahydrofolate) as "rescue agents,"[18] enzymatic cleavage of the drug, and removal of the drug by hemodialysis and charcoal filtration,[24] although the latter method appears to be of limited value.[25] Studies of methotrexate toxicity to the small intestine in mice have shown that methotrexate accumulates in intestinal mucosa and appears to be transported into cells by a carrier-mediated system; the drug reaches much higher levels in the intestine, compared with tumor cells, and has a

Table 12–4. Chemotherapeutic Agents with Prominent Gastrointestinal Toxicity

Drug	Route of Administration	Mechanism of Action	Cell Cycle Specific	Activation	Gastrointestinal Toxicity		Deactivation	Treatment
					Acute	*Delayed*		
Alkylating Agents								
Cyclophosphamide (Cytoxan)	PO/IV	Alkylates DNA	No	Converted to active intermediates in liver (and plasma)	Nausea and vomiting, pain, bleeding, jaundice		Excreted in urine as a metabolite	High fluid intake
Mechlorethamine (nitrogen mustard; Mustargen)	IV	Alkylates DNA	No	None	Nausea and vomiting	Sore throat, bleeding	Metabolized rapidly	Prochlorperazine, 10–20 mg, barbiturate before administration
Busulfan (Myleran)	PO	Alkylates DNA	No	None	Pain, sore throat, bleeding	Bleeding		High fluid intake
Carmustine (BCNU, (BiCNU)	IV	Alkylates DNA	No	None	Mouth, lip, and throat sores			
Chlorambucil (Leukeran)	PO				Pain, mouth and throat sores	Sore throat, bleeding		High fluid intake
Cisplatin (Platinol)	IV	Alkylates DNA	No	None	Pain, sore throat, nausea, and vomiting			High fluid intake
Estramustine (Emcyt, Estacyt)	PO	Alkylates DNA in cells with estrogen receptors	No	None	Pain, nausea, and vomiting	Diarrhea, bleeding		
Lomustine (CeeNu, CCNU)	PO				Mouth, lip, and throat sores	Sore throat, bleeding		Cessation
Melphalan (Alkeran, phenylalanine, mustard)	PO	Alkylates DNA	No	None	Diarrhea, jaundice, bleeding, unsteadiness	Sore throat, bleeding		Cessation
Streptozotocin (Zanosar)	IV	Alkylates DNA	No	None	Sore throat and mouth, lip and throat sores; diarrhea, jaundice	Sore throat, bleeding		High fluid intake
Antimetabolites								
Cytarabaine hydrochloride (arabinosyl cytosine; Cytosar-U)	IV	Inhibits DNA polymerase	Yes	None	Sore throat, bleeding, jaundice			Cessation
Floxuridine (FUDR)	IV				Nausea, vomiting, mouth sores	Diarrhea, pain, bleeding	Metabolized in liver	Cessation
Fluorouracil (5-FU, FU, Adrucil)	IV	Competitive inhibition of synthetase	Yes	None	Nausea	Oral and GI ulceration, stomatitis and diarrhea	Metabolized in liver	Cessation
Mercaptopurine (6-MP, Purinethol)	PO	Inhibits enzymes of purine metabolism	Yes	Converted to 5′phosphate ribonucleotides; toxicity increased by xanthine oxidase allopurinol	Occasional nausea and vomiting	Occasional hepatic damage	Metabolized in liver and excreted in urine	Cessation
Methotrexate (amethopterin; Mexate, MTX)	PO/IV	Competitive inhibition of dihydrofolate reductase	Yes	None	Occasional diarrhea, hepatic necrosis	Oral and GI ulceration, cirrhosis	Excreted in urine and bile	Leucovorin; $NaHCO_3$; hemodialysis
Thioguanine (6-TG)		Inhibits enzymes of purine metabolism	Yes	Converted to 5′phosphate ribonucleotides	Occasional nausea and vomiting	Mouth sores, diarrhea	Metabolized and excreted in urine	Cessation

Plant Alkaloids								
Vinblastine sulfate (Velban)	IV	Binds microtubular protein	Yes	None	Nausea and vomiting, anorexia, diarrhea	Constipation, paralytic ileus, stomatitis	Secreted in bile	Prophylactic laxatives
Vincristine sulfate (Oncovin)	IV	Binds microtubular protein	Yes	None		Constipation, paralytic ileus	Secreted in bile	Prophylactic laxatives
Antibiotics								
Doxorubicin (Adriamycin)	IV	Intercalates DNA base pairs	No	None	Pain; mouth, lip, and throat sores	Nausea, vomiting		
Bleomycin (Blenoxane)	IV/IM	Causes scission of DNA	Yes	None	Nausea	Bone marrow depression, cardiotoxicity, alopecia, stomatitis	Metabolized in liver	Cessation, hemodialysis
Dactinomycin (actinomycin D; Cosmegen)	IV	Forms complex with DNA that inhibits RNA synthesis	No	None	Nausea and vomiting	Stomatitis	Unknown	Cessation
Daunorubicin	IV	Intercalates DNA base pairs	No	None	Nausea and vomiting	Stomatitis, oral ulcers, diarrhea, bleeding	Excreted in urine and bile	Cessation
Mitomycin C (Mutamycin)	IV	Alkylates DNA and RNA	No	Cleaved to aziridine ring	Nausea and vomiting	Sore throat, bleeding	Excreted in urine	Cessation
Plicamycin (mithramycin, Mithracin)		Binds DNA	No	None	Nausea and vomiting	Sore throat, bleeding	Metabolized by liver and other tissues and excreted in urine	Cessation
Other Synthetic Agents								
Dacarbazine (DTIC-Dome; DIC)	IV	Purine analogue with alkylating properties	No	None	Nausea and vomiting	Sore throat, bleeding	Excreted in urine	May subside after several days of therapy
Hydroxyurea (Hydrea)	PO	Inhibits ribonucleoside diphosphate reductase	Yes	None	Mild nausea and vomiting	Nausea, vomiting, abdominal pain	Excreted in urine	Cessation
Mitotane (o,p′-DDD; Lysodren)	PO	Inhibits adrenal steroid synthesis	No	None	Nausea and vomiting	Nausea, vomiting, diarrhea	Excreted in urine and bile	Cessation
Procarbazine hydrochloride (methylhydrazine; ibenzmethyzin; Matulane, Natulan)	PO	Inhibition of DNA, RNA, and protein synthesis	No	None	Nausea and vomiting	Pain, nausea, vomiting	Metabolized and excreted in urine	Administer drug in gradually escalating doses
Prednisone (Deltasone, Meticorten, Orasone)	PO	Lymphocytolytic and interacts with glucocorticoid receptors	No	Converted to prednisone in tumor cells	Bleeding, pain, burning	Pain, nausea, vomiting		Cessation
Tamoxifen (Nolvadex)	PO	Estrogen antagonist		None	None	None		High fluid intake
Asparaginase (Elspar)	IV	Hydrolysis of serum asparagine, thus depriving leukemia cells of this essential amino acid		None	Pain, nausea, vomiting	Pain, nausea, vomiting, jaundice		High fluid intake
Etoposide (VP-16, VePesid)	IV	Podophyllum derivative	Yes	None	Mouth, lip, and throat sores	Diarrhea		Cessation

IM, intramuscularly; IV, intravenously; PO, orally; GI, gastrointestinal.

substantially longer duration of inhibition of DNA synthesis.[26] Methotrexate doses of greater than 3 mg/kg or concentrations in plasma of 5×10^{-9} M inhibit DNA synthesis in the intestine, and cell death occurs when inhibition of DNA synthesis lasts for more than 25 to 30 hours.[26] In humans, plasma levels of methotrexate of approximately 1×10^{-6} M for more than 48 hours lead to appreciable toxicity. Intestinal toxicity, at least in mice, appears to be related to the duration of inhibition of DNA synthesis, which reflects the persistence of exchangeable amethopterin levels in tissue adequate for complete inhibition of dihydrofolate reductase. Consequently, both the duration of exposure and suprathreshold concentrations of drug rather than the peak levels of drug achieved are responsible for the intestinal toxicity.

In humans, methotrexate is well absorbed from the GI tract, and its toxicity via the oral route is no greater than when it is administered parenterally. Absorption appears to occur by a saturable mechanism. After intravenous injection, methotrexate disappearance from plasma is triphasic. The initial half-life (distribution) is 0.65 to 0.85 hours; the second half-life (clearance) is 2 to 3.5 hours; and the third (enterohepatic circulation) is 9 to 12 hours. The terminal half-life, which is perpetuated by the enterohepatic circulation, is responsible for the majority of intestinal toxicity. Methotrexate is concentrated 4- to 8-fold in the liver and further concentrated 200-fold in bile to that of plasma concentrations. The amount of drug secreted in bile after intravenous administration of 30 mg/m^2 is 5% to 10% per 24 hours. Fifty to 70% of the drug binds to albumin and lesser amounts (0% to 17%) to protein in interstitial fluids.[27] The mechanisms by which methotrexate enters normal intestinal epithelial cells are not fully characterized, but energy-coupled, carrier-mediated, and passive systems operate in different cell systems.[28, 29]

Methotrexate is metabolized to polyglutamates by the liver and probably other organs and to other metabolites by tissue and intestinal bacterial enzymes. Metabolites account for as much as a third of the total plasma levels during the terminal plasma disappearance of high-dose therapy. Because the terminal phase of methotrexate disappearance determines the severity of amethopterin toxicity, metabolism, as well as the enterohepatic circulation, may be important in the origin of this toxicity. Methotrexate excretion occurs primarily by renal glomerular filtration (110 mL/min per square meter), and at high concentrations the drug is actively secreted by tubular cells. One to 2% of the drug is excreted in stool, indicating that most of the drug secreted in bile is reabsorbed by the intestinal mucosa. Fecal excretion increases as the methotrexate dose increases, as predicted by the limitations of the absorptive mechanisms.

The interaction of chemotherapeutic agents with other drugs is a critical factor in the poison potential. Methotrexate interacts with various other drugs, as described *in vivo* and *in vitro* using human tumor cells, including the following ways: displacement from plasma albumin (salicylate, sulfisoxazole), decrease in renal tubular transport (probenecid, salicylates, other organic acids), decrease in human leukemia cell uptake (cephalothin, hydrocortisone), and inhibition of intestinal absorption (oral broad-spectrum nonabsorbable antibiotics). Azathioprine and its metabolite, 6-mercaptopurine, both used in testing for inflammatory bowel disease, suppress the bone marrow and should not be used concomitantly. Trimethoprim, including trimethoprim-sulfa combinations, has antifolate activity, which potentiates the methotrexate effect, and is considered contraindicated.[19]

The intestinal response to subtoxic doses of methotrexate is characterized by a decrease in the number of mitoses in the crypts. This decrease is detectable within 3 hours and returns to normal within 96 hours; the villous pattern and epithelial length remain normal.[30] Toxic doses lead to a sustained reduction in mitoses with loss of surface absorptive cells without replacement cells. This desquamation of the epithelial cell lining is associated with extensive leukocytic infiltration of the lamina propria. Large areas of ulceration develop, and bleeding eventually occurs. The mucositis may involve the tongue, buccal mucosa, esophagus, stomach, small intestine, or colon. The pathology is not specific for methotrexate and may be seen with various poisonous or otherwise noxious agents, a fact that contributes to the intestine's notoriety for its limited response to injury. Experimental data indicate important time- and concentration-dependent relationships that may be specific for different organs. The critical time and plasma concentration thresholds for GI epithelium are approximately 42 hours and 2×10^{-8} M, respectively, both of which must be exceeded for toxicity to occur. The severity of toxicity is more closely associated with the duration of methotrexate exposure beyond the time threshold than the magnitude above the concentration threshold.

GI symptoms include nausea, vomiting, abdominal pain, diarrhea, and in severe cases hematemesis and melena. An assessment of the toxicity must bear in mind toxicity to other organs and toxicity of other agents that may be used in combination with methotrexate. The rapidly dividing cells of the bone marrow have a short cell cycle time similar to that of intestinal epithelium and are frequent recipients of methotrexate toxicity.

Primary physicians need to recognize both acute dose-related damage to rapidly dividing tissue and unpredictable idiosyncratic reactions. Experimental and controlled studies of low-dose methotrexate treatment have shown that fewer toxic effects occur when doses of 7.5 to 30 mg are given 1 day a week rather than the same total dose spread over 7 days. Both intramuscular and oral routes are tolerated equally. Predictable side effects of low-dose treatment include anorexia, nausea, vomiting, and diarrhea. Painful stomatitis may be a recurring event. This toxicity is reduced by supplementation with folic acid, 1 mg/d. Hepatotoxicity, cirrhosis, hypersensitivity pneumonitis, and *Pneumocystis carinii* and herpes zoster infections are reflections of long-term methotrexate use. They usually do not develop until a patient has received a cumulative dose of more than 1.5 g. Alcohol use is a determinant for hepatotoxicity.

Prevention

Methotrexate and other powerful chemotherapeutic agents should be restricted to prescription by physicians who are specifically trained in their use and to institutions prepared to deal with the complications of toxicity. Experienced staff, trained laboratory personnel, intensive care facilities, and renal dialysis should be available. The hazards of potent cytotoxic therapy are too numerous for use outside specialized centers.

The example of methotrexate therapy can be carried further to illustrate how prevention of toxicity can be accomplished.[18] An infusion of saline or 5% glucose (1.5 L/m^2) with 100 mEq HCO_3^- and 20 mEq KCl/L should be given 8 to 12 hours before high-dose therapy and continued until urine pH is 7.0 or greater. Extremely high initial plasma concentrations of methotrexate of 10^{-4} to 10^{-3} M may occur, especially after high-dose therapy used for osteogenic sarcoma or lung or breast cancer. Plasma levels of methotrexate are determined by a dihydrofolate reductase inhibition assay. Patients destined to have toxicity can be suspected by 24 hours and identified definitively by 3 to 4 days.[31] Thus, at 4 days all patients with plasma levels of amethopterin greater than 2×10^{-7} M are expected to have serious toxicity, and those with lower levels are not. This finding has led to earlier and more aggressive use of antidotes in patients with slow plasma disappearance of this drug.

Treatment

Outlines for treatment of intestinal toxicity from chemotherapeutic agents in wide use are included in Table 12–4. To continue with the illustration of methotrexate toxicity, the effects of this drug can be offset by administering leucovorin (5-formyltetrahydrofolate, folinic acid), 100 to 200 mg/m^2 every 6 hours for 72 hours or longer if needed. In fact, this antidote is frequently administered as a part of the treatment protocol and has acquired the distinguished term *rescue therapy.* The use of leucovorin rescue is guided by the plasma levels of methotrexate and continued until the level is less than 1×10^{-8} M. In addition, patients are well hydrated, and urine is alkalized by infusion of $NaHCO_3$, 45 mEq every 6 hours, to increase the solubility of methotrexate and to facilitate its excretion by the kidneys. Renal dialysis may be needed by patients in whom glomerular filtration rate is reduced for any reason; in patients treated with high-dose methotrexate, the drug actually may precipitate in renal tubules and lead to obstructive nephropathy. This latter complication is usually reversible after alkalization of the urine and temporary dialysis. Nausea and vomiting resulting from methotrexate or other chemotherapeutic agents may be relieved by prochlorperazine, 10 mg orally three times per day, or ondansetron, 4 to 8 mg every 4 to 8 hours. Despite leucovorin rescue, methotrexate is an occasional cause of anticancer drug–associated death.[25]

This example of treatment of toxicity due to methotrexate, a widely used but potentially lethal drug, illustrates the complexities involved in the assessment and treatment of poisoning by drugs used therapeutically and exemplifies the multitude of measures that may be available and needed for patients receiving chemotherapeutic poisons. Treatment of toxicity on a recurring basis preferably should be managed by physicians who are trained in oncology and who are knowledgeable about treatment of poisonous side effects of cancer chemotherapy. The importance of prevention of toxicity, if at all possible, cannot be overemphasized.

CHEMICAL POISONS

Chemical injury to the GI tract can result from various agents, including heavy metals, especially iron, lead, arsenic, and mercury; laxatives; colchicine; nonsteroidal anti-inflammatory drugs (NSAIDs); isotretinoin, loperamide; acids and alkalis (Fig. 12–1); lithium and fluoride; bacterial, plant, and mushroom

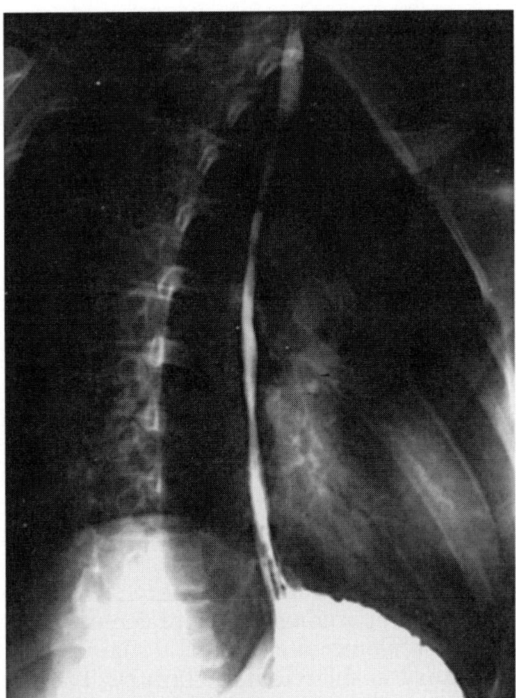

Figure 12–1. Lye stricture of the esophagus. The patient ingested lye accidentally as a child. She had persistent dysphagia, and a colon interposition was performed in early adulthood. (Courtesy of Dr. L. Goldberger.)

Table 12–5. Classification of Laxatives* and Representative Examples†

Stimulant (or irritant)
Ricinoleic acid (castor oil)
Dehydrocholic acids (Decholin)
Bisacodyl (Dulcolax)
Phenolphthalein (Ex-Lax; Correctol)
Oxyphenisatin (Lavema)‡
Aloe
Cascara sagrada
Senna (Senokot)
Danthron (Modane)
Stool softener (emollient)
Dioctyl sodium sulfosuccinate (DSS)
Dioctyl calcium sulfosuccinate (Surfak)
Kondremul
Saline
Magnesium hydroxide (milk of magnesia)
Magnesium sulfate
Sodium sulfate
Sodium phosphate (Fleet Phospho-Soda)
Sodium chloride
Osmotic
Polyethylene glycol (GoLYTELY, Colyte)
Lactulose (Chronulac, Duphalac)
Bulk
Psyllium seed derivatives (Konsyl, Metamucil, LA formula, Effer-Syllium, Serutan, Hydrocil)
Methylcellulose (Citrucel)
Bran products
Lubricant
Mineral oil (Agoral, Kondremul)

*Based on the report of the Food and Drug Administration panel on laxatives and antidiarrheal, antiemetic, and emetic products.
†More than 100 laxatives are listed in the *1996 Physicians' Desk Reference* and *Physicians' Desk Reference for Nonprescription Drugs.*
‡Withdrawn from distribution by the FDA because of its association with chronic active hepatitis.

toxins; phosphorus; radiation injury; endoscope-transmitted hydrogen peroxide and glutaraldehyde; and miscellaneous drugs.

Laxatives and certain drugs that injure the esophagus are discussed here. The other agents are discussed in specific chapters.

Laxative Abuse

Acute Laxative Poisoning

Excess ingestion of laxatives may result in acute or chronic poisoning. Cases of acute poisoning are usually accidental, but laxatives are occasionally used in suicide attempts. Most laxatives have a wide margin of safety, and large doses must be consumed to be fatal. A classification of laxatives and representative examples for each group are presented in Table 12–5.

Acute poisoning may lead to watery or bloody diarrhea (with accompanying water and electrolyte abnormalities), abdominal and rectal pain, vomiting, and respiratory and circulatory failure. The diagnosis is usually apparent from the history. The severity of magnesium intoxication can be assessed by measuring serum magnesium levels; toxicity begins at levels of 4 mEq/L and worsens as the concentration rises. Principles of management of acute laxative ingestion include gastric decontamination and supportive care as outlined in Chapter 1.

Chronic Laxative Abuse

Chronic laxative abuse occurs in three forms. One is exemplified by constipated patients who take laxatives continually and wittingly, another is exemplified by bulimic patients who use laxatives for weight loss, and the third is exemplified by surreptitious laxative abusers.

Cathartic colon is a consequence of prolonged laxative abuse. Clinically, the abnormality is discovered by barium enema and is primarily a radiologic diagnosis (Fig. 12–2). Almost all cases occur in patients who have taken irritant laxatives for 15 or more years. The major historical features are chronic constipation and laxative use. Diarrhea, fever, and blood in the stool are not encountered with cathartic colon. The rectal mucosa is not friable, and findings on proctosigmoidoscopy are normal. If the laxative taken contained anthracene derivatives such as cascara, aloes, and senna, melanosis coli may be present. The earliest and mildest changes are found in the cecum and ileocecal valve; these appear shortened and atrophic. More extensive changes are associated with a tubular colon with diminished or absent haustrations, which may extend to the distal descending colon (Fig. 12–2). Ulcerations and rigidity are absent. The differential diagnosis of the radio-

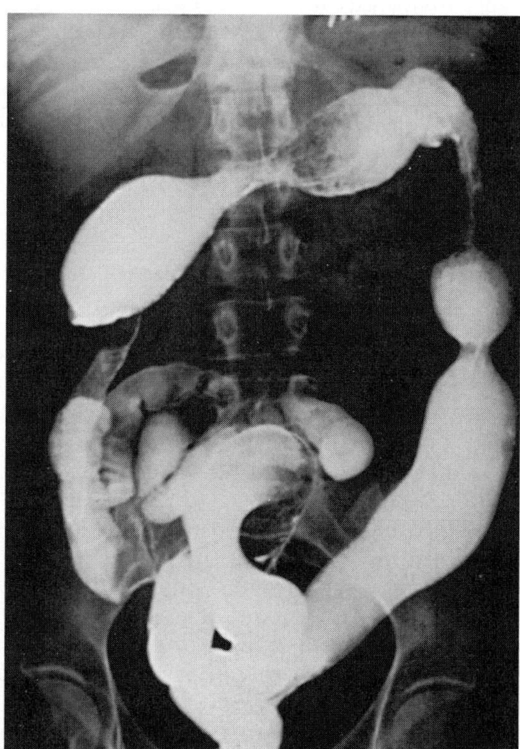

Figure 12–2. Cathartic colon due to chronic laxative abuse. The patient, a 53-year-old woman, had taken laxatives daily for the preceding 30 years for relief of chronic constipation. (Courtesy of Dr. L. Goldberger.)

logic findings includes inflammatory bowel disease (chronic ulcerative colitis and Crohn's disease) and amebiasis, but the diagnosis of cathartic colon can usually be made without difficulty. Systemic effects of chronic laxative abuse result from the increased fecal loss of sodium and potassium.[32] Patients may present to the emergency department with potassium depletion, muscle weakness, metabolic alkalosis, hyperaldosteronism, and chronic thirst. Cessation of excessive use is usually satisfactory treatment. Most of the laxatives in the stimulant category are too irritating for harmless, continuous use and should be avoided.

The second and emerging group of laxative abusers are patients with bulimia nervosa, especially women age 12 to 25 years, who eat in binges and then use cathartics in an effort to lose or control weight.[33–36] This disorder is usually practiced in secrecy and may present only in the form of one of its complications. An estimated 10% to 15% of adolescent girls and young women have anorexia nervosa or bulimia nervosa, and as many as 19% of college women have bulimia nervosa. Bulimia is distinct from anorexia and is characterized by secretive binge eating followed by various methods of purging, including cathartics, diuretics, and self-induced vomiting. An intense preoccupation with food is common to both syndromes. Persons who are in occupations for which thinness is considered a virtue or necessity (e.g., models, actors and actresses, jockeys, dancers, wrestlers, gymnasts) are at risk as well. These patients may develop severe metabolic disturbances and ventricular tachyarrhythmias. Sudden death may occur and may be heralded by prolongation of the QT interval.[37] Very careful heart and electrocardiographic monitoring is essential for these patients. Long-term therapy with medical, psychologic, and nutritional professionals may be required.

The third and most trying group with chronic laxative abuse includes those people who use laxatives surreptitiously and present with diarrhea of unknown cause or with metabolic abnormalities related to long-term laxative misuse.[38] A key feature of the disorder is denial by the patient that he or she takes laxatives, and this denial may continue well beyond the time that *prima facie* evidence has proved the point. Although clinical clues abound to alert a physician about laxative abuse, patients often attract at least an initial medical workup designed to rule out infectious, inflammatory, metabolic, and neoplastic diseases before abusive behavior is considered. These studies usually include stool sampling for bacterial culture, ova and parasite examinations, proctosigmoidoscopy, and barium radiographs, all of which may yield results within normal limits. Metabolic abnormalities showing dehydration and hypokalemia are common but are encountered in many diarrheal illnesses and are not specific.

It is less labor intensive and less costly to examine a patient's blood and urine for signs of laxatives than to launch into a barrage of additional tests looking for occult malabsorptive diseases and exotic tumors with secretory hormone production if any lingering doubt remains about a patient's veracity. A very simple examination is accomplished by alkalizing stool with sodium hydroxide; if phenolphthalein (a common ingredient in over-the-counter laxatives) is present, the stool becomes bright red. Urine containing aloes becomes red if alkalized. Clinical laboratories offer a laxative abuse screen of urine for bisacodyl and danthron. Proctosigmoidoscopy itself may be diagnostic by showing a darkened to black mucosa. Mucosal pigmentation results from melanin accumulation in macrophages in the lamina propria and may begin within 4 months of chronic laxative abuse. A trained sigmoidoscopist can detect color changes at an early stage. Pigmentation is seen most often with use of anthracene derivatives, including cascara, aloes, and senna. The barium enema results may be abnormal as well. The characteristic features are shown in Figure 12–2.

If neither stool, urine, proctosigmoidoscopy, nor barium enema results are abnormal and the diagnosis is still suspect, the patient should be admitted to the hospital for further evaluation. A room search is indicated, but it should be performed by an impartial participant and with the patient's consent in order to avoid an invasion of privacy. If the suspicion is well grounded but nothing is found, the symptoms should improve while the patient is under direct observation. Meanwhile, stool can be collected while the patient fasts and receives intravenous glucose and fluids. A large volume of 500 to 1000 mL or more suggests a secretory diarrhea, and the stool is evaluated for sodium, potassium, and osmolality. In secretory diarrhea, the osmolality is accounted for by twice the sodium plus potassium concentration and may be simulated by secretagogue laxatives such as senna, bisacodyl, and phenolphthalein. Osmotic diarrhea is characterized by a wide ion gap that may be caused by magnesium, sulfate, or other laxative ions, and these can be measured in the stool.

Laxatives by nature are not addictive. Persons who use them surreptitiously have a serious psychologic condition, usually anxiety or depression or both. The psychologic category most specific for this entity is chronic factitious disease with physical symptoms, also known as Munchausen's syndrome. Patients' apparent goal is to assume the role of a patient. They usually have no other secondary gain as do persons who are malingering. Physicians must realize that recognizing laxative abuse is only half the battle. These patients may prove very difficult to treat and may continue to use laxatives while under continued medical care.

Drug-Induced Esophageal Injury

Chemical injury to the esophagus by drugs is more common than generally supposed.[39] The drugs implicated in esophageal damage include antibiotics

Table 12–6. Common Agents That Have an Acid- or Alkali-Like Effect

Corrosive	Use	Common Names
Acids		
Sulfuric	Industrial	Oil of vitriol
Nitric	Industrial	Aquafortis
Hydrochloric	Industrial	Muriatic acid
Hydrofluoric	Industrial	
Oxalic	Industrial, bleach	Ethandioic acid
Carbolic	Antiseptic	Phenol
Lactic	Antiseptic, industrial	
Silver nitrate	Antiseptic	
Iodine	Antiseptic	
Ammonium chloride	Antiseptic	Anchlor
Boric	Antiseptic, industrial	Borofax
Mercuric chloride	Antiseptic	
Alkalis		
Sodium hydroxide	Drain cleaner	Lye, DrānO
Potassium hydroxide	To make soap, paint remover	Potash
Sodium hypochlorite	Bleach	Clorox, soda lye
Sodium bicarbonate	Baking powder, nonphosphate detergent	Baking soda
Potassium carbonate	Industrial	
Ammonia water	Detergent	
Calcium oxide	Building material	Lime

(tetracycline, doxycycline, clindamycin, lincomycin), 5-fluorouracil, NSAIDs (aspirin, indocin, phenylbutazone, others), oral potassium supplements, emepronium bromide, iron, quinidine, carbachol, ascorbic acid, cromolyn inhalant, cimetidine, and biphosphonates. The mechanism of injury for medications and household chemicals appears to be direct corrosion, either through acid or alkali effect (Table 12–6). Tetracycline and doxycycline are known to be highly acidic in solution. Although the injury is more likely in patients with mechanical or peristaltic abnormalities, drug injury may occur in a normal esophagus, especially if the agent is taken with insufficient liquid and the person immediately lies down.

The most common symptoms are chest pain and dysphagia. In patients with an underlying esophageal disease, the symptoms may be mistaken for the primary disease. The pathology varies from diffuse inflammation to ulceration or necrotizing esophagitis and hemorrhage. Perforation and stricture have occurred as complications. Treatment includes cessation of the offending drug and management of the complications. Recognition of this disorder is critical because the disease is usually reversible if discovered early. Caustic alkali (see Chapter 62) and acid (see Chapter 63) ingestions are discussed later in greater detail.

POISONING OF DIGESTIVE-ABSORPTIVE FUNCTION

Interference with nutrient digestion and absorption results from the toxic effect of a wide variety of exogenous agents. These agents not only interfere with nutrient absorption but often also affect the absorption of therapeutic drugs. The mechanisms leading to maldigestion and malabsorption include (1) alteration of environmental pH, (2) chemical binding of nutrients, (3) inhibition of digestive enzymes and inhibition of transport processes requiring membrane proteins, and (4) direct toxic injury to the epithelium. The steps involved in digestion and absorption of most nutrients were previously reviewed in the section on GI epithelial cell function.

The most-studied toxin of the small intestine is gluten.[40, 41] Gluten-sensitive enteropathy or celiac sprue is a nonallergic sensitivity to wheat, specifically the gliadin fraction of wheat protein. The enteropathy is characterized by flattening of the villi, cuboidal epithelial cells in disarray, elongation of the crypts, and inflammation of the lamina propria. The results of these changes, at their worst, include malabsorption of fat, protein, carbohydrate, salt, water, minerals, and water-soluble and fat-soluble vitamins. Selective malabsorption of individual food components may occur; for example, iron deficiency anemia secondary to iron malabsorption may be the presenting feature of the enteropathy. Epithelial cells arising from the crypts do not become susceptible to the cytotoxic process characteristic of the disease until they cross the crypt-villus junction and become mature (see the normal epithelial cell cycle in the section on GI epithelial cell renewal). In other words, the absorptive cells must be exposed to gluten in the intestinal lumen.

The pathophysiologic mechanism underlying gluten-sensitive enteropathy is not known for certain, but two main theories exist: (1) Cells at the crypt-villus junction show one or more surface antigens, including gluten, and become targets of a local immunologic effector mechanism; and (2) the absorptive cell is deficient in a peptidase or protease. As a result, gluten digestion is impaired and thus gluten or its particular digestive products accumulate, with resulting tissue toxicity. Gluten-sensitive enteropathy occurs only in susceptible persons, and the enteropathy subsides on a gluten-free diet. The reaction of the susceptible intestine to gluten represents the relatively limited pathologic response of the intestine to injury.

Numerous drugs adversely affect the digestion and absorption of nutrients. The most commonly used drugs for which reasonable evidence exists for their adverse effect are listed in Table 12–7. Removal of the drugs from a patient's treatment program and

Table 12–7. Commonly Used Drugs That Inhibit Digestive-Absorptive Mechanisms

Drug	Nutrient Malabsorbed	Putative Mechanisms
Neomycin	Fat, cholesterol, fat-soluble vitamins Glucose, amino acids, B_{12}, minerals	Precipitates fatty acids and bile acids[44] Histologic damage
Colchicine	Fat, glucose, B_{12}	Inhibits mitotic spindle[45]
Ethanol	Fat, glucose, amino acids, vitamins, minerals	Alters physical properties of the membrane. Inhibits Na^+-K^+-ATPase; stimulates cyclic AMP[46]
p-Aminosalicyclic acid	Fat, cholesterol, folate, B_{12}	Unknown[47]
Dilatin	Folate	Inhibits folate conjugase Alkalinizes intestinal contents[48]
Folate antagonists (methotrexate, aminopterin, trimethoprim)	Folate	Inhibit folate transport[49, 50] Inhibit cell proliferation
Oral contraceptives	Folate	Inhibit folate conjugase[51]
Sulfasalazine	Folate	Inhibits folate transport[52]
Biguanides	Glucose, amino acids, folate, B_{12}	Inhibit oxidative phosphorylation[53]
Aluminum hydroxide antacids	Phosphate, vitamin A	Intraluminal formation of insoluble complexes[54]
Anion exchange resins (cholestyramine, colestipol)	Water- and fat-soluble vitamins, bile salts, oxalate	Intraluminal binding[52, 55]
Cimetidine	B_{12} bound to food	Inhibits gastric acid and intrinsic factor secretion[56]
Somatostatin	Fat	Inhibits pancreatic lipase secretion[57]
Omeprazole	B_{12} bound to protein	Decreases intrinsic factor secretion[58]

restoration of nutrient deficiencies are usually sufficient treatment.

References

1. Whitehead R: Mucosal Biopsy of the Gastrointestinal Tract. Philadelphia, W.B. Saunders Co., 1979.
2. Crane RK: Intestinal structure and function related to toxicology. Environ Health Perspect *33*:3, 1979.
3. Alpers DH, Seetharam B: Pathophysiology of diseases involving intestinal brush-border proteins. N Engl J Med *296*:1047, 1977.
4. Norton L, Surbone A: Cytokinetics. *In* Holland JF, Frei E III, Bast RC, et al (eds): Cancer Medicine. Philadelphia, Lea & Febiger, p 598, 1993.
5. Williamson RCN: Intestinal adaptations. N Engl J Med *298*:1393, 1978.
6. Eastwood GL: Gastrointestinal epithelial cell renewal. Gastroenterology *72*:962, 1977.
7. Willems G: Factors controlling cell proliferation in gastroduodenal mucosa. Prog Gastroenterol *3*:29, 1977.
8. Nieburgs HE: Cytologic basis of gastrointestinal histopathology. *In* Haubrich WS, Schaffner F, Berk JE (eds): Bockus Gastroenterology, 5th ed. Philadelphia, WB Saunders, pp 370–393, 1995.
9. MacDonald WC, Trier JS, Everett NB: Cell proliferation and migration in the stomach, duodenum, and rectum of man: Radioautographic studies. Gastroenterology *46*:405, 1964.
10. Lipkin M, Sherlock P, Bell B: Cell proliferation kinetics in the gastrointestinal tract of man. II. Renewal in stomach, ileum, colon, and rectum. Gastroenterology *45*:721, 1963.
11. Bertalanffy FD, Nagy KP: Mitotic activity and renewal of the epithelial cells of human duodenum. Acta Anat *45*:362, 1961.
12. Shorter RG, Moertel CG, Titus JL, et al: Cell kinetics in the jejunum and rectum of man. Am J Dig Dis *9*:760, 1964.
13. Soll AH: Pathogenesis of peptic ulcer and implications for therapy. N Engl J Med *322*:909, 1990.
14. Turnberg LA, Riley SA: Digestion and absorption of nutrients and vitamins. *In* Sleisenger MH, Fordtran JS (eds): Gastrointestinal Disease. Philadelphia, W.B. Saunders Co., p 977, 1993.
15. Powell DW: Muscle or mucosa: The site of action of antidiarrheal opiates. Gastroenterology *80*:406, 1981.
16. Hofmann AF: Enterohepatic circulation of bile acids in health and disease. *In* Sleisenger MH, Fordtran JS (eds): Gastrointestinal Disease. Philadelphia, W.B. Saunders Co., p 127, 1993.
17. Jolivet J, Cowan KH, Curt GA, et al: Pharmacology and clinical use of methotrexate. N Engl J Med *309*:1094, 1983.
18. Bertino JR, Romanini A: Folate antagonists. *In* Holland JF, Frei E III, Bast RC, et al (eds): Cancer Medicine. Philadelphia, Lea & Febiger, p 698, 1993.
19. Egan LJ, Sandborn WJ: Methotrexate for inflammatory bowel disease: Pharmacology and preliminary results. Mayo Clin Proc *71*:69, 1996.
20. Feagan BG, Rochon J, Fedorak RN, et al: Methotrexate for the treatment of Crohn's disease. N Engl J Med *332*:292, 1995.
21. Roenigk HH Jr, Auerbach R, Maibach HI, et al: Methotrexate in psoriasis: Revised guidelines. J Am Acad Dermatol *19*:145, 1988.
22. Hausknecht RU: Methotrexate and misoprostol to terminate early pregnancy. N Engl J Med *333*:537, 1995.
23. Cronstein BN: Molecular mechanism of methotrexate action in inflammation. Inflammation *16*:411, 1992.
24. Djerassi I, Ciesielka W, Kim SJ: Removal of methotrexate by filtration-absorption using charcoal filters or by hemodialysis. Cancer Treat Rep *61*:751, 1977.
25. Winchester JF, Rahman A, Tilstone WJ, et al: Will hemoperfusion be useful for cancer chemotherapeutic drug removal? Clin Toxicol *17*:557, 1980.
26. Sirotnak FM, Moccio DM: Pharmacokinetic basis of differences in methotrexate sensitivity of normal proliferative tissue in the mouse. Cancer Res *40*:1230, 1980.
27. Liegler DG, Henderson ES, Hahn MS, et al: The effect of organic acids on renal clearance of methotrexate in man. Clin Pharmacol Ther *10*:849, 1969.
28. Zimmerman J: Methotrexate transport in the human intestine. Biochem Pharmacol *43*:2377, 1992.
29. Selhub J, Dhar GJ, Rosenberg IH: Gastrointestinal absorption of folates and antifolates. Pharmacol Ther *20*:397, 1983.
30. Trier JS: Morphologic alterations induced by methotrexate in the mucosa of human proximal intestine. Gastroenterology *42*:295, 1962.
31. Wallace CA, Bleyer WA, Sherry DD, et al: Toxicity and serum levels of methotrexate in children with juvenile rheumatoid arthritis. Arthritis Rheum *32*:677, 1989.
32. Gattuso JM, Kamm MA: Adverse effects of drugs used in management of constipation and diarrhea. Drug Safety *10*:47, 1994.

33. Comerci GD: Medical complications of anorexia nervosa and bulimia nervosa. Med Clin North Am *74*:1293, 1990.
34. Harris RT: Bulimarexia and related serious eating disorders with medical complications. Ann Intern Med *99*:800, 1983.
35. Diamond GA: Eating disorders. Ann Intern Med *105*:790, 1986.
36. Health and Public Policy Committee, American College of Physicians: Eating disorders, anorexia nervosa and bulimia. Ann Intern Med *105*:790, 1986.
37. Isner J, Roberts WC, Heymsfield SB, et al: Anorexia nervosa and sudden death. Ann Intern Med *102*:49, 1985.
38. Case Records of the Massachusetts General Hospital (Case 47-1985). N Engl J Med *313*:1341, 1985.
39. Collins FJ, Mathews HR, Baker SE, et al: Drug-induced esophageal injury. BMJ *1*:1673, 1979.
40. Trier JS: Celiac sprue. N Engl J Med *325*:1709, 1991.
41. Katz SI, Hall RP, Lowley TJ, et al: Dermatitis herpetiformis: The skin and the gut. Ann Intern Med *93*:857, 1980.
42. Lipkin M, Bell B, Sherlock P: Cell proliferation kinetics in the gastrointestinal tract of man. I. Cell renewal of colon and rectum. J Clin Invest *42*:767, 1963.
43. Cole JW, McKalen A: Observations of cell renewal in human rectal mucosa *in vivo* with thymidine-H^3. Gastroenterology *41*:122, 1961.
44. Lembcke B, Caspany WF: Malabsorption syndromes. Clin Gastroenterol *2*:329, 1988.
45. Stemmerman GN, Hayoshi T: Colchicine intoxication: A reappraisal of its pathology based on a study of three fatal cases. Hum Pathol *2*:321, 1971.
46. Wilson FA, Hoyumpa AM Jr: Ethanol and small intestinal transport. Gastroenterology *7*:387, 1979.
47. Longstreth GF, Newcomer AD, Westbrook P: Paraaminosalicylic acid-induced malabsorption. Dig Dis *17*:731, 1972.
48. Benn A, Swan CJ, Cooke WT, et al: Effect of intraluminal pH on the absorption of pteroylmonoglutamic acid. BMJ *10*:148, 1971.
49. Strum WB: A pH-dependent, carrier-mediated transport system for the folate analog, amethopterin, in rat jejunum. J Pharmacol Exp Ther *203*:640, 1977.
50. Strum WB: Enzymatic reduction and methylation of folate during pH-dependent, carrier-mediated transport in rat jejunum. Biochim Biophys Acta *554*:249, 1979.
51. Streiff RR: Folate deficiency and oral contraceptives. JAMA *214*:105, 1970.
52. Strum WB: Characteristics of the transport of pteroylglutamate and amethopterin in rat jejunum. J Pharmacol Exp Ther *216*:329, 1981.
53. Berchtold P, Dahlquist A, Gustafson A, et al: Effects of a biguanide (metformin) on vitamin B_{12} and folic acid absorption and intestinal enzyme activity. Scand J Gastroenterol *6*:751, 1971.
54. Spencer H, Lender M: Adverse effects of aluminum-containing antacids on mineral metabolism. Gastroenterology *76*:603, 1979.
55. Eusufzai S: Bile acid malabsorption in patients with chronic diarrhea. Scand J Gastroenterol *28*:865, 1993.
56. Steinberg WM, King CE, Toskes PP: Malabsorption of protein-bound cobalamin but not unbound cobalamin during cimetidine administration. Dig Dis Sci *25*:188, 1980.
57. Lembcke B, Creutzfeldt W, Schleser S, et al: Effect of somatostatin analogue sandostatin (SMS 201-995) on gastrointestinal, pancreatic and biliary function and hormone release in normal men. Digestion *36*:108, 1987.
58. Marcuard SP, Albernaz L, Khazanie PG: Omeprazole therapy causes malabsorption of cyanocobalamin (vitamin B_{12}). Ann Intern Med *120*:211, 1994.

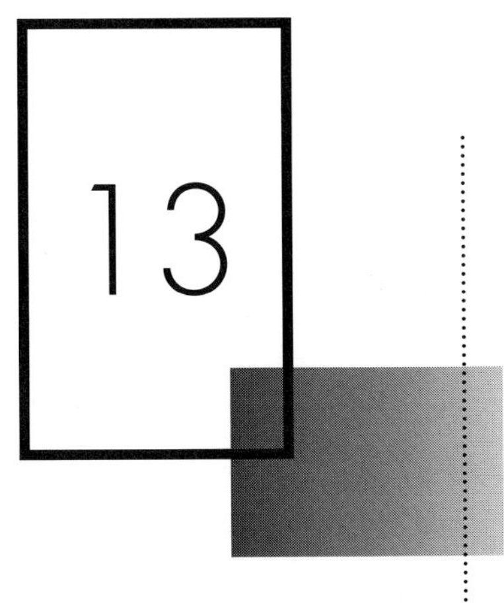

Hematologic Consequences of Poisoning

STEVEN C. CURRY, MD
MICHAEL W. CARLTON, MD

This chapter provides an overview of hematologic issues confronted by toxicologists caring for patients who are suffering from acute or chronic poisonings. Thousands of pharmaceutical agents produce adverse hematologic effects when given at therapeutic doses (e.g., agranulocytosis, aplastic anemia, and thrombocytopenia) or at intentionally toxic doses (e.g., chemotherapy); these agents are not the subject of this chapter. Details concerning specific agents are found in separate chapters in this text. The reader is also referred to Chapter 96 for discussion of thrombolytic agents and anticoagulants.

ERYTHROCYTES

Oxidant Stress

Oxidant stress, or the removal of electrons from molecules, results in three major disorders of toxicologic interest. The removal of electrons from the protein portion of hemoglobin produces *Heinz body hemolytic anemia*. The removal of electrons from iron found in hemoglobin produces *methemoglobinemia*. Finally, the oxidation of hemoglobin's porphyrin ring by sulfur produces *sulfhemoglobinemia*. These three disorders are intertwined with respect to the pathophysiology, occurrence,[1] diagnosis, and treatment of poisonings with oxidizing agents (Fig. 13–1).

In many instances, the parent drug or toxin producing hemolysis, methemoglobinemia, or sulfhemoglobinemia possesses no significant oxidizing potential *in vivo*. Oxidant stress in this setting is caused by electrophilic metabolites, which are frequently generated from metabolism by cytochrome P-450 enzymes. For example, dapsone and sulfonamides are metabolized to hydroxylamines that are responsible for the consequences of oxidant stress.

The mature erythrocyte lacks mitochondria and depends on glycolysis and the hexose monophosphate shunt for energy production (Fig. 13–2). Glycolysis fulfills the cell's adenosine triphosphate and NADH (nicotinamide-adenine dinucleotide, reduced form) requirements, the latter being essential to the maintenance of low fractions of methemoglobin. In contrast, the hexose monophosphate shunt mainly serves to facilitate the formation of NADPH (reduced NAD phosphate), which is used to protect against oxidant-induced hemolysis.[2]

Hemolysis

The mature erythrocyte continually undergoes oxidant stress from various sources, including food, infection, oxygen, drugs, and chemicals. Oxidation of the protein portion of hemoglobin (i.e., the removal of an electron from globin) results in denaturation of hemoglobin and attachment of damaged protein to the internal cell membrane. This denatured hemoglobin is visible as Heinz bodies on histologic examination of blood smears with special staining. Red cells containing denatured hemoglobin are removed from the circulation primarily by the spleen. The cells are trapped in the spleen's microcirculation, where they

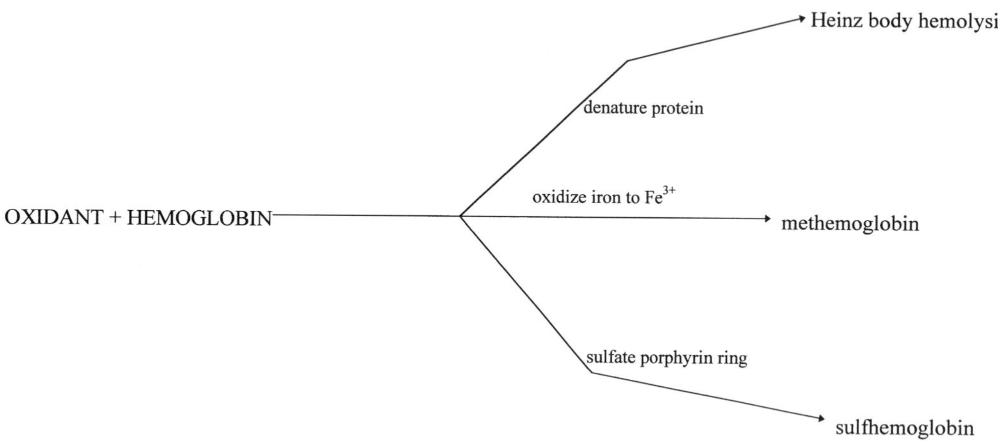

Figure 13–1. Results of oxidation of hemoglobin.

are destroyed; this produces mainly an extravascular hemolysis (nonspherocytic).[3] Oxidant stress may produce hemolysis by several additional mechanisms as well, including the depletion of intracellular glutathione stores with direct damage to the erythrocytic membrane, and the inactivation of several enzymes needed for erythrocyte integrity. Indeed, in the face of tremendous oxidant stress (e.g., arsine), hemolysis may occur intravascularly as well.

The main mechanism by which the erythrocyte protects itself against oxidant-induced hemolysis is to reduce oxidants before they have a chance to denature hemoglobin.[2] Reduced glutathione, both nonenzymatically and enzymatically with glutathione peroxidase, is responsible for most reducing capacity in this regard. Catalase also reduces hydrogen peroxide, and ascorbate serves as a mild reducing agent (Fig. 13–3).

Adequate stores of reduced glutathione are maintained within the erythrocyte through a conversion of NADPH to NADP (see Fig. 13–2). In turn, NADPH formation requires a properly functioning hexose monophosphate shunt. Patients with the various forms of congenital deficiency of glucose-6-phosphate dehydrogenase (G6PD), the first enzyme in the hexose monophosphate shunt, can be predisposed to hemolysis by sources of oxidant stress that would not affect the ordinary phenotype. The most common sources of oxidant stress in these patients are infection, drugs, and food. However, *Heinz body hemolysis can be produced in anyone (i.e., normal phenotypes) if oxidant stress is sufficiently severe* (i.e., after ingestion of dapsone or aniline).

Not surprisingly, substances capable of causing oxidant-induced hemolysis (Table 13–1) share the ability to produce methemoglobinemia and sulfhemoglo-

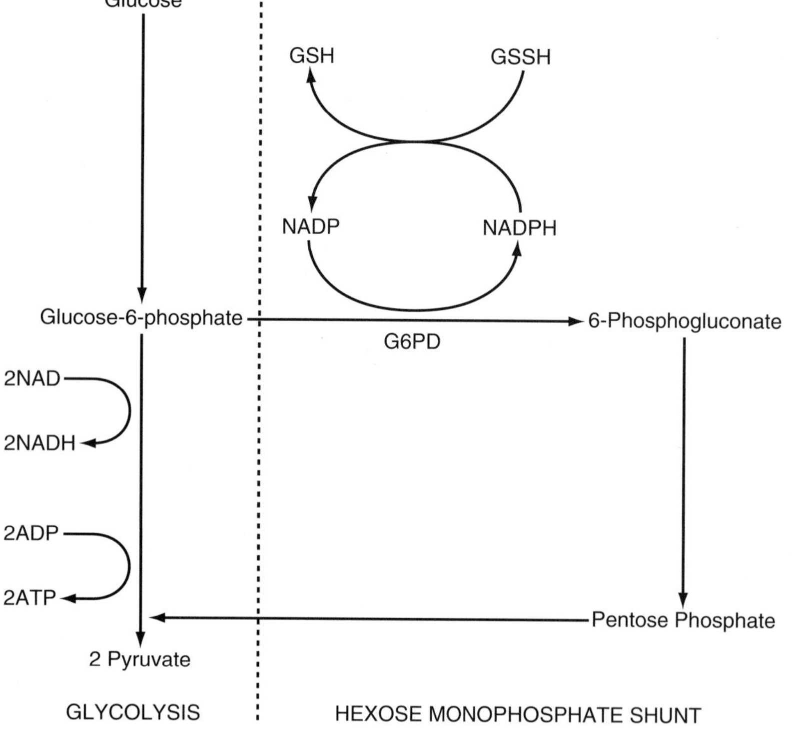

Figure 13–2. Metabolism in the erythrocyte. NAD, nicotine adenine dinucleotide; NADH, NAD; ADP, adenosine diphosphate; ATP, adenosine triphosphate; G6PD, glucose-6-phosphate dehydrogenase; NADP, nicotine adenine dinucleotide phosphate; NADPH, NADP; GSSH, oxidized glutathione; GSH, reduced glutathione.

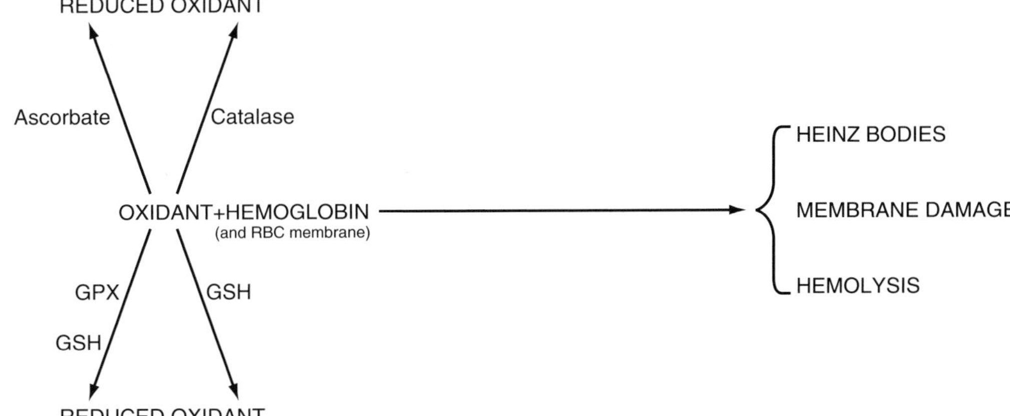

Figure 13–3. Inactivation of oxidants to prevent hemolysis. GPX, glutathione peroxidase.

binemia. However, some agents are better known for hemolytic activity that they induce than for accompanying dyshemoglobinemias. As examples, arsine and stibine produce massive hemolysis and death after inhalation. Ingestion of naphthalene results in the formation of an epoxide metabolite that is probably responsible for hemolysis. Patients ingesting, aspirating, or inhaling large amounts of gasoline also can experience significant hemolysis, although the exact cause of this outcome is not clear. Perhaps naphthalene, a component of gasoline, is also responsible for hemolysis in gasoline poisoning. Chlorates and chromates produce both severe hemolysis and methemoglobinemia.

The diagnosis of hemolysis is based on the demonstration of a decrease in blood hemoglobin concentration, an increase in plasma free hemoglobin concentration, and a decrease in serum haptoglobin concentration. Other diagnostic clues include hemoglobinuria (after plasma concentrations of hemoglobin

Table 13–1. Agents Producing Oxidant Stress*

Acetanilid	Dimethylaniline	Nitrosobenzene
Alloxans	Dimethyltoluidine	Pamaquine
α-Naphthylamine	Dinitrobenzene	Pentaerythritol tetranitrate
Aminophenols	Dinitrophenols	Phenacetin
p-Aminopropiophenone	Dinitrotoluene	Phenazopyridine
p-Aminosalicylic acid	Food additives	Phenetidine
Ammonium nitrate	Hydrazines	Phenols
Amyl nitrite	Hydroquinone	Phenylenediamine
Aniline dyes	Hydroxyacetanilid	Phenylhydrazine
Aniline and derivatives	Hydroxylamine	Phenylhydroxylamine
Anilinoethanol	Inks, marking	Piperazine
Antipyrine	Isobutyl nitrite	Plasmoquine
Aromatic amines	Lidocaine	Prilocaine
Arsine	Local anesthetics	Primaquine
Benzocaine	Menadione	Pyridine
Betanaphthol disulfonate	Menthol	Pyridium
Bismuth subnitrate	Methylacetanilid	Pyrogallol
p-Bromoaniline	Methylene blue	Quinones
Cetrimide	Metoclopramide	Resorcinol
Chloranilines	Monolinuron	Shoe dye or polish
Chlorates	Moth balls	Spinach
Chlorobenzene	Mushrooms	Sulfomethane
Chloronitrobenzene	Naphthalene	Sulfonamides
Chloroquine	Naphthol	Sulfones
Chromates	Naphthylamines	Tetralin
Cobalt preparations	Nitrates	Tetranitromethane tetronal
Copper sulfate	Nitrites	Toluenediamine
Corning extract	*p*-Nitroaniline	Toluidine
Crayons, wax (red/orange)†	Nitrobenzene and its derivatives	*p*-Toluidine
Dapsone	Nitroethane	Toluylhydroxylamine
Diaminodiphenylsulfone	Nitrofurans	Trichlorocarbanilide (TCC)
Diesel fuel additives	Nitrogen oxide	Trinitrotoluene
Dimethylamine	Nitroglycerin	Trional
Dimethylaminophenol	Nitrophenol	

*Poisoning by these agents variously produces Heinz body hemolytic anemia, methemoglobinemia, or sulfhemoglobinemia, or any combination of these. Agents best known for causing sulfhemoglobinemia are listed in Table 13–5.
†Children's crayons made in the United States are safe.

have become sufficiently elevated) and the presence of Heinz bodies (confirmed with special staining technique). Heinz bodies are not detectable on a routine Wright stain of blood, but "bite cells" may be noted.[4] Spherocytes are typically absent or only mildly increased in number. Reticulocytosis is delayed for several days after onset of hemolysis. Although hemolysis may occur early after poisoning (e.g., with chlorate toxicity), it may not become clinically apparent until several days after ingestion. Other complications of hemolysis include hyperkalemia, pigment nephropathy, and jaundice. In severe cases, impaired oxygen-carrying capacity results in metabolic acidosis, brain failure, and cardiovascular collapse. Methemoglobinemia and, occasionally, sulfhemoglobinemia may accompany Heinz body hemolytic anemia, and evidence for such a combination should be sought.

In general, treatment is supportive and includes blood transfusions, ensuring a brisk urine output, and monitoring for hyperkalemia. Specific therapies may be indicated in poisonings with specific toxins (e.g., exchange transfusions for arsine; D-penicillamine therapy for copper). Intravenous administration of *N*-acetylcysteine prevents severe decreases in whole blood glutathione concentration in cats suffering from acetaminophen-induced methemoglobinemia (this is not a problem in humans).[5] This finding suggests that *N*-acetylcysteine might be effective in preventing or lessening oxidant-induced hemolysis in humans with acute poisonings, but this conjecture has not been proved.

Methemoglobinemia

Pathophysiology

Reduced hemoglobin (deoxyhemoglobin) contains four heme groups, each with a ferrous (Fe^{2+}) ion capable of binding and transporting oxygen. Oxidation (removal of an electron) of iron to the ferric (Fe^{3+}) state produces *methemoglobin*. The fact that oxidant stress produces both denaturation of hemoglobin (Heinz body hemolytic anemia) and methemoglobin explains the common co-existence of hemolysis and methemoglobinemia (see Fig. 13–1).

Methemoglobin continuously forms in erythrocytes, to a large extent from the oxidizing power of oxygen. Methemoglobin most commonly is reported in percentages (fractions). These values represent the total percentage of hemoglobin pigments present as methemoglobin. Normally, methemoglobin fractions in circulating whole blood are less than 1% to 2%. When fractions exceed this value, methemoglobinemia is said to be present. Although the term "hemoglobinemia" refers to the presence of excess hemoglobin in plasma, the term "methemoglobinemia" refers to the presence of elevated circulating fractions of methemoglobin within erythrocytes.

Methemoglobin cannot transport oxygen and thus produces a functional anemia. Furthermore, ferric heme groups impair unloading of oxygen by ferrous heme on the same hemoglobin tetramer, shifting the oxyhemoglobin dissociation curve to the left and thereby further impeding oxygen delivery.[2] Thus, the signs and symptoms of methemoglobinemia result from the impairment of oxygen delivery to tissues.

Unlike hemoglobin, methemoglobin is dark brown. Five grams of normal reduced hemoglobin per deciliter of capillary blood produces visible cyanosis. However, only 1.5 g of methemoglobin per deciliter of blood produce noticeable discoloration. In a patient without anemia, methemoglobin fractions of approximately 10% to 15% produce cyanosis, even before the impairment of oxygen delivery becomes significant. As methemoglobin fractions increase to more than 20% in the nonanemic patient, cardiovascular and central nervous system signs develop and include headache, dyspnea, tachypnea, tachycardia, and mild hypertension. Further increases in methemoglobin fractions into the 40% to 50% range (without anemia) produce confusion, lethargy, and metabolic acidosis. Additional elevation results in coma, seizures, bradyrhythmias, ventricular dysrhythmias, and hypotension; when methemoglobin fractions approach 70%, death ensues. The anemic patient suffers more severe symptoms at given methemoglobin fractions than does the nonanemic patient. In addition, anemic patients exhibit less profound cyanosis at given methemoglobin fractions.

The inactivation of oxidants is relatively unimportant in maintaining methemoglobin fractions within the normal range. For example, patients with congenital glutathione deficiency, G6PD deficiency, catalase deficiency, and scurvy do not have elevated methemoglobin fractions. Rather, methemoglobin fractions are maintained within the normal range by immediate reduction back to ferrous hemoglobin after spontaneous formation.

Cytochrome-b_5 *reductase* is responsible for essentially all methemoglobin reduction *in vivo* (Fig. 13–4).[6] In the step mediated by this enzyme, electrons are transferred from NADH (from glycolysis) to cytochrome b_5, and then to methemoglobin to form deoxyhemoglobin. Thus, the normal functioning of this enzymatic reduction requires an intact glycolytic pathway, cytochrome b_5, and adequate activity of the reductase enzyme. Usually, the rate of the enzymatic reduction of methemoglobin exceeds the rate of spontaneous background methemoglobin formation by several hundred–fold. Patients who are heterozygous in this enzyme deficiency normally do not have elevated methemoglobin fractions but are predisposed to suffering methemoglobinemia in response to oxidant stress that would not otherwise affect a patient with a normal phenotype. Patients homozygous for this deficiency have congenital methemoglobinemia.[6]

A second enzyme, *NADPH methemoglobin reductase,* normally remains inactive. However, the addition of a cofactor such as methylene blue markedly accelerates NADPH methemoglobin reductase activity and serves as the basis for treating methemoglobinemia with methylene blue.[2] In this pathway (see Fig. 13–4), electrons are transferred from NADPH (from the hexose monophosphate shunt) to methyl-

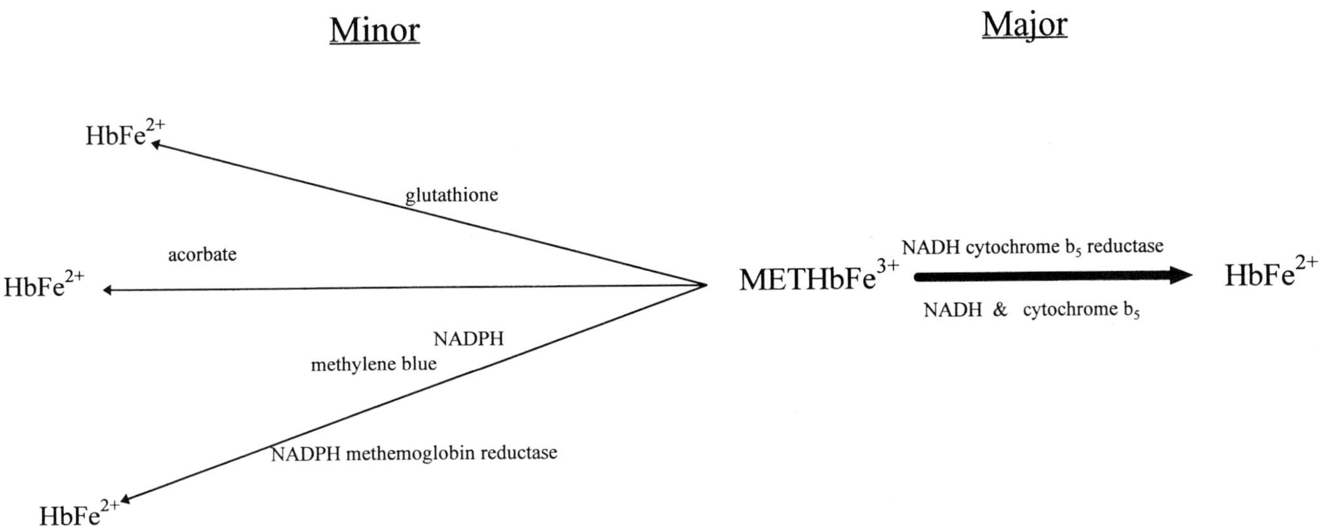

Figure 13–4. Reduction of methemoglobin. Essentially all methemoglobin reduction *in vivo* is catalyzed by cytochrome-b_5 reductase. Methylene blue markedly enhances methemoglobin reduction by acting as a cofactor for NADPH reduced methemoglobin reductase. $HbFe^{2+}$, normal ferrous hemoglobin; NADPH, reduced nicotine adenine dinucleotide phosphate; $METHbFe^{3+}$, methemoglobin.

ene blue and then to methemoglobin to produce deoxyhemoglobin. Thus, reduction of methemoglobin by this pathway requires an intact hexose monophosphate shunt, a cofactor such as methylene blue, and normal activity of the NADPH methemoglobin reductase enzyme. *In vitro,* some methemoglobin reduction can be demonstrated by glutathione and ascorbate; however, this activity is thought to be insignificant *in vivo*. Ascorbate generally is not considered an effective agent for the treatment of acute methemoglobinemia because of its slow action.

Infants are predisposed to methemoglobinemia because of their limited cytochrome-b_5 reductase activity and the low cytochrome b_5 concentrations in their erythrocytes. Oxidant stress resulting from infections such as gastroenteritis or urinary tract infections are by far the most common cause of acquired methemoglobinemia in patients of this age group.[7, 8]

Etiology

Congenital Causes.[3, 6] Homozygous deficiency for cytochrome-b_5 reductase produces congenital methemoglobinemia, which responds to oral methylene blue therapy. Several mutant hemoglobin species collectively termed "hemoglobin M" have been described in which the iron remains in the ferric form. Most patients with hemoglobin M suffer from congenital methemoglobinemia that is unresponsive to methylene blue therapy. Patients born homozygous for cytochrome-b_5 deficiency suffer from congenital methemoglobinemia. Finally, there exist mutant unstable hemoglobins that undergo denaturation to produce congenital Heinz body hemolytic anemias; some of these also oxidize to methemoglobin.

Acquired Causes. Most cases of methemoglobinemia are acquired and, except in neonates with infections, result from exposure to drugs or toxic agents (see Table 13–1). Oral overdoses of nitroglycerin and organic nitrates (which are esters of nitrite), as well as therapeutic doses of intravenous nitroglycerin are well known to produce methemoglobinemia.[9] The topical use of benzocaine spray, teething ointments, and hemorrhoidal creams, along with therapeutic doses of most other local anesthetics administered by injection or topical application (e.g., lidocaine spray for bronchoscopy) have produced this disorder. Methemoglobinemia is the rule following overdoses of phenazopyridine (Pyridium) or dapsone, and it occasionally results from the administration of therapeutic doses of the latter. The conversion of nitrates to nitrites by bacteria in the upper gastrointestinal tract has produced fatal methemoglobinemia in infants who ingested well water with high nitrate concentrations.[10] The recreational use of inhalable nitrites such as isobutyl nitrite has resulted in death. Aniline dyes are potent inducers of methemoglobinemia, and topical contact with these agents, which include components of printing ink on diapers, leather dyes in new shoes, and commercial marking crayons, has resulted in significant methemoglobinemia and death.[2]

As expected, many agents producing methemoglobinemia also produce oxidant-induced hemolysis. For example, profound hemolysis may accompany poisonings with chlorates, arsine, stibine, chromates, and dapsone.

Diagnosis

The diagnosis of methemoglobinemia is confirmed with multiple-wavelength co-oximetry. Other diagnostic clues, however, may be either helpful or misleading. Generalized cyanosis in the presence of a normal arterial oxygen tension almost always represents methemoglobinemia. Failure of cyanosis to resolve with oxygen therapy also is an important diagnostic clue. Many blood gas instruments do not actually measure per cent saturation, although they do report a value for saturation. This value is usually calculated from the oxygen tension and pH, and it represents what the saturation should be, assuming a lack of abnormal hemoglobin pigments. Therefore, in methemoglobinemia, the true per cent saturation as determined by co-oximetry is much lower than the calculated per cent saturation as reported by many blood gas instruments. The difference between these two values, or the *saturation gap,* should be less than 3% to 5% in arterial blood. Large saturation gaps in arterial blood are almost always due to methemoglobinemia or carboxyhemoglobinemia and less commonly result from sulfhemoglobinemia.

Most co-oximeters do not differentiate between methemoglobin and sulfhemoglobin and thus report elevated methemoglobin fractions in the presence of sulfhemoglobinemia. A simple screening method to help distinguish the two species is described later in the chapter in the section on sulfhemoglobinemia.

Pulse oximetry neither accurately nor reliably measures per cent saturation in the presence of methemoglobinemia.[11] Depending on the true oxygen saturation, pulse oximetry may yield falsely low or falsely high values, with the latter reported at high methemoglobin fractions. Once the diagnosis of methemoglobinemia has been made, the pulse oximeter should be disconnected from the patient so that medical personnel are not misled by unreliable readings.

Patients with significant methemoglobinemia may be observed to have chocolate-colored blood during blood sampling. A drop of this blood allowed to dry on filter paper appears noticeably brown when compared with venous blood from an asymptomatic patient when methemoglobinemia fractions exceed 10% to 15% in the nonanemic patient.[12] The presence of methemoglobinemia does not alter measurements of total hemoglobin concentration provided by the hematology laboratory. Because co-oximetry determines methemoglobin concentrations by measuring the absorption of light, substances that interfere with light absorption can produce false results on co-oximetry. Hyperlipidemia, such as that seen after the infusion of lipid emulsions or in patients with diabetes mellitus, interferes with the measurement of hemoglobin pigments by co-oximetry and results in the reporting of a falsely elevated fraction of methemoglobin.[13] Total blood and plasma free hemoglobin concentrations may also be falsely elevated in this situation. Immediately after a dose of methylene blue has been administered, co-oximetry may be unreliable for several minutes.[14] In the foregoing instances, it should be remembered that significant methemoglobinemia is not present in a patient with a normal hemoglobin concentration if he or she does not appear cyanotic.

Methemoglobin fractions commonly increase after death. Therefore, postmortem methemoglobin concentrations are not valid indicators of antemortem methemoglobinemia.[15]

Differential Diagnosis

Cyanosis caused by methemoglobinemia is most commonly confused with that accompanying hypoxia. However, in cases of isolated methemoglobinemia with or without hemolysis, the arterial oxygen tension remains unchanged from baseline values and, in the absence of other causes, is normal. Furthermore, the cyanosis from methemoglobinemia does not respond to oxygen therapy. An unusual and poorly characterized discoloration of skin and other organs has been reported in patients suffering from hydrogen sulfide poisoning. Rare cases of tellurium exposure are characterized by blue discoloration. Approximately one half of patients with severe cyanide poisoning experience cyanosis, and many other signs and symptoms of cyanide poisoning are similar to those of methemoglobinemia. Both carbon monoxide poisoning and sulfhemoglobinemia (described later in this chapter) produce saturation gaps in the presence of normal arterial oxygen tensions. Again, most co-oximeters measure and report sulfhemoglobinemia as methemoglobinemia. Skin contact with new clothing or towels that contain blue dyes may cause discoloration of the skin, but this discoloration is easily removed during washing. Excessive administration of methylene blue may also produce cyanosis that can be confused with continuing methemoglobinemia or cyanosis from other causes.

Treatment

Patients suffering from methemoglobinemia should receive oxygen to maximize the oxygen-carrying capacity of their remaining normal hemoglobin. Blood should be drawn and analyzed for evidence of hemolysis (hemoglobin measurement, blood smear, Heinz body staining, plasma free hemoglobin determination, and serum haptoglobin measurement). Patients should undergo arterial blood gas analysis and co-oximetry, and routine laboratory studies should be performed. An electrocardiogram should be obtained for ruling out myocardial ischemia.

Asymptomatic Patients. Most patients suffering from methemoglobinemia exhibit cyanosis but lack signs and symptoms and do not require specific treatment. Once exposure to the offending agent ends, methemoglobin levels usually return to normal within 36 hours. Most of these patients require admission to a hospital for clinical follow-up for worsening of signs and symptoms, monitoring for onset of hemolysis, and serial determination of methemoglobin levels. Assuming normal hemoglobin concentrations, asymptomatic patients usually have methemoglobin fractions between 10% and 15%.

Symptomatic Patients. Symptomatic patients suffering from methemoglobinemia (e.g., tachycardia, dyspnea, headache) are candidates for specific antidotal therapy with methylene blue, in the absence of a history of G6PD deficiency. Parenteral methylene blue is available as a 1% solution (10 mg/mL); it should be administered intravenously over 3 to 5 minutes at an initial dose of 2 mg/kg (0.2 mL/kg of a 1% solution). Resolution of cyanosis usually occurs within 15 to 20 minutes; more time may be required in some instances. If the patient is seriously symptomatic and no response occurs within 15 minutes, or if the patient remains moderately symptomatic without any improvement after 30 to 60 minutes, then repeat doses of 1 mg/kg (0.1 mL/kg of a 1% solution) may be given. If methemoglobin levels are readily available, repeat determinations of methemoglobin fractions should be performed before repeat dosing of methylene blue because large doses of methylene blue themselves produce discoloration of the skin. The total dose of methylene blue administered during the first few hours should not exceed 5 to 7 mg/kg.

Some methemoglobin-producing toxins have long half-lives. The classic example is dapsone, which may produce methemoglobinemia and hemolysis that last for days. In this situation, it may be necessary to administer methylene blue as a continuous infusion. Methylene blue may be dissolved in the crystalloid solution of choice and administered, on the basis of case reports in the literature, starting at 0.1 mg/kg per hour (0.01 mL/kg per hour of a 1% solution)[16]; however, the personal experience of the authors indicates that higher rates may be required. Serial methemoglobin fractions are followed in order to monitor therapy.

Methylene blue largely undergoes renal excretion unchanged (about 75%). Therefore, patients with renal insufficiency do not require changes in initial doses for the treatment of methemoglobinemia but should receive lower infusion doses of the drug determined on the basis of their creatinine clearance.

Adverse effects associated with large or rapidly administered doses of methylene blue in normal volunteers include dysuria, substernal chest pain, nausea, tachycardia, hypertension, and anxiety. Urine initially turns blue and then green as the drug undergoes excretion. Although the literature cautions that methylene blue may produce transient methemoglobinemia when given in large doses (e.g., 5 mg/kg over 35 to 70 minutes),[17] this has not been thought to be a significant problem in human beings receiving recommended doses and has been ascribed largely to an *in vitro* effect occurring in the presence of hypoxic conditions.[18, 19] Worsening hemolysis in methemoglobinemia patients has been ascribed to methylene blue therapy, even in those with normal G6PD activity. However, this finding has primarily been noted in case reports of patients in whom hemolysis was not unexpected from the agent producing methemoglobinemia, making causal relationships unclear. Importantly, neonates do seem sensitive to hemolytic actions of methylene blue.[20–22] Regardless of these concerns, the administration of methylene blue to a symptomatic patient with methemoglobinemia (without G6PD deficiency) has never been proved to worsen methemoglobinemia, and this explains why methylene blue continues to be the drug of choice for treating symptomatic patients. Furthermore, patients with methemoglobinemia should always be closely followed for evidence of hemolysis because hemolysis is common whether or not methylene blue is given.

Methylene blue should never be administered to someone with known G6PD deficiency. Such patients have low red cell NADPH concentrations; these low concentrations make augmentation of NADPH methemoglobin reductase by methylene blue limited. Importantly, methylene blue triggers hemolysis in such patients, which further impairs oxygen delivery to tissues.[2, 23] However, in a symptomatic patient, methylene blue should never be withheld simply because a history of G6PD deficiency cannot be obtained.

Cimetidine has been used to help control methemoglobinemia secondary to dapsone administration. By inhibiting cytochrome P-450 conversion to the oxidizing metabolite responsible for methemoglobinemia (dapsone hydroxylamine), the administration of 1200 mg of cimetidine per day orally to patients taking therapeutic doses of dapsone decreased circulating methemoglobin fractions by an average of 25%.[24]

During the care of patients with methemoglobinemia, one should always be careful to monitor total oxygen-carrying capacity by following both hemoglobin concentrations and methemoglobin fractions. For example, a decrease in the methemoglobin fraction from 30% to 15% will not result in improved oxygen delivery if accompanying hemolysis has resulted in a decrease of hemoglobin concentration from 15 to 5 g/dL. In fact, in this example, oxygen-carrying capacity has even worsened. Furthermore, the onset of anemia alone may result in the disappearance of cyanosis if total hemoglobin concentrations decrease to the point where significant amounts of methemoglobinemia do not produce discoloration. For example, a 10% methemoglobin fraction in combination with a hemoglobin concentration of 15 g/dL does produce visible cyanosis in most persons. However, a 20% methemoglobin fraction in a patient with a hemoglobin level of 5 g/dL produces no visible discoloration, yet it may be lethal. Therefore, caution must be taken in interpreting the disappearance of cyanosis to mean that methemoglobinemia has not worsened or that the patient's status has improved.

After initial signs and symptoms of methemoglobinemia have been addressed, then routine gastrointestinal and skin decontamination should be performed as indicated. If one does choose to use ascorbic acid in treating methemoglobinemia, a recommended dose is 0.5 to 1 g intravenously or orally every 6 hours. Again, ascorbic acid works slowly and generally is considered ineffective for the treatment of acute acquired methemoglobinemia.

Failure to Respond to Methylene Blue Therapy

When patients with methemoglobinemia do not improve with methylene blue therapy, several possibilities should be considered (Table 13–2). It may be they have been exposed to large amounts of drugs or chemicals that, even with methylene blue therapy, produce methemoglobin at rates greater than the rate of reducing capacity. However, this possibility remains the exception. Although there are certainly

Table 13–2. Possible Causes of Failure of Methylene Blue Therapy in Methemoglobinemia

Profound and overwhelming toxicity from oxidants (e.g., chlorates)
Glucose-6-phosphate dehydrogenase deficiency
NADPH methemoglobin reductase deficiency
Sulfhemoglobinemia
Discoloration from large doses of methylene blue

times when methemoglobin fractions do not return to normal because of continued methemoglobin formation, methylene blue therapy almost always results in at least a transient decrease in methemoglobin fractions.

The patient who does not respond to methylene blue therapy may also have an unrecognized G6PD deficiency. The rare patient with congenital lack of NADPH methemoglobin reductase also fails to respond to methylene blue treatment. Sulfhemoglobinemia can be mistaken for methemoglobinemia (see later in this chapter). Finally, repeated doses of methylene blue may result in blue discoloration of skin that is mistaken for methemoglobinemia.[25]

Treatment options for the patient who cannot receive or who fails to respond to methylene blue therapy remain somewhat limited. Blood transfusions and exchange transfusions may be life saving,[26] and they have been recommended whenever refractory methemoglobin fractions approach 70% in the nonanemic patient. Hyperbaric oxygenation can be a temporizing measure that provides adequate oxygen delivery during preparation for blood transfusion. However, a patient can only stay in a hyperbaric chamber for a relatively limited period of time without suffering from consequences of oxygen toxicity. Although not known to be effective, administration of large doses of ascorbic acid may also be indicated in this situation.

Sulfhemoglobin

Background and Characteristics

Sulfhemoglobin is a green molecule resulting from the incorporation of a sulfur atom into the porphyrin ring of hemoglobin by oxidant stress. Like methemoglobin, sulfhemoglobin cannot transport oxygen (Table 13–3). *Sulfmyoglobin,* the isomer of tetrameric sulfhemoglobin, has a 2500-fold lower affinity for oxygen than myoglobin.[27] Although small amounts of methemoglobin normally exist *in vivo,* no circulating sulfhemoglobin usually occurs. Unlike methemoglobin, sulfhemoglobin persists for the life of the erythrocyte and does not undergo conversion back to hemoglobin. Very little sulfhemoglobin causes typical slate-gray cyanosis. Only 0.5 g/dL of sulfhemoglobin produces noticeable skin discoloration (as compared with 1.5 g/dL of methemoglobin and 5 g/dL of deoxyhemoglobin).

During sulfhemoglobinemia (i.e., *in vivo*), hemoglobin tetramers usually contain only one or two sulfurated heme isomers. The affected molecules shift unaffected heme moieties toward the unliganded conformation. This reduces the oxygen affinity of the unmodified subunits and shifts the oxyhemoglobin dissociation curve to the right, enhancing oxygen delivery to tissues and partially ameliorating the effects of reduced oxygen-binding capacity.[28] In contrast, methemoglobin and carboxyhemoglobin shift the dissociation curve to the left, worsening the impairment of oxygen delivery to tissues.

Sulfhemoglobin, methemoglobin, and hemoglobin M possess similar light absorption spectra, and many early authors failed to distinguish between these three abnormal pigments. Most modern multiple-wavelength co-oximeters still report sulfhemoglobin as methemoglobin. Furthermore, early studies of "sulfhemoglobinemia" from hydrogen sulfide mixed with blood *in vitro* may have represented nothing more than a mixture of oxidized and denatured hemoglobin pigments that were unrelated to what is termed "sulfhemoglobin" today.[29] Readers interpreting the confusing medical literature on sulfhemoglobinemia must be aware that older literature describing sulfhemoglobin, which has been suggested to be better termed "pseudo-sulfhemoglobin,"[30] might represent true reports of sulfhemoglobinemia, methemoglobinemia, or hemoglobin M disease, or of various species of denatured hemoglobin from hydrogen sulfide mixed with blood *in vitro,* or perhaps other chemical compounds.

Formation and Etiology

Sulfhemoglobinemia is always acquired (Table 13–4), and chemicals capable of producing sulfhemoglo-

Table 13–3. Comparison of Hemoglobin Pigments

	Deoxyhemoglobin	Methemoglobin	Sulfhemoglobin	Carboxyhemoglobin
Color	Blue	Brown	Green	Bright red
Concentration when cyanosis appears	5 g/dL	1.5 g/dL	0.5 g/dL	—
Able to transport oxygen?	Yes	No	No	No
Shift in oxyhemoglobin dissociation curve	Rightward	Leftward	Rightward	Leftward
Response to methylene blue treatment	None	Decreases	None	None
Reported by most co-oximeters	—	Methemoglobin	Methemoglobin	Carboxyhemoglobin

Table 13–4. Clinical Substances Most Commonly Associated with "Sulfhemoglobinemia"*

Acetanilid	Naphthylamine
Aminophenol	Nitrites
p-Aminopropiophenone	*p*-Nitroaniline
Ammonium nitrite	Nitrobenzene
Amyl nitrite	Nitroglycerin
Aniline	Phenacetin
Anilinoethanol	Phenazopyridine
Bismuth subnitrite	Phenylenediamine
Dapsone	Phenylhydroxylamine
Dimethylamine	Sulfanilamide
Dinitrobenzene	Sulfapyridine
Ethyl nitrite	Sulfathiazole
Hydroxylacetylanilide	Toluenediamine
Hydroxylamine	Tolylhydroxylamine
Methylacetylanilide	Trinitrotoluene

*In some instances, it is not known whether "sulfhemoglobinemia" represents methemoglobinemia, sulfhemoglobinemia, or both.

binemia[31] usually are better known for their ability to produce methemoglobinemia and hemolysis. Thus, methemoglobinemia, sulfhemoglobinemia, and hemolysis may coexist. Why some patients develop sulfhemoglobinemia and others methemoglobinemia after exposure to the same agent remains a mystery.

Sulfhemoglobin forms when elemental sulfur binds to the β-pyrrole ring of the heme moiety (Fig. 13–5*A*). Based on studies of sulfmyoglobin, it has been suggested that an unstable episulfide bond forms (see Fig. 13–5*B*) that spontaneously converts to the stable conformation (see Fig. 13–5*C*), which persists for the life of the red blood cell.[32] In the past, authors had suggested that the source of sulfur responsible for the oxidation of hemoglobin to sulfhemoglobin was the offending chemical producing the oxidant stress. However, many drugs associated with sulfhemoglobinemia do not contain sulfur. It was also an older belief that an abnormally functioning gastrointestinal tract alone could produce hemolytic anemia, sulfhemoglobinemia, and methemoglobinemia ("enterogenous cyanosis") from the purported absorption of endogenously produced nitrites and sulfides. However, it appears that such patients were unknowingly ingesting analgesics known to cause such disorders.[33]

In an attempt to identify the source of the sulfur atom when exogenous sulfur was not supplied, Westphal and Azen[34] studied rats with jejunal pouches in which bacterial overgrowth occurred. Rats with jejunal pouches exposed to phenacetin were more likely to develop sulfhemoglobinemia than were the controls. In addition, erythrocytes from both control animals and those with pouches were more likely to become sulfurated when incubated in the urine of pouched rats than when incubated in the urine of controls. Finally, pouched rats were less likely to develop sulfurated hemoglobin when they were treated with neomycin. This suggests that bacterial metabolism in the gastrointestinal tract may serve as a source for sulfur found in sulfhemoglobin during times of oxidant stress induced by various chemicals. Endogenous sulfhydryl groups may act as sulfur donors during the production of sulfhemoglobin.

Laboratory Diagnosis

In an early attempt to discern what was being measured when "sulfhemoglobin" was reported to be present, Michel and Harris[35] reported that the addition of cyanide or dithionite (hydrosulfite) to blood bound methemoglobin eliminated its spectral absorption immediately, while that of sulfhemoglobin remained. However, this simple test did not exclude hemoglobin M (or perhaps other oxidation products of hemoglobin), which also remains after addition of these compounds. Carrico and colleagues[36] later demonstrated that carbon monoxide bound sulfhemoglobin to produce carbonmonoxysulfhemoglobin, a compound with enhanced spectral absorption and a down-field shift, whereas neither methemoglobin nor hemoglobin M bound carbon monoxide. Therefore, light absorption in the presence of cyanide (or dithionite) and carbon monoxide served for several years as laboratory tools to measure "sulfhemoglobin" fractions and concentrations, although it is not known that what we know today as sulfhemoglobin was always the species being measured. Most recently, Park and Nagel[28] reported that isoelectric focusing (a form of electrophoresis) reliably delineates the three pigments. Although this test is not widely available, it remains the most reliable way of distinguishing

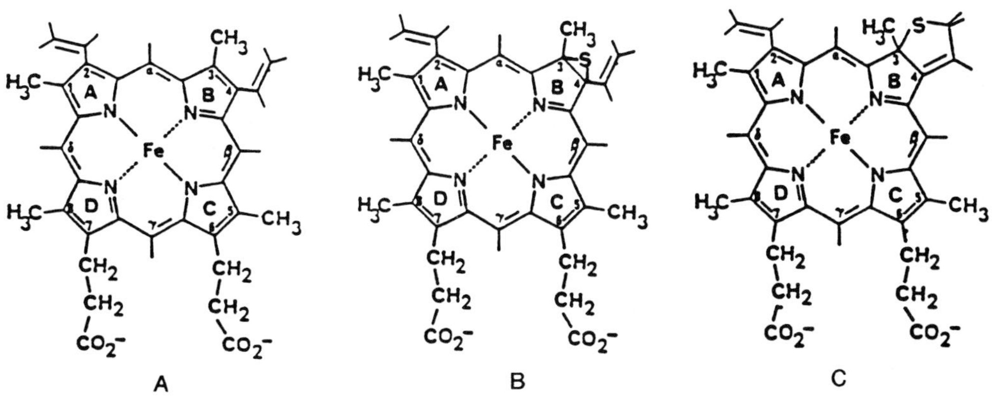

Figure 13–5. Proposed formation of sulfhemoglobin as illustrated in a single heme moiety (as in sulfmyoglobin). *A*, Native heme moiety. *B*, Initial episulfide bond across the β–β bond of β-pyrrole. *C*, Terminal sulfhemin in sulfmyoglobin. In sulfmyoglobin, no more than one to two heme moieties of a hemoglobin tetramer are oxidized to the sulfhemin state. (From Chatfield MJ, La Mar GN: 1H nuclear magnetic resonance study of the prosthetic group in sulfhemoglobin. Arch Biochem Biophys *295*:290, 1992.)

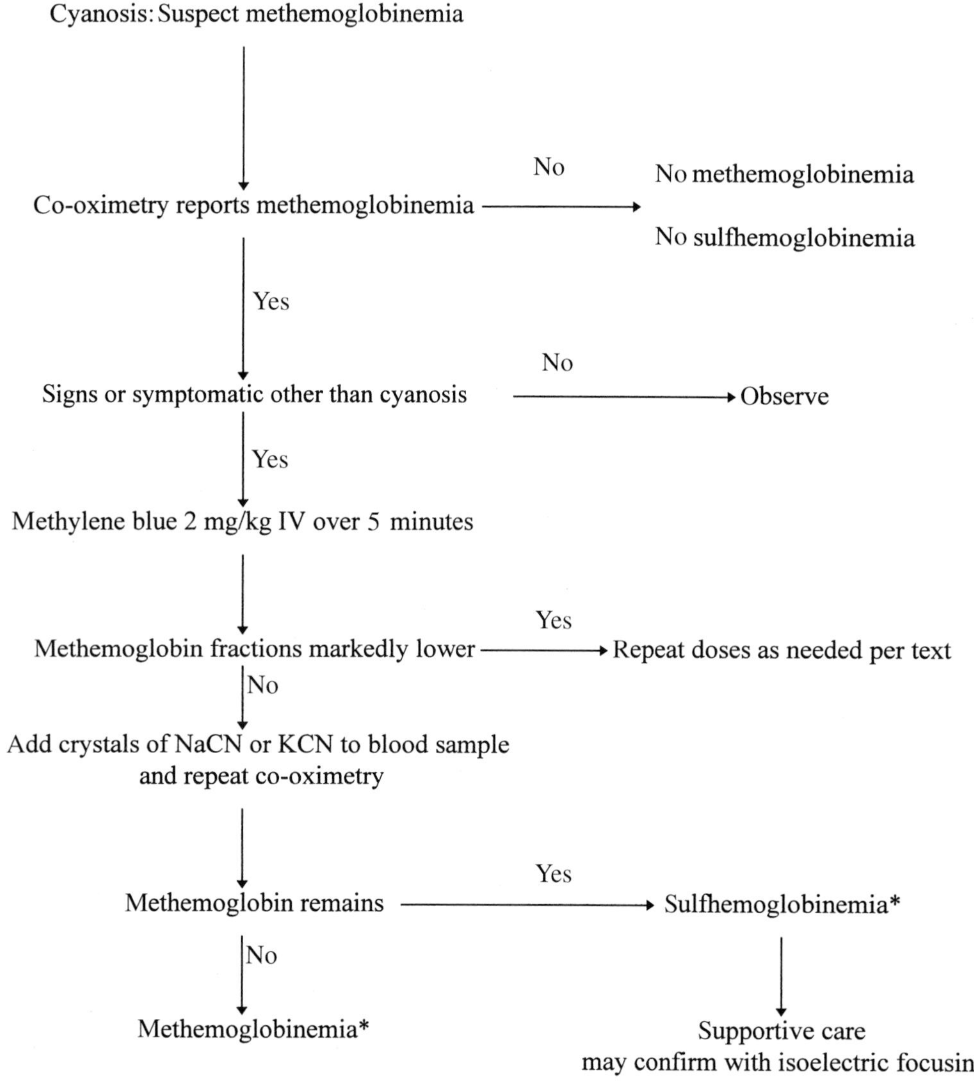

Figure 13–6. Initial diagnostic approach for sulfhemoglobinemia in the patient with suspected methemoglobinemia who does not respond to methylene blue therapy. Most co-oximeters measure and report sulfhemoglobin as methemoglobin. Cyanide combines with methemoglobin to produce cyanomethemoglobin. Cyanide has no effect on sulfhemoglobinemia.

sulfhemoglobin from methemoglobin and generally serves as the gold standard.

Diagnostic Strategy

When the clinician confronts a cyanotic patient in whom sulfhemoglobinemia is suspected (e.g., methemoglobinemia unresponsive to methylene blue therapy), blood should be sent for multiple-wavelength co-oximetry (Fig. 13–6). A positive result for methemoglobinemia may represent true methemoglobinemia, sulfhemoglobinemia, or a mixture of the two (excluding interfering conditions such as hyperlipidemia). Because the clinician frequently does not have the luxury of time to wait for the results of isoelectric focusing, a few crystals of potassium or sodium cyanide should then be added to the blood sample and co-oximetry repeated. If the co-oximeter reports that methemoglobinemia has disappeared, then the correct diagnosis is methemoglobinemia (cyanide combined with methemoglobin to produce bright red cyanomethemoglobin); if the co-oximeter reports that the methemoglobin fraction remains unchanged after the addition of cyanide, then the correct diagnosis usually is sulfhemoglobinemia (rare hemoglobin M disease is not distinguished from sulfhemoglobinemia by this method). If the co-oximeter reports that methemoglobin fractions have decreased but remain elevated, then both methemoglobin and sulfhemoglobin probably exist. Blood may be sent for hemoglobin electrophoresis by isoelectric focusing to confirm the presence of sulfhemoglobinemia. As with methemoglobin and carboxyhemoglobin, pulse oximetry does not reliably report true oxygen saturation in the presence of sulfhemoglobin.

Clinical Presentation

Because most co-oximeters do not distinguish between methemoglobin and sulfhemoglobin, the diagnosis of sulfhemoglobinemia is usually considered when the clinician is confronted with a cyanotic patient who (1) has a normal oxygen tension, (2) has what the laboratory reports to be elevated methemoglobin fractions, and (3) has failed to respond to methylene blue therapy (beware that G6PD deficiency also is a cause of this scenario). Except for cyanosis, most patients with sulfhemoglobinemia are not symptomatic unless other abnormal hemoglobins are present (e.g., methemoglobin) or there is accompanying anemia. The discoloration of cyanosis most often appears slate gray and may persist for weeks or even months owing to the irreversible nature of sulfhemoglobin. Only rarely is sulfhemoglobinemia severe enough to produce tachycardia, tachypnea, dyspnea, and altered level of consciousness due to impairment of oxygen delivery. The co-existence of methemoglobinemia and anemia, of course, may alter the discoloration of cyanosis and clinical symptoms. As with other hemoglobinopathies, arterial oxygen tension is normal unless co-existing disease is present.

To date, about 79 cases of "sulfhemoglobinemia" have been reported in the English literature, with the alleged causes of sulfhemoglobinemia being identified in 76. Only three papers reported confirmation of sulfhemoglobinemia by isoelectric focusing. In the past, the drugs most commonly causing sulfhemoglobinemia were acetanilide, phenacetin, and sulfonamides. Use of Bromo-Seltzer was the single most common cause, but acetanilid, the offending ingredient, has since been removed from this product's contents.

As examples of typical cases, Halvorsen[37] reported the case of an 85-year-old woman who received nitrofurantoin and phenazopyridine for a urinary tract infection. She was subsequently hospitalized when she complained of dizziness and was noted to exhibit cyanosis. Co-oximetry reported a methemoglobin fraction of 50.3%. The addition of cyanide to blood produced no change in the methemoglobin fraction. Methylene blue administration was given and repeated 1 hour later without effect. On the ninth day of hospitalization, co-oximetry reported a methemoglobin fraction of 26.5%. Her symptoms gradually resolved, but 9 months later she was inadvertently rechallenged with phenazopyridine in combination with co-trimoxazole. She was admitted to the hospital on the seventh day of therapy for cyanosis and what was reported to be a 30% methemoglobin fraction by co-oximetry. Again, methylene blue was given without effect, and cyanosis and reported methemoglobin fractions decreased over several weeks to months.

Basset and associates[38] reported the case of a 37-year-old man who was admitted with chronic anemia and cyanosis. For two weeks he had been taking an average of 100 tablets per week of aspirin, codeine, and phenacetin for headaches. Total hemoglobin concentration was 9 g/dL, the reticulocyte count was 12%, and Heinz body formation was observed. Diagnosis of sulfhemoglobinemia was made after identification of absorption spectra at 620 nm without change after addition of cyanide. Confirmation was performed with isoelectric focusing.

Chawla and co-workers[39] described a patient who ingested 3 g of dapsone in a suicide attempt and presented with cyanosis, tachycardia, and tachypnea. Laboratory studies revealed both methemoglobinemia (4.3 g/dL) and sulfhemoglobinemia (0.25 g/dL). Methylene blue therapy produced a resolution in cyanosis and methemoglobinemia and thus was continued for a total of 36 hours. Forty-eight hours later, the patient again became cyanotic, and repeat studies revealed that the methemoglobin concentration had decreased to 0.7 g/dL while the sulfhemoglobin level had risen to 0.39 g/dL.

Treatment

There is no specific antidote for sulfhemoglobinemia. Methylene blue does not confer any beneficial effect. Treatment centers on ensuring adequate oxygen delivery to tissues through the correction of coexistent methemoglobinemia and anemia (frequently from hemolysis) and on promoting maximal oxygen-carrying capacity with administration of oxygen when the patient is symptomatic. In the rare, severe case, transfusions have been performed, with a resultant increase in total hemoglobin concentration and a decrease in sulfhemoglobin fraction and concentration.

Other Erythrocyte Disorders

In addition to oxidant stress, anemia from other or unclear causes may occur in various acute or chronic poisonings (Table 13–5). Hemolysis from damaged red cell membranes may follow some poisonous snake bites or *Loxosceles* envenomations. Impaired heme or erythrocytic synthesis explains at least some of the anemias seen in those with toxicity produced by arsenic, lead, aluminum, colchicine, podophyllum, and nitrous oxide. Acute lead poisoning (from acute single ingestions of large amounts of lead) may be accompanied by profound hemolysis. The ingestion of zinc supplements prevents the absorption of copper and may lead to a sideroblastic anemia.[40]

Elevated values for mean erythrocytic cell volumes suggest the presence of several different toxins (Table 13–6). Refractory anemia seen in benzene-induced myelodysplastic syndromes may also be accompanied by an increased mean cell volume.

Carboxyhemoglobin is covered in detail in a separate chapter of this book. Like other dyshemoglobinemias, carboxyhemoglobin produces a per cent satu-

Table 13–5. Other Causes of Anemia in Acute and Chronic Poisoning*

Aluminum	*Loxosceles* spiders
Arsenic	Nitrous oxide
Benzene	Oxidizing agents (see Table 13–1)
Chemotherapeutic agents	Podophylum
Colchicine	Radiation
Ethanol	Snake envenomation
Lead	Zinc

*In many cases, the exact mechanism by which anemia occurs remains unknown.

Table 13–6. Agents That Elevate Erythrocytic Mean Cell Volume During Poisoning*

Arsenic
Benzene (myelodysplastic syndrome)
Methanol
Nitrous oxide

*Excluded are the multitude of agents that elevate erythrocytic mean cell volume when given at therapeutic doses.

ration gap. Like methemoglobin, carboxyhemoglobin does not carry oxygen and shifts the oxyhemoglobin dissociation curve to the left, further impairing oxygen delivery. Pulse oximetry does not detect low oxygen saturations that result from carboxyhemoglobin. Accurate diagnosis is made with the use of co-oximetry.

Porphyrias are diseases resulting from deficiencies of various enzymes involved in heme synthesis. Although a multitude of agents given at therapeutic doses have exacerbated or triggered onset of crises in patients with porphyrias, the chronic ingestion of grain treated with hexachlorobenzene (a fungicide) serves as the main example of a toxin's being primarily responsible for an outbreak of porphyria (porphyria cutanea tarda).[41] It is now recognized that most patients with idiopathic porphyria cutanea suffer from hepatitis C, and it is unclear whether hepatitis C played an important predisposing role in hexachlorobenzene-induced porphyria.

LEUKOCYTES

Although hundreds of pharmaceutical agents given at therapeutic doses produce leukopenia as an adverse effect, the presence of leukopenia in acute or chronic poisoning suggests only a few causes (Table 13–7). Leukopenia occurring after acute overdoses of chemotherapeutic drugs may not appear for several days, and commonly reaches a nadir in 1 to 3 weeks. In contrast, the leukopenia following colchicine poisoning is frequently severe and of rapid onset, with leukopenia appearing within 48 hours.[42] Leukopenia commonly accompanies the sideroblastic anemia seen in copper deficiency from the ingestion of excessive zinc supplements.[40] Some types of nonlymphocytic leukemias might result as part of a benzene-induced myelodysplastic syndrome after chronic exposure.

Table 13–7. Toxins Producing Leukopenia During Poisoning

Benzene (myelodysplastic syndrome)
Chemotherapeutic agents
Colchicine
Metals
Podophyllum
Radiation

PLATELETS

Thrombocytopenia may result from bone marrow suppression (e.g., by chemotherapeutic drugs, colchicine, or arsenic), increased destruction by enzymes (e.g., after snake bite), or an intoxication complicated by disseminated intravascular coagulation. In the authors' experience and in that of others, severe acetaminophen toxicity (with hepatic failure) may be accompanied by profound thrombocytopenia.[43] Most thrombocytopenia seen in patients who have received therapeutic doses of drugs is immune mediated.

Numerous pharmaceutical agents impair platelet function at therapeutic doses and, of course, at toxic doses. Examples include aspirin, nonsteroidal anti-inflammatory drugs, ticlopidine, dipyridamole, and nitroglycerin. Despite inhibition of platelet function, bleeding is a rare cause of serious morbidity or mortality after acute poisonings by these agents.

References

1. Evans AS, Enzer N, Eder HA, et al: Hemolytic anemia with paroxysmal methemoglobinemia and sulfhemoglobinemia. Arch Intern Med *86*:22, 1950.
2. Curry SC: Methemoglobinemia. Ann Emerg Med *11*:214, 1982.
3. Weatherall DJ, Clegg JB, Higgs DR, et al: The hemoglobinopathies. *In* Scriver CR, Beaudet AL, Sly WS, et al (eds): The Metabolic and Molecular Bases of Inherited Disease. 7th ed. New York, McGraw-Hill Book Co., pp 3417–3484, 1995.
4. Yoo D, Lessin LS: Drug-associated "bite cell" hemolytic anemia. Am J Med *92*:243, 1992.
5. Savides MC, Oehme FW, Leipold HW: Effects of various antidotal treatments on acetaminophen toxicosis and biotransformation in cats. Am J Vet Res *46*:1485, 1985.
6. Jaffe ER, Hultquist DE: Cytochrome b_5 reductase deficiency and enzymopenic hereditary methemoglobinemia. *In* Scriver CR, Beaudet AL, Sly WS, et al (eds): The Metabolic and Molecular Bases of Inherited Disease. 7th ed. New York, McGraw-Hill Book Co., pp 3399–3415, 1995.
7. Yano SS, Danish EH, Hsia YE: Transient methemoglobinemia with acidosis in infants. J Pediatr *100*:415, 1982.
8. Luk G, Riggs D, Luque M: Severe methemoglobinemia in a 3-week-old infant with urinary tract infection. Crit Care Med *19*:1325, 1991.
9. Curry SC, Arnold-Capell P: Toxic effects of drugs used in the ICU: Nitroprusside, nitroglycerin, and angiotensin-converting enzyme inhibitors. Crit Care Clin *7*:555, 1991.
10. Lukens JN: The legacy of well-water methemoglobinemia. JAMA *257*:2793, 1987.
11. Ralston AC, Webb RK, Runciman WB: Potential errors in pulse oximetry: III. Effects of interference, dyes, dyshaemoglobins and other pigments. Anaesthesia *46*:291, 1991.
12. Henretig FM, Gribetz B, Kearney T, et al: Interpretation of color change in blood with varying degree of methemoglobinemia. Clin Toxicol *26*:293, 1988.
13. Spurzem JR, Bonekat HW, Shigeoka JW: Factitious methemoglobinemia caused by hyperlipemia. Chest *86*:84, 1984.
14. Kirlangitis JJ, Middaugh RE, Zablocki A, et al: False indication of arterial oxygen desaturation and methemoglobinemia following injection of methylene blue in urological surgery. Mil Med *155*:260, 1990.
15. Reay DT, Insalaco SJ, Eisele JW: Postmortem methemoglobin concentrations and their significance. J Forensic Sci *29*:1160, 1984.
16. Berlin G, Brodin B, Hilden J-O: Acute dapsone intoxication: A case treated with continuous infusion of methylene blue, forced diuresis, and plasma exchange. J Toxicol Clin Toxicol *22*:537, 1985.

17. Lamont ASM, Roberts MS, Holdsworth DG, et al: Relationship between methaemoglobin production and methylene blue plasma concentrations under general anaesthesia. Anaesth Intensive Care *14*:360, 1986.
18. Way JL, Leung P, Sylvester DM, et al: Methaemoglobin formation in the treatment of acute cyanide intoxication. *In* Ballantyne B, Marrs TC (eds): Clinical and Experimental Toxicology of Cyanides. Bristol, England, IOP Publishing Ltd., pp 402–412, 1987.
19. Stossel TP, Jennings RB: Failure of methylene blue to produce methemoglobinemia *in vivo*. Am J Clin Pathol *45*:600, 1966.
20. Kirsch IR, Cohen HJ: Heinz body hemolytic anemia from the use of methylene blue in neonates. J Pediatr *96*:276, 1980.
21. Crooks J: Haemolytic jaundice in a neonate after intra-amniotic injection of methylene blue. Arch Dis Child *57*:872, 1982.
22. McEnerney JK, McEnerney LN: Unfavorable neonatal outcome after intraamniotic injection of methylene blue. Obstet Gynecol *61*(Suppl):35S, 1983.
23. Rosen PH, Johnson C, McGehee WG, et al: Failure of methylene blue treatment in toxic methemoglobinemia: Association with glucose-6-phosphate dehydrogenase deficiency. Ann Intern Med *75*:83, 1971.
24. Coleman MD, Rhodes LE, Scott AK, et al: The use of cimetidine to reduce dapsone-dependent methaemoglobinaemia in dermatitis herpetiformis patients. Br J Clin Pharmacol *34*:244, 1992.
25. Goluboff N, Wheaton R: Methylene blue–induced cyanosis and acute hemolytic anemia complicating the treatment of methemoglobinemia. J Pediatr *58*:86, 1961.
26. Harrison MR: Toxic methaemoglobinaemia: A case of acute nitrobenzene and aniline poisoning treated by exchange transfusion. Anaesthesia *32*:270, 1977.
27. Berzofsky JA, Peisach J, Blumberg WE: Sulfheme proteins: II. The reversible oxygenation of ferrous sulfmyoglobin. J Biol Chem *246*:7366, 1971.
28. Park CM, Nagel RL: Sulfhemoglobinemia: Clinical and molecular aspects. N Engl J Med *310*:1579, 1984.
29. Curry SC, Gerkin RD: A patient with sulfhemoglobin? Ann Emerg Med *16*:828, 1987.
30. Smith RP, Gosselin RE: Hydrogen sulfide poisoning. J Occup Med *21*:93, 1979.
31. Finch CA: Methemoglobinemia and sulfhemoglobinemia. N Engl J Med *239*:470, 1948.
32. Chatfield MJ, La Mar GN: 1H nuclear magnetic resonance study of the prosthetic group in sulfhemoglobin. Arch Biochem Biophys *295*:289, 1992.
33. Azen EA, Bryan GT, Shahidi NT, et al: Obscure hemolytic anemia due to analgesic abuse: Does enterogenous cyanosis exist? Am J Med *48*:724, 1970.
34. Westphal RG, Azen EA: Experimental enterogenous cyanosis and anaemia. Br J Haematol *22*:609, 1972.
35. Michel HO, Harris JS: The blood pigments: Properties and quantitative determination with special reference to spectrophotometric methods. J Lab Clin Med *25*:445, 1940.
36. Carrico RJ, Peisach RJ, Peisach J, Alben JO: The preparation and some physical properties of sulfhemoglobin. J Biol Chem *253*:2386, 1978.
37. Halvorsen SM: Phenazopyridine-induced sulfhemoglobinemia: Inadvertent rechallenge. Am J Med *91*:315, 1991.
38. Basset P, Bergerat JP, Lang JM, et al: Hemolytic anemia and sulfhemoglobinemia due to phenacetin abuse: A case with multivisceral adverse effects. Clin Toxicol *18*:493, 1981.
39. Chawla R, Gurnani A, Bhattacharya A: Acute dapsone poisoning. Anaesth Intensive Care *21*:349, 1993.
40. Fiske DN, McCoy HE III, Kitchens CS: Zinc-induced sideroblastic anemia: Report of a case, review of the literature, and description of the hematologic syndrome. Am J Hematol *46*:147, 1994.
41. Peters HA: Hexachlorobenzene poisoning in Turkey. Fed Proc *35*:2400, 1976.
42. Folpini A, Furfori P: Colchicine toxicity—Clinical features and treatment: Massive overdose case report. J Toxicol Clin Toxicol *33*:71, 1995.
43. Fischereder M, Jaffe JP: Thrombocytopenia following acute acetaminophen overdose. Am J Hematol *45*:258, 1994.

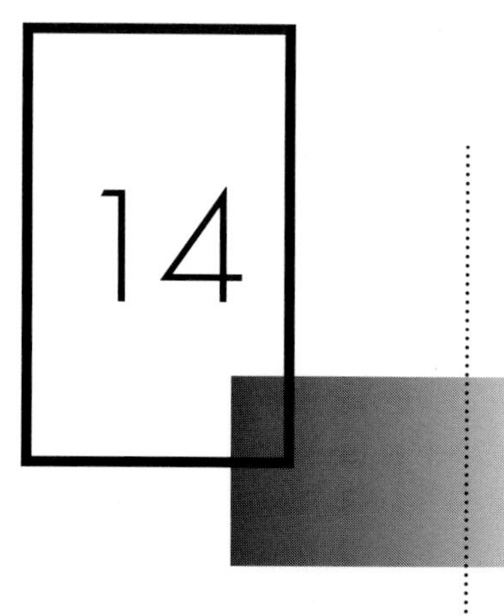

Toxic Injury to the Eye

ANGELA C. ANDERSON, MD

In 1994, 124,680 ocular toxic exposures were reported to national poison centers.[1] These exposures accounted for 6.2% of all poison center calls. Toxic injuries to the eye can result not only from direct contact with caustic substances, but also from systemic agents. This chapter reviews the more common and devastating caustic eye injuries and includes a brief discussion of potential abnormalities caused by toxins absorbed systemically.

Consequences of toxic eye injuries may range from minor eye irritation to total loss of vision. Understanding the mechanisms of injury of caustic substances requires an understanding of the anatomy, physiology, and repair mechanisms of the eye.

THE EYE

Anatomy

The anatomy of the eye is illustrated in Figures 14–1 and 14–2.[2, 3] The *conjunctiva* is the outermost layer of the globe. The portion that overlies the globe itself is called the bulbar conjunctiva, while that which lines the inner surfaces of the eyelids is the palpebral conjunctiva. The next layer is the *cornea,* which overlies the iris and the anterior chamber of the eye. It is continuous with the *sclera*—the white part of the eye. The bulbar conjunctiva covers both the cornea and the sclera. The cornea and sclera meet at the *limbus* (see Figs. 14–1 and 14–2). This area is also the location of the canal of Schlemm, which is the drainage system for aqueous fluid. Posterior to the cornea and anterior to the iris is a space called the *anterior chamber.* Behind the iris are the posterior chamber and the lens. Aqueous humor is secreted by the ciliary process into the posterior chamber, travels through the pupil into the anterior chamber, and drains into the canal of Schlemm. The vitreous and the retina are posterior to the lens.

Physiology of the Eye and Consequences of Injury

The cornea is normally transparent because it is avascular. It derives nutrition from the aqueous humor and oxygen from that which is dissolved in tears. The cornea comprises five layers. The outermost layer is the *epithelium,* which has three major purposes: (1) it provides a barrier to microbial pathogens, (2) it produces cytokines that inhibit collagenase production from fibroblasts, and (3) it produces superoxide dismutase, which scavenges free radicals.[4, 5] Alkali, acids, and other direct eye toxins can damage the epithelium and impair these functions.

The next layer is *Bowman's membrane.* It is not capable of regeneration if damaged. Injuries that extend through this layer always result in scar formation.[6]

The *stroma* is the third layer and makes up 90% of the cornea. It consists mostly of collagen. Binding of alkali cations to collagen causes stromal hydration; thickening and shortening of collagen meshwork occurs as well. Stromal hydration results in loss of corneal clarity; contracted meshwork causes increases in intraocular pressure (glaucoma).[4] The cellular components of the stroma are keratocytes, which are responsible for remodeling damaged stroma. Sensory nerve endings are located here as well; consequently, damage to the stromal layer may result in anesthesia of the eye.

The fourth layer of the cornea is *Descemet's membrane.* Injury to this layer produces corneal hydrops—a condition in which aqueous leaks from the anterior chamber into the stroma and causes corneal clouding.

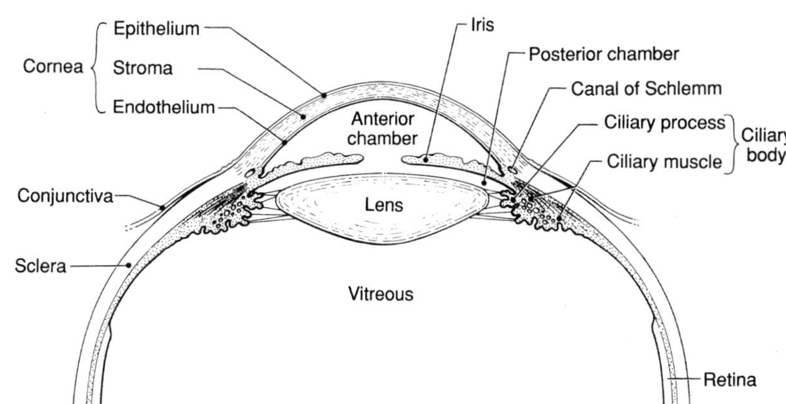

Figure 14–1. Anatomy of the anterior eye: transverse section. (From Sullivan J, Krieger G (eds): Acute Ocular Injury from Hazardous Materials. Baltimore, Williams & Wilkins, 1992.)

The *endothelium* is the innermost layer of the cornea. It is responsible for transporting aqueous back and forth between the anterior chamber and the cornea. Damage to this layer may result in permanent corneal edema.

Damage to the iris and ciliary body may cause either increased intraocular pressure secondary to impaired outflow of aqueous, or hypotony from decreased aqueous production or aqueous leakage. Lens injuries may result in cataract formation.

Mechanisms of Repair

Epithelium

Repair of the epithelium is a two-step process. *Re-epithelialization* is the first step: it involves replacement of lost or damaged epithelium. This is followed by *differentiation,* in which the newly formed epithelium undergoes further morphologic development. Small defects in the epithelium will be repaired in 1 to 3 days; large defects may take up to 2 weeks.[6] The rate of this process, and the ultimate morphology and physiology of the new epithelial layer, depends on the source of the migrating epithelium.[4] If portions of the corneal or limbal epithelium have remained intact following chemical injury, re-epithelialization is rapid and differentiation results in a normal, clear, and stable corneal epithelium. If the corneal and limbal epithelia have both been destroyed, resurfacing must depend on the conjunctival epithelium as a source for the new layer. This is a slower process, which may result in a normal epithelium if the injury was not severe. However, if damage was extensive, the new corneal surface will retain the characteristics of conjunctival epithelium, which will result in vascularization, fibrovascular pannus formation, and loss of clarity. This may cause significant vision loss. Additionally, severe damage to goblet cells may cause abnormal tear film production, leading to chronic ocular surface irritation. This may result in the formation of a *symblepharon*—an adhesion between the palpebral and tarsal conjunctiva.

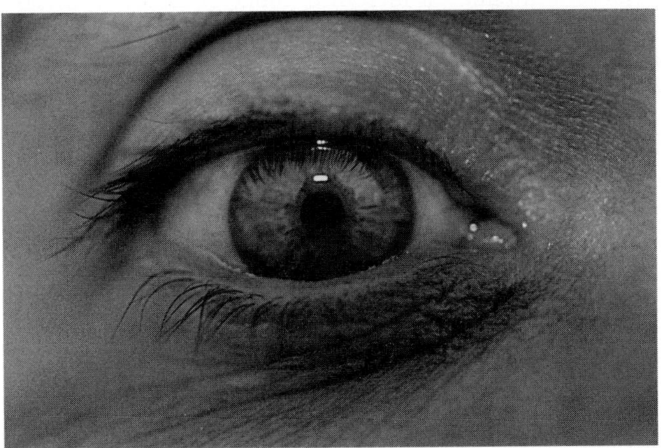

Figure 14–2. Anatomy of the anterior eye: surface view.

Stroma

Stromal keratocytes secrete collagen, collagenase and matrix mucopolysaccharides. If these cells are injured, balanced regulation of the healing cornea may be disturbed and collagen breakdown may exceed collagen synthesis. This causes sterile ulcerations of the cornea, which may progress to perforation.

CAUSTIC CHEMICALS

Alkalis

Chemical Identification and Structure

The most common and severely damaging alkalis are ammonium hydroxide (NH_4OH), sodium hydroxide ($NaOH$), potassium hydroxide (KOH), and calcium hydroxide ($Ca(OH)_2$) (see Table 14–1).

Pharmacodynamics/Mechanism of Action and Toxicity

Alkali burns commonly cause the most severe chemical injuries. By increasing the pH in tissue water, alkalis saponify fatty acids in cell membranes

Table 14–1. Alkalis: Characteristics, Uses, and Ocular Toxic Effects

Alkali	Chemical Composition	Domestic and Industrial Uses	Comments	Potential Complications
Ammonium hydroxide	NH_4OH	Fertilizer, refrigerant, cleaning agents	Highly soluble Extremely rapid penetration	Corneal anesthesia Cataract formation Glaucoma Permanent blindness
Sodium hydroxide	NaOH	Drain and oven cleaner Car airbags Acid neutralization Petroleum refining Treatment of cellulose, plastics and rubber	Second to NH_4OH in rate of penetration	Same as those of NH_4OH
Potassium hydroxide	KOH	Common laboratory reagent	Third highest rate of penetration of the alkalis	Similar to those of NaOH
Calcium hydroxide	CaOH	Mortar, plaster, cement, whitewash	Calcium soaps cause slower penetration than other alkali Particulate matter may provide reservoir for continued exposure	Superficial ground glass opacification

(see Fig. 14–3). This causes cell destruction and allows for further penetration of the substance into the deeper structures of the eye. The depth of destruction influences the potential complications caused by the exposure.

In animal studies in which rabbit corneas are *removed*, the degree of damage caused by various alkalis is dependent on the degree of elevation of the solution's pH, with irreversible damage occurring at a pH greater than 11.0.[7] However, when the corneal epithelium is intact, the extent of damage becomes dependent on the rate and manner of penetration through the epithelial barrier. The rate of epithelial penetration is highest for substances with the greatest fat solubility. Penetration rates of various alkalis (controlled for pH), listed from slowest to fastest, are as follows—calcium hydroxide, potassium hydroxide, sodium hydroxide, and ammonium hydroxide.[8]

Other factors important to the injury process include the concentration and amount of the chemical, the length of exposure, and binding of alkali cations (e.g. sodium, calcium) to corneal membranes.[8]

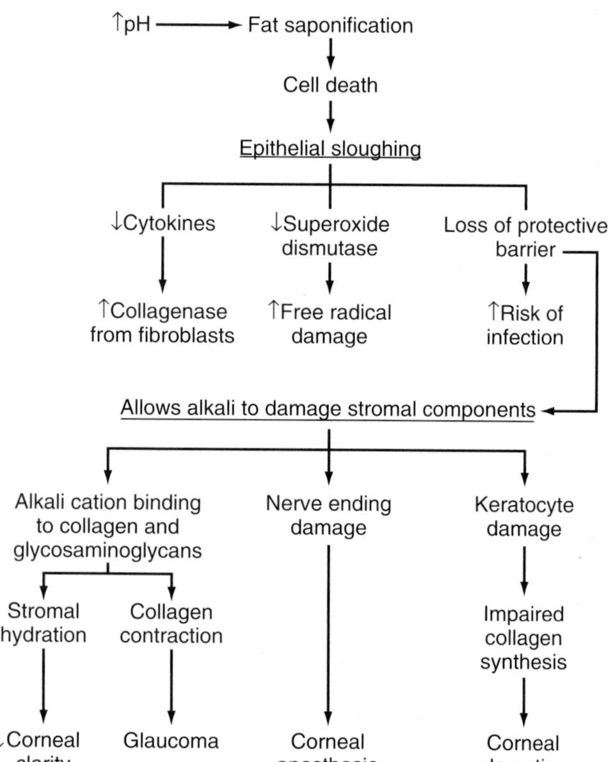

Figure 14–3. Alkali: mechanisms of action.

Clinical Presentation

Pain is the most common symptom associated with ocular injuries. Ironically, the absence of pain experienced in some exposures may yield a poorer prognosis, because some injuries destroy sensory nerves of the cornea, causing anesthesia. Injuries in which ocular sensation remains intact are more superficial and more painful. The patient may also complain of decreased visual acuity.

Specific Alkalis

Ammonia. Ammonia (NH_3) is a colorless gas used as a fertilizer, a refrigerant, and in the production of other chemicals. It is found most commonly in the household as a 7% solution used for cleaning. Available industrial solutions contain concentrations of ammonia as high as 29%.

Fumes of ammonia gas stimulate tearing, which dilutes the chemical and decreases its potential for injury. Consequently, ammonia gas is irritating to the eye, but it rarely causes significant damage without prolonged contact.

Ammonia liquefies under pressure to form ammonium hydroxide (NH_4OH). Aqueous ammonium hydroxide and liquid ammonia cause the most devastating eye injuries. These solutions are highly soluble in both liquid and water. High lipid solubility allows rapid penetration of ammonia into the deeper structures of the eye. The pH of the aqueous humor rises within seconds of exposure to ammonia, while similar increases from sodium hydroxide take 3 to 5 minutes.[4, 9] Aqueous pH returns to normal in 30 minutes to 3 hours, with or without irrigation.[10]

Because of its extremely rapid penetration, ammonia exposures are very difficult to ameliorate by rapid irrigation. As a result, ammonia burns to the eye are capable of causing *all* of the serious complications caused by strong alkalis, including (but not limited to) corneal opacification, corneal anesthesia, stromal edema, atrophy of the iris, dense cataract formation, persistent and recurrent glaucoma, and permanent blindness.[8]

Sodium Hydroxide. Sodium hydroxide (also termed lye, caustic soda, and sodium hydrate) is a white solid that dissolves in water to produce a strongly alkaline solution. Both the solid and liquid forms can cause severe injury to all tissues. It is most commonly found in the home as drain and oven cleaners in concentrations between 0.5% and 54%. Industrial uses include acid neutralization, petroleum refining, and treatment of cellulose, plastics, and rubber. Another, relatively new, potential source of exposure is in car airbags.[11]

The penetration rate of sodium hydroxide is second only to that of ammonium hydroxide; consequently, eye damage can be similarly devastating (see earlier discussion of ammonium hydroxide). Studies performed on rabbit eyes described severe injury and perforation following a 30-second exposure to a drop of 1N (4%) sodium hydroxide; some severe and some mild injuries following 15 to 20 seconds of exposure to a 2N solution; and mild burns from a 0.5N solution for 30 seconds.[8]

Potassium Hydroxide. Potassium hydroxide (caustic potash) causes the same degree of injury as sodium hydroxide.[8]

Calcium Hydroxide. Calcium hydroxide, or lime, is a common cause of alkali injury in the construction workplace. It is a white powdered or granular solid that is used to make plaster, cement, mortar and whitewash. Since calcium hydroxide exists in a particulate form, it is commonly retained in the eye (particularly beneath the upper eyelid) and provides a continuous source of exposure. Fortunately, it penetrates the eye much more slowly than ammonium hydroxide or sodium hydroxide, because it forms insoluble calcium soaps when it saponifies cell membrane fatty acids. The calcium soaps precipitate and make penetration of the cornea more difficult. Consequently, lime may cause many of the complications seen following other strong alkali injuries; however, the iris and lens are routinely spared.[8]

Although calcium hydroxide causes eye injuries that tend to be less severe than those of ammonium or sodium hydroxide, it promotes corneal opacification more quickly than other alkalis.[7] *Mild* lime burns typically cause a frosted or ground glass opacity superficially at the level of Bowman's membrane. They usually result in a significant loss of epithelium, but they rarely affect the underlying stroma. The opacifications in Bowman's membrane observed in mild exposures are secondary to precipitations of calcific material. Therefore, part of the management of these injuries involves the use of disodium edetate (EDTA) to extract the entrapped calcium (see Management).[12] More *severe* injuries occur when the pH is 12 or higher, and these result in stromal opacification and corneal anesthesia.[8] Stromal opacification is a result of actual damage to the structure of the stroma and is not responsive to EDTA treatment.

Acids

Chemical Identification and Structure

Acids can be classified as inorganic or organic (see Table 14–2). Strong inorganic acids include sulfuric, hydrochloric, hydrofluoric, and nitric acids, and liquid sulfur dioxide.[3, 13] These acids can cause significant ocular damage similar to that of alkalis. Common organic acids include acetic acid, formic acid, and phenol; common organic anhydrides include acetic anhydride and maleic anhydride. Typically, the organic acids destroy the conjunctiva and cause little damage to the cornea. However corneal opacification and complete vision loss have been occasionally described with these compounds.[14] Acid anhydrides usually cause more severe damage than their corresponding acids, because of their ability to penetrate the cornea more quickly.[14]

Pharmacodynamics/Mechanism of Action and Toxicity

In most acid burns to the eye, the hydrogen ion coagulates proteins of the corneal epithelium, forming a relative barrier to further penetration of the acid. Consequently, acids cause fewer stromal and intraocular complications and have a reputation of causing less severe eye injuries than alkalis. However, this is primarily true of weak or dilute mineral acids with concentrations of 10% or less. Although acid burns usually cause injury within a few hours of contact and tend to be less penetrating, the ocular surface injuries (vascularization and corneal scarring) can be as severe as those of alkali injuries.

Various factors enhance the severity of acid burns. Significant ocular injury does not occur unless the pH of the solution is 2.5 or less. If the protective epithelium of the cornea is removed or compromised, damage can occur with higher pH substances. Some acids react with water to produce an exothermic reaction. The heat liberated from this reaction damages the corneal epithelium and allows increased tissue penetration. Acids with strong solvent or lipophilic properties destroy cell membranes and penetrate the eye rapidly. Finally, prolonged contact with any acid increases the risk of significant ocular injury.

Clinical Presentation

As with most chemical eye injuries, pain or irritation are the most common presenting complaints.

Table 14–2. Acids: Characteristics, Uses, and Ocular Toxic Effects

Acid	Chemical Composition	Domestic and Industrial Uses	Comments	Potential Complications
Inorganic Acids				
Sulfuric acid	H_2SO_4	Automobile batteries Metal, chemical, fertilizer	Causes thermal and chemical injury	Globe perforation Corneal opacification
Hydrochloric acid	HCl	Metal refining, bleach, plumbing	Strong solvent properties promote cell membrane destruction	Corneal opacification
Hydrofluoric acid	HF	See Table 14–3	Free fluoride ion binds Ca^+ and Mg^+ to cause liquefaction necrosis Possible delayed toxicity	Globe perforation Total globe destruction
Nitric acid	HNO_3	Soda, engraving, metal, fertilizer	Causes yellow opacification of the cornea	Corneal opacification Symblepharon formation
Sulfur dioxide	SO_2	Refrigerant, bleach, fruit and vegetable preservative	Causes eye anesthesia Possible delayed toxicity	Symblepharon formation Conjunctival overgrowth of cornea
Organic Acids				
Acetic acid	CH_3OOH	Vinegar (10%) Essence of vinegar (80%) Glacial acetic acid (90%)	>10% needed to cause damage if exposure brief Severity of damage may be delayed	Minor injury unless concentrated solution or prolonged exposure
Formic acid	HCOOH	Airplane glue Cellulose, tanning, formate	Rapidly penetrating	Minor to severe damage
Phenol	C_6H_5O	Antiseptic, disinfectant, barn deodorant	Caustic to skin and eyes	Corneal hypesthesia and opacification Complete vision loss
Organic Anhydrides				
Acetic anhydride	CH_3COOH	Manufacture of acetyl compounds, cellulose acetates, glycerol Dehydrating agent	Severity of damage may be delayed More damaging than dilute acetic acid	Permanent opacification if delayed decontamination
Maleic anhydride	$C_4H_2O_3$	Manufacture of alkyd resins, pharmaceuticals Dye intermediate Agricultural chemicals	More damaging than maleic acid	Produces damage similar to that of alkali

Initial examination of patients with severe damage may reveal iritis, corneal opacification, or corneal anesthesia. Evidence of these abnormalities usually occurs within hours of acid contact, but they may be delayed, particularly following sulfuric acid and hydrogen fluoride injuries.

Specific Acids

Inorganic Acids

Sulfuric Acid. Sulfuric acid is used in fertilizing, metal, and chemical industries. It can be found in household drain cleaners in concentrations as high as 99.5%. However, most sulfuric acid burns to the eye result from exploding automobile batteries. The most common causes of battery explosions include improper use of battery cables, using a match to read the directions on the battery, smoking while working, and improperly connecting battery chargers.[14] When concentrated sulfuric acid reacts with water in the tear film of the cornea, heat is released, causing both thermal and chemical burns to the eye. Very severe burns may cause complete opacification of the cornea or perforation of the globe with loss of significant ocular fluid.[8] Complications include glaucoma and cataract formation.

Although the ocular damage caused by concentrated sulfuric acid may be devastating, diluted sulfuric acid causes much less damage because the oxygen and hydrogen molecules in the water that dilutes the acid partially satiate the acid's avidity for the same molecules in the eye. Consequently, diluted sulfuric acid produces less of an exothermic reaction on contact with the eye and behaves more like simpler acids, such as hydrochloric acid.[8]

Sulfur Dioxide. Sulfur dioxide exists in both gas and liquid forms. Sulfur dioxide gas is a common component of smog, but in concentrations thought to be too low to cause significant eye irritation.[8] Sulfur dioxide gas has a pungent smell and is irritating to the respiratory tract at concentrations lower than those that cause eye irritation. Exposure to sulfur dioxide gas does not cause significant eye injury because of the body's protective mechanisms.

The most damaging form of sulfur dioxide is sulfurous acid, which is formed when sulfur dioxide is combined with water. Sulfurous acid is thought to be more toxic than sulfuric, hydrochloric, or phosphoric acids, because it is highly lipid-soluble and therefore penetrates the corneal epithelium quickly.[8, 15]

Liquid sulfur dioxide is responsible for all significant eye burns. It is used in fruit and vegetable preservatives and in bleach, but it is most commonly encountered in domestic refrigerators. Eye damage from the refrigerant is attributable to the direct action of the acid itself and not to freezing.[15] The solution is often combined with oil, which causes prolonged contact with the eye.

Symptoms may be minimal following liquid sulfur

dioxide exposure because the acid damages corneal nerves, causing anesthesia of the eye.[15] The patient may not become aware of the extent of the injury until vision becomes impaired, which may develop over hours or days. Initially, the corneal epithelium becomes opacified but remains adherent to the stroma—similar to acid burns. Later, the opaque corneal epithelium sloughs, which may transiently afford the patient improved vision and allows for a better examination of deeper injury. Slit lamp evaluation may then reveal stromal edema, corneal opacity, interstitial vascularization, and damage to the endothelium. This deeper damage is similar to that encountered in alkali burns. Vascularization and opacification may continue for months causing severe vision impairment. Frequent complications include symblepharon formation and conjunctival overgrowth of the cornea.

Hydrochloric Acid (Muriatic Acid). Hydrochloric acid is a weak acid, however it has strong solvent properties that promote cell membrane destruction. Concentrated solutions of hydrochloric acid (36%) are used primarily in the metal refining, chemical manufacturing, and plumbing industries. More dilute concentrations (8.5% to 15%) are found in bleaching agents and toilet bowl cleaners.

Exposure to hydrochloric acid vapors in concentrations greater than 10 ppm causes immediate eye and mucous membrane irritation.[16] A concentration of 1350 ppm for 1.5 hours has caused corneal clouding in animals.[8] Strong protective responses in humans usually limit the degree of exposure so that serious injury from hydrochloric acid gas is rare.

Damage to the eye from hydrochloric acid solutions only occurs when the pH is below 3.[8] The severity of the injury can range from conjunctival irritation to total opacification of the cornea. A 2% solution of hydrochloric acid applied to human eyes for a few seconds has caused no significant injury. An application of a 10% solution to rabbit corneas resulted in corneal scarring 2 weeks following exposure.[8]

Nitric Acid. Nitric acid is one of the most commonly used industrial chemicals. It is found in the soda making, engraving, metal refining, electroplating, and fertilizer manufacturing industries. It is also a common laboratory reagent. Nitric acid exists as a colorless liquid that can cause yellow opacification of the corneal epithelium.[3] It causes tissue damage by binding to complex proteins to form a yellow substance called xanthoproteic acid.[17] Accidental applications of nitric acid to the eyes of newborn babies, given in lieu of dilute silver nitrate, has caused corneal opacification, symblepharon formation, and globe shrinkage.[8] In less severe cases, the opacified corneal epithelium may slough off in 1 or 2 days, and the eye may return to normal as the epithelium regenerates. Nitric acid causes eye injuries similar to those caused by hydrochloric acid burns and is less corrosive than sulfuric acid.

Hydrofluoric Acid. Hydrofluoric acid is formed when hydrogen fluoride is combined with water. Hydrogen fluoride can be a devastating eye, skin, and systemic toxin in both gaseous and liquid states. It has multiple industrial uses and is also available for household use (see Table 14–3).

The damage caused by hydrofluoric acid is related not only to the pH and concentration of the solution, but also to the dissociation of the fluoride ion. Because hydrofluoric acid is largely non-ionized, it can penetrate cell membranes easily. The fluoride ion is released on entry into deep tissues and forms insoluble complexes with calcium and magnesium. This results in liquefaction necrosis, hypocalcemia, and hypomagnesemia. Alterations in calcium concentrations result in an increase in potassium permeability, which causes spontaneous neuronal depolarization and pain. The onset of pain is immediate following exposure to high-concentration liquids, but it may be delayed for a number of days for less concentrated solutions.[18]

Penetration of the fluoride ion may continue for 24 hours, causing progressive damage to the corneal epithelium and underlying structures.[19] Reported ocular complications include tearing, conjunctival irritation and scarring, corneal opacification, uveitis, glaucoma, lid deformities, keratitis sicca, blindness, and globe perforation.[20] Anhydrous hydrogen fluoride has caused total eye destruction that necessitated enucleation.[8]

Animal studies of hydrofluoric acid solutions have shown complete recovery 10 days after exposure to 0.5% solutions, and mild persistent stromal edema and vascularization 40 days following 2% solutions.[21] Instillation of 20% hydrofluoric acid caused total corneal opacification, conjunctival ischemia, corneal stroma edema, and necrosis of anterior ocular structures.[8]

Organic Acids

Formic Acid. Formic acid is found in the airplane glue, cellulose formate, and tanning industries in concentrations of about 60%. It is one of the most

Table 14–3. Uses of Hydrofluoric Acid

Industrial uses
Semiconductor production
Aluminum manufacturing
Glass polishing and etching
Electropolishing of metals
Ceramic glazing and etching
High-test gasoline production
Manufacture of refrigerants
Fertilizer production
Leather tanning
Control of fermentation in breweries
Plastic production
Germicide production
Rust removal in commercial laundries
Photographic etching
Dispensing agents for insecticides
Dispensing agents for aerosol propellants
Household uses
Rust remover
Wire cleaner

rapidly penetrating acids; consequently, immediate and thorough irrigation is tremendously important. A topical exposure to 90% formic acid, that *was irrigated immediately*, initially showed cells in the anterior chamber and loss of epithelium, but recovery was complete in 36 to 60 hours.[22] A solution of 80% formic acid and 2% orthophosphoric acid caused chemosis and epithelial damage that resolved in the eyes that were copiously irrigated, but caused eye perforation and necessitated enucleation in a patient whose eye was less well irrigated.[23]

Formic acid can also cause eye damage if ingested. It is one of the metabolites of methanol responsible for the visual changes that occur in response to methanol poisoning. When fed to dogs and rabbits, formic acid produced histopathology in the retina and optic nerve similar to that caused by methanol.[24]

Phenol. Phenol, also known as carbolic acid, is used primarily as an antiseptic, disinfectant, or barn deodorant. It is available as a pure crystal and in liquid forms in concentrations that range from 1% to 88%.[25] Ocular exposure to 12.5% phenol in 25% glycerol has been reported to cause minor corneal opacification and a temporary decrease in visual acuity that fully resolved in 4 days.[8] Exposure to concentrated phenol, however, can cause conjunctival chemosis, corneal hypesthesia and opacification, and complete vision loss. Phenol is also very caustic to the skin and has damaged eyelids so severely that plastic surgery was required.[8]

Acetic Acids. Acetic acid (CH_3COOH) is an organic acid that is found in the household as common vinegar. Other names include ethanoic acid, ethylic acid, methane carboxylic acid, and glacial acetic acid. Vinegar and most other commercial products contain 4% to 10% acetic acid. "Essence of vinegar" is 80% acetic acid; glacial acetic acid contains 90% acetic acid.

Vinegar routinely produces only minor ocular damage unless contact is prolonged. Consequences of typical exposures include immediate pain, conjunctival hyperemia, and mild, reversible injury to the cornea. Acetic acid, in the absence of very prolonged contact, requires concentrations greater than 10% to cause severe injury.[26] Permanent corneal opacification was described in a woman who fainted after having vinegar thrown in her face.[8] Severe, irreversible damage may result from essence of vinegar and glacial acetic acid.[8]

Trichloroacetic acid causes injury similar to that of low concentration acetic acid.[3, 8]

Organic Anhydrides

Acetic Anhydride. Acetic anhydride, in both liquid and gaseous forms, is necrotizing to tissues and is more damaging than dilute acetic acid. In its liquid form, acetic anhydride causes immediate burning of the eye, followed hours or days later by increasing corneal and conjunctival edema.[8] Permanent opacification can occur if decontamination is delayed. Acetic anhydride reacts with water to form acetic acid. The severity of injury of both acetic anhydride and acetic acid may not be evident until a few days after exposure.

Maleic Anhydride. Maleic acid is a crystalline substance that has the potential to cause severe ocular damage similar to that caused by alkalis. It has a very reactive double bond and may cause protein denaturation.[8]

Solvents

Organic solvents are routinely found in laboratories and in industry. Common solvents include ethyl alcohol, methyl alcohol, toluene, acetone, and butanol. Fortunately, they have no strong alkaline or acidic properties and cause almost no reaction with tissues; therefore, they rarely cause any significant injury to the eye.[8] Contact typically causes immediate pain and may result in partial or complete loss of the corneal epithelium. Usually little or no damage occurs to the underlying stroma.[27] The epithelium commonly regenerates in a few days without permanent sequelae.

Detergents and Surfactants

Detergents and surfactants cause injury that ranges from minor irritation to extensive injury. Detergents are divided into four categories—inorganic detergents, organic detergents, combination detergents, and oil-soluble detergents.

Inorganic detergents (sodium carbonate, sodium silicates, sodium metasilicate, and sodium phosphates) are used for laundering and dishwashing. Liquid and granular automatic dishwashing detergents contain combinations of these agents and have pH values that range from 9.7 to 12.7.[28, 29] The phosphate detergents routinely cause only transient irritation. The non–phosphate-containing detergents (sodium carbonate, sodium silicate, sodium metasilicate) are much more alkaline than phosphate-containing agents (e.g., sodium tripolyphosphate). Consequently, sodium carbonate, sodium silicates, and sodium metasilicate have caused significantly more damage, including total and permanent opacity and corrosion to the cornea.[30]

Organic detergents are composed of soaps and surfactants. Soaps cause tearing and pain, but they very rarely cause significant eye injury. The exception is commercial laundry soap that contains free alkali and has a pH of 12 or higher. These agents have caused permanent corneal opacification.[8]

Combination detergents are compounds that contain both organic and inorganic detergents. They include sodium dodecylbenzene sulfonate, sodium tripolyphosphate, sodium silicate, and sodium sulfate. These agents have caused corneal opacification that resolved in weeks or months in animals.[8]

Oil-soluble detergents are additives to lubricating oils and produce no known eye hazard.

Surfactants are synthetic organic compounds that

have hydrophilic properties at one end and lipophilic properties at the other end. They are used industrially for cleaning and are found in the household in cosmetics, ophthalmic solutions, shampoos, and detergents.

Surfactants can be classified as cationic, anionic, and non-ionic. *Cationic surfactants* are usually quaternary ammonium compounds (e.g., benzalkonium chloride and benzethonium chloride). They precipitate proteins and routinely cause more damage than either anionic or non-ionic agents. *Anionic surfactants* cause cell lysis. Soaps are included in this category. They tend to cause less damage but produce more pain and irritation than cationic agents. However irreversible damage has occurred from 10% docusate and 40% dodecyl sodium sulfate.[8] Non-ionic surfactants usually cause little or no damage but can cause local anesthesia of the cornea. Full-strength tetradecylheptaethoxylate and tridecylhexaethoxylate caused permanent damage in rabbits, and G1690 in concentrations less than 10% has caused severe irritation and corneal opacity.[8]

Cyanoacrylates

Cyanoacrylate adhesives are the components of common household glues such as Krazy Glue and Super Glue. A number of accidental applications to the eye have occurred because the bottle was mistaken for an ophthalmic solution.[31, 32] Childhood curiosity and ingenuity have resulted in a number of pediatric exposures. Applications to the eye have resulted in focal destruction of the epithelium and mild superficial stromal edema that resolved without sequelae.[31]

SYSTEMIC EYE TOXINS

Multiple agents taken systemically cause a variety of eye and vision abnormalities. A detailed description of these substances is beyond the scope of this chapter. However a partial list of various agents and their effects (noted in humans) is depicted in Table 14–4.

PATIENT EXAMINATION

A detailed examination must wait until a thorough irrigation has been performed. It should include an assessment of visual acuity, intraocular pressure, and corneal debris. The lids should be everted and also examined for the presence of debris, particularly in the fornices. A sterile fluorescein examination (using sterile, single-use strips) should be performed as it will allow evaluation of corneal epithelial defects; however, fluorescein examination alone will not provide adequate information about deeper damage. A slit lamp examination is essential to assess the depth of the burn, the degree of anterior chamber involvement, and the potential presence of corneal edema.

Table 14–4. Eye and Vision Abnormalities from Systemic Agents

Substances reported to cause papilledema when taken systemically	
Aspirin	Lead
Bee sting (venom)	Levothyroxine
Chloramphenicol	Minocycline
Chlordecone	Minoxidil
Cisplatin	Nalidixic acid
Contraceptive hormones	Nitrofurantoin
Corticosteroids	DL-Penicillamine
Dynamite	Penicillin
Ergotamine	Phosphorus
Ethylene glycol	Sulfonamides
Isoniazid	Tetracycline
Isotretinoin	Vitamin A
Ketoprofen	
Substances reported to cause nystagmus when taken systemically	
Barbiturates	Methocarbamol
Carbamazepine	Methyl bromide
Carbon disulfide	Methyl chloride
Diazepam	Methyl iodide
Dieldrin	Phenytoin
Ergot	Primidone
Ethchlorvynol	Streptomycin
Ethyl alcohol	Toluene
Glutethimide	
Substances reported to cause central scotomas when taken systemically	
Carbon disulfide*	Ethchlorvynol
Cassava*	Ethyl alcohol
Chloramphenicol*	Ethylene glycol
Chloroquine	Ibuprofen
Chlorpropramide*	Isoniazid*
Digitalis*	Lead*
Digitoxin*	Methanol
Digoxin	Minoxidil
Dinitrochlorobenzene*	Streptomycin
Dinitrotoluene*	Sulfonamides
Disulfiram*	Tetraethyl lead*
Ergotamine	Thallium*
Emetine	Wasp sting* (venom)
Ethambutol*	
Substances reported to cause peripheral visual field constriction when taken systemically	
Bee sting (venom)	Ethambutol
Botulism toxin	Methylmercury compounds
Carbon dioxide	Methanol
Carbon monoxide	Naphthalene
Carbon tetrachloride	Oxygen
Castor beans	Pheniprazine
Chloramphenicol	Quinine
Emitine	
Substances reported to cause cataracts when taken systemically	
Acetaminophen†	Deferoxamine
Allopurinol	Ergot
Busulfan	Lead
Corticosteroids	Trinitrotoluene
Substances reported to cause alopecia of the eyebrows and eyelids	
Dactinomycin	Triparanol
Thallium	Vitamin A

*Also reported to cause bulbar neuritis.
†Has been described in animals, not humans.

PROGNOSIS

The severity of the injury at initial presentation appears to determine the ultimate prognosis of visual acuity.[4, 33] The most widely used grading system for

Table 14–5. The Hughes Classification System

Grade	Description	Prognosis
I	Corneal epithelial damage	Good
II	Cornea hazy Iris details seen Less than a third of limbus ischemic	Good
III	Total loss of corneal epithelium Stromal haze blurring iris details A third to half of limbus ischemic	Guarded
IV	Cornea opaque, obscures iris or pupil More than half of limbus ischemic	Poor

ocular alkali injuries is the Hughes classification.[4, 34] It is based on the degree of corneal epithelial damage and the extent of limbal ischemia. Damage to conjunctival and episcleral blood vessels will cause ischemia and pallor in the area of the limbus.[8, 13, 35] The degree of ischemia in this area is the most important prognostic sign following alkali injury. The Hughes classification divides injuries into the four groups listed in Table 14–5.

MANAGEMENT

Immediate Treatment

The initial management of all chemical ocular injuries requires immediate decontamination by irrigation. A topical anesthetic, such as 0.5% proparacaine, may aid compliance. Occasionally, a lid block may be necessary to relieve severe orbicularis spasm and allow irrigation.[36] The upper and lower eyelids should be retracted, inspected for retained solid material and injury, and irrigated. Contact an ophthalmologist immediately for all severe burns.

Type of Irrigation Solution

Any, *readily available*, sterile, non-irritating solution is appropriate for irrigation. The most commonly available solutions include sterile water, normal saline, and lactated Ringer's. Ordinary tap water is also appropriate, however, normal saline (pH 4.5–6.0) and lactated Ringer's solution (pH 6.0 to 7.5) are preferred because they are isotonic. Balanced saline solution plus (BSS Plus, Alcon Laboratories, Fort Worth, TX) or normal saline buffered with sodium bicarbonate are attractive because they cause less discomfort than the other solutions mentioned.[38] However, BSS Plus must be reconstituted prior to use and costs more than $100 per bottle. Normal saline can be buffered to a pH near 7.4 by adding 0.2 mL of bicarbonate (1 mEq/mL) to 500 mL of normal saline.[37] However, initiating immediate irrigation is again paramount; therefore, the use of special solutions is not appropriate unless they are readily available. Warmed solutions (available in most emergency departments) and the application of topical anesthesia prior to irrigation may also obviate the need for special formulations.

Duration of Irrigation

Prolonged irrigation appears to improve outcome; therefore, irrigation should be performed for at least 30 minutes or until the pH of the eye returns to normal (7.3 to 7.7).[23, 36, 38] Severe acid and alkali burns require at least 1 to 2 hours of irrigation regardless of normal ocular pH.[24] Severe injuries require immediate ophthalmologic consultation. A brief irrigation period (1 to 2 minutes) is needed for most solvent injuries.[8] An irrigation device may facilitate irrigation but is not required.[40]

Special Management Considerations

A few substances deserve special management considerations. Table 14–6 includes a summary of the potential treatments for these compounds.

Ocular Calcium Hydroxide Burns

Irrigation with sterile water or saline should begin promptly. Following irrigation, attention must be

Table 14–6. Special Management Considerations

Chemical	Concerns	Management
Calcium hydroxide	Embedded particulate matter Opacification secondary to calcium binding to Bowman's membrane	Swab soaked in 0.3–1.86% disodium edetate *or* 15 minute irrigation with 0.3–1.86% disodium edetate
Hydrofluoric acid	Binding of free fluoride ions Do *not* irrigate with benzethonium chloride or benzalkonium chloride Do *not* use subconjunctival injections of $CaCl_2$, $MgCl_2$ or calcium gluconate	Irrigate with water, normal saline, lactated Ringer's solution, or isotonic magnesium chloride Consider 1% calcium gluconate drops
Phenol	Decontamination may be difficult	Consider irrigation with 1% diethylenetriamine or 30–50% polyethylene glycol
Cyanoacrylates	Eyelid adhesions	Consider mineral oil or wet compress applied overnight Antibiotic ointment applied overnight may be somewhat helpful Acetone is effective but may cause transient corneal abrasions

paid to identification and removal of solid material, because particulate matter usually accompanies calcium hydroxide ocular burns. It may be necessary to double-evert the upper eyelid and swab or brush away lodged material, looking especially in the fornices, where particles are frequently hidden. Application of a topical anesthetic followed by a 15-minute irrigation with a 0.01 to 0.05M (0.3% to 1.86%) solution of EDTA (at a pH between 4.6 and 7.0) may help loosen and dissolve solid matter.[8] A cotton-tipped applicator soaked in EDTA may also facilitate particle removal. To prepare a 0.05M neutral solution of EDTA, dilute 20 mL of Endrate disodium (150 mg/mL) (Abbott Laboratories, North Chicago, IL) with 180 mL of sterile 0.9% sodium chloride.[8] Disodium edetate may also clear the corneal opacification caused by the binding of calcium to Bowman's membrane (see Calcium Hydroxide above).[12]

Ocular Hydrofluoric Acid Burns

Management of ocular hydrofluoric acid (HF) burns deserves special attention for two reasons. First, in addition to simple decontamination measures, treatment of HF burns is targeted at prevention of further penetration of the fluoride ion. Second, application of some of the methods used to treat cutaneous hydrochloric acid burns may cause damage to the eye.

Because the onset of severe symptoms may be delayed, patients with even minor symptoms following hydrogen fluoride exposure may develop significant pain and damage later. Immediate and copious irrigation is imperative, as with all chemically induced ocular injuries. Irrigation with benzethonium chloride solutions (0.2% or 0.5%) or benzalkonium chloride solution (0.05%) has been recommended for treatment of HF *skin* burns, because these compounds deactivate the free fluoride ion. However, these solutions are potentially damaging to the corneal epithelium of the normal eye and provide no benefit for patients with ocular hydrofluoric acid burns.[8, 20] Multiple irrigations also appear to be deleterious. A single, thorough irrigation with 1 to 2 L of sterile normal saline, water, or isotonic magnesium chloride is recommended.[21]

Injection of divalent cations (e.g., calcium or magnesium salts) binds free fluoride and is also commonly recommended for HF skin burns. Subconjunctival injections with $CaCl_2$, $MgCl_2$, and 10% calcium gluconate can induce significant eye damage and are contraindicated in the treatment of ocular hydrogen fluoride injuries.[20]

Finally, the instillation of 2 to 3 drops of 1% calcium gluconate solution every 3 hours appears to be effective in ocular HF burns. This solution, when used with topical cycloplegia and antimicrobial agents, provided complete resolution of signs and symptoms in a patient with ocular burns from 49% HF seen at a 3-month follow-up visit.[20]

Ocular Phenol Burns

Although isopropyl alcohol is commonly recommended for skin decontamination of phenol, water remains the solution of choice for eye irrigation. The use of 1% diethylenetriamine or 30% to 50% polyethylene glycol has been recommended for eye irrigation, but further investigation is necessary.[8, 40]

Ocular Cyanoacrylate Exposure

When faced with the task of managing ocular cyanoacrylate exposure, eyelid adhesions are usually the greatest source of aggravation for both the patient and the health care provider. The initial management should include warm fluid irrigation through any available eye opening, as this may decrease the likelihood of corneal abrasions (especially if performed within 15 minutes of exposure).[41]

Following irrigation, a few methods have proved to be instrumental in releasing eyelid adhesions. Chloramphenicol ophthalmic ointment applied into the conjunctival sac through a small defect for 24 hours, was followed by cutting the lashes and cutting the adhesions between the margins. This allowed for a hardened shell of glue to be removed.[32] Acetone has also been successfully utilized to loosen glue from the lashes as well as the cornea itself.[42] However, acetone is irritating to the eye and may cause temporary loss of corneal epithelium.[8]

Although these methods may be beneficial, easier methods have also been successful. The application of mineral oil has resulted in immediate softening of adhesions.[41] A wet compress applied overnight also allowed for easier separation.[43]

Final Considerations

After irrigation, re-inspect for particulate matter and other injuries. Check the ocular pH intermittently over the following hour to ensure that the pH remains neutral. An ophthalmic antimicrobial agent should be applied to prevent secondary infection, and a cycloplegic drug may be added to prevent painful ciliary spasms and the development of posterior synechiae. Application of a pressure patch may improve patient comfort and inhibit damage to the healing epithelium caused by blinking. Administer systemic analgesics rather than topical anesthetics for additional pain control. It is also advisable to arrange a 24-hour follow-up with an ophthalmologist, especially if one was not contacted initially. Finally, tetanus prophylaxis should be administered if the patient's tetanus immunization is not up to date.

Special Agents

Many other agents have been found to aid in the healing process following chemical injuries. These therapies are geared toward correcting impediments

Table 14–7. Medical Therapy for Chemical Injuries to the Eye

Agent	Mechanism of Action	Comments
Tear substitutes and lubricating ointments	Lubricant Minimizes trauma of eyelid movement	Use only nonpreserved medications
Topical corticosteroids[45]	Reduces inflammation Anticollagenolytic effects	Impairs the stromal repair process that occurs ~14 d after alkali injuries; should not be continued beyond 10–14 d
Medroxyprogesterone[2] (Provera 1%)	Reduces inflammation without affecting corneal wound repair	Can be used after 10–14 d
Ascorbate[2, 46] (topical and systemic)	Necessary for collagen synthesis Replaces ascorbate depletion that accompanies keratocyte damage	Reduces incidence of ulcer formation following alkali injury
Citrate[46]	Decreases polymorphonuclear neutrophils infiltration	
Retinoic acid[46] (vitamin A analogue)	Promotes corneal epithelial differentiation	Requires further investigation
Fibronectin[45]	Facilitates adhesion of migrating epithelium	Not currently available for clinical use
Epidermal growth factor[45]	Promotes epithelial mitosis	Not currently available for clinical use

to re-epithelialization and improving transdifferentiation (see Mechanisms of Repair). Factors that impair re-epithelialization include damage to the basement membrane, abnormal tear production, and infiltration by polymorphonuclear neutrophils.

Toxin-induced damage to the epithelial basement membrane may cause a decrease in fibronectin, which is needed to help the adherence of the advancing epithelium. If fibronectin is decreased, recurrent epithelial erosions can occur. Abnormal tear film production may lead to chronic ocular surface irritation, making re-epithelialization difficult. Finally, polymorphonuclear neutrophil infiltration will slow the epithelial migration process. Polymorphonuclear neutrophils also produce collagenase and other enzymes that interfere with corneal differentiation. Substances known or currently used to improve corneal healing are listed in Table 14–7.

SUMMARY

Toxic injuries to the eye may be permanent and debilitating. Rapid irrigation is essential to enhance the potential for full recovery after chemical injuries. Consultation with an ophthalmologist is required for all but the most trivial burns.

References

1. Litovitz T, Felberg L, Soloway R, et al: The 1994 annual report of the American Association of Poison Control Centers Toxic Exposures Surveillance System. Am J Emerg Med *13*:551, 1995.
2. Stein H, Slatt B, Stein R: Ophthalmic Terminology. 3rd ed. St. Louis, Mosby–Year Book, 1992.
3. Chernow S: Acute ocular injury from hazardous materials. *In* Sullivan J, Krieger G (eds): Hazardous Materials Toxicology. Baltimore, Williams & Wilkins, pp 433–440, 1992.
4. Wagoner M, Kenyon K: Chemical injuries. *In* Singleton B, Hersh P, Kenyon K (eds): Eye Trauma. St. Louis, Mosby–Year Book, pp 79–94, 1991.
5. Johnson-Wint B, Gross J: Regulation of connective tissue collagenase production: Stimulation from adult and fetal epidermal cells. Proc Natl Acad Sci USA 77:5531, 1984.
6. Onofrey B: Injury to the cornea. Optom Clin *3*:1, 1995.
7. Grant W, Kern H: Action of alkalis on the corneal stroma. Arch Ophthalmol *54*:931, 1955.
8. Grant W: Toxicology of the Eye. 4th ed. Springfield, IL, Charles C. Thomas, 1995.
9. Millea T, Kucan J, Smoot E: Anhydrous ammonia injuries. J Burn Care Rehabil *10*:448, 1989.
10. Paterson C, Pfister R, Levinson R: Aqueous humor pH changes after experimental alkali burns. Am J Ophthalmol *79*:414, 1975.
11. Smally A, Binzer A, Dolin S, et al: Alkaline chemical keratitis: Eye injury from air bags. Ann Emerg Med *21*:139, 1992.
12. Oosterhuis J: Treatment of calcium deposits in the cornea by irrigation and by application of EDTA. Ophthalmologica *145*:161, 1963.
13. Stern A, Pamel G, Benedetto L: Physical and chemical injuries of the eyes and eyelids. Dermatol Clin *10*:785, 1992.
14. Sullivan J, Krieger G (eds): Hazardous Materials Toxicology. Baltimore, Williams & Wilkins, 1992.
15. Minatoya H: Eye injuries from exploding car batteries. Arch Ophthalmol *96*:477, 1978.
16. Grant W: Ocular injury due to sulfur dioxide. Arch Ophthalmol *38*:755, 1947.
17. Finkel A, Hamilton A, Hardy H: Hamilton and Hardy's Industrial Toxicology. 4th ed. Boston, John Wright & Sons Ltd., 1983.
18. Patnaik P: A comprehensive guide to the hazardous properties of chemical substances. New York, Van Nostrand Reinhold, 1992.
19. Hatai J, Weber J, Doizaki K: Hydrofluoric acid burns of the eye: Report of possible delayed toxicity. J Toxicol Cutan Ocular Toxicol *5*:179, 1986.
20. Ellenhorn M, Barceloux D: Medical Toxicology. 1st ed. New York, Elsevier, 1988.
21. Bentur Y, Tannenbaum S, Yaffe Y, et al: The role of calcium gluconate in the treatment of hydrofluoric acid eye burn. Ann Emerg Med *22*:161, 1993.
22. McCulley J, Whiting D, Petitt M, et al: Hydrofluoric acid burns of the eye. J Occup Med *25*:447, 1983.
23. Sudarsky D: Ocular injury due to formic acid. Arch Ophthalmol *74*:805, 1965.
24. Saari K, Leinonen J, Aine E: Management of chemical eye injuries with prolonged irrigation. Acta Ophthalmol Suppl *161*:52, 1984.
25. Fink W: The ocular pathology of methyl alcohol poisoning. Am J Ophthalmol *26*:694, 1943.
26. Gosselin R, Smith R, Hodge H: Clinical Toxicology of Commercial Products. 5th ed. Baltimore, Williams & Wilkins, 1984.
27. McCulley J: Chemical Agents. *In* Smolin G, Thoft A (eds): The Cornea. 3rd ed. Boston, Little, Brown & Co., pp 617–633, 1994.
28. Teir H: Toxicologic effects of the eyes at work. Acta Ophthalmol Suppl *161*:60, 1984.

29. Krenzelok E: Liquid automatic dishwashing detergents: A profile of toxicity. Ann Emerg Med *18*:61, 1989.
30. Winter M, Ellis M: Automatic dishwashing detergents: Their pH, ingredients, and a retrospective look. Vet Hum Toxicol *28*:536, 1986.
31. Scharpf L, Hill I, Kelly R: Relative eye-injury potential of heavy-duty phosphate and non-phosphate laundry detergents. Food Chem Toxicol *10*:829, 1972.
32. Margo C, Trobe J: Tarsorraphy from accidental instillation of cyanoacrylate adhesive in the eye. JAMA *247*:660, 1982.
33. Morgan S, Astbury N: Inadvertent self administration of Superglue: A consumer hazard. BMJ *289*:226, 1984.
34. Saini J, Sharma A: Ocular chemical burns—clinical and demographic profile. Burns *19*:67, 1993.
35. Hughes W: Alkali burns of the cornea: II. Clinical and pathologic course. Arch Ophthalmol *36*:189, 1946.
36. Reim M: The results of ischemia in chemical injuries. Eye *6*:376, 1992.
37. Belin M, Catalano R, Scott J: Burns of the eye. *In* Catalano R, Belin M (eds): Ocular Emergencies, Philadelphia, W.B. Saunders Co., pp 179–197, 1992.
38. Herr R, White G, Bernhisel K, et al: Clinical comparison of ocular irrigation fluids following chemical injury. Am J Emerg Med *9*:228, 1991.
39. Onofrey B: Management of corneal burns. Optom Clin *4*:31, 1995.
40. Fernandes C: Eye irrigating lenses. Arch Emerg Med *8*:274, 1991.
41. Brown V, Box V, Simpson B: Decontamination procedures for skin exposed to phenolic substances. Arch Environ Health *30*:1–6, 1975.
42. Dean B, Krenzelok E: Cyanoacrylates and corneal abrasions. Clin Toxicol *27*:169, 1989.
43. Turss U, Turss R, Refojo M: Removal of isobutyl cyanoacrylate adhesive from the cornea with acetone. Am J Ophthalmol *70*:725, 1970.
44. Raynor L: Treatment for inadvertent cyanoacrylate tarsorrhaphy. Arch Ophthalmol *106*:1033, 1988.
45. Wagoner M, Kenyon K: Chemical injuries of the eye. *In* Albert D, Jakobeic F, Robinson N (eds): Principles and Practice of Ophthalmology. Philadelphia, WB Saunders, pp 234–244, 1994.
46. Pfister R, Haddox J, Yuille-Barr D: The combined effect of citrate/ascorbate treatment in alkali-injured rabbit eyes. Cornea *10*:100–104, 1991.

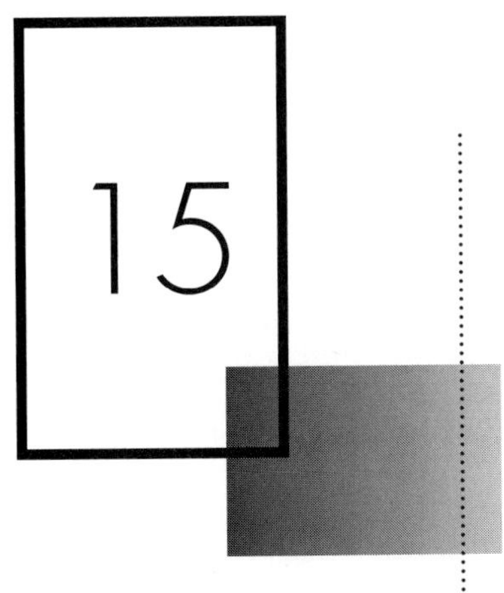

Endocrine Agent Toxicity

K. PATRICK OBER, MD

Endocrine systems are regulatory in nature, aimed at maintaining and preserving the stability and consistency of functions that are essential to the entire organism. The regulatory hormonal systems are a vast array of receptor mechanisms that continuously assess changes in the input of diverse signals of both internal and external origin. (These signals may range from photons of light to variations in nutrient availability, alterations in blood pressure, and a multitude of other stimuli.) The information gleaned by these receptor mechanisms is coupled to output mechanisms (the secretion of hormones) that act to compensate for the newly recognized changes in the environment and thereby maintain stability of function.

An *endocrine agent* may be readily defined as either a hormone or a drug that is used to alter a hormone level or a hormone effect. However, the definition of a *toxic* action of an endocrine agent is not quite as clear; all endocrine factors follow a steady continuum from physiologic to toxic effects, with no clear-cut demarcations. A metabolic response that is totally appropriate and reasonable in one situation can yield very deleterious and life-threatening results in another setting.[1] For example, a physiologic dose of insulin that maintains a normal glucose level when a patient with insulin-dependent diabetes eats a meal becomes a toxic dose if the meal is forgotten and a hypoglycemic seizure ensues. A dose of propylthiouracil that initially restores a severely thyrotoxic patient to euthyroid status could eventually render that same patient severely myxedematous. Similarly, administration of a high dose of a glucocorticoid may be life sustaining in an addisonian patient after a severe automobile accident, but continued use of the same dose for many years may lead to the complications of steroid-induced diabetes mellitus and osteoporosis. Thus, the difference between a physiologic effect and a toxic action of an endocrine agent is frequently situational and is commonly more a quantitative than a qualitative issue. Additionally, a time element is frequently a factor in the development of endocrine toxicity, and much of the toxicity of endocrine agents may not be acute and flagrant; instead, a substantial amount of the potential toxicity from endocrine agents may be chronic, gradual, and subtle in its development.

HYPOTHALAMIC AGENTS

Oxytocin is an octapeptide produced in the hypothalamus and stored in the posterior pituitary. It has uterine stimulatory action, a vasopressive effect, and an antidiuretic effect. It also stimulates the milk letdown reflex. Oxytocin is primarily used for medical induction of labor or for augmentation of uterine contractions, as well as for prevention of postpartum uterine atony and hemorrhage. Its adverse effects are primarily related to exaggerated expression of its physiologic properties. Adverse actions from oxytocin use include overstimulation of the uterus, with potential for fetal distress or uterine rupture, hypertension, or water intoxication (Table 15–1). Careful monitoring during intravenous infusion is essential for prevention of these problems, and the infusion must be discontinued immediately at the first evidence of adverse effect on the mother or her fetus. Hyponatremia, resulting from the intrinsic antidiuretic action of the molecule, can lead to various neurologic consequences, including convulsions. Management of oxytocin toxicity is the same as that for vasopressin toxicity (discussed next).

Table 15–1. Actions and Adverse Effects of Hypothalamic Agents

Agent	Physiologic or Pharmacologic Actions	Adverse Effects
Oxytocin	Uterine contraction; milk letdown	Fetal distress, uterine rupture Hypertension Water intoxication
Vasopressin	Free water retention	Water intoxication
Thyrotropin-releasing hormone	TSH stimulation	Minimal, transient
GH-releasing hormone	GH stimulation	Same as GH (see Table 15–2)
Corticotropin-releasing hormone	ACTH stimulation	Minimal, transient
Gonadotropin-releasing hormone	FSH/LH stimulation (with episodic pulsing: gonadorelin)	Ovarian hyperstimulation
	FSH/LH suppression (with sustained delivery: goserelin, histrelin, leuprolide, nafarelin)	Hypogonadism related (e.g., osteoporosis)

TSH, thyroid-stimulating hormone; GH, growth hormone; ACTH, adrenocorticotropic hormone; FSH, follicle-stimulating hormone; LH, luteinizing hormone.

Vasopressin and its analogues *(desmopressin, lypressin)* are used primarily for hormone replacement therapy in patients with central diabetes insipidus. As with any hormone replacement, toxic effects are uncommon if the agent is used in appropriate dosage, and the major adverse effects are related to the expected physiologic action of the molecule in question. Desmopressin (DDAVP) has emerged as the most commonly used vasopressin analogue for several reasons, including its convenient forms of administration and its prolonged half-life with enhanced antidiuretic and decreased vasopressor effects compared with the parent arginine vasopressin molecule.[2] Because of the drug's physiologic action, hypertension might also be anticipated as a possible adverse effect of vasopressin administration, but this is also very uncommon (particularly with desmopressin). Hyponatremia is the most likely adverse result of vasopressin administration but is a relatively uncommon problem, because hyponatremia cannot develop unless the vasopressin-stimulated decrease in renal tubular free water clearance is combined with an increase in free water intake. If it develops, hyponatremia is effectively treated by restriction of free water intake and a decrease in (or discontinuation of) vasopressin administration. As with any state of severe hyponatremia or hypo-osmolality, the use of hypertonic saline may be a consideration if the decrease in sodium concentration has been abrupt, is associated with neurologic abnormalities, and has not responded promptly to removal of the precipitating causes. The hypothalamic releasing hormones include thyrotropin-releasing hormone (TRH, or protirelin), gonadotropin-releasing hormone (GnRH, or gonadorelin), growth hormone–releasing hormone (GHRH), and corticotropin-releasing hormone. For the most part, these drugs are used as investigative or diagnostic agents, and toxic effects are limited and transient (and may include flushing, nausea, vomiting, brief abdominal discomfort, and occasional hypotension). No therapy is usually required in view of the brief duration of these effects. If hypotension persists, administration of intravenous fluids corrects the problem. In addition to their diagnostic use, two of the releasing hormones (GHRH and GnRH) have potential therapeutic uses.

GnRH is used for treatment of infertility in women who have hypothalamic disease with intact pituitary function, enabling them to respond to the hypothalamic agent. Treatment involves episodic pulsatile delivery of the peptide by an infusion pump.[3] Side effects include a potential for ovarian hyperstimulation (described further in the discussion on gonadotropins); because of this potential, this agent should be used only by reproductive endocrinologists who are well trained in its application. Sustained (nonpulsatile) delivery of GnRH analogues (so-called "superagonists") suppresses gonadotropin production (through down-regulation of the GnRH receptor), and thus these analogues (*goserelin, histrelin, leuprolide,* and *nafarelin*) are used when inhibition of gonadal function is desired (such as in patients with precocious puberty or carcinoma of the prostate or endometrium). Side effects are minor, with the major effects due to the expected suppression of gonadal function (osteoporosis).

GHRH is an investigational agent that may eventually have utility in therapy of individuals who have growth failure due to hypothalamic dysfunction but who maintain normal pituitary function. No significant toxicity has been described.

PITUITARY

Pituitary Hormones

The toxicity of growth hormone (GH) can be related to two different factors: (1) contaminants that might be inadvertently administered with the hormone and (2) the metabolic and physiologic effects of the hormone per se (Table 15–2). With the current era of recombinant DNA-produced GH (somatropin, somatrem), the former consideration is not a realistic concern. However, before the advent of the technology that led to biosynthetic GH production, the only available GH into the mid-1980s was derived from human cadavers, and cases of transmission of the devastating Creutzfeldt-Jakob infection have been described.[4] Because of the long incubation period for this slow virus, it is possible that more cases will develop in the future in patients who previously received virus-contaminated hormone preparations. Patients who have received these human cadaver–based GH injections are at continued risk and should be monitored for neurologic problems; unfortunately, no effective treatment is currently available.

Otherwise, problems with GH occur predominantly in situations in which the agent is used in excessive doses, thereby causing medical problems that are similar to the problems encountered in acromegaly.[5] Long-term administration can cause edema, hypertension, carpal tunnel syndrome, and arthralgias. Insulin resistance and impaired glucose tolerance are also metabolic consequences of GH administration, especially when the drug is used at supraphysiologic doses. Whether GH administration to adults might increase the risk of cardiovascular disease is a concern, based on the observation that acromegalic patients are at increased risk for hypertension and cardiomyopathy. It is not totally clear whether the cardiomyopathy reflects the cardiac response to acromegaly-associated hypertension or is instead evidence of an anabolic effect of GH on cardiac tissue. Whether GH might be a promoter of tumor growth is also speculated, because GH has been shown to exert mitogenic effects in some animal systems, and

Table 15–2. Actions and Adverse Effects of Pituitary Agents

Agent	Physiologic or Pharmacologic Actions	Adverse Effects
Growth hormone	Anabolic effects Growth promotion	Hyperglycemia Arthralgias Carpal tunnel syndrome Creutzfeldt-Jakob infection (from contaminated pituitary tissue) Hypertension? Cardiomyopathy? Promotion of tumor growth?
Gonadotropins (human chorionic gonadotropin and human menopausal gonadotropin)	Stimulation of gonadal steroidogenesis and ovulation	Ovarian hyperstimulation
Adrenocorticotropic hormone	Stimulation of adrenocortical steroidogenesis	Same as glucocorticoid excess (see Table 15–3)
Somatostatin (octreotide)	Suppression of hormone secretion (growth hormone, insulin, and others) Inhibition of gastrointestinal secretion and motility	Glucose intolerance Gallstone formation Malabsorption?
Bromocriptine	Suppression of prolactin Suppression of growth hormone (in acromegaly)	Orthostatic hypotension (especially first dose) Vasospasm Nausea Central nervous system effects

acromegaly has been associated with an increased risk of premalignant colonic polyps and colon cancer. It has also been suggested that GH therapy in children may be associated with increased risk of leukemia. Despite this speculation, GH therapy has no established association with any malignancy at this time.

Gonadotropin therapy is used in individuals with secondary gonadal dysfunction, primarily as treatment for infertility. *Human chorionic gonadotropin (hCG)* binds to luteinizing hormone receptors and thereby stimulates gonadal function. hCG promotes gonadal steroidogenesis and stimulates the aromatase enzyme that converts testosterone to estradiol; as a result, males have a disproportionate increase in estradiol compared with the increase in testosterone, and gynecomastia may develop. Acne, weight gain, and fluid retention can also occur. In order to achieve fertility in males with secondary hypogonadism, simply stimulating testosterone production with hCG is not sufficient; stimulation of spermatogenesis is also needed, and this requires the use of an agent with follicle-stimulating hormone effect; *human menopausal gonadotropin (hMG)* is used for this purpose. Because this product contains both follicle-stimulating hormone and luteinizing hormone, the same side effects of weight gain, edema, acne, and gynecomastia are noted.[3] Women who are treated with gonadotropins for infertility can also develop weight gain, edema, and acne. However, of greater clinical concern, women are at risk of ovarian hyperstimulation. This syndrome, which can occur in as many as 15% of hMG-treated patients, consists of cystic ovarian enlargement and fluid shifts (including ascites and pleural effusions), with more severe cases characterized by severe hemoconcentration, electrolyte imbalance, thromboembolism, and even death. The basis of the disorder appears to be increased capillary permeability with major fluid shifts that lead to hemoconcentration, prerenal azotemia, and development of a hypercoagulable state. Mild or moderate ovarian hyperstimulation can be monitored conservatively, with discontinuation of gonadotropin therapy. More severe cases require hospitalization with monitoring of fluid and electrolyte status, weight, fluid intake and output, hematocrit, and renal function. Sodium restriction may also be required, as well as cautious use of plasma expanders or albumin to maintain urine output. The likelihood of hyperstimulation syndrome can be minimized by careful monitoring of serum estradiol levels; if the estradiol level becomes excessively elevated during hMG stimulation, subsequent hCG administration should be postponed for that cycle.[6]

Adrenocorticotropic hormone (ACTH) is used for its action of stimulating the adrenal cortex. It is used in disorders that respond to glucocorticoid treatment. ACTH is used infrequently because of undesirable properties, which include the need for parenteral administration and an inability to titrate dosage to a specific glucocorticoid level. The unwanted simultaneous stimulation of mineralocorticoid and androgen activity also makes its use undesirable. In patients with disorders that respond to glucocorticoid effect, it is preferable to administer a known amount of glucocorticoid directly rather than to stimulate uncertain glucocorticoid levels through ACTH administration. Furthermore, the ACTH used for therapeutic purposes is derived from bovine pituitary glands and can produce allergic reactions. ACTH is also used for diagnostic evaluation of adrenal gland function; for this short-term purpose, a synthetic but fully bioactive analogue, composed of the first 24 amino acids of the 39-amino-acid human ACTH molecule (*cosyntropin*), is commonly used; this analogue is devoid of adverse effects.

Pituitary Hormone Inhibitors

Octreotide (a *somatostatin* analogue) is used in the therapy of acromegaly because of its ability to lower GH levels and potentially to reduce the mass of the pituitary adenoma.[7] Somatostatin also has a suppressive effect on many other hormone systems; therefore, octreotide is also used in treatment of other active hormone-producing tumors such as carcinoid tumors and vasoactive intestinal polypeptide–secreting tumors (vipomas). As an agent that has an inhibitory action on a number of physiologic processes, it is also used in a number of nonendocrine conditions, including the treatment of various diarrheal states. It is usually well tolerated. Gastrointestinal symptoms are among the most common problems, with nausea and cramps usually being short-term problems. Steatorrhea may occur as a transient problem, although malabsorption with long-term use has been a concern. The formation of gallstones during long-term treatment is also of concern because of stasis caused by inhibition of gallbladder contractility. Effects on glucose homeostasis are complex. The lowering of GH in acromegalic patients would be expected to improve glucose metabolism, but the simultaneous inhibition of insulin can have a diabetogenic effect. These changes largely appear to offset each other in acromegalic patients treated with octreotide.

The major control of secretion of prolactin secretion by the pituitary gland is by the suppressive action of hypothalamic prolactin inhibitory factors, of which dopamine is the most important. *Bromocriptine,* an ergot alkaloid, is a dopaminergic drug that is used to treat hyperprolactinemic states, acromegaly, and some nonendocrine disorders (Parkinson's disease). Its side effects range from minor nuisances to life-threatening cardiovascular changes.[8] At initiation of therapy, adverse effects include nasal stuffiness, lightheadedness, and orthostatic hypotension. Most of these symptoms improve with continued use of the drug. Orthostatic hypotension, which occurs in 1% to 2% of patients, can be particularly severe, and patients should be advised to take their first dose in circumstances where this does not expose them to danger if they should have a significant reduction in blood pressure. The drug also has vasospastic properties, although not as severe as other ergot alkaloids. Digital vasospasm, at times extremely severe, is the most common example, and possible coronary artery vasospasm has also been a concern. It is largely because of such concerns about potentially fatal vascular complications that use of the agent for stopping postpartum lactation is no longer an approved indication. Constipation can occur, and other gastrointestinal symptoms, such as nausea, can be persistent and severe. Most likely related to the first-pass effect of the drug on the liver, nausea can be avoided or minimized with intravaginal administration of the drug, which provides serum levels considerably higher than oral administration at the same dose. Central nervous system effects and neuropsychiatric problems are infrequent but can be severe, including headaches, dizziness, insomnia, sedation, confusion, hallucinations, and psychosis. The psychiatric side effects (as well as most other adverse effects) are dose related and thus are more common in patients with Parkinson's disease (which requires a higher dose than that typically used in prolactinomas or acromegaly). Discontinuation of the agent when pregnancy is diagnosed is a standard recommendation, but no harmful effect on pregnancy has been described in women who have continued to take the drug through their entire pregnancy.

THYROID

Thyroid Hormones

Levothyroxine (T_4), the major product of the thyroid gland, is the prohormone for triiodothyronine (T_3) and is the most appropriate and physiologic replacement form of thyroid hormone.[9] T_4, which has a lengthy half-life of about 1 week, is slowly converted to T_3 (which is the physiologically active thyroid hormone). Because of its short half-life, considerable elevation and fluctuation in T_3 levels can occur in patients who are treated with pure T_3 or combined T_4/T_3 products. Intermittent peaking to supraphysiologic levels can have adverse effects, especially in older patients with cardiovascular disease. As a result, a number of combined T_4/T_3 preparations have been taken off the market in recent years. Nonetheless, the traditional but outdated standard of an earlier era (desiccated thyroid hormone) is still available and used with surprising frequency (despite well-documented problems with inconsistent absorption and bioavailability and despite the fact that its safe use is problematic owing to its disproportionately high content of potentially cardiotoxic T_3 compared with T_4). Use of this T_3-heavy product can result in frequent overdosing and resultant T_3 toxicity.[10]

Long-term physiologic effects of excessive T_4 administration include cardiac changes (shortening of systolic time intervals and increased nocturnal heart rate), elevated levels of liver enzymes, and increased bone resorption; the last is of particular concern in postmenopausal women who already have a high risk of osteoporosis.[9, 11] More overt thyroid hormone excess can be associated with various toxic effects, as suggested by one of the synonyms for hyperthyroidism, *thyrotoxicosis.* The hypermetabolic consequences of hyperthyroidism can include weight loss, tremor, heat intolerance, loss of muscle mass and muscle strength, palpitation, and cardiac rhythm disorders (especially supraventricular dysrhythmias). Cases of true factitious hyperthyroidism are usually encountered in paramedical personnel, although anyone who has access to thyroid hormone can potentially be at risk. In recent years, it has become clear that the previously recommended T_4 doses of 0.2 to 0.3 mg or more daily are excessive. Additionally, some practitioners' continued use of desiccated thyroid hormone (with erratic and inconsistent potency and bioavailability and relative excess of T_3) also can lead to iatrogenic thyrotoxicosis.

In addition to the toxic effects associated with long-term ingestion of excessive doses of thyroid hormone, acute toxic symptoms can occur in the setting of accidental or intentional ingestion of large quantities of thyroid hormone. Excessive thyroid hormone intake is surprisingly well tolerated by young people, who represent the largest group of patients with acute thyroid hormone poisoning; they may have no more problem than some tachycardia and an increase in systolic blood pressure. The clinical course is almost always benign in young children, who may ingest as much as 18 mg with full recovery. The outcome is much worse in the elderly, in whom cardiovascular problems, cerebral embolism, and psychiatric disturbances have been reported.[11] The scope of thyroid hormone–associated toxicity can include sudden death, apparently on the basis of cardiac disease (presumably ventricular fibrillation). Personality disorders and ready access to thyroid hormone are risk factors for sudden death due to thyroid hormone.

In patients who have ingested massive amounts of thyroid hormone, a close correlation between serum hormone levels and severity of clinical illness is not observed, and treatment should be guided by clinical features rather than by laboratory test results.[12] Treatment of excess thyroid hormone ingestion has not been standardized and is largely anecdotal. To a great extent, therapy is symptomatic and supportive.[12] For recent ingestion, induced emesis and gastric lavage are used. Most of the cardiovascular consequences of thyroid hormone excess are mediated through the β-adrenergic receptor, and thus β-blockers are traditionally used to control tachycardia and dysrhythmias. The oral cholecystographic agents iopanoic acid (Telepaque) and sodium ipodate (Oragrafin) are extremely potent inhibitors of the conversion of T_4 to T_3 and have been used to treat patients with hyperthyroidism caused by T_4 ingestion.[12] Extractive techniques such as charcoal hemoperfusion and plasmapheresis have been reported to lower the half-life of total T_4 by 50% to 60% in patients with massive intake of T_4[13]; the ultimate clinical benefit of these procedures is still unclear, and they should be considered only in life-threatening situations.[12] In less acutely ill patients with excessive thyroid hormone ingestion, administration of cholestyramine (which absorbs the thyroid hormone cycled in the enterohepatic circulation) appears to lower thyroid hormone levels faster than the normal clearance mechanisms and may be a useful adjunct when excessive thyroid hormone levels pose an acute risk to a patient.[14]

Antithyroid Agents

Radioactive iodine is a frequently used first-line agent in the treatment of Graves' disease and toxic nodular thyroid disease.[15] There has been long experience with this agent, which is extremely safe. The eventual development of hypothyroidism is an expected outcome of the agent, although not universal. Radiation thyroiditis can occur within the first 2 weeks of treatment, with neck pain, swelling, and transient worsening of the hyperthyroidism. This can be effectively treated with analgesic agents and β-adrenergic blockers, as would be used in other types of painful thyroiditis. Whether radioactive iodine can provoke or worsen the ophthalmopathy of Graves' disease (perhaps by releasing thyroid antigens that stimulate the immune response in the orbit) is debated. Radioactive iodine has not been associated with increased risk of malignancy, nor is there evidence for any teratogenic effect in offspring of mothers who were previously treated with radioactive iodine. Pregnancy is an absolute contraindication to the use of radioactive iodine because of the risk of ablation of the fetal thyroid and subsequent congenital hypothyroidism. Because thyroid destruction becomes a risk only after the fetal thyroid has developed (which occurs at 10 weeks of gestation), radioactive iodine is safe and appropriate therapy for women of childbearing age (despite persisting medical folklore to the contrary) after a negative pregnancy test has been documented; advice to avoid pregnancy for the following 4 to 6 months is typically given.

The thionamide derivatives *propylthiouracil* and *methimazole* are commonly used to treat hyperthyroidism, and they have a generally good track record of limited toxicity.[15] These agents inhibit the organification of iodide and the coupling of iodothyronines, and thyroid hormone synthesis is thus reduced. Propylthiouracil also inhibits the peripheral deiodination of T_4 to T_3. Propylthiouracil crosses the placenta to a lesser degree than methimazole and can be used safely during pregnancy and by breast-feeding patients. In pregnancy, fetal exposure should be limited by using the lowest necessary dose to keep the free thyroxine index in the high-normal range, and monitoring of thyroid hormone levels in the infant of a breast-feeding woman is advocated to ensure that no effect of drug exposure occurs through the mother's milk.[16]

By far the most serious side effect of these drugs is agranulocytosis (frequently defined as granulocyte counts of 250/mm^3 or less), which occurs in about 3 of every 1000 treated patients. This is an idiosyncratic reaction that is more common in patients older than 40 years, but can occur regardless of a patient's age, the duration of therapy, or the drug dose.[17] The fall in granulocyte count is abrupt and precipitous, and thus no benefit is derived from periodic monitoring of blood counts. Most patients with drug-induced agranulocytosis present with fever, sore throat, or other features of infection, and patients taking thionamides should be advised to discontinue their medication immediately and arrange for blood count measurements at the first evidence of an infectious process. The hematologic abnormalities usually resolve within 7 to 10 days; in the meantime, inpatient hospitalization with intravenous antibiotics is usually recommended.[16] The simultaneous use of corticosteroids or granulocyte-stimulating factors has been suggested, but these are not proven interventions and thus are not recommended at this time.[16] Further thionamide therapy (even with another agent) should be avoided in patients who have experienced agranulocytosis from one of these drugs.

Liver disease is also a major potential toxic effect of the thionamides.[17] Drug-related hepatotoxicity seems to be a problem predominantly with propylthiouracil, whereas cholestatic jaundice has been associated with methimazole.[18] Propylthiouracil-related hepatic injury has been fatal in some cases.[19] The presentation is similar to that of viral hepatitis, and most patients recover with withdrawal of the drug. Mild abnormalities in liver function tests are common in patients who are treated with propylthiouracil,[20] and mild abnormalities on liver biopsy have also been demonstrated. This subclinical liver injury is considered to be transient and asymptomatic, and it has been suggested that therapy can be cautiously continued in patients who are symptom free and not jaundiced.[20]

SKELETON AND CALCIUM METABOLISM

Calcitonin, an inhibitor of bone resorption, is used in the treatment of Paget's disease, osteoporosis, and hypercalcemia. Both salmon and human calcitonin are available, and administration is by injection or nasal spray. Local effects are common, including itching and irritation at the injection site. Systemic symptoms are also frequent, including flushing, nausea, vomiting, and anorexia. A slight but asymptomatic decrease in serum calcium levels may occur after injection of calcitonin in patients with Paget's disease. Loss of efficacy is common; this may be related to down-regulation of calcitonin receptors or perhaps development of neutralizing antibodies to the salmon form of this peptide. The use of calcitonin has been limited by the availability of the bisphosphonates, which have similar actions with fewer undesirable effects.

Although not approved for use in treatment of metabolic bone disease, *sodium fluoride* is undergoing investigation (with occasional unlabeled use) as a therapeutic agent for osteoporosis because of its ability to stimulate osteoblast activity and promote new bone formation.[17] Concerns about its use have centered around the potential for abnormal bone formation with increased fracture risk, as well as other adverse effects such as gastric irritation.

Toxicity from *vitamin D (cholecalciferol [vitamin* D_3*], ergocalciferol [vitamin* D_2*]),* its metabolites *(calcifediol [25-OH vitamin* D_3*], calcitriol [1,25-(OH)*$_2$ *vitamin* D_3*],* and their analogues *(dihydrotachysterol)* is uncommon. Although vitamin D is a component of most over-the-counter multiple vitamin preparations, it is present in doses (typically 400 U per tablet) that are too small to cause toxicity. Vitamin D toxicity results from the use of much larger doses (such as the 50,000 U vitamin D_2, or ergocalciferol, capsules) or much more potent vitamin D products (such as 1,25-[OH]$_2$ vitamin D_3, or calcitriol), which are available only by prescription and are typically used for treatment of hypoparathyroidism, other hypocalcemic disorders, and some forms of metabolic bone disease, such as renal osteodystrophy. A more occult cause of vitamin D intoxication is unintentional oversupplementation of dairy products with vitamin D; deaths have resulted from this phenomenon.[21] The toxicity of vitamin D is essentially that of hypercalcemia. Symptoms tend to be vague and nonspecific (including malaise, lethargy, weakness, nausea, and vomiting), but routine laboratory testing identifies the hypercalcemia without difficulty. Management involves intravenous fluid administration (with isotonic saline being the preferred agent for volume restoration and induction of natriuresis, which promotes calciuresis), and discontinuation or decreasing the dose of the vitamin D product. If the responsible agent is calcitriol, the hypercalcemia should resolve fairly quickly (within days) because of the short half-life of this agent. With parent vitamin D (ergocalciferol, or vitamin D_2), the hypercalcemia may persist for many weeks owing to the accumulation of this fat-soluble substance in adipose stores, and additional therapy might include reduction of dietary calcium intake and use of glucocorticoids (which impair vitamin-dependent gastrointestinal calcium absorption) until the vitamin D stores have been depleted.

Bisphosphonates (including *etidronate, pamidronate,* and *alendronate*) are analogues of inorganic pyrophosphate. On administration, these compounds localize to the skeletal surface, where they inhibit bone resorption. This action leads to their use in treatment of Paget's disease, osteoporosis, and hypercalcemic disorders. These drugs, which are poorly absorbed orally, have limited toxicity.[22] Gastrointestinal symptoms such as nausea, diarrhea, esophagitis, and gastritis have been reported. In addition to inhibition of bone resorption, etidronate (but not the other bisphosphonates) can impair bone mineralization, and patients are at risk of developing osteomalacia with chronic etidronate use; as a result, the agent is usually prescribed in a cyclic regimen. Any of the bisphosphonates can transiently worsen bone pain. Other uncommon reactions include a self-limited acute phase response with fever and myalgia, inflammatory eye reactions, skin lesions, erythroderma, and bronchospasm (in a patient with known asthma).

ADRENAL CORTEX

Glucocorticoids

Glucocorticoids (which include *betamethasone, cortisone, dexamethasone, hydrocortisone, methylprednisolone, prednisolone, prednisone,* and *triamcinolone*) are commonly used in the treatment of various medical disorders associated with an immunologic or inflammatory component. Use of these agents is clearly a double-edged sword, however, because the immunosuppressive and anti-inflammatory effects of these agents can have adverse effects on a patient's normal response to infection. Furthermore, the catabolic effects of glucocorticoids can ultimately result in problems such as poor wound healing, easy bruising, and metabolic bone disease. In addition, the metabolic dysfunction associated with glucocorticoid therapy can include insulin resistance and development of overt diabetes mellitus. Long-term use of pharmacologic glucocorticoid doses results in suppression of the hypothalamic-pituitary-adrenal axis. Adrenal insufficiency may ensue if the steroid dose is lowered too quickly or if an intercurrent illness causes a need for higher endogenous steroid levels than the suppressed adrenal glands can deliver. All of these problems are related in general to the dose and duration of glucocorticoid therapy, as well as the mode of delivery. Unfortunately, there is no useful nor reliable algorithm to predict the exact degree to which each patient is at risk for the adverse effects of glucocorticoid therapy, and in any given patient the degree of suppression of the hypothalamic-pituitary-adrenal axis cannot be reliably estimated from the dose of glucocorticoid or duration of therapy.[23] Although inhaled glucocorticoids are considered to be relatively free of systemic effects, even this route of delivery can be associated with the same problems that occur with ingested or injected glucocorticoids.[24] The unpredictability of individual response must be taken into account when dealing with patients who are undergoing long-term steroid treatment, and these patients may be very fragile because of superimposition of the effects of steroid treatment on their underlying steroid-requiring medical disorder; a thoughtful, conservative, and prudent approach to their care is essential. Specifically, stress level steroid coverage is mandatory in acutely ill steroid-treated patients if there is any question of possible adrenal suppression.[25] With severe stress (such as abdominal surgery or major trauma), it is estimated that approximately 200 to 300 mg of hydrocortisone daily, in divided doses, reasonably mimics the response of normally functioning adrenals to a major illness (in contrast to the basal physiologic production of no more than 12 to 15 mg/m^2 per day for nonstressed individuals). In patients who are committed to long-term glucocorticoid treatment, efforts to prevent predictable complications are extremely important; this includes prescribing prophylactic therapies (described later) to block the osteopenic action of steroids, rather than waiting for the first fracture to occur.

The major complications of glucocorticoid therapy (Table 15–3) can be divided into those that are related to acute and relatively short-term steroid administration and those that pertain to long-term use.[26]

For many of the steroid-related complications, there are no specific nor unique antidotes. The generally made recommendations of limiting steroid use to the lowest possible effective dose for the shortest possible interval are inherently logical but may be of little practical use in the management of a specific

Table 15–3. Complications of Systemic Corticosteroids

Acute
Central nervous system
Mood swings (euphoria to depression)
Insomnia, jitteriness
Psychosis (rare)
Pseudotumor cerebri (rare)
Metabolic
Insulin resistance, hyperglycemia
Increased appetite
Edema
Chronic
Muscular: proximal myopathy
Skeletal: osteoporosis, aseptic necrosis
Endocrine
Cushing's syndrome: skin atrophy, acne, striae, hirsutism, childhood growth retardation
Pituitary-adrenal axis suppression
Immunologic: immunosuppression with increased opportunistic infection risk
Ophthalmologic: cataract formation
Gastrointestinal: peptic ulcer (controversial)

Adapted from Claman HN: Glucocorticosteroids II: The clinical responses. Hosp Pract *18*:143–146, 149–151, 1983.

patient who has a clear-cut need for high-dose glucocorticoid therapy for a prolonged interval.

Neuropsychiatric disturbances related to glucocorticoid therapy are fairly common and at times may be very difficult to control.[27] Steroid-induced problems can range from mood disorders to confusion and overt psychosis. The most common problems are emotional lability, anxiety, insomnia, and memory disturbances. Euphoria or psychosis has been reported in 3% of steroid-treated medical inpatients. Symptoms usually start within 5 to 14 days of the onset of glucocorticoid treatment and appear to correlate with dose. The pathogenesis of steroid-related mental changes is unknown, although it has been suggested that steroids affect energy metabolism in the hippocampus and other limbic structures. The diagnosis is made on clinical criteria. The behavioral changes usually last less than 2 months. Although recovery is usually complete, some patients have recurrent episodes, and suicide has been reported in patients with steroid-induced emotional disturbances. Treatment consists of tapering the steroids and using antipsychotic agents such as chlorpromazine.

Increased intracranial pressure (pseudotumor cerebri) has recurrently been associated with steroid use, but its nature and etiology continue to be enigmatic.[27] With use of either systemic or topical steroids, the symptoms usually occur after discontinuation or tapering of steroids (even with a slow taper). Manifestations of the increased intracranial pressure include headache, nausea, vomiting, and papilledema and less often diplopia and abducens (sixth) nerve palsies. Evaluation should include studies to preclude other causes of elevated intracranial pressure, particularly masses. The disorder is usually self-limited, and therapy is empirical (and, unfortunately, recommendations in the medical literature are contradictory—both lowering and increasing steroid doses have been advised). Other suggested approaches have included changing the specific type of steroid, performing lumbar punctures to lower pressure, or using the specific diuretic acetazolamide. Based on papilledema, headache, and vomiting in a patient with Addison's disease, the possibility of steroid withdrawal with rebound edema has been suggested as a mechanism for development of pseudotumor cerebri, in which case increased steroid doses would be logical. However, patients with pseudotumor cerebri typically do not have other features of steroid withdrawal, and a number of reports have correlated the resolution of symptoms of pseudotumor cerebri with the opposite maneuver (i.e., a rapid taper or discontinuation of the glucocorticoid).[27] The papilledema usually resolves in 8 days to 2 months, and headaches clear earlier. In the absence of any true understanding of pathogenesis, a rational approach to management is not available.

Spinal cord compression or nerve root compression can result from glucocorticoid-induced epidural lipomatosis.[27] In some patients, epidural fat deposition (lipomatosis) can cause myelopathy, cauda equina syndrome, or radiculopathy. The majority of patients have received long-term glucocorticoids at relatively high doses and are cushingoid in appearance. The lipomatosis can be seen with myelography, computed tomography, or magnetic resonance imaging. Laminectomy is the treatment of choice.

Osteoporosis is one of the most devastating complications of long-term glucocorticoid therapy.[28] All patients treated with more than 10 mg/day of prednisone have significant bone loss. At lower steroid doses, premenopausal women seem to be relatively protected from bone loss, whereas men of all ages are very sensitive to skeletal loss. The initial rapid early bone loss appears to slow somewhat after 6 months of treatment, but continued skeletal loss is undoubtedly persistent when therapy is continued. Trabecular bone is affected to a greater extent than cortical bone, and thus vertebral compression fractures may be the first sign of steroid-related bone loss.

The mechanism of bone loss related to glucocorticoid therapy is multifactorial.[28] Defects in calcium homeostasis are a major component of the pathology: Glucocorticoid-related impairment of intestinal calcium absorption as well as decreased renal calcium reabsorption (with resultant hypercalciuria) results in secondary hyperparathyroidism. Glucocorticoids also suppress the levels of anabolic factors, which are important in skeletal dynamics, and directly decrease bone formation and enhance bone resorption.

Clear-cut and straightforward data on optimal management of glucocorticoid-induced bone loss are scarce. The best approach undoubtedly is preventive. Dual-energy bone absorptiometry is a sensitive method of accurately assessing skeletal status and can be an excellent method for monitoring bone status in steroid-treated patients (especially important are the spine and femoral neck because of the particular sensitivity of trabecular bone to steroids). Limitation of steroid treatment to the lowest effective dose for the shortest possible interval is always a primary consideration. The choice of the specific glucocorticoid may also be a consideration, because some early evidence suggests that *deflazacort* (not available in the United States) has a less deleterious effect on bone metabolism than prednisone at doses that have comparable anti-inflammatory effects. Avoiding the use of systemic steroids whenever possible is critical, although inhaled agents can also exert systemic effects, which include adverse actions on skeletal mass and impairment of growth in children. Efforts to improve calcium balance are appropriate. Calcium supplements alone can reduce bone turnover, and intake of approximately 500 mg of elemental calcium three times per day is reasonable, along with maintenance of serum 25-OH vitamin D levels at the upper limits of normal (usually accomplished with 400 IU of vitamin D daily) to ensure adequate calcium absorption. The use of higher (pharmacologic) doses of vitamin D, including 1,25-$(OH)_2$ vitamin D_3 (or calcitriol), is risky (because of possible hypercalcemia and hypercalciuria) and of unproven benefit. Some have advocated the use of thiazide diuretics to lower urinary loss of calcium, but this must be done in combination with dietary sodium restriction, and the adverse actions of thiazides may argue against this approach. Hypogonadism should be treated, including supplementation of estrogen (and progesterone if appropriate) in postmenopausal women and in premenopausal women who have steroid-related menstrual disturbances. In men with lowered testosterone levels caused by steroid therapy, testosterone replacement has positive effects on both skeletal mass and muscle mass. Recombinant human growth hormone may eventually have a defined role because of its anabolic effect. Increasing information, however, supports the use of antiresorptive agents, particularly the bisphosphonates. Cyclic use of etidronate has been shown to be beneficial, as has pamidronate (either orally or intravenously). Etidronate once was the only available oral bisphosphonate in the United States, but its use has been limited by its propensity to impair mineralization. The introduction of alendronate provides an alternative with fewer adverse skeletal effects. Because of the lack of toxicity of the bisphosphonates and the increasingly persuasive data supporting their effectiveness, it is very reasonable to use these agents for skeletal protection in all patients who are going to be treated with pharmacologic steroids for any extended interval. Periodic monitoring of bone density on an annual basis is a reasonable way of assessing the effectiveness of treatment.

Osteonecrosis, or aseptic (avascular) necrosis, is a very serious complication of glucocorticoid treatment.[28] It usually presents with pain, and the hip is most commonly involved, although the head of the humerus and the distal femur can also be affected. The process is often bilateral and almost always progressive. The risk of this disorder increases with the duration and the dose of glucocorticoid therapy. The mechanisms of this process are uncertain. Hypotheses about etiology have included the possibility of fat emboli, fatigue fractures through the epiphysis due to osteoporosis, and impairment of vascular bed perfusion caused by increased intraosseous pressure (as a result of steroid-induced fat accumulation). The only definitive treatment for severe osteonecrosis of the hip or knee is prosthetic replacement of the involved joint; in early osteonecrosis of the hip, prolonged avoidance of weight bearing may be helpful.

Steroid myopathy is another problematic complication of glucocorticoid therapy.[27, 28] Patients present with proximal muscle weakness and atrophy, generally painless and symmetric, that affect proximal muscle before distal muscle and involve the lower extremities before the upper extremities. Symptoms may begin several weeks to several months after starting therapy, and higher steroid doses are more likely to cause myopathy. Even brief treatment with steroids can cause myopathy, which may be difficult to distinguish from the muscle weakness of the underlying disease process (such as polymyositis) by clinical criteria; measurement of muscle enzymes such as creatine kinase and aldolase can make the distinction, however, because these levels are not elevated with steroid myopathy. Treatment consists of tapering and discontinuing the responsible steroid. Clinical recovery can occur in 2 to 5 weeks, and physical therapy is helpful in the recovery process; steroid-treated patients should be encouraged to exercise.

In addition to the systemic effects of systemic glucocorticoids, local adverse effects can occur with the inhaled corticosteroids that are used for treatment of asthma.[24] These include an increased incidence of oropharyngeal candidiasis, dysphonia (possibly related to myopathic effects of the steroids), and reflex cough and bronchospasm (presumably related to upper airway irritation by propellants or detergents rather than the steroid itself). There is no evidence of significant change in the bronchial mucosa nor increased risk of acute viral or bacterial respiratory tract infections in patients treated with inhaled glucocorticoids.

Glucocorticoid Inhibitors/ Antagonists

A number of drugs are used in the therapy of Cushing's syndrome and adrenocortical carcinoma. These are not definitive treatments but are instead used for reversal of some of the severe consequences of Cushing's syndrome in preparation for surgery, while awaiting the effects of radiation therapy, or in ameliorating the more devastating effects of Cushing's syndrome in patients with malignancy. Adrenocortical insufficiency is the most obvious adverse effect, although each available agent also has the potential to cause other toxic effects.[29]

Aminoglutethimide inhibits the conversion of cholesterol to pregnenolone, the first step in steroid synthesis. Thus, in addition to lowering cortisol levels, it also inhibits production of other steroids, including aldosterone and estrogen. Iodine-concentrating abilities of the thyroid are also impaired. Adverse effects can therefore include hypoaldosteronism and hypothyroidism in addition to cortisol deficiency. Frequent nonendocrine toxic effects include lethargy, somnolence, and a fairly common maculopapular rash (often associated with fever, within 2 weeks of initiation of therapy, and frequently self-resolving).

Ketoconazole, used primarily as an antimycotic agent, is a potent inhibitor of a number of enzymes of steroidogenesis and has been used effectively to normalize cortisol production in patients with Cushing's syndrome, using doses between 200 and 1200 mg daily. Adrenal insufficiency has been reported with its use. It also lowers androgen production, and this decrement can lead to gynecomastia and reversible loss of libido and impotence in men, as well as a teratogenic effect in male fetuses. Hepatotoxicity is ketoconazole's most significant toxic action, and reversible transient abnormalities in liver function occur in about 10% of patients. Occasional fatal hepatotoxicity is reported. The need to monitor liver function with this agent is obvious.

Metyrapone blocks the final enzymatic step in cortisol synthesis (11β-hydroxylation). In addition to lowering cortisol levels, it also causes steroidogenesis to be shifted toward increased androgen production, which causes hirsutism and mild acne in women. Gastrointestinal symptoms occur with use of the drug but predominantly when overtreatment (and thus adrenal insufficiency) is a factor. Adrenal insufficiency is in fact the most serious adverse effect of metyrapone and can occur when an intercurrent illness develops (with an associated physiologic need for greater production of cortisol, which cannot be delivered in the presence of the agent) or with excessive metyrapone dosage. Monitoring is problematic and potentially misleading from the standpoint that the immediate precursor to cortisol, 11-deoxycortisol, accumulates to high levels with the use of metyrapone; the 11-deoxycortisol cross-reacts to various extents with most cortisol assays, which can give a false sense of security about the appropriateness of cortisol levels.

o,p′-DDD (mitotane) is a congener of the notorious insecticide DDT and an isomer of another insecticide, p,p′-DDD. It blocks cortisol synthetic enzymes and has an adrenolytic effect that results in its use in adrenocortical carcinoma. At the high doses required to treat malignancy (8 to 12 g daily), gastrointestinal side effects (nausea, vomiting, and diarrhea) are common, as are severe neurologic disturbances (lethargy and neuropathy). Because of concern about adrenocortical insufficiency, a glucocorticoid is commonly given simultaneously to lower concern about effects of excessive doses. Dosing is made more difficult by the fact that this drug accumulates in fat and thus continues to exert its effects for weeks after it is discontinued.

Trilostane is an inhibitor of 3β-hydroxysteroid dehydrogenase and is less effective in inhibition of adrenal function than the other agents described. Significant side effects occur in half of the patients who are treated with this drug, with abdominal pain, diarrhea, nausea, and vomiting being the most common.[30]

Mifepristone (RU 486) is a glucocorticoid receptor antagonist that until recently was banned in the United States. It is effective in reversing the manifestations of Cushing's syndrome by blocking the tissue effects of cortisol. The nature of its action makes it a difficult agent to monitor, because the circulating cortisol levels remain high and therefore misleadingly may be reassuring in patients who are overtreated. Patients must be monitored for clinical features of adrenal insufficiency to determine the appropriateness of dosage. (This agent is later discussed further as an antiprogestin.)

Mineralocorticoid

Fludrocortisone is an oral mineralocorticoid agent, free of glucocorticoid activity. Its use is typically for patients with aldosterone deficiency (Addison's disease or other hypoaldosterone states) or for situations in which volume expansion may be desirable, as in patients with idiopathic orthostatic hypotension. The toxic effects of this agent are related to the expected physiologic effects of a mineralocorticoid and tend to be dose related. Thus, excessive volume expansion and hypokalemia are the most likely problems with this agent.

Mineralocorticoid Antagonist

Spironolactone is a very useful endocrine agent. Classically used for its action as a competitive inhibitor at the aldosterone receptor, it is also a fairly potent antiandrogen (because it is also a competitive inhibitor at the dihydrotestosterone receptor and may be an inhibitor of androgen synthesis to some extent), and it also has progestin action. Its potential for toxicity is related to these endocrine effects. Thus, hyperkalemia is a risk in predisposed patients (such as those with renal insufficiency or long-standing diabetic patients who may have hypoaldosteronism); men can experience impaired libido, impotence, and gynecomastia due to the antiandrogen effects (and a theoretic risk, never documented, of impaired genital tract development in the male fetus); women frequently experience menometrorrhagia and mastodynia. These problems all are dose related.[31]

GLUCOREGULATORY

Hypoglycemic Agents

Hypoglycemia, the most common endocrine emergency, can be a result of a vast array of medical and metabolic disorders[32, 33]; of the many potential causes, medications and toxins are the most common causes of acute hypoglycemia.[34]

The immediate therapy for hypoglycemia is fairly straightforward and simply requires administration of glucose to the patient,[32] with the specific cause of hypoglycemia a secondary issue at the time (although simultaneous measurement of insulin and C peptide levels at the time of hypoglycemia eventually provide critical diagnostic information about patients for whom the cause of the low blood sugar level is unknown). For adults who are confused, combative, or comatose, glucose should be administered intravenously, with a dose of 25 g being effective in most cases. Attempts to administer glucose solutions orally to such patients are strongly discouraged because of the very real risk of tracheal aspiration. Another option with comparable efficacy in most patients is the use of 1 mg of intravenous glucagon.[35] Glucagon use should be considered only for patients with a strong likelihood of available glycogen stores in the liver; otherwise, the agent has no effect. Practically speaking, this use is restricted to known insulin-treated patients (in whom the glucagon overrides the insulin-induced interference with hepatic glycogenolysis). In patients who have no hepatic glycogen stores (e.g., patients who are hypoglycemic after a prolonged alcoholic binge or patients who have extensive displacement of liver parenchyma by metastatic carcinoma), the use of glucagon is futile.

Insulin is probably the most obvious cause of hypoglycemia. This is a particularly common problem in hospitalized diabetic patients who have decreased caloric intake due to illness and hospital routine.[36] As noted previously, the treatment of insulin-induced hypoglycemia is administration of either glucose or glucagon. Most patients recover without sequelae, although seizures are not uncommon and a small percentage of deaths in diabetic patients can be attributed to hypoglycemia.[32] Insulin has also been used as a means of suicide and homicide.[37] A concern is whether patients with recurring episodes of hypoglycemia experience any impairment of intellectual or cognitive function; some evidence suggests that this may occur, although the data are not consistent or clear-cut.[32] It should be noted that insulin is metabolized by the kidneys, and patients with frequent hypoglycemia or decreasing insulin requirements should be assessed for possible renal insufficiency. Addison's disease should also be considered as a possible contributor to hypoglycemia.

Insulin-induced hypoglycemia can also occur in patients who do not have diabetes. In this difficult situation, the differential diagnosis includes insulinoma and surreptitious insulin self-administration. The classic evaluation includes a prolonged fast (up to 72 hours) and requires demonstration of nonsuppressed insulin levels in combination with documented and symptomatic hypoglycemia. Measurement of C peptide at the same time is a critical determination. C peptide and insulin, the two breakdown products of proinsulin, are produced in equimolar amounts; therefore, elevated measurements of both insulin and C peptide are expected with an insulinoma, compared with the findings in a patient who surreptitiously uses exogenous insulin. The simultaneous finding of increased insulin and C peptide does not absolutely confirm the presence of insulinoma or preclude absolutely the possibility of drug-related hypoglycemia, however; ingestion of sulfonylureas, which stimulate pancreatic β-cell activity, also results in elevation of both insulin and C peptide.

All sulfonylureas *(acetohexamide, chlorpropamide, tolazamide, tolbutamide, glipizide, glyburide, glimepiride)* work through the same mechanism of stimulating insulin production by pancreatic β-cells. Thus, it is not surprising that all sulfonylureas have been associated with hypoglycemia,[38] with a frequency related to the half-life of each drug and its metabolites. Chlorpropamide, with the longest half-life, 35 hours, is responsible for the largest number of incidents of reported hypoglycemia and associated deaths. Because this drug is excreted primarily by the kidneys, the half-life (and thus the drug toxicity) increases considerably in patients with renal impairment. Some physicians preferentially choose chlorpropamide for its low cost in generic forms, but this practice can be particularly problematic in some elderly patients in whom inconsistent caloric intake combined with renal disease and long drug half-life presents a very substantial risk factor for hypoglycemia. The second-generation sulfonylureas (glyburide, glipizide, and glimepiride) currently account for the vast majority of sulfonylurea use; of these, glyburide is second only to chlorpropamide in the number of reported cases of severe hypoglycemia and death; these events reflect the drug's relatively long half-life and the frequency with which it is prescribed. Because of the duration of drug effect with the longer-acting agents (especially chlorpropamide), it may be prudent to admit some patients for further observation (and continued glucose infusion) even after their glucose level has been restored by glucose administration, especially if the patient is an elderly individual. (Chlorpropamide's toxicity also includes a propensity to cause hyponatremia, in addition to a disulfiram-like reaction if the drug is used in conjunction with ethanol.)

As in other situations involving drug toxicity, the issue of sulfonylurea-induced hypoglycemia is particularly difficult if the hypoglycemia is factitious. In some cases, the patient can be the innocent victim of a prescription or dispensing error, receiving a sulfonylurea instead of a drug with a similar name: Patients have received Diabinese (chlorpropamide) instead of Diamox (acetazolamide), Tolinase (tolazamide) instead of Tolectin (tolmetin),[37] or Diamox (acetazolamide) in place of Dymelor (acetohexamide).[38]

Many other agents are capable of causing hypoglycemia. *Ethanol* is by far the most common cause of severe and life-threatening hypoglycemia in the United States.[37] The mechanisms of ethanol-related hypoglycemia require a combination of inadequate calorie ingestion during the drinking spree, the eventual depletion of liver glycogen stores, and hepatic conversion of nicotine-adenine dinucleotide (NAD) to its reduced form (NADH) as alcohol is metabolized (thus rendering the liver incapable of providing new glucose formation through the NAD-dependent process of gluconeogenesis).[34] In the absence of hepatic glycogen stores, these patients cannot respond to administration of glucagon, and therefore the hypoglycemia must be treated by glucose administration. *Salicylate* poisoning has been associated with hypoglycemia (with most reports in children).[38] In addition, β-*blocking drugs* (particularly the nonselective agents *propranolol, pindolol,* and *nadolol*) have been implicated as causes of hypoglycemia, probably because of inhibition of hepatic glucose production. Other drugs that have been associated with hypoglycemia include *pentamidine, disopyramide* (Norpace), *ritodrine* (a β-sympathomimetic drug used to inhibit premature labor, with hypoglycemia reported in either mother or baby), and *quinine*; most of these agents seem to have variable effects in stimulating insulin release from the islet cells. *Haloperidol* is also associated with hypoglycemia, and in the setting of renal failure both *trimethoprim-sulfamethoxazole* and *propoxyphene* have been implicated.[33] The rodenticide *Vacor* is particularly toxic to pancreatic β-cells, inducing a massive release of stored insulin that may result in profound hypoglycemia; β-cell destruction eventually occurs, with resultant diabetes (similar to streptozocin). Hypoglycemia can also result from ingestion of naturally occurring substances, such as unripened Caribbean *akee fruit.*[34]

Antihyperglycemic Agents

Metformin is a biguanide that is used in the treatment of non–insulin-dependent diabetes mellitus but is not typically associated with a potential for causing hypoglycemia.[39] Unlike the sulfonylureas, it does not increase insulin production by the pancreatic β-cells but instead acts through nonpancreatic mechanisms that are not fully understood. Its major toxic effect is the potential development of lactic acidosis, a complication that is shared by another biguanide, phenformin (and which resulted in the removal of phenformin from the market in the 1970s). Metformin is eliminated exclusively by the kidneys, and impairment of renal function can lead to metformin accumulation and predisposition to lactic acidosis, which has an overall mortality rate in the range of 50%. Many patients with metformin-associated lactic acidosis have other factors that predispose to tissue hypoxia and clinical shock (including hepatic dysfunction, cardiac disease, and renal impairment). Therapy of lactic acidosis consists of removal of the precipitating agent, treatment of superimposed disorders (such as infections), vascular support, and administration of large amounts of bicarbonate.

Hyperglycemic Agents

Diazoxide, used infrequently as a parenteral agent in hypertensive crisis, is an inhibitor of insulin secretion and can be used as an oral agent in the therapy of patients with insulinomas. It causes sodium and fluid retention, with associated edema, and simultaneous use of a loop diuretic is a frequent need. In addition to being monitored for development of hyperglycemia related to excessive insulin suppression, patients should be monitored for complications that include gastrointestinal distress, pancreatitis, thrombocytopenia or leukopenia, impairment of renal function, and proteinuria.

Glucagon is used as a hyperglycemic agent in insulin-treated patients who become hypoglycemic and are too obtunded to take oral carbohydrates; nonendocrine uses have included therapy of β-blocker overdose, cardiovascular emergencies, and relaxation of the gastrointestinal tract for diagnostic procedures. Its toxicity is limited; nausea and vomiting are frequent consequences of its use. The expected increase in glucose does not occur in patients who are depleted of glycogen stores; for example, patients with alcohol-related hypoglycemia show no response, and delaying more effective therapy (such as glucose administration) poses a risk in such a setting. In a patient with an insulinoma, the initial beneficial increase in glucose levels may be followed by a subsequent precipitous glucose drop due to stimulation of further insulin production by the glucagon.

GONADAL

Androgens

Androgens are endocrine agents commonly used for legitimate purposes such as the treatment of male hypogonadism but are also very commonly obtained through illegal pathways for purposes that are much more controversial (frequently related to athletes' desire to increase muscle mass, stamina, strength, and endurance).[34] The common use of unsupervised black market androgens leads to a potential for the use of excessive doses and subsequent toxic actions that would not occur with medical therapy, which is administered at physiologic doses with appropriate supervision.

Many of the androgens that are clinically available are chemically altered versions of the testosterone molecule; without these modifications, effective androgen replacement would be difficult. Unmodified *testosterone* is quickly absorbed and very quickly metabolized by the liver, and oral administration of testosterone is therefore not a useful therapeutic approach. It is now possible to administer unmodified testosterone transdermally. Outside of the United States, testosterone implants are also available as a method for delivery of unmodified testosterone. Otherwise, the androgens that are available for administration can be divided into two major categories, based on the way in which the testosterone molecule has been modified for clinical use. Esterification of the 17β-hydroxyl group decreases the molecule's polarity and increases fat solubility. These testosterone esters, *testosterone enanthate* and *testosterone cypio-*

nate, are administered in oily injection vehicles and function as depot agents with long half-lives; once absorbed, the esters are hydrolyzed to free testosterone, with subsequent physiologic actions that are no different from those of endogenously produced testosterone.[3] In an effort to produce an androgen that can be given by the oral route, testosterone derivatives have been developed in which the molecule has been alkylated at the 17α position, sometimes in association with modification of the ring structure. These changes lead to a slowing of hepatic metabolism, which results in effective drug levels after oral administration. These 17α-*alkylated androgens* (*fluoxymesterone, methyltestosterone, oxandrolone, oxymetholone,* and *stanozolol*) have been associated with severe hepatic toxicity, including cholestasis, liver tumors (adenomas, hepatocellular carcinoma, and hepatic angiosarcoma), and peliosis hepatis (pooling of blood in the liver sinusoids). Because of these problems, it is generally recommended that these oral androgens should not be used for therapy of male hypogonadism[3]; nonetheless, they can still be prescribed, and their illicit use continues.

Other than the hepatic toxicity of the 17α-alkylated forms, the adverse effects of androgens (as with other hormones) tend to be related to the physiologic effects that result from the interaction of the hormone molecule with the hormone receptor. In the case of the androgens, the prostate gland is a major target organ for androgen action, with prostate cancer and benign prostatic hyperplasia being disorders of particular concern in patients who are treated with androgens.[40] Neither prostate cancer nor benign prostatic hyperplasia develops in the absence of testosterone exposure.[40, 41] Prostatic cancer arises by a two-step process. The first component is the development of microscopic (preclinical) disease, and animal studies suggest that androgens are promoters of this step. The second step is the progression to clinical cancer, and it is not known whether androgens promote this phase of the disease. The androgenic effect on benign prostatic hyperplasia is clearly demonstrated by the finding that prostate size can be reduced (and urinary obstructive symptoms improved) by agents that decrease androgen levels or androgen effect. Testosterone replacement in elderly men is associated with an increase in prostate-specific antigen.[41]

Testosterone administration does not cause excessive stimulation of libido or potency, except in prepubertal boys and young men with long-standing androgen deficiency[3]; in such patients, the possibility of severe and prolonged problems with priapism dictates that very small initial doses of testosterone be used (e.g., a testosterone ester dose of 50 to 100 mg every month, in contrast to the full adult replacement dose of approximately 200 mg every 2 weeks).

The effects of androgens on classic androgen-sensitive tissues are particularly of concern in athletes who take large and supraphysiologic doses of androgens. In male athletes, suppression of spermatogenesis, subsequent infertility, and testicular atrophy can occur. Female athletes can become virilized, and some of these changes (such as effects on deepening of the voice caused by androgen action on the larynx) can be irreversible. Children and adolescents can experience accelerated skeletal maturation and early epiphyseal closure, which ultimately inhibits their final height.[34]

In what may seem to be a paradoxical side effect, administration of testosterone can at times cause gynecomastia. This is related to the conversion of testosterone to estradiol in peripheral tissues by aromatase enzymes and appears to be more common in young boys who are treated with testosterone for induction of puberty and in men with underlying disorders such as hepatic cirrhosis; in these situations, an elevation of the ratio of estradiol to testosterone is the likely mechanism.[3]

Androgen effects on nonreproductive tissues include androgen-dependent changes in serum lipoproteins. Men have lower levels than women of the protective high-density lipoprotein (HDL) cholesterol, with the disparity in HDL cholesterol level developing at the time of puberty. A 10% to 15% drop in HDL cholesterol level occurs during testosterone therapy.[3] This androgen-driven decrement in HDL cholesterol may be a major contributor to the increased male risk for cardiovascular disease, although other factors such as a direct protective effect of estrogen on vascular tissue may also be important. The cardiovascular risk of androgens may depend on the particular type of androgen used. Orally administered 17-alkylated steroids cause a much more pronounced lowering of HDL cholesterol level than the testosterone esters,[3] as well as an elevation of LDL cholesterol level that is not noted with the parenteral testosterone products.[40] The oral agents may have a greater effect on lipids because of the first-pass effect through the liver; furthermore, the effect of testosterone may be attenuated by its conversion to estrogen (which cannot occur with the 17-alkylated agents).

The initiation of androgen therapy can be associated with modest weight gain, which reflects the anabolic effects of testosterone and a component of sodium retention. Patients with disorders such as congestive heart failure and cirrhosis can have worsening of their edema with testosterone treatment.[3] In combination with other risk factors such as obesity, chronic obstructive lung disease, and advancing age, testosterone administration to hypogonadal men appears to increase the incidence of sleep-related breathing disorders.[40] Androgens are also known to increase erythropoiesis, and elderly men who receive testosterone replacement can develop hematocrit levels above the upper limit of normal.

An ongoing controversy is whether or not androgens, when used in high doses, can induce pathologically aggressive and violent behavior or even psychotic symptoms.[42] It is difficult to separate fact from conjecture, because most reports are anecdotal and do not take into account the pretreatment ("premorbid") characteristics of the androgen user or consider possible concurrent use of other substances of abuse.[34] However, psychologic effects are suggested by the findings of a full affective disorder (major depression or mania) in more than 20% of athletes who used 10 to 100 times the usual therapeutic doses of these drugs, with psychotic symptoms appearing in 12% (consistent with the concept of androgen-related fluctuations in mood and increased levels of aggressiveness, which have been called " 'roid rage"[42, 43]). At less pronounced androgen excess (testosterone doses of double the physiologic replacement dose), little change in sexual and aggressive behaviors occurs, and the suggested concerns of adverse effects of exogenous testosterone on male sexual and aggressive behavior thus may be overstated.[44]

The question has also arisen about whether androgens can produce a psychologic dependence syndrome.[42] Evidence shows that in some individuals, androgen abuse can develop into a psychoactive substance dependence disorder with features that are similar to those seen with cocaine, alcohol, or opioid abuse. The features of psychologic dependence include a preoccupation with the use of androgens, drug craving, and difficulty in discontinuing the agent despite psychologic side effects; withdrawal effects are said to include mood swings, violent behavior, and profound depression.

Antiandrogens

Flutamide is an antiandrogen that is used to treat prostate cancer.[31] It is metabolized to active and inactive metabolites by the liver and is primarily excreted by the kidneys. The major risk from flutamide is a potentially fatal drug-induced hepatitis, occurring in fewer than 0.5% of treated patients. Because the drug might be considered for therapy of hirsutism, concern is expressed about the potential for ambiguity of the genitalia of male offspring of women who receive the agent.

Megestrol is discussed in the later section on antiprogestins.

Spironolactone is discussed in the earlier section on mineralocorticoid antagonist.

Finasteride, used for therapy of benign prostatic hyperplasia, is an inhibitor of the 5α-reductase enzyme that converts testosterone into the active metabolite dihydrotestosterone.[45] Although testosterone has a direct action in some tissues, it must be converted to dihydrotestosterone to exert an effect on the prostate and skin. Finasteride is relatively free of adverse effects; because libido and potency are related to testosterone (rather than dihydrotestosterone) effect, sexual dysfunction is relatively uncommon with use of this drug. Serum lipids and bone density are not affected. The drug is not approved for use in treatment of hirsutism, because its use in women would be associated with a theoretic risk of impaired virilization of the genitalia of male offspring.

Estrogens

The use of estrogen as medical treatment can be divided into at least three categories, depending on the purposes for the estrogen administration (which to some extent also reflects the specific estrogenic compounds that are used). Estrogen use is perhaps the most straightforward as a physiologic hormone replacement therapy in estrogen-deficient women. It becomes somewhat more complicated when used in premenopausal women for nonphysiologic (contraceptive) purposes. The most controversial situations occur when it is used for other purposes (such as the use of diethylstilbestrol [DES] in years past in the hope of improving pregnancy outcome but with the eventual discovery of unpredicted adverse effects).

Estrogen replacement therapy has become very popular for postmenopausal women (who might otherwise spend one third of their lives in an estrogen-deficient state[46]). The risks of estrogen deficiency are well described and include the discomfort of vasomotor instability, changes in estrogen-sensitive tissues, increased risks of osteoporosis, and adverse effects on lipoprotein metabolism and other cardiovascular factors.

However, the use of estrogen replacement in postmenopausal women also has potential risks. An increased risk of endometrial cancer was one of the first described complications of long-term estrogen therapy, with a 2- to 10-fold increase in risk compared with untreated women. This risk is present only in women who are treated with unopposed estrogen (e.g., without concurrent use of a progestational agent); it is generally recommended that all women who are estrogen treated and who have not had a hysterectomy should also be treated with a progestational agent. Options include the use of medroxyprogesterone acetate, 10 mg for 12 to 14 days monthly, in addition to daily estrogen, with resultant withdrawal bleeding from endometrial sloughing and complete abrogation of the risk from estrogen treatment. An alternate approach, which avoids menstrual bleeding, is to add medroxyprogesterone, 2.5 mg daily, to the daily estrogen therapy. The progestin reduces the nuclear concentration of estrogen receptors, causing involution of the endometrium; breakthrough bleeding may occur in the first several months.[46]

The question of whether postmenopausal estrogen therapy leads to an increased risk of breast carcinoma continues to be one of the most controversial concerns with estrogen treatment. Some studies have not shown any increase in risk, others have demonstrated some increased risk (which in some studies is related to duration of use), and some have shown even a decreased risk.[47] When increased risk has been demonstrated, it appears that survival from breast cancer in estrogen-treated patients may be better than that in non–estrogen-treated women; whether this is related to closer medical supervision and monitoring in estrogen-treated women, biologic differences in the cancers, or other unidentified factors is uncertain. The risk question is further complicated by a large number of other variables, including the variety of estrogen products that have been used and the possibility of bias in the selection of patients who take estrogen. Even though at least one meta-analysis has concluded that postmenopausal estrogen therapy does not increase the risk of breast cancer, it is premature to conclude that this issue is settled.[46] In particular, the contemporary tendency to combine estrogen and progestin may negate strict interpretation of earlier studies that evaluated estrogen-only therapy. Further studies will undoubtedly continue to provide more data on this topic; in light of the many conflicting results that have been reported thus far,[47, 48] no conclusive or final answer can be given to the breast cancer question at this time, and this will continue to be a topic of concern.

Postmenopausal estrogen therapy usually does not affect blood pressure. If it has any effect, it may cause somewhat of a reduction in blood pressure in both normotensive and hypertensive women,[48] with blood pressure elevation being an unusual finding (in contrast to the effects of oral contraceptive therapy, as noted later). Similarly, although oral contraceptive therapy is associated with increased risk of thrombosis, no epidemiologic data demonstrate an increased risk of thrombosis with standard postmenopausal replacement doses of estrogen. The risk for gallbladder disease, however, is approximately doubled with estrogen treatment,[47, 48] related to changes in the composition of bile. In addition, estrogen can trigger migraine headaches in susceptible women.[47]

Postmenopausal estrogen replacement is usually administered as either oral conjugated equine estrogens, oral estradiol, or transdermal estradiol. Transdermal therapy results in direct absorption of the estrogen into the systemic circulation and avoids the first-pass effect of estrogen on the liver (which stimulates production of various liver-derived proteins). The physiologic relevance of this is uncertain; however, in some settings (such as in patients with a prior history of thromboembolic disease), the use of transdermal estrogen should minimize risks related to stimulation of hepatic protein production. Otherwise, the choice between oral and transdermal estrogen is an issue of individual patient preference.

The current *oral contraceptive agents* used in the United States are combination pills that contain *ethinyl estradiol* and one of five possible progestational agents, all of which are 19-nortestosterone derivatives (*norethindrone, norethynodrel, norethindrone acetate, ethynodiol diacetate,* and *levonorgestrel*).[49] The risk of estrogen use in these products is a complex issue because of the varying doses of estrogen and the combinations with various progestational agents. All of the data on oral contraceptive risks should be considered to be somewhat of a "moving target," because the earlier agents were relatively rich in estrogen content compared with contemporary agents, and many of the problems described with the earlier products may not necessarily correlate strongly with the use of current formulations. Although increased cardiovascular risk was a concern with the initial oral contraceptives, the risk of death due to coronary artery disease does not appear to be increased in present or past birth control pill users in the absence of other cardiovascular risk factors. However, additional risk factors such as hypertension, diabetes, and hypercholesterolemia are synergistic with birth control pills as risk factors for myocardial infarction, and cigarette smoking in particular is the greatest single factor. In studies that show an increased risk of myocardial infarction with use of oral contraceptives, the finding of a concurrent smoking history is a dominant association. Birth control pills might influence cardiovascular risk factors in a number of ways (most of which have been minimized with the lowering of doses and improved formulations through the years). All estrogen-containing pills increase fasting triglyceride levels, and patients with underlying hypertriglyceridemia have an increased risk of pancreatitis if the triglyceride level exceeds the 800 to 1000 mg/dL range. Various effects on cholesterol metabolism are noted, depending on the dose of the estrogen and the particular progestin that is used.[49] The addition of progestin may tend to attenuate mildly the generally favorable effects of estrogen on lipoprotein levels (which include a decrease in low-density lipoprotein [LDL] cholesterol and an increase in HDL cholesterol), with further variables that include the androgenicity of the progestin, its dose, and the specific regimen. In the various formulations of triphasic pills, changes in total cholesterol, LDL, and HDL are generally very slight. Pills containing only progestin seem to have the least effect on lipids, and it has been suggested that progestin-only pills, implantable *levonorgestrel* (Norplant), or pills containing newer progestins such as *desogestrel* may be the best choice for patients who have a higher than usual risk for coronary artery disease but who would benefit from an effective contraceptive agent.[49] Because of the relatively slight changes in lipid levels with any oral contraceptive agent, all of this may be a moot point in terms of cardiovascular risk, and the most important cardiovascular consideration may be the use of the lowest estrogen dose to minimize changes in clotting factors.[49]

Before the 1990s, virtually all oral contraceptive pills caused some degree of insulin resistance, with some increase in serum glucose and insulin levels. Both the estrogenic and progestational agents are responsible for the insulin resistance in a dose-dependent manner, and the same effects are less apparent with current oral contraceptives.[49] In a practical sense, the changes in insulin and glucose metabolism are so small that they have no significance for normal women. However, in women with latent diabetes (such as normoglycemic patients with a history of gestational diabetes), periodic glucose monitoring is reasonable.

Of all the metabolic changes that are related to oral contraceptive use, the changes in liver protein metabolism are the most important, in particular, the hepatic proteins associated with coagulation, which increase in proportion to the estrogen content of the oral contraceptive. An increased risk of coagulation disturbances (particularly thrombophlebitis and pulmonary embolus) are the most serious complications related to the use of birth control pills.[49] The vascular venous complications do not seem to be related to age, parity, obesity, smoking, or other apparent factors. Levels of these serum proteins return to normal within 2 months or so of discontinuation of the pills; the increased risk of thrombophlebitis decreases sooner.

Blood pressure elevation has also been linked to oral contraceptive use. Combined oral contraceptives cause hypertension in 4% to 5% of women with normal blood pressure and an increase in blood pressure in 9% to 16% of women with previously established hypertension.[50] An estrogen-related effect on hepatic protein production (increased synthesis of angiotensinogen) has been invoked as a possible mechanism. In most patients, a compensatory decrease in renin levels seems to prevent the development of hypertension. Ethinyl estrogen at the typical doses of 30 or 35 μg has minimal effects on blood pressure, even in those individuals who may be predisposed to hypertension. Blood pressure is not influenced by progestin-only preparations,[49] and some of the new third-generation progestins may even have an antimineralocorticoid effect that lowers the risk of hypertension.[51] With the triphasic pills, mean blood pressure in groups of patients does not change, although individual patients may have some increase.[49]

DES is a synthesized stilbene with the estrogenic properties of naturally occurring estrogens. It was used for many years because of its effectiveness with oral administration and its low cost of production. DES was eventually banned from use in pregnancy in 1971 because of associated adverse medical effects.[51] The drug was commonly used in pregnancy (with an estimated 5 to 10 million American women exposed) because of its purported effectiveness in preventing miscarriages and premature births. In the early 1970s, clear association of clear cell vaginal carcinoma was observed in young women who had been exposed to DES *in utero.* These women also seem to be at greater risk for anatomic anomalies of the reproductive tract. It is not clear whether males exposed *in utero* have any increased risk of comparable problems. Daughters exposed *in utero* should have careful cervical and vaginal examinations, using half-strength Lugol's solution to stain the entire vaginal wall. If annual Papanicolaou's test results are suspicious, vaginal cytologic tests and colposcopy are recommended. When pregnant, these DES-exposed daughters should be followed as high-risk obstetric patients because of their increased risk of spontaneous abortions, ectopic pregnancies, and premature labor. Although no clear association with testicular cancer has been noted, routine genital examination is also suggested for DES-exposed sons (especially those with the risk factor of cryptorchidism, which does appear to be more prevalent with a DES exposure history).[51]

Antiestrogens

Antiestrogens (*clomiphene* and *tamoxifen*) are used for therapy of reproductive disorders and for treatment of estrogen-dependent malignancies. These agents are not pure antagonists but have both estrogen antagonist and estrogen agonist effects, a situation that complicates understanding of their action and controversy about their toxicity.[52] Tamoxifen's estrogen antagonist action is reflected by improved survival of tamoxifen-treated patients with breast cancer and lowered risk of contralateral breast cancer. The expected estrogen deficiency symptoms (vasomotor instability and vaginal dryness) are common; however, the estrogen agonist effects of tamoxifen seem to predominate over antagonistic action at the skeleton (where the drug increases bone density), in the metabolism of lipoproteins (it has an estrogen-like action in increasing triglycerides and lowering LDL cholesterol), and at the endometrium (an increased incidence of endometrial carcinoma has been noted with the agent). The other agent used for its antiestrogenic effects, clomiphene, has traditionally been used to induce ovulation in anovulatory women; by "masking" the estrogen receptor at the hypothalamic-pituitary level, gonadotropin secretion is augmented, with subsequent stimulation of ovarian function. Side effects are infrequent and fairly mild and include occasional pelvic cramping, hot flashes, nausea, and breast tenderness, as well as some visual symptoms. The most significant side effect is ovarian hyperstimulation, with formation of luteinized ovarian cysts; patients with severe periovulatory or postovulatory pain should undergo pelvic examination or ultrasound evaluation to confirm that the ovaries are of normal size before proceeding with further therapy.

Progestins

Many of the effects of progestin therapy were reviewed in the earlier section on oral contraceptives. Because progestins are commonly used in conjunction with estrogens, distinguishing the effects of progestins from those of estrogen has been difficult (especially for long-term health considerations such as cardiovascular disease risk). It is clear that more information is needed about the consequences, positive and negative, of combining estrogen with progesterone.

Progestins are at times used as sole agents (without concomitant estrogen therapy) for contraceptive purposes. Implantable levonorgestrel may not completely suppress gonadotropins, and the subsequent irregularity of estrogen secretion can result in irregular bleeding, which may necessitate removal. No consistent effects on blood pressure, lipoproteins, or coagulation have been noted with this agent. Injectable depot *medroxyprogesterone acetate (Depo-Provera)* has also been associated with irregular bleeding. Infertility may persist for months after its use. Despite gonadotropin suppression, bone density does not seem to be affected. Decreases in triglycerides and HDL cholesterol may occur without change in total cholesterol or LDL cholesterol.

Megestrol is a progestational agent that suppresses gonadotropin production, lowers testosterone levels, and thus functions as an antiandrogen. It has been used in treatment of prostate carcinoma, and its antigonadotropic activity has also led to its use in treatment of breast carcinoma and endometrial carcinoma. It has been observed that cancer victims who are treated with megestrol acetate tend to gain weight, leading to its use for the cachexia associated with malignancy and AIDS. At high doses, progestins appear to cross-react with receptors for other steroids, and thus these agents may also have a glucocorticoid effect. Adrenal suppression due to ACTH inhibition after abrupt discontinuation of megestrol in a patient with AIDS has been described.[53]

Specific progestin side effects, which are dose dependent, can include breast tenderness, bloating, irritability, and depression.[54]

Antiprogestin

Mifepristone (RU 486) is a somewhat notorious antiprogestin and antiglucocorticoid that is neither produced nor available in the United States,[48] largely because of its use in inducing abortions. As a competitive inhibitor of the progesterone receptor, it has potential use as a contraceptive as well as for induction of abortions. Effects related to its antiprogestin effect include heavy vaginal bleeding after a single dose and cessation of menses and intermittent hot flashes with long-term use. Men may experience impaired libido and gynecomastia, probably because of binding of the drug to androgen receptors. As noted previously, its ability to block the glucocorticoid receptor results in its effective use in treatment of Cushing's syndrome. The drug has some seemingly nonspecific side effects, which include fatigue, anorexia, nausea, and abdominal symptoms; however, it has been suggested that these may be manifestations of adrenal insufficiency, with improved symptoms in some patients after administration of dexamethasone. It is important to note, however, that the antiglucocorticoid effect of mifepristone occurs at a higher dose than does the antiprogestin effect.

LIPID METABOLISM

Lipid-lowering agents are commonly used medications. They can be classified into several distinct groups, and overall they have fairly limited toxic effects[55]; the long-term effects of lipid-lowering agents have yet to be elucidated.

The bile acid sequestrants (*cholestyramine* and *colestipol*) are effective in lowering LDL cholesterol but have a tendency to increase triglyceride levels and thus lead to worsening of triglyceride-related problems (such as acute pancreatitis) if not used appropriately. By virtue of the fact that these agents are not absorbed, systemic toxic effects are not an issue with their use. Constipation is a common problem with these substances and limits compliance in many cases. They also have a tendency to interfere with the absorption of a number of drugs (including digoxin, thyroxine, and anticoagulants) unless doses are appropriately spaced.

Fibrinic acid derivatives (*gemfibrozil* and *clofibrate*) are most effective in lowering levels of triglycerides and have a relatively small effect on lowering LDL cholesterol levels. These drugs can predispose to gallstone formation. Their use should be avoided in patients with renal insufficiency in order to avoid an increased risk of myopathy.

The hydroxymethylglutaryl-CoA inhibitors (including *lovastatin, simvastatin, pravastatin,* and *fluvastatin*) are used commonly and are very potent agents for lowering LDL cholesterol. Liver function abnormalities are occasionally encountered in patients who use these drugs; periodic monitoring of liver function is recommended. Drug-induced myopathy has also been reported, especially with lovastatin. Patients with renal insufficiency or patients who simultaneously take cyclosporine, gemfibrozil, or nicotinic acid are particularly at risk; periodic monitoring of muscle enzymes is recommended for these patients, and muscle enzyme values should be monitored in patients with muscle pain or weakness.

Nicotinic acid is a very effective agent in lowering LDL cholesterol and triglycerides while increasing HDL cholesterol levels. Severe flushing and pruritus after drug administration are problematic for many patients and may prevent achievement of the relatively high doses (1500 mg or more daily) that are required to obtain the optimal lipid-lowering effect. Pretreatment with salicylates may make the agent more tolerable. Use of nicotinic acid, in the doses needed to lower lipid levels, also results in insulin resistance, and susceptible patients may experience some increase in blood sugar level (or may even develop florid uncontrolled diabetes mellitus) with initiation of nicotinic acid use. Although nicotinic acid is considered by some to be contraindicated for use in patients with known diabetes, such a stance removes a very powerful therapeutic option from the very individuals who are likely to benefit most from an effective lipid-lowering agent, and a more reasonable approach might include readiness to initiate insulin therapy in patients who develop increasing glucose measurements on nicotinic acid therapy. Use of long-acting slow-release forms of nicotinic acid has been associated with liver function abnormalities.

Probucol is an agent used infrequently, probably because it lowers both LDL and HDL cholesterol levels. It has been suggested that its antioxidant effect may be its most important property and may lead to cardiovascular protection despite the decrease in HDL levels, but this is far from being resolved. In addition to the questions surrounding its overall efficacy in decreasing cardiovascular disease, it prolongs the QT interval on electrocardiogram and has been associated with polymorphic ventricular tachycardia.

References

1. Rolih CA, Ober KP: The endocrine response to critical illness. Med Clin North Am *79*:211–224, 1995.
2. Richardson DW, Robinson AG: Desmopressin. Ann Intern Med *103*:228–239, 1985.
3. Matsumoto AM: Hormonal therapy of male hypogonadism. Endocrinol Metab Clin North Am *23*:857–875, 1994.
4. Hintz RL: The prismatic case of Creutzfeldt-Jakob disease associated with pituitary growth hormone treatment. J Clin Endocrinol Metab *80*:2298–2301, 1995.
5. Corpas E, Harman SM, Blackman MR: Human growth hormone and human aging. Endocr Rev *14*:20–39, 1993.
6. Miller MM, Hoffman DI: Ovulation induction. *In* Becker KL (ed): Principles and Practice of Endocrinology and Metabolism. 2nd ed. Philadelphia, J.B. Lippincott Co., pp 900–906, 1995.
7. Lamberts SWJ, Reubi J-C, Krenning EP: Somatostatin analogs in the treatment of acromegaly. Endocrinol Metab Clin North Am *21*:737–752, 1993.
8. Jaffe CA, Barkan AL: Treatment of acromegaly with dopamine agonists. Endocrinol Metab Clin North Am *21*:713–735, 1993.
9. Mandel SJ, Brent GA, Larsen PR: Levothyroxine therapy in patients with thyroid disease. Ann Intern Med *119*:494–502, 1993.
10. Jackson IMD, Cobb WE: Why does anyone still use desiccated thyroid USP? Am J Med *64*:284–288, 1978.
11. Roti E, Minelli R, Gardini E, Braverman LE: The use and misuse of thyroid hormone. Endocr Rev *14*:401–423, 1993.
12. Cohen JF, Ingbar SH, Braverman LE: Thyrotoxicosis due to ingestion of excess thyroid hormone. Endocrine Rev *10*:113–124, 1989.
13. Binimelis J, Bassas L, Marruecos L, et al: Massive thyroxine intoxication: Evaluation of plasma extraction. Intensive Care Med *13*:33–38, 1987.
14. Shakir KMM, Micheals RD, Hays JH, Potter BB: The use of bile acid sequestrants to lower serum thyroid hormones in iatrogenic hyperthyroidism. Ann Intern Med *118*:112–113, 1993.
15. Franklyn JA: The management of hyperthyroidism. N Engl J Med *330*:1731–1738, 1994.
16. Klein I, Becker DV, Levey GS: Treatment of hyperthyroid disease. Ann Intern Med *121*:281–288, 1994.
17. Pak CYC, Sakhaee K, Adams-Huet B, et al: Treatment of postmenopausal osteoporosis with slow-release sodium fluoride. Final report of a randomized controlled trial. Ann Intern Med *123*:401–408, 1995.
18. Arab DM, Malatjalian DA, Rittmaster RS: Severe cholestatic jaundice in uncomplicated hyperthyroidism treated with methimazole. J Clin Endocrinol Metab *80*:1083–1085, 1995.
19. Hanson JS: Propylthiouracil and hepatitis. Two cases and a review of the literature. Arch Intern Med *144*:994–996, 1984.
20. Liaw Y-F, Huang M-J, Fan K-D, et al: Hepatic injury during propylthiouracil therapy in patients with hyperthyroidism. Ann Intern Med *118*:424–428, 1993.
21. Blank S, Scanlon KS, Sinks TH, et al: An outbreak of hypervitaminosis D associated with the overfortification of milk from a home-delivery dairy. Am J Public Health *85*:656–659, 1995.
22. Singer FB, Minoofar PN: Bisphosphonates in the treatment of disorders of mineral metabolism. Adv Endocrinol Metab *6*:259–288, 1995.
23. Schlaghecke R, Kornely E, Santen RT, et al: The effect of long-term glucocorticoid therapy on pituitary-adrenal responses to exogenous courticotropin-releasing hormone. N Engl J Med *326*:226–230, 1992.
24. Hanania NA, Chapman KR, Kesten S: Adverse effects of inhaled corticosteroids. Am J Med *98*:196–208, 1995.
25. Christy NP: Pituitary-adrenal function during corticosteroid therapy. N Engl J Med *326*:266–268, 1992.
26. Claman HN: Glucocorticosteroids II: The clinical responses. Hosp Pract *18*:143–146, 149–151, 1983.
27. Lacomis D, Samuels MA: Adverse neurologic effects of glucocorticosteroids. J Gen Intern Med *6*:367–377, 1991.
28. Lukert BP, Raisz LG: Pathogenesis and management of glucocorticoid-induced osteoporosis. Adv Endocrinol Metab *5*:97–135, 1994.
29. Trainer PJ, Besser M: Cushing's syndrome. Therapy directed at the adrenal glands. Endocrinol Metab Clin North Am *23*:571–584, 1994.
30. Sarne DH: Medical treatment of pituitary tumors and hypersecretory states. *In* Becker KL (ed): Principles and Practice of Endocrinology and Metabolism. 2nd ed. Philadelphia, J.B. Lippincott Co., pp 223–229, 1995.
31. Rittmaster RS: Medical treatment of androgen-dependent hirsutism. J Clin Endocrinol Metab *80*:2559–2563, 1995.
32. Service FJ: Hypoglycemia. Med Clin North Am *79*:1–8, 1995.
33. Service FJ: Hypoglycemic disorders. N Engl J Med *332*:1144–1152, 1995.
34. Rogol AD, Yesalis CE III: Anabolic-androgenic steroids and athletes: What are the issues? J Clin Endocrinol Metab *74*:465–469, 1992.
35. Collier A, Steedman DJ, Patrick AW, et al: Comparison of intravenous glucagon and dextrose in treatment of severe hypoglycemia in an accident and emergency department. Diabetes Care *10*:712–715, 1987.
36. Fischer KF, Lees JA, Newman JG: Hypoglycemia in hospitalized patients. N Engl J Med *315*:1245–1250, 1986.
37. Service FJ: Factitial hypoglycemia. Endocrinologist *2*:173–176, 1992.
38. Seltzer HS: Drug-induced hypoglycemia. Endocrinol Metab Clin North Am *18*:163–131, 1989.
39. Lalau JD, Lacroix C, Compagnon P, et al: Role of metformin accumulation in metformin-associated lactic acidosis. Diabetes Care *18*:779–784, 1995.
40. Bardin CW, Swerdloff RS, Santen RJ: Androgens: Risks and benefits. J Clin Endocrinol Metab *73*:4–7, 1991.
41. Tenover JS: Effects of testosterone supplementation in the aging male. J Clin Endocrinol Metab *75*:1092–1098, 1992.
42. Hallagan JB, Hallagan LF, Snyder MB: Anabolic-androgenic steroid use by athletes. N Engl J Med *321*:1042–1045, 1989.
43. Pope HG Jr, Katz DL: Psychiatric and medical effects of anabolic-androgenic steroid use. A controlled study of 160 athletes. Arch Gen Psychiatry *51*:375–382, 1994.
44. Bagatell CJ, Heiman JR, Matsumoto AM, et al: Metabolic and behavioral effects of high-dose, exogenous testosterone in healthy men. J Clin Endocrinol Metab *79*:561–567, 1994.
45. Rittmaster RS: Finasteride. N Engl J Med *330*:120–125, 1994.
46. Barrett-Conner E: Risks and benefits of estrogen replacement therapy. Adv Endocrinol Metab *2*:169–182, 1991.
47. Belchetz PE: Hormonal treatment of postmenopausal women. N Engl J Med *330*:1062–1071, 1994.
48. Spitz IM, Bardin CW: Mifepristone (RU 486)—a modulator of progestin and glucocorticoid action. N Engl J Med *329*:404–412, 1993.
49. Sondheimer SJ: Update on the metabolic effects of steroidal contraceptives. Endocrinol Metab Clin North Am *20*:911–923, 1991.
50. Baird DT, Glasier AF: Hormonal contraception. N Engl J Med *328*:1543–1549, 1993.
51. Giusti RM, Iwamoto K, Hatch EE: Diethylstilbestrol revisited: A review of the long-term health effects. Ann Intern Med *122*:778–788, 1995.
52. Davidson NE: Tamoxifen—panacea or Pandora's box? N Engl J Med *326*:885–886, 1992.
53. Leinung MC, Liporace R, Miller CH: Induction of adrenal suppression by megestrol acetate in patients with AIDS. Ann Intern Med *122*:843–845, 1995.
54. Grady D, Rubin SM, Petitti DB, et al: Hormone therapy to prevent disease and prolong life in postmenopausal women. Ann Intern Med *117*:1015–1037, 1992.
55. Garg A: Management of dyslipidemia in IDDM patients. Diabetes Care *17*:224–234, 1995.

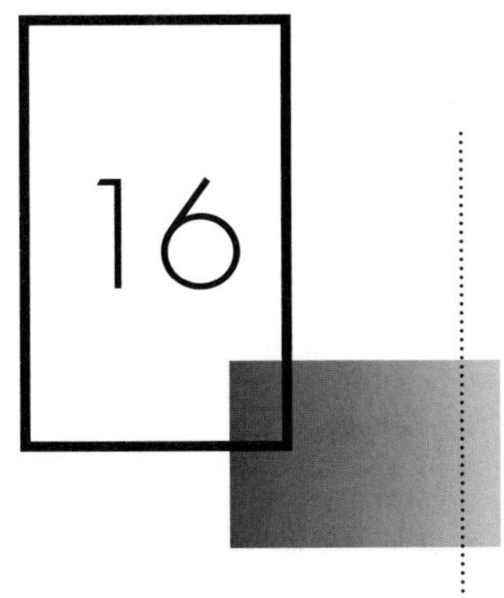

16 Management Principles of Overdose in Pregnancy

TIMOTHY B. ERICKSON, MD
VALERIE D. NEYLAN, MD

The obstetric patient can suffer from various toxicities resulting from acute intentional drug overdose, recreational drug abuse, accidental exposure to industrial or environmental toxins, and, finally, iatrogenic causes. Suicide attempts during pregnancy frequently involve intentional drug overdoses, which represent a more common means than self-mutilation, gunshot wounds, or jumping from high places.[1] Although an uncommon cause of maternal mortality as a whole (1% to 5%), suicide attempts and gestures can account for significant obstetric morbidity. According to one study, the incidence of attempted suicide for pregnant women ranged from 1% to 22%. Of women who actually committed suicide, 2% to 12% were pregnant.[2] Before abortion became legalized, the success rate was reported as 1 in every 88,000 to 400,000 live births; now, it is believed to be much less common.[1] Suicidal gestures are typically impulsive, being a result of untimely pregnancy, interpersonal conflicts, or broken homes. Additionally, pregnant women may take overdoses of an abortifacient with no intent of effecting self-harm. Attempts are most common during the early stages of pregnancy and early in the third trimester; half of all attempts are by primigravid mothers. Personality disorders are often present in these women, but true mental illness is infrequent, with neurotic depression being the most commonly diagnosed psychiatric disorder.[1]

Pregnant women have significant access to multiple medications. According to one study of prescription use in a population receiving Medicaid benefits, pregnant women received an average of 3.1 prescriptions for medications (excluding vitamins).[3] Another study of drug utilization by pregnant females revealed a median of 4.7 prescriptions; most commonly, the prescriptions were for vitamins, iron preparations, analgesics, antipyretics, anti-inflammatory agents, antiemetics, antacids, and antibiotics.[4] Illicit drug use also is reported to have an incidence rate between 10% and 25% among pregnant patients. It is the opinion of some that substance abuse during pregnancy is the most frequently missed diagnosis in perinatal medicine.[5] Thus, in the modern setting, the obstetric patient risks exposing her fetus to an unprecedented number of chemicals and drugs.

The Food and Drug Administration has assigned risk factors (Categories A, B, C, D, and X) to all drugs on the basis of the level of potential risk to the fetus (Table 16–1). However, it is beyond the scope of this text to cover all poisonings and their teratogenicity. Instead, this chapter focuses on the more common toxins to which pregnant patients may be exposed and those requiring special consideration in the obstetric setting. In addition, the altered physiology, pharmacokinetics, and general management of pregnant patients as they relate to poisoning are discussed.

The same principle of care applies to both healthy and poisoned obstetric patients—that is, optimum treatment of the mother results in optimum treatment of the fetus. Conversely, if treatment is delayed or withheld because of concern about inducing fetal harm and the mother's care is compromised, then both maternal and fetal outcome can be jeopardized. Therefore, the well-being of the mother should be the foremost concern in the treatment of a toxic exposure in a pregnant patient.

Table 16–1. Food and Drug Administration's Pregnancy Categories

Category A
Controlled studies in women fail to demonstrate a risk to the fetus in the first trimester (and there is no evidence of a risk in later trimesters), and the possibility of fetal harm appears remote.
Category B
Either animal reproduction studies have not demonstrated a fetal risk, but there are no controlled studies in pregnant women, or animal reproduction studies have shown an adverse effect (other than a decrease in fertility) that was not confirmed in controlled studies in women in the first trimester, and there is no evidence of a risk in later trimesters.
Category C
Either studies in animals have revealed adverse effects on the fetus (teratogenic or embryocidal effects or other) and there are no controlled studies in women, or studies in women and animals are not available. Drugs should be given only if the potential benefit justifies the potential risk to the fetus.
Category D
There is positive evidence of human fetal risk, but the benefits from use in pregnant women may be acceptable despite the risk (e.g., if the drug is needed in a life-threatening situation or for a serious disease for which safer drugs cannot be used or are ineffective). There will be an appropriate statement in the "warnings" section of the labeling.
Category X
Studies in animals or human beings have demonstrated fetal abnormalities, or there is evidence of fetal risk based on human experience, or both, and the risk of the use of the drug in pregnant women clearly outweighs any possible benefit. The drug is contraindicated in women who are or may become pregnant. There will be an appropriate statement in the "contraindications" section of the labeling.

Modified from Millstein LG: FDA's pregnancy categories. N Engl J Med *303*:706, 1980. Modified, with permission, from *The New England Journal of Medicine.*

PHARMACOLOGY AND PATHOPHYSIOLOGY OF PREGNANCY

Many of the physical and physiologic changes that occur during pregnancy alter the pharmacokinetics of drugs and therefore affect maternal exposure and toxic response.[6, 7] These physiologic changes of pregnancy are summarized by organ system in Table 16–2.

Absorption

Gastrointestinal absorption is altered secondary to delayed gastric emptying, decreased gastrointestinal motility, and prolonged transit time through the gastrointestinal tract. The gastrointestinal absorption of drugs in pregnancy is delayed but more complete. Increased minute ventilation, increased tidal volume, and decreased residual lung volume may increase absorption. Dermal absorption also may be enhanced because of increased total body surface area and increased blood flow to the skin.

Distribution

The apparent volume of distribution of drugs may be increased by increases in mean plasma volume, extracellular fluid volume, and body fat stores. The volume of distribution is variable in pregnancy because physiologic changes are dynamic throughout the gestational period. An increase in the serum concentrations of many drugs has been documented. Decreased plasma albumin, protein binding, and hepatic biotransformation as well as increased binding competition may all increase free drug concentration. The increased concentration of unbound or free drug results in larger volumes of distribution and the unbound drug is free to move into tissues. Free fractions of drug also may account for increased clearance rates as they are available for metabolism or elimination.

Metabolism

Hepatic alterations during pregnancy may include changes in hepatic blood flow, bile excretion, and enzyme induction. There appears to be no clinically significant change in hepatic blood flow or bile excretion. Enzyme induction can be variable. Overall hepatic elimination patterns are inconsistent and difficult to predict.

Renal Excretion

Increased renal blood flow and glomerular filtration may result in increased renal elimination. Drugs excreted by the kidney are more rapidly excreted during pregnancy.

Placental-Fetal Blood Flow

The maternal-fetal unit is complex in terms of drug disposition and pharmacokinetics. Increased lipid solubility and low molecular weight promote the transplacental passage of specific compounds. Additionally, drugs that are highly ionized tend to be more protein bound, and this limits their transport across the placenta. As a result, with certain drugs, the placenta can act as a barrier that protects the fetus from a toxic insult. Conversely, it may prevent the passage of a beneficial antidote in an overdose setting.

TREATMENT

Supportive Measures

The general management principles in the poisoned pregnant patient are the same as those in the nonpregnant patient, with the exception of the

Table 16–2. Physiologic Changes of Pregnancy by Organ System (Time of Detected Change)

Overall Physiologic Changes

- ↑ body mass 25% by term
- ↑ body water 7–8 L
- ↑ body fat 3–4 kg; 21%
- ↑ body temperature 0.5°C

Specific Organ Physiologic Changes

Renal

- ↓ Urine concentration (5 d)
- Ureteral dilation due to hormonal relaxation, mechanical compression
- ↑ Aldosterone secretion
- ↑ Antidiuretic hormone secretion
- ↑ Plasma volume 45–50% with 70% increase in volume of extracellular fluid space
- ↑ Renal plasma flow 25–85%
- ↓ Serum creatinine; blood urea nitrogen

Gastrointestinal

- ↑ Nausea and vomiting
- Relaxed cardiac sphincter
- ↑ Gastrointestinal reflux
- ↓ Gastric acidity 30–50% (0–4 mo)
- ↓ Mucous secretion
- ↓ Gastric motility
- ↓ Small bowel motility
- ↑ Stomach emptying time 0–160%
- Hepatic metabolism ↑ or ↓

Neurologic

- ↓ Plasma cholinesterases 20%

Cardiovascular

- ↑ Cardiac output (6 wk)
  - 35% by 10 wk
  - 48% by 25 wk
- ↑ Heart rate 20% or 15 bpm
- ↑ Stroke volume 10–32% or 17 mL
- ↓ Peripheral vascular resistance due to low resistance placental circulatory shunt
- ↑ Peripheral blood flow
- ↑ Perfusion of skin, mucosa, epidural space
- ↓ Oxygen extraction
- ↑ Oxygen consumption 15–20%

Urogenital

- ↑ Weight of uterus
  - 400% by 10 wk
  - 2000% by term

Pulmonary

- ↑ Ventilatory response to CO_2
- ↑ Arterial Po_2 10 mm Hg
- ↓ Arterial Pco_2 10 mm Hg
- ↑ Minute ventilation 40–50%
- ↑ Alveolar ventilation
- ↔ Vital capacity
- ↑ Respiratory rate 0–15%
- ↑ Tidal volume 40%
- ↓ Functional residual capacity 20%
- ↓ Expiratory reserve volume 20%
- ↓ Residual volume 20%
- Subjective dyspnea
- ↓ Airway resistance 36%
- Pulmonary blood flow

Blood

- ↑ Blood volume 35–40%
- ↑ Plasma volume 50%
- ↑ Red blood cell volume 18–20% 300–400 mL
- ↓ Hematocrit 15%
- ↓ Serum hemoglobin
- ↓ Serum iron
- ↑ White blood count 66%
- ↓ Total serum proteins 18% (3rd trimester)
- ↓ Serum albumin 14–30%
- ↑ α_1, α_2 globulins 0–20%
- ↑ Serum fibrinogen 40–200%
- ↑ Phospholipids
- ↑ Cholesterol
- ↑ Free fatty acids

concern for fetal well-being. As with all overdose patients, initial stabilization measures should address ventilatory and hemodynamic status. If the patient is hypotensive, as in the trauma setting, she should be placed in the left lateral decubitus position with aggressive intravenous fluid administration. A thorough history-taking and physical examination should be performed, with the time of and reason for exposure, type and quantity of the toxin, stage of pregnancy, and symptomatology being addressed. The physical examination should include fetal monitoring if the fetus is at an appropriate level of development. If the mother is experiencing altered mental status, assessment of her glucose status is indicated; if she is hypoglycemic, 50% dextrose solution should be administered. In the comatose pregnant patient with suspected opioid intoxication, the benefit of giving naloxone in the presence of respiratory compromise outweighs the potential risks of inducing narcotic withdrawal in mother and fetus.[8]

Decontamination Principles

Decontamination principles in pregnant patients are similar to those in general overdose patients, with a few caveats. On the basis of the most recent trends in the poison decontamination literature, use of the emetic agent syrup of ipecac is discouraged in pregnancy.[9, 10] This agent is absolutely contraindicated if the patient has altered mental status, seizures, and toxin-induced vomiting. Additionally, there are potential teratogenic concerns associated with the use of ipecac.[11] Although there are currently no studies addressing the utility and safety of gastric lavage in the pregnant patient, this procedure may be indicated following the recent ingestion of a potentially life-threatening or fetotoxic drug.[9] However, because the pregnant patient has physiologic delayed gastric emptying and decreased gut motility, delayed lavage may be appropriate after massive ingestions. Furthermore, the literature is unclear regarding the timing and indications for evacuation of drugs that slow gut motility (anticholinergics and opioids) or of those toxins that are known to form concretions (salicylates and iron). Activated charcoal, the most efficacious gastric decontamination modality, is not systemically absorbed from the gastrointestinal tract and is considered safe in the pregnant patient, with no cases of fetal toxicity having been reported.

Cathartic agents such as magnesium citrate or sorbitol should be used with caution in the pregnant patient, particularly in the later stages of pregnancy. Overzealous use of these agents may stimulate preterm labor or produce electrolyte imbalance.[12] Whole-bowel irrigation with an osmotically safe, high-molecular-weight polyethylene glycol solution has been shown to be efficacious and can be safely administered in iron, button battery, cocaine packet, lead, and sustained-released product ingestions.[13] Although reported cases are anecdotal, it has been safely used in the pregnant overdose patient.[14, 15]

Antidotes

Literature on the use of antidotes in the pregnant overdose patient is limited largely to animal studies and to isolated case reports or retrospective case series. No adequate or well-controlled clinical trials have been reported. Thus, definitive conclusions regarding the use of antidotes in obstetric patients cannot be made.[6] In general, the use of antidote therapy in pregnancy is indicated for the reversal of toxic manifestations in the mother, if needed. Several case studies in the literature have reported both maternal and fetal death when a potentially life-saving antidote was withheld because of fear of causing harm to the fetus.[16, 17] As with general poison management, if the mother is treated appropriately, then the fetus also is treated.

Enhanced Elimination

Literature regarding the use of hemodialysis and hemoperfusion in the poisoned pregnant patient is limited. However, if indicated, their implementation is recommended, as few adverse effects have been reported in women requiring their use in the acute overdose setting.[18, 19] Additionally, routine use of dialysis in pregnant patients with chronic renal failure is reported to be relatively safe. Premature labor and growth retardation have been described; however, these effects have been attributed to the chronic disease state and have not been considered a consequence of dialysis.[20, 21]

Disposition

The specific disposition of the poisoned pregnant patient depends on the type of toxin, symptomatology, stage of pregnancy, and intent of exposure. Unstable overdose patients should be closely monitored in an intensive care setting. Under certain circumstances, emergent delivery of a mature or term fetus may prove beneficial for the specific treatment of both the mother and newborn. When the poisoned mother is deemed stable, admission to a general obstetric, labor and delivery, or medical ward with close fetal monitoring is appropriate. If the toxic exposure is intentional, the patient, once medically stabilized, should undergo psychiatric evaluation. If the patient is medically stable and not mentally impaired, she may be discharged home with close outpatient prenatal care.

ACETAMINOPHEN

Acetaminophen (paracetamol) is readily available to the pregnant patient, as numerous over-the-counter preparations such as cold remedies, antipyretics, and analgesics contain this compound. Acetaminophen has been cited as the drug most frequently taken in an acute overdose by pregnant patients.[1]

In an acute overdose, the sulfonation and glucuronidation metabolic pathways become saturated; this causes an increased shift to the cytochrome P-450 pathway. As a result, glutathione stores are depleted, and this leads to hepatotoxicity via central lobular necrosis. Because acetaminophen crosses the placental barrier, the fetus is at risk from poisoning.[22, 23] Evidence of placental transfer has been documented in both animals[24] and humans.[23] The cytochrome P-450 system is present in the fetus by the 14th week of gestation.[25] Early in fetal development, cytochrome P-450 activity is only 10% of adult activity and develops in a linear fashion throughout gestation.[11] As a result, in the later stages of pregnancy, the fetus is more susceptible to toxicity because it is able to form the toxic metabolite of acetaminophen. This finding has been observed clinically in selected studies in which the fetal outcome was worse if the overdose had occurred during the third trimester, particularly if the mother demonstrated concomitant signs of hepatotoxicity.[11, 25–27]

In an acute ingestion, an acetaminophen level should be determined and plotted on the Rumack-Matthew nomogram to assess the risk of hepatotoxicity. Peak serum levels and pharmacokinetics of acetaminophen in the pregnant patient are unchanged when the drug is given in standard doses but have not yet been determined in the overdose setting.[28] In addition, baseline liver function tests and coagulation profiles should be drawn and followed in a serial manner, as indicated.

If the time of ingestion is unknown or if it is chronic in nature, determination of serum level is still recommended for documentation of the ingestion. Subsequent levels should be followed, as hepatic damage prolongs the half-life ($t_{1/2}$) of the drug. The mean $t_{1/2}$ of acetaminophen given in therapeutic doses has been shown to be 3.7 hours in the pregnant patient, compared with 3.1 hours in the nonpregnant patient.[28]

In acute acetaminophen overdose, general stabilization and decontamination measures should be implemented. If the nomogram indicates that the acetaminophen level is hepatotoxic or if more than 140 mg/kg has been ingested acutely, administration of the antidote *N*-acetyl-L-cysteine (NAC) is indicated. NAC acts by replenishing hepatic glutathione stores and is most effective when given within 8 hours after ingestion.[29]

In a study of 60 pregnant patients, Riggs and coworkers demonstrated a significant positive correlation between the time to initial administration of NAC and pregnancy outcome.[25] The incidence of spontaneous abortion or fetal demise was increased when the treatment was delayed. In a large series describing 48 cases, the authors observed no birth defects associated with first-trimester NAC therapy.[30] However, animal studies of whether NAC crosses the placental barrier are controversial. Although shown to undergo placental transfer in pregnant rats,[31] an ovine model documented negligible transfer.[32]

If the ingestion is deemed hepatotoxic on the basis of the history, the nomogram, or the results of liver function tests, the standard oral loading dose of NAC, 140 mg/kg followed by 70 mg/kg every 4 hours for 17 doses, should be administered *as soon as possible.* Some sources advocate use of the intravenous route in pregnant patients because the oral form of the drug produces lower plasma levels, may induce vomiting, and undergoes maternal first-pass hepatic metabolism, lessening its availability to the fetus.[10, 11, 32] The latest literature also supports treatment with NAC in chronic or delayed acetaminophen-induced hepatotoxicity, as the drug may rescue hepatocytes by acting as a free radical scavenger.[33]

Any pregnant patient presenting with a potentially hepatotoxic ingestion of acetaminophen should be admitted for both maternal observation and fetal monitoring. In general, the maternal-fetal outcome is good following an acetaminophen overdose.[25, 30, 34, 35] Thus, acetaminophen poisoning by itself should not be an indication for termination of a pregnancy.[30, 36] However, because the risk of significant fetal toxicity is greatest in the third trimester, some support emergent delivery of a mature fetus to allow direct extrauterine NAC therapy if the mother has documented toxic levels of acetaminophen.[11] If the mother demonstrates signs of hepatic failure or hepatic encephalopathy, she should be admitted to an intensive care unit. In this setting, consultation with a gastroenterologist or hepatologist is recommended for potential maternal liver transplantation.

IRON

As a result of its widely prescribed use in prenatal care, iron preparations are readily available to the obstetric patient and are documented as being the second most common drugs of overdose during pregnancy.[1] Iron normally does not diffuse through the placenta but is actively transported against a gradient into the fetal circulation.[37] As a result, the placenta acts as a barrier to protect the fetus from iron toxicity.[11] Animal studies have demonstrated that acutely elevated maternal serum iron concentrations are not accompanied by significant elevations in fetal serum iron levels.[37] In general, the mother suffers more than the fetus from the insult of iron. Fetal compromise probably results from maternal instability rather than from the direct toxic effects of iron. Although elevated iron levels in the fetus may be detrimental, there are no known reports of anomalies or adverse outcomes in the neonate in cases of maternal toxicity if the mother has survived the overdose.[38]

In pregnancy, peak serum iron levels have been reported to appear within 2 to 4 hours after ingestion; this interval is similar to that for nonpregnant patients.[39] The laboratory hallmark of toxicity is the attainment of serum iron levels exceeding the measured total iron-binding capacity of serum. However, these laboratory findings have not been consistently observed in the poisoned pregnant patient. In one reported case, iron levels in a third-trimester patient with toxicity did not exceed the total iron-binding capacity nor did they correlate with the severity of the poisoning.[10, 40]

Therapeutic interventions in iron toxicity begin with general decontamination principles. Specifically, gastric decontamination with lavage may be indicated in any potentially toxic overdose after recent ingestion. Use of syrup of ipecac is discouraged and contraindicated if the patient has already vomited, has altered mental status, or is presenting later than 1 hour after ingestion. Activated charcoal, although considered safe in the pregnant patient, is not efficacious in iron poisoning because of the drug's small ionic size.[10] However, activated charcoal may be administered if multiple drugs were ingested or if the history is unclear. Whole-bowel irrigation may be indicated in the setting of an iron overdose, particularly if multiple radiodense pills are observed on an abdominal flat plate radiograph.[15] Alternatively, if avoiding the minimal radiation exposure of an abdominal radiograph is desired, ultrasonography can be used for detection of the presence of pill fragments in the gastrointestinal tract as well as for assessment of the status of the fetus.[41]

Deferoxamine (DFO) is the specific chelating antidote for iron poisoning. DFO acts by binding to free circulating iron. Unlike elemental iron, the DFO-iron complex can be excreted through the kidneys. DFO therapy is recommended in the pregnant patient who has ingested more than 30 mg/kg of elemental iron or who has acute serum iron levels greater than 350 μg/dL.[38] The usual dose is 15 mg/kg per hour intravenously, not to exceed a daily dose of 6 g.[38, 42] Although some practitioners recommend that chelation therapy be given until after the urine clears of its vin rose color, others continue therapy until the acidosis and symptoms resolve. At present, establishing a specific endpoint of therapy remains a subject of controversy.

Chelation is critical in significant maternal iron toxicity, and its use should always override theoretic concerns of fetal teratogenicity.[16, 43] Cases of maternal death have been reported when DFO was withheld because of this concern.[16, 17] Reports of two animal studies documented fetal skeletal abnormalities during exposure to high doses of DFO during early gestation.[42, 43] However, limited case reports suggest that

DFO can be administered to a pregnant patient with iron toxicity without concern about producing adverse fetal effects.[38, 40] A more recent animal study with an ovine model demonstrated that maternal infusion of DFO resulted in a rapid decrease in maternal serum iron concentrations but had minimal effect on fetal serum iron levels; this supports the theory that DFO does not cross the placenta.[37] To date, infants delivered after DFO therapy appear to have tolerated the antidote well.[40, 43] Therefore, pregnancy should not be considered a contraindication to the use of DFO if its administration to the mother is indicated.[17, 44–45]

The largest known study addressing the effect on the outcome of pregnancy in iron overdose was a retrospective investigation involving 49 pregnant patients who had mild to moderate iron overdoses.[46] Twenty-five of these patients (51%) were treated with DFO. Of these, 21 had normal outcomes, and the authors found no evidence to suggest that DFO given for iron overdose caused toxicity in either the mother or the baby. Any malformations were not considered to be directly related to the DFO administration by the authors because all of the patients were treated after the first trimester.

Any pregnant patient who presents following a serious acute iron ingestion should be aggressively managed, should receive chelation therapy with DFO, and should be admitted to the medical intensive care unit for both maternal and fetal monitoring. If the patient is medically stable and has only a potentially toxic ingestion, admission to a general medical or obstetrical ward is appropriate, with close observation of serial iron levels and, possibly, chelation therapy. If the mother receives chelation therapy with DFO, particularly in later stages of pregnancy, pediatric postpartum monitoring of the infant's serum iron levels is recommended.[38, 42, 43] Finally, when the mother recovers from a significant iron ingestion, gastroenterologic consultation is recommended for diagnosis of any subsequent gastrointestinal scarring in the weeks after ingestion.

SALICYLATES

Salicylate use is extremely common in pregnancy because of the ubiquitous nature of the drug in over-the-counter preparations. It has been reported in numerous studies as one of the drugs most commonly taken during pregnancy.[2, 4, 47] Many pregnant women have taken salicylate-containing medications, both with and without medical supervision.[48] In therapeutic doses, salicylates appear to be safe in early pregnancy but should be avoided in the third trimester because they may affect neonatal coagulation and cause premature closure of the ductus arteriosus.[6]

Maternally ingested salicylates freely cross the placenta and can be detected in fetal serum. The toxicity of salicylates stems from the parent compound and not from its metabolites (as is the case with acetaminophen).[11] Particularly in later stages of pregnancy, the fetus appears to be at greater risk for toxicity than the mother for several reasons. First, salicylate concentrations at a given maternal level are greater in the fetus.[49] Second, a greater proportion of salicylates enters the fetal central nervous system than the mother's. Third, compared with the mother, the fetus has reduced buffering capacity in the face of the ensuing acidosis. Finally, the fetus has reduced metabolism and excretion of the drug compared with the mother.[11, 50] Several studies have documented the characteristic platelet abnormality caused by salicylates—namely, a loss of the secondary phase of platelet aggregation in babies born to mothers who had ingested salicylates just prior to delivery.[51] There have been several reports of petechiae, purpura, cephalohematoma, and severe gastrointestinal and intracranial bleeding in infants whose mothers had taken salicylates late in the third trimester.[51, 52] Salicylates also have been found to displace bilirubin from albumin-binding sites and may lead to hyperbilirubinemia in the neonatal period. One study of 144 infants chronically exposed to salicylates *in utero* revealed significantly lower birth weights and increased perinatal mortality but no significant difference in rate of congenital anomalies.[53] These infants were found to have elevated cord blood salicylate levels but demonstrated no clinical evidence of bleeding or hypoglycemia. In comparison with children, neonatal hypoglycemia has not been commonly observed.[49, 54] Pregnant women who ingest salicylates on a frequent basis are reported to have longer gestational periods, prolonged labor, more hemorrhage, and a higher frequency of cesarean section.[49] All of these are believed to be attributed to the antiprostaglandin properties of salicylates.[54]

The treatment guidelines for salicylate poisoning in the pregnant mother are deficient in the literature. The current recommendation is to treat the mother in the same fashion as the nonpregnant patient. Initial stabilization, supportive care, fluid management, and electrolyte and glucose monitoring are essential. Gastric lavage and administration of activated charcoal should be undertaken when indicated. Because salicylates may form gastric concretions, late gastric lavage may prove beneficial; however, this has not been proved. In addition, because of delayed absorption, serial determination of serum salicylate levels is essential until peak and declining levels have been documented. Enhanced elimination with sodium bicarbonate alkalization appears to be safe and efficacious in the pregnant patient, particularly if the mother is acidotic. As with any salicylate overdose, the effectiveness of alkalization is dependent on adequate potassium supplementation. Hemodialysis is indicated in the mother with salicylate toxicity, and the inclusion criteria are the same as those in the nonpregnant patient. However, these treatment methods generally may not be as effective in the fetus as in the mother; therefore, prompt delivery of a mature fetus should be considered for the outcome of treatment to be optimal.[11]

The obstetric patient manifesting signs of severe

salicylism (metabolic acidosis, pulmonary edema, or seizures) should be admitted to the intensive care unit, and close maternal and fetal monitoring should be conducted. In this setting, the nephrologist should be consulted for emergent hemodialysis. In the stable maternal patient with a potentially toxic ingestion, admission to an obstetric or medical ward is recommended for serial determination of salicylate levels. If the overdose occurs in the later stages of gestation, a pediatrician should be alerted to the potential for bleeding complications in the newborn.

COCAINE

Cocaine abuse is reported to be increasing among women of all socioeconomic groups in the United States. Cocaine abuse by women is most widespread during the childbearing years, and this age group has shown the greatest increase in recreational use since the mid-1980s.[6, 55] In fact, 20% of all women between the ages of 26 and 34 years have used cocaine at least once.[56] In addition, cocaine use is on the increase among pregnant women. In one study, 17% of urban women enrolled in prenatal care were found to have used cocaine at least once during pregnancy.[57] It is estimated that as many as one fetus out of every ten is exposed to cocaine via maternal use.[58] Smoking of crack cocaine has become the predominant route of exposure in pregnant women.[59] Unfortunately, an estimated 60% of pregnant women who use crack cocaine receive no prenatal care.[60] Many addicted women do not discover they are pregnant until well into gestation. Although some seek treatment, others assume that the fetus has already been harmed and therefore continue to abuse.[61] Finally, there exists a false perception in the lay population that cocaine use speeds up the labor and delivery process; in fact, it may actually intensify the awareness of pain and prolong delivery time.[62]

Symptoms and adverse effects of cocaine toxicity in the mother can include agitation, tachycardia, hyperthermia, hypertension, seizures, myocardial ischemia, cerebral vascular accidents, and intracranial bleeding and result in significant morbidity and mortality.[59] Maternal concentrations of serum cholinesterases are diminished during pregnancy; this results in more sustained cocaine blood levels than occur in nonpregnant users.[63] Fetal cholinesterase level is relatively deficient when compared with adult levels. Cocaine readily crosses the placental barrier; thus, the fetus is at risk following maternal use of cocaine by any route. Cocaine is biotransformed by the human placenta, presumably by cholinesterase activity. Therefore, the placenta may provide a moderate degree of protection from cocaine-induced morbidity by converting the cocaine into less active metabolites.[58] Cocaine administration in the pregnant ovine model increased uterine vascular resistance, decreased uterine blood flow, increased fetal heart rate and arterial blood pressure, and decreased fetal oxygen content.[64, 65] This animal study also showed that pregnancy itself increased the cardiovascular toxicity to cocaine; this effect is thought to be mediated by progesterone.[65] Maternal exposure can cause preterm labor, abruptio placentae, decreased fetal growth, prematurity, urinary congenital anomalies, neonatal neurobehavioral deficits, and fetal death.[66–68] However, assessing maternal and fetal risks of cocaine use is difficult because this patient population may abuse other illicit drugs, alcohol, and cigarettes. In addition, studies are limited by inconsistent cocaine detection methods, confounding socioeconomic factors, and reporting bias.[67]

Any pregnant patient suspected to have cocaine toxicity should undergo a toxicologic screen for confirmation. Urinary toxicologic screens detect cocaine metabolites for only 48 to 72 hours; therefore, an accurate prenatal history may prove more reliable. However, in one urban study, 24% of pregnant women denied using cocaine at the time of their interview but tested positive for the drug on urinary screens.[57] More recent studies have advocated the use of neonatal hair[69] or meconium tests for the measurement of cumulative intrauterine exposure.[70]

Numerous studies in the medical literature address the epidemiology, maternal-neonatal outcome, and detoxification efforts of the cocaine-abusing pregnant patient. However, specific treatment recommendations in the acutely intoxicated pregnant patient are lacking. As with other poisonings, optimal treatment of the mother ultimately benefits the fetus. The agitation, hypertension, tachycardia, and myocardial ischemia experienced by the acutely cocaine-intoxicated mother can often be controlled by the administration of benzodiazepines alone. Clinical experience supports use of these drugs as a first-line treatment for cocaine-intoxicated patients. Benzodiazepines have effective anxiolytic properties, and they reduce blood pressure, heart rate, and myocardial oxygen demand in the face of myocardial ischemia.[56] Although controversial, according to one authority, no specific fetal malformations have been attributed to the administration of benzodiazepines during pregnancy.[6] However, late in gestation or soon after delivery, the newborn can have transient central nervous system and respiratory depression. In this setting, the benefit of giving benzodiazepines to a pregnant patient with acute cocaine toxicity may outweigh the potential risks to the fetus. When presenting with chest pain, the mother should undergo baseline electrocardiography with continuous maternal and fetal monitoring. The presence of cardiac ischemia may also require the administration of nitroglycerin.[56] Cocaine-induced seizures should be treated with intravenous benzodiazepines. If seizure activity is refractory, phenobarbital loading may be an alternative therapy.[6] The use of phenytoin should be avoided because it is well documented to be neurotoxic to the fetus.[6] With seizures occurring during the third trimester of pregnancy, the diagnosis of eclampsia should also be entertained and usual intravenous doses magnesium administered, if indicated. One of the most critical treatment interventions is the rapid cooling of the acutely hyperthermic patient, as temperature duration and level can have a negative effect on both maternal and fetal mortality.[71] Finally, in a patient presenting with ingestion of cocaine packets (body packers and stuffers), activated charcoal and whole-bowel irrigation is recommended. In general, both modalities have been shown to be safe and efficacious in the pregnant patient.

Any pregnant patient presenting with severe cocaine toxicity should be monitored in the intensive care setting. If the patient manifests cardiotoxicity, a cardiologist should be consulted. If the mother and fetus survive the acute intoxication, prenatal care should focus on drug rehabilitation and education. If the cocaine exposure occurred throughout the prenatal period, the pediatrician should be aware that the newborn may manifest signs of cocaine withdrawal.

CARBON MONOXIDE

Carbon monoxide (CO) is the leading cause of poison-induced deaths in the United States.[72] The clinical presentation of CO poisoning can be subtle in the pregnant patient; if not approached with a high index of suspicion, misdiagnosis and significant maternal-fetal morbidity can result. During pregnancy, endogenous CO levels increase about 20% above normal nonpregnant values secondary to increased fetal production, increased red cell mass, and the action of progesterone on hepatic microsomal enzymes.[73] Additionally, at a given CO exposure, the pregnant patient is more susceptible to toxicity because of her increased minute ventilation. Cigarette smoking also results in higher than normal maternal and fetal CO levels.

In the mother, the affinity of CO to bind to hemoglobin is 240-fold that of oxygen; thus, CO exposure results in cellular hypoxia. CO decreases the capacity of blood to transport oxygen. CO shifts the oxyhemoglobin saturation curve to the left and alters the shape so that it appears more hyperbolic (Fig. 16–1).[73]

Fetal carboxyhemoglobin exacerbates this shift to the left, impairing the release of oxygen to the tissues. Under normal circumstances, the fetal carboxyhemoglobin level is approximately 10% to 15% greater than that of the mother.[73] With maternal exposure, the fetal carboxyhemoglobin level increases more slowly than does the maternal level but continues to increase for several hours after acute exposure until an equilibrium is reached.[72]

CO readily crosses the placenta by simple diffusion, and fetal hemoglobin has a greater affinity for CO than does adult hemoglobin.[74] As a result, unlike in the majority of poisonings, the fetus is at greater risk of toxicity and mortality than is the mother. This has been documented in several case reports in which the mother survived a significant CO exposure but fetal demise ensued.[72, 75, 76] As with the general population, maternal blood CO levels often do not correlate with the severity of symptoms. Maternal symptoms at the scene of exposure are a better predictor of fetal toxicity than are CO levels.[72, 74, 77] These symptoms may include altered mental status, neurologic deficits, seizures, and coma.

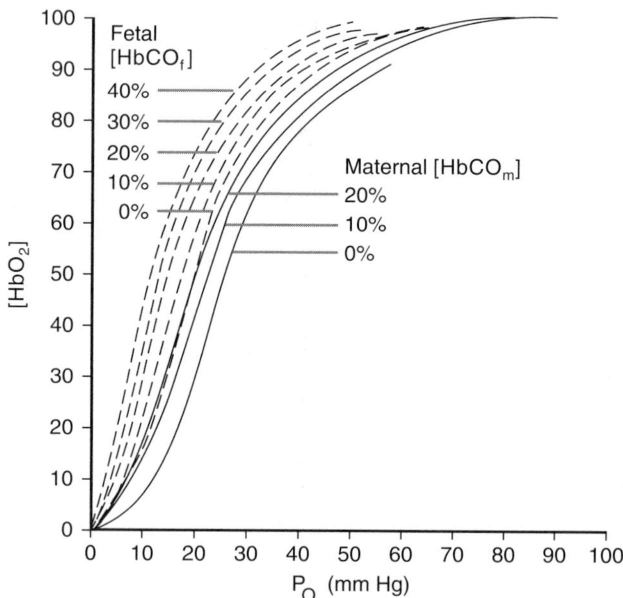

Figure 16–1. Human maternal and fetal oxyhemoglobin saturation curve showing the effects of carbon monoxide.

In addition to removal of the patient from the site of exposure, oxygen therapy is paramount. Oxygen acts by competing with the CO for hemoglobin binding sites. When the patient breathes room air, the half-life of CO is 5 to 6 hours; when she breathes 100% oxygen, it is 90 minutes, and when hyperbaric oxygenation (HBO) is used, the half-life decreases to 20 minutes. Because the fetal hemoglobin binds CO much more readily than does maternal hemoglobin, it is recommended that pregnant patients receive 100% oxygen 5 times longer than normal adults to ensure adequate reduction of CO in the fetus.[72, 74, 77] In the past, controversy existed with respect to the treatment of the pregnant patient with HBO because of the adverse effects of high partial pressures of oxygen on the fetus observed in animal investigations.[78] However, in several human studies, the majority of which are case reports,[74, 77–79] the use of HBO in pregnant patients exposed to CO is advocated.[10, 78, 80] Although no definitive guidelines have been established, it has been recommended that more liberal HBO treatment be initiated in pregnant patients because of the enhanced vulnerability of the fetus to CO, hypoxia, and permanent brain damage. The safety of HBO was documented in a prospective study in which 44 pregnant patients with CO poisoning tolerated HBO without any fetal or obstetric morbidity.[81] Human clinical experience indicates that the short duration of high-dose oxygen exposure used during HBO therapy can be tolerated by the fetus in all stages of pregnancy and can reduce the risk of death or deformity to the mother and fetus.[78] Indications for HBO in pregnancy include:

1. Any unfavorable neurologic findings in the mother
2. Signs of fetal distress
3. Pregnancy and CO levels greater than 20%

All pregnant patients with suspected CO poisoning should be removed from the source of exposure and transported to an emergency facility for evaluation, fetal monitoring, CO level measurement, and oxygen therapy. If symptoms or CO levels indicate the need for HBO, the patient should be transported to a facility able to provide HBO. With exposures occurring in the early stages of pregnancy, consultation should be obtained regarding potential fetal neurotoxicity. However, one case reported significant first-trimester CO exposure with subsequent normal outcome in the newborn.[82] If the mother presents in late-stage pregnancy and delivery is eminent, the pediatric intensivist should be advised of the need for aggressive oxygen delivery to the neonate.

LEAD

Lead poisoning is a major public health problem and a significant maternal and fetal toxicity. It is well documented that the fetus is at risk from maternal lead exposure. In fact, lead has historically been used as an abortifacient.[83] Pregnant women can suffer from environmental[84] or occupational lead exposure.[85, 86] The mother also may unknowingly ingest lead from containers coated with lead glaze[87] or demonstrate increased pica behavior during the prenatal period.[88, 89] In addition, because of the hormonal changes that occur during pregnancy, chronic maternal lead stores obtained prior to pregnancy may be mobilized from the bone and transferred to the fetus.[90] Placental transfer of lead has been demonstrated in the human fetus at 12 to 14 weeks' gestation, with fetal tissue lead stores increasing as gestational age advances.[84] This heavy metal has been shown to induce spontaneous abortion, teratogenesis, and neurodevelopmental delays in the newborn.[11] One study measured umbilical cord blood lead levels in over 5000 consecutive deliveries of over 20 weeks' gestation. Lead was found to be associated in a dose-related fashion with an increased risk of minor congenital anomalies such as hemangiomas, lymphangiomas, hydrocele, skin tags, and undescended testicles. This study controlled for other covariables and found no characteristic anatomic defect.[91] Although currently the subject of debate, the highest acceptable lead level in young children is 10 μg/dL. However, according to one investigative report, the fetus appears to be adversely affected at low blood lead concentrations, and the authors cautioned against the application of any level toward the fetus.[92] The primary treatment of maternal and congenital lead poisoning is discovery and removal of the mother from the source of exposure.

Data on chelation in obstetric patients with elevated blood lead levels are limited. In the past, there was concern that chelating agents may be teratogenic or toxic to the fetus because of their nonspecific action on metal binding and subsequent excretion.[90] According to one leading authority, maternal toxicity should be the primary reason for initiating chelation for lead poisoning during pregnancy.[11] Calcium ethylenediaminetetraacetic acid (EDTA) has been used with some success in the later stages of the third trimester of pregnancy.[86, 88, 90] In one case, a maternal blood lead level of 86 μg/dL was documented. The mother was given a 3-day chelation course with calcium EDTA. Eight days later, at delivery, her level had decreased to 26 μg/dL, but the cord blood level remained elevated at 79 μg/dL.[88] Based on this and other studies, it is unlikely that EDTA crosses the placenta and would therefore be an ineffective fetal chelator.[11] In addition, newborn infants have required continued chelation therapy with calcium EDTA, dimercaprol (British antilewisite), and d-penicillamine for weeks after delivery because lead levels have been noted to rebound.[87, 88] This demonstrates that a short intrauterine course of chelation therapy with these agents may not be adequate for fully treating congenital lead toxicity.

Because intramuscular dimercaprol penetrates the central nervous system tissues, it theoretically should cross into fetal tissues, although no data describing its use in pregnant humans with lead poisoning exist. However, this drug may be of limited value in the pregnant patient because of its known side adverse effects such as hypertension, febrile reactions, tachycardia, and nephrotoxicity. The new oral lead chelator dimercaptosuccinic acid (DMSA, succimer) is structurally related to dimercaprol but produces fewer severe side effects and may be the agent of choice for treating maternal lead toxicity.[11] However, no adequate, well-controlled studies exist regarding its use in the obstetric patient. Recent animal studies have documented that DMSA is not toxic to fetal development.[93] In one investigation, DMSA was administered to pregnant rodents. On day 20 of gestation, no gross external abnormalities, visceral or skeletal abnormalities, or teratogenicity at any dosage level was noted in the fetal rats.[94]

A pregnant patient exhibiting signs of acute lead intoxication with encephalopathy should be admitted to the hospital, with institution of chelation therapy and close fetal monitoring. When the blood lead levels are elevated but the mother is asymptomatic, removal of the patient from the source is essential, as are serial monitoring of levels and possible institution of outpatient chelation therapy. If maternal toxicity is documented at any time during the prenatal period, the newborn should be monitored for initial and rebounding lead levels.

ORGANOPHOSPHATES

Insecticide ingestions are uncommon in pregnancy; however, insecticides are widely available to an expectant mother with suicidal intentions. Pregnant females may also be occupationally or environmentally exposed to pesticides (organophosphates, carbamates, and pyrethrins). In addition, there has been a case report of its use in conjunction with substance abuse. Because of "street knowledge" that lowering one's cholinesterase activity may prolong the euphoric effects of cocaine, a near-term pregnant woman took an organophosphate with her cocaine and presented in both cholinergic and sympathomimetic crisis.[95] In general, the patient with acute organophosphate poisoning can present with maternal cholinergic crisis (diarrhea, urination, miosis, bradycardia, bronchosecretions, emesis, lacrimation, and salivation) along with nicotinic symptoms of central nervous system depression and muscle fasciculations.[96]

Few data account for the transplacental passage of specific organophosphate compounds.[11] In a case report describing both maternal and fetal fatalities from an organophosphate ingestion, the authors documented fetal levels of the insecticide on autopsy, indicating that these agents cross the placental barrier.[97] Regarding cholinesterase enzyme levels, studies have noted 50% to 70% decreases in the activity of red blood cell cholinesterase in normal neonatal plasma.[98, 99] This would intuitively make the fetus more susceptible to the effects of anticholinesterase insecticides.[11]

As with any organophosphate poisoning, the mother should be managed with gastric and skin decontamination, when indicated, along with aggressive airway control to maintain adequate maternal and fetal oxygenation. There have been cases in which organophosphate poisonings in the second and third trimesters of pregnancy have been successfully treated with appropriate doses of atropine (for the cholinergic effects) and pralidoxime (2-PAM) for the nicotinic manifestations.[100] In two of the cases, the women delivered normal, full-term infants. In one investigation using a chick embryo model, supplemental use of oxime cholinesterase reactivators such as pralidoxime reduced the incidence and severity of developmental defects to specific organophosphate teratogens such as parathion and dicrotophos (bidrin). The protective effect noted was dose related.[101]

Another case report described a woman at 35 weeks' gestation who presented with an unknown overdose in cholinergic crisis.[102] Organophosphate toxicity was presumed and confirmed by markedly depressed serum and erythrocyte cholinesterase levels. Moderate doses of atropine in the mother resulted in maternal improvement but also in profound fetal tachycardia, which led the treating physicians to stop the infusion; worsening of the mother's condition resulted. An emergent cesarean section was performed, and a hypotonic infant with low Apgar scores was delivered. The mother went on to require 8 days of assisted ventilation and 11 days of atropine infusion. The newborn required mechanical ventilation for 2 days and atropine therapy for 8 days. Neither patient received pralidoxime. Compared with that of the the baby, it took longer for the mother's cholinesterase activity to recover to normal. Of interest, the mother presented with more serious symptoms of poisoning, requiring doses of atropine that proved toxic or intolerable to the fetus. However, it is difficult to ascribe the cause of the fetal distress in this one case. Several factors may have contributed to both maternal and fetal distress, such as fetal hypoxia secondary to maternal respiratory distress, or the direct transplacental fetal action of the atropine.

Any pregnant patient with organophosphate poisoning manifesting acute cholinergic or nicotinic manifestations should be managed in an intensive care setting, with close maternal and fetal monitoring and administration of appropriate doses of atropine and pralidoxime.[96] Additionally, it may prove efficacious to deliver a mature or term fetus in distress for initiation of extrauterine therapy.[11]

CONCLUSION

Pregnant women have a significant risk of toxic exposures and may present a diagnostic and therapeutic dilemma. Unfortunately, few adequate or well-controlled studies addressing treatment guidelines for the poisoned obstetric patient have been published in the medical literature. The most critical issue in managing the pregnant patient who has been exposed to any toxin is stabilization and treatment of the mother, as this has a beneficial effect on the maternal and fetal outcomes. If questions concerning potential toxins and exposure to the pregnant patient arise, regional poison control centers and several resources on teratogens are available.

References

General

1. Rayburn W, Aronow R, DeLancey B, et al: Drug overdose during pregnancy: An overview from a metropolitan poison control center. Obstet Gynecol *64*:611–614, 1984.
2. Kleiner GJ, Gretson WM: Suicide during pregnancy. *In* Cherry SH, Merkatz IR (eds): Complications of Pregnancy: Medical, Surgical, Gynecologic, Pyschosocial, and Perinatal. 4th ed. Baltimore, Williams & Wilkins, pp 269–289, 1991.
3. Piper JM, Baum C, Kennedy DL: Prescription drug use before and during pregnancy in a Medicaid population. Am J Obstet Gynecol *157*:148–156, 1987.
4. Bonassi S, Magnani M, et al: Factors related to drug consumption during pregnancy. Acta Obstet Gynecol Scand *73*:535–540, 1994.
5. Chasnoff IJ: Drug use and women: Establishing a standard of care. Ann N Y Acad Sci *562*:208–210, 1989.
6. Koren G: Maternal-Fetal Toxicology: A Clinician's Guide. 2nd ed. New York, Marcel Dekker, 1994.
7. Ellenhorn MH, Barceloux DG: Toxic exposure during pregnancy. *In* Ellenhorn MJ, Barceloux DG (eds): Medical Toxicology: Diagnosis and Treatment of Human Poisoning. New York, Elsevier, pp 131–152, 1988.
8. Fine JS: Reproductive and perinatal principles. *In* Goldfrank LF, Flomenbaum NE, Lewin NA, et al (eds): Goldfrank's Toxicologic Emergencies. 5th ed. Norwalk, CT, Appleton-Century-Crofts, pp 421–437, 1994.
9. Graves HB, Smith EE, Braen CR, et al: Clinical policy for the initial approach to patients presenting with acute toxic ingestion or dermal or inhalation exposure. Ann Emerg Med *25*:570–585, 1995.

10. Ford MD, Olshaker JS: Concepts and controversies in toxicology. Emerg Med Clin North Am *12*:285–299, 1994.
11. Tenenbein M: Poisoning in pregnancy. *In* Koren G (ed): Maternal-Fetal Toxicology: A Clinician's Guide. 2nd ed. New York, Marcel Dekker, pp 223–252, 1994.
12. D'Ascoli P, Gall SA: Common poisons. *In* Gleicher N (ed): Principles of Medical Therapy in Pregnancy. New York, Plenum Press, 1985.
13. Howland MA: Whole bowel irrigation. *In* Goldfrank LR, Flomenbaum NE, Lewin NA, et al (eds): Goldfrank's Toxicologic Emergencies. 5th ed. Norwalk, CT, Appleton & Lange, pp 74–75, 1994.
14. Turk J, Aks SE, Ampuero F, et al: Successful therapy of iron intoxication in pregnant with intravenous deferoxamine and whole bowel irrigation. Vet Hum Toxicol *35*:441–444, 1993.
15. Van Ameyde KJ, Tenenbein M: Whole bowel irrigation during pregnancy. Am J Obstet Gynecol *160*:646–647, 1989.
16. Strom RL, Schiller P, Seeds AT, et al: Fatal iron poisoning in a pregnant female. Minn Med *59*:483–489, 1976.
17. Manoguerra AS: Iron poisoning: Report of a fatal case in an adult. Am J Hosp Pharm *59*:1088–1090, 1976.
18. Kurtz GG, Michael UF, Morosi HJ, et al: Hemodialysis during pregnancy: Report of a case of glutethimide poisoning complicated by acute renal failure. Arch Intern Med *118*:30–32, 1966.
19. Vaziri ND, Kumar KP, Mirahmadi K, et al: Hemodialysis in the treatment of acute chloral hydrate poisoning. South Med J *7*:377–378, 1977.
20. Trebbin WM: Hemodialysis in pregnancy. JAMA *241*:1811–1812, 1979.
21. Hou S: Pregnancy in women requiring dialysis for renal failure. Am J Kidney Dis *9*:368–373, 1987.

Acetaminophen

22. Ley G, Garrettson LK, Soda DM: Evidence of placental transfer of acetaminophen. Pediatrics *55*:895, 1975.
23. Roberts I, Robinson MZ, Mughal JG, et al: Paracetamol metabolites in the neonate following maternal overdose. Br J Pharmacol *18*:201–206, 1984.
24. Wang LH, Rudolph AM, Benet LZ: Pharmacokinetic studies of the disposition of acetaminophen in the sheep maternal-placental unit. J Pharmacol Exp Ther *238*:198–205, 1986.
25. Riggs BS, Bronsteine AC, Kulig K, et al: Acute acetaminophen overdose during pregnancy. Obstet Gynecol *74*:247–253, 1989.
26. Haibach H, Akhter JE, Muscato MS, et al: Acetaminophen overdose with fetal demise. Am J Clin Pathol *82*:240–242, 1984.
27. Kurzel RB: Can acetaminophen excess result in maternal and fetal toxicity? South Med J *83*:953–954, 1990.
28. Rayburn W, Skukla U, Stetson P, et al: Acetaminophen pharmacokinetics: Comparison between pregnant and nonpregnant women. Am J Obstet Gynecol *155*:1353–1356, 1986.
29. Smilkstein MJ, Knapp GL, Kulig KW, et al: Efficacy of oral *N*-acetylcysteine in the treatment of acetaminophen overdose. N Engl J Med *319*:1557–1562, 1988.
30. McElhatton PR, Sullivan FM, Volans GN, et al: Paracetamol poisoning in pregnancy: An analysis of the outcomes of cases referred to the Teratology Information Service of the National Poisons Information Service. Hum Exp Toxicol *9*:147–153, 1990.
31. Ansai N, Kimura T, Chida S, et al: Studies on the metabolic fate of *N*-acetylcysteine in rats and dogs. Pharmacometrics *26*:249–260; 1983.
32. Seldon BS, Curry SC, Clark RF, et al: Transplacental transport of *N*-acetylcysteine in an ovine model. Ann Emerg Med *20*:1069–1072, 1991.
33. Harrison PM, Keays R, Bray GP, et al: Improved outcome of paracetamol-induced fulminant hepatic failure by late administration of acetylcysteine. Lancet *335*:1572–1573, 1990.
34. Stokes IM: Paracetamol overdose in the second trimester of pregnancy: Case report. Br J Obstet Gynecol *91*:286–288, 1984.
35. Ludmir J, Main DM, Landon MB, et al: Maternal acetaminophen overdose at 15 weeks of gestation. Obstet Gynecol *67*:750–751, 1986.
36. Janes J, Routledge PA: Recent developments in the management of paracetamol (acetaminophen) poisoning. Drug Safety *7*:170–177, 1992.

Iron

37. Curry SC, Bond GR, Raschke R, et al: An ovine model of maternal iron poisoning in pregnancy. Ann Emerg Med *19*:632–638, 1990.
38. Lacoste H, Goyert GL, Goldman LS, et al: Acute iron intoxication in pregnancy: Case report and review of the literature. Obstet Gynecol *80*:500–501, 1992.
39. Rotham JL, Lietman PS: Acute iron poisoning: A review. Am J Dis Child *134*:875–879, 1980.
40. Olenmark M, Biber B, Dottori O, et al: Fatal iron intoxication in late pregnancy. Clin Toxicol *25*:347–359, 1987.
41. Anderson AC, Share JC, Woolf AD: The use of ultrasound in the diagnosis of toxic ingestions. Vet Hum Toxicol *32*:355, 1990.
42. Blanc P, Hryhorczuk DO, Danel I: Deferoxamine treatment of acute iron intoxication in pregnancy. Obstet Gynecol *64*:12S–14S, 1984.
43. Rayburn WF, Donn SM, Wulf ME: Iron overdose during pregnancy: Successful therapy with deferoxamine therapy. Am J Obstet Gynecol *147*:717–718, 1983.
44. Czeizel A, Szentesi I, Szekeres, et al: Pregancy outcome and health conditions of offspring of self-poisoned women. Acta Pediatr Hung *25*:209–236, 1984.
45. Perucca E: Drug metabolism in pregnancy, infancy and childhood. Pharmacol Ther *34*:129–143, 1987.
46. McElhatton PR, Roberts JC, Sullivan FM: The consequences of iron overdose and its treatment with deferoxamine in pregnancy. Hum Exp Toxicol *10*:251–259, 1991.

Salicylates

47. Corby DG: Aspirin in pregnancy: Maternal and fetal effects. Pediatrics *62*(Suppl):930–937, 1978.
48. Palmisano PA, Cassady G: Salicylate exposure in the perinate. JAMA *209*:556–558, 1969.
49. Levy G, Procnal JA, Garrettson LK: Distribution of salicylate between neonatal and maternal serum at diffusion equilibrium. Clin Pharmacol Ther *18*:210–214; 1975.
50. Levy G, Garrettson LK: Kinetics of salicylate elimination by newborn infants of mothers who ingested aspirin before delivery. Pediatrics *53*:201–210, 1974.
51. Haslam RH, Ekert H, Gillam GL: Hemorrhage in a neonate possibly due to maternal ingestion of salicylate. J Pediatr *84*:556, 1974.
52. Karlowicz MG, White LE: Severe intracranial hemorrhage in a term neonate associated with maternal acetylsalicylic acid ingestion. Clin Pediatr *32*:740–743, 1993
53. Turner G, Collins E: Fetal effects of regular salicylate ingestion in pregnancy. Lancet *3*:338–339, 1975.
54. Collins E: Maternal and fetal effects of acetaminophen and salicylates in pregnancy. Obstet Gynecol *58*:57S–62S, 1981.

Cocaine

55. Richardson GA, Day NL: Maternal and neonatal effects of moderate cocaine use during pregnancy. Neurotoxicol Teratol *13*:455–460, 1991.
56. Hollander JE: The management of cocaine-associated myocardial ischemia. N Engl J Med *333*:1267–1272, 1995.
57. Frank DA, Amaro H, Bauchner H, et al: Cocaine use during pregnancy: Prevalence and correlates. Pediatrics *82*:888–895, 1988.
58. Roe DA, Little BB, Bawdon RE, et al: Metabolism of cocaine by human placentas: Implications for fetal exposure. Am J Obstet Gynecol *163*:715–718, 1990.
59. Bandstra ES, Burkett G: Maternal-fetal and neonatal effects of *in utero* cocaine exposure. Semin Perinatol *15*:288–301, 1991.

60. Cherukui R, Minkoff H, Feldman J, et al: A cohort study of alkaloidal cocaine "crack" in pregnancy. Obstet Gynecol *72*:147–151, 1988.
61. Little DR: Cocaine addiction and pregnancy: Education in primary prevention. Res Staff Physician *39*:79–81, 1993.
62. Dombrowski MP, Wolfe HM, Welch RA, et al: Cocaine abuse is associated with abruptio placentae and decreased birth weight, but not shorter labor. Obstet Gynecol *77*:139–141, 1991.
63. Hoyme HE, Jones KL, Dixon SD, et al: Prenatal cocaine exposure and fetal vascular disruption. Pediatrics *85*:743–747, 1990.
64. Moore TR, Sorg J, Miller L, et al: Hemodynamic effects of intravenous cocaine on the pregnant ewe and fetus. Am J Obstet Gynecol *155*:883–888, 1986.
65. Woods JR, Plessinger MA, Clark KE: Effect of cocaine on uterine blood flow and fetal oxygenation. JAMA *257*:957–961, 1987.
66. Meeker JE, Reynolds PC: Fetal and newborn death associated with maternal cocaine use. J Anal Toxicol *14*:379–382, 1990.
67. Slutsker L: Risks associated with cocaine use during pregnancy. Obstet Gynecol *79*:778–789, 1992.
68. MacGregor SN, Keith LG, Chasnoff IJ, et al: Cocaine use during pregnancy: Adverse prenatal outcome. Am J Obstet Gynecol *157*:686–690, 1987.
69. Graham K, Koren G, Klein J, et al: Determination of gestational cocaine exposure by hair analysis. JAMA *262*:3328–3330, 1989.
70. Ostrea E, Brady M, Parks P, et al: Drug screening of meconium in infants of drug dependent mothers: An alternative to urine testing. J Pediatr *115*:474–483, 1989.
71. Brent RL: Relationship between uterine vascular disruption syndrome, and cocaine teratogenicity. Teratology *41*:757–760, 1990.

Carbon Monoxide

72. Farrow JR, Davis GJ, Roy TM, et al: Fetal death due to nonlethal carbon monoxide poisoning. J Forensic Sci *35*:1448–1452, 1990.
73. Longo LD: The biological effects of carbon monoxide on the pregnant woman, fetus, and newborn infant. Am J Obstet Gynecol *129*:69–103, 1977.
74. Koren GK, Sharav T, Garrettson LK, et al: A multicenter prospective study of fetal outcome following accidental carbon monoxide poisoning in pregnancy. Reprod Toxicol *5*:397–403, 1991.
75. Cramer CR: Fetal death due to accidental maternal carbon monoxide poisoning. J Toxicol Clin Toxicol *19*:297–301, 1982.
76. Muller GH, Graham S: Intrauterine death of the fetus due to accidental carbon monoxide poisoning. N Engl J Med *252*:1075–1078, 1955.
77. Caravati EM, Adams CJ, Joyce SM, et al: Fetal toxicity associated with maternal carbon monoxide poisoning. Ann Emerg Med *17*:714–717, 1988.
78. Van Hoesen KB, Camporesi EM, Moon RE, et al: Should hyperbaric oxygen be used to treat the pregnant patient for acute carbon monoxide poisoning? A case report and review of the literature. JAMA *261*:1039–1043, 1989.
79. Brown DB, Mueller GL, Golich FC: Hyperbaric oxygen treatment for carbon monoxide poisoning in pregnancy: A case report. Aviat Space Environ Med *63*:1011–1014, 1992.
80. Hollander DI, Nagey DA, Welch R, et al: Hyperbaric oxygen therapy for the treatment of acute carbon monoxide poisoning in pregnancy: A case report. J Reprod Med *32*:615–617, 1987.
81. Elkharrat D, Raphael JC, Jars-Guincestre MC, et al: Acute carbon monoxide intoxication and hyperbaric oxygen in pregnancy. Intensive Care Med *17*:289–292, 1991.
82. Copel JA, Bowen F, Bolognese RJ: Carbon monoxide intoxication in early pregnancy. Obstet Gynecol *59*:26S–28S, 1982.

Lead

83. Satin KP, Neutra RR, Guirguis G, et al: Umbilical cord blood lead levels in California. Arch Environ Health *46*:167–173, 1991.
84. Singh N, Donovan CM, Hanshaw JB: Neonatal lead intoxication in a prenatally exposed infant. J Pediatr *93*:1019–1021, 1978.
85. Ryu JE, Ziegler EE, Fomon SJ: Maternal lead exposure and blood concentration in infancy. J Pediatr *93*:476–478, 1978.
86. Angle CR, McIntire MS: Lead poisoning during pregnancy. Am J Dis Child *108*:436–439, 1964.
87. Ghafour SY, Khuffash FA, Ibrahim HS, et al: Congenital lead intoxication with seizures due to prenatal exposure. Clin Pediatr *23*:282–283, 1984.
88. Timpo AE, Amin JS, Casalino MB, et al: Congenital lead intoxication. J Pediatr *94*:765–767, 1979.
89. Horner RD, Lackey CJ, Kolasa K, Warren K: Pica practices of pregnant women. J Am Diet Assoc *91*:34–38, 1991.
90. Ernhart CB: A critical review of low-level lead prenatal lead exposure in the human: I. Effects on the fetus and newborn. Reprod Toxicol *6*:9–19, 1992.
91. Needleman HL, Rabinowitz M, Leviton A, et al: The relationship between prenatal exposure to lead and congenital anomalies. JAMA *251*:2956–2959, 1984.
92. Bellinger D, Leviton A, Waternaux C, et al: Longitudinal analyses of prenatal lead exposure and early cognitive development. N Engl J Med *316*:1037–1043, 1987.
93. Bosque MA, Domingo JL, Corbella J, et al: Developmental toxicity evaluation of monoisoamyl meso-2,3-dimercaptosuccinate in mice. J Toxicol Environ Health *42*:443–450, 1994.
94. Domingo JL, Ortega A, Paternain JL, et al: Meso-2,3 dimercaptosuccinic acid in pregnant Sprague-Dawley rats: Teratogenicity and alterations in mineral metabolism. J Toxicol Environ Health *30*:181–190, 1990.

Organophosphates

95. Aaron CK, Hirschman Z, Smilkstein M: Street pharmacology: A dangerous new way to prolong the high. Vet Hum Toxicol *31*:375, 1989.
96. Tafuri J, Roberts J: Organophosphate poisoning. Ann Emerg Med *16*:193–202, 1987.
97. Padadopoulou-Tsoukali H, Njau S: Mother-fetus postmortem toxicologic analysis in a fatal overdose with mecarbam. Forensic Sci Int *35*:249–252, 1987.
98. Zsigmond EK, Downs JR: Plasma cholinesterase activity in newborns and infants. Can Anesth Soc J *18*:278–285, 1971.
99. Karlsen RL, Sterri S, Lyngaas S, et al: Reference values for erythrocyte acetylcholinesterase and plasma cholinesterase activities in children: Implications for organophosphate intoxication. Scand J Clin Lab Invest *41*:301–302, 1981.
100. Karalliedde L, Senanayaka N, Ariaratam A: Acute organophosphate insecticide poisoning during pregnancy. Hum Toxicol *7*:363–364, 1988.
101. Landauder W: Cholinomimetic teratogens: The effect of oximes and related cholinesterase reactivators. Teratology *15*:33, 1977.
102. Weis OF, Müller FO, Lyell H, et al: Materno-fetal cholinesterase inhibitor poisoning. Anesth Analg *62*:233–235, 1983.

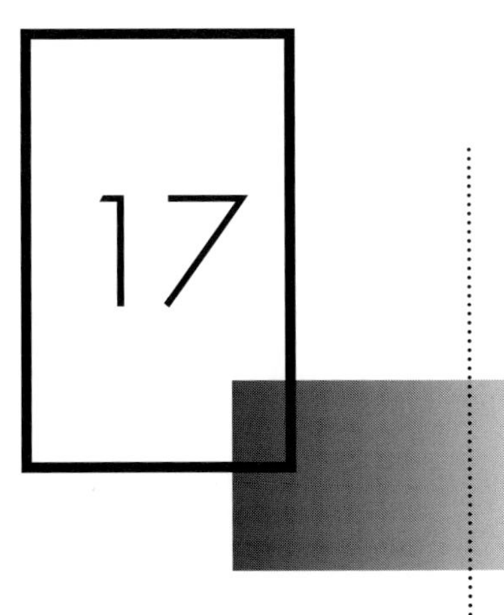

Toxic Emergencies in the Neonate

JAMES G. LINAKIS, PhD, MD

Since the late 1960s, technology has advanced to such a degree that premature and critically ill neonates who would have previously had no hope for survival can be saved, often with remarkably good outcome. With the advent of neonatal intensive care facilities, aggressive pharmacologic intervention has become the norm. Not surprisingly, the increasing use of potent pharmaceuticals in neonates has paved the way for occasional toxic reactions in this age group. This has been demonstrated on several occasions since the mid-1950s. In 1956, an increased incidence of kernicterus and excessive mortality were reported in premature infants receiving a sulfonamide antibiotic.[1] In 1959, high-dose chloramphenicol was implicated in the cardiovascular collapse of three neonates.[2] Similar outbreaks have been described with the use of benzyl alcohol as a preservative in bacteriostatic saline[3] and intravenous α-tocopherol[4, 5] in newborns. In addition, the escalating ubiquity of toxins in everyday life has also placed the neonate at risk for inadvertent exposure to environmental toxins.

This chapter reviews current knowledge regarding the causes of toxic reactions in the neonate and discusses those toxins that are most commonly responsible for neonatal toxic emergencies. It is by no means a comprehensive summary of the many toxic drug reactions reported to date in neonates. In addition to the descriptions provided in the text, further summary information on neonatal drug toxicity can be found in Table 17–1.

Neonatal toxicology does not entirely represent an extension of the previously established knowledge base of clinical toxicology. The physiology of the newborn is unique, and organs that have an important role in susceptibility to and the moderation of toxic reactions, such as the liver and kidney, are immature in their function. As a result, the manner in which the neonate handles a toxic exposure is frequently quite different from the response of an older child or adult. The basis for understanding these differences is dependent on knowledge of that which is unique to neonatal pharmacology and pharmacokinetics.

NEONATAL PHARMACOKINETICS

The term *pharmacokinetics* describes the various processes by which drugs are absorbed, distributed, metabolized, and excreted. Several of these processes are markedly different in the neonate than in the adult or even the older child. In many cases, the peculiarity of these processes in the neonate predisposes to the development of toxicity. This, combined with the fact that many infants in the neonatal intensive care unit suffer from diseases that may also alter the disposition of medications, places these infants at high risk for drug toxicity.[6]

Absorption

Drug absorption differences in the neonate are notable risk factors for the development of toxicity. Since gastrointestinal absorption of many drugs is pH dependent, the continuous changes that occur in gastric pH from birth through the second year of life complicate predictions of drug absorption.[7, 8] Furthermore, because gastric emptying is slower in the neonate and infant than in the adult, absorption of drugs may undergo considerable delay; this delay leads to a slowing in the time to peak concentration and in

Table 17–1. Commonly Used Drugs and Their Potential Toxicity in Neonates

Drug	Toxicity
Amikacin	Nephrotoxicity, ototoxicity
Aminophylline	Tachycardia, abdominal distention, GI hemorrhage, jitteriness, or seizures
Amoxicillin	Nephrotoxicity, vitamin K depletion, distal renal tubular acidosis
Ampicillin	Rare; increased transaminase; eosinophilia; irritability
Atropine sulfate	Tachycardia, urine retention, hyperthermia
Belladonna, tincture of	Hyperthermia, dry secretions, flushing
Bicarbonate	Transient hyperosmolarity, alkalosis, hypernatremia
Caffeine citrate	Tachycardia, seizures, abdominal distention
Calcium gluconate	Bradycardia, sloughing and calcification with IV infiltration; potentiates digitalis effect
Carbenicillin	Hypernatremia, sloughing with IV infiltration; transaminase elevation, platelet dysfunction
Cephalothin	Nephrotoxicity, neutropenia, false-positive Coombs' test results, allergic rash, poor passage through blood-brain barrier
Cefazolin	Neutropenia, thrombocytopenia, false-positive Coombs' test results, transient transaminase elevation
Chloral hydrate	Gastric irritation, paradoxic excitement
Chloramphenicol	May cause "gray baby syndrome" with toxic level; potentiates phenytoin effect, reversible bone marrow depression
Chlorothiazide	Hyperglycemia, hypokalemia, hyponatremia, alkalosis
Cholestyramine	Steatorrhea, GI dysfunction, malabsorption of fat-soluble vitamins; metabolic acidosis
Diazepam	Sodium benzoate diluent, competes with bilirubin for albumin binding sites; respiratory depression, hypotension
Diazoxide	Hypotension, hyperglycemia, sodium and water retention
Digoxin	Bradycardia, vomiting, arrhythmias, poor feeding
Epinephrine	Tachycardia, arrhythmia
Furosemide	Hypokalemia, hyponatremia, hypochloremia, alkalosis, dehydration, ototoxicity with aminoglycosides, renal calcifications; enhances nephrotoxicity of cephaloridine
Gentamicin	Nephrotoxicity, ototoxicity
Glucagon	Rebound hyperglycemia
Hydralazine HCl	May cause hypotension or tachycardia
Indomethacin	Transient renal and liver dysfunction, decreased platelet aggregation, hyponatremia, hypoglycemia
Isoproterenol	Marked inotropic effect, hypotension, arrhythmia
Kanamycin	Nephrotoxicity, ototoxicity
Lidocaine HCl	Hypotension, seizures, respiratory arrest, asystole
Magnesium sulfate	Hypotension, CNS depression
Mannitol	Rebound edema and/or circulatory overload
Moxalactam	Thrombocytopenia, platelet dysfunction, hypothrombinemia
Naloxone HCl	Tachycardia, hypertension, tremors, seizures
Nitroprusside	Hypotension, tachyphylaxis, thiocyanate toxicity with long-term use
Oxacillin	Penicillin sensitivity, nephrotoxicity
Paraldehyde	Cardiopulmonary depression, CNS depression, pulmonary edema
Phenobarbital	CNS depression with respiratory arrest with overdose
Phenytoin	Bone marrow depression, nystagmus
Prostigmine	Respiratory failure, cardiovascular collapse
Streptomycin sulfate	Nephrotoxicity, ototoxicity, cardiovascular collapse
Thorazine	Hypotension, hypothermia rare, liver disease and bone marrow depression
Ticarcillin	Bleeding problems, hypernatremia
Tobramycin sulfate	Nephrotoxicity, ototoxicity
Vancomycin	Nephrotoxicity, ototoxicity, histamine-like response

GI, gastrointestinal; IV, intravenous; CNS, central nervous system.
Modified from Harper RG, Jing JY: Handbook of Neonatology. 2nd ed. Chicago, Year Book Medical Publishers, 1987.

the achievement of a lower peak concentration.[7, 8] If these factors are not taken into account when medications are initially dosed in the neonate, supplemental dosing may be necessary, with a consequent increase in potential toxicity.

Absorption of drugs administered by the intramuscular route is also altered in the neonate. Because the relative blood flow of the various muscle groups changes dramatically, particularly in the first 2 weeks of postnatal life, and because muscle activity also may undergo alterations, intramuscular administration of medications may be notably unreliable in both premature and term infants.[7–9]

Transdermal absorption of drugs may also lead to toxicity in the neonate. The comparatively reduced thickness of the stratum corneum, particularly in the premature infant, permits more effective absorption by the cutaneous route.[8, 9] Indeed, the literature contains several reports of toxicity in neonates resulting from percutaneous absorption (see later).[10–14]

Distribution

Drug distribution in the neonatal period varies considerably from that occurring in later life. The differences are due to a number of factors—most notably, variations in protein binding at different ages, and variations in the relative contributions of extracellular and intracellular fluid volume to body weight with age.[8, 9] Overall, protein binding of drugs is reduced in the neonate. This may result in an

Table 17–2. Drug Disposition in Infants Compared with Adults: Potential Influence of Pharmacokinetics

Disposition Parameter	Newborn Versus Adult	Possible Pharmacokinetic Result	Example Drug
Absorption	↓	↓ AUC	Penicillins, sulphonamides
Volume of distribution	↑	↓ Peak	Gentamicin, digoxin
Protein binding (%)	↓	↑ Free fraction	Clindamycin, theophylline
Metabolism	↓	↓ Clearance	Chloramphenicol, theophylline
Excretion	↓	↑ AUC ↑ $t_{1/2}$	Gentamicin, furosemide

↓, less in newborns than in adults; ↑, greater in newborns than in adults; AUC, area under the concentration-versus-time curve; $t_{1/2}$, elimination half-life.
From Blumer JL, Reed MD: Principles of neonatal pharmacology. *In* Yaffe SJ, Aranda JV (eds): Pediatric Pharmacology: Therapeutic Principles in Practice. 2nd ed. Philadelphia, W.B. Saunders Co., p 175, 1992.

increase in the apparent volume of distribution of drug, with the potential for a consequent increase in the elimination half-life of the drug. Furthermore, the reduction in protein binding may result in an increased concentration of free (unbound, and therefore, active) drug, with a potentially augmented pharmacologic response for a given drug concentration in the plasma.[8, 9]

Metabolism

Drug metabolism in the neonate is a complex topic that is currently only partially understood. Nevertheless, there is sufficient information to indicate that, at birth, the activity of many of the enzymes catalyzing the nonsynthetic phase I metabolic functions of the liver (e.g., cytochrome P-450–dependent mixed-function oxidases) is markedly lower than that in adults. Postnatally, these systems appear to mature at varying rates, and by a few months of age, the activity of several of these systems may increase to levels greater than those observed in adults. The synthetic phase II reactions are also thought to be reduced at birth and to evolve more slowly (often over several years) postnatally.[7–9]

Renal clearance of drugs is also reduced in the neonate. Consequently, renally excreted drugs such as the aminoglycoside antibiotics undergo markedly reduced clearance. Furthermore, the various renal functions (e.g., glomerular filtration and tubular secretion) appear to develop at different rates.[9, 15]

Tables 17–2 and 17–3 outline the differences between newborns and adults with respect to several pharmacokinetic processes.

TOXIC EXPOSURES THROUGH BREAST MILK

Although breast milk offers a nearly ideal source of nutrients for the newborn, there is now considerable evidence that, under certain circumstances, human milk may become a route of exposure to potentially toxic substances.[16] Neubert has listed three circumstances by which "undesired chemicals" might be

Table 17–3. Differences in Specific Pharmacokinetic Processes Between the Neonate and Adult

Variable	Neonate	Adult
Absorption		
Stomach acidity	Premature: pH, 4.7; Full-term: pH, 2.3–3.6	pH, 1.4–2.0
Gastric emptying time	Prolonged; depends on maturity and gestational age	Adult levels at about 6 mo
Gastrointestinal motility	Irregular and unpredictable	
Percutaneous absorption	Increased in neonate	
Distribution		
Fat content	Premature: 3–12%; Full-term: 12%	18%
Skeletal muscle content	25%	43%
Extracellular water	60%	20%
Total body water	75%	50%
Plasma protein binding	Decreased binding due to decreased plasma proteins	Adult levels at about 1 y
Metabolism		
Microsomal tissue	26 mg/g of liver	35 mg/g of liver
NADPH–cytochrome *c* reductase	49% of adult activity	
Cytochrome P-450	25–50% of adult activity	
Glucuronidation	Low at birth	Adult level at 3 y
Excretion		
Glomerular filtration rate	Premature: 0.7–2 mL/min Full-term: 2–4 mL/min	130 mL/min
Tubular secretion	20–30% of adult function	Adult level at 5–7 mo

From Warner A: Drug use in the neonate: Interrelationships of pharmacokinetics, toxicity, and biochemical maturity. Clin Chem *32*:722, 1986.

Table 17–4. Excretion of Drugs in Human Milk

Drug	Maternal Dose	Peak Concentration in Milk	Milk/Plasma Ratio at Peak	Time of Peak Concentration in Milk	$t_{1/2}$ in Milk*	Amount Secreted in Milk 24 h after Single Dose†	Maternal Dose (%)‡
Acetaminophen	650 mg PO	10–15 μg/mL	0.8	1–2 h	2.3 h	0.88 mg	0.14
Antipyrine	18 mg/kg PO	20–30 μg/mL	1.0	10 min	6–22 h	7–25 mg	0.5–2.4
Caffeine	35–336 mg PO as beverage	2–7 μg/mL	0.6–0.8	½–1 h	6.1 h	0.57 mg	0.53
Cefazolin	2 g IV	1.51 μg/mL	0.023	3 h		1.5 mg	0.075
	500 mg IM tid	0		Not detected in milk		0	
Chlorothiazide	500 mg PO	0		Not detected in milk		<1 mg/d	
Diazepam	Not stated	0.27 μg/mL	0.68	3 d	3 d	0.27 mg (peak) on day 3	
Digoxin	0.25 mg PO	0.6–1.0 ng/mL	0.8–0.9	4 h	12 h	0.18–0.36 μg/d	0.07–0.14
Ethanol	0.6 g/kg PO	777 μg/mL	0.93	90 min	2.9 h	300 mg	1
Isoniazid	300 mg PO	16.6 μg/mL	1.6	3 h	5.9 h	7 mg	2.3
Lithium	Chronic: dose not specified PO	0.1–0.6 mmol/L	0.5	Levels fairly constant			
Methadone	70 mg/d PO	0.36 μg/mL 0.51 μg/mL	0.83 1.89			300 μg	0.4
Metronidazole	2.0 g PO	50–57 μg/mL		2–4 h	9 h	21.8 mg	1.1
Nicotine	1 pack/d (400 mg)	91 ng/mL Range: 20–512 ng/mL		No correlation		0.68 mg	0.17
Prednisolone	5 mg PO	26 ng/mL		1 h	8.2 h	6 μg	0.12
Prednisone	120 mg PO	154 ng/mL (prednisone)		2 h	1.8 h	47 μg (as both prednisone and prednisolone)	0.04
		473 ng/mL (prednisolone)		2 h	1.1 h		
Propranolol	20 mg	10 ng/mL	0.56	3 h		0.6 μg	0.03
	160 mg	150 ng/mL	0.65	3 h		90 μg	0.05
Salicylate	20 mg/kg						0.18–0.36
Sulfasalazine	2 g/d PO	9–15 mg/mL	0.6	Constant		1.4–2.1 mg	0.16
Sulphone	5 g IM sulphetrone or 500 mg PO dapsone	14 μg/mL	0.16	4–6 h		10 mg	2
Theophylline	4.25 mg/kg	4 μg/mL	0.7	2 h	4.0 h	8 mg	4
Verapamil	80 mg PO tid		0.6	1–2 h	4.3 h	31 μg	0.01

PO, perorally; IV, intravenously; IM, intramuscularly.

*$t_{1/2}$ is calculated from the elimination (β) phase.

†Amount excreted in 24 h is estimated by assuming that the infant ingests 90 mL of milk every 4 h.

‡The percentage of maternal dose is calculated by dividing the amount secreted in 24 h by the maternal dose (single dose or 24-h total maternal dose).

From Berlin CM Jr: The excretion of drugs and chemicals in human milk. *In* Yaffe SJ, Aranda JV (eds): Pediatric Pharmacology: Therapeutic Principles in Practice. Philadelphia, W.B. Saunders Co., p 208, 1992.

transferred to a neonate via the mother's milk: (1) when the nursing mother uses particular medications, (2) when the nursing mother uses "recreational" drugs or drugs of abuse, and (3) when certain environmental toxins have been stored within the maternal adipose tissue.[17]

There are a number of routes by which toxins might be transported into breast milk from the maternal tissues. According to Berlin, the most probable of these are transcellular diffusion, intercellular diffusion, passive diffusion, and ionophore diffusion.[18] Because diffusion represents the primary mechanism by which drugs enter breast milk, factors such as pH and pK_a, protein binding, and lipid solubility of the substance have an important role in the final concentration of the drug or toxin in breast milk.

For most substances, the concentration of the drug or toxin in breast milk is considerably lower than that in the maternal serum[19] (Table 17–4). However, some medications have been shown to be concentrated in breast milk to a level greater than that in maternal serum. These include iodine 131, propylthiouracil, erythromycin, and gentamicin.[17]

In addition to medications, several environmental substances have been found to accumulate in breast milk. Indeed, there has been increasing concern that milk expression may be the only significant path of elimination from the human body for lipophilic toxins such as the organochlorine insecticides, polychlorinated biphenyls, and polybrominated biphenyls.[18] Because of the continuing uncertainty regarding the actual degree of toxicity of these substances (see later) and the variability in level of exposure, it has been suggested that the breast milk of women exposed to these substances be tested before the initiation of breast-feeding.[20]

Table 17–5 lists a number of substances of maternal exposure that are thought to be contraindications to breast-feeding.

TOXIC EFFECTS OF MATERNAL DRUG DEPENDENCE

The use and abuse of drugs during pregnancy may have lasting implications for the neonate. The fetal alcohol syndrome resulting from maternal prenatal alcohol abuse has been well documented.[21] In addition to teratogenic effects, the use during pregnancy of a number of drugs has been found to result in neonatal abstinence syndromes, and occasionally, in long-term neurodevelopmental effects. Opiates, cocaine, barbiturates, benzodiazepines, and phencyclidine have all been associated with neonatal withdrawal symptoms. Because of the large number of users, opiates and cocaine represent the largest contributors to iatrogenic neonatal toxicity.

Opiates

An estimated 10,000 women who are addicted to opiates give birth each year.[22] Of the neonates, as many as 90% may show evidence of opiate withdrawal.[23] Methadone and heroin represent the most commonly implicated opiates, although chronic use of virtually any opiate risks perinatal addiction, including codeine-containing cough preparations.[23]

The time of abstinence symptom onset is related to the half-life of the narcotic. Thus, withdrawal is commonly first noted between 24 and 72 hours after delivery in heroin-addicted neonates, and it dissipates within about 2 weeks. For methadone-addicted infants, withdrawal symptoms typically begin between 3 and 7 days after birth, but the delay of symptoms for as long as 32 days post partum has been reported.[24] Signs of neonatal withdrawal include irritability, hypertonia, tremors, tachypnea, tachycardia, and high-pitched cry. In addition, diarrhea, yawning, increased sneezing, nasal congestion, poor feeding, and occasionally, low-grade fever and vomiting frequently occur. In rare instances, seizures have been reported.[23, 24] Jitteriness and hypertonicity may persist for several months post partum.

Early diagnosis of neonatal abstinence syndromes is important not only for determining the need for pharmacologic intervention, but also for ensuring that appropriate steps are taken to institute proper monitoring and provide social services. Opiate-addicted neonates are more commonly born prematurely and are more frequently small for gestational age than are normal newborns. Therefore, monitoring and supportive care must be particularly directed at the provision of ample fluid and calories as well as at the correction of possible hypoglycemia, polycythemia, and other problems ensuing from prematurity.[23]

Determination of the need for pharmacologic intervention in the neonate undergoing opiate withdrawal is frequently a difficult process. Many nurseries use scoring systems similar to those suggested by Kahn and associates[25] to dictate therapeutic interventions. In that system, newborns with grade I withdrawal (symptoms that are mild but obviously abnormal) are treated nonpharmacologically with environmental interventions such as gentle handling and swaddling. In grade II withdrawal, the neonate is symptomatic only when disturbed and again is treated primarily with environmental manipulations. The newborn who is repeatedly symptomatic even when undisturbed and whose symptoms interfere with his or her well-being (grade III) is a candidate for pharmacologic intervention.[23]

At the present, several pharmacologic agents are used for the management of opiate withdrawal in neonates.[26] The more common ones are listed in Table 17–6. When pharmacologic intervention is required, medication is started at the smallest recommended dose; the dose is titrated upward as required to achieve the desired level of well-being in the neonate. Once the infant has been asymptomatic for 2 to 3 days, the drug dose is tapered, first by lowering the dose and subsequently by increasing the dosing interval. This process is continued every 2 to 3 days until the symptoms of withdrawal have been com-

Table 17–5. Exposures Considered to Contraindicate Breast-Feeding

Antimetabolites (cancer chemotherapy drugs, including amethopterin, cyclophosphamide, doxorubicin, and methotrexate)	‡Marijuana
Androgens (e.g., testosterone)	§Mercury, methylmercury
*Bromides (high dose)	*Methimazole
†Bromocriptine	Metronidazole
Chloramphenicol	Nalidixic acid
*Cimetidine	Nitrofurantoin
*Clemastine	‡Phencyclidine (PCP)
Cocaine	†Phenelzine
Ergot alkaloid (high dose)	*Phenindione
Gold salt	§Pesticides
Heroin	§Polybrominated biphenyls
*Indomethacin	§Polychlorinated biphenyls
Iodides	§Polychlorinated terphenyls
Lead (if mother intoxicated)	Radiopharmaceuticals
Lithium	§Strontium 89, strontium 90
	Sulfonamides (for neonates)
	§Tetrachloroethylene
	*Thiouracil

*Although use of these agents during nursing should not result in excessive infant exposure (at usual doses), alternative therapeutic agents exist that do not share the same risk of serious adverse effects or case reports of adverse occurrences.

†May suppress lactation.

‡Use of these substances as drugs of abuse results in uncontrolled infant exposure because of unknown quality and purity of street drugs. Abstinence should be encouraged.

§Testing of milk indicated if mother is known to be exposed in excess to environmental chemicals for which infant sensitivity is not defined.

pletely ameliorated.[23] The total duration of treatment is dependent on a number of factors, including the specific opiate to which the mother is addicted, the severity of maternal addiction, and the medication used for treating withdrawal in the neonate.

Cocaine

Cocaine readily crosses the placenta and the blood-brain barrier. Its use prenatally has been associated with preterm labor and delivery, strokes, abruptio placentae, and poor fetal growth.[24] Postnatally, intrauterine cocaine exposure has been associated with several neurobehavioral abnormalities as measured by the Neonatal Behavioral Assessment Scale.[27] These abnormalities include altered interactive behavior in the cocaine-exposed neonate and an abnormal response to environmental stimuli.[28] Postnatal symptoms of hypertonia and coarse tremor have also been described.[29] In addition, these infants may manifest a syndrome that comprises jitteriness, sleep difficulties, poor sucking, and a generally labile state.[24] There has been disagreement as to the extent that these symptoms represent an abstinence syndrome rather than a direct effect of cocaine.[23, 30, 31] Lester and colleagues have suggested that many of the observed cocaine effects can, in fact, be categorized into two neurobehavioral syndromes: an "excitable" syndrome, and a "depressed" syndrome.[32] It is suggested that these two syndromes are the result of the direct neurotoxic effects of cocaine (excitable) and the indirect effects, such as poor fetal growth (depressed). Evidence also exists that cocaine metabolites, which can continue to be eliminated for more than 1 week in the neonate, may also contribute directly to the production of a clinical syndrome.[33] Fortunately, postnatal effects of intrauterine cocaine exposure require pharmacologic intervention relatively infrequently.

Cocaine also readily passes into breast milk, and maternal use of cocaine in the breast-fed infant has been reported to result in signs and symptoms of cocaine intoxication, including tachycardia, hypertension, irritability, and tremulousness.[23]

TOXIC ENVIRONMENTAL EXPOSURES IN THE NEONATE

Heavy Metals

Although acute neonatal exposure to heavy metals is rare, such exposures to both lead and mercury have been reported. Perhaps a more common mechanism for heavy metal intoxication in the neonate is prenatal placental transfer of the metal. This mechanism has been reported for a number of heavy metals, including lead, mercury, and cadmium.[34–36] Mercury and lead are also secreted into the breast milk of exposed mothers.[16]

Until recently, it was believed that the consequences of prenatal exposure to lead were primarily limited to an increased risk of minor anomalies.[6, 37] Cases of serious neurodevelopmental injury postnatally in infants whose mothers had high blood lead levels during pregnancy have been reported.[38–40] Fur-

Table 17–6. Medications Used to Treat Neonatal Opiate Withdrawal

Drug	Dose	Dosing Interval	Comments
Paregoric	0.05–0.1 mL/kg per dose, PO	q4h	Constituents can cause local mucosal irritation and CNS stimulation
Tincture of opium, USP (diluted 25-fold)	0.05–0.1 mL/kg per dose, PO	q4h	No irritating CNS stimulating constituents
Phenobarbital	1–2 mg/kg per dose, PO or IM	q6h	Does not control diarrhea; may result in poor suck
Chlorpromazine	0.4–0.7 mg/kg per dose, IM or PO	q6h	May cause extrapyramidal symptoms
Clonidine	0.5–1.0 μg/kg per dose, PO	q6h	Experience is limited in neonates

thermore, there is also significant evidence that low-level fetal lead exposure (maternal levels, ≤25 μg/dL) may lead to mild developmental delay for at least the first few years of life.[41] Although this delay often appears to be reversible by the time the child is of school age, it is not yet clear whether this is universally true. In any case, it is clear that infants of mothers with the potential for high-level exposures are at greatest risk. These include pregnant women residing near industrial point sources of lead (e.g., smelters), women with lead-related hobbies (e.g., manufacture of jewelry, stained glass, fishing sinkers), and women involved in construction, particularly in the rehabilitation of older, lead-based paint–containing dwellings. Chelation therapy for lead poisoning during pregnancy is controversial partly because of the apparent teratogenic potential of such therapy.[42] Similarly, the blood lead level at which a newborn should be chelated is also undecided, although most authorities agree that chelation is appropriate for levels greater than 40 to 45 μ/dL, with some arguing for chelation at even lower levels.[43, 44] Further discussion of the treatment of lead poisoning can be found in Chapter 57.

As mentioned above, mercury, particularly methylmercury compounds, also readily crosses the placental barrier, and numerous cases of fetal toxicity secondary to maternal exposure to this metal have been reported. It is thought that all of the mercury compounds are capable of producing fetal toxicity but that methylmercury is the most toxic. Of the reported cases of fetal mercury poisoning, most have been the result of maternal occupational exposure to mercury compounds or of substantial ingestion of contaminated fish.[45]

Postnatal exposure to toxic doses of mercury is much less common, although reports of acrodynia in neonates dates back to at least the 1920s.[46] In 1981, several hundred infants in Argentina were poisoned when their commercially laundered diapers were contaminated with mercury.[47] The mercury thermometers in infant incubators have been demonstrated to be a source of unacceptably high levels of mercury vapor exposure,[48, 49] although few if any cases of serious toxicity from this source have been reported. In addition, toxic exposure to mercury through breast-feeding has been well documented, particularly in relation to the Iraqi epidemic of 1971 and 1972. In that incident, methylmercury-contaminated grain was used to make bread; the contamination resulted in more than 6500 hospitalizations and over 450 deaths associated with mercury poisoning. Numerous infants developed severe toxicity via exposure to breast milk alone.[50] Toxicity included progressively worsening hyperreflexia and delayed motor development,[51] as well as mental retardation and impaired motor, sensory, and autonomic function in several infants.[52] Other rarer sources of mercury poisoning in infants also have been reported.[53, 54]

Treatment of mercury poisoning depends on a number of factors, including the duration of exposure and the form of mercury responsible for the poisoning (metallic, organic, inorganic). British antilewisite, ethylenediaminetetra-acetic acid (EDTA), and *d*-penicillamine are the most commonly used chelating agents. A more complete discussion of the management of mercury poisoning is found in Chapter 55.

Halogenated Hydrocarbons

Polychlorinated biphenyls (PCBs), dioxins, and furans have been postulated to produce a wide range of toxicities. Because of their persistence in the environment and their secretion in breast milk, concerns about these compounds' potential toxicity in the neonate have been raised.[55–58] To date, however, there have been few, if any, reports of acute toxicity due to these substances in newborns. It seems more probable that any toxicity due to these materials is likely to occur only after chronic exposure. Studies are currently being conducted to determine whether such toxicity does occur in infancy.[55, 56, 58]

Concern has also been expressed about the potential toxicity of chlorinated hydrocarbon pesticides in neonates. These compounds, which include dichlorodiphenyltrichloroethane (DDT), have well-described toxicities. They persist indefinitely in human tissues and are secreted in the milk of exposed mothers. As with PCBs and dioxin, it is clear that neonates are being exposed to chlorinated hydrocarbon pesticides.[59] The consequences of such exposure are presently unknown. Carbamate pesticides have also been shown to be transmitted across the placenta.[60]

IATROGENIC POISONING IN THE NEONATE

Dermatologic Exposures

The newborn infant may be exposed to a large number of chemicals and drugs through topical exposure.[12] Low-molecular-weight substances are particularly well absorbed, and the skin of the premature infant is especially vulnerable.[13] Over the past 100 years, there have been abundant accounts of toxicity caused by transcutaneous absorption of drugs and chemicals in the neonate. Exposure through contamination of diapers has led to outbreaks of methemoglobinemia (due to the aniline dyes previously used to mark new cloth diapers).[61, 62]

Hexachlorophene is a trichlorophenol antiseptic that was formerly used in nurseries to prevent staphylococcal infections. Frequently, it was used for the total-body bathing of newborns. However, after having been considered safe for nearly 20 years, hexachlorophene was implicated as the cause of central nervous system depression, seizures, and death in several infants in France. Subsequently, a distinct histologic lesion was found to be present in animal models of hexachlorophene poisoning and at autopsy in preterm infants regularly bathed in hexachlorophene solutions.[13] Iodine has also been shown to be absorbed systemically when repeatedly administered topically in neonates, and associated goiter and hypothyroidism have been reported.[63]

Alcohols also are frequently used topically in newborns, again primarily as antiseptic agents. Hemorrhagic necrosis of the skin in preterm infants who have been lying in alcohol-soaked bedding has been well described.[13] In addition, isopropyl alcohol has been reported to have systemic effects when used topically as part of umbilical cord care.[14] Similarly, methanol poisoning leading to metabolic acidosis and visual changes has been reported after the use of topical methanol.[64] It also is believed that isopropyl alcohol can cause systemic toxicity when used for sponging for fever reduction, although such toxicity is thought to arise from inhalation of the isopropyl vapor.[65]

Adhesive tape remover pads, which often contain solvents such as methylchloroform, have been used in numerous intensive care nurseries. Although systemic toxicity as a result of their use has apparently been rare, there have been associated cases of toxic epidermal necrolysis.[66] One study has shown that use of these pads also is associated with accumulation of detectable levels of methylchloroform in incubator air.[67]

Topical corticosteroids have been associated with the development of Cushing's syndrome in the neonate.[68] In addition, there is concern that extended administration of these agents may lead to depression of the hypothalamic-pituitary-adrenal axis; in this circumstance, withdrawal of the steroid should be carried out by tapering of the dosage.

Methemoglobinemia

Neonates are susceptible to the same methemoglobin-producing toxins that older children and adults are (see Chapter 13). However, there is evidence that neonates may be sensitive to significantly lower levels of the toxin. In addition, this problem is complicated by the high concentration of fetal hemoglobin in the neonate, which further restricts oxygen availability at the tissue level. Toxin-induced methemoglobinemia has been reported after inhalation exposures,[69] as well as after administration of local anesthetic agents.[70, 71] Because local anesthetics are known to cross the placenta, their use during labor and delivery may result in effects on the newborn infant. In addition to methemoglobinemia, intoxication with these agents may result in hypotonia, bradycardia, apnea, and seizures.[6]

Neonatal methemoglobinemia is relatively uncommon, but when it does occur its treatment must be undertaken with caution. It has been shown that doses of methylene blue (the medication used to treat methemoglobinemia) only slightly higher than those recommended are toxic in the neonate.[72]

Alcohols

In addition to the transcutaneous and inhalation exposures already discussed, accidental or intentional ethyl alcohol exposures occasionally occur in infants and may result in severe intoxication. Associated hypoglycemia may be particularly problematic in this age group. Similarly, accidental administration of methanol in infant formula has resulted in systemic toxicity,[73] which must be treated with ethanol, as described in Chapter 35.

In the early 1980s, administration of intravascular flush solutions containing benzyl alcohol as a preservative was found to result in a complex of symptoms, including metabolic acidosis, gasping respirations, and central nervous system depression progressing to coma and death. This "gasping syndrome" was attributed to the benzyl alcohol, which also is used as a preservative in a number of parenteral medications frequently administered in neonatal intensive care units.[6] Subsequently, use of intravascular fluids containing benzyl alcohol was discontinued in this setting.

Antibiotics

Antimicrobials are among the most commonly used medications in neonates. Adverse effects secondary to the use of these agents are not uncommon and thus must be considered as the potential basis for toxic reactions in the newborn. Perhaps the best described of the antibiotic-induced toxicities is that produced by chloramphenicol. During the first 2 weeks of life, the activity of clearance pathways for chloramphenicol is significantly less than that in later life. Consequently, chloramphenicol may accumulate to toxic levels resulting in what has been referred to as the "gray syndrome." This syndrome is manifest by lethargy, abdominal distention, hypotension, hypoxemia, and acidosis.[2] Careful attention to dosing and monitoring of drug levels contributes to prevention of this disorder. When this syndrome does occur, exchange transfusion appears to be the treatment of choice.[74]

Several other antibiotics pose a potential threat to the newborn, and particularly the premature infant. As noted earlier, sulfonamide therapy has been associated with an increased incidence of kernicterus,[1] and tetracycline with calcification disturbances. In addition, aminoglycoside antibiotics pose an increased risk of nephrotoxicity and ototoxicity to the neonate. Although not unique to infants, neonates are theoretically at greater risk for these adverse events because they exhibit a prolonged elimination and thus have an increased risk of drug accumulation during treatment. Vancomycin administration has been associated with adverse effects in neonates as well—most notably, shock and rash.[75] As with chloramphenicol, it appears that mindful attention to dose considerations and drug levels generally prevents these toxic effects.

Theophylline

Theophylline is commonly used for the treatment of apnea of prematurity. It is metabolized by methylation to caffeine, which contributes to theophylline's pharmacologic effect and, in some institutions, is used primarily in place of theophylline. When theophylline is used, both serum theophylline and caffeine levels should be monitored. Again, prolonged half-life and reduced clearance contribute to the risk of drug accumulation and adverse effects. The latter include hyperreflexia, tachycardia, cardiac dysrhythmias, tremors, jitteriness, vomiting, and seizures.[6, 76] Arrhythmias and seizures should be managed in the standard fashion. Although charcoal hemoperfusion is the recommended therapy for older children and adults, it has not been tested in infants for this indication. Nasogastric activated charcoal and exchange transfusion have been effective at eliminating theophylline.[77]

Ophthalmic Drops

Because of the risk of retinopathy of prematurity in low-birth-weight infants who have required oxygen therapy, frequent fundoscopic examinations are often required. To facilitate these examinations, mydriatic and cycloplegic agents must be instilled into the infants' eyes. The potential toxic effects of these agents include hypertension, tachycardia, ventricular dysrhythmias, and subarachnoid hemorrhage.[78] Premature infants are especially sensitive to these side effects, and a fatal outcome has been reported.[78] Consequently, current recommendations are to dilate infants' pupils with a single drop of 0.5% cyclopentolate, one drop of 2.5% phenylephrine, and one drop of 1% tropicamide. Further dilution to 1% phenylephrine and 0.2% cyclopentolate is recommended for premature infants.

THERAPY FOR NEONATAL POISONINGS[15]

The priorities for management of the poisoned neonate are similar to those for patients of any age with a suspected poisoning: supportive care, decontamination, enhancement of elimination, and administration of any available antidote. Not surprisingly, little research has been conducted to examine the latter three issues in the newborn population. Supportive care is the first priority, and cardiorespiratory status of the infant should be considered particularly fragile in the face of a toxic insult. Once airway, breathing, and circulation have been stabilized, decontamination should be undertaken in an appropriate fashion whenever acute exposures have occurred. Often, because of the frequency of dermal exposure to toxins, bathing may be the only decontamination required. When exposure has occurred through the gastrointestinal route, decontamination must be carried out with particular attention to the frailty of the neonate. Few data exist on the safety of syrup of ipecac in this age group, and thus its routine use cannot be advocated. Nasogastric tubes can be inserted in even the premature neonate with relative ease, although lavage should be conducted with normal saline rather than with water and in aliquots of approximately 25 mL to avoid fluid and electrolyte shifts. Furthermore, cathartics may represent a risk to the neonate's osmotic balance and, therefore, should be avoided. The use of activated charcoal is somewhat controversial in the newborn because of the vulnerability of the gastrointestinal tract. Nevertheless, it has been used successfully in patients of this age group.[77] Consequently, the use of activated charcoal may be a viable treatment option under certain conditions.

Enhancement of the elimination of toxins in neonates has also been relatively untested. The use of forced diuresis—a technique commonly used in older children and adults—may represent a serious risk to even the healthy neonate owing to immature renal function. Furthermore, when the infant has pulmonary or cardiac disease, the risks of this technique are obvious; thus, it is not commonly used. Similarly, hemodialysis and hemoperfusion are technically complex, in even full-term infants, and these techniques can be carried out by only a few specialized medical centers. Exchange transfusion, which is performed with comparative facility, is one potential means of eliminating toxins in the neonate. Its use is restricted to instances in which the toxin is primarily confined to the vascular space (low volume of distribution).

CONCLUSION

Toxic exposures in the neonate may be particularly difficult to diagnose because the signs and symptoms frequently are similar to those that occur in other neonatal ailments, including sepsis and cardiac disease. Although the incidence of such exposures is presumably quite rare, it is imperative that the all who care for newborns maintain a high index of suspicion for the diagnosis.[73] In instances in which a toxic exposure is suspected, the clinical toxicologist must work in concert with the neonatologist or pediatrician, using their knowledge of the unique aspects of neonatal physiology to establish a diagnosis and institute appropriate therapy.

References

1. Silverman WA, Anderson DH, Blanc WA, et al: A difference in mortality rate and incidence of kernicterus among premature infants allotted to two prophylactic antibacterial regimens. Pediatrics *18*:14, 1956.
2. Sutherland JM: Fatal cardiovascular collapse of infants receiving large amounts of chloramphenicol. Am J Dis Child *97*:461, 1959.

3. Menon PA, Thach BT, Smith CH, et al: Benzyl alcohol toxicity in a neonatal intensive care unit: Incidence, symptomatology and mortality. Am J Perinatol *1:*288, 1984.
4. Bodenstein CJ: Intravenous vitamin E and deaths in the intensive care unit. Pediatrics *66:*733, 1984.
5. Lorch V, Murphy D, Hoersten LR, et al: Unusual syndrome among premature infants: Association with a new intravenous vitamin E product. Pediatrics *75:*598, 1985.
6. Elhassani SB: Neonatal poisoning: Causes, manifestations, prevention and management. South Med J *79:*1535, 1986.
7. Morselli PL: Clinical pharmacokinetics in neonates. Clin Pharmacokinet *1:*81, 1976.
8. Routledge PA: Pharmacokinetics in children. J Antimicrob Chemother *34:*19, 1994.
9. Blumer JL, Reed MD: Principles of neonatal pharmacology. *In* Yaffe SJ, Aranda JV (eds): Pediatric Pharmacology: Therapeutic Principles in Practice. 2nd ed. Philadelphia, W.B. Saunders Co., pp 164–177, 1992.
10. Pyati SP, Ramamurthy RS, Krauss MT, et al: Absorption of iodine in the neonate following topical use of povidone iodine. J Pediatr *91:*825, 1977.
11. Tyrala EE, Hillman LS, Hillman RE, et al: Clinical pharmacology of kerochlorophene in newborn infants. J Pediatr *91:*481, 1977.
12. Cetta F, Lambert GH, Ros SP: Newborn chemical exposure from over-the-counter skin care products. Clin Pediatr *30:*286, 1991.
13. Rutter N: Percutaneous drug absorption in the newborn: Hazards and uses. Clin Perinatol *14:*911, 1987.
14. Vivier PM, Lewander WJ, Martin HF, et al: Isopropyl alcohol intoxication in a neonate through chronic dermal exposure: A complication of a culturally-based umbilical care practice. Pediatr Emerg Care *10:*91, 1994.
15. Banner W Jr: Clinical toxicology in the neonatal intensive care unit. Med Toxicol *1:*225, 1986.
16. Oskarsson A, Palminger Hallen I, Sundberg J: Exposure to toxic elements via breast milk. Analyst *120:*765, 1995.
17. Neubert D: Significance of pharmacokinetic variables in reproductive and developmental toxicity. Xenobiotica *18*(Suppl 1):45, 1988.
18. Berlin CM Jr: The excretion of drugs and chemicals in human milk. *In* Yaffe SJ, Aranda JV (eds): Pediatric Pharmacology: Therapeutic Principles in Practice. Philadelphia, W.B. Saunders Co., pp 205–211, 1992.
19. Kunka RL, Venkataramanan R, Stern RM, et al: Excretion of propoxyphene and norpropoxyphene in breast milk. Clin Pharmacol Ther *35:*675, 1984.
20. Marx CM, Pope JF, Blumer JL: Developmental toxicology. *In* Haddad LM, Winchester JF (eds): Clinical Management of Poisoning and Drug Overdose. 2nd ed. Philadelphia, W.B. Saunders Co., pp 388–436, 1990.
21. Jones KL, Smith DW, Ulleland CN, et al: Pattern of malformation in offspring of alcoholic mothers. Lancet: *1:*1267, 1973.
22. Hans SL: Developmental consequences of prenatal exposure to methadone. Ann N Y Acad Sci *562:*195, 1989.
23. Srinivasan G: Infants of drug-dependent mothers. *In* Yeh TF (ed): Neonatal Therapeutics. 2nd ed. St. Louis, Mosby-Year Book, pp 32–39, 1991.
24. Mast J: Toxic encephalopathy in the newborn. Semin Neurol *13:*66, 1993.
25. Kahn EJ, Neumann LL, Polk GA: The course of the heroin withdrawal syndrome in newborn infants treated with phenobarbital or chlorpromazine. J Pediatr *75:*495, 1969.
26. Anand KJ, Arnold JH: Opioid tolerance and dependence in infants and children. Crit Care Med *22:*334, 1994.
27. Zuckerman B, Bresnahan K: Developmental and behavioral consequences of prenatal drug and alcohol exposure. Pediatr Clin North Am *38:*1387, 1991.
28. Chasnoff JJ, Burns WJ, Schnoll SH, et al: Cocaine use in pregnancy. N Engl J Med *313:*666, 1986.
29. Chiriboga CA, Bateman DA, Brust JC, et al: Neurologic findings in neonates with intrauterine cocaine exposure. Pediatr Neurol *9:*115, 1993.
30. Ellis JE, Byrd LD, Sexson WR, et al: *In utero* exposure to cocaine: A review. South Med J *86:*725, 1993.
31. King TA, Perlman JM, Laptook AR, et al: Neurologic manifestations of *in utero* cocaine exposure in near-term and term infants. Pediatrics *96:*259, 1995.
32. Lester BM, Corwin MJ, Sepkoski C, et al: Neurobehavioral syndromes in cocaine-exposed newborn infants. Child Dev *62:*694, 1991.
33. Konkol RJ, Murphey LJ, Ferriero DM, et al: Cocaine metabolites in the neonate: Potential for toxicity. J Child Neurol *9:*242, 1994.
34. Alessio L, Dell'Orto A, Calzaferri G, et al: Cadmium concentrations in blood and urine of pregnant women at delivery and their offspring. Sci Total Environ *34:*261, 1984.
35. Sikorski R, Paszkowski T, Slawinski P, et al: The intrapartum content of toxic metals in maternal blood and umbilical cord blood. Ginekol Pol *60:*151, 1989.
36. Plockinger B, Dadak C, Meisinger V: Blei, Quecksilber und Cadmium bei neugeborenen und deren Müttern [Lead, mercury and cadmium in newborn infants and their mothers]. Z Geburtshilfe Perinatol *197:*104, 1993.
37. Needleman HL, Rabinowitz M, Leviton A, et al: The relationship between prenatal exposure to lead and congenital anomalies. JAMA *251:*2956, 1984.
38. Ghafour S, Khuffash F, Ibrahim H, et al: Congenital lead intoxication with seizures due to prenatal exposure. Clin Pediatr *23:*282, 1984.
39. Sensirivatana R, Supachadhiwong O, Phancharoens S, et al: Neonatal lead poisoning: An unusual clinical manifestation. Clin Pediatr *22:*582, 1983.
40. Grandjean P, Weihe P, Nielsen JB: Methylmercury: Significance of intrauterine and postnatal exposures. Clin Chem *40:*1395, 1994.
41. Dietrich KN: Low-level lead exposure during pregnancy and its consequences for fetal and child development. *In* Pueschel SM, Linakis JG, Anderson AC (eds): Lead Poisoning in Childhood. Baltimore, Paul H. Brookes Publishing Co., pp 117–139, 1996.
42. Liebelt E, Shannon MW: Oral chelators for childhood lead poisoning. Pediatr Ann *23:*616, 1994.
43. Chisolm JJ Jr: Medical management. *In* Pueschel SM, Linakis JG, Anderson AC (eds): Lead Poisoning in Childhood. Baltimore, Paul H. Brookes Publishing Co., pp 141–162, 1996.
44. Linakis JG: Childhood lead poisoning. R I Med *78:*22, 1995.
45. Koos BJ, Longo LD: Mercury toxicity in the pregnant woman, fetus, and newborn infant: A review. Am J Obstet Gynecol *126:*390, 1976.
46. Bilderback JB: Group of cases of unknown etiology and diagnosis. Northwest Med *19:*263, 1920.
47. Anonymous. Mercury poisoning in Argentine babies linked to diapers. New York, *The New York Times,* January 20, 1981.
48. Waffarn F, Hodgman JE: Mercury vapor contamination of infant incubators: A potential hazard. Pediatrics *64:*640, 1979.
49. McLaughlin JF, Telzrow RW, Scott CM: Neonatal mercury vapor exposure in an infant incubator. Pediatrics *66:*988, 1980.
50. Amin-Zaki L, Elhassani S, Majeed MA, et al: Perinatal methylmercury poisoning in Iraq. Am J Dis Child *130:*1070, 1976.
51. Amin-Zaki L, Majeed MA, Greenwood MR, et al: Methylmercury poisoning in the Iraqi suckling infant: A longitudinal study over five years. J Appl Toxicol *1:*210, 1981.
52. Bakir F, Rustam H, Tikriti S, et al: Clinical and epidemiological aspects of methylmercury poisoning. Postgrad Med J *56:*1, 1980.
53. Meme JS, Brown JD, Kagia J, et al: Mercury poisoning as a cause of acrodynia in Kenya children—a preliminary report. East Afr Med J *58:*641, 1981.
54. Moutinho ME, Tompkins AL, Rowland TW, et al: Acute mercury vapor poisoning: Fatality in an infant. Am J Dis Child *135:*42, 1981.
55. Koppe JG: Dioxins and furans in the mother and possible effects on the fetus and newborn breast-fed baby. Acta Paediatr Scand Suppl *360:*146, 1989.
56. Koppe JG, Pluim HJ, Olie K, et al: Breast milk, dioxins and the possible effects on the health of newborn infants. Sci Total Environ *106:*33, 1991.
57. Koopman-Esseboom C, Huisman M, Weisglas-Kuperus N, et al: Dioxin and PCB levels in blood and human milk in relation

to living areas in The Netherlands. Chemosphere *29*:2327, 1994.
58. Sauer PJ, Huisman M, Koopman-Esseboom C, et al: Effects of polychlorinated biphenyls (PCBs) and dioxins on growth and development. Hum Exp Toxicol *13*:900, 1994.
59. Siddiqui MK, Saxena MC, Bhargava AK, et al: Chlorinated hydrocarbon pesticides in blood of newborn babies in India. Pestic Monit J *15*:77, 1981.
60. Sarkar S, Narang A, Singh S: Transplacentally acquired carbamate insecticide (Baygon) poisoning in a neonate. Indian Pediatr *31*:343, 1994.
61. Scott EP, Prince GE, Rotondo CC: Dye poisoning in infancy. J Pediatr *28*:713, 1946.
62. Howarth BE: Epidemic of methaemoglobinaemia in newborn infants. Lancet *1*:934, 1951.
63. Chabrolle JP, Rossier A: Goitre and hypothyroidism in the newborn after cutaneous absorption of iodine. Arch Dis Child *53*:495, 1978.
64. Kahn A, Blum D: Methyl alcohol poisoning in an eight-month-old boy: An unusual route of intoxication. Pediatrics *94*:841, 1979.
65. Lacouture PG, Wason S, Abrams A, et al: Acute isopropyl alcohol intoxication: Diagnosis and management. Am J Med *75*:680, 1983.
66. Ittman PI, Bozynski MEA: Toxic epidermal necrolysis in a newborn infant after exposure to adhesive remover. J Perinatol *13*:476, 1993.
67. Gallagher JS, Kurt TL: Neonatal exposure to methyl chloroform in tape remover. Vet Hum Toxicol *32*:43, 1990.
68. Gemme G, Ruffa G, Borioli F, et al: Cushing's syndrome due to topical corticosteroids. Am J Dis Child *138*:987, 1984.
69. Montoya Cabrea MA, Hernandez Zamora A, Palacios Trevino JL: Methemoglobinemia caused by inhalation of aniline vapors by a newborn. Bol Med Hosp Infant Mex *37*:1021, 1980.
70. Lloyd CJ: Chemically induced methaemoglobinaemia in a neonate. Br J Oral Maxillofac Surg *30*:63, 1992.
71. Heber G, Hasenburg A, Jaspers V, et al: Methemoglobinemia in the newborn infant—caused by prilocaine?—A case report. Zentralbl Gynakol *117*:105, 1995.
72. Sills MR, Zinkham WH: Methylene blue–induced Heinz body hemolytic anemia. Arch Pediatr Adolesc Med *148*:306, 1994.
73. Weinstock MS, Hartnett L: Toxic emergencies in the neonate. *In* Haddad LM, Winchester JF (eds): Clinical Management of Poisoning and Drug Overdose. 2nd ed. Philadelphia, W.B. Saunders Co., pp 436–444, 1990.
74. Smith AL: Chloramphenicol. *In* Yaffe SJ, Aranda JV (eds): Pediatric Pharmacology: Therapeutic Principles in Practice. Philadelphia, W.B. Saunders Co., pp 276–286, 1992.
75. Lacouture PG, Epstein MF, Mitchell AA: Vancomycin-associated shock and rash in newborn infants. J Pediatr *111*:615, 1987.
76. Banner W Jr, Czajka PA: Acute caffeine overdose in the neonate. Am J Dis Child *134*:495, 1980.
77. Shannon M, Amitai Y, Lovejoy FH Jr: Multiple dose activated charcoal for theophylline poisoning in young infants. Pediatrics *80*:368, 1987.
78. Bauer CR, Trottier MCT, Stern L: Systemic cyclopentolate (Cyclogyl) toxicity in the newborn infant. J Pediatr *82*:501, 1973.

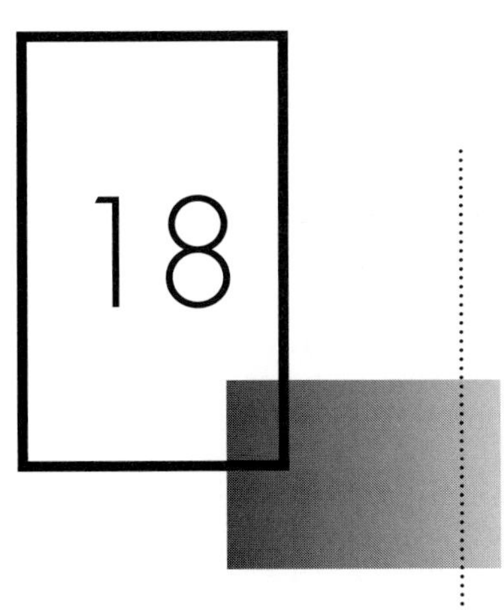

Introduction to Geriatric Toxicology

JAMES RAYMOND, MD
TIMOTHY MADER, MD

Age-dependent changes in the body's physiologic functions often result in unpredictable and eccentric responses to administered drugs. This chapter reviews these consequences of aging and their effects on drug pharmacology and toxicity. Acute poisoning and its treatment are discussed, and strategies for the prevention of drug toxicity are outlined.

THE DIMENSIONS OF AGING

The United States, like many technologically advanced nations, consists of an aging population. Twelve per cent of our population is older than 65 years, and this proportion is steadily growing. It is expected to more than double by the year 2040.[1] Geriatric patients, by their very numbers and their many medical problems, present serious logistic challenges to the health care system. They also constitute the most medicated group in society; nearly 40% of all prescription medicines go to the elderly, and many of these drugs tend to be hazardous.[2, 3]

Many factors complicate drug therapy in geriatric patients. The most important of these include the physiologic alterations of aging, associated disease states, and diminished patient compliance. When evaluating an older polymedicated patient with several chronic illnesses, the clinician is faced with determining whether a particular complaint represents a consequence of normal aging, a manifestation of disease, or an adverse reaction to a medication. Adding to the challenge, some symptoms occur so commonly among the elderly that their diagnostic importance is lost.

Michocki and Lamy[4, 5] have advocated an approach to this dilemma based on a division of the aging process into primary (physiologic), secondary (pathophysiologic), and tertiary (sociogenic) aging. *Primary aging* is the normal physiologic alterations in body function and composition that occur with growing old. These age-related changes affect all organ systems to various degrees and are discussed briefly in the following sections. *Secondary aging* refers to pathophysiologic deviation from the normal process and has been termed *chronic disease.* The heterogeneity of the elderly population is largely attributable to secondary aging. *Tertiary aging,* the effect of imposed socioeconomic factors on the condition of older patients, is often overlooked as a contributor to aging dynamics. It is an important determinant, however, of the success or failure of elderly patients' treatment plan.

AGE-RELATED PHYSIOLOGIC CHANGES AND DRUG DISPOSITION IN THE ELDERLY

Normal aging has important implications for the absorption, distribution, and elimination of drugs (see Chapter 4). This section discusses these age-related physiologic changes and how they affect body composition, organ function, and drug disposition (Table 18–1).

Body Composition

Significant changes occur in body composition during aging. Elderly persons have a general decrease in lean body mass and a proportionate increase in adipose tissue.[6] This shift to adiposity, independent of accompanying obesity, occurs in both active and sedentary individuals. Associated with this are decreases in intracellular and extracellular water. Plasma albumin concentration also declines as a consequence of decreased synthesis, increased catabolism, or both.[7]

Table 18–1. Age-Related Physiologic Changes

Body Composition
Decreased lean body mass
Increased fat
Decreased plasma volume
Decreased total-body water
Decreased total plasma albumin
Cardiovascular System
Heart
Decreased cardiac output
Hypertrophy
Decreased response to stress
Circulation
Increased systolic blood pressure
Decreased blood vessel resilience
Increased thickness of vessels
Decreased perfusion to organs, especially kidneys but also liver, brain, muscles, and gastrointestinal tract
Kidneys
Decreased glomerular filtration rate and renal blood flow
Serum creatinine same but decreased creatinine clearance
Decreased tubular maximum for many substances
Gastrointestinal Tract
Decreased gastric secretions
Increased gastric pH
Decreased active transport
Decreased amplitude of esophageal peristalsis
Decreased rate of stomach emptying
Liver
Decreased size
Decreased number of hepatocytes
Altered phase I drug metabolism
Decreased protein synthesis

Modified from Lamy PP: Comparative pharmacokinetic changes and drug therapy in an older population. J Am Geriatr Soc *30*:11, 1982.

Changes in body composition have important implications for drug metabolism. The decrease in total-body water results in higher drug concentrations. The increased ratio of fat to lean body mass alters the volume of distribution for lipophilic and hydrophilic drugs. Finally, the relative decrease in serum albumin levels influences a drug's free concentration through reduced protein-binding sites.[8]

Cardiovascular System

Occult cardiovascular disease occurs frequently in the elderly and makes defining normal aging difficult. The influence of diet, smoking, activity, and genetic factors further confuses the distinction. Nevertheless, certain age-related changes occur regularly, and primary aging is thus suggested as their basis. Hypertrophy of the left ventricle develops independently of clinical cardiovascular disease, and overall it appears that cardiac output declines with age.[9, 10] Blood vessels generally become thickened and less resilient. These changes may lead to decreased perfusion of the kidneys and liver, and delivery of drugs to other tissues, such as the central nervous system, may be reduced.

Kidneys

Renal mass, plasma flow, glomerular filtration rate, creatinine clearance, and renal tubular function decline with age.[11] Despite these decrements, the serum creatinine level does not predictably increase owing to the diminished muscle mass with aging. The creatinine level is, therefore, an unreliable guide to renal excretory capacity.

These changes in the kidneys influence the clearance of drugs. Alterations in body composition and cardiac output also affect drug excretion through decreased delivery to the kidneys. Secondary aging factors (heart and renal diseases) may accentuate this excretory impairment.[12]

Gastrointestinal Tract

Gastric mucosal changes result in altered secretory function and an increased incidence of achlorhydria, which reaches 20% to 30% by the eighth decade.[13, 14] Evidence also shows that gastric emptying becomes progressively delayed with age. These observations have important implications with respect to the rate of delivery of drugs to the small intestine, their major site of absorption. Impaired active transport of selected nutrients in the gut has also been documented. These observations may reflect a general reduction in all intestinal active transport, including medications.[15]

Because most drugs are administered orally, these changes might be expected to impair absorption of many medications. The longer transit time may lead to food-drug interactions, which further decrease absorption. Reduced splanchnic blood flow and active transport may also retard drug absorption and thereby alter the substance's pharmacokinetic properties.

Liver

In general, hepatic mass and blood flow decrease with advancing age. These decrements correlate histologically with a loss of functioning hepatocytes.[16] Accompanying these gross and microscopic changes are ultrastructural and biochemical alterations that have implications for drug detoxification and metabolism. These latter changes appear to alter phase I metabolism while having little effect on phase II metabolism.[17] This is of minor importance, however, compared with the metabolic decrease prompted by diminished hepatic blood flow and loss of functioning hepatocytes.

SPECIAL CONSIDERATIONS IN GERIATRIC TOXICOLOGY

Adverse Drug Reactions

Whether adverse drug reactions (ADRs), noxious or unintended responses to the usual doses of drugs, occur more frequently with aging is a subject of considerable controversy. Early studies demonstrated a positive correlation,[18, 19] whereas more recent ones have concluded that age alone is not an independent risk factor.[20, 21] More attention has focused on ADRs as a cause of hospitalization, and drug-related admissions appear to increase with advancing age.[22] As many as 8% or more of the elderly's admissions may be a direct result of ADRs, although one cannot infer from this that the elderly are necessarily more susceptible.[23, 24]

Factors other than age alone appear to be more important as a cause of ADRs. These include multiple-drug therapy, chronic illnesses, altered pharmacokinetics and pharmacodynamics, and the types of drugs prescribed. The increased incidence of ADRs with aging may be explained by the confluence of many of these factors in older patients.

Polypharmacy

The average number of prescription medications taken by an elderly outpatient is two to three, and a small subset take five or more.[25] In addition, as many as three nonprescribed medications are consumed by the typical patient older than 65 years. The highest incidence of polypharmacy is in chronically institutionalized patients, who receive an average of seven daily drugs.[26, 27]

The incidence of ADRs increases exponentially with the number of drugs taken, indicating that these reactions are not merely additive.[18] A major reason for this nonlinear relationship is that patients taking large numbers of medications are often severely ill and thereby may be predisposed to ADRs. Drug doses are also likely to be higher in the severely ill, and thus the probability of ADRs is increased.[28] Finally, drug-drug interactions are more common as the number of medications increases. All of these factors present a hazard in the elderly, and elimination of even one or two drugs from their formulary may substantially reduce this risk.

Multiplicity and Severity of Disease

The diseases necessitating drug therapy in the elderly tend to be more serious and often require aggressive medical management. This may involve the use of potent drugs that have a potential for untoward effects. The low therapeutic index of many of these (digoxin, warfarin, insulin, antiarrhythmics, and antihypertensives) creates a situation conducive to toxicity and ADRs.

With aging, chronic diseases have their onset and become long-term illnesses. These illnesses, along with their escalating drug therapy, also increase the likelihood of ADRs and drug-disease interactions.

Drug-Drug Interactions

Administration of two or more drugs within a relatively short time may result in potentiation of action, accumulation of side effects, antagonism, or indifference.[29] *Potentiation* refers to the enhancement of one drug's action by another. *Antagonism* is the reduction in a drug's action by another. *Accumulation* of side effects occurs when drugs with similar side effects are given together. The elderly are at risk for all of these possible reactions because they are usually taking several medications. Over-the-counter medications can possess serious side effects and can be another source of potential drug-drug interactions.

Drug-Disease Interactions

Secondary aging effects (i.e., chronic illness) influence drug disposition in important ways. Congestive heart failure, for instance, through reduced organ perfusion, may hamper absorption and distribution of some drugs. Hepatic dysfunction, an accompaniment of some chronic illnesses, may interfere with drug metabolism and clearance. Renal impairment also has predictable reductive effects on drug excretion.

Certain drugs used to treat one disease may exacerbate another. The use of β-adrenergic blockers for hypertension or angina pectoris can exacerbate asthma or existing cardiac disease. Nonsteroidal anti-inflammatory drugs used in musculoskeletal disorders may worsen or precipitate renal dysfunction. It is likely that these drug-disease interactions occur with more frequency in the elderly than do drug-drug interactions.

Drug-Nutrition Interactions

Malnutrition, the state of many elderly patients, increases the risk for ADRs. Inadequate intake of essential nutrients can alter the pharmacokinetics of many drugs.[30] Certain foods may reduce the bioavailability of drugs, and some medicines can influence food absorption. Gastrointestinal uptake of ingested drugs is thus modified. The elderly are at risk for many of these interactions.

Drug-Alcohol Interactions

Alcohol interacts with a significant number, possibly half, of the most commonly prescribed medications taken by the elderly.[31] Examples include increased anticoagulation (when taken with anticoagulants), hypotension (when taken with antianginal agents), increased sedation (when taken with any sedative), and a disulfiram-like reaction and hypoglycemia (when taken with antidiabetic agents). In addition, alcohol interferes with the absorption of certain nutrients (thiamine and folic acid) and can lead to drug-nutrition interactions. These and other alcohol effects are often overlooked when prescribing for the elderly.

ACUTE POISONING IN THE ELDERLY

Unintentional Poisoning

Most acute poisonings are unintentional. Although the majority of these involve children 5 years old or younger, the most serious ones occur in adults and account for 90% of fatalities.[32] Thirteen per cent of accidental poison deaths are in patients 65 years or older, and the highest death rate for any age group is among those older than 80 years.[33]

The elderly receive nearly 40% of all prescription drugs dispensed, and these account for the majority of unintentional poisonings.[34] The most common classes of drugs implicated, in decreasing order of frequency, are cardiovascular medications, analgesics, antidepressants, respiratory medications, anticonvulsants, and sedative-hypnotics. The predominance of exposures involving cardiovascular agents and analgesics is understandable because these are the two medications most often used by persons 65 years of age and older.[35] Although most of these mishaps occur in the home, a smaller yet significant number (up to 14% of the total) occur in institutional settings.[36]

The majority of these accidental poisonings in the elderly are a result of senility or confusion, improper use or storage of a product, or mistaking one agent for another.[35] Prevention efforts should take these precipitants into consideration.

Intentional Poisoning

Although suicide is a serious, although infrequent, problem among geriatric patients, it has received little attention as a public health issue. Ageist attitudes among physicians and the lay public that it is somehow a rationally "understandable" phenomenon may contribute to this neglect.[37] In fact, however, suicide is a more preventable cause of death in old age than are many acute and chronic medical conditions.

A discernible worldwide increase in suicides among the elderly has occurred during the past two decades. Since 1980, in the United States, the suicide rate has increased 17% for those older than 65 years.[38] Elderly white men are particularly susceptible, and they commit suicide at a rate four times the national average. An unsuccessful serious attempt by an older individual leads to a successful one within a year of the initial incident in a third of patients.[39]

An array of suicidal risk factors has been identified in the aging population. These range from association with assorted medical conditions to considerations of day of the month.[40–43] Recent bereavement, solitary living conditions, and economic adversities may also contribute. The most consistent medical associations, however, are chronic and painful physical conditions (50%), depression (75%), and alcohol abuse (10% to 20%).[44–46] The importance of depressive illness in association with elderly suicide cannot be overstated. Estimates of depression ranging from 60% to 90% have been reported, and nearly half of these individuals consulted their physician in the month preceding death.[47] Depression remains an underdiagnosed and undertreated condition in the elderly.

After gunshots and other violent methods, drug ingestion is the most popular method of suicide in the aged; one third involve prescription drugs.[48] A majority of patients ingested two or more agents. It is probable that the spectrum of ingested drugs will change as new pharmaceuticals reach the market and physicians' prescribing habits change.

As the percentage of aging individuals grows, their incidence of suicide is likely to increase, and prevention will assume even greater significance. As noted, a substantial number of these individuals have unrecognized or untreated depressive illness, and many visit their primary care physician in the weeks before successful suicide. The potential role of physicians in prevention thus becomes central. In this regard, systematic continuing education programs to improve the recognition and treatment of depression in the elderly have shown encouraging results.[49]

Table 18–2. Selected Agents and Their Geriatric Toxicologic Syndromes

Anticholinergic Medications
Tachycardia
Elevated temperature
Delirium
Lethargy
Mydriasis
Flushed skin
Dry mucous membranes
Diminished peristalsis
Urinary retention
Antihypertensive Medications (Central α-Adrenergic Agonist)
Lethargy
Miosis
Respiratory depression
Bradycardia
Hypotension
Cardiac Glycosides
Disorientation
Syncope
Nausea
Vomiting
Bradycardia
Hypotension
Atrioventricular nodal block
Ventricular dysrhythmia
Salicylates
Tachycardia
Hyperpnea
Elevated temperature
Nausea
Vomiting
Tinnitus
Delirium
Lethargy
Respiratory alkalosis
Metabolic (anion gap) acidosis

Modified from Elliott SK, Wang DO: Toxicologic syndromes in the elderly: Recognition and management of drug-related adverse events. Emerg Med Rep *16*:49, 1996.

Recognition and Management of Acute Ingestions in the Elderly

Because of the varied manifestations of toxic ingestions in the elderly, recognition can be problematic. This difficulty is compounded by the fact that many diseases in the elderly present with similar features. Despite these difficulties, certain toxicologic syndromes ("toxidromes") may occur and provide a clue to the class of drug(s) involved (Table 18–2).[50] Toxidromes, however, must be diagnosed with caution in the elderly, because normal aging, chronic disease, and polypharmacy may obscure expected findings and thus may lead to misdiagnosis.

With two major caveats, the principles of management are identical to those for younger patients (see Chapter 1). First, most elderly patients are suffering from at least one chronic disease. Treatment of the ingestion should not exacerbate concomitant illness if at all possible. Second, many geriatric patients are taking several medications. The superimposed acute ingestion can give rise to ADRs and drug-drug interactions that may complicate management. After a patient has made a satisfactory recovery, psychiatric evaluation is imperative in cases of intentional ingestion.

Old age itself should never be a deterrent to aggressive therapy. In acute overdose, a complete history is often unavailable. Although a patient may have an underlying terminal illness or a severely debilitating one, these facts may not come to light until the initial resuscitation has been completed. There is usually time enough after a patient's admission to decide how intensive subsequent management should be. The ethical arguments surrounding these issues continue to be discussed and debated.

DRUG TOXICITY PREVENTION IN THE ELDERLY

Prevention of drug toxicity is a major responsibility facing physicians who care for older patients. Unfortunately, few busy physicians take the time required

Table 18–3. Recommendations for Drug Prescribing and the Prevention of Drug Toxicity in the Elderly

Carefully evaluate the need for drug therapy.
Obtain a detailed drug history.
Use the safest drug and begin with the lowest effective dose.
Avoid prescribing several drugs when possible.
Provide the patient (or caregiver) with a prescription diary or medication cards.
Educate the patient (or caregiver) about the drug's side effects and interaction potentials, particularly with alcohol and nonprescription medications.
Review the drug regimen frequently.

to give adequate information about the drugs they are prescribing and to monitor patients' compliance.

As a first step, physicians need a detailed drug history; this should not be restricted to current prescription medications and drug allergies but must include information about the use of over-the-counter drugs, a patient's reliability in taking scheduled drugs, diet, the use of alcoholic beverages, and the ability to pay for medications. Patients must then receive clear information from the physician about prescribed drugs. A drug's action should be explained in simple, nonscientific terms, and the dosing regimen carefully detailed. Side effects should be discussed, as well as the interactions of the drug with food, alcohol, or other medications. Finally, the use of generic substitutes should be explained, as well as the storage and handling of all medications.

Several investigators have developed suggestions to help reduce the potential for ADRs (Table 18–3).[31] By following these straightforward prescribing recommendations, physicians may prevent some of the serious consequences of drug toxicity in the elderly.

References

1. Cessna CB, Landes A, Foster CD (eds): Growing Old in America: The Information Series on Current Topics. Wylie, TX, Information Plus, p 2, 1990.
2. Lamy PP: New dimensions and opportunities. Drug Intell Clin Pharm *19*:399, 1985.
3. Lamy PP: Comparative pharmacokinetic changes and drug therapy in an older population. J Am Geriatr Soc *30*:11, 1982.
4. Michocki RJ, Lamy PP: A "risk" approach to adverse drug reactions. J Am Geriatr Soc *36*:79, 1988.
5. Lamy PP: Renal effects of nonsteroidal anti-inflammatory drugs. Heightened risk of the elderly? J Am Geriatr Soc *34*:586, 1986.
6. Bruce A, Anderson M, Arvidsson B: Body composition. Prediction of normal body potassium, body water and body fat in adults on the basis of body height, body weight and age. Scand J Clin Lab Invest *40*:461, 1980.
7. Greenblatt DJ: Reduced serum albumin concentration in the elderly: A report from the Boston Collaborative Drug Surveillance Program. J Am Geriatr Soc *27*:20, 1979.
8. Lamy PP: Geriatric pharmacology. Geriatrics *36*:41, 1986.
9. Port S, Cobb FR, Coleman E: Effect of age on the response of the left ventricular ejection fraction to exercise. N Engl J Med *303*:1133, 1980.
10. Gerstenblith G, Lakatta EG, Weisfeldt ML: Age changes in myocardial function and exercise response. Prog Cardiovasc Dis *19*:1, 1976.
11. Lindemann RD, Tobin J, Shock NW: Longitudinal studies on the rate of decline in renal function with age. J Am Geriatr Soc *33*:278, 1985.
12. Thomson NM: Drugs and the kidney in the elderly. Med J Aust *162*:543, 1995.
13. Andrews GR, Haneman B, Arnold BJ: Atrophic gastritis in the aged. Aust Ann Med *16*:230, 1967.
14. Geokas MC, Haverback BJ: The aging gastrointestinal tract. Am J Surg *17*:881, 1969.
15. Montgomery R, Hazney MR, Ross IN: The aging gut: A study of intestinal absorption in the relation to nutrition in the elderly. Q J Med *47*:197, 1978.
16. Wynne HA, Cope LH, Mutch E, et al: The effect of age upon liver volume and apparent liver blood flow in healthy man. Hepatology *9*:297, 1989.
17. Schmucker DL: Drug disposition in the elderly: A review of the critical factors. J Am Geriatr Soc *32*:144, 1984.
18. Nolan L, O'Malley K: Prescribing for the elderly. Part I: Sensitivity of the elderly to adverse drug reactions. J Am Geriatr Soc *36*:142, 1988.
19. Brawn LA, Castleden CM: Adverse drug reactions: An overview of special considerations in the management of the elderly patient. Drug Safety *5*:421, 1990.
20. Chrischilles EA, Segar ET, Wallace RB: Self-reported adverse drug reactions and related resource use. Ann Intern Med *117*:634, 1992.
21. Gurwitz JH, Avorn J: The ambiguous relation between aging and adverse drug reaction. Ann Intern Med *114*:956, 1991.
22. Lin SH, Lin MS: A survey on drug-related hospitalization in a community teaching hospital. Int J Clin Pharmacol Ther Toxicol *31*:66, 1991.
23. Beard K: Adverse reactions as a cause of hospital admissions in the aged. Drugs Aging *2*:356, 1992.
24. Chan TYK, Chan JGN, Tomlinson B, Critchley JAJH: Adverse reactions to drugs as a cause of admissions to a general teaching hospital in Hong Kong. Drug Safety *7*:235, 1992.
25. Nolan L, O'Malley K: Prescribing for the elderly. Part II: Prescribing patterns: Differences due to age. J Am Geriatr Soc *36*:245, 1988.
26. Segal JL, Thompson JF, Floyd RA: Drug utilization and prescribing patterns in a skilled nursing facility: The need for a rational approach to therapeutics. J Am Geriatr Soc *27*:117, 1979.
27. Bergman HD: Prescribing of drugs in a nursing home. Drug Intell Clin Pharm *9*:365, 1975.
28. Steel K, Gertman PM, Crescenzi C, Anderson J: Iatrogenic illness on a general medical service at a university hospital. N Engl J Med *304*:638, 1981.
29. Lamy PP: The elderly and drug interaction. J Am Geriatr Soc *34*:586, 1986.
30. Lamy PP: The elderly, undernutrition and pharmacokinetics. J Am Geriatr Soc *30*:560, 1983.
31. Stein BE: Avoiding drug reactions: Seven steps to writing safer prescriptions. Geriatrics *49*:28, 1994.
32. Litovitz TL, Hohn KC, Bailey KM, Schmitz BF: 1991 Annual report of the American association of poison control centers national data collection system. Am J Emerg Med *10*:452, 1992.
33. Oderda GM, Klein-Schwartz W: Poison prevention in the elderly. Drug Intell Clin Pharm *18*:183, 1984.
34. Lamy PP: Pharmacotherapeutics in the elderly. Md Med J *38*:144, 1989.
35. Kroner BA, Scott RB, Waring ER, Zanga JR: Poisoning in the elderly: Characterization of exposures reported to a poison control center. J Am Geriatr Soc *41*:842, 1993.
36. Klein-Schwartz W, Odera GM, Booze L: Poisoning in the elderly. J Am Geriatr Soc *31*:195, 1983.
37. Draper BM: Prevention of suicide in old age. Med J Aust *162*:533, 1995.
38. Meehan PJ, Saltzman LE, Sattin RW: Suicide among older United States residents: Epidemiologic characteristics and trends. Am J Public Health *81*:1198, 1991.
39. Hawton K, Fagg J: Deliberate self-poisoning and self-injury in older people. Int J Geriatr Psychiatry *5*:367, 1990.
40. Fawcett J, Scheftner W, Clark D, et al: Clinical predictors of

suicide in patients with major affective disorders: A controlled prospective study. Am J Psychiatry *144*:35, 1987.
41. Lester D, Yang B: Social and economic correlates of the elderly suicide rate. Suicide Life Threat Behav *22*:36, 1992.
42. Canetto SS: Gender and suicide in the elderly. Suicide Life Threat Behav *22*:80, 1992.
43. Haight BK: Suicide risk in frail elderly people relocated to nursing homes. Geriatr Nurs *16*:104, 1995.
44. Frierson RL: Suicide attempts by the old and very old. Arch Intern Med *151*:141, 1991.
45. Draper B: Suicidal behavior in the elderly. Int J Geriatr Psychiatry *9*:655, 1994.
46. Conwell Y, Rotenberg M, Caine ED: Completed suicide at age 50 and over. J Am Geriatr Soc *38*:640, 1990.
47. Cattell H, Jolley DJ: One hundred cases of suicide in elderly people. Br J Psychiatry *166*:451, 1995.
48. Benson RA, Brodie DC: Suicide by overdoses of medicines among the aged. J Am Geriatr Soc *23*:304, 1975.
49. Rutz W, Von Knorring L, Walinder J: Frequency of suicide on Gotland after systematic postgraduate education of general practitioners. Acta Psychiatr Scand *80*:151, 1989.
50. Elliott SK, Wang RY: Toxicologic syndromes in the elderly: Recognition and management of drug-related adverse events. Emerg Med Rep *16*:49, 1995.

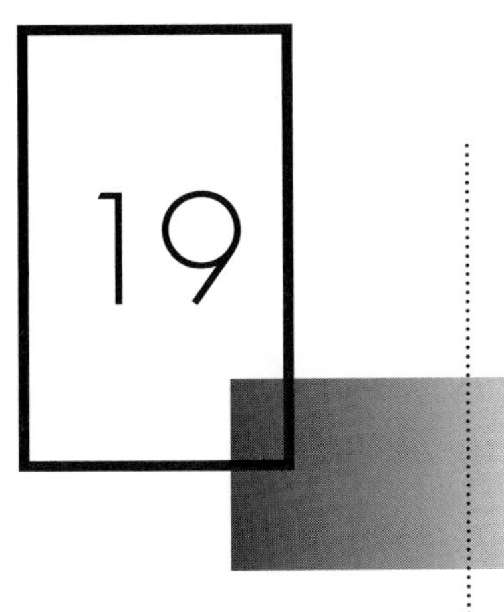

Psychiatric Evaluation of the Suicidal Patient

JOSEPH J. ZEALBERG, MD

Evaluation of a suicidal patient presents a difficult problem for the psychiatrist, emergency physician, or others.[1–5] Suicide is a devastating act that can touch the lives of poor, wealthy, male, female, young, or elderly people, those who are unemployed, or those who have professional jobs.

Statistical and epidemiologic data help clinicians understand the risk factors critical in identifying the prototype of a patient who may be at risk for completed suicide. However, statistics may not always help the crisis clinician with an *individual* emergency patient, and local statistics on suicide may vary from community to community. Therefore, physicians must understand the patient's individual risks, as well as how that individual may fit into the prototypical epidemiologic profile for suicide risk.

Patients may often give only indirect clues about their suicidal ideation, such as by making vague references to ending their life, giving away valuable possessions, or making out a will. Such clues or threats must always be taken seriously and must always be evaluated for their meaning and intent. At other times, families and friends may be unaware of a person's suicidal thoughts and the suicidal intention will be unknown. *Physicians should always assume that a person with suicidal ideation is serious and must thoroughly evaluate any mention of suicidal thoughts.* Physicians need to understand and use statistical, epidemiologic, and diagnostic information in the assessment of suicidal patients. A patient may not always be truthful with an examining clinician, and thus other historians must also be contacted. Patients who may wish to die are often too ashamed or hopeless to share their real feelings. Despair may hide truth. Physicians must always contact others who can verify a patient's story. A patient sometimes says, "This is merely a misunderstanding—I've never wanted to hurt myself." However, another historian, such as a family member or friend, might share information about the patient's going out to buy a gun, leaving a suicide note, or engaging in other alarming thoughts or actions. Astute clinicians can be fooled if others are not contacted. A patient's desire for confidentiality may be overlooked if information from outside sources might make a difference between life and death. Even if a suicidal patient protests, a clinician may contact others if the information is clinically indicated for assessing a patient's true lethality potential. Of course, everything must be done in the service of treating a patient's emergency presentation. Clinicians should never share confidential information if it is not essential for managing a life-threatening situation.

RISK FACTORS

The National Center for Health Statistics estimates that 32,410 suicides occurred in the United States during 1994, a rate of approximately 12.4 per 100,000 persons (to compare this as a public health issue, 23,730 homicides occurred in the United States during that same year). This estimate represents an increase in suicides from 1993, when the number of completed suicides totaled approximately 31,230, a rate of 12.1 per 100,000. Suicide is currently the eighth leading cause of death in the United States. For young American males ages 15 to 24 years, the suicide rate is 26 per 100,000, a rate that has tripled since the 1950s. The rate for females of that age in 1994 was 3.2 per 100,000. Table 19–1 lists the risk factors for suicide.

Table 19–1. Factors in Suicide

- More males than females complete suicide (approximately 4:1 ratio).
- Females make more suicide *attempts* than males.
- Racial risk: Whites > Native Americans > blacks > Hispanic Americans.
- Marital status risk: Divorced, widowed, separated > married.
- Age risk: Highest rate in the elderly. However, adolescent rates have tripled in the past 30 years (but overall completion is still lower than for older groups).
- Patients with mood disorders: About 15% of people with mood disorders (i.e., depression and bipolar disorder) commit suicide.
- Patients with schizophrenia: 10% of people with schizophrenia die by suicide.
- Patients who are drug or alcohol users: Alcohol and cocaine are frequently involved in suicide completion.
- Several studies imply that panic attacks or panic disorder may be predictive for suicide completion, especially in depressed patients or in patients with borderline personalities.
- Isolated people without support systems may be at higher risk.
- Recent unemployement, especially being fired or laid off, can be a risk factor.
- Recent loss of a significant relationship. This risk may be particularly great in depressed alcoholics who have lost their last important relationship (i.e., who have "burned their last bridge"). Such losses in the previous 2 months may pose a risk for suicide completion.
- A history of past significant attempts may predict completion.
- A family history of completed suicide may predict behavior modeling or may indicate a genetic propensity toward suicidal behaviors.

ASSESSMENT OF RISK

Patients with suicidal ideation may present to an emergency department or other clinical setting. Specific questions must be asked if it is to be understood whether a patient is simply having thoughts of self-harm, whether the patient is in control of such thoughts, or whether the patient has more than passive suicidal ideation—that is, a suicide plan, a means to complete the plan, and the intent to carry out that particular plan. The further a patient is beyond mere ideation, the higher is the probability of a future suicidal act.

Physicians must be good detectives when assessing suicidal patients. Clinicians should gather as much data and history as possible from both patients and others. If a patient is receiving mental health treatment, that patient's treating professional (e.g., doctor, therapist, or case manager) should be contacted for valuable information. If treatment is not progressing well, especially if the patient is receiving intensive counseling or dynamic psychotherapy, the suicidal crisis may be related to this issue.

Critical questions must always be addressed to quickly assess potential lethality and need for hospitalization.

A Patient Who Presents After an Actual Suicide Attempt

- If a patient has made a suicide attempt, the clinician must determine the circumstances by which the patient's action was discovered. These facts may be the most important pieces of information to be gathered. The exact details of the discovery of a potential suicide must be known. If police, an emergency medical service, a friend, or family member brings the patient in for evaluation, every effort must be made to find out what happened. Did the patient make earnest efforts to reach out to someone before, during, or after the attempt at self-harm? Did the patient call a friend, family member, therapist, emergency medical service, police, hotline, co-worker, psychiatric emergency service, emergency department, poison-control center, or mental health clinic? If so, this might indicate ambivalence and a wish to live, and thus the degree of lethal intent would be diminished. Similarly, if the patient harmed himself or herself in front of another person or loved one, the patient may have had a desire (although it may have been "unconscious") for someone to stop him or her from causing self-harm. Exercise great caution if the patient was *accidentally discovered* by someone—that is, if the suicide attempt was discovered only by chance or coincidence. This implies an extreme degree of lethality and a real wish for death. A period of inpatient observation and evaluation is *always* indicated in such cases.
- Ask the person who made a suicide attempt the following question: "How do you feel about not

having died?" Some patients might believe that their gesture of self-harm was not potentially lethal. For example, many patients are unaware that an overdose of acetaminophen may be toxic to the liver and potentially lethal. After medical treatment, a psychiatric evaluation, and the use of crisis intervention techniques, many patients feel better and less hopeless. Thus, their suicidal intent or wish may pass. If the patient still expresses the wish for death after clinical psychologic intervention, this is a true lethal wish and hospitalization is indicated.

- If a patient picked up a gun and fired it, one should assume that this is the highest degree of potential lethality. Similarly, patients who barricade themselves in with weapons or who climb to heights such as bridges or rooftops should be assumed to be potentially lethal, and hospitalization should be mandated.

A Patient Who Presents with Suicidal Ideation Only

Clinicians should investigate several issues (Table 19–2) when assessing patients who present with suicidal ideation.

Clinicians should surmise whether a patient is in a high- or low-risk demographic group. The aforementioned risk factors should be assessed and considered in the formulation of the best treatment for a patient with suicidal ideation. Determine whether the patient has a major psychiatric disorder (e.g., major depression, bipolar disorder, or schizophrenia) or has a comorbid occurrence of both a major psychiatric disorder and a personality disorder. For example, a depressed patient with bipolar disorder and a fragile narcissistic personality disorder may be at higher risk than another patient without those vulnerabilities. Similarly, a suicidal patient who has a borderline personality disorder and panic disorder and who is using alcohol and cocaine has a higher degree of risk for suicidal behaviors.

A clinician must further determine whether a patient made serious suicide attempts before, the type of attempts, and whether they were serious or were not considered lethal. If the attempts were serious, is the patient in the same psychologic condition or state as before? If so, this may predict another serious attempt. If a patient attempted suicide before, was the patient's previous attempt truly lethal? Were previous attempts made by firing a gun, by hanging, by carbon monoxide poisoning, or by a lethal, well-thought-out overdose attempt (e.g., a patient who read the *Physicians' Desk Reference* to find the lethal dose requirement of a tricyclic antidepressant). Does the patient have a family history of completed suicide, which might predict behavioral modeling or genetic predisposition to suicide or impulsivity? Data suggest that low levels of 5-hydroxyindoleacetic acid (5-HIAA) in cerebrospinal fluid assays of patients may be predictive of impulsive behaviors such as suicide attempts.

Table 19–2. Assessment of Suicidal Ideation

1. Is the patient in a high-risk or low-risk demographic group?
2. Does the patient have a major psychiatric axis I disorder (e.g., major depression, bipolar disorder, or schizophrenia) or does the patient have a comorbid occurrence of two or more major psychiatric disorders?
3. Has the patient made serious suicide attempts before? What type? Were they serious or not considered lethal? If the attempts were serious, is the patient in the same psychologic condition or state as before? If so, this may predict another serious attempt.
4. Was the patient's previous attempt truly lethal (i.e., firing a gun, hanging, carbon monoxide poisoning, or a lethal, well-thought-out drug overdose attempt)?
5. Is the patient suffering from command hallucinations that order him or her to harm or kill himself or herself? If the patient always hears command hallucinations, have these hallucinations changed in character and have they become more acute and threatening?
6. Is the patient experiencing dramatically failing health or a severe chronic illness or is the patient terminally ill?
7. Does the patient have a family history of completed suicide, which might predict a behavioral modeling or genetic predisposition to suicide or impulsivity? (Low levels of 5-hydroxyindoleacetic acid in cerebrospinal fluid of patients may be predictive of impulsive behaviors such as suicide attempts.)
8. Has the patient been significantly embarrassed or humiliated?
9. After clinical evaluation and crisis intervention, does the patient continue to feel hopeless? Does the patient feel better after clinical intervention, or is intense psychologic pain still present?
10. Is the patient's behavior a wish for death, or is the patient wanting to obtain psychologic relief by cutting or battering his or her body? Some patients may suffer from deliberate self-harm syndromes or parasuicidal behaviors. Patients with severe personality disorders (e.g., borderline personality) may have a need to cut or beat themselves when they feel extremely dysphoric, anxious, or upset. Such self-harm behaviors can at times actually bring a sense of relief and diminished tension. Such behaviors do not always mean that the patient wants to die. At times, however, these patients may also wish for death. The clinician must explore such behaviors carefully.

Overall, there is good news for physicians: Only 1% of all patients who attempt suicide will complete it within the next year; 99% will not.

Some patients suffer from *command hallucinations* that order them to harm or kill themselves. If a patient always hears command hallucinations (and some patients with psychotic disorders may), then one must inquire whether their usual hallucinations have changed in character and whether their hallucinations have become more acute and threatening.

Does the patient have dramatically failing health or a severe chronic illness, such as severe chronic obstructive pulmonary disease or end-stage renal disease? Is the patient terminally ill? These severe disease states may make people feel depressed, hopeless, and more likely to wish for death.

Has the patient been significantly embarrassed or humiliated? Undergoing arrest or public exposure of illegal or immoral activity can fill a patient with extreme levels of guilt and shame. Expulsion from school or loss of a job can likewise cause an immediate assault on a person's sense of self. These intense levels of frustration, humiliation, and shame may lead to suicidal behaviors owing to a sudden loss of self-esteem.

After clinical evaluation and crisis intervention, does the patient continue to feel hopeless? Does the patient feel better after clinical intervention, or is intense psychologic pain still present? A lack of psychologic improvement, with little resolution of psychologic suffering, suggests that the patient's ideas of self-harm may still be imminent.

Is the patient's behavior a wish for death, or is the patient wanting to obtain psychologic relief by cutting or battering his or her body? Some patients may suffer from deliberate self-harm syndromes or parasuicidal behaviors.[6] Patients with severe personality disorders (e.g., borderline personality) may have a need to cut or hurt themselves when they feel extremely dysphoric, anxious, or upset. Such self-harm behaviors can at times actually bring a sense of relief and diminished tension to these patients. These patients must sometimes feel a painful stimulus in order for their internal anxiety and dysphoria to diminish or abate. Such behaviors do not always mean that the patient wants to die. At times, however, these patients may also wish for death. Clinicians must carefully explore such behaviors with these difficult patients.

Adolescents with Suicidal Thoughts

Psychiatric evaluation of suicidal adolescents differs inherently from the treatment of adult psychiatric patients.[7–26] With adult patients, families are involved minimally or sometimes not at all. With a suicidal child or adolescent, suicidal thoughts or dysfunctional behaviors may be the product of a biologic mental illness or may be secondary to various dynamics operating within a family system.

Life at the end of the twentieth century is different from that in the fifties, the sixties, or even the seventies. Adults may mistakenly think, "Well, when I was a kid, I felt this way," or "I know what kids go through. I was a teenager once." This type of thinking may be fallacious. Divorce was unusual in earlier decades. Suicide among adolescents was a rare event. Schools did not need metal detectors. AIDS was not a problem. Alcohol use among children and teenagers was not as common. Few teenagers had direct access to guns. Physicians must help parents see the current dangers of living in a fast-changing world. Teenagers need lots of love and lots of limits. One without the other can bring disaster.

By engaging the family of a suicidal youth in the history-taking process, physicians give the indirect message that they are interested in everyone's welfare. Clinicians must quickly form an alliance with all parties—that is, the suicidal teenager and the parents or guardians. *No one should be accused or should be seen as being at fault.* The family history not only illustrates the context from which the family operates but also provides information on familial mental illness, substance abuse, and completed suicide. Suicidal ideation (particularly suicide pacts or recent completed suicides of close friends or peers) should be explored. Homicidal ideation should also be precluded. Guns, rifles, knives, other weapons, and pills should be removed or secured in the homes of severely depressed adolescents—especially those who have made threats or past attempts.

The group at highest risk for successful suicide is older adolescent males who suffer from depression, who have made previous suicide attempts, and who abuse alcohol or other substances. The breakup of a romance or being "kicked out of the family" can also be a precipitant of a suicide attempt by a depressed teenager. Suicide by a friend or close acquaintance can induce the so-called cluster suicide phenomenon, in which more suicide attempts or completions may follow. Group identification among teens is very powerful and may lead to imitative behaviors such as cluster suicide among friends or acquaintances.

Adolescents are often impulsive and have difficulty expressing powerful emotions in an appropriate or controlled manner. A suicide attempt can represent a maladaptive means of demonstrating and conveying to others one's internalized experience or pain. The availability of firearms may be associated with adolescent suicide even in the absence of psychiatric diagnosis, owing to the extreme moodiness and impulsivity of teenagers under stress. It should be clear that in every serious crisis or psychiatric emergency, the presence of firearms must be assessed and guns *must* be secured.[27–28]

In addition to the usual information about a possible suicide attempt, another important question that should be asked is, How did the family respond to the attempt, and can they monitor the adolescent's safety and provide a supportive environment until follow-up is initiated? Parents sometimes feel so powerless and frustrated that they "just don't care what happens." Even if they do not mean this literally, the teenager can often believe that it is so. If a family member is apathetic or hostile about an adolescent's suicide attempt, this should be seen as a potential danger sign, and if the adolescent is not going to be hospitalized, extreme caution should be used. Undue tension in the home may warrant an alternative placement (e.g., with another relative or in a temporary foster care setting). Clinicians should remember that even if adults have an impulse to harm themselves, they still have some ability to think before carrying out that impulse. This is often not true of adolescents, whose psychologic self and nervous system have not yet matured to that level of capability and forethought.

Alcohol-Intoxicated Patients with Suicidal Ideation

It is not unusual for intoxicated patients to present with acute suicidal ideation. Substance-induced mood disorders are quite common in patients who present to the emergency department. For the most part, the risk of behavior is short lived and is limited by the degree of alcohol intoxication that a patient experiences. In general, it is not possible to conduct a complete and effective psychiatric or clinical evaluation with an out-of-control, inebriated patient. It is important to hold such a patient temporarily in a secure setting until the acute effects of the intoxicating substance wear off. Many patients who present to the emergency department with acute suicidal ideation while intoxicated are no longer suicidal on reaching sobriety. A good general rule with a patient who is suicidal and under the influence of alcohol is to get the patient to a secure, monitored area and allow that patient to be observed until sober (or at least until his or her alcohol level is less than 0.100). If suicidal ideation persists after the patient reaches a reasonable state of sobriety, the patient may have an underlying depressive disorder, and hospitalization should be considered.

Because of the acute central nervous system effects of alcohol, patients with chronic alcohol dependence or acute high alcohol levels feel and often experience severe temporary symptoms of depression. On reaching sobriety or on completing a detoxification program, the majority of these patients are no longer depressed or suicidal. However, a small percentage of these patients have major psychiatric illnesses such as major depression, schizophrenia, or panic or bipolar disorder and need inpatient evaluation and treatment of these disorders. An intoxicated patient who continues to have strong suicidal ideation with a suicide plan and suicidal intent should be hospitalized if these thoughts continue despite reaching sobriety. Transient suicidal ideation that clears with sobriety can often be dealt with on an outpatient basis if the patient agrees to follow-up recommendations and has a support system available (e.g., a shelter, home, or Alcoholics Anonymous sponsor).

TREATMENT OF SUICIDAL PATIENTS

After the aforementioned risk factors and clinical considerations are reviewed, the patient may be judged to be at a high or low degree of risk. High-risk patients should be hospitalized.

Suicidal patients often may not have immediate intent to kill themselves, but they may not feel that they are in control of their impulses. Many patients feel unsafe if they leave the emergency department or clinic, because of persistent suicidal ideation. Similarly, a patient may not be able to guarantee his or her physical safety owing to ongoing impulsivity, depression, or dysphoria. Patients who present with suicidal ideation should not be sent home alone; rather, a support system should be created for them. Friends, supportive family members, and community agencies can sometimes be used to help support patients while they are awaiting definitive outpatient mental health follow-up. In other cases, when the patients are believed to be imminently dangerous or are unwilling to accept recommended treatment or when a support system is unavailable, it may be necessary to hospitalize them or to provide a crisis residential setting or holding bed where they can be safely monitored by professional mental health staff. Table 19–3 lists examples of criteria that would warrant admission. Please note that even when every precaution is taken, because of the unpredictability of these highly impulsive patients, a few patients are released and complete suicide. No current biologic or psychologic markers can always reliably predict the likelihood of suicide completion.

In general, if low-risk patients are able to guarantee or verbally contract for their own safety and the aforementioned factors have been thoroughly reviewed and considered, they may possibly be treated on an outpatient basis. However, it is important to make certain that patients have a support system available and agree to stay in touch with the emergency department or clinical evaluation service if suicidal thoughts recur. If a patient is asked, "Do you agree to call us right away if any suicidal thoughts come back to your mind?" the clinician must hear a definite yes from the patient. Patients must also agree to any recommended follow-up procedures, such as scheduling and attending outpatient appointments, taking medicines, getting rid of firearms, or agreeing to follow-up visits to the clinic setting or emergency department (follow-up house calls by mo-

Table 19–3. Indications for Admission

- Patients who fired a gun in an attempt to commit suicide.
- Patients who jump from a significant height.
- Patients who barricade themselves in and have a standoff with police.
- Patients with multiple previous lethal attempts.
- Psychotic or paranoid patients who, when acutely ill, arm themselves because of extreme fear.
- Patients with a lethal plan or patients who were only accidentally discovered after an attempt.
- Patients who are experiencing acute command hallucinations to kill themselves.
- Patients who cannot assure the clinician of their safety.
- Patients who have no support system to return to or one cannot be created (e.g., with family, clergy, friends, Alcoholics Anonymous sponsors, boss, co-workers, shelters, or other resources).
- Suicidal persons who feel no sense of psychologic relief after crisis intervention.
- Patients who have not been truthful. If patient has not shared truthful feelings and facts, the clinician cannot be assured of the validity and reliability of any information from the patient.
- Patients who will not agree to outpatient treatment recommendations for immediate follow-up care (e.g., patients who refuse to take medicine or to go to an outpatient visit or refuse to call if thoughts of harming themselves recur).

Remember: There are many other indications for hospitalization. A clinician's emotional and cognitive decisions should be congruent. When a decision is made NOT to hospitalize a patient, the clinician's "gut" and "head" should be in agreement about the decision. The clinician's cognitive and intuitive sense should be that both the patient and the treatment plan can be trusted.

bile crisis teams are also ideal, where such interventions are available). Clinicians should also ask patients if they have firearms at home, and if they do, every attempt should be made to sequester those weapons by contacting family, friends, neighbors, or the police. If a patient who presented with suicidal ideation or a suicide attempt is to be discharged, follow-up calls to the patient and to the agency to which the patient is being referred for treatment should be a routine part of every clinical service's aftercare procedure. The people involved in the patient's support system must be given explicit, clear instructions on how to watch the patient and what to do if any difficulties recur. Phone numbers of crisis hotlines, outpatient clinics, and emergency services should be provided to all parties.

SUICIDE AND HOMICIDE

Suicide and homicide often occur together. As mentioned earlier, patients who exhibit impulsive behaviors (such as harm to themselves or violence toward others) may have low levels of the serotonin metabolite 5-HIAA in their cerebrospinal fluid. This is indirect biochemical evidence of a common link between violent behaviors toward the self and violence toward others. Newspaper and media reports of people who shoot their families and then shoot themselves are not infrequent. These people are often depressed and hopeless. Severely suicidal people often think, "I must leave the world and take my loved ones with me. This is too much hell for them to live through." Also, some depressed patients may experience such severe mood swings, irritability, or anger that they cannot control their rage. Every suicidal patient must be asked about issues of homicidality. If homicidal ideas are coming to the patient's mind, clinicians must find out about any means, plan, or intent.

If a patient has clear homicidal thoughts with *intent* to carry out the act, that patient must be hospitalized or placed in a secure setting. If homicidality is directed toward a specified person or group of persons, a professional clinician has a duty to protect those potential victims from imminent harm. In such cases, the patient must be hospitalized, potential victims must be warned, and the patient must be told that this is mandated by law for everyone's protection. The Tarasoff rulings mandate that the police should be involved if a clinician cannot locate and warn a particular potential victim. Careful documentation of such clinical procedures is essential.[29]

OTHER TREATMENTS

Pharmacologic treatment may diminish a patient's suicidal thoughts. For extreme dysphoria, the physician or consulting psychiatrist may administer an anxiolytic or sedative drug such as lorazepam (2 mg by mouth for mild agitation or administered sublingually or via intramuscular injection for extreme agitation) to relieve the patient's discomfort. If the patient remains agitated or is still extremely dysphoric, hospitalization may be indicated.

Patients with dysphoric feelings secondary to psychotic disorders benefit from rapid tranquilization with high-potency antipsychotic drugs such as haloperidol or fluphenazine hydrochloride (5 mg intramuscularly or 10 mg orally). Extremely agitated individuals can be made more comfortable with intramuscular injections of 5 mg of haloperidol plus 2 mg of lorazepam or by administering droperidol (2.5 to 5.0 mg) intramuscularly.

If a patient presents with major depression and suicidal ideation, it appears appropriate for emergency departments to administer antidepressant medications for treatment in certain cases. This would be appropriate only for patients who are not believed to be at imminent risk of harm. A patient sometimes may not be able to obtain an intake appointment in a mental health setting for several weeks. Physicians should not prescribe tricyclic antidepressants from the emergency setting because of their high potential for lethal cardiotoxicity when taken in even small overdoses (e.g., 20 50-mg tablets of a tricyclic antidepressant can be lethal). The newer agents—that is, the selective serotonin reuptake inhibitors, drugs such as fluoxetine (Prozac), sertraline (Zoloft), paroxetine (Paxil), or some newer agents such as venlafaxine (Effexor), fluvoxamine (Luvox), or nefazodone (Serzone)—are considered to be relatively safe for the cardiac system. Patients, however, should not be given medication unless a follow-up plan has been arranged and they are able to assure the clinician of their safety.

Every crisis or emergency setting should have a close relationship with its community's mental health care system. If necessary, some physicians bring patients back for a clinic or emergency department visit before their first definitive outpatient visit in the mental health care setting. Careful follow-up may thus be provided. Ideally, however, psychiatric or mental health care centers should give priority to those cases that present the greatest emergency.

Proper assessment of suicide includes evaluation of risk factors, history taking from the patient and family, and appraisal of support systems. Hospitalization is mandated when indicated. Proper documentation of the medical record is essential.

FINAL RECOMMENDATIONS

Clinicians should ascertain if patients (1) are not imminently dangerous by clinical history and facts, (2) are willing to follow the recommendations for immediate and short-term treatment, and (3) have a support system. Favorable answers to these questions may allow a clinician to treat a patient on an outpatient basis. Negative responses to these general questions most often mandate emergency hospitalization.[30]

Once again, we offer a note of caution about weapons.[31] Clinicians should always inquire whether a patient with suicidal ideation has any firearms. If firearms are present in a patient's home, emergency clinicians should make every attempt to have those weapons secured by relatives or close friends. If a patient has no reliable supports, the police can be used and are most often willing to secure the weapons of persons who are potentially harmful to themselves or others.

References

1. Blumenthal SJ, Kupfer DJ (eds): Suicide Over the Life Cycle. Washington, DC, American Psychiatric Association Press, 1990.
2. J Clin Psychopharmacol *12*(2): Entire supplement, 1992.
3. Stanford EJ, Goetz RR, Bloom JD: The no harm contract in the emergency assessment of suicidal risk. J Clin Psychiatry *55*:344–348, 1994.
4. Weissman MM, Klerman GI, Markowitz JS, et al: Suicidal ideation and suicide attempts in panic disorder and attacks. N Engl J Med *321*:1209–1214, 1989.
5. Fawcett J, Scheftner WA, Fogg L, et al: Time related predictors of suicide in major affective disorder. Am J Psychiatry *147*:1189–1194, 1990.
6. Pies RW, Popli AP: Self injurious behavior: Pathophysiology and implications for treatment. J Clin Psychiatry *56*:580–588, 1995.
7. Bland R, Neuman S, Orn H: Recurrent and nonrecurrent depression. A family study. Arch Gen Psychiatry *43*:1085–1089, 1986.
8. Brent D, Perper J, Moritz G, et al: Stressful events, psychopathology and adolescent suicide: A case control study. Suicide Life Threat Behav *23*:179–187, 1993.
9. Delga I, Heinssen R, Fritsch R, et al: Psychosis, aggression, and self-destructive behavior in hospitalized adolescents. Am J Psychiatry *146*:521–525, 1989.
10. Goodyer I, Cooper P, Vize C, Ashby L: Depression in 11–16 year old girls: The role of past parental psychopathology and exposure to recent life events. J Child Psychol Psychiatry *34*:1103–1115, 1993.
11. Goodyer I, Ashby L, Anthem M, et al: Temperament and major depression in 11–16 year olds. J Child Psychol Psychiatry *34*:1409–1423, 1993.
12. Goodyer I, Cooper P: A community study of depression in adolescent girls. II. The clinical features of identified disorder. Br J Psychiatry *163*:374–380, 1993.
13. Henggeler SW, Schoenwald SK, Pickrel SG, et al: The contribution of treatment research to the reform of children's mental health services: Multisystemic family preservation as an example. J Ment Health Adm *21*:229–239, 1994.
14. Henry B, Feehan M, Mcbee R, et al: The importance of conduct problems and depressive symptoms in predicting adolescent substance use. J Abnorm Child Psychol *21*:469–481, 1993.
15. Inamdar SC, Lewis DO, Siomopoulos G: Violent and suicidal behavior in psychotic adolescents. Am J Psychiatry *139*:932–935, 1982.
16. King C, Raskin A, Gdowski C, et al: Psychosocial factors associated with urban adolescent female suicide attempts. J Am Acad Child Adolesc Psychiatry *29*:289–294, 1990.
17. Low B, Andrews S: Adolescent suicide. Med Clin North Am *74*:1251–1261, 1990.
18. Lewinsohn P, Rohde P, Seeley J: Psychosocial risk factors for future adolescent suicide attempts. J Consult Clin Psychol *62*:297–305, 1994.
19. Miller K, King C, Shain B, Naylor M: Suicidal adolescents' perceptions of their family environment. Suicide Life Threat Behav *22*:227–239, 1992.
20. Northcutt C: Interaction patterns in families with suicidal and nonsuicidal adolescents. Diss Abstr Int *49*:2868b, 1989.
21. Paluszny M, Davenport C, Kim W: Suicide attempts and ideation. Adolescence *26*:209–215, 1992.
22. Puig-Antich J: Depression and conduct disorder in prepuberty. J Am Acad Child Psychiatry *21*:118–128, 1982.
23. Rich C, Sherman M, Fowler R: San Diego suicide study: The adolescents. Adolescence *25*:854–865, 1990.
24. Shaffer D: The epidemiology of teen suicide: An examination of risk factors. J Clin Psychiatry *49*:36–41, 1988.
25. Shaffer D, Garland A, Gould M, et al: Preventing teenage suicide: A critical review. J Am Acad Child Adolesc Psychiatry *27*:675–687, 1988.
26. Adams D, Overholser J, Lehnert K: Perceived family functioning and adolescent suicidal behavior. J Am Acad Child Adolesc Psychiatry *33*:498–507, 1994.
27. Rosenberg M, Mercy J, Houk V: Guns and adolescent suicides. JAMA *266*:3030, 1991.
28. Brent D, Perper J, Moritz G, et al: Firearms and adolescent suicide. Am J Dis Child *147*:1066–1071, 1993.
29. Mill MJ, Sullivan G, Eth S: Protecting third parties: A decade after Tarasoff. Am J Psychiatry *144*:68–74, 1987.
30. Bengelsdorf H, Levy LE, Emerson RL, Barile FA: A crisis triage rating scale: Brief dispositional assessment of patients at risk for hospitalization. J Nerv Ment Dis *172*:424–430, 1984.
31. Kellerman AL, Rivara FP, Soures G, et al: Suicide in the home in relation to gun ownership. N Engl J Med *327*:467–472, 1992.

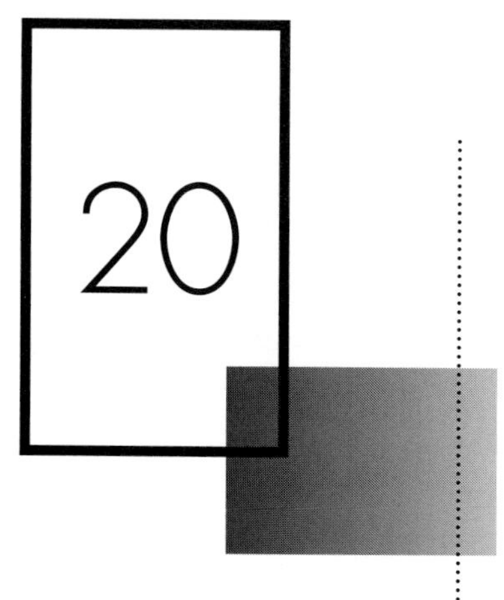

20 Prevention of Childhood Poisonings

ALAN DAVID WOOLF, MD, MPH
FREDERICK H. LOVEJOY, JR, MD

During the past 30 years, childhood morbidity and mortality due to poisoning have decreased as a result of new prevention strategies, along with improved triage and management techniques. Poisoning nevertheless remains a threat to the health of young children. More than 1 million poison exposures in children age 5 years and younger were reported by 67 reporting poison centers in the United States in 1995.[1] An analysis of more than 3.8 million United States childhood poisonings during a 5-year period from 1985 to 1989 revealed that hazardous medications (e.g., iron preparations, cardiovascular medications, antidepressants, and methylsalicylates) and household products (e.g., gun bluing, pesticides, and hydrocarbons) still cause many preventable deaths among preschoolers.[2] The researchers calculated a *hazard factor* for each toxic agent on the basis of the frequency and the extent of injuries following poisonings involving the agent (Table 20–1). Such a ranking could potentially help in developing more focused strategies for poisoning prevention.

Although the prevention of poisonings might be broadly defined to include the prevention of excessive morbidity and mortality due to the injury once a poison exposure has taken place, in this chapter the definition is restricted to those measures that attempt to avert the poisoning exposure itself. Indeed, targeted education, improved technology, and more effective government regulations in the interests of poisoning prevention all have served as models for efforts to prevent other types of injuries.

PASSIVE VERSUS ACTIVE STRATEGIES

Poisoning prevention strategies can be divided conceptually into passive and active interventions. *Passive* interventions are those measures that do not depend on behavioral changes by the public for their success. Examples include federal regulations prohibiting the retail sale of caustic agents in household products in concentrations higher than those regarded as safe for home use. Because highly caustic agents have become less accessible to the public, the probability that they will cause poisoning is automatically reduced.

Another example of a passive safety strategy is packaging potentially dangerous medications in child-resistant containers. Such packaging limits a young child's chance of exposure to a toxic dose of a drug before being discovered by a supervising adult. Because the child-resistant cap is automatically part of the packaging, a parent does not need to make an active decision to implement this safety measure.

Active poisoning prevention strategies, on the other hand, are those that require sustained behavioral change in the target population if they are to be effective. For example, counseling parents to poison-proof their household requires continued vigilance to ensure proper handling of potential toxins entering the household and a sustained and repeated effort to ensure that those household products that might be poisonous to toddlers are stored safely.

Table 20–1. Agents with High Hazard Factors Associated with Poisonings of United States Children Younger Than 6 Years (1985-1989)

Substance*	Total Pediatric Exposures†	Hazard Factor‡
Pharmaceuticals		
Amphetamines	6409	4.5
Acetaminophen and propoxyphene	2171	4.5
Aspirin	10002	3.1
Amitriptyline	2897	22.8
Antiarrhythmics	1203	4.0
Anticholinergics	6516	3.2
Antihypertensives	8099	27.6
Barbiturates (long acting)	4475	13.3
Barbiturates (short acting)	1051	6.1
Carbamazepine	4113	32.5
Cardiac glycosides	3846	10.9
Cocaine	546	59.0
Cyclic antidepressant and phenothiazine	832	19.4
Desipramine	935	27.6
Diphenoxylate and atropine	2500	12.2
Doxepin	887	14.5
Imipramine	2503	20.0
Iron	11234	8.5
Lithium	1054	10.7
Marijuana	694	7.0
Oral hypoglycemics	2609	6.8
Phenothiazines	7451	12.8
Phenytoin	3619	9.3
Propoxyphene	514	6.3
Theophylline	8622	7.7
Valproic acid	1197	6.7
Nonpharmaceuticals		
Alkali	10267	3.8
Alkali drain cleaners	1474	21.9
Alkali industrial cleaners	938	29.2
Alkali oven cleaners	4619	3.5
Carbon monoxide	3103	31.1
Chlorinated hydrocarbons	9694	4.8
Chlorine gas	2208	4.4
Ethanol	2622	8.0
Ethylene glycol	2321	3.5
Hydrochloric acid	784	6.2
Kerosene	10751	7.9
Lighter fluid	8865	4.4
Methane, natural gas	700	9.2
Methanol	1883	5.1
Mineral seal oil	6564	3.2
Organophosphate alone	16560	5.6
Organophosphate and other pesticides	1806	3.6

*Specific substances only—broader categories are not all included; bites and envenomations are not included.

†Only substances with more than 500 exposures included.

‡Only hazard factors > 3.0 included.

Adapted from Comparison of pediatric poisoning hazards: An analysis of 3.8 million exposure incidents—a report from the American Association of Poison Control Centers. Pediatrics *89*:1002–1004, 1992.

THE ETIOLOGY OF POISONING

Children living in families whose system of supervision has broken down are at high risk for poisoning. Some particular stress such as a recent move, family loss, or financial hardship can cause parents to relax their vigilance. Poisonings often occur when a parent is distracted—for example, around mealtime or when entertaining guests. Many poisonings occur when the parent-child interaction is not in the "business-as-usual" routine of everyday life. For example, at holiday time, new hazards are introduced into a child's environment (e.g., Christmas trees and ornaments), and the parents may be distracted from their usual supervisory activities by parties and family social gatherings. Previous studies have suggested that many childhood poisonings occur when a product is in use,[3] and the occurrences reinforce the idea that lack of supervision is what places a child at high risk.

Considerable evidence shows that complex family dynamics sometimes underlie poisoning incidents. Families of childhood poisoning repeaters are characterized as disorganized, socially isolated, and operating under the stress of poor housing, frequent moves, or the psychiatric or physical illness of family members.[4–6] Sobel and Margolis have suggested that children who repeatedly poison themselves use such incidents as tactics in an ongoing power struggle with their parents.[7] They found that the mothers of such poisoning repeaters often came from broken homes and had poor parental role models. The children were often products of an unwanted pregnancy and tended to be hyperactive and negativistic. The importance of such disordered family relationships in poisoning causation is reinforced by Baltimore and Meyer's findings that the poisoning recognition and storage habits of parents of 52 poisoned children were no different from those of parents of 52 control children.[8] Thus, the environmental hazards present seemed to be the same; what differed between families that had experienced childhood poisoning events and those that had not seemed to be psychosocial and behavioral factors.

Poisoning prevention strategies that fail to address important moderators such as the behavior of the child, the organization and structure of the family, and the nature of the child-parent interaction have little chance for success. Although child-proofing changes in the house may remain static, the circumstances in which the threshold to a poisoning injury is breached are dynamic (e.g., opened household products or medications, poor supervision, altered family routines). Modification of these circumstances requires patience, counseling, increased social supports, and behavioral adaptations by both children and parents. These goals are somewhat elusive and are part of the challenge in the development of new poisoning prevention strategies.

GENERAL POISONING PREVENTION STRATEGIES

Model poisoning prevention strategies have sought to combine improved technologic advances with enlightened government regulations and effective public education to reduce the risk of a poisoning injury. Baker and colleagues[9] enumerated such general injury prevention strategies, when applied to poisonings, as follows:

1. Banning or reducing the manufacture or sale of an injurious toxin
2. Decreasing the concentration of a poison or the total amount of a poison available to the individual to subinjurious levels
3. Preventing access to the substance
4. Creating barriers between the host and agent during the use of the toxin
5. Substituting products with less inherent toxicity but equal efficacy for more dangerous products
6. Changing the formulation of a product to make it less injurious

Each of these various principles has been successfully applied to various causes of poisoning among adults as well as children. The banning of dichlorodiphenyltrichloroethane (DDT) exemplifies legislation targeted at preventing environmental toxic exposures. Limiting the number of baby aspirin to 36 tablets per bottle reduces the likelihood that toddlers can ingest an injurious dose. Child-resistant containers, blister packs for medication, and safe storage of hazardous products prevent access or create a barrier between the child and an injurious dose of the drug or household product. The substitution of acetaminophen for propoxyphene gives equal analgesia while avoiding propoxyphene's considerable toxicity in the event of overdose. The reformulation of children's cough and cold preparations and mouthwashes to exclude alcohol removes a potential source of toxicity to young children and infants.

Although a number of excellent poisoning prevention strategies have been implemented to reduce adult injuries due to exposure to occupational or environmental poisons, strategies to prevent injuries to children due to environmental toxins are equally compelling if not more so. Such strategies often include regulatory measures. (Regulations limiting pesticide residues in children's food are beyond the scope of this chapter.) This chapter addresses only those specific prevention strategies effective in reducing acute home poisoning among children. The following strategies to prevent home poisonings are discussed:

1. Product packaging changes
2. Sticker trials
3. Community-wide programs
4. Clinic-based counseling
5. Creation of poison control centers

SPECIFIC POISONING PREVENTION STRATEGIES

Product Packaging Changes

As early as 1960, the federal government began to take regulatory steps to reduce the incidence of poisoning in the United States by passing the Federal Hazardous Substance Labeling Act. This consumer-oriented legislation required proper labeling of products but did not attempt to regulate their packaging, sale, or use.[10] During the next 15 years, better designs of child-resistant containers were developed and field tested. The rationale for such technology was developmental—that children at highest risk for accidental poisoning (i.e., those 18 to 36 months old) lacked the ability to combine gross motor skills (the palmar exertion of a sufficient straight vector force) simultaneously with fine motor skills (the finger-exerted twisting of sufficient torque) to open easily products secured by child-resistant containers.

The technologic advances in the engineering of child-resistant containers, combined with enough education of the public to convince them of the potential worth of such packaging changes, culminated in passage of the Poison Prevention Packaging Act in 1970.[11] This legislation established standards for special packaging of household products and pharmaceuticals, defined appropriate testing procedures and those products that were subject to the regulation, and set a timetable for gradually phasing in the regulations during an 8-year period. The first products to be regulated were those containing aspirin. The products covered and the dates of implementation are listed in Table 20–2. This regulation provides that if a consumer product presents a serious danger to children and special packaging is both technically feasible and practical, then a safety closure design must be submitted before the product is approved for marketing. Premarketing tests must demonstrate that 85% of a panel of 200 children younger than 5 years fail to open the package in a 5-minute period. A panel of adults is also allowed a single 5-minute period in which 90% must be able to open the safety closure after reading the opening instructions on the package.

The purpose of child-resistant caps is to separate the child physically from the potential poison by providing a barrier between the two. The intent of the regulation was not to poison-proof the container but simply to delay children long enough in their attempts to get at a poison for an adult to discover and correct the hazardous situation. Follow-up studies suggest that the effectiveness of child-resistant containers has been dramatic. Accidental ingestion of aspirin by children younger than 5 years accounted for 26% of all accidental ingestions in 1965 but only 4.7% by 1974.[9] Overall poisoning-related death rates among preschool children declined dramatically between 1960 and 1980. Other studies have shown that poisoning by safety-packaged products decreased nationally by 38% from 1973 to 1976 among the age group between birth and 4 years. Poisonings by unregulated products increased by 20% during the same period among children of the same age group.[12]

As a result of child-resistant packaging, an estimated 86,000 poisoning injuries were averted between the years 1974 and 1981.[13] Walton's study

Table 20–2. Products Covered by the Poison Prevention Packaging Act

PPPA Regulation	Effective Date	Characteristics of Products Regulated
Aspirin	8/14/72	Products for oral human use
Furniture polish	9/13/72	Nonemulsion liquid form, low viscosity, containing ≥ 10% mineral seal oil or petroleum distillates
Methylsalicylate	9/21/72	Liquid products containing ≥ 5% by weight
Controlled drugs	10/24/72	For oral human use
Sodium and/or potassium hydroxide	4/11/73	Dry forms ≥ 10% by weight; other forms ≥ 2% by weight
Turpentine	7/1/73	Liquid form ≥ 10% by weight
Kindling and/or illuminating preparations	10/29/73	Prepackaged liquid, low viscosity, containing ≥ 10% petroleum distillates
Methyl alcohol	7/1/73	Liquids containing ≥ 4% by weight
Sulfuric acid	8/14/73	Substances containing ≥ 10% by weight
Prescription drugs	4/16/74	For oral human use
Ethylene glycol	6/1/74	Liquids containing ≥ 10% by weight
Paint solvents	4/23/77	Solvents for paints that contain ≥ 10% by weight of benzene, toluene, xylene
Iron-containing drugs	10/17/78	Noninjectable animal and human drugs containing 250 mg or more elemental iron (total package)
Dietary supplements	10/17/78	Dietary supplements containing 250 mg or more elemental iron (total package)
Acetaminophen	2/27/80	Preparations for oral human use with 1 g or more acetaminophen (total package)

From Walton W: An evaluation of the Poison Prevention Packaging Act. Pediatrics *69*:364, 1982.

during a 6-year period (1972 to 1978) demonstrated a decline from 7500 to 2300 ingestions during the first 6-year period after the regulations took effect, whereas ingestions of various unregulated products either increased or stayed the same.[14]

In one public survey, more than 98% of parents could describe safety packaging or safety caps.[15] An overwhelming 85% of the 636 families surveyed approved of the idea of safety packaging, and 89% had safety packages in the home. Only 3% of respondents had discontinued use of a product because of difficulty with the package. The Poison Prevention Packaging Act is a model of well-crafted legislation brought about by successful combination of physician advocacy, improved technology, and effective public education. The fact that many childhood poisonings occur with open products already in use[16] tempers the gains realized by the implementation of child-resistant packaging.

More recent product changes have included the use of unit dosing with blister packs. Such dispensers are expensive but accomplish the dual purposes of lowering the risk of unintentional drug overdoses because of misinterpretation of dosing instruction and decreasing the risk of an accidental overdose by children, who must spend more time unwrapping each individual pill and thus, it is hoped, cannot ingest a harmful quantity before being discovered.

The advent of tamper-resistant containers with protective plastic-wrapped seals has also decreased the risk that a product might be intentionally altered without being noticed by an unwary consumer. Such an outer wrap theoretically imposes yet another barrier to children as well. The success of such tamper-proof packaging in preventing poisonings has yet to be fully evaluated.

Sticker Trials

Older children can be educated to recognize hazardous agents and to avoid them. Such education usually includes the use of warning stickers that parents affix to hazardous household products to alert children to the danger. These stickers, picturing a skull and crossbones, angry serpent, or frowning face (Mr. Yuk), are meant to evoke psychologically unpleasant or fearsome images in a child's mind so that she or he will be deterred from sampling the poisonous contents. Braden found that such a method of discriminating hazardous agents was necessary; preschool children incorrectly identified 40% of poisonous products with which they were confronted.[17] When children were exposed to an educational program on products labeled with warning stickers, their accuracy of recognition improved to 86%. Krenzelok and Garber introduced poison recognition teaching aids into a daycare center program serving 3285 children 30 to 60 months old and tested 195 randomly selected children 6 weeks later.[18] The children showed improvements in their recognition of the warning symbol, Mr. Yuk, and in their understanding of which products were poisonous.

No decrease in the incidence of poisonings has been associated with exposure to such a program, however. When Fergusson's group performed a controlled field trial that distributed labels to 583 families with 543 matched controls, no significant differences in poisoning rates could be appreciated.[19] More than 40% of the parents thought Mr. Yuk labels were not useful, had misgivings about the program, or did not use the warning labels to cover all the poisons in the home. The success of an educational effort using warning stickers probably is contingent on reinforcement of the learning; continuity of medical care and repetition of the advice may improve the effectiveness of such a program.[20] Other concerns have been expressed about the use of warning stickers on household products. Some researchers and parents fear that young children may be attracted instead of repulsed by the warning stickers or may not be able to understand what a poison means.[21] Furthermore, many poisons (e.g., plants) cannot be labeled with a warning. Finally, those poisoning incidents occurring outside the household, which may represent as many as 13% of all poisonings in children younger than 5 years,[22] cannot be effectively forestalled by a home-centered program.

Community-Wide Educational Efforts

Relatively few programs have attempted to implement poisoning prevention on a community-wide basis. The health department or a poison control center has usually spearheaded such projects with the cooperation of local government officials, health professionals, community action groups, and even businesses and merchandisers. Fisher and colleagues[23] introduced one such intervention, which included community outreach seminars, school curriculum changes, point-of-purchase education efforts by retailers, and mass media and educational material distribution activities in Monroe County, New York. As a result, the number of poisonings requiring emergency department treatment in area hospitals declined 66% and poisoning admissions diminished 71%, whereas hospitalization rates in comparable control communities remained stable. Maisel and associates[24] organized a poisoning prevention project in Charleston County, South Carolina, involving education of the public about the recognition of potential poisons and techniques for their safe storage. Activities such as programs for community groups, poster contests, mass media presentations, and group discussions were used. Results of preintervention versus postintervention surveys suggested that 88% of parents had been reached by the educational campaign and had implemented the recommendations. Researchers noted that the number of children hospitalized in Charleston County for poisoning declined. Both of these model programs have demonstrated that community awareness about poisoning prevention can be increased and can lower the rate of poisoning. How long such educational efforts can be sustained remains unclear; whether a more modest but self-perpetuating program of education can be as effective a deterrent needs to be tested.

Clinic-Based Educational Programs

One strategy for promoting the prevention of poisonings among young children is clinic-based education for their parents. Such education invariably includes information about the recognition of hazardous chemicals in the home environment; elimination of the hazard by not purchasing the poison, safely storing it in the home, and disposing of partially used products; readiness for a poisoning event by the home storage of syrup of ipecac and use of telephone stickers with emergency telephone numbers; and the appropriate first response (first aid) if a toxic exposure occurs in the home.

The success of such programs has been found to depend on a number of factors (Table 20–3):

1. Content: The educational message must be clear, readable at the fifth grade level, succinct, and targeted at the intended audience in terms of sophistication.
2. Timeliness: Education is most effective when the audience is addressed during a window of receptivity to such a message—that is, when they recognize its importance, are not distracted, and are personally motivated enough to take action.
3. Relevance: The message must be important to the audience and perceived as crucial to their well-being. They must be motivated by its relevance to their own health or that of their family in order to take action.
4. Lack of barriers: The education must give information that is practical and for which compliance is not too difficult or beset with barriers (interposed tasks the parent must complete to make the effort effective).
5. Repetitiveness: The most effective educational modules are repeated to reinforce the message, if it is intended for the parent to carry out active safety behaviors routinely (e.g., checking labels for toxic ingredients and containers for child-resistant caps).
6. Educator: The professional stature of the educator has been found to relate to the success of the compliance with educational recommendations. Parents are much more likely to value their physician's personal suggestions than they are a written summary or slide show, for example. Other cultural, ethnic, and social forces may

Table 20–3. Attributes of Ideal Poisoning Prevention Education

Clear content
Timeliness
Relevance
Recommendations easy to implement
Repetitive intervention
Effective educator
Brief format

also enhance or detract from the educator's effectiveness in delivering the message.

7. Attention span: The educational program cannot be so abbreviated that the parent does not recognize its importance. Conversely, the education should not be preachy and should not tax the attention or time constraints of the audience. A program that engages parents in an active and collaborative learning experience is more effective.

Previous investigations of clinic-based educational programs have been limited by structural or research design problems. Alpert and Heagarty developed a program that used coupons that parents could redeem for poison prevention packs at their local pharmacy.[25] This multistep program proved to be too cumbersome for parents, however, and the expected results were not achieved. Fewer than 3% of the coupons were turned in; thus, parents did not receive the intended ipecac or the poisoning prevention message. Dershewitz and Williamson failed to show an effect when a safety counseling program to childproof a home was instituted in the clinic setting.[26]

Several studies have shown that a more focused message directed at a specific population might be more effective. Dershewitz and colleagues, by means of a short poisoning prevention message delivered to mothers by a physician during the well childcare visit, demonstrated that parents would remember a simple message and would implement the suggested safety measures at home.[27] Because these mothers were attending the clinic in a health maintenance organization, the universal efficacy of such a program may be questionable.

Ipecac kept in the home has been shown to be an effective part of family readiness for a poisoning, and it can prevent injury and reduce the need to seek medical assistance.[28–30] In a follow-up study of 202 families counseled in an emergency clinic setting, Woolf and colleagues showed that such counseling could increase the availability of ipecac 6 months later such that 68% of families had ipecac in their houses.[31] Thus, a clinic-based counseling program, combined with other prevention measures, can substantially improve family safety practices and readiness in the event of an emergency. A meta-analysis of 20 studies of injury prevention counseling in primary care settings showed positive effects in 18 such studies.[32]

Poison Control Centers

Regionalization of poison control centers across the United States has contributed to the remarkable progress in poisoning prevention and improvements in poisoning management.[33] This success is derived from the leadership that poison control centers have provided in four different areas:

1. Accuracy of toxicologic information and advice for the management of human poisonings
2. Advocacy as a lead agency in poisoning prevention
3. Training for health professionals
4. Research into the etiology, management, and prevention of poisonings

Access to a regional poison control center undoubtedly improves the medical triage and management of a toxic exposure, thus preventing excessive morbidity and mortality. Studies of the use of health services in states with and without poison control centers demonstrate remarkable improvements in telephone triage patterns, avoidance of excess emergency department visits, and improved quality and quantity of pertinent information given for those poisonings in states with regional poison control centers.[34–36]

It is perhaps underappreciated that poison control centers also serve a focusing role as the lead agency in the community for poisoning prevention programs. Poison control centers are a valuable resource for providing public and professional information about the identification of toxic compounds, acceptable exposure levels, and safe storage and use. One study demonstrated that poison centers could develop poisoning prevention strategies aimed at high-risk families using the information hotline.[37] Poison control centers also have increasingly expanded their role to service those calls requesting information about occupational or environmental exposures and toxicology. Poison control centers serve as a highly visible networking resource that can make referrals to other community facilities with more specialized knowledge about teratogenicity, public health implications of specific exposures, and plant or animal identifications.

Poison control centers also serve in poisoning prevention by improving the toxicology training of health professionals through tutorials, staff lectures, in-service programs, and regional workshops and symposia. Additionally, poison control centers can serve to alert health professionals, through surveillance of adverse drug reactions, of changes in prescribing style or precautions that must be taken. By pursuing active public education goals via newsletters, public service announcements, health fairs, and media campaigns (e.g., National Poison Prevention Week), poison control centers help to keep the public alert to the principles of poisoning prevention.

Finally, poison control centers often serve as the stimulus to develop new techniques in poisoning prevention. The centers accumulate a dynamic clinical poisoning experience from which epidemiologic trends in poisoning types and circumstances can be identified. Ideally, such an early warning surveillance system regarding a community's specific toxic exposure problems can lead to directed programs aimed at averting microepidemics of poisoning injuries. Because poison control centers are respected by the public and by health professionals for possessing a particular type of expertise, they can stimulate interest in new research and regulations for poisoning prevention.

THE PHYSICIAN'S RESPONSIBILITY

Physicians have a dual role in the prevention of poisonings, as advocates for their patients' families and as influential and respected community leaders. Physicians must recognize those circumstances that pose a higher than usual potential risk for a poisoning and must take corrective action. This action may include diverse recommendations, such as changing or simplifying a prescribed drug or recommending or advocating daycare, nursing home care, other social supports, psychiatric evaluation, or family counseling. Physicians must give adequate attention to poisoning prevention topics that they discuss with patients as part of their routine health care.

Physicians, in their capacity as community leaders, have an obligation to advocate changes necessary to decrease the risk of poisoning and to alert the community to new or previously unrecognized toxic hazards. Such advocacy includes support for the local or regional poison control service serving the community and for its programs in poisoning prevention. Physicians might also make use of public forums to change the public perceptions of poisoning prevention strategies (e.g., the need for child-resistant containers, the importance of following directions for the use of medications, and the dangers of drug abuse). Physicians can also be influential consultants to legislative bodies considering new initiatives restricting or regulating the use and disposal of drugs and toxins.

Dedicated health professionals must make a concerted effort to continue the momentum and consolidate the gains that have been made in poisoning prevention and to advance new aspects of the field.

References

1. Litovitz TL, Felberg L, White S, et al: 1995 Annual report of the American Association of Poison Control Centers Toxic Exposure Surveillance System. Am J Emerg Med *14*:487–537, 1996.
2. Litovitz T, Manoguerra A: Comparison of pediatric poisoning hazards: An analysis of 3.8 million exposure incidents—a report from the American Association of Poison Control Centers. Pediatrics *89*:999–1006, 1992.
3. Jensen G, Wilson W: Preventive implications of a study of 100 poisonings in children. Pediatrics *65*:490–496, 1960.
4. Sibert R: Stress in families who have ingested poisons. BMJ *3*:87–89, 1975.
5. Beautrais A, Fergusson D, Shannon T: Accidental poisoning in the first three years of life. Aust Paediatr J *17*:104–109, 1981.
6. Bithoney B, Snyder J, Michalek J, Newberger E: Childhood ingestions as symptoms of family distress. Am J Dis Child *139*:456–459, 1985.
7. Sobel R, Margolis J: Repetitive poisoning in children: A psychosocial study. Pediatrics *35*:641–651, 1985.
8. Baltimore C, Meyer R: A study of storage, child behavioral traits, and mother's knowledge of toxicology in 52 poisoned families and 52 comparison families. Pediatrics *44*:816–820, 1969.
9. Baker S, O'Neill B, Karpf R: Poisonings. *In* The Injury Fact Book. Lexington, MA, Lexington Books, 1984.
10. McIntire M: Safety packaging: A model for successful accident prevention. Pediatr Ann *6*:706–708, 1977.
11. Title 16—commercial practices. Consumer Product Safety Commission, Subchapter E—Poison Prevention Packaging Act of 1970 Regulations (1973). August 7, 1973; *38*:21247–21250.
12. Fisher L: An integrated model for childhood preventive programs. Vet Hum Toxicol *23*:261–264, 1981.
13. Centers for Disease Control: Update: Childhood poisonings—United States. MMWR Morb Mortal Wkly Rep *34*:117, 118, 1985.
14. Walton W: An evaluation of the poison prevention packaging act. Pediatrics *69*:363–370, 1982.
15. McIntire M, Angle C, Sathees K, Lee P: Safety packaging—what does the public think? Am J Public Health *67*:169–171, 1977.
16. Jackson R, Walker J, Wynne N: Circumstance of accidental poisoning in childhood. BMJ *4*:245–248, 1968.
17. Braden B: Validation of a poison prevention program. Am J Public Health *69*:942–944, 1979.
18. Krenzelok E, Garber R: Teaching poison prevention to preschool children, their parents, and professional educators through child care centers. Am J Public Health *71*:750–752, 1981.
19. Fergusson D, Horwood L, Beautrais A, Shannon F: A controlled field trial of a poisoning prevention method. Pediatrics *69*:515–520, 1982.
20. Phillips W, Little T: Continuity of care and poisoning prevention education. Patient Counsel Health Educ *2*:170–173, 1980.
21. Vernberg K, Culver-Dickson P, Spyker D: The deterrent effect of poison-warning stickers. Am J Dis Child *138*:1018–1020, 1984.
22. Polakoff J, Lacouture P, Lovejoy F: The environment away from home as a source of potential poisoning. Am J Dis Child *138*:1014–1017, 1984.
23. Fisher L, Van Buren J, Nitzkin J, et al: Highlight results of the Monroe County poison prevention demonstration project. Vet Hum Toxicol *22*(Suppl 2):15–17, 1980.
24. Maisel G, Langdoe B, Jenkins M, Aycock E: Analysis of two surveys evaluating a project to reduce accidental poisoning among children. Public Health Rep *82*:555–560, 1967.
25. Alpert J, Heagarty M: Evaluation of a program for distribution of ipecac syrup for the emergency home management of poison ingestions. J Pediatr *69*:142–146, 1960.
26. Dershewitz R, Williamson J: Prevention of childhood household injuries: A controlled clinical trial. Am J Public Health *67*:1148–1153, 1977.
27. Dershewitz R, Posner M, Paichel W: The effectiveness of health education on home use of ipecac. Clin Pediatr *22*:268–270, 1983.
28. Amitai Y, Mitchell A, Carrel J, et al: Patterns of calling time and ipecac availability among poison center callers. Am J Dis Child *141*:622–625, 1987.
29. Bond GR: Home use of syrup of ipecac is associated with a reduction in pediatric emergency department visits. Ann Emerg Med *25*:338–343, 1995.
30. Amitai Y, Mitchell AA, McGuigan MA, Lovejoy FH: Ipecac-induced emesis and reduction of plasma concentrations of drugs following accidental overdose in children. Pediatrics *80*:364–367, 1987.
31. Woolf A, Lewander W, Filippone G, Lovejoy F: Prevention of childhood poisoning: Efficacy of an educational program carried out in an emergency clinic. Pediatrics *80*:359–363, 1987.
32. Bass JL, Christoffel KK, Widome M, et al: Childhood injury prevention counseling in primary care settings: A critical review of the literature. Pediatrics *92*:544–551, 1993.
33. Lovejoy FH, Robertson WO, Woolf AD: Poison centers, poison prevention, and the pediatrician. Pediatrics *94*:220–224, 1994.
34. Thompson D, Trammel H, Robertson N, Reigart J: Evaluation of regional and nonregional poison centers. N Engl J Med *308*:191–194, 1983.
35. Chafee-Bahamon C, Caplan D, Lovejoy F: Patterns in hospital's use of a regional poison information center. Am J Public Health *73*:396–400, 1983.
36. Chafee-Bahamon C, Lovejoy F: Effectiveness of a regional poison center in reducing excess emergency room visits for children's poisonings. Pediatrics *72*:164–169, 1983.
37. Woolf AD, Saperstein A, Forjuoh S: Poisoning prevention knowledge and practices of parents after a childhood poisoning incident. Pediatrics *90*:867–870, 1992.

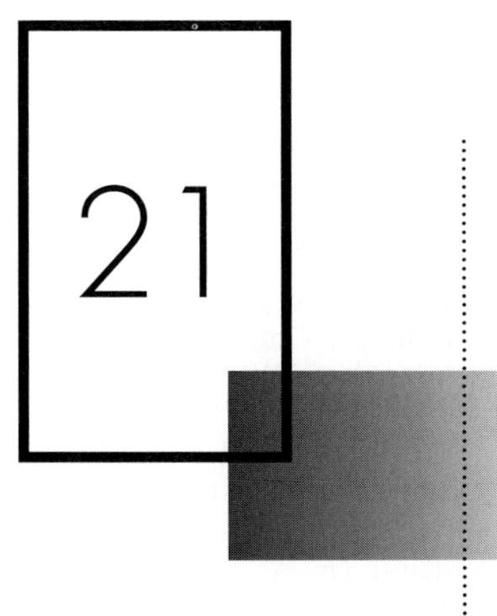

Drug-Drug Interactions

MICHAEL D. REED, PharmD
JEFFREY L. BLUMER, PhD, MD

Despite the introduction of drugs with increasing potency and pleiotypic effects, clinically important drug interactions are relatively infrequent. Nevertheless, the potential for drug interactions remains great, and as a result, practitioners are inundated with anecdotal reports and poorly designed studies that are often accepted with an uncritical eye. Part of the problem is that in the current definition of a drug interaction, the clinical importance of the effect is assumed rather than proved. Furthermore, many important drug-drug interactions remain unidentified during initial clinical evaluations because the vast majority of "controlled" clinical studies of possible drug interactions are performed in healthy adult volunteers and do not reflect circumstances encountered when the drug is used clinically. If the definition of drug-drug interactions were limited to those interactions resulting in new or unexpected effects that complicate clinical management, a better perspective might be obtained. This would limit the consideration of interactions to certain types of drugs and certain types of patients (Table 21–1). Nevertheless, the importance of such interactions cannot be overstated.

Clinically important interactions among drugs administered with therapeutic intent are an often overlooked component of clinical practice.[1, 2] Individual patients' lifestyle components, including diet, alcohol and tobacco use, and environmental exposures, also may not receive adequate consideration but are factors in the therapeutic efficacy and safety of these agents. Despite this relative complacency on the part of many health care practitioners, the potential for drug interactions to occur is limitless. In 1975, Robinson estimated that a drug formulary containing only 200 drugs theoretically possesses an astounding 19,900 pair combinations.[3] Furthermore, the increasing prevalence of polypharmacy further predisposes patients to the possibility of adverse drug interactions.[2, 4]

Drugs may interact through a number of different mechanisms, which may be classified on a pharmaceutical, pharmacokinetic, or pharmacodynamic basis (Table 21–2). Any or all of these interactions may result in unpredictable clinical effects or toxicologic responses. Pharmaceutical interactions include those resulting in drug inactivation when compounds are physically mixed together before administration in syringes, infusion tubing, or parenteral fluid preparations. Inactivation of aminoglycosides by certain β-lactam antibiotics, when these drugs are mixed together in the same intravenous fluid, represents one of the more common clinically relevant examples of this type of interaction.[5] Pharmacokinetic interactions can occur when the disposition characteristics of one compound (i.e., absorption, distribution, metabolism, or excretion) are influenced by those of

Table 21–1. Characteristics of Drugs and Patients at Risk for Drug Interactions

Drugs
Potent
Widely used
Affect vital organ functions—i.e., clotting mechanisms, cardiac rhythms, glucose homeostasis, renal/hepatic function
Narrow therapeutic index
Saturable hepatic metabolism
Extensive plasma protein binding (>90%)
Patients at Risk
Critically ill
Receiving polypharmacy
With impaired hepatic or renal function
With hypoxemia
With metabolic disturbances
Elderly

Table 21–2. Primary Mechanisms of Clinically Important Drug Interactions

Pharmaceutical
Drug compatibility
Drug stability
Pharmacokinetic
Absorption
Distribution
Metabolism
Excretion
Pharmacodynamic
Mechanism of action
Receptor binding
Receptor reactivity
Safety profile

another. This type of interaction may involve one or more specific aspects of a drug's pharmacokinetic profile. For example, one drug may reduce the rate but not the overall extent of absorption; in another case, a compound may displace a drug from its protein-binding sites while concomitantly retarding its elimination from the body. Finally, drugs may interact pharmacodynamically (i.e., compete for the same receptor or physiologic system) and thus may alter a patient's response to drug therapy.[6]

The number of known, clinically important drug interactions, combined with the ever increasing number of available pharmacologic agents, underscores the need to understand the pharmacologic basis of drug interactions. A number of excellent texts[7] and reviews[2, 3, 6, 8–13] have been published on the subject of drug interactions, and these emphasize both their importance and the clinical neglect of the issue. This chapter reviews and specifically evaluates the pharmacokinetic and pharmacodynamic mechanisms of drug interactions by using clinically important interactions as examples when appropriate. Also incorporated, when available, are data obtained from reports of drug overdose or toxic exposure.[14, 15]

EPIDEMIOLOGY

Drug interactions are a common event in medical practice and occur more frequently than is clinically recognized.[1, 2, 6] In 1972, the Boston Collaborative Drug Surveillance Program,[16] reporting on 9900 consecutively monitored hospitalized patients who collectively had 83,200 drug exposures, identified 3600 reported adverse drug reactions, of which 234 (6.9%) were attributed to drug interactions. In another series, 22% of the adverse drug reactions recognized on medical wards were attributed to drug interactions.[17] Durrence and co-workers[18] determined that 17% of 1825 general surgical patients received potentially interacting drug combinations. Further experience has extended these observations beyond hospitalized patients to patients receiving care in both ambulatory settings and extended care facilities.

A number of epidemiologic evaluations have clearly demonstrated that the incidence of adverse drug reactions increases as the number of simultaneously prescribed drugs increases.[3, 10, 13, 19, 20] This problem is further compounded by potential complications arising from self-medication with over-the-counter (OTC) products and alcohol or tobacco use.[6, 12, 20] The authors' laboratory undertook a prospective evaluation of adverse drug reactions among 193 noninstitutionalized residents of Cuyahoga County who were 65 years of age or older.[20] A total of 1204 medications were taken by the study subjects; 37% of these agents were OTC medications. Moreover, 57% of subjects reported that they had experienced at least one adverse drug reaction to their medications. Not surprisingly, a significant correlation ($P < .005$) was observed between the number of prescription drugs taken and the incidence of adverse drug reactions.[20] The significance of these data and the risks for serious drug-drug interactions are further emphasized by the increasing number of formerly prescription-only medications that continue to be released for OTC use.

PHARMACOKINETIC MECHANISMS OF DRUG INTERACTIONS

Gastrointestinal Absorption

Absorption is defined as the translocation of drug from its site of administration into the systemic circulation. Drugs administered extravascularly, by the oral, sublingual, or intramuscular routes, must cross several membranes to reach the systemic circulation before distribution to their sites of action. The process of absorption can be divided, for pharmacokinetic purposes, into two distinct domains: rate and extent. Both of these domains are influenced by the physicochemical properties of the drug as well as various host factors. The physicochemical properties of a drug that affect absorption include molecular weight, degree of lipid solubility, extent of ionization at physiologic pH, and type of formulation administered (e.g., tablet, capsule, and suspension). Independent of the site of administration, a drug must be in solution to be available for absorption. Thus, for a drug administered orally in a solid dosage form (e.g., tablet or capsule), the dissolution rate, or the rate at which a drug dissolves into solution, is the rate-limiting step in the absorption process.

A number of potential types of interactions between two or more compounds may clearly influence directly the rate or amount of drug absorbed (Table 21–3). Foods or drugs capable of altering gastrointestinal pH could theoretically modify the absorption characteristics of a compound by changing the proportion of drug that is in the un-ionized (more lipid-soluble) state. Thus, coadministration of antacids, histamine$_2$ (H_2)-receptor antagonists, or the newer H^+ ion proton pump inhibitors, which alter gastrointestinal pH, may substantially influence the amount of drug—particularly a weak base—that is absorbed

Table 21–3. Mechanisms Involved in Interactions That Affect Drug Absorption

Alteration of gastric emptying rate or gastrointestinal motility
Modification of volume, composition, or viscosity of gastrointestinal secretions
Effects of pH on drug ionization and dissolution
Effects of mucosal and bacterial drug metabolism
Interactions with active transport systems
Alterations of splanchnic blood flow
Complexation and chelate formation
Toxic effects on gastrointestinal mucosa

Adapted from Pond SM: Pharmacokinetic drug interactions. *In* Benet LZ, Massoud N, Gambertoglio JG (eds): Pharmacokinetic Basis for Drug Treatment. New York, Raven Press, pp 195–220, 1984.

from the stomach. In practice, however, this is generally not the case because the majority of drugs, independent of their pK_a values, are absorbed from the small intestine.[21] Conversely, these drugs, by decreasing gastric acid secretion, might promote an increase in the absorption of acid-labile drugs (e.g., penicillin G). Again, few data evaluating the clinical relevance of these potential pharmacokinetic interactions are available.[21, 22]

In contrast, because drug chelates with food or other compounds,[22] decreased absorption (e.g., tetracycline plus divalent cations; ferrous sulfate plus calcium carbonate, sucralfate, and quinolones, and so on) would appear to be the more common and clinically relevant interactions (Table 21–4). Concomitant administration of antacids with other medications is common and leads to frequent, clinically important interactions arising from the gastrointestinal and

Table 21–4. Selected Clinically Important Interactions Due to Alteration of Drug Absorption

Drug	Compound Affected	Effect on Absorption (Pharmacokinetic Parameter Estimates)
Antacids*	Captopril	AUC
	Clorazepate	AUC
	Ketoconazole	AUC
	Quinolone antibiotics†	AUC
	Isoniazid	Peak serum concentration
Cholestyramine	Digitalis glycosides	AUC
	Thyroid hormone	AUC
Kaolin	Lincomycin	AUC
Sucralfate	Aminophylline	AUC
	Digoxin	AUC
	Phenytoin	AUC
	Quinolone antibiotics†	AUC
	Tetracycline	AUC
	Theophylline	AUC

AUC, area under the serum concentration time curve.

*Interaction may be dependent on specific ion(s) (e.g., Cl^{2+}, Ca^{2+}, Mg^{2+}) present in antacid formulation.

†Includes ciprofloxacin, enoxacin, fleroxacin, lomefloxacin, norfloxacin, and ofloxacin.

chemical effects of the aluminum, calcium, and magnesium ions liberated from the particular antacid preparation.[22] The recognized, clinically relevant interaction between aluminum- or magnesium-containing antacids and sucralfate, which reduces the bioavailability of quinolone antibiotics (see Table 21–4), underscores the significance of antacid drug interactions. Patients who require antacid medications and a quinolone antibiotic should be instructed to separate the administration of these two agents by at least 6 hours for ciprofloxacin and norfloxacin and by approximately 3 hours for other quinolone analogues.[22] Moreover, gastric complexation with orally administered activated charcoal, which markedly inhibits the systemic absorption of numerous compounds, remains the mainstay of clinical toxicology practice. Coadministration of cholestyramine resin also has been shown to reduce the systemic absorption of a limited number of compounds and may be a viable alternative to oral charcoal administration in selected intoxications.

Drugs that affect gastrointestinal motility may influence the gastrointestinal absorption of orally administered drugs by controlling the rate of drug delivery to the major absorptive surfaces, as well as the duration of contact with these surfaces.[23] For example, coadministration of the anticholinergic agent propantheline has been shown to increase the rate and extent of digoxin absorption, whereas digoxin absorption was decreased after metoclopramide administration. In many instances, coadministration of the gastroprokinetic agents metoclopramide, cisapride, or domperidone may decrease the time to peak serum drug concentration (T_{max}) and increase the peak serum drug concentration (C_{max}) but in general have no appreciable effect on the drugs' overall extent of bioavailability.[23] Thus, the clinical significance of this probable drug interaction would appear to be very limited. Moreover, the magnitude of the effect of gastroprokinetic agents on the T_{max} and C_{max} of orally administered drugs appears to be much greater and to occur more frequently when the gastroprokinetic agent is administered by the intravenous route rather than orally.

Distribution

Drug distribution describes the movement of a pharmacologically or toxicologically active moiety from the systemic circulation into various body compartments, tissues, and cells. The pharmacokinetic parameter estimate, volume of distribution (Vd), is an apparent value that attempts to describe the relationship between the amount of drug in the body and its serum concentration. The process of distribution depends on the partition coefficient of a drug between blood and tissue, regional blood flow, and the extent of binding to plasma protein or tissues.

Alterations in drug distribution most commonly result from the displacement of bound drug from circulating plasma proteins. Acidic compounds bind most often to albumin, whereas basic compounds bind predominantly to α1-acid glycoprotein.[6, 24, 25] It is assumed that the free or non–protein-bound fraction of a compound is the pharmacologically active moiety capable of diffusing into tissues, traversing cellular membranes, and binding to receptors.[6, 24] As such, changes in drug binding that result in an increase in the amount of free drug may increase the amount of drug available for tissue distribution and may possibly increase the drug's concentration at the site of action.[24] The displacement of dicumarol-like oral anticoagulants (e.g., warfarin) from serum albumin-binding sites by other highly protein-bound compounds (e.g., aspirin, phenylbutazone, and so forth) represents a classic example of such an interaction.[6] This more traditional view as a simple competitive displacement reaction is based on a number of assumptions, however, many of which defy physiologic validation (discussed later). Moreover, it is important to recognize that protein displacement interactions have been evaluated primarily *in vitro* and, in fact, have been very difficult to corroborate *in vivo*.[6, 25]

A number of variables may directly influence the physiologic impact of a drug displacement interaction. For such reactions to be important clinically, both compounds must be at least 80% to 90% bound to the same protein species. In addition, the displaced compound must exhibit capacity-limited body clearance or must have a relatively small apparent Vd, less than 0.15 L/kg.[6, 24–26] This last factor is likely to be the most important, because as the Vd increases, less of the total amount of drug in the body is present in the plasma compartment. Thus, with proportionately less compound to displace and a larger "space" in which to distribute, the effect of a displacement interaction would be, at best, only transient. Finally, it is important to recall that increasing the amount of free drug concurrently increases the amount of compound available for metabolism or excretion.[6]

The physiologic impact of drug-drug protein displacement reactions clearly depends on the balance among a large number of variables. In an overdose situation, this is compounded further because very little is known about the impact of a single large dose of a displacing agent on the overall biodisposition of the displaced agent. The result depends largely on whether exposure to the displacing agent occurs under single- or multiple-dose conditions. Moreover, the magnitude and duration of the interaction are determined by the clearance rate of the displacing agent. Nevertheless, case reports describing saturable protein binding for some highly protein-bound drugs in overdose situations such as with valproic acid[27] underscore the probable clinical significance of protein displacement interactions in poisoned patients. These preliminary reports confirm the importance of more aggressive clinical investigation to define probable changes in the extent of protein binding for highly protein-bound drugs in cases of acute overdose. Any imbalance in the amount of free, unbound drug could affect the timing and severity of associated symptoms and the treatment approach.

Despite the perception that these displacement reactions are of clinical importance, very few have actually been documented.[6, 25, 26] The traditionally cited interaction between oral anticoagulants and salicylates leading to an increased hypoprothrombinemic effect is most likely due to a combination of mechanisms rather than simple drug displacement.[6] First, acetylation of the platelet by salicylates and their derivatives inhibits adenosine diphosphate–induced platelet aggregation. Second, oral salicylate administration increases gastrointestinal blood losses. Finally, long-term administration of aspirin may interfere with warfarin protein binding by actually altering the structure of the serum albumin molecule. Another example in which a combination of mechanisms rather than simply a protein displacement reaction more clearly accounts for a clinically important drug interaction involves phenylbutazone. This highly protein-bound drug may displace warfarin from albumin but also decreases the body clearance of the more potent warfarin S isomer, which leads to an accumulated hypoprothrombinemic effect.[6] A similar interaction has been suggested for sulfonamides combined with oral sulfonylurea hypoglycemic agents.

In contrast to the interactions just discussed, changes in Vd resulting from altered tissue binding, although rare, are exemplified by the now well-known interaction between digoxin and quinidine.[28] The decrease observed in quinidine Vd and the concurrent increase in serum digoxin concentrations are most likely due to digoxin tissue-binding displacement by quinidine. These changes in digoxin pharmacokinetics have been noted to occur after administration of a single dose of quinidine. In addition to causing tissue displacement, quinidine also decreases the renal and nonrenal clearance of digoxin. Quinine, the S isomer of quinidine, has also been shown to interfere with nonrenal clearance of digoxin.[29]

Metabolism

Although a number of organs, including the adrenal glands, kidneys, lungs, placenta, and gut, are capable of drug metabolism, the liver is the primary organ involved in the biotransformation of endogenous and exogenous substances. Most compounds are hepatically biotransformed by the mixed-function oxidase (cytochrome P-450) system. Considering the large number of endogenous and exogenously administered compounds that are partially or completely metabolized by the liver, it is easy to recognize the vulnerability of this site relative to drug interactions. A large number of drug-drug, drug-disease, and drug-nutrient interactions have been described in the literature as a result of one agent or process influencing the metabolism of another. This influence could obviously involve either an increase or a decrease in the metabolic clearance rate of a given compound. For drugs that are completely eliminated from the body via hepatic biotransformation, total-body clearance is a function of liver blood flow and the ability of the liver to extract the drug.[30–32] Thus, in addition to metabolic capacity, liver blood flow may be an important determinant of a drug's clearance, most notably for those drugs with high hepatic extraction ratios (e.g., lidocaine, propranolol).[30] All of these variables can be influenced to variable extents in an acutely intoxicated patient.

Drugs well known to be potent and predictable inducers of hepatic cytochrome P-450 activity[9, 10, 30–32] include the barbiturates,[33] glutethimide,[33] carbamazepine,[34] rifampin,[35] and griseofulvin. In addition, it is important to recognize that other agents such as phenytoin,[33] ethanol (chronic use/abuse),[36] environmental pollutants including tobacco smoke,[37] organochlorine insecticides, polychlorinated phenols,[38] foods such as Brussels sprouts and cabbage,[39] and charcoal broiling[40] all can stimulate the hepatic metabolism of drugs. Interactions of potential clinical importance with selected metabolic inducers are outlined in Tables 21–5 and 21–6.

The clinical impact of enzyme induction on drug action has been recognized for decades[41] and is exemplified by the now classic interaction involving the decrease in the hypoprothrombinemic effect of warfarin by coadministration of phenobarbital.[33] Induction, or the stimulation of cytochrome P-450 activity, appears to be a result of an increase in the absolute number of cytochrome P-450 molecules. This increase in P-450 molecules also appears to involve the many forms of P-450, the various isoforms that together form the P-450 drug-metabolizing enzyme system.

Agents capable of inducing the hepatic cytochrome mono-oxygenase system represent a wide array of differing chemical moieties, including drugs, hormones, and environmental pollutants (see Table 21–6).[32, 38] In addition, the time course of induction varies with both the type and dose of the inducing agent.[41–44] Potent inducing compounds such as phenobarbital and rifampin may begin to induce enzyme activity after only 1 to 2 days of therapy.[43, 44] Return to constitutive enzyme activity after withdrawal of the inducing agent appears variable but would be influenced by the inducer's body clearance rate combined with the microsomal enzyme turnover rate.[41] Dossing and associates,[44] using the antipyrine saliva test and the aminopyrine breath test in an elaborate investigation involving four healthy subjects, described enhanced clearance occurring after 1 week and persisting for 10 days after cessation of phenobarbital administration.

As previously stated, a number of drugs are also capable of inhibiting hepatic microsomal mono-oxygenase activity[31, 32, 41]; thus, the metabolism of another compound is partially or completely inhibited (Tables 21–6 and 21–7). This inhibition can decrease

Table 21–6. Commonly Prescribed Drugs That Can Induce or Depress the Activity of Hepatic Drug-Metabolizing Enzymes

Inducers
Carbamazepine
Oral contraceptives
Phenobarbital
Phenytoin
Rifampin
Inhibitors
Cimetidine
Chloramphenicol
Erythromycin
Quinolone antibiotics
Ethanol (acute consumption/intoxication)
Valproic acid

Table 21–5. Selected Clinically Important Interactions Due to Induction of Drug Metabolism

Inducer	Compound Affected	Pharmacokinetic Parameter Measured (U)	Change: Before	Change: After
Phenobarbital	Alprenolol	AUC (ng/mL per h)	706	154
	Digitoxin	$t_{1/2}$ (d)	7.8	4.5
	Doxycycline	$t_{1/2}$ (h)	15.3	11.1
	Quinidine	$t_{1/2}$ (h)	4	1.6
	Warfarin	Css (mg/L)	0.73	0.18
	Nortriptyline	Css (ng/mL)	28	18
Rifampin	Disopyramide	AUC (μg/mL per h)	20	8
	Metoprolol	AUC (μg/mL per h)	930	624
	Warfarin	AUC (μg/mL per h)	600	258
	Digitoxin	$t_{1/2}$ (d)	12	3.2
	Tolbutamide	$t_{1/2}$ (h)	5.4	3.3
	Oral contraceptive	$t_{1/2}$ (h)	7.5	3.3
Tobacco smoke	Lidocaine	$t_{1/2}$ (min)	96*	88†
	Propranolol	Mean Css (mg/L)	—	>200
	Theophylline	$T_{1/2}$ (h)	11.5	7.4

AUC, area under the serum concentration time curve; $t_{1/2}$, elimination half-life; Css, steady-state serum concentration.
*Nonsmoker
†Cigarette smoker.
Adapted from Pond SM: Pharmacokinetic drug interactions. *In* Benet LZ, Massoud N, Gambertoglio JG (eds): Pharmacokinetic Basis for Drug Treatment. New York, Raven Press, pp 195–220, 1984.

Table 21–7. Selected Clinically Important Interactions Due to Inhibition of Drug Metabolism

Inhibitor	Compound Affected	Pharmacokinetic Parameter Measured (U)	Change	
			Before	*After*
Chloramphenicol	Dicumarol	$t_{1/2}$ (h)	8.7	25
	Phenytoin	$t_{1/2}$ (h)	12	28
	Tolbutamide	$t_{1/2}$ (h)	5.2	14.1
Phenylbutazone	Phenytoin	$t_{1/2}$ (h)	13.7	22
	Tolbutamide	$t_{1/2}$ (h)	8	23
	Antipyrine	Cl (mL/kg per min)	37.7	26.6
Oral contraceptives	Nitrazepam	Cl (mL/min)	459	323

$t_{1/2}$, elimination half-life; Cl, body clearance.
Adapted from Pond SM: Pharmacokinetic drug interactions. *In* Benet LZ, Massoud N, Gambertoglio JG (eds): Pharmacokinetic Basis for Drug Treatment. New York, Raven Press, pp 195–220, 1984.

the hepatic clearance of drugs, and this decreased clearance consequently prolongs the total-body clearance rate of a compound and thus the time the drug remains in the body. Drugs commonly used in a clinical setting that are capable of inhibiting cytochrome P-450 activity are listed in Table 21–6. Interactions of potential clinical importance involving some of these agents are listed in Table 21–7. Table 21–8 outlines the effects of cimetidine on various drugs.[9, 10, 21, 36, 41] Exaggerated clinical effects and duration of activity would clearly be expected in patients who are receiving any of these drugs therapeutically and who then become involved in an acute overdose with a competitive compound (Tables 21–6 to 21–9). Further, the ability of a compound to influence its own metabolic rate in large doses (e.g., theophylline) also requires more study.

The histamine H_2-receptor antagonists cimetidine, famotidine, nizatidine, and ranitidine are among the most widely prescribed drugs today. The availability of many of these agents as OTC medications only adds to their frequent use. Of these four agents, cimetidine is a potent inhibitor of hepatic microsomal enzyme activity.[30] Concurrent cimetidine administration has been reported to inhibit the metabolism of more than 25 different compounds (see Table 21–8). Dossing and colleagues[44] found that the inhibitory effect of cimetidine on microsomal enzyme activity occurred 24 hours after drug initiation and subsided within 2 days after the last dose. In rodents, inhibition of microsomal enzyme activity by cimetidine has been shown to decrease the hepatotoxicity of certain drugs,[30] such as acetaminophen[45, 46] and cocaine.[46] Some researchers have thus been led to suggest a possible therapeutic value for this metabolic interaction, particularly in the overdose setting. However, the variability in the time course of the inhibitory effect of cimetidine on hepatic microsomes[42] and the uncertainty of the dose relative to the magnitude of enzyme inhibition appear to limit the drug's clinical utility as an adjunct in the treatment of drug intoxications. In addition, cimetidine, more so than other H_2-receptor antagonists, is capable of reducing hepatic blood flow; this further compromises the metabolism of high-extraction ratio drugs.

Table 21–8. Influence of Cimetidine on the Disposition of Selected Drugs

Drug Affected	Pharmacokinetic Parameter Measured	Change	
		Before	*After*
Diazepam	Cl (mL/min)	19.9	11.4
Imipramine	$t_{1/2}$ (h)	10.8	22.7
Lidocaine	Cl (mL/min)	776	576
Meperidine	Cl (L/kg per h)	0.6	0.47
Procainamide	$t_{1/2}$ (h)	2.9	3.7
Propranolol	AUC (μg/L per h)	450	727
Theophylline	$t_{1/2}$ (h)	11.5	14.1
Triamterene	Renal Cl (mL/min)	71	27

$t_{1/2}$, elimination half-life; Cl, body clearance; AUC, area under the serum concentration time curve.
Data from the following: Pond SM: Pharmacokinetic drug interactions. *In* Benet LZ, Massoud N, Gambertoglio JG (eds): Pharmacokinetic Basis for Drug Treatment. New York, Raven Press, pp 195–220, 1984; Somogui A, Muirhead M: Pharmacokinetic interactions of cimetidine 1987. Clin Pharmacokinet *9*:493–510, 1984; and Powell JR, Donn KH: Histamine H-2 antagonist drug interactions in perspective: Mechanistic concepts and clinical implications. Am J Med 77(Suppl 5B):57–84, 1984.

Cimetidine has also been shown to decrease the renal clearance of a number of cationic drugs, including procainamide, *N*-acetylprocainamide,[47] and triamterene, by inhibition of renal proximal tubule cationic secretion.[30, 48] In contrast to cimetidine, clinically significant drug interactions with ranitidine, famotidine, or nizatidine are rare[21, 30, 49, 50] and are described in only a few case reports.[21] Although ranitidine has been shown to bind cytochrome P-450,[21, 30, 50] the drug's binding affinity is approximately 10-fold lower than that described for cimetidine.[21, 30, 51] Similar observations have been reported for both famotidine and nizatidine.

Viral infections and vaccines have been shown to decrease the clearance of a number of drugs, including theophylline, phenytoin, and warfarin.[52–54] In 1982, Kraemer and colleagues[53] described theophylline toxicity in 11 children who were stabilized on oral theophylline for several months during an influenza B outbreak. Two of these 11 children had seizures as the primary manifestation of theophylline toxicity. Similar observations have been described after influenza vaccine administration and respiratory tract infections due to influenza A and adenovirus. The mechanism by which certain viral infections alter drug metabolism is unknown but appears to be

Table 21–9. Clinically Important Drug-Drug Interactions: The Importance of Hepatic Cytochrome P-450 Isozyme Activity

Cytochrome	Polymorphism	Substrate	Inhibitors	Inducers
1A2	Possible	Caffeine, phenacetin, tacrine, theophylline	Cimetidine Fluvoxamine Quinolones	Cigarette smoke Cruciferous vegetables Omeprazole Rifampin
2C9	Yes	Diclofenac, ibuprofen, naproxen, phenytoin, piroxicam, S-warfarin, tolbutamide	Azoles Chloramphenicol Isoniazid Sulfaphenazole	Rifampin
2D6	Yes	Captopril, codeine, debrisoquine, D-methorphan, ecainide, flecainide, fluoxetine, norfluoxetine, haloperidol, imipramine, nortriptyline, paroxetine, risperidone, thioridazine	Cimetidine Fluoxetine/norfluoxatine Paroxetine Quinidine Sertraline	Rifampin (?)
2C19	Yes	Diazepam, imipramine, omeprazole, propranolol, S-mephenytoin		Rifampin
2E1	No	Dapsone, theophylline?	Isoniazid	
3A3/3A4	Possible	Astemizole, cisapride, cyclosporine, erythromycin, itraconazole, lidocaine, loratadine, lovastatin, midazolam, quinidine, tacrolimus, taxol, terfenadine, verapamil	Azoles Macrolides Naringenin Protease inhibitors Steroids	Carbamazepine Phenobarbital Phenytoin Rifampin Steroids

Coadministration of drugs that are metabolized via the same primary cytochrome isozyme have the potential of precipitating a clinically important drug-drug interaction.

Adapted from DeVane CL: Pharmacogenetics and drug metabolism of newer antidepressant agents. J Clin Psychiatry *55*(Supl 12):38, 1994; and Polk R: Rational approach to investigate antimicrobial drug-drug interactions. J Infect Dis Pharmacother *1*:45, 1995.

a result of endogenous interferon synthesis. Drugs known to induce endogenous interferon production have been shown to interfere with hepatic drug metabolism.[54] The interactions between specific viruses or vaccines and hepatic microsomal enzyme activity continue to be the subject of active investigation.

Our understanding of the mechanism(s) involved in metabolically based drug-drug interactions has advanced greatly with the delineation of the importance of specific cytochrome P-450 isozymes in the metabolism of specific substrates. Moreover, recognizing which cytochrome P-450 isozymes are responsible for the metabolism of which substrates (e.g., parent drug/metabolite, and so on) permits the *a priori* prediction of certain interactions before they are described in the literature as a clinical catastrophe. The cytochrome P-450 isozymes considered to represent the most important isozymes involved in human hepatic drug metabolism with representative, clinically relevant substrates are outlined in Table 21–9.

Last, a number of compounds can interfere with or directly inhibit hepatic drug metabolism via nonmicrosomal pathways. Allopurinol, a xanthine oxidase inhibitor used to decrease endogenous uric acid production, also inhibits the metabolism of other xanthine analogues, most notably 6-mercaptopurine and its pro-drug azathioprine. Although this drug combination has been used for its therapeutic potential, it has also led to serious adverse drug effects, of which enhanced myelosuppression is the most notable. Disulfiram (Antabuse) is a potent inhibitor of acetaldehyde dehydrogenase, the enzyme primarily responsible for the metabolism of ethanol to acetic acid. Concurrent ethanol consumption and disulfiram administration leads to acetaldehyde accumulation and the classic Antabuse reaction, characterized by the following unpleasant symptoms: flushing, throbbing headache, nausea, vomiting, sweating, palpitations, hypotension, and syncope. Another frequently cited reaction mediated via a nonmicrosomal pathway is the hypertensive crisis resulting from administration of sympathomimetic amines and consumption of tyramine-containing foods (cheese, red wine) by patients receiving drugs that inhibit monoamine oxidase activity.[7, 9, 55]

Elimination

The most common pathway by which drugs or their metabolites are eliminated from the body is via the kidneys. Interactions that influence renal clearance of a compound primarily involve the physiologic processes of glomerular filtration, tubular reabsorption, or active tubular secretion. Additionally, agents that alter renal blood flow may also influence renal elimination. Consequently, alterations in renal clearance represent an important mechanism of drug interactions. Nevertheless, for such interactions to be of clinical importance, the overall elimination of active drug must depend primarily on renal mechanisms. As discussed in the earlier section on distribution, displacement interactions (i.e., displacement from protein-binding sites) may transiently increase the amount of free drug in the vascular compartment and the result is an increase in the amount of drug available to be filtered by the glomeruli and cleared. However, to our knowledge this has not been reported as the sole mechanism responsible for a clinically important drug interaction.

In contrast to displacement interactions, a number of drugs can directly influence glomerular filtration through another mechanism. The nonsteroidal anti-inflammatory drugs (NSAIDs)—aspirin, fenoprofen, ibuprofen, indomethacin, naproxen, and others—all have been shown to reversibly depress renal function in certain patients.[56, 57] This drug-induced decrease in renal function is most likely a result of NSAIDs' inhibition of renal prostaglandin synthesis[56] and has resulted in increased side effects because of accumulation of other concurrently administered drugs. The dienoic prostaglandins PGI_2, PGE_2, and PGF_2, produced by the medullary interstitial cells of the kidneys, are important vasodilators responsible for maintaining vascular balance and renal blood flow. Their synthesis and secretion appear to occur as a result of renal vascular ischemia. Individuals predisposed to NSAID-induced renal toxicity would be patients who have pre-existing renal disease, hypertension, and congestive heart failure. In intoxications involving NSAIDs, this secondary renal effect would appear to be of primary clinical importance in those patients with some degree of pre-existing renal compromise (e.g., the elderly), because it is in these patients that prostaglandins exert an important role in maintaining renal function. Moderate to severe NSAID intoxications in younger patients, including children, are most often associated with mild, transient, rapidly reversible decreases in glomerular filtration as evidenced by moderate elevations in the patients' serum creatinine concentration.

In clinical practice, interactions that influence renal tubular function are observed frequently and can result in serious consequences (Table 21–10). Tubular secretion of organic acids and bases is an active process that most likely involves distinct pathways.[58] The classic uricosuric agents probenecid and sulfinpyrazone[59] are among the most potent inhibitors of organic acid secretion by the proximal tubule. Probenecid has been shown to inhibit the renal clearance of a number of drugs including sulfinpyrazone and indomethacin and has been used clinically to maintain serum penicillin (β-lactam) concentrations for the treatment of uncomplicated gonorrhea and other systemic infectious processes. Although interactions involving organic bases would similarly be expected, those of clinical importance primarily involve those already described after chronic cimetidine administration.[47, 48]

Table 21–10. Clinically Important Interactions of Drug Elimination Due to Alteration in Renal Excretion

	Compound Affected	Effect on Excretion
Probenecid	β-lactam antibiotics	Secretion
	Indomethacin	Secretion
	Sulfinpyrazone	Secretion
Urinary alkalization (sodium bicarbonate)	Salicylate	Reabsorption
	Phenobarbital	Reabsorption
Urinary acidification (ammonium chloride)	Amphetamine	Reabsorption
	Chloroquine	Reabsorption
	Lidocaine	Reabsorption

Modification of the passive distal tubular reabsorption of weak acids and bases is another mechanism by which drugs may interact and represents a potentially important therapeutic modality in the treatment of certain intoxications (see Table 21–10). An inverse relationship exists between the compound's degree of ionization and the overall amount of a compound reabsorbed from the urine—that is, the greater the amount of compound present in the urine in the non-ionized, more lipid-soluble state, the greater the amount reabsorbed. In general, for renal clearance to be sensitive to changes in urine pH, acidic and basic drugs must have pK_a values that range between 3 to 7.5 and 7 to 11, respectively.[58] This principle of altering urinary pH has been used in the management of a number of drug intoxications, including those by salicylates, phenobarbital, amphetamine, and phencyclidine.[9, 10] Alkalization of urine by either intermittent or continuous intravenous infusion of sodium bicarbonate can dramatically decrease distal tubular reabsorption of salicylates and phenobarbital.

Intraluminal trapping of acids in their ionized form appears to be greatest when urine pH exceeds 7.5.[58] Conversely, urinary acidification with either ammonium chloride administered orally or intravenously or dilute hydrochloric acid administered intravenously can markedly augment the renal clearance of amphetamine and phencyclidine. Although the manipulation of urinary pH to promote ion trapping and to augment renal clearance appears desirable, it is not without risk. Needless to say, rapidly raising or lowering urinary pH requires alteration of the blood pH, a change that may be undesirable and possibly detrimental in certain instances. Furthermore, clinicians must carefully weigh the associated risks of pH manipulation and the time necessary to achieve effective changes in urinary pH with the effectiveness of other therapeutic modalities and, most important, with the anticipated duration of serious symptoms.

Last, the bile represents an often overlooked but relatively important means for the elimination of a number of drugs and substrates. Parent compounds or their metabolites (pharmacologically active or inactive) excreted via the bile may be reabsorbed/absorbed, respectively, into the systemic circulation from the intestine. This process of enterohepatic circulation is an important mechanism responsible for delayed and prolonged drug absorption and elimination of a number of commonly used drugs including phenothiazines, phenobarbital, carbamazepine, spironolactone, and others. Increasing the total-body clearance of many of these compounds by interfering with the enterohepatic circulation process underscores the importance of administering repeated doses of oral activated charcoal to patients who experience intoxications involving compounds that undergo substantial enterohepatic circulation.[60]

Drug-Nutrient Interactions

Nutritional habits may dramatically influence the response to pharmacologic intervention. The type and quantity of food consumed as well as the overall nutritional status of a patient may directly or indirectly alter drug disposition characteristics. For decades, it has been recognized that malnutrition and starvation can suppress a number of important endogenous enzymatic processes responsible for drug biotransformation and elimination.[36, 55, 61] These nutrient-drug effects may result from simple cofactor (e.g., vitamin, trace metal/mineral) deprivation leading to inhibition of specific enzymatic reactions to modifying renal function[62] or the quantity and functional activity of the hepatic mixed-function oxidase system.[63] The impact of these effects obviously is difficult to predict and would appear to be at least partially responsible for the interindividual variation frequently observed in many pharmacologic evaluations. Moreover, certain drugs may directly alter or impair a patient's underlying nutritional status (e.g., electrolyte and mineral depletion following chronic diuretic therapy).

The specific composition of a meal as well as one's overall diet can markedly alter drug absorption (Table 21–11). The most notable example of food-associated inhibition of drug absorption involves the complexation of tetracycline compounds when coadministered with divalent cation-containing compounds (e.g., milk, cheese, antacids, vitamins).[9, 10] Such an interaction's resulting in decreased systemic bioavailability is unusual. What occurs more frequently is that the rate but not the overall extent of drug absorption is decreased when the drug is administered in the presence of food. The intestinal absorption of some commonly administered drugs, such as acetaminophen, digoxin, levodopa, many penicillin and cephalosporin analogues, and phenytoin, may be delayed or reduced when these agents are given in the presence of food. Conversely, the bioavailability of some orally administered drugs including spironolactone, griseofulvin, and cefuroxime axetil can be increased when the drugs are administered in the presence of food (see Table 21–11).

Table 21–11. Influence of Food on the Bioavailability of Selected Drugs

Total Amount of Drug Absorbed	
Increased	*Decreased*
Cefuroxime axetil	Azithromycin
Diazepam	Captopril
Erythromycin ethylsuccinate and estolate	Erythromycin stearate
Griseofulvin (↑fat)	Isoniazid
Hydralazine	Levodopa
Hydrochlorothiazide	Methyldopa
Lovastatin	Rifampin
Misoprostol	Tetracyclines
Nitrofurantoin	
Spironolactone	

Coadministration of certain medications with enteral nutrition formulas has resulted in decreased drug absorption and poor therapeutic effect. Subtherapeutic patient responses have been noted in patients receiving carbamazepine, phenytoin, or warfarin when these drugs have been coadministered with enteral formulas.[55] The mechanism of this drug-nutrient interaction is unknown but clearly exceeds simple drug adherence to the feeding tubing. To minimize the effect that enteral nutrition formulas may have on the bioavailability of these drugs, the tube feeding should be stopped and the tubing flushed approximately 1 to 2 hours before drug administration. Tube feeding is resumed 1 to 2 hours later.

Both hepatic drug metabolism and renal elimination can be influenced by the type and quantity of nutrient consumed. Cabbage, Brussels sprouts, and cauliflower all have been shown to contain certain indoles that are potent inducers of intestinal and hepatic drug-metabolizing enzymes.[39] Conversely, compounds present in grapefruits (e.g., naringenin) are capable of inhibiting the activity of cytochrome P-450 3A3/3A4 activity (see Table 21–9). Diets high in protein (e.g., >40% of total calories) have been shown to increase the metabolic capacity of the hepatic mixed-function oxidase system; this results in increased clearances of a number of drugs, including antipyrine, theophylline, and propranolol.[39, 40, 61, 64] This increase in body clearance is not observed when similar quantities of either carbohydrate or fat are substituted for protein.[63, 64] In addition, diets deficient in protein are associated with altered renal hemodynamics, a condition that leads to marked decreases in glomerular filtration,[62] which further influences a drug's body clearance and pharmacodynamics.

Pharmacodynamic Mechanisms of Drug Interactions

In patients receiving multiple drugs, the overall effects manifested are a summation of the similar or opposing but independent actions of these multiple agents on a given cell or organ system.[1] These interactions have not historically been considered drug interactions, yet many are of extreme clinical importance. These interactions are properly termed *pharmacodynamic drug interactions* and are thought to involve drug-receptor interactions either directly or indirectly.

The types of interactions that might occur at the receptor level are varied. Moreover, the understanding of these interactions is often confounded because simple potentiation or antagonism is distinctly uncommon. Most of these interactions occur through an interplay of receptor mechanisms controlling the function of a given tissue or organ system. In a similar fashion, drugs may interact with physiologic or biochemical control loops, a process that leads to alterations in response to normal stimuli and input signals. Finally, one drug may prevent access of another to its site of action, and thus the pharmacodynamic process is abrogated.

Direct Receptor Effects

In a few instances, drug interactions occur through direct receptor site antagonism. Consider, for example, an asthmatic patient receiving a β_2-adrenergic agonist bronchodilator (e.g., albuterol, terbutaline) who develops angina and is treated with propranolol. The nonselective blocker propranolol clearly has the potential to inhibit the bronchodilator effect of the β_2-adrenergic agonist drug. This risk continues to be great in today's climate of medical practice in which patients continue to see subspecialists for care, and prescriptions provided by one clinician to ameliorate symptoms in one system may unwittingly interfere with drugs prescribed by another physician who is focusing on another organ system. The use of specific agonists or antagonists (e.g., naloxone) represents specific interactions at the receptor level that are of immense clinical importance, particularly in the treatment of poisoned patients.

Another example of direct pharmacodynamic interaction can occur during therapy with the coumarin anticoagulants. The effects of these agents may be potentiated by dextrothyroxine[65] and antimicrobial agents containing a thiomethyltetrazole ring.[66] In addition, quinidine appears to augment the cellular uptake of warfarin, and thus warfarin's effective concentration at the site of action is increased. Finally, certain broad-spectrum antibiotics may enhance the efficacy of warfarin through the eradication of gut bacteria responsible for vitamin K_1 synthesis.

Indirect Receptor Effects

Pharmacodynamic interactions associated with indirect receptor effects are those side effects of one drug that mimic the pharmacologic effects of another. Augmentation of the hypoglycemic effects of insulin and oral hypoglycemic agents by nonselective blocking agents is an example of agents with differing mechanisms of action that produce the same clinical effects.

The use of drugs with actions on the myocardium, cardiac conduction system, or capacitance and resistance vessels predisposes to a large number of pharmacodynamic interactions. Calcium channel blockers and β-adrenergic receptor antagonists often augment the myocardial depressant, bradycardiac, and hypotensive effects of one another when used in concert. Other effects augmented by the simultaneous administration of vasoactive drugs and β-adrenergic blocking agents include exacerbation of first-dose hypotensive effects of prazosin, enhancement of the hypertensive response during clonidine withdrawal, and peripheral ischemia associated with ergotamine administration.

The importance and proliferation of NSAIDs (prescription and OTC) have focused attention on a number of serious interactions that may occur with these agents.[56, 57] The sodium and water retention that result from long-term use of these agents may blunt the antihypertensive effects of angiotension-converting enzyme inhibitors (e.g., captopril, enalapril, and others), thiazide diuretics, and β-adrenergic blocking agents. These effects may also offset the benefits of diuretic therapy in mild to moderate congestive heart failure. Moreover, the gastrointestinal ulcerations often found in patients receiving these agents may predispose those patients receiving concomitant anticoagulant therapy to hemorrhage.

Other examples of drugs associated with indirect pharmacodynamic effects include the following: coadministration of spironolactone and potassium chloride, resulting in life-threatening hyperkalemia; various antibiotic combinations that show synergy or antagonism; and enhanced neurotoxicity of neuroleptics when coadministered with lithium.

Cellular Transport Mechanisms

A number of classic drug interactions involve the uptake and release of neurotransmitters at the nerve terminal. These include interactions between tricyclic antidepressant agents and certain antihypertensive agents. Fortunately, the use of newer antidepressant drugs, in particular the selective serotonin reuptake inhibitors, has largely eliminated these effects as clinically important problems.

SUMMARY

Drug interactions remain an important consideration in the assessment of a patient's response to pharmacologic intervention. It is clear that the pharmacologic response of a drug can be markedly influenced by concurrent administration of another therapeutic agent or food. These interactions may result in a decreased therapeutic effect or in an increase in the amount and extent of untoward reactions. Despite the well-described and real clinical consequences of certain drug interactions,[1, 7, 9, 10] this aspect of patient care continues to be too often overlooked.

Drugs can interact via a number of mechanisms but most notably on a pharmaceutical, pharmacokinetic, or pharmacodynamic basis. These interactions may occur as a result of concurrently prescribed therapeutic modalities, environmental variables, or the patient's specific habits, such as diet and alcohol and tobacco use or abuse. The unpredictable nature of drug interactions underscores how important it is for all health care practitioners to understand the mechanisms of interaction and to be suspicious of their occurrence.

Generally, pharmacodynamic drug interactions result in adverse effects either through the augmentation of the effects of one drug by another having similar effects (Table 21–12) or, less frequently,

Table 21–12. Pharmacodynamic Augmentation of Drug Effects

Effect	Combined Agents
Central nervous system depression	Benzodiazepines, alcohol, opioids, propofol, antidepressants, anticonvulsants, neuroleptics
Bleeding diathesis	Coumarin anticoagulants, heparin, streptokinase, tissue plasminogen activator, nonsteroidal anti-inflammatory drugs, salicylates, antineoplastic agents, certain antibiotics (e.g., moxalactam)
Hyperglycemia	Corticosteroids with diuretics
Hypoglycemia	Sulfonylureas with salicylates, phenytoin
Hypokalemia	Corticosteroids or amphotericin B with diuretics
Hyperkalemia	Potassium chloride with potassium-sparing diuretics or angiotensin-converting enzyme inhibitors
Hypotension	Antihypertensives with tricyclic antidepressants, phenothiazines, antianginals, vasodilators

Adapted from McInnes GT, Brodie MJ: Drug interactions that matter: A clinical reappraisal. Drugs *36*:83, 1988.

through the antagonism of the effects of one drug by the side effects of another. As our therapeutic armamentarium increases in size as well as in potency and efficacy, the potential for these adverse reactions increases. The seriousness of this issue is compounded by medical subspecialization and the attendant independent prescribing practices of various physicians, with patients' increasing self-medication with more potent OTC medications.

References

1. Faich GA, Knopp D, Dreiss M, Turner W: National adverse drug reaction surveillance: 1985. JAMA *257*:2068–2070, 1987.
2. Quinn DI, Day RO: Drug interactions of clinical importance. An updated guide. Drug Safety *12*:393–452, 1995.
3. Robinson DS: The application of basic principles of drug interaction to clinical practice. J Urol *113*:101–107, 1975.
4. May FE, Stewart RB, Cluff LE: Drug interactions and multiple drug administration. Clin Pharmacol Ther *22*:322–328, 1977.
5. Pickering LK, Rutherford I: Effect of concentration and time upon inactivation of tobramycin, gentamicin, netilmicin and amikacin by azlocillin, carbenicillin, mecillinam and piperacillin. J Pharmacol Exp Ther *217*:345–349, 1981.
6. Frazee LA, Reed MD: Warfarin and nonsteroidal anti-inflammatory drugs: why not? Ann Pharmacother *29*:1289–1291, 1995.
7. Hansten PD, Horn JR: Drug Interactions and Updates. 6th ed. Vancouver, WA, Applied Therapeutics, Inc., 1993.
8. Gilette JR, Pang KS: Theoretic aspects of drug interactions. Clin Pharmacol Ther *22*:623–639, 1977.
9. Pond SM: Pharmacokinetic drug interactions. *In* Benet LZ, Massoud N, Gambertoglio JG (eds): Pharmacokinetic Basis for Drug Treatment. New York, Raven Press, pp 195–220, 1984.
10. McInnes GT, Brodie MJ: Drug interactions that matter. A clinical reappraisal. Drugs *36*:83–110, 1988.
11. Rider MJ: Mechanisms of unpredictable adverse drug reactions. Drug Safety *11*:196–212, 1994.
12. Honig PK, Gillespie BK: Drug interactions between prescribed and over-the-counter medications. Drug Safety *13*:296–303, 1995.
13. Freedman MD: Drug interactions: Classification and systematic approach. Am J Ther *2*:433–443, 1995.
14. Rosenberg J, Benowitz NL, Pond S: Pharmacokinetics of drug overdose. Clin Pharmacokinet *6*:161–192, 1981.
15. Drew RH: Applying pharmacokinetic principles to the management of drug poisoning. Pediatr Ann *16*:913–924, 1987.
16. Boston Collaborative Drug Surveillance Program: Adverse drug interactions (editorial). JAMA *220*:1238–1239, 1972.
17. Borda IT, Slone D, Jick H: Assessment of adverse reactions within a drug surveillance program. JAMA *205*:645–647, 1968.
18. Durrence CW, DiPiro JT, May JR, et al: Potential drug interactions in surgical patients. Am J Hosp Pharm *42*:1553–1556, 1985.
19. Smith JW, Seidl LG, Cliff LE: Studies on the epidemiology of adverse drug reactions. V. Clinical factors influencing susceptibility. Ann Intern Med *65*:629–640, 1977.
20. Reed MD, Amer MK, Blumer JL: Drug Use in the Elderly. Cleveland, OH, The Cleveland Foundation Report, 1985.
21. Kirch W, Hoensch H, Janisch HD: Interactions and non-interactions with ranitidine. Clin Pharmacokinet *9*:493–510, 1984.
22. Sadowski DC: Drug interactions with antacids, mechanisms and clinical significance. Drug Safety *11*:395–407, 1994.
23. Greiff JMC, Rowbothom D: Pharmacokinetic drug interactions with gastrointestinal motility modifying agents. Clin Pharmacokinet *27*:447–461, 1994.
24. Svensson CK, Woodruff MN, Baxter JG, Lalka D: Free drug concentration monitoring in clinical practice. Rationale and current status. Clin Pharmacokinet *11*:450–469, 1986.
25. Sansom LN, Evans AM: What is the true clinical significance of plasma protein binding displacement interactions? Drug Safety *12*:227–233, 1995.
26. Sellers EM: Plasma protein displacement interactions are rarely of clinical significance. Pharmacology *18*:225–227, 1979.
27. Farrar HC, Herold DA, Reed MD: Acute valproic acid intoxication: Enhanced drug clearance with oral activated charcoal. Crit Care Med *21*:299–301, 1993.
28. Schenck-Gustafsson K, Jogestrand T, Nordlander R, Dahlqvist R: Effect of quinidine and digoxin concentration in skeletal muscle and serum in patients with atrial fibrillation. Evidence for reduced binding of digoxin in muscle. N Engl J Med *305*:209–211, 1981.
29. Wandell M, Powell JR, Hager WD, et al: Effect of quinine on digoxin kinetics. Clin Pharmacol Ther *28*:425–430, 1980.
30. Powell JR, Donn KH: Histamine H-2 antagonist drug interactions in perspective: Mechanistic concepts and clinical applications. Am J Med *77*(Suppl 5B):57–84, 1984.
31. Murray M: P450 enzymes: Inhibition mechanisms, genetic regulation and effects of liver disease. Clin Pharmacokinet *23*:132–146, 1992.
32. Wrighton SA, Stevens JC: The human hepatic cytochromes P450 involved in drug metabolism. Crit Rev Toxicol *22*:1–21, 1992.
33. MacDonald MG, Robinson DS, Sylwester D, Jaffe JJ: The effects of phenobarbital, chloral betaine and glutethimide administration on warfarin plasma levels and hypoprothrombinemic responses in man. Clin Pharmacol Ther *10*:80–84, 1969.
34. Rapeport WG, McInnes GT, Thompson GG, et al: Hepatic enzyme induction and leucocyte delta-aminolaevulinic acid synthase activity: Studies with carbamazepine. Br J Clin Pharmacol *16*:133–137, 1983.
35. Baciewicz AM, Self TM: Rifampin drug interactions. Arch Intern Med *144*:1667–1671, 1984.
36. Hoyumpa AM, Schenker S: Major drug interactions: Effect of liver disease, alcohol and malnutrition. Annu Rev Med *33*:113–149, 1982.
37. Jusko WJ: Role of tobacco smoking in pharmacokinetics. J Pharmacokinet Biopharm *6*:7–39, 1978.
38. Alvares AP: Interactions between environmental chemicals and drug biotransformation in man. Clin Pharmacokinet *3*:462–477, 1978.
39. Pantuck EJ, Pantuck CB, Anderson KE, et al: Effect of brussel sprouts and cabbage on drug conjugation. Clin Pharmacol Ther *35*:161–169, 1984.

40. Kappas A, Alvares AP, Anderson KE, et al: Effect of charcoal-broiled beef on antipyrine and theophylline metabolism. Clin Pharmacol Ther *21*:445–450, 1978.
41. Park BK, Breckenridge AM: Clinical implications of enzyme induction and enzyme inhibition. Clin Pharmacokinet *6*:1–24, 1981.
42. Breckenridge A, Orme MLE, Davies L, et al: Dose-dependent enzyme induction. Clin Pharmacol Ther *14*:514–520, 1971.
43. Ohnhaus EE, Park BK: Measurement of urinary 6-β-hydroxy-cortisol excretion as an *in vivo* parameter in the clinical assessment of the microsomal enzyme-inducing capacity of antipyrine, phenobarbitone and rifampin. Eur J Clin Pharmacol *15*:139–145, 1979.
44. Dossing M, Pilsgaard H, Rasmussen B, Enghusen-Poulsen H: Time course of phenobarbital and cimetidine mediated changes in hepatic drug metabolism. Eur J Clin Pharmacol *25*:215–222, 1983.
45. Abernethy DR, Greenblatt DJ, Divoll M, et al: Differential effect of cimetidine on drug oxidation (antipyrine and diazepam) vs conjugation (acetaminophen and lorazepam): Prevention of acetaminophen toxicity by cimetidine. J Pharmacol Exp Ther *224*:508–513, 1983.
46. Peterson FJ, Knodell RG, Lindemann NJ, Steele NM: Prevention of acetaminophen and cocaine hepatotoxicity in mice by cimetidine treatment. Gastroenterology *85*:122–129, 1983.
47. Somogyi A, McLean A, Heinzow B: Cimetidine-procainamide pharmacokinetic interaction in man: Evidence of competition for tubular secretion of basic drugs. Eur J Clin Pharmacol *25*:339–345, 1983.
48. van Crugten J, Bochner F, Keal J, Somogyi A: Selectivity of the cimetidine-induced alterations in the renal handling of organic substrates in humans. Studies with anionic, cationic and zwitteronic drugs. J Pharmacol Exp Ther *236*:481–487, 1986.
49. Wormsley KG: Safety profile of ranitidine: A review. Drugs *46*:976–985, 1993.
50. Echizen H, Ishizaki T: Clinical pharmacokinetics of famotidine. Clin Pharmacokinet *21*:178–194, 1991.
51. Rendic S, Kajfez F, Ruf H-H: Characterization of cimetidine, ranitidine and related structures interaction with cytochrome P-450. Drug Metab Disp *11*:137–142, 1983.
52. Meredith CG, Christian CD, Johnson RF, et al: Effects of influenza virus vaccine on hepatic drug metabolism. Clin Pharmacol Ther *37*:396–401, 1985.
53. Kraemer MJ, Furukawa CT, Koup JR, et al: Altered theophylline clearance during an influenza B outbreak. Pediatrics *69*:476–480, 1982.
54. Azhary RE, Mannering GJ: Effects of interferon inducing agents on hepatic hemoproteins, heme metabolism and cytochrome P450-linked monooxygenase system. Mol Pharmacol *15*:698–707, 1979.
55. Kirk J: Significant drug-nutrient interactions. Am Fam Physician *51*:1175–1182, 1995.
56. Dunn MJ: Nonsteroidal anti-inflammatory drugs and renal function. Annu Rev Med *35*:411–428, 1984.
57. Brouwers JRBJ, deSnet AGM: Pharmacokinetic-pharmacodynamic drug interactions with nonsteroidal anti-inflammatory drugs. Clin Pharmacokinet *27*:462–485, 1994.
58. Peterson RG, Peterson LN: Cleansing the blood: Hemodialysis, periotoneal dialysis, exchange transfusion, charcoal hemoperfusion, forced diuresis. Pediatr Clin North Am *33*:675–689, 1986.
59. Perel JM, Dayton PG, Snell MM, et al: Studies of interactions among drugs in man at the renal level: Probenecid and sulfinpyrazone. Clin Pharmacol Ther *10*:834–840, 1969.
60. Park GD, Spector R, Goldberg MJ, Johnson GF: Expanded role of charcoal therapy in the poisoned and overdosed patient. Arch Intern Med *146*:969–973, 1986.
61. Krishnaswamy K: Drug metabolism and pharmacokinetics in malnutrition. Clin Pharmacokinet *3*:216–240, 1978.
62. Fernandez-Repollet E, Tapia E, Martinez-Maldonado M: Effects of angiotensin-converting enzyme inhibition on altered renal hemodynamics induced by a low protein diet in the rat. J Clin Invest *80*:1045–1049, 1987.
63. Pantuck EJ, Pantuck CB, Weissman C, et al: Effect of parenteral nutritional regimens on oxidative drug metabolism. Anesthesiology *60*:534–536, 1984.
64. Fagan TC, Walle T, Oexmann MJ, et al: Increased clearance of propranolol and theophylline by high-protein compared with high carbohydrate diet. Clin Pharmacol Ther *41*:402–406, 1987.
65. Solomon HM, Shiogie JJ: Change in receptor site affinity: A proposed explanation for the potentiating effect of D-thyroxine on the anticoagulant response to warfarin. Clin Pharmacol Ther *2*:797–799, 1967.
66. Lipsky JJ: Antibiotic associated hypoprothrombinaemia. J Antimicrob Chemother *21*:281–300, 1988.

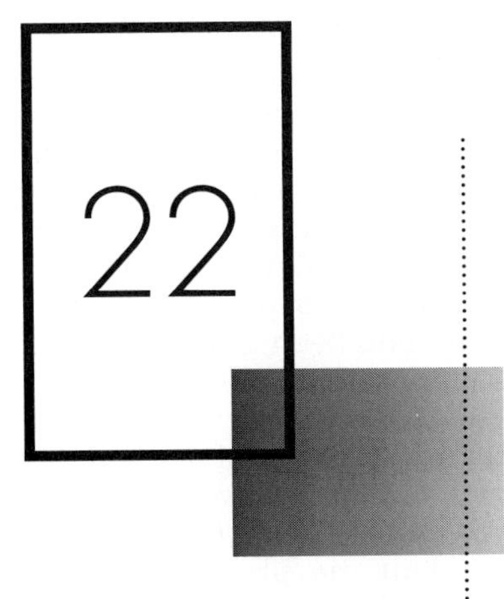

Disaster Management of Massive Toxic Exposure

CONSTANCE J. DOYLE, MD
JAMES CISEK, MD
MARK J. UPFAL, MD

Exposure to hazardous materials is unfortunately as much a fact of modern life as are such things as vehicular accidents and poisonings. The term *hazardous material* is used here to mean any substance that can be harmful to humans, animals, or the environment when released in any uncontrolled manner. This chapter focuses on the management principles applicable to acute exposure to hazardous materials, including large-scale incidents. It does not address the issues surrounding chronic lower-level exposure.

Fixed industrial and storage sites account for the largest amount of hazardous materials. Seventy-seven per cent of all accidents involving the release of hazardous materials occur in stationary facilities. According to the Occupational Safety and Health Administration (OSHA), 575,000 chemicals are used in the workplace.

One need not live near a chemical manufacturing plant, heavy industry, or a chemical dump site to be at risk for exposure to hazardous materials. A source of potential exposure is the nearest road, railroad track, or waterway. Several billion tons of hazardous materials are transported in the United States each year, with approximately 40% being shipped via truck. This represents more than 40,000 motor carriers and an additional 60,000 shippers via other routes. In 1992, 9,294 hazardous materials incidents were reported to the U.S. Department of Transportation. During 1995, CHEMTREC logged over 189,000 telephone calls for hazardous materials emergency assistance. Most of these voluntary calls were informational, with medical emergencies representing only 5% of the calls.[1–4]

A brief hypothetical example illustrates the complexity involved in a hazardous materials incident: a train derails near a populated suburb next to the river that is the source of the city's water supply. Multiple chemical tank cars are damaged, and the accident involves a moderate number of human casualties. Someone who has seen the wreck calls for help. Immediately, several issues are apparent. First and foremost, what are the chemicals and how can one identify them? Is it safe to approach the train to remove the wounded? Is a fire or explosive hazard present? Is the water supply to the city in danger, and, if so, what can be done about it? Do rescuers need respiratory and skin protection? Can victims be brought to the hospital emergency department without exposing the emergency department personnel and patients to chemical hazards? Which hospitals have the ability to manage physical trauma, burns, and systemic poisoning? Should nearby residents be evacuated and if so, how far from the site? How do you know if the overturned tank cars are leaking? Who should be notified? Who is in charge? Who is responsible? Who will pay for the cleanup?[5–7]

THE BHOPAL EXPERIENCE[8–19]

The events in Bhopal, India, represent an example of a mass toxic exposure. On the night of Dec 3, 1984, a cloud of methyl isocyanate gas leaked from a storage tank at the Union Carbide plant in Bhopal, Madhya Pradesh, India. Approximately 500 people in the surrounding area were killed before reaching medical treatment, and the total death count was approximately 2,500. One hospital alone treated 25,000 patients in the first 24 hours.

Immediate respiratory problems consisted of severe coughing, dyspnea, pharyngitis, and pulmonary edema. Severe conjunctival irritation and corneal ulceration developed. Gastrointestinal symptoms consisted of increased salivation, nausea, vomiting, abdominal pain, and defecation; increase in urination was also noted. Central nervous system symptoms were manifested by coma, seizures, dizziness, limb weakness, and tremors.

Methyl isocyanate is used in the manufacture of carbamate insecticides. It is a liquid that has a low boiling point and is heavier than air in its gaseous form. It has a strong odor and is irritating to the eyes, skin, and respiratory tract. It may be toxic both by inhalation and cutaneous exposure. At the time of the Bhopal incident, there was a paucity of toxicologic data in the literature about exposure to this chemical.

A crowded shantytown existed immediately outside the Union Carbide plant. Residents were sleeping, and no warning was sounded at the time of the gas release. The hutlike dwellings provided little protection against the gas. Ninety to 95% of the dead and severely injured came from this area. A crowded railway station situated 1 km from the plant had more than 100 dead: 200 people were unconscious and 600 were lying about injured. Several studies of survivors were undertaken 3.5 months after the incident. Patients in these studies were categorized according to their distance from the plant on the night of the accident. Group 1 consisted of those 0.5 to 2 km from the plant, and group 2 was composed of those at least 8 km from the plant. The groups were similar socioeconomically and demographically. One hundred per cent of the group 1 sample and 42% of group 2 had symptoms at the time of the incident. At the time of the study, 80% of group 1 and 28% of group 2 had continued respiratory complaints consisting of cough, with or without sputum production; breathlessness; and chest pain. Fifty-seven per cent of group 1 had abnormal chest radiographs, 49% had documented restrictive defects, and 21% had obstructive defects. Smokers constituted 12%. It is unclear whether previous pulmonary disease was present or whether some patients had both restrictive and obstructive pulmonary disease.

In a group of children categorized in the same manner, most symptoms occurred in the immediate area of the plant, although the more remote group was not without symptoms. Ninety-five per cent of children from group 1 had immediate cough and 74% experienced breathlessness. Three months later, 84% noted persistent cough and 48% suffered from continued breathlessness. Abnormal radiographs were found in 66% of group 1 children, compared with 8.1% of group 2 children. Pulmonary testing was performed on children older than 7 years. Obstructive defects were found in 28 of 33 children. Persistent abdominal pain and anorexia were found in the group 1 children only. Group 1 children experienced persistent conjunctivitis, and 10% demonstrated visual abnormalities. No persistent eye abnormalities were found in group 2. Persistent neurobehavioral symptoms consisted of poor memory and weakness. Comprehensive psychological testing was not performed. Some children who later developed obvious psychic disturbances had been classified as dead at the time of the accident and had been initially placed in morgues. Others had witnessed the deaths of parents or siblings.

The local lake had measurable levels of isocyanates for 9 months after the incident. Such levels were not detectable, however, 1 year after the incident.

At the time of the incident, no plans existed to alert the local population in the event of a disaster. Methods of protection or routes of evacuation were not publicized. The plant was located in a densely populated area, with a shantytown around the plant. Widespread knowledge of the hazardous materials being used or the products manufactured was lacking, and there were no standard operating practices and few engineering controls. It is estimated that approximately 50,000 lb of methyl isocyanate in liquid and vapor form were released into the atmosphere when a valve on a storage tank opened for approximately 2 hours. Light winds prevented rapid dispersal of the heavier-than-air cloud. The accident happened at night, when most of the residents were asleep. Because of the rapid onset of symptoms and the large numbers of people affected, local hospitals were rapidly overwhelmed. Many patients were treated in the hospital garden. Local citizens helped each other in the initial rescue attempt. No local medical authority on methyl isocyanate was immediately available.

In summary, methyl isocyanate is used in the manufacture of carbamate pesticides. The major acute effects resulting from the exposures at Bhopal were related to irritation of the respiratory tract and eyes. Data regarding the chronic effects of methyl isocyanate are lacking, and the long-term effects of this incident may not become apparent for many years. One might expect to see cases of reactive airways, chronic obstructive pulmonary disease, bronchiolitis, and restrictive lung disease resulting from pulmonary fibrosis.

THE CHERNOBYL EXPERIENCE

On April 26, 1986, the fourth reactor at Chernobyl, U.S.S.R. (now the Ukraine), exploded and caught fire after an experiment to test the reactor's emergency systems failed. The cause was intense generation of steam, fuel-channel rupture, and a thermal explosion after some of the graphite control rods were removed from the radioactive core.[20] Thankfully, only 3 to 5% of the core amount of radiation was released. Thirty-one people were killed and various sources cite acute radiation syndrome in 237 to 299 persons. One hundred twenty-nine patients were sent to specialized hospitals in Kiev and Moscow. Thirty bone marrow transplants and six human embryonic liver cell transplants were carried out over the ensuing several weeks to months.[21, 22]

Fifty thousand people were evacuated from the nearby town of Pripyat after a delayed public announcement a day and a half after the release. It is estimated that a total of 135,000 persons were evacuated and permanently rehoused; in addition, 500,000 mothers and children from the surrounding area were reportedly sent to resorts along the Black Sea, and another 300,000 were sent to other locations.

It was estimated that 30 to 60 km^2 of topsoil and road surfaces would have to be removed to properly decontaminate the area.[22]

Winds carried radiation into Scandinavia, eastern Europe, parts of western Europe, and surrounding Russia. The initial international detection came from Sweden, when radiation alarms went off 2 days after the accident. The accident was announced that evening by the Soviet Union. Many countries had radioactive fallout, and milk from grass-fed cows was banned, vegetables were destroyed, and children were kept indoors and were given iodine to block the effects of ^{131}I. Estimates of cancer increases were initially said to be "no more than 1000" and have risen in the past 10 years since the accident. Most of the pilots who helped to entomb the reactor are dead or have leukemia. More and more of the cleanup workers have required treatment for radiation-induced diseases. Thyroid cancer has increased a hundredfold in Belarus. More recent estimates put the number of new cancer cases resulting from the Chernobyl accident at 50,000. Other genetic changes that might occur over the next several decades are virtually inestimable.[20–23]

DISASTER PLANNING

Lessons Learned

In planning for chemical, radiation, and biologic disasters, one must consider all of the possibilities from human error, to employee sabotage, to mentally ill workers, to terrorism. Planners for the 1996 Olympic Games in Atlanta considered such possibilities, as well as natural and structural disasters, in their disaster plan. Evacuation routes, resources, and methods in case of a disaster must be evaluated. In the Soviet Union, Chernobyl was 50 miles from large population centers, yet evacuation was difficult. Sources indicate that 177 Communist Party members failed to do their duty in the evacuation of Pripyat and surrounding areas. Others were compliant on the threat of being shot. In more western countries with less political, social, and police control, it is possible that some workers will take care of themselves and their families first, and then attend to duty.

Planning for chemical disasters is essential for all communities, as no location is exempt from risk. International efforts at information sharing and preparedness are addressed by the United Nations, the World Health Organization (WHO), and other multinational groups. In the medical management of chemical exposure emergencies, numerous simultaneous considerations are paramount. Although individual patient care issues must be considered, personal protection and safety for the rescuer takes precedence. Decontamination precedes emergency care or can occur simultaneously with proper rescuer respiratory and skin protection. Plans to coordinate and define contaminated areas, decontamination and triage procedures on scene, resource and information management, and transportation to definitive medical care require preplanning. Each community should have developed and put into place an emergency contingency plan that details specific actions and responsibilities of various community services in the event of a crisis situation.

A specific hazardous materials appendix to a disaster plan should be identified. This contingency plan, which should be updated yearly, will contain detailed instructions to follow, including emergency response operations; a roster of emergency assistance phone numbers; a description of each service's legal authority and responsibility during an emergency; a description of the structure and responsibility of the designated response organization; a section on resource laboratories for analysis of chemical and patient data; and a cleanup and disposal equipment resource section. In addition to community disaster planning, industrial sites using hazardous materials must also have a disaster site plan. Industry and the local hospitals should work together to plan for emergency response. Ideally, patients should be transported to the department along with copies of the appropriate materials safety data sheets (MSDSs).

Hospitals must plan for major *chemical* incidents. Large amounts of antidotes specific to the potential exposures must be available. Most hospitals in the United States do not have enough atropine (hundreds of milligrams, or even grams, may be required) to treat large numbers of organophosphate-poisoned patients. Treatment locations must be planned. Twenty-five thousand patients would overwhelm even the largest hospital system. In some geographic locations, inclement weather may preclude the treatment of patients on the hospital grounds. Plans would need to include large, sheltered treatment areas. Hospitals in the path of a chemical cloud may need to be evacuated, unless indoor air quality could be maintained. Any emergency department could be faced with a large-scale hazardous materials emergency resulting from a transportation accident or a nearby manufacturing site from raw, stored, or finished materials. Little regulation exists to limit the routes and times of day that may be used for hazardous materials transportation.[24–26]

Most chemical substances do not fall under the regulation of the Toxic Substances Control Act of

1976 (TOSCA), which requires that *new* chemicals be reviewed. The Clean Air Act allows the Environmental Protection Agency (EPA) to regulate emissions from plants under *normal* conditions, rather than in emergency conditions, such as at Bhopal.

Multiple manufacturing facilities have located in third world countries to utilize inexpensive labor and to be closer to those markets. Technologic support is sparse and unevenly distributed. Maintenance of equipment may be poor, and manufacturing standards and controls are a far cry from those in the developed world. Regulations governing plant site planning and the manufacture of chemicals are few. In third world countries, very dense residential areas spring up around manufacturing facilities, allowing poor workers easy and inexpensive commutes.

Neither Bhopal nor a similar facility in Institute, West Virginia, had evacuation plans at the time of the Bhopal disaster. The Institute plant had recorded 84 "escapes" of methyl isocyanate and phosgene during the 5-year period between 1980 and 1985. Some of these were not "reportable" under current regulations, because the amounts were too small. Prevention issues were not even addressed.

Since the Bhopal incident, many chemical industries in the United States have reviewed their safety standards. Site plans are now required for all facilities using hazardous materials and Material Safety Data Sheets must be on site. In addition, computerized site plans with maps of local areas may be available. Local emergency planning committees (LEPCs) are mandated by the Superfund Amendments and Reauthorization Act (SARA, title III). These committees are responsible for developing and implementing plans for hazardous materials emergency response in the local community.

Local medical authorities should be familiar with the hazardous materials used in various manufacturing processes so that they can plan treatment in the event of an emergency. Sheltered off-site locations for treatment should be available if a hospital is overwhelmed or must be evacuated. Warning mechanisms and a plan for early evacuation will minimize injuries. Hazardous materials training of first responders is paramount. Rescuers must be trained in the use of protective equipment and in decontamination procedures to minimize contamination of medical personnel, vehicles, medical facilities, and the environment. Local haz-mat response units with special training and equipment are being formed in many communities. These units, with trained personnel, would be responsible for evaluation and management of scene hazards and decontamination before transport. With multiple casualties, the real possibility exists that some patients will present to triage at local hospitals while still contaminated. All medical facilities should have plans to identify contaminated patients, protect personnel and the emergency environment, and provide for decontamination with protective equipment.[27–29]

Table 22–1 lists a few of the known hazardous materials incidents worldwide.

Table 22–1. Known Hazardous Materials Incidents

April 26, 1986—Chernobyl, USSR

Explosion and fire and radiation leak from nuclear power plant reactor number 4 kills 31, ~250 injured immediately from the radiation. Score of cleanup workers and pilots who helped entomb the reactor affected over the next decade. Multiple evacuations and many incidences of new cancers are emerging (see text).

December 1984—Bhopal, India

2500 deaths and 250,000 injuries result from a leak of methyl isocyanate at a Union Carbide plant (see text).

November 1984—Mexico City, Mexico

More than 400 deaths and 4000 injuries result from a liquified gas explosion

March 28, 1979—Three Mile Island, PA

Loss of coolant leads to a partial meltdown. A small amount of radioactive material escapes. Iodine given to block thyroid gland uptake of ^{131}I. Multiple self-evacuations by concerned citizens.

July 1976—Seveso, Italy

A chemical plant explosion results in a massive release of dioxin (2,3,7,8-tetrachlorodibenzo-para-dioxin) in an urban area, resulting in many cases of chloracne (primarily in children and young adults) but no deaths.

July 1975—Hopewell, VA

Life Science Products plant closed after 16 months operation, having exposed 150 employees to exceedingly high levels of kepone (an organophosphate pesticide) and polluted the surrounding environment, creating a major community health problem and millions of dollars in damage. Approximately 30 employees hospitalized for acute poisoning.

June 1974—Flixborough, Humberside, England

28 workers killed when a chemical plant pipe ruptures and an explosion results. Every building on a 60 acre site is destroyed.

May 1971—Times Beach, MO

18,000 gallons of industrial waste liquid and used motor oil sprayed in barns and stables and roads. Birds, rats, and mice die in weeks; 48 horses die in months. A flood in 1982 further spreads contamination of dioxin. Levels reached 300 ppm. Levels of 1 ppb considered toxic. 2000 residents evacuated and permanently moved (after 10 years' exposure).

July 1948—Ludwigshafen, Germany

Dimethylether explosion of a rail car, kills more than 200 and wounds 4000 people.

Legislation

As required by the OSHA Hazard Communication Standard, "hazards of all chemicals produced or imported by chemical manufacturers or importers [must be] evaluated, and information concerning their hazards [must be] transmitted to affected employers and employees within the manufacturing sector. This transmittal of information is to be accomplished by means of comprehensive hazard communication programs, which are to include container labeling and other forms of warning, material safety data sheets, and employee training" (29 CFR §1910.1200). Workers must know the hazards of the chemicals with which they work and methods to protect themselves in the event of an accident or incident. There should also be some training in first aid and decontamination procedures at the plant.

In addition to the worker's "right to know" law, a community's "right to know" is also mandated by the Comprehensive Environmental Response, Compensation and Liability Act (CERCLA) amendments of 1986, otherwise known as SARA, title III. A balance must be achieved between worker safety, community safety, and production for profit.

Title III of SARA required that a state emergency response commission be established by April 1987 in each state. This commission, appointed by the governor of the state, must coordinate community emergency planning committees in the development of plans for emergency response to hazardous materials emergencies. A list of 402 extremely hazardous materials, published in the Federal Register (Nov 17, 1986), gave threshold planning quantities. If these materials are produced, used, or stored in quantities exceeding the thresholds, they become subject to the emergency planning requirements. Additionally, requirements were set for emergency notification whenever a release of hazardous material exceeded a reportable quantity. The community "right to know" provisions of SARA require facilities to provide MSDSs and chemical inventories to local emergency planning committees, local fire departments, and state emergency response commissions.

DISASTER MANAGEMENT

In a disaster, needs outstrip the resources to deal with the emergency in an appropriate time frame. *The primary theme of disaster management is information management. Timely information can change the entire character of the disaster.* For example, if it is known immediately that a leaking tank car contains a particular poisonous gas, then rescuers would not approach the scene without respiratory and skin protection. If it is known immediately that a certain spilled chemical can contaminate the water supply but is otherwise innocuous, then immediate containment is in order. If the local emergency facility knows that all casualties have incurred carbon monoxide exposure, they can arrange for auxiliary oxygen sources as well as transportation for hyperbaric oxygen treatment, if indicated. If the emergency department receives large numbers of casualties with identical chemical injuries, the resources needed to treat that injury might be depleted. However, when many of these questions cannot be answered in an appropriate time frame, a potential disaster can turn into a true disaster.

The emergency department must also have rapid access to information about the management of exposures to exotic materials that rarely present to the physician. For example, arsine, a highly toxic gas used in the semiconductor industry, requires a specific protocol for management. However, since exposures are fortunately rare, few physicians will have had the opportunity to treat arsine poisoning prior to an acute incident. Thus, information about proper workup and treatment must be readily available. One excellent source of this information is the Poisindex. Another source of information about the ingredients, toxicologic features, and other hazardous properties of specific chemicals and mixtures, as well as very limited first aid information, is the MSDSs. The MSDS is available from the manufacturer of the chemical product and is required to be present and available in all industrial plants using the product. It has very limited medical information. First aid information and levels of protection are specified, as are flammability and explosion hazards. The major use of the MSDS is the proper spelling of the chemical names so that toxicity data can be accessed from other sources.[30]

The second principle of proper disaster management is that of procurement of resources in a time frame appropriate to the situation. For example, a dozen people with moderate carbon monoxide poisoning could be handled by most emergency departments. However, 100 casualties would overwhelm the system if they arrived unannounced. With sufficient time and planning to procure the necessary supplies, even this number could be handled in a large area adjacent to the emergency department or in a community facility. Few, if any, could handle a large number of serious chemical or radiation burn victims. Even with extra supplies and personnel, some prioritization may have to take place, with resultant delay in decontamination and treatment for some victims.[31–33]

The third principle of disaster management is planning. It is said that once a disaster is planned for, the disaster no longer exists. Each community should have developed and put into place an emergency contingency plan that details specific actions and responsibilities of various community services in the event of a crisis situation. The plan may contain a specific hazardous materials annex. This contingency plan, which should be brought up to date yearly, will contain detailed instructions to follow, including emergency response operations; a roster of emergency assistance telephone numbers; a description of each service's legal authority and responsibility during an emergency; a description of the structure and the responsibility of the designated response organization; a section of spill cleanup techniques; a section on resource laboratories for analysis of chemical and patient data; and a cleanup and disposal equipment resource section.

In addition to community disaster planning, industrial sites using hazardous materials must also have a disaster site plan. Plants using large quantities of hazardous materials (e.g., chemical companies) or unusually toxic materials (e.g., semi-conductor manufacturers) and local hospitals should work together to plan for emergency response. Information about all significant hazards should be made available to the emergency facility. Ideally, a plant's MSDSs should be on file in the emergency department, and emergency physicians should be familiar with them. Additionally, patients should be transported from the plant to the department along with copies of the appropriate MSDSs.

In general terms, the sequence of events in a disaster is as follows: An accident occurs. Knowledge of it is transmitted to appropriate agencies; these agencies respond and gather more data. They may activate other resources. Fire and the haz-mat team assume charge and direct law enforcement to control and secure the scene. The scope of the problem is defined. The necessary plans for the solution of the problem are activated, and follow-up and evaluation are accomplished.

First and foremost is notification of appropriate agencies—that is, police, fire department, haz-mat team, emergency medical system, local disaster coordinator, county and state officials, and federal agencies. It is beyond the scope of this chapter to indicate who must be notified in any given incident. This varies with the incident and with local and state regulations. Various local and state agencies may have jurisdiction over a particular kind of hazard. These interests may overlap, depending on the nature of the chemical, the location of a spill, and the various laws in a state. Local government sources are probably the best initial resource concerning all the possible agencies that might be involved.

The fire chief and the haz-mat team assume charge and usually have the police set up perimeters and evacuate the surrounding area, if necessary. Crowd control and control of access to the site are also the responsibility of the police agency. A fire agency has responsibility to respond to the chemical or fire hazard and to initiate extrication, decontamination, and first aid to casualties. An emergency medical service (EMS) agency is responsible for medical decisions and treatment. Other agencies may have jurisdiction and authority or serve in an advisory capacity such as the Agency for Toxic Substances and Disease Registry (ATSDR), the Centers for Disease Control and Prevention (CDC), the EPA, OSHA, the Federal Emergency Management Agency (FEMA), and the state health department (Table 25–2). Local municipal authorities must know how to gain access to other sources of help, including state and federal agencies. At all times, it is critical for all responders to know who is in control. The agency that assumes control may change as more information concerning the exact nature of the hazard becomes available or during different phases of the entire operation, including cleanup. It is obvious that obtaining information in an appropriate time frame is critical in all phases of response to a hazardous material emergency. Planning guides are available from the ATSDR and from FEMA, as well as multiple other resources, to help in the planning phase.

Plans at the local and hospital levels should include local sources of expertise that can be contacted for technical assistance. Sources may include an emergency physician, a medical toxicologist, a pharmacologist, an industrial hygienist, an occupational medicine specialist, testing laboratories, and chemists. Plans should include potential sources of specialized equipment that may be needed for a given hazard—e.g., equipment for extrication and diking, decontamination showers, oxygen, protective gear, and transportation vehicles.

Table 22–2. Agencies Potentially Involved in Hazardous Materials Emergencies

Local EMS, police, and firefighters
City or county emergency management
Local hospitals/emergency departments
Regional hospitals or specialty hospitals (e.g., burn units, dialysis units, radiation units)
Local emergency planning committees (LEPCs)
State emergency planning commission
Regional poison control centers
Agency for Toxic Substances and Disease Registry (ATSDR)
Occupational Safety and Health Administration (OSHA)
National Institute for Occupational Safety and Health (NIOSH)
Nuclear Regulatory Commission
Military/National Guard
Coast Guard (contamination of any stream that empties into a navigable body of water)
Department of National Resources
Fish and Game Commission
Highway/transportation department
Flood control authority
Harbor Commission/Port Authority
Conservation agencies
Water resources
Public works
Federal Emergency Management Agency (FEMA)

Prehospital Site Management

Plan

Planning for the treatment of persons exposed to chemicals involves all levels of the health care team, from emergency medical services personnel to emergency department physicians. It is essential to ensure that exposure is limited to the smallest number of people possible.

Equipment

Equipment to handle spills and protective equipment for rescuers must be strategically located in the community, and its location must be known to all responders. An adequate supply of air tanks and self-contained breathing apparatuses (SCBAs) or equipment to refill tanks with adequate-quality breathing air must be available. Persons utilizing SCBAs must be properly trained in their use and understand the limitations of the equipment. Specifically, the time limitations of the supply tank and the reserve tank must be understood so that egress from the contaminated area can be accomplished prior to loss of supply air. The nature of the hazard and the necessary protective equipment must be determined *before* first responders enter an area of chemical spill.

Many first responders (police and fire personnel, EMS people, and even physicians and nurses) have been so thoroughly trained to aid an injured victim immediately that a hazard to their own health may be disregarded. As a result, the rescuer entering the contaminated area also may become contaminated and thus become a victim. Although rescue of any injured or ill victims who are unable to leave the spill site is of paramount importance, rescue should be attempted only after one ascertains that any rescuers will not themselves become victims.

Identification of the Spill

Identification of the hazardous material should be attempted prior to approach of the spill. One can read the placarding on the truck or train car from afar. *Be aware that placarding may be wrong 40% of the time and manifest papers may be wrong 35% of the time.* Binoculars are an invaluable aid. The bill of lading (cargo manifest) is located in the cab of a truck, but it may not be accessible without full protective gear. The diamond-shaped placard on the side of a tank or rail car with the Department of Transportation (DOT) number on it will identify the specific material, and the *DOT Emergency Response Guidebook* will provide the hazard class and general emergency information as well as evacuation distances. Some states also have numbered placards with emergency telephone numbers to call. These telephone numbers are a good first resource. Follow-up continues by contacting the shipper and confirming materials that are in the container or vehicle. The various symbols within the diamond-shaped placard (Fig. 22–1) should identify the general class of material being shipped. *The absence of a placard should not lead one to believe that danger is absent. An empty tank car is considered to be one that contains less than 300 gallons of material. One should treat a chemical spill and injuries from an unplacarded vehicle with the same caution.* Identification of the shipper may be possible by reading the markings on the truck or train car from a distance. The shipper may be contacted to assist in chemical identification and provision of resources. On a train, the waybill can be found with the conductor. Call the nearest company trainmaster, relaying the number of the car and the location, who can get information and handling information from the tracking computer. The waybill contains a standard transportation code (STC) number that identifies the specific chemical. Chemicals whose numbers begin with 49 are classified as hazardous. The waybill contains specific chemical names and handling information. With train cars numbered from engine to caboose, one can thus learn what chemical the car may contain.

Rapid emergency information can be obtained by calling CHEMTREC at 1–800–424–9300 in an emergency situation and giving the name of the compound (Table 25–3). In an emergency, CHEMTREC will connect emergency personnel with the manufacturer's and/or shipper's personnel, who can advise on emergency handling. CHEMTREC can then advise what sort of rescue gear may be needed and what decontamination, if any, is needed at the site. Most manufacturing plants have a site plan showing the location of hazardous material. Physician advice is not available through CHEMTREC.

Police are needed to secure an area or initiate evacuation when danger from fumes, fire, or explosion exists. They must control crowds so that others do not become casualties. When evacuation is necessary, those downwind from the hazard should be evacuated first.

In the event that the chemical is unknown, the safest way to rescue any victim is for rescuers to enter the area in fully encapsulated suits with positive-pressure SCBA. Firefighters are trained in use of similar gear, whereas many EMS rescue teams are not. In many locations firefighters who complete special training serve as the local haz-mat team. Some localities have access to special acid-resistant or fully encapsulated suits and other protective gear. Under medical guidance, the firefighters begin decontamination and rescue of casualties and begin first aid. The fire department is the most qualified to assess the potential for fires and explosions and to advise medical personnel of such.

The smallest number of rescuers possible should enter the contaminated area. At least two should go in together, employing a buddy system, to ensure each other's safety. A backup person with a similar level of protective gear should remain at the boundary to assist the rescuers in the event of an accident.[34]

Table 22–3. Sources of Information and Assistance for Emergency Response

ATSDR (Agency for Toxic Substances and Disease Registry): Public health agency for response to releases in the environment. Provides emergency response assistance on a 24-hour basis: (404) 639–0615. Information number: (404) 639–6360.

Physician and toxicologist help with chemical emergencies.

Local and regional poison control centers are staffed with a toxicologist and have access to multiple databases, including detailed medical treatment. Lists of numbers of local and regional poison centers should be kept where they can be accessed on an emergent basis. Local physicians with toxicology and haz-mat backgrounds and local industrial hygienists and chemical experts may also serve as resources.

CHEMTREC (Chemical Transportation Emergency Center); telephone: (800) 424–9300 (continental United States) or (800) 483–7616 (outside continental United States or Washington, DC). Can help identify ingredients of a product, help with MSDS information, field information on safe distances, first aid, explosion and fire hazards, and can put one in touch with manufacturer's and shipper's representatives. Some decontamination personal protective gear information and environmental information is available.

Chemical Referral Center (this is CHEMTREC's nonemergency line): (800) 262–8200 (9 AM–6 PM EST, Monday through Friday) or (800) 887–1255 (Washington, DC, same hours, same days).

REAC/TS (Radiation Emergency Assistance Center/Training Site): (423) 481–1000 (ask for REAC/TS assistance). This 24-hour response number can provide information and resource assistance in dealing with radiation emergencies, including decontamination, health care, and monitoring.

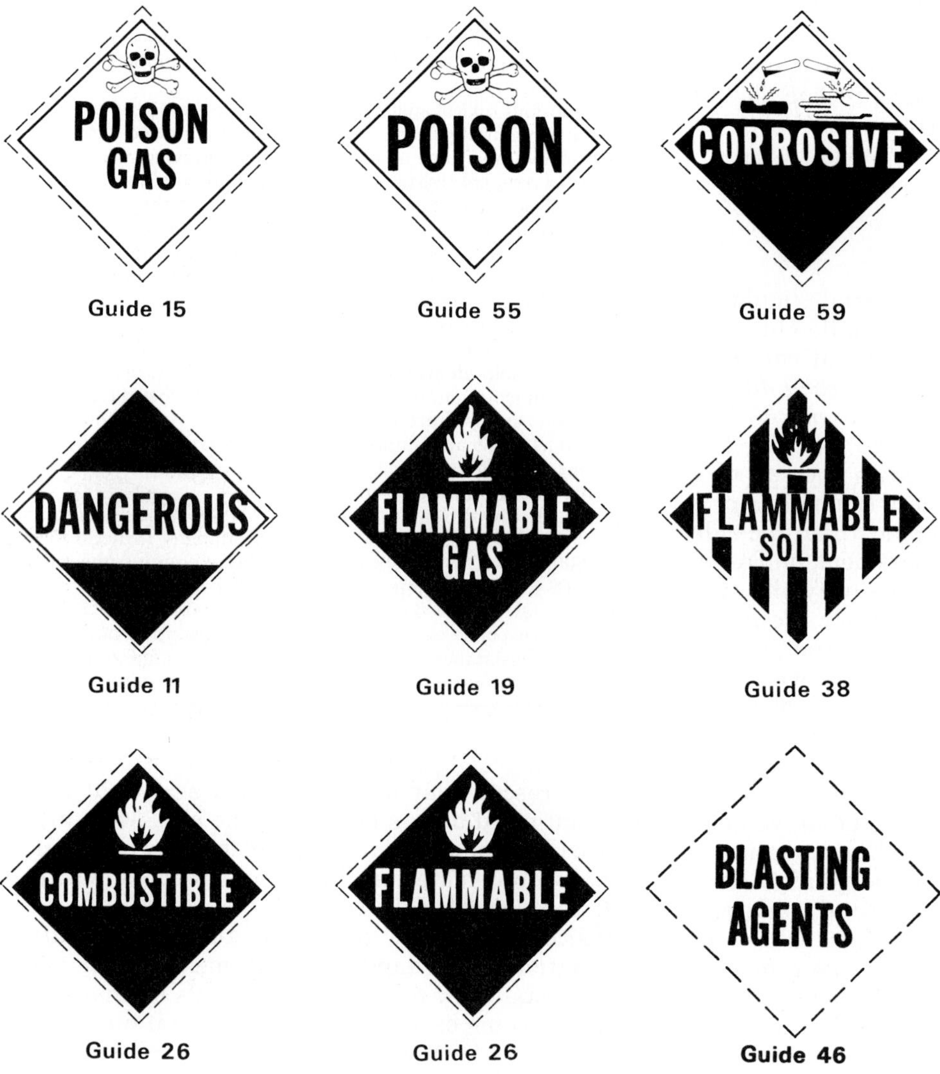
USE ONLY IF MATERIALS CANNOT BE SPECIFICALLY IDENTIFIED
THROUGH SHIPPING PAPERS OR MARKINGS.
POISON GAS
Guide 15
POISON
Guide 55
CORROSIVE
Guide 59
DANGEROUS
Guide 11
FLAMMABLE GAS
Guide 19
FLAMMABLE SOLID
Guide 38
COMBUSTIBLE
Guide 26
FLAMMABLE
Guide 26
BLASTING AGENTS
Guide 46

Figure 22–1. Table of placards and applicable response guide pages.(From Office of Hazardous Materials Regulation: Emergency Response Guidebook. Washington, DC, Materials Transportation Bureau, US Department of Transportation, 1980.)

Exposure Assessment

In general, the assessment of exposure risks in the industrial setting requires equipment and methods from the field of industrial hygiene. The industrial hygienist can perform qualitative and quantitative studies both on site and in the laboratory. Before discussing actual monitoring methods, however, it would be useful to define some terms and review some fundamental industrial hygiene concepts.

First, any chemicals can be handled safely *if* proper precautions are taken. In an uncontrolled release, this means that if there is no fire, explosion, or hazardous reaction, chemical releases can be approached with proper personal protective equipment. In most major incidents and in some minor incidents, this includes full-body suits that are impermeable to the hazardous material, and a positive-pressure demand style of SCBA. Personnel wearing an SCBA must be fully trained in its use, limitations, and what to do if the equipment fails. These persons must be medically cleared for SCBA use to be part of an emergency response team. The SCBA must have been properly inspected, maintained, and cleaned at regular intervals A full respirator program as required by OSHA (29 CFR §1910.134) must be in place. This includes periodic medical monitoring.

Second, any chemical, no matter now nontoxic, can be hazardous if handled inappropriately. For example, a release of methane or nitrogen in an enclosed space can cause asphyxiation. Numerous reports have been published of attempted rescues in such "nontoxic" environments, in which the initial victim and the rescuers all died of simple asphyxiation.

The identity of the specific agent is only one of a number of factors affecting the actual hazard. Other factors include the air concentration, potential for skin contact, duration of exposure, temperature of

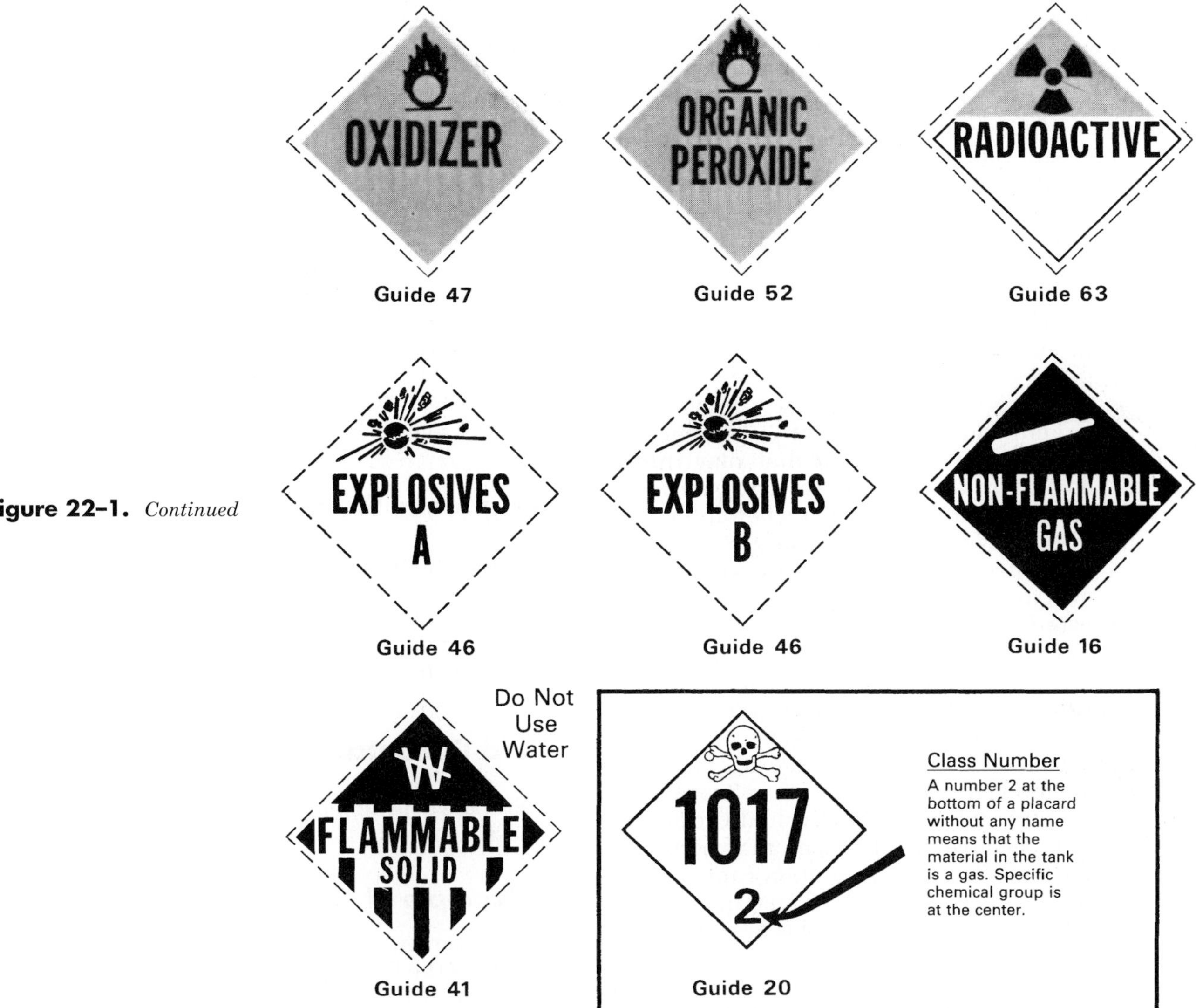
USE ONLY IF MATERIALS CANNOT BE SPECIFICALLY IDENTIFIED
THROUGH SHIPPING PAPERS OR MARKINGS.
OXIDIZER
Guide 47
ORGANIC PEROXIDE
Guide 52
RADIOACTIVE
Guide 63
EXPLOSIVES A
Guide 46
EXPLOSIVES B
Guide 46
NON-FLAMMABLE GAS
Guide 16
Do Not Use Water
FLAMMABLE SOLID
Guide 41
1017
2
Class Number
A number 2 at the bottom of a placard without any name means that the material in the tank is a gas. Specific chemical group is at the center.
Guide 20
Class Numbers: 1. Explosive 2. Gases 3. Flammable and Combustible Liquids 4. Flammable Solids 5. Oxidizers and Organic Peroxides 6. Poisons 7. Radioactive Material 8. Corrosives

Figure 22–1. *Continued*

the material, and individual susceptibility of the exposed persons.

Inhalation of air contaminants is the most frequent route of exposure for hazardous materials. Air contaminants may be found in a variety of forms, such as gases, vapors (the gaseous form of a substance that is primarily liquid or solid at room temperature), dusts (solid particles entrained in air), fumes (tiny solid particles often formed when a metal is heated, as in welding), mists (liquid particles entrained in air), and smoke (carbon or soot particles from incomplete combustion). Fumes, dusts, and smokes are measured in mass units of contaminant per volume unit of air (e.g., milligrams per cubic meter or parts per million). These two units can be easily interconverted if molecular weight, temperature, and altitude are known. Because fumes are minute solid particles, respirators designed for protection against fumes will have no efficacy against vapors or gases, and vice versa.

Once an air concentration is determined, several criteria exist for assessing the risk of exposure. The level that is immediately dangerous to life and health (IDLH) "represents a maximum concentration from which, in the event of respirator failure, one could escape within 30 minutes without experiencing any escape-impairing or irreversible health effects."[25] The IDLH level is used to determine the unquestionable need for a reliable positive-pressure demand SCBA. Standby personnel with full protective gear and a lifeline should be available when the IDLH level is exceeded. Specific IDLH values can be found in the *National Institute for Occupational Safety and Health (NIOSH) Pocket Guide to Chemical Hazards.*

The most widely used criteria for assessing exposure levels are the threshold limit values (TLVs) for hundreds of common industrial chemicals, which are updated and published annually by the American Conference of Governmental Industrial Hygienists. They "represent conditions under which it is believed that nearly all workers may be repeatedly exposed day after day without adverse effect."[25, 28] Most TLVs are established for 8-hour time-weighted average exposures (TWAs). In general, these values protect against the effects of a lifetime of chronic exposure. However, short-term exposure limits and ceiling limits for some substances are also included in the TLV list.

TLVs are designed to protect a population of healthy workers and are not meant to be applied to a general community population that may include infants, the elderly, and the infirm. Thus, an industrial hygienist should be consulted when interpretations based on TLVs are to be made. In addition to TLVs, a set of legally enforceable workplace standards, known as permissible exposure limits (PELs), has been established.

A common fallacy is the use of odor as a measure of exposure. Information about odor may sometimes by helpful in the qualitative identification of agents or as a crude guide to the exposure level. Odor thresholds for a wide variety of materials have been published. However, wide variations between reference sources and considerable individual variation in the ability to perceive specific odors may occur. For example, up to 40% of the population cannot detect the almond-like odor of cyanide. Thus, quantitative assessments based on odor thresholds are quite unreliable.

Some materials have excellent warning properties. For example, if the odor or irritation of ammonia is absent, one can be sure that there will be no toxic sequelae due to exposure to this agent. However, some materials, such as carbon monoxide, are odorless at lethal levels. Other agents, such as hydrogen sulfide, have a characteristic odor initially but induce olfactory fatigue. As a result, lethal exposures may result as exposed individuals perceive levels to be diminishing.

Air concentrations can be measured at specific locations and computer models can sometimes be used to predict worst-case ambient concentrations at downwind locations. Environmental monitoring can be performed with direct reading instruments providing real-time measurements of levels, or it can be performed by taking air samples that can be analyzed subsequently. Direct reading instruments include photoionization detectors, portable gas chromatographs, portable infrared spectrophotometers, portable carbon monoxide detectors, flammable gas detectors, and oxygen detectors. A simple direct reading method for instantaneous levels is the colorimetric detector tube.

In addition to monitoring the environment, it is important to provide medical surveillance for exposed victims and rescuers, both to assess potential health effects and to provide information about the exposure. Excellent documentation is essential, because many of these incidents result in litigation. The physician's initial charting may be a deciding factor in determining whether or not someone gets their deserved compensation. It may also determine whether or not abuses of the system occur, which cost public and private organizations large sums of money.

It is important to document subjective complaints and objective findings and assessments thoroughly and carefully. One should not document that symptoms are all due to a "toxic exposure" unless this is clearly the case. Describe actual clinical findings as they are manifest.

Diagnostic Studies

The diagnostic studies for each patient will depend on the clinical presentation and the specific agents to which they have been exposed. Please refer to specific chapters in this textbook for the discussion of specific toxins.

Field Decontamination and Triage

Standard principles of triage apply in a chemical disaster.

Example of Field Decontamination

The sequence for field decontamination is illustrated by the following example: A truck transporting a concentrated liquid chemical turns over on a highway, and the tank begins to leak. A large pool of chemical is rapidly filling a low section of roadway, and a hazy cloud begins to form over the pool. The driver and companion, who are both injured, begin to move away under their own power. They begin to cough and choke, and then they pass out. Several bystanders enter to help and are overcome and lose consciousness. In the meantime, all of the victims have chemical on their clothing (Fig. 22–2). Without going into specific details of particular chemicals, how might rescue be effected?

The first responders must attempt to identify the chemical from the placard on the truck. Especially note the logo W̶, which means USE NO WATER. The chemical may ignite, explode, or produce toxic fumes with water. The responders should notify central dispatching for fire department, police, and EMS backup and indicate that specialized resources or expertise may be required for a hazardous materials incident. If the placard can be read, the dispatcher can call CHEMTREC for specific handling informa-

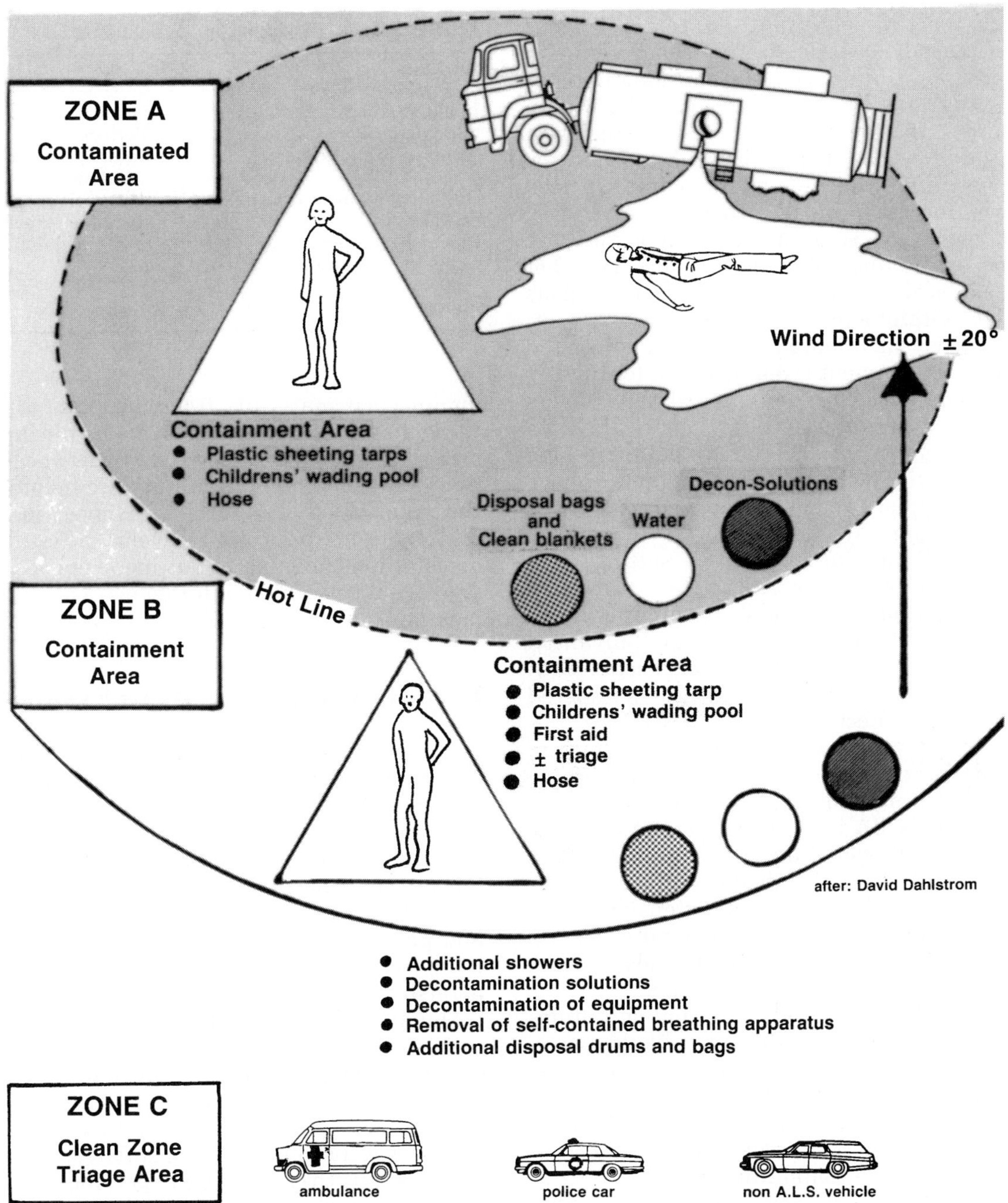

Figure 22–2. Sequence for field decontamination.

tion. Police, fire department, or EMS personnel should have access to the DOT *Emergency Response Guide: Emergency Handling of Hazardous Materials in Surface Transportation*. Access to other guides, Poisindex, or a poison control center for further information should be available, if possible. A triage or medical station should be set up upwind from the site at a "safe" distance. Distances are listed in the DOT Emergency Response Guidebook. An area designated as contaminated or hot should be defined (Fig. 22–2). An intermediate or containment area should be established. Rescuers can continue decontamination and emergency treatment in this area.

Rescuers should enter the contaminated area with full protective gear unless the hazard assessment indicates otherwise. Information is contained in several guides available to rescue personnel or from CHEMTREC. If the details of the release are uncertain, then level A protective gear is essential.

Only a minimum of first aid, such as attention to the cervical spine and exsanguinating hemorrhage, should be attempted in a highly toxic environment. Do not intubate or establish intravenous access in a highly toxic environment. Move victims from the immediate area of the spill. Remove all clothing. In general, wash the entire body, including the hair, quickly with water: Exceptions to this rule include contaminants that are elemental metals, such as sodium, which react violently with water. All of the wash water must be contained. This can be done in a number of ways. Children's plastic wading pools or plastic sheeting may be used with an earthen dam or brick border to prevent used wash water from entering ground water. Three fire ladders may be laid sideways in a triangle and tarpaulins placed over them to form a pool. All waste water, hoses, tarpaulins, pools, and so on are left inside the "hot line" for the environmental cleanup team. The "hot line" defines a border between the toxic or hazardous area and the containment area (see Fig. 22–2).

The victims may then move or be moved across the hot line to the containment reduction area for further decontamination. Rescuers then discard outer layers of gloves, boot covers, and suits and place these in disposal containers in the "hot" area before crossing the line. SCBAs may need to be left on, and are the last piece of equipment removed. In the containment area, more thorough washing should take place. This may be done in a similar manner by setting up a hose or some type of shower. All waste water must be contained so as not to spread contamination.

More thorough attention to injuries and advanced airway management can be given in this zone. With very toxic materials, rescuers still will be hampered in their efforts by protective suits and SCBA.

The victims are wrapped again in clean blankets as they move from zone B (containment area) to zone C (clean area). Rescuers discard additional protective clothing, and the SCBA is removed last, on entering the clean zone. All contaminated equipment and clothing is placed in bags and drums for later decontamination or disposal. Here, more extensive triage can take place, and intravenous lines and other advanced life support treatment can take place. Note that all movement is upwind from the spill.

Since one cannot be absolutely sure that decontamination is complete in the field, one should use a non–advanced life support (ALS) vehicle if possible. Decontamination of an ALS vehicle is time-consuming and costly and availability is extremely limited. To have one out of service for decontamination imposes a hardship on the community.

The selection of receiving hospitals must be based on the number of victims and the hospital's ability to manage concomitant trauma, burns, contamination, and systemic toxicity (Table 22–4).

All equipment and gear in vehicles and in the emergency department should be protected from any contamination by layers of plastic and blankets, if possible.

Decisions about evacuation are based on the identification of the chemical, information from the transporter or manufacturer, chemical characteristics, explosive characteristics, danger of fire, means of safe evacuation, and weather conditions.

Additional community planning for chemical hazards involves surveying local industries for products manufactured and products imported into the community that are used in the manufacturing process. As previously mentioned, MSDSs should be available for all such materials from the plant that is using the materials. Surveying for major pipelines in one's area and knowing major road, rail, and water shipping routes in one's community are helpful. Enlisting the support of all agencies involved in a chemical disaster and instituting several mock disasters or disaster drills can point out inefficiencies in the plan and areas in which interagency communication is lacking.

Table 22–4. Antidotes for Systemic Toxins

Antidote	Toxin
Lilly Cyanide Antidote Kit	Cyanide
Methylene blue	Methemoglobin
Atropine/Pralidoxime	Organophosphates/ carbamates
Oxygen/hyperbaric oxygen	Carbon monoxide/cyanide
Calcium	Hydrofluoric acid
Chelators (dimercaprol, dimercaptosuccinic acid, ethylenediametetraacetic acid)	Heavy metals

Regional Assessment of Exposure

A major hazardous spill may raise fears in the general population of possible long-term toxic effects. Patients and workers immediately exposed to the chemical hazard, such as firefighters, EMS personnel, and police, may require ongoing medical surveillance. The long-term environmental impact also must be assessed. If a survey of the immediate area and patient population shows no significant hazard, then the public may be reassured. In the event a persistent hazard is determined to exist, local and national authorities may need to expand testing in concentric circles from the exposure site.

The physician, however, also must be aware of the mass psychogenic component that is commonly present in perceived environmental exposures. Whether or not patients are suffering toxic effects, it is likely that they also will experience symptoms and signs of catecholamine release. Some persons may have nonspecific symptoms such as headaches, nausea, vomiting, hyperventilation, chest pain, and paresthesias. Objective signs other than tachycardia, tachypnea, mild hypertension, and respiratory alkalosis are generally lacking when symptoms are caused only by this syndrome. However, secondary cardiac ischemia, seizures, and other acute emergency conditions may present in the absence of toxic exposure, precipitated by the panic condition.

Hospital Management

Cutaneous decontamination is not required for all patients exposed to a hazardous material. Exposure to an inhaled toxin (e.g., carbon monoxide or arsine gas) poses little risk for secondary contamination, and decontamination is not required. Many gases (e.g., isocyanates, chlorine) can cause skin and mucous membrane injury and necessitate formal decontamination. Any liquid or solid material must be removed promptly. If uncertainty exists, then decontamination is mandatory.

Surface swipes before and after dermal cleansing can provide valuable information on the extent of contamination and efficacy of removal. Portable radiation detectors guide the duration and intensity of decontamination. Assessing the adequacy of chemical decontamination is more difficult in that the analysis takes more time. The physician will often not know "how clean is clean?" and will be forced to terminate decontamination based on less objective criteria.

Decontamination is *always* best performed prior to hospital arrival. A patient is never too unstable to have clothing removed and a brief decontamination performed in the field. Decontamination in the field must be repeated at the hospital. Initial decontamination will be required at the hospital for those patients not evaluated at the scene.

Decontamination may occur inside the hospital in specially designed facilities equipped with a separate ventilation system that will provide adequate air flow. Air return from this room must never enter the hospital. Many specialized sites will have floor drains leading to holding tanks that are easily accessed by hazardous waste contractors for toxin removal. An expenditure of large amounts of money is not necessary for the safe, efficient management of patients. The majority of hospitals will decontaminate patients outside the emergency department. Portable curtains will provide privacy and warm water can be delivered outside in all weather. Portable decontamination stretchers allow for synchronous decontamination and resuscitation. Portable wading pools are an inexpensive means of containment of irrigation fluid for ambulatory patients. Contaminated patients must always be decontaminated prior to entry into the main emergency department.

Protection of hospital personnel is of primary importance. The medical team must always be equipped with a level of protection consistent with the contamination of the victim. Patient care must never be initiated prior to the donning of appropriated protection. An SCBA is probably not required if the decontamination occurs outside. Chemically resistant clothing and gloves are vital for the safe management of patients. Local hazardous materials teams often provide initial decontamination at the hospital for patients not evaluated in the field.

Water irrigation, mild soap, and gentle washing is the initial approach for all toxins except elemental metals (e.g., sodium, lithium). These metals explode on contact with water and should be removed by other methods prior to the application of water. Occasionally detergents, dilute bleach, or the addition of corn meal will be required. The irrigation of contaminated wounds should take priority. Care must be taken not to allow irrigation runoff to contaminate clean skin.

A small number of dermal toxins require special attention. Phenol is best removed with 200 to 400 molecular weight polyethylene glycol or isopropanol. Small amounts of water increase dermal absorption. "Deluge" quantities of water are required when polyethylene glycol is not available. Limited data indicate that hexavalent chromium may be treated with topical ascorbic acid to allow reduction to the trivalent (less toxic) state. White phosphorus will fume or flame spontaneously on contact with air. Prior to debridement, the phosphorus should be covered with a moistened gauze. A Wood's lamp allows visualization of phosphorus in tissues. Copper sulfate irrigation of wounds for phosphorus visualization can cause copper toxicity and provides little benefit over a Wood's lamp. Calcium gluconate is the antidote in hydrofluoric acid (HF) exposures (Table 22–4). HF is a weak acid but causes systemic and local toxicity through its strong affinity for calcium and magnesium ions. Severe exposure to concentrated HF is associated with rapid hemodynamic compromise. Intravenous calcium must be administered early in these cases to control arrhythmias and shock. Dilute HF (<20%) typically causes delayed pain and tissue injury presenting as late as 24 hours postexposure. Topical application of a 2.5% calcium gluconate gel and parenteral narcotics constitute the initial management of dermal injury. If this fails to relieve pain, then calcium gluconate can be infiltrated into the wounds at a dose of .5 mL/cm^2. Hand wounds with persistent pain that do not respond to topical therapy are best managed with an intra-arterial infusion of calcium gluconate (10 mL of a 10% solution mixed with 40 mL of saline infused over 4 hours) until pain is resolved. Patients should not be discharged home with persistent pain.[35]

References

1. Levitin HW, and Task Force on Hazardous Materials: Hospital Based Hazardous Materials: Emergency Preparedness. White Paper from the Disaster Section of American College of Emergency Physicians, Dallas, 1996.
2. Hall IH, Dara VR, Price-Green PA, et al: Surveillance for Emergency Events Involving Hazardous Substances—United States, 1990–1992. MMWR *43*:ss-2, July 22, 1994.
3. Sauer H: CHEMTREC data: Personal communication, 1994.
4. Kirk MA, Cisek J, Rose SR: Emergency department response to hazardous materials incidents. Emerg Clin North Am *12*:461–481, 1994.
5. Agency for Toxic Substances and Disease Registry: Managing Hazardous Materials Incidents: vol 1. Emergency Medical Systems. Washington, DC, US Department of Health and Human Services, 1993.
6. ACEP Disaster Planning Interogatory. Dallas, American College of Emergency Physicians, 1995.
7. Baxter PJ: Review of major chemical incidents and their medical management: Major chemical disaster—medical aspects of management. *In* Murray V (ed): International Congress and Symposium Series, No. 155. London, Section of Occupational Medicine, Royal Society of Medicine Services, 1990.
8. Aydelotte C: Bhopal tragedy focuses on changes in chemical industry. Occup Health Safety 54:33–35, 1985.
9. Bhopal Working Group: The public health implications of the Bhopal disaster. Am J Public Health 77:230–235, 1987.

10. Irani SF, Mahashur AA: A survey of Bhopal children affected by methyl isocyanate gas. J Postgrad Med 32:195–198, 1986.
11. Deutsch PV, Adler J, Richter ED: Sentinel markers for industrial disasters. Israel J Med Sci 28:526–533, 1992.
12. Kamat SR, Mahashur AA, Twari AK, et al: Early observations on pulmonary changes and clinical morbidity due to the isocyanate gas leak at Bhopal. J Postgrad Med 31:63–72, 1985.
13. Marwick C: Bhopal tragedy's repercussions may reach American physicians. JAMA 253: 2001–2004, 1985.
14. Lorin, HG, Kuling PE: The Bhopal tragedy: What has Swedish disaster medicine planning learned from it? J Emerg Med 4:311–316, 1986.
15. Naik SR, Acharya VN, Bhalerao RA, et al: Medical survey of methyl isocyanate gas–affected population of Bhopal: Part I. J Postgrad Med 32:175–184, 1986.
16. Haddad LM: Acute poisoning. *In* Bennett JC, Plum F (eds): Cecil Textbook of Medicine, 20th ed. Philadelphia, WB Saunders, pp 503–510, 1996.
17. Klaassen CD, Amdur MO, Doull J: Casarett and Doull's Toxicology. 3rd ed. New York, Macmillan, 1986.
18. Rumack BH, Hall AH: Methyl Isocyanate Management: Tomes Information System, vol 55. Denver, Micromedex, 1988.
19. Das JJ: The Bhopal tragedy. J Indian Med Assoc 83:73–74, 1985.
20. Carpenter D: Chernobyl, Ukraine 10 years later. Ann Arbor News, April 18, 1996.
21. Mould RF: Chernobyl: The Real Story. Oxford, England, Pergamon Press, 1988.
22. Gale RP: Final Warning: The Legacy of Chernobyl. New York, Warner Books, 1988.
23. Greenwald J: Chernobyl: May 12, 1986. New York, Time Inc and Compact Publishing, 1994.
24. Agency for Toxic Substances and Disease Registry: Managing Hazardous Materials Incidents: vol 2. Hospital Emergency Departments. Washington DC, US Department of Health and Human Services, 1993.
25. National Institute for Occupational Safety and Health (NIOSH): Pocket Guide to Chemical Hazards, NIOSH publication No. 85–114. Washington, DC, US Department of Health and Human Services, 1985.
26. Organisation for Economic Cooperation and Development (OECD): Health Aspects of Chemical Accidents: OECD environment monograph No. 81, UNEP IE/PAC technical report No. 19. Paris, 1994.
27. Leonard RB: Hazardous Materials Accidents: Initial Scene Assessment and Patient Care. Aviat Environ Med 64:546–551, 1993.
28. Borak J, Callan M, Abbott W: Hazardous Materials Exposure. Englewood Cliffs, NJ, Brady, 1991.
29. Binder S: Deaths, injuries, and evacuations from acute hazardous materials releases. Am J Public Health 79:1042–1044, 1989.
30. Agency for Toxic Substances and Disease Registry: Managing Hazardous Materials Incidents: vol 3. Medical management guidelines for acute chemical exposures. Washington, DC, US Department of Health and Human Services, 1994.
31. Doyle CJ: Resources for Toxicology: Critical Decisions in Emergency Medicine. vol 6. Dallas, ACEP Publishing, 1993.
32. Proctor NH, Hughes JP: Chemical Hazards of the Workplace, 2nd ed. Philadelphia, JB Lippincott, 1988.
33. US Department of Transportation: Hazardous Material-Emergency Response Guidebook. Washington, DC, US Department of Transportation, 1994.
34. Doyle CJ: Hazardous chemicals. Emerg Med Clin North Am 1:653, 1983.
35. Upfal M, Doyle CJ: Medical Management of Hydrofluoric Acid Exposure. J Occup Med 32:726, 1990.

Suggested Reading

Burgess WA: Recognition of Health Hazards in Industry: A Review of Materials and Processes. New York, John Wiley & Sons, 1981.

Noji EK, Kelen GD: Manual of Toxicologic Emergencies. Chicago, Year Book Medical Publishers, 1989.

Rorison DG, McPherson SJ: Acute toxic inhalations. Emerg Med Clin North Am 10:2, 1992.

Rumack BH, Hall AH, et al: Poisonindex. Denver, Tomes, Micromedec (updated every 3 months), Aug 31, 1995.

Sullivan JB Jr, Krieger GR (eds): Hazardous Materials Toxicology. Baltimore, Williams & Wilkins, 1992.

National Transportation Statistics Annual Report. Washington, DC, US Department of Transportation, Sept 1993.

Walter RA, DiGregorio RC, Kooyoomjian KJ, et al: A Statistical Analysis of Hazardous Material Releases Reported to the National Response Center: Proceedings of the 1986 Hazardous Materials Spills Conference. St Louis, 1986, pp 163–171.

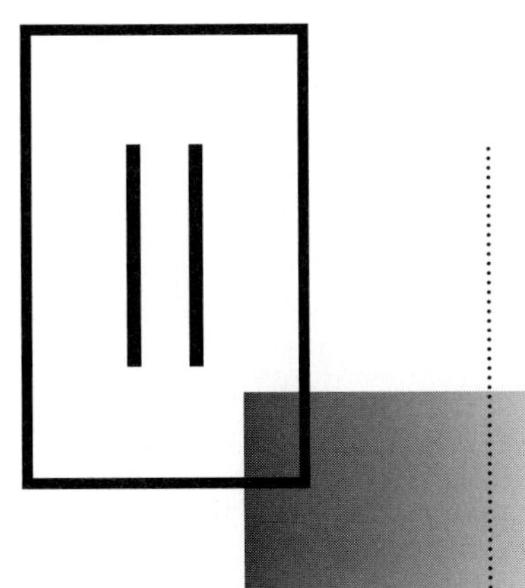

II

Specific Poisons

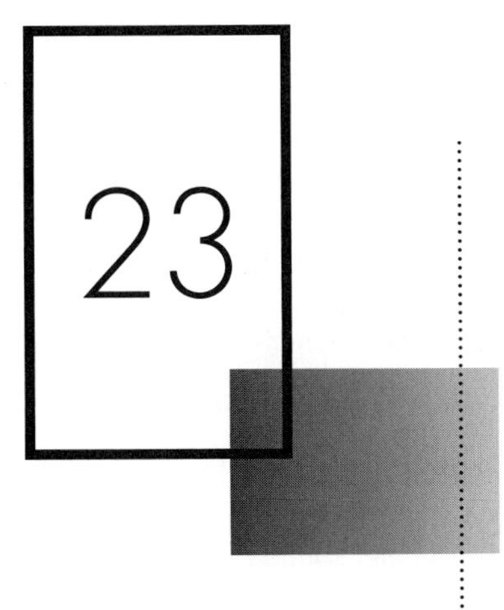

SECTION **A**

NATURAL AND ENVIRONMENTAL TOXINS

North American Venomous Snakebite

FRANK G. WALTER, MD
MIGUEL C. FERNÁNDEZ, MD
LESTER M. HADDAD, MD

ETIOLOGY

Venomous snake classification remains as controversial as the treatment of snakebite. Some experts regard the Crotalidae as a distinct family,[1–5] whereas others regard the Crotalidae as a subfamily of the Viperidae.[6, 7] Some experts regard the Laticaudae as a distinct family,[1] whereas others regard the Laticaudae as a subfamily of the Hydrophiidae.[6] Table 23–1 lists some of the important poisonous snakes of the world, some of which are maintained as exotic snakes in our national zoos (see Color Figs. 23–1 through 23–6).

In North America, two snake families have venomous members, the Crotalidae and Elapidae.[2] At least one species of indigenous snake is found in every state of the United States except Alaska, Hawaii, and Maine.[3]

North America has three genera of Crotalidae, *Crotalus*, *Sistrurus*, and *Agkistrodon* (Table 23–2).[7] Rattlesnakes are members of the genera *Crotalus* and *Sistrurus*.[2, 7] Members of the genus *Agkistrodon* lack rattles. North America has 17 species of Crotalidae and numerous subspecies (see Table 23–2).[7]

North America has two genera of Elapidae, *Micruroides* and *Micrurus*.[7] *Micrurus fulvius* consists of two subspecies, *Micrurus fulvius fulvius*, the eastern coral snake and *Micrurus fulvius tenere*, the Texas coral snake (see Table 23–1).[7]

EPIDEMIOLOGY

The 1994 report of the American Association of Poison Control Centers documented 1,328 venomous North American snakebites (Table 23–3).[8] Of these, 59% were by rattlesnakes, 32% by copperheads, 4% by cottonmouths, 4% by coral snakes, and 1% by unspecified crotalids (see Table 23–3).[8] In this case series, 85% of victims were treated in health care facilities (see Table 23–3).[8] In this series, 2 patients died, 1,279 patients suffered morbidity, and 47 patients had no significant health effects and could be considered to have had "dry bites" (i.e., bites from venomous snakes that do not result in signs or symptoms of envenomation[2]) (see Table 23–3).[8] This 4% dry bite incidence is in contradistinction to the 20% to 25% dry bite incidence quoted by many authors.[9] Russell estimated 20% of crotalid bites were dry bites and Parrish found 27% of bites were dry bites; however, Wingert and Chan found a low incidence of dry bites (1%).[2, 3, 10]

Snakebite is most common in school-age children, adolescents, and young adults.[3, 10, 11] Two studies found the highest snakebite rates in 5- to 19-year-olds.[3, 11] Another study found that 55% of victims were 17 to 27 years old, with a mean age of 24 years and a median age of 22 years.[10]

Most snakebite victims are male. Two studies reported 2:1 male-to-female ratios.[3, 11] One study reported a 9:1 male-to-female ratio.[10]

Snakebites occur most frequently in the Southeastern, South Central, and Southwestern United States (Table 23–4).[3] The ten states with the highest incidence of snakebite are detailed in Table 23–4.[3]

Snakebite varies not only by geographic region, but also by anatomic region. In one study, 58% of victims were bitten in a lower extremity; 38% in an

Table 23–1. Classification of Some Important Poisonous Snakes of the World

Family	Common Name	Scientific Name	World Region
Colubridae	Boomslang	*Dispholidus typus*	Central and Southern Africa
Elapidae	Coral		
	Eastern coral*	*Micrurus fulvius fulvius*	Southeast US
	Texas coral	*Micrurus fulvius tenere*	South Central US
	Arizona or Sonoran	*Micruroides euryxanthus*	Southwest US
	Cobra		
	Egyptian	*Naja haje*	Egypt, Arabia, and the Sahara
	Indian	*Naja naja naja*	India
	King	*Ophiophagus hannah*	India, China, Malay archipelago, Philippines
	Cape	*Naja nivea*	Southern Africa to the Cape
	Mamba		
	African green	*Dendroaspis angusticeps*	Central and Southern Africa
	African black	*Dendroaspis polylepis*	Central and Southern Africa
	Krait		
	Malayan	*Bungarus candidus*	Malaysia and Indonesia
	Banded	*Bungarus fasciatus*	India, Indochina, Malay archipelago
	Blue	*Bungarus caeruleus*	India, Bangladesh, Sri Lanka
	Australian-Pacific		
	Common death adder	*Acanthophis antarcticus*	Australia
	Tiger snake	*Notechis scutatis*	Australia
	Taipan	*Oxyuranus scutellatus*	Australia and New Guinea
Hydrophiidae	Yellow-bellied sea snake	*Pelamis platurus*	All of Pacific and Indian oceans
	Common sea snake	*Enhydrina schistosa*	Western Pacific Ocean
	Yellow-lipped sea brait	*Laticauda colubrina*	Tropical coasts of Eastern Indian, Western Pacific oceans
	Stoke's sea snake	*Astrotia stokesi*	Pacific, near Australia
	Banded sea snake	*Hydrophis spiralis*	Pacific, near Malaya
Viperidae	Asp viper	*Vipera aspis*	Elba and Sicily, Spain, France, and Italy
	Russell's viper	*Vipera russelli*	Thailand, Burma, India, China, and Indonesia
	European viper (adder)	*Vipera berus*	Great Britain and Europe through Bosnia to Asia
	Long-nosed viper	*Vipera ammodytes*	Bosnia, southeastern Europe to Middle East
	Carpet (saw-scaled) viper	*Echis carinatus*	Middle East to India, and northwest Africa
	Desert horned viper	*Cerastes cerastes*	Sahara to Arabian peninsula
	Puff adder	*Bitis arietans*	Africa
	African gaboon viper	*Bitis gabonica*	Africa
Crotalidae	Agkistrodon (see Table 23–2)		
	Mamushi	*Agkistrodon halys*	Japan and Korea
	Malayan pit viper	*Agkistrodon calloselasma*	Malaya, Indochina, Sumatra
	Bothrops		
	Barba amarilla	*Bothrops atrox*	Central America
	Fer-de-lance	*Bothrops lanceolatus*	Martinique
	Jararaca	*Bothrops jararaca*	Amazon region of South America
	Crotalus (see Table 23–2)		
	Cascabel	*Crotalus durissus terrificus*	South America
	Central American rattler	*Crotalus durissus durissus*	Central America
	Lachesis		
	Bushmaster	*Lachesis mutus mutus*	Amazon region of South America
	Sistrurus (see Table 23–2)		
	Trimeresurus		
	Habu	*Trimeresurus flavoviridis*	Ryukyu islands and Okinawa

*See Color Figs. 23–1 through 23–6 at the beginning of the book.

upper extremity; 0.7% in the torso; 0.5% in the head, face, or neck; and in 2.8% of bites, the site was not clearly specified.[3] This study also found more victims were bitten on the right side of their bodies (55%) than the left.[3] In another study, 87% of victims were bitten in an upper extremity, 12% in a lower extremity, and 1% in the torso.[10]

The bite site is related to the victim's activity at the time of the bite. In one study, victims were engaged in the following activities when they were bitten, in descending order of frequency: playing, working, or walking in their own yards; working on a farm or ranch; playing outside their own yards; hunting or fishing; pursuing other outdoor recreational activities; handling a venomous snake; walking on or near a highway; working or playing inside a barn or henhouse; picking up logs or lumber; picking berries; reaching into obscure places; and engaging in mili-

Table 23–2. Some Crotalidae of North America*

Genus	Species	Subspecies	Common Name	U.S. Location
Crotalus	*adamanteus*		Eastern diamondback rattlesnake*	Southeast U.S.
	atrox		Western diamondback rattlesnake	Southwest U.S.
	cerastes		Sidewinder	Southwest U.S.
	horridus		Timber rattlesnake*	North and Eastern U.S.
	lepidus		Rock rattlesnake	Southwest U.S.
	mitchelli		Speckled rattlesnake	Southwest U.S.
	molossus		Black-tailed rattlesnake	Southwest U.S.
	pricei		Twin-spotted rattlesnake	Southwest U.S.
	ruber		Red diamond rattlesnake	California
	scutulatus	*scutulatus*	Mojave rattlesnake*	Southwest U.S.
	tigris		Tiger rattlesnake	Arizona
	viridis	*abyssus*	Grand Canyon rattlesnake	Grand Canyon
		cerberus	Arizona black rattlesnake	Arizona
		concolor	Midget faded rattlesnake	Colorado, Utah
		helleri	Southern Pacific rattlesnake	California
		lutosus	Great Basin rattlesnake	Western U.S.
		nuntius	Hopi rattlesnake	Arizona
		oreganus	Northern Pacific rattlesnake	Northwest U.S.
		viridis	Prairie rattlesnake	Rocky Mountains
	willardi		Ridge-nosed rattlesnake	Arizona, New Mexico
Sistrurus	*catenatus*		Massasauga	Midwest to Southwest
	miliarius		Pigmy rattlesnake	Southeast U.S.
Agkistrodon	*contortrix*		Copperhead*	Massachusetts to Texas
	piscivorus		Cottonmouth*	Virginia to Texas

*See Color Figs. 23–1 through 23–6 at the beginning of the book.

tary maneuvers.[11] Only 4% of patients were handling a venomous snake.[11] This correlates with more lower extremity bites (63%) and fewer upper extremity bites (34%) in this study.[11] This is in contradistinction to another study in which 57% of victims were handling a venomous snake, 28% were clinically intoxicated with ethanol, and 87% were bitten in an upper extremity.[10]

Snakebites occur most commonly during the warmest months of the year when snakes are most active and people are out-of-doors more often. In one study, 94% of snakebites occurred from April through October.[3] In another study, 73% of snakebites occurred from April through September.[10]

Snakebites occur most commonly during the morning, afternoon, and evening hours when people are most active out-of-doors. In one study, 77% of victims were bitten between 9 AM and 9 PM.[3] In another study, 88% of victims were bitten between 10 AM and 10 PM.[10]

CROTALIDAE SNAKEBITE

Clinical Presentation

Pathophysiology

Crotalid venom has multitudinous chemical constituents that act in concert to produce snake venom poisoning in a specific victim.[2] The clinician must always remember to treat the patient, not the snake, the venom, or the known or suspected venom constituents.[2]

Venom is 70% water by weight.[12] Lyophilized or desiccated venom is 90% protein and polypeptides by dry weight.[12]

The main functions of crotalid venom are immobilization, death, and digestion of prey.[2] Not only do crotalids use venom offensively to obtain food, but also defensively as protection against predators and aggressors.[2] Most crotalid venoms do not produce

Table 23–3. Epidemiology of Bites from Venomous North American Snakes

Type of Snake	No. (%) of Patients	No. (%) of Patients Treated in Health Care Facility	No. (%) with No Morbidity	No. (%) with Life-Threatening Morbidity	No. (%) of Deaths
Rattlesnake	782 (59)	654 (84)	26 (3)	61 (8)	2 (0.3)
Copperhead	419 (32)	377 (90)	9 (2)	10 (2)	0 (0)
Coral	62 (4)	51 (82)	7 (11)	2 (3)	0 (0)
Cottonmouth	59 (4)	47 (80)	4 (7)	2 (3)	0 (0)
Unspecified crotalid	6 (1)	2 (33)	1 (17)	0 (0)	0 (0)
Total	1328 (100)	1131 (85)	47 (4)	75 (6)	2 (0.2)

From Litovitz TL, Felberg L, Soloway RA, et al: 1994 annual report of the American Association of Poison Control Centers toxic exposure surveillance system. Am J Emerg Med *13*:551, 1995.

Table 23–4. Geographic Distribution of Snakebite in the United States

State	Incidence per 100,000 People/yr
North Carolina	18.79
Arkansas	17.19
Texas	14.70
Georgia	13.44
West Virginia	11.29
Mississippi	10.83
Louisiana	10.25
Oklahoma	8.85
Arizona	7.83
South Carolina	7.72

From Parrish HM: Incidence of treated snakebites in the United States. Pub Health Rep *81*:269, 1966.

immobilization through neuromuscular blockade.[2] Immobilization is usually due to polypeptide, lethal venom components that produce hypovolemic shock so prey cannot escape.[2] These polypeptide, lethal venom components ultimately kill prey due to hypovolemic shock.[2] Digestion is mediated via numerous proteolytic and other enzymes.[1, 2] This digestive function is critical to snakes because they swallow prey whole and do not masticate their food.[2] The digestive ability of crotalid venom is facilitated by injection into live prey while some perfusion continues to distribute venom.[2] The venom's polypeptide, lethal components damage endothelial cells and allow plasma to exude and blood to extravasate into surrounding tissues, producing hypovolemic shock due to third-spacing.[2] Leaky capillaries also allow delivery of digestive components of snake venom to tissues; this speeds digestion.[2] When live prey was fed to the crotalid, *Bothrops jararacussu*, digestion time was 4 to 5 days versus 12 to 14 days for dead prey.[2]

The Mojave rattlesnake, *Crotalus scutulatus scutulatus,* with venom A, is the classic exception to the fact that most crotalids immobilize prey with polypeptide, lethal venom components that produce hypovolemic shock.[13–20] Mojave rattlesnakes with venom A have Mojave toxin that immobilizes prey by neuromuscular blockade.[13–20] Mojave toxin is an acidic protein that consists of a basic phospholipase A_2 subunit and an acidic peptide subunit.[13–17] Some other North American crotalid species (e.g., *Crotalus tigris, C. viridis concolor, C. horridus, C. atrox*) have been shown to have some amounts of Mojave toxin in their venoms; however, Mojave rattlesnake venom A has the most Mojave toxin and the lowest median lethal dose (LD_{50}) values of any North American crotalid venom.[13–23] Other populations of Mojave rattlesnakes with venom B lack Mojave toxin and immobilize prey by producing hypovolemic shock from third-spacing similar to other crotalids.[18–25] Mojave rattlesnakes with venom B are located predominantly in areas surrounding and between Phoenix and Tucson, Arizona.[18–20]

Clinical Manifestations

Pathophysiologic, clinical manifestations of crotalid envenomation can be thought of in a familiar "A,B,C,D,E" paradigm.[26] The cardiovascular and neuromuscular systems are primarily at risk because these primary toxic targets are fundamentally affected by venom (Table 23–5).[2, 5, 27] Secondary toxic targets can be affected by indirect complications from crotalid venom's primary effects (see Table 23–5).[27]

The primary toxic target of most crotalid venoms is the cardiovascular system, especially vascular endothelial cells.[2, 5, 28] Crotalid venom produces capillary endothelial cell damage, resulting in endothelial cell swelling and rupture, which leave large gaps in the microvasculature that allow third-spacing of plasma and extravasation of erythrocytes.[28] Endothelial cell damage is due to relatively low-molecular-weight polypeptides.[1, 29] These polypeptides have molecular weights between about 4,500 and 6,000 daltons.[1] They produce shock with intravascular hemoconcentration and hypoproteinemia due to exudation of plasma through the damaged capillary endothelium.[1] This correlates clinically with profound edema that does not necessarily involve extravasation of large numbers of erythrocytes; therefore, hypovolemia can result from third-spacing of plasma.[1, 2]

While endothelial cells are damaged by lower-molecular-weight nonenzymatic polypeptides, vascular basement membranes and perivascular extracellular matrices are destroyed by hemorrhagic metalloproteinases (zinc-containing enzymes with molecular weights between 20,000 and 100,000 daltons) that allow extravasation of erythrocytes.[30] This correlates clinically with hemorrhage into envenomated parts of the body.[1, 30] This extravasation of plasma and erythrocytes leads to shock and death in prey animals and can lead to shock and death in severely envenomated humans.

Other significant cardiovascular effects of venom are its direct actions on the clotting ability of blood.[1, 2] Crotalid venom characteristically causes a disseminated intravascular coagulation (DIC)-like syndrome through fibrinogenolysis by thrombin-like, enzymatic venom glycoproteins with molecular weights between 29,000 and 35,000 daltons. These thrombin-like glycoproteins produce fibrin monomers, either fibrinopeptide A, most commonly, or fibrinopeptide B, rarely, depending on the specific venom, without utilizing the victim's own thrombin.[1, 2, 31–36]

These thrombin-like venom glycoproteins do not activate factor XIII to produce cross-linked fibrin, whereas thrombin *does* activate factor XIII in true

Table 23–5. Targets of Crotalid Venom's Toxic Effects

Body Components at Risk	Primary Targets	Secondary Targets
Airway		X
Breathing		X
Cardiovascular system	X	
Disability (neuromuscular system)	X	
Elimination (kidneys and liver)		X

DIC to produce cross-linked fibrin that yields D-dimer on fibrinolysis. Non–cross-linked fibrin formed from thrombin-like crotalid enzymes is rapidly lysed to fibrin degradation (split) products, but not D-dimer, and the intravascular thrombosis with microangiopathic hemolytic anemia and intravascular consumption of platelets that is typical of true DIC does not occur.[1, 2, 31–36] Exsanguination is rare from crotalid envenomations because the victim's ability to form thrombin, and thereby cross-linked fibrin, remains intact, and hemostasis can occur.[1, 2, 31–36]

The fundamental difference between true DIC and DIC-like syndromes from crotalid venoms is that true DIC always involves pathologic generation and activity of the victim's endogenous thrombin, whereas DIC-like syndromes do not.[1, 2, 31–36] Other differences between true DIC and DIC-like syndromes from crotalid venoms are outlined in Table 23–6.[1, 2, 31–36] The pathophysiologic differences between true DIC and DIC-like syndromes from crotalid venoms have important therapeutic implications.[1, 2, 31–36] Crotalid antivenin is effective for crotalid, venom-induced coagulopathies, but heparin and blood products are not.[1, 2, 31–36] Heparin is ineffective for crotalid, venom-induced coagulopathies because crotalid, thrombin-like enzymes are not inhibited by antithrombin III (heparin cofactor).[1, 2, 31–36] Transfused blood product coagulation factors and platelets are ineffective for crotalid venom–induced coagulopathies because they are destroyed by circulating venom.[1, 2, 31–35] Therefore, administration of blood products to patients with crotalid venom–induced coagulopathies may expose patients to the risks of blood product therapy without the benefits, unless they are actively exsanguinating despite copious antivenin administration and intensive supportive care.[1, 2, 4, 5, 31–35, 37]

Table 23–6. Comparison of True DIC with DIC-Like Syndromes from Crotalid Venoms

Manifestations and Therapy	DIC	DIC-Like Syndromes
Pathologic thrombin production and activity	Yes	No
Pathologic activation of factor XIII by thrombin	Yes	No
Thrombin production of both fibrinopeptides A and B	Yes	No
Production of either fibrinopeptide A or B, but not both	No	Yes
Production of cross-linked fibrin	Yes	No
Production of fibrin degradation (split) products	Yes	Yes
Production of D-dimer	Yes	Uncommon
Antithrombin III depletion	Yes	No
Thrombocytopenia	Almost always	Sometimes
Active bleeding	Commonly	Rarely
Intravascular thrombosis	Commonly	Rarely
Heparin therapy helpful	Possibly	No
Crotalid antivenin therapy helpful	No	Yes

DIC, disseminated intravascular coagulation.

Crotalid venom results in platelet aggregation without serotonin release.[33, 34] Investigators isolated a timber rattlesnake toxin, a serine protease termed Crotalocytin, that aggregates platelets.[38]

Although a characteristic DIC-like syndrome from crotalid venoms is described, crotalid venom–induced coagulopathies often vary markedly from case to case.[2, 31] Many crotalid envenomations are accompanied by no significant laboratory abnormalities.[2] Others demonstrate isolated hypofibrinogenemia, isolated thrombocytopenia, or some combination of these, with or without prolongation of the prothrombin time, partial thromboplastin time, or elevated fibrin degradation (split) products.[2, 31, 33] In general, certain species of crotalids may produce characteristic coagulopathies in their victims.[31] For example, the Southern Pacific rattlesnake (*Crotalus viridis helleri*) characteristically produces severe thrombocytopenia without significant hypofibrinogenemia.[31, 39] Despite generalizations, exceptions always exist; although 90% of victims of pigmy rattlesnake (*Sistrurus miliarius*) bites had no defibrination, 10% did.[31] One pigmy rattlesnake envenomation even resulted in true DIC, a rare and reportable event.[31, 40] Not only do venom constituents vary within and between crotalid species, but they also vary in the same snake depending on its age and the season of the year.[41, 42]

Fibrinolysis due to DIC-like syndromes from crotalid venom is due to indirect activation of plasminogen by release of tissue plasminogen activator from damaged vascular endothelial cells.[34]

Crotalid envenomation can also cause thrombocytopenia.[1, 2, 4, 5, 31–37] Thrombocytopenia is predominantly due to consumption of platelets at the envenomation site, where disrupted microvasculature exposes platelets to collagen in basement membranes, producing local platelet deposition and aggregation.[28, 30, 35]

The major clinical problems encountered in caring for victims of crotalid envenomations are local tissue destruction due to digestive enzymes, edema due to exudation of plasma, hemorrhage due to destruction of the microvasculature, shock due to hypovolemia, and neuromuscular blockade in some victims (see Table 23–5). Although the cardiovascular and neuromuscular systems are primarily at risk in snake venom poisoning, airway and breathing can be at risk due to massive orofacial or neck edema when the victim is envenomated in the mouth, face, or neck.[43, 44] Airway and breathing can also be at risk due to neuromuscular blockade as a result of Mojave toxin's effect on muscles involved in airway patency and ventilation.[23] Airway and breathing can also be compromised as a result of coma from intravenous or perivenous envenomations or coma from shock with decreased ability to maintain airway patency and ventilation.[45, 46] Elimination via the kidneys can be disrupted because of acute tubular necrosis due to shock or myoglobinuric renal failure due to rhabdomyolysis.[23, 45] The most common clinical manifestations from crotalid bites in one case series are reported in Table 23–7.[2]

Table 23–8. Crotalid Envenomation: Minimal-Moderate-Severe Scoring Method

Minimal Envenomation	Moderate Envenomation	Severe Envenomation
Local swelling Other local changes No systemic signs or symptoms Normal laboratory values	Swelling beyond bite site Systemic signs and/or symptoms Abnormal laboratory values	Marked local response Severe systemic signs and symptoms Markedly abnormal laboratory values

From Dart RC, Hurlbut KM, Garcia R, et al: Validation of a severity score for the assessment of crotalid snakebite. Ann Emerg Med *27*:321, 1996.

Diagnosis

Differential Diagnosis

The differential diagnosis of snakebite includes puncture wounds and abrasions from other causes, wound infections, cellulitis, deep venous thrombosis, DIC, thrombocytopenia from other causes, inherited bleeding disorders, septicemia, hypovolemic shock from other causes, and weakness as a result of neuromuscular blockade from other causes.

The diagnosis of snake venom poisoning is usually simple because the patient, family, or friends tell the clinician that the patient has been bitten by a snake. However, it is important to consider snake venom poisoning in the differential diagnosis of preschool children, developmentally delayed patients, patients with ethanol or drug intoxication, or unconscious patients who present with puncture wounds, abrasions, edema, or ecchymoses, with or without coagulopathies, shock, or fasciculations. Snake envenomation must be considered in the patient with an *unknown* bite. This is especially true in areas in which a high incidence of snakebites occurs (see Table 23–4).[3] Numerous cases of snakebites have been noted in small children who came in crying after playing in the yard.[11]

It is essential to completely undress and examine all nonspeaking patients and patients with altered sensoria to search for snakebite punctures or abrasions, and to search for other local, regional, or systemic signs of envenomation.[46] The authors have cared for diabetic patients with poor vision due to diabetic retinopathy and poor lower extremity sensation due to diabetic neuropathy who were unaware of a snakebite but presented with wounds in edematous, ecchymotic legs and had crotalid venom–induced coagulopathies.

Clinical Diagnosis

Diagnosis of envenomation from a snakebite is a clinical diagnosis. A *history* of snakebite is the most helpful diagnostic tool. This history can be obtained from the patient, family, friends, or prehospital care personnel. Signs and symptoms of crotalid envenomation are detailed in Tables 23–7 through 23–11.[2, 27, 47]

Table 23–7. Clinical Manifestations of Crotalid Bites

Signs or Symptoms	% of Patients
Fang marks (punctures or abrasions)	100
Edema	74
Weakness	72
Pain	65
Diaphoresis	64
Oral, perioral, scalp, or feet paresthesias	63
Abnormal pulse rates	60
Light-headedness, faintness, dizziness	57
Ecchymoses	51
Nausea, vomiting, or both	48
Abnormal blood pressures	46
Paresthesias near the envenomation site	42
Fasciculations	41
Regional lymphadenopathy	40
Abnormal respiratory rates	40
Bullae	40
Thirst	34
Abnormal body temperatures	31
Local tissue necrosis at bite site	27
Cyanosis	16
Hematemesis, melena, or hematuria	15
Unconsciousness	12
Seizures	1

From Russell FE: Snake Venom Poisoning. 2nd ed. Great Neck, NY, Scholium International, p 281, 1983.

Table 23–9. Crotalid Envenomation: Grade 0–IV Scoring Method

Grade	Characteristics
0	No envenomation: fang marks and minimal pain
I	Minimal envenomation: fang marks, pain, 1 to 5 in. of edema and erythema during the first 12 hr; no systemic symptoms
II	Moderate envenomation: fang marks, pain, 6 to 12 in. of edema and erythema in the first 12 hr; systemic symptoms may be present along with rapid progression of signs from grade I; may be bloody ooze at bite site
III	Severe envenomation: fang marks, pain, edema >12 in. in first 12 hr; systemic symptoms, including coagulation defects after crotalid bites; signs of grades I and II appear in rapid progression, with immediate systemic signs and symptoms
IV	Very severe envenomation; local reaction develops rapidly; edema may involve ipsilateral trunk; ecchymoses, necrosis, blebs, and blisters develop; at tightly restrictive fascial planes, tension may become great enough to obstruct venous or even arterial flow

From Dart RC, Hurlbut KM, Garcia R, et al: Validation of a severity score for the assessment of crotalid snakebite. Ann Emerg Med *27*:321, 1996.

Table 23–10. Crotalid Envenomation: The Snakebite Severity Score

Criteria	Points*
Pulmonary system	
No symptoms/signs	0
Dyspnea, minimal chest tightness, mild or vague discomfort, or respirations of 20 to 25/min	1
Moderate respiratory distress (tachypnea, 26 to 40 breaths/min; accessory muscle uses)	2
Cyanosis, air hunger, extreme tachypnea, or respiratory insufficiency/failure	3
Cardiovascular system	
No symptoms/signs	0
Tachycardia (100 to 125 beats/min), palpitations, generalized weakness, benign dysrhythmia, or hypertension	1
Tachycardia (126 to 175 beats/min) or hypotension, with systolic blood pressure >100 mm Hg	2
Extreme tachycardia (>175 beats/minute), hypotension with systolic blood pressure <100 mm Hg, malignant dysrhythmia, or cardiac arrest	3
Local wound	
No symptoms/signs	0
Pain, swelling, or ecchymosis within 5–7.5 cm of bite site	1
Pain, swelling, or ecchymosis involving less than half the extremity (7.5–50 cm from bite site)	2
Pain, swelling, or ecchymosis involving half to all of the extremity (50–100 cm from bite site)	3
Pain, swelling, or ecchymosis extending beyond affected extremity (>100 cm from bite site)	4
Gastrointestinal system	
No symptoms/signs	0
Pain, tenesmus, or nausea	1
Vomiting or diarrhea	2
Repeated vomiting, diarrhea, hematemesis, or hematochezia	3
Hematologic signs	
No signs or symptoms	0
Coagulation parameters slightly abnormal: PT, <20 sec; PTT, <50 sec; platelets, 100,000–150,000/mL; or fibrinogen, 100–150 µg/mL	1
Coagulation parameters abnormal: PT, 20 to 50 sec; PTT, 50 to 75 sec; platelets, 50,000–100,000/mL; or fibrinogen, 50–100 µg/mL	2
Coagulation parameters abnormal: PT, 50 to 100 sec; PTT, 75 to 100 sec; platelets, 20,000 to 50,000/mL; or fibrinogen, <50 µg/mL	3
Coagulation parameters markedly abnormal, with serious bleeding or the threat of spontaneous bleeding: unmeasurable PT or PTT; platelets, <20,000/mL; or undetectable fibrinogen; severe abnormalities of other laboratory values also fall into this category	4
Central nervous system	
No symptoms/signs	0
Minimal apprehension, headache, weakness, dizziness, chills, or paresthesia	1
Moderate apprehension, headache, weakness, dizziness, chills, paresthesia, confusion, or fasciculation in area of bite site	2
Severe confusion, lethargy, seizures, coma, psychosis, or generalized fasciculation	3

PT, prothrombin time; PTT, partial thromboplastin time.
*Points are assessed on the basis of manifestations caused by the venom itself (antivenom reactions not included). Ranges given are for adults; appropriate compensation should be made for age.
From Dart RC, Hurlbut KM, Garcia R, et al: Validation of a severity score for the assessment of crotalid snakebite. Ann Emerg Med 27:321, 1996.

Table 23–11. Crotalid Envenomation: Determining the Degree of Envenomation

Degree of Envenomation	Contiguous Manifestations	Systemic Manifestations	Laboratory Abnormalities
None or trivial ("dry bite")	Punctures or abrasions; pain and tenderness at bite	None	None
Mild or minimal	Punctures or abrasions; pain, tenderness, edema, and erythema at and adjacent to bite	Perioral paresthesias	None
Moderate	Punctures or abrasions; pain, tenderness, edema, and erythema beyond area adjacent to bite	Perioral paresthesias; peripheral paresthesias; gustatory changes; nausea; emesis; diarrhea; weakness; light-headedness; diaphoresis; chills	↑ PT; ↑ PTT; ↓ platelets; ↓ fibrinogen; ↑ hemoglobin
Severe	Punctures or abrasions; pain, tenderness, edema, and erythema of entire extremity	Ventilatory insufficiency; hypotension; shock; bleeding; altered mental status; fasciculations; seizures	↑ ↑ PT; ↑ ↑ PTT; ↓ ↓ Platelets; ↓ ↓ fibrinogen; ↑ ↑ hemoglobin

PT, prothrombin time; PTT, partial thromboplastin time

The most important aspects of clinical diagnosis of crotalid envenomation are determining the degree of envenomation on presentation (see Tables 23–8 through 23–11) and determining whether progression of the envenomation syndrome (i.e., worsening of clinical signs and symptoms) is occurring over time. Three common systems are used to determine the degree of envenomation on presentation: (1) the minimal-moderate-severe scoring method, (2) the grade 0 through IV scoring method, and (3) the snakebite severity score (see Tables 23–8 through 23–10).[47] The snakebite severity score (see Table 23–10) is a recently published research tool and is not intended for clinical use at this time. The authors use a modified minimal-moderate-severe scoring method that integrates portions of all three systems; this is detailed in Table 23–11.[27]

Serial physical examinations and assessment of vital signs and clinical status, searching for tissue edema, induration and tenderness, progression of swelling, and development of systemic signs and symptoms, *are essential to proper diagnosis and management of the snakebite victim.*

Laboratory Diagnosis

Laboratory diagnosis of snake venom poisoning focuses predominantly on detection of the following: coagulopathies; hemoconcentration due to third-spacing of plasma; anemia due to extravasation of erythrocytes or other sources of bleeding; rhabdomyolysis as indicated by elevated creatine phosphokinase values, elevated creatinine levels not attributable to renal failure, and myoglobinuria; and hematuria or hemoglobinuria on urinalysis. Laboratory tests to detect these potential abnormalities should be obtained on presentation and periodically thereafter. The authors recommend obtaining a complete blood count with platelets, prothrombin time, partial thromboplastin time, fibrinogen, and fibrin degradation (split) products on presentation and every 4 hours thereafter for at least the first 12 hours of hospitalization. This is recommended because laboratory evidence of coagulopathy may not be evident initially or can worsen after initial presentation. Frequency of obtaining these laboratory data should be determined by the clinician depending on the patient's clinical course, the results of the laboratory tests, and whether and when the patient receives antivenin. After administering antivenin, the authors prefer to obtain these laboratory data every 4 hours until values have returned to normal or to stable near-normal levels. *Obtaining blood for typing and screening prior to giving antivenin is critical, because blood typing can be more difficult after antivenin administration.*

The authors often screen for laboratory abnormalities due to concurrent illnesses that may confound the care of envenomated patients. This also helps to determine whether coagulopathies are the result of an envenomation or of underlying severe liver disease.

Chest radiography and electrocardiograms should be obtained for patients with preexisting cardiopulmonary diseases and for patients with cardiopulmonary signs or symptoms. The authors do not routinely obtain these for all patients with crotalid envenomations. All snakebitten patients should receive an intravenous lifeline, continuous cardiac monitoring, frequent automated blood pressure measurements, and pulse oximetry.

Treatment

Poisoning Treatment Paradigm

Care of envenomated patients can be thought of in a familiar "A,B,C,D,E" paradigm.[26] Basic resuscitation is similar for all envenomated patients. This includes a primary survey and resuscitation consisting of management of airway and breathing; cardiovascular resuscitation, including administration of intravenous fluids; treatment of any disability (i.e., preserving neuromuscular function); and complete exposure of the patient with environmental control.[26] In addition to the primary survey and resuscitation, the "A,B,C,D,E" mnemonic can be modified to organize care of envenomated patients by utilizing the poisoning treatment paradigm (Table 23–12).[27] The poisoning treatment paradigm organizes therapy of poisoned patients by considering whether kinetic aspects of a toxin can be modified, by determining whether the effects of the toxin can be modified pharmacodynamically with an antidote, and by reemphasizing basic care of the patient (i.e., the primary survey and resuscitation) (see Table 23–12).[27]

Immediate Measures: First Aid and Prehospital Care

In 1994 and 1995, some North American snakebite authorities published their viewpoints regarding first aid for crotalid bites.[48, 49] These authorities agreed on most aspects of first aid and prehospital care; however, some differences of opinion still existed, based on individual clinical experiences and lack of large prospective clinical studies.[48, 49] These viewpoints are summarized in Table 23–13 with modifications re-

Table 23–12. Poisoning Treatment Paradigm

General Paradigm	Specific Therapy for Crotalid Envenomation
Alter absorption	The Extractor Sling
Antidote	Wyeth polyvalent crotalid antivenin
Basics	Resuscitation basics (A,B,C,D,E) IV isotonic crystalloid Cleanse and dress wounds Tetanus immunization No antibiotics
Change catabolism	None
Distribute differently	None
Enhance elimination	None

Table 23–13. Immediate Snakebite Treatment

First Aid and Prehospital Care	No	Yes	Controversial
Capture snake	X		
Incise fang marks	X		
Oral suction	X		
Electric shock to denature venom	X		
Ice	X		
Tourniquet	X		
Constriction bands	X		X
Splint	X		X
The Extractor		X	X
Sling		X	
Isotonic IV in other extremity		X	
EMS activation with a cellular phone		X	
Rapid transport		X	

IV, intravenous; EMS, emergency medical services.

flecting the authors' clinical experiences and review of the literature.[48, 49]

The most important principle of first aid for snakebite victims is, *"Primum non nocere"* (first, do no harm). First aid measures have never been proven to decrease morbidity or mortality from crotalid envenomations. A large case series of victims of rattlesnake bites found no differences in clinical courses between patients who did and did not receive first aid.[10]

Another important "first aid" principle is to realize that its name means no more than it says. First aid is the first step in beginning a treatment process that includes definitive care with antivenin, if indicated. In other words, first aid should never be considered a substitute for definitive medical care and should never delay in-hospital administration of antivenin if it is indicated.

First aid and prehospital measures for snakebite can be considered to fall into three categories: (1) those that may be helpful and are unlikely to be harmful, (2) those that may be helpful but may become harmful, and (3) those that are unhelpful or harmful. *All patients who may have been bitten by a venomous snake should be taken to an appropriate health care facility as soon as possible.* Any delay can be fraught with danger. The most helpful first aid tool is a cellular phone, which allows the rapid summoning of emergency medical services (EMS) without moving the victim. Walking has been shown to increase transit time of ersatz venom in a human study.[50] Rapid EMS transport is the safest form of first aid and prehospital care for snakebite.

Other first aid and/or prehospital care that is likely to be helpful, or at least not harmful, includes applying a sling to bitten upper extremities and keeping the bite site in a neutral position (i.e., at heart level). Another reasonable prehospital EMS intervention is to start a large-bore intravenous line in a nonbitten extremity to infuse isotonic crystalloid. This serves as an intravenous lifeline to allow administration of isotonic crystalloids if noticeable swelling begins.

Snake identification is helpful. For example, knowing the patient was bitten by a Mojave rattlesnake is useful, because aggressive antivenin therapy and supportive care is necessary and often life saving. Identifying a copperhead is helpful because antivenin is generally unnecessary. Harmless snakes characteristically have round pupils, rows of teeth that leave imprints on the skin, a double caudal plate, and the absence of a pit. Although snake identification is helpful, it is unnecessary to capture or kill the snake for identification.[48, 49] Attempts to capture or kill the snake could result in more bites to the victim and bites that could turn potential rescuers into victims.[48, 49] Administration of antivenin (Crotalidae) polyvalent (Wyeth-Ayerst, Philadelphia) is effective for all crotalid envenomations and does not require definitive identification of the envenomating crotalid.[5, 48, 49]

Controversial crotalid bite first aid and prehospital measures that may be helpful but also may be potentially harmful include use of constriction bands, splints involving constriction bands, and The Extractor (Sawyer Products, Safety Harbor, FL). Published data on The Extractor are limited.[51, 52] Radiolabeled crotalid venom was injected into rabbits and The Extractor was applied 3 minutes after injection.[51] After 3 minutes of suction (i.e., 6 minutes after venom injection), 23% of the injected venom was removed by The Extractor.[51] Thirty-four per cent of radiolabeled venom was removed after suction for 30 minutes (i.e., 33 minutes after injection).[51] The only published data on use of The Extractor in patients is an abstract describing three people bitten by rattlesnakes.[52] Two of the three patients exhibited clinical signs of envenomation and venom was recovered from the wounds of these two patients with The Extractor.[52] The Extractor was left in place until its cup filled with serosanguineous fluid; this was repeated five times in each patient.[52] The largest portion of venom was recovered during the initial application of The Extractor.[52] The clinician should be aware that both of these references are to abstracts and include small numbers of subjects.[51, 52] There are unanswered questions regarding use of The Extractor. Does removal of some portion of injected venom improve the patient's clinical course? Does The Extractor concentrate venom at the bite site and result in more bite site necrosis? In summary, use of The Extractor is not unreasonable, but it remains unproven and controversial.[53–55]

Use of constriction bands is also controversial. Most authors use the term *constriction band* to describe a device that impairs efflux of superficial venous and lymphatic flow from bitten extremities.[4, 48–50, 56–58] Although some studies with envenomated animals and one human study with ersatz venom indicated decreased efflux from extremities with constriction bands, no human clinical studies have shown proven safety or efficacy.[50, 56–58] An animal study showed that systemic absorption of crotalid venom was decreased with constriction band therapy using a sphygmomanometer cuff with the pressure maintained at 45 mm Hg.[56] Continual adjustments, allowing air to escape from the cuff, were necessary to avoid limb-threatening constriction as the envenomated animal's leg swelled.[56] Continual cuff adjustments would be difficult in first aid and prehospital care. In addition, the 45 mm Hg cuff pressure exceeds normal capillary perfusion pressure of about 30 mm Hg. Another animal study found that elastic wrapping of an envenomated extremity at 55 mm Hg and splinting decreased systemic absorption of Australian elapid venom; however, Australian elapid venom causes minimal tissue edema.[57] This study also showed that splinting alone or pressure wrapping alone did not limit systemic venom absorption.[57] Both techniques had to be used simultaneously to limit venom absorption.[57] Another study used similar elastic wrapping and splinting and showed decreased systemic absorption of Eastern diamondback rattlesnake venom; however, the high pressure (initially 55 mm Hg) could cause extreme pain in a swollen envenomated extremity and could cause limb-threatening ischemia as swelling increased.[58] Splinting the envenomated limb is also controversial because splinting involves circumferential elastic wrapping that could also compromise limb perfusion as swelling increases due to crotalid envenomation. In summary, constriction bands have not been studied clinically in North American patients with crotalid envenomations; therefore, their safety and efficacy are unproven and the authors do not recommend them. A constriction band could turn what is uncommonly a life-threatening event (6%) into a limb-threatening event (see Table 23–3).[8]

The remaining first aid and prehospital measures are mentioned only to condemn them, because they are either ineffective or dangerous:[4, 5, 48, 49]

1. Do not incise fang marks.[5, 48, 49] Incision by persons without training or experience can result in damage to deep structures and can introduce infection and exacerbate tissue necrosis.[5, 48, 49]
2. Do not use oral suction.[5, 48, 49] Oral suction can introduce human oral flora and carries the theoretical possibility of causing a human bite infection.[5, 48, 49] Oral suction can also result in envenomation of the lips and/or mouth if the lips are cracked or have lesions or if there is a break in the oral mucosa.
3. Do not apply ice or immerse the envenomated extremity in ice, ice water, or snow.[2, 5, 48, 49, 59] So called cryotherapy can result in profound tissue necrosis due to further vasoconstriction and ischemia in marginally perfused tissues.[2, 5, 48, 49, 59]
4. Do not apply a tourniquet that would result in obstruction of deep venous or arterial flow.[2, 5, 48, 49] This will exacerbate ischemia, infarction, and necrosis in a limb that already may have marginal perfusion due to envenomation. A tourniquet also endangers a limb on which a patient has received a dry bite, without any envenomation or risk of morbidity.[2, 5, 48, 49]
5. Do not use electric shock to treat snakebites.[4, 5, 48, 49, 60–64] Studies have shown that electric shocks are ineffective and clinical experience has shown that they can be dangerous.[4, 5, 48, 49, 60–64]

Hospital Care

When a snakebitten patient arrives at the hospital, the clinician should perform a standard primary survey and resuscitation ("A,B,C,D,E").[26] Most patients will not require airway or breathing interventions such as oxygen administration or endotracheal intubation, because most crotalid envenomations are not life-threatening.[8] However, patients with signs or symptoms of dyspnea or hypoxia should receive oxygen and assisted ventilation, if necessary. Endotracheal intubation should be performed for the usual indications.[26] Prompt endotracheal intubation is necessary for any patient with any signs of envenomation to the lips, tongue, head, or neck.[43, 44] Endotracheal intubation must be done as soon as possible, before massive swelling of the airway occurs, which would make endotracheal intubation difficult or impossible. It is critical that endotracheal intubation be done as soon as possible, because cricothyroidotomy would be extremely difficult in the presence of a swollen neck and venom-induced coagulopathy. Not only are airway patency and breathing in danger of being compromised as a result of head and neck envenomations, they also may be compromised as a result of rare occurrences of anaphylactoid, angioedematous reactions involving the upper airway secondary to intravenous or perivenous envenomations and as a result of rare envenomations associated with adult respiratory distress syndrome (ARDS).[45, 46, 65, 66]

Cardiovascular resuscitation is critical in moderate and severe crotalid envenomations with marked third-spacing of plasma into subcutaneous tissue and extravasation of erythrocytes through damaged microvasculature. Intravascular volume resuscitation should be guided by the usual clinical parameters (e.g., administering enough intravenous isotonic crystalloids to relieve the patient's thirst and to produce urine output of at least 1 mL/kg per hour).[45, 65–67]

Basic neuromuscular resuscitation involves endotracheal intubation with mechanical ventilation for those uncommon patients with moderate to severe Mojave toxin envenomations that produce neuromuscular blockade and ventilatory insufficiency.[13–21, 23] Ventilatory insufficiency can also develop because of a decreased level of consciousness due to shock and hypoperfusion of the brain,[45] in rare cases of snakebite complicated by seizures,[2] and in rare cases of intravenous or perivenous envenomations associated with coma.[46]

Basic resuscitation to preserve the organs of elimination (i.e., the liver and kidneys) is directed primarily at preserving renal perfusion and urine output. The liver is rarely damaged by crotalid venom poisoning. Occasionally, the kidneys are damaged due to acute tubular necrosis from hypoperfusion and hypovolemia or myoglobinuric renal failure from rhabdomyolysis.[10, 23, 40, 45, 66–69]

Other basic supportive care for crotalid snakebites

includes cleansing the wound and keeping it clean and dry. We usually recommend application of a dry 4 × 4 gauze pad to the wound itself, without tape. Taping the dressing in place can result in vesiculation and formation of bullae due to shearing forces from the tape on the skin as the affected extremity swells. Tetanus immunization should be given if needed.

Prophylactic antibiotics are not mandatory for snakebite because there is no evidence that they are effective.[70, 71] Routine use of prophylactic antibiotics is no longer recommended.[9, 70, 71] Broad-spectrum antibiotics are indicated only if signs of wound infection are present.[9, 70, 71] Older recommendations to prophylactically administer antibiotics to patients with snakebite were based on studies of the oral flora of snakes and not on the incidence of wound infection following North American snakebites.[72]

Administration of the Antidote

Antivenin (Crotalidae) polyvalent has been commercially available in the United States since 1954.[73] Wyeth polyvalent crotalid antivenin is manufactured by immunizing horses with venom from four crotalid species, *Crotalus adamanteus* (Eastern diamondback rattlesnake), *C. atrox* (Western diamondback rattlesnake), *C. durissus terrificus* (South American or tropical rattlesnake), and *Bothrops atrox* (fer-de-lance).[74] This polyvalent antivenin is capable of neutralizing venom from all North, Central, and South American crotalids.[73, 74] Because this antivenin is derived from immunization of horses it is of equine origin and can cause true anaphylaxis (type I hypersensitivity), anaphylactoid reactions, and serum sickness, i.e., immune-complex disease (type III hypersensitivity).[4, 5, 9, 73, 74]

Prior to administration of any medication, the clinician must ask a five-part question: What are the indications, contraindications, complications, dosage, and route of administration for the medication?[27] Answers to the five elements of this general question are summarized for Wyeth polyvalent crotalid antivenin in Table 23–14.[27]

Wyeth polyvalent crotalid antivenin is the mainstay of therapy for snake venom poisoning from North American crotalids, especially the rattlesnake.[4, 73, 75–78] It is critical to remember to treat the patient, not the snake.[2]

Antivenin therapy shows regional differences within the United States. Identification of the specific North American crotalid that bit the patient is not necessary in the Western United States, where crotalid snakebite envenomation is often serious and life-threatening, and Wyeth polyvalent crotalid antivenin is usually administered.

However, in the Eastern United States, where the most common culprit of venomous snakebite is the copperhead, observation and supportive care may be all that is indicated, as antivenin therapy is usually not necessary. Antivenin therapy is almost always necessary for the Eastern diamondback rattlesnake, and is generally indicated for the cottonmouth, or water moccasin.

Table 23–14. Guidelines for Use of Wyeth Polyvalent Crotalidae Antivenin

5 General Questions	Answers for Use of Wyeth Crotalidae Antivenin	
Indications	Mild, moderate or severe crotalid envenomations	
Contraindications	Relative contraindications: Horse product allergy Inability to manage anaphylactoid reactions and anaphylaxis (life-threatening envenomations) Absolute contraindications: Refusal after informed consent Inability to manage anaphylactoid reactions and anaphylaxis (non–life-threatening envenomations)	
Complications	Anaphylactoid reactions Anaphylactic reactions (type I hypersensitivity, IgE-mediated) Serum sickness (type III hypersensitivity; antigen-antibody, immune complex–mediated)	
Dosage*	*Degree of Envenomation*	*Initial No. of Vials**
	Dry bite (no envenomation)	0
	Mild	0–10
	Moderate	10–20
	Severe	20
Route	Intravenous in an intensive care setting, in the emergency department or intensive care unit	

*Depends on the region of the country, type of snake, and clinical presentation (see text).

Polyvalent crotalid antivenin is indicated in severe cases of crotalid envenomation and in mild to moderate crotalid envenomations with progression (worsening) of clinical signs and symptoms. Some experts recommend that all patients with progressive worsening of signs and symptoms from crotalid envenomations receive antivenin immediately.[4] Progression is defined as worsening of the local injury, laboratory abnormalities, or systemic manifestations.[4]

The clinician should never be lulled into a false sense of security just because the patient and/or clinician knows the envenomation is from a copperhead bite. Fatal copperhead bites have been reported.[79] The authors recently consulted on an intravenous or perivenous copperhead bite to a patient's medial malleolus that resulted in shock, ventilatory failure, seizure, and coma that required immediate endotracheal intubation, mechanical ventilation, massive intravenous fluid administration, and antivenin therapy. Ultimately, the patient recovered without permanent sequelae.

Any medication has relative and absolute contraindications. Relative contraindications to Wyeth polyvalent crotalid antivenin include a history of horse product allergy, a history of previous allergic reaction to Wyeth polyvalent crotalid antivenin, and inability of the clinician to manage an anaphylactic or anaphylactoid reaction in a patient with a life-threatening envenomation (see Table 23–14).[27] An absolute contraindication to Wyeth polyvalent crotalid antivenin is the patient's refusal after informed consent, if he is awake, alert, fully oriented, with a clear sensorium, without clinical signs of drug or ethanol intoxication, and reiterates and understands the risks and benefits of antivenin therapy. Another absolute contraindication is inability of the clinician to manage an anaphylactic and/or anaphylactoid reaction in a patient without a life-threatening envenomation.

The main complications of Wyeth polyvalent crotalid antivenin are anaphylactic reactions (type I hypersensitivity), anaphylactoid reactions, and serum sickness (type III hypersensitivity).[4, 5, 9] Anaphylactic or anaphylactoid reactions are immediate complications of antivenin therapy that occur during antivenin administration. Serum sickness, an immune-complex disease, is a delayed complication of antivenin administration.

Anaphylactic and anaphylactoid reactions are indistinguishable clinically.[80–82] Despite their indistinguishable clinical appearances, anaphylactic and anaphylactoid reactions differ on the basis of pathogenesis.[80–82] An anaphylactic reaction is a type I hypersensitivity reaction, an anamnestic reaction, which requires initial exposure to an antigen that results in production of IgE antibody that attaches to mast cells via its Fc portion.[80–82] After this initial sensitization step, reexposure to even the smallest concentrations of the inciting antigen elicits an anaphylactic reaction due to the antigen binding to preformed IgE attached to mast cells, resulting in degranulation of mast cells with release of histamine and other mediators.[80–82]

Anaphylactoid reactions also result in release of histamine and other mediators from mast cells, but this release is not dependent on IgE.[80–82] Another important distinction between anaphylactic and anaphylactoid reactions is that the smallest concentrations of the antigen will elicit an IgE-dependent anamnestic response in true anaphylactic reactions; however, substances that elicit anaphylactoid reactions are not acting as antigens for preformed IgE, and therefore the smallest concentrations of these substances will not necessarily elicit an anaphylactoid reaction.[80–82] In other words, anaphylactoid reactions are elicited in a fashion that is concentration-, rate-, and dose-dependent. This has important therapeutic implications, especially when administering heterologous proteins such as Wyeth polyvalent crotalid antivenin. By maximally diluting the Wyeth polyvalent crotalid antivenin and administering it slowly, anaphylactoid reactions may be modulated or avoided. True IgE-mediated anaphylactic reactions cannot be avoided with dilution or slower administration.

Anaphylactoid reactions to antivenin are called *anticomplement reactions* by some experts.[5, 83, 84] This anticomplement reaction is thought to result from immunoglobulin and other protein aggregates that directly activate the complement cascade with formation of the anaphylatoxins, C3a and C5a.[5, 73, 82–84] One study showed a 23% incidence of anaphylactic or anaphylactoid reactions in patients treated with Wyeth polyvalent crotalid antivenin.[85] Half of these patients manifested only cutaneous signs and symptoms, whereas half of the affected patients manifested systemic signs and symptoms.[85] Treatment of these antivenin reactions were uniformly effective with no mortality, minimal morbidity, and no permanent sequelae.[85] Another study found that 14% of antivenin-treated patients developed urticaria, 10% developed pruritus, 6% suffered hypotension, 1% suffered bradycardia, and 1% suffered apnea that investigators thought was related to antivenin administration.[10] No patient in this study suffered permanent sequelae from any of these complications.[10] Another study found that 14% of antivenin-treated patients developed a rash, 4% developed a rash and fever, and 14% suffered hypotension and/or respiratory distress.[86]

Serum sickness, a subtype of type III hypersensitivity, is an immune-complex disease due to antigen-antibody complexes.[87] These immune complexes trigger a wide variety of inflammatory processes, including activation of the complement cascade to generate C3a and C5a (anaphylatoxins), which stimulate release of vasoactive amines such as histamine and serotonin and also stimulate release of chemotactic factors from mast cells and basophils.[73, 87, 88] The C5a complement component is also chemotactic for basophils, eosinophils, and neutrophils.[87]

The incidence of serum sickness seems dose related. One study found an 83% incidence of serum sickness in patients who received more than 8 vials of Wyeth polyvalent crotalid antivenin versus a 38% incidence in patients who received less than 8 vials; however, due to the small sample size, this difference was not statistically significant.[85]

Clinically, serum sickness may manifest the following signs and symptoms: fever, malaise, urticaria, lymphadenopathy, myalgias, arthralgias, and, rarely, vasculitis, glomerulonephritis, or neuritis.[73, 87] These signs are due to deposition of antigen-antibody complexes in susceptible tissues. Under nonpathologic conditions, antigen-antibody complexes are cleared by the reticuloendothelial system without sequelae; however, under pathologic conditions, with increased microvascular permeability and slight antigen excess, these antigen-antibody complexes diffuse between damaged endothelial cells and deposit along the basement membrane. These immune complexes trapped in microvascular walls activate complement, exacerbate the inflammatory response, and release vasoactive mediators. Signs and symptoms are commonly manifest in the skin and synovia. Onset of serum sickness after Wyeth polyvalent crotalid antivenin administration usually occurs between 3 days and 3 weeks after administration, with an average onset of about 1 week.

Dosage of Wyeth polyvalent crotalid antivenin is determined by the victim's degree of envenomation and has nothing to do with the victim's age or weight.[2, 27, 47] This is because antivenin neutralizes a specific amount of venom. Clinically, the amount of venom is estimated by the effect of the venom on the patient. This can be estimated by various grading systems (see Tables 23–8 through 23–11).[27, 47]

When the decision for antivenin therapy has been made, it is important to note that the recommended dose of antivenin has increased over the years.[4] Although regional differences have been noted, from 5 to 10 vials (given intravenously) of Wyeth polyvalent crotalid antivenin may be required as the *initial* dose in all treated rattlesnake envenomations.[4, 27] In rapidly progressive envenomations or in those with hemodynamic instability, up to 20 vials of antivenin may be required *initially,* in addition to aggressive resuscitation.[4, 9, 27] After the initial antivenin administration, obtain serial laboratory data every 4 hours and do serial physical examinations at least hourly for evidence of continuing progression (i.e., worsening of clinical signs and/or laboratory data). Repeat antivenin therapy, usually in the range of 5 to 10 vials at a time, may be necessary, until the patient's condition becomes stable.[4, 9]

Some parameters indicating an end-point for administration of antivenin include cardiovascular stability, manifested by an increase in blood pressure or diminution of pulse rate in a patient in shock; a rise in platelet count or fibrinogen level, a halt in muscle fasciculation, or the advance of swelling; an improvement in the patient's sense of well-being; or a general improvement in the patient's condition.[45]

The route of antivenin administration is always intravenous.[4, 9, 27] Intravenous administration allows systemic antivenin distribution to counteract systemic venom effects and allows precise titration of antivenin to help prevent or modulate anaphylactoid reactions that are concentration-, rate-, and dose-dependent. Wyeth polyvalent crotalid antivenin should not be administered intramuscularly or into the wound area.

Prior to intravenous administration of Wyeth polyvalent crotalid antivenin, a skin test should be administered.[4, 5, 9, 27, 74, 86] The skin test should only be given after the physician has decided to administer antivenin, based on progression of signs or symptoms in mild to moderate crotalid envenomations or based on a severe envenomation at presentation (see Tables 23–8 through 23–11).[4, 5, 9, 27, 47, 74, 86] This should be done after the patient has given informed consent, if possible, and before any antihistamines are given. This is because skin testing can sensitize patients to horse antigens by inducing IgE antibody formation, because skin testing has resulted in life-threatening anaphylactic and anaphylactoid reactions. Skin testing should be done before administration of any antihistamines because antihistamines can mask the signs of a positive skin test, which can include a wheal and/or flare response >10 mm in diameter, urticaria, and systemic anaphylactic or anaphylactoid reactions.[4, 5, 9, 27, 74] A wheal and/or flare reaction >10 mm in diameter is all that is necessary to declare a skin test positive.[4, 5, 9, 27, 74] Prior to the administration of the skin test, the clinician should read the package insert and call a consultant in medical toxicology or a regional poison center, unless he or she has extensive experience in administering the skin test and treating crotalid-envenomated patients. All equipment and drugs necessary to manage anaphylactic and anaphylactoid reactions must be at the bedside.[4, 5, 9, 27] A clinician who is able to manage anaphylactic and anaphylactoid reactions must also be at the bedside.[27] Two intravenous lines with isotonic crystalloid should be in place. The patient should be attached to a cardiac monitor, a pulse oximeter, and a blood pressure monitor.[27] After these precautions are taken, 0.02 mL of a 1:10 dilution of normal horse serum is injected intradermally into one shoulder and 0.02 mL of normal saline control is injected into the other shoulder.[74] The 1:10 diluted normal horse serum is already packaged, premixed, and ready for injection.[74] The control and horse serum sites should be observed for 30 minutes to see if wheal, flare, urticaria, or systemic anaphylactic or anaphylactoid reactions develop.[4, 5, 9, 27, 74]

If the skin test is positive, the clinician should reconsider using antivenin in mild and moderate envenomations and discuss the therapeutic pros and cons with the patient in light of the positive skin test.[27, 86] If antivenin will be given, the authors suggest pretreating the patient with diphenhydramine, 1 mg/kg, intravenously, or 50 mg in the average adult, and cimetidine, 6 mg/kg, intravenously, or 300 mg in the average adult.[27] Steroids are not necessarily indicated. Steroids have not been proven safe or effective in treatment of crotalid envenomations.[2, 59]

During the 30-minute observation period for the skin test, the lyophilized Wyeth polyvalent crotalid antivenin should be mixed.[4, 5, 9] This lyophilized antivenin is diluted with 10 mL of bacteriostatic water, which comes in the Wyeth polyvalent crotalid antivenin package.[74] The authors have found that the most expedient method to solubilize this lyophilized antivenom is to place the vials on an automated blood vial rocker from the hospital laboratory and gently rock the vials back and forth.[89] This allows the health care provider to care for the patient rather than to try to solubilize antivenin by rolling the vials between the palms. This also prevents vigorous shaking of the antivenin, which denatures it.[74] Foaming within the vial indicates that some denaturation has occurred.[74]

After solubilizing the lyophilized antivenom in 10 mL of bacteriostatic water, the authors prefer to dilute the antivenom 10:1 (i.e., dilute 10 vials of antivenin in 1 L of normal saline).[27, 74] Although this differs from more concentrated solutions recommended by some experts, it is the most dilute solution suggested in the *Physicians' Desk Reference,* and this more dilute solution may help prevent anaphylactoid reactions that are concentration-, rate-, and dose-dependent.[4, 5, 74] For children, we dilute the initial dose of antivenin in enough normal saline so the patient will receive an antivenin infusion that does not exceed 20 mL/kg, the usual resuscitation bolus dose for crystalloid infusions in pediatric resuscitation.[26, 27]

The dilute antivenin infusion should be started slowly and gradually increased over time to help prevent anaphylactoid reactions that are concentration-, rate-, and dose-dependent.[4, 5, 9, 27, 74] The authors use the antivenin infusion guidelines detailed in Table 23–15.[27] The guidelines are based on an integration of product information from the *Physicians' Desk Reference*, our own clinical experience, and guidelines from other experts.[4, 5, 9, 27, 74] These are reasonable guidelines, but they have never been validated by a clinical trial. Although life-threatening anaphylactic or anaphylactoid reactions can occur at any time during antivenin infusion, they usually occur while the infusion rate is gradually increased to the maximum of 960 to 1000 mL/h (see Table 23–15).[27] Therefore, the authors' usual practice is to have a clinician at the bedside who is able to manage all aspects of anaphylaxis, until the maximum infusion rate of 960 to 1000 mL/h has been achieved without complications.

If signs or symptoms of an anaphylactic or anaphylactoid reaction occur during antivenin infusion, immediately stop the infusion and treat the patient with intravenous diphenhydramine and cimetidine. If stopping the infusion and administering diphenhydramine and cimetidine do not achieve the desired result, treat the anaphylactic or anaphylactoid reaction with epinephrine and steroids (and glucagon in patients on β-blocker therapy), as in any anaphylactic or anaphylactoid reaction, regardless of the cause.[4, 5, 9, 27] If the clinician has not yet consulted with a regional poison control center or medical toxicologist, he or she may do so at this time.

Life-threatening crotalid envenomations complicated by anaphylactic and/or anaphylactoid reactions to antivenin have been treated with concomitant antivenin and intravenous epinephrine infusions.[4, 5, 9, 27, 85, 90] Intravenous epinephrine is titrated to effect during antivenin infusions in which the risk-benefit ratio seems to favor administration of antivenin. The authors are involved in a handful of such cases each snakebite season. To date, the authors' patients have suffered no permanent sequelae from this treatment.

Surgery is rarely necessary for crotalid envenomation. Twenty years ago, surgery was recommended by some as the primary treatment for crotalid envenomations,[91, 92] with early excisional débridement or fasciotomy; however, animal and human studies do not support this position.[75, 77, 93–95]

Table 23–15. Antivenin Infusion

Start the antivenin infusion at no more than 60 mL/h (1 mL/min)
If no adverse reactions occur in 3 min, increase the drip rate to 120–125 mL/h
If no adverse reactions occur in 3 min, increase the drip rate to 240–250 mL/h
If no adverse reactions occur in 3 min, increase the drip rate to 480–500 mL/h
If no adverse reactions occur in 3 min, increase the drip rate to 960–1,000 mL/h

Fasciotomy should *only* be performed when clinical signs and symptoms of compartment syndrome are present and hourly, serially measured compartment pressures exceed 30 mm Hg despite elevation of the affected limb and administration of 20 vials of antivenin after an elevated compartment pressure has been documented.[4, 5, 9, 27] This 30 mm Hg pressure limit is based on the fact that capillary perfusion pressure is usually about 30 mm Hg.[96–98] Compartment perfusion pressure is also dependent on the patient's blood pressure.[97, 99–101] One study showed significant decreases in compartmental perfusion when compartment pressures rose to within 30 mm Hg of the diastolic blood pressure.[99] Another study found compartment muscle hypoperfusion and anaerobic metabolism when compartment pressures were within 30 mm Hg of the mean arterial pressure (MAP) in nontraumatized muscles.[100] In traumatized muscles, compartment hypoperfusion and anaerobic metabolism occurred when compartment pressures were within 40 mm Hg of the MAP.[100]

The duration of clinical signs and symptoms of compartment syndrome also relates to prognosis. If compartment syndrome signs or symptoms are allowed to persist for 12 hours or more, residual functional deficits almost always occur.[97, 102] Series of patients who undergo fasciotomy within 12 hours of onset of signs or symptoms of compartment syndrome have from 0% to 17% incidence of residual functional deficits.[97, 102]

To allow for maximum antivenin dosing and effect, it is reasonable to obtain a few hourly serial compartment pressures if the patient has signs or symptoms of compartment syndrome and the initial pressure was elevated.[4, 5, 9, 27] Consider fasciotomy if the compartment pressure stays pathologically elevated after infusion of at least 20 vials of Wyeth polyvalent crotalid antivenin and elevation of the affected extremity, and well before the patient has had symptoms or signs of compartment syndrome for 12 hours.[4, 5, 9, 27, 97, 102] Guidelines for management of potential compartment syndromes from crotalid envenomations have been published.[4]

Some experts advocate intravenous mannitol to decrease compartment pressures.[4, 5, 9] The authors are unaware of any published experimental or clinical data on mannitol therapy for suspected compartment syndrome from crotalid envenomations and have not used this therapy to date. When considering whether to administer mannitol, the clinician must realize that an antivenin infusion is hyperosmolar and a large volume load. If mannitol, 1 to 2 g/kg, were administered in addition to this, the patient would receive a significant osmotic and volume challenge that could compromise patients with tenuous cardiopulmonary or kidney function. In addition, both crotalid antivenin and mannitol have been associated with anaphylactoid reactions, believed to be related in part to their hyperosmolarity. This is similar to anaphylactoid reactions that occur with hyperosmolar radiographic contrast media.

Surgical débridement of frankly necrotic tissue is reasonable. However, it is difficult to determine which tissue is frankly necrotic and which tissue may still be viable early in the course of snake venom poisoning. In addition, necrosis occurs in a minority of patients with snake venom poisoning.[2] In the series of Russell of 100 snakebitten patients in Southern California, 27% developed some necrosis of local tissue.[2] Bullae are usually left intact unless they are on digits and are circumferential or are becoming circumferential and appear to compromise digital perfusion as evidenced by lower skin temperatures measured with a thermistor, by narrower pulse volume amplitude measurements from a Doppler flowmeter, or by lower oxygen content on pulse oximetry.[27, 94] Digital dermotomy has been recommended by some.[103] Potential complications of any surgical procedure include infection, scarring, and anesthetic complications.

Patients who may have had a snakebite from a North American crotalid require medical observation for at least 12 hours.[9, 104, 105] This is because signs and symptoms of envenomation can be delayed in onset and develop insidiously.[9, 104, 105] During this observation period, hemoglobin, hematocrit, prothrombin time, partial thromboplastin time, fibrinogen, fibrin split products, and platelets should be assayed on presentation and every 4 hours thereafter to assess for development of venom-induced coagulopathies that can be delayed in onset. Every 15 to 60 minutes, the patient's affected extremity should be palpated on both the medial and lateral aspects, starting proximally at the torso and gently moving distally until the leading edge of induration, edema, and tenderness is felt.[4, 5, 9] This leading edge of induration, edema, and tenderness should be marked on the skin with the corresponding time of observation.[4, 5, 9, 27] If proximal progression of the leading edge of induration, edema, and tenderness occurs, the patient should be admitted and treated with antivenin after his or her informed consent is obtained.[4, 5, 9, 27] Antivenin administration requires an intensive care setting within the emergency department or intensive care unit.[4, 5, 9, 27] If the patient has a coagulopathy on initial presentation or develops one during observation, he or she should be admitted and receive antivenin after informed consent has been given.[4, 9, 27] If after 12 hours of close clinical observation and serial laboratory tests the clinician is certain that the snakebite was of crotalid origin, and the patient has no sign of snakebite other than punctures or abrasions (i.e., no signs of envenomation and no coagulopathy), a reliable patient can be sent home with instructions to return immediately if he or she notes any of the following: increase in pain; onset of redness, swelling, fever, or pus formation; bruising; bloody nose; red or dark urine; weakness; nausea or vomiting; faintness; dyspnea; diaphoresis; or any sign or symptom other than the mildest pain at the bite site.[4, 5, 9, 104, 105]

Prognosis

Although any significant snakebite is potentially lethal, death is unusual after North American crotalid bites (0.2% in cases reported to the AAPCC; see Table 23–3).[8] in cases reported to the American Association of Poison Control Centers. The Western Envenomation Database, a consecutive case series of crotalid bites in which the Arizona Poison Control Center was consulted by clinicians from throughout the United States, reported a mortality rate of 1.4%.[106] This 1.4% mortality rate may be artifactually high because the Arizona Poison Control Center commonly receives calls from throughout the United States for consultation on severe or unusual crotalid envenomations.[106] Therefore, a selection bias for more severe envenomations may be present in the Western Envenomation Database.[106] Selected details from the three (1.4%) fatal cases are contained in Table 23–16.[106] Common characteristics of these fatal cases include more proximal bite sites, bites due to *Crotalus* spp., little or no intravenous fluid infusion in two patients, minimal or no antivenin administration, and nonaccidental upper extremity envenomations in two patients.[106] One treating physician thought that one patient's bite was from a nonvenomous snake prior to the patient's fatal cardiorespiratory arrest 5 hours after the bite.[106]

The Western Envenomation Database also tabulated nonfatal sequelae from crotalid envenomations (Table 23–17).[106] Long-term morbidity (i.e., permanent sequelae) are more common in upper extremity and face bites (see Table 23–17).[106] This may be due to the circumstances of these bites. Most patients with upper extremity or facial bites were handling the snake at the time of the bite. Snakes that feel threatened from handling may inject larger amounts of venom. The complexity of fine motor functions and sensation in the face and upper extremities may also be more easily impaired due to venom effects, and disability would be more apparent.[106] Most long-term morbidity involved weakness, pain, decreased range of motion, hypesthesia, paresthesia, anesthesia, or skin discoloration.[106] The most common long-term morbidity was decreased range of motion.[106] Only one amputation was necessary.[106] This was an amputation of an envenomated finger.[106] These data suggest that a patient's physical therapy should begin as soon as possible after antivenin administration has halted progression of signs of envenomation and no further antivenin therapy is needed.[4, 106]

Research and Development of a New Crotalid Antivenin

A new, experimental polyvalent, crotalid, ovine-derived, fragment antibody (Fab) antivenin has been developed (Crotab, Therapeutic Antibodies, Inc., Nashville, TN).[107] This new polyvalent antivenin was developed by immunizing sheep with the venom from four North American crotalids: *Crotalus atrox* (western

Table 23–16. Fatal Crotalid Envenomations

Study Parameters	Patient 1	Patient 2	Patient 3
Age (y)	2	7	32
Sex	F	M	M
Bite site	Shoulder	Knee	Forearm
Snake	*Crotalus viridis*	*Crotalus*, unknown species	*Crotalus atrox*
Time to hospital	30 min	30 min	40 min
IV Fluids	Very slow rate	No	Several liters
Antivenin	1 vial	No	4 vials, hours after shock ensued
Other therapy	No	No	Fasciotomy, steroids
Initial assessment by physician	Severe envenomation	Nonvenomous bite	Severe envenomation
Course	Cardiorespiratory arrest at 3 h	Cardiorespiratory arrest at 5 h	Prolonged hypotension and death at 16 h
Circumstances	Nonaccidental; adult placed snake around child	Accidental, while playing	Nonaccidental; rattlesnake roundup

IV, intravenous.
From Dart RC, McNally JT, Spaite DW, et al: The sequelae of pitviper poisoning in the United States. *In* Campbell JA, Brodie ED (eds): Biology of the Pitvipers. Selva Press, Tyler, TX, pp 395–404, 1992.

diamondback rattlesnake), *C. adamanteus* (eastern diamondback rattlesnake), *C. scutulatus scutulatus* (Mojave rattlesnake with venom A), and *Agkistrodon piscivorus piscivorus* (eastern cottonmouth).[107] These venoms were chosen on the basis of their clinical importance in snakebites occurring in the United States and northern Mexico, the geographic ranges of the snakes, genetic dissimilarities of the four immunizing venoms, and cross-antigenicity with venoms from other clinically important crotalids.[107] An animal study showed that Crotab was very effective.[107]

ELAPIDAE SNAKEBITE

All three coral snake species found in the United States are venomous. There have been very few published reports of envenomations by the Sonoran or Arizona coral snake (*Micruroides euryxanthus euryxanthus*). North American coral snakes are brightly colored but are rarely noticed due to their furtive nature; therefore, encounters with coral snakes are relatively uncommon.[108] When they do occur, it is often due to deliberate handling or by accidentally reaching into piles of leaves or around rocks. United States coral snakes are most active in the early morning and late afternoon.[2, 108] Envenomation by coral snakes differs from the Crotalidae in that coral snakes have a pair of short, fixed, grooved, anterior fangs, which carry venom along the grooves from ducts located at the base of the fangs. For an effective envenomation to occur, the coral snake must usually chew or hang onto its victim for at least several seconds, because its venom is not injected directly, as is the venom of crotalids.[109]

Table 23–17. Bite Location and Sequelae After Crotalid Envenomations

Bite Sites	Total No.	Total %	Permanent Sequelae No.	Permanent Sequelae %
Finger	40	30.5	16	40
Hand	8	6.1	4	50
Arm/shoulder	2	1.5	1	50
Torso	1	0.8	0	0
Head/face/neck	1	0.8	1	100
Thigh/knee	9	6.9	0	0
Calf/ankle	35	26.7	4	11
Foot	24	18.3	3	12
Toe	11	8.4	0	0
Total	131	100.0	29	22

From Dart RC, McNally JT, Spaite DW, et al: The sequelae of pitviper poisoning in the United States. *In* Campbell JA, Brodie ED (eds): Biology of the Pitvipers. Selva Press, Tyler, TX, pp 395–404, 1992.

Pathophysiology

Elapid snake venom contains a complex mixture of polypeptides, and it may also contain cholinesterase or acetylcholine. The neurotoxic components are thought to be small polypeptides devoid of enzymatic activity that act primarily by binding postsynaptically at the neuromuscular junction. This competitive, nondepolarizing blocking of acetylcholine receptor sites is distinct from the action of curare in that it has a slow onset and a markedly prolonged duration of effect.[113, 114] Enzyme components of North American coral snake venom are thought to be of minor importance causing no or minimal tissue edema in most cases.[2, 109, 117, 118]

Clinical Manifestations

Coral snake envenomations differ clinically from crotalid envenomations in two major ways. With crotalid envenomations, the onset of signs and symptoms is usually, but not always, apparent within the first few hours after the bite. However, in elapid envenomations, *the onset of signs and symptoms may be delayed for 13 or more hours,*[109, 110] *but then they may occur precipitously.*[109, 111] Coral snake envenomations can occur with or without visible fang marks.[109, 112]

Coral snake envenomations also differ from most crotalid envenomations in that envenomation primarily produces neurotoxic effects with very few local tissue toxic effects.[109, 110]

Victims of Sonoran coral snakebite have reported local paresthesia, weakness, hand discoordination, nausea, and drowsiness. Envenomation by Eastern and Texas coral snakes can produce far more severe neurotoxic effects.

The venom of the Eastern coral snake has lower LD_{50} values than any other North American snake except the Mojave rattlesnake (*Crotalus scutulatus scutulatus*) with venom A.[115] A large coral snake may store up to four or five lethal doses of venom within its venom glands.[116] Signs and symptoms of Eastern coral snake envenomations can include local swelling (40%), paresthesias (35%), nausea (30%), vomiting (25%), euphoria (15%), weakness (15%), dizziness (10%), diplopia (10%), dyspnea (10%), diaphoresis (10%), muscle tenderness (10%), fasciculations (5%), and confusion (5%).[109] Seizures have also been reported, particularly in children, although it is unclear whether these were related to hypoxia.[117] Ventilatory failure is the immediate cause of death and is usually, but not always, preceded by signs of cranial nerve dysfunction, including ptosis, blurry vision, myosis, dysarthria, hypersalivation, and dysphagia. Abdominal pain has also been reported with *Micruroides euryxanthus euryxanthus* envenomation.[2, 117]

Diagnosis

Clinical diagnosis of coral snake envenomation can be difficult. Although several snakes' coloration resembles the bright red-, yellow-, and black-banded coloration of the coral snakes, the mnemonic "red next to yellow, kill a fellow" is still useful in identifying a coral snake. The patient and clinician may not realize that a coral snake envenomation has occurred without positively identifying the snake and because of the possibility of delayed onset of symptoms.

Unlike crotalid envenomations, significant hematologic abnormalities have not been reported with North American coral snake envenomations. No significant laboratory abnormalities have been noted.[2]

Treatment

Any patient with a potential coral snakebite should be admitted to the hospital for 24 to 48 hours of observation because of the potential for delayed onset of neurotoxicity. Some aspects of prehospital management of elapid snakebite are controversial. Because venom can still be present on the skin's surface and can enter through abrasions, remove any remaining venom with a vigorous water rinse and soap scrub, if possible.[110] Venous rather than lymphatic routes of absorption of the active neurotoxic polypeptide venom components may be more significant in coral snake envenomations.[119, 124] In general, proximal constricting bands are felt to be ineffective. However, an Australian study showed that application of a tight (55 mm Hg) crepe bandage the entire length of the envenomated extremity, combined with splint immobilization, resulted in delayed proximal movement and limited systemic absorption of radiolabeled venom and neurotoxin in monkeys envenomated with tiger snake venom, an elapid relative of the North American coral snakes.[57] There are no studies on use of constriction bands, compressive dressing, or splints in North American coral snakebite.

The Extractor (Sawyer Products, Safety Harbor, FL) has not been studied in North American coral snakebite envenomation; however, no harm would be expected to result from its use. Studies are necessary to investigate its effectiveness. *No first aid should delay rapid transport to a medical facility.* As in crotalid envenomations, incision of the wound, oral suction, cryotherapy, and electric shock treatment are not supported by the literature and are contraindicated.

If the airway is compromised and airway support is available in the field, it should be initiated as soon as possible.[109] A prehospital intravenous lifeline should also be established.

Antivenin (*Micrurus fulvius*) (equine origin) (Wyeth-Ayers Laboratories, Philadelphia) is available for Eastern and Texas coral snake envenomations, but not for Sonoran or Arizona coral snake envenomations.[121, 124] Antivenin use in the prehospital setting is not advisable due to the risks of anaphylactic and anaphylactoid reactions. EMS notification with a cellular phone and rapid transport to a medical facility are the most effective prehospital care.

On arrival at a medical facility, a rapid primary survey and resuscitation should be performed and the best possible history obtained.[26] Although it is generally not advisable to capture a venomous snake because of the risk of further envenomations, a positive identification is helpful in determining the length of patient observation in a potential coral snakebite. If a positive identification has been made, or if there are signs or symptoms of coral snake envenomation, then coral snake antivenin treatment is indicated, even in the absence of gross physical evidence of a bite, such as fang marks or obvious abrasions.[2, 109–112]

Prior to administration of antivenin, a skin test should be performed. Wyeth *Micrurus fulvius* antivenin skin testing and administration involves similar risks and requires similar precautions as use of the Wyeth polyvalent crotalid antivenin, because both are of equine origin. The recommended initial dose of Wyeth *Micrurus fulvius* antivenin varies among authors.[109, 122] One vial of antivenin can neutralize 2 mg of venom.[2]

The authors recommend a minimum of 5 vials of antivenin administered over 1 to 2 hours. First, the antivenin should be reconstituted in the diluent that accompanies the lyophilized antivenin, with precautions similar to those used in reconstituting Wyeth polyvalent crotalid antivenin. This should be added to 250 to 500 mL of normal saline. The antivenin infusion should begin slowly at 1 to 2 mL over 3 to 5 minutes; the patient should be observed for evidence of hypersensitivity. If hypersensitivity ensues, stop the infusion and give intravenous diphenhydramine and cimetidine. Administration of epinephrine, steroids, and glucagon may be necessary if diphenhydramine and cimetidine are unsuccessful; treat this response as you would treat an anaphylactic or anaphylactoid reaction due to any other agent. In the absence of an adverse reaction, the rate of infusion may be gradually increased over the next 5 to 10 minutes with the goal of eventually infusing the initial dose of antivenin within 1 to 2 hours. Before or after complications ensue, it is advisable to contact a regional poison center or medical toxicologist for a toxicology consultation.[122]

Coral snake antivenin is best given *early* (if available) in coral snake envenomation *before* the onset of neurotoxic effects. Once neurotoxic signs or symptoms develop, they may progress despite adequate doses of antivenin.[109] Good supportive care is paramount, including early endotracheal intubation, prior to progression of paralytic symptoms.[2] In one study, three patients who received elective endotracheal intubation before ventilatory failure did not develop aspiration pneumonia, whereas three other patients who were intubated during progression of ventilatory insufficiency all developed aspiration pneumonia.[109]

A new bovine-derived fragment-antibody (Fab) antivenin to treat Eastern coral snake envenomation has been produced and compared, in vitro and in vivo, with the Wyeth *Micrurus fulvius* antivenin.[123] In mice, the bovine Fab antivenin was approximately four times more effective than the equine product in protecting mice after envenomation with twice the LD_{50} of *Micrurus fulvius fulvius* venom.[123]

As with other bites, administer tetanus prophylaxis if indicated. As previously noted, prophylactic antibiotics are not mandated.

Disposition

Patients should be admitted to the hospital for 24 to 48 hours for potential North American coral snakebites, even in the absence of bite marks or other signs or symptoms. Patients may be discharged after this period if no signs of toxicity ensue. Prognosis is excellent in most cases; however, some patients have required prolonged supportive care, as they did not recover from paralysis for up to 2 months. Death occurs early in most cases as a result of ventilatory failure from neuromuscular blockade.[109] Aspiration pneumonia can be a major complication.[109] About 10% of treated patients developed serum sickness in one case series.[109] Important points in management of North American coral snakebite include recognizing the potential for envenomation when coral snakebite is likely, administering antivenin early, giving adequate doses of antivenin, and avoiding inappropriate first aid, such as tourniquet application or cryotherapy.[2, 110]

References

1. Russell FE: Toxic effects of animal toxins. *In* Klaassen CD (ed): Casarett and Doull's Toxicology: The Basic Science of Poisons. 5th ed. New York, McGraw-Hill, pp 801–839, 1996.
2. Russell FE: Snake Venom Poisoning. 2nd ed. Great Neck, NY, Scholium International, pp 1–343, 1983.
3. Parrish HM: Incidence of treated snakebites in the United States. Pub Health Rep *81*:269, 1966.
4. Dart RC, Gomez HF: Reptile bites and scorpion stings. *In* Tintinalli JE (ed): Emergency Medicine: A Comprehensive Study Guide. 4th ed. New York, McGraw-Hill, pp 864–867, 1996.
5. Sullivan JB, Wingert WA, Norris RL: North American venomous reptile bites. *In* Auerbach PS (ed): Wilderness Medicine: Management of Wilderness and Environmental Emergencies. 3rd ed. St. Louis, Mosby–Year Book, pp 680–709, 1995.
6. Warrell DA: Animal toxins. *In* Cook GC (ed): Manson's Tropical Diseases. 20th ed. Philadelphia, W.B. Saunders, pp 468–515, 1996.
7. Behler JL, King FW: National Audubon Society Field Guide to North American Reptiles and Amphibians. 2nd ed. New York, Alfred A. Knopf, pp 680–698, 1995.
8. Litovitz TL, Felberg L, Soloway RA, et al: 1994 annual report of the American Association of Poison Control Centers toxic exposure surveillance system. Am J Emerg Med *13*:551, 1995.
9. Russell FE, Dart RC: Snakes, Crotalidae. *In* POISINDEX. Denver, Micromedex, 1996.
10. Wingert WA, Chan L: Rattlesnake bites in Southern California and rationale for recommended treatment. West J Med *148*:37, 1988.
11. Parrish HM, Goldner JC, Silberg SL: Comparison between snakebites in children and adults. Pediatrics *36*:251, 1965.
12. Iyaniwura TT: Snake venom constituents: Biochemistry and toxicology (parts 1 and 2). Vet Hum Toxicol *33*:468, 1991.
13. Cate RL, Bieber AL: Purification and characterization of Mojave (*Crotalus scutulatus scutulatus*) toxin and its subunits. Arch Biochem Biophys *189*:397, 1978.
14. Castilonia RR, Pattabhiraman TR, Russell FE: Neuromuscular blocking effects of Mojave rattlesnake (*Crotalus scutulatus scutulatus*) venom. Proc West Pharmacol Soc *23*:103, 1980.
15. Gopalakrishnakone P, Hawgood BJ, Holbrooke SE, et al: Sites of action of Mojave toxin isolated from the venom of the Mojave rattlesnake. Br J Pharmacol *69*:421, 1980.
16. Ho CL, Lee CY: Presynaptic actions of Mojave toxin isolated from Mojave rattlesnake (*Crotalus scutulatus*) venom. Toxicon *19*:889, 1981.
17. Valdes JJ, Thompson RG, Wolff VL, et al: Inhibition of calcium channel dihydropyridine receptor binding by purified Mojave toxin. Neurotoxicol Teratol *11*:129, 1989.
18. Glenn JL, Straight R: Mojave rattlesnake (*Crotalus scutulatus scutulatus*) venom: Variation in toxicity with geographical origin. Toxicon *16*:81, 1978.
19. Glenn JL, Straight RC, Wolfe MC, et al: Geographical variation in *Crotalus scutulatus scutulatus* (Mojave rattlesnake) venom properties. Toxicon *21*:119, 1983.
20. Glenn JL, Straight R: Intergradation of two different venom populations of the Mojave rattlesnake (*Crotalus scutulatus scutulatus*) in Arizona. Toxicon *27*:411, 1989.
21. Weinstein SA, Minton SA, Wilde CE: The distribution among ophidian venoms of a toxin isolated from the venom of the Mojave rattlesnake (*Crotalus scutulatus scutulatus*). Toxicon *23*:825, 1985.

22. Huang SY, Perez JC, Rael ED, et al: Variation in the antigenic characteristics of venom from the Mojave rattlesnake (*Crotalus scutulatus scutulatus*). Toxicon *30*:387, 1992.
23. Jansen PW, Perkin RM, Van Stralen D: Mojave rattlesnake envenomation: Prolonged neurotoxicity and rhabdomyolysis. Ann Emerg Med *21*:322, 1992.
24. Hardy DL: Envenomation by the Mojave rattlesnake (*Crotalus scutulatus scutulatus*) in Southern Arizona, USA. Toxicon *21*:111, 1983.
25. Hardy DL: Fatal rattlesnake envenomation in Arizona: 1969–1984. Clin Toxicol *24*:1, 1986.
26. American College of Surgeons Subcommittee on Advanced Trauma Life Support: Initial assessment and management. *In* Advanced Trauma Life Support Instructor Manual. 5th ed. Chicago, American College of Surgeons, pp 17–37, 1993.
27. Walter FG: Envenomations. Dallas, TX, American College of Emergency Physicians, 1995.
28. Ownby CL, Kainer RA, Tu AT: Pathogenesis of hemorrhage induced by rattlesnake venom: An electron microscope study. Am J Pathol *76*:401, 1974.
29. Dubnoff JW, Russell FE: Isolation of lethal protein and peptide from *Crotalus viridis helleri* venom. Proc West Pharmacol Soc *13*:98, 1970.
30. Bjarnason JB, Fox JW: Hemorrhagic metalloproteinases from snake venoms. Pharmacol Ther *62*:325, 1994.
31. Kitchens CS: Hemostatic aspects of envenomation by North American snakes. Hematol Oncol Clin North Am *6*:1189, 1992.
32. Kitchens CS, Van Mierop LHS: Mechanism of defibrination in humans after envenomation by the Eastern diamondback rattlesnake. Am J Hematol 14:345, 1983.
33. Hasiba U, Rosenbach LM, Rockwell D, et al: DIC-like syndrome after envenomation by the snake, *Crotalus horridus horridus*. N Engl J Med 292:505, 1975.
34. Budzynski AZ, Pandya BV, Rubin RN, et al: Fibrinogenolytic afibrinogenemia after envenomation by Western diamondback rattlesnake (*Crotalus atrox*). Blood *63*:1, 1984.
35. Simon TL, Grace TG: Envenomation coagulopathy in wounds from pit vipers. N Engl J Med 305:443, 1981.
36. Mosher DF: Disorders of blood coagulation. *In* Bennett JC, Plum F (eds): Cecil Textbook of Medicine. 20th ed. Philadelphia, W.B. Saunders, pp 987–1003, 1996.
37. Burgess JL, Dart RC: Snake venom coagulopathy: Use and abuse of blood products in the treatment of pit viper envenomation. Ann Emerg Med *20*:795, 1991.
38. Schmaier AH, Colman RW: Crotalocytin: Characterization of the timber rattlesnake platelet activating protein. Blood *56*:1020, 1980.
39. Ruiz CE, Schaeffer RC, Weil MH, et al: Hemostatic changes following rattlesnake (*Crotalus viridis helleri*) venom in the dog. J Pharmacol Exp Ther *213*:414, 1980.
40. Ahlstrom NG, Luginbuhl W, Tisher CC: Acute anuric renal failure after pigmy rattlesnake bite. South Med J *84*:783, 1991.
41. Reid HA, Theakston RDG: Changes in coagulation effects by venoms of *Crotalus atrox* as snakes age. Am J Trop Med Hyg *27*:1053, 1978.
42. Gregory VM, Russell FE, Brewer JR, et al: Seasonal variations in rattlesnake venom proteins. Proc West Pharmacol Soc *27*:233, 1984.
43. Gerkin R, Sergent KC, Curry SC, et al: Life-threatening airway obstruction from rattlesnake bite to the tongue. Ann Emerg Med *16*:813, 1987.
44. Lewis JV, Portera CA: Rattlesnake bite of the face: Case report and review of the literature. Am Surg *60*:681, 1994.
45. Curry SC, Kunkel DB: Death from a rattlesnake bite. Am J Emerg Med *3*:227, 1985.
46. Banner W, Russell F, Barton B, et al: Fatal rattlesnake bite in a child. Abstract. Vet Hum Toxicol *26*:400, 1984.
47. Dart RC, Hurlbut KM, Garcia R, et al: Validation of a severity score for the assessment of crotalid snakebite. Ann Emerg Med *27*:321, 1996.
48. Forgey W, Norris RL, Blackman J, et al: Viewpoints: Rattlesnake bite. J Wilderness Med *5*:216, 1994.
49. Walter FG, Olson KR: First aid for snakebite. Am Acad Clin Toxicol Update *8*(2):1, 1995.
50. Howarth DM, Southee AE, Whyte IM: Lymphatic flow rates and first-aid in simulated peripheral snake or spider envenomation. Med J Aust *161*:695, 1994.
51. Bronstein AC, Russell FE, Sullivan JB, et al: Negative pressure suction in field treatment of rattlesnake bite. Abstract. Vet Hum Toxicol *27*:297, 1985.
52. Bronstein AC, Russell FE, Sullivan JB, et al: Negative pressure suction in the field treatment of rattlesnake bite victims. Abstract. Vet Hum Toxicol *27*:485, 1986.
53. Gellert GA: Snake-venom and insect-venom extractors: An unproved therapy. Letter. N Engl J Med *327*:1322, 1992.
54. Forgey WW, Gellert GA: More on snake-venom and insect-venom extractors. Letter. N Engl J Med *328*:516, 1993.
55. Gold BS: Snake venom extractors: A valuable first aid tool. Letter. Vet Hum Toxicol *35*:255, 1993.
56. Burgess JL, Dart RC, Egen NB, et al: Effects of constriction bands on rattlesnake venom absorption: A pharmacokinetic study. Ann Emerg Med *21*:1086, 1992.
57. Sutherland SK, Coulter AR, Harris RD: Rationalisation of first-aid measures for elapid snakebite. Lancet *1*:183, 1979.
58. Sutherland SK, Coulter AR: Early management of bites by the eastern diamondback (*Crotalus adamanteus*): Studies in monkeys (*Macaca fascicularis*). Am J Trop Med Hyg *30*:479, 1981.
59. Clark RW: Cryotherapy and corticosteroids in the treatment of rattlesnake bite. Mil Med *136*:42, 1971.
60. Dart RC, Lindsey D, Schulman A: Snakebite and shocks. Letter. Ann Emerg Med *17*:1262, 1988.
61. Russell FE: A letter on electroshock for snakebite. Letter. Vet Hum Toxicol *29*:320, 1987.
62. Johnson EK, Kardong KV, MacKessy SP: Electric shocks are ineffective in treatment of lethal effects of rattlesnake envenomation in mice. Toxicon *25*:1347, 1987.
63. Howe NR, Meisenheimer JL: Electric shock does not save snakebitten rats. Ann Emerg Med *17*:245, 1988.
64. Dart RC, Gustafson RA: Failure of electric shock treatment for rattlesnake envenomation. Ann Emerg Med *20*:659, 1991.
65. Davidson TM: Intravenous rattlesnake envenomation. West J Med *148*:45, 1988.
66. Hardy DL: Fatal rattlesnake envenomation in Arizona: 1969–1984. Clin Toxicol *24*:1,1986.
67. Kitchens CS, Hunter S, Van Mierop LHS: Severe myonecrosis in a fatal case of envenomation by the canebrake rattlesnake (*Crotalus horridus atricaudatus*). Toxicon *25*:455, 1987.
68. Bush SP, Jansen PW: Severe rattlesnake envenomation with anaphylaxis and rhabdomyolysis. Ann Emerg Med *25*:845, 1995.
69. Cruz NS, Alvarez RG: Rattlesnake bite complications in 19 children. Pediatr Emerg Care *10*:30, 1994.
70. Clark RF, Selden BS, Furbee B: The incidence of wound infection following crotalid envenomation. J Emerg Med *11*:583, 1993.
71. Weed HG: Nonvenomous snakebite in Massachusetts: Prophylactic antibiotics are unnecessary. Ann Emerg Med *22*:220, 1993.
72. Goldstein EJC, Citron DM, Gonzalez H, et al: Bacteriology of rattlesnake venom and implications for therapy. J Infect Dis *140*:818, 1979.
73. Horowitz RS, Dart RC: Antivenins and immunobiologicals: Immunotherapeutics of envenomation. *In* Auerbach PS (ed): Wilderness Medicine: Management of Wilderness and Environmental Emergencies. 3rd ed. St. Louis, Mosby–Year Book, pp 731–741, 1995.
74. Antivenin (Crotalidae) polyvalent (equine origin). *In* Physicians' Desk Reference. 49th ed. Montvale, NJ, Medical Economics Data Production Co., pp 2643–2644, 1995.
75. Garfin SR, Castilonia RR, Mubarak SJ, et al: The effect of antivenin on intramuscular pressure elevations induced by rattlesnake venom. Toxicon *23*:677, 1985.
76. Dart RC, Goldner AP, Lindsey D: Efficacy of delayed administration of crotalid antivenom and crystalloid fluids. Toxicon *26*:1218, 1988.
77. Stewart RM, Page CP, Schwesinger WH, et al: Antivenin and fasciotomy/debridement in the treatment of the severe rattlesnake bite. Am J Surg *158*:543, 1989.

78. Russell FE, Ruzic N, Gonzalez H: Effectiveness of antivenin (Crotalidae) polyvalent following injection of *Crotalus* venom. Toxicon *11*:461, 1973.
79. Parrish HM, Carr CA: Bites by copperheads (*Agkistrodon contortrix*) in the United States. JAMA *201*:107, 1967.
80. Kaplan AP: Anaphylaxis. *In* Bennett JC, Plum F (eds): Cecil Textbook of Medicine. 20th ed. Philadelphia, W.B. Saunders, pp 1417–1420, 1996.
81. Zull DN: Anaphylaxis. *In* Harwood-Nuss AL (ed): The Clinical Practice of Emergency Medicine. 2nd ed. Philadelphia, Lippincott-Raven, pp 929–932, 1996.
82. Brostoff J, Hall T: Hypersensitivity—type I. *In* Roitt I, Brostoff J, Male D (eds): Immunology. 4th ed. St. Louis, Mosby–Year Book, pp 22.1–22.17, 1996.
83. Sutherland SK: Serum reactions—an analysis of commercial antivenoms and the possible role of anticomplementary activity in de-novo reactions to antivenoms and antitoxins. Med J Aust *1*:613, 1977.
84. Waldesbuhl M, Renata A, Meylan A: Anticomplementary activity of gamma-globulins and their subunits. Immunochemistry *7*:185, 1970.
85. Jurkovich GJ, Luterman A, McCullar K, et al: Complications of Crotalidae antivenin therapy. J Trauma *28*:1032, 1988.
86. Spaite DW, Dart RC, Hurlbut K, et al: Skin testing: Implications in the management of pit viper envenomation. Abstract. Ann Emerg Med *17*:389, 1988.
87. Hay F: Hypersensitivity—type III. *In* Roitt I, Brostoff J, Male D (eds): Immunology. 4th ed. St. Louis, Mosby–Year Book, pp 24.1–24.12, 1996.
88. de Shazo RD: Immune complex diseases. *In* Bennett JC, Plum F (eds): Cecil Textbook of Medicine. 20th ed. Philadelphia, W.B. Saunders, pp 1421–1424, 1996.
89. Iserson KV: Verbal communication, 1993.
90. Loprinzi CL, Hennessee J, Tamsky L, et al: Snake antivenin administration in a patient allergic to horse serum. South Med J *76*:501, 1983.
91. Huang TT, Lynch JB, Larson DL, et al: The use of excisional therapy in the management of snakebite. Ann Surg *179*:598, 1974.
92. Glass TG: Early débridement of pit viper bites. JAMA *235*:2513, 1976.
93. Garfin SR, Castilonia RR, Mabarak SJ, et al: Rattlesnake bites and surgical decompression: Results using a laboratory model. Toxicon *22*:177, 1984.
94. Curry SC, Kraner JC, Kunkel DB, et al: Noninvasive vascular studies in management of rattlesnake envenomations in extremities. Ann Emerg Med *14*:1081, 1985.
95. Garfin SR, Castilonia RR, Mubarak J, et al: Role of surgical decompression in treatment of rattlesnake bite. Surgical Forum *30*:502, 1979.
96. Ganong WF: Review of Medical Physiology. 16th ed. Norwalk, CT, Appleton & Lange, pp 521–537, 1993.
97. Van Ryn DE: Compartmental syndrome. *In* Roberts JR, Hedges JR (eds): Clinical Procedures in Emergency Medicine. 2nd ed. Philadelphia, W.B. Saunders, pp 859–866, 1991.
98. Hargens AR, Akeson WH, Mubarak SJ, et al: Fluid balance within canine anterolateral compartment and its relationship to compartment syndromes. J Bone Joint Surg Am *60*:499, 1978.
99. Whitesides TE, Haney TC, Morimoto K, et al: Tissue pressure measurements: A determinant for the need for fasciotomy. Clin Orthop *113*:43, 1975.
100. Heppenstall RB, Sapega AA, Scott R, et al: The compartment syndrome: An experimental and clinical study of muscular energy metabolism. Clin Orthop *226*:138, 1988.
101. Zweifach SS, Hargens AR, Evans KL, et al: Skeletal muscle necrosis in pressurized compartments associated with hemorrhagic hypotension. J Trauma *20*:941, 1980.
102. Matsen FA: Compartmental Syndromes. New York, Grune & Stratton, 1980.
103. Watt CH: Treatment of poisonous snakebite with emphasis on digit dermotomy. South Med J *78*:694, 1985.
104. Guisto JA: Severe toxicity from crotalid envenomation after early resolution of symptoms. Ann Emerg Med *26*:387, 1995.
105. Hurlbut KM, Dart RC, Spaite DW, et al: Reliability of clinical presentation for predicting significant pit viper envenomation. Abstract. Ann Emerg Med *17*:438, 1988.
106. Dart RC, McNally JT, Spaite DW, et al: The sequelae of pitviper poisoning in the United States. *In* Campbell JA, Brody ED (eds): Biology of the Pitvipers. Tyler, TX, Selva Press, pp 395–404, 1992.
107. Consroe P, Even NB, Russell FE, et al: Comparison of a new ovine antigen binding fragment (Fab) antivenin for United States Crotalidae with the commercial antivenin for protection against venom-induced lethality in mice. Am J Trop Med Hyg *53*:507, 1995.
108. Ernst CH, Barbour RW: Snakes of eastern North America. Fairfax, VA, George Mason University Press, 1989.
109. Kitchens CS, Van Mierop LHS: Envenomation by the eastern coral snake (*Micrurus fulvius fulvius*): A study of 39 victims. JAMA *258*:1615–1618, 1987.
110. Parrish HM, Khan MS: Bites by coral snakes: Report of 11 representative cases. Am J Med Sci *253*:561–568, 1967.
111. Moseley T: Coral snake bite: Recovery following symptoms of respiratory paralysis. Ann Surg *163*:943–948, 1966.
112. Norris RL, Dart RC: Apparent coral snake envenomation in a patient without visible fang marks. Am J Emerg Med *7*:402–405, 1989.
113. Lee CY: Elapid neurotoxins and their mode of action. Clin Toxicol *3*:457–472, 1970.
114. Pettigrew LC, Glass JP: Neurologic complications of a coral snakebite. Neurology *35*:589–592, 1985.
115. Russell FE, Puffer HW: Pharmacology of snake venoms. Clin Toxicol *3*:433–444, 1970.
116. Fix JD: Venom yields of the North American coral snake and its clinical significance. South Med J *73*:757–741, 1980.
117. McCollough NC, Gennaro JF Jr: Coral snake bites in the United States. J Fla Med Assoc *49*:968–972, 1963.
118. Watt CH: Poisonous snakebite treatment in the United States. JAMA *240*:654–656, 1978.
119. Russell FE: Prevention and treatment of venomous animal injuries. Experentia *30*:8–12, 1974.
120. Russell FE, Carlson RW, Wainschel J, Osborne AH: Snake venom poisoning in the United States: Experiences with 550 cases. JAMA *233*:341–344, 1975.
121. Olin BR (ed): Drug Facts and Comparisons. 49th ed. St. Louis, MO, Wolters Kluwer Company, p 452, 1995.
122. Soskis JE: Snakebite assessment and treatment in the eastern United States. 2nd ed. Midway, FL, Snakebite Publishing, 1994.
123. Rawat R, Laing G, Smith DC, et al: A new antivenom to treat eastern coral snake (*Micrurus fulvius fulvius*) envenoming. Toxicon *32*:185–190, 1994.
124. Russell FE: Verbal communication, 1996.

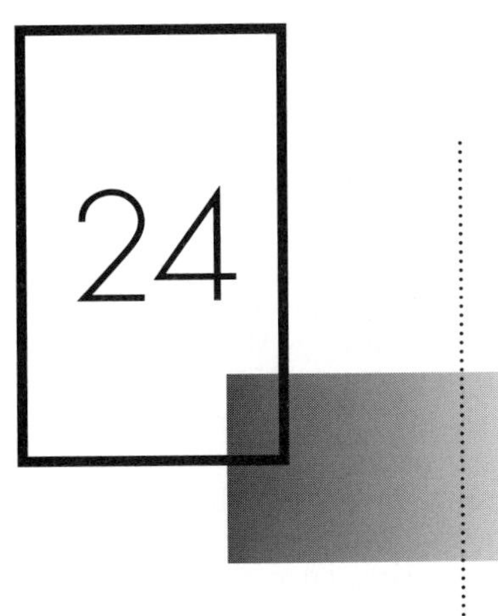

Poisonous Arthropods

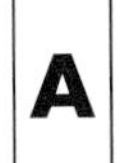

A Spiders

CHRISTIAN TOMASZEWSKI, MD

The arthropods are a diverse group of organisms that can cause painful and even necrotic bites, but these bites usually are not life threatening. All arthropods have a chitinous exoskeleton and jointed bodies and legs. They account for more than 1.5 million different species. Many are venomous, and among the most clinically important venomous arthropods are the spiders, scorpions, and hymenopterans. All can cause painful local reactions that are not limb threatening. Systemic symptoms can also result, however, most commonly associated with allergic reactions to hymenopteran stings, which can be life threatening.

Almost all spiders, except for those of two families, are venomous, and they use their venom to kill and digest their live prey. Of the 20,000 or more species found in the United States, only about 50 of these have fangs that can penetrate human skin.[1] Fortunately, even fewer cause clinical problems because either their venom is too weak or their mouth parts cannot penetrate human skin. In the 1995 annual report of the American Association of Poison Control Centers, black widow and the brown recluse spiders were the two most common spiders inflicting bites for which patients sought medical treatment at a health care facility, with 689 and 1051 cases, respectively.[2] Venomous spiders are found throughout the world, and they show a preference for human dwellings as much as for the wild environment. Therefore, it is not surprising that they are blamed for most "bug" bites, although 80% of bites in one series of 600 were attributable to nonspider arthropods (i.e., ticks, mites, fleas, flies, beetles and hymenoptera), and another 10% were determined not to be bites at all.[3] If the offending organism is available for identification, it is characterized as a spider if it has a body divided into a nonsegmented abdomen and a cephalothorax, to which eight legs are attached.

Initial therapy for any presumed spider bite is essentially supportive, including tetanus prophylaxis. The preferential use of heat or cold has not been studied, and their injudicious use could potentially cause damage. Commercial suction devices may remove venom if used within minutes of a bite.[4] A loose constriction band may delay venom absorption.[5] None of these measures can be routinely recommended, however, because of lack of evaluation in actual spider envenomations.

BLACK WIDOW *(LATRODECTUS)*

The black widow spider inflicts painful bites on unwary victims throughout the United States (except Alaska) and most of the world. In most species, the large, glossy black female, 1 to 1.5 cm in length, has a large bulbous abdomen and a distinctive red hourglass mark ventrally. Only the female causes a clinically significant bite, mainly because of its larger size relative to the diminutive male, which is often consumed after mating.

Five species have been found in the United States, and *Latrodectus mactans* is the most common. Other species include *L. hesperus,* found more commonly in the west, and *L. variolus.* One notable variant is the brown widow spider of Florida, *L. geometricus,* which is actually red, black, and yellow.

The female black widow spider creates webs near the ground in secluded dark areas such as barns, garages, abandoned burrows, sheds, and even the notorious outhouse.[6] Because of the similarity of their venom, all species cause comparable clinical syndromes with envenomation.[7, 8] The most dramatic consequence is the painful, sustained muscle spasms caused by the neurotoxic component.

Pathophysiology. Black widow spider venom contains a neurotoxin, α-latrotoxin, which is more potent by volume than pit viper venom.[9] The venom binds to the synaptic membranes and leads to calcium-dependent release of massive amounts of acetycholine at neuromuscular junctions.[10–12] Amplifying this effect is the fact that the venom prevents presynaptic neuronal reuptake of acetylcholine and amines.[13] In addition, it results in stimulation of the autonomic nervous system through the depletion of catecholamines at adrenergic nerve endings.[14]

Clinical Presentation. The initial bite of the black widow spider is often a mild pinprick-like sensation followed by a dull ache 20 minutes later. All that may be visible is one or two puncture wounds 1 to 2 mm apart. Local erythema and in some cases a diffuse erythematous maculopapular rash extending beyond the bite site may occasionally be noted.

Systemic symptoms can start 30 minutes to 3 hours after the initial bite and can last for 24 to 48 hours and occasionally days. The most common symptoms in Clark and colleagues' series of 163 patients was abdominal or back pain in more than half of cases.[15] This muscle tightness can be confused with an acute abdomen, especially in children who cannot relate the story of the initial bite. Other but less common symptoms are local pain, hypertension, diaphoresis, chest pain, nausea and vomiting, and tachycardia.[15–18] Moderate hypertension occurs in 20% to 60% of cases but rarely is sufficient to cause stroke or cardiac side effects.[15–23] Hypertension may be indirect owing to central nervous stimulation of the adrenals or may result from direct vasoconstriction.[24] In severe cases, because of pain or direct venom effects, patients have a characteristic facies showing flushing, periorbital edema, and conjunctivitis.[7, 17, 22, 25] Rarely, death has been reported in series dating from the 1950s, particularly in the southeastern United States.[26]

Treatment. The mainstay of treatment for symptomatic black widow spider bites is symptomatic relief of the muscle spasms. This is done initially with intravenous administration of narcotics and benzodiazepines. In Clark and associates' series, 55% of the patients treated with morphine or meperidine attained relief, and this was increased to 70% in those treated with narcotics plus benzodiazepines.[15] The most common combination used is parenteral meperidine and diazepam, which often requires cardiac monitoring in cases requiring repetitive dosing. Other muscle relaxants such as methocarbamol, once advocated, have been found to be less efficacious than calcium.[27]

Calcium is a specific antidote recommended for black widow envenomation. It is purported to antagonize the venom's stimulation of neurotransmitter release at nerve endings.[28] Calcium is particularly useful for severe muscle spasms, especially in patients with respiratory embarrassment or intractable pain. Because the effect of intravenous calcium may last only 15 to 20 minutes, repeated intravenous administration of 10 mL of 10% calcium gluconate may be indicated.[29]

The role of calcium has come into question. In Clark and co-workers' series, only 1 of 24 patients with systemic symptoms had relief when given calcium; however, the mean dose in this series was only 1400 mg, which is generally an inadequate amount.

Antivenin (Merck & Co., Inc.) is generally reserved for severe recalcitrant cases due to the bite of any *Latrodectus* species. It is extracted as a horse serum product. Therefore, its risks include *immediate* hypersensitivity with potential respiratory and cardiovascular compromise and death. Indications for antivenin include severe symptoms, pain, or hypertension unresponsive to routine care with maximal administration of intravenous narcotics and muscle relaxants. In one series, one vial of antivenin was completely effective in 50 of 58 patients, with mean time to relief being 30 minutes.[15] No patient required more than two vials for relief. An additional benefit is that in this series, the admission rate was 52% for patients who did not receive antivenin versus 12% for those who did. In severe cases that do not respond completely within 1 hour, use of a second vial may be considered.

Because of the danger of anaphylactic death with antivenin,[15] it is emphasized that *antivenin should be used only for severe, recalcitrant cases.* Although not extremely reliable, a skin test with the actual reconstituted antivenin, diluted 1:10, 0.01 to 0.02 mL subcutaneously, should be performed before antivenin administration. Cardiopulmonary resuscitation equipment should be available, and patients should be watched for at least 30 minutes for any allergic response. One should keep in mind that allergic reactions have occurred in as many as one third of patients who were given snake antivenin and who had negative skin test results initially.[30, 31] If the skin test result is negative, one vial of antivenin can be given cautiously, with cardiac monitoring, by infusing one vial in 50 to 100 mL of 5% dextrose in water or normal saline over 30 minutes.

Late presentation or pregnancy is not a contraindication to antivenin administration. Although most pregnant women fare well after envenomation, antivenin has been used successfully in a bitten woman who was 20 weeks pregnant and had muscle cramps. She subsequently had a normal term delivery.[27, 32] As for late treatment, antivenin usefulness 1 to 2 days after the bite has been reported.[21, 33–35] In fact, treatment has been successful several days (80 hours in one case and 14 days in another) after bites of the Australian subspecies of *L. mactans,* the redback spider.[36–39]

BROWN RECLUSE SPIDER (*LOXOSCELES*)

In the United States, the *Loxosceles* species of spiders are notorious for local wound necrosis and in rare cases systemic illness. These brown spiders are small (6 to 22 mm) and have a distinctive violin-shaped marking on the dorsum of the cephalothorax. They are found throughout the southern United States but are rarely seen because of their shy, reclusive nature. These spiders form small, inconsequential webs and are often encountered in home storage areas or outdoors, typically in woodpiles.

In a survey of South Carolina physicians, patients seeking medical treatment for presumed brown recluse spider bites outnumbered those seeking treatment for black widow spider bites, 478 to 143 for the year 1990.[40] The true *Loxosceles reclusa* is found only in the southeastern United States, except for Florida. Bites by other spiders can become necrotic wounds; *Chiracanthium* species (the clubionid spiders), *Phidippus* (the jumping spider), *Argiope,* and *Tegenaria* (the hobo spider) are often the actual culprits when the brown recluse is mistakenly blamed.

The venom of the brown recluse spider contains various cytotoxic enzymes. Sphingomyelinase D, the primary dermatonecrotic factor, disrupts cellular membranes.[41, 42] Sphingomyelinase D also causes serotonin release, which is associated with platelet aggregation and thus thrombosis of small capillaries.[43–46] The venom can later cause local endothelial changes that attract neutrophils, which in turn release more destruction enzymes and promote further platelet aggregation and thrombosis.[47–49] The essential role of polymorphonuclear leukocytes in the cutaneous lesion was shown in a rabbit model in which pretreatment with nitrogen mustard decreased the cutaneous effects of the venom.[47] The venom can also cause erythrocyte hemolysis, which contributes to systemic effects.[50]

Clinical Presentation. A brown recluse spider bite is usually a mild bite that a patient often cannot even recall. Within 24 hours, the patient presents for treatment of a painful purple papule. This erythematous lesion is often surrounded by a blanched ischemic zone, which can coagulate and become thrombosed. A necrotic, ulcerating wound results and may progress for as long as a week after the initial bite.[51] The eschar may slough, and the lesion may extend into subcutaneous fat and create a disfiguring ulcer that can take weeks to heal and occasionally requires surgical grafting.[52] In addition, an occasional patient presents with systemic loxoscelism, which can include fever, chills, nausea, arthralgias, a morbilliform rash, and even red blood cell hemolysis.[51] One 12-year-old girl even required a red blood cell transfusion 6 days after a bite.[53] In rare cases, patients can develop disseminated intravascular coagulation, renal failure, and even seizures.[54, 55]

Laboratory. Diagnosis of a brown recluse bite is usually presumptive, partly because the bite is not very painful and the spider is rather shy. Patients usually present late with necrotic effects already evident. Experimentally, various serologic tests and biopsy techniques are used for confirming the bite.[56–59] However, none of these are readily available, and none is 100% sensitive. Apart from confirmatory tests, some routine laboratory work is indicated in severe envenomations. Blood cell count, urinalysis, and renal function tests may be indicated in patients with systemic symptoms of loxoscelism. In most cases, however, patients show only a local lesion without any significant systemic effects.

Treatment. Generally, all that is required for most presumed brown recluse spider bites is routine wound care, including tetanus prophylaxis. This can include débridement of necrotic tissue as well watching for late infection; routine prophylactic antibiotics are not indicated. If a patient appears ill, blood and urine tests can be performed to preclude systemic hemolysis. Treatment for hemolytic anemia would be supportive, with red blood cell replacement provided as needed.

Several experimental therapies have been advocated for patients with brown recluse spider bites, especially for those with the threat of a disfiguring scar. The most popular has been the use of dapsone. The theoretic basis of this agent lies in inhibiting the polymorphonuclear leukocytes from aggregating at the wound site and causing tissue necrosis. In a poorly described study of dermal envenomation, pretreatment of guinea pigs with oral dapsone resulted in skin lesions less than 50% the size of those seen in control animals.[60] Post-treatment in a similar model showed smaller necrotic lesions with the use of dapsone.[61] However, two recent studies were unable to reproduce these favorable results.[62, 63] Clinical experience, although uncontrolled, has been favorable; Rees and co-workers[64] showed that patients had smaller scars and better healing if they were administered dapsone.

Because of the lack of controlled randomized studies, dapsone should be considered an experimental treatment for presumed brown recluse spider bites. If it is to be used, the potential adverse effects of this drug must be acknowledged. The most serious are hemolysis and methemoglobinemia, occurring most commonly in patients with glucose-6-phosphate dehydrogenase deficiency.[64] Short-term therapy can result additionally in dizziness, fatigue, shortness of breath, and nervousness. Longer treatment courses have caused agranulocytosis, rashes including erythema nodosum and toxic epidermal necrolysis, and even nephrotoxicity and hepatotoxicity. Adverse effects have been reported with use of dapsone for brown recluse spider bites, including hypersensitivity reactions, methemoglobinemia, and hemolysis.[65–67] In summary, because of the lack of proven clinical efficacy for dapsone, dapsone should probably be offered only for bites in cosmetically sensitive areas. (The beginning dose is 25 mg two to three times a day, increasing the dose in increments with periodic complete blood counts to 50 to 100 mg twice a day for 1 to 2 weeks.[68])

Other treatments, such as antivenin, steroids, electric shock, cyproheptadine, colchicine, and even nitroglycerin either have been disappointing in controlled trials or have not been studied at all. Intralesional injection of experimental antivenin in patients resulted in little or no scarring, just as in the dapsone group.[51] Electric shock was shown to be of no value in a guinea pig envenomation model.[61] Cyproheptadine, a serotonin antagonist, was of no benefit in a rabbit model.[62] Surgical excision guarantees a scar at a site that could potentially heal without any disfigurement.[64, 69] Surgical débridement may be reserved for days to weeks later as dictated by local wound care.

Hyperbaric oxygen was previously used in brown recluse bites with purported successes but no controls.[70, 71] More recent controlled studies of animal models have yielded equivocal results. Maynor reported that a single hyperbaric oxygen treatment as long as 48 hours later caused a 50% reduction in lesion size after experimental envenomation in rabbits.[72] However, two other studies failed to show any beneficial effects of hyperbaric therapy on gross lesion appearance in similar animal models.[62, 63, 73] Risks to patients include barotrauma and the expense of an unproven therapy. Potential beneficial effects of hyperbaric oxygen in recluse bites are multifaceted, including inactivation of the venom, reoxygenation of the wound, and sequestration of polymorphonuclear leukocytes away from the wound.[74] Although the Undersea and Hyperbaric Medical Society has yet to approve routine hyperbaric treatment for brown recluse bites, one might want to use it in cases of severe necrotic ulcers. In one clinical series, Maynor and colleagues were able to show good outcomes in such a series of patients.[75]

OTHER SPIDERS

Although the black widow and brown recluse are the most important spiders clinically, occasional bites by other species are notable. Necrotic arachnidism cannot always be assumed to be due to *Loxosceles.* In fact, several other United States spiders have been associated with direct tissue damage, including *Chiracanthium* (the clubionid spider),[76] *Phidippus* (the jumping spider),[77] and *Tegenaria* (the hobo spider).[78] The hobo spider, imported to the Pacific Northwest, can cause identical local and systemic symptoms and signs as seen with *Loxosceles.* Other spiders usually cause only local painful reactions and swelling, most notably *Argiope* (golden orb weaver) and *Lycosa* (wolf spider). In one series of wolf spider bites, only one patient developed a necrotic wound, possibly complicated by infection.[79] Tarantulas, members of the primitive mygalomorph suborder of spiders, can inflict a histamine-like reaction either by a painful bite or by brushing hairs toward their prey. Treatment for all of these envenomations is supportive, with the possible exception of tarantula encounters, which can be treated with oral antihistamines and topical steroids as needed.

None of the other spiders rival the number of medical problems inflicted by the black widow and brown recluse spider species. Fortunately, deaths from spider bites are rare in the United States. One death has been caused by black widow antivenin.[15] Therefore, clinicians should be comfortable with supportive care of any presumed spider bite, knowing that in almost all cases no life- or limb-threatening condition exists.

References

1. Horen WP: Arachnidism in the United States. JAMA *185*:839–843, 1983.
2. Litovitz TL, Felverg L, White S, et al: 1995 Annual report of the American Association of Poison Control Centers Toxic Exposure Surveillance System. Am J Emerg Med *14*:487–537, 1996.
3. Russell FE: Venomous animal injuries. Curr Probl Pediatr *3*:1–47, 1973.
4. Bronstein AC, Russell FE, Sullivan JB: Negative pressure suction in field treatment of rattlesnake bite. Abstract. Vet Hum Toxicol *25*:297, 1995.
5. Burgess JL, Dart RC, Egen NB, et al: Effects of constriction bands on rattlesnake venom absorption: A pharmokinetic study. Ann Emerg Med *21*:1086–1093, 1992.
6. Wong RC, Hughes SE, Voorhees JJ: Spider bites. Arch Dermatol *123*:98–104, 1987.
7. Maretic Z: Latrodectism: Variations in clinical manifestations provoked by *Latrodectus* species of spiders. Toxicon *21*:457–466, 1983.
8. McCrone JD, Netzloff ML: An immunological and electrophoretical comparison of the venoms of the North American *Latrodectus* species. Toxicon *3*:107–110, 1965.
9. Rosenthal L, Meldolesi J: Alpha-latrotoxin and related toxins. Pharmacol Ther *42*:115–134, 1989.
10. Baba A, Cooper JR: The action of black widow spider venom on cholinergic mechanisms in synaptosomes. J Neurochem *34*:1369–1379, 1980.
11. Fesce R, Segal JR, Ceccarelli B, Hurlbut WP: Effects of black widow spider venom and Ca^{2+} on quantal secretion at the frog neuromuscular junction. J Gen Physiol *88*:59–81, 1986.
12. Petrenko AG, Larayeva VD, Geppart M, et al: Polypeptide composition of the alpha-latrotoxin receptor. J Biol Chem *268*:1860–1867, 1993.
13. Rothlin RP, Pardal JF, Pardal MMF: Supersensitivity to norepinephrine induced *in vitro* by crude *Latrodectus mactans* venom in the rabbit ear artery. Toxicon *15*:71–74, 1977.
14. Granata F, Paggi P, Frontali N: Effects of chromatographic fractions of black widow spider venom on *in vitro* biological systems. Toxicon *10*:551–555, 1972.
15. Clark RF, Wethern Kestner S, Vance MV, Gerkin R: Clinical presentation and treatment of black widow spider envenomation: A review of 163 cases. Ann Emerg Med *21*:782–787, 1992.
16. Moss HS, Binder LS: A retrospective review of black widow spider envenomation. Ann Emerg Med *16*:188–192, 1987.
17. Muller GJ: Black and brown widow spider bites in South Africa. A series of 45 cases. S Afr Med J *83*:399–405, 1993.
18. Artaza O, Fuentes J, Schindler R: Latrodectismo: Evaluation clinico-therapeutica de 89 cases. Rev Med Chile *110*:1101–1105, 1982.
19. Visser LH, Khusi SN: Pulmonary oedema from a widow spider bite. A case report. S Afr Med J *75*:338–339, 1989.
20. Timms PK, Gibbons RB: Latrodectism—effects of the black widow spider bite. West J Med *144*:315–317, 1986.
21. Mead HJ, Jelinek GA: Red-back spider bites to Perth children, 1979–1988. J Paediatr Child Health *29*:305–308, 1993.
22. Sutherland SK, Trinca JC: Survey of 2144 cases of red-back spider bites. Med J Aust *2*:620–623, 1978.
23. Istell R, Bodmer EJ, Buchbinder E: Black widow spider *(Latrodectus mactans):* Bite of the foot. J Am Podiatr Assoc *69*:562–563, 1979.
24. Sampayo RRLT: Pharmacological action of the venom of *Latrodectus mactans* and other *Latrodectus* spiders. J Pharmacol Exp Ther *80*:309–322, 1994.
25. Kobernick M: Black widow spider bite. Am Fam Physician *29*:241–245, 1984.

26. Parrish HM: Analysis of 460 fatalities from venomous animals in the United States. Am J Med Sci *24*:35–47, 1963.
27. Key GF: A comparison of calcium gluconate and methocarbamol (Robaxin) in the treatment of latrodectism (black widow spider envenomation). Am J Trop Med Hyg *30*:273–277, 1981.
28. Pardal JF, Granata AR, Barrio A: Influence of calcium on 3H-noradrenaline release by *Latrodectus antheratus* (black widow spider) venom gland extract in arterial tissues of the rat. Toxicon *17*:455–465, 1979.
29. White RDD, Goldsmith RS, Rodrigues R, et al: Plasma ionic calcium levels following injection of chloride, gluconate, and gluceptate salts of calcium. J Thorac Cardiovasc Surg *71*:609, 1976.
30. Jurkovich GJ, Luterman A, McCullar K, et al: Complications of Crotalidae antivenin therapy. J Trauma *28*:1032–1037, 1988.
31. Malasit P, Warrell DA, Chanthavdnith P, et al: Prediction, prevention, and mechanism of early (anaphylactic) antivenin reactions in victims of snake bites. BMJ *292*:17–20, 1986.
32. Russell FE, Marcus P, Streng JA: Black widow spider envenomation during pregnancy. Report of a case. Toxicon *17*:188–189, 1979.
33. Brown AF: Delayed diagnosis of red-back spider envenomation: A timely reminder. Med J Aust *151*:705–706, 1989.
34. Suntorntham S, Roberts JR, Nilsen GJ: Dramatic clinical response to the delayed administration of black widow spider antivenin. Letter. Ann Emerg Med *24*:1198–1199, 1994.
35. Allen RC, Norris RL: Delayed use of widow spider antivenin. Ann Emerg Med *26*:393–394, 1995.
36. Banham ND, Jelinek GA, Finch PM: Late treatment with antivenom in prolonged red-back spider envenomation. Med J Aust *161*:379–381, 1994.
37. Pincus DR: Response to antivenom 14 days after red-back spider bite. Letter. Med J Aust *161*:226, 1994.
38. Weiner S: Red-back spider bite treated with antivenin. Med J Aust *1*:858, 1956.
39. Southcott RV: Red-back spider bite (latrodectism) with response to antivenin therapy given eighty hours after the injury. Med J Aust *1*:669–682, 1961.
40. Schuman SH, Caldwell ST: 1990 South Carolina Physician Survey of tick, spider and fire ant morbidity [see comments]. J S C Med Assoc *87*:429–432, 1991.
41. Geren CR, Chan TK, Howell DE, Odell GV: Isolation and characterization of toxins from brown recluse spider venom *(Loxosceles reclusa)*. Arch Biochem Biophys *174*:90–99, 1976.
42. Rees RS, Nanney LB, Yates RA, King LEJ: Interaction of brown recluse spider venom on cell membranes: The inciting mechanism? J Invest Dermatol *83*:270–275, 1984.
43. Gates CA, Rees RS: Serum amyloid P component: Its role in platelet activation stimulated by sphingomyelinase D purified from the venom of the brown recluse spider *(Loxosceles reclusa)*. Toxicon *28*:1303–1315, 1990.
44. Rees RS: Platelet activation stimulated by the toxin of the brown recluse spider requires serum amyloid P component, not C-reactive protein. Toxicon *27*:953–954, 1989.
45. Kurpiewski G, Campbell BJ, Forrester LJ, Barrett JT: Alternate complement pathway activation by recluse spider venom. Int J Tissue React *3*:39–45, 1981.
46. Rees RS, Gates C, Timmons S, et al: Plasma components are required for platelet activation by the toxin of *Loxosceles reclusa*. Toxicon *26*:1035, 1988.
47. Smith CW, Micks DW: The role of polymorphonuclear leukocytes in the lesion caused by the venom of the brown spider, *Loxosceles reclusa*. Lab Invest *22*:90–93, 1970.
48. Patel KD, Modur V, Zimmerman GA, et al: The necrotic venom of the brown recluse spider induces dysregulated endothelial cell-dependent neutrophil activation. Differential induction of GM-CSF, IL-8, and E-selectin expression. J Clin Invest *94*:631–642, 1994.
49. Futrell JM: Loxoscelism. Am J Med Sci *304*:261, 1992.
50. Hufford DC, Morgan PH: C-reactive protein as a mediator in the lysis of human erythrocytes sensitized by brown recluse spider venom. Proc Soc Exp Biol Med *167*:493, 1981.
51. Rees R, Campbell D, Rieger E, King LE: The diagnosis and treatment of brown recluse spider bites. Ann Emerg Med *16*:945–949, 1987.
52. Gendron BP: *Loxosceles reclusa* envenomation. Am J Emerg Med *8*:51–54, 1990.
53. Murray LM, Seger DL: Hemolytic anemia following a presumptive brown recluse spider bite. J Toxicol Clin Toxicol *32*:451–456, 1994.
54. Majeski JA, Durst GG: Bite by the spider *Herpyllus ecclesiasticus* in South Carolina. Toxicon *13*:377, 1975.
55. Vorse H, Seccareccio P, Woodruff K, Humphrey GB: Disseminated intravascular coagulopathy following fatal brown spider bite (necrotic arachnidism). J Pediatr *80*:1035–1037, 1972.
56. Barrett SM, Romine Jenkins M, Blick KE: Passive hemagglutination inhibition test for diagnosis of brown recluse spider bite envenomation. Clin Chem *39*:2104–2107, 1993.
57. Cardoso JL, Wen FH, Franca FO, et al: Detection by enzyme immunoassay of *Loxosceles gaucho* venom in necrotic skin lesions caused by spider bites in Brazil [see comments]. Trans R Soc Trop Med Hyg *84*:608–609, 1990.
58. Berger RS: A critical look at therapy for the brown recluse spider bite. Arch Dermatol *107*:298, 1973.
59. Rees RS, King LE: Therapy for brown recluse spider bites is dependent on venom persistence. Clin Res *33*:302, 1985.
60. King LE, Rees RS: Dapsone treatment of a brown recluse bite. JAMA *250*:648, 1983.
61. Barrett SM, Romine Jenkins M, Fisher DE: Dapsone or electric shock therapy of brown recluse spider envenomation? Ann Emerg Med *24*:21–25, 1994.
62. Phillips S, Kohn M, Baker D, et al: Therapy of brown spider envenomation: A controlled trial of hyperbaric oxygen, dapsone, and cyproheptadine. Ann Emerg Med *25*:363–368, 1995.
63. Hobbs G, Anderson A, Greene T, et al: Comparison of hyperbaric oxygen and dapsone therapy for *Loxosceles* envenomation. Acad Emerg Med *3*:758–761, 1996.
64. Rees RS, Altenbern DP, Lynch JB, King LEJ: Brown recluse spider bites. A comparison of early surgical excision versus dapsone and delayed surgical excision. Ann Surg *202*:659–663, 1985.
65. Wille RC, Morrow JD: Case report: Dapsone hypersensitivity syndrome associated with treatment of the bite of a brown recluse spider. Am J Med Sci *296*:270–271, 1988.
66. Iserson KV: Methemoglobinemia from dapsone therapy for a suspected brown spider bite. J Emerg Med *3*:285–288, 1985.
67. Hansen RC, Russell FE: Dapsone use for *Loxosceles* envenomation treatment. Vet Hum Toxicol *26*:260, 1984.
68. Wasserman GS: Wound care of spider and snake envenomations. Ann Emerg Med *17*:1331–1335, 1988.
69. DeLozier JB, Reaves L, King LE, Jr, Rees RS: Brown recluse spider bites of the upper extremity. South Med J *81*:181–184, 1988.
70. Svendsen FJ: Treatment of clinically diagnosed brown recluse spider bites with hyperbaric oxygen: A clinical observation. J Ark Med Soc *83*:199–204, 1986.
71. Kendall TE, Caniglia RJ: Hyperbaric oxygen in the treatment of clinically diagnosed brown recluse spider bites: A review of 48 cases. Abstract. Undersea Biomed Res *16*(Suppl):21, 1989.
72. Maynor ML, Moon RE, Kiltzman B, et al: HBO and the effect of brown spider venom in rabbits. Undersea Hyperb Med *20*(Suppl):45, 1993.
73. Strain GM, Snider TG, Tedford BL, Cohn GH: Hyperbaric oxygen effects on brown recluse spider *(Loxosceles reclusa)* envenomation in rabbits. Toxicon *29*:989–996, 1991.
74. Tomaszewski CA, Thom SR: Use of hyperbaric oxygen in toxicology. Emerg Med Clin North Am *12*:437–459, 1994.
75. Maynor ML, Abt JL, Osborne PD: Brown recluse spider bites: Beneficial effects of hyperbaric oxygen. J Hyperbaric Med *7*:89–102, 1992.
76. Spielman A, Levi HW: Probable envenomation by *Chiracanthium mildei*: A spider found in houses. Am J Trop Med Hyg *19*:729, 1970.
77. Russell FE: Bite by the spider *Phidippus formosus*: Case history. Toxicon *8*:193–194, 1970.
78. Vest DK: Necrotic arachnidism in the northwest United States and its probable relationship to *Tegenaria agrestis* (Walckenaer) spiders. Toxicon *25*:175–184, 1987.
79. Campbell DS, Rees RS, King LE: Wolf spider bites. Cutis *39*:113–114, 1987.

B Scorpions

MARY BETH MILLER, DO
DONALD B. KUNKEL, MD

Scorpions are invertebrate arthropods that have existed for longer than 400 million years. Because they have eight legs, they belong to the class Arachnida, along with spiders. A scorpion has an elongated, segmented body similar to that of a shrimp and a relatively long, segmented, and highly mobile "tail." The last segment of the tail, or *telson,* is a bulbous structure called the *vesicle,* which contains the venom apparatus. The stinger is attached to the telson. Prey is seized by a set of pincers located anterior to the legs, and the tail is thrust over the body so that the stinger may inject the victim.

Approximately 650 species of scorpions have been identified; 40 of these are found in the continental United States. Almost all toxic species belong to the family Buthidae. Although scorpions live in desert or semi-arid climates, envenomations have been reported in such places as Michigan, where a scorpion was imported to the area in a patient's luggage.[1] The only American species of clinical consequence is *Centruroides sculpturatus* Ewing (also known as *C. exilicauda*). This small, slender species is indigenous to Arizona, with a range into Mexico, and colonies are found in California, Texas, New Mexico, and southern Nevada.[2]

SCORPION VENOM AND ITS CLINICAL EFFECTS

Scorpion venoms are low-molecular-weight proteins whose various actions depend on the species.[3] A hyperadrenergic state with high levels of circulating catecholamines, hypertension, cholinergic signs, pulmonary edema, myocardial injury, cardiac dysrhythmia, cardiovascular collapse, and death can result from stings by the yellow scorpion *Leiurus quinquestriatus* (range: Lebanon, Turkey, Syria, Jordan, and northern Africa).[4] Similar effects occur with stings by the common North African *Androctonus* species[4] and the *Mesobuthus* species found in India.[5] Hypertension, cholinergic symptoms, convulsions, coma, and death can follow stings by the South American *Tityus* species.[4] Hemolysis, renal failure, bleeding disorders (including disseminated intravascular coagulation), tissue necrosis, pancreatitis, and neurotoxicity have also been described as a result of stings by non-American scorpions.[4–6] Effective antivenins are produced in Israel, Egypt, Algeria, South Africa, Brazil, and Turkey for the aforementioned species.[4] For a current summary of the physiology of these scorpion venoms and various proposed pharmacologic treatments, readers are referred to the excellent review by Ismail.[6]

In contrast to non-American scorpions, the effects of *Centruroides* venom seem to be entirely neurotoxic. Because the venom contains no enzymes that cause tissue destruction, the usual inflammatory findings do not occur at the sting site. A first group of protein neurotoxins bind neuronal sodium channels to cause incomplete sodium channel activation; a second type causes or enhances repetitive firing of axons.[3] Clinical findings are consistent with this increased presynaptic activity at the neuromuscular junction, parasympathetic nerves, and possibly adrenergic nerve endings and adrenal medulla (Table 24B–1). Symptoms begin immediately after the sting and usually reach maximum severity within 5 hours.

The stings of other American species, including *Vejovis* species (stripe-tailed scorpion) and *Hadrurus* species (giant hairy scorpion), may produce local swelling, edema, and pain. Although envenomations by non-American scorpions still cause fatalities,[4] no deaths have been reported in the United States since 1968.[7] Improved eradication methods, skillful supportive care, and the use of antivenin have contributed to this advance.

EVALUATION AND MANAGEMENT OF *CENTRUROIDES* ENVENOMATIONS

The Samaritan Regional Poison Center in Phoenix, Arizona, was consulted in more than 3400 cases of

Table 24B–1. Grades of *Centruroides sculpturatus* Envenomation

Grade I	Local pain and/or paresthesias at the site of envenomation
Grade II	Pain and/or paresthesias remote from the site of envenomation, in addition to local findings
Grade III	*Either* cranial nerve *or* somatic skeletal neuromuscular dysfunction: 1. Cranial nerve dysfunction: blurred vision, wandering eye movements, hypersalivation, trouble swallowing, tongue fasciculations, problems with upper airway, slurred speech 2. Somatic skeletal neuromuscular dysfunction: jerking of extremities, restlessness, severe involuntary shaking and jerking, which may be mistaken for seizure activity (but are not)
Grade IV	*Both* cranial nerve *and* somatic skeletal neuromuscular dysfunction

scorpion envenomation in 1994 and manages significant envenomations directly in the emergency department. In an extensive 1984 review of experiences there, Curry and associates devised a grading system of severity of *C. sculpturatus* envenomation, based on clinical signs and symptoms, that is used to guide therapy (Table 24B–1).[2] Patients with grade I and grade II envenomations are usually treated at home with cautious application of ice to the sting site for pain relief and with oral analgesics. Although patients with grades III and IV envenomations may be treated with supportive care, antivenin administration is usually recommended in severe cases. Its careful administration results in resolution of symptoms within 1 to 3 hours and may avoid the morbidity associated with sedation, intubation, or pharmacologic paralysis.

Specific *Centruroides* antivenin derived from goat serum is available from Antivenom Production Laboratories, Arizona State University, Tempe, Arizona. It is not approved for general use by the Food and Drug Administration but is available within the state of Arizona by special action of the Arizona State Board of Pharmacy.

Administration of antivenin requires careful preparation and constant observation. Aggressive airway management is crucial to patient outcome, because increased secretions and impaired cranial nerve function may lead to respiratory compromise (reversal of neuromuscular impairment by antivenin may take 15 to 30 minutes or longer). Patients should be placed on a cardiac monitor with pulse oximetry. Medications and equipment used to treat anaphylaxis should be prepared and available for immediate use.

A skin test is performed by diluting 0.1 mL of reconstituted antivenin in 1 mL of normal saline; 0.2 mL of the test solution is used to raise a small intradermal wheal. After 10 minutes, the site is checked for the presence of erythema or urticarial wheal. It is important to remember that the skin test may not always predict those patients who will have an immediate adverse reaction.

One vial of reconstituted antivenin is diluted in 50 mL of crystalloid solution and administered at a few microdrops per minute. Patients are monitored for any signs of adverse reaction such as rash, dyspnea, or change in vital signs. If this is well tolerated for 5 minutes, the rate can be cautiously increased until the infusion is completed. Total infusion time is 15 to 30 minutes. If severe symptoms persist 1 hour after the infusion is completed, a second vial may then be administered. In the absence of complicating factors, patients may be discharged once symptoms have resolved.

Complications of antivenin therapy may be immediate or delayed. Only three series report the rate of immediate (anaphylactic/anaphylactoid) reactions. In the first, Curry and colleagues report that only 1 patient in 22 developed a reaction consisting of a single urticarial wheal. This rapidly cleared with epinephrine, and the patient then received the complete infusion.[2] The second reports no acute reactions in a series of 12 patients.[8] In another series, 8% of patients manifested reactions ranging from a wheal at the site of injection to localized rash or edema. All patients were able to receive the complete infusion.[9] The incidence of delayed hypersensitivity (serum sickness) has ranged from zero in earlier reports to 58% in more recent literature,[2, 8] and thus the need for follow-up in these patients is emphasized.

References

1. Trestrail JH: Scorpion envenomation in Michigan. Vet Hum Toxicol *23*:8, 1971.
2. Curry SC, Vance MV, Ryan PJ, et al: Envenomation by the scorpion *Centruroides sculpturatus*. J Toxicol Clin Toxicol *21*:417–449, 1983–1984.
3. Wang GK, Strichartz GR: Purification and physiological characterization of neurotoxins from venoms of the scorpions *Centruroides sculpturatus* and *Leiurus quinquestriatus*. Mol Pharmacol *23*:519–533, 1983.
4. Keegan HL: Scorpions of Medical Importance. Jackson, MS, University Press of Mississippi, 1985.
5. Conner DA, Seldon BS: Scorpion envenomation. *In* Auerbach PS (ed): Wilderness Medicine—Management of Wilderness and Environmental Emergencies. St. Louis, Mosby–Year Book, pp 831–842, 1995.
6. Ismail M: The scorpion envenomation syndrome. Toxicon *33*:825–858, 1995.
7. Likes K, Banner W, Chavez M: *Centruroides exilicauda* envenomation in Arizona. West J Med *141*:634–637, 1984.
8. Bond GR: Antivenin administration for *Centruroides* scorpion sting: Risks and benefits. Ann Emerg Med *21*:788–791, 1992.
9. Gateau T, Bloom M, Clark R: Response to specific *Centruroides sculpturatus* antivenom in 151 cases of scorpion stings. Clin Toxicol *32*:165–170, 1994.

C Stinging Insects

FRANCIS X. TUNNEY, MD

TAXONOMY AND EPIDEMIOLOGY

The stinging insects responsible for causing systemic reactions in humans constitute the order Hymenoptera of the class Insecta (Fig. 24C–1). Within the Hymenoptera, three families of importance are the Vespidae (yellow jackets, hornets, and wasps), Apidae (honeybees and bumblebees) and Formicidae (fire ants). Fire ants are discussed separately at the end of this chapter. Most sting reactions in the United States are secondary to stings by vespids, especially yellow jackets. Unlike other vespids such as wasps

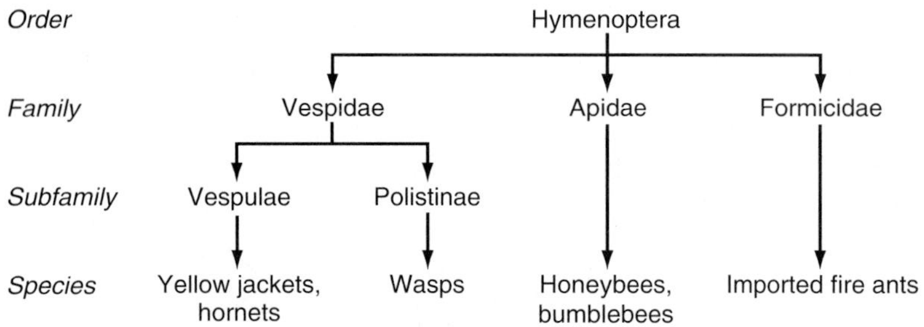

Figure 24C–1. Taxonomy of Hymenoptera.

and hornets, which build their nests in trees or under awnings, yellow jackets are primarily ground dwellers and as such are often in contact with humans, especially during warm months with outdoor activities such as gardening, lawn mowing and walking barefoot. All vespids are attracted to sugary substances and fragrances, and they often become aggressive when exposed to scents from outdoor cooking, trash cans, picnics, or perfumes. Honeybees and bumblebees, on the other hand, tend to build their nests away from humans, are quite passive, and attack only if provoked. Most stings by honeybees occur as a consequence of professional beekeeping. Within families of the Hymenoptera, venoms are often similar in composition and share similar antigenic properties. Thus, patients allergic to yellow jackets often are also allergic to hornets. The stinging mechanism of hymenopterans resides in the abdomen and is a modified ovipositor. This structure consists of a venom sac attached to a barbed stinger. The barbs serve to hold the stinger within the victim while the venom sac contracts and venom is injected. Apid stingers have several barbs, which usually cause the stinger to remain embedded in the skin of the victim and to detach from the body of the insect; thus apids inflict single stings. Vespids, having stingers with few barbs, are capable of multiple stings.

Honeybees are not native to the Western Hemisphere but in fact were imported from Europe. Having few natural predators in Europe, with temperate climates and little competition, these species developed docile behaviors. By contrast, African bees evolved under extreme conditions with variable rainfall, intense competition, and many predators. Thus, these species developed intense, aggressive swarming and stinging behaviors, often in response to minimal disturbance. In the 1950s, scientists in Brazil imported bees from Africa for the purpose of interbreeding with existing honeybee populations, in the hope of improving adaption to the tropical climate of equatorial South America. Unfortunately, a few queens with swarms escaped, and these aggressive "Africanized" bees have since made a steady northward expansion. In the early 1990s, Africanized bees were discovered in Texas and have since appeared in Arizona and California. The health risk of Africanized bees lies not in the toxicity of their venom, which is nearly identical to that of their European cousins (along with their appearance), but in the marked persistence of their pursuit and the massive numbers, even thousands, of stings they are capable of inflicting.[2]

In the United States, an average of 40 deaths directly attributable to Hymenoptera stings are reported annually, approximately three times the number caused by poisonous snakes. However, the actual number is almost certainly higher. Autopsy findings of patients who succumb to insect stings often are nonspecific and may or may not reveal laryngeal or pulmonary edema, vascular engorgement, or atherosclerosis. Postmortem studies have detected the presence of immunoglobulin E (IgE)-antibodies to Hymenoptera venom in 50% of patients experiencing sudden unexplained death outdoors, compared with only 6% in the general population.[3] Published case reports have described patients' awakening from resuscitation for acute cardiac arrest and recalling being stung as an initiating event.

Certainly, when determining the cause of a sudden unexpected death occurring outdoors during warm months, anaphylaxis due to Hymenoptera sting should be considered. Tryptase level determination may be helpful in diagnosis, because tryptase is produced only by mast cell degranulation, and elevated levels can be detected in the sera of patients sustaining anaphylaxis due to insect stings.

Most fatalities due to insect stings occur in individuals who are older than 40 years, usually male, and who often have coexistent cardiovascular or respiratory disease. Although yellow jackets cause most systemic sting reactions, bees inflict more fatalities, possibly because of the larger quantities of venom injected by bees. Most deaths due to Hymenoptera stings occur within 1 hour of the stinging, usually before patients reach a hospital, and rarely from more than five stings. In approximately 50% of deaths, victims have no prior known history of Hymenoptera hypersensitivity.[4]

PATHOPHYSIOLOGY AND IMMUNOLOGY

The prevalence of Hymenoptera allergy in the general population is 1% to 3%. Although death tends to occur in older individuals, severe systemic reactions with significant morbidity occur at any age. Frequency of exposure tends to be a major determinant in developing Hymenoptera sensitivity; thus, beekeepers are more frequently allergic to bee venom than is the general population. Interestingly, excessive exposure tends to confer protection, because beekeepers who sustain large numbers (more than 50) of stings annually develop the opposite—less sensitivity.[5] Although it is generally agreed that atopy does not increase the risk of Hymenoptera sensitivity, atopic patients typically have more severe reactions, especially bronchospasm. The timing of insect stings may also have a role, because those individuals who sustain subsequent stings within months develop anaphylaxis more frequently than those stung again several years later.

Classically, systemic Hymenoptera reactions are examples of IgE-mediated immediate hypersensitivity. On initial sensitization, IgE antibodies to a protein or polypeptide antigen are produced. These immunoglobulins subsequently become bound to mast cell membranes, whereupon re-exposure to the inciting allergen induces a series of events leading to degranulation of mast cells and release of histamine, prostaglandins, leukotrienes, platelet-activating factor, tryptase, and heparin. However, nearly 10% of patients with Hymenoptera sting reactions (and half of fatal cases) have no prior history of sustaining an insect sting, and this finding supports the concept that other pathways of direct non-IgE mast cell stimulation may occur, possibly involving complement and kinin pathways, as well as direct mast cell stimulation independent of IgE by specific components of insect venom.[6] Mast cells are concentrated throughout the body, especially in the airways, lungs, heart, and skin; this explains some of the local effects noted in allergic reactions to insect stings.

Mast cell mediators of primary importance in insect sting reactions are histamine, prostaglandins, and leukotrienes. These all have similar local effects, including smooth muscle contraction, increased vascular permeability, vasodilatation, and increased mucus production. Thus, many of the symptoms of insect sting anaphylaxis can be attributed to these mediators. In addition, secondary mediators from inflammatory cells recruited by mast cell stimulation, such as eosinophils and macrophages, may further directly induce degranulation. Thus, delayed or biphasic reactions are occasionally seen.

Hymenoptera venoms consist of various substances of known toxicity as well as allergenic proteins and polypeptides. Potential allergens include phospholipase A, hyaluronidase, acid phosphatase, mellitin (a major bee venom antigen) and antigen 5, a vespid allergen of unknown function. Vespid venoms share much more similarity in these allergens with other vespids than with bee venoms, and this explains the cross-sensitivity between vespid species. Additional compounds include apamin, mast cell–degranulating peptide, dopamine, serotonin, and kinins.[7]

CLINICAL PRESENTATION

Unlike venomous spider bites, all Hymenoptera stings cause some degree of local pain and swelling, and therefore, unless cognition is impaired, all patients know they have been stung. These small local reactions of erythema and edema at the sting site are self-limited and non–IgE mediated and resolve spontaneously in 24 hours. Some patients may develop more extensive large local reactions. These are more severe reactions of local edema and erythema sometimes involving most or all of an extremity. These reactions are often delayed in appearance, occurring 1 to 2 days after the sting and lasting for as long as a week. The cause of large local reactions is not clear, but they are believed to occur via local mast cell degranulation. These reactions are often misdiagnosed as cellulitis; in fact, infection rarely complicates insect stings. Of interest, marked local reactions have been reported as causes of significant morbidity. Fatalities have resulted from total airway occlusion secondary to stings occurring inside the oral cavity, and optic neuritis, retinal damage, and stroke have also been reported to occur secondary to severe local reactions.[8]

Systemic anaphylactic symptoms due to insect stings are no different from other anaphylactic reactions. Onset may be rapid, often within 10 minutes of being stung, and serious, life-threatening symptoms may occur rapidly and unexpectedly. The most common anaphylactic symptoms due to Hymenoptera sting are cutaneous and mild in nature, such as urticaria, pruritus, or angioedema. Non–life-threatening gastrointestinal symptoms also are common, including nausea, vomiting, diarrhea, and cramping pain. More serious systemic symptoms involve the respiratory and cardiovascular systems. Bronchorrhea and bronchoconstriction may occur, leading to cough, wheezing, and dyspnea, with possible subsequent hypoxia and respiratory failure. Local edema of the upper airway may cause congestion of the larynx, epiglottis, and surrounding tissues. Patients may relate a sensation of having a lump in their throat, stridor may ensue, and total upper airway obstruction can occur. More than 60% of insect sting fatalities occur secondary to respiratory complications.

Cardiovascular symptoms of systemic reactions to Hymenoptera stings may range from mild hypotension and tachycardia to profound circulatory collapse and shock. Differentiating anxiety reactions with vasovagal symptoms from anaphylaxis may be difficult, and although bradycardia is more commonly encountered in the former, the presence of bradycardia does not rule out anaphylaxis. Severe left ventricular dysfunction, malignant arrhythmias, ischemia, and myocardial infarction all have been described in patients with systemic reactions to insect stings. Although other factors may account for some of these symptoms, including hypoxia, hypotension, and therapeutic use of epinephrine, the concept of "cardiac anaphylaxis" has gained favor.[9] Many cases of fatal insect stings are secondary to direct cardiac events, and as previously stated, a number of unexplained sudden deaths may have Hymenoptera sting as a direct cause. Cardiac tissue is rich in concentrations of mast cells, and their numbers are increased in diseased, atheromatous arteries. Mast cell mediators, especially histamine, leukotrienes, and prostaglandins, can induce a number of potentially dangerous cardiac events, including coronary vasoconstriction and spasm, local platelet aggregation with thrombus formation, left ventricular dysfunction, and increased automaticity. Myocardial infarction has been documented in patients who were experiencing anaphylaxis due to insect stings but who subsequently were demonstrated to have normal coronary arteries.[10]

Unusual delayed reactions have also been reported, including serum sickness, vasculitis, glomerulonephritis, neuropathy, disseminated intravascular coagulation, and arthritis. These are believed to be immune mediated, because elevated venom-specific IgG and IgE levels have been detected in these patients. Also, direct toxic effects of Hymenoptera venom have been reported, independent of any immune mechanism. These are dose-dependent reactions, often occurring in patients sustaining multiple stings by Africanized bees. Rhabdomyolysis, hemolysis, and acute renal failure from direct tubular toxicity have been described in patients without coexistent hypoxia or hypotension.[11]

TREATMENT

Prehospital Management

Because most deaths due to insect stings occur within 1 hour of being stung, early aggressive stabilization and transport are mandatory, especially for patients with histories of severe reactions. Emergency kits for self-medication may include 0.3 mg (EpiPen) or 0.15 mg (EpiPen Jr.) of epinephrine alone or in a kit with an oral antihistamine (Ana-Kit). The use of self-administered inhaled epinephrine (Medihaler-Epi) has gained favor in Europe, and studies have demonstrated its superiority over subcutaneous epinephrine in certain subgroups of patients, especially those with primarily airway or respiratory symptoms.[12] Patients with known histories of moderate or severe reactions should carry these kits with them and self-medicate after stings at the earliest sign of reaction. All patients with anaphylactic symptoms should receive emergent hospital treatment.

Emergency Department Management

Patients with isolated local reactions often respond well to conservative treatment with antihistamines, elevation, and cool compresses. Steroids may be of some benefit, especially in large local reactions. For patients with systemic symptoms, as for any patient with life-threatening illness, immediate attention to the ABC's of emergency management is paramount. Time and personnel should not be spent meticulously removing embedded stingers, because 100% of bee venom is delivered within 60 seconds of being stung.[13] Because patients with anaphylaxis can deteriorate rapidly and without warning, intravenous access, cardiac monitoring, and supplemental oxygen should be in place and airway and crash cart equipment immediately available. Specific pharmacologic therapy for systemic sting reactions includes the following:

Epinephrine. Many investigators recommend the use of epinephrine as first-line treatment for all systemic reactions, including angioedema and urticaria.[14] For these and moderate reactions such as laryngospasm, bronchospasm, and hypotension, aqueous epinephrine given subcutaneously or intramuscularly (1:1000 concentration) in doses of 0.01 mL/kg for children, 0.3 to 0.5 mL for adults, should be administered. In severe reactions, such as shock, total airway obstruction, or respiratory arrest, 1 to 5 mL of intravenous epinephrine (1:10,000 concentration), further diluted 10:1 with saline, may be cautiously administered slowly intravenously while carefully observing for signs of improvement or adverse reactions (e.g., arrhythmia), along with aggressive airway management if needed. Unlike all other medications used in the treatment of systemic reactions, with the exception of glucagon, epinephrine stabilizes mast cells and thereby terminates continued propagation of anaphylaxis. Epinephrine should be used with caution (or not at all) in patients older than 40 years and those who are pregnant, use β-blockers, or have coronary artery disease.

Glucagon. In those patients for whom epinephrine is contraindicated (e.g., on β-blockers), glucagon may prove beneficial, especially in the presence of hypotension. The usual dose is 1 mg for adults, 0.5 mg for children, intravenously and may be given as repeated injections or continuous infusion if necessary. Side effects such as nausea may be prevented by injecting slowly.

Volume Expansion. An intravenous bolus of normal saline is certainly indicated in the presence of hypotension, especially in anaphylactic patients. Continued infusion to ensure continuous urine outflow is also generally indicated. Pressor agents other than repeated administration of epinephrine are generally not necessary.

Antihistamines. Although not as efficacious as epinephrine, H_1 antagonists may provide additional relief of pruritus, urticaria, and bronchospasm associated with insect sting reactions. Diphenhydramine (Benadryl) or hydroxyzine (Atarax) may be used by slow intravenous push or intramuscularly; the dose is generally titrated, beginning with 25 mg intravenously in adults and progressing up to a total of 1 to 2 mg/kg if necessary, with careful monitoring of vital signs. The H_2 blocker cimetidine (4 mg/kg intravenously) may also be indicated. The combined use of H_1 and H_2 antagonists is more effective than either used alone, especially for hypotension.[15]

Corticosteroids and Other Agents. Although corticosteroids have no documented effect in acute reactions, their use is generally indicated because they may prevent late phase reactions. Intravenous

Solu-Medrol, 125 to 250 mg for adults, is generally administered. Nebulized β-adrenergic agonists such as albuterol are often useful in the presence of wheezing. Aminophylline is rarely if ever used today.

PATIENT DISPOSITION

Patients with local reactions or urticaria alone can often be discharged after symptoms have resolved. Because a small percentage of patients with systemic anaphylactic symptoms have a biphasic course, with recurrent symptoms of equal severity occurring a few hours after initial symptoms have cleared, all patients with moderate systemic anaphylactic symptoms need to be observed for 8 to 12 hours for signs of recurrence. Any patient with severe reactions should be hospitalized.

All patients sustaining systemic symptoms after Hymenoptera stings should receive the following before discharge: (1) provision of epinephrine for self-medication (Ana-Kit, EpiPen or Medihaler-Epi) with instructions and demonstration of its use, (2) specific avoidance instructions (Table 24C–1), (3) provision for obtaining an anaphylaxis identification bracelet, (4) arrangements to adjust medications such as β-blockers; and (5) referral to an allergist. Unfortunately, all too often this is not done. A California survey found that only 50% of physicians provided specific avoidance instructions, and most failed to refer patients to allergists or provide identification bracelets.[16] β-blockers are withdrawn because subsequent sting reactions may be more severe than those occurring in patients not on β-blockers, owing to increased risk of bronchospasm, continued mast cell degranulation, and unopposed α-adrenergic receptor–mediated hypertension due to endogenous and exogenous cathecholamines.

VENOM IMMUNOTHERAPY

Patients with systemic reactions from Hymenoptera stings may be candidates for Venom Immunotherapy (VIT). After skin testing with pure venom extracts of the five known vespids and apids in the United States, those venoms eliciting positive reactions are injected in gradually increasing doses, culminating in a maintenance dose, every 6 to 8 weeks for a 3- to 5-year period. Although the exact mechanism for successful VIT is not known, it is believed that patients are desensitized by production of venom-specific IgG (so-called blocking antibodies), which acts to prevent IgE-induced mast cell degranulation or IgE production. IgE levels decrease over time with VIT, and it is this IgG-to-IgE ratio of venom-specific antibody that confers protection against future reactions.

Controversy exists, however, about how best to determine who should receive VIT. Based on earlier studies that indicated that most patients with generalized reactions to insect stings would have reactions of similar type and severity when stung again at a later date, most children with severe symptoms and adults with moderate or severe symptoms were encouraged to undergo VIT. Immunotherapy has been very successful, with an overall desensitization or "cure" rate of 98% after 3 to 5 years of treatment. Studies in Europe, however, have altered this approach. By directly challenging patients with histories of Hymenoptera anaphylaxis presenting for VIT, using live insects under controlled in-hospital settings, Van der Linden and colleagues were able to demonstrate that only 28% had repeat reactions to subsequent stings. These findings suggest that more than two thirds of patients who may be candidates for VIT under current criteria may not need it.[17] Until more controlled studies of this issue are undertaken, most patients with moderate or severe reactions will be candidates for VIT.

Table 24C–1. Avoidance Instructions for Patients Allergic to Insect Stings

Always wear shoes outdoors.
Avoid wearing brightly colored clothes or floral prints.
Refrain when possible from eating outdoors and keep foods tightly covered.
Always have your epinephrine emergency self-administration kit available.
Wear pants and snug-fitting long-sleeved shirts when outside.
Avoid scented lotions, soaps, and perfumes.
Always have a professional remove insect nests.
Keep garbage cans tightly closed and away from outdoor living areas.
Avoid freshly fallen fruit or brightly colored flowers outside.
Keep windows screened and doors to the house closed.
If confronted by stinging insects, avoid sudden movements and walk away slowly. If swarms of bees attack, move away quickly and seek shelter.
Seek medical attention immediately if stung.

FIRE ANTS

Since arriving in the United States in the early 1900s in Alabama, the imported fire ant (IFA) has spread throughout the southeast. The black IFA, *Solenopsis richteri,* has been contained in a small area of central Alabama and Mississippi. The red IFA, *Solenopsis invicta,* is now well entrenched in more than 160 million acres in 13 states, from Texas to North Carolina. A highly adaptive insect, the IFA has both supplanted and interbred with local ant populations and now accounts for more than 90% of ants of southern states. New hybrids display tolerance for cold and drought that may enable the IFA to spread much farther into the United States. Their spread will surely create a significant public health problem, because as many as 60% of individuals in ant-infested areas will be stung annually. In the southeastern United States, the IFA is now the leading cause of insect sting hypersensitivity.

The IFA is small, 3 to 6 mm, black or red, and similar in appearance to ordinary house or garden ants. These ants inhabit conspicuous mounds of loose dirt or sand, up to 50 cm in diameter, and typically form colonies with a single queen and more than 100,000 individuals, although colonies with several queens exist as well. Underground side channels can extend as far as 20 m from the mound. Fire ants tend to build mounds in sunny areas; thus, valuable farm and residential land is encroached on and the risk of encounters with humans is increased. When the mound is disturbed, communication via pheromones induces an aggressive outpouring of ants that latch onto the skin of the victim, usually the foot. Stinging is a two-part maneuver: The ant uses its powerful mandible to bite and anchor itself to the victim and then injects venom through its abdominal stinger in a series of stings rotating in a circle around its head. Unlike the venom of other stinging insects, which are high in protein (allergen) content, IFA venom is composed primarily of alkaloids, especially piperadines, which have local necrotic and hemolytic effects. This property helps explain the unique local reactions of IFA stings as well as the difficulty in isolating purified IFA venom protein for skin testing and immunotherapy.

In most individuals, IFA stings result in a local wheal and flare reaction, with subsequent development of a sterile pustule at the location of the bite, which is nearly pathognomonic for IFA stings. These sterile pustules may last 2 to 3 weeks before spontaneously involuting and often are accompanied by significant pruritus. These pustules occasionally become secondarily infected and can progress to cellulitis or sepsis. A minority of patients (17%) also develop extensive local reactions adjacent to the bite, with induration and erythema that may last as long as 7 days. Systemic reactions occur in 1% to 2% of individuals, and direct toxic effects of IFA venom have included disseminated intravascular coagulation, seizures, mononeuritis monoplex, and rhabdomyolysis. Severe anaphylactic reactions to IFA stings occur in 0.1% of individuals stung. The annual mortality from IFA stings is not known.[18]

To date, no therapy has proved beneficial in preventing or resolving local reactions, including pustules. Many therapies may proved symptomatic relief, however, including use of antihistamines or topical steroids, application of ice or alcohol, or topical treatment with camphor and menthol (Sarna lotion). Severe local reactions may benefit from steroids. Secondary infections and unusual systemic reactions should be treated accordingly, and anaphylactic reactions are managed as previously described.

Reactions to IFA stings can best be prevented by avoidance. Yards and playing fields should be regularly inspected for mounds, and appropriate measures taken at eradication. The IFA is notoriously difficult to eradicate, but significant breakthroughs in recent years predict that control will be possible. For those individuals with anaphylactic reactions to IFA stings, immunotherapy with whole-body extract has been successful.

References

1. Reisman RE: Insect Stings. N Engl J Med *331*:523, 1994.
2. Winston ML: The Africanized "killer" bee: Biology and public health. Q J Med *87*:263, 1994.
3. Charpin D, Birnbaum J, Vervloet D: Epidemiology of hymenoptera allergy. Clin Exp Allergy *24*:1010, 1994.
4. Barnard J: Studies of 400 Hymenoptera sting deaths in the United States. J Allergy Clin Immunol *52*:259, 1973.
5. Reisman RE: Venom hypersensitivity. J Allergy Clin Immunol *94*:651, 1994.
6. Valentine MD: Anaphylaxis and stinging insect hypersensitivity. JAMA *268*:2830, 1992.
7. Valentine MD: Insect venom allergy: Diagnosis and treatment. J Allergy Clin Immunol *73*:299, 1984.
8. Berrios R, Serrano L: Bilateral optic neuritis after a bee sting. Am J Ophthalmol *117*:677, 1994.
9. Wasserman S: The heart in anaphylaxis. J Allergy Clin Immunol *77*:663, 1986.
10. Wagdi P, Mehan V, Burgi H, et al: Acute myocardial infarction after wasp stings in a patient with normal coronary arteries. Am Heart J *128*:820, 1994.
11. Beccari M, Castiglione A, Cavaliere G, et al: Unusual case of anuria due to African bee stings. Int J Artif Org *15*:281, 1992.
12. Heilborn H, Hjemdahl P, Daleskog M, et al: Comparison of subcutaneous injection and high-dose inhalation of epinephrine—implications for self-treatment to prevent anaphylaxis. J Allergy Clin Immunol *78*:1174, 1986.
13. Schumacher M, Tveten M, Egen N: Rate and quantity of delivery of venom from honeybee stings. J Allergy Clin Immunol *93*:831, 1994.
14. Muller U, Mosbech H, Blaauw P: Emergency treatment of allergic reactions to Hymenoptera stings. Clin Exp Allergy *21*:281, 1991.
15. Mayumi H, Kimura S, Asano M, et al: Intravenous cimetidine as an effective treatment for systemic anaphylaxis and acute allergic skin reactions. Ann Allergy *58*:447, 1987.
16. McDougle L, Klein G, Hoehler F: Management of hymenoptera sting anaphylaxis: A preventive medicine survey. J Emerg Med *13*:9, 1995.
17. Van der Linden PW, Struyvenberg A, Kraaijenhagen R, et al: Anaphylactic shock after insect-sting challenge in 138 persons with a previous insect-sting reaction. Ann Intern Med *118*:161, 1993.
18. Tracy J, Demain J, Quinn J, et al: The natural history of exposure to the imported fire ant (*Solenopsis invicta*). J Allergy Clin Immunol *95*:824, 1995.

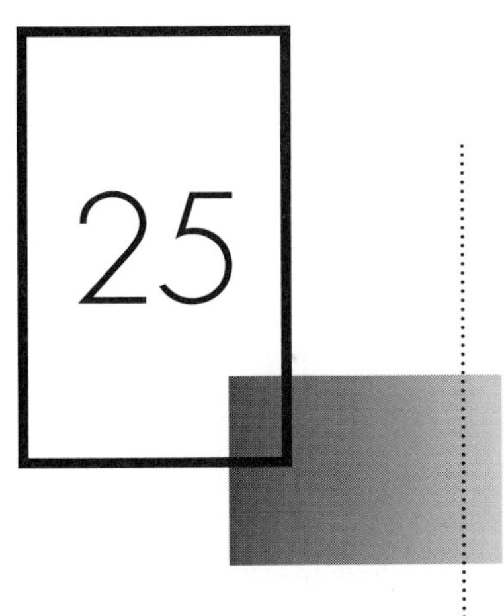

Mushrooms

JEFFREY BRENT, MD, PhD
KENNETH KULIG, MD

Mushrooms are the sexual organs, or fruiting bodies, of fungi. The word *mushroom* derives from an early Greek term roughly translated into "mucus," the stuff that the ancients thought to be the substance of origin of mushrooms as well as frogs.[1] Of the possibly 10,000 species of mushrooms worldwide, only about 50 to 100 are known to be toxic. For most mushrooms, little is known about the effects of their ingestion.

Mushroom poisonings most frequently result from the growing trend worldwide of foraging for edible fungi. They are used for food, in religious ceremonies, and even as medication by herbal healers. They are most commonly identified by experience, through guidebooks, or simply by feeding them to domestic animals as a bioassay of toxicity. Of the earliest reports of mushroom poisoning, the most notable was the tragic account of the Greek poet Euripides, who described the death of his wife and three children due to the ingestion of poisonous mushrooms.[2]

It is probably easiest to understand mushroom toxicology by categorizing mushrooms into groups based on the toxins they contain and the symptoms and signs they may cause. For a patient with a history of mushroom ingestion, the clinical picture should help to determine to which group the mushroom belonged, pending definitive identification. In the majority of cases, the actual identification of the offending mushroom is unknown. Analysis of exposures reported to poison control centers in the United States indicates that the precise species of mushroom is identified in only 3.4% of all exposures.[3] However, even in the absence of this identification, the clinical syndrome being treated may be identified and appropriate therapeutic measures may be undertaken. In the majority of cases, no illness results from mushroom ingestion.[3] The possible mushroom-associated syndromes and the typical causative species are listed in Table 25–1. This determination of the types of mushrooms ingested based on the presenting syndrome is quite similar to what is encountered daily in the clinical practice of medical toxicology, when patients are often seen after overdosing on unknown medications.

GENERAL MANAGEMENT

As with all poisonings, supportive care is of primary importance. Airway management and cardiopulmonary resuscitation, along with maintenance of vital signs, should take priority over identification of the toxin and concern about antidotes. Our concepts of the treatment of mushroom poisoning are to this day evolutionary and dynamic, thus fraught with debate and controversy.

Guidelines for initial management are listed in Table 25–2. Most patients with symptoms after mushroom ingestion have prominent gastrointestinal (GI) complaints: vomiting, diarrhea (possibly bloody), and abdominal pain. It is of crucial importance to determine the time course of the development of symptoms after ingestion. If they developed later than 6 hours after ingestion, it can be assumed that the mushrooms belonged either to the cyclopeptide (commonly the deadly *Amanita*), gyromitrin, or orelline group. With mushrooms from the orelline group, symptoms may develop later than 24 hours after ingestion. It is emphasized, however, that GI symptoms occurring within a few hours of ingestion do not rule out poisoning by these mushrooms; a patient may also have ingested a number of different mushrooms, including ones that cause early symptoms.

Activated charcoal may be of benefit in adsorbing any toxin remaining in the gut. If a patient presents within 1 hour of the time of ingestion and has not

Table 25–1. Summary of Common Mushroom-Associated Syndromes*

Syndrome	Clinical Course	Toxin(s)	Typical Causative Mushroom(s)
Delayed gastroenteritis followed by hepatorenal syndrome	Stage 1: 24 h after ingestion: onset of nausea, vomiting, profuse cholera-like diarrhea, abdominal pain, hematuria Stage 2: 12–48 h after ingestion: apparent recovery; levels of hepatic enzymes are rising during this stage Stage 3: 24–72 h after ingestion: progressive hepatic and renal failure, coagulopathy, cardiomyopathy, encephalopathy, convulsions, coma, death	Cyclopeptides, principally amatoxins	"Deadly *Amanitas,*" *Galerina* spp.
Hyperactivity, delirium, coma	30 min–2 h after ingestion: delirium, hallucinations, and coma	Muscimol, ibotenic acid	*Amanita muscaria, A. pantherina*
Delayed gastroenteritis with central nervous system abnormalities	6–24 h after ingestion: nausea, vomiting, diarrhea, abdominal pain, muscle cramps, delirium, convulsions, coma; hemolysis and methemoglobinemia may occur	Gyromitrin	*Gyromitra esculenta* ("false morel")
Cholinergic syndrome	30 min–2 h after ingestion: bradycardia, bronchorrhea, bronchospasm, salivation, perspiration, lacrimation, convulsions, coma	Muscarine	*Boletus* spp., *Clitocybe* spp., *Inocybe* spp., *Amanita* spp.
Disulfiram-like reaction with ethanol	30 min after drinking ethanol (may occur up to 1 wk after eating coprine-containing mushrooms): flushing of skin of face and trunk, hypotension, tachycardia, chest pain, dyspnea, nausea, vomiting, extreme apprehension	Coprine	*Coprinus atramentarius*
Hallucinations	30 min–3 h after ingestion: hallucinations, euphoria, drowsiness, compulsive behavior, agitation	Psilocybin and psilocyn	*Psilocybe* spp.
Delayed gastritis and renal failure	Abdominal pain, anorexia, vomiting starting over 30 h after ingestion, followed by progressive renal failure 3 to 14 d later	Orelline, orellanine	*Cortinarius* sp.
Immune-mediated hemolytic anemia	Syncope, gastroenteritis, oliguria, hemoglobinuria, back pain, hemolysis	Immunoglobulin mediated	*Paxillus involutus*
General gastrointestinal irritants	30 min–2 h after ingestion: nausea, vomiting, abdominal cramping, diarrhea; may recover without treatment	Unidentified, probably multiple	*Chlorophyllum molybdites,* backyard mushrooms ("little brown mushrooms"), many others

*See Table 25–3 for an extensive list of mushrooms causing these syndromes.

spontaneously vomited, it may be useful to lavage the stomach with a large-bore tube. Any gastric contents obtained by either spontaneous emesis or lavage should be saved and examined for spores. To examine for spores, the gastric aspirate or emesis sample should be filtered through cheesecloth and centrifuged for 10 minutes. The heavier layer at the bottom of the test tube contains the spores, and a sample is carefully removed with a pipette. A drop of water is then added, a coverslip placed, and the slide examined under oil immersion. Mushroom spores, in general, are similar in size to red blood cells (8 to 20 μm). Spores found in either the gastric contents or the lamellae of the mushroom should be examined under the microscope for (1) general appearance, (2) shape, (3) color, (4) thick or thin walls, and (5) the presence of pores.[4]

A spore print can be helpful in identifying the mushroom in question. This is formed by placing the cap of the mushroom on a white piece of paper (Fig. 25–1) and allowing the spores to fall on the paper, imparting a characteristic color. An example of a spore print is shown in Figure 25–2. Because an adequate spore print generally takes several hours to develop, one should be started as soon as possible. It is usually helpful to cover the cap with a glass or bowl while the spore print is being formed to prevent the dispersion of spores by drafts.

Because even veteran mushroom hunters occasionally make an error, many have adopted the practice of eating only one kind of mushroom at a time and saving a sample in case unanticipated effects occur.

If you have a professional mycologist in your area, he or she should be able to tell you the principal

Table 25–2. General Management of Mushroom Ingestion

1. Determine history of ingestion: how many types of mushrooms ingested, what time, if anyone else ate them, and what symptoms are present.
2. Attempt to determine which of the possible syndromes (see Table 25–1) the patient may have. For example, gastrointestinal symptoms occurring more than 6 hours after ingestion strongly suggest cyclopeptide, gyromitrin, or *Cortinarius* poisoning.
3. Administer activated charcoal. If the patient has diarrhea, do not give a cathartic. If a cathartic is used, give it only with the first dose of activated charcoal. Use repeated doses of activated charcoal for suspected amatoxin poisonings.
4. If feasible and when indicated, send gastric aspirate or emesis, along with any remaining mushrooms, to a mycologist for identification.
5. Try to perform a preliminary identification of mushroom and spores. Start to develop a spore print as soon as possible.
6. Maintain supportive measures, including airway support, intravenous fluids, and vasopressors (if needed). Monitor volume status.
7. Avoid antispasmodics for gastrointestinal symptoms.
8. Anticipate the clinical course (see Table 25–1).

types of mushrooms in your region and assist in mushroom identification. Local or regional poison centers should know how to reach mycologists in their region. When a patient is seen after a mushroom ingestion, ask a family member or friend to bring in a similar mushroom (if possible) for identification purposes. Keep the specimen under refrigeration, wrapped in wax paper, and stored in a paper bag (a thorough discussion of mushroom identification may be found in appropriate references).[5]

The greatest concern is about the ingestion of deadly *Amanita* species. Many antidotes and treatments have been suggested for this kind of poisoning, most of them unproven. If vomiting and diarrhea are severe enough to result in significant fluid loss, intravenous replacement of volume and electrolytes is important. The intravenous solution should contain glucose.

By consulting Table 25–1, the group to which the ingested mushrooms may belong should be apparent. For ease of discussion, further management recommendations are described under the specific toxins. Common mushroom species containing the toxins discussed are listed in Table 25–3.

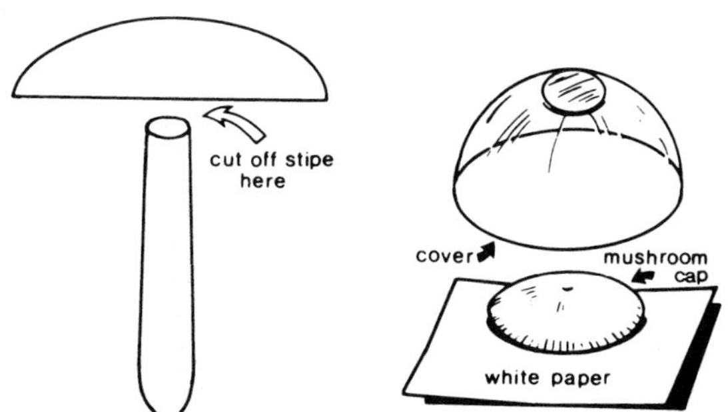

Figure 25–1. Technique of developing a spore print. (From Rumack BH, Salzman E (eds): Mushroom Poisoning: Diagnosis and Treatment. West Palm Beach, FL. CRC Press, 1978. Copyright The Chemical Rubber Company, CRC Press, Inc.)

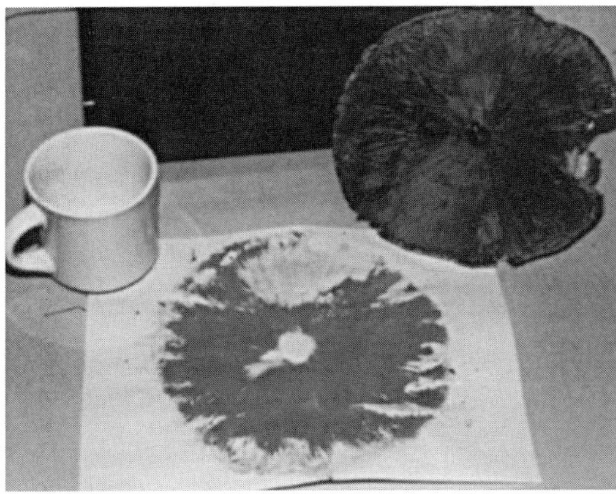

Figure 25–2. Spore print of *Chlorophyllum molybdites*. (Courtesy of Lynn Augenstein, M.D., and the Rocky Mountain Poison Center, Denver.)

CYCLOPEPTIDES

(Figs. 25–1 to 25–4 [see Color Plates])

The cyclopeptide-containing mushrooms are responsible for more than 90% of all deaths due to mushroom poisonings in the Western world. Although the group contains various mushrooms (see Table 25–3), almost all fatalities and serious poisonings are caused by the deadly cyclopeptide-containing *Amanita,* particularly *Amanita phalloides* (see Fig. 25–3). Ingestion of deadly *Amanita* most commonly occurs after misidentification of the mushroom by foragers. These mushrooms are most commonly found during the late summer or autumn in well-forested areas. The cyclopeptides consist primarily of amatoxins, which contain eight amino acids, and phallotoxins, which contain seven. More than 15 cyclopeptides have been isolated from the genus *Amanita.* Note, however, that not all mushrooms of the *Amanita* species contain significant quantities of amatoxin. *Amanita muscaria* and *Amanita pantherina,* for example, contain no amatoxin and do not cause hepatotoxicity.

The phallotoxins are extremely potent hepatotoxins but are not well absorbed from the GI tract and therefore contribute little to *Amanita* toxicity. They may contribute to the initial gastroenteritis-like picture, although this has been questioned.[6] Laboratory animals cannot be poisoned by oral administration of the phallotoxin phalloidin, whereas they die within hours after intravenous injection.

Amatoxins are actively absorbed and are extremely potent hepatotoxins. Nine cyclic octapeptide amatoxins, of approximately 900 daltons, have been identified. α-Amanitine is the principal toxin in this group. Nucleoli of liver cells disintegrate soon after exposure to α-amanitine, which interferes with transcription of deoxyribonucleic acid (DNA) by inhibiting ribonucleic acid (RNA) polymerase II. They accomplish this by binding to the 140,000-dalton subunit of the enzyme. Because the primary action of amatoxins is inhibition of DNA transcription, tissues that are highly dependent on protein synthesis—namely, the GI tract and

Table 25–3. Some Mushroom Species, by Clinical Grouping of Toxins

Cyclopeptides (Amatoxins, Phallotoxins)

Amanita phalloides ("death cap" or "green death cap")
A. verna ("death angel")
A. virosa ("destroying angel" or "white destroying angel"
A. bisporigera ("white destroying angel")
A. ocreata
A. suballiacea
A. tenuifolia
Galerina autumnalis
G. marginata
G. venenata
Lepiota helveola
L. brunneoincarnata
L. chlorophyllum
L. vosserandii
Conocybe filaris

Muscimol, Ibotenic Acid

Amanita muscaria ("fly agaric")
A. pantherina
A. gemmata
A. cokeri
A. cothurnata
A. regalis

Monomethylhydrazine

Gyromitra esculenta ("false morel")
G. gigas
G. amabigua
G. infula
G. caroliniana
G. brunnea
G. fastigiata
Paxina spp.
Sarcosphaera coronaria
Cyathipodia macropus

Muscarine

Boletus calopus
B. luridus
B. pulcherrimus
B. satanas
Clitocybe cerrusata
C. dealbata
C. illudens
C. riuulosa
Inocybe fastigiata
I. geophylla
I. lilacina
I. patuoillardi
I. purica
I. rimosus
*Amanita muscaria**
*A. pantherina**

Coprine

Coprinus atramentarius ("inky cap")
Clitocybe clavipes

Indoles

Psilocybe cubensis
P. caerulescens
P. cyanescens
P. baeocystis
P. fimentaria
P. mexicana
P. pelluculosa
P. semilanceata
P. silvatica
Conocybe cyanopus
Gymnopilus aeruginosa
G. spectabilis
G. validipes
Panaeolus foenisecii ("mower's mushroom")
P. subbalteatus
Stropharia coronilla

Orelline/Orellanine

Cortinarius orellanus
C. speciosissinus
C. splendoma
C. gentilis
Mycena pura
Omphalatus orarius

General Gastrointestinal Irritants

Many species from diverse genera
"Little brown mushrooms" (backyard mushrooms)
Chlorophyllum molybdites
Omphalates illudens ("jack-o-lantern")

*Typically contain only trace amounts of muscarine.

liver—are most sensitive to this poisoning. Once absorbed through the gut, amatoxins are transported into hepatocytes by a nonspecific transport system. Circulating amatoxin is excreted by the biliary system and the kidneys; however, enterohepatic recirculation of amatoxins excreted through the bile is significant.

Circulating amatoxins can be detected for hours after ingestion.[7] Most of the ingested α-amanitine is excreted renally, and urine levels tend to be higher than serum levels. Although amatoxins can be detected by very sensitive radioimmunoassay or high-pressure liquid chromatographic methods, these are not usually clinically available. The Meixner test is a bedside assay that can detect amatoxins. In this test, gastric material or pulverized mushroom juice is spotted on pulp paper (e.g., newspaper) and allowed to dry. A blue response developing within 1/2 hour of applying several drops of concentrated (10 to 12N) hydrochloric acid to the spot constitutes a positive test result. If the mushroom has been dried, it should be extracted with methanol and then tested as just described. Because false-positive results occur, a section of paper on which no mushroom material has been applied should also be tested. Psilocybin can give a positive Meixner test result.[4]

The cyclopeptides are not denatured by boiling, and hence cooking deadly *Amanita* mushrooms does not render them nontoxic. It has been estimated that one *A. phalloides* cap may be lethal to an adult.

Identifying deadly *Amanita* mushrooms in the field should not be difficult, but for various reasons even those who have picked and consumed mushrooms for many years with impunity are not immune to making that fatal mistake. Figure 25–3 demonstrates the maturation of a typical *Amanita* mushroom and how the classic annulus and "death cup" develop. These structures are not always obvious, however, and may be obliterated in the act of picking the mushrooms out of the ground. The immature "buttons" in many ways resemble edible puffballs. It is useful to remember that all species of deadly *Amanita* have white gills and spore prints.

The classic clinical presentation of *Amanita* poisoning consists of three stages. Patients do not have GI symptoms for at least 6 hours after ingestion, and then they develop colicky abdominal pain, vomiting, and severe diarrhea (stage 1). The diarrhea may contain blood and mucus and may be so severe that it has been termed cholera-like.

Even without treatment, patients may apparently recover (stage 2), although their hepatic enzyme levels may be rising. Two to 4 days after ingestion, patients may then suffer fulminant hepatic, cardiac, and renal failure (stage 3). Pancreatitis, diffuse intravascular coagulation, convulsions, and death may then occur in the subsequent 2 to 4 days.

The pathologic picture of hepatic necrosis tends to be most marked in the centrilobular areas. In series of treated patients, the death rate due to *A. phalloides* poisoning ranges from 10% to 30%. Although many patients with cyclopeptide-induced hepatotoxicity recover fully, approximately 20% develop immune complex–mediated chronic active hepatitis with antismooth muscle antibodies.

A wide variety of antidotes to *Amanita* poisoning have been touted to be beneficial, but clinical reports have for the most part been anecdotal. The use of thioctic acid has been lauded in the literature on the basis of anecdotal reports. Being a dithiol compound, it has been postulated to function as a free radical scavenger. However, there is no convincing human evidence of its efficacy.

Intravenous penicillin has also been recommended on the theory that it inhibits the uptake of amatoxin by hepatocytes. Various other protective mechanisms for penicillin have also been proposed. Animal data and retrospective human data suggest that benzylpenicillin (penicillin G) in a dose range of 300,000 to 1,000,000 units/kg per day is hepatoprotective; however, this could not be demonstrated in a prospective study.

Silibinin, a water-soluble preparation of silymarin, an abstract of thistle, has been shown to be effective in animals in reducing hepatotoxicity by inhibiting amatoxin uptake by hepatocytes. It has also been postulated to act as a free radical scavenger. However, no convincing data show that it is useful in humans, and its routine use therefore cannot be recommended.

Anecdotal reports and preliminary animal data suggest a number of additional antidotes, including hyperbaric oxygen, cimetidine, ascorbic acid, cephalosporins, corticosteroids, cytochrome C, bile salts, heavy metal salts, D-penicillamine, and diethyldithiocarbamate. However, no firm clinical data indicate that any of these are useful.

Although it is unclear if any of these specific antidotes are of value in the management of amatoxin poisoning, there is little doubt that optimization of a patient's fluid status is of great importance.

Charcoal hemoperfusion, hemodialysis, or plasma exchange[8] may be theoretically useful in enhancing elimination early after ingestion. However, this has never been proved to be beneficial and may be impractical because most patients present late. Antiamatoxin Fab fragments have been studied in animal models, but these strongly enhance the observed toxicity.

Liver transplantation has been successfully performed on patients with severe cyclopeptide-induced hepatotoxicity. Because most patients with amatoxin poisoning recover with aggressive supportive care, transplantation should not be considered to be standard treatment for hepatotoxicity. However, if a patient shows signs of severe hepatotoxicity, transfer to a transplantation center may be beneficial to facilitate the procedure should it become necessary. Although no universally agreed on criteria exist for transplantation, encephalopathy is generally consid-

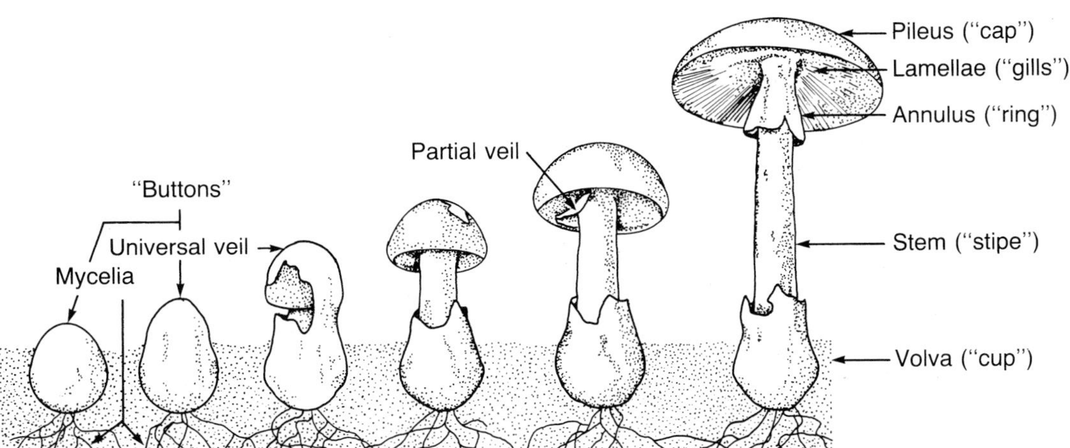

Figure 25–3. Maturation of *Amanita* species. The early stages ("buttons") may resemble nontoxic puffballs. The lamellae and spores are white in all *Amanita* species, whereas the pileus may be white, as in *A. phalloides, A. Verna,* or *A. virosa,* or bright orange-red, as in *A. muscaria.* The distinguishing features of all amanitas include the annulus and volva ("death cup"); however, these are frequently destroyed in the process of picking and preparing the mushroom. Poisonous *Amanita* mushrooms are toxic during all stages of development. (Adapted from Litten W: The most poisonous mushrooms. Sci Am *232*:90, 1975.)

ered such a poor prognostic sign that liver transplantation should be considered.

Because amatoxins have been reported to undergo enterohepatic recirculation, it may be useful to administer multiple doses of activated charcoal for at least 48 hours after ingestion. Duodenal suction is also of theoretic benefit during this period.

Although several other genera of mushrooms contain the toxic cyclopeptides (see Table 25–3), *Amanita* (see Color Figs. 25–1 to 25–3) is by far the most commonly ingested genus that results in significant clinical toxicity. Several species of *Galerina* (see Color Fig. 25–4) contain amatoxin, but these mushrooms are quite small; approximately 15 to 20 *Galerina* mushrooms contain the same amount of toxin as 1 mature *A. phalloides.*

One of the common errors made in identification of mushrooms of the *Amanita* species is confusing them with *Chlorophyllum molybdites* mushrooms, which also possess an annulus and a swelling at the base resembling a cup. Persons ingesting *C. molybdites* mushrooms, however, usually develop severe vomiting and diarrhea within 2 hours, although many are able to consume these mushrooms without becoming symptomatic. Differentiating between *C. molybdites* and *Amanita* spp. should not be difficult. *Chlorophyllum* spp. are the only mushrooms with greenish gills and spores, and the spores are thick walled and contain pores. The mushroom itself stains reddish orange where it is injured, and the annulus is movable; in *Amanita,* the annulus is fixed.

As noted in Table 25–3, several species of *Galerina* and *Lepiota* contain cyclopeptides and are therefore capable of causing similar symptoms.[9–11] *Lepiota helveola* contains more cyclopeptides than *A. phalloides. Galerina* spp. are common, indiscreet, small brown mushrooms. They may be ingested by crawling children or by those seeking psychoactive mushrooms. *Galerina* tends to contain small amounts of amatoxins, and it is commonly believed although not empirically verified that one to two dozen are required for toxicity.

MUSCIMOL, IBOTENIC ACID

(see Color Figs. 25–5 and 25–6)

Mushroom species of this group contain the closely related isoxazoles muscimol (a hallucinogen) and ibotenic acid (a potent insecticide). Muscimol and ibotenic acid may be assayed in mushrooms using high-performance liquid, gas, or thin-layer chromatography.[15]

Although the pathophysiology of muscimol poisoning is imperfectly understood, its central nervous system effects seem to derive from its action as a γ-aminobutyric acid (GABA) agonist. Ibotenic acid acts at excitatory glutamic acid receptors.[13]

Mushrooms in this class tend to have a relatively low concentration of psychoactive substances; thus, large numbers of these mushrooms typically must be ingested before a toxic effect is manifested.[14]

Many cases of *A. muscaria* poisoning occur in individuals who deliberately seek and ingest the mushroom for its hallucinogenic properties, and so the history is very important. Purposeful ingestion of urine from people who have eaten these mushrooms has been reported as a way to elicit the psychoactive effects of the excreted muscimol.

Both *A. muscaria* and *A. pantherina* are very common mushrooms with a wide geographic distribution. *A. muscaria* is commonly known as the "fly agaric" because it attracts and kills flies that land on it. These mushrooms have been used for at least 3000 years in the rituals of many Asian and Indian tribes. Within 30 minutes of ingestion, intoxication with ataxia, euphoria, visual perceptual changes, and hallucinations occurs. If the amount is not carefully titrated, however, frank psychosis, convulsions, and coma can develop. It appears that seizures are more common in pediatric patients.[12]

Muscarine was first extracted from *A. muscaria* in 1869, and its use as a pharmacologic research tool has enhanced our knowledge of the muscarinic receptors of the parasympathetic nervous system. Paradoxically, most patients poisoned by *A. muscaria* do not have cholinergic findings. In fact, poisoning by this group of mushrooms has been described as causing anticholinergic manifestations. However, despite some similarities to a classic anticholinergic syndrome, neither the pathophysiology nor clinical manifestations of poisoning by this group of mushrooms are truly anticholinergic.

Identification of *A. muscaria* should be relatively easy. The cap is bright orange or red and is covered with small white plaques, which are remnants of the universal veil (see Fig. 25–3). As in all *Amanita* species, the annulus and volva are prominent, and the spores are hyaline, thin walled, and without pores.

A. pantherina, another member of this group, may be confused with edible agarics ("meadow mushrooms") by inexperienced collectors. Despite its toxic effects, *A. pantherina* is used as a food, mostly in the Pacific Northwest. This requires peeling off the skin of the cap, which contains the highest concentration of isoxazoles, and parboiling the remaining parts. Because the isoxazoles are water soluble, they are extracted by this process. Needless to say, the water should be discarded.

Treatment of this group of poisonings consists of appropriate supportive care and GI decontamination. There is little to suggest, based on either pathophysiology or published clinical experience, that the once touted antidote physostigmine is effective in controlling any toxic manifestation of ibotenic acid or muscimol poisoning.

GYROMITRIN

(see Color Figs. 25–7 and 25–8)

The *Gyromitra* spp., or false morels, are an extremely interesting genus toxicologically. Many species of *Gyromitra* contain the hydrazone gyromitrin and small amounts of other hydrazones. Gyromitrin is metabolized to monomethylhydrazine (CH_3NHNH_2).

Monomethylhydrazine poisoning causes symptoms and signs similar to those of isoniazid overdose. Both agents inhibit the formation of GABA in the brain by inducing a state of pyridoxine (vitamin B_6) deficiency.

Six to 48 hours after ingestion of mushrooms from the *Gyromitra* spp., patients develop vomiting, diarrhea, dizziness, fatigue, and muscle cramps.[16] These symptoms are usually mild, but delirium, coma, and convulsions may occur. Methemoglobinemia and hemolysis may be life threatening, and in parts of Eastern Europe, fatalities due to *Gyromitra esculenta* are common. Hepatic and renal failure may occur with large ingestions. Mortality rates as great as 10% have been reported.[17]

Treatment consists of supportive care, administration of methylene blue for significant methemoglobinemia, blood transfusions if required, and intravenous pyridoxine for monomethylhydrazine-induced seizures. Pyridoxine, which is depleted in poisoning by hydrazines, is a cofactor in the synthesis of GABA. Pyridoxine also forms a chemical complex with hydrazines, and this may have a role in its antidotal effect in treating monomethylhydrazine poisoning. Hydrazines also inhibit the metabolism of folic acid to tetrahydrofolate, its active form, and supplementation with folinic acid has been suggested on theoretic grounds.

High doses of pyridoxine are known to cause peripheral neuropathy, and thus its excessive use should be avoided. If a patient is having seizures, a dose of 5 g administered intravenously is generally regarded as appropriate. This should be repeated only for recurrent seizures or coma. Pyridoxine does not reverse the other aspects of poisoning by these mushrooms.[18]

The *Gyromitra* spp. are nongilled fungi, the spores of which develop is asci, or microscopic sacs, on the surfaces of the fruiting bodies. The bodies of *Gyromitra* are extremely convoluted, hence the nickname "brain fungi." Many species of *Gyromitra* are edible, but determining which ones may be ingested is best left to experts.

In post–World War II Poland, death due to ingestion of *G. esculenta* exceeded that caused by *A. phalloides.*[19] Poisoning by this mushroom occurs in the spring, in contrast to poisoning by *A. phalloides,* which tends to be common in the autumn. The hydrazones in these mushrooms may be destroyed and volatilized by cooking; however, this should not be considered to be a foolproof strategy for rendering them edible. Gas-liquid, gas mass spectrometry, and thin-layer chromatography may be used to identify hydrazone and hydrazine compounds in mushrooms.

MUSCARINE

(see Color Figs. 25–9 and 25–10)

Mushrooms in this group predictably cause symptoms and signs of poisoning by the cholinergic alkaloid muscarine. Muscarine is structurally similar to acetylcholine and causes depolarization of neurons by binding to the acetylcholine receptor. Because muscarine does not possess an ester bond,[20] it is not hydrolyzed by cholinesterases. Thus, the cholinergic effect of muscarine is prolonged.

Minutes to an hour after ingestion, patients may develop the classic cholinergic syndrome consisting of diaphoresis, bradycardia, bronchospasm, profuse bronchorrhea, miosis, seizures, salivation, lacrimation, involuntary loss of urine and stool, and vomiting. Unlike the cholinergic crisis occurring after poisoning by organophosphate insecticides, the syndrome in these cases is usually mild and seldom life threatening. This may be at least partially due to the poor GI absorption of muscarine. Unlike organophosphates, muscarine does not stimulate nicotine receptors. Muscarine is heat labile, so vigorous cooking of these mushrooms may prevent their cholinergic effects.

Treatment consists of GI decontamination, supportive care, and administration of atropine. Although activated charcoal is theoretically beneficial in preventing absorption of muscarine, it is important to emphasize that cathartics should not be administered to patients with diarrhea syndromes. Atropine has been recognized as a treatment for this poisoning since the mid-1800s.[21] The antidote should be given as frequently as necessary to dry pulmonary secretions. The muscarinic syndrome typically resolves within 24 hours.

More than 30 species of *Inocybe* and 6 species of *Clitocybe* contain muscarine. These inconspicuous mushrooms commonly grow in lawns and public parks. *A. pantherina* and *A. muscaria* contain muscarine (hence the name) but usually in quantities that are insufficient to cause a cholinergic syndrome. Muscarine was initially isolated from *A. muscaria.*[21] The best analytic method for detecting muscarine in mushrooms is high-performance thin-layer chromatography.[22] Although of theoretic utility, this technique has not been applied to body fluids.

COPRINE

(see Color Fig. 25–15)

Coprine poisoning is most commonly associated with ingestion of *Coprinus atramentarius,* or the "inky cap." It is so called because the mature specimens have lamellae that deliquesce into an inky black fluid that is obvious on examination of the mushroom. The mushrooms themselves are edible. However, they contain coprine, which is a glutamic acid derivative that induces hyperacetaldehydemia in the presence of ethanol by inhibiting acetaldehyde dehydrogenase. Coprine itself is not an inhibitor of this enzyme.[23, 24] However, it has been speculated that a metabolite of coprine, like disulfiram (Antabuse), inhibits the metabolism of ethanol at the acetaldehyde dehydrogenase step, resulting in clinical symptoms.[25]

The disulfiram-like reaction may occur after the ingestion of alcohol several days after consumption of *C. atramentarius*. The symptom complex engendered by this interaction has been referred to as "Clayton's hangover."[26] This syndrome consists of flushing of the face and trunk, palpitations, dyspnea, chest pain, and diaphoresis. Hypotension may occur secondary to peripheral vasodilatation.[25, 27–29]

Treatment of the coprine syndrome consists primarily of symptomatic and supportive care. There are no specific antidotes, although several have been suggested.[25] No specific antidote has been studied. The coprine syndrome usually abates within several hours. No fatalities have been reported to result from this syndrome.

Coprine may be detected by thin-layer chromatography. Because coprine is an amino acid, a coprine-containing spot stains when sprayed by ninhydrin.[23, 29, 30] Because of its disulfiram-like effect, coprine has been suggested as a potential agent for chemoprevention of alcohol abuse. However, the mutagenic, carcinogenic, and male gonadotoxic effects render it inappropriate for this use.[25]

INDOLES

(Figs. 25–13 and 25–14 [see Color Plates])

The psilocin-psilocybin–containing mushrooms have been used by Aztec and American Indians in religious ceremonies for thousands of years.[31] They are frequently referred to as "magic mushrooms." The *Psilocybe* genus contains more than 100 species of small brown, slender-stalked mushrooms. They are commonly but not exclusively found growing in piles of horse and cow dung and fertilized grasses, especially after a spring rain. Also growing in a similar environment and with a similar appearance is the cyclopeptide-containing mushroom *Conocybe filaris*. Indole-containing mushrooms are found in moist areas all over the United States, most commonly in the South. The spores are smooth purple and contain pores. A classic feature of the *Psilocybe* mushrooms is the blue-green areas where it has been injured or handled. Although this color usually derives from the oxidation of psilocin,[30] this color change is not specific for hallucinogenic mushrooms.

Thirty to 60 minutes after the psychotropic *Psilocybe* is ingested, a feeling of euphoria develops, followed by perceptual distortions and hallucinations that are usually but not always considered pleasant.[32] These effects are caused by the indoles psilocybin and psilocyn, which are chemically related to both lyseric acid and serotonin. Psilocybin was first isolated in 1958 by Albert Hoffman, the discoverer of lysergic acid diethylamide (LSD). Intravenous use of these mushrooms has been reported.[33, 34] Because of the small amounts of psychoactive indoles in these mushrooms, ingestion of several caps is usually required to elicit a hallucinogenic effect. Although use of this mushroom is generally limited by its supply, these mushrooms tend not to be expensive.[35] Tachycardia, mydriasis, and paresthesias are common effects. Seizures have been reported.[36] The experience generally lasts 4 to 6 hours. Flashbacks may occur.[35] Among connoisseurs of the psychoactive effects of indoles, these mushrooms are often preferred over LSD.[35, 37] Patients who require medical care usually need reassurance only,[38] but sedation may be required. Benzodiazepines are generally considered the drugs of choice in this case. As with any illicitly purchased substance, the actual material used may not be what is suspected by history. In a study of 886 samples sold as psilocybin mushroom, only 28% contained psilocybin. An additional 31% contained LSD or phencyclidine, and in 37%, no psychoactive substances could be identified.[39]

Many analytic techniques have been described for the identification of psilocybin and other psychoactive indoles.[15]

ORELLANINE

(see Color Figs. 25–11 and 25–12)

Some mushrooms of the genus *Cortinarius* contain the bipyridyl toxin orellanine.[40] The syndrome of poisoning by these mushrooms was first described after a large outbreak of cases in Poland in 1952. Ingestion of these mushrooms may result in the development of gastroenteritis, thirst, polyuria, chills, headaches, and myalgias, after a hiatus of several days. A small percentage of these cases evolve to renal failure, evident days to weeks later.[40–43] Few cases of *Cortinarius* poisoning have been reported in the United States, but many occurrences have been documented in Europe and Japan. Some species of *Cortinarius* are edible, creating a dangerous temptation to seasoned yet adventurous mushroom hunters. Mushrooms of this genus are distinguished by their rusty-brown spores. *Cortinarius* is the largest genus of mushrooms, containing more than 800 species, making the differentiation between the edible and poisonous varieties extremely difficult. Although orellanine is the primary nephrotoxin in these fungi, some species appear to contain other related nephrotoxins known as *cortinarines*.[44, 45] These nephrotoxins appear to require activation by cytochrome P-450.[46]

Orellanine is a heat-stable toxin that is chemically closely related to the herbicides paraquat and diquat. Poisoning by these compounds results in tubulointerstitial nephritis and fibrosis.[42] There are no antidotes for poisoning by these mushrooms. Because patients tend to become symptomatic more than 24 hours after ingestion, activated charcoal is unlikely to be of much benefit. Treatment therefore consists of aggressive fluid management and close monitoring of renal function. In the majority of cases, renal failure improves over time.[42] Orellanine may be detected by thin-layer or high-performance liquid chromatography.[15]

A similar syndrome of delayed renal failure has also been recently attributed to the mushroom *Amanita smithiana*.

PAXILLUS SYNDROME

(see Color Fig. 25–16)

Paxillus involutus ("brown rim-roll" mushroom) is, for most people who ingest it, a simple GI irritant.[42, 48] However, a small proportion of those eating this mushroom develop immune-mediated hemolytic anemia, referred to as the *Paxillus syndrome.*[47, 49] This syndrome typically follows long periods of ingestion of these mushrooms and is manifested, once started, as progressively worsening reactions.[47, 49] Given these characteristics, it is of little surprise that the *Paxillus* syndrome is rarely encountered clinically. The *Paxillus* syndrome is typically manifested 1 to 2 hours after ingesting the fungi. Clinical features generally reported are syncope, gastroenteritis, decreased urine output, hemoglobinuria, decreased haptoglobins, and low back pain. Treatment consists primarily of aggressive fluid management and, if the mushroom was recently ingested, oral activated charcoal. Plasmapheresis has been used in severe cases,[50] but no convincing evidence shows that this technique provides any therapeutic benefit.

The precise mechanism defining the pathophysiology of the *Paxillus* syndrome is unknown. It appears to be an immunoglobulin-mediated hemolysis provoked by exposure to a yet unidentified antigen. A hemagglutination test in which a mushroom extract, the patient's serum, and erythrocytes are incubated together has been described.[47, 50–52] Although the *Paxillus* syndrome is generally described as occurring after repeated ingestion of the brown roll-rim mushroom, one case was reported after ingestion of *Suillus luteus* ("slippery Jack"),[53–55] a bolete generally regarded as edible, although this has been questioned.[56, 57] The clubfoot mushroom, *Clitocybe clavipes,* has also been suggested as a possible cause of the *Paxillus* syndrome,[44] but it is more likely that any observed reactions to this mushroom derive from its disulfiram-like effect.[58]

GASTROINTESTINAL IRRITANTS

This group has traditionally been a catchall for mushrooms that (1) usually produce vomiting and diarrhea shortly after ingestion and (2) do not produce other significant systemic symptoms or signs. The number of species considered in this classification is so great that to list them would be unproductive. Not all species of this group of mushrooms cause symptoms in all people. The same species may cause symptoms in one person at one time and not at another time. The toxins responsible for the GI symptoms are, for the most part, unidentified.

Among the most common species causing acute gastroenteritis is *Chlorophyllum molybdites.*[59] In its juvenile form, it resembles the "shaggy mane," and it is quite often mistaken for this edible mushroom. It is, however, easily distinguished from virtually all other mushrooms by its green gills and spore print (see Fig. 25–2). However, sterile forms of this mushroom are known to exist. These produce no spores.[59]

Many common backyard mushrooms or "little brown mushrooms" can be considered to be in this group. When these mushrooms are ingested by children or in large quantities by adults, it is still safest to presume them to be toxic and to have them identified.

Generally, no therapy is required for ingestion of these mushrooms. If symptoms are significant or if signs of volume depletion are evident, it is advisable to provide hydration and GI decontamination with activated charcoal. However, it must be emphasized that administration of cathartics with activated charcoal is very likely to exacerbate the condition being treated and thus should be avoided.

Table 25–4. Possible Pitfalls in the Treatment of Mushroom Poisoning

- Forgetting that "mushroom poisoning" may actually be an allergic reaction or food poisoning secondary to bacteria
- Forgetting that "mushroom poisoning" may actually be secondary to pesticides sprayed on the mushroom or edible mushrooms laced with drugs (e.g., phencyclidine) or from a concomitant medical or surgical disease
- Assuming that all persons ingesting the same mushroom must become ill
- Assuming that if symptoms occur before 6 hours after ingestion, deadly *Amanita* species could not have been eaten
- Discharging patients when they appear to have recovered from their gastrointestinal symptoms when those symptoms developed more than 6 hours after ingestion and therefore may have been due to a potentially very toxic mushroom
- Forgetting the principles of supportive care while concentrating on toxin identification and antidotes

CONCLUSION

The management of mushroom poisoning is best thought of by dividing mushrooms into clinical syndromes based on the toxins they contain. The treatment of mushroom poisoning is not significantly different from that for drug overdose; supportive care must take highest priority pending identification of the toxin.

Common pitfalls in the management of mushrooms poisoning are listed in Table 25–4. By avoiding these common errors and emphasizing supportive care and continued monitoring, the outcome in most cases of mushroom poisoning should be favorable.

References

1. Baker T: Origins of the word *mushroom.* Mycologist *3:*88–90, 1990.
2. Klein AS, Hart J, Brems JJ, et al: *Amanita* poisoning: Treatment and the role of liver transplantation. Am J Med *86:*187–193, 1989.
3. Trestrail JH: Mushroom poisoning in the United States—An analysis of 1989 United States Poison Center data. Clin Toxicol *29:*459–465, 1991.
4. Lampe KF, McCann MA: Differential diagnosis of poisoning by North American mushrooms, with particular emphasis on

Amanita phalloides–like intoxication. Ann Emerg Med *16:*956–963, 1987.
5. Rumack BH, Salzman E (eds): Mushroom Poisoning: Diagnosis and Treatment. West Palm Beach, FL, CRC Press, p 263, 1978.
6. Duffy TJ, Vergeer PP: *Amanita* poisoning: Treatment and role of liver transplantation. Letter. Am J Med *87:*244, 1989.
7. Jaeger A, Jehl F, Flesch F, et al: Kinetics of amatoxins in human poisoning: Therapeutic implications. Clin Toxicol *31:*63–80, 1993.
8. Ponikvar R, Drinovec J, Kandus A, et al: Plasma exchange in management of severe acute poisoning with *Amanita phalloides.* Prog in Clin Biol Res *337:*327–329, 1990.
9. Meunier BC, Camus CM, Houssin DP, et al: Liver transplantation after severe poisoning due to amatoxin-containing *Lepiota*—report of three cases. Clin Toxicol *33:*165–171, 1995.
10. Paydas S, Kocak R, Erturk F, et al: Poisoning due to amatoxin-containing *Lepiota* species. Br J Clin Pharmacol *44:*450–453, 1990.
11. Ramirez P, Parrilla P, Bueno FS, et al: Fulminant hepatic failure after *Lepiota* mushroom poisoning. J Hepatol *19:*51–54, 1993.
12. Benjamin DR: Mushroom poisoning in infants and children: The *Amanita pantherina/muscaria* group. Clin Toxicol *30:*13–22, 1992.
13. DeFeudis FV: Binding studies with muscimol: Relation to synaptic γ-aminobutyrate receptors. Neuroscience *5:*675–688, 1980.
14. Hatfield GM, Brady LR: Toxin of higher fungi. Lloydia *38:*36–55, 1975.
15. Bresinsky A, Besl H: Giftpilze. Stuttgart, Wissenschaftliche Verlagsgesellschaft, 1985.
16. Hanrahan J, Gordon M: Mushroom poisoning: Case reports and review of therapy. JAMA *251:*1057–1061, 1984.
17. Gerault A, Girre L: Mise au point sur les intoxications par les champignons superieurs. Bull Soc Mycol Fr *93:*373–405, 1977.
18. Braun R, Greeff U, Netter KJ: Liver injury by the false morel poison gyromitrin. Toxicology *12:*155–163, 1979.
19. Grymala S: Les recherches sur la frequence des intoxications par les champignons. Bull Med Leg Toxicol Med *2:*200–210, 1965.
20. Kogl F, Salemink CA, Schouten H, et al: Uber Muscarin III. Rec Trav Chim Pays-Bas *76:*109–127, 1957.
21. Schmiedeberg O, Koppe R: Das Muskarin, das giftige Alkaloid des Fliegenpilzes (*Agaricus muscarius* L.) Leipzig, Vogel, 1869.
22. Stijve T: High performance thin layer chromatographic determination of the toxic principles of some poisonous mushrooms. Mitt Geb Lebensmittelunters Hyg *72:*44–54, 1981.
23. Hatfield GM, Schaumberg JP: Isolation and structural studies of coprine, the disulfiram-like constituent of *Coprinus atramentarius.* Lloydia *38:*489–496, 1975.
24. Herrmann M: Der Rettichhelmling-Mycena pura (Pers. Ex Fr.) Kum.-ist giftig! Mykol Mitt Bl *17:*17–18, 1973.
25. Michelot D, Toth B: Poisoning by *Gyromitra esculenta*—a review. J App Toxicol *11:*235–243, 1991.
26. Barbato MP: Poisoning from accidental ingestion of mushrooms. Med J Aust *158:*842–847, 1993.
27. Hatfield GM, Schaumberg JP: The disulfiram-like effects of *Coprinus atramentarius* and related mushrooms. *In* Rumack BH, Salzman C (eds): Mushrooms. New York, CRC Press, pp 181–186, 1978.
28. Iten PX: Antialkohol-Wirkstoff des Faltentintlings (*Coprinus atramentarius*) Aufgeklart, Schweiz. Z Pilzkd *55:*1–9, 1977.
29. Lindberg P: Coprine, a Cyclopropanone-Related Disulphiram-like Constituent of *Coprinus atramentarius.* Thesis. University of Lund, Lund, Sweden, p 109, 1977.
30. Levine W: Formation of blue oxidation product from psilocybin. Nature *215:*1292–1293, 1967.
31. Ott J: A brief history of hallucinogenic mushrooms. *In* Ott J, Bigwood J (eds) Teononacatl: Hallucinogenic Mushrooms of North America. Seattle, Madrona Press, pp 5–22, 1978.
32. Preden NR, Bissett AF, Macaulay KEC, et al: Clinical toxicology of "magic mushroom" ingestion. Postgrad Med J *57:*543–545, 1981.
33. Curry SC, Rose MC: Intravenous mushroom poisoning. Ann Emerg Med *14:*900–902, 1985.
34. Sivyer G, Dorrington L: Intravenous injection of mushroom. Letter. Med J Aust *140:*182, 1984.
35. Schwartz RH, Smith DE: Hallucinogenic mushrooms. Clin Pediatr *27:*70–73, 1988.
36. McCrawley EL, Brummett RE, Dana GW: Convulsions from *Psilocybe* mushroom poisoning. Proc West Pharmacol Soc *5:*27–33, 1962.
37. Thompson JP, Anglin MD, Emboden W, et al: Mushrooms usage by college students. J Drug Educ *15:*111–124, 1985.
38. Peden NR, Pringle SD, Crooks J: The problem of psilocybin mushroom abuse. Hum Toxicol *1:*417–424, 1982.
39. Renfroe C, Messinger TA: Street drug analysis: An eleven-year perspective on illicit drug alteration. Semin Adolesc Med *1:*247–258, 1985.
40. Schumacher T, Hoiland K: Mushroom poisoning caused by species of the genus *Cortinarius fries.* Arch Toxicol *53:*87–106, 1983.
41. Marichal JF, Triby F, Wiederkehr JL, et al: Insuffisance renale chronique apres intoxication par champignons de type *Cortinarius orellanus Fries, Nouv.* Presse Med *6:*2973–29975, 1977.
42. Bouget J, Bousser J, Pats B, et al: Acute renal failure following collective intoxication by *Cortinarius orellanus.* Intensive Care Med *16:*506–510, 1990.
43. Delpech N, Rapior S, Cozette AP, et al: Evolution d'une insufficiance renale aigue par ingestion volontaire de *Cortinarius orellanus.* Presse Med *19:*122–124, 1990.
44. Koppel C: Clinical symptomatology and management of mushroom poisoning. Toxicon *31:*1513–1540, 1993.
45. Tebbett IR, Caddy B: Mushroom toxins of the genus *Cortinarius.* Experientia *40:*441–446, 1984.
46. Nieminen L: Effects of drugs on mushroom poisoning induced in the rat by *Cortinarius speciosissimus.* Arch Toxicol *35:*235–238, 1976.
47. Schmidt J, Hartmann W, Wurstlin A, et al: Akutes Nierenversagen durch immunhamolytische Anamie nach Genuss des Kahlen Kremplings (Paxillus involutus). Dtsch Med Wochenschr *96:*1188–1191, 1971.
48. Flammer R: Hamolyse bei Pilzvergiftungen: Fakten und Hypothesen. Schweiz Med Wochenschr *113:*1555–1561, 1983.
49. Deicher H, Stangel W: Akute immunhamolytische Anamie nach Genuss des Kahlen Kremplings, Verh Dtsch Ges Inn Med *83:*1606–1609, 1977.
50. Winkelmann M, Stangel W, Schedel I, et al: Severe hemolysis caused by antibodies against the mushroom *Paxillus involutus* and its therapy by plasma exchange. Klin Wochenschr *64:*935–938, 1986.
51. Lefevre H: Immunhamolytische Anamie nach Genuss des Kahlen Krempling (*Paxillus involutus*). Dtsch Med Wochenschr *107:*1374, 1982.
52. Winkelmann M, Borchard F, Stangel W, et al: Todlich verlaufene immunhamolytische Anamie nach Genuss des Kahlen Kremplings (*Paxillus involutus*). Dtsch Med Wochenschr *107:*1190–1194, 1982.
53. Bobrowski H: Ostra niewydolnosc nerek w przebiegu ostrego nabytego zespolu hemolitycznego u osoby uczulonej na grzyb maslak (*Boletus luteus*) (Acute renal failure in the course of an acute haemolytic reaction in a subject sensitive to *Boletus luteus*). Pol Tyg Lek *21:*1864–1865, 1966.
54. Albrecht W: Gibt es enzymabhangige und blutgruppenspezifische Pilzvergiftnungen. Sudwestdeutsche Pilzrundschau *19:*11–14, 1983.
55. Hausen BM: Unerwunschte Nebenwirkungen beim Genuss essbarer Pilze. Mat Med Nordm *29:*230–253, 1977.
56. Lincoff GH: The Audubon Society Field Guide to North American Mushrooms. New York, Knopf, p 926, 1981.
57. Prager MH, Goos RD: A case of mushroom poisoning from *Suillus luteus.* Mycopathologia *85:*175–176, 1984.
58. Christiansen AL, Rasmussen KE, Tonnesen F: Determination of psilocybin in *Psilocybe semilanceata* using high-performance liquid chromatography on a silica column. J Chromatogr *210:*163–167, 1981.
59. Lehmann PF, Khazan U: Mushroom poisoning by *Chlorophyllum milybdites* in the midwest United States. Mycopathologia *118:*3–12, 1992.

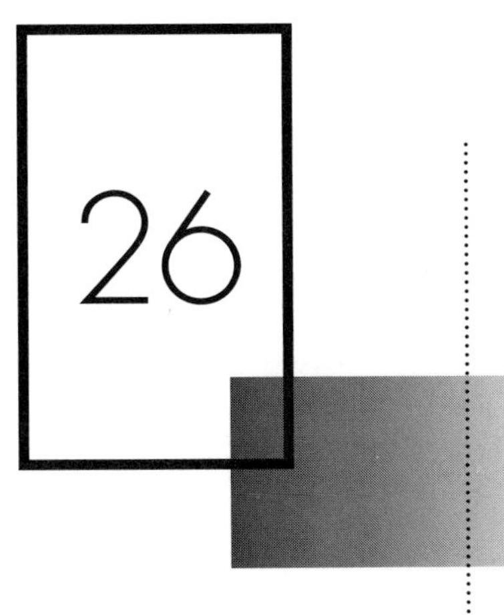

Poisonous Plants

DONALD B. KUNKEL, MD
GEORGE BRAITBERG, MB, BS

The toxic properties of some plants are well known, but those of many are relatively obscure and difficult to ascertain. The list of plants known to cause adverse effects in human beings and other animals is overwhelming and is constantly being expanded. It is of interest to practitioners that so few cases of human death occur after exposure to poisonous plants, because the exposures are many and result in a great number of inquiries to poison control centers. It is estimated that 5% to 10% of all such telephone calls concern plants, yet hospitalizations are rare. It seems there might be "much ado about nothing" in this virtual jungle of toxins, yet the concerns are real, and the offending plants may be capable of producing serious intoxication.

PLANT IDENTIFICATION

A significant problem in dealing with a plant exposure inquiry is proper identification of the plant itself, especially over the telephone. Surprisingly few of us are aware of even the common local names, let alone botanic names, of many plants regularly encountered. Attempting to ascertain the identity of the ubiquitous "little red berry" by means of a telephone conversation with a distraught mother whose child has just feasted on one can be a frustrating experience.

The problem of absolute lack of knowledge about the plant is compounded by difficulties in the nomenclature of plants, which exist at several levels. Names for plants tend to vary geographically, and one plant may have several common names depending on locality. For example, yellow oleander *(Thevetia peruviana)* is also known as "lucky nut" and "be still tree." Botanists have not made the identification of plants easier for practitioners, because botanic names tend to change occasionally, sometimes for obscure reasons.

It is wise to become an amateur botanist if one is dealing often with plant inquiries. A general knowledge of poisonous and nonpoisonous plants in a particular locale can be time saving and realistically can provide better patient care, because more than a few children and adults are given an emetic to cause vomiting to err on the side of caution if the plant is not identified. Local experts are usually agreeable to becoming involved in the medical system as informal consultants, and even nursery people can be quite helpful.

It is advisable to have relatives or friends of the patient bring in specimens of the consumed plant when any question exists about the identity of the plant. Specimens of vomitus containing plant material should be saved for possible use in determining the type of plant ingested.

The references at the end of this chapter are especially helpful in plant identification and in the treatment of exposures.

PROBLEMS IN CLINICAL EVALUATION

To treat or not to treat, that is the question. Once ingested plant material is properly identified as part of a poisonous plant, can one with consistency predict toxicity? Many factors enter into an evaluation of potential toxicity; some are listed here.

Human Versus Animal Data. Much of the literature concerning poisonous plants is abstracted from veterinary experience, especially livestock studies. This information is of undoubted interest to clinicians but must be interpreted with care. What is relevant to a herd of sheep may not indicate treatment of a child.

Geographic and Seasonal Variables. Plants known to be toxic in one part of the world may not be so very toxic in other areas. An example of this phenomenon is the chinaberry tree, which is known to cause central nervous system (CNS) stimulation and death in its native Africa but seems to cause only gastroenteritis in the United States. Soil conditions and climate most likely account for these variances.

Plant Part Ingested. A plant may be listed as poisonous, but certainly all parts of the plant are not consistently toxic in each case. The common garden tomato, a solanine alkaloid-containing plant, has perfectly edible fruit, but stems and leaves are known to be toxic. Likewise, peaches and apricots contain a cyanide-producing principle, amygdalin glycoside, within the fruit kernel and the leafy portions of the tree, but the fruits are common edibles.

Absorbability of Toxins. Some plant products listed as extremely toxic, such as castor beans, many times are limited in toxicity because of factors that impede absorption across the gut wall. Castor beans have a very tough seed coating that inhibits release of the active principles unless the bean is chewed. Dieffenbachia usually presents no problem with systemic absorption of oxalates because of the violent oropharyngeal reaction after the leaf is chewed.

Controversies. The available literature is inconsistent in regard to the potential toxicity of some plants. Evolving evidence is constantly changing the toxic or nontoxic status of some plants. Controversies rage in respect to the true poison potential of some plants. Pyracantha is listed in some texts as a poisonous plant, yet delicious jellies made of pyracantha berries are commercially available. Because of a 1919 report of a child's death after ingestion of wild poinsettia, hybrid poinsettias were previously labeled as very poisonous but are now thought to cause only mild gastroenteritis after ingestion, if any symptoms occur at all.

A physician must take into consideration the factors just mentioned and, above all, the patient's presenting and continuing clinical picture when formulating a treatment plan. The sage warning "Just don't do something, stand there!" is probably cogent in many cases of plant ingestion.

MECHANISMS OF EXPOSURE

Poisonous plant contacts are generated in the following ways in declining frequency:

"Accidental" Childhood Exposures. These usually are no "accident," actually. Children are attracted to bright berries and shiny leaves and ingest plant parts as an expression of their own innate inquisitiveness and the desire to feel the texture of a new substance as a form of learning. Most childhood ingestions (usually in the 2- to 3-year-old age group) are nontoxic or relatively benign episodes, and simple reassurance of the parent is indicated after the plant is reasonably well identified. On occasion, home emesis or other measures, such as milk administration for dieffenbachia ingestions, may be advised, followed by careful home management protocols established by the physician or poison control center. On rare occasions, referral to a physician or hospital emergency department may be necessary.

Accidental Dermal Exposures. Fairly frequent calls are received concerning skin rashes (some with systemic sequelae) and punctures caused by plants. Some rashes may be due to applied pesticides, but most can be managed safely at home. Severe neurologic and shocklike clinical presentations have occasionally been caused by punctures by palm fronds and century plant blades.

Use of Plants as Drugs of Abuse. A number of plants containing psychoactive principles are rather commonly abused, some with treacherous sequelae. Jimsonweed is used fairly commonly but usually not more than once because of the severe hallucinations and peripheral anticholinergic effects, which usually prompt an evaluation in an emergency department. Many of the common street drugs are plant derivatives (heroin) or intact plant products (marijuana), and deliberate consumption of poisonous plants borders on drug abuse. Some psychostimulant plants have become part of the culture in which they are found. Their uses in these circumstances are governed by traditional mores. When taken outside these social values, abuse potential is high. An example is the evergreen tree khat *(Catha edulis)* and the synthetic derivative of its active alkaloid, cathinone. Khat chewing is a pastime of men in societies in Northern Africa and has not posed an abuse problem for centuries. Methcathinone, a synthetic street drug derivative, has been available in Russia and the United States and is abused for its amphetamine-like properties.

Foraging Incidents. Serious plant intoxications occur through experimenting, for food-gathering purposes, and in tasting and ingesting unknown plants or plants morphologically similar to known edible wild plants. This sometimes fatal mistake seems to occur repeatedly with umbellifers, plants that are represented by not only the common carrot but also the water hemlock, which elaborates cicutoxin and causes seizures. Similarly, toxic mushrooms can be mistaken for edible ones (see Chapter 25).

Use of Herbs as Medication and Food Supplements. The use of a wide variety of plants as home remedies, beverages, and food supplements is certainly not new. Indeed, many modern drugs are either derivatives of plants or modifications of known plant chemical products. Twenty-five per cent of today's pharmacopeia is estimated to be of natural origin. Various ethnic groups have contributed herbal lore that is spread by word of mouth and popular publications. Commercialization of herbal products has resulted in therapeutic alternatives to traditional medicine. Unfortunately, perhaps largely because of misidentification of plants and their overzealous use, illness and death have resulted. Striking recent examples have been the tragic results of the use of amygdalin (Laetrile), pennyroyal, and groundsel instead of gordolobo yerba.

ADVICE FOR THERAPY

Reassurance. Most plant exposures require only well-informed explanations after the plant is identified. The reassurance must be firmly given and reasonably stated, for the fixation on poisonous plants is strong.

Decontamination. General principles of any poisoning episode are to be followed, with some minor exceptions:

1. *Ingestion*: It is very difficult to remove leafy material, twigs, large berries, and so on from the gut with a tube, even a large-bore orogastric hose. Likewise, it may be somewhat hazardous to induce emesis in a situation of ingestion of *large* amounts of leafy plant product (possible glottic obstruction). The use of activated charcoal is recommended. Cathartics may be of benefit to hasten elimination.
2. *Injection (puncture wounds)*: Penetrating wounds by thorns, cactus spikes, palm fronds, and so on are notoriously prone to early inflammatory reaction and secondary infection. Careful removal of embedded foreign material with meticulous cleansing is important. Tetanus prophylaxis is recommended, and antibiotics may be necessary for infectious complications. Deep punctures into joint spaces may be especially troublesome.

Elimination of Absorbed Toxin. Most plants contain complex mixtures of organic and inorganic (e.g., selenium) compounds. Attempts at speeding renal elimination by forced diuresis or the use of extracorporeal devices seem to be futile and potentially harmful in most cases of intoxication by plant material. The use of *repeated* oral doses of activated charcoal in plant ingestions has not been studied sufficiently.

Antidotes. Physiologic antagonists do exist for the effective treatment of physiologic effects of some plant intoxications. These are discussed later. Emphasis always should be on basic resuscitation and accurate diagnosis before use of potentially harmful drugs as antidotes.

Supportive Care. As in any intoxication, general supportive care is paramount. Careful attention to airway, ventilation, cardiovascular status, control of seizures, management of body core temperature, and so on is essential. Remember that plant poisonings may be complex and not well delineated in the existing literature, and multisystem problems may be anticipated, even though the plant may be in a specific toxin category.

SYMPTOM COMPLEXES AND APPROACHES TO SPECIFIC THERAPY

As noted, most plant poisonings are complex in clinical presentation. Numerous structural variants of the same general class of toxins may be present within a plant (e.g., the various alkaloids of jimsonweed), or totally different toxins may be present in the same plant (e.g., castor oil and ricin in castor beans). Gastrointestinal (GI) symptoms occur almost universally, but other organ systems may also be affected. As more experience with plant poisonings is documented, these syndromes undoubtedly will become better defined, but many plant intoxications remain confusing. Table 26–1 lists symptomatic responses to common poisonings.

The following discussion is an attempt to organize the toxicity and basic management of ingestion of some of the better-recognized poisonous plants into a "target organ" scheme. It is recognized that such a delineation may be misleading in that many toxic plants affect more than one organ system, as any single drug might do.

Gastrointestinal/Mucous Membrane. The organ system probably most often affected by plant ingestion, the GI system, including here the buccal cavity and the liver, may be solely affected or may be only an early target followed by other organ toxicity.

Buccal/Pharyngeal Irritation. Many of the oxalate-containing plants, such as dieffenbachia, contain spicule-like crystals of oxalic acid, which probably act in concert with plant enzymes to produce severe irritation that may cause upper airway compromise (thus the common name, *dumb cane*, as a result of aphonia). Chewing of the rosary pea (jequirity bean) may cause a reaction described as caustic in nature. Patients may be advised to drink milk for limited topical irritation. Watch for upper airway obstruction.

Gastroenteritis. Nausea, vomiting, or diarrhea may be the only clinical finding in a particular plant poisoning, or it may be a premonitory sign of systemic involvement. The numbers of plants known to cause GI disturbance are overwhelming. Local irritation, for example, may follow the ingestion of wisteria seeds or pods and the pods of the Mexican bird of paradise (poinciana). A common pediatric plant ingestion is chinaberry *(Melia azedarach)*. The berries turn color from green to yellow or brown as they age and look like candy. After ingestion of as little as one berry, gastroenteritis and bloody diarrhea may ensue. Onset of symptoms is variable. GI symptoms that may be an early indication of systemic toxicity are observed in the ingestion of oleander parts and castor bean seeds. Management is by aggressive replacement of intravascular fluid and electrolytes, with symptomatic treatment of bowel cramping and hypermotility in severe cases. Of course, if absorbable toxins affecting other organ systems potentially are present, attention must be paid to progressive

Text continued on page 384

Table 26–1. Some Toxic Plants Found in the United States

Common Name	Scientific Name	Toxic Parts	Poisonous Principles	Symptoms
Akee	*Blighia sapida*	Fruit, except ripe aril, which is edible	Hypoglycins A and B	Vomiting ("Jamaican vomiting sickness"), convulsions, coma; may be lethal. Severe hypoglycemia possible
Apricot (also applies to parts of other fruits whose kernels or seeds contain amygdalin glycoside, e.g., peach, apple, pear)	*Prunus* spp.	Fruit kernels, foliage	Amygdalin glycoside (cyanogenic—produces free cyanide ion after hydrolysis in the gut)	Symptoms and findings of cyanide poisoning, such as shock, hyperpnea, and coma. Breath may have bitter almond odor. Metabolic acidosis usually marked. Deaths have been reported from ingestion of these natural products or the purified amygdalin glycoside (Laetrile)
Autumn crocus or meadow saffron	*Colchicum autumnale*	All parts	Colchicine alkaloid	Burning pain and rawness in mouth and throat. Vomiting, diarrhea, shock, renal failure. Symptoms usually appear 2–6 h after ingestion. Death may occur during relapse after period free of symptoms
Azalea—see Rhododendron				
Bird of paradise (Mexican bird of paradise or poinciana)	*Casesalpinia gilliesii*	Pods	Unknown	Vertigo, severe vomiting and diarrhea, dehydration (symptoms may persist for 24 h)
Black locust	*Robinia pseudoacacia*	Inner bark, young leaves, and seeds	Robin (phytotoxin) and robitin (glycoside)	Vomiting, diarrhea, shocklike picture, CNS depression
Bleeding heart	*Dicentra formosa,* other species	Foliage, roots	Several isoquinoline-type alkaloids, including apomorphine, protoberberine, and protopine	Tremors, staggering gait, labored breathing, salivation, convulsions. Death may be due to paralysis
Buckeye	*Aesculus* spp.	Leaves, flowers, and seeds	Esculin (glycoside)	Vomiting, diarrhea, pupillary dilation, muscle twitching, weakness, ataxia, CNS depression, and paralysis
Burn bean—see Texas moutain laurel				
Caladium—see Philodendron				
Castor bean (see Color Figure 26–1)	*Ricinus communis*	All parts, mainly seeds	The phytotoxins—ricin and ricinine (toxalbumins)	Nausea, vomiting, violent purging, burning sensation in mouth and throat, hemolysis of red blood cells, kidney failure, death. 2–4 seeds produce serious poisoning in adults. 1–3 seeds in a child could be lethal if chewed. Hard seed coating is protective
Century plant (see Color Figure 26–2)	*Agave americana*	Sap	Unknown	Skin exposure to sap may cause severe dermatitis, sometimes hemorrhagic. Rash may be associated with fever and leukocytosis
Chinaberry (see Color Figure 26–3)	*Melia azedarach*	Fruit	Probably a resinoid	Has caused serious poisoning in certain animals (hogs and sheep), including dyspnea, sluggish movements, weak and fast pulse, vomiting. 6–8 fruits may be lethal to a child, but human exposures in the USA seem limited to severe gastroenteritis
Christmas holly—see Holly				
Christmas rose	*Helleborus niger*	Rootstocks and leaves	Two very toxic glycosides, helleborin and belleborein	Juice produces inflammation and numbing sensations in mouth. Vomiting, diarrhea, and possible convulsions; affects CNS

Daffodil—see Narcissus				
Daphne	*Daphne mezereum* and other species	Berries, bark, leaves	Daphnin and vesicant resin, mezerenic acid anhydride	Plant intensely acrid, producing vesication when rubbed on skin; ingestion produces burning sensation in mouth. Vomiting, diarrhea with blood and mucus, stupor, kidney failure, weakness, convulsions, and death. Mortality is about 30%
Desert potato	*Jatropha macrorhiza*	Plant root	Phytotoxins	Nausea, vomiting, abdominal cramps, profuse watery diarrhea that may lead to dehydration
Dieffenbachia, dumb cane (see Color Figure 26–4)	*Dieffenbachia sequine* or *picta*	All parts, including sap	Calcium oxalate crystals, toxic proteins	Burning of mouth, tongue, lips; inflammation of larynx, may affect breathing. Juice in the eye causes marked burning and inflammation; direct eye contact may cause corneal opacity
Digitalis—see Foxglove				
Dutchman's breeches	*Dicentra cucullaria*	See Bleeding heart		
Elephant ear—see Philodendron				
Fava bean	*Vicia faba*	Bean or plant pollen	Sensitivity to beans or inhaled pollen noted in individuals deficient in glucose-6-phosphate dehydrogenase	Sensitive persons may experience headache, nausea, vomiting, abdominal pain, and hyperthermia. More severe reactors may develop sudden hemolytic anemia with secondary hemoglobinuria and icterus. Occurs in persons of Mediterranean extraction
Four-o'clock	*Mirabilis jalapa*	Root, seed	The alkaloid trigonelline	Irritant to skin, mouth, and throat. Causes purgation
Foxglove (see Color Figure 26–5)	*Digitalis purpurea*	Leaves and seeds	Several glycosides, mainly digitoxin, digitalin, digitonin	One of the sources of the drug digitalis, used to stimulate the heart. In large amounts, the active principles cause atrioventricular block and slow pulse and other cardiac arrhythmias) (see Chapter 85)
Golden chain	*Laburnum anagyroides*	Beanlike capsules in which the seeds are suspended	The quinolizidine alkaloid cytisine	Dysphagia, possible pupil dilation, excitement, incoordination, vomiting, renal failure, convulsions, coma, and death through asphyxiation. Considered very poisonous shrub or tree in Britain. Action similar to that of nicotine
Gordolobo—see Threadleaf				
Goundsel—see Threadleaf				
Holly	*Ilex* spp.	Berries	Ilicin	Nausea, abdominal pain, severe vomiting and diarrhea
Hyacinth	*Hyacinthus orientalis*	Bulb	Probably narcissine-like alkaloids	Intense digestive upset, vomiting, diarrhea; severe purgation
Hydrangea	*Hydrangea* spp.	Entire plant	A cyanogenic glycoside (hydrangin)	See Apricot
Indian licorice—see Rosary pea				
Indian tobacco	*Lobelia inflata*	Entire plant	Alkaloids of lobeline, lobelamine, etc.	Nausea, vomiting, weakness, tremors, convulsions, coma, and death
Iris (blue flag)	*Iris versicolor*	Leaves and root stalks	Acrid resinous substances irisin, irigenin, iridin	Acts on GI tract, liver, and pancreas, causing purging and congestion of the intestinal tract. Can also cause dermatitis
Jack-in-the-pulpit (Indian turnip)	*Arisaema triphyllum*	Rhizome	Calcium oxalate crystals	Intense irritation of mouth and throat; burning pain; inflammation of larynx (resembles dumb cane)
Jasmine—see Yellow jessamine				
Jequirity bean—see Rosary pea (see Color Figure 26–6)				

Table continued on following page

Table 26–1. Some Toxic Plants Found in the United States *(Continued)*

Common Name	Scientific Name	Toxic Parts	Poisonous Principles	Symptoms
Jerusalem cherry	*Solanum pseudocapsicum*	Berries	Solanine and related alkaloids	Headache, abdominal pain, vomiting, diarrhea, circulatory collapse, convulsions, CNS and respiratory depression
Jimsonweed (thorn apple) (see Color Figure 26–7)	*Datura stramonium, D. metel, D. inoxia, D. suaveolens,* and other species	All parts, especially seeds	The solanaceous alkaloids atropine, hyoscyamine, and scopolamine	Symptoms include intense thirst, urinary retention, dryness of mouth, rapid pulse, delirium, incoherence; later, slow respiration, high temperature, convulsions or coma preceding death. Handling leaves or seeds followed by rubbing eyes can cause dilation of pupils
Laburnum—see Golden chain				
Lantana (see Color Figure 26–8)	*Lantana camara*	Berries (unripe)	A polycyclic triterpenoid named lantadene A	Extreme muscle weakness, GI irritation, lethargy, cyanosis, and circulatory collapse. Syndrome resembles atropine poisoning in some respects.
Larkspur	*Delphinium ajacis* and other species	Young plant, seeds	Poisonous alkaloids, mainly delphinine	Ingestion produces digestive upset, respiratory depression, paresthesias, salivation, headache, hypotension, and cardiac arrhythmias
Laurel—see Texas mountain laurel *or* Mountain laurel. (Caveat: Many "laurels" are nontoxic)				
Lily of the valley (see Color Figure 26–9)	*Convallaria majalis*	Leaves, flowers, roots	The cardiac glycosides convallarin, convallamarin, and convallatoxin	Cardiac effects similar to those of digitalis glycosides. Dizziness and vomiting may occur in 1–2 h if large quantities are eaten
Locust—see Black locust				
Mescal—see Peyote				
Mescal bean (see Color Figure 26–10)—see Texas mountain laurel				
Mistletoe	*Phoradendron* spp.	Berries	β-Phenylethylamine and tyramine, choline	Several deaths among children have been attributed to eating the berries. Tea brewed from berries has caused fatality. Death occurred about 10 h after onset of symptoms of acute gastroenterititis and cardiovascular collapse. Acute GI symptoms of nausea, vomiting, diarrhea; respiratory difficulties, bradycardia, delirium, hallucinations, cardiovascular collapse, and coma
Monkshood	*Aconitum napellus* and other species	Roots, seeds, leaves	Poisonous alkaloids, mainly aconitine, a polycyclic diterpene	Alkaloids cause vagal stimulation and bradycardia. Also, tingling and numbing sensation of the lips and tongue; irregular pulse; dimness of vision; GI upset with nausea, vomiting, and diarrhea; respiratory failure
Morning glory (heavenly blue, pearly gates, flying saucer varieties)	*Ipomoea violacea*	Seeds	The olavine alkaloids ergine, isoergine, elymoclavine, and others; all chemically related to LSD	From 50–200 ingested powdered seeds are capable of inducing psychotomimetic effects for several hours (hallucinations). Used by thrill seekers because of LSD-like effects. Produce nausea, uterine stimulation, euphoria

Mountain laurel	*Kalmia latifolia* and *angustifolia*	All parts	Andromedotoxin, a resinoid substance	Curare-like effect on skeletal muscles. Stimulation of skeletal muscle followed by paralysis. Inhibitory action on heart tissues. Depresses the CNS, causing respiratory failure and ultimately death
Narcissus or daffodil	*Narcissus* spp.	Bulb	Narcissine, lycorine, and other alkaloids	Severe gastroenteritis, vomiting, purging, trembling, convulsions, hypotension, possible hepatic degeneration
Nightshade family (includes many wild and cultivated plants, such as black nightshade, potato, tomato, eggplant, and some jasmines) (see Color Figure 26–15)	*Solanum* spp.	Variable with species; some have edible fruit (tomato, eggplant) or tubers (potato)	Solanine alkaloids (see Jerusalem cherry)	See Jerusalem cherry
Oleander (see Color Figure 26–11)	*Nerium oleander*	All parts, green or dry. Single leaf, well chewed, reportedly lethal	Cardiac glycosides; oleandroside, oleandrin, nerioside	Local irritation of mucous membranes, mouth, and stomach. Nausea, vomiting, diarrhea, slow and irregular pulse changing to rapid and thready pulse, and ventricular fibrillation and death
Pencil tree	*Euphorbia tirucalli*	Leaves, stems, milky sap	Irritant in sap	Irritation to lips, tongue, and mouth. Sap may blister skin and irritate eyes
Peyote (see Color Figure 26–12)	*Lophophora williamsii* and *L. diffusa*	All parts, usually cactus "button" used	Various alkaloids, of which mescaline is only one	Sensory distortion, hallucinations (primarily visual)
Philodendron	*Philodendron* spp.	Entire plant	Calcium oxalate	Location irritation of mucous membranes, swelling of lips and tongue, along with excessive salivation, may lead to difficulty in swallowing. Excessive swelling of tongue and pharyngeal edema may inhibit respiration. No systemic effects have been reported
Caladium	*Caladium bicolor*	Entire plant	Calcium oxalate	
Elephant ear	*Colocasia antiquorum*	Entire plant	Calcium oxalate	
Poison hemlock (see Color Figure 26–13)	*Conium maculatum*	All parts	Coniine (alkaloid)	Nausea, vomiting, early CNS stimulation, followed by severe CNS depression, associated muscle paralysis, and respiratory failure
Poison ivy (erroneously called poison oak)	*Toxicodendron radicans* or *Rhus toxicodendron*	All parts, even the smoke from burning it	An oily resin called urushiol, which is made up of phenolic substances like 3-*N*-pentadecylcatechol	Produces a severe allergic response causing dermatitis on contact, resulting in inflammation, blistering, and vesicles. As skin breaks, a liquid exudes and scabs of crusts form
Pokeweed (pigeonberry, inkberry)	*Phytolacca americana, P. decandra*	Roots and leaves; fruit is least toxic but has also caused poisoning	A resinous material and a water-soluble saponin, glycoprotein, and possibly two other alkaloids—phytolaccine and phytolaccotoxin	Produces burning sensation in mouth, GI cramps, vomiting, diarrhea (also amblyopia and tremors). Later, visual disturbance, perspiration, salivation, lassitude, prostration, and weakened respiration and pulse. If recovery does not occur in 24 h, may be fatal
Privet	*Ligustrum japonicum*	All parts	Perhaps andromedotoxin. Most sources state the principle is unknown	Poisoning seems to be rare in USA, but in Europe children have died from eating fruit. In animals it causes severe vomiting, colic, and diarrhea
Red squill	*Urginea maritima*	Bulb	Cardiac glycosides	Similar to those for oleander
Rhododendron (also azalea)	*Rhododendron* spp.	All parts	Andromedotoxin	Salivation, nasal discharge, nausea, vomiting, diarrhea, muscle weakness, labored breathing, coma (based on animal studies), dullness of vision, paralysis, hypotension, lacrimation, anorexia

Table continued on following page

Table 26–1. Some Toxic Plants Found in the United States *(Continued)*

Common Name	Scientific Name	Toxic Parts	Poisonous Principles	Symptoms
Rhubarb (see Color Figure 26–14)	*Rheum rhaponticum*	Leaf *blade* (not the petiole, which is edible)	Oxalic acid	Severe intermittent abdominal pains, vomiting, diarrhea, headache, weakness, and hemorrhages. Muscle cramps and tetany due to hypocalcemia may occur. Large amounts of raw and cooked leaves can cause convulsions and coma, followed rapidly by death associated with renal failure
Rosary pea (crab's eye, precatory bean, jequirity bean, Indian licorice)	*Abrus precatorius*	Seeds	The phytotoxin abrin and the tetanic glycoside abric acid	Seed is caustic. Causes burns to mouth and esophagus. Less than one seed, if chewed, may be fatal. Symptoms resemble those of castor bean poisoning. Nausea, vomiting, severe diarrhea, weakness, shock, trembling of hands, oliguria, hemolytic anemia, hallucinations in children, and fatal uremia
Star-of-Bethlehem (snowdrop)	*Ornithogalum umbellatum*	All parts	Alkaloids (related to colchicine)	Nausea, nervous symptoms, and general disturbances of the intestinal tract
Sweet pea	*Lathyrus odoratus*	Seeds	Aminopropionitrile	Skeletal deformity and growth suppression; muscle paralysis (from animal studies)
Texas mountain laurel	*Sophora secundiflora*	Entire plant	Cytisine	Increased salivation, nausea, vomiting, headache, vertigo, confusion, hallucinations, excessive thirst, muscle fasciculation, convulsion, and respiratory stimulation followed by failure
Thorn apple—see Jimsonweed				
Threadleaf groundsel (Senecio)	*Senecio longilobus*	Entire plant	Pyrrolizidine alkaloids	Chronic ingestion may cause enlarged liver, ascites, abdominal pain, nausea, vomiting, diarrhea, headache, apathy, and emaciation. Poisoning usually results from drinking certain herbal teas. Senecio is a major cause of hepatic veno-occlusive disease (see Chapter 9)
Tobacco (and wild tobacco, tree tobacco) (see Color Figure 26–16)	*Nicotiana* spp.	Probably all parts	Nicotine and related alkaloids	Nausea, vomiting, muscular fasiculation; early CNS stimulation followed by severe CNS depression in association with muscle paralysis and respiratory failure

Water hemlock (cowbane) (see Color Figure 26–17)	*Cicuta maculata* and other species	All parts, mostly the roots	Resin-like substance called cicutoxin	Symptoms appear in 15 min and include severe stomach pain, great mental excitation and frenzy, vomiting, salivation, and violent spasmodic convulsions alternating with periods of relaxation. Pupils dilate, and delirium is common. Death may occur within 15 min after ingestion of lethal amount
Wisteria (see Color Figure 26–18)	*Wisteria floribunda* (Japanese) and *W. sinensis* (Chinese)	Seeds or pods	Poisonous resin and a glucoside, wisterin	Mild to severe gastroenterititis with repeated vomiting, abdominal pain, and diarrhea
Yellow jasmine (Carolina jasmine)	*Gelsemium sempervirens*	Whole plant, berries	Toxic alkaloids gelsemine and gelseminine	The alkaloids chiefly depress and paralyze motor nerve endings. Depression of the motor neurons of the brain and spinal cord results in respiratory arrest
Yellow oleander (be still tree) (see Color Figure 26–19)	*Thevetia peruviana*	All parts; fruit ("lucky nut") most attractive to children	Cardiac glycosides (thevetin A and B, thevetoxin)	See Oleander
Yew (see Color Figure 26–20)	*Taxus baccata* and *T. canadensis*	All parts, especially *seed* if chewed; fleshy red pulp of fruit least harmful	Taxine, an alkaloid	Nausea, vomiting, diarrhea, abdominal pain, circulatory failure, and difficulty in breathing. The alkaloid depresses heart function. Can cause dermatitis

CNS, central nervous system; GI, gastrointestinal.

Gratitude is extended to Alan Barreuther, Pharm.D., and Albert L. Picchioni, Ph.D., for allowing abstraction from *Toxic Plants,* a compendium released by the Arizona Poison and Drug Information Center of the Arizona Poison Control System. Special recognition to the late Jay M. Arena, M.D., of Duke University, whose compendia appear in many publications and whose foresight brought us to the present state of the art.

All figures are from the private collection of the chapter author Donald B. Kunkel, M.D.

findings and specific treatment anticipated, if available.

Hepatic Involvement. Direct hepatic involvement by plant materials is rare. Recognized liver toxins include groundsel *(Senecio longilobus)*, which contains a pyrrolizidine alkaloid that can be mistakenly substituted in herbal tea for the harmless herb gordolobo yerba, which it closely resembles. Senecio contains the alkaloid retronecine, which is capable of producing both acute hepatitis and chronic veno-occlusive disease of the liver, with tragic results. Pennyroyal oil, used as an abortifacient, contains the active component pugelone, which can cause centrilobular liver necrosis after ingestion of as little as 5 to 10 mL. Various bulb plants (iris, daffodil, narcissus) have been implicated in hepatic complications following ingestion. Hepatic failure may occur after prolonged shock and renal failure as a secondary effect of poisoning. Care is largely supportive.

Renal. Deposition of products of intravascular hemolysis, as in castor bean intoxication due to absorption of toxalbumins, or deposition of oxalate crystals, reported to occur after cooking and eating rhubarb leaves, may result in renal failure. In the former, urinary alkalization may be of benefit. In the latter, attention must be turned to correction of hypocalcemia and to maintenance of urine output. Hemodialysis as supportive care may be necessary. Ingestion of the autumn crocus (colchicine poisoning) may cause primary renal failure. A French study reported the successful use of colchicine antibodies in life-threatening poisoning. Further information is required before recommendation can be made.

Hematopoietic. As noted, certain plants contain phytotoxins (toxalbumins), which may cause hemagglutination, hemolysis, and renal failure. Included in this group are such plant materials as castor beans and jequirity beans. If hemolysis should occur (apparently a very rare event), exchange transfusion may be considered, along with renal care as just noted. Favism in glucose-6-phosphate dehydrogenase–deficient individuals is well known as a cause of hemolysis. Some plants contain excessive amounts of nitrates, depending on types of agricultural fertilizers used. Methemoglobinemia in infants has been traced to feeding vegetables with high nitrate content and subsequent intraluminal conversion to absorbable nitrite. Treatment is supportive, with consideration of methylene blue infusion in a severe situation.

Cardiovascular. A number of plants can have various effects on the heart and peripheral vascular system, as a result of direct or indirect causes. Plants and fungi are the sources of some commercial cardiac/vascular preparations (e.g., digitalis, ergot). The group of plants containing the cardiac glycosides (digitalis-like compounds) deserves special attention. Foxglove, oleander, yellow oleander, lily of the valley, and others contain glycosides capable of causing intoxication associated with GI symptoms, followed by progressive atrioventricular block. Cardiac glycosides contain haptens that cross-react with digoxin and that demonstrate various degrees of digoxin-like activity. Cardiac toxicity develops as a result of enhancement of vagal tone and inhibition of the sodium-potassium–adenosine triphosphatase pump, leading to bradycardia, conduction block, increased automaticity, and decreased contractility. Hyperkalemia is a result of inhibition of the adenosine triphosphate cellular pump. Therapy is directed at decontamination similar to that previously noted and correction of electrolyte imbalance. Bradycardia can be treated with atropine or isoproterenol. If these measures fail or the patient shows signs of significant poisoning, treatment with digoxin-specific Fab antibodies should reverse foxglove toxicity and may reverse oleander toxicity. Failure at this juncture would require continued inotropic support and the insertion or application of a cardiac pacemaker.

Grayanotoxins are found in such plants as rhododendrons, mountain laurel, and azaleas. Toxicity most commonly results after ingesting contaminated honey. Symptoms include hypotension and bradycardia (arrhythmias uncommonly), although neurologic effects such as paresthesia and incoordination may occur. The condition is self-limiting (<24 hours), and there is no specific treatment.

Ergot alkaloids are discussed in Chapter 94.

Respiratory. Plant pollens account for the seasonal miseries of a significant portion of the population. Although these reactions are not considered a true poisoning problem in the context of this book, nonetheless, more human morbidity undoubtedly results from hypersensitivity reactions than from classic plant intoxications.

Cellular respiration may be impaired by cyanide intoxication secondary to gut hydrolysis of ingested plant parts containing amygdalin glycoside. Treatment is supportive, and use of the Lilly cyanide kit is necessary in severe poisoning. (For antidotal therapy with amyl nitrite, sodium nitrite, and sodium thiosulfate, see Chapter 71).

Central Nervous System. Many sources refer to a plant as causing CNS “stimulation” or “depression.” This differentiation may be somewhat artificial, because a person who is agitated initially may become comatose. Likewise, seizure activity may not be a primary result of CNS stimulation but may reflect cerebral hypoxia secondary to depressive effects. Plants have been used therapeutically primarily for sedation and analgesia but have been used selectively for religious and recreational purposes for many effects, including arousal (coca leaf), hallucinations (peyote cactus), and sedation (opium poppy). Therapy, of course, varies widely depending on clinical presentation and knowledge of the pharmacologic action of the plant used or abused.

Autonomic Nervous System. Many naturally occurring substances, particularly those affecting the CNS, also affect the autonomic nervous system. One outstanding group of plants in this regard is those that produce atropine-like alkaloids, which act on muscarinic receptors. The prime plant of current concern is jimsonweed. The clinical presentation of intoxication by this plant is that of central and peripheral anticholinergic effect: hallucinations, tachyarrhythmias, hypertension, elevated body temperature, dilated pupils, dry and flushed skin, decreased bowel activity, and urinary retention. Treatment is largely supportive, although physostigmine may be used cautiously for life-threatening conditions, as a diagnostic tool, and for control of hallucinations and hyperactivity in select situations.

Nicotinic receptor stimulation results in a biphasic response of stimulation followed by depression. Stimulation of the sympathetic nervous system produces diaphoresis, tachycardia, and hypertension. Central effects include nausea, vomiting, agitation, seizure, and hypotension. Cholinergic stimulation may cause bronchorrhea and bronchoconstriction. In addition, somatic nicotinic receptor stimulation causes an initial motor hyperactivity followed by weakness, hypotonia, decreased tendon reflexes, fasciculations, and finally motor paralysis. Plants that may cause nicotinic receptor stimulation include the tobacco plants, golden chain tree, lupine, mescal bean bush, and poison hemlock *(Conium maculatum)*.

Skin and Eyes. Topical irritation of exposed skin or mucous membranes may be caused by contact with the sap of some plants. Severe hemorrhagic rash has developed immediately after exposure to the sap of the century plant (an agave). In most cases, dermatitis following plant exposure seems to be based on a hypersensitivity reaction, with poison ivy and poison oak being prime offenders. Treatment is usually symptomatic, although severe reactions may require antihistamines and corticosteroid therapy. Conjunctival irritation following direct contact with dieffenbachia sap is a known phenomenon. Allergic conjunctivitis and corneal abrasions following contact with many plants are more common manifestations of plant exposure.

Further Reading

Botanic References

Brenzl KN (ed): Sunset Western Garden Book. Menlo Park, CA, Sunset Publishing Co., 1995. (Excellent color plates and line drawings with helpful cross-referencing to common and botanic names.)

Muenscher WC: Poisonous Plants of the United States. New York, Collier Books (Macmillan), 1975. (Illustrative line drawings.)

Perry F (ed): Complete Guide to Plants and Flowers. New York, Simon & Schuster, 1974. (Helpful color plates.)

Standard Medical Texts

Auerbach PS (ed): Wilderness Medicine. 3rd ed. St. Louis, C.V. Mosby Co., 1995. (Plants plus.)

Hardin JW, Arena JM: Human Poisoning from Native and Cultivated Plants. Durham, NC, Duke University Press, 1974. (Medically oriented.)

Kingsbury HM: Poisonous Plants of the United States and Canada. Englewood Cliffs, NJ, Prentice-Hall, 1964. (Excellent coverage of plant toxins and nomenclature; oriented toward veterinarians.)

Lampe KF, McCann MA: AMA Handbook of Poisonous and Injurious Plants. Chicago, American Medical Association, 1985. (Highly recommended.)

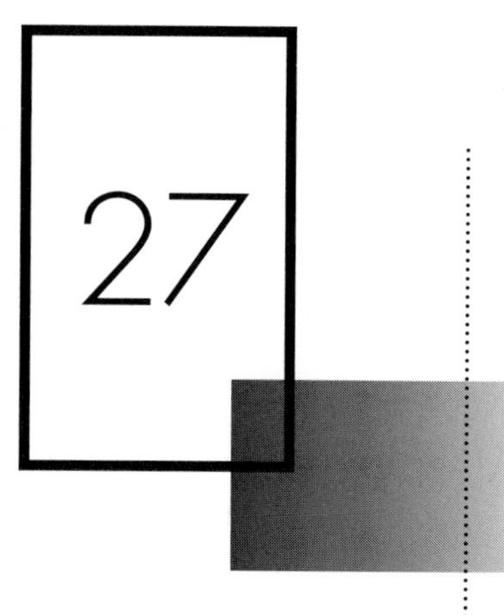

Toxic Marine Life

LESTER M. HADDAD, MD
RICHARD F. LEE, PHD

The sea invites feelings of inner peace and joy to one's soul. Long a source of inspiration and fear, the sea has also proved to be a source of human morbidity and mortality. Reference to poisonous and venomous marine animals dates back to ancient Greek and Roman times. In the Bible[1] (Deut. 14:9–10), Moses cautions the Israelites: "Of all that are in the waters you may eat whatever has fins and scales. And whatever does not have fins and scales you shall not eat; it is unclean." Moses gave his people sound medical advice: The puffer fish and venomous marine animals such as the jellyfish (see Color Figs. 27–1 and 27–2), the sea snake, sea wasp, moray eel, stingray, sea urchin, Portuguese man-of-war, and blue-ringed octopus (see Color Fig. 27–3) all lack fins and scales.

Some of the substances known to be most toxic to human beings are found in marine organisms (Table 27–1). Toxins injected by an animal into its prey are usually high-molecular-weight proteinaceous substances known as *venoms.* Toxins that produce clinical symptoms after consumption are called *poisons;* they are generally low-molecular-weight molecules.

Marine life is toxic to humans[2, 3] through (1) *envenomation* by stinging (jellyfish, corals, and sea anemones), by spinous puncture injury (stingray, catfish, scorpion fish, weever fish, sea urchin, cone shell, and sponges), and by bites by the sea snake and the neurotoxic Australian blue-ringed octopus, *Octopus maculosa;* through (2) *infection* of wounds or of seafood, as by the marine organism *Vibrio vulnificus;* and (3) through *poisoning* by ingestion (paralytic shellfish poisoning, amnesic shellfish poisoning, scombroid fish poisoning, puffer fish poisoning, and ciguatera). Shark bite is the most obvious example of marine trauma. This chapter reviews the more common marine toxins that have clinical significance (Table 27–2).

The three most common marine organisms causing emergency department visits in the mainland United States are stingrays, catfish, and jellyfish.

ENVENOMATION

Jellyfish and the Coelenterates

The phylum Coelenterata is composed of invertebrates that have the dominant characteristic of tentacles equipped with nematocysts. The phylum[2] is divided into three classes:

1. *Hydrozoa.* This group includes *Physalia physalis,* or the Portuguese man-of-war (blue bottle) and its Pacific relative, *Physalia utriculus,* found off Hawaii and in the Indo-Pacific; and the hydroid corals, which are commonly found growing in tufts on rocks, seaweed, and dock pilings. Examples include *Millepora alcicornus,* the stinging fire coral; and *Lytocarpus philippinus,* the feather hydroid, usually attached to the sea floor.
2. *Scyphozoa.* This group includes the jellyfish, such as the Chesapeake sea nettle, *Chrysaora quinquecirrha;* the deadly sea wasp or box jellyfish of Australian waters, *Chironex fleckeri* Southcott; the deadly sea wasp of Philippine waters, *Chiropsalmus quadrigatus* Haeckel; and *Carukia barnesi* Southcott, the cause of "Irukandji stings" to swimmers around Queensland, Australia.
3. *Anthozoa.* This group includes the sea anemones and the corals. Venomous sea anemones of the anthozoan class include *Anemonia sulcata, Actinodendron plumosum, Triactis producta,* the rosy anemone *Sagartia elegans, Radianthus paumotensis,* and others.

Table 27–1. Relative Toxicities of a Selected Group of Toxic Substances

Toxin	Minimum Lethal Dose (μg/kg)*	Source
Botulinum toxin A	0.00003	Bacterium: *Clostridium botulinum*
Tetanus toxin	0.00010	Bacterium: *Clostridium tetani*
Ricin	0.02000	Plant: castor bean, *Ricinus communis*
Palytoxin	0.15000	Zoanthid: *Palythoa* spp.
Crotalus toxin	0.20000	Snake: The rattlesnake, *Crotalus atrox*
Diphtheria toxin	0.30000	Bacterium: *Corynebacterium diphtheriae*
Cobra neurotoxin	0.30000	Snake: *Naja naja*
Kokoi venom	2.7	Frog: *Phyllobates bicolor*
Tarichatoxin	8	Newt: *Taricha torosa*
Tetrodotoxin	8	Fish: *Sphoeroides rubripes*
Saxitoxin	3.4–9	Produced by the dinoflagellate *Gonyaulax catenella* transvected by shellfish
Bufotoxin	390	Toad: *Bufo vulgaris*
Curare	500	Plant: *Chondodendron tomentosum*
Strychnine	500	Plant: *Strychnos nux-vomica*
Muscarin	1100	Mushroom: *Amanita muscaria*
Samandarin	1500	Salamander: *Salamandra maculosa*
Diisopropyl fluorophosphate	3000	Synthetic nerve gas
Sodium cyanide	10,000	Inorganic poison

*Minimal lethal dose refers to mouse, except for ricin, in which it refers to guinea pig, and for bufotoxin and muscarin, in which it refers to cat.
From Mosher HS, Fuhrman FA, Buckwald HD, Fisher HG: Tarichatoxin-tetrodotoxin: A potent neurotoxin. Science *144*:1103, 1964. Copyright 1964 by The American Association for the Advancement of Science.

The coelenterates produce human injury by firing off their nematocysts on contact. Nematocysts, or stinging cells, are actually cell organoids in specialized epithelial cells. At least 17 types of nematocysts are found in coelenterates. In general, they consist of a capsule wall enclosing a tightly coiled hollow tube that bursts forth like a dart on contact with a human being or animal (Fig. 27–1). The fluid in the capsules is the venom. Nematocysts range from 5 μm to 1.12 mm in length.

Table 27–2. Representative Toxic Marine Life

Envenomation

Jellyfish and the coelenterates
- Hydrozoa
  - Portuguese man-o'-war *(Physalia physalis)*
  - Stinging fire coral (*Millepora alcicornus*)
- Scophozoa
  - Jellyfish
  - Sea wasp (*Chironex fleckeri, Chiropsalmus quadrigatus, Carukia barnesi*)
- Anthozoa
  - Sea anemones (*Actinodendron plumosum*)
  - Corals

Stingrays
Catfish
Sea urchins
Weever fish
Scorpion fish and stonefish
The blue-ringed octopus and cone shells
Sea snakes

Infection

Vibrio vulnificus

Poisoning

Paralytic shellfish poisoning
Amnesic shellfish poisoning
Scombroid fish poisoning
Puffer fish poisoning
Ciguatera

When activated, the nematocysts discharge forcibly. During discharge, the coiled internal tubule everts progressively, bringing its armament of chitinous spikes and spines to the external surface. Actual penetration of the prey is facilitated by the continuously renewed crest of spines created at the tip of the everting tubule when spines that were previously internal reach the tip and become superficial.[4] The venom in the capsule is conveyed to the victim through the thread. Although all coelenterates have nematocysts, most are not injurious to humans.

The severity of the stinging in human beings depends on the type of nematocysts, their penetrating power, the area of the victim's skin exposed, and the sensitivity of the victim to the venom. Injurious effects resulting from an encounter with coelenterate nematocysts range from mild dermatitis to instant death.[5]

Portuguese Man-of-War

The Portuguese man-of war (see Color Fig. 27–4) is characterized by a floating stem with several tentacles dangling from the underside of the float. One or more of the tentacles are markedly elongated and are called *fishing tentacles. Physalia* is pelagic—it inhabits the surface of the sea—and is found worldwide in warmer waters. One fishing tentacle may contain almost a million nematocysts. The sting of a Portuguese man-of-war is far more severe than that of the common jellyfish and often produces intense local pain extending up the extremity, similar to an electric shock. Generalized symptoms such as headache, urticaria, shock, muscle cramps, nausea, and vomiting may occur. Two confirmed deaths due to *Physalia* have been reported in the literature.[6, 7]

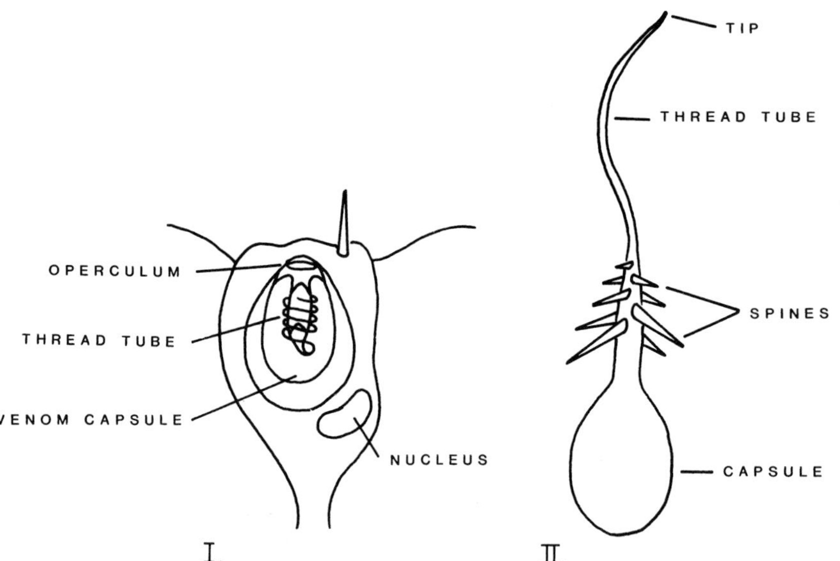

Figure 27–1. Generalized coelenterate nematocyst. I, Undischarged. II, Discharged. (Modified from Halstead BW: Poisonous and Venomous Marine Animals of the World. Revised ed. Princeton, NJ, Darwin Press, 1980.)

Hydroid Corals

Hydroid corals are upright, clavate, bladelike, or branching calcareous growths or encrustations that are important in the development of reefs. The stinging coral is not a true coral but a hydroid characterized by an exoskeleton of calcium carbonate, the surface of which is covered with numerous minute pores. Hydroid corals vary in color from white to yellow-green and are widely distributed throughout tropical seas in shallow water. *Millipora* is the best-known genus, the most famous being the fire coral *M. alcicornus,* a nuisance to divers off the Florida Keys and in the Caribbean.

Jellyfish

Jellyfish are the most common of the coelenterates that produce clinical injury and account for a significant number of emergency department visits in coastal areas of the United States, Australia, and worldwide, especially during the summer.

Jellyfish are marine, and most are pelagic. They display a wide variety of shapes, sizes, and colors. Many appear semi-transparent or glassy, and they often have brilliantly colored gonads, tentacles, or radial canals. They may vary in size from a few millimeters to more than 2 m across the bell (top), with tentacles up to 36 m in length. Because the tentacles in some species are long, it is possible to encounter them without seeing the bell. After a storm during which jellyfish have been broken up and washed ashore, one can be stung while walking along a beach by stepping on tentacles containing undischarged nematocysts. Even when dry, the nematocysts retain the capacity to discharge and produce typical symptoms.

Sea wasps (see Color Fig. 27–5) are the lethal cubomedusans, *C. fleckeri* of Australia and *C. quadrigatus* Haeckel of the Philippines. In Australian waters, the box jellyfish were responsible for more than 50 deaths from 1950 to 1970. Death in less than 3 minutes has been caused by stings of *C. fleckeri.* Another cubomedusan from the family Carybdeidae, *C. barnesi,* has been described by Southcott[8] as the causative agent of the Irukandji syndrome or type A stinging, described by Flecker[9] in swimmers in northern Queensland, Australia. Type A stinging is said to occur in swimmers who suffered severe generalized symptoms but no wheals after a sting. Type B stinging refers to urticaria but no generalized symptoms.

Stings by *C. fleckeri* and *C. quadrigatus* are dangerous. The effects usually consist of extremely painful localized areas of wheal, edema, and vesiculation, which later result in necrosis involving the full thickness of the skin. The initial lesions, caused by the structural pattern of the tentacles, are multiple linear wheals with transverse barring. The purple or brown tentacle marks form a whiplike skin lesion. Painful muscle spasms, shock, and pulmonary edema rapidly ensue. The pain is excruciating,[10] and victims frequently scream and become irrational. Death usually occurs in less than 15 minutes.

Sea Anemones and Corals

Sea anemones are some of the most abundant seashore animals. Commonly known is the Hell's Fire sea anemone, *Actinodendron plumosum.* Anemones are sessile and range in size from a few millimeters to a half meter in diameter. Anemones have a flowerlike appearance under water when their tentacles are extended. When anemones are irritated or when the water recedes, the tentacles invaginate and the body contracts rapidly. In addition to having stinging nematocysts, some sea anemones are poisonous if eaten.

Corals are the major constituent of living reefs, such as the Great Barrier Reef off the northeastern shore of Queensland, Australia. They are composed of an external calcium carbonate skeleton that houses small anemone-like polyps. The actual stinging ability of true corals is probably exaggerated. More dangerous are the cuts and lacerations one can suffer from handling coral or brushing against it.

Coral stings have been described as a distinct stinging sensation, followed by weeping of the lesion, wheal formation, and itching. If coral cuts or stings are left untreated, a superficial scratch may within a few days become an ulcer, with a septic sloughing base surrounded by a painful zone of erythema. Cellulitis, lymphangitis, enlargement of the local lymph glands, fever, and malaise commonly ensue. The ulcer may be quite disabling, and the pain is usually out of proportion to the physical signs. If the ulcer occurs in a lower extremity, the patient may be unable to walk for weeks or months after the injury. Relapses, which occur without warning, are common.

Diagnosis

A jellyfish sting can be identified by the patient or a companion. When a patient experiences an unknown sting, the diagnosis is usually made by observing a row of urticarial lesions or the presence of a tentacle adherent to the patient's skin. Stingrays leave a penetrating wound, and snakes leave fang marks. Catfish leave a barb, and this occurs only in handling the catfish.

A differential diagnosis with respect to the type of coelenterate is not so important in the United States, but where lethal coelenterates exist, as in Australia, identification of nematocysts—if time permits—on the patient by examining the skin wheals on the victim may be important. Halstead[2] suggests that the wheal should be scraped with the edge of a microscope slide or scalpel and the material examined microscopically for the presence of nematocysts. Nematocysts may also be obtained by microscopic examination of a strip of transparent tape that has been pressed against the surface of the wheal. The nematocysts adhere to the sticky side of the tape. Identification of nematocysts from the skin of the victim yields positive identification of coelenterate sting but does not provide positive information about species identification. *Clinical assessment is essential.*

Treatment

Treatment of coelenterate stings is symptomatic and supportive. Advanced cardiac life support may be necessary for patients who sustain cardiac arrest, either from toxic effects of the venom (e.g., *C. fleckeri*) or from anaphylaxis. Unfortunately, it is not uncommon for patients with sea wasp stings to be beyond resuscitation by the time medical help arrives. For those who are fortunate enough to be alive after a *Chironex* sting, rapid intravenous (IV) administration of sheep-derived sea wasp antivenin (Commonwealth Serum Laboratories, Melbourne, Australia) may be life saving. Tentacles should also be safely removed using a hemostat.

For anaphylactic shock, IV epinephrine, oxygen, IV fluids, dopamine, diphenhydramine, and a glucocorticoid such as Solu-Medrol may be indicated.

For asthma-like attacks, epinephrine, oxygen, normal saline, IV fluids, a bronchodilator such as albuterol, and perhaps a steroid may be considered, generally depending on the patient's presentation and response to treatment. Tetanus prophylaxis and treatment should be provided as indicated.

Considerable success has been achieved by using the following steps in management of jellyfish and Portuguese man-of-war stings in the United States.[3]

1. At the scene, advise the emergency medical service personnel or available family member or companion to remove any jellyfish tentacles that may be adhering to the skin, using sand held by a bath towel. Do not rub off the tentacles, rather pull them off. Care must be taken not to expose the treating individual, who also might be stung. As long as the tentacles are on the skin, they will continue to discharge their nematocysts.
2. In the United States, the wound should be washed with alcohol to fix the remaining nematocysts, thus preventing them from discharging. In Australia, vinegar is recommended in case of *C. fleckeri* stings but is not recommended for Portuguese man-of-war stings.[11]
3. A paste of baking soda (sodium bicarbonate) should be applied to the wound, affording considerable local relief. After an hour, moisten the baking soda with water and scrape it off with a dull object, like a spoon, to remove any remaining nematocysts.
4. Jellyfish often cause allergic reactions, and generalized urticaria and intense pruritus are common. Parenteral diphenhydramine (Benadryl), 50 mg IV in an adult, or a steroid, such as Solu-Medrol, 125 mg IV, or both may be indicated. Patients should be discharged with a prescription for an antihistamine or a steroid or both, to use as an outpatient. For as long as 1 to 4 weeks after the initial sting, it is not uncommon for patients to return for recurrence of urticarial lesions at the site of the sting. These should be treated symptomatically with antihistamines. For this reason, follow-up is recommended to all patients with jellyfish stings.
5. Patients who incur Portuguese man-of-war stings may have severe radiating pain and generalized symptoms. Morphine may be necessary to relieve pain. Generalized symptoms, including hypotension, may be present, and IV fluid therapy with normal saline and general supportive measures may be indicated. Patients who present in serious condition may require hospitalization.

Stingrays

Stingrays are a common cause of emergency department visits. Three common stingrays are the round stingray, *Urolophus halleri,* found along the

Pacific coast from California to Panama; the blunt-nosed stingray, *Dasyatis sayi,* found along the eastern Atlantic coast of North, Central, and South America; and the spotted eagle ray, *Aetobatus narinari,* found throughout tropical waters from the Atlantic to the Pacific.

Rays and sharks belong to the same marine vertebrate class and are collectively called elasmobranchs. The order *Rajiformes* includes both rays and skates. There are several families of rays, such as the manta rays, the electric rays, and sting rays. The electric ray, *Torpedo marmorata,* is able to generate an electric discharge capable of temporarily disabling an adult man.[2, 12] Table 27–3 lists some venomous stingrays. Some stingrays display an interesting characteristic: They have a sense of territory and usually do not stray too far from their claimed "turf." The *Dasyatis* stingrays (see Color Fig. 27–6) are difficult to detect because of their habit of lying buried in the mud or sand with only a portion of the body exposed.

Accidents usually occur when bathers step on a buried ray. The ray then whips its tail up and forward, driving the stinger into the foot or leg. Shuffling the feet in murky water causes stingrays to swim away from the immediate area. Commercial fisherman are sometimes stung in the hand or arms when emptying nets. Divers may be stung on the chest or abdomen.

The tail is armed with one or more venomous spines. The spine has a sharp, arrow-like tip and backward-pointing serrations along the sides so that after penetration the barb is difficult to remove and lacerates the tissues as it is withdrawn. The venom apparatus consists of a spine, integumentary sheath, and associated venom glands. When this is torn, the venom is released, and a violent tissue reaction is produced.

Pharmacology

The venom is primarily protein, and extracts contain serotonin and enzymes such as 5′-nucleotidase and phosphodiesterase.[12–15]

Stingray venom is one of the most powerful vasoconstrictors found among natural toxins. Coronary artery spasm, with resultant ST changes on the electrocardiogram and actual myocardial injury with subsequent decrease in cardiac output and hypotension, as well as arrhythmias, including cardiac standstill, have been observed.[12] The venom is highly unstable and is markedly heat labile.

Clinical Aspects

Most stings occur on the ankle or foot. The stingray spine is very sharp, and by virtue of the mechanism of injury, it is common for a patient to receive a laceration rather than a puncture wound.[3] Patients who present to the emergency department may describe walking in the ocean and feeling a fluttering under their foot and then a sudden stabbing pain.

Table 27–3. Some Important Venomous Stingrays

Family and Common Name	Proper Name	Geographic Distribution
Dasyatidae		
Blunt-nosed stingray	*Dasyatis sayi*	Atlantic coast of the Americas
Southern stingray	*Dasyatis americanus*	Cayman Islands, U.S. Atlantic coast to Brazil
Caribbean stingray	*Himantura scmarde*	Caribbean
Atlantic stingray	*Dasyatis sabina*	Chesapeake Bay to Gulf of Mexico
Diamond stingray	*Dasyatis brevis*	California to Peru and Galapagos Islands
Red stingray	*Dasyatis akajei*	China, Japan, Korea
Common stingray	*Dasyatis pastinaca*	Mediterranean Sea
Porcupine ray	*Urogymosus africanus*	Indian Ocean from Africa to Australia
Feathertail stingray	*Hypolophus sephen*	Indian and Pacific oceans
Ribbontail ray	*Taeniura lymna*	Indian Ocean, Red Sea to Australia
Thorntail stingray	*Dasyatis thetidis*	New Zealand and Australia
Tahitian stringray	*Himantura fai*	Tahiti, Polynesia, to Thailand
Urolophidae		
Round stingray	*Urolophus halleri*	U.S. Pacific coast to Panama
Yellow stingray	*Urolophus jamaicensis*	U.S. Atlantic, Gulf of Mexico and Caribbean
Crossback stingaree	*Urolophus cruciatus*	Australia, Tasmania
Common stingaree	*Trygonoptera testaceus*	Australia
Myliobatidae		
Spotted eagle ray	*Aetobatus narinari*	Tropical oceans from Atlantic to Indo-Pacific
Bat stingray	*Myliobatis californicus*	U.S. Pacific coast, California to Sea of Cortez
Bull ray	*Myliobatis aquila*	Mediterranean Sea
Southern bat ray	*Myliobatis tentuicaudatus*	Australia and New Zealand
Rhinopteridae		
Cownose ray	*Rhinoptera bonasus*	U.S. Atlantic coast to Brazil
Flapnose ray	*Rhinoptera javanica*	Pacific, Indonesia to Japan

Adapted from Halstead BW: Poisonous and Venomous Marine Animals of the World. Revised ed. Princeton, NJ, Darwin Press, 1978; and Michael SW: Reef Sharks and Rays of the World. Monterey, CA, Sea Challengers Publications, 1993.

The usual presenting symptom is severe shooting pain that increases in intensity during the first hour.

Systemic symptoms, such as chest pain, syncope, and other neurologic sequelae, have been described. Death has been reported but is uncommon and is usually related to chest or abdominal injuries. One highly unusual fatality occurred in a 12-year-old boy who was riding in a boat when a manta ray leaped out of the water and impaled him in the chest.[15]

Treatment

The key to therapy involves care of the wound, relief of pain, hot water immersion, observation, and hospitalization in severe cases.

Therapy should begin immediately, with irrigation of the wound with salt water. The wound should then be immersed continuously in hot water for at least 60 minutes; this deactivates the heat-labile venom and relieves the pain. *The use of hot water immersion is based on extensive clinical experience and is a standard of care.*[3]

In the emergency department, hot water immersion should be continued. Hot water immersion alone often provides pain relief, and pain medication is not necessary. After an hour of continuous hot water immersion, have the patient take the foot or affected part out of the water. If he or she suffers no pain, then one can stop treatment. Extremity wounds should then be irrigated, cleansed, débrided, and explored if necessary to remove any foreign body. A radiograph to rule out a foreign body may be useful. Lacerations may then be surgically closed, although leaving the wound open with follow-up may be preferable, depending on the clinical situation. Observation in the emergency department for 4 hours from the time of injury to rule out systemic involvement is generally indicated.

Patients with systemic symptoms should be observed, and patients with chest pain, irregular pulse, or hypotension should have an electrocardiogram and should be placed on a cardiac monitor. Hospitalization may be necessary when symptoms persist. Supportive therapy may be indicated. Patients who suffer a wound on the chest or abdomen may require surgical exploration.

Most cases respond to treatment in the emergency department. Tetanus prophylaxis is necessary. Antibiotics such as ciprofloxacin are usually required, because these wounds are prone to infection. Serious wounds require outpatient follow-up.

Catfish

Marine catfish are abundant silvery fishes with a smooth, scaleless skin. They have four to five barbels or "whiskers" around the mouth, giving them their name. The dorsal and pectoral spines of many species, especially juvenile catfish, are venomous and capable of inflicting very painful wounds. Stinging usually results from handling the fish, such as when removing the fish from the net or taking a hook out of its mouth. The venom of one species, the Indo-Pacific catfish, *Plotosus lineatus,* is often lethal.[2] The candiru or *Urinophilus*, a small Amazonian catfish, can penetrate the urethral orifice of mammals, including humans.[2] The Egyptian catfish, *Malapterus,* can transmit an electric shock.[2]

Catfish stings are common and painful and often become secondarily infected. Irrigation to remove venom, cleansing, hot water immersion, débridement, and removal of the catfish barb are essential to management.[3] A patient often has a painful, swollen, and infected wound days after the initial result. The typical history is that the person was stung while handling a catfish but thought that the barb had been removed. X-ray films are indicated, because catfish barbs are radiopaque. If the foreign body is seen on the radiograph, the wound should then be opened and explored and the catfish spine removed.

Both tetanus and antibiotic coverage are indicated; in our experience, cephalexin (Keflex) or ciprofloxacin (Cipro) are the preferred antibiotics.

Sea Urchins

The invertebrate phylum Echinodermata[2] includes the venomous sea urchins (see Color Fig. 27–7), such as the black sea urchin *Diadema setosum, Toxopneustes pileolus,* and *Echinothrix calamaris;* starfish, such as *Acanthaster planci,* the crown-of-thorns starfish; and sea cucumbers, such as *Pentacta australis.* Both venomous sea urchins and the venomous starfish have venomous spines. The Tam O'Shanter urchin of Australia, *Araeosoma thetidis,* has venom organs on the tips of the spines; these introduce the potent venom.[16] The sea urchins *T. pileolus* and *Tripneustes gratilla* contain pedicellariae that can envenomate with pincer jaws.[2, 16]

Sea urchin stings are extremely painful, and the spines often become embedded in the patient. The sea urchin spines of *D. setosum* contain purplish dye, which may temporarily stain the skin and give the false impression of a retained foreign body.[16] Stings by the sea urchin *Tripneustes* may produce neurologic symptoms.[16]

Sea urchin (and starfish) toxin is remarkably heat labile, and hot water immersion therapy[14] is indicated for pain relief and deactivation of the venom. Surgical removal, especially of the thick calcium-containing spines, is indicated, as well as tetanus prophylaxis. Antibiotic therapy and follow-up wound care are often necessary.

Weever Fish

The weever fish, or Trachinidae, is found in the Mediterranean Sea, along the Atlantic coast of Europe and North Africa, and up to the North Sea. *Trachinus draco,* or dragon fish, or aranha, has five dorsal and two opercular spines that can inflict on unwary fishermen one of the most painful venoms known.[2] Weever fish often hide in mud or sand with only the head exposed,[2] only then to dart out to attack their prey.[17] Weever fish can survive out of the water for hours.[2] A puncture wound by a weever fish produces instantaneous, often crippling pain so severe that the patient often loses consciousness. Local ischemia, secondary infection at the wound site, and systemic involvement may occur.[17] Hot water immersion[14, 16–18] is effective early in treatment for pain relief and deactivation of the venom; intravenous calcium is useful for pain relief.[18] Exploration of the wound is often necessary. Supportive therapy and long-term wound care are generally indicated.

Scorpion Fish and Stonefish

The scorpion fish and stonefish (*Synanceja* spp.) belong to the family Scorpaenidae.[2] Examples of venomous fish in this family include the butterfly fish, *Pterois lunulata,* the zebra fish, *Dendrochirus zebra* (see Color Fig. 27–8); the lionfish *Pterois volitans* (see Color Fig. 27–9); sculpin (*Scorpaena* spp.); and rockfish (*Sebastes* spp.). Most venomous Scorpaenidae are found in tropical water, but a somewhat less venomous species of scorpion fish lives along the coast of California and the southeastern coast of the United States. Most scorpion fish stings occur when handling the fish in home aquariums. Venomous dorsal spines, which cause the injury, are characteristic of these fish. The stonefish *Synanceja horrida* (see Color Fig. 27–10) is a master of disguise, resembling a rock, and is the most venomous of the group.

Intense pain results from stings by this group, but systemic symptoms, including headache, seizures, paralysis, abdominal pain, and hypotension, generally result only from stonefish envenomation.[2, 10, 14]

Treatment of scorpion fish injury is similar to stingray injury. Hot water immersion,[2, 19] wound debridement, and supportive care are indicated. An antivenin for stonefish envenomation is available from the Commonwealth Serum Laboratories in Melbourne, Australia.[2, 10] Several deaths have been attributed to stonefish injury, dating back to antiquity.

Blue-Ringed Octopus and Cone Shells

Venomous mollusks include the Australian blue-ringed octopus (see Color Fig. 27–3), *Hapalochlaena maculosa* or *O. maculosa,* and cone shells.

The Australian blue-ringed octopus rarely exceeds 8 inches in full extension and can fit in the palm of the hand. The octopus is brown with yellow bands and blue rings; when it becomes excited, the blue rings take on an iridescent glow.[20] The octopus bites with its beak and secretes tetrodotoxin from its posterior salivary gland. Tetrodotoxin has an unusual distribution in nature, also found in such diverse life as puffer fish, the California newt *Taricha,* and the central American frog *Atelopus.*[20] Tetrodotoxin blocks the movement of sodium ions by inhibiting the sodium channel, thus causing failure of nerve conduction and subsequent paralysis. Envenomation is described as painless, but the patient rapidly succumbs, becoming weak and unconscious, and develops respiratory arrest, often within 15 minutes. Cardiac arrest and death follow. In a case report of two patients[21] who survived after cardiopulmonary arrest due to the bite of the blue-ringed octopus, early resuscitative efforts were determined critical to survival, because the toxin has a short duration of action.

Cone shells are carnivorous snails that have a harpoon-like venom apparatus. They can fire a detachable radular tooth into their prey, and this paralyzes the victim.[2, 10] Envenomation is uncommon in humans and usually occurs on the fingers when an unwary person picks up the attractive shells. Treatment is supportive.

Sea Snakes

Sea snakes belong to the family Hydrophiidae and have evolved from the Elapid family of snakes. They are aquatic and mostly helpless on land. Their anatomy has been highly adapted for marine life: The body and particularly the tail are vertically compressed to provide swimming ability, the nostrils are located on top of the head rather than on the side, and specialized glands secrete salt in order to permit life in a saline environment.[2, 22]

Sea snakes inhabit the Indian and Pacific oceans from the Arabian Sea to Malaysia south to Australia and New Zealand. A common sea snake is *Pelamis platurus,* or the yellow-bellied sea snake. This snake has the widest distribution and has been found from the Indian Ocean all the way to the Pacific coast of Central America. No venomous sea snake has ever been found in the Atlantic Ocean or Caribbean Sea. The most highly toxic sea snake is the beaked sea snake, *Enhydrina schistosa* (see Color Fig. 27–11). Included in this group are the sea kraits, such as *Laticauda colubrina,* the yellow-lipped sea brait, which lives in coastal waters and at night rests on land. Table 27–4 lists some important venomous sea snakes.

Sea snake bites are often painless. The fangs are often small, frequently only 2 to 3 mm in length; thus, bites are often difficult to detect, because there may only be one or multiple small puncture wounds.[2, 3, 13, 16] Perhaps from one third to one half of bites do not result in envenomation.[2] Divers and fishermen are the usual victims, and symptoms may occur within 2 hours of the bite, generally within 6 to 8 hours, but are often delayed for 24 hours. Sea snake venom is neurotoxic,[2, 3, 16, 22–24] similar to that of the coral snake, and symptoms include weakness and visual disturbances, including double vision, progressing to paralysis and respiratory distress.[22–24]

Table 27–4. Important Venomous Sea Snakes (Family Hydrophiidae)

Common Name	Scientific Name	Geographic Distribution
Common sea snake	*Enhydrina schistosa*	Indian and western Pacific
Annulated sea snake	*Hydrophis cyanocinctus*	Arabian Gulf to Indonesia
Yellow-bellied sea snake	*Pelamis platurus*	All of Pacific and Indian oceans
Banded sea snake	*Hydrophis spiralis*	Pacific, near Malaya
Jerdon's snake	*Kerilia jerdoni*	Indian Ocean
Yellow-lipped sea brait	*Laticauda colubrina*	Tropical coasts of Indo-Pacific
Stoke's sea snake	*Astrotia stokesi*	Pacific, near Australia
Shaw's sea snake	*Lapemis curtus*	Persian Gulf and Arabian Sea
Hardwick's sea snake	*Lapemis hardwickii*	Pacific, Japan to Indonesia
Samoan sea snake	*Laticauda semifasciata*	Samoa, Philippines to China sea
Dubois sea snake	*Aipysurus duboisii*	Coral Sea to New Guinea

From Department of the US Navy: Important Snakes of the World. Washington, DC, United States Government Printing Office, 1966.

Rhabdomyolysis, myoglobinuria, and subsequent renal failure may ensue.[22–24]

Sea snake antivenin is produced by Commonwealth Serum Laboratories of Melbourne, Australia, and contains horse antiserum against *E. schistosa* (sea snake) and *Notechis scutatus* (terrestrial tiger snake) venoms[23, 24] and is effective for most sea snake envenomations. Monovalent sea snake antivenin for *E. schistosa* is also produced by the Halfkine Institute of Bombay, India, and is also effective for most sea snake envenomations in that region.[13] If these are unavailable, the Commonwealth Serum Laboratories monovalent tiger snake *(Notechis scutatus)* antivenin may be used.[10, 13, 14, 16] As with coral snakes, intravenous antivenin should be administered *early,* at the first onset of symptoms, in order to be most effective.

INFECTION

Infection by marine organisms may occur by ingestion of contaminated seafood or by infection of wounds. One particularly virulent infection is *V. vulnificus.*

Vibrio vulnificus

V. vulnificus is a halophilic (salt-loving) marine organism that has become the major cause of mortality due to food poisoning in Florida, particularly along the Gulf Coast. From 1981 to 1992, 72 cases of *V. vulnificus* infection due to eating raw oysters were reported in Florida; of these, 36 (50%) ended in death.[25]

V. vulnificus occurs naturally in the marine environment and causes infections in two ways: by contamination of raw oysters and by infection of wounds while bathing in salt water or handling seafood, such as picking crabs or peeling shrimp.[26, 27] Infection occurs especially during the warmer months of the year.[28, 29] This calls to mind the custom in the South of eating raw oysters during only the months that contain an *r,* September through April.

V. vulnificus is a gram-negative lactose-fermenting rod that elaborates a toxin that is both hemolytic and cytotoxic, as well as extracellular proteins such as protease, collagenase, and phospholipases.[26, 27]

After ingestion of contaminated shellfish, especially raw oysters, primary septicemia occurs with abrupt onset of chills, fever, hypotension, and skin eruption.[26–31] Vomiting and diarrhea affect fewer than half of the victims. Hypotension occurring within the first 12 hours has been associated with a 90% mortality rate.

Skin manifestations are dramatic. They begin as hemorrhagic bullae on the trunk and extremities, and these often develop into necrotic ulcers. Necrotizing fasciitis and myositis with obvious purulence may develop. Gangrene has resulted, requiring amputation.[26, 27, 29–31]

Wound infections occurred either by exposure of a pre-existing wound to salt water or by sustaining a puncture wound or laceration while handling seafood.[30] Localized infection and cellulitis began at the wound site and then rapidly progressed to the full-blown picture of septicemia and extensive skin and soft-tissue involvement.

V. vulnificus infection is highly lethal to patients with underlying liver disease.[25–32]

Treatment must be aggressive and includes antibiotic therapy and surgical débridement. Tetracycline and chloramphenicol are the most effective antibiotics; third-generation cephalosporins and aminoglycosides may also be effective.[30, 31] Resuscitation with IV fluids, supportive care, and admission to an intensive care unit are necessary.

POISONING

Marine life include species containing one or more toxins that produce poisoning, such as paralytic shellfish poisoning, amnesic shellfish poisoning, scombroid fish poisoning, puffer fish poisoning (*fugu*), and ciguatera.

Evaluation for ingestion of toxic marine organisms should include the patient's history (including the actual seafood consumed), physical examination, available laboratory test results, clinical manifestations, emergency care, and course of the illness. Critical poisoning by toxic marine ingestion may occur in remote areas where IV fluid resuscitation, mechanical ventilation, and emergency and supportive care may be required; transfer to a medical center after initial management may be indicated for those who survive. In divers, air embolism, decompression sickness (the bends), and other diving emergencies must also be considered.

Paralytic Shellfish Poisoning

Blooms of toxic algae appear to be increasing worldwide as coastal pollution increases.[33] Outbreaks of paralytic shellfish poisoning occur worldwide. Paralytic shellfish poisoning results from consumption of mollusks such as mussels, clams, oysters, and scallops that have fed on certain toxic *Gonyaulax* species. The dinoflagellates primarily responsible for outbreaks of paralytic shellfish poisoning (PSP) include *Gonyaulax catenella*, which is found along the Pacific Coast from Alaska and California to Venezuela and west to Japan; *G. tamarensis* var. *excavata*, which is found on the Atlantic Coast from Massachusetts and Nova Scotia to the North Sea; and *Pyrodinium bahamense* var. *compressa*, which is found from Central America to the Philippines.[40] Mollusks feed by filtering seawater that contains phytoplankton. The shellfish are not adversely affected by the algal toxins.[34–40]

There is no known antidote to the potent toxins[38–43] which include saxitoxin and analogues. These toxins block action potentials by preventing the flow of sodium, thus impeding nerve conduction. Immunity is not engendered through antibody production after exposure to sublethal doses. Poisonous shellfish cannot be recognized by appearance, odor, or any method other than chemical analysis and (mouse toxicity) bioassay. Cooking, frying, and baking only partially ameliorate toxicity.[42] A victim's prognosis may[41] or may not[42] relate to the quantity ingested.

The best prevention of paralytic shellfish poisoning in humans is strict adherence to public health agency guidelines on harvesting, processing, and consumption of shellfish.[34] The sporadic and unpredictable nature of red tides and paralytic shellfish poisoning further argues for stringent compliance with quarantine regulations.

Red tides result from excessive growth (bloom) of particular unicellular algae (phytoplankton), giving the water a red-brown appearance due to the pigments contained in the algae. Factors involved in the initiation, subsequent development, and continuation of a red tide are not totally understood. Red tides occur sporadically and are usually of short duration. In general, the abundance and seasonal distribution of dinoflagellates are intimately related to temperature, salinity, light, nutrients, and hydrographic conditions, including currents and water column stability in the sea. However, toxic red tides are essentially a coastal phenomenon.

Poisonings related to ingestion of shellfish were described in the time of Moses, about 1491 BC. Blooms or red tides of oceans are mentioned in the Bible in Exodus 7:20–21: "And all the waters that were in the river were turned to blood. And the fish that was in the river died; and the river stank, and the Egyptians could not drink the water of the river."[1] Because of the red tide in 208 BC, the name Red Sea was given by the ancient Greeks to all coasts of Arabia. The red tides were mentioned in the *Iliad* as well as in the writings of Tacitus. As early as 1689, the first case of paralytic shellfish poisoning was described.

Medical history gives accounts of incidents of shellfish poisoning in many parts of the world between 1827 and 1909. The great Wilhelmshaven outbreak that took place in Germany in 1885 attracted scientific attention to the red tide as a health hazard.[34]

The first large epidemic recorded in the United States was in San Francisco in 1927; 102 persons became ill, and 6 died.[43]

The work of Sommer and his associates in the 1930s proved that the California mussel *Mytilus californianus* lost its toxicity in filtered water but regained it in seawater taken from a red tide area.[43] These same scientists correlated an increase in toxicity of mussels with the number of *Gonyaulax catenella* present in their environment.

It was first demonstrated that the toxin of *Gymnodinium breve,* which causes red tide off the Florida coast, could act as an upper respiratory tract irritant to people along the coast. Death of large numbers of fish became associated with blooms of this microorganism, now named *Ptychodiscus brevis,* as did seabird fatalities and shellfish poisoning.[44]

Paralytic shellfish poisoning originates from red tides, with filter-feeding bivalve mollusks as transvectors, especially mussels and clams—for example, *Mytilus edulis* (mussel), *Mytilus californianus* (mussel), *Saxidomus giganteus* (Alaskan butter clam), *Clinocardium nuttalli* (cockles), *Siliqua patula* (razor clams), and *Protothaca staminea* (littleneck clams) in northeastern Pacific Ocean coastal waters; and *Mya arenaria* (soft-shell clam), *Placopecten magellanicus* (sea scallop), and *Mytilus edulis* in northwestern Atlantic Ocean coastal waters.[42]

Although shellfish include mollusks such as clams, mussels, and scallops and crustaceans such as shrimp, lobsters, and crabs, mollusks that have a hard shell are particularly prone to cause paralytic shellfish poisoning. Crustaceans can have softer shells; however, where an outbreak of paralytic shellfish poisoning occurs, much of the marine life can be involved, and fish, shellfish, and other seafoods may be poisonous or restricted.

Rates of accumulation and loss of toxin differ among species. In mussels, for example the *Mytilus* species, the toxins are concentrated in the digestive glands ("hepatopancreas," "liver," or "dark glands"). Toxicity is usually lost within weeks from mussels in seawater that does not contain toxic dinoflagellates. In the Alaskan butter clam (*S. giganteus*), for example, the principal storage sites of the toxin after the initial accumulation in the digestive glands are the gills and siphons. Butter clams can remain toxic for as long as 2 years after initial accumulation of toxin from a red tide.

Fortunately, the muscle tissues (white meat) of mollusks (mantle muscle, adductor muscles, foot, and body—exclusive of digestive glands) tend to store relatively small amounts of poison. These are the tissues most commonly eaten by people.

Crustacean shellfish such as lobsters are only rarely transvectors of paralytic shellfish poisoning.

Toxicology

The toxic principles of *Gonyaulax* species, of which mollusks are transvectors, are substituted tetrahydropurine structures that include saxitoxin 1, neosaxitoxin 2, gonyautoxin 3, and at least 15 more analogues.[37, 40] The chemical and physiologic characteristics of saxitoxin 1 and analogues are very similar. Saxitoxin is among the most potent human poisons known, and was quantitated by Sommer into mouse units.[43] A mouse unit is the amount of toxin that kills a 20-g mouse in 15 minutes by intraperitoneal injection, which equals 0.18 μg of saxitoxin.[40] A dose of purified saxitoxin or analogues lethal to humans is 0.1 mg.[2] A quarantine limit for closure of fisheries or interstate trade of mussels is 80 μg or 400 mouse units of saxitoxin per 100 mg of shellfish.[40–42, 45, 46]

Clinical Presentation

Patients with paralytic shellfish poisoning may develop neurologic symptoms and, in severe cases, respiratory paralysis and motor paralysis. A case review[42] reported that in 113 of 117 patients, the initial manifestation of poisoning consisted of *paresthesia*—specifically, numbness and tingling around the lips, mouth, upper airway, and fingers—which may become apparent within a few minutes after eating poisonous shellfish. These sensations are followed by a feeling of numbness in other parts of the body.[46] Nausea, vomiting, and diarrhea can occur. Floating sensations may be reported by the patient. Until proven otherwise, paralytic shellfish poisoning is a life-threatening emergency. As the illness progresses, respiratory distress and muscle paralysis become more severe. Death results from respiratory paralysis within 2 to 12 hours. Children are more susceptible to mortality.[41] If a patient survives for 24 hours, the prognosis is favorable, and there appears to be no lasting effect.[46]

Diagnosis

Without an adequate history, diagnosis can be and often is most puzzling. A complete history is essential for proper diagnosis—a presumptive diagnosis of paralytic shellfish poisoning should be made in a patient who develops neurologic symptoms after ingestion of mussels during seasons of risk in areas where paralytic shellfish poisoning occurs. Other causes of neurologic illness may appropriately have to be ruled out. Obtaining saxitoxin from the implicated shellfish, identifying the toxin in the patient, and identifying the toxin in an algal organism such as *G. catenella* may be helpful. Analyses of toxic shellfish and toxic dinoflagellate algal organisms for toxins have helped establish a diagnosis in patients involved in certain outbreaks of shellfish poisonings, particularly because the seawater is not always pigmented abnormally or may not appear pigmented until late in the outbreak. It is preferable that all the toxins be rapidly identified in the patient's blood or urine.

Management

The treatment of paralytic shellfish poisoning is symptomatic and supportive. Gastric lavage and activated charcoal are indicated because saxitoxin is readily adsorbed on charcoal. An alkaline diuresis with sodium bicarbonate may be of value, because saxitoxins are reportedly unstable in an alkaline medium. Steroids such as hydrocortisone may be indicated. Endotracheal intubation, respiratory support, cardiac monitoring, and maintenance of blood pressure are often necessary, because these patients are usually in critical condition.

Amnesic Shellfish Poisoning

A unique illness occurred in Canada in November and December of 1987. It was characterized by acute onset of gastrointestinal symptoms within 24 hours of eating mussels, followed by rapid onset of confusion, disorientation, and memory loss within 48 hours.[47] In a month, more than 250 cases were reported to the Health Department in Canada. Of these, 109 patients met the case definition; 19 patients required hospitalization; and 12 patients required intensive care because of serious neurologic impairment such as seizures, coma, mutism, and purposeless chewing and grimacing.[48] Three elderly patients died.[47–49]

Health officials in Canada expertly tracked the outbreak to mussel cultivation beds primarily from the Cardigan River estuary of Prince Edward Island, and an embargo on mussel shipments was quickly placed.[47, 49]

Domoic acid, an amino acid neuroexcitatory transmitter,[47–50] was identified as the causative toxin, the source of which was *Nitzschia pungens,* a form of marine vegetation.[47] Chronic residual memory deficits result from domoic acid intoxication.[48] Treatment is supportive. As of this writing, no other outbreaks of amnesic shellfish poisoning have been reported.

Scombroid Fish Poisoning

Scombroid fish poisoning is a clinical syndrome produced by histamine[51–54] release from spoiled fish of the family Scombroidae, which include tuna and mackerel, skipjack, albacore, and bonito.[51] Other fish implicated include mahi-mahi, herring, sardine, anchovy, amberjack, and the Japanese saury.[52, 53]

Fish left in the sun after being caught are invaded by bacteria such as *Escherichia coli, Klebsiella, Aerobacter,* or *Proteus,* which produce histidine decarboxylase and convert histidine in the muscle of the fish to histamine.[51]

Patients who have eaten significant quantities of these spoiled fish (even when cooked) often report a peppery taste[52, 54] and then present with signs and symptoms of histamine intoxication, often within 30 minutes. Flushing, erythema, and urticaria predominate, and generalized symptoms such as headache, chills, vomiting, diarrhea, and abdominal cramps also occur. Conjunctival erythema may be frequent.[52] Erythema is often confined to the face, neck, and upper chest. Severe cases that include bronchospasm and hypotension have been reported. Illness may be more severe in patients taking isoniazid, which inhibits histaminase.[52]

Because this syndrome is often confused with seafood allergy, it is important to consider this diagnosis. Patients who present with this syndrome should be asked if they have eaten any of the previously listed fish and if they noted a peppery taste. Otherwise, the physician may wrongly advise the patient or family they are allergic to seafood and must avoid seafood forever.

Administration of antihistamines such as the H_2 blocker cimetidine or the H_1 blocker diphenhydramine is key to treatment, as well as intravenous fluids, steroids, and general supportive care. Epinephrine may be indicated in the presence of bronchospasm or hypotension. The syndrome is usually self-limited and usually resolves within a few hours.

This syndrome is completely preventable if freshly caught fish are immediately placed on ice and then refrigerated on reaching shore.

Puffer Fish Poisoning

Puffer fish poisoning is a highly lethal form of fish poisoning.[55] The puffer fish toxin tetrodotoxin can produce a prolonged state of suspended animation resembling death.[2] Fugu in Japan and the tambor puffer in Cuba are popular fish eaten by some persons in some cultures. In Japan, a 59% mortality was reported in 6386 cases of puffer fish poisoning during a 78-year period.[2] At least three deaths due to eating puffer fish have been reported in Florida.

Puffer fish (see Color Fig. 27–12) are named for their ability to inflate themselves to a nearly spheric shape when disturbed. Some common tetrodotoxic puffers in various areas of the world are blowfish (United States), akeke (Hawaii), tambores (Cuba), fugu (Japan), West Indian swellfish, tinga tinga (Philippines), mamaiacu (Brazil), qarrad (Red Sea), kend (India), buntal pisang (Malaysia), tetraodon, porcupine fish, globefish, tiger puffer, rabbit fish, and botete.[2]

Toxicology

The toxin that causes puffer fish poisoning is tetrodotoxin. Tetrodotoxin is a basic compound that is readily soluble in water. It is *not* heat labile, and boiling or heating the fish does not deactivate the poison.[55–57] Tetrodotoxin is a specific inhibitor of sodium channels, blocking conductance of nerve cells.[55, 56, 58, 59]

Social Aspects

In Japan, fugu is considered a delicacy, and all cooks and restaurants handling fugu must be specially licensed to prepare fugu. The muscle of the fish is the part that is eaten, usually during the winter months (during the nonreproductive season for puffers). Even with extensive regulations, fugu is still the major cause of death due to food poisoning in Japan.

Tetrodotoxin has been suggested as the causative agent in Haitian voodoo potions that produce a zombie-like state.

Clinical Presentation

The clinical manifestations of puffer poisoning include paresthesia about the lips, fingertips, and elsewhere; diaphoresis, hyperemesis, dysphonia, floating sensations, progressive muscle paralysis, cyanosis, and often seizures, coma, and respiratory arrest.[2, 55, 56]

A most unusual phenomomen has been described: patients may be completely paralyzed, have absent corneal reflexes, and have dilated fixed pupils but on recovery are found to have had complete retention of consciousness while in such a state.[2, 55]

Treatment

Management is symptomatic and supportive. Airway management, endotracheal intubation, and mechanical ventilation may be required in apneic patients, who may have extensive respiratory and muscle paralysis. Atropine or a cardiac pacemaker or both may be useful in managing symptomatic bradycardia.[56] Cardiac arrhythmias should be managed appropriately. Normal saline IV infusion and perhaps dopamine may be helpful in managing symptomatic hypotension. Gastric lavage may be performed with a 2% solution of sodium bicarbonate, followed by activated charcoal.

Considerable caution is urged when pronouncing death due to puffer fish poisoning, because the toxin may produce a deceptive state of suspended animation.

Ciguatera

Numerous species of coral reef fish have been linked to ciguatera.[60–63] Toxins from the photosynthetic benthic dinoflagellate *Gambierdiscus toxicus* pass up the food chain when herbivorous fishes consume the organism in algae that contain toxin.[60–65] These are eaten by carnivorous fishes, which are then consumed by humans. Sensitized persons, who are susceptible to small amounts of toxic fish, can become quite ill and may require aggressive treatment. Although rarely lethal, ciguatera fish poisoning is unique in that chronic relapsing symptoms can occur and are often difficult to manage.[60, 65]

Barracuda, amberjack, dolphin fish, the moray eel, surgeonfish, and even such delicacies as grouper and red snapper are among the approximately 300 species that have at various times been implicated in causing ciguatera.[60–66] Sixty per cent of the cases reported in the Miami study followed ingestion of grouper.[63] So many reports of ciguatera followed the ingestion of barracuda that its sale is prohibited in southern Florida.[63] Common causes of ciguatera in Hawaii[60, 66] include the kingfish ulua (*Caranx ignobilis*), the jack papio (*Caranx sexfasciatus*), and the amberjack kahala (*Seriola dumerili*). A common cause of ciguatera in the Indo-Pacific, including Hawaii, is the surgeonfish *Ctenochaetus strigosus,* also known as maito in Tahiti.[66]

Toxicology

The principal toxin is ciguatoxin-1, a lipid-soluble polyether that is highly stable and is *not* inactivated by heating, drying, cooking, smoking, or freezing.[67, 68] The toxin induces membrane depolarization in nerve tissue by opening voltage-dependent sodium channels.[68] Maitotoxin has also been isolated from *G. toxicus,* a water-soluble toxin that opens calcium channels. A third toxin, scaritoxin,[60] is postulated to cause the delayed neurotoxic effects that prove so troublesome to ciguatera victims.

Clinical Presentation

The clinical syndrome of ciguatera occurs after eating a ciguatoxic fish and includes both gastrointestinal and neurologic symptoms.[60, 61, 69–72] Characteristic features of ciguatera include *paresthesia of the perioral region and distal extremities, especially of the palms and soles, and a cold-to-hot sensory reversal dysesthesia—patients usually describe a burning hot sensation while picking up a cold drink.*

Bagnis and associates reviewed 3009 cases of ciguatera in the South Pacific and noted paresis involving the extraocular muscles or the lower extremities in 10.5% of patients, paralysis of the lower extremities in 0.6% of patients, and only three deaths, or 0.1% of the total group.[61]

Ataxia, headache, arthralgias, and vertigo are also common complaints. Pruritus is present. Another unusual feature is that patients may complain that their teeth feel loose and may fall out of their sockets or are painful. Oropharyngeal paresthesia, acral paresthesia, and even total body paresthesia can develop. Nausea, vomiting, and diarrhea may be severe. Hypotension, including postural hypotension, and symptomatic bradycardia (including heart blocks) can develop.

Paresthesia, pruritus, and prolonged weakness after the acute phase may persist for several weeks to months.[60, 65] It has also been noted that repeated episodes of ciguatera may be more severe in character.

Diagnosis

The diagnosis of ciguatera is made on clinical grounds. The history of consumption of fish such as grouper, barracuda, or amberjack with subsequent gastrointestinal symptoms and the unique characteristic neurologic findings of cold-to-hot sensory reversal dysesthesia, a sensation of loose teeth, and paresthesias of the perioral region and the extremities confirm the clinical diagnosis.

Treatment

A promising new treatment of acute ciguatera in appropriate patients is intravenous mannitol.[73] After an IV infusion of normal saline or lactated Ringer's solution is established, 20% mannitol is given as a piggyback (IV) solution. The dose of mannitol is calculated to a maximum of 1 g/kg of body weight and given at a rate of 500 mL/h. Thus, a 70-kg man would receive 70 g of 20% mannitol, or 350 mL over 42 minutes.[73] Symptomatic and supportive therapy may also be indicated.

Some patients feel well before the infusion is completed. However, patients should still be placed on a ciguatera diet avoiding fish, shellfish, alcoholic beverages, nuts or nut products, and seeds or seed products for 6 to 12 months, because these dietary products exacerbate symptoms.

Chronic ciguatera may be bothersome, because symptoms may wax and wane with mood swings, the weather, and even sexual activity.[60, 65] The most success in treatment has been with the use of amitriptyline,[60, 65, 70, 74–75] which also affects sodium channels. Treatment is generally begun with amitriptyline 25 mg twice a day. Remissions and exacerbations may occur.

References

GENERAL

1. The New American Bible, St. Joseph's Edition. New York, Catholic Publishing Company, 1992; or The Authorized King James Version of the Holy Bible. Gordonsville, TN, Mid America Bible Society, 1993; or The Holy Scripture. Philadelphia, Jewish Publications Society, 1993.
2. Halstead BW: Poisonous and Venomous Marine Animals of the World. Revised ed. Princeton, NJ, Darwin Press, 1978.
3. Haddad LM, Lee RF, McConnell OJ, Targett NK: Toxic marine life. In Haddad LM, Winchester JF (eds): Clinical Management of Poisoning and Drug Overdose. Philadelphia, W. B. Saunders, Co. pp 303–317, 1983.

JELLYFISH

4. Lane CE: Nematocyst toxins of Coelenterates. In Humm HJ, Lane CE (eds): Bioactive Compounds from the Sea. New York, Marcel Dekker, p 123, 1974.
5. Ellis MD: Dangerous Plants, Snakes, Arthropods, and Marine Life. Drug Intelligence Publications, Hamilton, IL, 1978.
6. Burnett JW, Gable WD: A fatal jellyfish envenomation by the Portuguese man-o'-war. Toxicon *27:*823–824, 1989.
7. Stein MR, Marracini JV, Rothschild NE, Burnett JW: Fatal Portuguese man-o'-war (Physalia physalis) envenomation. Ann Emerg Med *18:*312–315, 1989.
8. Southcott RV: Revision of the Irukandji syndrome. Aust J Zool *15:*651, 1967.
9. Flecker H: Irukandji stings to N. Queensland bathers. Med J Aust *2:*89, 1952.
10. Gurry D: Marine stings. Aust Fam Physician *21:*26–34, 1992.
11. Fenner PJ, Williamson JA, Burnett JW, Rifkin J: First aid treatment of jellyfish stings in Australia. Med J Aust *158:*498–501, 1993.

STINGRAY

12. Michael SW: Reef Sharks and Rays of the World Monterey, CA, Sea Challengers Publications, 1993.
13. McGoldrick J, Marx JA: Marine envenomations. J Emerg Med *9:*497–502, 1991.
14. Auerbach PS: Marine envenomations. N Engl J Med *325:*486–493, 1991.
15. Fenner PJ, Williamson JA, Skinner RA: Fatal and non-fatal stingray envenomation. Med J Aust *151:*621–625, 1989.

SEA URCHIN, WEEVER FISH, AND SCORPION FISH

16. Auerbach PS: Marine envenomation. In Auerbach PS (ed): Wilderness Medicine. 3rd ed. St. Louis, C.V. Mosby Co., pp 1327–1374, 1995.
17. Cain D; Weever fish sting: An unusual problem. BMJ *287:*406–407, 1983.
18. Brown CK, Shepherd SM: Marine trauma, envenomations, and intoxications. Emerg Med Clin North Am *10:*385–408, 1992.
19. Kizer KW, McKinney HE, Auerbach PS: Scorpaenidae envenomation: A five-year poison center experience. JAMA *253:*807–810, 1985.

BLUE-RINGED OCTOPUS AND SEA SNAKES

20. Williamson JAH: The blue-ringed octopus bite and envenomation syndrome. Clin Dermatol *5:*127–133, 1987.
21. Walker DG: Survival after severe envenomation by the blue-ringed octopus (Hapalochlaena maculosa). Med J Aust *2:*663–665, 1983.
22. Reid HA: Diagnosis, prognosis, and treatment of sea-snake bite. Lancet *1:*399–402, 1961.
23. Warrell DA, Fenner PJ: Venomous bites and stings. Br Med Bull *49:*423–439, 1993.
24. Mercer HP, McGill JJ, Ibrahim RA: Envenomation by sea snakes in Queensland. Med J Aust *137:*130–132, 1981.

VIBRIO VULNIFICUS

25. Hlady WG, Mullen RC, Hopkins RS: Vibrio vulnificus from raw oysters. J Fl Med Assoc *80:*536–538, 1993.
26. Blake PA, Merson MH, Weaver RE, et al: Disease caused by a marine vibrio. N Engl J Med *300:*1–5, 1979.
27. Morris JG, Black RE: Cholera and other vibrioses in the United States. N Engl J Med *312:*343–350, 1985.
28. Kizer KW: Vibrio vulnificus infections and raw oysters. Am J Prev Med *10:*123–124, 1994.
29. Bonner JR, Coker AS, Berryman CR, Pollock HM: Spectrum of *Vibrio* infections in a Gulf Coast community. Ann Intern Med *99:*464–469, 1983.
30. Tacket CO, Brenner F, Blake PA: Clinical features and an epidemiological study of Vibrio vulnificus infections. J Infect Dis *149:*558–561, 1984.
31. Chuang Y, Yuan C, Liu C, et al: Vibrio vulnificus infection in Taiwan. Clin Infect Dis *15:*271–276, 1992.
32. Dayal HH, Trieff NM, Dayal V: Preventing Vibrio vulnificus infections. Am J Prev Med *9:*191–193, 1993.

RED TIDE

33. Anderson DM: Red tides. Sci Am *271:*62–68, 1994.
34. Ahles MD: Red tide: A recurrent health hazard. Am J Public Health *64:*807, 1974.
35. Todd E, Avery G, Grant GA: An outbreak of severe paralytic shellfish poisoning in British Columbia. Can Commun Dis Rep *19:*99–102, 1993.
36. Bond RM, Medcof JC: Epidemic shellfish poisoning in New Brunswick, 1957. Can Med Assoc J *19:*19, 1978.
37. Collins M: Algal toxins. Microbiol Rev *42:*725, 1978.
38. Meyer KF: Food poisoning (in 3 parts). N Engl J Med *249:*765 (I), 804 (II), 843 (III), 1953.
39. Hughes JM, Merson MH: Fish and shellfish poisoning. N Engl J Med *295:*1117–1120, 1976.
40. Halstead BW, Schantz BJ: Paralytic shellfish poisoning. WHO Offset Publ *79:*1–59, 1984.
41. Rodrigue DC, Etzel RA, Hall S, et al: Lethal paralytic shellfish poisoning in Guatemala. Am J Trop Med Hyg *42:*267–271, 1990.
42. Gessner BD, Middaugh JP: Paralytic shellfish poisoning in Alaska: A 20 year retrospective analysis. Am J Epidemiol *141:*766–770, 1995.
43. Sommer H, Meyer KF: Paralytic shellfish poisoning. Arch Pathol *24:*560, 1937.
44. Pierce RH: Red tide (Ptychodiscus brevis) toxin aerosols: A review. Toxicon *24:*955–965, 1986.
45. Hartigan-Go, K, Bateman DN: Red tide in the Philippines. Hum Exp Toxicol *13:*824–830, 1994.
46. Centers for Disease Control: Paralytic shellfish poisoning—Massachusetts and Alaska, 1990. MMWR *40:*157–161, 1991.

AMNESIC SHELLFISH POISONING

47. Perl TM, Bedard L, Kosatsky T, et al: An outbreak of toxic encephalopathy caused by eating mussels contaminated with domoic acid. N Engl J Med *322:*1775–1780, 1990.
48. Teitelbaum JS, Zatorre RJ, Carpenter S, et al: Neurologic sequelae of domoic acid intoxication due to the ingestion of contaminated mussels. N Engl J Med *322:*1761–1767, 1990.
49. Kosatsky T: Improving epidemic control: Lessons from the 1987 toxic mussels affair. Can Med Assoc J *147:*1769–1772, 1992.
50. Cendes F, Andermann F, Carpenter S, et al: Temporal lobe epilepsy caused by domoic acid intoxication. Ann Neurol *37:*123–126, 1995.

SCOMBROID FISH POISONING

51. McInerney J, Sahgal P, Vogel M, et al: Scombroid poisoning. Ann Emerg Med *28:*235–238, 1996.
52. Sanders WE: Intoxications from the seas: Ciguatera, scombroid, and paralytic shellfish poisoning. Infect Dis Clin North Am *1:*665–676, 1987.
53. Morrow JD, Margolies GR, Rowland J, Roberts LJ: Evidence that histamine is the causative toxin in scombroid fish poisoning. N Engl J Med *324:*716–720, 1991.
54. Muller GJ, Lamprecht JH, Barnes JM, et al: Scombroid poisoning. S Afr Med J *81:*427–430, 1992.

PUFFER FISH POISONING

55. Torda TA, Sinclair E, Ulyatt DB: Pufferfish (tetrodotoxin) poisoning. Med J Aust *1:*599–602, 1973.
56. Sims JK, Ostman DC: Pufferfish poisoning: Emergency diagnosis and management. Ann Emerg Med *15:*1094–1098, 1986.
57. Mills AR, Passmore R: Pelagic paralysis. Lancet *1:*161–164, 1988.

58. Tibballs J: Severe tetrodotoxic fish poisoning. Anaesth Intensive Care *16*:215–217, 1988.
59. Sun K, Wat J, So P: Pufferfish poisoning. Anaesth Intensive Care *22*:307–308, 1994.

CIGUATERA

60. Gollop JH, Pon EW: Ciguatera: A review. Hawaii Med J *51*:91–99, 1992.
61. Bagnis R, Kuberski T, Laugier S: Clinical observations on 3009 cases of ciguatera in the South Pacific. Am J Trop Med Hyg *28*:1067–1073, 1979.
62. Lewis ND: Disease and development: Ciguatera fish poisoning. Soc Sci Med *23*:983–993, 1986.
63. Lawrence DN, Enriquez MB, Lumish RM, Maceo A: Ciguatera fish poisoning in Miami. JAMA *244*:254, 1980.
64. Gillespie NC, Lewis RJ, Pearn JH, et al: Ciguatera in Australia—occurrence, clinical features, pathophysiology and management. Med J Aust *145*:584, 1986.
65. Lange WR, Snyder FR, Fudala PJ: Travel and ciguatera fish poisoning. Arch Intern Med *152*:2049–2053, 1992.
66. Katz AR, Terrell-Perica S, Sasaki DM. Ciguatera on Kauai. Am J Trop Med Hyg *49*:448–454, 1993.
67. Losacker W: Ciguatera fish poisoning in the Cook Islands. Bull Soc Pathol Exot *85*:447–448, 1992.
68. Lewis RJ, Holmes MJ: Origin and transfer of toxins involved in ciguatera. Comp Biochem Physiol *106C*:615–628, 1993.
69. Chretien JH, Fermaglich J, Garagusi VF: Ciguatera poisoning—presentation as a neurologic disorder. Arch Neurol *38*:783, 1981.
70. Lange WR: Ciguatera fish poisoning. Am Fam Physician *50*:579–584, 1994.
71. Engleberg NC, Morris JG, Lewis J, et al: Ciguatera fish poisoning: A major common source outbreak in the U. S. Virgin Islands. Ann Intern Med *98*:336, 1983.
72. Morris JG, Lewin P, Hargrett N, et al: Clinical features of ciguatera fish poisoning. A study of the disease in the U. S. Virgin Islands. Arch Intern Med *142*:1090, 1982.
73. Palafox NA, Jain LG, Pinano AZ, et al: Successful treatment of ciguatera fish poisoning with intravenous mannitol. JAMA *259*:2740, 1988.
74. Bowman PB: Amitriptyline and ciguatera. Med J Aust *140*:802, 1984.
75. Davis RT, Villar LA: Symptomatic improvement with amitriptyline in ciguatera fish poisoning. Letter. N Engl J Med *315*:65, 1986.

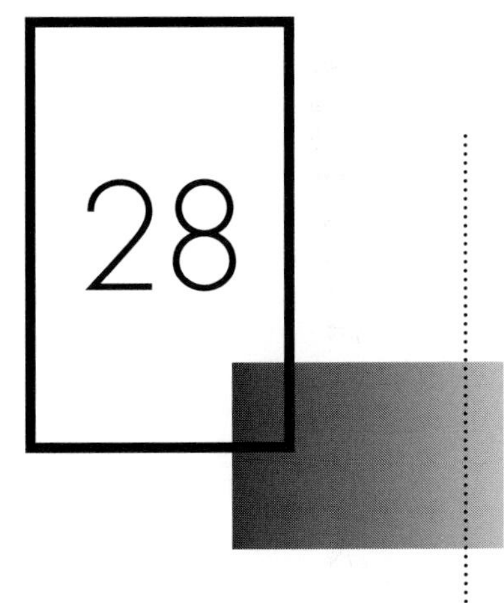

Botulism and Food Poisoning

COREY M. SLOVIS, MD
IAN D. JONES, MD

Many different organisms and toxins are capable of causing food poisoning. This chapter is devoted primarily to food-borne botulism, the most deadly food-related toxicologic disease known. The chapter also contains a review of the other forms of botulism and information on the food-borne toxicologic syndromes of *Clostridium perfringens,* cholera and noncholera vibrios, *Bacillus cereus, Salmonella, Shigella, Campylobacter, Escherichia coli,* and Jamaican vomiting sickness.

BOTULISM

Botulism is probably the best-known rare disease in both the United States and Canada.[1, 2] Botulism is the clinical syndrome that results from the actions of the botulinum toxin, a neurotoxin. The neurotoxins produced by the anaerobic, spore-forming, gram-positive rod *Clostridium botulinum* are the most potent acute toxins known.[2, 3] Despite the toxin's potency, the unique actions of the toxin have made it useful in the treatment of various conditions.[2]

The four distinct forms of botulism are (1) food-borne botulism, (2) infant botulism, (3) wound botulism, and (4) botulism, classification undetermined.[3] Food-borne botulism is the best-known form of botulism. Fortunately, food-borne botulism is rare in the United States, with an average of only 32 cases a year reported in the years 1973 to 1990.[4] It occurs when an individual consumes food contaminated with preformed toxin.[1, 3] Infant botulism, as opposed to classic botulism, occurs when an infant consumes foods contaminated with spores of *C. botulinum.* Disease occurs when the spores germinate and proliferate in an infant's gastrointestinal (GI) tract and produce toxin.[5, 6] Wound botulism is an extremely rare form of the disease; a total of fewer than 100 cases are reported in the literature.[7] It occurs when wounds become contaminated with spores of *C. botulinum,* which germinate and produce toxin that is absorbed systemically.[3] The final category of botulism is classification undetermined. It comprises cases of botulism that occur in patients who are older than 1 year and in whom no obvious food or wound source can be identified.[1, 3]

BACTERIOLOGY

C. botulinum is a ubiquitous organism found in the soil and in marine sediments worldwide. The species is subdivided into seven antigenically distinct serologic types (A to G), which produce disease in either humans or animals.[3, 8] The botulinum toxin is produced after the botulinum spore germinates and begins cell growth. Toxin is released when the mature cell wall lyses.[8] The dormant spores of *C. botulinum* are highly resistant to heating, freezing, aerobic and anaerobic conditions, ionizing radiation, and exposure to various chemical agents. Spores are able to withstand boiling, and temperatures greater than 120°C for at least 30 minutes are required to destroy them.[3, 9] Although spores may remain viable under various harsh conditions, germination requires the presence of a number of factors: the organic acids alanine or cysteine, lactate or bicarbonate, a pH of 4.6 to 7.0, and a temperature between 4 and 70°C.[2, 8] An alkaline medium prevents spore germination.[10] Once germination occurs, continued organism growth requires even more specific conditions, which include the presence of nine amino acids, three vitamins, an anaerobic environment, a low redox state, a neutral pH, and a temperature in the range of 15 to 45°C.[3] Not all types of botulism are so fastidious; growth of E-type organisms has been reported at temperatures as low as 3°C and in nonanaerobic environments.[3]

THE BOTULINUM TOXIN

The botulinum toxin is the most powerful and lethal toxin known, and the lethal dose is as small as 0.5 μg.[1] Although botulinum spores are relatively heat resistant, the toxin itself is heat sensitive.[3] Heating at 80°C for 30 minutes or 100°C for 10 minutes destroys active toxin.[10, 11] Boiling under pressure is required at higher altitudes. If the organism is allowed to mature in a food substance, it synthesizes a protoxin that can be released before and during cell lysis. Ingestion allows the stomach's proteases to cleave portions of the protoxin into the active form, which is then rapidly absorbed in the small bowel. Once the toxin has been absorbed, it spreads via blood and the lymphatic system to nerve terminals and neuronal tissue throughout the body.[9] A three-step process occurs once the toxin arrives at the nerve terminal. In the initial step, the toxin binds to a receptor on the presynaptic nerve terminal. During the second step, the toxin crosses the cell membrane by receptor-mediated endocytosis. The final step occurs when the toxin enters the cell and blocks the release of acetylcholine from the nerve terminal.[2, 3]

The exact mechanism by which botulinum toxin blocks acetylcholine release remains unclear, as does the toxin's exact site of action. The toxin appears to block neurotransmitter release by some form of enzymatic activity after calcium influx at the nerve terminal.[2] The toxin's blockade of acetylcholine occurs at four separate sites: (1) the neuromuscular junction, (2) ganglionic nerve endings, (3) postganglionic parasympathetic nerve endings, and (4) postganglionic sympathetic nerve endings that use acetylcholine.[8] At high toxin concentrations, adrenergic systems may also be affected.[12] The toxin affects only the release of acetylcholine and does not affect acetylcholine's synthesis, storage, or metabolism.[8] Botulinum toxin does not affect impulse conduction down nerves or impulse conduction at nerve terminals.[9, 13]

FOOD-BORNE BOTULISM

Clinical Presentation

Food-borne botulism usually presents within 12 to 48 hours of ingestion of contaminated foods.[2, 14–16] Onset of symptoms may be delayed, however, as long as 14 days after ingestion. Delay in onset of symptoms may make diagnosis difficult, especially in type B botulism, which appears to progress more slowly and be less severe than type A.[14] The initial symptoms of botulism are GI; nausea, vomiting, diarrhea, and abdominal distention are common.[14–17] Abdominal pain and distention and patients' increasing anxiety may falsely suggest the diagnosis of an acute abdomen. As the disease progresses, approximately 70% of patients develop constipation. Although GI complaints are common, they do not occur in approximately one third of patients.[3]

Patients may also present with neurologic symptoms due to cholinergic blockade. Visual disturbances, dysarthria, dysphagia, and dry mouth are the four most specific neurologic symptoms.[3, 15, 16, 18] Additional nonspecific neurologic symptoms associated with botulism include malaise, generalized weakness, headache, dizziness, and paresthesias.[3, 15, 18, 19] As the disease progresses, oculobulbar signs, descending paralysis, and progressive respiratory weakness often leading to respiratory failure evolve.

Oculobulbar symptoms are exceedingly common findings in botulism.[3, 17, 20] Blurring of vision, lateral rectus palsy, ptosis, dilated pupils, and external ophthalmoplegia occur in most patients who develop neurologic symptoms.[15, 18, 19] Fixed or dilated pupils are seen in almost half the patients who present in botulism epidemics. Sixth nerve palsy and accommodative paresis are frequent early ophthalmic signs of botulism.[19, 20] Third nerve palsy, if seen, may indicate a higher likelihood of respiratory failure and the need for mechanical ventilation.[19, 20] Because botulism is so rare and is associated with nonspecific symptoms, the Centers for Disease Control (CDC)[3] and others[18] have suggested various constellations of signs and symptoms to help clinicians consider the diagnosis of botulism early in its presentation (Table 28–1).

Most patients in whom disease is suspected are found not to have botulism, and as many as half these patients with suspected cases either have no illness or receive no final diagnosis.[3] The disease is most commonly confused with Guillain-Barré syndrome. Approximately 10.5% of persons with suspected cases of botulism reported to the CDC are ultimately diagnosed as having Gullain-Barré syndrome. Other diseases commonly confused with botulism include carbon monoxide poisoning (3.4% of reported cases of botulism), food poisoning of unknown etiology, (3.2%), and food poisoning due to staphylococcal organisms (3.0%).[3] Table 28–2 presents a comprehensive list of the diseases cited in the differential diagnosis of botulism.[1–3] Physicians should always consider botulism whenever a patient presents with weakness of any kind such as generalized, ocular, or oropharyngeal.

Diagnosis

When botulism is clinically suspected, a definite diagnosis is best made by confirming the presence of botulinum toxin in the patient's serum.[3] Unfortunately, only one third of patients with botulism are found to have the toxin in their serum. False-negative results are especially common when a patient's serum is examined late in the course of illness.[3] Examination of the stool and gastric aspirate for preformed toxin and botulinum organisms may be very helpful in the early diagnosis of botulism. Postmortem diagnosis may be aided by detecting toxin or organisms in autopsy specimens of the small intestines, large intestines, or liver.[12] When both stool and serum testing are used, the diagnosis of botulism may be confirmed by the laboratory in approximately 75% of the cases. Stool should be obtained without the use of enemas and before institution of antibiotic therapy.[3]

In the absence of positive diagnostic test results, diagnosis of botulism may be difficult. Epidemiologic association with confirmed cases, along with laboratory findings of preformed toxin or organisms in food ingested by the affected patient, is supportive evidence of the diagnosis.[3] An electromyogram (EMG) may also be useful in correctly differentiating botulism from myasthenia gravis, Guillain-Barré syndrome, and Eaton-Lambert syndrome.

The EMG of a patient suffering from botulism shows a decrease in the evoked action potential at slow-frequency stimulation (2 Hz/s), whereas at rapid stimulation (50 Hz/s) an increase is noted in the evoked action potential.[21] Post-tetanic potentiation may also be observed with repetitive high-frequency stimulation.[21] The EMG findings in myasthenia gravis show decreased evoked muscle responses at both slow and fast stimulation, and these EMG findings improve with the use of edrophonium chloride.[21] A decrease in evoked potential is usually noted as the muscle is repetitively stimulated, the opposite of what is found in botulism.[21] The EMG findings in a patient who has Eaton-Lambert syndrome are very similar to those in a patient suffering from botulism.[21, 22] EMG findings for botulism, however, are very dissimilar between different muscle groups and evolve over time, whereas EMG findings between different muscles for Eaton-Lambert syndrome are very similar and stay relatively stable over time. EMG findings for Guillain-Barré usually show patchy slowing, which is indicative of demyelination.

EMG findings alone should never be used to differentiate any disease from botulism, because (1) as many as 15% of patients with botulism may have normal findings on EMG and (2) improvement with edrophonium may be noted in as many as 25% of patients with proven cases of botulism, and low-frequency findings supportive of myasthenia gravis may be observed in as many as 20% of patients who suffer from botulism.[14]

In summary, the diagnosis of botulism may be difficult to make on a patient's initial presentation. The common presenting symptoms (see Table 28–1), the keys for differential diagnosis (see Table 28–2), and a patient's EMG findings should be helpful. Until

Table 28–1. Most Common Presentations of Food-Borne Botulism

Presenting complaints	Dry mouth and/or dysphagia Abdominal symptoms
Initial appearance	Anxious Normal mental status Weak
Medical history	Previously well
Vital signs	Afebrile Slow or normal pulse
Physical examination	Dysphonia Dysarthria Symmetric ocular weakness Symmetric neurologic abnormalities

Table 28–2. Differential Diagnosis in Botulism

Disease or Condition	Differential Manifestations
Neurologic Diseases	
Guillain-Barre syndrome	Usually ascending paralysis Elevated CSF protein Paresthesias Preceding viral illness common Absent deep tendon reflexes
Myasthenia gravis	Lack of autonomic findings Increased fatigability Improvement with edrophonium EMG findings
Eaton-Lambert syndrome	Underlying malignancy, especially oat cell carcinoma Progression much slower Predominant thigh and pelvic muscle involvement Extraocular muscle involvement rare Pupillary findings almost never present EMG findings
Cerebrovascular accident	Asymmetric Unilateral Vascular distribution Asymmetric deep tendon reflexes
Biologic Infections and Toxins	
Bacterial food poisons (staphylococcal, clostridial, and so forth)	Rapid onset Gastrointestinal complaints predominate No paralysis No cranial nerve involvement
Diphtheria	Pseudomembrane Pharyngitis Schick's test Limb paralysis occurs weeks after cranial nerve involvement
Poliomyelitis	Fever Meningeal signs Crampy muscle pain Asymmetric distribution CSF may show encephalitis pattern
Tick paralysis	More common in children Tick(s) found on physical examination Paralysis usually ascending Deep tendon reflexes may be absent
Encephalitis	Altered mental status Fever Meningeal signs Abnormal CSF
Saxitoxin	Symptoms within 1 hour of fish ingestion
Trichinosis	Paresthesias of face predominate Tachycardia Vertigo Fever
Amanita	Myositis Periorbital edema Eosinophilia
Tetanus	Coma Violent vomiting Hepatic failure Trismus Risus sardonicus Neck and jaw stiffness Muscle spasms
Poisoning and Overdose	
Phenothiazine reaction	Spastic muscle contractures Resolution with antihistamines
Carbon monoxide poisoning	Headache Altered mental status Elevated carbon monoxide level
Organophosphate overdose	Fasciculations Cholinergic symptoms Resolution with atropine
Anticholinergic poisoning	Fever Altered mental status Tachycardia and vasodilation No cranial nerve involvement Medication history
Aminoglycoside-induced paralysis	Postanesthesia History of renal impairment Serum levels Exposure history
Heavy metal exposure	Rapidity of onset Serum or urine levels Medication history
Hypermagnesemia	Renal impairment Serum magnesium level
Medical Conditions and Emergencies	
Acute myocardial infarction Appendicitis Bowel obstruction Bowel infarction	Classic signs and symptoms should evolve over time
Acute intermittent porphyria	History or family history Cranial nerve involvement rare Prior psychiatric or CNS complaints Urinary test abnormalities
Carcinomatous invasion of the base of the skull	Cranial nerves V and VIII involvement only Meningeal signs and symptoms
Hysteria	Variable, inconsistent findings No objective findings
Sepsis	Fever Leukocytosis Localized sites of infection Abnormal CSF findings Positive blood cultures

EMG, electromyography; CSF, cerebrospinal fluid; CNS, central nervous system.

absolutely certain of another diagnosis, the physician should always consider botulism in the differential diagnosis of any patient who presents with a neurologic or neuromuscular complaint.

Epidemiology and Types of Botulism

Toxin types A, B, and E account for almost all cases of human botulism.[3, 10] Types F and G are very rare in humans, although type G has been implicated in the sudden deaths of one cluster of five patients.[10] Toxin types C and D are associated with botulism in mammalian animals and birds.[10] Between 1975 and 1988, 48% of cases reported to the CDC were caused by type A toxin.[23] In that same period, types B and E were responsible for 29% and 23% of cases, respectively.[23] Geographic distribution of spore types parallels the toxin type identified in outbreaks. In the western United States, type A spores predominate in the soil and the majority of disease is due to type A toxin.[3, 12] Type B spores predominate in the central and eastern United States, and the majority of cases in these areas are due to type B toxin.[3, 12] Type E spores are less ubiquitous but are most commonly found in damp locations including sediments around the Great Lakes and the coasts of Washington and Alaska. These coastal areas are the same locations where type E botulism occurs.

Food Types

The name *botulism* originally comes from the Latin word *botulus,* meaning "sausage." Improperly prepared blood sausage was first implicated in causing the disease in the late 18th century. The organism was first reported to be associated with the disease in 1897 after it was isolated from uncooked ham after an outbreak of 23 cases at a music club in Belgium. Although poorly preserved meat was the cause of most cases of botulism in the past, most present-day cases of types A and B botulism in the United States result from improper home canning of vegetables. Home-canned asparagus, green beans, and peppers account for most outbreaks in the United States.[24] In certain parts of the world, meat and fish are responsible for the majority of cases. In Poland, for example, meats were the most commonly implicated food source in more than 1000 outbreaks reported during a 3-year period.[12] The majority of recent cases of botulism in the United States have involved only one or two people.[3, 11] Although restaurant-acquired botulism accounts for only 4% of the total number of outbreaks, restaurant-associated outbreaks account for 40% of the total number of cases of botulism.[11] The largest outbreak in the United States involved 59 people and occurred because of improper home canning of jalapeño peppers for a restaurant hot sauce.[17] Before making the hot sauce, many of the home-canned jars exploded on the restaurant's shelves. Unfortunately, the contaminated but yet unexploded portions were used in the hot sauce.

Although poor home canning or food preparation techniques cause most cases, several large outbreaks have been caused by onions and potatoes that were left at warm temperatures for more than 12 hours in incubator-like conditions.[11, 18, 25] Either insufficient heating to kill the spores or introduction of spores to the food after cooking led to proliferation of the organism with subsequent toxin production. Anaerobic conditions may exist especially if the food is immersed in a liquid or is covered. The onions, which were immersed in butter, were used in patty melt sandwiches and resulted in 28 cases.[11, 18] The potatoes were wrapped in aluminum foil and later used in potato salad and caused 34 cases.[25] A similar incubation process has been implicated in other outbreaks involving beef and chicken pot pies, turkey loaf, and beef stew, all of which were kept warm and left to stand for longer than 12 hours without reheating.[11, 24, 26]

Cases of type E botulinum food poisoning result from either poor vacuum packing or improper home preparation or preservation techniques.[27] Common foods in the Inuit Eskimo communities are urraq (uncooked seal flipper in seal oil), muktuk (chunks of white whale skin, blubber, and meat), and fermented salmon eggs; these foods allow growth of the botulinum organism when left to ferment at room temperature because the foods are low in carbohydrates and thus do not become acidic.[27] The largest outbreak of type E botulism to date recently occurred in Egypt and involved at least 91 people. It resulted from the consumption of faseikh, which is a traditional ungutted, salted fish that was placed in a barrel and kept in a warm environment.[4] Additional outbreaks have involved consumption of kapchunka, another uneviscerated salted fish. Conditions present in the fish intestines during preservation allowed for type E spores to proliferate in both of these situations.[28]

Treatment

The treatment of botulism requires early and aggressive stabilization with meticulous attention to airway and ventilatory status. Most early deaths result from respiratory failure before a patient has presented for health care or from the failure of health care workers to recognize early signs of respiratory impairment once a patient has presented.[18, 29]

If the diagnosis of botulism is suspected, patients should have their ABC's secured—that is, their airway patency, ability to breathe, and cardiovascular status should be rapidly assessed and stabilized. Patients should be placed in a well-observed treatment area on an electrocardiogram monitor and should have continuous pulse oximetry monitoring. An intravenous line should be established, and equipment necessary for intubation should be available nearby. Patients suspected of having botulism should be carefully and calmly interviewed. They should be asked if any of their family or friends have similar symptoms. Although any food ingested during the prior 8 days could possibly cause botulism, food consumption during the past 2 to 3 days is of most importance. Patients should be asked if they have eaten any home-canned foods, eaten in a restaurant, or eaten any unusually prepared meats.

Pulmonary function tests are required for all patients with suspected botulism.[30] Although arterial blood gas measurements may be helpful in the complete assessment of any patient, they are not helpful in predicting a declining respiratory reserve.[29, 31] Hypercarbia due to respiratory muscle weakness usually develops very late in the course of botulism, just before respiratory arrest.[29] In an effort to predict those patients who will experience a declining ventilatory status, vital capacity and forced inspiratory volume should be measured regularly at 2- to 4-hour intervals. In one study, all adult patients with a vital capacity less than one third that predicted eventually required mechanical ventilation.[29] Elective intubation before respiratory arrest dramatically decreases the mortality in botulism.[15]

After a patient's ventilatory status has been assessed, assuming mechanical ventilation is not required, the next step is to call the state health department consultant.[30] The CDC maintains a 24-hour telephone number to provide callers with their state's on-call consultant (404-639-2888). This telephone number provides 24-hour access to consultation regarding suspected cases of botulism. Information is also provided about the nearest location for obtaining the antitoxin, which is usually at or near regional airports and quarantine stations. After the state health officer is notified, serum and stool samples should be obtained for processing by the CDC.[30] These samples should be kept refrigerated but not frozen.[3] It is preferable to obtain serum before antibiotic administration and to obtain the stool sample spontaneously rather than after an enema.[3] If this cannot be accomplished, it should be appropriately noted on the specimen label.

Because botulism has anticholinergic effects, unabsorbed toxin-containing food may still be present in a patient's stomach or lower GI tract. Upper and lower gastric decontamination with an orogastric tube and high enemas should be performed. The efficacy of an oral gut lavage solution in suspected cases of botulism is yet to be evaluated. After gastric decontamination has been performed, patients should be admitted to a monitored area where close observation is possible.

In all but asymptomatic patients, a trivalent (A, B, E) antitoxin should be administered. Very few studies have critically evaluated the efficacy of antitoxin.[3, 11, 29, 32] Hypersensitivity reactions occur in approximately 1 in 10 patients treated with the horse serum–prepared antitoxin.[34] More than half of these reactions are nonfatal acute hypersensitivity reactions ranging from urticaria to true anaphylaxis; the remainder are delayed serum sickness–type hypersensitivity reactions.[34] Skin testing before treatment does not reliably distinguish those patients who will or will not have immediate or delayed allergic reaction.[33] Serum sickness is more likely to occur in patients treated with more than four vials (40 mL) of the trivalent antitoxin.[34] Because of the incidence of side effects and the fact that not all patients who have eaten the same foods develop botulism, physicians must use their judgment in administering the antitoxin to asymptomatic patients. It is probably most prudent to monitor patients closely and to give the toxin only if some GI symptoms, neurologic complaints, or cranial nerve findings develop.

Once a patient has been stabilized in an intensive care unit, numerous telephone calls should be made to alert all neighboring emergency departments.[16] Similarly, local and state health departments should be mobilized, and in proven cases or epidemics, the media should be used to help to alert any potential victims.

The mortality for botulism has declined dramatically during the past 40 years, from more than 60% to between 5% and 15%.[3, 11, 15, 29] There are many reasons for this, including more widespread media coverage, more aggressive early care, availability of an antitoxin, and accumulated intensive care expertise by physicians. Botulism cases should be cared for by experts in ventilator management and intensive care medicine. In recent reports, almost all in-hospital deaths have been due to pulmonary and ventilator-related complications.[15, 29, 36]

Severity of disease appears to be related to the type of toxin. Cases of type A botulism have had a significantly higher incidence of respiratory failure requiring intubation and mechanical ventilation than have cases of types B and E.[11, 15, 23] Type E botulism has the lowest incidence of intubation but has a shorter incubation period; almost all individuals have symptoms within 24 hours of ingestion.[23] Type B is intermediate in severity between types A and type E and has the longest incubation period.

Recovery from botulism may be delayed for months.[21] Patients are often weak and tire easily for as long as a year after the acute phase of their disease. Guanidine has been used to increase nonrespiratory muscle strength but has many side effects.[1] This agent may be helpful for selected patients but is not believed to be curative.[3, 25, 29] A vaccine developed from a recombinant fragment of *C. botulinum* neurotoxin serotype A has protected mice against intraperitoneal doses of toxin 10 million times the normal lethal dose.[33]

Infant Botulism

Infant botulism, first reported in 1976, is now by far the most common form of botulism in the United States. In one 12-year period, 57 cases were reported at the Children's Hospital of Pennsylvania alone.[6] Infant botulism has also been implicated as a possible occult cause of the sudden infant death syndrome. Two nonbotulinum *Clostridium* organisms, *C. butyri-*

cum and *C. barati,* have been shown to cause infant botulism by elaboration of botulism toxins type E and F, respectively.[35, 36] At present, more than 1000 cases of infant botulism have been reported to the CDC.[6]

Unlike classic adult botulism, which results from ingestion of preformed toxin, infant botulism is due to *in vivo* germination of botulism spores with concomitant toxin production. The human colon is believed to be the site of bacterial colonization, and symptoms occur when released toxin is absorbed from the gut.[5] Botulism spores do not germinate in the presence of high acidity, a complex mix of aerobic and anaerobic bacteria, or a mature GI immune system.[37] Infants are at risk until about 4 to 6 months of age because of the unique characteristics of their GI tract, including a more alkaline gastric environment, a paucity of normal flora, and a lack of mature mucosal immunologic defenses including lysozyme, complement, and secretory IgA.[37, 38, 40] In infants, the median age at presentation is generally 2 to 4 months, and cases of infant botulism after 6 months of age are very uncommon.

Breast-feeding remains a controversial risk factor in the development of infant botulism. A study has shown that before 2 months of age, there is no significant difference between the number of breast-fed and formula-fed infants diagnosed with the disease.[39] The severity of disease in formula-fed infants younger than 2 months appears to be greater, however, and more formula-fed infants require intubation. In infants older than 2 months, those who have been breast-fed have a significantly higher chance of being diagnosed with infant botulism. The true reason for this is unclear, but it has been hypothesized that breast milk confers some degree of immunity and that formula-fed infants older than 2 months may be dying before presenting for medical attention.[5, 39] Other risk factors for infant botulism include residence in regions that have a high soil load of botulism spores. The high spore load in local soils of California, Utah, and Pennsylvania parallels the frequency of disease, and more than half of the reported cases of infant botulism come from these regions.[5] Additional risk factors for infant botulism include alkaline soil, nearby construction, high dust counts, and ingestion of corn syrup or honey.[39, 40] Natural honey is one of the causes of infant botulism. As many as 25% of samples have botulism spores. The CDC recommends that natural honey not be given to children younger than 12 months.[39]

The symptoms of infant botulism are well described.[5, 38, 39] The syndrome usually begins with constipation in infants 6 weeks to 6 months in age.[3] Constipation may precede other symptoms by weeks.[5] Numerous nonspecific symptoms then develop, including weakness or hypotonia, poor feeding, lethargy, irritability, and weakened cry.[5, 38, 39] Parents may report that the baby has been floppy.[38] Infants may not present, however, until the more severe signs and symptoms of ptosis, impaired gag reflex, generalized hypotonia, absent deep tendon reflexes, and respiratory distress are present. Respiratory distress is usually a late finding, but clinicians should be aware that symptoms and rates of progression vary widely. Rapid progression leading to death may take only hours in some cases.[5] A significant percentage of affected infants ultimately require intubation and mechanical ventilation.[5, 6] Atelectasis, the syndrome of inappropriate secretion of antidiuretic hormone, autonomic instability, apnea, and urinary tract infections are fairly common complications of infant botulism.[5, 6, 39] Symptoms are usually most pronounced between 2 and 3 weeks into the disease and, like classic food-borne botulism, may take several months to resolve.[5, 6]

The diagnosis of infant botulism should initially be based on the aforementioned clinical symptoms. Assays for toxin in the serum rarely yield positive results in infant serum samples, and a definitive diagnosis may be confirmed by isolation of toxin or organisms from the stool.[3] EMG may be a helpful test and may reveal brief small abundant motor unit action potentials.[5] Normal EMG findings do not rule out the disease.

The mortality for infant botulism is very low as long as health care is obtained and the diagnosis is made before the development of respiratory insufficiency. Overall mortality rates have been estimated to be less than 5%. Of note, no deaths were reported in 57 cases during a 12-year period at the Children's Hospital of Pennsylvania.[5, 6] Care is mainly supportive and centers on close attention paid to respiratory and nutritional status and careful observation for complications. Anticlostridial antibiotics such as penicillin have not been shown to be of benefit, and aminoglycoside antibiotics are contraindicated because they may potentiate neuromuscular blockade.[5, 39] Trivalent antitoxin has no role, because only very low levels of circulating toxin are found in the serum and antitoxin has numerous side effects.[39] Clinical trials are currently under way to evaluate the efficacy of human-derived botulism immunoglobulin, which would be considerably safer than horse serum–derived antitoxin.

Wound Botulism

Wound botulism is a very rare form of botulism; fewer than 100 cases are reported in the literature. First reported in 1951, it presents exactly like classic food-borne botulism, with only few exceptions: Nausea, vomiting, and other GI complaints are much less common; fever may occur occasionally; and the incubation period is longer (4 to 18 days).[7, 41] A diagnosis relies on clinical symptoms of botulism with no history suggestive of food-borne illness and a positive history of some form of trauma. Laboratory findings that confirm the diagnosis include isolation of the toxin from the wound or serum, culture of the organism from the wound, or both. Serotypes A and B of *C. botulinum* are the two types so far reported in wound botulism.[7] Mortality has been reported to be 10%.[7, 41]

Although often thought of as being caused by dirty wounds, wound botulism has been reported postoperatively in surgical incisions as well as in various other clean wounds.[41] It is most common in wounds due to direct trauma or as a result of inoculation of subcutaneous tissues in intravenous drug abusers.[41, 42] Wound botulism has also occurred in one case of a tooth abscess and in at least two cases of sinusitis secondary to intranasal cocaine abuse.[42, 43] A significant number of cases of wound botulism due to both intravenous and subcutaneous (skin popping) injection of black tar heroin have been seen. In California, 19 cases of wound botulism due to black tar heroin were reported in the first 11 months of 1995 alone.[44] The majority of patients who develop wound botulism are young to middle-aged adults, although several cases in children younger than 8 years have been reported.[41]

Wound botulism should be suspected in any postoperative or wounded patient who develops any of the signs or symptoms of botulism. It should also be suspected in patients who develop unexplained weakness or declining respiratory effort, especially if they have received treatment with aminoglycosides. The management of suspected wound botulism is debridement and drainage of the wound with both aerobic and anaerobic cultures of wound material. Even minor-appearing wounds should be thoroughly debrided.[41]

Patients suspected of having wound botulism should be admitted to an intensive care unit, with close monitoring of respiratory status and early intubation and mechanical ventilation if needed. Blood should be cultured and serum sent for botulinum toxin analysis because trivalent antitoxin should be administered as soon as possible, as antitoxin is ineffective once the toxin has bound to the nerve terminal.[7, 41] Along with antitoxin, patients should receive tetanus prophylaxis.

Antibiotic therapy has not yet been proved to be efficacious in treating wound botulism, most likely because of the minimal delivery of drug to hypoperfused anaerobic wound sites where *C. botulinum* organisms proliferate.[41, 42] Intravenous anticlostridial antibiotic therapy in the form of high-dose penicillin is controversial in proven cases of wound botulism. Penicillin along with other broad-spectrum antibiotics is appropriate, however, until a definitive diagnosis can be made.[41] Aminoglycoside antibiotics, which may enhance neuromuscular blockade, should be avoided in all suspected cases.

Wound botulism has been reported with increasing frequency since the early 1980s, especially in intravenous drug abusers. A number of these patients have not had prominent skin infections but presented because of cranial nerve dysfunction. Patients with suspected wound botulism should undergo careful skin examinations and should have both wound material and serum cultured and analyzed for the presence of the organism and the toxin, respectively.

Botulism, Classification Undetermined

A fourth form of botulism, classification undetermined, was established by the CDC in 1978.[3] By definition, patients in this group must be older than 1 year and no foodstuff or wound can be suspected as the source of their disease. It is possible that patients in this group may represent an adult variant of infant botulism. Evidence suggests that in certain cases of adult botulism, *in vivo* toxin production may occur.[45] In a significant number of cases of botulism, viable organisms are cultured from the stool. In one case, toxin was detected in the serum of an individual 47 days after ingestion of the suspected food, which was contaminated with organisms but did not test positive for preformed toxin.[45] This suggests continued production of toxin by organisms colonizing the gut. In another case, organisms were cultured from the stool 119 days after the onset of illness.[45] Predisposing risk factors for this variant of infant botulism in adults have included the lack of normal GI barrier mechanisms including intestinal surgery, gastric achlorhydria, and prior antibiotic therapy.[45]

ADDITIONAL SELECTED FOOD-RELATED TOXINS (Table 28–3)

Staphylococcal Food Poisoning

Staphylococcal food poisoning is one of the most common causes of food poisoning in the United States.[46] Seven distinct, preformed, heat-stable enterotoxins are known to exist.[47] The vast majority of cases of staphylococcal food poisoning are attributed to enterotoxins produced by *Staphylococcus aureus,* but one study of a large outbreak in California and Nevada has implicated enterotoxin-producing *S. intermedius.*[48] *S. hyicus* and several coagulase-negative staphlococci are also known to produce enterotoxin but have not yet been proved to cause human disease.[48]

S. aureus grows and produces enterotoxin under a wide variety of conditions. Optimum temperature for bacterial growth is 35 to 40°C, but the organism can grow and produce toxin at temperatures between 3 and 60°C.[46, 49] Various protein-rich foodstuffs are associated with staphylococcal food poisoning, including ham and other pork products, meats, poultry, fish, and shellfish. Milk and other dairy products, eggs, potato salad, and desserts containing cream or custard filling are also commonly implicated.[46, 49, 50] Improper food handling is the cause of most outbreaks.

Humans are the natural reservoir for *S. aureus.* Studies show that between 20% and 50% of healthy individuals are asymptomatic carriers.[51] Of these, between 12% and 50% carry enterotoxigenic strains.[51] Contamination with enterotoxin occurs when food that is mishandled and comes into contact with con-

Table 28–3. Most Common Sources and Incubation Periods of Selected Food Toxins

Disease	Incubation Period	Source of Toxins
Botulism		
Types A and B	1–2 d	Home-canned, low-acidity vegetables (asparagus, green beans, peppers)
Type E	1–2 d	Fermented fish and fish products (seal meat, whale meat, salmon eggs)
Bacillus cereus		
Emetic type	1–6 h	Fried rice
Diarrheal type	12–16 h	Reheated meats
Cholera and other vibrios	12–14 h	Raw shellfish (especially oysters and crabs)
Clostridium perfringens	12–24 h	Meats and poultry, meat stew
Staphylococcus aureus	1–6 h	Foods stored at room temperature (ham, meats, potato and egg salads, and baked goods with cream fillings), milk, meats, and poultry
Shigella	24–48 h	Fecal-oral, contaminated water
Campylobacter	24–48 h	Fecal-oral, unpasteurized milk, meat and poultry
E. coli 0157:H7	1–14 d	Raw or undercooked ground beef
Jamaican vomiting sickness	1–3 h	Unripe akee fruit
Salmonella	5–72 h	Fecal-oral, raw eggs, unpasteurized foods

taminated food handlers or equipment is stored at temperatures at which *S. aureus* can grow. Data show that consumption of as little 1 ng of enterotoxin may produce symptoms of food poisoning.[51]

The molecular mechanism by which staphylococcal enterotoxin causes food poisoning is not well understood. Evidence in the past several years has shown that staphylococcal enterotoxin acts as a superantigen in systemic infection and stimulates intense cytokine production inducing a toxic shocklike illness. It is not believed, however, that the GI symptoms in staphylococcal food poisoning are related to this mechanism.[52]

The symptoms associated with staphylococcal food poisoning are the classic triad of abdominal pain and nausea, followed by vomiting and often diarrhea.[46, 50] Dehydration, hypotension, and bloody diarrhea can also occur. Symptoms usually present between 2 and 6 hours after ingestion. Most cases of the disease are mild and self-limited. Death, though rare, may affect the elderly and debilitated.[46, 50]

Clostridium perfringens

C. perfringens food poisoning is another very common, underreported cause of enterotoxin-related food poisoning. The bacterium is known to produce at least 13 distinct toxins and can be classified into five types (types A to E), of which type A is implicated in most food-borne disease.[53]

C. perfringens is an anaerobic spore-forming bacterium that is ubiquitous in the environment and is part of the normal intestinal flora of humans and many other organisms. Only those organisms capable of producing enterotoxin lead to diarrheal disease, however. Elaboration of enterotoxin occurs during spore formation, and at least one study has shown that more than 1000 times more enterotoxin is produced by sporulating organisms than by vegetative cells.[53] The enterotoxin is thought to be a component of the spore coat. Sporulation usually occurs under harsh conditions such as those in the GI tract or in certain high-protein foods such as meats, stews, and gravy that have been stored at room temperature for many hours. Investigation has shown that nonanimal protein sources such as beans, peas, and legumes may also serve as a suitable medium for proliferation of *C. perfringens.*[54] The optimal temperature for sporulation has been shown to be 35 to 40°C.[53] Clostridial enterotoxin is heat labile and is inactivated at temperatures greater than 75°C. The toxin has also been shown to be inactivated by freeze-thawing. Improper food handling is the usual source for many food poisoning outbreaks. Retrospective studies have shown that outbreaks are often associated with institutional settings and banquets where food is often cooked many hours before being served and is not reheated to temperatures high enough to inactivate the toxin.[55–57]

The molecular mechanism by which *C. perfringens* enterotoxin causes disease involves the enterotoxin's binding to a receptor on the intestinal epithelium. This results in the formation of a membrane complex that allows leakage of small molecules such as amino acids and ions.[53] This ultimately leads to death and sloughing of the intestinal epithelium. The resultant fluid losses lead to the diarrheal disease occurring in cases of food poisoning.[53]

Symptoms of *C. perfringens* food poisoning usually develop within 12 to 24 hours of ingestion. Diarrhea and abdominal cramps most commonly occur, nausea occurs occasionally, and rarely, fever, chills, and vomiting.[55–57] Death is rare and more often occurs in elderly debilitated patients. A more serious hemorrhagic enteritis associated with toxins other than enterotoxin has been associated with *C. perfringens* type C in both Germany and New Guinea.[55] Care is generally supportive, with appropriate volume and electrolyte replacement.

Vibrio

Vibrios are halophilic, motile, gram-negative rods endemic to many coastal areas worldwide, including coastal areas of the western and more commonly the southern United States. Thirteen species have the potential to cause human disease. Diseases commonly associated with vibrio infections include gastroenteritis, wound infections, and septicemia.

Vibrio cholerae is still associated with large-scale morbidity and mortality in several parts of the world. Cholera, although historically significant in the United States, now occurs only periodically in small outbreaks usually due to the El Tor strain. More common strains associated with GI illness in the Unites States include non-01 serotype *V. cholerae, V. parahaemolyticus, V. mimicus, V. fluvialis,* and *V. hollisae.*[58, 59] Symptoms usually occur within 24 hours of ingestion of organisms. In the case of cholera, an intense watery diarrhea may develop with profuse fluid losses that may be as great as 1 L/h.[60] Severe cases (cholera gravis) often result in profound dehydration and death if not aggressively treated. Patients have noncrampy rice water–like grayish stools and in some cases develop vomiting.[60] The symptoms of noncholera vibrio-associated gastroenteritis almost always include diarrhea; vomiting, abdominal cramps, and fever are also common.[58] Bloody stool can also occur, and as many as 86% of patients with *V. fluvialis* and 35% with *V. parahaemolyticus*–associated gastroenteritis produced bloody stool.[58]

In addition to gastroenteritis, certain vibrios are capable of causing severe systemic disease. Nearly all of the cases of vibrio-associated GI disease in the United States are a result of ingestion of raw oysters. A particular hazard involves *V. vulnificus* infection in persons with compromised immune systems or liver disease. Individuals who have predisposing liver disease and who consume raw oysters are 80 times more likely to contract disease and 200 times more likely to die of infection with *V. vulnificus* than individuals without liver disease.[61]

The mechanism by which *V. cholerae* causes illness is well understood. Ingested organisms adhere to the intestinal mucosa and secrete an enterotoxin known as the *cholera toxin.* The cholera toxin blocks sodium absorption and enhances secretion of chloride by directly stimulating adenylate cyclase in the gut epithelial cells. A direct product of this is the intense watery diarrhea characteristic of the disease. Noncholera vibrios produce disease by various molecular mechanisms that are beyond the scope of this discussion.

Treatment of gastroenteritis due to both cholera and noncholera vibrio infections is generally supportive. Aggressive oral rehydration or intravenous fluids with isotonic saline, glucose, and electrolyte replacement are required.[60] Administration of drugs that interfere with adenylate cyclase or electrolyte fluxes across gut epithelial cells may significantly decrease volume losses. Chlorpromazine, aspirin, indomethacin, and nicotinic acid all have been shown to be effective in treating cholera.[60]

Bacillus cereus

B. cereus is a relatively common, underreported cause of food poisoning that may mimic staphylococcal, clostridial, or vibrio food-borne illness.[62] *B. cereus* is an aerobic, gram-negative rod that is ubiquitous in the environment and has the capacity to form endospores that are highly resistant to extremes of cold and heat.[63] Illness due to *B. cereus* is via the elaboration of two distinct enterotoxins, a heat-labile diarrheal enterotoxin and a heat-stable emetic enterotoxin. Spores of *B. cereus* are very commonly found in cereals, rice, vegetables, spices, and pasteurized fresh and powdered milk.[63–65] In one study, 70% of ready-to-eat foods tested in different cafeterias around Washington, D.C., were positive for *B. cereus.*[63]

The upper GI or emetic form of the disease has a more rapid onset and shorter clinical course than the diarrheal form. Patients usually become ill within 1 to 6 hours of ingestion and recover within 24 hours.[62] This form of the disease closely resembles staphlococcal food poisoning. Diarrhea and abdominal cramps may occur but are not the prominent feature of the emetic form.

Fried rice is the foodstuff usually associated with the emetic form of *B. cereus* infection, and Chinese food was implicated in 24 of 58 separate outbreaks in the United States between 1973 and 1987.[63] The heat-resistant spores germinate when already cooked rice is left to cool and is unrefrigerated for 2 or more hours.[65] The diarrheal form of *B. cereus* food poisoning is often associated with the consumption of contaminated meats and vegetables.

The emetic form of the disease is caused by a toxin that has been shown to cause vacuole formation and mitochondrial swelling *in vitro* and might also uncouple oxidative phosphorylation.[66]

Because *B. cereus* food poisoning may mimic other forms of food poisoning, diagnosis can be confirmed only by detecting 10^5 organisms per gram of food.[62] Stool examination and culture are generally not useful in aiding in the diagnosis. Treatment is supportive only, and most cases of *B. cereus* food poisoning are mild and self-limited.

Salmonella, Shigella, and *Campylobacter*

Salmonella, Shigella, and *Campylobacter* comprise the most common forms of acute bacterial diarrheal illness in the United States.[67] The three genera are remarkably similar in many ways including source of infection, symptoms of illness, localized invasion of the bowel epithelium, and duration of disease. There are a number of differences between the three, however, and thus they are discussed separately.

Salmonella

Salmonellae are motile, gram-negative rods that are ubiquitous in nature and are known to colonize the intestinal tracts of a wide variety of organisms including mammals, reptiles, and even insects.[68] The organism is resistant to freezing and drying but is rapidly killed by high temperatures. More than 2000 serovars of *Salmonella* have been identified, but the majority of human diarrheal infections are caused by either *S. enteridis* or *S. typhimurium*.[68]

The two most common sources of disease are food or water contaminated with the organism and transmission via the fecal-oral route. Food sources commonly associated with outbreaks include raw or undercooked eggs, unpasteurized milk, and various meats, especially poultry.[68] Homemade eggnog, hollandaise sauce, and caesar salad dressing all have been implicated as causes of *Salmonella* infection.[69] Sources implicated in the fecal-oral route include household dogs and cats and occasionally other infected humans, particularly children in daycare situations.[67] In the past, a number of infections were associated with pet turtles, and these led to a prohibition of their sale in the United States.[67]

Salmonella gastroenteritis has an incubation period of 5 to 72 hours. Symptoms of disease generally last from 2 to 5 days, but in certain cases, an asymptomatic carrier state may persist for as long as a year.[68, 70] Nausea and vomiting are the most common symptoms and are usually followed by low-grade fever, chills, abdominal pain, and diarrhea.[68] The course of the disease is more severe and protracted in the very young, the elderly, and immunocompromised patients. Patients with AIDS and patients with certain hemolytic anemias such as sickle cell anemia are at a much higher risk for developing *Salmonella* bacteremia. Enteric fever, commonly associated with *S. typhi* and *S. paratyphi,* is a more severe form of disease associated with a longer incubation period (1 to 2 weeks), sustained fever, malaise, weakness, fever and chills, diarrhea, bacteremia, and occasionally multiple organ dysfunction.[67, 68]

The diagnosis of *Salmonella* gastroenteritis is based on a patient's history, and confirmation of diagnosis requires stool culture. Microscopic examination of the stool usually reveals leukocytes, and the stool may contain occult blood.

Once ingested, the *Salmonella* bacterium must survive the host defenses including gastric acidity and competition with normal flora. Once past the gastric barrier, the organisms multiply in the small intestine and penetrate the intestinal mucosa, where they proliferate within mesenteric lymphoid tissue.[70] The majority of infections do not spread beyond the local lymphoid tissue. The actual mechanism by which *Salmonella* causes diarrhea is not well understood but may involve local infiltration of polymorphonuclear leukocytes and release of prostaglandins, which increase intestinal fluid secretion.[70] It has been demonstrated that *S. typhimurium* produces a cholera-like enterotoxin, but its role *in vivo* is not clear.[70]

The treatment in most cases is supportive, with fluid and electrolyte replacement as needed. Antibiotics are not recommended in uncomplicated cases because they do not alter the severity of disease and may prolong the carrier state. Antibiotics are reserved for more serious cases such as enteric fever, focal infections, or bacteremia.[67, 68] Antimotility agents, which slow intestinal transport times, may lead to intestinal perforation and are not recommended in cases of invasive diarrheas such as salmonellosis.

Shigella

Members of the genus *Shigella* are small, nonmotile, gram-negative rods that are very similar morphologically and biochemically to *E. coli.* Four different species are associated with human infection: *S. dysenteriae, S. flexneri, S. sonnei,* and *S. boydii. S. sonnei* and *S. flexneri* are responsible for the bulk of cases in the United States.[70, 71] A more severe form of infection, bacillary dysentery, is often associated with *S. dysenteriae* infection. The organism has a very low infectious dose, and disease can develop in some volunteers fed as few as 100 organisms.[71]

The fecal-oral route is the primary mode of transmitting *Shigella* infection. Humans and monkeys are the only known natural hosts for *Shigella* bacilli.[71] The majority of infections are spread by consumption of food or water contaminated with fecal material from an infected individual. *Shigella* infections commonly occur in daycare centers, mental institutions, prisons, and nursing homes, where overcrowding, poor hygiene, and unsanitary conditions may exist.[67, 71] Of interest, a significant percentage of troops in operation Desert Shield who developed diarrhea were found to have enteric pathogens in their stool.[72] Of this group, 26% yielded cultures for *Shigella* species.[72] Outbreaks have been associated with various contaminated foods, and reports indicate that *Shigella* can live for many days on certain foods outside of its normal human host.

The incubation period in shigellosis is usually 24 to 48 hours. The clinical presentation has a wide spectrum, some individuals have nonspecific symptoms and a short course of watery diarrhea only.[67, 71] More severe forms of the disease may progress to true dysentery, including high fever, tenesmus, nausea, abdominal pain, and profuse watery diarrhea that evolves over hours to a few days to mucoid, bloody stools.[67, 71] Untreated shigellosis is usually self-limited, and the illness usually persists for 1 week. An individual may continue to shed organisms in the stool for several weeks after clinical infection subsides. As with salmonellosis, a diagnosis of shigellosis is made primarily by history and is confirmed with stool culture. Laboratory findings may include leukocytosis and the presence of fecal leukocytes in addition to occult or grossly bloody stool. Complications include seizures (especially in children), dehydration, and death in the very elderly or in children younger than 1 year.[67, 73]

Shigella organisms possess a high degree of acid resistance and as such are able to survive passage through the acidic gastric barrier quite well.[74] Once ingested, the organisms invade the epithelial lining of the intestine, multiply intracellularly, and spread to surrounding cells. Local damage to intestinal epithelium and superficial erosion of the intestinal mucosa are responsible for the clinical picture.[70] A number of separate gene products are responsible for the virulence of *Shigella,* including the Shiga toxin and other Shiga-like toxins. These toxins, similar to those of enterotoxigenic *E. coli* (ETEC), are cytotoxic and are known to inhibit protein synthesis in infected cells.

Treatment for shigellosis is initially supportive, with attention to correcting fluid and electrolyte abnormalities. Antibiotic therapy has been shown to improve the clinical course of the disease, but patients are often already improving when culture results become available. Antibiotics are therefore reserved for patients who are not showing signs of improvement or who have more severe forms of infection. All individuals who have culture-proven *S. dysenteriae* or those with other species who are high risk of infecting others should receive antibiotics. As in the case of *Salmonella, Shigella* infection is an invasive enteritis, and as such, antimotility agents are not recommended. Recommendations for children in daycare centers with culture-proven *Shigella* require antibiotic therapy and repeat negative follow-up cultures before returning to daycare.[67]

Campylobacter

Campylobacter species are small, motile, curved or S-shaped, gram-negative bacteria. *Campylobacter* enteritis is today one of the most commonly identified bacterial causes of diarrhea. Human disease is most commonly caused by *Campylobacter jejuni,* which is a part of the normal flora of a wide variety of animals including cattle, sheep, pigs, and poultry.[67, 75] Infection has also been traced to household pets including dogs and cats. *Campylobacter* may also be found in unpurified drinking water such as that in rural areas or in contaminated springs.[75] The source of contamination in these cases is usually the feces of wild animals and birds.

The primary mode of transmission of *Campylobacter* is fecal-oral. In addition to infection from contaminated water, various foods are associated with infection. Food may become contaminated with organisms at slaughterhouses whenever improper handling occurs or when intestinal spillage comes into contact with animal carcasses. Contaminated meat and poultry products are commonly associated with infection. Raw milk, often consumed by children during youth activities such as visits to dairy farms, is another common source of *Campylobacter* enteritis.[76] *Campylobacter* does not proliferate on foods that it has contaminated as do other organisms such as *Salmonella* species or *S. aureus.*[75] The organism may actually survive longer if refrigerated and can survive in water or unpasteurized milk for weeks.[75]

Fever, headache, malaise, myalgias, and cramping abdominal pain usually occur in the first 48 hours after ingestion of an infectious dose of organisms.[67, 75, 77] The abdominal pain of *Campylobacter* infection may mimic that of appendicitis. Diarrhea usually presents within 24 hours after the onset of abdominal pain and may be described as watery, bile stained, mucoid, or grossly bloody.[67, 77] Clinical disease usually does not persist for more than a week. Relapse is not uncommon, and the organism may be shed for several weeks in the stools of asymptomatic individuals.

Campylobacter causes disease by invasion of the colonic and small bowel epithelium in a fashion similar to that of *Shigella.* The resultant loss of small and large bowel epithelium produces the clinical picture.

As in the case of *Salmonella* and *Shigella* infection, the diagnosis of *Campylobacter* infection is confirmed by stool culture. A direct microscopic examination of stool stained with either carbolfuchsin or Gram's stain may also be helpful. The characteristic curved, gram-negative rods may be seen in profusion in the stool specimen.[67] Administration of antibiotics shortens the course of infection and decreases the relapse rate and the period of excretion of organisms after infection. The American Academy of Pediatrics Committee on Infectious Disease recommends giving erythromycin to decrease the duration of excretion.[67] GI antimotility agents are not recommended, because *Campylobacter* infection is an invasive enteritis and agents that decrease GI motility may lead to more serious complications including intestinal perforation.

Escherichia coli

E. coli organisms are gram-negative rods that are part of the normal flora of all warm-blooded animals. A number of different pathogenic mechanisms are known to exist. At least four different categories of diarrheal illness producing *E. coli* have been described. Both enterotoxigenic (ETEC) and enteropathogenic *E. coli* (EPEC) produce a noninflammatory form of diarrhea, the former due to enterotoxin release.[79] Enteroinvasive *E. coli* (EIEC) and enterohemorrhagic *E. coli* (EHEC) cause inflammatory diarrheas characterized by either direct invasion or cytotoxic damage to the colonic epithelium.[79] A number of the virulence factors in the preceding categories are encoded on plasmids that express gene products giving the differing serotypes variable degrees and mechanisms of virulence.

Enteropathogenic, enterotoxigenic, and enteroinvasive *E. coli* infections are more common in underdeveloped countries with poorer sanitary conditions than exist in the United States. These infections are often spread through contaminated drinking water or through person-to-person contact. EPEC infection, most commonly affecting children, is characterized by fever, watery diarrhea, and vomiting. ETEC, the common agent in many cases of traveler's diarrhea, is caused by two separate enterotoxins and is characterized by the abrupt onset of watery diarrhea. It usually has a fairly mild clinical picture.[79] A significant number of cases of diarrheal disease in Operation Desert Shield were due to ETEC.[72] EIEC causes disease by invasion of intestinal epithelial cells in a manner similar to that of *Shigella*. As a result of intestinal epithelial invasion, infection may present exactly like shigellosis, with fever, abdominal pain, and watery diarrhea that may progress to true dysentery.[79]

A great deal of attention has recently been paid to the EHEC, specifically *E. coli* serotype 0157:H7. This serotype, first isolated in 1982, has been increasingly reported as a cause of gastroenteritis in the United States.[78, 80] Infection is more common in children, and *E. coli* 0157:H7 accounts for a majority of cases of the hemolytic-uremic syndrome in children.[78] The organism is primarily transmitted by consumption of contaminated raw or undercooked ground beef. Outbreaks have also been associated with milk, cheese, unpasteurized apple cider, other meats, and even swimming pool water.[78]

The spectrum of infection with *E. coli* 0157:H7 may range from asymptomatic infection to a relatively mild case of nonbloody diarrhea only to more severe symptoms with low-grade fever, abdominal cramps, vomiting, and grossly bloody diarrhea. The incubation period ranges from 1 to 14 days, depending on the setting and symptoms, and diarrhea lasts from 6 to 10 days.[78, 79] Death is uncommon but can occur in the very young, the elderly, and persons with underlying disease or immunosuppression. Extraintestinal manifestations are not uncommon and may include neurologic and cardiac abnormalities, thrombotic thrombocytopenic purpura, and the hemolytic-uremic syndrome.[78]

EHEC causes disease not by intestinal epithelial invasion but by the elaboration of two distinct Shiga-like toxins, so named because of their biochemical similarities to the Shiga toxin.[78] These toxins are cytotoxic and are known to inhibit protein synthesis in mammalian cells. Toxin-induced epithelial death results in the clinical picture of hemorrhagic colitis seen in *E. coli* 0157:H7 infection.

The diagnosis of disease caused by E. *coli* 0157:H7 is based on clinical manifestations along with stool culture and detection of Shiga-like toxin. Many laboratories do not routinely screen for *E. coli* 0157:H7 as is done for other organisms such as *Salmonella, Shigella,* and *Campylobacter.* It is therefore important to inquire about laboratory's capability to assay for *E. coli* 0157:H7 and to request this specific screening if necessary. The treatment of *E. coli* 0157:H7 infection is supportive only, with attention to management of fluid and electrolyte imbalances and extraintestinal complications. Antibiotics are not recommended, and it is postulated that antibiotics may actually increase mortality. Antimotility agents are not recommended.

Akee Fruit Poisoning (Jamaican Vomiting Sickness)

Jamaican vomiting sickness is a relatively rare disease characterized by the acute onset of vomiting within 2 to 3 hours of eating a meal. The disease is caused by the ingestion of the unripe akee fruit, a fruit that is not usually available or eaten outside of Jamaica.[81] Seizures, coma, and even death may occur in severe cases.[81, 82]

The aril and seeds of the unripe akee fruit contain the amino acids hypoglycin A and B (L-α-aminomethylene cyclopropionic acid and its γ-glutamyl conjugate, respectively).[81] Hypoglycin A (or hypoglycin) is more potent than hypoglycin B. The amino acids in hypoglycin A and B cause their toxicity by blocking long-chain fatty acid metabolism and subsequent gluconeogenesis at the mitochondrial level.[81, 83] Blockade is accomplished by inhibition of several cofactors including acyl coenzyme A and carnitine.[81] The result is profound hypoglycemia at levels as low as 3 mg/dL.[81, 82] Hypoglycin itself may cause vomiting and central nervous system depression in the absence of significant hypoglycemia. Hepatotoxicity similar to that of Reye's syndrome has been found at postmortem study.[81, 84]

Intravenous glucose and supportive care are the mainstays of therapy in treating Jamaican vomiting sickness. In untreated persons who develop hypoglycemic coma, the mortality may be as high as 80%.

References

1. Sellin LC: Botulism—an update. Mil Med *149:*12–16, 1984.
2. Hambleton P: *Clostridium botulinum* toxins: A general review of involvement disease, structure, mode of action, and preparation for clinical use. J Neurol *239:*16–20, 1992.
3. Centers for Disease Control (CDC): Botulism in the United States, 1899–1977: Handbook for Epidemiologists, Clinicians, and Laboratory Workers. CDC, Washington, DC, pp 1–49, 1979.
4. Webber JT, Tauxe RV, Weber JT, et al: A massive outbreak of type E botulism associated with traditional salted fish in Cairo. J Infect Dis *167:*451–454, 1993.
5. Wiggington JM, Thill P: Infant botulism: A review of the literature. Clin Pediatr *32:*669–674, 1993.
6. Shreiner MS, Field E, Ruddy R: Infant botulism: A review of 12 years experience at The Children's Hospital of Philadelphia. Pediatrics *87:*159–165, 1991.
7. Burningham MD, Walter FG, Crawford M, et al: Wound botulism. Ann Emerg Med *24:*184–187, 1994.
8. Simpson LL: The origin, structure, and pharmacological activity of botulinum toxin. Pharmacol Rev *33:*155–188, 1981.
9. Simpson LL: The action of botulinal toxin. Rev Infect Dis *1:*656–662, 1979.
10. Dowell VR Jr: Botulism and tetanus: Selected epidemiologic and microbiologic aspects. Rev Infect Dis *6*(Suppl 1):202–207, 1984.
11. Macdonald KL, Cohen ML, Blake PA: The changing epidemiology of adult botulism in the United States. Am J Epidemiol *124:*794–799, 1986.
12. Dodds KL: *Clostridium botulinum. In* Hui YH, Gorham JR, Murrell KD, Oliver DO (eds): Foodborne Disease Handbook. New York, Marcel Dekker, pp 97–132, 1994.
13. Sellin LC, Thesleff S, Dasgupta BR: Different affects of types A and B botulinum toxin on transmitter release at the rat neuromuscular junction. Acta Physiol Scand *119:*127–133, 1983.
14. St. Louis ME, Peck SH, Bowering D, et al: Botulism from chopped garlic: Delayed recognition of a major outbreak. Ann Intern Med *108:*363–368, 1988.
15. Hughes JM, Blumenthal JR, Mersom MH, et al: Clinical features of types A and B food-borne botulism. Ann Intern Med *95:*442–445, 1981.

16. Ruthman JC, Hendricksen DK, Bonefield R: Emergency department presentation of type A botulism. Am J Emerg Med *3:*203–205, 1985.
17. Terranova W, Bremen JC, Locey RP, Speck S: Botulism type B: Epidemiologic aspects of an extensive outbreak. Am J Epidemiol *108:*150–156, 1978.
18. MacDonald KL, Spengler RF, Hathaway CL, et al: Type A botulism from sauteed onions: Clinical and epidemiologic observations. JAMA *253:*1275–1278, 1985.
19. Terranova W, Bremen JG, Palumbo JN: Ocular findings in botulism type B. JAMA *241:*475–477, 1979.
20. Simcock PR, Kelleher S, Dunne JA: Neuro-ophthalmic findings in botulism type B. Eye *8:*646–648, 1994.
21. Cherington M: Botulism: Ten-year experience. Arch Neurol *30:*432–437, 1974.
22. Sanders AB, Seifert S, Kobernick M: Botulism: Clinical review. J Fam Pract *16:*987–1000, 1983.
23. Woodruff BA, Hatheway CL, Griffin PM, et al: Clinical and laboratory comparison of botulism from toxin types A, B, and E in the United States, 1975–1988. J Infect Dis *166:*1281–1286, 1992.
24. CDC: Foodborne botulism—Oklahoma, 1994. MMWR Morb Mortal Wkly Rep *44:*200–202, 1995.
25. Mann JM, Martin S, Hoffman R, et al: Patient recovery from type A botulism: Morbidity assessment following a large outbreak. Am J Public Health *71:*266–269, 1981.
26. CDC: Botulism and commercial pot pie—California. MMWR Morb Mortal Wkly Rep *32:*39–40, 45, 1983.
27. Hauschild AHW, Gavreau L: Food-borne botulism in Canada, 1971–84. Can Med Assoc J *133:*1141–1146, 1985.
28. CDC: Fish botulism—Hawaii, 1990. JAMA *266:*324, 327, 1991.
29. Schmidt-Nowara WW, Samet JM, Rosario PA: Early and late pulmonary complications of botulism. Arch Intern Med *143:*451–456, 1983.
30. CDC: Release of botulism antitoxin. MMWR Morb Mortal Wkly Rep *35:*490–491, 1986.
31. Hughes JM, Tackett CO: Sausage poisoning revisited. Editorial. Arch Intern Med *143:*425–427, 1983.
32. Tacket CO, Shandera WX, Mann JM, et al: Equine antitoxin use and other factors that predict outcome in type A foodborne botulism. Am J Med *76:*794–798, 1984.
33. Clayton MA, Clayton JM, Brown DR, Middlebrook JL: Protective vaccination with a recombinant fragment of *Clostridium botulinum* neurotoxin serotype A expressed from a synthetic gene in *Escherichia coli.* Infect Immun *63:*2738–2742, 1995.
34. Black RE, Gunn RA: Hypersensitivity reactions associated with botulinal antitoxin. Am J Med *69:*567–570, 1980.
35. Arnon SS: Infant botulism: Anticipating the second decade. J Infect Dis *154:*201–206, 1986.
36. Aureli P, Fencia L, Pasolini B, et al: Two cases of type E infant botulism caused by neurotoxigenic *Clostridium butyricum* in Italy. J Infect Dis *154:*207–211, 1986.
37. Arnon SS: Breast feeding and toxigenic intestinal infections: Missing links in crib death? Rev Infect Dis *6*(Suppl 1):193–201, 1984.
38. Long SS, Gajewski JL, Brown LW, Gilligan PH: Clinical, laboratory, and environmental features of infant botulism in southeastern Pennsylvania. Pediatrics *75:*935–941, 1985.
39. Schmidt RD, Schmidt TW: Infant botulism: A case series and review of the literature. J Emerg Med *10:*713–718, 1992.
40. Istre GR, Compton R, Novotny T, et al: Infant botulism: Three cases in a small town. Am J Dis Child *140:*1013–1014, 1986.
41. Mechem CC, Walter FG Wound botulism. Vet Hum Toxicol *36:*233–237, 1994.
42. Weber JT, Hewitt C, Taxue RV, et al: Wound botulism in a patient with a tooth abcess: A case report and review. Clin Infect Dis *16:*635–639, 1992.
43. Kudrow DB, Henry DA, Mathisen GE, et al: Botulism associated with *Clostridium botulinum* sinusitis after intranasal cocaine abuse. Ann Intern Med *109:*984–985, 1988.
44. CDC: Wound botulism—California, 1995. MMWR Morb Mortal Wkly Rep *44:*889–892, 1995.
45. McCroskey LM, Hatheway CL: Laboratory findings in four cases of botulism suggest colonization of the intestinal tract. J Clin Microbiol *26:*1052–1054, 1988.
46. Holmberg SD, Blake PA: Staphlococcal food poisoning in the United States: New facts and old misconceptions. JAMA *251:*487–489, 1984.
47. Tranter HS: Foodborne staphlococcal illness. Lancet *336:*1044–1046, 1990.
48. Khambaty FM, Bennett RW, Shah DB: Application of pulsed field gel electrophoresis to the epidemiological characterization of *Staphlococcus intermedius* implicated in a food-related outbreak. Epidemiol Infect *113:*75–81, 1994.
49. CDC: Staphlococcal food poisoning from turkey at a country club buffet—New Mexico. MMWR Morb Mortal Wkly Rep *35:*715–716, 721–722, 1986.
50. Weineke AA, Roberts D, Gilbert JR: Staphlococcal food poisoning in the United Kingdom, 1969–90. Epidemiol Infect *110:*519–531, 1993.
51. Martin SE, Myers ER: *Staphlococcus aureus. In* Hui YH, Gorham JR, Murrell KD, Oliver DO (eds): Foodborne Disease Handbook. New York, Marcel Dekker, pp 345–394, 1994.
52. Cantor H, Crump AL, Glimcher LH, et al: Immunoregulatory effects of superantigens: Interactions of staphylococcal enterotoxins with host MHC and non-MHC products. Immunol Rev *131:*27–39, 1993.
53. McClane B: *Clostridium perfringens* enterotoxin acts by producing small molecule permeability alterations in plasma membranes. Toxicology *87:*43–67, 1994.
54. Roach RL, Sienko D: *Clostridium perfringens* outbreak associated with minestrone soup. Am J Epidemiol *136:*1288–1291, 1992.
55. Shandera WX, Tacket CO, Blacke PA: Food poisoning due to *Clostridium perfringens* in the United States. J Infect Dis *147:*167–170, 1983.
56. Lowenstein MS: Epidemiology of *Clostridium perfringens* food poisoning. N Engl J Med *286:*1026–1028, 1972.
57. Peterson LR, Mshar R, Cooper GH Jr, et al: A large *Clostridium perfringens* foodborne outbreak with an unusual attack rate pattern. Am J Epidemiol *127:*605–611, 1988.
58. Levine WC, Griffin PM: *Vibrio* infections on the Gulf Coast: Results of first year of regional surveillance. J Infect Dis *167:*479–483, 1993.
59. Desenclos JC, Hoecher S, Klontz C, Wolfe LE: The risk of vibrio illness in the Florida raw oyster eating population, 1981–1988. Am J Epidemiol *134:*290–297, 1991.
60. Morris JG, Black RE: Cholera and other vibrioses in the United States. N Engl J Med *312:*343–350, 1985.
61. CDC: *Vibrio vulnificus* infections associated with raw oyster consumption—Florida 1981–1992. MMWR Morb Mortal Wkly Rep *42:*405–407, 1993.
62. Terranova W, Blake PA: *Bacillus cereus* food poisoning. N Engl J Med *298:*143–144, 1978.
63. Schultz FJ, Smith J: *Bacillus:* Recent advances in *Bacillus cereus* food poisoning research. *In* Hui YH, Gorham JR, Murrell KD, Oliver DO (eds): Foodborne Disease Handbook. New York, Marcel Dekker, pp 29–62, 1994.
64. CDC: *Bacillus cereus*—Maine. MMWR Morb Mortal Wkly Rep *35:*408–410, 1986.
65. Blakely LJ, Priest FG: The occurrence of *Bacillus cereus* in some dried foods including pulses and cereals. J Appl Bacteriol *48:*297–302, 1980.
66. Sakurai N, Koike KA, Irie Y, Hayashi H: The rice culture filtrate of *Bacillus cereus* isolated from emetic-type food poisoning causes mitochondrial swelling in a Hep-2 cell. Microbiol Immunol *38:*337–343, 1994.
67. Stutman HR: *Salmonella, Shigella,* and *Campylobacter:* Common causes of infectious diarrhea. Pediatr Ann *23:*538–543, 1994.
68. Baird-Parker AC: Foodborne salmonellosis. Lancet *336:*1231–1235, 1990.
69. CDC: Update: *Salmonella enteritidis* infection and shell eggs—United States 1990. MMWR Morb Mortal Wkly Rep *39:*909–912, 1990.
70. Finlay BB: Molecular and cellular mechanisms of *Salmonella* pathogenesis. Curr Top Microbiol Immunol *192:*163–185, 1994.
71. Maurelli AT, Lampell KA: Shigella. *In* Hui YH, Gorham JR, Murrell KD, Oliver DO (eds): Foodborne Disease Handbook. New York, Marcel Dekker, pp 319–344, 1994.

72. Hyams KC, Bourgeois AL, Merrell BR, et al: Diarrheal disease during operation Desert Shield. N Engl J Med *325:*1423–1425, 1991.
73. Bennish ML, Harris JR, Wojtyniak BJ, et al: Death in shigellosis: Incidence and risk factors in hospitalized patients. J Infect Dis *161:*500–506, 1990.
74. Gorden J, Small PL: Acid resistance in enteric bacteria. Infect Immun *61:*364–367, 1993.
75. Franco DA, Williams CE: *Campylobacter jejuni. In* Foodborne Disease Handbook. New York, Marcel Dekker, pp 71–96, 1994.
76. Wood RC, Macdoward KL, Osterholm KL: Campylobacter enteritis outbreaks associated with drinking raw milk during youth activities: A ten year review of outbreaks in the United States. JAMA *268:*3228–3230, 1992.
77. Blaser MJ, Berkowitz ID, LaForce MF, et al: *Campylobacter* enteritis: Clinical and epidemiologic features. Ann Intern Med *91:*179–185, 1979.
78. Chinyu S, Brandt LJ: *Escherichia coli* 0157:H7 infection in humans. Ann Intern Med *123:*698–713, 1995.
79. Neill MA, Tarr PI, Taylor DN, Trofa AF: *Escherichia coli. In* Hui YH, Gorham JR, Murrell KD, Oliver DO (eds): Foodborne Disease Handbook. New York, Marcel Dekker, pp 169–214, 1994.
80. CDC: *Escherichia coli* 0157:H7 outbreak at a summer camp—Virginia, 1994. JAMA *274:*19–20, 1995.
81. Tanaka K, Kean EA, Johnson B: Jamaican vomiting sickness. N Engl J Med *295:*461–467, 1976.
82. Bressler R: The unripe akee—the forbidden fruit. N Engl J Med *295:*500–501, 1976.
83. Billington D, Osmundsen H, Sherratt HSA: The biochemical basis of Jamaican akee poisoning. N Engl J Med *295:*1482, 1976.
84. Tanaka K, Isselbacher KJ: Isovaleric and methylbutyric acidemias induced by hypoglycin A: Mechanism of Jamaican vomiting sickness. Science *175:*69–71, 1972.

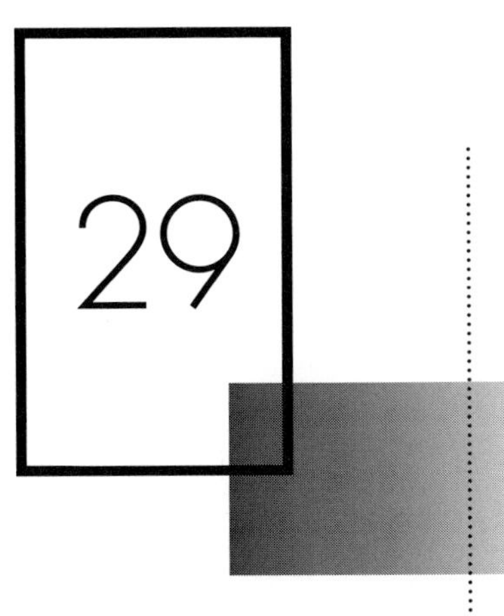

Radiation Poisoning

RICHARD Y. WANG, DO
WILLIAM K. CHIANG, MD

On September 13, 1987, in the town of Goiania, Brazil, a radiation therapy device containing cesium 137 (^{137}Cs) was removed from a clinic and sold to a junkyard as scrap.[1] The object was broken open out of curiosity. Its green luminescent content enthralled all those that gathered. The cesium chloride mass was divided into smaller pieces and distributed among the crowd. Children were attracted by the mass's brilliance and carried it all around town while playing with it; some even ingested the pieces. In a short period of time, significant radiation contamination resulted in many people throughout the town. The accident became known 15 days later, when 22 people arrived ill at the local hospital and were later diagnosed with acute radiation syndrome. All of these patients required intensive care, and 10 were considered in critical condition. These 10 patients were exposed to radiation doses from 3 to 7 Gy (300 to 700 rad). After 5 weeks had passed, 4 patients had died, having received doses between 4.5 and 6 Gy (450 to 600 rad). One of those who died was a 6-year-old child who had ingested powdered cesium. The town was extensively decontaminated; a total of 12,500 drums and 1470 boxes were filled with contaminated debris. The radiation accident at Goiania was the most severe of its kind, having resulted in a total of 244 exposures and 54 hospital admissions. Management efforts were complicated by the combined external and internal exposures in some individuals. The impact of this event continued to affect the town for several months.

RADIATION ACCIDENTS

The Radiation Emergency Assistance Center/Training Site (REAC/TS) has an extensive registry of radiation accidents.* Between 1947 and 1984, about 290 significant accidental exposures have occurred around the world, involving 136,607 people.[2] A significant exposure is defined as a whole-body exposure greater than 0.25 Sv (25 rem); as skin dose equal to or exceeding 6 Sv (600 rem); an absorbed dose equal to or exceeding 0.75 Sv (75 rem) to other tissues or organs from an external source; internal contamination equal to or exceeding half the maximal permissible body burden as defined by the International Commission on Radiological Protection (ICRP); and medical misadministrations resulting in a dose equal to or exceeding those given in the preceding criteria.[3]

Sources of radiation exposure are numerous and include nuclear reactors, transportation of nuclear materials, research laboratories, medical facilities, and nuclear weapons. Radiation accidents or events resulting from these accidents can be divided into two types: (1) those that occur on a large scale and involve many people, and (2) those that involve few individuals. Large-scale occurrences have been well publicized and include the accident at Chernobyl in the former Soviet Union in 1986, the accident at Three Mile Island, Pennsylvania, in 1979, and the accident on the Marshall Islands in the Pacific Ocean in 1954. Catastrophes of this scale are few and uncommon. Significant exposures that occur on a smaller scale and affect few individuals are more common and more likely to go unreported. These tend to occur in industry, medicine, research, and military settings. These exposures are classified as "criticality" accidents, sealed source exposures, or reactor accidents.

Criticality accidents occur when enough fissionable material (e.g., plutonium or uranium) is brought together to generate enough energy to produce a nuclear reaction. Many of these events occur in research reactors and at testing sites (e.g., Los Alamos Laboratory, New Mexico, 1958) and are responsible for the greatest number of deaths for accidents of this type.[2]

Sealed source exposures (i.e., radiation devices) are most commonly found in industrial and medical settings. They usually occur over a prolonged period of time because initially they are unrecognized. The majority of these events occur in the industrial setting and involve crystallography or radiography. Industrial radiographs are used to evaluate the integrity of metallic structures (e.g., pipewells, airplane propellers). Commonly exposed areas of the body are the extremities (especially the hands). Whole-body exposure from penetrating radioisotopes (e.g., cobalt 60 [^{60}Co], iridium 192) can result in death. The medical setting accounts for only 10% to 20% of sealed exposure incidents.[2] The radiation devices are used to sterilize supplies and chemicals. They are stationary and large units possessing stronger radiation sources than their industrial counterparts. Thus, a brief exposure to a medical source is more likely to result in a significant exposure than that to an industrial source. The causes of accidents are usually failure to observe safety procedures, technical malfunctions, and the use of complicated systems by personnel not familiar with their operation.

Another cause of radiation device exposure is the recovery of radiation-producing items by unsuspecting individuals. The Goiania incident is an example of this, and it was the most severe of the sealed source events. Not only was an entire town exposed, but also 22 people required critical care support. In another case, a ^{60}Co radiation therapy unit was processed into scrap metal and used to make reinforcing brackets for tables.[3]

In 1994, 194 exposures to radioisotopes were reported to the American Association of Poison Control Centers.[4] Many of these events involved the transport of radioactive material or spillage of these agents in either medical or scientific facilities. Usually, a facility's radiation physicist is able to respond and provide initial recommendations; however, in some instances (e.g., in large exposures with many victims), the poison center and medical toxicologist may be required to initiate care. The approach is a combined effort, and its plan must have been prepared in advance. The role of the toxicologist is not to provide definitive care, but rather to be sufficiently familiar with its principles to initiate care.

RADIATION PRINCIPLES

Radiation is energy transmitted as either particles or rays. When this energy is strong enough to cause the disruption of cellular atoms or molecules, it is referred to as *ionizing radiation*. Particles (e.g., α (alpha)-particles, β (beta)-particles, neutrons, and positrons), roentgen rays (i.e., x-rays), and γ (gamma)-rays are examples of this type of radiation. *Nonionizing radiation* forms are low-frequency electromagnetic waves; they include ultraviolet, infrared, microwave, ultrasound, and electrical energies.

Matter is considered radioactive if it can emit energy. Atoms containing an excess number of protons or neutrons release energy to achieve a more stable structure. Those that undergo this process in a spontaneous fashion are termed *radioisotopes*. The amount of radioactivity from the isotope is measured in units of becquerel (Bq). The curie (Ci) was the former unit of measure for radioactivity. One curie equals 37 billion Bq. The Chernobyl event released about 50 million Ci of radioactivity.[5] Objects exposed to the energy source are irradiated, or in clinical terms, *radiation poisoned*. When cells are radiation poisoned, atoms and molecules are excited, chemical bonds break, and ions and free radicals are formed and cause further damage.[6] *It is extremely uncommon for irradiated objects to become radioactive.* An exception is an object that has been exposed to neutrons.

The energy released by a particular matter is determined by its kinetic energy, which is a function of its mass and speed. Thus, objects that are heavy and move quickly are the most injurious to humans.

*The REAC/TS is located in Oak Ridge, Tennessee, and can be reached for assistance at (615) 576-1004.

α-Particles are heavy (containing two protons and two neutrons) and can cause a high number of ionizing events as they travel. When α particle–emitting substances are absorbed internally, a significant health risk is posed because of the α particles' proximity to sensitive cellular structures. However, as an external radiation source, α particles are not of concern to humans because they can travel only a few centimeters in air and can be easily stopped by a sheet of paper or by the epidermis. α-Particles are only a threat to humans when present internally. Radium is an example of a radioisotope that emits α particles. *β-Particles* are electrons and can traverse several meters in air. They can penetrate up to 5 mm of tissue and are of concern as external and internal sources of contamination. β-Particles can be stopped by a thin piece of metal. Carbon 14, hydrogen 3 (tritium), strontium 90, and iodine 131 (^{131}I) are some of the substances that emit β particles. β-Particles present both an external and internal threat to humans. *Neutrons* are found in nuclear fission reactions and can penetrate deep into tissue. These particles can pass through 30 cm of water. Uniquely, when traveling neutrons are finally stopped, they are captured by the nuclei of the material through which they are passing and thus make it radioactive. Sodium, phosphorus, and chloride are some of the atoms that may become radioactive in the body. Care must be exercised in removing metal objects (e.g., belt buckles) from individuals who have been exposed to neutrons because these items are extremely susceptible to becoming radioactive.

γ-Rays are a significant threat to humans as an external source of contamination. They travel quickly and contain a high level of energy. γ-Particles have no mass, and they dissipate less energy in their travel and penetrate more than do α particles. They can penetrate up to 50 cm of tissue, and several centimeters of lead. These electromagnetic waves are emitted by radium, ^{137}Cs, and ^{60}Co. *X-rays* are produced by the bombardment of an anode with a high-speed electron beam. Although x-rays travel slowly, they can still pass through tissue. Depending on their intensity, x-rays can travel up to 120 to 240 m in air, and 0.3 to 1.5 mm of lead are required to stop them. Common sources of this wave are medical diagnostic and therapeutic devices.

When a radioisotope undergoes decay, both particles and waves may be emitted. The specific type of activity is different for each radioisotope and determines the level of risk to humans. Radium emits α particles and γ-rays; it is the combination of these components that determines a person's dose of radiation exposure.[7]

RADIATION SOURCES

Artificial sources of radiation can be found in industry, medicine, and the military. Professionals at risk for radiation exposure include aircraft pilots, astronauts, dentists, electron microscopists, luminous dial painters, nuclear submarine workers, oil well workers, physicians, underground miners, and radiography technicians. The occupational limit of exposure as set by the International Commission on Radiological Protection (ICRP) is 100 man-Sv over 5 years; the limit for any 1 year is 50 man-Sv.[8] In the United States, the average occupational exposure is less than 20 man-Sv per year.

Radiopharmaceutical agents include gold 198, which is used for irradiating serosal and peritoneal surfaces in the treatment of malignancies such as carcinoma of the ovary; phosphorus 32 for polycythemia vera; sulfur 35 for chondrosarcoma; and ^{131}I for hyperthyroidism and thyroid carcinoma.[9] Bone marrow depression is expected when more than 300 mCi of ^{131}I is administered. The usual ^{131}I dose is 20 mCi.[10] Another use for radioisotopes is in nuclear imaging; agents used for this purpose are gallium 67, indium 111, and technetium 99m.

Natural, or background, sources of radiation are the earth and the cosmos. People living in mountainous regions may receive twice the natural radiation exposure compared with those living at sea level because of the additional effect of cosmic rays. The earth's crust contain several radioisotopes, including uranium, thorium, and potassium. The average exposure to background radiation per person is about 100 mrem per year.[11] The source of most of this radiation is radon. *Radon* is the product of the radioactive decay of radium 226, which is a daughter of uranium. Uranium, radium, and radon are present in varying concentrations in rock and soil. Houses situated over land masses emitting radon often contain high levels of this agent. Air carries the radon into houses, and the radon remains in the houses if they are inadequately ventilated.[12] Radon concentrations are greatest in the basement, being three- to fivefold those on the upper-level floors.

The current interest in radon concerns its role as a lung carcinogen. This association was clearly demonstrated in uranium miners[13]; however, whether this risk also exists for environmental exposure (at lower levels for longer periods of time) remains an unresolved issue. The true carcinogen of radon is its daughter, polonium, which is an α-particle emitter. The route of internal exposure to polonium is the respiratory tract. Particles of polonium that are inhaled and deposited along the bronchial epithelium induce cancer. Passive inhalation of tobacco smoke increases the dose delivered to the bronchial tissues and thus presents a risk for radon-induced lung cancer.[14]

DETERMINANTS FOR TOXICITY

Several factors affect the likelihood of occurrence of significant radiation poisoning after an exposure. Already mentioned have been the route of exposure and the specific activity of the agent. The type of matter being emitted from the radioisotope determines whether an external exposure is a threat. In contrast, almost all internal exposures (e.g., via inhalation, ingestion, and absorption through open wounds) are to be considered worrisome. The radiation dose, the rate of administration, and the area of involvement are other issues important in the evaluation of an exposure.

The *radiation dose* is the amount of radiation delivered to the tissue. The greater the dose, the more severe the clinical manifestations and the shorter their time to onset. The unit used for measuring the radiation deposited in tissue is the *radiation absorbed dose (rad)*. One rad is equivalent to 100 ergs of energy deposited in 1 g of tissue. The absorbed dose is considered the essential indicator of the anticipated clinical course of an irradiated person.[9] The Système International unit for radiation dose measurement is the *gray (Gy)*. One gray equals 100 rad. A skin dose from chest radiography is about 0.4 mGy (40 mrad), that from a cardiac catheterization procedure may be as high as 300 Gy (30,000 rad), and that from computed tomography can vary from 10 to 50 mGy (1000 to 5000 mrad).[15] The term *committed dose* is reserved for the description of internal exposure because removal of the offending agent and decontamination of the patient are very difficult in this situation. For acute exposures, the LD50/60 (the median radiation dose leading to death in 60 days) is about 2.5 to 3.5 Gy (250 to 350 rad) when only first aid is available.[16] With the availability of antibiotics and reverse isolation, this lethal threshold increases to 4.5 Gy (450 rad). Survival can be expected after exposure to 6 Gy (600 rad) if critical care support is given. The LD50 value is useful in triaging patients and allocating resources.

Because some radioactive agents are more densely ionized than others, the radiation doses that they deliver can produce various biologic effects. Thus, the unit *roentgen equivalent man (rem)* was developed. This is a dose-equivalent unit that expresses the health effects of all types of radiation on a common scale. One rem of radiation emitted from any matter is expected to produce approximately the same biologic effect. The Système International dose-equivalent unit is the *sievert (Sv)*. One sievert equals 100 rem. When an exposure to a population is considered, the term *collective dose* is used. The appropriate unit in this setting is the *person-sievert (person-Sv)*. One sievert of radiation delivered to each of 100 people is expressed as 100 person-Sv.

The rate at which the dose is administered (the *dose rate*) also is important in determining toxicity. A dose that is lethal when administered within a matter of minutes may be tolerable if it were delivered over days to weeks because exposures sustained over a prolonged period of time allow cells to repair their damaged nuclear material. An example of a unit of measure used to express dose rate is rem per hour (rem/h). Background radiation (e.g., cosmic and terrestrial radiation) is about 100 mrem/y per person.[11]

Factors governing the risks associated with internal exposures to radioactive agents are several. The size of the particle affects its ability to be dispersed in the respiratory tract upon inhalation. Heavy (atomic weight) radioisotopes are less well absorbed from the gastrointestinal tract than lighter ones.[7] The bioavailability of the isotope is also determined by the body's store of the element and the presence of other elements with similar structures that may serve as competitors.[17] Solubility of the agent also affects absorption from the respiratory and gastrointestinal tracts. Although poorly soluble agents may not be well absorbed from the lungs, they may present a significant risk for local damage.

The chemical nature of the radioisotope also is an important factor in determining its toxicity. Certain agents can be incorporated into biochemical pathways and result in not only specific organ toxicity, but also delayed elimination from the body. Strontium, plutonium, radium, and calcium are "bone seekers." Iodine has an affinity for the thyroid gland. The bone seeker isotopes tend to be more hazardous biologically than any other radioisotope because of their slow elimination from the body.

Radium is of historical interest because it was an accepted form of oral and parenteral therapy for rheumatism, gout, syphilis, anemia, epilepsy, and multiple sclerosis from 1913 to 1930.[18] The product was marketed by William J.A. Bailey under the brand name Radithor, and it contained a mixture of radium 226, mesothorium (radium 228), and triple-distilled water. Each half-ounce bottle had 37 kBq of radium activity, and it was administered in unit doses ranging from 370 to 3700 kBq. The toxicity of radium was soon realized when a wealthy industrialist, Eben M. Byers, died after he had used Radithor for only 2 years. The medical examiner's report of the body described necrosis of the jaw similar to that seen in radium dial painters, a swollen renal cortex, cerebral abscesses, a hyperplastic regenerative bone marrow, and bronchopneumonia. When absorbed internally, radium behaves like calcium. It is deposited on the surfaces of bone, has a long half-life, and is recognized to cause osteogenic sarcoma.[19]

The half-life of a radioisotope is determined by the time it takes for it to lose 50% of its activity. This period is termed the *physical half-life* and is important in the assessment of the health risk posed by an external contaminant to the general public. When the agent is absorbed internally, the time required for the body to eliminate half of the absorbed amount is termed the *biologic half-life*. The *effective half-life* reflects both factors and is more important in the individual setting. It is the time required for a radioactive agent in the body to be diminished by 50% as a result of the combined effects of biologic elimination and physical decay.[15] Typically, the biologic half-life is shorter than the physical half-life.

TYPES OF EXPOSURES

There are four types of exposures, and each is different with respect to the risks it poses to patients and health care providers.[20] *External contamination* is the adherence of radioactive agents to clothing and skin. This is only of risk to the skin and contamination of rescue workers and facility. *Internal contamination* results when the agent is inhaled, ingested, or in contact with an open wound. Such contamination requires immediate attention because certain radioisotopes can be incorporated into tissues and have a sustained effect. Internal exposures usually present too low a dose to cause acute radiation sickness; however, the tissue in proximity to the agent may be at significant risk for damage. Affected patients usually do not pose a significant risk to health care workers and the facility because the amount of radioactivity in the bodily fluids is very small.[21] *External irradiation* occurs when an individual is exposed to the energy emitted from a radioactive source but does not come into contact with the source itself. This type of exposure does not render the patient radioactive, and thus it presents no health threat to others. The patient may develop acute radiation sickness if the amount of exposure is sufficiently large. *Localized exposure* occurs when radiation affects only a part of the body. The risk of localized exposure is usually limited to the skin.

CLINICAL MANIFESTATIONS

The clinical effects of radiation are due to the excitation or ionization of essential biomolecules. This leads to damage of DNA and other macromolecules that affect chemical and physiologic reactions; the altered reactions translate into clinical manifestations. Cells with high metabolic and reproductive rates are susceptible to radiation poisoning and manifest changes early. These include bone marrow, gastrointestinal, and reproductive cells. The later effects of radiation poisoning are carcinogenesis, cataract formation, sterility, and hereditary defects.[22] Some of these effects may take years to become apparent. Immature spermatogonia are the most radiosensitive cells in the body.[22] Temporary depression in sperm count occurs with a dose equivalent to 0.15 Sv (15 rem). Permanent sterility may result from exposure to greater than 4 Sv (400 rem). With respect to the ovaries, the risk for temporary sterility occurs at 1.5 to 2.0 Sv (150 to 200 rem); that for permanent sterility occurs at 2 to 3 Sv (200 to 300 rem). The appearance of gonadal effects is often delayed by 2 months and may last for 1 to 2 years after exposure. After the sixth week of human gestation, the risk for malformations from radiation exposure decreases except for cerebral and gonadal development. From the atomic bomb experience in Japan, the peak incidence of microcephaly and mental retardation was in infants who were exposed during their 8th to 15th week of gestation.[23] Important factors contributing to the severity of radiation poisoning are the dose, the dose rate, the pattern of distribution, and individual susceptibility.

Localized Exposures

Localized external exposures are most common in the occupational setting. The duration of exposure is chronic, and the professionals at risk include radiologists and nuclear medicine technicians. The extremities are frequently affected by dryness and atrophy of the skin.[24] Acute localized exposures to β particles and γ-rays may occur among workers at nuclear reactor sites. The damage to the skin can present as a mild dermatitis or a severe burn. Generally, the time of onset of radiation burns is longer than that for thermal burns.[21] A high index of suspicion is necessary in identifying these injuries because patients initially may complain only of a burning sensation in the absence of an apparent lesion. The lesion presents later—with low level exposures, usually after 1 to 2 weeks. The subcutaneous tissue also can be affected. α-Particles are not of concern as external agents because of their poor ability to penetrate the epidermis.

Erythema is the initial manifestation of skin damage from irradiation, and its time of onset is dependent on the dose of exposure.[25] The erythema is caused by vasodilation. At high doses (greater than 50 Gy [5000 rad]), erythema, pain, and a sensation of heat can be experienced within a few minutes to half an hour. The physical manifestations can resemble those of chemical burns. Moderate exposures of 2 to 3 Gy (200 to 300 rad) can cause symptoms within 2 to 3 hours. With moderate exposures, a re-emerging redness with blistering and desquamation may occur after a latency period of 2 to 3 weeks. In high-dose exposures, this second phase can progress very quickly, and underlying tissues can be affected.

Subcutaneous tissue damage involving nerves, sweat glands, and hair follicles presents later, and initially the extent of injury usually is underestimated.[21] Progressive tissue necrosis may continue for months after the exposure because of small vessel disease.[24] Alopecia occurs at 2 to 3 weeks after exposure to doses greater than 2 to 4 Gy (200 to 400 rad). At exposure levels greater than 7 Gy (700 rad), hair follicles are destroyed and permanent hair loss may result. The intensity of irradiation required for loss of limbs and digits is even greater than the amount necessary to cause acute radiation syndrome.[24]

Whole-Body Exposure

Generalized or whole-body exposures are an uncommon occurrence. Victims of the atomic bomb explosions in Japan, the radioactive fallout from nuclear testing in the Marshall Islands, and the nuclear reactor accident in Chernobyl sustained this degree of contamination. Exposures of this type affect multiple organ systems and can cause death. Thirty-one deaths resulted from the Chernobyl accident—nearly equal the number of deaths that have occurred since the atomic bomb incidents.[5] The time of onset of the systemic manifestations of radiation poisoning depends on the dose and can vary from hours to years. Those manifestations that present rapidly are known as *acute radiation syndrome,* and those that occur later (years) are known as *long-term effects.* Acute radiation syndrome is a risk when whole-body exposure is greater than 1 Gy (100 rad) and occurs over a short time interval (i.e., within 2 days).[9]

Acute radiation syndrome is determined not only by the aforementioned factors, but also by individual susceptibility. The very young and the very old are at greatest risk for the development of this disorder.[9] Children are generally more susceptible than adults. Levels of exposure greater than 1 Gy (100 rad) are likely to cause significant symptoms. Levels less than this cause minor symptoms and can be managed with supportive care. The symptoms affect the gastrointestinal, hematologic, central nervous, and cardiovascular systems. The syndrome is classically described in four stages that start at the time of exposure.[26]

The early phase is characterized by nausea, vomiting, and anorexia, and is similar to a viral syndrome. This prodromal phase may include diarrhea, abdominal cramps, salivation, diaphoresis, and hypotension. These symptoms are attributed to parasympathetic stimulation and may be occur with exposures to as little as 1 Gy (100 rad); they may be seen at 2 to 6 hours after exposure.[27] For exposures to less than 4 Gy (400 rad), these symptoms usually last for less than 2 days. Laboratory manifestations are detectable at approximately 1 Gy (100 rad).[9] The time of onset of gastrointestinal symptoms is a rough gauge of severity of illness and exposure. At greater than 6 Gy (600 rad), the time to onset may be as short as 2 hours. If vomiting develops within 1 to 5 hours, then a significant exposure has occurred. If vomiting is present in 1 hour, then death is likely; if it occurs within minutes, then death is most certain.[9] Other possible clinical findings during this phase include weakness, fatigue, erythema, diaphoresis, paresthesias, and conjunctivitis.

The patient's symptoms may subside, and he or she may begin to feel well; however, weakness and fatigue may persist. The duration of this second phase is indirectly related to the amount of exposure—that is, the greater the level of exposure, the shorter its duration. The second phase usually lasts 1 to 2 weeks with exposures of 6 to 8 Gy (600 to 800 rad) and only hours with exposures of greater than 15 Gy (1500 rad). Hair loss and mucosal ulceration present 13 to 20 days after a significant exposure.

The third phase of acute radiation syndrome represents the true damage of the exposure and begins at about the third to fifth week after contamination.[26] The organ systems affected are several, and their presentation is determined by the radiation dose. The gut and bone marrow are primarily involved, and the disorder can last for weeks to months. At a dose of 7 Gy (700 rad), gastrointestinal manifestations appear first and include anorexia, vomiting, and diarrhea. Mucosal ulcerations and dysentery occur at 10 Gy (1000 rad). Significant complications of fluid and electrolyte imbalances and enteric sepsis are to be expected and are the focus of management. The bone marrow response is pancytopenia and occurs later. Death at this stage is usually the result of an overwhelming infection. Patients who survive the sixth week after exposure are expected to recover.

Lymphocytopenia is observed initially; granulocytopenia, thrombocytopenia, and anemia follow.[9] This order follows the duration of survival of the respective cell type. The dose of exposure necessary to affect the bone marrow is 1 Gy (100 rad), which is less than that for the gastrointestinal system. An acute dose of 3 to 5 Gy (300 to 500 rad) is sufficient to kill enough hematopoietic cells to cause a profound drop in leukocyte and platelet counts and to necessitate transfusion. The lymphocytes may disappear within 24 hours, the granulocytes within days, and the platelets within 1 to 2 weeks. If there are more than 1000 lymphocytes per cubic millimeter at 48 hours after exposure, then the prognosis for survival is good. Fewer than 500 lymphocytes at this time portends a poor prognosis. Other useful prognostic indicators are the severity of reticulocytopenia, granulocytopenia, and thrombocytopenia. The granulocyte count may increase temporarily in the first 5 days and then again at 10 to 15 days after exposure to a dose of 2 to 5 Gy (200 to 500 rad).[9] With exposures greater than 5 Gy (500 rad), the second increase in granulocyte count is absent. Infections resulting from granulocytopenia are most likely to occur from 15 to 30 days after exposure.

The duration of pancytopenia can be protracted with significant bone marrow toxicity. The nadir of the period of lymphocytopenia is about 25 to 45 days after exposure.[9] The anemia from bone marrow toxicity is not as serious as the disorders of the lymphocytes and platelets because of the long period of red blood cell survival. The most common cause of anemia is gastrointestinal bleeding.[9] Complete bone marrow recovery is expected at 6 months after exposure; however, lymphocyte recovery may take longer.[9]

Another manifestation of generalized radiation poisoning that may present in this phase is the central nervous system syndrome. It occurs at exposures greater than 10 Gy (1000 rad) and is characterized by neurologic and cardiovascular findings. Its true existence in humans is debated, as it has only been demonstrated to occur in animals and in limited clinical situations.[28, 29] The clinical course is rapid and consists of hypotension, ataxia, seizure, coma, and death within 2 days. Pathologic specimens have demonstrated cerebral vasculitis, meningitis, encephalitis, cerebral edema, and cardiac necrosis.[29] At this level of exposure, severe dermal burns are to be expected, and death is inevitable.

The prognosis of an exposed patient is best determined on the basis of careful monitoring of the clinical manifestations. Although the course of acute radiation syndrome is described in stages, individual organ systems may dominate, depending on the degree of radioactive exposure. Exposures to greater than 50 Gy (5000 rad) result in neurovascular toxicity and lead to death within 24 to 48 hours. Exposures to between 2 to 20 Gy (200 to 2000 rad), the classic four-phase course would be expected, and survival is strongly dependent on aggressive therapy, including bone marrow transplantation.

Long-Term Effects

Some of the effects of radiation poisoning may present years after exposure and involve multiple organ systems. The data compiled on exposures to atomic bomb radiation in Japan and to nuclear fallout from detonations have demonstrated that these long-term consequences may affect both germ and somatic cells. Furthermore, these effects may be stochastic or nonstochastic. *Nonstochastic effects* are dose dependent and uniform; they included hypothyroidism, ocular cataract formation, growth retardation, and sterility. Long-term *stochastic effects* include neoplasm, teratogenic effects, and genetic effects. The most important and concerning of these are neoplasms that occur secondary to chromosomal damage.

The two most common neoplasms related to radiation exposure are leukemia and thyroid cancer.[30, 31] The thyroid gland is the organ most commonly affected in a nuclear accident because of the abundance of radioiodines (^{125}I, ^{131}I) present in nuclear reactors. Although the radioiodines have a relatively short physical half-life (8 days for ^{131}I), they are concentrated by the thyroid gland to cause hypothyroidism and neoplasm. The best examples of thyroid abnormalities resulted from the Bravo hydrogen bomb detonation on the Bikini Atoll of the Marshall Islands in 1954. Hypothyroidism, thyroid nodularity, and thyroid carcinoma were discovered within 11 years after the event.[32] Other epidemiologic studies confirm the increased risk of thyroid cancer from radiation exposure.[32–35] The peak incidence of cancer occurs approximately 25 years after exposure. Recent reports from the Chernobyl accident in 1986 have demonstrated that this time interval may be as short as 4 years in children.[34, 35] Almost all of the lesions of radiation-induced thyroid cancer are papillary thyroid carcinomas.

Leukemia may be the most commonly recognized neoplasm associated with radiation exposure, particularly when the exposure exceeds several grays.[31, 36] Excessive leukemia rates were previously demonstrated in radiologists, atomic bomb survivors, and radiotherapy patients. The lifetime risk for leukemia is estimated to be 2×10^{-5} per 0.01 Gy (or 2×10^{-5} per rad).[37] All types of leukemias except chronic lymphocytic leukemia have been associated with radiation exposure. The latency period for the development of leukemia is approximately 10 years, with the minimum period being as short as 2 to 3 years. Young children are at greatest risk for the development of leukemia, and they also have the shortest latency period. On the basis of the atomic bomb survivor data, it appears that by 30 years after exposure, the risk of leukemia reverts to that of the general population.[36]

Various solid organ tumors also are associated with radiation exposure. In fact, the number of all radiation-induced solid tumors is about fivefold that of leukemia cases. Some of the organs that are most susceptible to radiation-induced neoplasm include the salivary glands, the breast, the bladder, the colon, the stomach, the liver, the lung, the ovary, and the skin.[37]

An increased incidence of microcephaly and mental retardation in children was documented from *in utero* exposure after the atomic bomb detonations in Japan.[23] The risk for the development of these abnormalities is nonstochastic and is greatest when the exposure is between 8 and 15 weeks of gestation. The threshold for these injuries appears to be 0.1 to 0.2 Gy (10 to 20 rad). The estimated risks for mental retardation are 40% per 1 Gy (or 40% per 100 rad) and 10% per 1 Gy (or 10% per 100 rad) for *in utero* exposures at 8 to 15 weeks and 16 to 25 weeks, respectively. No known risk is associated with exposure at less than 8 weeks of gestation.[23, 38, 39]

Radiation-induced cataracts have been documented in both animal studies and in atomic bomb survivors. The opacity begins in the posterior pole of the lens (as opposed to the anterior pole in senile cataracts). The pathophysiology is associated with radiation-induced damage to the epithelial cells of the anterior lens, which leads to the migration and degeneration of these cells in the posterior pole of the lens. The average latency period for the development of cataracts is approximately 2 to 3 years, but it may be delayed up for to 30 years.[40] The risks for cataracts are dose, time, and age dependent (young children at greatest risk).[37]

Patients receiving repeated localized fractionated radiation therapy with cumulative doses exceeding 40 to 50 Gy (4000 to 5000 rad) also may sustain delayed effects. These include strictures, fibrosis, enteric fistulae, nephritis, and aseptic necrosis of the femoral head and mandible. These types of organ disorders are not usually seen with single-dose total-body exposure because such a dose is not commensurate with survival.[37]

MANAGEMENT

The management of radiation injuries requires a multidisciplinary approach. These strategies include assessment for the type of radiation and degree of exposure, determining the need for decontamination, protecting medical personnel, and providing initial and follow-up care to the patients (Table 29–1).[41–43]

Fortunately, the chance of occurrence of a radiation accident is small. However, also small is the number of physicians and medical personnel who have adequate experience and knowledge to manage victims' care were such an event to occur. Although it may be foolhardy to believe that any one center can handle a major nuclear disaster, it is quite possible for most

Table 29–1. Emergency Management of Radiation Poisoning*

1. Determine nature and extent of radiation accident.
2. Radiation protocol: Secure emergency department and designate treatment room(s).
3. Isolate and decontaminate patients.
4. Measure radioactivity with a Geiger-Müller counter before and after decontamination.
5. Draw blood for at least a complete blood count, HLA typing, and thyroid studies.
6. Undertake emergency management of thermal burns and associated injuries.
7. Provide chelation therapy.
8. Admit patients for observation and treatment, as indicated, for:
   - Determination of the extent of exposure
   - Fluid resuscitation
   - Hyperalimentation
   - Antibiotic therapy
   - Treatment of associated injuries and complications
   - Bone marrow transplantation
   - Supportive care

*At medical centers with appropriately equipped emergency departments.

medical facilities, with adequate training and preparation, to handle a small radiation accident. Only one emergency department in the entire United States is specially designed and prepared to handle a radiation accident: the REAC at the Methodist Medical Center in Oak Ridge, Tennessee. Currently, the Joint Committee on Accreditation of Hospital requires hospitals to have a written protocol for the management of patients involved in such accidents. Appropriate equipment, adequate personnel, and proper training are key to handling a radiation accident. Some of the essential resources, such as specialty equipment (e.g., Geiger-Müller counter, scintillation counter, and personal film badges) and a nuclear physicist, are available in the nuclear medicine department of many hospitals. A detailed list of the necessary equipment and a plan of management have been provided by Pons and Sullivan.[43]

In the event of a radiation accident, the first step is to determine the nature and extent of the radiation exposure. This delineates the precautions that the medical personnel must take, as well as the need for decontamination. Immediate life-threatening conditions (e.g., burns, trauma, smoke inhalation, and airway compromise) are to be addressed initially. Symptoms of radiation exposure are often delayed. The most serious immediate medical problem resulting from the Chernobyl accident was thermal burns.[44] Patients who have been exposed to radiation are not radioactive and pose no contamination risk to health care providers. The exception would be the rare scenario in which the victim has been irradiated with a high dose of neutrons. Radionuclide contamination, whether external or internal, requires that precautions be taken by medical personnel and that the patient be decontaminated.

The notification of a nuclear accident to a hospital should automatically activate an established protocol of response. All patients must be cleared from the ambulance entrance to the emergency department. A safety officer is designated to maintain the flow of traffic and monitor for contamination to other areas. A separate room or area for the management of these patients must be properly demarcated with tape and signs. Many hospitals have a special hazardous material management room that has appropriate showers and a self-contained drainage storage system for wastes. If such a room is not available, then plastic sheets must be placed on the floor, taped, and sealed to catch all the contaminated effluent for disposal. All essential equipment, drawers, and cabinets must be properly covered to prevent contamination. Appropriate personnel must be available and designated to control the flow of patients, secure the area, assess the degree of contamination, and manage the patients. Finally, proper protective clothing such as masks, waterproof gowns, gloves, caps, and shoe covers, as well as personal dosimeter badges to monitor exposure, are to be available to hospital personnel.

A direct measurement of contamination is useful for determining the efficacy of the decontamination process. The Geiger-Müller counter, when used by a qualified experienced operator, can assess for $\gamma\beta$ radiation. The use of an α radiation counter requires greater expertise and should be available but is not essential. α-Radiation has limited tissue penetration, and its measurement is useful for evaluating environmental and external contamination. Once contamination has been confirmed, immediate decontamination procedures should be implemented.

All clothing should be removed and contained. Saline swabs of the ear, nose, and open wounds are to be collected and analyzed for radioactive contamination prior to any cleansing. Irrigation of the eyes, ears, nose, and mouth with water or saline is to be performed carefully and in such a manner that any cross contamination and swallowing of the effluent are avoided. Mild soap and water, along with a soft sponge or brush, can be used to wash the skin. The hair also should be washed and rinsed. If contamination persists, the hair should be removed by cutting and not shaving, so that further contamination through dermal abrasions is prevented. All open wounds must be promptly and copiously irrigated with saline to prevent internalization of any radionuclides. Repeated washing with monitoring of the hair, skin, and effluent may be necessary to achieve complete external decontamination. When external decontamination is completed, the body can be completely dried.

Internal contamination can be assessed by the analysis of nasal swabs (suggesting inhalation or pulmonary contamination) or gastric lavage fluid. Significant pulmonary contamination with nonsoluble radionuclides can be mitigated with pulmonary alveolar lavage through a double-lumen endotracheal tube (to isolate each lung). Consultation with REAC or a radiation expert is recommended before this procedure. Gastric lavage can be performed for oral ingestions. Cathartics may be used to enhance the movement of the radionuclides through the gastrointestinal tract. Magnesium sulfate can form insoluble salts with certain radionuclides and decrease absorption. Aluminum-containing antacids (e.g., Maalox and Mylanta) form insoluble salts with strontium and thus prevent systemic absorption. The use of whole-bowel irrigation has not been reported for internal radionuclide decontamination, but it may have a role in enhancing the gut's elimination of these substances.

Assessment

Once initial resuscitation, stabilization, and decontamination have been accomplished, the patient's radiation exposure dose should be assessed to determine potential toxicity and prognosis. There are three possible means of estimating the total-body irradiation dose: theoretic calculations, physical measurements, and biologic dosimetry. *Theoretic calculations* can be performed with the use of computer simulations for estimating the radiation field. However, such methods are seldom helpful for accurately determining an individual's exposure. *Physical measurements* can be performed if the victim is wearing a dosimeter or a film badge; also, a paramagnetic resonance analysis of dental enamel or clothing can be performed. Internal and external contamination can be assessed by whole-body scintillation with the use of equipment available in the nuclear medicine department.

The most practical technique for estimating the amount of exposure is biologic dosimetry. Predictable biologic responses to levels of radiation are used for estimating exposure. Trends of lymphocyte, reticulocyte, granulocyte, platelet, and erythrocyte counts are followed to predict toxicity. Lymphocytes are particularly sensitive to radiation, and their counts can be expected to decline within 2 to 3 days after a significant exposure. Because of the potential for loss of essential blood elements, it is important to obtain blood samples as soon as possible for HLA typing for future bone marrow matching.[45] In the Chernobyl accident, HLA typing was difficult to perform in some patients because of rapid and profound lymphocytopenia. Although the other hematologic parameters are less predictive in the early phase after exposure, they are helpful later when combined with assessments of lymphocyte counts (Fig. 29–1).[42] Other injuries (e.g., burns) can also account for lymphocytopenia and granulocytopenia and should be considered in the evaluation. More sophisticated analysis on dicentric chromosomes and other cytogenetic abnormalities can be used for estimating the radiation dosage.[46, 47]

The early onset of nausea and vomiting and their lasting longer than 2 days are also findings predictive

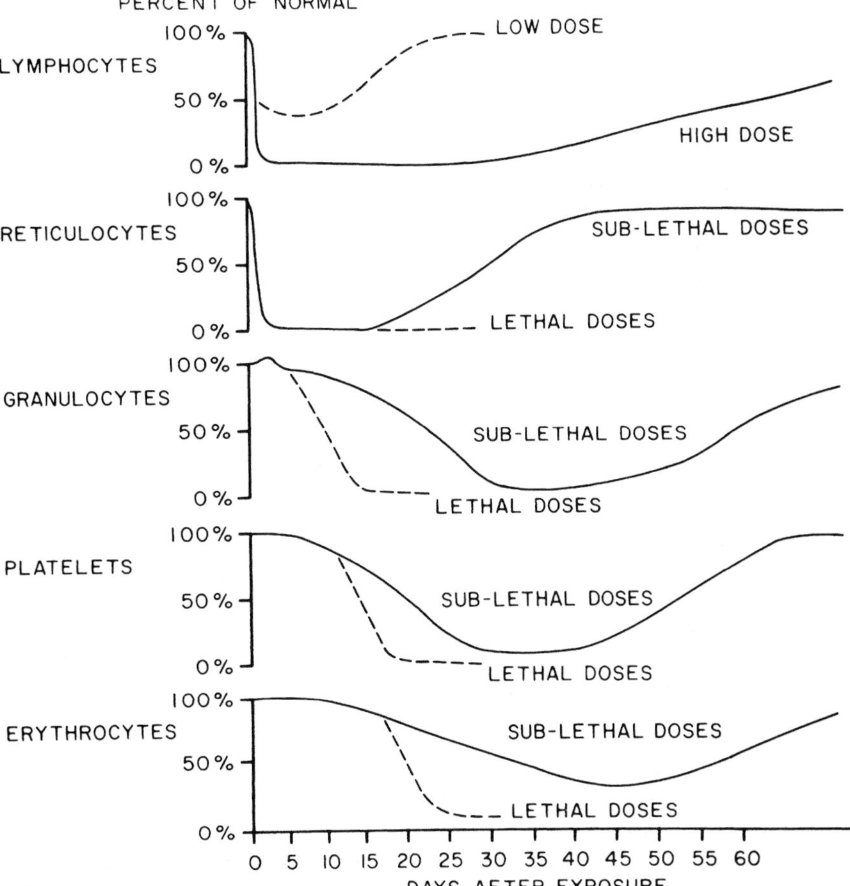

Figure 29–1. Hematologic response to acute whole-body irradiation. (From Milroy WC: Management of irradiated and contaminated casualty victims. Emerg Med Clin North Am *2*:667–686, 1984.)

of a significant exposure. A simple and practical method for estimating total-body radiation exposure is to assess gastrointestinal symptoms and the lymphocyte count on the third day after exposure (see Table 29–1).[41] *If a significant decline in lymphocyte count is not observed at day 3, and if the duration of nausea and vomiting is 2 days or shorter, then the amount of exposure is probably less than 2 Gy (200 rad).* However, if the duration of the nausea and vomiting is longer than 2 days and a significant decline in lymphocyte count is noted, then the exposure dose is approximately 2 to 4 Gy (200 to 400 rad). Any significant decline in the lymphocyte count (to less than 800 to 900/mm^3, or to less than 50% of normal) suggests an exposure greater than 4 Gy (400 rad). The additional presentation of diarrhea with a significant decline in lymphocyte count suggests a radiation dose greater than 6 Gy (600 rad).

Just as knowing the radiation dose is important, so too is determining the pattern of exposure on the body. For example, the shielding of an extremity may save a quantity of hematopoietic progenitor cells adequate to prevent complete bone marrow failure, even when the exposure is exceedingly large. An analysis of the distribution of cytogenetic abnormalities is useful for estimating the uniformity of the exposure.[46] This usually requires the involvement of technical expertise from outside resources.

Table 29–2. Simple Biologic Dosimetry for Estimating Total-Body Radiation Exposure

Decline in Lymphocyte Count	Nausea and Vomiting	Diarrhea	Estimated Dose*
No	≤2 d	No	≤2 Gy
No	>2 d	No	2–4 Gy
Yes	>2 d	No	4–6 Gy
Yes	>2 d	Yes	6 Gy

*1 Gy = 100 rad.

Specific Measures: Chelation and Organ Protection

Other means of organ protection must also be considered in the event of a nuclear accident. They are blocking the concentration of the radionuclide presented to the target organ, altering the tissue distribution of the radionuclide, and enhancing the radionuclide's elimination with the use of selected chelators (Table 29–3). In a nuclear accident, common radionuclides released are ^{125}I, ^{131}I, and ^{137}Cs. Radioactive iodine can be concentrated in the thyroid gland, causing hypothyroidism and thyroid and parathyroid cancer. The administration of potassium iodide (KI), concurrent with or before the radioiodine exposure, can block up to 97% of the radioiodine uptake into the thyroid gland. The efficacy of KI decreases rapidly if it is administered after the radioiodine exposure. At 6 hours after the radioiodine exposure, KI is minimally effective, if at all. The potential adverse effects of KI are the precipitation of hypothyroidism and hyperthyroidism. The decision to administer KI must be made in consideration of the significance of the exposure and of the safety and rapidity with which KI can be given. If the thyroid-absorbed dose of radioiodine is expected to exceed 0.30 Gy (30 rad), KI is recommended as blocking therapy.[48] The dose for KI is 100 mg for adults and 50 mg for children younger than 1 year of age. The administration of KI should be continued for 2 to 3 days, or until the radiation exposure has been terminated. Potassium iodide was administered following the Chernobyl accident; under such circumstances, the benefits of KI therapy would outweigh the potential risks.

During the Goiania accident, Prussian blue (potassium ferricyanoferrate) was used to enhance the elimination of cesium. Prussian blue given orally exchanges potassium for cesium; this exchange forms an insoluble complex that is eliminated through the gastrointestinal tract. This therapy also interrupts the enteral circulation of cesium. Toxic effects associated with Prussian blue are minimal, but include constipation. The expected biologic half-life of ^{137}Cs is approximately 50 to 150 days. In the patients treated with Prussian blue at Goiania, total radiation dose was reduced by greater than 50%.[49]

The elimination of certain radioisotopes can be enhanced through the use of heavy metal chelators such as diethylenetriaminepentaacetic acid (DTPA), dimercaprol (BAL or British antilewisite), 2,3-dimercaptosuccinic acid (DMSA), dimercaptosulfonate (DMPS), penicillamine, calcium disodium ethylenediaminetetraacetic acid ($CaNa_2EDTA$), and deferoxamine (Table 29–2).[43] The data on the clinical efficacy of chelation therapy in this setting are limited. Nev-

Table 29–3. Chelating Agents for Radioactive Material

Chelating Agent	Radioisotope
Diethylenetriaminepentaacetic acid (DTPA)	Plutonium, americium, curium, neptunium, californium, cerium, yttrium, lanthanum, scandium, promethium, niobium, lutetium, zirconium, zinc
Calcium disodium ethylenediaminetetraacetic acid ($CaNa_2$ EDTA)	Lead, zinc, copper, nickel, chromium, manganese
Penicillamine	Copper, mercury, lead, gold
Dimercaptosuccinic acid (DMSA)	Mercury, arsenic, lead, copper, cadmium, zinc, nickel, gold
Dimercaprol and DTPA	Cadmium
Dimercaptosulfonate (DMPS)	Cadmium, gold, chromium
Dimercaprol (British antilewisite)	Mercury, arsenic, lead, copper, cadmium, zinc, nickel, gold, bismuth
Deferoxamine	Iron

From Pons P, Sullivan JB Jr: Radiation and radioactive emergencies. *In* Sullivan JB Jr, Krieger GR (eds): Hazardous Material Toxicology. Clinical Principles of Environmental Health. Baltimore, Williams & Wilkins, pp 441–449, 1992.

ertheless, chelation is recommended, and treatment should be started as soon as possible after exposure.

Animal investigations demonstrate the potential clinical benefit of some new agents in protecting against radiation-induced tissue injuries when these agents are administered before or concomitant with radioactive exposure.[50] The mechanisms of action of these radioprotectants are several and include scavenging for superoxide and hydroxyl free radicals, donating hydrogen atoms to repair damaged macromolecules, and binding to macromolecules to promote their stabilization. These agents can be classified into three categories: aminothiols (e.g., cysteine, cystamine, amifostine); antioxidants and free radical scavengers (e.g., glutathione, catalase, superoxide dismutase, cytochrome C); and immunomodulators (e.g., interferons, endotoxins, azimexon). Data regarding the efficacy of these agents in humans are limited.[51]

Supportive Measures

The quality of supportive therapy has a significant role in enhancing the survival of radiation-poisoned victims. Treatment includes fluid and parenteral nutritional support for patients with gastrointestinal tract injuries and burns, wound care, and therapy for other associated injuries. Primary therapy is aimed at preventing the complications associated with infections and bleeding and at stimulating or replenishing the hematopoietic system. Complications from infections and bleeding are the leading cause of morbidity and mortality, which generally occur within 14 to 28 days after the exposure. The risk of infections from the skin and gastrointestinal tract flora increases as the granulocyte count drops below 0.5×10^9/L.[45, 52] Oral antibiotics are used to alter the intestinal bacterial flora. Broad-spectrum systemic antibiotics should be administered immediately to febrile patients. Common regimens are combination therapy with a third-generation cephalosporin with *Pseudomonas* coverage and a semisynthetic penicillin with gram-positive bacteria coverage, or imipenem. Patients with persistent fever despite appropriate antibiotic coverage should also be treated with an antifungal agent such as amphotericin B or with azoles. Recrudescent herpetic infections may occur after radiation exposure and can be managed with an antiviral agent (e.g., acyclovir). Reverse isolation is often implemented to prevent infectious transmissions from other patients. However, this practice has not been proved to be beneficial because most bacterial infections are caused by the patient's own skin and gastrointestinal flora.

Thrombocytopenia of less than 20×10^9 cells/L may lead to spontaneous bleeding, and platelet transfusion should be carried out to maintain counts above this level. Genetically related donors can increase the chance for subsequent bone marrow rejection; thus, they are best not used as platelet donors until the possibility of bone marrow transplantation has been excluded.[45] Erythrocyte transfusion should also be instituted for significant anemia in order to maintain a hematocrit of 30%. The irradiation (15 Gy) of all cellular blood products prior to transfusion is recommended for preventing any type of graft-versus-host disease. Unfortunately, granulocyte transfusions are not protective for granulocytopenic patients. Hematopoietic growth factors such as *granulocyte-macrophage colony-stimulating factor* and *granulocyte-colony stimulating factor* may be administered to speed up bone marrow recovery.[45, 53] Platelet colony-stimulating factor may be available in the future for thrombocytopenic patients. The use of hematopoietic growth factors assumes that some bone marrow germ cells survived the radiation exposure. Current evidence substantiates this assumption in most patients. With proper supportive therapy, most patients may survive total-body irradiation of up to 4 to 5 Gy (400 to 500 rad).[45]

Beginning at a total-body radiation dose of greater than 5 Gy (500 rad), mortality increases dramatically. Patients with such exposures have significant fluid and nutritional requirements because of gastrointestinal tract and dermal injuries. Intravenous hyperalimentation usually is necessary. Most patients succumb to infections and bleeding disorders before the bone marrow can recover. Because autologous bone marrow recovery is unpredictable and incomplete, bone marrow transplantation has been advocated. Bone marrow transplantations have been successful in the treatment of very-high-dose total-body irradiation in both animal models and in patients with leukemia and other neoplasms (up to 15 Gy [1500 rad]).[52] Although the reconstitution of the hematopoietic system from transplantation may only be temporary, the time afforded may be sufficient to allow for spontaneous recovery of the endogenous hematopoietic system. Significant adverse effects are associated with bone marrow transplantation. Graft rejection is a primary concern. The immunity of patients receiving a total-body radiation dose of less than 10 Gy (1000 rad) may be sufficient to induce a graft-versus-host rejection.[54] Other potential adverse effects include graft-versus-host reaction, immunosuppression, and toxicity from immunosuppressive agents. Some of these adverse effects can be minimized if the donor is an identical twin. At higher total radiation doses (greater than 10 Gy [1000 rad]), the success of bone marrow transplantation increases because of host immunosuppression, which decreases the risk of host-versus-graft disease. At these doses, however, bone marrow transplantation may not ensure or improve survival because most patients with such radiation poisoning succumb to other organ toxicities.[47, 52, 54]

The exact benefits of bone marrow transplantation for patients exposed to high levels of radiation (greater than 5 Gy [500 rad]) are difficult to define because of the small number of experiences and of the presence of associated injuries that may affect outcome. The decision for transplantation remains complex and is probably limited to a small subset of patients with significant radiation exposure. Even in the Chernobyl accident, transplants were performed in only 13 of the more than 200 victims. The estimated dosimetric values in these patients based on lymphocyte kinetics and analysis of dicentric chromosomes were 4.7 to 13.4 Gy (median, 7) and 4.4 to 11.9 Gy (median, 8.3), respectively. Seven of the 13 transplant recipients died within 3 weeks because of dermal burns, gastrointestinal toxicity, and infections. Four more died later because of graft-versus-host disease, infections, interstitial pneumonia, and renal failure, leaving only 2 survivors.[47] Some of the factors to consider in making this decision are the estimated dosimetry, the uniformity of exposure in the body, the significance of associated injuries, and the compatibility of available donors. In general, supportive care is sufficient for patients receiving less than 2 Gy (200 rad) of total-body radiation. Granulocyte colony-stimulating factors should be given to patients with exposures greater than 2 Gy (200 rad), and bone marrow transplantation should be considered for those who received doses greater than 5 to 8 Gy (500 to 800 rad).[52, 54] These decisions are best made for each patient on an individual basis.

Disposition

Patients with minimal or no symptoms who are suspected to have received total-body irradiation of less than 2 Gy (200 rad) may be discharged after appropriate assessment and decontamination. Close follow-up within 2 to 3 days that includes repeated lymphocytic measurement is necessary for ensuring that the patient is properly triaged. Further follow-up is necessary for assessing the subacute and long-term consequences of the radiation exposure.

CONCLUSION

In recent years, the medical community has made significant strides in the treatment of severely radiation-poisoned patients. Some of the survivors of the Chernobyl accident sustained levels of exposure previously thought to be lethal. However, the limitations of the heroic therapies also were made apparent. The care of these patients continues to require a multidisciplinary approach, and continued research for radioprotective agents, such as free radical scavengers, may yield additional benefits in the future.

May mankind remember the past so that future nuclear accidents can be prevented.

References

1. Roberts L: Radiation accident grips Goiania. Science *238*:1028, 1987.
2. Nenot JC: Overview of the radiological accidents in the world, updated December 1989. Int J Radiat Biol *57*:1073, 1990.
3. Mettler RA, Ricks RC: Historical aspects of radiation accidents. *In* Mettler FA, Kelsey CA, Ricks RC (eds): Medical Management of Radiation Accidents. Boca Raton, FL, CRC Press, pp 18–26, 1990.
4. Litovitz TL, Felberg L, Soloway RA, et al: 1994 Annual report of the American Association of Poison Control Center toxic exposure surveillance system. Am J Emerg Med *13*:551, 1995.
5. Behar A, Cohen-Boulakia F, Othmani S: Chernobyl three years later: Radiobiologic evaluation of a radioactive contamination. J Environ Pathol Toxicol Oncol *10*:281, 1990.
6. Cole A, Meyn RE, Chen R, et al: Mechanisms of cell injury. *In* Meyn R, Withers HR (eds): Radiation Biology in Cancer Research. New York, Raven Press, pp 33–58, 1990.
7. Little JB: Environmental hazards: Ionizing radiation. N Engl J Med *275*:929, 1966.
8. Exposure of the U.S. Population from Occupational Radiation. Bethesda, MD, National Council on Radiation Protection and Measurement Report No. 101, 1989.
9. Mettler RA: Effects of whole body irradiation. *In* Mettler FA, Kelsey CA, Ricks RC (eds): Medical Management of Radiation Accidents. Boca Raton, FL, CRC Press, pp 80–87, 1990.
10. Halnan KE, Pochin EE: Symposium on the thyroid: II. Aspects of the radio-iodide treatment of thyroid carcinoma. Metabolism *6*:49, 1957.
11. Ionizing Radiation Exposure of the Population of the United States. Bethesda, MD, National Council on Radiation Protection and Measurement Report No. 93, 1987.
12. Samet JM, Nero AV: Indoor radon and lung cancer. N Engl J Med *320*:591, 1989.
13. Sevc J, Junz E, Placek V: Lung cancer in uranium miners and long term exposures to radon daughter products. Health Phys *30*:433, 1976.
14. Muller J, Kusiak R, Ritchie AC: Factors modifying lung cancer risk in Ontario uranium miners, 1955–1981. Ontario Ministry of Labour Report. Toronto, Ontario, Ministry of Labour, 1989.
15. Mettler FA, Kelsey CA: Fundamentals of radiation accidents. *In* Mettler FA, Kelsey CA, Ricks RC (eds): Medical Management of Radiation Accidents. Boca Raton, FL, CRC Press, pp 2–16, 1990.
16. Management of Persons Accidentally Contaminated with Radionuclides. Bethesda, MD, National Council on Radiation Protection and Measurement Report No. 65, 1980.
17. Voelz GL: Evaluation and treatment of persons exposed to internally deposited radionuclides. *In* Mettler FA, Kelsey CA, Ricks RC (eds): Medical Management of Radiation Accidents. Boca Raton, FL, CRC Press, pp 151–168, 1990.
18. Maklis RM: Radithor and the era of mild radium therapy. JAMA *264*:614, 1990.
19. Chemelevsky D, Kellerer AM, Spiess H, et al: A proportional hazards analysis of bone sarcoma rates in German radium 224 patients. *In* Gossner W, Gerber GB (eds): The Radiobiology of Radium and Thorotrast. Munich, Urban and Schwarzenberg, 1986.
20. Rosenberg R, Mettler FA: Emergency room management of radiation accidents. *In* Mettler FA, Kelsey CA, Ricks RC (eds): Medical Management of Radiation Accidents. Boca Raton, FL, CRC Press, pp 184–198, 1990.
21. Andrews GA, Cloutier FJ: Accidental acute radiation injury. Arch Environ Health *10*:498, 1965.
22. Nonstochastic Effects of Ionizing Radiation. International Commission on Radiological Protection (ICRP) Publication 41. Annals of the ICRP. Vol. 14, No. 3. Oxford, Pergamon Press, 1984.
23. Yamazaki JN, Schull WJ: Perinatal loss and neurological abnormalities among children of the atomic bomb. JAMA *264*:605, 1990.
24. Mettler FA: Assessment and management of local radiation injury. *In* Mettler FA, Kelsey CA, Ricks RC (eds): Medical Management of Radiation Accidents. Boca Raton, FL, CRC Press, pp 128–148, 1990.
25. Jamnet H, Daburon F, Gerber GB, et al: Radiation damage to the skin: Fundamental and practical aspects. Fr Br J Radiol *19*(Suppl):1, 1986.
26. Finch SC: Acute radiation syndrome. JAMA *258*:664, 1987.
27. Saenger EL: Radiation accidents. Ann Emerg Med *15*:1061, 1986.
28. Shipman TL, Lushbaugh CC, Peterson DF, et al: Acute radia-

tion death resulting from an accidental nuclear critical excursion. J Occup Med *1*:421, 1959.
29. Fanger H, Lushbaugh CC: Radiation death from cardiovascular shock following a criticality accident. Arch Pathol *83*:446, 1967.
30. Nagataki S, Shibata Y, Inoue S, et al: Thyroid diseases among atomic bomb survivors in Nagasaki. JAMA *272*:364, 1994.
31. Shimizu Y, Schull WJ, Kato H: Cancer risk among atomic bomb survivors. JAMA *264*:601–609, 1990.
32. Dobyns BM, Hyrmer BA: The surgical management of benign and malignant thyroid neoplasms in Marshall Islanders exposed to hydrogen bomb fallout. World J Surg *16*:126, 1992.
33. Hamilton TE, van Belle G, LoGerfo JP: Thyroid neoplasia in Marshall Islanders exposed to nuclear fallout. JAMA *258*:629–636, 1987.
34. Kazakov VS, Demidchik EP, Astakhova LN: Thyroid cancer after Chernobyl. Nature *359*:21, 1992.
35. Baverstock K, Egloff B, Ponchera A, et al: Thyroid cancer after Chernobyl. Nature *359*:21–22, 1992.
36. Ichimaru M, Ishimaru J, Belsky JL, et al: Incidence of leukemia in A-bomb survivors by dose, years after exposure, age and type of leukemia, 1950–71. RERF Technical Report 10–76. Hiroshima, Japan, Radiation Effects Research Foundation, 1976.
37. Mettler FA Jr, Upton AC: Medical Effects of Ionizing Radiation. 2nd ed. Philadelphia, W.B. Saunders Co., 1995.
38. Otake M, Schull WJ: *In utero* exposure to A-bomb radiation and mental retardation: A reassessment. Br J Radiol *57*:409–414, 1984.
39. Otake M, Yoshimaru H, Schull WJ: Severe mental retardation among the prenatally exposed survivors of the atomic bombing in Hiroshima and Nagaski: A comparison of the T65DR and DS86 dosimetry systems. RERF Technical Report 16–87. Hiroshima, Japan, Radiation Effects Research Foundation, 1987.
40. Sinskey RM: The status of lenticular opacities caused by atomic radiation. Am J Ophthalmol *39*:285–293, 1955.
41. Kumar P, Jagetia GC: A review of triage and management of burn victims following a nuclear disaster. Burns *20*:397–402, 1994.
42. Milroy WG: Management of irradiated and contaminated casualty victims. Emerg Med Clin North Am *2*:667–686, 1984.
43. Pons P, Sullivan JB Jr: Radiation and radioactive emergencies. *In* Sullivan Jr JB, Krieger GR (eds): Hazardous Material Toxicology: Clinical Principles of Environmental Health. Baltimore, Williams & Wilkins, pp 441–450, 1992.
44. Linnermann RE: Soviet medical responses to the Chernobyl nuclear accident. JAMA *258*:637–643, 1987.
45. Gale RP, Butturini A, Baranov A: Radiation accidents: Primum non nocere. Bone Marrow Transplant *11*:421–424, 1993.
46. Gale RP: Immediate medical consequences of nuclear accidents. JAMA *258*:625–628, 1987.
47. Baranov A, Gale RP, Guskova A, et al: Bone marrow transplantation after the Chernobyl nuclear accident. N Engl J Med *321*:205–212, 1989.
48. Becker DV: Reactor accidents: Public health strategies and their medical implications. JAMA *258*:649–654, 1987.
49. Melo DR, Lipsztein JL, de Oliveira CAN, et al: ^{137}Cs internal contamination involving a Brazilian accident, and the efficacy of prussian blue treatment. Health Phys *66*:245–252, 1994.
50. Durakovic A: Radioactive agents in medicine. Arh Hig Rada Toksikol *44*:331, 1993.
51. Kligerman MM, Turrisi AT, Urtasan RC, et al: Final report on Phase I trial of WR-2721 before protracted fractionated radiation therapy. Int J Radiat Oncol Biol Phys *14*:1119, 1988.
52. Gale RP, Butturini A: Medical response to nuclear and radiation accidents. Occup Med *6*:581–596, 1991.
53. Brandao-Mello CE, Oliveira AR, Valverde NJ, et al: Clinical and hematological aspects of ^{137}Cs: the Goiania radiation accident. Health Phys *60*:31–39, 1990.
54. Champlin R: Treatment for victims of nuclear accidents: The role of bone marrow transplantation. Radiat Res *113*:205–210, 1988.

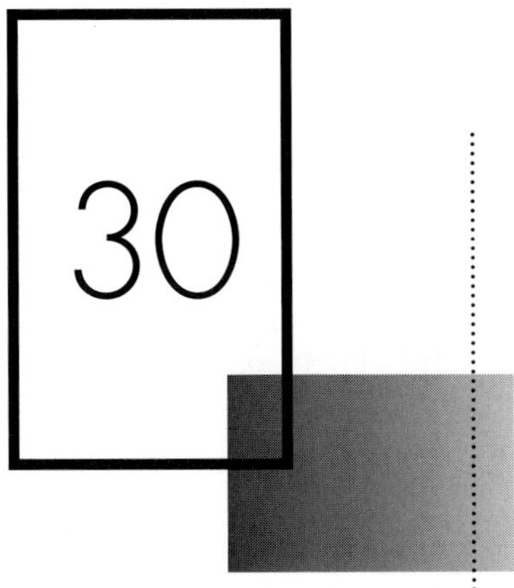

Environmental Toxicology

SCOTT D. PHILLIPS, MD

Environmental medicine is a discipline that has emerged out of the interface of people with their surroundings. Many professionals have traditionally dealt with this area, including occupational medicine specialists, internal medicine physicians, family practitioners, emergency physicians, medical toxicologists, public health practitioners, and others. Relevant government agencies include the Environmental Protection Agency (EPA), the Agency for Toxic Substance Disease Registry (ATSDR), other United

States public health agencies such as the Centers for Disease Control and Prevention, and state and local agencies. Nonmedical professionals are commonly involved. Hydrologists, engineers, ecologists, agronomists, environmental lawyers, and others frequently participate in this field. This discipline has arisen during our century partly as a result of environmental contamination during the World Wars. Many notable examples include Love Canal; Times Beach, Missouri; the Exxon oil tanker spill in Valdez, Alaska; the explosion of the Union Carbide plant in Bhopal, India; and the Chernobyl disaster.

The signs and symptoms of illness that may occur are not unlike those in other fields of medicine. It is the process of evaluating patients, determining causation, and preventing further exposures that makes this field unique. Environmental medicine has developed into a specialty that focuses on environmental sources of illness rather than on illness of occupational origin. These types of exposures tend to affect large segments of the population by means of air, water, and soil pollution; thermal illness; radiation poisoning; noise exposure; chemical carcinogenesis; and others.

Chemical exposures in environmental toxicology are similar to those in the occupational setting. Treatment may be different, in that the typical dose incurred is less in patients with environmental illness. Environmental toxicology is also characterized by a greater length of exposure and a larger population exposed in a poorly controlled setting. The total dose may be lower. Because of this, the paucity of data limits clinicians' attempts to demonstrate causation. As this area grows, more subjects will be adopted by this discipline.

Physicians tend to have limited formal training in the field of environmental toxicology. Because the lay public have a heightened sense of environmental awareness, they are frequently willing to participate in environmental risk assessment and community action committees. Public awareness of the possible health effects of contamination has been increased by coverage in the lay press. Depending on the toxin, some substances have a very substantial biologic persistence, which may increase the public's concern. The goal of environmental toxicologists is to integrate aspects of these various disciplines in order to provide accurate and reliable risk communication to the public.

Physicians are trusted individuals and may be called on to communicate risks to the public. They may recommend breast self-examination for cancer or explain the health effects of ground water contamination. Physicians are usually comfortable communicating about medical risks, yet when unfamiliar chemicals are found in soil samples, they often have more difficulty conveying the real risk to the public. How to communicate risk is one of the most important skills that a practitioner in the field of environmental toxicology can learn. It is important to recognize that people never face zero risk. Putting risk in perspective in a rational, caring, open manner is a skill that develops only with much effort.

The risk of environmental contamination may come from the air, water, soil, or food supply. Pollutants move between phases, or media, in the environment. These include the air, water, and soil. Pollutants discharged into water may move into the soil or may evaporate into the air. One cannot think of exposures as resulting from only one medium. In evaluating a patient with a potential exposure, it is important to consider also the work and home as other important environments. Consider exposures from all media when evaluating a patient. Environmental and occupational toxicology, not unlike occupational medicine, is an arena that lends itself as a form of preventive medicine.

The dearth of information about environmental exposures frequently handicaps toxicologists. Chronic low-dose exposure makes it difficult to establish causation in many cases. Physicians may serve as risk communicators, attempting to provide answers to those potentially exposed. Because antidotes for environmental exposures seldom exist, information becomes the most important asset that a toxicologist has to offer. It is difficult if not impossible to obtain accurate scientific information on the long-term health consequences and the potential for carcinogenesis from low-level exposures.

This section provides an overview of environmental toxicology. Specific evaluations of air pollution, including ozone, particulates, oxides of nitrogen, and others, are reviewed. Ozone and oxides of nitrogen may cause oxidative damage to the respiratory tract, whereas acid aerosols and sulfates may result in more respiratory complaints from a direct irritative action. People exposed to these pollutants make more frequent emergency department visits on days with high levels in the air. Particulates have also been shown to be responsible for an increase in respiratory disease patterns. The current Clean Air Act (CAA) standard restricts the National Ambient Air Quality Standards (NAAQS) to the mass concentration of inhalable particles ≤ 10 μm aerodynamic diameter (PM_{10}). This may not be sufficient to prevent pulmonary complaints. This chapter examines each of these toxicants and their contribution to the health effects of air pollution.

This chapter also discusses the role of chemicals in the development of cancer. Chemicals may directly alter gene characteristics or affect gene regulation. New tumor suppressor genes and proto-oncogenes are identified daily. Each new gene discovery foretells the promise of beneficial therapy and the potential for ethical conflict. Cancers in certain industries result from various chemicals. Chemicals tend to cause specific tumors in specific sites, and this chapter elucidates how this varies from one species to another. An important point to remember is that the types of cancer that are increasing in our society tend to be preventable. Most notable are those due to ultraviolet light, diet, and smoking. It is estimated that 30% of cancers are preventable. This translates into tens of thousands of lives potentially saved each year. An in-depth discussion of cancer biology follows. Chemicals may cause cancer and other maladies, such as effects on reproductive health, behavioral abnormalities, chronic lung diseases, and birth defects.

Finally, any benefits and the potential for harm from medical monitoring programs are discussed. These programs evaluate populations exposed to some level of a substance, usually with cancer as the endpoint, the hope being that early detection will result in a cure. Such measures initially appear useful when screening for cancer, but each test we perform has a risk and a benefit. The risks sometimes outweigh the advantage of a test. For example, chest surgery for a false-positive lesion in the lung carries a 1% to 2% mortality. A screening chest radiograph in a nonsmoker, which has only a 1% to 25% positive predictive value, is still safer. Clearly, one must approach this area with caution when recommending a medical monitoring program to a group.

The field of environmental medicine is growing. As with any new area of medicine, it will have its stumbling blocks. The American College of Occupational and Environmental Medicine and the American Academy of Clinical Toxicology recognize environmental medicine as an important discipline.

AIR POLLUTION

Perhaps the exposure medium that reaches the largest portion of the population is the air we breathe. Enactment of the CAA occurred in 1963 in response to a growing air pollution problem. The CAA is regulated under the auspices of the United States Environmental Protection Agency (EPA), which is the primary federal agency responsible for enforcing the mandates of the act. However, input from state and local authorities regarding the control of air pollution makes this a multifaceted regulatory framework. The most recent amendment to the CAA of 1990 provided new goals for attaining required air standards. This federal statutory process primarily outlined the responsibility of individual states to achieve the necessary emission reductions. Should the states not be able to meet these statutes, the EPA will assume the task of meeting the mandated objectives. One of the more important aspects of the CAA is the mandate to establish standards for air contamination. These are defined in the NAAQS. The NAAQS standards determine the airborne concentration of pollutants, called *criteria pollutants* (Table 30–1), that may exist but create no adverse effect level. In addition to the primary standards, secondary standards provide a measure of protection to plants and animals within the environment. Within the United States, individual areas are designated by the amount of air pollution in their area relative to the standard. These include attainment, nonattainment, or unclassifiable within the standard. For areas of the country that are in attainment, the act requires them to prevent significant deterioration (PSD). These are the PSD requirements. Obviously, the primary concerns within the NAAQS are about areas within the country that are in nonattainment of the standards. In an area of nonattainment, standards are devised for local municipalities to bring them into compliance with the CAA. For areas of nonattainment, further inquiry determines the degree of air pollution control that is required. This is in part determined by the population statistics and the United States census bureau in that area. A significant population lives in areas of nonattainment (Fig. 30–1). Criteria pollutants may have different levels of severity. For example, oxides of sulfur and nitrogen and lead require control strategies in

Table 30–1. National Ambient Air Quality Standards of the Criteria Pollutants

Pollutant	Primary Standard*	Type of Average
Ozone	0.12 ppm† (235 μg/m³)	Maximum daily 1 h
PM_{10}	50 μg/m³	Annual arithmetic mean‡
	150 μg/m³	24-h mean‡
Sulfur dioxide	0.03 ppm	Annual arithmetic mean‡
	80 μg/m³	24 h§
Nitrogen dioxide	0.053 ppm	Annual arithmetic mean
	100 μg/m³	
Carbon monoxide	9 ppm (10 mg/m³)	8 h§
	35 ppm (40 mg/m³)	1 h§
Lead	1.5 μg/m³	Maximum quarterly average

*The primary standard is to protect against adverse health effects.

†The ozone standard is attained when the expected number of days per calendar year with a maximum hourly average concentration >0.12 ppm is ≤1 (averaged over the previous 3 y).

‡Particulate standards use PM_{10} (particles ≤10 μm in diameter) as the indicator pollutant. The annual standard is attained when the expected annual arithmetic mean concentration is ≤50 μg/m³; the 24-h standard is attained when the expected number of days per calendar year >150 μg/m³ is ≤ 1.

§Maximum quarterly average.

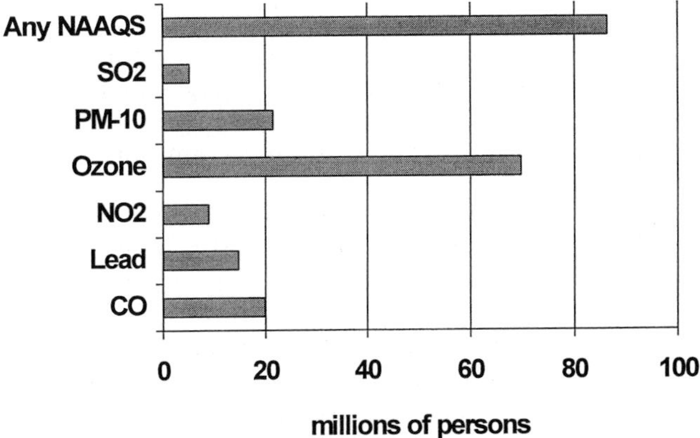

Figure 30–1. Number of people living in counties with measured air quality above primary National Ambient Air Quality Standards (NAAQS). Figures based on 1991 air quality data. (From Document No. 450-12-92-001 of the U.S. Environmental Protection Agency Office of Air Quality Planning and Standards.)

order to meet required standards, whereas carbon monoxide and particulate matter (PM) have two levels of classification. One of the more complicated criterion pollutants is ozone, which has five levels of classification. Discussions of air pollution usually consider only the individual components. However, it is the combined effect of these pollutants and their interrelations that ultimately determine health effects.

Research into air pollutants has provided many interesting findings. Pollutants may act as incitors or triggers when the airways are hyper-responsive and may result in transient airway narrowing. They may act as inducers increasing airway inflammation or may have a direct toxic effect on the airways, leading to asthma. They may affect the immune system, resulting in sensitization or increased allergic responses.

Dockery and colleagues[1] estimated the effects of air pollution on mortality in a follow-up study in six United States cities. The results suggest mortality rates most strongly associated with cigarette smoking, but after adjusting for this, the investigators observed a statistically significant association between air pollution and mortality. Air pollution is associated with death due to lung cancer and cardiopulmonary disease but not with death due to other causes. Mortality was most strongly associated with air pollution with fine particulates including sulfates but less so with others. The study also included evaluations of particles, aerosol acidity, sulfur dioxide (SO_2), nitrogen dioxide, and ozone. The six cities included Watertown, Massachusetts; Harriman, Tennessee (including Kingston); St. Louis, Missouri; Steubenville, Ohio; Portage, Wisconsin (including Wyocena and Pardeeville); and Topeka, Kansas. Total particulates were not associated with mortality. Small differences in ozone levels that range from 19.7 to 28 ppb limited the power of the study to detect any association between mortality and ozone level. Mortality relates levels of inhaled fine and sulfate particles with levels of either total particles, SO_2 levels, nitrogen dioxide levels, or aerosol activity. Total concentrations of particulates declined during the study period, whereas concentrations of fine particles and sulfate particles were relatively stable. The researchers believed they were unable to differentiate the influence of historical exposure from that of more recent exposure and the effect on mortality.

Sulfur Dioxide

When levels of SO_2 are especially high, asthmatic individuals may have increased symptoms after exertion. Because SO_2 is an irritant gas, it may trigger bronchial hyperreactivity. Inducers such as SO_2 are agents that increase airway inflammation or airway narrowing, leading to increased asthmatic episodes. In addition to SO_2, other nonspecific spasmogens include histamine, methacholine, exercise, hyperventilation, drying of the airway mucosa, fog, metabisulfite, and bradykinin. Air pollutants have effects on the airways of asthmatic subjects in several ways. SO_2 causes chest tightness and immediate bronchial constriction, but the concentration required depends to some extent on the degree of airway hyper-responsiveness. In asthmatic patients, bronchial constriction develops at concentrations greater than 1 ppm. With moderate exercise, however, bronchial constriction occurs in asthmatic patients at concentrations of 0.25 ppm.

Oxides of Nitrogen

Nitrogen oxide is a reddish-brown gas with an irritating odor. It combines with water to form nitric acid in the airways or atmosphere. Because of its low water solubility, its effects escape initial appreciation as it penetrates deep into the airways. Nitrogen oxides are responsible, in concentrated form, for silo filler's disease. A normal subject's exposure to high concentrations of nitrogen oxide has caused significant pulmonary injury; however, when at usual ambient air levels, nitrogen oxide causes small and inconsistent effects. Exposures to concentrations of less than 1 ppm have not had any significant effects. Long-term exposure of asthmatic patients, including patients with severe asthma, to nitrogen oxide in concentrations of 0.3 and 0.6 ppm and to ambient air in Los Angeles with a nitrogen oxide content of 0.09 ppm had no effect on airway function.[2] Even in patients with severe asthma, no significant evidence showed that nitrogen oxide effects are potentiated by other pollutants. However, nitrogen oxide concentrations of 0.4 ppm for 6 hours cause increased interleukin-8 and tumor necrosis factor-α (TNFα). Small increases in airway responsiveness have been reported at TNFα concentrations of 0.1 to 0.3 ppm. The responsiveness of normal and asthmatic subjects does not appear to differ. Reportedly, concentrations of 0.08 to 0.12 ppm for more than 6 hours increased airway hyper-responsivity in normal subjects. The long-term effects are difficult to evaluate, but because this compound is an oxidizer, potential adverse health effects may exist.

Ozone

Ozone, the major active product of photochemical smog, is a potent oxidant and an irritant to the respiratory system. This is a major component of the brown cloud that affects many large urban areas of the east and southern California. Levels of ozone and other oxidants such as nitrogen dioxide contribute to the air pollution in Mexico City. In the past, this effect of ozone was tempered by its short atmospheric persistence. Ozone concentrations would steadily increase throughout the morning to peak at midday and later decline. This pattern has changed in recent years. In areas of high traffic and ample sunlight, such as Los Angeles and Atlanta, the ambient ozone level frequently reaches 0.2 to 0.3 ppm. These levels may persist for several hours.

Ozone, unlike other criteria pollutants, has five classification levels: marginal, moderate, serious, severe, and extreme. In order to effect compliance, the EPA created time tables for November 1993 to November 2007. Ironically, the most polluted areas have the longest time in which to meet compliance. Individuals exposed at the highest levels have the longest exposure time and potentially receive the highest dose. This may result in a greater dose for those exposed.

Ozone is a secondary pollutant because it is generated photochemically. There are no emission sources for ozone. The contribution of ozone as a secondary pollutant was first recognized in southern California more than 40 years ago. Ozone results from the interaction between the effects of ultraviolet light on organic compounds and oxides of nitrogen emitted by traffic and industry (Fig. 30–2). Ozone is one of the main concerns in air pollution, and tens of millions of people are exposed.

Because of ozone's low water solubility, it tends to exert most of its pulmonary effects on the lower respiratory tract. Several studies have addressed the link between ozone concentration in the ambient atmosphere and hospital visits for asthma or other respiratory problems. These studies have had variable results; most show an association.[3] White and colleagues[4] evaluated emergency department visits by children with asthma at an inner city hospital in Atlanta, Georgia, during the summer of 1990 and found that hospital visits were significantly more numerous on days when the 1-hour maximum ozone level exceeded 0.11 ppm. No relationship was noted when the level of ozone was less than 0.11 ppm or with the mean 8-hour daily maximum of ozone. Asthmatic individuals and patients with chronic obstructive pulmonary disease do not appear to be more sensitive to ozone than is the general population.[5]

In 1971, the NAAQS set the level of photochemical oxidants at 0.08 ppm. This led the EPA in 1979 to re-establish an ozone-only standard of 0.12 ppm—a significant weakening of the standard. The CAA has set a schedule to tighten the ozone standard for those cities that are in nonattainment. The current ozone standard is 0.12 ppm. At this level, children experience increases in respiratory disease, loss of lung function, and greater bronchoreactivity, and mediators of inflammation occur. These effects occur at 0.08 ppm with prolonged exposure. This fact may be especially important in areas of the country that

$$NO_2 \xrightarrow{UV} NO^{\cdot} + O^{\cdot}$$
$$O^{\cdot} + O_2 \rightarrow O_3$$
$$O_3 + NO^{\cdot} \rightarrow NO_2$$

Figure 30–2. Generation of ozone photochemically by the action of ultraviolet radiation on nitrogen dioxide. Note the regenerating nature of the reaction.

commonly exceed 0.08 ppm of ozone for several hours a day.

The present NAAQS for ozone is 0.12 ppm (as a 1-hour maximum concentration), and the American Conference of Governmental Industrial Hygienists 8-hour threshold limit value–time-weighted average (TLV-TWA) is 0.1 ppm. A large proportion of the United States is in nonattainment of these standards. Atmospheric ozone levels tend to be highest in the late morning or afternoon. Ozone concentrations less than the NAAQS have caused pulmonary symptoms and functional abnormalities suggestive of bronchoconstriction.[6] Animal[7] and human[8] studies suggest that chronic exposure to ozone may cause permanent decline in pulmonary function.

Exposure of asthmatic subjects to 0.12 ppm of ozone for 1 hour caused a small increase in airway response to inhaled allergens but no increase in exercise-induced bronchial constriction. Ozone with high concentrations of 0.4 ppm for 4 hours has increased the eosinophilic inflammatory response to internasally applied allergens in atopic subjects. Most studies suggest that those ozone concentrations that may be present during the summer months may have a small effect on airway responsiveness.

Ozone is a strong oxidizing agent that can react with unsaturated lipids or other biomolecules to form free radicals, peroxides, and aldehydes. The role of ozone in pulmonary inflammation appears to be its ability to release leukotrienes, prostaglandins, and cytokines. Mediators released from macrophages and epithelial cells lining the respiratory tract may enhance inflammation.[9] In addition to its local effects, ozone appears to modulate the immune response[10] in a manner that depends on the time course and the dose. The function of natural killer lymphocytes is impaired.[11] Ozone may lead to enhanced susceptibility to bacterial growth, possibly through its effect on altered immune function. Researchers have found that ozone can cause sustained elevation of intracellular calcium.[12] This effect is blocked by verapamil, which causes intracellular storage release and blocks influx of calcium from the extracellular fluid. Studies are under way to establish the nature of the secretagogue that may be resulting in the influx of calcium. Studies examining the effects on bronchoalveolar lavage fluids have found that levels of neutrophils, albumin, and other serum proteins increased after exposure to 0.4 ppm of ozone.[13] This response of increased neutrophils suggests that ozone provokes the inflammatory response that is present for as long as 18 hours after exposure. The long-term effects of ozone in animals produce more centriacinar damage than the diffuse alveolar destruction occurring with emphysema. Although collagen may be deposited in the distal airways with significant exposures, this tends to result in more of a restrictive than obstructive defect. Many of the effects of ambient ozone exposure dissipate after 24 hours.

Efforts to reduce photochemical air pollution have not been as successful as with SO_2 emissions. SO_2 is emitted from point sources such as power plants, whereas photochemical air pollution is related to the volume of traffic. Efforts to reduce ozone have not been successful owing to the increase in vehicular travel.

Acid Aerosols

Acid rain is an air pollution issue that affects mostly the northeastern region of the United States. Inhalation of sulfuric acid fog at relevant concentrations has little or no effect on airway function in either normal or asthmatic individuals. Three classic episodes of major air pollution were associated with cold weather and still wind that caused polluted air to become trapped or inverted. These occurred in the Meuse Valley in Belgium in 1930; in Dondora, Pennsylvania, in 1948; in London, England, in 1952; and more recently in Mexico City. Findings of studies of the health effect of air pollution are difficult to interpret owing to confounders such as socioeconomic factors, coexistent aeroallergens, cigarette smoking, and others. In a large survey in Switzerland, no relationship was found between levels of air pollutants and respiratory symptoms in children apart from the association with total suspended particles. Also, considering the extent of air pollution in Los Angeles, no evidence shows that the prevalence of asthma is higher there than in any other areas of the United States.

Schwartz[14] compared patterns of death in the Harvard Six City Study and the London, England, smog epidemic of 1952. He examined death certificates from Philadelphia, Pennsylvania, on 5% of the days with the highest particulate of air pollution and 5% of the days with the lowest particulate of air pollution during the years 1973 to 1980. He found little difference in weather between the high- and low-pollution days, but total suspended particulate matter concentrations averaged 141 mg/m^3 on high-pollution days versus 47 mg/m^3 on low-pollution days. The relative risk of dying on high-pollution days was 1.08 ($P < .001$). The relative increase was higher for chronic obstructive pulmonary disease (1.25) and pneumonia (1.13). This pattern paralleled that in London in 1952, and the age pattern of relative risk of deaths was also similar.

Particulates

Particulate air pollution is a complex mixture of substances. These include carbon particles from fossil fuel combustion, dust, and acid aerosols. Particulate air pollution was originally referred to as total suspended particulate matter or PM. Particle size is a major determinant of the depth of penetration of inhaled particulates into the lungs. The toxicity of particles is a function of their surface-to-mass ratio, which increases with diminishing size. Particles are described by their size in micrometers. The term PM_{10} is used to describe particles that are less than 10 μm in diameter. Particles less than 10 μm in aerodynamic diameter may be inhaled into the alveoli, where mucociliary clearance is slow. The upper respiratory tract scavenges larger PM.

Two categories of particulates are described in the air pollution literature, depending on particle size. Larger (nonrespirable) particles result from erosion and abrasion nonpoint sources (agricultural tilling, dirt roads, and so on). Smaller respirable particles are generated by both stationary and mobile point sources. These include fossil fuel combustion engines, power plants, and so on. The smaller particles also tend to be acidic, which alters their toxicity.

The current 24-hour NAAQS for PM_{10} is 150 μg/m^3. The annual arithmetic mean standard is 50 μg/m^3. California has the most stringent PM standard in the United States, 50 μg/m^3. It is estimated by the EPA that 45% of the United States population reside in counties where the PM_{10} exceeds 50 μg/m^3.[15]

Data suggest that the PM_{10} (NAAQS) standard may not be protective, and a smaller particulate size standard may have more health benefits.[16] Another particulate measure that appears to be more protective is the $PM_{2.5}$. This designation refers to all particles with a diameter of equal to or greater than 2.5 μm. A prospective cohort study found an association between particulates and mortality.[17] A study of children in the Utah Valley, elevation of more than 4500 feet with frequent thermal inversions, found that particulates were associated with more frequent hospital admissions.[18] This occurred in 23% to 41% of healthy children. Emergency room visits and asthma medication use in Seattle[19] were associated with increased particulates even at levels below the PM_{10}. Small impairments in lung function do not occur in patients with obstructive lung disease.[17] These findings lend support to the movement toward lowering the particulate cutoff to $PM_{2.5}$.

Lead

Leaded gasoline is no longer widely available in the United States. Airborne lead has been a product of the combustion of alkyl lead fuel additives. The elimination of leaded gasoline resulted in a marked reduction in ambient levels of airborne lead.[20] Leaded gasoline is still available for agricultural equipment and in countries outside the United States. Average blood lead levels have correlated closely with airborne lead levels.[21] As ambient lead levels continue to decline, airborne lead may cease to be a major concern related to air quality. More information on lead poisoning is available in Chapter 57.

Carbon Monoxide

Carbon monoxide is a byproduct of incomplete combustion of carbon-based fossil fuels. In 1983 to 1984, the EPA conducted an exposure survey on population-based samples of nonsmoking adults from Washington, D.C., and Denver, Colorado.[22] In this study, the activity contributing most to overall exposure of nonsmokers to carbon monoxide was motor vehicle travel. Travel time exposures averaged 5 ppm, and average subjects spent a mean of 2 hours/day in transit. Automobile exhaust continues to be the major source of carbon monoxide. However, carbon monoxide is produced by cigarette smoking, manufacturing, wildfires, power equipment, barbecuing, and space heating. In workers who spend a significant amount of time in and about traffic (tunnel workers, police officers) or near combustion sources (concrete cutters and power equipment operators), long-term carbon monoxide exposure may result in a lowering of the angina threshold. The long-term neuropsychiatric sequelae are not well known. The rate of accumulation of carbon monoxide is dependent on the inspired concentration of carbon monoxide, the minute ventilation of the subject, and the diffusing capacity into the blood stream.

Carbon monoxide is one of the few inhaled pollutants that is not responsible for local effects in the lungs and appears to exert its effect through systemic dissemination only. Studies have demonstrated increased cardiovascular effects in patients with angina.[23] Chapter 70 offers a more in-depth discussion of carbon monoxide.

Other Air Pollutants

Studies of the health effects of multiple air pollutants have not been able to reproduce true air pollution because of the complexity of the task. Results have been variable but suggest an overall decrement in lung function. These imperfect studies require complex statistical methods to assess outcome. They are crucial to our understanding of air pollution, in that it is the mixture of pollutants that causes the real health concern.

The increased prevalence of asthma may be related to an increase of latex particles in the atmosphere.[24] Latex antigens are extractable from rubber tires and are abundant in air samples. The particles shed from radial tires are smaller than those from bias tires.[25] They may contribute to allergic responses directly or in conjunction with other particulates. Further studies are ongoing to evaluate this causal link. Many other air pollutants that exist in ambient air can reflect local industry.

Conclusions

Increasing evidence clearly suggests that ambient air pollution is responsible for an increase in respiratory disease exacerbation. The American Lung Association supports the reduction of the ozone standard to 0.07 ppm, or one-exceedance level. Consideration is needed for a more stringent particulate standard such as the $PM_{2.5}$. Efforts to reduce SO_2 emissions have been successful. This is proof of our ability to make significant changes in air quality. Ozone and nitrogen dioxide levels will continue to rise unless alternative fuels and mass transportation become acceptable.

CHEMICAL CARCINOGENESIS

First reports of chemical carcinogenesis are attributed to Paracelsus. By the 16th century, miners of Europe developed a chronic illness termed *bergkrankheiten*, later believed to be due to radon. Later studies identified excess bladder tumors in dyestuff workers. The attribution to synthetic dyes occurred in 1938. Later, bladder cancer due to the aromatic amines was noted in experimental animals. In 1775, Pott[26] described cancer of the scrotum in English chimney sweeps. This was attributed to polycyclic aromatic hydrocarbons. These substances are recognized by various organizations as human carcinogens.

The public fears that environmental chemical contamination may result in cancer. Although cancer-causing compounds are found in the environment, overall trends in new cases of cancer do not suggest that all types of cancer are increasing. Some believe that only the cancers related to tobacco, such as lung cancer,[27] are becoming more common.

Toxicologists become involved in cancer causation and prevention issues. Mutagenesis and tumor formation can be a type of end-organ response to chemicals in our environments and workplaces owing to sufficient exposure to toxic substances in susceptible hosts. These may be either benign or malignant. Benign tumors typically end in the suffix *-oma*. Examples include neuromas, fibromas, and lipomas. Malignant tumors occur in either the epidermis (ectoderm and endoderm) or the mesenchyma. Epithelium-derived malignant tumors are referred to as *carcinomas*, whereas tumors of mesenchymal origin are called *sarcomas*.

Several organizations are involved in the evaluation of chemical carcinogenesis. They attempt to determine if a substance is a carcinogen from *in vitro*, animal, and human experience. They then assign a rating of substances according to their ability to induce cancers. These organizations include the International Agency for Research on Cancer (IARC) of the World Health Organization, the EPA, and the National Toxicology Program (NTP) of the United States Public Health Service. These agencies categorize chemicals into groups according to their ability to cause malignant transformation. Carcinogenicity information is not available for all chemicals, because their review is a slow and tedious process. Ratings as either a 1 or A signify ample evidence to implicate the chemical as a carcinogen in humans. Benzene is a recognized human carcinogen according to all three organizations. Chemicals believed to be carcinogenic are listed in Table 30–2. Chemotherapeutic agents and ionizing radiation were purposefully omitted. Certain environmental scenarios or oc-

Table 30–2. Carcinogen Ratings by Several Organizations

Chemical	Recognized Human Carcinogens*		
	EPA	*IARC*	*NTP*
Aflatoxins		1	A
4-Aminobiphenyl		1	A
Arsenic	A	1	A
Asbestos	A	1	A
Benzene	A	1	A
Benzidine	A	1	A
Bis(chloroethyl)ether	A	1	A
Coal tars		1	A
Coke production		1	A
Chromium (VI)	A	1	A
Diethylstilbestrol	A	1	A
Direct black 38	A		B
Direct blue 6	A		B
Direct brown 95	A		
Estrogens		1	A
Methylhydrazine	A		
2-Naphthylamine		1	A
Nickel	A	1	A
Tobacco (smoke)		1	
Vinyl chloride	A	1	A

EPA, Environmental Protection Agency; IARC, International Agency for Research on Cancer; NTP, National Toxicology Program.
*Chemotherapeutic agents omitted.

cupations associated with certain forms of cancer are listed in Table 30–3.

Cancer Biology

A multistep model of carcinogenesis was proposed[28] as a two-stage process more than 50 years ago. This led to the terms *initiation* and *promotion*. This model is an oversimplified approach by our current standards. Many steps within these stages are required for tumors to progress. Carcinogenesis is currently described by a three-step model. These steps include initiation, promotion, and progression.

Chemicals may cause genetic damage by single base pair substitutions or gross chromosomal changes. These may lead to either altered gene expression or a change in the chemical function of the gene.[29] Genes of particular importance are those involved in the proliferation and differentiation of cells. These types of genes are known as proto-oncogenes or tumor suppressor genes.

Proto-oncogenes are normal cellular genes that when activated inappropriately as cancer genes, or *oncogenes*, cause altered regulation of growth and differentiation pathways enhancing the probability of neoplastic transformation by the cell. Tumor suppressor genes are normal cellular genes that when inactivated may allow dysregulation and enhance the probability of neoplastic transformation. It is now becoming clear that the development of tumors common in adults, those of the lung and breast, involve the loss or inactivation of multiple tumor suppressor genes or the activation of proto-oncogenes. The best-characterized example of this human tumor is that of the colon, in which three tumor suppressor genes (MCC, p53, DCC) and one proto-oncogene, K-*ras*, are frequently altered.[30]

These findings support a multistage model of tumor development. Chemicals, in the occupational setting, have long been known to be responsible for cancers. Tumors probably descend from a single altered cell, referred to as *monoclonal* in origin. Cells must undergo many changes after modification to result in a tumor. These steps are illustrated in Figure 30–3. A cell may be attacked by an electrophilic

Table 30–3. Occupational Cancers

Industry or Material	Carcinogen	Site of Associated Cancer*
Asbestos	Asbestos	Lung
Brewing	Alcohol	Liver
Commercial fishing	Ultraviolet light	Skin
Demolition	Asbestos	Lung
Furniture manufacturing	Wood dusts	Nasal
Glue factories	Benzene	Leukemia
Insulation	Asbestos	Lung
Ion-exchange resin production	Bis(chloromethyl)ether	Lung
Isopropyl alcohol manufacturing	Isopropyl alcohol	Lung
Mineral oil	Polycyclic hydrocarbons	Lung
Nickel refining	Nickel	Respiratory
Ore manufacturing	Chromium	Lung
Outdoor occupations	Ultraviolet light	Skin
Pesticides—arsenic	Arsenic	Lung, skin
Petroleum production	Polycyclic hydrocarbons	Lung
Pigment manufacturing	Chromium	Lung
Rubber manufacturing	Aromatic amines	Bladder
Shipyards	Asbestos	Lung
Smelters	Arsenic	Lung, skin
Uranium mining	Ionizing radiation	Lung, others
Varnish	Benzene	Leukemia
Vinyl chloride	Vinyl chloride	Liver

From Costanza ME, Li FP, Greene HL, et al: Cancer Manual. 8th ed. Framingham, MA, American Cancer Society, Massachusetts Division, p 44, 1990.

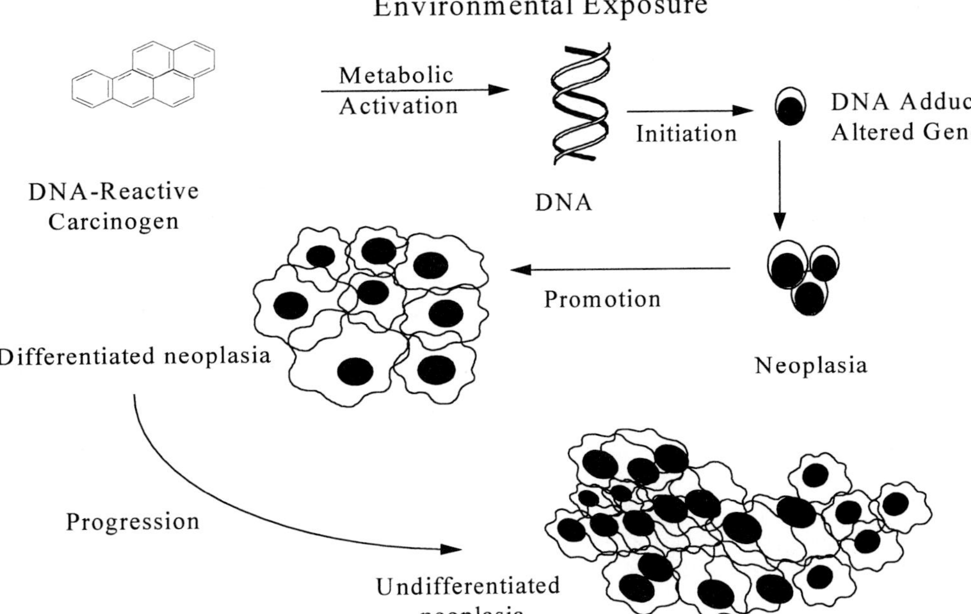

Figure 30–3. Pathway of possible environmental carcinogenesis. A DNA reactive molecule forms a substrate-DNA adduct causing initiation. Promoters result in tumor formation, which can evolve to a metastatic tumor mass.

chemical that can covalently bind to the cell's DNA. This forms a DNA adduct, which may result in initiation. In the presence of a promoter, this process may lead to tumor development. Repair mechanisms are in place to combat the constant barrage of chemical attacks on the genome, such as free radical scavengers or tumor suppressor genes. Attempts to categorize the carcinogens according to the mechanisms of action are not always possible because a single carcinogen may have many effects and hence may be perceived as operating by several mechanisms.

Genetic changes induced by chemical carcinogens could include gene mutations, gene amplifications, chromosomal rearrangement, and aneuploidy. Specific examples are identified for each of these genetic changes. One such example is the observation of point mutations activating proto-oncogenes or inactivating tumor suppressor genes in certain cancers. Chromosomal rearrangements leading to activation of proto-oncogenes or inactivation of tumor suppressor genes are also documented.

Chemical carcinogen binding to DNA can be noted using radiolabeled carcinogens. Carcinogen-DNA adducts differ quantitatively and qualitatively in their mutagenic potential. Moreover, the adduct concentrations obtained with some carcinogens may vary widely among cell types of given tissues.[31] The carcinogen-derived adducts and adducted bases in cells and tissues can be eliminated spontaneously by DNA repair processes.

Historically, carcinogenesis can be divided into two to four phases. These have included initiation, promotion, and progression. The first interaction of chemical with DNA is initiation. Tumor promoters facilitate clonal expansion. Those initiated divide to form increased numbers of cancer cells. Progression is the process that allows the cells to become malignant cancers.

Carcinogenesis is a multistage process of induction followed by promotion and progression. The concept of a multistage process in carcinogenesis was first recognized during skin cancer experiments in mice. Polycyclic aromatic hydrocarbons (inducer) applied to the skin in extremely low doses resulted in tumors. No skin tumors developed during the rodents' lifetime. This application was followed by weekly topical doses of croton oil, a promoter, which resulted in multiple skin tumors. Significant delays of as much as a year before application of the promoter resulted in a similar amount of tumors.[32] Initiators alter the genetic material of the cell and do not result in cancer after a single exposure. These chemicals are genotoxic and bind to DNA. Multiple applications of an initiator may result in tumor formation. Promoters, on the other hand, are not carcinogenic and do not bind to DNA as do initiators; rather, they permit the initiated cell to develop into a neoplasia. Rarely, a chemical may be both an initiator and promoter. When both properties are attributed to one substance, the substance is described as a complete carcinogen. Carcinogens may be termed either *primary carcinogens* or *procarcinogens*. The former directly act with DNA as a genotoxin, and the latter require metabolic activation before they can interact with the genome.

Most xenobiotics that cause cancer require some type of metabolic alteration. Typically this is conversion to highly reactive electrophils,[33] as was discovered more than 20 years ago with the metabolism of azo dyes. The enzyme most likely to result in activation of the substrate is of the P-450 enzyme system. Distinct P-450s are involved in the activation of specific types of chemical carcinogen processes. For example, Koop and colleagues[34] have shown that P-450IIE1 metabolizes benzene, and Hammons and associates[35] have shown that P-450IA2 metabolizes 4-aminobiphenyl–hemoglobin adduct formation.

Chemicals may be activated in one region of the body yet result in cancer in another. For example, certain direct-acting chemicals such as *N*-methylnitrosourea are activated in the liver. Certain chemical carcinogens show target organ specificity. A chemical that requires metabolic activation but results in distant carcinogenesis is acrylonitrile. This conversion to cyanoethylene oxide occurs in the liver and is distributed throughout the body. After this distribution, cancer may develop in the brain without evidence of cancer at other sites. Elimination routes are important in terms of the location of cancer. Some metabolites excreted in the urine result in bladder cancer. Chemical carcinogenesis tends to be site specific.

Carcinogenic compounds apparently bind covalently to DNA or RNA, resulting in induction. This covalent binding to DNA results in chemical-DNA adducts. These may function either as inducers or as promoters. Certain genes, targeted by chemical carcinogens, can be linked to disturbances of growth and differentiation. These *proto-oncogenes* are numerous. They may alter growth or differentiation by one of several mechanisms, including point mutations, chromosome translocations, or gene amplification. Inactivation of tumor suppressor genes may also occur, resulting in expression of tumorigenic processes.

Carcinogens may act on cellular constituents including proteins, lipids, or nucleic acids or may act directly with the genetic material within the cell. Certain carcinogens require "activation," whereas others may directly interact with those cellular components resulting in the cascade of chemical carcinogenesis. Chemicals that require metabolic activation are termed *indirect acting*. They are generally stable in an environment and are commonly encountered by the general population. Metabolic activity is affected by many factors including species, gender, age, diet, enzyme-inducing substances, and other factors. Indirect-acting carcinogens may be known as *precarcinogens* or *procarcinogens*. Most indirect-acting xenobiotics, including those that are carcinogens, are detoxified by oxidation to result in the ultimate carcinogen. These reactions typically are through the P-450 system. A theoretic example of indirect carcinogenesis from benzo[*a*]pyrene is shown in Figure 30–3.

Relatively few carcinogens are direct acting because, by their nature, they are chemically unstable. An example of this would include ethylene diamine, β-propiolactone, bis(chlormethyl)ether, bis(2-chloroethyl)sulfide, diepoxybutane, ethylene oxide, methyl methane sulfonate, and nitrogen mustard (e.g., cyclophosphamide). Many of these compounds are alkylators of cellular macromolecules. These generally act at the seven positions of guanine and cytosine. By definition, direct-acting carcinogens do not require metabolic activation for this interaction to occur. Direct-acting carcinogens may not be as potent because these species are so reactive, and intervening metabolic processes occur before they reach their final receptor. Compounds that have less reactivity may in fact be more potent. However, most direct-acting carcinogens do not represent an appreciable hazard to the general population except for those involved in the treatment of patients with chemotherapeutic agents.

Rarely are we exposed to a single chemical. Rather, mixtures tend to be the usual source of exposure. One substance may predominate. Examples of these would include tobacco smoke and diesel exhaust fumes. The interactions of various mixtures may result in enhanced, reduced, or no significant effect on carcinogenesis. Mixtures may provide both inducers and promoters, resulting in an augmented effect.

It is unknown whether carcinogens act as initiators by causing point mutations activating oncogenes, cause deletions in growth suppressor genes, act on elements that regulate transcription, or induce changes in DNA amplification. Carcinogens are generally classified as either genotoxic or epigenetic; however, this distinction is complicated by the absence of a clear-cut criterion for defining genotoxicity.

Genotoxic carcinogens are those that either react with genetic material or are converted by metabolism to react as intermediates forming adducts with genetic material, the cell. Direct- and indirect-acting carcinogens are considered to be genotoxic carcinogens. Nongenotoxic or epigenetic carcinogens do not appear to bind to DNA of the cell but may form adducts with other cellular constituents. Materials such as films and fibers are epigenetic carcinogens. Also, certain physiochemical factors such as osmolarity or abnormal pH induced by some nonphysiologic condition may lead to the development of cancer by epigenetic mechanisms. This may be especially true in the bladder. Certain conditions that allow the formation of crystals and calculi in the bladder, especially in male rats, have led to bladder tumors with lifetime high-level exposure. This occurs with saccharine.

It has long been known that specific chemicals cause tumor in specific organs. This is termed *organotropism*.[36] The organ specificity of chemicals has significant interspecies similarity. For example, vinyl chloride induces angiosarcomas of the liver in rats, mice, hamsters, and humans.[37] Certain carcinogens have species-dependent organ specificity. 2-Naphthylamine causes bladder cancer in dogs, monkeys, and humans and is known to produce hepatomas in mice but has not been shown to be carcinogenic in cats or rabbits.[38] Factors that determine tissue specificity include species strain, route of exposure, pharmacokinetics, DNA modification repair, promotion, and specific target genes. Examples of organ-specific carcinogens include many familiar agents. A more complete list appears in Table 30–4.

Animal Carcinogenicity Tests

Long-term carcinogenicity studies are conducted on various agents believed to induce cancers. Rodent

Table 30–4. Chemical Carcinogens and Their Selected Sites

Site	Carcinogen
Lung	Asbestos, arsenic, chloromethyl ethers, chromium, mustard gas, nickel, polyaromatic hydrocarbons, radon
Hematopoietic system	Ionizing radiation, benzene
Urinary tract	Benzidine, 4-biphenylmeamine, 2-naphthylamine, 2-naphthylamine; *N,N*-bis(2-chloroethyl)-2H-1,3,2-oxazakphosphorine; 2-(bis)2-chloroethyl (amino), tetrahydro-,2-oxide, purine; 6-(1-methyl-4-nitroimidazol-5-yl), thyo- + ; polycyclic aromatic hydrocarbons, asbestos, ionizing radiation
Gastrointestinal system	Aflatoxins, hemangiosarcoma, Thiotrast (thorium dioxide), steroids (both antibiotic and estrogen types of steroids), vinyl chloride, arsenic
Endocrine system	Ionizing radiation (breast cancer)
Germ cell	Ionizing radiation, asbestos, dimethylformamide, chromates
Central nervous system	Vinyl chloride, acrylonitrile, nitrosoureas, lead acetate, diethyl and dimethyl sulfate, ethylene oxide, 1,3-propane sulfone, ionizing radiation
Skin	Ultraviolet radiation, arsenic, polycyclic aromatic hydrocarbons

studies are commonly conducted for a defined period. This typically is two species in two sexes for 2 years. With these techniques, chemical carcinogens lead to a significant increase in incidence of neoplasias of one or more tissue types in the exposed animals when compared with an appropriate control group. To determine the appropriate dose for the long-term assay, information is obtained from short-term 90-day exposures. Doses are then decreased from the 90-day dose typically to a dose that does not alter the normal growth or survival patterns in these animals. Results obtained from these types of long-term assays do provide information about common and uncommon neoplasias. Evidence includes progression of tumors, latency of tumors, multiplicity, metastases, dose-response relationships, and structure-activity relationships.

An evolving approach is the use of transgenic testing. This can be performed either in vitro or in vivo. Transgenic cells are created when a specific gene is introduced along with a promoter into a cell to determine tumor induction when exposed to a specific chemical or substrate. Transgenic animals are used as a way of studying the consequences of introduction of various proto-oncogenes and activated oncogenes into specific tissue sites. This is a very exciting field because transgenic mice respond within weeks to months when exposed to a carcinogen. With this method, a great deal of information can be collected in a relatively short period.

Short-term tests for mutagenicity typically are *in vitro* studies. The basis for these tests is the assumption that all carcinogens are mutagenic. Many agents known to be carcinogenic in humans are also mutagenic. A number of short-term tests are available. Each has in common the use of genetic damage as an endpoint. The most widely known is the mutagenicity assay developed by Ames and colleagues.[39] In this test, bacterial cells that are deficient in DNA repair lack the ability to grow without histidine. The bacterial cells are treated with several dose levels of the chemical compound. They revert to a histidine-positive phenotype. This causes the bacteria, typically *Salmonella typhimurium*, to mutate away from histidine. Mammalian mutation assays include the mouse lymphoma L5178Y assay, the Chinese hamster ovary assay, and the V79 fibroblast assay, as well as others. Tests may investigate the indirect incorporation of radiolabeled thymidine into DNA as a repair mechanism.

Human Biomarkers

Two general types of biomarkers for cancer have been identified. These include genetic and nongenetic tests. Certain tumor markers are measured in biologic fluids. We are familiar with the nongenetic forms of biomarkers. These include prostate-specific antigen, carcinoembryonic antigen, 5′-nucleotidase, and many others. A complete listing of these and their uses may be found in current oncology texts. Genetic biomarkers are now being investigated. The most notable are the *BRCA1* and *BRCA2* cancer susceptibility genes. The *BRCA1* gene was first localized in 1990 by Hall and associates at the University of California at Berkeley.[40] Using linkage analysis, they mapped these genes to an area on the long arm of chromosome 17 (q12-q21). *BRCA1* codes for a protein of 1863 amino acids. Most mutations (±70%) of the *BRCA1* gene involve truncation of the protein. Some researchers have suggested that women who are heterozygous for mutations of these genes may have as much as a 90% lifetime risk for cancer of the breast, colon, and other sites.[41–43]

Researchers reported that one in six people in the United States lack the gene *GSTT1*, which appears to be responsible for detoxification of chemical carcinogens. Lack of this gene is associated with an increased risk of myelodysplastic syndrome.[44]

The prospects of having these cancer susceptibility genes raise important and difficult questions in the area of industry and pre-employment testing. Will people who lack a tumor suppressor gene be prohibited from participating in an industry with adequate safeguards?

CONCLUSIONS

Our knowledge of chemical-induced carcinogenesis is rapidly progressing. The genome has been mapped, and each year many new genes are identified as being linked to cancer, such as the *GSTT1* gene and chemical detoxification and the *BRCA1* gene and breast cancer.

The prevention of environmental and occupational cancers can best be obtained by elimination of tobacco products. Tobacco use reportedly accounts for as many as 30% of all cases of newly diagnosed cancers in the United States. In fact, according to Doll and Petro,[27] no recent dramatic increased risk of cancers has occurred in the United States except for those due to asbestos in tobacco products. This implies that cancer risk can be effectively controlled in various workplaces and that some cancers thus can be eliminated. Studies on population or case-specific screening are not beneficial.

References

1. Dockery DW, Pope CA, Xu X, et al: An association between air pollution and mortality in six U.S. cities. N Engl J Med *329*:1753–1759, 1993.
2. Bauer MA, Utell MJ, Morrow PE, et al: Route of inhalation influences airway responses to 0.30 ppm nitrogen dioxide in asthmatic subjects. Abstract. Am Rev Respir Dis *133*:A171, 1985.
3. Lipfert FW, Ammerstrom TH: Temporal patterns in air pollution and hospital admissions. Environ Res *59*:374–399, 1992.
4. White MC, Etzel RA, Wilcox WD, Lloyd C: Exacerbations of childhood asthma and ozone pollution in Atlanta. Environ Res *65*:56–68, 1994.
5. Kreit JW, Gross KB, Moore TB, et al: Ozone-induced changes in pulmonary function and bronchial responsiveness in asthmatics. J Appl Physiol *66*:217–222, 1989.
6. Folinsbee LJ, McDonnell WF, Hortsman DH: Pulmonary function and symptom responses after 6.6 hour exposure to 0.12 ppm ozone with moderate exercise. J Air Pollut Control Assoc *38*:28–35, 1988.
7. Johnson DA: Ozone inactivation of human $alpha_1$-antiprotease inhibitor. Am Rev Respir Dis *121*:1031–1038, 1980.
8. Detels R, Tashkin DP, Sayre JW, et al: The UCLA population studies of chronic obstructive lung disease. 9. Lung function changes associated with chronic exposure to photochemical oxidants; a cohort study among never-smokers. Chest *92*:594–603, 1987.
9. Salari H, Wong A: Generation of platelet activating factor (PAF) by a human lung epithelial cell line. Eur J Pharmacol *175*:253–259, 1989.
10. Jakab GJ, Spannhake EW, Canning BJ, et al: The effects of ozone on immune function. Environ Health Perspect *103* (Suppl 2):77–89, 1995.
11. Burleson GR, Keyes LL, Stutzman JD: Immunosuppression of pulmonary natural killer activity by exposure to ozone. Immunopharmacol Immunotoxicol *11*:715–735, 1989.
12. Qu QS, Chen LC: Modulation of Ca^{2+} influx by a mediator released from human tracheal epithelial cells exposed to ozone *in vitro*. Am J Physiol *268*:L558–L564, 1995.
13. Koren HS, Devlin RB, Graham DE, et al: Ozone-induced inflammation in the lower airways of human subjects. Am Rev Respir Dis *139*:407–415, 1989.
14. Schwartz J: What are people dying of on high pollution days? Environ Res *64*:26–35, 1994.
15. Current Estimates from the National Health Interview Survey—United States, 1991. US Department of Health and Human Services, Washington, DC, 1992.
16. Lipfert FW, Malone RG, Daum ML, et al: A Statistical Study of the Macroepidemiology of Air Pollution and Total Mortality. Upton, NY, Brookhaven National Laboratories, 1988.
17. Wichmann HE, Mueller W, Alhoff P, et al: Health effects during a smog episode in West Germany in 1985. Environ Health Perspect *79*:89–99, 1989.
18. Pope CA, Dockery DW, Xu X, et al: Mortality risks of air pollution: A prospective cohort study. Am Rev Respir Dis *147*:A13, 1993.
19. Schwartz J, Slater D, Larson TV, et al: Particulate air pollution and hospital emergency room visits for asthma in Seattle. Am Rev Respir Dis *147*:826–831, 1993.
20. U.S. Environmental Protection Agency: Air Quality Criteria for Lead. Vols. VII and XI. Research Triangle Park, NC, US Environmental Protection Agency, 1986. EPA Publication EPA-600/8-83/028.
21. Mahaffey KR, Annest JL, Roberts J, Murphy RS: National estimates of blood lead levels: United States, 1976–1980. Association with selected demographic and socioeconomic factors. N Engl J Med *307*:573–579, 1982.
22. Akland GG, Hartwell TD, Johnson TF, Whitmore RW: Measuring human exposure to carbon monoxide in Washington, DC, and Denver, Colorado, during the winter of 1982–1983. Environ Sci Technol *19*:911–918, 1985.
23. Allred EN, Bleecker ER, Chaitman BR, et al: Short-term effects of carbon monoxide exposure on the exercise performance of subjects with coronary artery disease. N Engl J Med *321*:1426–1432, 1989.
24. Williams PB, Buhr MP, Weber RW, et al: Latex allergen in respirable particulate air pollution. J Allergy Clin Immunol *95*:88–95, 1995.
25. Bogdan L, Albrechinski TM: Characterization of tire wear particles. Washington, DC, US Department of Commerce, 1981. EPA Publication PB82-153586.
26. Pott P: Cancer Scroti. *In* The chirurgical works of Percival Pott. London, Hawes, Clarke, Collins, pp 734–736, 1775.
27. Doll R, Petro R: The causes of cancer: Quantitative estimates of avoidable risks of cancer in the United States today. J Natl Cancer Inst *66*:1191–1308, 1981.
28. Mottram JC: The origin of tar tumours in mice, whether from single cells or many cells. J Pathol *40*:407–409, 1935.
29. Bishop JM: The molecular genetics of cancer. Science *235*:305–311, 1987.
30. Fearon ER, Vogelstein B: The genetic model for colorectal tumorogenesis. Cell *61*:759–767, 1990.
31. Belinsky SA, White CM, Devereux TR, et al: Cell selective alkylation of DNA in rat lung following low dose exposure to the tobacco specific carcinogen 4-(*N*-Methyl-*N*-Nitrosamino)-1-(3-pyridyl)-1-butanone. Cancer Res *47*:1143–1148, 1987.
32. Peraino C, Jones CA: The multistage concept of carcinogenesis. *In* Sirca AE (ed): The Pathobiology of Neoplasia. New York, Plenum Publishing Corp., pp 131–148, 1989.
33. Miller EC: Some current perspectives on chemical carcinogenesis in humans and experimental animals: Presidential address. Cancer Res *38*:1479–1496, 1978.
34. Koop DR, Laethem CL, Schnier GG: Identification of ethanol-inducible P450 isozyme 3a (P450IIE1) as a benzene and phenol hydroxylase. Toxicol Appl Pharmacol *98*:278–288, 1989.
35. Hammons GJ, Dooley KL, Kadlubar FF: 4-Aminobiphenyl-hemoglobin adduct formation as an index of *in vivo* *N*-oxidation by hepatic cytochrome P-450IA2. Chem Res Toxicol *4*:144–147, 1991.
36. Rice JM, Frith CH: The nature of organo specificity chemical carcinogenesis. *In* Langebach R, Nes S, Rice JM (eds): New York, Plenum Publishing Corp., pp 1–22, 1983.
37. Etoni C, Lefemine G: Carcinogenicity bioassay of vinyl chloride: Current results. Ann N Y Acad Sci *246*:185–218, 1975.
38. Dong Z, Jeffrey AM: Mechanisms of organs specificity and chemical carcinogenesis. Cancer Invest *8*:523–533, 1990.
39. Ames BN, Durston WE, Yamasaki E, Lee FD: Carcinogens are mutogens: A simple test system combining liver homogenates for activation in bacteria for detection. Proc Natl Acad Sci U S A *70*:2281–2285, 1973.
40. Hall JM, Lee MK, Newman B, et al: Linkage of early-onset familial breast cancer to chromosome 17q21. Science *250*: 1684, 1990.
41. Hoskins KF, Stopfer JE, Calzone KA, et al: Assessment and counseling for women with family history of breast cancer. A guide for clinicians. JAMA *273*:577–585, 1995.

42. Offit K, Brown K: Quantitating familial cancer risk: A resource for clinical oncologists. J Clin Oncol *12*:1724–1785, 1994.
43. Marcus JN, Watson P, Page DL, et al: Hereditary breast cancer: Pathobiology, prognosis, and BRCA1 and BRCA2 gene linkage. Cancer *77*:697–709, 1996.
44. Chen H, Dandler DP, Taylor JA, et al: Increased risk for myelodysplastic syndromes in individuals with glutathione transferase theta (GSTT1) gene defect. Lancet *347*:295–297, 1996.
45. Weisburger EK: Chemical carcinogenesis in experimental animals and humans. *In* Sirica AE (ed): The Pathobiology of Neoplasia. New York, Plenum Publishing Corp., pp 39–56, 1989.

SECTION B

CENTRALLY ACTIVE AGENTS

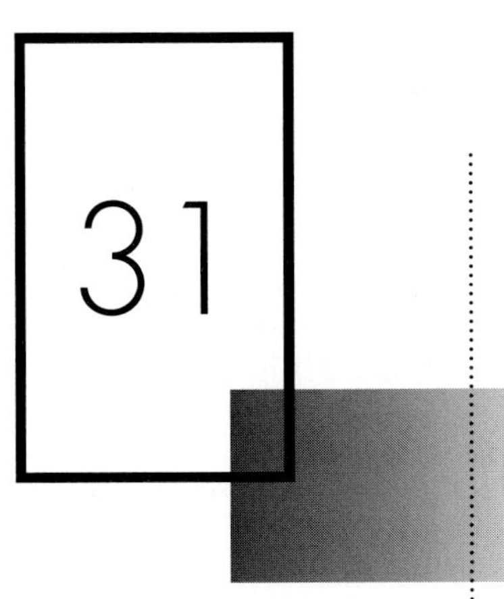

Tricyclic Antidepressants and Selective Serotonin Reuptake Inhibitors

PAUL R. PENTEL, MD
DANIEL E. KEYLER, PHARMD
LESTER M. HADDAD, MD

EPIDEMIOLOGY

Tricyclic antidepressants (TCAs) are the most common cause of death due to prescription drug overdose in the United States and are a leading cause worldwide. Despite the continuing introduction of new selective serotonin reuptake inhibitors (SSRIs) and their remarkable popularity as antidepressants, the number of deaths due to TCAs has remained essentially constant for the past 10 years.[1, 2] The SSRIs are also commonly involved in overdoses but are much less toxic than the TCAs, and deaths are quite rare. Monoamine oxidase inhibitor overdose (see Chapter 32) may also have serious consequences but is far less common than poisoning with either TCAs or SSRIs (Table 31–1). Factors contributing to the large number of deaths due to TCA overdose include the widespread availability of TCAs to depressed patients at high risk for suicide by drug ingestion, the severity of cardiovascular and central nervous system effects associated with overdose, and the limited efficacy of available treatments for overdose.[3, 4]

TRICYCLIC ANTIDEPRESSANTS

TCAs (sometimes called *cyclic antidepressants* in deference to the additional ring structures present in maprotiline and amoxapine) may be classified as secondary or tertiary amines (Fig. 31–1). Several of the tertiary amines (imipramine, amitriptyline) are demethylated *in vivo* to active secondary amine metabolites (desipramine, nortriptyline), which are also available for clinical use. At therapeutic doses, the clinically available TCAs may be distinguished from one another by their relative abilities to inhibit the reuptake of neurotransmitters (norepinephrine, dopamine, serotonin), their anticholinergic and antihis-

Table 31–1. Principal Toxic Effects of Antidepressants

*Tricyclic Antidepressants (TCAs)**
Cardiovascular
Intraventricular conduction delay (QRS prolongation)
Sinus tachycardia
Ventricular arrhythmias
Hypotension
Central nervous system
Coma
Myoclonus
Seizures
Other
Hyperthermia
Ileus
Urinary retention
Selective Serotonin Reuptake Inhibitors (SSRIs)
Tremor
Sinus tachycardia
Nausea and vomiting
Obtundation
Seizures
Serotonin syndrome
Monoamine Oxidase Inhibitors†
Hypertension or hypotension
Muscular rigidity
Myoclonus
Seizures
Hyperthermia

*Cardiovascular toxicity is less common and central nervous system toxicity is more common with amoxapine and maprotilene than with other TCAs.
†Discussed in Chapter 32.

taminic potencies, and their tendencies to sedate.[5] At toxic doses, these differences are unimportant, and the toxicities of most TCAs are qualitatively and quantitatively similar. Some epidemiologic studies have suggested that certain TCAs are more toxic than others in overdose (desipramine, dothiepin, amitriptyline), but other factors such as selectively prescribing these drugs to high-risk patients or even the size of the tablets available (milligrams per tablet) may contribute to this impression.[6, 7] One exception is the tertiary amine lofepramine, which is itself inactive but is slowly metabolized to desipramine. Because of the limited rate at which desipramine is formed, lofepramine appears to be less toxic than other TCAs after acute overdose.[8]

Amoxapine is structurally related to the TCAs and has similar therapeutic actions, but acute overdose is characterized by a higher incidence of seizures, and cardiovascular toxicity is rare.[9] Maprotiline is also more likely than other TCAs to produce seizures but may be associated with cardiovascular toxicity at sufficient doses.[10]

Pharmacokinetics (Table 31–2)

Peak serum TCA concentrations occur 2 to 8 hours after administration of a therapeutic dose. After overdose, the anticholinergic properties of the TCAs may slow gastric emptying and further delay drug absorption. Nevertheless, the onset of toxicity after overdose is typically rapid, and most deaths occur within several hours of presentation. This time course probably reflects the potencies of the TCAs such that absorption of even a fraction of the ingested dose may prove toxic or fatal. First-pass hepatic metabolism of therapeutic doses of TCAs is extensive (23% to 73% for imipramine) but may become saturated with overdose, resulting in increased bioavailability.[11]

All TCAs have a large volume of distribution (10 to 20 L/kg), and in some tissues drug concentrations are 10 to 100 times that of blood. Distribution of TCAs to tissues is rapid, and less than 1% to 2% of the ingested dose is present in blood even in the early hours after overdose. Serum TCA levels typically decline biexponentially.[12, 13] The initial or distribution half-life is quite short (1 to 2 hours) and corresponds to the substantial improvement typically noted in patients with TCA overdose in the first 4 to 8 hours after presentation. Elimination half-lives for therapeutic doses of TCAs average 8 to 30 hours (55 to 127 hours for protriptyline), with longer half-lives in the elderly.[12, 14] The elimination half-life after overdose may be somewhat longer owing to saturable metabolism but is still generally within the range reported for therapeutic doses.[15]

Elimination of TCAs is almost entirely due to hepatic metabolism; renal excretion of these drugs, which are weak bases, is negligible even when urine is acidified. Most TCAs are first converted to demethylated or hydroxylated metabolites that are similar in toxicity to their parent compounds. The serum

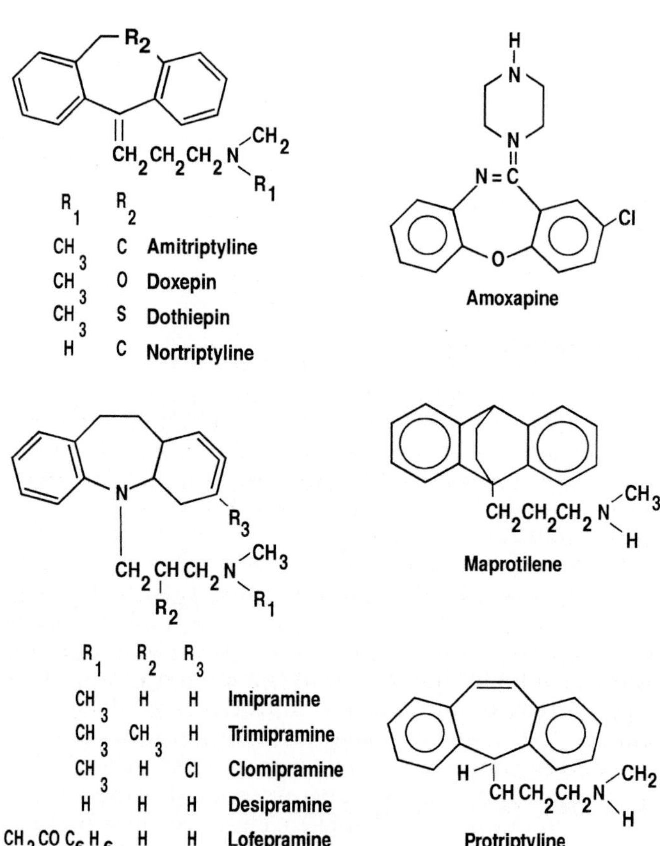

Figure 31–1. Structures of some tricyclic antidepressants.

Table 31–2. Pharmacokinetic Parameters of Some Antidepressants

Drug	Volume of Distribution (L/kg)	Elimination Half-Life (h)	Daily Dose (mg)	Therapeutic Level* (ng/mL)	Principal Active Metabolites
TCAs					
Amitriptyline	10–19	10–25	50–300	125–150†	Nortriptyline 10-OH amitriptyline 10-OH nortriptyline
Amoxapine	—	8	50–300	160–800‡	8-OH amoxapine 7-OH amoxapine
Clomipramine	7–20	19–37	50–300		Desmethylclomipramine
Desipramine	2–59	12–30§	50–300	50–300	2-OH desipramine
Dothiepin	11–78	14–24	75–150	50–150	Dothiepin-*S*-oxide
Doxepin	9–33	8–24	50–300	75–200†	Desmethyldoxepin
Imipramine	20–40	18–34§	50–300	150–300†	Desipramine 2-OH imipramine 2-OH desipramine
Lofepramine		1.5–2.5	140–210		Desipramine
Maprotiline	15–28	47	50–300	50–300	Desmethylmaprotiline
Nortriptyline	21–57	16–36	30–100	50–150	10-OH nortriptyline
Protriptyline	19–26	55–127	15–60	50–150	
Trimipramine	—	—	50–300	30–170	Desmethyltrimipramine
SSRIs					
Fluoxetine	14–100	48–96	5–40	100–800*	Norfluoxetine
Fluvoxamine	5–20	15–25	50–300		
Nefazodone		2–4	100–600	500–4000	Hydroxynefazodone
Paroxetine	12–16	12–21	10–50		
Sertraline	20	26	50–200		
Trazodone	1–2	5–9	100–400	700–1600	
Venlafaxine	4	6–10	30–600	50–400	*O*-desmethylvenlafaxine
Other					
Bupropion	19–21	10–14	150–300	20–75	Hydroxybupropion

TCAs, tricyclic antidepressants; SSRIs, selective serotonin reuptake inhibitors.
*Most numbers refer to usual serum concentrations because therapeutic concentrations are not established.
†Parent compound plus demethylated metabolite.
‡Parent compound plus metabolite.
§Longer for slow hydroxylators.

concentration of active metabolites in the first few hours after overdose is generally low, but metabolites may contribute to toxicity after the first 12 to 24 hours.[13, 16] Active metabolites undergo further demethylation or conjugation to inactive compounds that are excreted in urine. There is little biliary excretion of TCAs as parent drug or active metabolite.[17]

Hydroxylation of some TCAs by hepatic microsomes displays genetic polymorphism at the CYP2D6 allele. In the United States, 90% to 95% of patients are rapid hydroxylators and have a much shorter desipramine half-life (13 to 23 hours) than slow hydroxylators (81 to 131 hours).[18] Cases of slow recovery from desipramine overdose[19] and toxicity from therapeutic dosing[20] have been reported in slow hydroxylators.

The TCAs are weak bases and so are extensively bound to α1-acid glycoprotein in serum. Changes in the serum α1-acid glycoprotein concentration or pH may markedly affect the bound fraction of TCAs, but changes in binding are unlikely to affect overdose toxicity (see the later discussion of protein binding).

Mechanisms of Tricyclic Antidepressant Toxicity

Overview. The most important toxic effects of TCA overdose are hypotension, arrhythmias, coma, seizures, and hyperthermia. Cardiovascular toxicity results primarily from effects on the cardiac cell action potential, direct effects on vascular tone, and indirect effects mediated by the autonomic nervous system (Table 31–3). Hyperthermia is due to exces-

Table 31–3. Mechanisms of Tricyclic Antidepressant Cardiovascular Toxicity

Toxic Effect	Mechanism
Conduction Delays, Arrhythmias	
QRS prolongation, atrioventricular block	Cardiac sodium channel inhibition → slowed depolarization in atrioventricular node, His-Purkinje fibers, and ventricular myocardium
Sinus tachycardia	Cholinergic blockade, inhibition of norepinephrine reuptake
Ventricular tachycardia	
Monomorphic	Cardiac sodium channel inhibition → re-entry
Torsades de pointes	Cardiac potassium channel inhibition → prolonged repolarization
Ventricular bradycardia	Impaired cardiac automaticity
Hypotension	
Vasodilation	Vascular α-adrenergic receptor blockade
Decreased cardiac contractility	Cardiac sodium channel inhibition → impaired excitation-contraction coupling

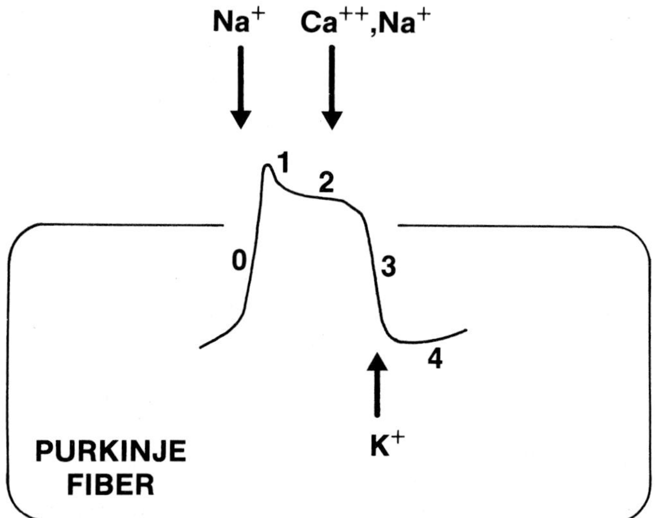

Figure 31–2. Normal Purkinje's fiber action potential. Phase 0 depolarization is due to activation of the fast sodium channel and the resulting inward sodium current. Depolarization is maintained during phase 2 by an inward current of calcium and sodium. Repolarization (phase 3) is due in part to an outward potassium current. In cells with intrinsic automaticity, spontaneous depolarization during phase 4 initiates phase 0 depolarization when the threshold voltage is reached. (From Pentel PR, Benowitz NL: Tricyclic antidepressant poisoning: Management of arrhythmias. Med Toxicol *1*:101–121, 1986.)

sive muscular activity in the presence of high anticholinergic tone. Central nervous system toxicity is less well understood; blockade of cholinergic, histaminic, and γ-aminobutyric acid (GABA) receptors and inhibition of neuronal sodium channels may contribute. Deaths are most often due to refractory hypotension.

Cardiac Cell Action Potential. The principal features of the action potential in cardiac cells are shown in Figure 31–2. The most important effect of the TCAs is inhibition of the fast sodium channel and the slowing of phase 0 depolarization in His-Purkinje tissue and ventricular myocardium. In this respect, the TCAs resemble class I antiarrhythmic agents (e.g., quinidine, procainamide, encainide, and flecainide).[21] Impaired depolarization of cells within the His-Purkinje system slows the propagation of ventricular depolarization and appears on the electrocardiogram as prolongation of the QRS interval, the hallmark of TCA overdose (Fig. 31–3). If such slowing occurs nonuniformly, it may cause unidirectional block and re-entry analogous to that occurring in ischemic myocardium and resulting in ventricular tachycardia.[22]

Impaired phase 0 depolarization may also contribute to hypotension after TCA overdose. The movement of sodium into cells during phase 0 is closely coupled to the entry of calcium and the subsequent triggering of myocardial contraction. Impaired entry of sodium into cardiac cells may therefore impair myocardial contractility.

Sodium channel inhibition *in vitro* is sensitive to pH, and increasing the extracellular pH minimizes TCA-induced slowing of phase 0 depolarization. Elevating blood pH has been shown to have a beneficial effect in various animal models of TCA overdose, resulting in improvement in intraventricular conduction delays, hypotension, and ventricular arrhythmias.[23–25] Conversely, acidosis may aggravate TCA cardiotoxicity.[25] Increasing the extracellular sodium concentration also minimizes the effects of TCAs on phase 0 depolarization.[26] Together with increasing blood pH, increasing the serum sodium concentration appears to mediate the therapeutic effect of hypertonic [1 molar (1M)] sodium bicarbonate on TCA cardiotoxicity.[25, 27] The mechanism of these effects is not clear. The binding of the class IC antiarrhythmic drug flecainide to sodium channels on Purkinje's cells *in vitro* is reduced by high concentrations of sodium[28]; whether sodium (or high pH) acts in a similar manner on TCA binding to sodium channels is not known.

The TCAs also slow repolarization and phase 4 (spontaneous) depolarization.[29] Prolongation of repolarization results in prolongation of the QT interval and is a feature of both therapeutic and toxic doses. QT prolongation predisposes to the development of torsades de pointes, which has been reported in pa-

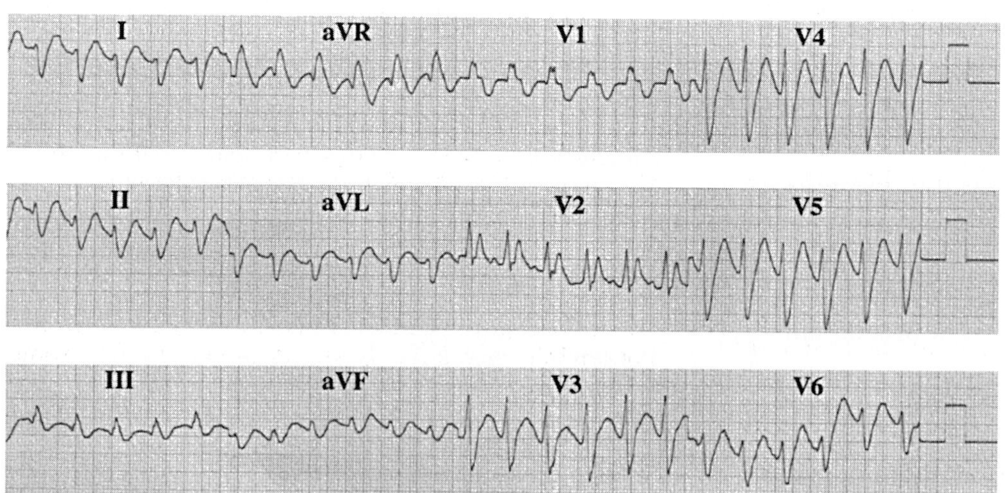

Figure 31–3. Electrocardiogram of a 23-year-old woman 2 hours after ingestion of 3 g of imipramine, demonstrating the typical features of tricyclic antidepressant overdose. QRS complex duration is markedly prolonged (0.21 sec), and the QRS axis is rightward (+174 degrees). The rhythm in most leads could easily be mistaken for ventricular tachycardia, but P waves are visible in lead V_2, identifying the rhythm as sinus tachycardia. Note the unusual QRS morphology in lead V_2, giving the impression of a normal QRS duration and illustrating the importance of obtaining a 12-lead ECG.

tients taking therapeutic doses of TCAs. Torsades de pointes typically occurs when the ventricular rate is slow. Because the underlying rhythm in patients with TCA overdose is most often sinus tachycardia, torsades de pointes is an uncommon feature of overdose. Slowing of phase 4 depolarization inhibits ventricular automaticity. At toxic doses, impaired automaticity may suppress ventricular escape rhythms and cause bradycardia. The TCAs also inhibit L-type calcium channels, but it is not clear if this contributes to TCA toxicity.

Neurotransmitter Reuptake. Inhibition of neuronal neurotransmitter reuptake (norepinephrine, dopamine, serotonin) and the resulting increase in synaptic neurotransmitter levels are thought to be important in mediating the antidepressant effect of TCAs.[5] With overdose, increases in cardiac or vascular concentrations of catecholamines may contribute to sinus tachycardia or to the early and typically transient hypertension occasionally observed.[30] Increased concentrations of catecholamines might also contribute to ventricular arrhythmias, but data on this question are limited. It has also been suggested that profound or prolonged inhibition of norepinephrine reuptake could cause hypotension by depleting neuronal reserves of the neurotransmitter. The limited efficacy of high doses of catecholamines in correcting severe TCA-induced hypotension argues against this being the predominant mechanism for hypotension.

Cholinergic Blockade. The anticholinergic actions of TCAs contribute to the development of sinus tachycardia, hyperthermia, ileus, urinary retention, pupillary dilatation, and probably coma. Of these, the most important is hyperthermia, which is caused by impaired sweating and is most often observed in patients who are generating excessive heat owing to repetitive seizures, myoclonus, or agitation.[31] It has been suggested that seizures are also anticholinergic in origin, but this question has not been adequately investigated, and inhibition of neuronal sodium channels, GABA, or *N*-methyl-D-aspartate receptors might also contribute to seizures.[32]

Alpha Blockade. At therapeutic doses of TCAs, α-adrenergic blockade causes vasodilation and postural hypotension. At toxic doses, vasodilation is invariably an important contributor to hypotension.[33]

Protein Binding. The serum protein binding of TCAs is enhanced *in vitro* by increasing pH.[34] It has therefore been postulated that the beneficial effect of sodium bicarbonate ($NaHCO_3$) on TCA cardiotoxicity might be due to increasing blood pH, enhancing protein binding, and reducing the concentration of unbound (pharmacologically active) drug. The very small fraction of the total dose present in serum and the failure of exogenously administered α1-acid glycoprotein to ameliorate TCA toxicity in rats despite markedly increasing its binding in serum argue against this hypothesis.[35]

Presentation

General. Life-threatening overdose is usually associated with ingestion of more than 1 g of TCA. Of patients who reach the hospital, many deaths occur within the first few hours of presentation and most occur within the first 24 hours.[36] It is not uncommon for a patient's clinical condition to deteriorate rapidly with progression from no symptoms to life-threatening cardiotoxicity or seizures in less than 1 hour.[37]

Cardiovascular

QRS Morphology. QRS interval prolongation is the most distinctive feature of serious TCA overdose (see Fig. 31–3).[38] QRS morphology is usually that of a nonspecific intraventricular conduction delay, and discrete bundle branch block is less common. TCA-induced conduction delay is rate dependent, and tachycardia exaggerates QRS prolongation.[39] The QRS axis is typically shifted to the right, as is the axis of the terminal 40 msec of the QRS complex, and R wave amplitude in lead aV_R is increased.[40–42] Because baseline values for these parameters vary considerably and clinical experience with their use is limited, it is unclear if any is more useful than QRS prolongation for the diagnosis of TCA overdose or assessment of the risk of complications.

QRS prolongation is not in itself harmful but rather serves to identify patients at risk of developing further complications.[42] In one study, a QRS duration of greater than 0.16 second identified patients at greatest risk of ventricular arrhythmias, and a QRS duration of greater than 0.10 second identified patients at greatest risk of seizures.[43] However, these and other complications may occur with a lesser degree of QRS prolongation, and patients with any degree of QRS prolongation are considered at risk for developing life-threatening TCA toxicity.

Atrioventricular Block. The PR interval in TCA overdose is often prolonged, but second- or third-degree atrioventricular block is rare.[44]

QT Interval. The QT interval is mildly prolonged with therapeutic doses of TCAs and is more prolonged with overdose.[45] However, the degree of QT prolongation is not a useful predictor of complications. Nonspecific changes in ST-T wave morphology are common.

Sinus Tachycardia. The most common rhythm associated with TCA overdose is sinus tachycardia, which is present in more than 50% of patients. The sinus rate is usually modest (<160 beats per minute) and does not cause hemodynamic compromise. The severity of sinus tachycardia is not a useful predictor of other complications. Sinus tachycardia may be aggravated by concurrent hypoxia, hypotension, hyperthermia, or the use of β1-adrenergic agonists.

Ventricular Arrhythmias. Ventricular tachycardia is the most common ventricular arrhythmia in patients with TCA overdose. However, it may be quite difficult to distinguish from sinus tachycardia when QRS prolongation is marked and P waves are not visible (see Fig. 31–3). It is likely that some cases of ventricular tachycardia (and its treatment) described in the literature are actually cases of supraventricular rhythms. The present discussion of ventricular tachycardia should be interpreted with this limitation in mind.

Ventricular tachycardia most often occurs in patients with marked QRS prolongation or hypotension[43, 46] and may be precipitated by seizures.[47, 48] Other predisposing factors include hypoxia, hyperthermia, acidosis, and the use of β1-adrenergic agonists. Mortality in patients with ventricular tachycardia is high.

Premature ventricular beats are uncommon in patients with TCA overdose. Ventricular fibrillation is usually a terminal rhythm that occurs as a complication of ventricular tachycardia or hypotension. Torsades de pointes has been reported with TCA overdose[49] but is rare and more often complicates therapeutic use of TCAs. A number of cases of sudden death in children taking TCAs therapeutically have been reported, and QT prolongation with resultant torsades de pointes has been speculated to be a potential mechanism.[50] Slow ventricular rhythms may occur with massive TCA overdose.

Wide-Complex Tachycardia Without P Waves. One of the most difficult diagnostic problems in patients with TCA overdose is classifying the cardiac rhythm when P waves are not visible (see Fig. 31–3). The most common underlying rhythm in this situation is sinus tachycardia with QRS prolongation. P waves may be obscured by the preceding T wave because of the prolonged PR and QT intervals and rapid heart rate. When QRS duration is markedly prolonged, this rhythm may be indistinguishable from ventricular tachycardia. A 12-lead electrocardiogram (ECG) may reveal P waves not visible on a rhythm strip. If time allows, an ECG obtained using an esophageal electrode or an intra-atrial pacemaker as a sensing lead may help by revealing P waves that the standard 12-lead ECG does not. When patients present soon after overdose, serial observation of the ECG is often helpful. A gradual evolution of QRS morphology before the loss of P waves suggests that the wide-complex rhythm is supraventricular. The observation of atrioventricular dissociation or fusion beats would, as in other settings, suggest that the rhythm is ventricular in origin. Other criteria commonly used to differentiate ventricular and supraventricular rhythms, such as QRS morphology and duration, have not been tested in patients with TCA overdose and may not be applicable in this setting.

Late Arrhythmias. TCA toxicity usually resolves in 24 to 48 hours,[36] although slower recovery has been reported in slow hydroxylators.[19] Maximal toxicity and almost all deaths occur within 24 hours of presentation.[37, 45] A few cases of arrhythmias or sudden death 2 to 5 days after TCA ingestion have been described. Most involved patients with residual TCA toxicity or coexisting disease, although one report described a patient with apparently full resolution of cardiac toxicity 24 hours before a bradycardiac arrest.[51] Several retrospective reviews specifically addressing this question have failed to find any cases of late, unexpected deterioration or death.[45, 52] Moreover, the pharmacokinetics of the TCAs offer no theoretic basis for the late reappearance of toxicity. If late arrhythmias are in fact a feature of TCA overdose, their incidence must be quite low.

Hypotension. Refractory hypotension is the most common cause of death due to TCA overdose. Hypotension is due to vasodilation or impaired cardiac contractility.[33, 53] Because vasodilation occurs even with modest doses of TCAs, it is almost always a factor in overdose, and hypotension can occur in the absence of signs of cardiac toxicity such as QRS prolongation.[46] Other factors contributing to hypotension include very fast or very slow heart rates, intravascular volume depletion, hypoxia, hyperthermia, acidosis, seizures, or the coingestion (or therapeutic use) of other cardiodepressant or vasodilating drugs.

Central Nervous System

Coma. Central nervous system depression is usually present in patients with QRS prolongation but may also occur when QRS duration is normal, particularly when other central nervous system depressant drugs are coingested.

Delirium. Delirium may occur with the ingestion of modest doses of TCAs or early in the course of more massive TCA overdose. It is characterized by agitation, disorientation, or psychotic behavior. The presumed mechanism is cholinergic blockade in the central nervous system, and other anticholinergic signs (such as hyperthermia, dry skin, mydriasis, sinus tachycardia, ileus, and urinary retention) may be present.

Seizures and Myoclonus. Seizures are most common in patients with QRS prolongation but may also occur in those with a normal QRS duration.[43, 54] Maprotiline and amoxapine are more likely than other cyclic antidepressants to cause seizures.[9] Seizures due to TCAs most often occur within 1 to 2 hours of presentation and are usually generalized, brief, and single and subside before an anticonvulsant can be administered. Seizures may result in acidosis, hyperthermia, or rhabdomyolysis but are usually well tolerated.[54] In several series, however, 10% to 20% of patients with seizures abruptly developed cardiovascular deterioration (hypotension, ventricular arrhythmias) during or within minutes after the seizure.[48, 54] Patients with more severe cardiovascular toxicity before the seizure were at highest risk. Cardiovascular deterioration may have been due to seizure-induced acidosis.

A further illustration of the potential consequences of seizures is provided by amoxapine overdose. Although this drug has little cardiovascular toxicity, one study found amoxapine overdose to have a substantially higher incidence of seizures and higher mortality than other TCAs.[9]

Myoclonus is less common than seizures, although the reported incidence varies. Potential complications are the same as for seizures but are less likely to occur.

Hyperthermia. Hyperthermia in TCA overdose results from excessive heat generation (seizures, myoclonus, or agitation) in the presence of impaired heat dissipation (decreased sweating). Death or permanent neurologic sequelae have been reported in patients with drug overdose (including TCA overdose) when core temperature exceeds 105°F for periods as brief as several hours.[31] The unusually high morbidity and mortality associated with overdose-induced hyperthermia may be due to the coexistence of multiple cerebral insults such as hyperthermia, hypotension, and hypoxia.

Other. Urinary retention and ileus are common in TCA overdose. Pupil size is variable owing to the opposing influence of cholinergic and α-adrenergic blockade. Pupils nonreactive to light have been reported but are rare.[55] Pulmonary complications include aspiration pneumonitis and the adult respiratory distress syndrome.[56] These are most likely secondary to coma, hypotension, pulmonary infection, or excessive fluid administration rather than primary toxic effects of the TCAs. A case of pancreatitis has been reported.[57]

Differential Diagnosis

Overdoses most likely to be confused with TCA toxicity are those that produce QRS prolongation. TCA cardiotoxicity may be indistinguishable from overdose with class IA (quinidine, procainamide, disopyramide) or class IC (flecainide, encainide, propafenone) antiarrhythmic agents. Other drugs that may prolong QRS duration if given in overdoses include cocaine, propranolol, quinine, chloroquine, hydroxychloroquine, high-dose antipsychotics (thioridazine, chlorpromazine, mesoridazine), propoxyphene (via the norpropoxyphene metabolite), and digoxin (with hyperkalemia). Very rarely, diphenhydramine and lithium have been reported to cause QRS prolongation. Nondrug causes of QRS prolongation include hyperkalemia, cardiac ischemia, cardiomyopathy, and disease of the cardiac conduction system.

Management

While many controlled animal studies of TCA toxicity are available, data regarding overdoses in humans are derived primarily from case reports and patient series.

Initial Measures. Because of the risk of rapid deterioration, patients with known or suspected TCA overdose should have an intravenous line started for access and cardiac rhythm should be monitored. Prompt administration of activated charcoal with sorbitol is probably the single most important intervention in patients with TCA overdose. Although ileus is common with TCA overdose, decreased or absent bowel sounds are generally not contraindications to the administration of activated charcoal. It is common practice to perform gastric lavage via a large-bore tube if TCA ingestion was within 1 hour of presentation or to administer charcoal followed by lavage and then additional charcoal, but the benefit of doing so is unproven[58] and some clinicians now omit this step in favor of administering activated charcoal as quickly as possible. Syrup of ipecac is contraindicated because vomiting may occur during seizures or when the patient's level of consciousness has deteriorated. Monitoring of vital signs should include frequent measurement of temperature, particularly in patients with agitation or seizures. A 12-lead ECG should be obtained because it may reveal QRS prolongation that is not evident on the single lead of a cardiac monitor (see Fig. 31–3).

Admission Criteria. Patients who have ingested TCAs but show no signs of toxicity during 6 hours of observation (and have received oral activated charcoal) require no further medical monitoring.[36, 37] Psychiatric evaluation should be obtained. Patients with sinus tachycardia alone have a low incidence of other complications but are generally admitted for observation.[59]

Laboratory Evaluation. Measurement of serum electrolytes, blood urea nitrogen, hemoglobin, and prothrombin time is indicated to screen for coingested drugs or other complicating diagnoses. Arterial blood gas determinations are indicated for intubated patients or when acid-base status or ventilatory adequacy is in question.

TCAs can be detected qualitatively in urine by thin-layer chromatography or liquid chromatography, or quantitatively in serum by liquid or gas chromatography. Active demethylated metabolites are usually measured by these methods, but hydroxylated metabolites are not. Therapeutic TCA concentrations are generally in the range of 50 to 300 ng/mL (see Table 31–2). Bedside immunoassays are available but have not been extensively tested.[60]

The correlation of serum TCA concentrations with toxicity is imprecise,[36, 43] and their measurement adds little to the management of TCA overdose. Serum concentrations of less than 1 μg/mL are usually associated with minimal toxicity, although even these concentrations may prove toxic with mixed drug ingestions.[45] Life-threatening toxicity is usually accompanied by a serum concentration of greater than 1 μg/mL, and concentrations of greater than 3 to 5 μg/mL are often fatal.[38] The serum TCA concentration may increase up to fivefold post mortem. When using TCA levels to determine cause of death, the measurement of liver drug concentrations or parent-to-metabolite drug ratios is preferable.[61]

Duration of Monitoring. Cardiac monitoring of patients after TCA overdose is generally recommended until all signs of toxicity are absent for 24 hours.[3, 52] QRS duration may be considered normal if it is less than 0.10 second or similar to the duration before overdose. When QRS duration is marginally prolonged (0.10 to 0.12 second) and no baseline ECG is available, it may be unclear whether the observed QRS duration is normal for that patient or prolonged from the overdose. In this situation, measurement of the serum TCA concentration may be helpful. A clearly elevated TCA concentration would suggest that the QRS prolongation is drug induced and that continued cardiac monitoring is indicated. Patients who receive activated charcoal and remain free of signs or symptoms of TCA overdose for 6 hours require no further medical monitoring other than psychiatric evaluation.[62]

Hypertonic Sodium Bicarbonate. Hypertonic $NaHCO_3$ administered intravenously is effective in treating each of the most important manifestations of TCA cardiotoxicity: QRS prolongation, ventricular arrhythmias, and hypotension (Fig. 31–4). It is also one of the safest therapies available for TCA toxicity, provided that excessive alkalemia is avoided.[63, 64] The formulation used is a 1 molar solution (1M, 1 mEq/mL), usually supplied as a preloaded syringe of 50 mEq/50 mL.

When TCAs were introduced into clinical use, TCA overdose was noted to share many of the features of quinidine toxicity, for which hypertonic sodium lactate (which is rapidly metabolized to bicarbonate) had been reported to be of benefit. Subsequent case reports and uncontrolled series suggested that hypertonic sodium lactate or bicarbonate was of benefit for TCA cardiotoxicity as well.[65] Subsequent controlled studies in animals clearly established that hypertonic $NaHCO_3$ is effective in reducing QRS prolongation, increasing blood pressure, and suppressing ventricular ectopy due to TCA toxicity.[23, 25, 66] Controlled studies in patients have not been reported, but a large body of anecdotal data continues to support its use.[64, 67, 68]

Because acidosis aggravates TCA cardiotoxicity, the beneficial effect of $NaHCO_3$ lies partly in the correction of acidosis. It is clear, however, that $NaHCO_3$ is effective even when blood pH is normal. This beneficial effect appears to be mediated by increases in both blood pH and sodium concentration,[26] although the relative contribution of each differs in various animal models.[23–25, 27]

Few data comment on the optimal dose of hypertonic $NaHCO_3$ in TCA overdose. It is common practice to administer 50 mEq of $NaHCO_3$ (1 mEq/mL) as an initial intravenous bolus, with repeat doses as needed for cardiotoxicity or until the arterial blood pH is 7.50 to 7.55.[4, 64] Because marked alkalosis can precipitate ventricular arrhythmias even in the absence of TCAs, the safety of increasing blood pH further is not known.[63] If increasing the serum sodium concentration is important in humans, then administering hypertonic $NaHCO_3$ as a bolus may be preferable to diluting it in intravenous fluids before administration (after which it is no longer hypertonic). No evidence shows that hypertonic $NaHCO_3$ is effective for treating TCA-induced seizures.

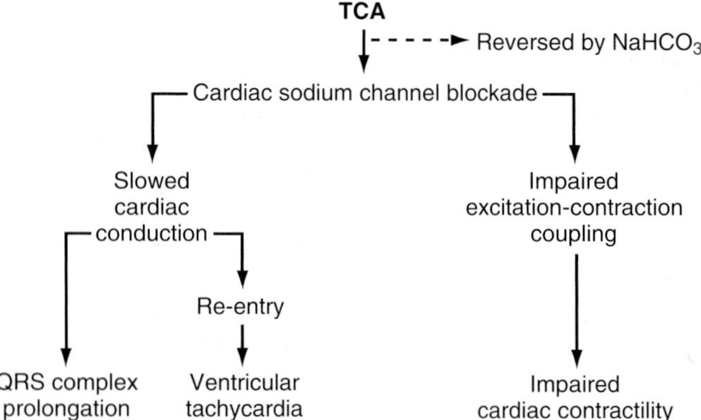

Figure 31–4. Role of cardiac sodium channel inhibition in mediating tricyclic antidepressant (TCA) cardiotoxicity.

Hyperventilation. Hyperventilation has been reported to benefit patients with TCA-induced cardiotoxicity,[69, 70] but clinical data are less abundant than data on the use of $NaHCO_3$. The efficacy of hyperventilation for ventricular ectopy has been demonstrated in dogs.[23] Hyperventilation, however, is less effective than use of $NaHCO_3$ for cardiotoxicity in rats, possibly because $NaHCO_3$ increases the serum sodium concentration whereas hyperventilation does not.[25] Because hyperventilation in other clinical settings mayprovoke seizures, the possibility that it might aggravate TCA-induced seizures has been raised. $NaHCO_3$ is therefore generally preferred to hyperventilation for TCA cardiotoxicity. Nevertheless, hyperventilation may be useful if use of $NaHCO_3$ is relatively contraindicated, such as in a patient with pulmonary edema.

Phenytoin. Use of phenytoin was reported to improve QRS duration in an uncontrolled series of patients, and one preliminary report that noted more rapid improvement of cardiovascular toxicity in patients randomized to phenytoin.[71, 72] Controlled animal studies have not confirmed a beneficial effect, and possible aggravation of ventricular ectopy was noted in one report.[62, 73, 74] These data do not support the clinical use of phenytoin for TCA cardiotoxicity.

Phenytoin has also been used in TCA overdose as an anticonvulsant, although its efficacy for this purpose is not established. When administered as a pretreatment, phenytoin has been reported to reduce the incidence of amoxapine-induced seizures in dogs.[69] However, phenytoin was not effective for imipramine-induced seizures in rats in one study, whereas diazepam and phenobarbital were.[75]

Physostigmine. The cholinesterase inhibitor physostigmine may antagonize some anticholinergic features of TCA overdose, such as sinus tachycardia and coma,[76] but these complications can generally be treated supportively. Physostigmine is otherwise ineffective for treating TCA cardiotoxicity and may even exacerbate it. Severe bradycardia and asystole have been reported with its use in TCA overdose.[77] Physostigmine has also been used to terminate TCA-induced seizures and myoclonus. Although efficacy has been reported anecdotally, physostigmine may also precipitate seizures, even when administered at recommended doses. In view of this toxicity, physostigmine has no role in the management of TCA overdose.

β-Blockers. β-Blockers have been reported to reduce QRS prolongation in patients with TCA overdose.[78] Because QRS prolongation is rate dependent, this effect may be secondary to slowing of the heart rate. The possibility of hemodynamic deterioration with β-blockers argues against their use.

Enhancing Elimination. Enhancing elimination of the TCAs is difficult owing to their large volume of distribution and the small fraction of the absorbed dose that is present in blood. Several uncontrolled case reports note shorter than expected elimination half-lives for TCAs with the use of repeated doses of activated charcoal, but these data are of limited value because early sampling may have overlapped the TCA distribution phase with its much shorter half-life. In controlled studies, repeated oral doses of activated charcoal have been reported to have either no effect on the clearance of subtoxic doses of imipramine[79] or to shorten the elimination half-life of doxepin or amitriptyline by 20%.[80] Because most deaths due to TCA overdose occur within hours of drug ingestion, a small increase in clearance is not likely to alter outcome. It is possible, however, that repeated doses of charcoal might shorten the duration of toxicity in slow hydroxylators who have very long TCA half-lives. Little active TCA is excreted in urine, and measures to enhance urinary TCA excretion have a negligible effect on total clearance.[80]

Hemodialysis is ineffective in enhancing the elimination of TCAs because of their extensive protein binding and lipid solubility. Hemoperfusion overcomes these limitations but is relatively ineffective because of the large volume of drug distribution.[81] One case report noted removal of less than 2% of the ingested dose of imipramine as parent drug or active metabolite during 6 hours of hemoperfusion.[13] Nevertheless, rapid improvement in cardiotoxicity after TCA overdose has been anecdotally reported during hemoperfusion.[82–84] Because these reports are based on uncontrolled observations, it is possible that improvement was coincidental with hemoperfusion rather than a consequence of it. In support of this possibility, serum TCA levels often decrease rapidly in the first few hours after admission even without hemoperfusion, because of drug distribution.[85] Animal data are not available. There is, therefore, little support for the use of hemoperfusion in the management of TCA overdose.

Mechanical Support of the Circulation. Because TCA toxicity is reversible, temporary mechanical support of the circulation might be useful in hypotensive patients who are unresponsive to other measures. Serum TCA levels often decline rapidly after overdose owing to distribution of drug to tissues. A temporary period of mechanically assisted circulation might therefore allow time for spontaneous improvement. Isolated reports of a child who survived 2.5 hours of cardiopulmonary resuscitation during nonperfusing ventricular tachycardia due to imipramine overdose[86] and an adult treated successfully with femoral-femoral extracorporeal circulation for refractory hypotension[87] support this possibility. Preliminary data in swine suggest that cardiopulmonary bypass may allow survival after a fatal dose of TCA.[88] Although further study is needed, it seems reasonable to consider these or similar measures for viable patients who cannot be otherwise supported.

Investigational Therapies. The use of TCA-specific antibody Fab fragments for the treatment of TCA overdose, analogous to those used to treat digoxin overdose, has been studied in rats. Fab doses capable of binding 10% to 30% of the TCA body burden rapidly reverse QRS prolongation and hypotension and prolong survival.[89, 90] The toxic dose of TCAs is more than 100 times higher than that of digoxin, however, and the Fab dose required to reverse toxicity is also much higher (1 to 3 g/kg). Whether these very high Fab doses are safe enough for human use is not yet clear.

Specific Complications (Table 31–4)

QRS Prolongation. QRS prolongation identifies patients at risk for developing arrhythmias, hypotension, or seizures. In the absence of these complications, it is not known whether there is any benefit to treating the QRS duration per se with hypertonic $NaHCO_3$. The potential adverse effects of prophylactic therapy include pulmonary edema due to large doses of $NaHCO_3$ (50 mEq sodium/50-mL ampule)

Table 31–4. Treatment of Tricyclic Antidepressant Toxicity

Toxic Effect	Treatment
Cardiovascular	
QRS prolongation	$NaHCO_3$* if QRS prolongation is marked or progressing. Not clear if treatment is needed in the absence of hypotension or arrhythmias
Hypotension	Intravascular volume expansion, $NaHCO_3$ Vasopressors (norepinephrine) or inotropic agents (dopamine) Correct hyperthermia, acidosis, seizures Consider mechanical support
Ventricular tachycardia	$NaHCO_3$, lidocaine, overdrive pacing Correct hypotension, hyperthermia, acidosis, seizures
Torsades de pointes	Overdrive pacing
Ventricular bradycardia	Chronotropic agent (epinephrine), pacemaker
Sinus tachycardia	Treatment rarely needed
Atrioventricular block—type II second or third degree	Pacemaker
Hypertension	Rapidly titratable antihypertensive agent (nitroprusside)
Central Nervous System	
Delirium	Restraints, benzodiazepine Neuromuscular blockade for hyperthermia, acidosis
Seizures	Benzodiazepine Neuromuscular blockade for hyperthermia, acidosis
Coma	Intubation, ventilation if needed
Other	
Hyperthermia	Control seizures, agitation Cooling measures
Acidosis	$NaHCO_3$ Correct hypotension, hypoventilation

*Hypertonic (1 molar, 1 mEq/mL) $NaHCO_3$.

and aggravation of arrhythmias or seizures due to excessive alkalosis. A possible approach to patients with QRS prolongation is to correct any factor that might aggravate toxicity (acidosis, hypoxia, dehydration) and institute further therapy only if the QRS duration is markedly prolonged (≥0.14 second), QRS prolongation is worsening, or complications are present (hypotension or ventricular arrhythmias). Use of phenytoin is not indicated as a treatment for QRS prolongation.

Sinus Tachycardia. Treatment for sinus tachycardia is not generally needed. β-Blockers may slow the sinus rate but can also impair cardiac output and cause hypotension. Physostigmine can also slow the sinus rate but may precipitate seizures, bradycardia, or asystole and is therefore contraindicated.

Atrioventricular Block. First-degree atrioventricular block requires no treatment. Second- (type II) or third-degree atrioventricular block is usually managed with a pacemaker or isoproterenol. Owing to the rarity of these complications, data regarding the efficacy and safety of these interventions are lacking.

Ventricular Tachycardia. Predisposing factors such as acidosis, hypotension, and hyperthermia should be corrected. If a β1-adrenergic agonist is being used for inotropic support, the lowest effective dose should be used. The only measures that have been experimentally demonstrated as beneficial for ventricular arrhythmias are hypertonic $NaHCO_3$, hyperventilation, and lidocaine. $NaHCO_3$ may be administered until the arrhythmia subsides or arterial blood pH is 7.5 to 7.55. Lidocaine may be used if $NaHCO_3$ is ineffective but should be administered slowly to avoid precipitating seizures. The use of other antiarrhythmic agents is limited because class IA or IC drugs may worsen sodium channel inhibition and aggravate cardiotoxicity, and class III drugs might worsen QT prolongation. Direct current cardioversion may be useful if hypertension is present. Overdrive pacing has been used successfully in a patient with refractory ventricular tachycardia.[91]

Wide-Complex Tachycardia. Diagnostic strategies for differentiating ventricular tachycardia from sinus tachycardia with QRS prolongation were discussed earlier. When diagnosis of the rhythm is not possible, it is reasonable to correct potential aggravating factors and administer hypertonic $NaHCO_3$ as described previously for ventricular tachycardia. These maneuvers may correct ventricular tachycardia and are not likely to compromise the patient if the rhythm is supraventricular. It has been suggested that further measures be withheld if blood pressure is stable and that the rhythm be considered ventricular tachycardia (and treated as such) if the patient is hypotensive.[92]

Ventricular Bradycardia. This rhythm is often agonal, and there are no data regarding its management in TCA overdose. The usual therapy in other situations is a pacemaker, epinephrine, or isoproterenol.

Hypotension. Acidosis and hyperthermia should be corrected. A fluid challenge often corrects mild hypotension and may facilitate the management of more severe hypotension.[33] For hypotension unresponsive to fluids, both $NaHCO_3$ and sympathomimetic agents have been shown to be beneficial in animals. $NaHCO_3$ is generally used first because of its safety.

In animals, various inotropic and vasopressor agents have been reported to be useful for TCA-induced hypotension, including dopamine, norepinephrine, isoproterenol, and prenalterol.[93–95] It is not clear which agent is most effective, and no comparisons of these drugs have been made in patients. Because both vasodilation and impaired cardiac contractility may contribute to hypotension, the requirements of individual patients for inotropic or vasopressor drugs may differ. A pulmonary artery catheter may be helpful in tailoring therapy, but treatment must generally be initiated before such a catheter can be placed. One approach is to start with a vasopressor such as norepinephrine[53] or an inotrope such as dopamine and add the other drug if needed. Glucagon has been used in patients, but its efficacy relative to other inotropic agents is unknown.[32] Mechanical support of the circulation, discussed earlier, is an option if hypotension is refractory.

Hypertension. Hypertension generally is mild, is of short duration, and requires no treatment. If severe (blood pressure >170 mm Hg systolic or 110 mm Hg diastolic), a rapidly titratable drug such as nitroprusside should be used because TCA-induced hypotension may later supervene.

Seizures. Because seizures may aggravate cardiotoxicity, their early termination is important. Controlled studies of seizure management in patients are not available. However, anecdotal observations in patients suggest that *diazepam* is effective for terminating seizures and does not worsen hypotension or arrhythmias, even with repeated doses.[54] Whether other anticonvulsants such as phenytoin or phenobarbital are useful is not clear, but either may aggravate hypotension. Propofol was effective for one patient with seizures refractory to other agents,[96] but it can also cause hypotension.

In addition to anticonvulsant therapy, supportive management should address the consequences of seizures. Acidosis may be minimized by ensuring adequate ventilation during seizures (using manual bag ventilation if mechanical ventilation is ineffective). Prolonged seizures and the resulting lactic acidosis may also require administration of $NaHCO_3$. Core temperature should be measured and hyperthermia treated. In patients with frequent seizures or status epilepticus, conservative measures may fail to prevent acidosis or hyperthermia. Such patients may benefit from a brief period of neuromuscular blockade.[31] Prolonged paralysis should be avoided so that seizures are not obscured. As in other clinical situations, prolonged seizures (>2 hours) carry the risk of permanent brain injury.

Delirium. Mechanical restraint is usually sufficient, but other measures may be needed in agitated patients to allow tracheal intubation or control of hyperthermia. Sedation may precipitate respiratory depression. If sedation is required, a benzodiazepine is least likely to aggravate cardiotoxicity.[3, 54] Neuromuscular blockade has been useful in patients with severe agitation and hyperthermia. Physostigmine is useful for anticholinergic delirium due to other drugs but is contraindicated in TCA overdose because it may cause bradyarrhythmias or seizures.

Hyperthermia. Patients at highest risk for hyperthermia (those with agitation, myoclonus, seizures) should have their core temperature measured at least every 30 minutes because of the rapidity with which hyperthermia may develop. A core temperature of more than 105°F may cause neurologic damage.[31] Cooling should be initiated well before this temperature is reached. Cooling may be accomplished by standard measures, including external application of ice, evaporative cooling, or ice-water gastric lavage. If seizures or agitation cannot be adequately controlled, paralysis may be needed to facilitate cooling.

Drug Interactions

Pharmacodynamic interactions of importance in the setting of TCA overdose may be noted with drugs that have additive toxic effects such as impairment of cardiac contractility (β-blockers, calcium channel blockers), cardiac conduction (class IA, IC, or III antiarrhythmic agents), vasodilation (α-blockers, nitrates), sedation, or seizures (many drugs). Cholinergic agonists such as physostigmine may cause severe bradyarrhythmias or asystole. Flumazenil may precipitate seizures when administered to patients who have ingested both TCAs and benzodiazepines, possibly by reversing the anticonvulsant effect of the benzodiazepines.[97, 98] This possibility argues against the use of flumazenil for benzodiazepine overdose when a patient has co-ingested a TCA or when the identity of the drugs ingested is not known. Some TCAs inhibit neuronal reuptake of serotonin and can increase synaptic serotonin levels (e.g., clomipramine, amitriptyline). Either therapeutic or excessive doses of these drugs, in combination with other drugs that also increase synaptic serotonin levels (such as monoamine oxidase inhibitors), can cause a serotonin syndrome consisting of tremor, agitation, delirium, rigidity, myoclonus, hyperthermia, and obtundation.[99] This syndrome is discussed more fully in Chapter 32. Pharmacokinetic interactions caused by TCAs or affecting TCA disposition are discussed next, along with such interactions for SSRIs.

SELECTIVE SEROTONIN REUPTAKE INHIBITORS

General Features

SSRIs represent a structurally diverse group of drugs that share the ability to inhibit the presynaptic neuronal reuptake of serotonin, which results in increased synaptic serotonin levels. Various SSRIs have additional actions at therapeutic doses that may contribute to their antidepressant action or side effects, such as inhibition of norepinephrine or dopamine reuptake (venlafaxine), α-adrenergic blockade (trazodone, nefazodone), or serotonin 5-HT_2 receptor blockade (trazodone, nefazodone).

Despite these distinctions, the overdose effects of SSRIs tend to be generally similar and attributable to excessive synaptic serotonin. Death due to SSRI overdose alone is extremely rare. Nausea, vomiting, diarrhea, tremor, and a decreased level of consciousness are the most common features of overdose and have been reported with virtually all SSRIs in excessive doses. Bradycardia is a feature of therapeutic doses of many SSRIs, an effect that can be reproduced in animals with direct injection of serotonin into the brain and that is probably mediated by an increase in vagal tone. In overdose, a mild bradycardia or first-degree atrioventricular block may be observed, but tachycardia is more common. The principal toxic effect of massive doses of SSRIs in animals is seizures. Most SSRIs have been associated with seizures in overdose, but the incidence appears to be low. All SSRIs can produce the serotonin syndrome with either overdose or therapeutic use. The serotonin syndrome is most common when these drugs are used or ingested in combination with other drugs that increase synaptic serotonin levels, such as monoamine oxidase inhibitors (see Chapter 32), but may on occasion be produced by a single drug. The SSRIs may also cause a wide variety of pharmacokinetic drug interactions (discussed later).

Fluoxetine/Sertraline/Paroxetine

The most common features of fluoxetine overdose are nausea, vomiting, tremor, and a decreased level of consciousness.[100] Seizures may occur but are uncommon. Deaths due to fluoxetine alone are exceedingly rare.[101] Cardiac toxicity has been reported but with a very low incidence and often in patients who have ingested other drugs, and thus their relationship to fluoxetine is unclear. These reported cardiac effects include sinus tachycardia, junctional tachycardia, sinus bradycardia, atrial fibrillation, ventricular tachycardia, and QT interval prolongation. Therapeutic doses may cause a brief, self-limited syncope that is probably due to excessive vagal tone.[47] Therapeutic doses have been reported to prolong the bleeding time in one patient but did not do so in a larger study of this question. Because fluoxetine has a long elimination half-life and a long-acting active metabolite, prolonged toxicity might be anticipated but has not been reported. However, it is important to wait at least 3 to 4 weeks after discontinuing fluoxetine before starting therapy with a monoamine oxidase inhibitor because of the risk that an interaction might produce the serotonin syndrome.[102]

Overdose data for sertraline are more limited than

for fluoxetine. The most common reported effects include tremor, lethargy, and nausea. Less common are agitation, confusion, and vomiting.[103] Signs and symptoms suggestive of serotonin syndrome (tachycardia, hyperthermia, agitation, hallucinations) have also been reported after overdose.[104]

Few data are available regarding paroxetine overdose, but signs and symptoms would be expected to resemble those of fluoxetine and sertraline.

Venlafaxine

In addition to inhibiting the reuptake of serotonin, venlafaxine inhibits norepinephrine and to a lesser extent dopamine reuptake as well. These actions likely underlie the occasional finding of hypertension and tachycardia with overdose.[105] As with other SSRIs, a decreased level of consciousness and gastrointestinal symptoms are common, and seizures have been reported.[106]

Trazodone/Nefazodone

In addition to inhibiting neuronal serotonin reuptake, trazodone blocks the 5-HT_2 class of postsynaptic serotonin receptor. Thus trazodone both increases synaptic serotonin levels and alters the pattern of serotonin receptor activation. Nevertheless, overdose toxicity is similar to that of other SSRIs, consisting primarily of nausea, vomiting, and a decreased level of consciousness.[107–109] Although trazodone is an α-adrenergic blocker, hypotension is a relatively uncommon feature of overdose. Bradycardia and first-degree atrioventricular block have been reported.[110] Deaths have generally involved other sedating drugs in addition to trazodone. Priapism, usually a complication of therapeutic dosing, may also occur after overdose.[111] At therapeutic doses, a minimal but significant decrease in heart rate and prolongation of the QT interval have been reported.[112] Case reports have implicated trazodone in causing ventricular tachycardia,[113] eosinophilic pneumonia,[114] torsades de pointes,[115] and complete heart block, as well as in

Table 31–5. Selected Substrates and Inhibitors of Some Cytochrome P-450 Enzymes*

CYP Enzymes			
1A2	*2C19*	*2D6*	*3A4*
Substrates			
TCA†	**TCA**†	**TCA**‡	**TCA**†
Mexiletine	Phenytoin	**Trazodone**	Quinidine
Theophylline	Diazepam	**Fluoxetine**	Terfenadine
Caffeine	Indomethacin	**Paroxetine**	Cyclosporine
Estradiol	*S*-warfarin	**Venlafaxine**	Tamoxifen
Tacrine	Propranolol	Metoprolol	Lidocaine
R-warfarin	Omeprazole	Timolol	Cisapride
Amiodarone	Phenobarbital	Haloperidol	Rifabutin
	Carbamazepine	Clozapine	Midazolam
		Risperidone	Triazolam
		Thioridazine	Alprazolam
		Perphenazine	Carbamazepine
		Dextromethorphan	Dapsone
		Phenytoin	Lovastatin
Inhibitors			
Fluvoxamine	**Fluoxetine**	**Sertraline**	**Fluoxetine**
Cimetidine	**Fluvoxamine**	Quinidine	**Venlafaxine**
Erythromycin	**Sertraline**	Amiodarone	**Sertraline**
Ciprofloxacin	Citmetidine	Fluphenazine	**Nefazodone**
Enoxacin	Amiodarone	Moclobemide	**Fluvoxamine**
Meclobamine	Ketoconazole		Fluconazole
Disulfiram	Erythromycin		Ketoconazole
	Propoxyphene		Erythromycin
	Felbamate		Clarithromycin
			Amiodarone
			Saquinavir
			Cimetidine

TCA, tricyclic antidepressant; SSRIs, selective serotonin reuptake inhibitors.

*SSRIs and TCAs are indicated by bold type. Any two drugs that are substrates of the same cytochrome P-450 (CYP) enzyme may potentially compete with each other for that enzyme and thereby inhibit each other's metabolism. Some drugs may also inhibit a CYP enzyme without themselves being a substrate. Note that this table indicates potential interactions; not all have been demonstrated or are necessarily of clinical importance. Some drugs listed as inhibitors may actually be substrates for that particular CYP, but sufficient documentation is not available. Some drugs are substrates or inhibitors of more than one CYP enzyme.

†Demethylation of tertiary amine TCAs; imipramine, amitriptyline, clomipramine

‡Hydroxylation of desipramine, imipramine, clomipramine, amitriptyline, nortriptyline

Adapted from DeVane CL: Pharmacogenetics and drug metabolism of newer antidepressant agents. J Clin Psychiatry *55*(Suppl):38–47, 1994.

contributing to sinus arrest after electroconvulsive therapy,[116] but a causal role for trazodone in these instances is not established. Little overdose information is available regarding nefazodone, but in view of its pharmacologic similarities to trazodone, signs and symptoms would be expected to be similar.

Bupropion

Bupropion is not an SSRI but is included here because it is an atypical antidepressant. Its mechanism of action is not clear, but it does inhibit the neuronal reuptake of dopamine and to a lesser extent norepinephrine. Like SSRIs, overdose toxicity is generally mild and characterized by sinus tachycardia, tremor, and a decreased level of consciousness.[117] Seizures may be observed even with therapeutic dosing. The occurrence of four seizures in 55 bulimic patients in one study led to a delay in the marketing of bupropion, but the incidence of seizures with therapeutic dosing in other populations appears to be similar to that of other antidepressants (0.1% to 1.0%). Seizures are, however, relatively common with overdose (12 of 58 cases in one series).[117] Deaths are rare but have been reported, including one case in which no other drugs were detected.[118]

Treatment

Treatment of SSRI overdose is supportive. Activated charcoal is indicated but repeated doses are not, in view of the large volumes of distribution of these drugs. Use of the 5-HT_3 blocker ondansetron for nausea seems reasonable, but data on its efficacy in this setting are not available. Seizures are generally self-limited, and there are no specific data on their treatment. In view of the excellent outcome of SSRI overdose, measures other than general supportive care would seem unnecessary.

Interactions

Many TCAs and SSRIs are either substrates or inhibitors of cytochrome P-450 (CYP) enzymes.[119] CYP is a family of isoenzymes with different specificities, some of which are listed in Table 31–5. Any two drugs that are substrates of a given isoenzyme CYP may compete with each other for the enzyme and thereby inhibit each other's metabolism. For example, many antipsychotics increase serum TCA levels when administered concurrently. In addition, some drugs can inhibit or induce the activity of a particular CYP even though they themselves are not substrates. Some examples of such drugs are given in Table 31–5. Several SSRIs are potent inhibitors of CYP enzymes and can markedly increase serum levels of other drugs. Of particular importance is the inhibition of TCA metabolism due to SSRI (fluoxetine, sertraline, paroxetine) inhibition of CYP2D6. Note also that some drugs (not listed in Table 31–5) can induce CYP enzymes and enhance drug metabolism. Thus, cigarette smoking induces CYP1A2, and smoking cessation may lead to reduced TCA metabolism.

References

1. Litovitz TL, Normann SA, Veltri JC: 1985 Annual Report of the American Association of Poison Control Centers National Data Collection System. Am J Emerg Med *4*:427, 1986.
2. Litovitz TL, Felberg L, Soloway RA, et al: 1994 Annual Report of the American Association of Poison Control Centers Toxic Exposure Surveillance System. Am J Emerg Med *13*:551, 1995.
3. Frommer DA, Kulig KA, Marx JA, Rumack B: Tricyclic antidepressant overdose. JAMA *257*:521, 1987.
4. Dziukas LJ, Vohra J: Tricyclic antidepressant poisoning. Med J Aust *154*:344, 1991.
5. Richelson E: Pharmacology of antidepressants—characteristics of the ideal drug. Mayo Clin Proc *69*:1069, 1994.
6. Buckley NA, Dawson AH, Whyte IM, Henry DA: Greater toxicity in overdose of dothiepin than of other tricyclic antidepressants. Lancet *343*:159, 1994.
7. Henry JA, Alexander CA, Sener EK: Relative mortality from overdose of antidepressants. BMJ *310*:221, 1995.
8. Lancaster SG, Gonzalez JP: Lofepramine: A review of its pharmacodynamic and pharmacokinetic properties, and therapeutic efficacy in depressive illness. Drugs *37*:123, 1989.
9. Litovitz TL, Troutrman WH: Amoxapine overdose—seizures and fatalities. JAMA *250*:1069, 1983.
10. Wedin GP, Odera GM, Klein-Schwartz W, Gorman R: Relative toxicity of cyclic antidepressants. Ann Emerg Med *15*:797, 1986.
11. Brosen K, Gram LP: First-pass metabolism of imipramine and desiprarnine: Impact of the sparteine oxidation phenotype. Clin Pharmacol Ther *43*:400, 1988.
12. Schultz P, Turner-Tamiysay K, Smith G, et al: Amitriptyline disposition in young and elderly normal men. Clin Pharmacol Ther *33*:360, 1983.
13. Pentel PR, Bullock ML, DeVane CL: Hemoperfusion for impiramine overdose: Elimination of active metabolites. J Toxicol Clin Toxicol *19*:239, 1982.
14. Dawling S, Crome P, Graithwaite R: Pharmacokinetics of single oral doses of nortriptyline in depressed elderly hospital patients and young healthy volunteers. Clin Pharmacokinet *5*:394, 1980.
15. Nelson JC, Jatlow PI: Nonlinear desipramine kinetics: Prevalence and importance. Clin Pharmacol Ther *41*:666, 1987.
16. Gram LF, Bjerre N, Kragh-Sorenson P, et al: Imipramine metabolites in blood of patients during therapy and after overdose. Clin Pharmacol Ther *33*:335, 1983.
17. Breyer-Pfaff U, Prox A, Wachsmith H, Yao P: Phenolic metabolites of amitriptyline and nortriptyline in rat bile. Drug Metab Dispos *15*:882, 1987.
18. Brosen KD, Otton V, Gram LF: Imipramine demethylation and hydroxylation: Impact of the sparteine oxidation phenotype. Clin Pharmacol Ther *40*:543, 1986.
19. Spina E, Henthorm TK, Eleborg L, et al: Desmethylimipramine overdose: Nonlinear kinetics in a slow hydroxylator. Ther Drug Monit *7*:239, 1985.
20. Bluhm RE, Wilkinson GR, Shelton R, Branch TA: Genetically determined drug-metabolizing activity and desipramine-associated cardiotoxicity: A case report. Clin Pharmacol Ther *53*:89, 1993.
21. Connolly SJ, Mitchell LB, Swerdlow CD, et al: Clinical efficacy and electrophysiology of imipramine for ventricular tachycardia. Am J Cardiol *53*:516, 1984.
22. Wit AL, Cranefield PF, Hoffman BF: Slow conduction and reentry in the ventricular conducting system. Circ Res *30*:11, 1972.
23. Nattel S, Mittleman M: Treatment of ventricular tachyar-

rhythmias resulting from amitriptyline toxicity in dogs. J Pharmacol Exp Ther *231*:430, 1986.
24. Stone CK, Kraemer CM, Carroll R, Low R: Does a sodium-free buffer affect QRS width in experimental amitriptyline overdose. Ann Emerg Med *26*:58, 1995.
25. Pentel PR, Benowitz NL: Efficacy and mechanism of action of sodium bicarbonate in the treatment of desipramine toxicity in rats. J Pharmacol Exp Ther *230*:12, 1984.
26. Sasyniuk BI, Jhamandas V: Mechanism of reversal of toxic effects of amitriptyline on cardiac Purkinje fibers by sodium bicarbonate. J Pharmacol Exp Ther *232*:387, 1984.
27. McCabe JL, Emegazzo JJ, Cobaugh DJ, Auble TE: Recovery from severe cyclic antidepressant overdose with hypertonic saline/dextran in a swine model. Acad Emerg Med *1*:111, 1994.
28. Ranger S, Sheldon R, Fermini B, Nattel S: Modulation of flecainide's cardiac sodium channel blocking actions by extracellular sodium: A possible cellular mechanism for the action of sodium salts in flecainide cardiotoxicity. J Pharmacol Exp Ther *264*:1160, 1993.
29. Tamargo J, Rodriguez S, Garcia De Jalon P: Electrophysiological effects of desipramine on guinea pig papillary muscles. Eur J Pharmacol *55*:171, 1979.
30. Merigian KS, Hedges JR, Kaplan LA, et al: Plasma catecholamine levels in cyclic antidepressant overdose. Clin Toxicol *29*:177, 1991.
31. Rosenberg J, Pentel PR, Pond S, Benowitz N: Hyperthermia associated with drug intoxication. Vet Hum Toxicol *26*:413, 1984.
32. Sener EK, Gabe S, Henry JA: Response to glucagon in imipramine overdose. Clin Toxicol *33*:51, 1995.
33. Langou RA, VanDyke C, Tahan SR, Cohen LS: Cardiovascular manifestations of tricyclic antidepressant overdose. Am Heart J *100*:458, 1980.
34. Levitt A, Sullivan J, Owens M, et al: Change in amitriptyline plasma protein binding with increase in plasma pH over 7.4. Vet Hum Toxicol *26*:399, 1984.
35. Pentel PR, Keyler DE: Effects of high dose alpha-1-acid glycoprotein on desipramine toxicity in rats. J Pharmacol Exp Ther *246*:1061, 1988.
36. Hulten BA, Heath A: Clinical aspects of tricyclic antidepressant poisoning. Acta Med Scand *213*:275, 1982.
37. Callaham M, Kassel D: Epidemiology of fatal tricyclic antidepressant ingestion: Implications for management. Ann Emerg Med *14*:1, 1985.
38. Biggs JT, Spiker DG, Petit JM, Ziegler VE: Tricyclic antidepressant overdose: Incidence of symptoms. JAMA *238*:135, 1977.
39. Nattel S: Frequency-dependent effects of amitriptyline on ventricular conduction and cardiac rhythm in dogs. Circulation *72*:898, 1985.
40. Lavoie FW, Gansert GG, Weiss RE: Value of initial ECG findings and plasma drug levels in cyclic antidepressant overdose. Ann Emerg Med *19*:696, 1990.
41. Liebelt EL, Francis PD, Woolf AD: ECG lead a V_R versus QRS interval in predicting seizures and arrhythmias in acute tricyclic antidepressant toxicity. Ann Emerg Med *26*:195, 1995.
42. Caravati EM, Bossart PJ: Demographic and electrocardiographic factors associated with severe tricyclic antidepressant toxicity. Clin Toxicol *29*:31, 1991.
43. Boehnert MT, Lovejoy FH: Value of the QRS duration versus the serum drug level in predicting seizures and ventricular arrhythmias after an acute overdose of tricyclic antidepressants. N Engl J Med *3Z3*:474, 1985.
44. Thorstrand C: Clinical features in poisonings by tricydic antidepressants with special reference to ECG. Acta Med Scand *Z99*:337, 1976.
45. Pentel P, Sioris L: Incidence of late arrhythmias following tricyclic antipressant overdose. Clin Toxicol *18*:543, 1981.
46. Shannon M, Merola J, Lovejoy FH: Hypotension in severe tricyclic antidepressant overdose. Am J Emerg Med *6*:439, 1988.
47. Ellison JM, Milofsky JE, Ely E: Fluoxetine-induced bradycardia and syncope in two patients. J Clin Psychiatry *51*:385, 1990.
48. Taboulet P, Michard F, Muszynski J, et al: Cardiovascular repercussions of seizures during cyclic antidepressant poisoning. Clin Toxicol *33*:205, 1995.
49. Davidson ET: Amitriptyline-induced torsades de pointes: Successful therapy with atrial pacing. J Electrocardiol *18*:299, 1985.
50. Alderton HR: Tricyclic medication in children and the QT interval: Case report and discussion. Can J Psychiatry *40*:325, 1995.
51. McAlpine SM, Calabro JJ, Robinson MD, Burkle FM: Late death in tricyclic antidepressant overdose revisited. Ann Emerg Med *15*:1349, 1986.
52. Goldberg RJ, Capone RJ, Hunter JD: Cardiac complications following tricyclic antidepressant overdose. JAMA *254*:1772, 1985.
53. Teba L, Schiebel F, Dedhia HV, Lazzell VA: Beneficial effect of norepinephrine in the treatment of circulatory shock caused by tricyclic antidepressant overdose. Am J Emerg Med *6*:566, 1988.
54. Ellison DW, Pentel PR: Clinical features and consequences of seizures due to cyclic antidepressant overdose. Am J Emerg Med *7*:5, 1989.
55. Nosko MG, McLean DR, Chin WDN: Loss of brain stem and pupillary reflexes in amoxapine overdose: A case report. Clin Toxicol *26*:117, 1988.
56. Shannon M, Lovejoy FH: Pulmonary consequences of severe tricyclic antidepressant ingestion. Clin Toxicol *25*:443, 1987.
57. Roberge RJ, Martin TG, Hodgman M, Benitez HG: Case reports: Acute chemical pancreatitis associated with a tricyclic antidepressant (clomipramine) overdose. Clin Toxicol *32*:425, 1994.
58. Bosse GM, Barefoot JA, Pfeifer MP, Rodgers GC: Comparison of three methods of gut decontamination in tricyclic antidepressant overdose. J Emerg Med *13*:203, 1995.
59. Foulke GE, Albertson TE, Walby WF: Tricyclic antidepressant overdose: Emergency department findings as predictors of clinical course. Am J Emerg Med *4*:496, 1986.
60. Schwartz JG, Hurd IL, Carnahan JJ: Determination of tricyclic antidepressants for ED analysis. Am J Emerg Med *12*:513, 1994.
61. Apple FS, Bandt CM: Liver and blood postmortem tricyclic antidepressant concentrations. J Clin Pathol *89*:794, 1988.
62. Callaham M, Schumaker H, Pentel P: Phenytoin prophylaxis of cardiotoxicity in experimental amitriptyline poisoning. J Pharmacol Exp Ther *245*:216, 1988.
63. Wrenn K, Smith B, Slovis C: Profound alkalemia during treatment of tricyclic antidepressant overdose: A potential hazard of combined hyperventilation and intravenous bicarbonate. Am J Emerg Med *10*:553, 1992.
64. Hoffman JR, Votey SR, Bayer M, Silver L: Effect of hypertonic sodium bicarbonate in the treatment of moderate-to-severe cyclic antidepressant overdose. Am J Emerg Med *11*:336, 1993.
65. Bismuth CR, Peray-Peyroula F, Frejaville JP, et al: Nouveaux cas d'intoxication aigue par les derives tricycliques: Traitement par les sels de sodium. J Eur Toxicol *6*:285, 1969.
66. Nattel S, Keable H, Sasyniuk BL: Experimental amitriptyline intoxication: Electrophysiologic manifestations and management. J Cardiovasc Pharmacol *6*:83, 1984.
67. Brown TCK, Barker GA, Dunlop ME, Loughnan PM: The use of sodium bicarbonate in the treatment of tricyclic antidepressant-induced arrhythmias. Anaesth Intensive Care *1*:203, 1973.
68. Hoffman JR, McElroy CR: Bicarbonate therapy for dysrhythmia and hypotension in tricyclic antidepressant overdose. West J Med *134*:60, 1981.
69. Bessen HA, Niemann JT, Haskell RJ, Tothshein RJ: Effect of respiratory alkalosis in tricyclic antidepressant overdose. West J Med *139*:373, 1983.
70. Kingston ME: Hyperventilation in tricyclic antidepressant poisoning. Crit Care Med *7*:550, 1979.
71. Hagerman GA, Hanashiro PK: Reversal of tricyclic antidepressant-induced cardiac conduction abnormalities by phenytoin. Ann Emerg Med *10*:82, 1981.
72. Boehnert M, Lovejoy FH Jr: The effect of phenytoin on car-

diac conduction and ventricular arrhythmias in acute tricyclic antidepressant (TCA) overdose. Vet Hum Toxicol *27*:297, 1985.

73. Kulig K, Bar-or D, Marx J, et al: Phenytoin as treatment for tricyclic antidepressant cardiotoxicity in a canine model. Vet Hum Toxicol *26*:399, 1984.
74. Mayron R, Ruiz E: Phenytoin: Does it reverse tricyclic antidepressant induced cardiac conduction abnormalities? Ann Emerg Med *14*:505, 1985.
75. Beaubien AR, Carpenter DC, Mathieu LF, et al: Antagonism of imipramine poisoning by anticonvulsants in the rat. Toxicol Appl Pharmacol *38*:1, 1976.
76. Slovis TL, Ott JE, Teitelbaum DT, Lipscomb W: Physostigmine therapy in acute tricyclic antidepressant poisoning. Clin Toxicol *4*:451, 1971.
77. Pentel P, Peterson CD: Asystole complicating physostigmine treatment of tricyclic antidepressant overdose. Ann Emerg Med *9*:588, 1980.
78. Freeman IW, Loughhead MG: Beta blockade in the treatment of tricyclic antidepressant overdosage. Med J Aust *1*:1233, 1973.
79. Goldberg MJ, Park GD, Spector R, et al: Lack of effect of oral activated charcoal on imipramine clearance. Clin Pharmacol Ther *38*:350, 1985.
80. Karkkainen S, Neuvonen PJ: Pharmacokinetics of amitriptyline influenced by oral charcoal and urine pH. Clin Pharmacol Toxicol *24*:326, 1986.
81. Heath A, Wickstrom I, Martensson E, Ahlmen J: Treatment of antidepressant poisoning with resin hemoperfusion. Hum Toxicol *1*:361, 1982.
82. Diaz-Buxo JA, Farmer CD, Chandler JT: Hemoperfusion in the treatment of amitriptyline intoxication. Trans Am Soc Artif Intern Organs *24*:699, 1978.
83. Marbury T, Mahoney J, Foller T, et al: Treatment of amitriptyline overdosage with charcoal hemoperfusion. Kidney Int *12*:485, 1978.
84. Pedersen RS, Jorgensen KA, Olesen AS, Christensen KN: Charcoal hemoperfusion and antidepressant overdose. Lancet *1*:719, 1978.
85. Bramble MG, Lishmen AH, Purdon J, et al: An analysis of plasma levels and 24-hour ECG recordings in tricyclic antidepressant poisoning: Implications for management. Q J Med *56*:357, 1985.
86. Southall DP, Kilpatrick SM: Imipramine poisoning: Survival of a child after prolonged cardiac massage. BMJ *4*:508, 1974.
87. Williams JM, Hollingshed MJ, Vasilakis A, et al: Extracorporeal circulation in the management of severe tricyclic antidepressant overdose. Am J Emerg Med *12*:456, 1994.
88. Larkin GL, Graeber GM, Hollingsed MJ: Experimental amitriptyline poisoning: Treatment of severe cardiovascular toxicity with cardiopulmonary bypass. Ann Emerg Med *23*:480, 1994.
89. Dart RC, Sidki A, Sullivan JD Jr, et al: Ovine desipramine antibody fragments reverse desipramine cardiovascular toxicity in the rat. Ann Emerg Med *27*:309, 1996.
90. Pentel PR, Scarlett W, Ross CA, et al: Reduction of desipramine cardiotoxicity and prolongation of survival in rats with the use of polyclonal drug-specific antibody fab fragments. Ann Emerg Med *26*:334, 1995.
91. Peters RW, Buser GA, Kim HJ, Gold MR: Tricyclic overdose causing sustained monomorphic ventricular tachycardia. Am J Cardiol *70*:1226, 1992.
92. Pentel PR, Benowitz NL: Tricyclic antidepressant poisoning: Management of arrhythmias. Med Toxicol *1*:101, 1986.
93. Follmer CH, Lum BK: Protective action of diazepam and of sympathomimetic amines against amitriptyline induced toxicity. J Pharmacol Exp Ther *222*:424, 1982.
94. Sangster B, de Groot G, Borst C, de Wildt D: Dopamine and isoproterenol in imipramine intoxication in the dog. Clin Toxicol *23*:407, 1985.
95. Knudsen K, Abrahamsson J: Effects of epinephrine and norepinephrine on hemodynamic parameters and arrhythmias during a continuous infusion of amitriptyline in rats. Clin Toxicol *31*:461, 1993.
96. Merigian KS, Browning RG, Leeper KV: Successful treatment of amoxapine-induced refractory status epilepticus with propofol (Diprivan). Acad Emerg Med *2*:128, 1995.
97. Haverkos GP, DiSalvo RP, Imhoff TE: Fatal seizures after flumazenil administration in a patient with mixed overdose. Ann Pharmacother *28*:1347, 1994.
98. Lheureux P, Vranckx M, Leduc D, Askenasi R: Flumazenil in mixed benzodiazepine/tricyclic antidepressant overdose: A placebo-controlled study in the dog. Am J Emerg Med *10*:184, 1992.
99. Mills KC: Serotonin toxicity: A comprehensive review for emergency medicine. Top Emerg Med *15*:54, 1993.
100. Borys DJ, Setzer SC, Ling LJ, et al: Acute fluoxetine overdose: A report of 234 cases. Am J Emerg Med *10*:115, 1992.
101. Kincaid RL, McMullin MM, Crookham SB, Rieders F: Report of a fluoxetine fatality. J Anal Toxicol *14*:327, 1990.
102. Feighner JP, Boyer WF, Tyler DL, Neborsky RJ: Adverse consequences of fluoxetine-MAOI combination therapy. J Clin Psychiatry *51*:222, 1990.
103. Lau GT, Horowitz BZ: Sertraline overdose. Acad Emerg Med *3*:132, 1996.
104. Kaminski CA, Robbins MS, Weibley RE: Sertraline intoxication in a child. Ann Emerg Med *23*:1371, 1994.
105. Fantaskey A, Burkhart KK: A case report of venlafaxine toxicity. Clin Toxicol *33*:359, 1995.
106. Garnier R, Azoyan P, Chataigner D, et al: Acute fluvoxamine poisoning. J Int Med Res *21*:197, 1993.
107. Gamble DE, Peterson LG: Trazodone overdose: Four years of experience from voluntary reports. J Clin Psychiatry *47*:544, 1986.
108. Henry JA, Ali CJ, Caldwell R, Flanagan RJ: Acute trazodone poisoning: Clinical signs and plasma concentrations. Psychopathology *17*:77, 1984.
109. Ali CJ, Henry JA: Trazodone overdosage: Experience over 5 years. Neuropsychobiology *15*:44, 1986.
110. Richardson JW, Pichelson E: Antidepressants: A clinical update for medical practitioners. Mayo Clin Proc *59*:330, 1984.
111. Scher M, Krieger JN, Sjergens JN, Juergens S: Trazodone and priapism. Am J Psychiatry *140*:1362, 1983.
112. Burgess CD, Hames TK, George CF: The electrocardiographic and anticholinergic effects of trazodone and imipramine in man. Eur J Clin Pharmacol *23*:417, 1982.
113. Vitullo RN, Wharton JM, Allen NB, Pritchett ELC: Trazodone-related exercise-induced nonsustained ventricular tachycardia. Chest *98*:247, 1990.
114. Salerno SM, Strong JS, Roth BJ, Sakata V: Eosinophilic pneumonia and respiratory failure associated with a trazodone overdose. Am J Respir Crit Care Med *152*:2170, 1995.
115. Augenstin WL, Smolinske SC, Kulig KW, Rumack BH: Traodone overdose and severe cardiac toxicity. Vet Hum Toxicol *29*:478, 1987.
116. McCracken J, Radoslav K: Trazodone administration during ECT associated with cardiac conduction abnormality. Am J Psychiatry *141*:1488, 1984.
117. Spiller HA, Ramoska EA, Krenzelok EP, et al: Bupropion overdose: A 3-year multi-center retrospective analysis. Am J Emerg Med *12*:43, 1984.
118. Freil PN, Logan BK, Fligner CL: Three fatal drug overdoses involving bupropion. J Anal Toxicol *17*:436, 1993.
119. DeVane CL: Pharmacokinetics and drug metabolism of newer antidepressant agents. J Clin Psychiatry *55*(Suppl):38, 1994.

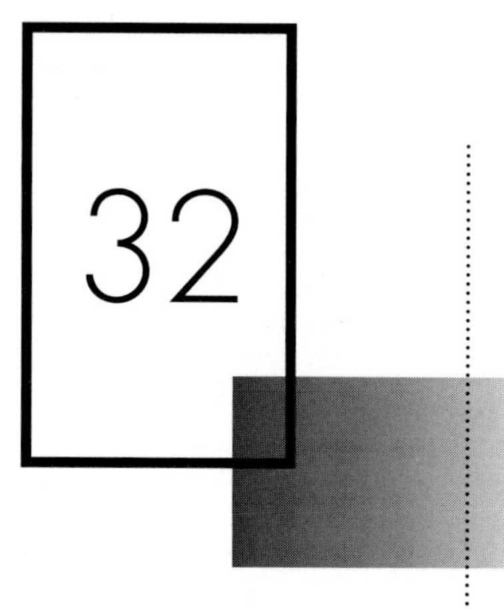

32 Monoamine Oxidase Inhibitors and the Serotonin Syndrome

JEFFREY BRENT, MD, PhD

The monoamine oxidase inhibitors (MAOIs) are a diverse group of agents that have been the center of considerable controversy during the past 40 years in terms of their place in therapy. This controversial position is largely caused by the many toxic reactions and interactions for which MAOIs are responsible. This chapter reviews the biochemistry of the enzyme monoamine oxidase (MAO), the pharmacology of the MAOIs, and the diagnosis, pathophysiology, and treatment of the various toxic reactions associated with these agents.

HISTORY

In 1951, isoniazid and its isopropyl derivative, iproniazid (Marsilid), were introduced for the treatment of tuberculosis. Although the latter antibiotic is no longer marketed, it was quickly noted that patients treated with it exhibited signs and symptoms of elevated mood. This psychotropic effect was found to result from iproniazid's ability to inhibit MAO. Shortly thereafter, MAOIs began to be used in the treatment of depression and thus became the first true specific antidepressant agents. Enthusiasm for their use was tempered in 1962 when a fatality associated with Stilton cheese ingestion in a patient taking an MAOI was reported.[1] The realization of the potential seriousness of adverse MAOI interactions caused considerable retrenchment from their use, a situation that has only recently been reconsidered. The mood-elevating properties of MAOIs are attributable to the inhibition of an MAO isoenzyme family referred to as MAO type A (MAO-A). This is in distinction to the MAO isoenzyme, which is referred to as MAO type B (MAO-B).

In 1989, several reports[2, 3] suggested that an inhibitor of MAO-B, known as L-deprenyl (selegiline), had a marked effect in the treatment of Parkinson's disease. Since that time, interest in the role of inhibitors of the B isoenzyme in the treatment of this disease has been growing.

PLACE IN THERAPY

MAOIs are used today for various psychiatric indications. One of their most common uses is in the treatment of depression refractory to therapy with standard cyclic antidepressants. MAOIs have assumed this secondary role presumably because of the reluctance to use these agents as a first-line drug, given the concerns about major toxic interactions. They are also used for the treatment of several other assorted conditions such as vascular headaches, narcolepsy, panic disorders, phobias, obsessive-compulsive disorder, eating disorders, and post-traumatic stress syndrome. For a full description of the uses of MAOIs, readers are referred to several of the excellent references on this topic.[2, 4–6]

Inhibitors of MAO-B used in the treatment of Parkinson's disease appear to slow the progression of the disease and extend the time before it is necessary to treat patients with this condition with L-dihydroxyphenylalanine.[7]

THE PHYSIOLOGY OF MONOAMINE OXIDASE

MAO (EC 1.4.3.4) is an intracellular enzyme tightly bound to the outer mitochondrial membrane. The intracellular location of MAO is a critical factor in understanding the pathogenesis of toxic reactions associated with MAOIs. Because MAO is intracellular, inhibition of MAO raises levels of its biogenic amine substrates only if they are themselves intracellular. Exogenous biogenic amines that act directly at extracellular receptors are therefore little influenced by MAO. Thus, inhibition of MAO does not result in toxic reactions with these directly acting agents.

MAO oxidatively deaminates biogenic amines such as epinephrine, norepinephrine, dopamine, 5-hydroxytryptamine (5-HT, serotonin), and tyramine. The generic reaction of MAO on primary biogenic amines is as follows[8]:

$$RCH_2NH_2 + O_2 + H_2O \rightarrow RCHO + NH_3 + H_2O_2$$

Note that one of the products of the MAO reaction is hydrogen peroxide, which is a generator of highly toxic free radicals.[9] Examples of the specific reactions of MAO with several biogenic amines are shown in Figure 32–1.

MAO is a ubiquitous enzyme, found primarily in brain, peripheral noradrenergic neuronal axons, intestine, and liver. Virtually all tissues contain some small amounts of MAO, the exceptions being erythrocytes, blood serum, and skeletal muscle. In general, MAO levels tend to increase with age. The two isoenzymes of MAO are separate gene products. Both genes for MAO are found on the X chromosome.

MONOAMINE OXIDASE ISOENZYMES

The two families of MAO isoenzymes differ in both their anatomic distribution and their substrate specificities (Table 32–1). Because of these differences, their role in the pathophysiology of toxic syndromes associated with MAOIs must be considered separately.

The highest concentration of MAO is in the liver, which contains approximately equivalent amounts of both isoenzymes. Brain similarly contains an approximately equal amount of both isoenzymes, although type B is found primarily in glial cells.

Table 32–1. Monoamine Oxidase Isoenzymes

	Locations	**Substrate Specificity**
MAO-A	Intestinal mucosa Placenta Biogenic amine terminals Liver Brain*	Serotonin Dopamine Norepinephrine Tyramine Epinephrine
MAO-B	Brain* Platelets Liver	Dopamine Tyramine Phenylethylamine Epinephrine Norepinephrine

*Approximately equal quantities of both isoenzymes exist in the brain, but there are considerable differences in their regional distribution. In addition, MAO-B is found primarily in glial tissue.

The substrate specificities of the MAOs[10–12] are mostly quantitatively different, although qualitatively most substrates are oxidized by both (see Table 32–1). The K_m and V_{max} for epinephrine, norepinephrine, dopamine, and tyramine are similar for both isoenzymes. The major difference in substrate specificities is for 5-HT, which is almost exclusively metabolized by MAO-A. The opposite pattern obtains for 2-phenylethylamine, which is primarily metabolized by MAO-B. The latter substrate is the parent compound of amphetamines and amphetamine-derived hallucinogens.

PHARMACOLOGY OF MONOAMINE OXIDASE INHIBITORS

Although the pharmacokinetics of the various MAOIs have distinct differences, their similarities tend to overshadow their differences. These agents are available only as oral preparations. MAOIs are metabolized hepatically and are rapidly cleared from the blood. In general, MAOIs are transported into cells by the neurotransmitter amine reuptake system.

As can be seen in Table 32–2, MAOIs are generally classified according to their preferential effect on the isoenzyme they inhibit. For most of these agents, however, the selectivity is not complete and tends to be lost at higher doses.

The classic MAOIs irreversibly inhibit the enzyme. Their duration of action is prolonged out of proportion to their blood levels after the therapeutic use of these irreversible agents. Although serum levels of

5-HT —MAO→ 5-Hydroxyindoleacetaldehyde

Tryptamine —MAO→ Indoleacetic Acid

Epinephrine, norepinephrine —MAO→ 3,4-Dihydroxymandelic Acid

Figure 32–1. Representative reaction of monoamine oxidase. 5-Hydroxyindoleacetaldehyde is further metabolized to 3-methoxy, 4-hydroxy-mandelic acid (VMA) by catechol-*O*-methyl transferase. MAO, monoamine oxidase; 5-HT, 5-hydroxytryptamine.

Table 32–2. Characteristics of Monoamine Oxidase Inhibitors

Generic Name	Trade Name	Selectivity	Reversibility	Hydrazine
Clorgyline		A*	No	No
Isocaboxazid	Marplan	A§	No	Yes
Moclobemide	Aurorix	A*	Yes	No
Pargyline	Eutonyl	B‖	No	No
Phenelzine	Nardil	A§	No	Yes
Selegiline	Deprenyl, Eldepryl	B*	No	No
Tranylcypromine	Parnate	A§	No	No
Brofaromine	Consonar	A*	Yes	No
Iproniazid	Marsilid†	A§	No	Yes
Isoniazid		No‡	No	Yes
MDMA		A§	Yes	No
Fluoxetine	Prozac	B*	Probably	No

MDMA, 3,4-methylenedioxymethamphetamine ("ecstasy").
*electivity is lost at supratherapeutic doses.
†No longer manufactured.
‡Weak MAOI.
§Weak inhibitor of MAO-B.
‖Weak inhibitor of MAO-A.

the MAOIs decline rapidly after last use, their effects are long lived. It is generally believed that a period of weeks is necessary to regain MAO activity after the cessation of the administration of an irreversible inhibitor, because new enzyme must be synthesized.

A new class of MAOIs, which are reversible inhibitors of the enzyme,[13–19] the prototype of which is moclobemide, have been developed (see Table 32–2). The reversible inhibitors act primarily on MAO-A and are therefore referred to as *reversible inhibitors* of MAO-A (RIMAs). The effect of RIMAs is short lived, with MAO activity being reconstituted within hours to days of the last dose. Because of the reversible nature of the binding of RIMAs with MAO, adverse reactions such as the pressor effect with tyramine ingestion ("cheese reaction") are unlikely to occur, and it is possible that they do not occur.[17] Approximately 150 mg of tyramine is needed to cause an increase in blood pressure while taking moclobemide. This is the equivalent of eating approximately 300 g of a tyramine-containing cheese.[20] Thus, although a tyramine reaction is theoretically possible, it is extremely unlikely to occur given the doses required. The reason why MAO-A inhibition by moclobemide does not predispose to a tyramine reaction is that the latter displaces the RIMA from the enzyme and thus may be normally metabolized. Whether one can suffer a cheese reaction after RIMA ingestion under any circumstances is still unknown.

Several of the older MAOIs are derived from hydrazine (NH_2-NH_2) (see Table 32–2). These MAOIs tend to be metabolized into active products and, like the well-known hydrazine isoniazid, are inactivated at a genetically determined rate by acetylation. The human population can be broadly separated into fast and slow acetylators on the basis of the rate of this reaction. For example, approximately equal numbers of American and European Caucasians may be classified as fast versus slow acetylators. The rate of slow acetylators is higher in Asian populations. Various adverse effects are specifically associated with the hydrazine-derived MAOIs.[21] Most prominent among these are the inhibition of multiple enzyme systems, hepatotoxicity, and the induction of pyridoxine (vitamin B_6) deficiency and the associated problem of seizures. The hepatotoxicity of MAOI hydrazines has been well reviewed.[22–24]

Among the enzyme systems inhibited by hydrazine MAOIs, the most important are pyridoxal kinase, L-amino acid decarboxylase, diamine oxidase, and cytochrome P-450.[21] In addition, hydrazines tend to form soluble complexes with pyridoxine and thus cause a state of deficiency of this vitamin by virtue of enhancing its urinary excretion.

In addition to the induction of pyridoxine deficiency, hydrazines prevent the use of pyridoxine for important metabolic reactions. Pyridoxine is not active as an enzyme cofactor until it is phosphorylated to pyridoxal phosphate by the enzyme pyridoxal kinase. Among the reactions for which pyridoxal phosphate is a cofactor is the synthesis of γ-aminobutyric acid (GABA) by the decarboxylation of glutamic acid, catalyzed by L-amino acid decarboxylase. Reduced production of GABA may cause the development of profound seizures as a result of poisoning by hydrazine MAOIs. The specific treatment for these seizures is administration of pyridoxine.

Virtually all MAOIs have a terminal phenyl group attached to a short aliphatic side chain, thus mimicking the phenylethylamine structure of amphetamines. It is thus possible that excessive doses of these agents may cause amphetamine-like reactions. Conversely, amphetamine or its derivatives tend to have some inhibitory effects on MAO.

MAOIs enhance synaptic biogenic amine transmitter concentrations by various mechanisms (Table 32–3). By inhibiting the enzymatic degradation of these neurotransmitters, their cytoplasmic concentrations are increased. Thus, the tendency is for release of these biogenic amines by a mass action effect. In addition, the act of transporting the MAOI into the cell by the amine reuptake system causes the ligand-binding site of the membrane-bound transporter molecule to face inward, and it thus becomes available

Table 32–3. Factors Contributing to MAO-A Inhibitor Toxicity

Decreased biogenic amine degradation
Amphetamine-like effect and increased catecholamine release from intracellular vesicles
GABA deficiency (hydrazines)
Decreased amine reuptake
Depletion of biogenic amine stores
GABA antagonism (tranylcypromine, isocarboxazid)
Increased amine release
Metabolism to amphetamine (tranylcypromine)

GABA, γ- aminobutyric acid.

for the transport of neurotransmitter into the synapse or neuroeffector junction. By being transported into the cell by the amine reuptake pump, the MAOIs act as competitive inhibitors of bioactive amine transport out of the synapse by this system. All of these factors tend to increase both intracellular and extracellular amine levels.

Being amphetamine congeners, MAOIs provoke release of stored amines from presynaptic vesicles, and thus the free intracellular concentrations of these molecules are increased. Given the decreased degradation of these amines by virtue of inhibition of MAO, any free bioactive amine molecules resulting from either release from vesicles or from reuptake are relatively protected from catabolism.

As noted in Table 32–2, the MAOIs differ in their characteristics. Several of them, however, merit specific comment.

Although no longer available as a therapeutic agent, clorgyline is the prototypic inhibitor of MAO-A. By virtue of the fact that nanomolar concentrations of this agent irreversibly inhibit MAO-A in a selective manner, this particular isoenzyme was defined.

Moclobemide is the prototype RIMA.[13–19] Although not available in the United States, moclobemide is available in most other parts of the world. In general, it appears that moclobemide and other RIMAs are safer than the traditional MAOIs.

In addition to the MAOIs noted in Table 32–2, various other agents have weak inhibiting properties of this enzyme. For example, procarbazine (Matulane) is a chemotherapeutic agent used in regimens to combat Hodgkin's disease. It is a weak MAOI; however, this has no significant therapeutic implications.

Tranylcypromine is an MAOI with great structural similarity to amphetamine. It may be metabolized to amphetamine. This generation of amphetamine may have a role in some of the toxicity of this agent. In addition, tranylcypromine can inhibit the action of GABA at the $GABA_A$ receptor. By doing so, it prevents chloride influx, which is the mechanism by which GABA inhibits neuronal activity. This inhibition of GABA activity by tranylcypromine may be responsible for the seizures observed with therapeutic doses of this agent. A similar effect on GABA channels is possible with isocarboxazid.

OVERDOSE

Overdose with the classic irreversible inhibitors of MAO-A, although infrequent, is associated with extremely high morbidity and mortality. All classic MAO-A inhibitors can cause a similar severe toxic syndrome associated with overdose. Ingestion of these agents in amounts greater than approximately 2 mg/kg should in general be considered to be potentially life threatening.[25] Although many factors affect the course of poisoning by these agents, a general chronologic framework may be noted in the construct of MAOI overdose promulgated by Linden and Rumack,[25] which highlights the following four phases:

1. Asymptomatic (latent)
2. Neuromuscular excitation and sympathetic hyperactivity
3. Central nervous system (CNS) depression with the potential for cardiovascular collapse
4. Secondary complications for survivors of the above

As noted in this scheme, a relatively asymptomatic period may precede the clinical manifestations of MAOI poisoning. Although it is unusual for this latent period to last for greater than 6 to 12 hours, it is generally believed that patients ingesting these agents should be observed for a full 24 hours to adequately rule out significant toxicity.[25–28]

The clinical effects of MAO-A inhibitor overdose are varied. The early manifestations frequently include headache and mild agitation. These may progress to profound central and peripheral nervous system stimulation associated with increased agitation, hyperthermia, hyperreflexia, diaphoresis, tremor, myoclonus, seizures, and a general sympathetic type of state. More serious cases evolve to frank rigidity. This is often followed by obtundation and a sympatholytic syndrome, which may progress to cardiovascular collapse. Common in cases of acute overdose are manifold complications including adult respiratory distress syndrome, disseminated intravascular coagulation, multiple organ system failure, and rhabdomyolysis.[25, 26, 28–32]

The pathophysiology of MAO-A inhibitor overdose involves many factors (see Table 32–3). The exact weight of the contribution of each of these factors is unknown.

Inhibition of MAO-A is associated with various effects on the degradative metabolism of intracellular catecholamines, indoles, and histamine. Because MAO-A is the major enzyme for the degradation of these intracellular amines, its inhibition results in increased cytoplasmic levels of these substances. Normally stored in intracytoplasmic vesicles, these amines are generally inaccessible to MAO. However, any that is released from these vesicles, any that is metabolically generated, or free amines resulting from reuptake are substrates for MAO-A.

Catecholamines are metabolized by MAO and catechol-*O*-methyl transferase (COMT). The latter enzyme is extracellular and is responsible for the degradation of catecholamines that are extracellular—for example, in the synaptic cleft. However, MAO is the major enzyme for intracellular catabolism of bioactive amines.

Serotonin is the major biologically active indole metabolized by MAO-A (Fig. 32–2). Thus inhibition of MAO-A results in elevated levels of intracytoplasmic 5-HT.[33] It should be noted, however, 5-HT metabolism has alternative minor pathways.[33–35] Tryptamine is a seizurogenic indole derived from the decarboxylation of tryptophan.[36] MAO is the major enzymatic pathway for the catabolism of tryptamine, which is oxidatively deaminated to indoleacetic acid.[33, 37] After poisoning by MAO-A inhibitors, urinary excretion of unmetabolized tryptamine increases.[33] This inhibition of tryptamine catabolism may contribute to the CNS excitation and seizures that occur after overdoses of these agents.

Histamine is metabolized either oxidatively or by acetylation to acetylhistamine.[8] The oxidative metabolism of histamine is accomplished by either MAO or diamine oxidase. As already noted, hydrazine MAOIs inhibit both of these enzymes. Thus, overdoses with hydrazine MAOIs are expected to result in elevated histamine levels,[33] which would contribute to the flushing and hypotension.

All of these factors associated with an overdose of an MAO-A inhibitor may be anticipated to increase intracytoplasmic biologically active amine concentrations. However, the exact contribution of the inhibition of MAO to the toxidrome engendered by an acute overdose of these agents is unknown. Some doubt may be raised about the significance of the inhibition of MAO in an acute overdose, because at least at therapeutic doses, this takes approximately 1 week. It is of course possible that higher doses may cause faster inhibition of this enzyme.

The multiple manifestations of MAO-A inhibitor poisoning characterized by cardiovascular and central and peripheral nervous system excitation with significant hyperthermia can be a diagnostic dilemma in the absence of a history of ingestion. Other causes of this presentation that should be included in the differential diagnosis are neuroleptic malignant syndrome, sepsis, heatstroke, sympathomimetic syndrome, lithium toxicity, serotonin syndrome, and thyrotoxicosis.

TREATMENT

The treatment of MAO-A inhibitor overdose is primarily supportive. The early sympathomimetic component of MAO-A inhibitor poisoning may have associated hypertension, which can be severe. However, caution must be used in the treatment of this hypertension because this early sympathomimetic state may unpredictably and suddenly be replaced by a sympatholytic syndrome with hypotension. Thus, the treatment of MAOI-induced hypertension should involve a short-acting agent such as phentolamine or nitroprusside at titrated doses. Standard agents should be used to treat cardiac dysrhythmias. However, bretylium, because of its propensity for causing catecholamine release and a subsequent sympatholytic state, should theoretically be avoided.

Gastrointestinal decontamination for patients presenting after a MAOI overdose should include administration of activated charcoal. Given its relative inefficacy and the possibility of a sudden and severe deterioration in the patient's clinical status, syrup of ipecac should be considered contraindicated. Patients presenting very early after overdose may benefit from gastric lavage.

Although not systematically studied in a controlled trial, aggressive management of MAOI-induced hyperthermia is generally considered to be of paramount importance in favorably altering a patient's prognosis.

The muscular hyperactivity and CNS stimulation in MAOI overdoses contribute to catecholamine release,[38] hyperthermia, and rhabdomyolysis. Thus, sedation of agitated, rigid, or hyperactive patients is generally recommended, and either benzodiazepines

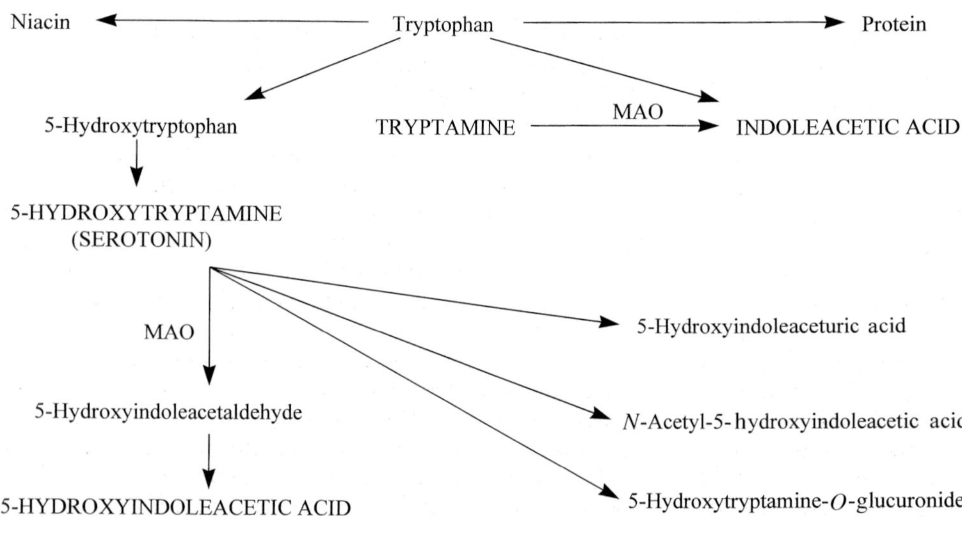

Figure 32–2. Metabolism of tryptophan. (From Baldridge ET, Miller LV, Haverback BJ, Brunjes S: Amine metabolism after an overdose of a monoamine oxidase inhibitor. N Engl J Med *267*:421–426, 1962. Reprinted, by permission, from *The New England Journal of Medicine*.)

or barbiturates are used. Although both types of agents have been used, benzodiazepines may be preferable because they have relatively fewer hemodynamic side effects. Linden and colleagues have suggested that amobarbital would be an appropriate barbiturate to use because of its short duration of effect and rapid onset of action.[25] If rigidity, agitation, or muscular activity cannot be controlled by simple pharmacologic maneuvers, then paralysis should be induced. It must be remembered, however, that paralyzing patients deprives a clinician of their most obvious marker for seizures, and thus paralyzed patients may be having CNS seizures that are unappreciated. It is therefore important either to use a short-acting paralytic agent, to induce a state of partial paralysis as measured by twitches, or to perform continuous electroencephalographic monitoring.

Blood pressure support should be accomplished using direct-acting sympathomimetic amines. These most prominently include epinephrine, norepinephrine, and phenylephrine. The direct agonists act at smooth muscle receptors on blood vessels and do not require intracellular metabolism to generate an active pressor amine. They are be catabolized by COMT. However, because of decreased reuptake of these amines and decreased degradation of any that is transported to the intracellular compartment, an exaggeration of their effect is a theoretic possibility.[39] Therefore, low and titrated doses should initially be used. The indirect-acting amines, the most significant one for blood pressure support being dopamine, are metabolized to active pressors (epinephrine and norepinephrine) intracellularly. MAO would normally prevent excessive amounts of these metabolites from being generated; however, this may not occur in the setting of its inhibition, and an exaggerated hemodynamic response may occur. Thus, the indirect pressor amines are generally considered to be contraindicated, a notion that is based primarily on theoretic considerations.

As already discussed, a hyperexcitable state or seizures in patients who have overdosed on a hydrazine type of MAOI (see Table 32–2) should be treated with pyridoxine. Because one component of the toxidrome scene following MAOI overdoses is an excess of 5-HT, it seems reasonable that a serotonin antagonist would be of benefit. However, this treatment approach has not been well studied in the setting of an MAOI overdose. Cyproheptadine is an antagonist at 5-HT_1 and 5-HT_2 receptors and is relatively devoid of potentially harmful effects; however, it is available only as an oral preparation. Methysergide is a 5-HT_1 and 5-HT_2 antagonist but is not available as a parenteral preparation. Ondansetron is a 5-HT_3 antagonist, and it is unlikely that this receptor is involved in the pathogenesis of the MAOI toxidrome. Procainamide, propranolol, and trazodone also have 5-HT antagonist properties; however, little is known about the effects of these agents in MAOI overdose. Bromocriptine is an ergot derivative that acts as a direct agonist at the dopamine receptor and can be beneficial in the MAOI toxidrome because it may blunt the effects of excess dopamine. Dantrolene sodium is an inhibitor of calcium release from the sarcoplasmic reticulum of skeletal muscle and thereby attenuates with excitation-contraction coupling. It may be of use in the muscle rigidity associated with MAOI poisoning. As noted earlier, hydrazine MAOIs (see Table 32–2) block histamine catabolism, and therefore it is theoretically useful to provide antihistamine (e.g., diphenhydramine) therapy in these cases.

The antihypertensives tolazoline, pentolinium, and clonidine have been touted as appropriate agents to treat the hypertension associated with the early stages of MAOI poisoning.[40, 41] However, no evidence shows that these agents are preferable to other antihypertensives.

Urinary acidification has a minor enhancing effect on the urinary excretion of tranylcypromine.[42] No data suggest that urinary acidification will further the clearance of other MAOIs. Given the almost inevitable rhabdomyolysis associated with the MAOI toxidrome and the lack of proven efficacy of urinary acidification, this treatment should be considered to be contraindicated.

The only RIMA that has been studied in overdose is moclobemide.[43, 44] Patients ingesting as much as 2 g have shown either gastrointestinal or no symptoms. In doses up to 5 g, depression of consciousness and slight increase in blood pressure may occur. At higher doses, fatigue, agitation, tachycardia, hypertension, and dilated slowly reacting pupils have been noted. No more serious side effects have been documented.[43] Plasma moclobemide concentrations as great as 30 times the therapeutic level are not associated with major toxic effects.[44] It therefore seems reasonable that routine gastrointestinal decontamination with activated charcoal and perhaps gastric lavage in selected early presenting cases are the major therapeutic interventions necessary. Because a delayed emergence of a RIMA toxidrome has not been observed, these patients should be observed until their toxic manifestations have resolved. Treatment is supportive.

INTERACTION OF MONOAMINE OXIDASE INHIBITORS WITH DIETARY AMINES

One of the greatest concerns in the therapeutic use of MAOIs is the potential hypertensive reaction associated with the ingestion of dietary amines. The amine most commonly implicated in these reactions is tyramine. Because 80% of all of these reactions and almost all of the reported deaths have been associated with the ingestion of tyramine-containing cheese,[45, 46] the name generally applied to this phenomenon is *cheese reaction*. Various cases have been associated with other dietary sources of amines. Spontaneous cases in the absence of any apparent exogenous amine have also been reported, in patients taking both classic MAOIs and RIMAs.[47, 48]

As already discussed, direct-acting sympathomimetic amines such as epinephrine (Sus-Phrine), norepinephrine, isoproterenol, albuterol, and metaproterenol are unlikely to cause a significantly exaggerated response because they do not require MAO for their metabolism. However, some exaggeration of their response is possible, for reasons previously discussed, and therefore doses of these direct acting amines should be carefully titrated. It is clearly the indirect-acting amines that are responsible for hypertensive cheese-type reactions. Of these, tyramine is the major dietary amine. Tyramine does not cross the blood-brain barrier, and therefore, the manifestations of the cheese reaction are due to its peripheral effects. Tyramine is an indirect-acting agonist that may provoke norepinephrine release from peripheral noradrenergic neurons. Therefore, the tyramine effect is the result of excessive norepinephrine secretion.

Dietary tyramine is normally metabolized by gastrointestinal MAO-A,[49–52] and therefore little gains access to the systemic circulation. That which does is further subject to degradation by neuronal MAO-A. Although tyramine is a substrate for both isoenzyme families of MAO, it is clearly the MAO-A that provides protection against the cheese effect. Patients taking MAO-B inhibitors are not vulnerable to a cheese reaction except at supertherapeutic doses of the inhibitor, in which case these agents may loose their isoenzyme selectivity.[53]

The literature contains considerable debate and misunderstanding about the potential dietary sources of tyramine and thus the restrictions required of patients being treated with MAO-A inhibitors. The various foods that have been implicated in hypertensive reactions associated with MAO-A inhibitors are prodigious (Table 32–4). Such an extensive list of dietary restrictions is both impractical and not justified by scientific data. Certain dietary restrictions do appear to be necessary, however.

The greatest concern with regard to food interactions with MAO-A inhibitors involves cheeses. Many aged cheeses are high in tyramine content and therefore should be restricted. However, some aged cheeses such as Brie, Emmenthal, and Gruyère contain little tyramine and can be eaten.[45] Cottage cheese, processed cheese slices, ricotta cheese, cream cheese, Havarti, Boursin, Parmesan cheese, bleu cheese dressing, Gorgonzola, feta, Muenster cheese, sour cream, and yogurt can likewise be eaten because of their low tyramine content.[45] Alcoholic beverages have been a source of concern, although none contain dangerously high levels of tyramine. Chianti wine has traditionally been singled out because of a 1964 report showing dangerously high tyramine levels.[54] However, more recent studies have failed to confirm this.[45]

The original reports of high levels of tyramine in pickled herring[55] have not been replicated by more recent studies.[45, 56] It has been suggested that the original report by Nuessle and colleagues in 1965[55] alleging a high level of tyramine in this fish was due to either an unreliable assay method or spoilage. Similarly, studies of smoked fish and caviar have also failed to demonstrate any significant tyramine content.[45]

Processed meat such as salami and some sausage have been shown to be high in tyramine.[45, 56] However, other meats such as liver, bologna, aged meat, corned beef, and pâtés have failed to demonstrate any significant tyramine content. Fruits and figs, including avocado, have virtually no tyramine content and should not be restricted. The one exception is banana peels, which contain approximately 1.4 mg of tyramine per peel. Therefore, preparations of whole banana should be eaten in moderation.

Concentrated yeast extracts (Marmite) contain significant amount of tyramine and should be restricted in patients taking MAO-A inhibitors.[45, 57] However various brewer's yeasts have low to nonexistent tyramine content and may be eaten without concern.[45] Sauerkraut contains nearly 14 mg of tyramine per 250-g serving and therefore should be considered contraindicated in patients who are taking MAO-A inhibitors, although there have been no case reports of a pressor response associated with this food.[45] Bouillon and soy sauce have been found to contain very low amounts of tyramine and therefore can be eaten without any concern.[45] Fava beans contain virtually no tyramine.[45] Italian green broad bean pods are

Table 32–4. Foods Implicated in Hypertensive Reactions with Monoamine Oxidase Inhibitors

Cheese	*Alcoholic beverages*	*Fish*	*Meat*	*Fruit*	*Yeast extracts*
All cheeses except cottage cheese and yogurt	Red wine (especially Chianti), sherry, vermouth, cognac, beer, liqueurs	Smoked fish, pickled herring, caviar	All fermented/aged meat including corned beef, salami, pepperoni, liver, sausage	Spoiled or overripe fruits, canned or overripe figs, stewed or whole bananas (including peeled)	Vitamin supplements (brewer's yeast)
Sauerkraut	*Bouillon*	*Soy sauce*	*Beans*		
			Broad bean pods (Italian green beans), fava beans		

not a concern with regard to their tyramine content, although they do contain the indirect-acting pressor dopa and therefore should not be eaten.[58] Given these data, it is clear many of the existing lists of food stuffs to be avoided by patients taking MAO-A inhibitors are unduly restrictive, and more liberalized and scientifically based suggestions have evolved.[6, 45, 59] It appears to be safe for patients using MAO-A inhibitors simply to avoid aged cheeses, concentrated yeast extract (Marmite), Italian broad bean pods, sauerkraut, salami, and sausage.

If a patient does have a hypertensive response associated with the ingestion of a dietary amine, treatment is generally considered to consist of pharmacologic control of blood pressure and management of any complications associated with the hypertensive episode. If the ingestion was recent, administration of activated charcoal may be considered on theoretic grounds. Although no controlled studies have investigated the appropriate management of these hypertensive responses, phentolamine in doses of 5 to 10 mg is generally recommended because it is an α-blocker and would be anticipated to antagonize the hypertensive effect of norepinephrine. However, no data suggest that other antihypertensive regimens would not be effective.

It is generally considered that there is a low risk of a cheese reaction with MAO-B inhibitors[17, 60, 61] except at high doses, which may cause these agents to loose their isoenzymes selectivity.[20, 53] However, a cheese reaction has been reported in a patient ingesting selegiline in therapeutic doses.[62] Cheese reactions should thus be considered to be a possibility in patients taking MAO-B inhibitors, and these patients should be aware of the dietary restrictions described earlier. However, it appears that these reactions are less likely to occur with these agents than with MAO-A inhibitors. Further experience with MAO-B inhibitors is required to verify this generally held impression.

Reversible inhibitors of MAO-A are unlikely to cause a pressor response from ingested cheese because tyramine can displace RIMAs from their binding site on MAO-A.[17, 18, 53] Very large doses of tyramine can cause an elevation in blood pressure in patients taking RIMAs[20]; however, hypertensive reactions with a dietary amine have not been reported to occur in patients taking these agents.

SEROTONIN SYNDROME

In 1959, a "fatal toxic encephalitis" was described in a patient who received meperidine while he was being treated for tuberculosis with iproniazid. Before the patient's demise, he exhibited severe muscular hyperactivity, rigidity, and clonus.[63] Shortly thereafter, Oates and Sjoerdsma[64] noted that tryptophan administered to patients who were taking an MAOI caused a phenomenon of unsteady gait, clonus, tremor, incoordination, feeling of lightheadedness, paresthesias, CNS excitation, dilated pupils, and hyperactive reflexes. Noting that tryptophan is a precursor in the biosynthetic pathway of both 5-HT and the neuroexcitatory transmitter tryptamine (see Fig. 32–2), the researchers concluded that inhibition of MAO caused an increase in levels of these molecules.[64] That these effects were indeed likely due to a derivative of tryptophan was verified by Smith and Prockop,[65] who showed that high doses of this amino acid can cause a similar effect. The following year, similar effects were observed when rhesus monkeys were fed high doses of tryptophan.[66] That these effects were likely not due to the tryptophan itself but to a metabolic derivative was shown in 1964 by Hodge and colleagues,[67] who demonstrated that they can be prevented by the administration of an inhibitor of the enzyme L-amino acid decarboxylase, which prevents the formation of tryptamine and 5-HT from tryptophan (see Fig. 32–2).

In 1971, Grahame-Smith[68] produced a similar phenomenon in rats, thus creating the animal model most commonly used to study the serotonin syndrome. That the observed syndrome is due to heightened levels of serotonin and not tryptamine was suggested by the clinical report by Beaumont,[69] which described four cases of a fatal interaction associated with similar symptoms as the prior reports, in patients taking an MAOI and the serotonergic antidepressant clomipramine (Anafranil). Although not specifically discussed in this report, this interaction suggests that it is 5-HT that is responsible for this syndrome. In 1982, Insel and associates[70] described a similar syndrome in patients taking clomipramine plus an MAOI and coined the term *serotonin syndrome*.

Diagnosis of the Serotonin Syndrome

Given the clinical presentation of the serotonin syndrome, the differential diagnosis to be entertained is quite broad and includes withdrawal states, tetanus, neuroleptic malignant syndrome, thyrotoxicosis, sepsis, and overdose of sympathomimetics, strychnine, MAOIs, or lithium. In 1991, Sternbach[71] proposed the following three diagnostic criteria for the serotonin syndrome:

A. Coincident with the addition of a known serotonergic agent to an established medication regimen or an increase in its dose, at least three of the following clinical features are present:
   1. Mental status changes (confusion, hypomania)
   2. Agitation
   3. Myoclonus
   4. Hyperreflexia
   5. Diaphoresis
   6. Shivering
   7. Tremor
   8. Diarrhea

9. Incoordination
10. Fever

B. Other causes (e.g., infectious, metabolic, substance abuse or withdrawal) have been ruled out.
C. A neuroleptic had not been started or increased in dose before the onset of the signs and symptoms listed earlier.

Insel[72] and Dursen[73, 74] and their colleagues have suggested modifications of Sternbach's criteria by replacing the 10 items under the first diagnostic criterion with the following, of which three were believed to be required:

1. Uncontrollable shivering
2. Incoordination
3. Restlessness in the feet while sitting
4. Initial involuntary contractions followed by myoclonus-like movements in the legs
5. Hyperreflexia
6. Frightened, diaphoretic hyperarousal state
7. Agitation
8. Oculogyric crisis
9. Diarrhea
10. Fear

Serotonin and the Pathophysiology of the Serotonin Syndrome

Since the mid-1930s, it has been known that a substance in intestinal enterochromaffin cells had a stimulating effect on bowel motility.[75] In 1948, a vasoconstrictor material was isolated from serum and named *serotonin*. This material was subsequently chemically characterized as 5-HT.[76] By 1952, it was known that the gut-stimulating material from the enterochromaffin cells was similarly 5-HT.[75]

It is now known that serotonin is synthesized from tryptophan (see Fig. 32–2) intracellularly and stored in vesicles by ion trapping. Any free 5-HT that is not so stored is metabolized by intracellular MAO.

Serotonin is found in high concentrations in platelets, enterochromaffin cells of the gastrointestinal tract, and the brain. Platelet 5-HT is important in hemostasis. Intestinal enterochromaffin cells contain approximately 90% of the total-body 5-HT. Tumors of these cells produce excess amounts of 5-HT and give rise to the carcinoid syndrome.

Serotonin acts by interaction with a specific family of receptors. The universe of serotonin-binding sites was originally thought to be composed of two separate receptors known as M and D.[77] However, by the early 1970s, studies of lysergic acid diethylamide (LSD) binding to serotonin receptors indicated that this scheme of two receptor types was too simple. Subsequently, multiple serotonin receptors, designated as 5-HT_1, 5-HT_2, 5-HT_3, and 5-HT_4 were demonstrated.[78] The 5-HT_1 receptor was found to be a family consisting of five different subtypes, designated 1A, 1B, 1D, 1E, and 1F.[79] We now know of some 13 separate serotonin receptors.[80] All of the 5-HT_1 receptors are neuronal and cause a decrease in intracellular cyclic adenosine monophosphate (cAMP). The three 5-HT_2 receptors (5-$HT_{2, A, B, C}$) are found in various tissues and act via intracellular phosphatidylinositol. The 5-HT_3, the two 5-HT_5, the 5-HT_6, and the 5-HT_7 receptors are neuronal. The 5-HT_3 receptor is cation channel related, whereas the others appear to raise intracellular cAMP levels. The 5-HT_{1A} receptor appears to be of importance in the pathogenesis of the serotonin syndrome. Agonists at this receptor, which include lysergic acid diethylamide (LSD) and 5-HT, inhibit the firing of raphe neurons. These neurons tend to modulate and attenuate sensory input. 5-HT_2 receptors, which also appear to be important in the pathophysiology of the serotonin syndrome, are excitatory and stimulate vascular smooth muscle and the CNS neurons. Serotonin is an indole compound structurally similar to LSD and psilocybin. The effects of these hallucinogens are mediated through interaction with the serotonin receptors. Because 5-HT_{1A} antagonists block some features of the serotonin syndrome, it has been hypothesized that this is the receptor most responsible for the various manifestations of 5-HT excess. However, some of the manifestations of the serotonin syndrome are also blocked by 5-HT_2 antagonists. Therefore, it has been theorized that this receptor as well has at least some role in the manifestations of the serotonin syndrome.

An alternative explanation for the serotonin syndrome derives from the similarity in clinical features between this condition and the neuroleptic malignant syndrome, which results from blockade of central dopamine effects. An excess of 5-HT inhibits brain dopaminergic neurons by blocking dopamine release or synthesis.[81–83] If this hypothesis is true, then some or all of the clinical features of the serotonin syndrome could potentially be blocked or attenuated by dopamine agonists. This has not been studied experimentally.

Clinical Manifestations

In 1991, Sternbach[71] reviewed 38 reported patients with the serotonin syndrome and used the observed clinical features to define his diagnostic criteria. The most common manifestations were, in decreasing order of frequency, restlessness, confusion, myoclonus, hyperreflexia, diaphoresis, shivering, tremor, hypomania, diarrhea, and incoordination. A later review found that the most common reported manifestations were, in order of decreasing frequency, hyperreflexia, altered mental status, myoclonus, ataxia, diaphoresis, fever, shivering, and diarrhea.[84] Mills conducted the most comprehensive analysis of reported cases and reported the signs and symptoms in 100 previously reported cases, dividing them into cognitive/behavioral, autonomic, and neuromuscular. The results of his analysis are shown in Table 32–5.

Table 32–5. Signs and Symptoms of Serotonin Syndrome (Review of 100 Cases)

Sign/Symptom	Frequency (%)
Cognitive-Behavioral Symptoms	
Confusion/disorientation	51
Agitation/irritability	34
Coma/unresponsiveness	29
Anxiety	15
Euphoria/hypomania	14
Headache	13
Drowsiness	13
Seizures	12
Insomnia	11
Hallucinations (visual and auditory)	6
Dizziness	5
Autonomic Nervous System	
Hyperthermia	45
Diaphoresis	45
Sinus tachycardia	36
Hypertension	35
Dilated pupils	28
Tachypnea	26
Nausea	23
Unreactive pupils	20
Flushing	16
Hypotension	15
Diarrhea	8
Ventricular tachycardia	6
Cyanosis	5
Abdominal cramps	4
Salivation	2
Neuromuscular	
Myoclonus	58
Hyperreflexia	52
Muscle rigidity	51
Restlessness/hyperactivity	48
Tremor	43
Ataxia/incoordination	40
Clonus	23
Babinski's sign (bilateral)	16
Nystagmus	15
Trismus	7
Teeth chattering	6
Opisthotonos	6
Paresthesias	6

Agents Causing the Serotonin Syndrome

Theoretically, any scenario in which 5-HT increases can result in the serotonin excess syndrome. However, with the exception of a very few instances, this syndrome results from a combination of serotonergic agents. This occurs most commonly when two agents that increase serotonin levels by different mechanisms are taken. The various serotonergic agents are listed in Table 32–6. It is an impossible exercise to attempt to memorize which combinations of these agents have been documented to cause a serotonin syndrome. Bodner and associates[86] compiled a six-page table documenting the various interactions of serotonergic agents that may cause a serotonin syndrome. It is wisest to assume that any two serotonergic agents in combination are at least theoretically capable of causing this syndrome. The most common drug combinations reported to cause the serotonin syndrome are MAOIs plus selective serotonin reuptake inhibitors (SSRIs).[71, 84–89] and MAOIs plus clomipramine.[86, 90] Another combination that has been frequently implicated in causing the serotonin syndrome is simultaneous administration of an MAOI and tryptophan.[64, 72, 86, 91–101]

One particular drug combination that has received considerable attention is the interaction between an MAOI and meperidine. In 1962, a woman who received meperidine in labor was reported to have developed coma and hypotension. It was subsequently noted that she had been self-administering phenelzine, and thus concern was raised about a possible drug interaction.[102] Shortly thereafter, a patient on pargyline therapy was reported to have developed rigidity, coma, and clonus after receiving Demerol.[103] Since then, several other cases of an interaction of a similar nature in patients taking meperidine in MAOIs have been reported.[84, 86] There are several unexplained curiosities about the serotonin syndrome generated by the interaction between meperidine and MAOIs. Despite the diverse group of serotonergic drugs in common clinical practice (see Table 32–6) and the frequent use of meperidine, no reports have described a serotonin syndrome with any other agent in combination with meperidine. Similarly, Ebrahim reported a series of 42 patients who were taking isocarboxazid and who were premedicated with meperidine for surgery; none of them had an adverse effect.[104]

Although in the overwhelming majority of instances the serotonin syndrome is caused by a combination of serotonergic agents, in occasional instances, a single drug has caused this symptom complex. These cases always involve excessive doses of the serotonergic agent. An animal model developed for this syndrome almost three decades ago involved the

Table 32–6. Serotonergic Agents

Agent	Mechanism
MAOIs	Inhibit serotonin breakdown
Clomipramine	Inhibits serotonin reuptake
Selective serotonin reuptake inhibitors	Inhibit serotonin reuptake
Tryptophan	Metabolized in serotonin
Lithium	Enhances serotonin release, potentiates effects of 5-HT_{1A} receptor
Amitryptyline/impramine	Inhibits serotonin reuptake
Meperidine	Inhibits serotonin reuptake
Dextromethorphan	Inhibits serotonin reuptake
Levodopa	Causes serotonin release
Trazodone	Inhibits serotonin reuptake
MDMA	MAOI, causes serotonin release
Amphetamines	Cause serotonin release
Cocaine	Causes serotonin release
Lysergic acid diethylamide (LSD)	5-HT_{1A} agonist

MAOI, monoamine oxidase inhibitor; 5-HT, 5-hydroxytryptamine; MDMA, 3,4-methylenedioxymethamphetamine.

sole administration of high doses of tryptophan to rats, which caused a unique constellation of tremors and movement abnormalities.[68] The same syndrome could be induced by simply administering high doses of an MAOI.[68] This observation provided evidence that some aspects of the clinical syndrome engendered by MAOI overdoses are related to serotonin excess. It is theoretically possible that a serotonin excess syndrome could occur after overdoses of SSRIs. However, this appears to occur extremely rarely and was not a feature in a series of fluoxetine overdoses.[105] A child ingested an excessive amount of sertraline and appeared to develop a serotonin syndrome manifested by tachycardia, hypertension, hallucinations, coma, hyperthermia, tremors, and skin flushing.[106]

A serotonin syndrome–like toxidrome has been reported to follow the ingestion of MDMA ("ecstasy").[107–115] These reports must be evaluated carefully, because MDMA has various potential pharmacologic actions. Being a phenylethylamine type of agent, it is structurally similar to amphetamines and likely affects dopaminergic as well as serotonergic neurons. Hence, it is theoretically capable of provoking a complex syndrome that may not be a pure serotonin syndrome. In addition, MDMA is frequently ingested in the context of a "rave," a gathering at which so-called smart drinks, which are amino acid supplements possibly containing significant amounts of tryptophan, are also ingested.[108, 116] Thus it is possible that the complex clinical syndrome noted after MDMA ingestion may often be a drug interaction between two serotonergic agents.

Although in general they appear to be safer than classic MAOIs, RIMAs are capable of causing a drug interaction resulting in a serotonin syndrome. All reported cases have involved the interaction of moclobemide and either clomipramine, citalopram, or another serotonin reuptake inhibitor, after both overdose[117–119] and therapeutic use.[120] Two of the fatalities involve purposeful taking of the combination to achieve a psychologic "high."[117]

As noted in Table 32–6, lithium has several serotonergic effects including stimulating 5-HT release[121] and enhancing the response to stimulation of 5-HT_{1A} receptors.[122, 123] Several case reports describe a serotonin syndrome caused by the therapeutic combination of lithium with SSRIs.[124–126] Given the frequency with which lithium is prescribed in combination with SSRIs, the relatively few cases of serotonin syndrome induced by these combinations suggest that this is an unusual interaction.

The use of MAOIs with tricyclic antidepressants has been the subject of considerable debate. Combining these two agents has been associated with a serotonin syndrome–like picture.[127, 128] However, given the frequency of the use of this combination and the rarity of adverse reports, it appears that the likelihood of an adverse effect from this combination is small.[129] However, particular caution must be exercised when using clomipramine, which is a tricyclic antidepressant (3-chloroimipramine) that has a significant effect on inhibiting serotonin reuptake (see Table 32–6). The combination of a TCA with a RIMA appears to be safe, with the exception of agents such as clomipramine, which have a significant effect on serotonin uptake.[130]

A body of literature suggests that the serotonergic effects of dextromethorphan (DM), in consort with other agents, may produce a serotonin syndrome. In 1970, Rivers and Horner described profound hyperthermia in a patient ingesting a DM-containing preparation while taking phenelzine.[131] Several reports have since described similar interactions.[132–134] A similar syndrome has been described in rabbits pretreated with MAOIs.[135] Whether DM can cause a serotonin syndrome in concert with an SSRI has been the subject of controversy. Two cases have been reported.[132–134] It has been proposed that the nature of the interaction in these two cases, involving paroxetine and fluoxetine, respectively, derives from an interaction at the level of the hepatic microsomal P-450 isoenzyme CYP2D6 (debrisoquin hydroxylase).[136–139] DM is metabolized by this enzyme to dextrorphan, in a genetically determined manner by one of two phenotypes, known as extensive and poor metabolizers. Administration of DM in subjects who have had this isoenzyme inhibited by quinidine results in profoundly elevated DM levels associated with signs and symptoms of a serotonin syndrome. Both paroxetine and fluoxetine are inhibitors of this isoenzyme,[138, 139] as are sertraline and fluvoxamine.[140, 141] However, the significance of this enzymatic inhibition in the generation of a serotonin syndrome associated with the administration of DM has been questioned on the basis of the small amounts of DM requisite to the formation of a manifestation of 5-HT in these combinations.[90]

Sandyk[142] reported an apparent serotonin syndrome in a patient with parkinsonism treated with bromocriptine in whom levodopa was started. The reported syndrome consisted of tremor, mild clonus, hyperreflexia, clonus, hypertension, tachycardia, diaphoresis, and diarrhea. Support that this was due to serotonin excess was suggested by its prompt response to the serotonin antagonist methysergide. Both bromocriptine and levodopa are serotonergic agents. Serotonergic neurons are capable of decarboxylating levodopa to dopamine, during which 5-HT may be released.[143, 144] Bromocriptine appears to increase brain levels of serotonin, inhibiting 5-HT catabolism[145, 146]; however, only one case of such an interaction has been described.[142]

Trazodone is an antidepressant with complex serotonergic effects. At low doses, it appears to be a serotonin antagonist.[147] At higher doses, however, it appears to be a mixed agonist/antagonist.[147] Low doses appear to be safe when trazodone is taken in combination with an MAOI.[148] One case of a serotonin syndrome has been reported after the combined administration of trazodone and the 5-HT_{1A} receptor partial agonist buspirone.[149]

Selegiline and MAO-B inhibitors have been reported to cause the serotonin syndrome. Although 5-

HT is metabolized by MAO-A, selegiline may cause an excess serotonin effect by virtue of its loss of MAO specificity at higher doses. Cases of the serotonin syndrome, including death, have been reported with the combination of selegiline and SSRIs[150–152] and tricyclic antidepressants.[84, 153]

Buspirone is an anxiolytic agent that is a partial agonist at the $5\text{-}HT_{1A}$ receptor. Its potential role in the generation of the serotonin syndrome is unclear but probably unlikely because animals treated with high doses do not develop a full-blown serotonin syndrome. The one case report[149] of an interaction with buspirone and trazodone involved primarily only mild clonus. It is likely that the relative inability of buspirone to induce a serotonin syndrome is related to its being a partial antagonist at the serotonin receptor.

Sumatriptan is a serotonergic antimigraine agent that has not been implicated in the etiology of the serotonin syndrome. It acts primarily on $5\text{-}HT_1$ receptors, although it is also a $5\text{-}HT_{1A}$ agonist. Sumatriptan does not cross the blood-brain barrier. Its antimigraine effect is on the basis of vasoconstriction of cephalic blood vessels.

Tramadol is a serotonergic agent that blocks 5-HT reuptake.[154, 155] It has not been implicated in the serotonin syndrome, although it was present in one patient who died of a fatal moclobemide-clomipramine interaction.[119]

Treatment of the Serotonin Syndrome

No prospective studies have investigated any specific treatment for the serotonin syndrome. Virtually all of the data that we have to rely on come from anecdotal case reports and animal studies. From these, it can be gleaned that discontinuation of the provoking agents and supportive care are the cardinal principles in the treatment of this syndrome.

Cyproheptadine, a general 5-HT receptor antagonist that is most potent at the $5\text{-}HT_2$ receptor,[156] is the most commonly touted antidote for the serotonin syndrome. The apparent utility of cyproheptadine is evidence suggesting that the $5\text{-}HT_2$ receptor is important in the pathophysiology of the serotonin syndrome. In addition to being a serotonin antagonist, cyproheptadine is antihistaminic and anticholinergic. Animal studies suggest that cyproheptadine can block the serotonin syndrome.[157]

Several anecdotal reports describe treatment of the serotonin syndrome with cyproheptadine.[126, 149, 158, 159] Unfortunately, cyproheptadine is available only as an oral preparation. A standard starting dose is 4 to 8 mg, typically followed by doses of 4 mg every 2 to 4 hours. Because of its antimuscarinic properties, anticholinergic side effects may occur; therefore, doses should not exceed more than 0.5 mg/kg per day.

Methysergide maleate is a nonspecific serotonin antagonist that appears to have some efficacy in animal studies in preventing the serotonin syndrome.[160] Clinical data evaluating the efficacy of methysergide in this toxidrome are sparse. In one case report, it appeared to be effective in the treatment of a serotonin syndrome induced by the therapeutic use of the combination of levodopa and bromocriptine.[142] Methysergide is available only as an oral preparation. It is usually given in doses of 2 to 6 mg, the latter being the typical total dose. It is frequently administered in a twice-a-day regimen.

β-Adrenergic receptor antagonists also tend to have some serotonin antagonist qualities. Propranolol is a $5\text{-}HT_{1A}$ blocker[161] that is effective in blocking the serotonin syndrome in animals.[160, 162] Responses to it have been inconsistent.[87, 99, 158]

Dantrolene has been mentioned as an agent that might inhibit the neuromuscular hyperactivity component of the serotonin syndrome; however, there has been little clinical experience with it in this setting.

Although phenothiazines are $5\text{-}HT_2$ antagonists, there has been little experience with them in the treatment of the serotonin syndrome. The few case reports studied have shown mixed results.[163–166]

References

1. Hemmelhoch JM: Monoamine oxidase inhibitors. *In* Kaplan HI, Saddock BJ (eds): Comprehensive Textbook of Psychiatry. 6th ed. Baltimore, Williams & Wilkins, pp 2038–2053, 1995.
2. Parkinson Study Group: Effect of deprenyl on the progression of disability in early Parkinson's disease. N Engl J Med *321*:1364–1371, 1989.
3. Tetrud JW, Langston JW: The effect of deprenyl on the natural history of Parkinson's disease. Science *245*:519–522, 1989.
4. Baldessarini RJ: Biomedical Aspects of Depression and Its Treatment. Washington, DC, American Psychiatric Press, 1983.
5. Baldessarini RJ: Chemotherapy in Psychiatry: Principles and Practice. 2nd ed. Cambridge, MA, Harvard University Press, 1985.
6. Larsen JK: MAO inhibitors: Pharmacodynamic aspects and clinical implications. Acta Psychiatr Scand *78*(Suppl 345):74–80, 1988.
7. Tipton KF: What is it that *l*-deprenyl (selegiline) might do? Clin Pharmacol Ther *56*:781–795, 1994.
8. Davidson AN: Physiological role of monoamine oxidase. Physiol Rev *38*:729–747, 1958.
9. Brent J, Rumack BH: The role of free radicals in toxic hepatic injury. 11. Are free radicals the cause or the consequences of toxin-induced injury? J Toxicol Clin Toxicol *31*:173–196, 1993.
10. O'Carroll A-M, Fowler CJ, Philips JP, et al: The deamination of dopamine by human brain monamine oxidase: Specificity of the two forms in seven brain regions. Naunyn Schmiedebergs Arch Pharmacol *323*:198–202, 1983.
11. O'Carroll A-M, Bardsley ME, Tipton KF: The oxidation of adrenaline and noradrenaline by the two forms of monoamine oxidase from human and rat brain. Neurochem Int *8*:493–500, 1986.
12. Kinemuchi H, Fowler CJ, Tipton KF: Substrate specificities of the two forms of monoamine oxidase. *In* Tipton KF, Dostert P, Strolin Benedetti M (eds): Monoamine Oxidase and Disease: Prospects for Therapy with Reversible Inhibitors. New York, Academic Press, pp 53–62, 1984.
13. DaPrada M, Keller H, Keller R, et al: Ro 11-1163, a specific short acting MAO inhibitor with antidepressant properties. *In* Kamito K, Usdin E, Nagatsu T (eds): Monoamine Oxidase.

Basic and Clinical Frontiers. Amsterdam, Excerpta Medica, pp 183–196, 1981.
14. Youdim MBH, Da Prada M, Amrien R (eds): The cheese effect and new reversibly MAO-A inhibitors. J Neural Transm Suppl 26: 1988.
15. Haefely W, Burkard WP, Cesura AM, et al: Biochemistry and pharmacology of moclobemide, a prototypical RIMA. Psychopharmacology *106*:56–514, 1992.
16. Haefely W, Burkard WP, Cesura A, et al: Pharmacology of moclobemide. Clin Neuropharmacol *16*(Suppl 2):58–518, 1993.
17. Youdim MBH: The advent of selective monoamine oxidase A inhibitor antidepressants devoid of the cheese reaction. Acta Psychiatr Scand *91*(Suppl 386):5–7, 1995.
18. Callingham BA: Possible drug interactions with reversible MAO inhibitors. Clin Neuropharmacol *15*(Suppl 1):339A–340A, 1992.
19. Amrein R, Allen SR, Guentert TW, et al: The pharmacology of reversible monoamine oxidase inhibitors. Br J Psychiatry *155*(Suppl 6):66–71, 1989.
20. Dallow S: Selective MAOIs. Lancet *345*:1055, 1995.
21. Tollefson GD: Monoamine oxidase inhibitors: A review. J Clin Psychiatry *44*:280–288, 1983.
22. Browne B, Linter S: Monoamine oxidase inhibitors and narcotic analgesics. A critical review of the implications for treatment. Br J Psychiatry *151*:210–212, 1987.
23. Ciraulo DA, Shader RI: J Clin Psychopharmacol *10*:48–50, 1990.
24. Dupont H, Davies DS, Strolin Benedetti M: Biochem Pharmacol *36*:1651–1657, 1987.
25. Linden CH, Rumack BH, Strehlke C: Monoamine oxidase inhibitor overdose. Ann Emerg Med *13*:1137–1144, 1984.
26. Matell G, Thorstrand C: A case of fatal nialamide poisoning. Acta Med Scand *181*:79–82, 1967.
27. Reid DD, Kerr WC: Phenelzine poisoning responding to phenothiazine. Med J Aust *2*:1214–1215, 1969.
28. Mawdsley JA. "Parstelin." A case of fatal overdose. Med J Aust *2*:292, 1968.
29. Platts MM, Usher A, Stentiford NH: Phenelzine and trifluoperazine poisoning. Lancet *2*:738, 1965.
30. Robertson JC: Recovery after massive MAOI overdose complicated by malignant hyperpyrexia, treated with chlorpromazine. Postgrad Med J *48*:64–65, 1972.
31. King J, Barnett PS, Kew MC: Drug-induced hyperpyrexia. A case report. S Afr Med J *567*:190–191, 1979.
32. Coulter C, Edmunds J, Pyle PO: An overdose of Parstelin. Anaesthesia *26*:500–501, 1971.
33. Baldridge ET, Miller LV, Haverback BJ, Brunjes S: Amine metabolism after an overdose of a monoamine oxidase inhibitor. N Engl J Med *267*:421–426, 1962.
34. Melsaac WM, Page IH: New metabolites of serotonin in carcinoid urine. Science *128*:537, 1958.
35. Davidson J, Sjoerdsma A, Loomis LN, Undenfriend S: Studies with serotonin precursor. 5-hydroxytryptophan in experimental animals and man. J Clin Invest *36*:1594–1599, 1957.
36. Tedeschi DH, Tedeschi RE, Fellows EJ: Effects of tryptamine on central nervous system including pharmacological procedure for evaluation of iproniazid-like drugs. J Pharmacol Exp Ther *126*:223–232, 1959.
37. Sjoerdsma A, Oates JA, Zaltzman P, Udenfriend S: Identification and assay of urinary tryptamine: Application as index of monoamine oxidase inhibition in man. J Pharmacol Exp Ther *126*:217–222, 1959.
38. von Euler US, Hellner S: Excretion of noradrenaline and adrenaline in muscular work. Acta Physiol Scand *26*:183–191, 1952.
39. Boakes AJ, Laurence DR, Teoh PC, et al: Interactions between sympathomimetic amines and antidepressant agents in man. BMJ *1*:311–315, 1973.
40. Reynolds JEF: Martindale, the Extra Pharmacopoeia. 28th ed. London, Pharmaceutical Press, p 28, 1982.
41. Cain NN, Cain RM: A compendium of antidepressants. Drug Ther *8*:114–150, 1978.
42. Turner P, Young JH, Paterson J: Influence of urinary pH on the excretion of tranylcypromine sulphate. Nature *215*:881–882, 1967.
43. Myrenfors PG, Eriksson T, Sandstedt CS, Sjoberg G: Moclobemide overdose. J Internal Med *233*:1–115, 1993.
44. Iwersen S, Schmoldt A: Three suicide attempts with moclobemide. Clin Toxicol *34*:223, 1996.
45. Shulman KI, Walker SE, MacKenzie S, Knowles S: Dietary restriction, tyramine and the use of monoamine oxidase inhibitors. J Clin Psychopharmacol *9*:397–402, 1989.
46. Livingston MG: Reply to Dallow. Letter. Lancet *345*:1056, 1995.
47. Fallon B, Foote B, Walsh BT, Roose SP: 'Spontaneous' hypertensive episodes with monoamine oxidase inhibitors. J Clin Psychiatry *49*:163–165, 1988.
48. Lavin MR, Mendelowita A, Kronig MH: Spontaneous hypertensive reactions with monoamine oxidase inhibitors. Biol Psychiatry *34*:146–151, 1993.
49. Blackwell B, Marley E: Interactions with cheese and its constituents with monoamine oxidase inhibitors. Br J Pharmacol Chemother *26*:120–141, 1966.
50. Ilett KF, George CF, Davies DS: The effect of monoamine oxidase inhibitors on "first pass" metabolism tyramine in dog intestine. Biochem Pharmacol *29*:2551–2556, 1980.
51. Davies DS, Yasuhara H, Boobis AR, George CF: The effects of reversible and irreversible inhibitors of monoamine oxidase on tyramine deamination by the dog intestine. *In* Tipton KF, Dostert P, Strolin Benedetti M (eds): Monoamine Oxidase and Disease; Prospects for Therapy with Reversible Inhibitors. London, Academic Press, pp 443–448, 1984.
52. Hasan F, McCrodden JM, Kennedy NP, Tipton KF: The involvement of intestinal monoamine oxidase in the transport and metabolism of tyramine. J Neural Transm *26*(Suppl):1–9, 1988.
53. Callingham BA: Drug interactions with reversible monoamine oxidase-A inhibitors. Clin Neuropharmacol *16*(Suppl 2):S42–S50, 1993.
54. Horowitz D, Lovenberg W, Engelman K, Sjoerdsma A: Monoamine oxidase inhibitors, tyramine, and cheese. JAMA *188*:1108–1110, 1964.
55. Nuessle WF, Norman FC, Mille HE: Pickled herring and tranylcypromine reaction. JAMA *192*:726–727, 1965.
56. Da Prada M, Zurcher G, Wuthrich I, et al: On tyramine food, beverages and the reversible MAO inhibitor moclobemide. J Neural Transm *26*:31–56, 1988.
57. Blackwell B, Mabbitt LA: Effects of yeast extract after monoamine oxidase inhibition. Lancet *1*:940–943, 1965.
58. Hodge JV, Nye ER, Emerson GW: Monoamine-oxidase inhibitors, broad beans and hypertension. Lancet *1*:1108, 1964.
59. Sweet RA, Brown EJ, Hemiberg RG, et al: Monoamine oxidase inhibitor dietary restrictions: What are we asking patients to give up? J Clin Psychiatry *56*:196–201, 1995.
60. Kalir A, Sabbagh A, Youdim MBH: Selective acetylenic "suicide" and reversible inhibitors of monoamine oxidase A and B. Br J Pharmacol *73*:55–64, 1981.
61. Finberg JPM, Tenne M, Youdim MBH: Tyramine antagonistic properties of AGN-1135, an irreversible inhibitor of monoamine oxidase B. Br J Pharmacol *73*:65–70, 1981.
62. McGrath PJ, Stewart JW, Quitkin FM: A possible deprenyl induced hypertensive reaction. J Clin Psychopharmacol *9*:310–311, 1989.
63. Mitchell RS: Fatal toxic encephalitis occurring during iproniazid therapy in pulmonary tuberculosis. Ann Intern Med *42*:417–424, 1955.
64. Oates JA, Sjoerdsma A: Neurologic effects of tryptophan in patients receiving a monoamine oxidase inhibitor. Neurology *10*:1076–1078, 1960.
65. Smith B, Prockop DJ: Central-nervous system effects of ingestion of L-tryptophan by normal subjects. N Engl J Med *267*:1338–1341, 1962.
66. Curzon G, Ettlinger G, Cole M, et al: The biochemical, behavioral and neurologic effects of high L-tryptophan intake in the rhesus monkey. Neurology *12*:431–438, 1963.
67. Hodge JV, Oates JA, Sjoerdsma A: Reduction of the central effects of tryptophan by a decarboxylase inhibitor. Clin Pharmacol Ther *5*:149–155, 1964.
68. Grahame-Smith DG: Studies *in vivo* on the relationship between brain tryptophan, brain 5-HT synthesis hyperactivity

in rats treated with a monoamine oxidase inhibitor and L-tryptophan. J Neurochem *18*:1053–1066, 1984.

69. Beaumont G: Drug interactions with clomipramine (Anafranil). J Intern Med Res *1*:480–484, 1973.
70. Insel R, Roy B, Cohen R, Murphy D: Possible development of the serotonin syndrome in man. Am J Psychiatry *139*:954–955, 1982.
71. Sternbach H: The serotonin syndrome. Am J Psychiatry *148*:705–713, 1991.
72. Insel TR, Roy BF, Cohen RM, et al: Possible development of the serotonin syndrome. Am J Psychiatry *139*:954–955, 1982.
73. Dursun SM, Mathew VM, Reveley MA: Toxic serotonin syndrome after fluoxetine plus carbamazepine. Lancet *342*:442, 1993.
74. Dursun SM, Burke JG, Reveley MA: Toxic serotonin syndrome or extrapyramidal side-effects? Letter. Br J Pharmacol *166*:401–402, 1995.
75. Erspamer V: Occurrence of indolealkylamines in nature. Handb Exp Pharmakol *19*:132–181, 1966.
76. Rapport MM, Green AA, Page IH: Serum vasoconstrictor (serotonin), IV: Isolation and characterization. Biol Chem *176*:1243–1251, 1948.
77. Gaddun JH, Hameed KA: Drugs which antagonize 5-hydroxytryptamine. Br J Pharmacol *9*:240–248, 1957.
78. Peroutka SJ, Snyder SH: Multiple serotonin receptors: Differential binding of [3H]-lysergic acid diethylamide and [3H]-spiroperidol. Mol Pharmacol *16*:687–699, 1979.
79. Pedigo BW, Yamamura HI, Nelson DL: Discrimination of multiple serotonin biding sites by the neurole spiperone in rat brain. J Neurochem *36*:220–226, 1981.
80. Saxena PR: Serotonin receptors: Subtypes, functional responses, and therapeutic relevance. Pharmacol Ther *66*:339–368, 1995.
81. Meltzer H, Young M, Metz J, et al: Extrapyramidal side effects and increased serum prolactin following fluoxetine, a new antidepressant. J Neural Transm *45*:165–175, 1979.
82. Baldessarini RJ, Marsh E: Fluoxetine and side effects. Letter. Arch Gen Psychiatry *47*:191–1, 1990.
83. Lappin R, Auchincloss E: Treatment of serotonin syndrome with cyproheptadine. N Engl J Med *331*:1021–1022, 1994.
84. Sporer KA: The serotonin syndrome. Drug Saf *13*:94–104, 1995.
85. Mills KC: Serotonin syndrome. Am Fam Physician *52*:1475–1482, 1995.
86. Bodner RA, Lynch T, Lewis L, Kahn D: Serotonin syndrome. Neurology *45*:219–223, 1995.
87. Ruiz F: Fluoxetine and the serotonin syndrome. Ann Emerg Med *24*:983–985, 1994.
88. Feighner JP, Boyer WF, Tyler DL, Nebrosky RJ: Adverse consequences of fluoxetine-MAOI combination therapy. J Clin Psychiatry *51*:222–225, 1990.
89. Corkeror MA: Serotonin syndrome—a potentially fatal complication of antidepressant therapy. Med J Aust *163*:481–482, 1995.
90. Nierenberg DW, Semprebon M: The central nervous system serotonin syndrome. Clin Pharmacol Ther *53*:84–87, 1993.
91. Price LH, Charney DS, Heninger GR: Serotonin syndrome. Letter. Am J Psychiatry *111*:116–117, 1992.
92. Pope HG, Jonas JM, Hudson JI, Kafka MP: Toxic reactions to the combination of monoamine oxidase inhibitors and tryptophan. Am J Psychiatry *142*:491–492, 1985.
93. Hodge JV, Oates JA, Sjoerdsma A: Reduction of the central effects of tryptophan by a decarboxylase inhibitor. Clin Pharmacol Ther *5*:149–155, 1964.
94. Baloh RW, Dietz J, Spooner JW: Myoclonus and ocular oscillations induced by L-tryptophan. Ann Neurol *11*:95–97, 1982.
95. Thomas JM, Rubin EH: Case report of a toxic reaction from a combination of tryptophan and phenelzine. Am J Psychiatry *141*:281–283, 1984.
96. Glassman AH, Platman SR: Potentiation of a monoamine oxidase inhibitor by tryptophan. J Psychiatr Res, pp 83–88, 1969.
97. Thomas JM, Rubin EH: Case report of a toxic reaction from a combination of tryptophan and phenelzine. Am J Psychiatry *141*:281–283, 1984.
98. Levy AB, Bucher P, Votolato N: Myoclonus, hyperreflexia and diaphoresis in patients on phenelzine-tryptophan combination treatment. Can J Psychiatry *30*:434–436, 1985.
99. Guze BH, Baxter LR Jr: The serotonin syndrome: Case responsive to propranolol. J Clin Psychopharmacol *6*:119–120, 1986.
100. Brennan D, MacManus M, Howe J, McLoughlin J: "Neuroleptic malignant syndrome" without neuroleptics. Br J Psychiatry *152*:578–579, 1988.
101. Kline SS, Mauro LS, Scala-Barnett DM, Zick D: Serotonin syndrome versus neuroleptic malignant syndrome as a cause of death. Clin Pharmacol *8*:510–514, 1989.
102. Cocks DP, Passmore-Towe A: Dangers of monoamine oxidase inhibitors. Br Med J *1*:1545–1546, 1962.
103. Vigran IM: Dangerous potentiation of meperidine hydrochloride by pargyline hydrochloride. JAMA *18*:163–164, 1964.
104. Ebrahim ZY, O'Hara J, Borden L, Tetzlaff J: Monoamine oxidase inhibitors and elective surgery. Cleve Clin J Med *60*:129–130, 1993.
105. Phillips SD, Heiligenstein J, Burkett M, et al: Fluoxetine vs tricyclic antidepressants: A prospective multicenter study of antidepressant drug overdoses. Abstract. Vet Hum Toxicol *36*:37, 1994.
106. Kaminski CA, Robbins MS, Weibley RE: Sertraline intoxication in a child. Ann Emerg Med *23*:1371–1374, 1994.
107. Demirkiran Y, Jankovic J, Dean JM: Ecstasy intoxication: An overlap between serotonin syndrome and neuroleptic malignant syndrome. Clin Neuropharmacol *19*:157–164, 1996.
108. Randall T: Ecstasy-fueled 'rave' parties become dances of death for English youths. JAMA *268*:1505–1506, 1992.
109. Iwerson S, Schmoldt A: Two very different fatal cases associated with the use of methylenedioxyethylamphetamine (MDEA): Eve as deadly as Adam. Letter. Clin Toxicol *34*:241–244, 1996.
110. Brown C, Osterloh J: multiple severe complications from recreational ingestion of MDMA (ecstasy). JAMA *258*:780–781, 1987.
111. Screaton GR, Singer M, Cairns HS, et al: Hyperpyrexia and rhabdomyolysis after MDMA ('ecstasy') abuse. Lancet *339*:677–678, 1992.
112. Singarajah C, Lavies NG: An overdose of ecstasy. Role for dantrolene. Anaesthesia *47*:686–687, 1992.
113. Chadwick IS, Curry PD, Linsley A, et al: 3,4-Methylenedioxymethamphetamine (MDMA), a fatality associated with coagulopathy and hyperthermia. J R Soc Med *84*:371, 1991.
115. Tehan B, Hardern R, Bodenham A: Hyperthermia associated with 3,4-methylenedioxyethamphetamine ('Eve'). Anaesthesia *48*:507–510, 1993.
116. Friedman R: Ecstasy, the serotonin syndrome, and neuroleptic malignant syndrome—a possible link. Letter. JAMA *269*:869–870, 1993.
117. Neuvonen PJ, Pohjola-Sintonen S, Tacke U, Vuori E: Five fatal cases of serotonin syndrome after moclobemide-citalopram or moclobemide-clomipramine overdoses. Lancet *342*:1419, 1993.
118. Kuisma MJ: Fatal serotonin syndrome with trismus. Letter. Ann Emerg Med *26*:108, 1993.
119. Hernandez AF, Montero MN, Pla A, Villanueva E: Fatal moclobemide overdose or death caused by serotonin syndrome? J Forensic Sciences *40*:128–130, 1995.
120. Spigset O, Mjorndal T, Lovhein O: Serotonin syndrome caused by a moclobemide-clomipramine interaction. BMJ *306*:248, 1993.
121. Treiser SL, Cascio CS, O'Donohue TL, et al: Lithium increases serotonin release and decreases serotonin receptors in the hippocampus. Science *231*:1529–1531, 1981.
122. Goodwin GM, De Souza RJ, Green AR, Heal DJ: The enhancement by lithium of the 5-HT_{1A} mediate serotonin syndrome produced by 8-OH-DPAT in the rat: Evidence for a post-synaptic mechanism. Psychopharmacology *90*:488–493, 1986.
123. Price LH, Charney DS, Delgado PL, Heninger GR: Lithium and serotonin function: Implications for the serotonin hypothesis of depression. Psychopharmacology *100*:2–12, 1990.
124. Salama AA, Shafey M: A case of severe lithium toxicity

induced by combined fluoxetine and lithium carbonate. Am J Psychiatry *148*:705–713, 1989.
125. Ohman R, Spigset O: Serotonin syndrome induced by fluvoxamine-lithium interaction. Pharmacopsychiatry *26*:263–264, 1993.
126. Muly EC, McDonald W, Steffens D, Book S: Serotonin syndrome produced by a combination of fluoxetine and lithium. Letter. Am J Psychiatry *150*:1565, 1993.
127. McDaniel KD: Clinical pharmacology of monoamine oxidase inhibitors. Clin Neuropharmacol *9*:207–234, 1986.
128. Brodribb TR, Downey M, Gilbar PJ: Efficacy and adverse effects of moclobemide. Lancet *343*:475, 1994.
129. Goldberg RS, Thornton WW: Combined tricyclic-MAOI therapy for refractory depression: A review, with guidelines for appropriate use. J Clin Pharmacol *18*:143–146, 1978.
130. Zimmer R, Gieschke R, Fischbach R, Gasic S: Interaction studies with moclobemide. Acta Psychiatr Scand *360* (Suppl):84–86, 1990.
131. Rivers N, Horner B: Possible lethal reaction between Nardil and dextromethorphan. Can Med Assoc J *103*:85, 1970.
132. Sovner R, Wolfe J: Interaction between dextromethorphan and monoamine oxidase inhibitor therapy with isocarboxazid. N Engl J Med *2*:850–851, 1988.
133. Shamsie SJ, Barriga C: The hazards of use of monoamine oxidase inhibitors in disturbed adolescents. Can Med Assoc J *104*:715, 1971.
134. Sauter D, Macneil P, Weinstein E, et al: Phenelzine sulfate dextromethorphan interaction: A case report. Vet Hum Toxicol *33*:365, 1991.
135. Sinclair JG, Lo GF: The blockade of serotonin uptake and the meperidine-monoamine oxidase inhibitor interaction. Proc West Pharmacol Soc *20*:373–374, 1977.
136. Skop BP, Finkelstein JA, Mareth TR, et al: The serotonin syndrome associated with paroxetine, an over-the-counter cold remedy, and vascular disease. Am J Emerg Med *12*:642–644, 1994.
137. Achamallah NS: Visual hallucinations after combining fluoxetine and dextromethorphan. Am J Psychiatry *149*:1406, 1992.
138. Harvey AT, Burke M: Comment on the serotonin syndrome associated with paroxetine, an over-the-counter cold remedy, and vascular disease. Letter. Am J Emerg Med *13*:605–606, 1995.
139. Bloomer JC, Woods FR, Haddock RE, et al: The role of cytochrome P-4502D6 in the metabolism of paroxetine by human liver microsomes. Br J Clin Pharmacol *33*:521–523, 1992.
140. Preskorn SH, Alderman J, Chung M, et al: Pharmacokinetics of desipramine coadministered with sertraline or fluoxetine. J Clin Psychopharmacol *14*:90–98, 1994.
141. Spina E, Pollicino AM, Avenoso A, et al: Effect of fluvoxamine on the pharmacokinetics of imipramine and desipramine in healthy subjects. Ther Drug Monit *15*:243–246, 1993.
142. Sandyk R: L-dopa induced "serotonin syndrome" in a parkinsonian patient on bromocriptine. Letter. J Clin Psychopharmacol *6*:194, 1986.
143. Klawans HL, Goetz C, Bergen D: Levodopa-induced myoclonus. Arch Neurol *32*:331–334, 1975.
144. Karobath M, Diaz JL, Huttunen M: The effect of L-dopa on the concentration of tryptophan, tyrosine and serotonin in rat brain. Eur J Pharmacol *14*:393–396, 1971.
145. Hutt CS, Snider SR, Fahn S: Interaction between bromocriptine and levodopa. Neurology *27*:505–510, 1977.
146. Snider SR, Hutt CS, Stein B, et al: Increase in brain serotonin produced by bromocriptine. Neurosci Lett *1*:237–241, 1975.
147. Palider Maj J, Rawlow A: Trazodone, a central antagonist and agonist. J Neurol Transm *44*:236–248, 1979.
148. Jacobsen FM: Low-dose trazodone as a hypnotic in patients treated with MAOI and other psychotropics—pilot study. J Clin Psychiatry *51*:298–302, 1990.
149. Goldberg RJ, Huk M: Serotonin syndrome from trazodone and buspirone. Psychosomatics *33*:235–236, 1992.
150. Suchowersky O, deVries JD: Possible interactions between deprenyl and Prozac. Can J Neurol Sci *17*:571–572, 1990.
151. Suchowersky O, deVries JD: Interaction of fluoxetine and selegiline. Can J Psychiatry *35*:571–572, 1990.
152. Jermain DM, Hughes PL, Follender AB: Potential fluoxetine-selegiline interaction. Ann Pharmacother *26*:1300, 1990.
153. U. S. Government Printing Office: Eldepryl and Antidepressant Interaction. FDA Medical Bulletin. U. S. Food and Drug Administration, Washington, DC, p 6, 1995.
154. Driessen B, Reimann W: Interaction of the central analgesic, tramadol, with the uptake and release of 5-hydroxytryptamine in the rat brain *in vitro*. Br J Pharmacol *105*:147–151, 1992.
155. Raffa RB, Friderichs E, Reimann W, et al: Opioid and nonopioid components independently contribute to the mechanism of action of tramadol, an atypical opioid analgesic. J Pharmacol Exp Ther *260*:275–285, 1992.
156. Peroutka SJ: Serotonin receptors. *In* Meltzer HY (ed): Psychopharmacology: The third generation of progress. New York, Raven Press, pp 303–311, 1987.
157. Gerson SC, Baldessarini RJ: Motor effects of serotonin in the central nervous system. Life Sci *27*:1435–1451, 1980.
158. Lappin RI, Auchincloss EL: Treatment of the serotonin syndrome with cyproheptadine. Letter. N Engl J Med *331*:1021–1022, 1994.
159. Beasley CM, Masica DN, Heiligenstein JH, et al: Possible monoamine oxidase inhibitor-serotonin uptake inhibitor interaction: Fluoxetine clinical data and preclinical findings. J Clin Psychopharmacol *13*:312–320, 1993.
160. Heal DJ, Luscombe GP, Martin KF: Pharmacological identification of 5-HT receptor subtypes using behavioral models. *In* Marsden CA, Heal DJ (eds): Central Serotonin Receptors and Psychotropic Drugs. Boston, Blackwell Scientific Publications, pp 56–99, 1992.
161. Sprouse JS, Aghajanian GK: Propranolol blocks the inhibition of serotonergic dorsal raphe cell firing by HT1A selective agonists. Eur J Pharmacol *128*:295–298, 1986.
162. Deakin JFW, Green AR: The effects of putative 5-hydroxytryptamine antagonists on the behaviors produced by administration of tranylcypromine and L-tryptophan or tranylcypromine and L-DOPA to rat Br J Pharmacol *64*:201–209, 1978.
163. Brodribb TR, Downey M, Gilbar PJ: Efficacy and adverse effects of moclobemide. Lancet *343*:475, 1994.
164. Graham PM, Potter JM, Paterson J: Combination monoamine oxidase inhibitor/tricyclic antidepressant interaction. Lancet *2*:440, 1982.
165. Grantham J, Neel W, Brown W: Reversal of imipramine-monoamine oxidase inhibitor induced toxicity with chlorpromazine. J Kans Med Soc *65*:279–280, 1964.
166. Tackley RM, Tregaskis B: Fatal disseminated intravascular coagulation following a monoamine oxidase inhibitor/tricyclic interaction. Anaesthesia *42*:760–763, 1987.

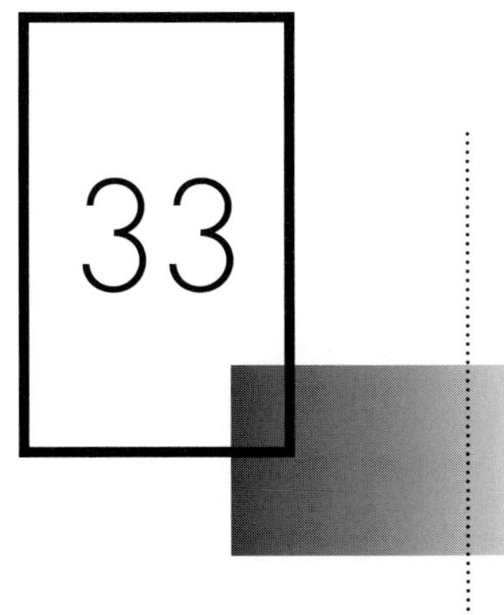

Lithium

JAMES F. WINCHESTER, MD

Lithium carbonate, in its various formulations (Table 33–1), is an indispensable psychiatric tool that has allowed many patients with manic-depressive illness to achieve almost total rehabilitation. In the United States alone, the savings in health care dollars have been estimated to be around 4 billion dollars in the first 10 years (1972 to 1982) that lithium was approved for restricted use by the Food and Drug Administration. These costs include savings in psychiatric care as well as increased economic production.

Despite an early suggestion that lithium might act on depression, it was not until 1949 that an effect on mania was observed; since then, lithium has become standard psychiatric treatment.[1, 2] It is difficult to determine the incidence of lithium intoxication, but approximately 250 cases have been reported.[3] Lithium has a narrow therapeutic index, and serum levels above well-defined ranges can result in toxicity. A gradual onset of intoxication is far more common than acute overdose. After cessation of lithium administration in an intoxicated patient, the symptoms may persist for some time and reflect the toxicokinetics of lithium. In many cases, predisposing factors and drug interaction have major roles.

Acute overdose carries a 25% mortality, whereas the mortality rate in patients intoxicated during maintenance treatment with lithium is around 9%. In addition, persistent central nervous system or renal damage or both occur in approximately 10% of patients.[3]

Before 1950, lithium had been used as a salt substitute and was the major constituent of 7-Up, a well-known American soft drink. The use of lithium in nonpsychiatric disorders (Table 33–2) results in a large number of patients being exposed to the potential toxicity of lithium.

Table 33–1. Some Available Lithium (Li) Preparations*

Trade Name	Chemical Formulation	Dosage Forms
United States		
Lithane (Miles Pharmaceutical)	Lithium carbonate	Tablets, 300 mg
Lithium carbonate USP	Lithium carbonate	Capsules, 150 mg, 300 mg, 600 mg; tablets, 300 mg
Lithium citrate syrup USP (Roxane)	Lithium citrate	Syrup, 8 mEq/5 mL—equivalent to 300 mg of lithium carbonate
Cibalith-S (CIBA)	Lithium citrate	Syrup, 8 mEq/5 mL—equivalent to 300 mg of lithium carbonate
Lithobid (CIBA)	Lithium carbonate	Tablets, 300 mg (sustained release)
Eskalith (SmithKline)	Lithium carbonate	Capsules and tablets, 300 mg
Eskalith CR (SmithKline)	Lithium carbonate	Tablets, 300 mg, 450 mg; capsules, 300 mg (sustained release)
Canada		
Carbolith (ICN)	Lithium carbonate	Capsules and tablets, 300 mg
Lithane (Pfizer)	Lithium carbonate	As above
Lithizine (Maney)	Lithium carbonate	As above
United Kingdom	Lithium carbonate	400 mg tablets also available
Scandinavia		
Litarex	Lithium carbonate	Sustained-release formulation

*Molecular mass = 73.89 daltons; atomic number, 3; atomic weight, 6.94; emission line on flame photometer, 671 nm.

Table 33–2. Therapeutic Uses of Lithium

Psychiatric Disorders	Nonpsychiatric Disorders
Manic-depressive (bipolar) illness*	Pain
Unipolar depressive illness	Premenstrual tension
Behavior disorders	Leukopenia/chemotherapy
Character disorders	Felty's syndrome
Pain	Thyrotoxicosis
Alcoholism/drug abuse	Tardive dyskinesia
Premenstrual tension	Huntington's chorea
Organic brain syndrome	? Pancreatic cholera syndrome
Cycloid psychosis	? Syndrome of inappropriate antidiuretic hormone secretion
Anorexia nervosa	
Schizoaffective disorders	
Steroid-induced psychosis	

*Only approved use for lithium in the United States; other uses are experimental.

In the United States, lithium carbonate is the principal formulation used, but lithium citrate is also available in syrup form. In other countries, different salts of lithium are available, but the predominant formulation in Canada, the United Kingdom, and Scandinavia is lithium carbonate. In the United Kingdom, 400-mg tablets are available; in Scandinavia, the United Kingdom, and the United States, sustained-release formulations may also be obtained (see Table 33–1). Lithium is the lightest of all the known metals and exists in nature in various ionized forms and salts. Lithium bromide was used in the past as a sedative-hypnotic agent, and lithium chloride at one time was used as a table salt substitute. Its molecular mass is approximately 74 daltons, its atomic number is 3, and atomic weight is 6.94. It is handled by the body very similarly to sodium, but it shows a different emission line than sodium on the flame photometer at around 671 nm. Although lithium chloride was introduced for treatment of manic-depressive psychosis, lithium carbonate was found to be a more stable compound and accordingly has come into widespread use.

Lithium produces many metabolic and neuroendocrine changes, but no conclusive evidence favors one particular mode of action. In terms of mineral metabolism, lithium competes for sodium, potassium, magnesium, and calcium, in that order, and displaces them from intracellular and bone sites in this progression. Lithium ions affect neurotransmitter impulses by several methods,[4] among which are (1) inhibition of release and augmentation of reuptake of norepinephrine at nerve endings and (2) inhibition of the hydro-osmotic effect of arginine vasopressin via reduction of receptor-mediated synthesis of cyclic adenosine monophosphate from inhibition of the enzyme adenylate cyclase (a mechanism probably responsible for the nephrogenic diabetes insipidus[5] and alterations in thyroid function occurring in some patients). In addition, long-term lithium administration stimulates release of endogenous serotonin from the hippocampus but not from the cortex in animal brains—data that are consistent with the concept that lithium stabilizes serotoninergic neurotransmission.[6] Regardless of its biochemical mechanisms, it is clear that lithium is able to affect receptor sensitivity and bring about changes in neurotransmission. Because of its chemical similarity to sodium, potassium, and calcium, it may interact or interfere with biochemical pathways for these substances at the cell membrane level and within the cell.

Gastrointestinal absorption is rapid and complete after oral administration of tablets or the liquid form of lithium. Peak serum levels are reached within 1 to 2 hours (with the exception of sustained-release formulations), and the drug is freely distributed in whole-body water but with slow uptake by and release from central nervous system tissue. In fact, it may take 24 hours for lithium to cross the blood-brain barrier effectively. Lithium is neither protein bound nor tissue bound, and with the usual oral doses of 900 to 1800 mg daily, steady-state plasma levels are reached within 5 to 6 days.[7] Blood samples for monitoring serum lithium levels are best taken 12 hours after the last dose.

Excretion is predominantly by the kidneys, and trace amounts are found in the stool. Approximately 80% of lithium is reabsorbed at the proximal renal tubule, and 20% is excreted in the urine.[8] The avid proximal tubular reabsorption explains the fact that distal tubular diuretics (thiazides and so on) may cause compensatory increases in proximal tubular reabsorption of both sodium and lithium,[9] and loop diuretics (furosemide and ethacrynic acid) cause continued sodium and lithium excretion.[10] It is of interest that the serum half-life of lithium is shorter in a young person than in an older person; values of 18 hours in the former and 36 hours in the latter have been reported.[11] On average, the half-life of elimination ($t_{1/2}$) is approximately 29 hours for an adult; thus, serum levels normally decrease by about 20% within 6 hours of stopping lithium therapy.[12] It is important that the $t_{1/2}$ correlates with the glomerular filtration rate (GFR), because renal lithium clearance is estimated to be approximately one fourth that of creatinine clearance.[10] In view of the pharmacokinetic handling of lithium in elderly patients and in those with diminished renal capacity, it is essential that levels in patients receiving lithium be monitored almost continuously. Lithium renal clearance (C_{Li}) is normally 10 to 40 mL/min, and the fractional excretion of lithium ($FE_{Li} = C_{Li}/C_{creatinine}$) is approximately 17% to 30%. The apparent volume of distribution of lithium is slightly greater than that of whole-body water—around 0.79 L/kg of body weight.

Renal elimination of lithium is influenced by several factors, including sodium and water balance, the presence of drugs that affect renal tubular reabsorption of sodium, and other phenomena. As discussed later, any condition leading to sodium and water imbalance may seriously affect the handling of lithium by the kidneys and consequently may predispose to toxicity. Another interesting phenomenon not fully explained is that manic patients may tolerate high levels of lithium during the initial control of their manic state, but after control, it has been observed that patients become less tolerant to high serum levels of lithium.[13] On the other hand, lithium toxicity may appear in elderly patients at lower serum levels than usual, and therapeutic levels in the elderly may be around 0.2 mEq/L.[4]

THERAPEUTIC USES

Table 33–2 outlines the therapeutic uses of lithium. In the United States, lithium is approved only for the treatment of manic-depressive (bipolar) illness, but as can be seen from Table 33–2, it has been used experimentally in a wide variety of psychiatric and nonpsychiatric disorders.

LITHIUM INTOXICATION

As noted, most cases of lithium intoxication arise during prolonged therapy,[3, 13, 14] although acute ingestion is recognized.[15] Small adjustments in dose or frequency of administration commonly give rise to toxic manifestations, and in only a minority of cases is self-poisoning responsible for the intoxication. In general, therefore, it follows that lithium toxicity may not present dramatic symptoms, and psychiatrists or other physicians treating patients may be unaware of the subtle changes occurring in the prodromal phase of lithium poisoning.

The *prodromal phase* lasts for several days to weeks and may be manifested by a combination of the following symptoms: vomiting, diarrhea, drowsiness, coarse muscle tremor, muscle twitching, lethargy, tinnitus, nystagmus, slurred speech, and, in severe cases, polyuria and polydipsia. It is not surprising that the symptoms can be mistaken for those of the primary depressive illness. Close correlation exists between the symptoms of lithium poisoning and the serum lithium concentration.[3] In the full-blown syndrome, the toxic manifestations can be graded on a scale of I to III, as shown in Table 33–3. The full syndrome of lithium toxicity may take many days to dissipate after cessation of lithium ingestion. As noted, the central nervous system manifestations may never completely regress,[16–19] even as long as 5 years after intoxication,[20] and in certain situations lithium toxicity has an appreciable mortality rate.

Table 33–3. Serum Lithium and Toxic Manifestations*

Severity of Symptoms	Toxic Stage†	Serum Lithium Concentration (mEq/L)
No toxicity (therapeutic)	0	0.4–1.3
Mild toxicity	I	1.5–2.5
Serious toxicity	II	2.5–3.5
Life-threatening toxicity	III	>3.5

*N.B.: Lithium toxicity may be manifested even at therapeutic levels, especially in the elderly, when the therapeutic level may be 0.2 mEq/L.

†Classification of Hansen and Amdisen.[3] (Stages I and II: apathy, tremor, weakness, ataxia, motor agitation, rigidity, fascicular twitching, nausea, vomiting, and diarrhea. Stage III: Latent convulsive movements, stupor, and coma.)

Systemic Manifestations

Central Nervous System

After a fine hand tremor is observed, the patient may develop muscular and reflex hyperirritability; spastic, dystonic, or choreiform movements; cogwheel rigidity; parkinsonism; confusion[21, 22] or mental lapses with prolonged memory impairment (the latter for 2 months in a patient acutely poisoned and treated with hemodialysis)[23]; neurologic asymmetry; cutaneous hyperalgesia; and polyneuropathy.[24] Other manifestations are anxiety, delirium, hyperpyrexia, and stupor progressing to coma. Findings on an electroencephalogram may well be abnormal, and some patients may show 2- to 5-Hz patterns with spikes and sharp waves. Cerebellar signs may predominate.[25] Paradoxically, in otherwise well-controlled patients, mania is the principal manifestation of toxicity.[26, 27]

Gastrointestinal System

Severe gastroenteritis often occurs initially after acute overdose of lithium.

Cardiovascular System

Arrhythmias, hypotension, circulatory failure, and interstitial myocarditis have been reported. The electrocardiogram may show depressed ST waves or T inversion in chest leads V_4 to V_6,[3] premature atrial contractions,[28] complete heart block,[29] or myocardial infarction.[30] In the latter case report, the patient had a plasma lithium concentration of 14.6 mmol/L, had a first hemodialysis of 17.5 hours, required four dialyses total because of a persistent plasma lithium level of 6 mmol/L for 48 hours, and made a complete recovery.[30] Myocytic degeneration and lymphocyte, histiocyte, and plasma cell infiltration, exacerbated by uremia, with severity closely correlated with plasma lithium levels, have been observed in rats chronically intoxicated with lithium.[31]

Miscellaneous

As mentioned, leukocytosis occurs with predominant neutrophilia in the peripheral blood and in bone marrow, with accompanying lymphocytopenia. Isolated cases of leukopenia also have been reported.[32] Increased calcium, magnesium, and parathyroid hormone levels may be observed in blood samples. Increases in serum calcium and parathyroid hormone within the normal range occur in 80% of patients in the early weeks of lithium therapy and exceed the normal range in 10% on long-term therapy.[33] In patients receiving long-term therapy, osteoporosis has been reported and disturbed iodine metabolism is common; 4% of patients develop a goiter but rarely hypothyroidism.[34] Rare cases of exophthalmos have occurred during lithium treatment, as has thyrotoxicosis.[35] Weight gain is also reported, but the mechanism is unknown. Lithium also affects glucose metabolism by enhancing uptake and use of glucose in muscle and stimulating the release of insulin from the pancreas. Other miscellaneous side effects are acne, exacerbation of psoriasis, production of other rashes, and hair loss. Reduction in body temperature also has been observed,[36] as has adult respiratory distress syndrome.[37, 38]

Teratogenicity

Long-term lithium treatment of pregnant women has been associated with fetal cardiac abnormalities, particularly of the tricuspid valve, in 11 of 13 offspring of patients exposed to lithium. In addition, congenital goiter has been reported. During pregnancy, lithium clearance increases by approximately 100% and decreases abruptly after delivery to prepregnancy levels. Breast milk contains lithium in concentrations of approximately half the maternal serum concentration. In view of this, bottle feeding is recommended, because lithium intoxication can occur in infants. Affected babies are described as hypotonic, floppy, and listless, but they revert to normal over time.

The Kidneys

Because the body's handling of lithium is so closely related to renal function, it follows that even subtle alterations of renal function may seriously affect lithium excretion and lead to toxicity.[39] Lithium competes with sodium and potassium at the renal tubular level; therefore, sodium and water balance influence not only the serum level of lithium but also its toxicity. Conditions that enhance proximal tubular reabsorption of lithium constitute a very significant hazard because they occur episodically and may go undetected. These conditions include volume depletion, congestive heart failure, hyponatremia, administration of diuretics that act on the distal tubules, low-salt or weight-reducing diets, and administration of nonsteroidal anti-inflammatory agents such as indomethacin, phenylbutazone, mefenamic acid, and piroxicam.[40–42] Loop diuretics have no direct effect on lithium reabsorption, but if they precipitate sodium depletion, a reduction in the fractional excretion of lithium, with retention of lithium by the kidneys, may occur. Proximal tubular diuretics such as acetazolamide, urea, and aminophylline can increase fractional lithium clearance.[39] Lithium itself may affect the thirst center, turn off the normal response to hyperosmolality, and promote dehydration.

Reports support the theoretic prediction that inhibition of angiotensin II–regulated maintenance of GFR (in congestive failure, volume depletion, and renal ischemia) by angiotensin-converting enzyme inhibitors results in lithium toxicity. Efferent glomerular arteriolar constriction maintained by angiotensin II is lost, and the result is lowered GFR and reduced lithium clearance.[43–45]

The predominant effect that lithium has on the kidneys, however, is the production of nephrogenic diabetes insipidus, with polyuria and polydipsia. This syndrome does not respond to exogenous antidiuretic hormone and is due to a vasopressin-insensitive defect in urine concentration at the tubular level. This is manifested by the fact that most patients have high endogenous vasopressin levels during the polyuric phase. Polyuria and polydipsia are present in about 30% of patients receiving lithium; in only 10% of all lithium recipients is the effect serious enough to lead to dehydration.[46] Urinary incontinence developed in 17% of women taking lithium and was ascribed to lithium-induced changes in bladder cholinergic-adrenergic balance.[47] As shown in Figure 33–1, sodium and water deficiency or renal impairment leads to a reduction of the fractional excretion of lithium and lithium clearance, which in turn may promote sodium loss by the kidneys. A vicious cycle may ensue and further complicate the lithium toxicity. Lithium itself may produce a urinary acidification defect, probably as a result of a distal renal tubular acidosis.[39] Lithium-induced urinary concentration defects are most often reversible when the drug is discontinued, although in some patients the concentration defect may persist for some time.[39] Several other renal effects of lithium have been observed. In patients with lithium intoxication, renal biopsy has revealed changes consistent with acute tubular necrosis; whether this is due to lithium or to the accompanying circulatory collapse of lithium poisoning has not yet been determined.[39] Acute renal failure, presumably from acute tubular necrosis, has been described.[48] Nephrotic syndrome due to minimal change disease *(lipoid nephrosis)* or focal segmental glomerular sclerosis also has been reported in patients receiving lithium; variable degrees of proteinuria (not in the nephrotic range) commonly are observed in lithium-treated patients.[39]

At present, the literature presents conflicting reports on the incidence of chronic interstitial nephropathy in patients receiving lithium, with or without accompanying changes in renal function, albuminuria, and urinary enzyme abnormalities.[39] The inci-

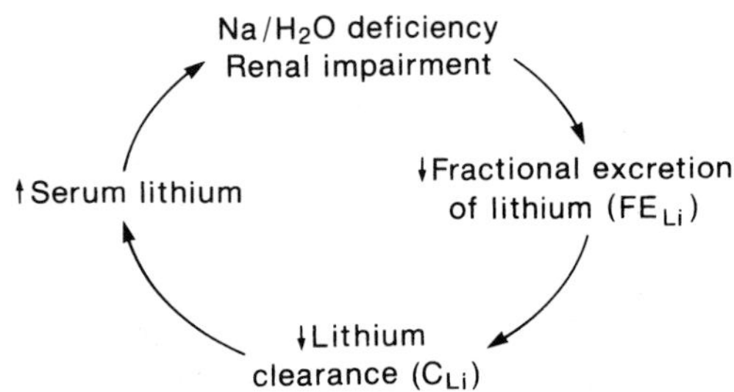

Figure 33–1. The vicious cycle of sodium and water depletion and lithium toxicity.

dence of chronic interstitial nephritis and renal insufficiency in patients receiving lithium therapy apparently is fairly low, however, and the etiologic role of lithium is in doubt.[39] It is of interest that patients with severe psychiatric illness may well be at greater risk for developing renal disease than normal individuals, and thus the etiologic role of lithium in induction of interstitial nephritis is further complicated.[49] Moreover, a prospective study of the GFR in patients before and after lithium treatment, with an average of 6 years of treatment, has shown no differences in renal function before and after therapy.[50] On the other hand, rats ingesting lithium for a prolonged period do develop renal interstitial fibrosis.[39]

Pathophysiology of Lithium Intoxication

As noted, lithium excretion depends on sodium and water balance and the GFR. Any increase in serum lithium level leads to toxicity, a reduction of lithium clearance, and a protracted $t_{1/2}$ owing to a reduced fractional excretion of lithium by the kidneys (see Fig. 33–1). In addition, increases in serum lithium level also promote natriuresis, with further obligatory water loss, and lead to the vicious cycle illustrated in Figure 33–1. Diabetes insipidus also may promote sodium and water loss, particularly if the polyuria leads to water loss in excess of water intake—a particular condition of patients whose manic-depressive illness is exacerbated.

Lithium toxicity may arise from several predisposing factors. The most important of these are dehydration, dietary restriction of sodium, anorexia, vomiting, diarrhea, and strenuous exercise—all of which produce sodium and water imbalance. Additionally, after parturition, the GFR and consequently renal lithium clearance decline precipitously to half the level during pregnancy. Certain drugs may affect the handling of lithium by the kidneys, whereas other drugs may interact with lithium in the central nervous system to produce toxic effects. These drugs are listed in Table 33–4. Finally, primary renal disease due to any cause predisposes to lithium intoxication. As noted, primary renal disease seems to be more common in patients with manic-depressive illness and may arise from other drug toxicity, such as excessive use of mixed analgesics and nonsteroidal anti-inflammatory agents.

Laboratory Manifestations

In general, the serum levels of sodium are within the normal (or low normal) range, whereas lower sodium concentrations may be encountered in the cerebrospinal fluid. A *low anion gap* may serve as a useful diagnostic aid when a history of lithium ingestion cannot be obtained. Such an observation was made in two severely intoxicated patients (serum lithium level > 4 mEq/L). It was corrected with dialysis and was not observed in patients with therapeutic lithium levels.[51] No changes are noted in potassium concentrations in blood or cerebrospinal fluid. Serum calcium and magnesium may occasionally be found in increased concentration in the blood, but the most important abnormality is a serum lithium concentration usually in the excessive range (see Table 33–3). Plasma concentrations of antidiuretic hormone (vasopressin), parathyroid hormone, thyroid-stimulating hormone, aldosterone, and renin may be increased.

Table 33–4. Known Drug Interactions with Lithium

Drug	Effects of Interaction
Haloperidol	Rigidity, ataxia, oral tardive dyskinesia, ↑ depression, ↑ haloperidol toxicity
Tricyclic antidepressants (TCA)	Additive antidepressant effect, hypotension, delirium, seizures, increase in blood pressure if hypotension secondary to TCA
Phenothiazines	↑ Lithium and phenothiazine toxicity, ↑ depression along with toxicity
Benzodiazepines	↑ Depression
Neuromuscular blockers	↑ Neuromuscular blockade
Methyldopa	↑ Parkinsonian syndrome
Nonsteroidal anti-inflammatory drugs: indomethacin, piroxicam, mefenamic acid, phenylbutazone	Partial reversal of nephrogenic diabetes insipidus and ↑ serum lithium, ↓ renal lithium clearance
Phenytoin	Polyuria, polydipsia, tremor
Calcium channel blockers: verapamil, nifedipine, diltiazem	Additive or synergistic action with lithium
Angiotensin-converting enzyme inhibitors (e.g., captopril, enalapril)	Reduced glomerular filtration rate, ↓ lithium clearance
Diuretics	
Thiazides	↑ Serum lithium
Osmotics, acetazolamide, sodium bicarbonate	↑ Urinary lithium excretion
Furosemide	No change in serum lithium, unless induces significant sodium loss
Potassium-sparing diuretics and potassium supplements	Abolish distal renal tubular acidosis and may prevent renal lithium toxicity

Treatment

By far the most important aspect of treatment of lithium poisoning is its anticipation *before* serious intoxication occurs. Regular serum lithium measurements should be taken in patients who are undergoing long-term treatment, and dosage adjustment should be made on the basis of the measurements. Five to 7 days may be required after dosage adjustment for serum lithium levels to fall within the desired range. It is most important that patients be cautioned to avoid sodium and water restriction, particularly in the early stages of treatment with lithium. Patients should promptly report any intercurrent illness with pyrexia in which sweating may become excessive, leading to sodium and water loss.

In certain situations, the urinary concentration defect resulting in severe polyuria may benefit from modest doses of a thiazide diuretic, which may allow continued treatment with lithium.[52] In addition, nonsteroidal anti-inflammatory agents such as indomethacin and phenylbutazone may help reduce lithium-induced polyuria.[53] It is of interest that potassium supplementation or potassium-sparing diuretics such as triamterene and amiloride may reverse the lithium-induced inhibition of water transport and may also restore urinary acidification, but in general these drugs have no effect on lithium clearance.[54] It follows, therefore, that serum potassium level also must be monitored during lithium treatment.

Definitive Steps to Be Taken

1. Whenever lithium toxicity is suspected, the patient should be *admitted to the hospital.* Although symptoms in general progress slowly, seizure activity may arise unexpectedly and may become life threatening.
2. In all cases, *lithium carbonate should be withdrawn* and any concomitant diuretic therapy such as thiazide diuretics should be withheld. If self-poisoning is the reason for the intoxication, *gastric lavage* should be performed. It is worth reiterating that symptoms may progress despite cessation of lithium or thiazide in view of the prolonged $t_{1/2}$ of lithium. Intestinal decontamination using polyethylene glycol solutions to clear bowel of its contents may also have a role,[55] as may the (experimental) administration of ion-exchange resins,[56] such as sodium polystyrene sulfonate (Kayexalate).
3. *Restore sodium and water balance.* In infected or dehydrated patients, appropriate attention to fluid balance and control of pyrexia must be maintained. In patients with nephrogenic diabetes insipidus, infusion of standard (normal) saline may induce a hypertonic state,[57] which itself raises the appreciable morbidity and mortality. In the latter situation, half-normal saline or other hypotonic fluid may be required, or thiazide diuretics may be reintroduced to control the diabetes insipidus. Amiloride, by inhibiting water transport in the collecting tubule, has been shown to reduce the mean urine volume from 4.7 to 3.1 L and to induce a rise in mean urinary osmolality from 575 to 699 mOsm/kg in a series of nine patients. It also avoided the need for potassium supplementation.[54]
4. *Forced diuresis/sodium infusion. Forced diuresis has no role*[3, 14] in the management of lithium intoxication unless the GFR is below normal, on restoration of which the serum lithium level should decline to around 1 mEq/L within 30 hours of stopping diuretic treatment. Sodium chloride had long been proposed as useful in enhancing excretion of lithium by the kidneys, but current evidence does not favor an effect of sodium chloride on lithium excretion, and the fractional excretion of lithium did not change consistently during sodium infusion.[3, 14] Only in the presence of reduction in GFR due to hypovolemia would sodium chloride infusions have any effect on increasing the fractional excretion of lithium, because such infusions are also accompanied by an increase in

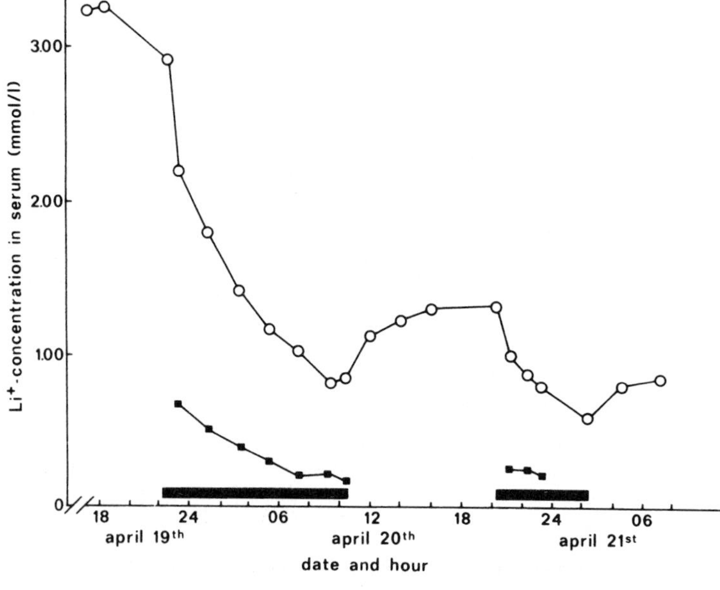

Figure 33–2. Serum lithium response to hemodialysis in a 66-year-old man. ○, Dialyzer inlet lithium concentration; ■, dialyzer outlet concentration; *bar,* hemodialysis periods. (From Hansen HE, Amdisen A: Lithium intoxication. Q J Med *47:*123, 1978.)

creatinine clearance due to volume expansion. It is recommended that fluid therapy or forced diuresis be used only when the serum lithium level has been elevated for a few days and not above 2.5 mEq/L; in this situation, frequent measurements of serum lithium level should be made. If serum lithium level fails to decline to 1 mEq/L within 30 to 36 hours of treatment, then dialysis should be considered (discussed later).

5. *Antidotes.* Direct adenylate cyclase stimulators, such as forskolin, have met with no success in a mouse model of lithium toxicity[58] and are not recommended until definitive studies have demonstrated their efficacy.
6. *Hemodialysis* is the *treatment of choice* for severe lithium intoxication.[3, 14, 59–61] When hemodialysis is not immediately available, peritoneal dialysis may first be instituted. Lithium is the most dialyzable toxin known, in view of its small molecular weight, negligible protein binding, and behavior similar to that of sodium. Extraction of lithium by hemodialysis, therefore, is greater than 90%. Hemodialysis has been shown to reduce the $t_{1/2}$ substantially and to reduce serum lithium levels rapidly[3] (Fig. 33–2). Several investigators recommend protracted hemodialysis (10 to 12 hours), which is repeated as necessary until the serum lithium level remains at less than 1 mEq/L 6 to 8 hours after dialysis.[3, 14, 15] Bicarbonate dialysis theoretically removes more intracellular lithium and helps reduce the organic anion–induced retention of lithium inside cells.[62] As with any drug intoxication, "rebound" in plasma levels occurs owing to lithium redistribution or continued gastrointestinal absorption. A 6-hour hemodialysis with modern high-surface-area hemodialyzers substantially reduces serum lithium level, but if continuous arteriovenous hemodialfiltration is used, this requires more time (14 hours versus a calculated hemodialysis time of 5.75 hours in one study),[63] but with the added advantage of convenience in the intensive care setting. A guide to the need for initial hemodialysis, arising from the known first-order elimination of lithium and suggested by several investigators,[3, 64] is depicted in Figure 33–3. Hemodialysis should be performed on unstable patients or if three or more serum lithium concentrations, plotted on a log-linear scale against time, predict that the lithium concentration will not decline below 0.6 mEq/liter within 36 hours or longer.
7. *Maintenance of water balance.* It must be appreciated that persistent sodium and water loss may occur for days to weeks after lithium intoxication, and patients require careful monitoring of fluid balance during this stage.[65, 66]
8. Finally, one of the most distressing features of lithium intoxication may be the persistent neurologic or renal defects that occur in approximately 10% of patients.[3, 16–19] Indeed, some of the classic descriptions of lithium poisoning pointed to the dreaded neurologic complications of lithium toxicity. Of particular note is the "coma vigil" of lithium poisoning, in which a patient presents in a catatonic state and the sole sign of activity is the eyes ever open and vigilant. In such cases, neurology consultation (or in the event of renal complications, nephrology consultation) may be indicated.

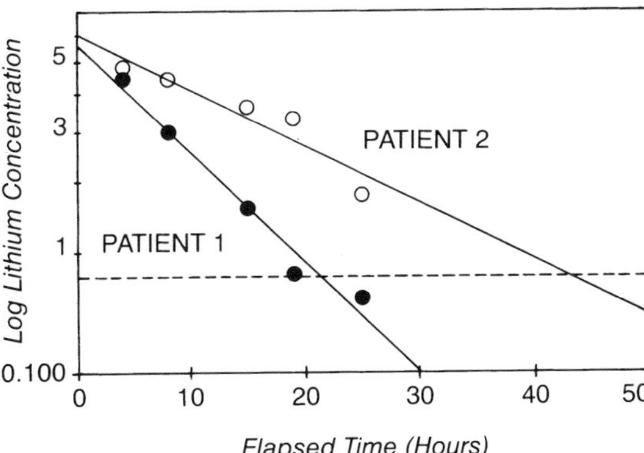

Figure 33–3. Log plasma lithium levels plotted against time in two patients. In patient 1 (●), the predicted level of 0.6 mEq/L occurs at 24 hours, whereas in patient 2 (○), the predicted level of 0.6 mEq/L occurs at 45 hours. Dialysis would be recommended for patient 2.

References

1. Cade J: Lithium salts in the treatment of psychotic excitement. Med J Aust *36:*349, 1949.
2. Schou M: Lithium treatment of manic-depressive illness. Past, present and perspective. JAMA *259:*1834, 1988.
3. Hansen HE, Amdisen A: Lithium intoxication. Q J Med *47:*123, 1978.
4. Rosenbaum AH, Maruta T, Richelson E: Drugs that alter mood. II. Lithium. Mayo Clin Proc *54:*401, 1979.
5. Jackson BA, Dousa TP: Lithium-induced nephrogenic diabetes insipidus. *In* Christensen S (ed): Lithium and the Kidney. Basel, S. Karger AG, pp 126–133, 1990.
6. Treiser SL, Cascia CS, O'Donohue TL, et al: Lithium increases serotonin release and decreases serotonin receptors in the hippocampus. Science *213:*1529, 1981.
7. Schou M: Lithium studies. 3. Distribution between serum and tissues. Acta Pharmacol Toxicol *15:*115, 1958.
8. Thomsen K, Schou M: Renal lithium excretion in man. Am J Physiol *215:*823, 1968.
9. Petersen V, Hvidt S, Thomsen K, Schou M: Effect of prolonged thiazide treatment on renal lithium clearance. BMJ *3:*143, 1974.
10. Jefferson JW, Kalin NH: Serum lithium levels and long-term diuretic use. JAMA *241:*1134, 1979.
11. Prien PF: Lithium in the treatment of affective disorders. Clin Neuropharmacol *3:*113, 1978.
12. Mason RW, McQueen EG, Keary PJ, James N: Pharmacokinetics of lithium: Elimination half-time, renal clearance and afferent volume of distribution in schizophrenia. Clin Pharmacokinet *3:*241, 1978.
13. Fyro B, Sedvall G: The excretion of lithium. *In* Johnson FN (ed): Lithium Research and Therapy. New York, Academic Press, p 287, 1975.
14. Amdisen A: Clinical features and management of lithium poisoning. Med Toxicol Adverse Drug Exp *3:*18, 1988.
15. Jacobsen D, Aasen G, Fredericksen P, Eisenga B: Lithium intoxication: Pharmacokinetics during and after terminated hemodialysis in acute intoxication. J Toxicol Clin Toxicol *25:*81, 1987.
16. Von Hartitszch B, Hoenich NA, Leigh RS, et al: Permanent

neurological sequelae despite haemodialysis for lithium intoxication. BMJ *4:*757, 1972.
17. Juel-Jensen P, Schou M: Permanent brain damage after lithium intoxication. BMJ *4:*673, 1973.
18. Nagaraja D, Taly AB, Sahu RN, et al: Permanent neurological sequelae due to lithium toxicity. Clin Neurol Neurosurg *89:*31, 1987.
19. Modestin J, Foglia A: Lithium poisoning with persistent neurological sequelae. Schweiz Med Wochenschr *118:*173, 1988.
20. Izzo KL, Brody R: Rehabilitation in lithium toxicity: Case report. Arch Phys Med Rehabil *66:*779, 1985.
21. Adityanjee A: The syndrome of lithium effectuated neurotoxicity. J Neurol Neurosurg Psychiatry *51:*1246, 1987.
22. Goetting MG: Acute lithium poisoning in a child with dystonia. Pediatrics *76:*978, 1985.
23. Saxena S, Mallikarjuna P: Severe memory impairment with acute overdose lithium toxicity. Br J Psychiatry *152:*853, 1988.
24. Chang YC, Yip PK, Chin YN, Lin HN: Severe generalized polyneuropathy in lithium intoxication. Eur Neurol *28:*39, 1988.
25. Tesio L, Porta GL, Messa E: Cerebellar syndrome in lithium poisoning: A case of partial recovery. J Neurol Neurosurg Psychiatry *50:*235, 1987.
26. El Mallakah RS, Kantesaria AN, Chaikovsky LI: Lithium toxicity presenting as mania. Drug Intell Clin Pharm *21:*979, 1987.
27. Nurnberger JI Jr: Diuretic-induced lithium toxicity presenting as mania. J Nerv Ment Dis *173:*316, 1985.
28. Dhillon AS, Adams JS: Lithium-related premature atrial contractions. J Clin Psychiatry *48:*305, 1987.
29. Salama AA: Complete heart block associated with mesoridazine and lithium combination. J Clin Psychiatry *48:*123, 1987.
30. Perrier A, Martin PY, Favre H, et al: Very severe self-poisoning lithium carbonate causing a myocardial infarction. Chest *100:*863, 1991.
31. Baandrup U, Bagger JP, Christensen B: Myocardial changes in rats with lithium-induced uremia. Acta Pathol Microbiol Immunol Scand [A] *93:*317, 1985.
32. Green ST, Dunn FG: Severe leucopenia in fatal lithium poisoning. BMJ *290:*517, 1985.
33. Mallette LE, Eichhorn E: Effects of lithium carbonate on human calcium metabolism. Arch Intern Med *146:*770, 1986.
34. Surks MI, Sievert R: Drugs and thyroid function. N Engl J Med *333:*1688, 1995.
35. McDermott MT, Burman KD, Hofeldt DT, Kidd GS: Lithium-associated thyrotoxicosis. Am J Med *80:*1245, 1986.
36. Follézou JY, Bleibel JM: Reduction of temperature and lithium poisoning. N Engl J Med *313:*1609, 1985.
37. Lawler PG, Cove-Smith JR: Acute respiratory failure following lithium intoxication. A report of two cases. Anaesthesia *41:*623, 1986.
38. Friedman BC, Bekes CE, Scott WE, Bartter T: ARDS following acute lithium carbonate intoxication. Intensive Care Med *18:*123, 1992.
39. Christensen S (ed): Lithium and the Kidney. Basel, Karger AG, 1990.
40. Frolich JC, Leftwich R, Ragheb M, et al: Indomethacin increases plasma lithium. BMJ *1:*1115, 1979.
41. Shelley RK: Lithium toxicity and mefenamic acid. A possible interaction and the role of prostaglandin inhibition. Br J Psychiatry *151:*847, 1987.
42. Walbridge DG, Bazire SR: An interaction between lithium and piroxicam presenting as lithium toxicity. Br J Psychiatry *147:*206, 1985.
43. Navis GJ, de Jong PE, de Zeeuw D: Volume homeostasis, angiotensin converting enzyme inhibition, and lithium therapy. Am J Med *86:*621, 1989.
44. Baldwin CM, Safferman AZ: A case of lisinopril-induced lithium toxicity. Drug Intell Clin Pharm *24:*946, 1990.
45. Correa F, Eiser A: Angiotensin converting enzyme inhibitors and lithium toxicity. Am J Med *93:*108, 1992.
46. Forrest JN, Cohen AD, Torretti J, et al: On the mechanism of lithium-induced diabetes insipidus in man. J Clin Invest *53:*1115, 1974.
47. Rosenbaum JF, Pollack MH: Treatment-emergent incontinence with lithium. J Clin Psychiatry *46:*444, 1985.
48. Fenves AZ, Emmett M, White MG: Lithium intoxication associated with acute renal failure. South Med J *77:*666, 1985.
49. Kincaid-Smith P, Burrows GD, Davies BM, et al: Renal biopsy findings in lithium and prelithium patients. Lancet *2:*700, 1979.
50. DePaulo JR, Correa EL, Sapir DG: Renal function and lithium: A longitudinal study. Am J Psychiatry *143:*892, 1986.
51. Keleher SP, Raciti A, Arbeit LA: Reduced or absent serum anion gap as a marker of severe lithium intoxication. Arch Intern Med *146:*1839, 1986.
52. Levy ST, Forrest JN, Heninger GR: Lithium-induced diabetes insipidus, manic symptoms, brain and electrolyte correlates and chlorothiazide treatment. Am J Psychiatry *130:*1014, 1973.
53. Rapoport J, Chiamovitz C, Alroy GG, Better OS: Lithium-induced nephrogenic diabetes insipidus: Studies of tubular function and pathogenesis. Isr J Med Sci *75:*765, 1979.
54. Batlle DC, von Riotte AB, Gaviria M, et al: Amelioration of polyuria by amiloride in patients receiving long-term lithium. N Engl J Med *312:*408, 1985.
55. Smith S, Ling L, Halstenson C: Whole-bowel irrigation as a treatment for acute lithium overdose. Ann Emerg Med *20:*536, 1991.
56. Watling SM, Gehrke JC, Gehrke CW, et al: *In vitro* binding of lithium using the cation exchange resin sodium polystyrene sulfonate. Am J Emerg Med *13:*294, 1995.
57. Verbov JL, Phillips JD, Fife DG: A case of lithium intoxication. Postgrad Med J *41:*190, 1965.
58. Kaplan Z, Schreiber G, Belmaker RH: Lack of effectiveness of forskolin or inositol as antidote in lithium toxicity. Short note. J Neurol Trans *72:*167, 1988.
59. Amdisen A, Skjoldborg H: Haemodialysis for lithium poisoning. Lancet *2:*213, 1969.
60. Winchester JF, Gelfand MC, Knepshield JH, Schreiner GE: Dialysis and hemoperfusion of poisons and drugs—update. Trans Am Soc Artif Intern Organs *23:*762, 1977.
61. Bismuth C, Baud FJ, Buneaux F, Du Fretay X: Spontaneous toxicokinetics of lithium during a therapeutic overdose with renal failure. J Toxicol Clin Toxicol *24:*261, 1986.
62. Szerlip HM, Heeger P, Feldman GM: Comparison between acetate and bicarbonate dialysis for the treatment of lithium intoxication. Am J Nephrol *12:*116, 1992.
63. Bellomo R, Kearly Y, Parkin G, et al: Treatment of life-threatening lithium toxicity with continuous arterio-venous hemodiafiltration. Crit Care Med *19:*836, 1991.
64. Simard M, Gumbiner B, Lee A, et al: Lithium carbonate intoxication. A case report and review of the literature. Arch Intern Med *149:*36, 1989.
65. Mann J, Branton LJ, Larkins RG: Hyperosmolality complicating recovery from lithium toxicity. BMJ *2:*1522, 1978.
66. Cairns SR, Wolman R, Lewis JG, Thakker R: Persistent nephrogenic diabetes insipidus, hyperparathyroidism, and hypothyroidism after lithium treatment. BMJ *290:*516, 1985.

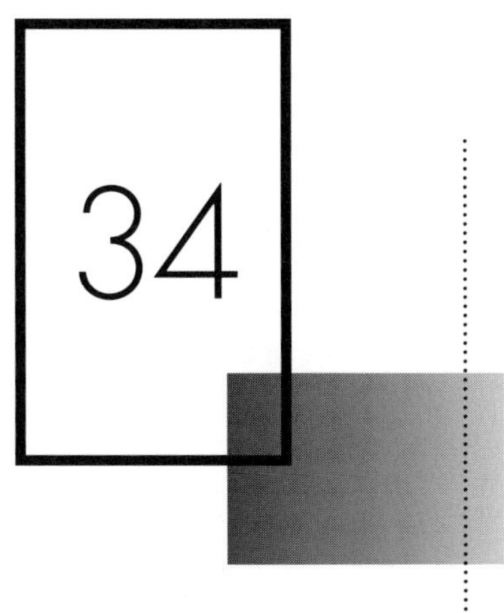

Ethanol

KURT C. KLEINSCHMIDT, MD
KATHLEEN A. DELANEY, MD

Ethanol is derived from fermentation of sugars in fruits, cereals, and vegetables. Valued for its medicinal and mood-altering effects, ethanol has had a significant historical role in mankind's medical, social, and religious rituals. Although its modern medical uses are limited, ethanol remains a popular "social lubricant" and is widely used in religious and social ceremonies. Ethanol is also frequently abused by both adults and adolescents, resulting in significant medical and social morbidity. Its widespread availability makes ethanol a common cause of accidental poisoning in children. In addition to alcoholic beverages, many household products such as perfumes, colognes, food extracts, mouthwashes, and cough preparations contain ethanol, often in large amounts (Table 34–1).[1, 2] Alcohol is the toxin identified most frequently in emergency department visits in the United States.

Ethanol is a clear, low-molecular-weight hydrocarbon that is highly soluble in water and lipids. It is rapidly absorbed by diffusion across the lipid membranes of the stomach and small intestine, reaching peak levels 20 to 60 minutes after ingestion.[3, 4] Its volume of distribution (0.6 L/kg) is roughly equivalent to that of total body water. The absolute dose of ethanol correlates directly with the resultant blood ethanol concentration (BEC) but not with the time to attainment of the peak level.[4] Various factors affect ethanol absorption (Table 34–2). Coingestion of food or decreased gastrointestinal motility produces a delay in absorption (which occurs primarily in the small intestine) and increases the gastric metabolism of ethanol.[3] Activated charcoal does not bind ethanol and thus does not decrease its absorption.[5]

Table 34–1. Alcohol Content of Common Products and Medications

Product	Ethanol Content (%)
After-shaves	15–80
Cold/allergy medications	5–16
Cough preparations	2–25
Glass cleaners	10
Mouthwashes	15–25
Perfumes/colognes	25–95

PHARMACOLOGY AND METABOLISM

The first step in the oxidation of ethanol involves its conversion from ethanol to acetaldehyde. Three hepatic enzyme systems can accomplish this step: the hydrogen peroxide–dependent peroxisome catalase system, the microsomal ethanol-oxidizing system (MEOS) located in the endoplasmic reticulum, and the cytosol enzyme alcohol dehydrogenase (ADH) (Fig. 34–1). The contribution of the peroxisome catalase system is minimal in most cases.[6]

In the nonalcoholic, 90% of the oxidation of ethanol to acetaldehyde is accomplished by ADH. Multiple isoenzyme forms of ADH occur with variable frequency in different human populations. These ADH isoenzymes have different affinities for ethanol, resulting in variations in ethanol elimination rates among individuals and racial groups. The activity of ADH does not change with chronic ethanol consumption.[7] However, liver ADH is degraded in the fasting state, which may result in as much as a 40% decrease in ADH activity.[8]

After ingesting equal amounts of alcohol, women attain higher BECs than do men. This is because women generally have a smaller body mass but more fat than men; this results in decreased total-body

Table 34–2. Absorption and Metabolic Factors Affecting Blood Ethanol Concentrations

Factor	Effect on Blood Ethanol	Reason
Adiposity	↑	Relative ↓ in Vd
Age	↑ in elderly	↓ Vd secondary to ↑ adipose/lean body mass ratio
	↓ in those < 13 y of age	↑ in metabolic rate
Chronic ethanol use	↑ ↓	If severe alcoholic liver disease present, ↑ in metabolic rate secondary to ↑ MEOS oxidation
Fasting state	↑	↑ Absorption secondary to faster gastric emptying and temporary ↓ in gastric ADH activity; decreased gastric metabolism
Delayed gastric emptying	↓	Longer exposure to gastric ADH
Increased lung tidal volume	↓	↑ in elimination from breath
Medications	Variable	Often secondary to change in MEOS activity
Sex	↑ in females	↑ in absorption secondary to ↓ gastric metabolism ↑ in adipose tissue ↓ in lean body weight
Cigarette smoking	↓	↑ in metabolic rate
Lean body weight (increased)	↓	Relative ↑ in Vd

↑, Increase; ↓, decrease; Vd, volume of distribution; MEOS, microsomal ethanol oxidizing system; ADH, alcohol dehydrogenase.

water volume and a decreased volume of distribution of ethanol.[9] In addition, the mucosa of the intestinal tract, particularly the stomach, also contains ADH, which causes a "first-pass" metabolism of up to 20% of ingested ethanol.[10] Women have a lower level of gastric ADH activity than do men, and this also contributes to their having higher BECs.[10]

The MEOS is a cytochrome P-450–dependent enzyme system that contributes less than 10% to the oxidation of ethanol in the moderate drinker; the specific member of this enzyme superfamily that oxidizes ethanol is CYP2E1 (the same enzyme that metabolizes acetaminophen). The K_m (the concentration of a substrate that yields one-half maximal enzyme activity) of ADH for ethanol is much lower than that of the MEOS. This is consistent with the observation that ADH is the primary oxidizer of ethanol. The contribution of the MEOS to the oxidation of ethanol increases as the BEC rises. The activity of the MEOS is significantly increased in chronic drinkers.[6] Unlike ADH, which requires oxidized nicotinamide-adenine dinucleotide (NAD^+) and generates reduced NAD (NADH), the MEOS requires the reduced form of NAD phosphate (NADPH) and yields the oxidized form of NAD phosphate ($NADP^+$). Oxidation of ethanol by ADH results in an increased $NADH/NAD^+$ ratio, which decreases the oxidative capacity of the liver. This creates an unfavorable "redox" state for oxidative metabolism and limits the rate of ADH activity. The activated MEOS in chronic alcoholics creates excess $NADP^+$, which improves the redox state of the liver and enhances ADH activity.[6]

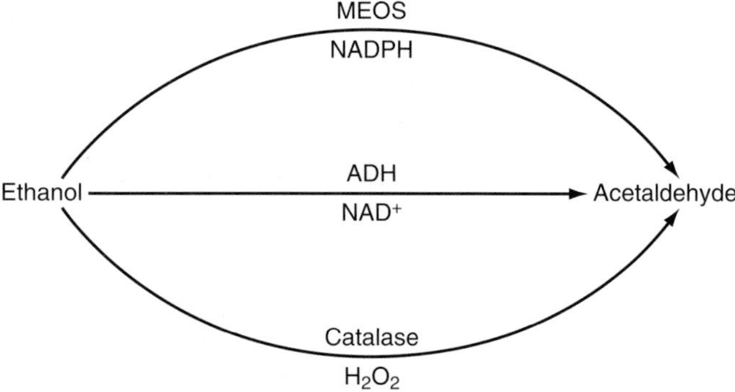

Figure 34–1. Pathways for ethanol oxidation to acetaldehyde. MEOS, microsomal ethanol oxidizing system; ADH, alcohol dehydrogenase; H_2O_2, hydrogen peroxide; NAD^+, nicotinamide-adenine dinucleotide, oxidized form; NADPH, nicotinamide-adenine dinucleotide phosphate, reduced form.

The next step in ethanol metabolism is the oxidation of acetaldehyde to acetate, which yields more NADH (Fig. 34–2). The reaction is catalyzed by various acetaldehyde dehydrogenase isoenzymes. These isoenzymes are very efficient, having a K_m approximately 1000 times lower than that of ADH for ethanol.[8] Fifty per cent of people of Japanese or Chinese origin have isoenzymes with decreased activity; this results in increased levels of acetaldehyde after ingestion of ethanol.[6, 8] This may be the cause of the increased incidence of facial flushing, vasodilation, and tachycardia (acetaldehyde syndrome) noted in some Japanese or Chinese after ethanol ingestion.[8] The increased acetaldehyde levels found in chronic alcoholics result from increased production rather than inadequate acetaldehyde dehydrogenase activity.[11, 12] Acetaldehyde is thought to be a mediator of alcoholic liver toxicity. It decreases cellular capacity to repair DNA, increases free radical–mediated lipid peroxidation, and augments hepatic collagen synthesis.[13]

Both environmental and genetic factors alter the absorption, metabolism, and elimination of ethanol, affecting the resultant BECs (see Table 34–2).[3, 11] The significance of some of these factors is difficult to determine owing to the large variations in elimination rates among different individuals and groups. For example, lung tidal volume affects levels because ethanol is excreted unchanged in the breath. The contribution of this mechanism may be significant when the BEC is high.[7] Alcoholics with severe liver

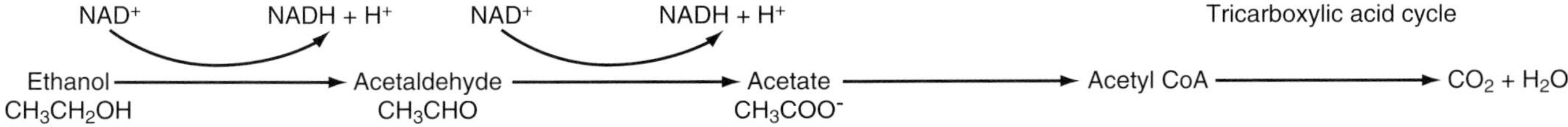

Figure 34–2. Ethanol metabolism. NADH, nicotinamide-adenine dinucleotide, reduced form; CoA, coenzyme A.

disease have decreased rates of ethanol metabolism that correlate with the severity of hepatic damage.[11] This mechanism may contribute to the loss of previously attained tolerance in some chronic alcoholics.[11, 12] Abnormalities of liver function test results are not associated with changes in BECs.[14]

Various studies have found ethanol elimination rates in nondrinkers to be 12 to 24 mg%/h; in social drinkers, 15 mg%/h and higher; and in alcoholics, 15 to 49 mg%/h. Not all studies have been able to demonstrate differences between chronic and intermittent drinkers.[14] It is clear that the only way to definitely know any one individual's elimination rate is to obtain serial BECs. It is reasonable to assume a metabolic rate of 20 mg%/h for unselected patients in an emergency department setting.[14] Ethanol elimination rates in children are typically 20 to 30 mg%/h.

The metabolism of ethanol has classically been considered to be linear, following zero-order kinetics—that is, an absolute amount of elimination occurs per unit of time. However, many studies suggest that the elimination kinetics of ethanol are not so easily defined. The elimination kinetics are difficult to evaluate because multiple enzyme systems with different K_m's are involved, different BEC ranges have been studied, and much individual variability exists in the rates of ethanol elimination. One case report described a patient with a BEC of 1500 mg% whose elimination followed first-order kinetics (an absolute percentage is eliminated per unit time) down to 400 mg%.[15] The elimination rate likely reflects a combination of different kinetic patterns. When BECs are high, the initial availability of free enzymes and the activation of the MEOS contribute to a rapid decline in ethanol concentration that is most consistent with a first-order process. The contribution of the MEOS decreases at moderate ethanol concentrations, when the more linear decline reflects saturation of ADH. Ethanol elimination slows even further at low concentrations, a pattern most consistent with the final phase of first-order kinetics. Thus, the elimination kinetics of ethanol are most accurately described by the Michaelis-Menten equation, with zero-order elimination across the usual range of BEC.

ACUTE INTOXICATION

It is unusual for alcoholics to present for acute care with intoxication as their only medical problem. In one urban emergency department series, only 26% of patients intoxicated with ethanol had intoxication as their sole problem.[14] Another urban hospital emergency department reported that 50% of 289 consecutive toxicologic screens that yielding positive results for ethanol revealed at least one other drug.[16] Fifty-three per cent of 116 consecutive motor vehicle accident victims admitted to an urban trauma service had BECs greater than 100 mg%.[17]

The BEC that defines legal intoxication in most states is 100 mg%, which is equivalent to 100 mg/dL, 0.1 g/dL, and 0.1%. However, lower levels may be significantly toxic in adults and, especially, in children. A toxic dose is considered to be 5 g/kg in an adult or 3 g/kg in a child. The ethanol content of popular beverages ranges from 3% to 6% for beers to as high as 90% for some distilled liquors. One ounce of whiskey (80 proof, or 40% ethanol), 12 oz of beer, and 4 oz of wine are approximately equipotent and raise the BEC by 25 mg% in the average adult.

Symptoms of intoxication vary, ranging from loss of fine motor control to coma and death. Although BECs typically correlate with symptoms in nondrinkers (Table 34–3), chronic drinkers require higher levels to reach similar states of intoxication.[18–21] The degree of intoxication also correlates with the rate of

Table 34–3. Signs and Symptoms of Intoxication and Blood Ethanol Concentrations in a Non–Alcohol-Dependent Population*

Ethanol Concentration (mg%)	Signs and Symptoms
<25	Sense of warmth Sense of well-being Talkativeness Self-confidence Mild incoordination
25–50	Euphoria Clumsiness Decreased judgment and control
50–100	Decreased sensorium Worsened coordination, ataxia Decreased reflexes/increased reaction time Emotional lability
100–250	Cerebellar/vestibular dysfunction (ataxia, diplopia, slurred speech, visual impairment, nystagmus) Severe emotional lability, confusion, stupor Nausea, vomiting
250–400	Stupor or coma Little response to stimuli Incontinence Respiratory depression
>400	Respiratory paralysis Loss of protective reflexes Hypothermia Death

*Correlation between signs and symptoms and blood ethanol levels show wide variability among individuals.

increase of the BEC. Slower ethanol ingestion results in less intoxication.[18] Acute tolerance has been demonstrated with a single large ingestion of ethanol. This manifests as a greater degree of intoxication at any BEC when the level is increasing compared with when the level is decreasing.[18] Levels as low as 47 mg% have been associated with motor vehicle accidents.[20] Visual tracking of objects is decreased as much as 25% when the BEC is 80 mg%.[22] Coma is unusual when the BEC is below 200 mg%.[19] The lethal level for 50% of the non–ethanol-dependent population is 450 mg%,[19] although individuals with BECs as high as 1500 mg% have survived.[15] Although most states use a BEC of 100 mg% as the legal level for intoxication, significant compromise can occur at lower levels. In recognition of this, the Surgeon General recently recommended that intoxication be defined as a BEC of 80 mg% and that this value be reduced to 40 mg% by the year 2000.[23]

LABORATORY EVALUATION

The patient's chief complaint and the data obtained on the history and physical examination should guide the selection of ancillary laboratory studies. The usefulness of routine measurement of the BEC in the emergency department is controversial. It is an appropriate part of the evaluation of a patient with an altered mental status. However, the BEC is less likely to affect management decisions in an intoxicated individual who is awake and alert. Determining the disposition of intoxicated patients involves clinical decision-making and should not be based on BECs. Controversy exists as to the correlation between initial BECs and the potential severity of withdrawal symptoms and the amount of detoxification medication required.[24]

The BEC may be approximated with the use of various body fluids; however, venous blood and breath samples are most commonly used. BECs are *not* affected by the use of ethanol in the skin preparation, despite theoretic concerns.[25] The accuracy of the breath ethanol analyzer (BEA) depends on the constant equilibrium of the ratio of the ethanol level in the blood to that of alveolar air at 2100:1.[26] BEA results are slightly lower than venous blood measurements, especially at higher levels of ethanol intoxication, and they may be affected by the patient's ability to cooperate.[26] BEA results are also consistently less than venous blood estimations in older patients or those with poor pulmonary function.[27] Testing within 15 to 20 minutes of the last drink or the presence of vomitus in the mouth may cause small false elevations in measured levels. False-negative results are rare.[26]

MANAGEMENT OF THE ACUTELY INTOXICATED PATIENT

Although ethanol intoxication is a common cause of altered mental status, a broad differential diagnosis should be considered in the patient who appears to be intoxicated. Other common causes of altered mental status in the alcoholic patient include hypothermia, hepatic encephalopathy, hypoglycemia, head trauma, sepsis, shock, and intoxication with substances other than ethanol. The threshold for performing computed tomography of the head must be low. Computed tomography of the head is indicated if a patient's sensorium does not clear during a period of observation. Steady improvement is the rule when a patient's mental status is depressed by ethanol.

Fluid administration is indicated because the intoxicated patient frequently has volume depletion secondary to ethanol-induced diuresis, vomiting, and poor oral intake. Alcoholic patients should also receive multivitamins, thiamine, and folate. Hypoglycemia must be excluded in patients who have altered mental status or use ethanol chronically. The routine administration of glucose to alcoholic patients is rational because of the significant incidence of ketoacidosis and glycogen deficiency in sick alcoholic patients. Studies have not consistently shown caffeine,[28] naloxone,[29] fructose,[30] or flumazenil[31] to have any benefit in reversing the effects of ethanol. Gastric emptying is ineffective at decreasing BECs because of ethanol's rapid absorption. Despite charcoal's inability to bind ethanol, its administration should be considered in patients who may have ingested other toxins.

OTHER CLINICAL EFFECTS

Endocrine, Nutritional, and Metabolic Effects

Ethanol alters many aspects of endocrine function, including gonadal activity and the metabolism of bones, minerals, glucocorticoids, fat, and carbohydrates. Some evidence suggests that these effects may be reversible with prolonged abstinence.[32] Ethanol directly and indirectly affects all levels of the hypothalamic-pituitary-testicular axis. Ethanol and its metabolites, acetaldehyde and acetate, directly decrease testosterone production.[32] Up to one half of alcoholics with cirrhosis have atrophic testes, and many have gynecomastia. Women who drink moderately have an increased incidence of anovulatory cycles. Amenorrhea occurs more frequently in women with cirrhosis than in those without cirrhosis.[32]

Alcoholism is associated with osteoporosis in both men and women. Ethanol is directly toxic to osteoblasts. Other factors contributing to osteoporosis include hypogonadism, decreased calcium intake and malabsorption, increased urinary calcium excretion, decreased exercise, and an altered parathyroid hormone response to hypocalcemia.[32] Even acute intoxication appears to result in an inverse correlation between the BEC and calcium levels.[33]

Acute and chronic ethanol ingestion are associated with stimulation of the hypothalamic-pituitary-adrenal axis. Elevated adrenocorticotropin hormone and cortisol levels in some alcoholics suggest Cushing's syndrome.[19, 32] These individuals have classic clinical stigmata such as central obesity and laboratory abnormalities that include altered dexamethasone suppression. One study found that up to one fifth of alcoholics in a detoxification ward had altered dexamethasone suppression.[32] The increased glucocorticoid secretion returns to normal within a few weeks of abstinence.[32]

Ethanol alters fat and carbohydrate metabolism. Hepatic lipogenesis is increased, and lipoprotein release is decreased. Peripheral fat mobilization is increased, as is hepatic uptake of circulating lipids. The increased $NADH/NAD^+$ ratio impedes the function of the tricarboxylic acid cycle and slows fatty acid oxidation.[13] These effects ultimately result in the accumulation of triglycerides in hepatocytes (steatosis) and in increased serum triglyceride levels. Hypoglycemia is common. Liver glycogen stores can be depleted within 12 hours, especially if fasting is present.[32] The altered redox ratio decreases gluconeogenic activity.[13, 32, 34]

Malnutrition leads to vitamin and electrolyte abnormalities. Vitamin deficiency disorders include pellagra, stomatitis, and scurvy. Thiamine deficiency is particularly common because the total-body supply of this nutrient can be depleted within 33 days.[35] Electrolyte disorders include hypokalemia, hypophosphatemia, and hypomagnesemia. The marked negative balance of potassium is also caused by gastrointestinal losses and urinary excretion owing to altered mineralocorticoid activity.[34, 36] Serum potassium levels often do not reflect the extent of the deficiency because of the extracellular migration of potassium resulting from a relative insulin deficiency in alcoholics.[34]

Various acid-base abnormalities occur in alcoholic patients. Ethanol itself does not cause significant lactic acidosis; thus, other pathologic processes should be considered if lactic acidosis is present. The anion-gap acidosis commonly seen in alcoholic patients is multifactorial and results from a combination of ketoacids and lactic acid. The increased $NADH/NAD^+$ ratio favors production of lactate over that of pyruvate (Fig. 34–3).[34, 37] A metabolic alkalosis secondary to vomiting and volume contraction is also frequently encountered.[34]

Alcoholic ketoacidosis may cause severe acidosis in chronic alcoholics. The process often begins with ethanol-associated abdominal pain (e.g., from gastric irritation, pancreatitis, or hepatitis) and vomiting. Volume-depletion occurs, and ethanol ingestion decreases as the patient becomes more ill. Comorbid

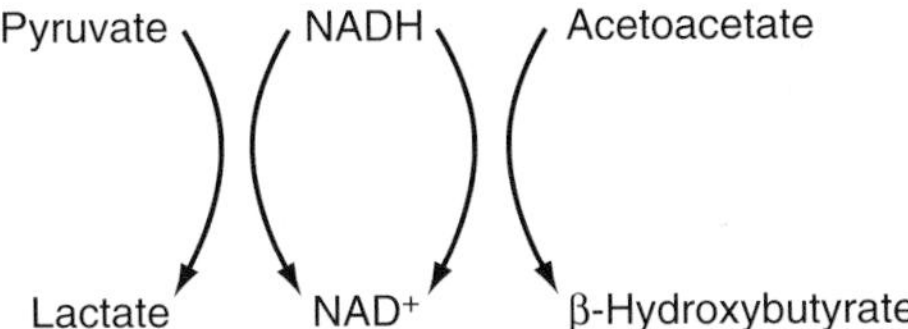

Figure 34–3. Some effects of the increased $NADH/NAD^+$ ratio.

Table 34–4. Alcoholic Ketoacidosis Presentation Summary

Source of Data	Findings
History-taking	Alcoholism Cessation or decrease of ethanol intake over prior 24–72 h Fasted state Abdominal pain Vomiting
Physical examination	Consciousness Status consistent with volume depletion Tachycardia Tachypnea
Laboratory	Anion-gap metabolic acidosis pH may be acidemic, normal, or alkalemic Acidemia secondary to ketoacidosis Alkalosis secondary to tachypnea and vomiting Hypokalemia Hypophosphatemia Glucose level mildly elevated, normal, or low Serum and urinary ketones increased (elevation may be underestimated with the nitroprusside test because this test only measures acetoacetate, whereas β-hydroxybutyrate is the primary ketoacid)

conditions often cloud the typical clinical characteristics of alcoholic ketoacidosis (Table 34–4). The stress-related catecholamine increase and the resurgent gluconeogenesis (occurring after cessation of drinking) result in normal to mildly elevated serum glucose levels. Multiple events contribute to the significant ketoacidosis, including acetyl coenzyme A shunting to ketone production, increased lipolysis and free fatty acid release, decreased peripheral tissue uptake and metabolism of ketones, and decreased urinary elimination of ketones (Fig. 34–4).[37] The primary ketoacids are β-hydroxybutyrate and acetoacetate. In alcoholic ketoacidosis, the increased $NADH/NAD^+$ ratio favors β-hydroxybutyrate production (see Fig. 34–3).

The treatment of alcoholic ketoacidosis should include volume resuscitation, administration of thiamine and glucose, and management of associated disorders. Glucose administration causes endogenous insulin release, which suppresses free fatty acid release and ketogenesis. Treatment of alcoholic ketoacidosis results in a decreased $NADH/NAD^+$ ratio, which decreases the β-hydroxybutyrate/acetoacetate ratio. Because the nitroprusside test for ketones measures only acetoacetate, the nitroprusside test result for ketones paradoxically will become increasingly positive.

Acute ethanol ingestion causes a dose-dependent suppression of pituitary antidiuretic hormone release, which results in the familiar diuretic effect. This causes free water loss without significant urinary electrolyte loss.[36] The effect of chronic ethanol intake on total-body water is the subject of debate. The ethanol-induced diuresis and periodic abdominal upset and vomiting may lead to dehydration in chronic alcoholics. However, there is also evidence

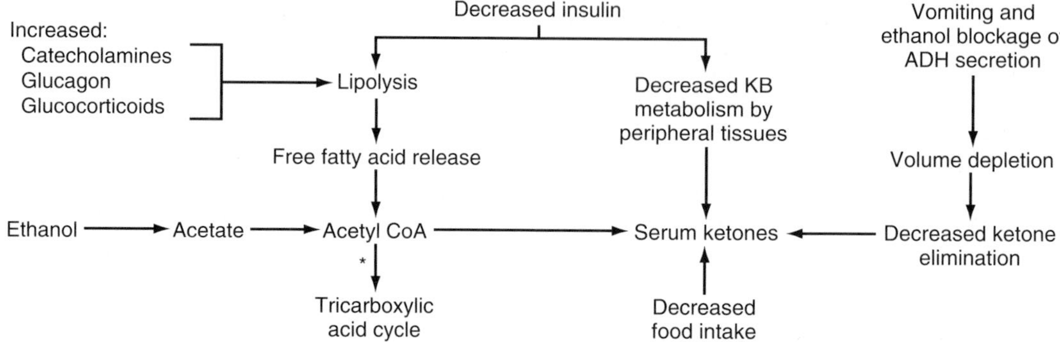

Figure 34–4. Factors causing ketonemia in alcoholic ketoacidosis. ADH, antidiuretic hormone. *The tricarboxylic acid cycle is significantly slowed due to intermediates' being used for gluconeogenesis.

that chronic ethanol use results in a lowering of the pituitary osmole receptor set-point; this lowering increases antidiuretic hormone secretion, and this in turn results in eventual volume overload.[36] Fluid supplementation should be based on the clinical evaluation findings.

Neuropsychiatric Effects

In addition to the neuropsychiatric effects of acute intoxication and withdrawal, chronic ethanol use is associated with polyneuropathy, Wernicke's encephalopathy, Korsakoff's psychosis, cerebellar degeneration, dementia, and central pontine myelinolysis. Controversy exists regarding the cause and management of these disorders and their relationships. Acute ingestion of ethanol also can cause the unusual temporary phenomenon known as a "blackout." Blackout is characterized by amnesia and the inability to form new memories but has no effect on immediate recall or long-term memories.[20]

The most common neurologic symptoms in alcoholics are those of polyneuropathy. Common findings include painful dysesthesia, anesthesia, weakness, decreased pain and temperature sensation, and decreased touch and vibration sense.[20, 21] Disease progression is gradual, bilateral, and symmetric. Symptoms are distal more often than proximal and involve the legs more than the arms.[20, 21] Physical examination reveals atrophy and decreased deep tendon reflexes. The cause remains unclear, but there is evidence of both nutritional effects and direct ethanol toxicity resulting in axonal degeneration and demyelination.[21] Abstinence may result in recovery that generally is slow and incomplete.[21]

Wernicke's encephalopathy (WE) results from a deficiency of vitamin B_1 (thiamine) and is characterized by the classic clinical triad of oculomotor abnormalities, ataxia, and global confusion. Thiamine is a cofactor with many enzymes, including pyruvate decarboxylase in the tricarboxylic acid cycle. Although WE generally is associated with alcoholism, thiamine deficiency can occur in any state of nutritional depletion.[20, 21, 38] Indeed, one autopsy series demonstrated that only 18% of the cases occurred in alcoholics.[38] Thiamine deficiency occurs in alcoholics for various reasons, including poor diet, reduced thiamine absorption and liver storage, and decreased conversion of thiamine to its active form.[21, 38] Another proposed cause of WE is glucose loading in thiamine-depleted individuals.[38] This has led to the medical adage that thiamine must be given before glucose is administered to patients with altered mental status. WE actually requires several days to develop, so administration of glucose and thiamine within a similar time frame prevents its occurrence. Only a minority of thiamine-deficient patients develop WE. The development of clinical disease in so few thiamine-deficient individuals reflects either a genetic contribution, unknown variables, or underdiagnosis.[35] A promising ancillary test is magnetic resonance imaging, which is used for assessing the mamillary body shrinkage associated with WE.[21, 38] A laboratory demonstration of low thiamine levels has poor specificity for the diagnosis of WE because most individuals with thiamine deficiency do not have WE.

WE may be more common than is generally perceived because the diagnosis can be difficult to establish. Autopsy series have demonstrated cerebral and cerebellar neuropathologic changes specific for WE in 0.8% to 2.8% of the general population and in 12% of alcoholics.[38] Reviews of premorbid symptoms from these series found stupor and coma to be the most common presentations, whereas WE was diagnosed in no more than 20% of the patients.[38, 39]

Pathologic studies and chart reviews indicate that the clinical presentation of WE with the classic triad occurs in only 10% to 33% of patients, and as many as one fifth of these have none of the three.[20, 38] The onset occurs over several days to many weeks. The hallmarks of WE are the extraocular movement abnormalities, with horizontal nystagmus noted in 85% of patients; bilateral lateral rectus paralysis in 54% of patients; and paresis of conjugate gaze in 44% of patients.[40] Loss of equilibrium is secondary to vestibular paresis and cerebellar dysfunction and typically produces ataxia of gait but not of the limbs.[40] The global confusional state consists of apathy, poor concentration, spatial and temporal disorientation, and slow and irrational thinking. Most patients have a normal level of consciousness. Impairment of memory and ability to learn is present in a majority but is often difficult to demonstrate because of the impairment of concentration.[18] Other manifestations include hypothermia and hypotension secondary to altered temperature regulation and decreased sympathetic outflow.[38] WE evolves over time, with mild, subclinical episodes progressing until the clinical triad is apparent.[38] The mortality for treated WE is 17% during the initial weeks after diagnosis. Pathologic evaluation of these patients reveals that the vast majority have significant associated diseases, including infections and cirrhosis.[40]

WE is reversible with the administration of thiamine. It should be considered a medical emergency because of the associated morbidity and mortality. Patients should be hospitalized and receive 100 mg of thiamine intravenously every day for at least 5 days.[20, 21] The ocular abnormalities reverse completely within hours to days except for a fine horizontal nystagmus on lateral gaze, which persists in 60% of patients.[40] Recovery from ataxia usually takes longer than 1 month and is complete in only one third of patients. Virtually all patients recover from the global confusion within 2 months, although most have persistent memory difficulties.[40]

Korsakoff's psychosis (KP) has been defined as "an abnormal mental state in which memory and learning are affected out of all proportion to other cognitive functions in an otherwise alert and responsive patient."[40] It is characterized by retrograde (recent events) and anterograde (events occurring now) amnesia, but retention of past memory is not impaired. Patients are alert and responsive and can interact well socially. However, they are often indifferent to their surroundings and are unaware of their disability.[40] Other less severe disorders of cognition and perception can be present, including mild disorientation. The term "psychosis" is confusing because patients with KP do not have the gross distortion of mental capacity typically associated with a psychosis. Eighty per cent of persons with WE demonstrate KP once the global confusion of WE has cleared after thiamine treatment.[40] Indeed, the memory impairment associated with WE is likely the beginning of KP, and at times differentiation of one from the other is difficult. However, not all patients with KP have had WE. Complete recovery from KP occurs over 1 to 3 months in 20% of afflicted patients. Twenty-five per cent of patients do not recover at all. Management includes routine nursing care, proper diet, and abstinence from alcohol. The contribution of thiamine to recovery from KP has not been defined.[40]

Alcoholic cerebellar degeneration affects chronic drinkers and is characterized by a gradual onset of ataxia that affects the trunk more than the limbs and the legs more than the arms.[20, 21] The symptoms and anatomic cerebellar abnormalities are similar to those found in WE, suggesting that the two diseases may actually be different aspects of the same process.[21] Although the gait ataxia is similar to that in WE, patients with cerebellar degeneration have more limb ataxia and dysarthria and much less nystagmus.[20] Various causes have been proposed, including thiamine deficiency, electrolyte abnormalities, and direct toxicity from ethanol.[21] The disease stabilizes or improves with the cessation of drinking.[21]

Alcoholic dementia likely has multiple causes, including the direct toxic effect of ethanol on the central nervous system. Cerebral atrophy is a common finding. Some researchers believe that the dementia is a manifestation of KP.[21] Central pontine myelinolysis, a rare disorder that evolves over days to weeks, is sometimes associated with alcoholism.[21] Frequently, there is also a history of hyponatremia. The pontine corticobulbar white fibers undergo demyelination, which causes dysarthria, dysphagia, facial and neck weakness, dysfunctional tongue movements, and gaze palsies. Mental confusion also is a prominent symptom.[20, 21] The pontine lesions are readily demonstrated by magnetic resonance imaging.[21]

Cardiac Effects

Cardiac abnormalities associated with ethanol use include alcoholic cardiomyopathy with congestive heart failure, dysrhythmias, hypertension, and coronary artery disease. The term "alcoholic heart disease" is slowly replacing the name "alcoholic cardiomyopathy" because a cardiomyopathy is technically a primary disease of cardiac muscle of unknown cause. Alcoholic heart disease is affected by genetic predisposition and the amount and length of ethanol abuse.[41] Once alcoholic heart disease is present, the prognosis is poor unless patients abstain from further ethanol intake.[41] The pathophysiology is not clear, but postulated effects include changes in the sarcolemma, the sodium/potassium–adenosine triphosphatase (Na^+/K^+ ATPase) pump, calcium homeostasis, and contractile proteins.[41] Changes in cardiac structure and function include four-chamber dilatation, reduced left ventricular compliance and ejection fraction, mild endocardial and valve leaflet scarring, and mural thrombi.[41] Early symptoms may include an exertional cough, nocturia, and reduced exercise tolerance. Eventually, more characteristic signs and symptoms of biventricular failure develop.[41] Young, healthy individuals with normal hearts may experience acute myocardial depression from the cardiotoxic effects of ethanol. The clinical significance of this is unclear.[42]

Moderate-to-heavy ethanol abusers have increased systolic and diastolic blood pressures.[41] The relationship between the degree of elevation and the amount and duration of ethanol exposure is not well defined.[41] Conversely, acute ethanol ingestion causes a decrease in blood pressure that may be due to a combination of decreased vascular resistance and cardiac function.[42] The effect of ethanol on coronary artery atherosclerotic disease is mixed. Epidemiologic studies have clearly related low-to-moderate ethanol consumption with a decrease in coronary artery atherosclerotic disease compared with abstinence and heavy consumption. This protective effect may be related to an increase in high-density lipoprotein levels and a decrease in low-density lipoprotein levels rather than to a direct protective effect of ethanol.[42, 43] Ethanol decreases coronary vascular resistance acutely; this leads to an increase in coronary blood flow that may have a protective effect or that may result in a coronary steal phenomenon that adversely affects the myocardial ratio of supply and demand.[43] Coronary artery disease has not been demonstrated to increase mortality in chronic ethanol abusers.

Dysrhythmias of both atrial and ventricular origin are associated with ethanol consumption. The classic paper of Ettinger and colleagues described the "holiday heart syndrome" in alcoholics without overt alcoholic heart disease who developed dysrhythmias. Atrial fibrillation and flutter were most common and resolved with abstinence.[44] The relationship between ethanol and atrial fibrillation was supported by a review finding that ethanol caused or contributed to 63% of admissions for atrial fibrillation. Eighty-nine per cent of patients with ethanol-related atrial fibrillation had conversion to sinus rhythm within 24 hours of admission, in contrast to only 42% of those with atrial fibrillation having a pulmonary or cardiac cause.[45] Conduction defects and rhythm disturbances have also been associated with alcoholic heart disease.[41]

Gastrointestinal Effects

The effects of ethanol on the gastrointestinal tract include esophagitis, gastritis, peptic ulcer disease, malabsorption, gastrointestinal bleeding secondary to numerous causes, and liver and pancreatic diseases. Ethanol-associated liver disorders include fatty infiltration, alcoholic hepatitis, and fibrosis (cirrhosis). Fatty infiltration of the liver can start within days of the onset of heavy drinking. It is due primarily to triglyceride deposition, but dietary fat intake also contributes.[9] Inflammation resulting from alcoholic hepatitis hastens the deposition of collagen. Inflammation associated with fatty infiltration results in the deposition of collagen, the primary protein of fibrous tissues. Liver lipocytes are eventually transformed into collagen-producing cells. Cirrhosis develops when collagen production (or fibrosis) outpaces collagen degradation.[9] The induction of the MEOS may also be associated with hepatic injury. The MEOS converts various xenobiotic compounds such as anesthetics and industrial solvents to toxic, "free radical" metabolites. The cytochrome P-450 system also activates carcinogens that may contribute to the increased incidence of upper alimentary and respiratory tract cancers in alcoholics. Acetaldehyde accumulation is associated with impairment of hepatic oxygen utilization, increased free radical production, lipid peroxidation, and fibrinogenesis.[13]

Hematologic and Infectious Effects

Both acute and chronic ethanol abuse suppress hematopoietic elements of the bone marrow. The causes include malnutrition-related vitamin deficiency and direct ethanol toxicity. Ethanol causes decreased bone marrow cellularity, vacuolization of marrow precursor cells, and a macrocytosis independent of folate deficiency. Chronic ethanol abuse causes thrombocytopenia that resolves with abstinence. Its effect on platelet function is not clear.[46]

Ethanol is associated with many types of anemia, including iron and folate deficiency, hemolytic, and sideroblastic anemias. Classic folate-dependent megaloblastic anemia occurs in 4% of ambulatory alcoholics and generally affects those who imbibe hard liquor because beer is actually a good source of folate.[46] Folate deficiency in alcoholics is caused by poor diet, malabsorption, disruption of the enterohepatic circulation, and the direct antifolate effect of ethanol. Infection in alcoholics is associated with increased morbidity. Immunosuppression occurs with acute and chronic ethanol abuse. Acute ingestion causes decreased neutrophil delivery to sites of infection and decreased adherence, whereas chronic abuse results in marrow suppression, decreased chemotaxis, and neutropenia. Neutrophil bactericidal and phagocyte activity are not affected by ethanol.[47] Abstinence results in reversal of leukopenia within a few days.[46] Ethanol is also associated with decreases in pulmonary macrophage mobilization, bactericidal activity, and reticuloendothelial system clearance.[46]

TOLERANCE, DEPENDENCY, AND WITHDRAWAL

Chronic ethanol use eventually results in tolerance, physical dependence, addiction, and alcoholism. Although these states are different, they likely represent a progression of disease. *Tolerance* is a condition in which larger and larger doses of an agent are required to obtain the same effect.[48] Tolerance is a manifestation of cellular adaptation to the effects of ethanol. *Physical dependence* is a physiologic state in which ethanol consumption is necessary for maintaining the desired psychologic effect or for preventing the symptoms of withdrawal. The withdrawal syndrome occurs in physically dependent individuals who reduce or abruptly cease their ethanol intake.[48] *Addiction* is a behavioral pattern reflecting a constant, powerful need for ethanol use. Addicted individuals often relapse after withdrawal periods.[48] *Alcoholism* is a complex disease consisting of social, behavioral, and medical disturbances. The social aspects relate to its effects on family, work, and community. The behavioral component is characterized by the continuation of drinking despite knowledge of the harm being done. The medical problems involve the management of the disease itself and the complications of the chronic drinking.

It has been observed that as alcoholics have more

and more episodes of withdrawal, they experience increasingly severe withdrawal symptoms. This phenomenon has been referred to as "kindling."[49] "Reinstatement" is another clinical entity in alcoholics that refers to the ever-shortening drinking bouts required before cycles of withdrawal.[49] Considering both phenomena, chronic alcoholics may slowly develop withdrawal episodes of ever increasing frequency and severity.

PATHOPHYSIOLOGY OF INTOXICATION AND WITHDRAWAL

The complex cellular mechanisms of ethanol intoxication, tolerance, dependence, and withdrawal are not completely clear. Ethanol is a relatively weak sedative. Much greater concentrations of ethanol than of agents such as benzodiazepines or barbiturates are required to induce the same effect. This likely reflects the absence of specific receptors for ethanol.[20] The effects of ethanol appear to be related to changes in cell membrane function. Ethanol alters membrane fluidity and the function of membrane structures involved in signal transduction, the binding of neurotransmitters, and the regulation of gene expression.[20, 21] Certain areas of the brain are more sensitive to ethanol than are others.[20, 21] Selective sites of toxicity include the receptor complex of the inhibitory neurotransmitter γ-aminobutyric acid (GABA), the areas regulating excitatory amino acids, calcium channels, the central adrenergic system, dopamine and adenosine receptors, and the hypothalamic-pituitary-adrenal axis.

The GABA receptor is part of a large membrane protein complex that includes a GABA-activated chloride channel and a closely linked benzodiazepine receptor whose effect is also mediated by the chloride channels.[20, 21] Ethanol causes GABA-like neuronal inhibition directly by having an effect on the chloride channel and indirectly by potentiating GABA.[20] The physical proximity of these receptors may explain the cross tolerance that occurs between ethanol and the benzodiazepines. Chronic ethanol use decreases the magnitude of GABA complex–mediated neuroinhibition, an effect that probably contributes to the development of tolerance.[20] Decreased GABA-activated chloride channel flux during abstinence contributes to the central nervous system hyperexcitability of ethanol withdrawal.[20] The sedating effect of benzodiazepines on patients with symptoms of ethanol withdrawal is likely due to the activation of these same channels. Although the exact mechanism is not clear, certain benzodiazepine antagonists—including picrotoxin and bicuculline—block the effect of ethanol on the chloride channels.[20, 21]

Calcium channels and their receptors also may contribute to cellular mechanisms of tolerance and withdrawal. A few days of ethanol use causes an increase in both calcium channel flux and binding site availability that persists for several hours after drinking has ceased. Calcium channel blockers decrease tremors, seizures, and death in ethanol-dependent rodents deprived of ethanol. Calcium channel blockers attenuate some of the sympathetic symptoms of withdrawal in humans; however, they have not been demonstrated to prevent seizures or delirium tremens (DTs).[21]

Ethanol has been shown to affect the activity of excitatory amino acids, particularly *N*-methyl-D-aspartate (NMDA), in certain areas of the brain.[21] Ethanol decreases both NMDA receptor–associated calcium channel flux and changes the cellular response to its activation. Of particular interest is ethanol's inhibition of NMDA receptors in the hippocampus, an area involved in learning and memory. This is a proposed mechanism of the cognitive defects and "blackouts" associated with ethanol use.[20, 21]

Adrenergic central nervous system effects appear to have a major role in withdrawal symptoms. The excitatory neurotransmitter norepinephrine is released by presynaptic vesicles. It interacts with various receptors and is then taken back up into the presynaptic terminal. Within the hypothalamus, intersynaptic norepinephrine is taken up by extraneuronal cells (possibly astrocytes) and converted to epinephrine that is then released back into the synapse. Phenylethanoamine-*N*-methyltransferase (PNMT) catalyzes this extraneuronal conversion of norepinephrine to epinephrine. Epinephrine activates presynaptic α_2-receptors, which inhibit norepinephrine release. Ethanol increases PNMT activity, and this leads to central adrenergic inhibition. Chronic ethanol ingestion leads to compensatory down-regulation of presynaptic α_2-receptors. Ethanol withdrawal is associated with decreased PNMT activity; this means that less epinephrine is available to stimulate the previously down-regulated α_2-receptors. Because the α_2-receptors provide negative feedback to the presynaptic neurons, the resultant loss of negative inhibition yields increased sympathomimetic activity.[49] This pathophysiologic mechanism accounts for the effect of the central α_2-agonist clonidine in decreasing the sympathomimetic activity associated with withdrawal.

Excess dopaminergic states have been associated with psychosis, hallucinosis, cravings, and the mechanisms of reward and reinforcement.[21] 5-Hydroxytryptamine$_3$ (serotonin) receptors stimulate dopamine release. Ethanol enhances dopamine release by potentiating serotonin receptor binding. The roles of serotonin and dopamine in ethanol intoxication and withdrawal are not clearly defined.[21] It has been noted that individuals who suffer blackouts appear to have a decrease in the serotonin precursor tryptophan; this suggests a possible role of altered serotoninergic transmission in this condition.[20]

Adenosine has also been linked to the development of physical dependence and tolerance.[21] Although not a neurotransmitter itself, adenosine is a modulator with significant impact on the effects of neurotransmitters. Acute ethanol ingestion inhibits intracellular transport of adenosine, leading to increased stimulation of extracellular membrane A_2 adenosine receptors. This stimulation of the A_2 receptors causes increased G protein–mediated adenylate cyclase activity and increased intracellular adenosine 3′,5′-cyclic phosphate (cyclic adenosine monophosphate [cAMP]). Chronic ethanol intake eventually results in an adaptive decrease in cAMP production mediated by decreased production of messenger RNA for G protein synthesis. These cells require the presence of ethanol to maintain adequate cAMP production; this represents a manifestation of "physical dependence" at the cellular level.[21] The adenosine nucleoside transporter also loses its sensitivity to ethanol inhibition with chronic ethanol use. Protein kinase A activity, which requires cAMP, is responsible for the decreased adenosine nucleoside transporter uptake. The decrease in available cAMP associated with chronic ethanol ingestion eventually results in increased adenosine transporter activity. This represents "tolerance" at the cellular level.[21]

WITHDRAWAL SYNDROMES

A classic study by Isbell and co-workers published in 1953 clearly convinced the medical community that delirium tremens (DTs) and other manifestations of withdrawal were actually caused by the cessation of drinking rather than by a toxic effect of ethanol.[50] In their study, ethanol was given daily to 10 healthy, former opiate addicts in controlled conditions that provided adequate diets and vitamins but prevented the introduction of other agents. Upon cessation of drinking, four subjects who drank for up to 34 days developed tremor, perspiration, gastrointestinal distress, and anorexia lasting 1 to 3 days. Three of these four drank for no longer than 16 days, a finding that reflected the little time needed for the development of physical dependence. The six subjects who drank between 48 and 87 days experienced 5 to 8 days of vomiting, diarrhea, insomnia, hyperreflexia, and fever in addition to the other symptoms. Five of these also had hallucinations, two had seizures, and three developed full-blown DTs.[50] Ethanol withdrawal developed as long as the amount of ethanol ingested remained large over time—even if the study participants did not become intoxicated. The authors concluded that three factors contributed to the development of physical dependence and the severity and duration of withdrawal: dose, duration of abuse, and frequency of administration.[50]

Symptoms of ethanol withdrawal range from mild anxiety and tremors to seizures, DTs, and death. Symptoms appear 6 to 8 hours after a significant drop in serum ethanol level. Sympathetic symptoms include tremors, tachycardia, hypertension, irritability, and hyperreflexia. Neuropsychiatric symptoms include anxiety, agitation, hyperalertness, susceptibility to startling, insomnia, craving for rest, self-preoccupation, inattention, and mild disorientation to time with no gross confusion.[18, 50] The absence of significant disorientation, confusion, and autonomic instability differentiates typical withdrawal from the more serious DTs. Tremors may be minimally noticeable (shaky inside) but worsen with activity or agitation and can become so coarse that the patient many not be able to talk, walk, or eat.[18] Symptoms often peak and begin to resolve within 24 hours but can last from days to longer than a week. Without treatment, the hyperalertness, shakiness, and insomnia can last as long as 10 to 14 days.[18] A mild symptom complex occurs in 70% to 80% of patients, whereas 15% to 20% become moderately ill if treatment is not provided.[51]

Hallucinations can be a prominent part of withdrawal, occurring in up to 25% of patients. In 75% of cases, hallucinations begin within 48 hours of cessation of drinking; however, they may not occur until 6 to 8 days thereafter.[18] Pure visual hallucinations occur fivefold more frequently than do auditory ones.[18] Rarely, they may be tactile or olfactory in nature. Other disorders of perception, such as illusions, are transient and rarely last longer than 3 days.[18]

Victor and Adams described an unusual manifestation of ethanol withdrawal termed "acute auditory hallucinosis," which occurred in 2% of their patients.[18] The patients did not have significant autonomic hyperactivity. The auditory hallucinations affected only chronic alcoholics, were usually threatening in nature, and lasted from a few days to 2 weeks. Patients were oriented during the hallucinatory events. Upon recovery, patients realized that the voices were imaginary but could vividly recall the events.[18]

Alcoholic withdrawal seizures, also known as "rum fits," are generalized and tonic-clonic. The onset of this disease is in adulthood, and this feature helps in differentiating it from idiopathic seizures. In one series, 94% of alcohol withdrawal seizures began in patients older than 30 years of age.[52] Electroencephalograms of patients with ethanol withdrawal seizures demonstrate diffuse slowing that normalizes after cessation of seizures. The situation is different in idiopathic seizure patients, whose baseline electroencephalograms are abnormal.[50, 52] The frequency of withdrawal seizures in patients with concomitant idiopathic epilepsy is increased relative to the frequency in those without epilepsy.[18] Three per cent to 12% of untreated withdrawal patients have seizures, with 50% occurring within 13 to 24 hours and 90% between 7 and 48 hours after cessation of drinking.[18, 52] Patients who have seizures that occur within 12 hours of the cessation of drinking often have other contributing factors, including prior ethanol tapering or head trauma.[18, 52] Fifty-four per cent of patients with alcohol withdrawal seizures have more than one seizure; all of their seizures occur within a few hours of each other.[18, 52] One third of patients who have convulsions develop DTs if not treated,[18, 52] whereas one third of those who have DTs will have had a seizure during the current withdrawal.[53] Seizures are unusual after the onset of DTs. Patients who have both withdrawal seizures and DTs experience the seizures first. The DTs begin during the postictal period in 25% of patients, and most episodes begin within 3 days of the seizures.[18] Seizures occur in 10% of patients with hallucinatory states.[18]

Although there is no question that ethanol withdrawal can cause seizures, some researchers have proposed that ethanol itself causes seizures. Ng and associates retrospectively evaluated 308 inner city patients with seizures of new onset. They noted that only 30% of the alcoholic patients had reduced or stopped their drinking during the 2 weeks before their seizures.[54] In an accompanying editorial, Simon[55] echoed these researchers' observations and noted that even patients reported in a series by Victor and colleagues[18, 52] had seizures outside the typical time frames. Ng and associates and Simon believe that seizures in the setting of ethanol use should be referred to as "ethanol-related seizures" because differentiating seizures due to direct ethanol toxicity from those due to withdrawal may be difficult.[54]

DTs is an infrequent but potentially fatal syndrome. It can occur in individuals who have drunk steadily for as few as 48 days[50] and develops in approximately 5% to 6% of patients with untreated ethanol withdrawal.[18, 56] It typically begins 3 to 5 days after ethanol intake has decreased but can start within 24 hours or as late as 14 days.[18] DTs is marked by severe autonomic hyperactivity (hypertension, tachycardia, fever, tremors, diaphoresis, dilated pupils) and significant disorientation. Excessive speech and motor activity may simply be responses to the altered perceptions and hallucinations that are generally present. Although it may be difficult to distract a patient in DTs who is fixed on some misperception, the patient also may be easily startled by the slightest environmental stimuli.[18] Patients may demonstrate brief moments of insight and reality if their attention can be obtained. Although 83% of patients recover within 3 days, 10% can have relapses, and the entire process for the latter group can last up to 31 days.[18] Survivors of DTs are typically amnesic for events during the delerium.[18]

Prior to the 1950s, the mortality associated with DTs was as high as 50% (average, 20% to 25%).[56] Victor and Adams' series conducted in the 1950s reported a 15% mortality rate.[18] The current mortality rate is still often quoted to be between 5% and 15% in treated patients.[51] However, mortality has not been well studied since the benzodiazepines became the mainstay of therapy. It is likely that mortality is actually quite low in patients with DTs who have received adequate doses of benzodiazepines and proper supportive care. The cause of death in those with DTs is most closely associated with the patients' underlying medical conditions. However, patients with DTs can also die abruptly and unexpectedly with coma and vascular collapse. On autopsy, these patients uniformly have extensive liver disease, pulmonary edema, or pneumonia.[53]

The historically high mortality associated with DTs has been linked to significant underlying illnesses, such as pancreatitis, subarachnoid hemorrhage, gastrointestinal hemorrhage, infection, and liver disease. Patients who died of DTs had hyperthermia, dehydration, seizure disorders, severe electrolyte abnormalities, and cardiac rhythm disturbances.[53, 56] Hyperthermia or seizures in patients with DTs are particularly associated with poor outcome. In one series, seizures occurred in 31% of those who died but in only 13% of those who survived. Even more significant was the finding that 51% of those with temperatures greater than 104°F died, whereas only 8% of those who survived had such high temperatures.[53]

MANAGEMENT OF WITHDRAWAL

The treatment goals for individuals with the withdrawal syndrome are to prevent the progression of withdrawal to seizures and DTs, allay symptoms, treat underlying disorders, and prepare for long-term rehabilitation. Both pharmacologic and nonpharmacologic approaches have been used. Benzodiazepines are the mainstay of pharmacologic therapy. Nonpharmacologic approaches include reassurance, reality orientation, frequent monitoring of signs and symptoms, personal attention, and general nursing care.[57] Although the effectiveness of nonpharmacologic therapy has been reasonable, this intervention has only been used in selected patients with mild withdrawal symptoms and without ethanol-related seizures or concomitant medical problems.[57, 58]

Patients in withdrawal should receive supplementary multivitamins, thiamine, glucose, and folate. Multivitamins are included because of the malnourishment resulting from the ingestion of "empty" ethanol calories. Thiamine can be given by the oral, intramuscular, or intravenous route. Wrenn and coworkers demonstrated the safety of intravenous thiamine administration in a prospective study of 989 consecutive patients.[59] Eleven of these patients had local irritation, and only 1 developed mild generalized pruritus. Dextrose should be routinely provided because hypoglycemia is common due to poor oral intake, glycogen depletion, and decreased carbohydrate production. Potassium, phosphate, and magnesium supplementation is also sometimes needed.

Patients with severe symptoms, altered mental status, or significant comorbid conditions should be hospitalized. Hayashida and associates demonstrated that outpatient management was effective, safe, and less costly in a population with mild to moderate symptoms, no comorbid disease, and access to daily follow-up.[60] Issues including homelessness and social support must also be considered when management decisions are being made.

Benzodiazepines are cross-tolerant with ethanol and are the drugs of choice in the treatment of withdrawal because of their sedative, anxiolytic, and anticonvulsive properties.[61] The efficacy of benzodiazepines was established initially in the classic papers of Sereny and Kalant[62] and Kaim and colleagues.[63] Sereny and Kalant performed a five-armed, randomized, double-blind study comparing two doses of chlordiazepoxide, two doses of promazine, and placebo. Chlordiazepoxide improved study parameters more consistently than did promazine; also, the latter agent was associated with an increased progression to DTs.[62] Kaim and colleagues compared chlordiazepoxide, chlorpromazine, hydroxyzine, thiamine, and placebo for the treatment of withdrawal. Chlordiazepoxide was clearly the best at preventing the progression of withdrawal.[63]

Benzodiazepine therapy should be started at the onset of withdrawal symptoms, regardless of the BEC. The amount of benzodiazepine required may be large. Although the exception, one patient received over 200 mg of diazepam intravenously initially and more than 1000 mg throughout the course of the withdrawal period. [19] Problems associated with the use of benzodiazepines include excessive sedation and minor cardiovascular and respiratory depression.[19]

Patients with severe symptoms of withdrawal, seizures, or DTs should be treated with intravenous benzodiazepine therapy titrated to effect. Intramuscular administration of lorazepam is appropriate if intravenous access initially cannot be obtained. Oral agents should not be used in significantly ill patients as titration is difficult and overdosing or underdosing may result.

The optimal choice of benzodiazepine for the treatment of withdrawal is debated, especially with regard to the desirability of drug characteristics such as half-life, lipid solubility, mechanism of metabolism, and the presence of active metabolites. Oversedation may be a problem, especially with oral dosing. Comparisons of the characteristics of benzodiazepines are shown in Table 34–5. Agents with long half-lives or active metabolites may accumulate and cause extended periods of sedation.[61] Excessive sedation should not occur with proper dosing. A lengthy drug effect may be advantageous as it provides more consistent activity at the GABA complex.[61] Severe liver dysfunction slows the metabolism of benzodiazepines eliminated by oxidation (e.g., diazepam and chlordiazepoxide) more than that of benzodiazepines eliminated by glucuronidation.[61] Patients with liver disease may become oversedated, especially with oral regimens, if dosing is not adjusted appropriately. The significance of lipophilicity is unclear. Although diazepam is more lipophilic and has a slightly more rapid onset of action than other drugs of this class, its redistribution also is faster, and this fact may affect its duration of action.[61] Cost is another consideration. The average wholesale price of oral generic tablets at our institution is $0.19 for 1 mg of lorazepam, $0.08 for 25 mg of chlordiazepoxide, and $0.07 for 5 mg of diazepam.

Two double-blind studies have compared oral diazepam with lorazepam. Miller and McCurdy used 5-day tapers and found no differences in symptom alleviation.[64] However, these authors recommended lorazepam over diazepam because of former's pharmacologic properties. They pointed out that diazepam's oxidative metabolism is decreased in the presence of cirrhosis and in chronic active hepatitis, as well as in the elderly, and that its half-life is increased by concomitant administration of disulfiram, cimetidine, or ethanol.[64] However, the blind 6-day study of Ritson and Chick comparing diazepam and lorazepam found that patients treated with lorazepam had significantly more anxiety and depression and performed worse with regard to some aspects of cognitive testing.[65] Solomon and colleagues compared chlordiazepoxide and lorazepam in a 5-day, double-blind trial that demonstrated them to be equally effective for treating withdrawal.[66] However, these authors recommended lorazepam because of theoretic concerns about the decreased capacity for oxidative metabolism of chlordiazepoxide in the alcoholic patient.[66] Massman and Tipton recommended oxazepam, which is detoxified by glucuronidation, as the agent of choice in the elderly or in those with liver disease.[67] None of these studies actually provided data supporting their recommendations for the use of a benzodiazepine metabolized primarily by glucuronidation. A review of 29 randomized controlled trials comparing various medications for the management of withdrawal demonstrated only that benzodiazepines were superior to placebo. Significant methodologic flaws in the studies prevented the drawing of other conclusions.[68]

Benzodiazepines can be dosed in various ways. One approach is the "loading dose technique," in which 20 mg of diazepam is given orally every 1 to 2 hours

Table 34–5. Comparison of Benzodiazepines Used for the Treatment of Withdrawal

Characteristic	Chlordiazepoxide	Diazepam	Lorazepam	Oxazepam
Routes	IV, IM*, PO	IV, IM*, PO	IV, IM, PO	PO
Initial dosing regimen	15–50 mg t.i.d/q.i.d.	5–20 mg t.i.d./q.i.d.	1–2 mg b.i.d./q.i.d.	15–30 mg t.i.d./q.i.d.
Liver metabolism	Oxidation	Oxidation	Glucuronidation	Glucuronidation
Active metabolites	Yes	Yes	No	No
Half-life (h)†	(Long) Range: 6–30 Average: 10	(Long) Range: 20–70 Average: 33	(Intermediate) Range: 5–25 Average: 15	(Intermediate) Range: 5–20 Average: 8
Cost (average generic wholesale price)	PO: $0.08 per 25-mg tab	PO: $0.07 per 5-mg tab Parenteral: $10.05 per 5 mg	PO: $0.19 per 1-mg tab Parenteral: $12.01 per 2 mg	PO: $0.35 per 15-mg tab

IM, intramuscular; IV, intravenous; PO, oral; tab, tablet.
*IM absorption is erratic, and thus this route of delivery should be avoided if possible. Inject in the deltoid muscle if administration must be IM.
†Chlordiazepoxide's and diazepam's active metabolites have half-lives from 25 to 100 h.

until the patient experiences symptom improvement or sedation. With this approach, patients on average received four doses over 12 hours, and thereafter were administered no further medications. The long half-lives of diazepam and its major active metabolite desmethyldiazepam (nordiazepam) facilitate this approach because therapeutic levels persist beyond 72 hours.[61] A pharmacokinetic study of the diazepam loading dose technique revealed that some patients did not reach T_{max} until 90 minutes after administration. The authors recommended that the intervals for dosing be at least 90 minutes in duration.[69]

The most commonly used benzodiazepine protocol in the United States is a fixed-dose, 3-day taper with chlordiazepoxide.[70] A slower taper should be considered when the glucuronidated benzodiazepines lorazepam and oxazepam are used.[19] Tapering should be carried out with decreases is dose and not with increases in the interval between doses.[19] Some recommend that tapering regimens should be individualized on the basis of the patient's symptoms.[70]

A randomized, double-blind study compared symptom-triggered versus fixed dose regimens of chlordiazepoxide in ethanol withdrawal patients. The symptom-triggered approach decreased both the benzodiazepine requirements and duration of treatment.[70] Symptom-triggered management has only been studied in patients with mild withdrawal and not in those who are more seriously ill or have had ethanol-related seizures.[67, 70, 71] The symptom-triggered approach may induce drug-seeking behavior, lead to undertreatment patients, and result in "kindling" sensitization.[71] The antipsychotic agents have no demonstrated role in the management of withdrawal. The use of phenothiazines should be avoided because these drugs lower the seizure threshold, modify the body's ability to regulate hyperthermia, and can produce hypotension.[19] The butyrophenones also have no demonstrated benefit over currently used therapies.

Therapy with sympatholytic agents such as the centrally acting α_2-agonists and β-blockers assists in the management of withdrawal. These agents' primary benefit is attenuation of hyperadrenergic symptoms such as tremor, tachycardia, and hypertension without an effect on normal cognitive function.[72, 73] However, because these drugs are usually used in conjunction with other agents, the problems associated with the use of multiple drugs potentially exist. These agents also do not prevent seizures or progression to DTs.[73] In seriously ill patients, the reduction of sympathetic symptoms has been shown to mask the progression to DTs or the worsening of associated medical problems.[72, 73] The use of β-blockers may also be contraindicated because of pre-existing medical problems, including hypoglycemia, cardiomyopathy, and chronic obstructive pulmonary disease.[72]

The use of magnesium in withdrawal has been proposed because many alcoholics are hypomagnesemic. However, no benefit of magnesium has been demonstrated. Possible indications include cardiac dysrhythmias or seizures that may occur secondary to hypomagnesemia.[73]

Patients with alcohol-related seizures should be treated with benzodiazepines. Phenytoin has no role in their management. Controlled series have failed to demonstrate phenytoin's superiority over placebo in patients without an underlying seizure disorder who have had alcohol-related seizures.[73] The efficacies of other anticonvulsants, including valproic acid, carbamazepine, and primidone, have either not been studied or demonstrated.[73] The inability to rapidly load these agents also precludes their use in the acute care setting.

MEDICATION INTERACTIONS

Ethanol has the potential to interact with many drugs because of its complex pharmacologic characteristics (Table 34–6). Because of the cross-tolorance between ethanol and barbiturates, alcohol-dependent individuals who are abstaining from ethanol require relatively large doses of barbiturates for induction of anesthesia.[74] Conversely, barbiturate and benzodiazepine metabolism is inhibited in actively drinking individuals because ethanol already occupies the microsomal P-450 oxidizing system. Ethanol-associated central nervous system sedation is additive to that produced by the benzodiazepines and other sedative-hypnotics such as chloral hydrate, ethylchlorvinyl, meprobamate, methaqualone, and glutethimide.[74] Sedation associated with phenothiazines, antihistamines, and narcotics also is enhanced by ethanol.[75] The long-term use of β-blockers by alcoholics may mask sympathomimetic symptoms associated with hypoglycemia or early withdrawal.[75] The significance of the interaction between the $histamine_2$ antagonists and ethanol is debated. All $histamine_2$ blockers except famotidine inhibit gastric ADH and have been associated with increased BECs.[76]

Disulfiram (Antabuse) irreversibly inhibits acetaldehyde dehydrogenase activity. If ethanol is ingested after pretreatment with disulfiram, a 5- to 10-fold increase in acetaldehyde level develops within 15 minutes. Patients experience flushing and throbbing pains of the head and neck secondary to vasodilatation. In addition, abdominal cramps, nausea, vomiting, chest pain, weakness, dizziness, dyspnea, hyperventilation, tachycardia, diaphoresis, and hypotension also occur.[48, 74, 75] Symptoms last from 30 minutes to several hours. This reaction develops even up to 2 weeks after the disulfiram exposure.[75] Toxicity can be precipitated by as little as 7 mL of ethanol.[48] Patients using disulfiram should be made aware of the presence of ethanol in over-the-counter products so that they can prevent unexpected reactions. Diethyldithiocarbamate, the major metabolite of disulfiram, chelates metals and thus inactivates metalloenzymes, including ADH and dopamine β-hydroxylase. The increased BECs sometimes associated with disulfiram therapy have been attributed to ADH suppression. The sometimes intractable hypotension

Table 34–6. Medications That Interact with Ethanol

Medications	Mechanism of Interaction	Final Effect
Acetaminophen Anesthetics Barbiturates Benzodiazepines Isoniazid Phenytoin Tolbutamide Warfarin	Chronic ethanol use enhances MEOS activity if (1) alcoholic is currently abstaining from drinking (2) alcoholic is currently drinking alcohol	Fulminant hepatic failure ↓ in medication levels ↑ in medication levels
Cimetidine Ranitidine	Inhibits gastric ADH, increasing ethanol bioavailability	↑ in blood ethanol concentration
Barbiturates Benzodiazepines Chloral hydrate Meprobamate	Effects are synergistic with those of ethanol	↑ in sedation ↑ in respiratory depression
Allopurinol Cephalosporins Chloramphenicol Griseofulvin Metronidazole Quinacrine Sulfonylurea oral hypoglycemics	Synergistic with the ↑ in serum uric acid levels secondary to ethanol Disulfiram-like reaction with inhibition of acetaldehyde dehydrogenase	↑ in gouty arthritis Acetaldehyde syndrome

MEOS, microsomal ethanol-oxidizing system; ADH, alcohol dehydrogenase.

associated with disulfiram reactions may be secondary to dopamine β-hydroxylase inhibition, which causes a decrease in nerve terminal norepinephrine production.[48] Long-term users of disulfiram have an increased incidence of depression, which may be secondary to altered dopamine metabolism due to suppression of central nervous system dopamine β-hydroxylase.[74] Although other medications have been associated with disulfiram-like reactions (see Table 34–6), their effects generally are inconsistent and mild.[74] Management of patients with disulfiram reactions generally is supportive. However, hypotension secondary to vomiting and vasodilation can be severe, and aggressive volume resuscitation may be needed. If vasopressor support is indicated, direct α-adrenergic agonists such as norepinephrine should be used because dopamine's effect is blocked by disulfiram's inhibition of dopamine β-hydroxylase. Antiemetics should be considered if vomiting is present.

Disulfiram itself generally is safe, but it can produce toxic reactions, even without coingestion of ethanol. Complications include allergic dermatitis, urticaria, fatigue, restlessness, tremor, headache, dizziness, a garlic-like or metallic taste in the mouth, and gastrointestinal discomfort. More serious but rare complications include peripheral neuropathies, hepatitis, and psychosis.[48]

Chronic ethanol use in combination with acetaminophen ingestion has been associated with a syndrome of fulminant hepatic failure and death (unless orthotopic liver transplantation is performed). Unlike classic acetaminophen hepatotoxicity, which is associated with acute single ingestions of greater than 150 mg/kg, cases of ethanol-acetaminophen–related hepatic injury have typically occurred in the context of long-term, supratherapeutic ingestions of acetaminophen (greater than 4 g/d). These cases of ethanol-acetaminophen–related hepatic failure are often inadvertent (i.e., not associated with attempts at suicide). Also, because ethanol alone is associated with hepatic injury, the diagnosis of combined toxicity is often overlooked. The mechanism of this synergistic hepatotoxicity is thought to be induction of cytochrome CYP2E1 by ethanol, which results in the increased formation of acetaminophen's hepatotoxic metabolite, *N*-acetylbenzoquinonimene. Further discussion of this interaction in found in Chapter 49.

CHILDREN AND THE ELDERLY

The metabolism of ethanol in the elderly is not significantly different from that in younger adults. However, age-related increases in adipose tissue and decreases in lean body mass result in a reduction in total-body water. This leads to higher BECs than those obtained by younger individuals who ingest equal amounts of ethanol.[77] Cognitive impairment and dementia also may be worsened by chronic ethanol use.[77] In addition, ethanol interacts with many medications commonly used by the elderly, including central nervous system depressants, analgesics, anticoagulants, and antidiabetic agents.[77]

Childhood exposure to ethanol is not unusual and represents approximately 3% of contacts with poison control centers.[2] Fortunately, reports of pediatric deaths due to ethanol consumption alone are rare. Unlike most childhood toxic exposures, the victims are often older (76% are older than 3 years of age).[2] Approximately 75% of the exposures reported to poison control centers involve perfumes, colognes, and after-shaves, whereas alcoholic beverages and mouthwashes represent 15% and 7% of the ingestions, respectively. Most emergency department visits and hospital admissions are associated with the drinking of alcoholic beverages.[2] Nonaccidental exposure must always be considered, and the appropriate child protection agencies must be contacted if this concern exists. Although the pharmacokinetics of ethanol metabolism are similar in children and adults, children younger than 13 years of age appear to metabolize ethanol more quickly than do nonalcoholic adults.[2] Children have more severe effects at lower BECs than do adults, and fatal complications have been reported when BECs were less than 50 mg%.[2] Children commonly present with marked sleepiness or coma and may also have vomiting, ataxia, and seizures.[2] Ethanol-induced hypoglycemia occurs more frequently in children than in adults and has occurred with a BEC level as low 20 to 30 mg%.[2] Hypoglycemia is usually associated with the ingestion of alcoholic beverages but does not appear to be dose dependent.[2] Seizures may occur and are often associated with hypoglycemia.[2] The pathogenesis of hypoglycemia in children compared with that in adults is not fully understood, but children's smaller glycogen stores may be a contributing factor.[2]

The clinician can estimate the potential BEC, using the relationship among the volume of distribution (Vd), the specific gravity of ethanol (SG), and the volume ingested (A):

$$\text{BEC (in mg/dL)} = \frac{\text{A (in mL)} \times \text{\%EtOH} \times \text{SG (0.80 g/mL)}}{V_d\,\text{(0.6 L/kg)} \times \text{Body weight (in kg)}}$$

For example, a concerned individual calls because a 20-kg toddler has ingested a half-ounce (15-mL) shot glass of 100-proof (50% ethanol) whiskey. The numerator determines the absolute amount of ethanol ingested (15 mL × 0.50 × 0.80 g/mL) and is divided by the volume in which it is distributed (0.6 L/kg × 20 kg). After correction for the units used, the expected BEC is 50 mg%. This is a potentially dangerous level in such a young child, and immediate evaluation in an emergency department is appropriate. Conversely, the formula can be rearranged to determine the amount ingested once the BEC has been calculated. This information may be used for verification of the history when the possibility of a nonaccidental exposure is being considered.

SUMMARY

Ethanol is a clear and rapidly absorbed hydrocarbon found in alcoholic beverages and in many household products. Its intoxicating effects include incoordination and alteration of mental status, and it can cause respiratory paralysis and death when it is ingested at very high concentrations. Chronic ethanol use is associated with many medical problems, including osteoporosis, electrolyte abnormalities, polyneuropathy, endocrine disorders, dementia, alcoholic heart disease, cardiac dysrhythmias, liver dysfunction, and suppression of all hematopoietic elements. Various vitamin deficiency disorders also are associated with chronic ethanol ingestion, including WE and KP. The metabolism of ethanol involves multiple biochemical pathways, including the cytochrome P-450–dependent MEOS. Ethanol withdrawal is common among chronic drinkers, and symptoms can range from mild (tremor, tachycardia, and restlessness) to severe (seizures and DTs). Treatment with benzodiazepines is the mainstay of therapy for all patients with symptoms of withdrawal.[78] The pathophysiology of ethanol withdrawal is complex and involves GABA receptors, various ion channels, and the central adrenergic system. Ethanol's complex metabolism results in many potential drug interactions, particularly in the chronic abuser whose MEOS has been induced. The elderly and children are more likely to experience ethanol's effects than are others.

References

1. Petroni NC, Cardoni AA: Alcohol content of liquid medicinals. Drug Ther *8*:72–93, 1978.
2. Vogel C, Caraccio T, Mofenson H, et al: Alcohol intoxication in young children. J Toxicol Clin Toxicol *33*:25–33, 1995.
3. Holt S, Stewart MJ, Adam RD, et al: Alcohol absorption, gastric emptying and a breathalyser. Br J Clin Pharmacol *9*:205–208, 1980.
4. Jones AW, Jonsson KA, Neri A: Peak blood-ethanol concentration and the time of its occurrence after rapid drinking on an empty stomach. J Forensic Sci *36*:376–385, 1991.
5. Minocha A, Herold DA, Barth JT, et al: Activated charcoal in oral ethanol absorption: Lack of effect in humans. J Toxicol Clin Toxicol *24*:225–234, 1986.
6. Crabb DW, Bosron WF, Li TK: Ethanol metabolism. Pharmacol Ther *34*:59–73, 1987.
7. Bogusz M, Pach J, Stasko W: Comparative studies on the rate of ethanol elimination in acute poisoning and in controlled conditions. J Forensic Sci *22*:446–451, 1976.
8. Li TK: Genetic variability of enzymes of alcohol metabolism in human beings. Ann Emerg Med *15*:997–1004, 1986.
9. Lieber CS: Seminars in medicine of the Beth Israel Hospital, Boston: Medical disorders of alcoholism. N Engl J Med *333*:1058–1065, 1995.
10. Caballeria J: First-pass metabolism of ethanol: Its role as a determinant of blood alcohol levels after drinking. Hepatogastroenterology *39*(Suppl I):62–66, 1992.
11. Panes J, Soler X, Pares A, et al: Influence of liver disease on hepatic alcohol and aldehyde dehydrogenases. Gastroenterology *97*:708–714, 1989.
12. Panes J, Caballeria J, Guitart R, et al: Determinants of ethanol and acetaldehyde metabolism in chronic alcoholics. Alcohol Clin Exp Res *17*:48–53, 1992.
13. Lieber CS: Hepatic and metabolic effects of ethanol: Pathogenesis and prevention. Ann Intern Med *26*:325–330, 1994.
14. Gershman H, Steeper J: Rate of clearance of ethanol from the blood of intoxicated patients in the emergency department. J Emerg Med *9*:307–311, 1991.
15. O'Neill S, Tipton KF, Prichard JS, et al: Survival after high blood alcohol levels. Arch Intern Med *144*:641–642, 1984.
16. Bailey DN: Comprehensive toxicology screening: The frequency of finding other drugs in addition to ethanol. J Toxicol Clin Toxicol *22*:463–471, 1984.
17. Fantus RJ, Zautcke JL, Hickey PA, et al: Driving under the influence—A level-I trauma center's experience. J Trauma *31*:1517–1520, 1991.
18. Victor M, Adams RD: The Effect of Alcohol on the Nervous System. Baltimore, Williams & Wilkins, 1953.
19. Adinoff B, Bone GHA, Linnoila M: Acute ethanol poisoning and the ethanol withdrawal syndrome. Med Toxicol *3*:172–196, 1988.

20. Charness ME, Simon RP, Greenberg DA: Ethanol and the nervous system. N Engl J Med *321*:442–454, 1989.
21. Diamond I, Messing RO: Neurologic effects of alcoholism. West J Med *161*:279–287, 1994.
22. Bittencourt P, Wade P, Richens A, et al: Blood alcohol and eye movements. Lancet *2*:981, 1980.
23. Coffman NB, Fernandes JJ: Blood ethanol testing. J Am Osteopath Assoc *91*:781–785, 1991.
24. Vinson DC, Menezes M: Admission alcohol level: A predictor of the course of alcohol withdrawal. J Fam Pract *33*:161–167, 1991.
25. McIvor RA, Cosbey SH: Effect of using alcoholic and non-alcoholic skin cleaning swabs when sampling blood for alcohol estimation using gas chromatography. Br J Clin Pharmacol *44*:235–236, 1990.
26. Gibb K: Serum alcohol levels, toxicology screens, and use of the breath alcohol analyzer. Ann Emerg Med *15*:349–353, 1986.
27. Wilson A, Sitar DS, Molloy WD, et al: Effect of age and chronic obstructive pulmonary disease on the breathalyzer estimation of blood alcohol level. Alcohol Clin Exp Res *11*:440–443, 1987.
28. Nuotto E, Mattila MJ, Seppala T, et al: Coffee and caffeine and alcohol effects on psychomotor function. Clin Pharmacol Ther *31*:68–76, 1982.
29. Nuotto E, Palva ES, Lahdenranta U: Naloxone fails to counteract heavy alcohol intoxication. Lancet *2*:167, 1983.
30. Brown SS, Forrest JAH, Roscoe P: A controlled trial of fructose in the treatment of acute alcoholic intoxication. Lancet *2*:898–899, 1972.
31. Fluckiger A, Hartmann D, Leishman B, et al: Lack of effect of the benzodiazepine antagonist flumazenil (Ro 15-1788) on the performance of healthy subjects during experimentally induced ethanol intoxication. Eur J Clin Pharmacol *34*:273–276, 1988.
32. Adler RA: Clinically important effects of alcohol on endocrine function. J Clin Endocrinol Metab *74*:957–960, 1992.
33. Petroianu A, Barquete J, de Almeida Plentz EG, et al: Acute effects of alcohol ingestion on the human serum concentrations of calcium and magnesium. J Int Med Res *19*:410–413, 1991.
34. Halperin ML, Hammeke M, Josse RG, et al: Metabolic acidosis in the alcoholic: A pathophysiologic approach. Metabolism *32*:308–315, 1983.
35. Wilson JD, Madison LL: Deficiency of thiamine (beriberi), pyridoxine, and riboflavin. *In* Isselbacher KJ, et al (eds): Harrison's Principles of Internal Medicine. 9th ed. New York, McGraw-Hill Book Co., pp 425–429, 1980.
36. Ragland G: Electrolyte abnormalities in the alcoholic patient. Emerg Med Clin North Am *8*:761–773, 1990.
37. Duffens K, Marx J: Alcoholic ketoacidosis: A review. J Emerg Med *5*:399–406, 1987.
38. Reuler JB, Girard DE, Cooney TG: Current concepts: Wernicke's encephalopathy. N Engl J Med *312*:1035–1039, 1985.
39. Naik P, Lawton J: Pharmacological management of alcohol withdrawal. Br J Hosp Med *50*:265–269, 1993.
40. Victor M, Adams RD, Collins GH: The Wernicke-Korsakoff Syndrome. Philadelphia, F.A. Davis Co., 1971.
41. Piano MR, Schwertz DW: Alcoholic heart disease: A review. Heart Lung *23*:3–17, 1994.
42. Lang RM, Borow KM, Neumann A, et al: Adverse cardiac effects of acute alcohol ingestion in young adults. Ann Intern Med *102*:742–747, 1985.
43. Ahlawat SK, Siwach SB: Alcohol and coronary artery disease. Int J Cardiol *44*:157–162, 1994.
44. Ettinger PO, Wu CF, DeLa Cruz C, et al: Arrhythmias and the "holiday heart": Alcohol-associated cardiac rhythm disorders. Am Heart J *95*:555–562, 1978.
45. Lowenstein SR, Gabow PA, Cramer J, et al: The role of alcohol in new-onset atrial fibrillation. Arch Intern Med *143*:1882–1885, 1983.
46. Girard DE, Kumar KL, McAfee JH: Hematologic effects of acute and chronic alcohol abuse. Hematol Oncol Clin North Am *1*:321–334, 1987.
47. MacGregor RR: Alcohol and immune defense. JAMA *256*:1474–1478, 1986.
48. Gilman AG, Rall TW, Nies AS, et al: The Pharmacological Basis of Therapeutics. 8th ed. New York, Pergamon Press, 1990.
49. Linnoila M, Mefford I, Nutt D, et al: Alcohol withdrawal and noradrenergic function. Ann Intern Med *107*:875–889, 1987.
50. Isbell H, Fraser HF, Wikler A, et al: An experimental study of the etiology of "rum fits" and delirium tremens. Q J Stud Alcohol *16*:1–33, 1953.
51. Lerner WD, Fallon HJ: The alcohol withdrawal syndrome. N Engl J Med *313*:951–952, 1985.
52. Victor M, Brausch C: The role of abstinence in the genesis of alcoholic epilepsy. Epilepsia *8*:1–20, 1967.
53. Tavel ME, Davidson W, Batterton TD: A critical analysis of mortality associated with delirium tremens. Am J Med Sci *242*:58–69, 1961.
54. Ng SKC, Hauser WA, Brust JCM, et al: Alcohol consumption and withdrawal in new-onset seizures. N Engl J Med *319*:666–673, 1988.
55. Simon RP: Alcohol and seizures. N Engl J Med *319*:715–716, 1988.
56. Moore M, Gray MG: Delirium tremens: A study of cases at the Boston City Hospital, 1915–1936. N Engl J Med *220*:953–956, 1939.
57. Sellers EM, Naranjo CA: New strategies for the treatment of alcohol withdrawal. Psychopharmacol Bull *22*:88–92, 1986.
58. Sullivan JT, Swift RM, Lewis DC: Benzodiazepine requirements during alcohol withdrawal syndrome: Clinical implications of using a standardized withdrawal scale. J Clin Psychopharmacol *11*:291–295, 1991.
59. Wrenn KD, Murphy F, Slovis CM, et al: A toxicity study of parenteral thiamine hydrochloride. Ann Emerg Med *18*:867–870, 1989.
60. Hayashida M, Alterman AI, McLellan AT, et al: Comparative effectiveness and costs of inpatient and outpatient detoxification of patients with mild-to-moderate alcohol withdrawal syndrome. N Engl J Med *320*:358–365, 1989.
61. Bird RD, Makela EH: Alcohol withdrawal: What is the benzodiazepine of choice? Ann Pharmacother *28*:67–71, 1994.
62. Sereny G, Kalant H: Comparative clinical evaluation of chlordiazepoxide and promazine in treatment of alcohol-withdrawal syndrome. BMJ *1*:92–97, 1965.
63. Kaim SC, Klett CJ, Rothfeld B: Treatment of the acute alcohol withdrawal state: A comparison of four drugs. Am J Psychiatry *125*:1640–1646, 1969.
64. Miller WC, McCurdy L: A double-blind comparison of the efficacy and safety of lorazepam and diazepam in the treatment of the acute alcohol withdrawal syndrome. Clin Ther *6*:364–371, 1984.
65. Ritson B, Chick J: Comparison of two benzodiazepines in the treatment of alcohol withdrawal: Effects on symptoms and cognitive recovery. Drug Alcohol Depend *18*:329–334, 1986.
66. Solomon J, Rouck LA, Koepke HH: Double-blind comparison of lorazepam and chlordiazepoxide in the treatment of the acute alcohol abstinence syndrome. Clin Ther *6*:52–58, 1983.
67. Massman JE, Tipton DM: Signs and symptoms assessment: A guide for the treatment of the alcohol withdrawal syndrome. J Psychoactive Drugs *20*:443–444, 1988.
68. Moskowitz G, Chalmers TC, Sacks HS, et al: Deficiencies of clinical trials of alcohol withdrawal. Alcohol Clin Exp Res *7*:42–46, 1983.
69. Heinala P, Piepponen T, Heikkinen H: Diazepam loading in alcohol withdrawal: Clinical pharmacokinetics. Int J Clin Pharmacol Ther *28*:211–217, 1990.
70. Saitz R, Mayo-Smith MF, Roberts MS, et al: Individualized treatment for alcohol withdrawal: A randomized double-blind controlled trial. JAMA *272*:519–523, 1994.
71. Sullivan JT: Individualized treatment of alcohol withdrawal. JAMA *273*:183–184, 1995.
72. Baumgartner GR, Rowen RC: Transdermal clonidine versus chlordiazepoxide in alcohol withdrawal: A randomized, controlled clinical trial. South Med J *84*:312–321, 1991.
73. Liskow BI, Goodwin DW: Pharmacological treatment of alcohol intoxication, withdrawal and dependence: A critical review. J Stud Alcohol *48*:356–370, 1987.
74. Seizas FA: Alcohol and its drug interactions. Ann Intern Med *83*:86–91, 1975.

75. Interactions of drugs with alcohol. Med Lett Drugs Ther *23*:33–36, 1981.
76. Gugler R: H_2-Antagonists and alcohol: Do they interact? Drug Saf *10*:271–280, 1994.
77. Dufour MC, Archer L, Gordis E: Alcohol and the elderly. Clin Geriatr Med *8*:127–141, 1992.
78. Rosenbloom A: Emerging treatment options in the alcohol withdrawal syndrome. J Clin Psychiatry *49*:28–31, 1988.

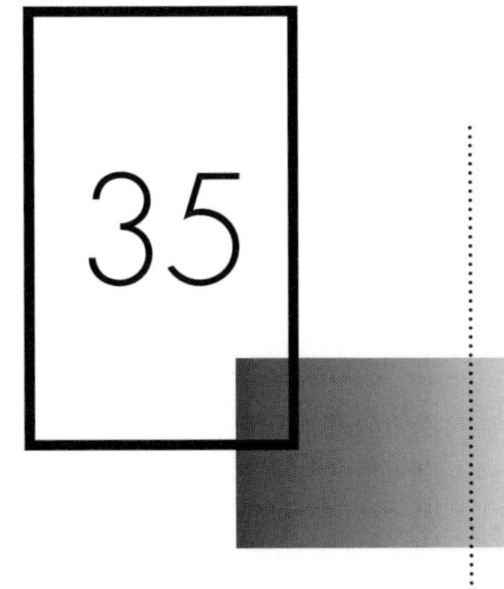

35 Methanol, Isopropyl Alcohol, Higher Alcohols, Ethylene Glycol, Cellosolves, Acetone, and Oxalate

JAMES F. WINCHESTER, MD

This chapter deals with substances that produce metabolic complications, particularly acidosis. Poisoning by several of these substances requires early intervention, in the case of methanol to prevent ocular and central nervous system (CNS) toxicity and in the case of ethylene glycol to prevent renal failure.

METHANOL

Methanol (methyl alcohol, wood spirits) is a widely used commercial, industrial, and marine solvent and paint remover as well as a solvent in paints, varnishes, shellacs, and photocopying fluid. It may be used alone as an antifreeze fluid (starting concentration 95%) and is commonly used in windshield-washing fluids (starting concentration 35% to 95%).[1] In addition, it can be formulated as a solid canned fuel (4%), along with ethanol and soap, or as a liquid fuel for heating small engines used in various hobbies.[2] In the United Kingdom, methanol is adulterated with a purple dye to distinguish it from ethanol. However, its high industrial production and its use in laboratories, schools, and industrial processes account for the fact that large volumes may be obtained and contribute to epidemic outbreaks of methanol poisoning (Table 35–1).[3]

Methanol is widely used in industry as a solvent and an adulterant to make ethyl alcohol unfit to drink when the latter is used for cleaning purposes. Because methanol can be purchased tax free and is considerably less expensive than normal alcoholic beverages, it is not surprising that chronic alcoholics may consume such compounds. Methanol has no therapeutic properties and is considered to be only a toxicant. Six per cent of all cases of blindness in the

Table 35–1. United States Production of Solvents (Millions of Pounds)*

	1981	1986	1991
Ethylene glycol	4143	4771	4930
Methanol	8577	7205	8654
Isopropyl alcohol	1669	1301	8654

*Data for 3 selected years in the past decade, Chem Eng News *70*:32, 1993.[3]

United States Armed Forces in World War II were caused by methanol ingestion. The fatal dose is said to be between 60 and 240 mL,[2] or 15 to 30 mL of a 40% solution. However, with aggressive treatment, survival may be achieved despite much higher intake.

Toxicology and Pharmacology

Although toxicity has been reported after inhalation or skin absorption,[4–6] the main route of toxicity is ingestion. Methyl alcohol is readily absorbed from the gastrointestinal (GI) tract after ingestion and reaches peak blood levels in 30 to 90 minutes. It is widely distributed in body tissues, with a distribution of 0.6 to 0.7 L/kg.[7–10] A small amount of methanol is found in the expired breath of normal persons, possibly because of endogenous metabolic production. In animals, most infused methanol is excreted by the respiratory tract (30% of the ingested dose), but this is not the prime mode of excretion in humans. The kidneys in untreated patients excrete less than 5% of unchanged methanol, and the remaining methanol (90% to 95%) is excreted by hepatic biotransformation to other compounds. The majority of methanol, therefore, is converted to breakdown products, principally in the liver, by the metalloenzyme alcohol dehydrogenase and produces formaldehyde. Thereafter, formaldehyde is converted to formate by such enzyme systems as aldehyde dehydrogenase, xanthine oxidase, glyceraldehyde-3-phosphate hydrogenase, catalases, peroxidase, aldehyde oxidase, and a glutathione-dependent formaldehyde dehydrogenase.[11] The elimination half-life of methanol is between 14 and 20 hours (mild intoxication) and 24 and 30 hours (severe intoxication) in untreated patients, and this is prolonged to 30 to 35 hours by the administration of ethanol.

Unlike poisoning by ingestion of formaldehyde, which does not produce retinal damage, local production of formaldehyde from methanol in the retina is believed to be responsible principally for optic papillitis and retinal edema with subsequent blindness,[12] although *continuous* infusion of formate may produce optic nerve edema.[13] The ability to oxidize methanol to formic acid and to oxidize formic acid varies considerably with different animal species. For instance, rabbits excrete only 1% of methanol as urinary formic acid, compared with 20% for dogs; the oxidation capabilities of humans are intermediate.[13] Oxidation of methanol, like that of ethanol, proceeds independently of the blood concentration but at a rate only one seventh that of ethanol. Complete oxidation and excretion of methanol thus requires several days. Although oxidation is achieved mainly within the liver, it also occurs within the kidneys.[13] The enzyme alcohol dehydrogenase, the principal enzyme involved in oxidation of ethanol, is also used in the oxidation of methanol. Ethanol is preferentially metabolized by this enzyme, however, and administration of ethanol delays methanol's clinical and biochemical effects. It is for this reason that ethyl alcohol is used clinically to slow down the metabolic transformation of methanol to the toxic product (formic acid), itself the product of oxidation. The metabolic pathways for the breakdown of methanol are shown in Figure 35-1.

Clinical Manifestations of Methanol Intoxication

Symptoms of methanol poisoning may be delayed for 12 to 36 hours, and this latent period is thought to result from the delayed metabolism of methanol to the principal toxic product, formic acid. The manifestations are as follows: a minor CNS intoxication similar to that of ethyl alcohol intoxication, a major acidosis due to the production of formic acid and lactic acidosis, and the most serious toxicity to the retinal cells by the local production of formaldehyde in the retina and optic disk,[12] enhanced by acidosis. In animals (monkeys and rats), it has been demonstrated that folate deficiency seems to promote the acidosis, and in animals folic or folinic acid enhances the breakdown of formic acid to carbon dioxide and water and may prevent ocular toxicity.[12, 14, 15] The fatal human dose is between 60 and 240 mL, although survival toward the upper end of this range has been reported. As little as 10 mL has been con-

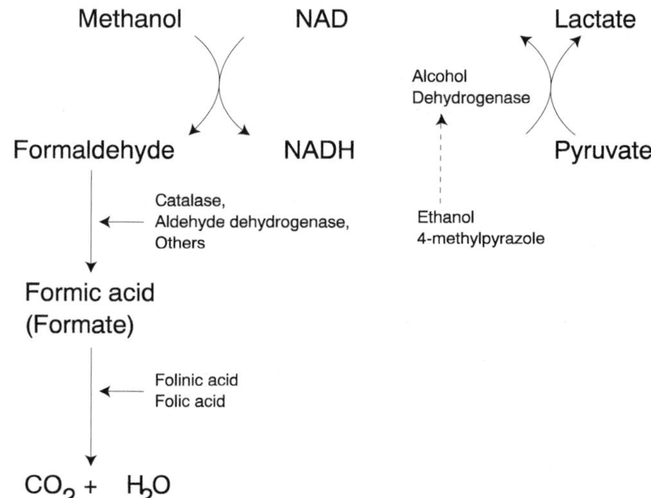

Figure 35–1. Metabolic degradation of methanol and treatment of toxicity. *Solid arrow,* promotes metabolic process; *broken arrow,* inhibits metabolic process.

sidered toxic; although death may be prompt, it is usually delayed for several days. Even before hemodialysis was used as specific therapy for this intoxication, *institution of therapy before visual disturbances occurred appeared to improve the prognosis.*[8] As mentioned, methanol may be consumed along with ethyl alcohol, but even when it is consumed alone, inebriation and subsequent drowsiness are noticed to be mild and somewhat transient.

The period of inebriation is characteristically followed by an asymptomatic period; then within 6 to 30 hours (which may be protracted if ethanol was also ingested) the characteristic symptoms and signs occur (Table 35–2). The major symptoms and signs of methanol poisoning consist of vertigo, vomiting, severe abdominal pain, diarrhea, back pain, dyspnea, motor restlessness, cold and clammy extremities, blurred vision, and hyperemia of the optic disk with occasional blindness. Blood pressure is usually well maintained, but severely ill patients may have a slow pulse; this confers a grave prognosis. Because the visual disturbance can proceed to blindness, pupillary light reactions may be absent. In very severe cases, restlessness and delirium may be marked features, and in the presence of severe acidosis, Kussmaul's respiration may or may not be noted. Death may be rapid or may occur many hours after the onset of coma. One modus of death is inspiratory apnea, terminal opisthotonos, and convulsions.[8] Another clinical manifestation is the finding of pancreatitis on autopsy of patients with severe cases of methanol poisoning,[16] a feature that might explain the severe abdominal pains accompanying acute methanol poisoning (hyperamylasemia [salivary] has been observed,[10] as has myoglobinuric acute renal failure). In the latter regard, a diagnosis of renal failure based on serum creatinine level alone may be false, because methanol interferes with creatinine determination.[17] Permanent optic nerve damage occurs in 25% of poisoned individuals. Other permanent neurologic features include parkinsonism and necrosis of the putamen, observed either at autopsy or on computed tomography of the brain.[18] Reversible cardiac failure has also been reported.[19]

Table 35–2. Methanol Intoxication

Major Symptoms/Signs	Laboratory Features
Early	
Inebriation Drowsiness	May have detectable serum ethanol and methanol levels
Delayed (6–30 h)	
Vomiting, vertigo	Systemic acidosis with low bicarbonate*
Upper abdominal pain (± pancreatitis)	Formic acidemia
Dyspnea	Lactic acidemia*
Acidosis (± Kussmaul's respiration)	↑ Hematocrit*
Blurred vision	↑ Anion gap
Hyperemia of optic disk	↑ Mean corpuscular volume*
Blindness	↑ Blood glucose
Dilated pupils → absent light reflex	↑ Serum amylase ↑ Osmolal gap
Urinary formaldehyde smell	Methanol > 30 mg/dL†

*More severe abnormalities correlate with poor outcome.
†Hemodialysis should be instituted at blood methanol concentrations > 50 mg/dL.

Factors in the Production of Acidosis

It has long been believed that formic acid was the prime metabolite responsible for the profound metabolic acidosis in methanol poisoning. Formic acid production, however, accounts for only half the anion gap in this condition. Trapping of nicotinamide-adenine dinucleotide in its reduced form in the liver from the oxidation of methanol to formic acid allows formate accumulation, which in turn inhibits cytochrome oxidase and leads to lactic acidosis.[20] McMartin and associates found that the increased level of blood formate correlated best with the anion gap increase.[21] On the other hand, Smith and co-workers found no such correlation in a single patient intoxicated with methanol.[22] Mild ketonuria may occasionally be observed. Swartz and colleagues[23] showed that acidosis (and particularly the low serum bicarbonate concentration) correlated more closely with the blood methanol level as well as with the GI and CNS symptoms. In addition, they showed that the red blood cell mean corpuscular volume in severely intoxicated patients was higher than in those patients with mild intoxication and that it correlated well with the degree of acidosis and symptoms. The changes in mean corpuscular volume were not related to hemodilution or hemoconcentration, nor was it believed that they were related to abnormalities in folic acid metabolism but rather they were produced by the direct toxic effect of formaldehyde on cellular ion transport.

It has been shown that formate accounts for more than 50% of the bicarbonate deficit and that mortality correlates better with the degree of acidosis than with the blood methanol concentration. It also appears that serum formate concentration may be a better guide to hemodialysis.[24]

Treatment of Methanol Intoxication

As shown in Table 35–3,[5, 11, 21, 23, 25–27] in the era before hemodialysis was demonstrated to be effective in removing methanol, formic acid, and formaldehyde, outbreaks of methanol intoxication were associated with very high mortality and morbidity due to permanent optic atrophy after a period of papilledema. Dialysis methods have largely centered on the more efficient method of hemodialysis; however, in certain situations, peritoneal dialysis, although less efficient than hemodialysis, may be of some benefit in the treatment of this disease. Not every pa-

Table 35–3. Methanol Poisoning and Outcome

Reference	No. of Patients	Survived	Died	Outcome Unknown	Normal Vision	Permanently Impaired Vision	Dialysis Used
Bennett et al[8]	323	282	41	—	7	2	No
Tonning et al[25]	49	49	—	—	49	—	No
Gonda et al[26]	9	7	2	—	4	3	Yes
McCoy et al[27]	2	?	—	—	2	—	Yes
McMartin et al[21]	2	2	—	—	1	—	Yes
Swartz et al[23]	46 total	44	2	—	22	2	No
	tertiary care	19	—	—	13	6	Yes
Frenia & Schauben[5]	4	3	1	—	2	1	Yes

tient requires hemodialysis for a successful outcome,[28] and this is discussed more fully in the section on management of an epidemic of methanol poisoning. Certain forms of dialysate regeneration for hemodialysis markedly decrease the efficiency of methanol and formate removal.

The following guidelines are suggested for the routine management of methanol intoxication:

1. If the patient is seen early, gastric lavage for the removal of residual gastric methanol should be instituted as rapidly as possible.
2. After this, ethanol (ethyl alcohol) should be administered to all patients while awaiting methanol determination. The usual dose to maintain a blood level of 100 mg/dL of ethanol should begin with a loading dose of 0.6 g/kg,[27] and this can be maintained with an ethanol infusion of 66 mg/kg per hour for nondrinkers (154 mg/kg per hour for chronic ethanol drinkers) in view of the increased hepatobiliary transformation of ethanol in the latter group. Ethanol alone may be all that is required for a blood concentration less than 50 mg/dL. Ethanol should be given as an intravenous infusion of 10% ethanol diluted in 5% dextrose in water.
3. Initial correction of the acidosis with bicarbonate is imperative, particularly if the serum bicarbonate concentration is less than 15 mEq/L and the plasma pH is less than 7.35 (see also Chapter 5). (Large quantities may be required.)
4. Extracorporeal hemodialysis that achieves a methanol clearance of approximately 150 mL/min using a blood flow of between 200 and 300 mL/min through a dialyzer of surface area 1.0 mL is associated with more rapid attenuation of blood methanol levels than with conservative management alone[23]; modern dialyzers and technology give clearance values in excess of this. It is imperative that ethanol be replaced for that removed during dialysis, and this can be achieved by increasing the ethanol infusion rate to 7.0 g/h or by adding ethanol to the hemodialysate. Hemodialysis should be instituted if the blood methanol concentration is greater than 50 mg/dL and should be continued until the serum methanol level is reduced to the range of 25 mg/dL. Ethanol removal is very similar to methanol removal in terms of clearance, and values are reported to be between 100 and 150 mL/min of ethanol clearance.

In one patient reported by Swartz and associates,[23] the addition of ethanol to the dialysate decreased the clearance of ethanol by approximately 30%, and the patient did not require more vigorous ethanol replacement during hemodialysis. Another interesting feature observed by these workers was that in seven of nine patients who underwent hemodialysis, the blood methanol level increased by as much as 20 mg/dL, even up to 36 hours after hemodialysis was terminated. Such rebound increases in methanol levels were previously reported[21] and are consistent with observations of other drugs removed with hemodialysis. These increases reflect the movement of methanol from tissues to the plasma compartment. It must be remembered, however, that dialysis must be continued, along with ethanol administration, until methanol levels are less than 25 mg/dL. Because profound acidosis is a common feature, it is prudent to use bicarbonate-based dialysate for methanol poisoning.

In monkeys, administration of 4-methylpyrazole (4-MP), which inhibits alcohol dehydrogenase, was used with some success for the treatment of methanol poisoning.[29] It has been tested in normal human volunteers[30] and for the treatment of ethylene glycol poisoning,[31] with only moderate side effects. Folinic or folic acid has also been administered to humans[28, 32] to promote catalase-mediated metabolism of formate to enhance the metabolism of formate to carbon dioxide and water. In addition, correction of the acidosis decreases lipophilicity of formate and enhances renal elimination of formate, which itself is even further enhanced by furosemide, which blocks the tubular formate-chloride exchange.[32]

The usual but not invariable[33] high anion gap acidosis is accompanied by an osmolal gap (Table 35–4), which can be used for identification of an alcohol poisoning and for calculation of the serum concentration of the alcohol involved.[10, 34]

Management of an Epidemic

As has been pointed out, sporadic cases of methanol poisoning are fairly rare, and the largest experi-

Table 35–4. Molecular Mass of Alcohols and Their Contribution to the Osmolal Gap

	MM (Daltons)	Osmolal Gap (mOsm/kg) at 100 mg/dL
Ethanol	46	22
Ethylene glycol	62	16
Isopropyl alcohol	60	17
Methanol	32	31

ences are generally gained from managing methanol intoxication epidemics. Swartz and colleagues investigated an epidemic at a Michigan state prison,[23] and their observations allow a few statements to be made about the triage management of such epidemics. Management of methanol intoxication comprises two different approaches for those patients who were referred for tertiary care in hospitals and those who were not. This division was based predominantly on manifestations in the CNS and the ocular and GI systems. Those who exhibited major symptoms in each of these systems were referred for further treatment. However, Swartz and colleagues pointed out that hemodialysis, although useful for enhancing elimination of methanol—especially when blood levels were greater than 100 mg/dL or the acidosis was refractory to standard management—was not always necessary.[23] When hemodialysis might be associated with a high risk, such as upper GI hemorrhage or hemodynamic instability, conservative treatment or peritoneal dialysis might suffice to stabilize the patient during the phase of slow but efficient pulmonary elimination of residual methanol. They also pointed out that in certain cases, the initial severe CNS complications might prove irreversible, even with aggressive treatment. This accounts for some of the deaths associated with methanol poisoning as reported in Table 35–3 and the permanent CNS manifestations.[18]

ISOPROPYL ALCOHOL

Isopropyl alcohol (2-propanol, isopropanol) is an important aliphatic alcohol widely used in industry and the home as a solvent and in medicine as a rubbing alcohol or sterilizing agent (see Table 35–4). In the home, isopropyl alcohol may be found in rubbing alcohol, skin lotion, hair tonics, aftershave lotions, and window-cleaning fluids.[35] Like methanol, isopropyl alcohol is ingested by debilitated or misguided alcoholics because it is cheaper than standard ethanol. Of the 76 alcohol-related deaths reported to the American Association of Poison Control Centers (AAPCC), only 4 were due to isopropanol.[36] However, certain features differentiate the ingestion of isopropyl alcohol from that of ethanol and methanol, principally the production of ketonuria, because approximately 15% of an ingested dose of isopropyl alcohol is metabolized to acetone.

Pharmacology and Toxicology

Isopropyl alcohol appears to be more toxic than ethyl alcohol but less toxic than methanol. It is about twice as potent as ethanol and is metabolized at a much slower rate than ethanol. The reported lethal dose in adults is 240 mL; intoxicating doses as low as 20 mL have been reported.[37] Within 30 minutes, 80% of an oral dose is absorbed, and complete absorption occurs within 2 hours.[37] The apparent volume of distribution is 0.6 to 0.7 L/kg, and the compound is excreted by first-order kinetics,[37] with an elimination half-life of 2.5 to 3.2 hours and a pulmonary alveolar clearance of 8 L/min.[38] The kidneys account for 20% to 50% of unchanged isopropanol excretion.[39] The oxidation of isopropanol to *acetone* probably involves the enzyme alcohol dehydrogenase; however, ethanol administration has not been used clinically. Although ingestion of isopropanol is the major route for intoxication, accidental inhalation of isopropanol vapor during massage or alcohol sponging of febrile patients in poorly ventilated areas has been reported to produce deep coma.[35] One disturbed individual administered isopropyl alcohol as an enema and became toxic, because the alcohol is readily absorbed from the bowel. The clinical signs of isopropyl alcohol use persist for two to four times the usual duration of those of ethanol; this again reflects the slower metabolism of the drug.[40]

The signs and symptoms of isopropyl alcohol poisoning are similar to those of ethanol. Patients may characteristically be in deep coma after an acute ingestion, with the coma preceding respiratory arrest—all taking place within a few hours of ingestion. Isopropyl alcohol, like ethanol, also leads to cardiomyopathy, which may be manifested as an arrhythmia or severe hypotension, an unfavorable prognostic sign.[39] Dehydration and hemorrhagic gastritis (a striking feature of isopropyl alcohol ingestion) may contribute to hypotension. As with all CNS depressants, aspiration of stomach contents into the lungs is a definite risk. Severe hypotension is an unfavorable prognostic sign; it may result in renal shutdown. Hepatic cellular damage also has been described as a result of isopropyl alcohol intoxication in animals; the fatty (triglyceride) content of the liver is increased significantly, as with ethanol. Because other ingredients such as menthol, camphor, methylsalicylate, and naphthalene may be ingested concomitantly, the CNS signs normally associated with isopropyl alcohol ingestion alone may be superseded by the central stimulatory effects of these ingredients. Other rare symptoms of isopropyl intoxication are hemolysis and myopathy (including myoglobinuria[41]); the mechanism for production of these symptoms is unknown. In coingestions with hydrocarbons, evidence shows that isopropanol enhances the toxicity of hydrocarbons.[42]

Diagnosis of Isopropyl Alcohol Poisoning

The principal features outlined previously should suggest the diagnosis. In alcoholic patients, the characteristic smell of rubbing alcohol on the breath, combined with acetonemia/acetonuria, in the absence of glycosuria and acidosis should alert the physician to the possibility of isopropanol ingestion. The symptoms and signs are similar to those of methanol and ethylene glycol intoxication and alcoholic ketoacidosis, however, although they lack the retinal toxicity of formaldehyde in methanol poisoning and the oxalate crystals in urine in ethylene glycol poisoning. Evidence of an osmolal gap (0.17 mOsm/kg for every 1 mg/dL isopropanol) is usually found, as in ethanol intoxication itself (see Table 35–4). Clues to the diagnosis of acidosis in alcoholic patients are given in Chapter 34. Renal dysfunction (and acidosis) may occur if coma and hypotension have been prolonged, and mild hepatic dysfunction may be evident. Increased cerebrospinal fluid protein has been recorded, but the etiology of this is unknown. Although tachycardia is common, bradycardia and other arrhythmias may be detected on clinical and electrocardiographic examinations. Hypoglycemia may also be a prominent feature. Isopropanol can be detected in both blood and gastric contents; serum levels of approximately 50 mg/dL indicate mild intoxication, whereas serum levels of 150 mg/dL have been associated with deep coma.[43] A pediatric patient recovered after treatment despite an isopropanol blood level of 520 mg/dL,[44] however, and adult recovery with blood levels of 346 to 560 mg/dL has been recorded.[45]

Treatment

As with most other ingested poisons, gastric lavage is one of the most important methods of treatment. Most isopropanol recovery from the stomach occurs within 2 hours of ingestion, but even when gastric lavage is delayed, a large amount of isopropyl alcohol can still be removed. Activated carbon adsorbs isopropanol at a rate of only 500 mg/g of carbon. Burkhart and Martinez showed that 87% to 92% of isopropyl alcohol could be removed if a 20:1 ratio of charcoal to alcohol was given.[46] As with other poisons, attention must be paid to preservation of a patent airway during gastric lavage. If a patient shows evidence of alveolar hypoventilation, oxygen administration and artificial respiration may be required. The main method of treatment for isopropyl alcohol poisoning is supportive therapy, with preservation of fluid balance and blood pressure, which may require the use of intravenous fluids and pressor drugs. Hemodialysis to reduce blood levels of isopropanol is rarely necessary.

Several investigators have now reported beneficial clinical outcomes with the institution of early hemodialysis in this uncommon condition. Friereich and associates demonstrated that isopropanol and its metabolite acetone were removed with hemodialysis,[47] whereas King and colleagues reported attenuation of blood isopropanol level from 440 to 100 mg/dL after 5 hours of hemodialysis.[48] In the latter report, the clinical response was dramatic; the patient was in stage 4 coma at the start of hemodialysis and became normotensive and responsive after a 5-hour hemodialysis. A report of successful recovery from nearly fatal isopropanol poisoning in a child treated with peritoneal dialysis has been published.[49]

As mentioned, although it is believed that isopropanol is metabolized through alcohol dehydrogenase, differences in the kinetics of elimination between isopropanol and ethanol or methanol elimination in dogs and rats exist. Alcohol administration has not been used in humans to inhibit the formation of the toxic metabolite to the same degree it is used clinically in methanol or ethylene glycol poisoning.

NORMAL PROPYL ALCOHOL

Normal propyl alcohol (propanol-1, *n*-propanol) is related to isopropyl alcohol but may be more toxic, although it appears to induce the same metabolic effects. A human fatality has been recorded.[50]

THE HIGHER ALCOHOLS

A full discussion of the higher alcohols is included to point out that the higher saturated aliphatic alcohols have some toxicity. The higher liquid alcohols are butyl, amyl, ethyl, hexyl, and so on, and the solid fatty alcohols include lauryl, myristyl, cetyl, and stearyl. The liquid alcohols are used as solvents, and the solid fatty alcohols are used in cosmetics. The butyl alcohols are generally less toxic than the amyl alcohols to the CNS, but they are two to five times more toxic than ethanol in rats. In general, however, the order of increasing toxicity by single oral doses is as follows: ethyl, isopropyl, *sec*-butyl, *n*-butyl, *tert*-butyl, isobutyl, and amyl alcohol. *n*-Butyl alcohol vapors have produced conjunctivitis and keratitis, and although skin irritation is common with the liquid alcohols, percutaneous absorption does not seem to occur. Vapor inhalation may, however, produce pulmonary injury. *n*-Butyl alcohol does not appear to produce ill effects after intravenous infusion. However, extrapolation of animal data to humans gives a calculated mean oral lethal dose of *n*-butyl alcohol of 90 to 210 mL.

The amyl alcohols are more toxic, and ingestion or rectal instillation of about 30 mL has proved lethal in human adults. In addition, glycosuria and methemoglobinemia may result from ingestion of isoamyl alcohol in the fermentative fusel alcohol.[51]

Animal data have established that the alcohols in this group are indeed toxic, but very few cases of human toxicity have been described. In general, the major clinical effects are in the CNS, particularly with vaporizing compounds, and include headache, muscle weakness, giddiness, ataxia, confusion, delirium, and coma. If these agents are ingested, GI effects are principally vomiting and diarrhea, and the odor of the alcohol is noted. Death is mainly due to respiratory failure but may also result from cardiac arrhythmias.

Treatment of Higher Alcohol Poisoning

The main method of treatment after ingestion is gastric lavage until all the alcohol is removed. Some have suggested mineral oil instillation into the stomach, although no clinical evidence supports its use. Because the primary alcohols—the group containing ethyl, isopropyl, butyl, and amyl alcohols—are oxidized to the aldehydes and acids, significant metabolic acidosis may result from their ingestion. The secondary alcohols are converted to ketone, which may also cause CNS depression, and should be managed appropriately. Fortunately, the tertiary alcohols are metabolized slowly and incompletely and excreted in the urine as glucuronides.

BENZYL ALCOHOL

Although benzyl alcohol is not reported to be an adult human toxic agent, some concern is expressed about the presence of benzyl alcohol concentrations in a stable dialysis population at levels significantly higher than those in normal controls.[52] The normal detoxification of benzyl alcohol is by way of oxidation to benzoic and hippuric acids, after which these compounds are rapidly excreted in the urine. In dialyzed patients, however, hippuric and benzoic acids can be removed in the absence of renal function.

Benzyl alcohol–preserved intravenous solutions have been associated with deaths of premature infants, given in an average dosage of 130 to 405 mg/kg per day. In these infants, high urine and serum benzoate levels were detected as well as high urinary hippurate levels. It has since been confirmed that a specific syndrome, the *gasping syndrome,* occurs in premature infants with progressive CNS depression and intraventricular hemorrhage when they are given large quantities of benzyl alcohol–preserved intravenous solutions. The syndrome is one of metabolic acidosis, bradycardia, skin breakdown, respiratory depression with gasping, hypotonia, hepatorenal failure, hypotension, and CNS depression. Use of benzyl alcohol–containing solutions should be avoided in premature infants.[53–55]

ETHYLENE GLYCOL

Ethylene glycol intoxication is one of the most serious and dramatic poisonings encountered in clinical toxicology. As with methanol and isopropanol, ethylene glycol is commonly ingested by debilitated or misguided alcoholic patients, but unlike methanol, ethylene glycol ingestion is sporadic. Intentional administration occasionally leads to poisoning.[56] In the 1994 AAPCC report, 36 of the 766 fatalities involved ethylene glycol, 4 involved isopropanol, and 8 methanol.[36]

Ethylene glycol is used in many chemical manufacturing processes, as a solvent, as a component of cosmetics, and as an antifreeze solution. A large group of glycols exists, and they vary in their toxicity, chemical structure, and metabolism (Fig. 35–2); ethylene glycol poisoning is the more common clinical entity and is discussed in some detail. Although sporadic cases are more common, epidemics have been reported.[57, 58]

Pharmacology and Toxicology

Ethylene glycol itself is nontoxic, although skin irritation, skin penetration, and iridocyclitis may occur after accidental eye contact. After ingestion, peak blood levels occur at 1 to 4 hours, and the unchanged compound undergoes glomerular filtration and passive reabsorption. The compound is highly toxic owing to its breakdown products and the induction of acidosis. Inhalation is not generally associated with toxicity, although cases of chronic poisoning with nystagmus and recurrent attacks of unconsciousness have been reported in factory workers exposed to vapors of ethylene glycol.[59] Although the accepted lethal dose of ethylene glycol ingestion in adults is 100 mL, recovery has been reported after ingestion of as much as 2000 mL.[60]

The major toxicity of ethylene glycol results from accumulation of its four major breakdown products (Fig. 35–3). Ethylene glycol is an odorless solution, and patients can appear to be inebriated as with methanol, although the absence of alcohol on the breath helps in the differential diagnosis, as does fluorescence of body fluids.[1] Ingestion is usually concomitant with ethyl alcohol, although the compound

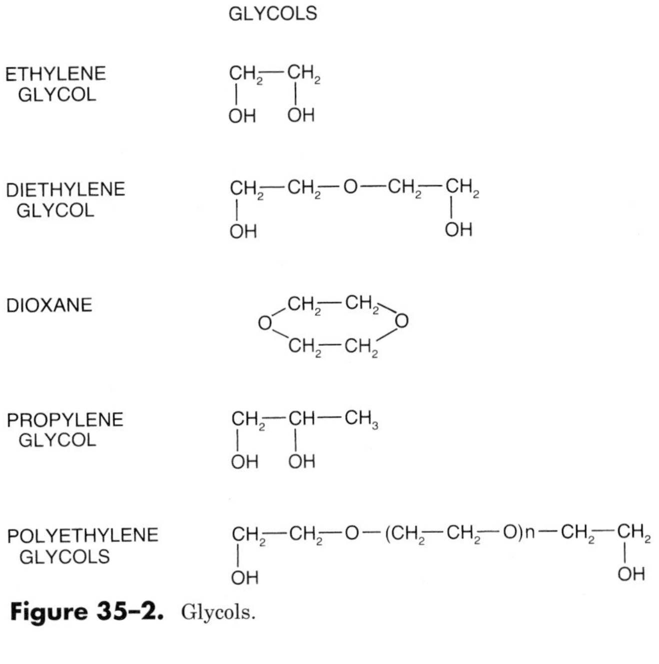

GLYCOLS

ETHYLENE GLYCOL: $CH_2(OH)—CH_2(OH)$

DIETHYLENE GLYCOL: $CH_2(OH)—CH_2—O—CH_2—CH_2(OH)$

DIOXANE: $O(CH_2—CH_2)_2O$ (ring)

PROPYLENE GLYCOL: $CH_2(OH)—CH(OH)—CH_3$

POLYETHYLENE GLYCOLS: $CH_2(OH)—CH_2—O—(CH_2—CH_2—O)n—CH_2—CH_2(OH)$

Figure 35–2. Glycols.

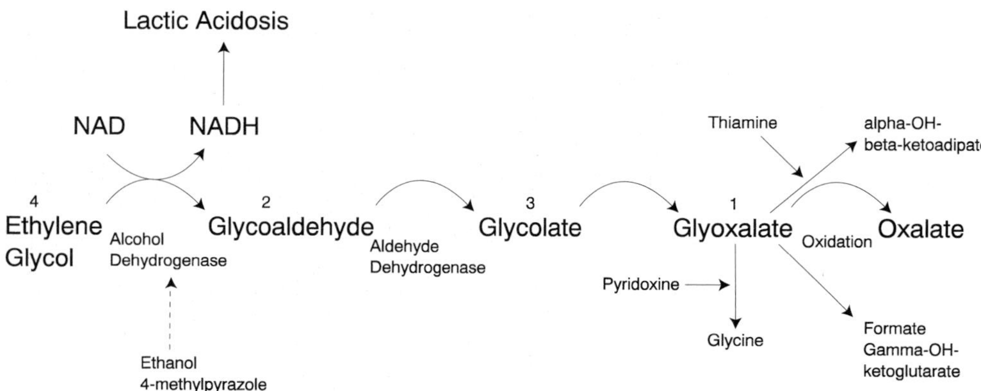

Figure 35–3. Metabolic degradation of ethylene glycol and treatment of toxicity. *Solid arrow,* promotes metabolic process; *broken arrow,* inhibits metabolic process. Toxicity rating, Beasley and Buck, 1980.[78]

has been taken alone in many cases. In the severest form of intoxication, accumulation of the four breakdown products (aldehydes, glycolate, oxalate, and lactate) accounts for all the symptoms. In the more fulminant form, patients are in profound coma with seizure activity, which in turn may be complicated by respiratory failure, cardiovascular collapse, pulmonary edema, adult respiratory distress syndrome,[61] and an increase in the existing severe metabolic acidosis.[62] Death may follow in 8 to 24 hours if the condition is not treated. Survivors of the acute phase experience renal failure. On renal biopsy or autopsy, extensive destruction of the renal substance is seen, caused by deposition of birefringent oxalate crystals in the renal tubules, with evidence of interstitial nephritis and focal hemorrhagic necrosis in the cortex as well as acute tubular necrosis.[63–65]

The underlying basis for the toxicity can be divided into two major categories: tissue destruction due to deposition of calcium oxalate crystals and severe acidosis due to aldehyde, glycolate, and lactate production. The changes just outlined in the renal substance are not limited to the kidneys but have been shown in the meninges of the brain, blood vessels, liver, and pericardium.[63] The tissue destruction is due to deposition of calcium oxalate crystals, as a consequence of which calcium ions are chelated and hypocalcemia may follow. Tissue destruction generally improves after the removal of ethylene glycol to remove or prevent the formation of calcium oxalate crystals. Although renal failure usually reverses, permanent renal, CNS, and cranial nerve damage have frequently been reported.[60] It is believed that the initial CNS depression is from glycol itself or the production of glycoaldehyde, which is maximal 6 to 12 hours after ingestion.

The metabolic acidosis is produced by the combination of lactic acidosis (resulting from trapping of nicotinamide-adenine dinucleotide during the breakdown of ethylene glycol) and the byproducts of glyoxalate metabolism, which inhibit the citric acid cycle; both increase lactic acid production (see Fig. 35–3). In addition, glycolate (and to a lesser extent glyoxalate) recondenses under the activity of pyridoxal phosphate and glyoxalate transaminase enzymes to form glycine and carbon dioxide; glycine production is associated with consumption of bicarbonate and accounts for the profound metabolic acidosis in this condition (see Chapter 5).

The metabolism of ethylene glycol (spontaneous half-life, 3 hours) depends on alcohol dehydrogenase contained in the hepatocytes. Only a small amount of glycol is excreted in the urine after an oral dose; rather, the production of the metabolites in the sequence outlined in Figure 35–3 accounts for the major toxicity,[66] and it appears that tissue damage occurs predominantly in those species that preferentially metabolize ethylene glycol to oxalate (including humans).

Urinary oxalate crystals of the dihydrate or monohydrate type are seen[64] (Fig. 35–4).

Clinical Presentation

The clinical presentation of ethylene glycol toxicity occurs in three fairly well-defined phases.[67] The first phase occurs within 3 minutes to 12 hours after ingestion of ethylene glycol. Patients appear to be drunk but do not have the alcohol smell on their breath and may experience nausea, vomiting, and hematemesis. The major effects, however, are on the CNS. Patients may be in a coma and may have seizure activity that is often focal in nature. Other CNS effects are nystagmus, paralysis of the external muscles of the eyes, depressed reflexes, myoclonic seizures, and tetany due to hypocalcemia.

In the second phase of intoxication, which begins 12 to 14 hours later, patients may experience tachycardia, mild hypertension, pulmonary edema, and congestive cardiac failure, all of which are believed to be due to the deposition of calcium oxalate crystals within the vascular tree, the myocardium, and the lung parenchyma.

The third phase of ethylene glycol poisoning, which begins between 24 and 72 hours after ingestion, is marked by the predominance of flank pain, with costovertebral angle tenderness and evidence of acute tubular necrosis, usually in the form of oliguric acute renal failure.

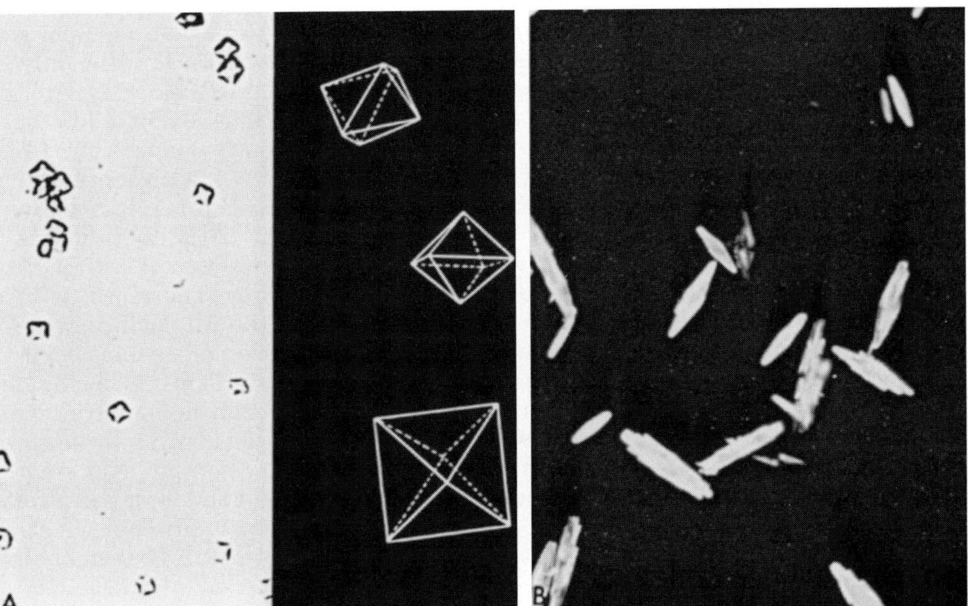

Figure 35–4. *A,* calcium oxalate dihydrate. (Courtesy of Dr. G.E. Schreiner.) *B,* calcium oxalate monohydrate crystals. (Courtesy of Dr. A. Terlinsky.)

Diagnosis of Ethylene Glycol Poisoning

Ethylene glycol poisoning should be strongly suspected in patients who appear to be inebriated but have no alcohol smell on their breath. Other diagnostic features of ethylene glycol poisoning include the presence of calcium oxalate crystals in the urine, either as dihydrate or monohydrate crystals (see Fig. 35–4). In addition, microscopic hematuria may occur during the third phase of the poisoning, and oliguria, proteinuria, and urine with a low specific gravity may be observed. Any evidence of renal failure is manifested by an increase in serum creatinine and blood urea nitrogen levels. The more profound features, however, are those associated with metabolic acidosis: Patients may have Kussmaul's respiration, with a large anion gap and evidence of an osmolal gap (0.2 mOsm/kg for every 1 mg/dL of ethylene glycol) (see Table 35–4). A persistent high osmolal gap with low ethylene glycol levels may be due to persistence of glycolate in plasma[68]; however, a normal osmolal gap may be encountered,[69] especially if a patient has metabolized most of the compound. In addition to these features, lactic acidosis complicates the picture. During the initial phase of toxicity, hypocalcemia may be observed in addition to the profound acidosis, and if renal failure supervenes, hyperkalemia may develop. Additionally, an increased white blood cell count is commonly found, and lumbar puncture may reveal high protein values. Ethylene glycol may be detected in gastric fluid as well as in urine and blood. Oxalic acid (oxalate) levels also may be extremely high.

Treatment

Aggressive treatment of the acidosis and institution of hemodialysis,[62, 65] variations of hemodialysis (hemodiafiltration),[70] and experimental use of 4-MP[31] form the mainstay of therapy.

Treatment should include gastric lavage for removal of residual ethylene glycol, correction of dehydration and shock, and management of fluid balance in the presence of pulmonary edema, which might be due to the toxic effects of ethylene glycol metabolites or the sodium overload. In addition, hypocalcemia should be corrected with calcium chloride, depending on serum calcium levels. The mainstay of treatment, however, is correction of the metabolic acidosis, which often requires administration of massive doses of sodium bicarbonate; such obligatory sodium administration requires early institution of hemodialysis.

As in methanol poisoning, ethyl alcohol is administered to act as a preferential substrate for the enzyme hepatic alcohol dehydrogenase, and administration of ethyl alcohol should be gauged to maintain a plasma ethanol level of 100 to 200 mg/dL. Also as in methanol poisoning, hepatic enzyme induction may be present in a habitually alcoholic patient, and thus more ethanol may be required than in a patient who has been abstinent from alcohol. Ethanol should be given as an intravenous infusion of 10% ethanol diluted in 5% dextrose in water.

In one study, blood ethylene glycol levels before dialysis were 50 mg/dL; the osmolal gap was 90 mOsm/kg, and the spontaneous elimination half-life of ethylene glycol during intravenous administration of 5% ethanol was 3 hours.[71] During oral administration of ethanol, the elimination half-life was prolonged to 17 hours, when the blood levels of ethanol ranged between 130 and 200 mg/dL. During dialysis and continued oral ethanol therapy, the half-life of ethylene glycol was reduced to 2.5 hours. Ethylene glycol removal was equivalent to urea clearance, and 111 g of ethylene glycol was removed with dialysis, compared with 10 g of ethylene glycol excretion in the urine during the same 6-hour hemodialysis period. It was recommended that in the management of ethylene glycol poisoning, an oral loading dose of 0.6 g of 50% ethanol per kilogram of body weight be given, followed by oral maintenance doses of 109 mg of 20% ethanol per kilogram per hour, and that dialysis be initiated. During hemodialysis, 230 mg of ethanol per kilogram per hour should be administered to maintain blood ethanol levels of 100 to 200 mg/dL. These measures should be continued until ethylene glycol has been eliminated from the blood (< 10 mg/dL). Most recommend intravenous administration of ethanol for unconscious patients. The enzyme alcohol dehydrogenase is 50% inhibited at an ethanol concentration of 2 mg/dL and more than 90% saturated at 50 mg/dL[72]; however, ethylene glycol requirements to saturate the enzyme by 50% are reported to be much higher at 326 mg/dL.[73]

Peterson and associates also pointed out that alcohol can be added to the dialysate bath to give a dialysate level of 100 mg/dL using 95% ethanol.[71] Stabilization of blood ethanol levels was easier than with intravenous or oral ethanol therapy. Bicarbonate dialysis is most appropriate. Dialysis is recommended at levels exceeding 50 mg/dL.[74] Glycolic acid concentrations are invariably elevated, lactic acidosis may be present, and glycolic acid is well dialyzed (105 mL/min at a blood flow rate of 200 mL/min measured in one of three patients).[66] Glycolic acid is the major contributor to the profound acidosis and has an elimination half-life of 7 hours (ethylene glycol itself had a half-life of 8.4 hours, which was prolonged more than 10-fold by ethanol).[75] Clearance of ethylene glycol by the kidneys was 27.5 ± 4.5 mL/min and a fractional renal clearance of 19.8 ± 1.5% (both lower than respective urea clearances), whereas hemodialyzer clearance was 156 mL/min.[75] It is well recognized that coingestion of ethyl alcohol may reduce symptoms due to ethylene glycol ingestion, but what is less well recognized is that the anion gap may be normalized with ingestion of exogenous anions (e.g., bromide).[76]

Hemoperfusion has been attempted in a single patient with ethylene glycol poisoning.[77] Because column saturation occurred and correction of acid-base changes was not possible, hemoperfusion is not recommended.

Pyridoxine (500 mg intramuscularly four times daily, which stimulates the metabolism of glyoxalate to glycine) and thiamine (100 mg intramuscularly four times daily, which stimulates glyoxalate to α-OH-β-ketoadipate) are cofactors for the metabolism of ethylene glycol and have been suggested as antidotes.[78]

In a protocol based on studies of 4-MP in animals, Baud and associates treated three patients with oral 4-MP (20 mg/kg per day or intermittent intravenous 4-MP, 9.5 mg/kg at 9 hours after glycol ingestion, decreasing to 0.6 mg/kg 57 hours after glycol ingestion) until plasma ethylene glycol determinations were negative.[31] No patient was treated with hemodialysis. A mild metabolic acidosis in two patients, a skin rash in one, and possible eosinophilia in the others were the only associations with treatment with 4-MP. More recent phase 1 studies of humans have shown that 4-MP has a low side effect profile.[79] It is not available for clinical use in the United States.

As with methanol poisoning, the primary ingested substance is not directly responsible for the toxicity; it is the metabolites that produce the serious consequences of both methanol and ethylene glycol poisoning. Therefore, it is mandatory not only to remove the intoxicating substance but to prevent the formation of the metabolites or remove them by hemodialysis. This is easily accomplished clinically and has been demonstrated in animals and humans to prevent both morbidity and mortality in ethylene glycol poisoning. Not only correction of acidosis but also diversion of the alcohol dehydrogenase enzyme activity to another substrate (ethanol), or its inhibition by 4-MP, is extremely important in this regard.

DIETHYLENE GLYCOL

Many of the derivatives of ethylene glycol are available in commercial and industrial settings. However, used as a 73% vehicle for the preparation of drugs, diethylene glycol did result in 105 deaths.[80] Diethylene glycol ingestion does not cause oxalate crystals to form, yet the renal pathology closely resembles ethylene glycol toxicity, as do the pathologic findings in the liver, lungs, heart, and meninges.[81] The structure of diethylene glycol (see Fig. 35–2) and the simple esters of diethylene glycol contain a stable ether linkage that is resistant to metabolism to oxalate or formate. This explains the fact that metabolic acidosis is encountered rarely and has been reported only in diethylene glycol poisoning in children. However, the ether linkage in diethylene glycol, dipropylene glycol, dioxane, and monomethyl and butyl ethers of diethylene glycol is associated with a far higher degree of renal damage.[82]

The simple ethers of ethylene glycol and diethylene glycol appear to be more toxic than the parent alcohol and produce severe nephrotoxicity partly compounded by the intravascular hemolysis that occurs with several of these compounds, in addition to the production of CNS depression, liver damage, and pulmonary edema.

Management of the ethers of ethylene glycol poisoning is similar to management of intoxication with the parent compound. The use of ethanol is recommended in view of the metabolism by alcohol dehydrogenase. In one series, however, observation after ingestion of ethylene glycol butyl ether was all that was required.[83]

CELLOSOLVES

Cellosolves, used as solvents for resins, paints, inks, and industrial coatings and cleaners, are the monoalkyl ethers of ethylene glycol and principally consist of methyl cellosolves and butyl cellosolves. Toxicity arises from these compounds by inhalation of their vapors, which produces toxic encephalopathy and bone marrow depression without hemolysis. However, in rats but not in canine species, hemoglobinuria has been observed, particularly with butyl cellosolves rather than ethyl or methyl cellosolves. As with the simple ethers of ethylene glycol, pulmonary, renal, and hepatic changes that resemble toxicity from diethylene glycol have been observed. Severe metabolic acidosis also has been reported after ingestion of the monomethyl ether of ethylene glycol.[84] Management of cellosolve poisoning is essentially similar to that of diethylene glycol, but particular attention must be paid to correction of the acidosis and the occasional renal failure.

POLYGLYCOLS AND PROPYLENE GLYCOL

Triethylene glycol, the lowest-molecular-weight polymer to be derived from the series of ethylene and diethylene glycols, has a molecular mass of approximately 200 daltons and is a liquid; such polymers remain liquid up to a molecular mass of 1000 daltons, after which they become solid and are termed *carbowaxes*. The toxicity decreases with ascending molecular mass, but as a class this group of compounds is in general of very low toxicity. Reported deaths appear to result from renal injuries rather than CNS depression. Chronic toxicity may arise from chronic ingestion of the polyethylene glycols ranging in molecular mass from 200 to 6000 daltons, but evidence shows that compounds with a molecular mass greater than 6000 daltons have less toxicity. Polyethylene glycol of a molecular mass of 400 daltons is recovered in the urine in about 80% of the ingested dose. However, these remarks apply to experiments using rats and dogs; it appears that even compounds with a molecular mass of 6000 daltons are excreted to a high degree in human urine after intravenous administration.

Propylene glycol, however, has been reported to be completely innocuous and as such has been allowed by the Food and Drug Administration for use in cosmetics and foods and as a solvent for certain drugs. In a patient who had renal failure and who was unable to excrete propylene glycol in the urine, such retention caused severe CNS depression. In addition, lactic acidosis was a prominent feature in this patient, with a large anion gap and a lactic acid level of 80 mEq/L. The patient rapidly responded to use of intravenous fluids and sodium bicarbonate and on recovery volunteered a history of "gas" exposure. Propylene glycol levels of 70 and 60 mg/dL were found in blood and urine, respectively.[85] Two previous cases of childhood poisoning with propylene glycol have been recorded: Stupor and seizures developed, and the symptoms regressed on cessation of propylene glycol exposure.[86, 87] Propylene glycol contamination of intravenous nitroglycerin preparations has been associated with hyperosmolar coma and a high osmolal gap without acidosis; the patient responded to hemodialysis.[88]

Propylene glycol appears to be metabolized to lactic acid, which subsequently enters the glycolytic pathway.[85] Cate and Hedrick believed that propylene glycol probably accumulated in blood because of impaired renal clearance, with resultant lactic acidosis and stupor. Management of such toxicity should include the use of sodium bicarbonate and intravenous fluids.

In lithograph workers, myeloid hypoplasia has been observed as well as birth defects and testicular damage after exposure to glycol ether and methyl cellosolves, and it has been suggested that ethoxyacetic acid, the major urinary breakdown product, be measured as a means of monitoring industrial exposure.[89]

ACETONE

Acetone is included in this chapter because of its relationship to isopropyl alcohol metabolism and its important toxicity. Although not commonly reported, acetone ingestion does produce certain clinical effects. Acetone (dimethylketone, β-ketopropane, propanone, and pyroacetic ether) is a component of a large number of industrial and household cleaners, glues, and solvents and is commonly found in the household as nail polish remover. Other ketone derivatives, such as ethyl butyl ketone, isobutyl ketone, and methyl ethyl ketone in addition to such solvents as chloroform, carbon tetrachloride, and so on, are found in paint and varnish removers, industrial metal cleaners, carburetor cleaners, and shoe polish. Acetone is relatively nontoxic, and ingestions of 200 to 400 mL may not be serious.[90] Acetone has a characteristic odor, and it has narcotic properties.

The compound may be inhaled or ingested, and the recommended threshold limit for industrial hygiene is 1000 ppm for workers exposed 8 hours a day. With inhalation, recent reports suggest that acetone also may be a solvent abused for recreational purposes by young people, although it appeared at one time that industrial exposure was more prevalent. Ingested acetone, which produces significant blood levels equal to those of toxic ethanol concentrations, is said to produce similar symptoms although its anesthetic potency is greater.[91] The pharmacokinetics of acetone indicate that the half-life in plasma is between 19 and 31 hours, with a mean half-life of 28 hours. The major excretory route is through the lungs, and the fruity odor of the breath is characteristic of acetone poisoning. The kinetics of elimination indicate that because the volume of distribution is 0.82 L/kg of body weight, with an average minute ventilation, several days are required for complete elimination of acetone from the breath.

Clinical symptoms of acetone inhalation include cough, bronchial irritation, headache, and fatigue; after oral ingestion, GI symptoms of vomiting and nausea occur. In severe cases, CNS depression similar to that encountered with alcohol occurs. Patients may appear drunk,[90] but the progression to coma appears to be more rapid than with ethanol. Other reported symptoms are a red and swollen pharynx with erosions of the soft plate, lethargy, stupor, and coma. In addition, acidosis has been reported,[90] although it is not clear whether this was because of CNS depression or the toxicity of acetone itself.

Treatment

A person who has inhaled acetone should be moved into an area of fresh air, and oxygen administered as required. If a patient has ingested acetone, gastric lavage should be performed or an emetic given. Attention to correction of acidosis and maintenance of respiration is extremely important, and patients should not be expected to recover rapidly. As Ramu and associates have pointed out, 2 to 3 days are required for a progressive but slow improvement in consciousness.[90] A concentration of acetone in blood (measured by gas chromatography) at the height of toxicity in the patient described by Ramu and associates was 0.25 g/dL,[90] and at levels greater than 1 g/dL, the elimination of acetone is determined by the respiratory route; no acidosis was observed even with such concentrations. At lower levels, saturable metabolism of acetone also has been documented, with conversion of acetone into glucose.

OXALATE

Oxalic acid is included in this chapter because of its relationship to ethylene glycol poisoning; however, it is a dangerous poison in its own right. Oxalic acid is found in bleaches, metal cleaners, and many plant substances such as rhubarb leaves, *Dieffenbachia* leaves (dumb cane), citrus fruit, beet, mangold, halogeton, sorrel, purslane, dock, greasewood, and Russian thistle.[92] Oxalate formation may also occur spontaneously *in vivo* in primary oxalosis. Ascorbic acid ingestion in high doses is associated with oxalate deposition in tissue in dialysis recipients.[93] The poisoning mainly relates to the oxalic acid and its soluble salts, which have corrosive activity on the alimentary tract with production of severe gastroenteritis and hypotension, the former of which may last for 1 week. Prolonged inhalation of fumes produced by boiling oxalic acid solutions also may lead to oxalic acid poisoning with renal impairment. Gangrene of the hands has been reported after immersion of the hands in oxalate solutions. Absorption in less severe cases of oxalate poisoning produces chelation of calcium and thus symptoms related to hypocalcemia, such as muscle twitching, cramps, and CNS depression, the severity of which may provoke cardiac arrhythmias. As with ethylene glycol poisoning, oxalate is deposited in the blood vessels, kidneys, liver, heart, and lungs. The mean lethal dose is between 15 and 30 g, and death usually follows within a few hours.[93] If the patient survives, the picture is almost identical to that of corrosive acid poisoning, with the almost invariable occurrence of acute renal failure. Urinalysis may reveal oxalate crystals as well as hematuria and albuminuria (see Fig. 35–4).

Symptoms include pain in the throat, esophagus, and stomach, and the mucous membranes take on a whitish opaque appearance. Hematemesis is possible, and extreme diarrhea also has been reported, often leading to shock. Tetany, convulsions, stupor, coma, and death also may result from hypocalcemia, and renal failure is noted.

Treatment

Treatment should be rapidly instituted by giving a dilute solution of calcium lactate, limewater, finely pulverized chalk, plaster, or milk to supply large amounts of calcium to inactivate oxalate by forming an insoluble calcium salt in the stomach. Gastric lavage is controversial because it may compound an already severe corrosive lesion in the esophagus or stomach. If used, however, gastric lavage should be carried out with limewater (calcium hydroxide). Intravenous gluconate or calcium chloride solutions should be given to prevent hypocalcemic tetany; in severe cases, parathyroid extract also has been given. Strictures may develop in the survivors, as well as other GI lesions. Additionally, acute renal failure should be anticipated, and careful fluid management is necessary.

Removal of oxalate (in primary oxalosis) with hemodialysis is on the order of 650 mg/4.5 h, whereas long-dwelling peritoneal dialysis using four 2-L exchanges in 24 hours approximates 300 mg/day of oxalate removal. For this reason, although hemodialysis or peritoneal dialysis has never been suggested in the past for oxalate poisoning, it is possible that oxalate removal with these techniques might prevent acute renal failure and certainly helps correct the hypocalcemia because dialysate calcium concentrations are approximately 6.4 mg/dL*. Hemoperfusion with activated charcoal has been attempted in primary oxalosis for the removal of oxalate. Maggiore and associates demonstrated a 44% decrease in plasma oxalate levels during a 2-hour hemoperfusion.[94]

The total quantity of oxalate removed, however, is approximately 150 mg with a 4-hour charcoal hemoperfusion, but saturation of the charcoal is observed at 2 hours.*

References

1. Winter ML, Ellis MD, Snodgrass WR: Urine fluorescence using a Wood's lamp to detect the antifreeze additive sodium fluorescein. A qualititative adjunctive test in supporting ethylene glycol ingestion. Ann Emerg Med *19*:663, 1990.

*Personal observation of the author.

2. Gosselin RE, Smith RP, Hodge HC (eds): Methyl alcohol. *In* Clinical Toxicology of Commercial Products. 5th ed. Baltimore, Williams & Wilkins, pp 111–275, 1984.
3. Facts and figures from the chemical industry. Chem Eng News *70:*32, 1992.
4. Kahn A, Blum D: Methyl alcohol poisoning in an 8 month old boy. An unusual route of intoxication. J Pediatr *94:*841, 1979.
5. Frenia ML, Schauben JL: Methanol inhalation toxicity. Ann Emerg Med *22:*1919, 1993.
6. Aufderheide TP, White SM, Brady WJ, Steuven HA: Inhalational and percutaneous methanol toxicity in two firefighters. Ann Emerg Med *22:*1916, 1993.
7. Eriksen SP, Kulkarni AB: Methanol in normal human breath. Science *141:*639, 1963.
8. Bennett IL, Carey FH, Mitchell GL, Cooper MN: Acute methyl alcohol poisoning: A review based on experiences in an outbreak of 323 cases: Medicine *32:*431, 1953.
9. Axelrod J, Daly J: Pituitary gland: Enzymic formation of methanol from 5-methyl adenosine. Science *150:*892, 1965.
10. Becker CE: Methanol poisoning. J Emerg Med *1:*51, 1983.
11. Cooper JR, Kim MM: Biochemical aspects of methanol poisoning. Editorial. Biochem Pharmacol *11:*405, 1962.
12. Martin-Amat G, Tephly TR, McMartin KE, et al: Methyl poisoning. II. Development of a model for ocular toxicity in methanol poisoning using the rhesus monkey. Arch Ophthalmol *95:*1847, 1977.
13. Ritchie JM: The aliphatic alcohols. *In* Gilman AG, Goodman LS, Gilman A (eds): The Pharmacological Basis of Therapeutics. 6th ed. New York, Macmillan Publishing Co., p 376, 1980.
14. McMartin KE, Makar AB, Martin-Amat G, et al: Methanol poisoning. I. The role of formic acid in the development of metabolic acidosis in the monkey and the reversal by 4-methylpyrazole. Biochem Med *13:*319, 1975.
15. Baumbach GL, Cancilia PA, Martin-Amat G, et al: Methyl alcohol poisoning. IV. Alterations of the morphological findings of the retina and optic nerve. Arch Ophthalmol *95:*859, 1977.
16. Kaplan K: Methyl alcohol poisoning. Am J Med Sci *244:*170, 1982.
17. Grufferman S, Morris D, Alvarez J: Methanol poisoning complicated by myoglobinuric acute renal failure. Am J Emerg Med *3:*24, 1985.
18. McLean DR, Jacobs H, Mielke BW: Methanol poisoning: A clinical and pathological study. Arch Neurol *8:*161, 1980.
19. Cavalli A, Volpi A, Maggioni AP, et al: Severe reversible cardiac failure associated with methanol intoxication. Postgrad Med J *63:*867, 1987.
20. Liesivuori J, Savolainen H: Methanol and formic acid toxicity: Biochemical mechanisms. Pharmacol Toxicol *69:*157, 1991.
21. McMartin KE, Ambre JJ, Tephly TR: Methanol poisoning in human subjects. Am J Med *68:*414, 1980.
22. Smith SR, Smith SJM, Buckley BM: Combined formate and lactic acidosis in methanol poisoning. Lancet *2:*1295, 1981.
23. Swartz RD, Millman RP, Billi JE, et al: Epidemic methanol poisoning: Clinical and biochemical analysis of a recent episode. Medicine *60:*373, 1981.
24. Osterloh JD, Pond SM, Grady S, Becker CE: Serum formate concentrations in methanol intoxication as a criterion for hemodialysis. Ann Intern Med *104:*200, 1986.
25. Tonning DJ, Brooks DW, Harlow CM: Acute methyl alcohol poisonings in 49 naval ratings. Can Med Assoc J *74:*20, 1956.
26. Gonda A, Gault H, Churchill D, Hollomby D: Hemodialysis for methanol intoxication. Am J Med *64:*749, 1978.
27. McCoy HG, Cipolle RJ, Ehlers SM, et al: Severe methanol poisoning. Am J Med *67:*804, 1979.
28. Brent J, Lucas M, Kulig K, Rumack BH: Methanol poisoning in a 6-week old infant. J Pediatr *118:*644, 1991.
29. Blomstrand R, Ostling-Wintzell IT, Lot A, et al: Pyrazoles as inhibitors of alcohol oxidation and as important tools in alcohol research: An approach to therapy against methanol poisoning. Proc Natl Acad Sci USA *76:*3499, 1979.
30. Jacobsen D, Sebastian CS, Barron SK, et al: Effects of 4-methylpyrazole, methanol/ethylene glycol antidote, in healthy humans. J Emerg Med *8:*455, 1990.
31. Baud EJ, Galliot M, Astier A, et al: Treatment of ethylene glycol poisoning with intravenous 4-methylpyrazole. N Engl J Med *319:*97, 1988.
32. Moore DF, Bentley AM, Darling S, et al: Folinic acid enhances renal elimination in formic acid intoxication. J Toxicol Clin Toxicol *32:*199, 1994.
33. Palmisano J, Gruver C, Adams NA: Absence of anion gap acidosis in methanol poisoning: A case report and review of the literature. Am J Kidney Dis *9:*441, 1987.
34. Smith M: Solvent toxicity: Isopropanol, methanol and ethylene glycol. Ear Nose Throat J *62:*126, 1983.
35. Gosselin RE, Smith RP, Hodge HC (eds): Isopropyl alcohol. *In* Clinical Toxicology of Commercial Products. 5th ed. Baltimore, Williams & Wilkins, pp 111–217, 1984.
36. Litovitz TL, Felberg L, Soloway RA, et al: 1994 Annual report of the American Association of Poison Control Centers Toxic Exposure Surveillance System. Am J Emerg Med *13:*551, 1995.
37. Lacouture PG: Isopropyl alcohol. Clin Toxicol Rev *3:*3, 1980.
38. Brugnone F, Perbellini L, Apostoli P, et al: Isopropanol exposure. Environmental and biological monitoring in a print works. Br J Ind Med *40:*160, 1983.
39. Daniel DR, McAnally BIT, Garriott JC: Isopropyl alcohol metabolism after acute intoxication in humans. J Anal Toxicol *5:*110, 1981.
40. Williams RT: Detoxication Mechanisms. 2nd ed. New York, John Wiley & Sons, 1959.
41. Kulig K, Duffy JP, Linden CH, et al: Toxic effects of methanol, ethylene glycol and isopropyl alcohol. Top Emerg Med *6:*14, 1986.
42. Traiger GJ, Plaa GC: Chlorinated hydrocarbon toxicity: Potentiation by isopropyl alcohol and acetone. Arch Environ Health *28:*276, 1976.
43. McCord WM, Switzer PK, Brill HH: Isopropyl alcohol intoxication. South Med J *41:*639, 1948.
44. Visudhiphan P, Kaufman IT: Increased cerebrospinal fluid protein following isopropyl alcohol intoxication. N Y State J Med *71:*887, 1971.
45. Alexander CB, McBay AJ, Hudson RP: Ispopropanol and isopropanol deaths—ten years experience. J Forensic Sci *27:*541, 1982.
46. Burkhart KK, Martinez MA: The adsorption of ispropanol and acetone by activated charcoal. J Toxicol Clin Toxicol *30:*371, 1992.
47. Freireich AW, Cinque TJ, Xanthaky G, Landau D: Hemodialysis for isopropanol poisoning. N Engl J Med *277:*699, 1967.
48. King LH, Bradley KP, Shires DL: Hemodialysis for isopropyl alcohol. JAMA *211:*1855, 1970.
49. Depner TA, Mecckalsic MD: Peritoneal dialysis for isopropanol poisoning. West J Med *137:*322, 1981.
50. Durwald W, Degen W: Eine todliche Vergiftung mit *N*-Propyl-Alkohol. Arch Toxikol *16:*85, 1956.
51. Treon JF: Alcohols. *In* Irish DD, Fassett DW (eds): Patty's Industrial Hygiene and Toxicology. 2nd ed. New York, Interscience Publishers, p 1409, 1963.
52. Bowen D, Cowburn D, Renekamp M, Sullivan J: Benzyl alcohol: High levels found in plasma of uremic patients on hemodialysis. Clin Chim Acta *61:*399, 1975.
53. Brown WJ, Buist NRM, Gipson HTC, et al: Fatal benzyl alcohol poisoning in a neonatal intensive care unit. Lancet *1:*1250, 1982.
54. Gershanik J, Boecker B, Ensley H, et al: The gasping syndrome and benzyl alcohol poisoning. N Engl J Med *307:*1384, 1982.
55. Hiller JC, Benda GI, Rahatzad M, et al: Impact on mortality and intraventricular hemorrhage among very low birth weight infants. Pediatrics *77:*500, 1986.
56. Woolf AD, Wynshaw-Boris A, Rinaldo P, Levy HL: Intentional infantile ethylene glycol poisoning presenting as inherited metabolic disorder. J Pediatr *120:*421, 1992.
57. Geiling EMK, Cannon PR: Pathologic effects of elixir of sulfanilamide (diethylene glycol) poisoning. JAMA *111:*919, 1938.
58. Karlson-Stiber C, Persson H: Ethylene glycol poisoning: Experiences from an epidemic in Sweden. Clin Toxicol *30:*565, 1992.
59. Troisi FM: Chronic intoxication with ethylene glycol vapour. Br J Ind Med *1:*65, 1950.
60. Ethylene Glycol. Denver, Poisindex, Micromedex Inc., 1996.
61. Catchings TT, Beamer WC, Lundy L, et al: Adult respiratory

distress syndrome secondary to ethylene glycol ingestion. Ann Emerg Med *14:*594–596, 1985.
62. Friedman EA, Greenberg JB, Merrill JP, Dammin GJ: Consequences of ethylene glycol poisoning: Report of four cases and review of the literature. Am J Med *32:*891, 1962.
63. Pons CA, Custer RP: Acute ethylene glycol poisoning: A clinicopathologic report of eighteen fatal cases. Am J Med Sci *211:*544, 1946.
64. Terlinsky AS, Grochowski J, Geoly KL, et al: Identification of atypical calcium oxalate crystalluria following ethylene glycol ingestion. Am J Clin Pathol *76:*223, 1981.
65. Schreiner GE, Maher JF, Marc-Aurele J, et al: Ethylene glycol—two indications for hemodialysis. Trans Am Soc Artif Intern Organs *5:*81, 1959.
66. Gabow PA, Clay K, Sullivan LB, Lepoff R: Organic acids in ethylene glycol intoxication. Ann Intern Med *105:*16, 1986.
67. Schreiner GE, Maher JF: Toxic nephropathy. Am J Med *38:*409, 1965.
68. Hewlett TP, McMartin RE: Ethylene glycol intoxication: The value of glycolic acid determination for diagnosis and treatment. Clin Toxicol *24:*389, 1986.
69. Steinhart B: Case report: Severe ethylene glycol intoxication with normal osmolal gap—"a chilling thought." J Emerg Med *8:*583, 1990.
70. Walder AD, Tyler CK: Ethylene glycol antifreeze poisoning. Three case reports and a review of treatment. Anaesthesia *49:*964, 1994.
71. Peterson CD, Collins A, Himes JM, et al: Ethylene glycol poisoning. Pharmacokinetics during therapy with ethanol and hemodialysis. N Engl J Med *304:*21, 1981.
72. Pietruszko R, Crawford K, Lester D: Comparison of substrate specificity of alcohol dehydrogenase from human liver, horse liver and yeast towards saturated and 2-enoic alcohols and aldehydes. Arch Biochem Biophys *159:*50, 1973.
73. Pietruszko R, Voigtlander K, Lester D: Alcohol dehydrogenase from human and horse liver: Substrate specificity with diols. Biochem Pharmacol *27:*1296, 1978.
74. Stokes JB, Averon F: Prevention of organ damage in massive ethylene glycol ingestion. JAMA *243:*2065, 1980.
75. Cheng JT, Beysolow TDf, Kaul B, et al: Clearance of ethylene glycol by kidneys and hemodialysis. J Toxicol Clin Toxicol *25:*95, 1987.
76. Heckerling PS: Ethylene glycol poisoning with a normal anion gap due to occult bromide intoxication. Ann Emerg Med *16:*1384, 1987.
77. Sangster B, Prenen JAC, DeGroot G: Ethylene glycol poisoning. N Engl J Med *302:*465, 1980.
78. Beasley VR, Buck WB: Acute ethylene glycol toxicoses: A review. Vet Hum Toxicol *22:*255, 1980.
79. McMartin KE, Heath A: The treatment of ethylene glycol poisoning with intravenous 4-methylpyrazole. N Engl J Med *320:*125, 1989.
80. Geiling EMK, Cannon PR: Pathoiogic effects of elixir sulfanilamide (diethylene glycol) poisoning; clinical and experimental correlations: Final report. JAMA *111:*919, 1938.
81. Leech PN: Elixir of sulfanilamide—Massengill. Chemical, pharmacologic, pathologic and necropsy reports; preliminary toxicity reports on diethylene glycol and sulfanilamide. JAMA *109:*1531, 1937.
82. Kesten HD, Mullinos MC, Pomerantz L: Pathologic effects of certain glycol and related compounds. Arch Pathol *27:*447, 1939.
83. Dean BS, Krenzelok EP: Clinical evaluation of pediatric ethylene glycol monobutyl ether poisonings. J Toxicol Clin Toxicol *30:*557, 1992.
84. Nitter-Hauge S: Poisoning with ethylene glycol monomethyl ether. Acta Med Scand *188:*277, 1970.
85. Cate JC, Hedrick R: Propylene glycol intoxication and lactic acidosis. N Engl J Med *303:*1237, 1980.
86. Martin G, Finberg L: Propylene glycol: A potentially toxic vehicle in liquid dosage form. J Pediatr *77:*877, 1970.
87. Arulanantham K, Genel M: Central nervous system toxicity associated with ingestion of propylene glycol. J Pediatr *93:*515, 1978.
88. Demey H, Daelemans R, De Broe ME, Bossaert L: Propylene glycol intoxication due to intravenous nitroglycerin. Lancet *1:*1361, 1984.
89. Hardin BD, Lvon JP: Summary and overview of NIOSH symposium on toxic effects of glycol ethers. Environ Health Perspect *57:*273, 1984.
90. Ramu A, Rosenbaum J, Blaschke TF: Disposition of acetone following acute acetone intoxication. West J Med *129:*429, 1978.
91. Oliver JS, Watson JM: Abuse of solvents "for kicks." A review of 50 cases. Lancet *1:*84, 1977.
92. Gosselin RE, Smith RP, Hodge HC (eds): Oxalate. *In* Clinical Toxicology of Commercial Products. 5th ed. Baltimore, Williams & Wilkins, pp 111–326, 1984.
93. Balcke P, Schmidt P, Zaggornik J, et al: Ascorbic acid aggravates secondary hyperoxalemia in patients on chronic hemodialysis. Ann Intern Med *101:*344, 1984.
94. Maggiore W, Poggi A, Parlongo S, Cerrai T: Oxalate removal by dialysis and hemoperfusion. Proc Eur Dial Transplant Assoc *16:*717, 1979.

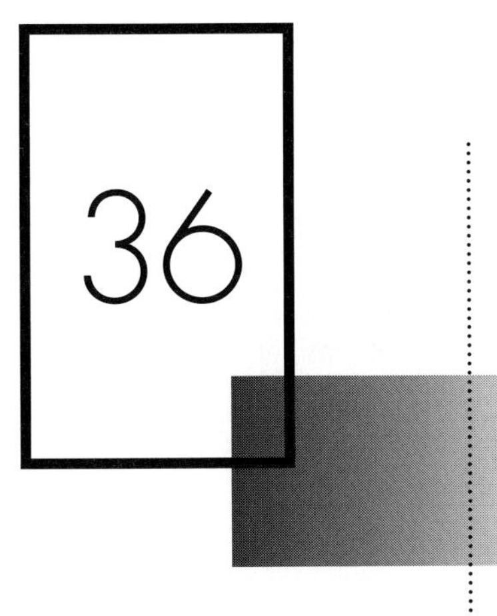

Opiates and Narcotics

MICHAEL SCHWARTZ, MD

Opium is derived from the Greek word "opus," for juice or sap, and has become identified specifically with the juice of the opium poppy, *Papaver somniferum.*[1] Opium sap, recovered from the heads of immature poppies, contains morphine, codeine, and numerous other related alkaloids.

The term *opiate* initially referred to all naturally occurring alkaloids derived from opium. The development of numerous synthetic derivatives brought with it a need to provide a more specific terminology. *Opioid* refers to all drugs, natural or synthetic, with morphine-like actions or actions mediated through binding to opioid receptors.[2] The term *narcotic* is derived from the Greek word for stupor or "numbness" and is applied to any drug that induces sleep. For a number of years it was used to refer to morphine-like analgesics. More recently, *narcotic* has been designated, for legal purposes, as the illicit form of this group of drugs.

HISTORY

Opium has been harvested through the ages for recreational, religious, and medicinal purposes. Shakespeare, acknowledging both faces of opium, wrote: Within the infant rind of this small flower, Poison hath residence, and medicine power."[3]

Opium use dates back to earliest recorded history.[4] The Sumerians, who occupied what is now Iraq, were the first to isolate and use opium for religious purposes around 3000 BC. Opium was brought by Arab traders to India and China and eventually made its way to Europe. During the 17th century, opium abuse was well recognized in China, where there were unsuccessful efforts to suppress its rampant use. The Chinese, who attempted to restrict opium production and trade, were ultimately defeated by the British and French in a series of conflicts known as the Opium Wars.

It was not until 1806 that Friedrich Sertürner, a German pharmacist, isolated the alkaloid morphine from poppies. This milestone offered the potential for parenteral use. Until that time, only a relatively crude preparation was utilized from poppies. Morphine was soon recognized to be as addictive as opium. In 1898, Dreser synthesized diacetylmorphine (heroin), in hopes of finding a safer and less addicting opiate. As history bears out, this has not been the case.[5]

Over the years, additional agents with agonist, antagonist, and combined activities have been synthesized, each with its own therapeutic potential. More recently, the discovery of opiate receptors and endogenous ligands has led to an explosion of research aimed at improving our understanding of their biopharmacology, with efforts to manipulate the beneficial effects of opioids while eliminating the undesirable consequences.

Although the analgesic benefits of opioids are indisputable, there are countless ways in which opioid abuse takes its toll on society. The complications and issues span the boundaries of medicine, exemplified most notably by the intravenous (IV) drug user who may suffer from the immediate effects of parenteral heroin use and its secondary infectious (e.g., localized abscesses, endocarditis, hepatitis B, and AIDS) and noninfectious (e.g., addiction, potential for withdrawal) complications. Related to this category is the unfortunate neonate with the neonatal abstinence syndrome born to an IV drug-using or methadone-using mother, with attendant developmental problems and HIV risk. Presentations of other common problems include the suicidal patient with a history of intentional polypharmaceutical ingestion or the accidental pediatric overdose.

This chapter focuses on the clinical issues concerning the acute and chronic toxicology of opioids and appropriate treatment relevant to current clinical practice.

EPIDEMIOLOGY

Various methods have been used to estimate opioid use in our society. In 1993, the National Household Survey on Drug Abuse (NHSDA) reported that approximately 1% of those interviewed reported heroin use in their lifetime, with approximately 0.1% of respondents reporting use in the prior year. The NHSDA data are probably conservative figures, given the possible limitations of self-reporting and the exclusion of institutionalized and homeless persons.[5]

Another source has been the Drug Abuse Warning Network (DAWN). DAWN data are based on drug-related emergency department visits (acute and chronic issues) including requests for detoxification from a selected group of hospitals nationwide. Emergency department visits related to opioid use have continued to rise since the inception of the DAWN survey in the late 1970s. Heroin-related visits specifically have continued to increase since the early 1980s. During the period from 1990 to 1992, mention of heroin-related issues in emergency department evaluations increased by approximately 50%. This may reflect increased heroin use, a greater number of individuals seeking detoxification, or perhaps an older population of chronic heroin-using patients suffering from complications. This trend continued through the first half of 1993.[6]

Worldwide opium production has increased significantly since the 1980s. Southeast Asia produces the majority share, providing approximately 76% of the world's supply. Higher production, increasing purity, and lower prices have contributed considerably to the heroin problem. The higher purity enables users to smoke and snort heroin rather than to only inject it. This may also contribute to its more widespread use.[7]

PHARMACOLOGY

Chemical Identification and Structure

Opioids can be divided into five structural classes: phenanthrenes, diphenylheptanes, phenylpiperidines, benzomorphans, and morphinans (Table 36–1). The agents within each class share certain structural similarities but differ regarding chemical substitutions at specific sites (Fig. 36–1). For example, members of the phenanthrene group share similarities around their ring moiety and the N17 position, which have been demonstrated to confer opioid agonist activity. Substitutions at position 3 and 6 of the molecule may therefore play a role in explaining differences in potency of these agents. Similarly, additions

Table 36–1. Structural Classification of Opioid Agents

Phenanthrenes	Diphenylheptanes
Morphine	Methadone
Heroin	L-α-Acetylmethadol (LAAM)
Codeine	Propoxyphene
Hydrocodone	Phenylpiperidines
Hydromorphone	Meperidine
Oxycodone	Diphenoxylate
Oxymorphone	Fentanyl
Nalorphine	Sufentanil
Naloxone	Alfentanyl
Naltrexone	Fentanyl derivatives
Nalbuphine	Alphaprodine
Buprenorphine	Anileridine
Morphinan	Loperamide
Butorphanol	Profadol
Levorphanol	Benzomorphans
	Pentazocine

of a methyl group at the 3 or α carbon on fentanyl also dramatically increase the potency of the resulting molecule. These types of substitutions are critical in determining the amount of agonist, antagonist, or combined interaction with the various opioid receptors.[8, 9]

Endogenous Opioids

Any understanding of opioid toxicology requires a knowledge of the effects and activities of endogenous opioids at the molecular and cellular level. Endogenous opioids are naturally occurring peptides with various types of opioid activity. Although there are several types of endogenous opioids, they may be divided into three principal categories: (1) the enkephalins (methionine enkephalin and leucine enkephalin,[10] (2) the endorphins, and (3) the dynorphins. These are derived from proenkephalin, pro-opiomelanocortin, and prodynorphin, respectively,[11] and are found at various sites and in differing quantities throughout the central and peripheral nervous system. Complex interactions with multiple opioid receptors results in modulation of the response to painful stimuli.

Opioid Receptors

The development of synthetic opioid analogues has assisted in the characterization of opiate receptors and subtypes with which naturally occurring and exogenous opioids interact. Several of these receptors have been identified. These include mu, kappa, and delta (each with its own set of subtypes), along with the lesser known sigma and epsilon (Table 36–2).

Mu receptors were the first opioid binding sites described. The earliest agonists were related to morphine and were noted to have a high affinity for the mu receptor. Mu receptors are further classified into mu_1 and mu_2 subclasses. Mu_1 receptors have a high affinity for morphine and are postulated to have supraspinal analgesic properties. Mu_1 receptors are

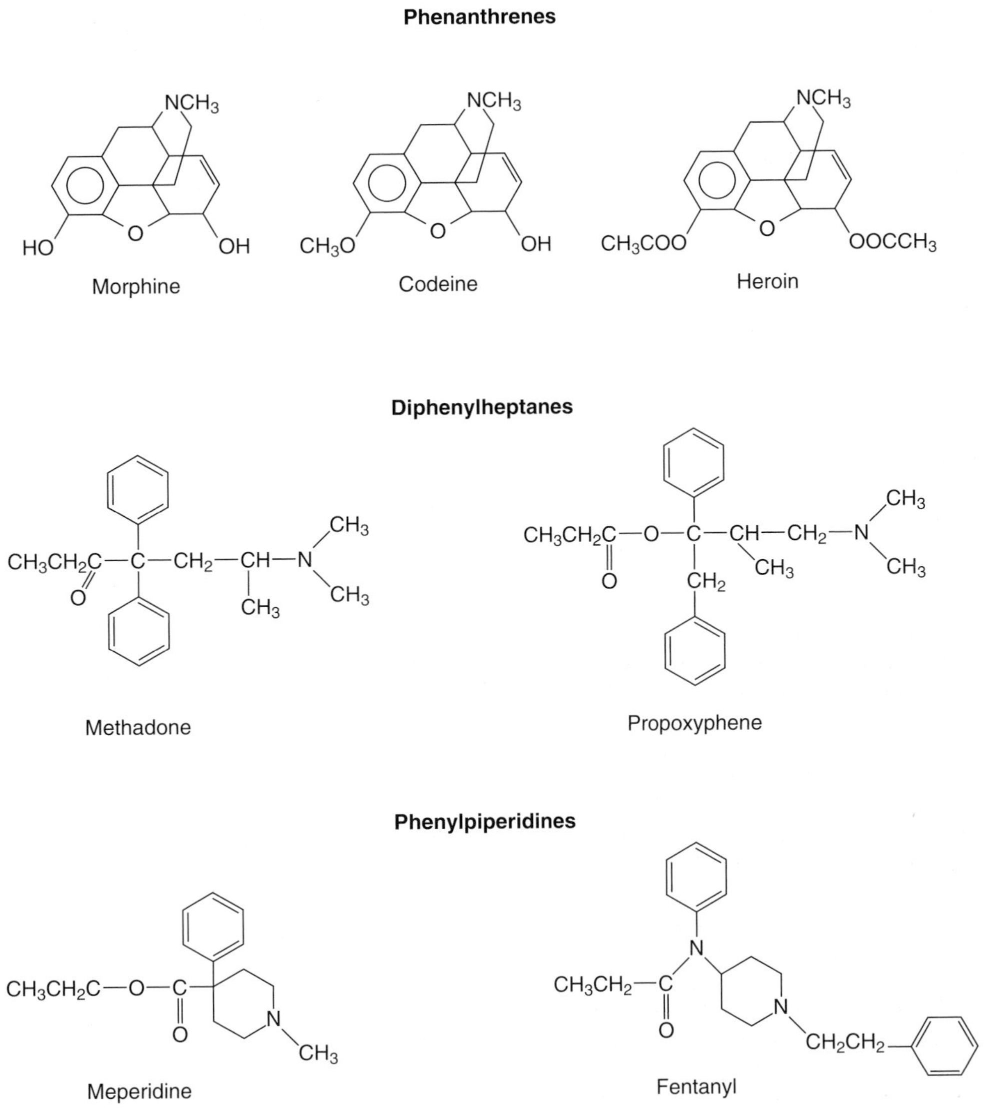

Phenanthrenes

NCH3 HO O OH Morphine

NCH3 CH3O O OH Codeine

NCH3 CH3COO O OOCCH3 Heroin

Diphenylheptanes

CH3CH2C—C—CH2—CH—N CH3 CH3 O CH3 Methadone

CH3CH2C—O—C—CH—CH2—N CH3 CH3 CH3 O CH2 Propoxyphene

Phenylpiperidines

CH3CH2C—O—C O N CH3 Meperidine

N CH3CH2—C O N CH2CH2 Fentanyl

Figure 36–1. Chemical structures of common opioids.

found in the peri-aqueductal gray matter, the nucleus raphe magnus, and the locus caeruleus. In fact, almost all analgesic properties of opiates are derived from this subclass. Stimulation of the mu_1 receptors causes almost none of the unwanted side effects of the opioids. Mu_2 receptors were noted to have a lower affinity for opioids than mu_1. Most of the untoward side effects of opioids can be attributed to stimulation of mu_2 receptors. These include respiratory depression, delayed gastrointestinal motility (leading to nausea, vomiting, and constipation), urinary retention, bradycardia, miosis, euphoria, and physical dependence.[12, 13]

Kappa agonists produce analgesia that is unaffected by tolerance or antagonists to mu receptors. $Kappa_1$ receptors appear to be concentrated in the spinal cord, whereas $kappa_3$ receptors appear to predominate in the supraspinal region. They may even outnumber mu receptors in that region. Agonists include pentazocine. Untoward effects of kappa stimulation include respiratory depression (less than mu), miosis, dysphoria, and psychotomimetic effects.[13, 14]

Delta receptors mediate spinal analgesia, specifically via thermal nociception. Both enkephalins and β-dynorphin bind to this class. Delta receptors also have a cortical distribution and may have a role interacting with centrally located mu receptors. Untoward side effects include respiratory depression via decreased respiratory rate.[14]

Sigma receptors have no role in analgesia. Stimulation of the sigma receptor may play a role in addictive side effects of opiates. Additional untoward effects include dysphoria and hallucinations. Beneficial effects include respiratory stimulation. Agonists include pentazocine and heroin.

The receptor epsilon has not yet been well elucidated. It apparently has a high affinity for β-endorphin, no affinity for enkephalin, and little analgesic activity.

Activation of these receptors results in inhibition of synaptic transmission in both the central nervous system and neural plexus in the periphery. An understanding of the various receptor types and their actions permits logical explanation of the activity of

Table 36–2. Classification of Opioid Receptor Subtypes and Actions from Animal Models

	Receptor Subtype	Agonists	Antagonists*
Analgesia			
Supraspinal	Mu_1, $kappa_3$, $delta_1$, $delta_2$	Analgesic	No effect
Spinal	Mu_2, $delta_2$, $kappa_1$	Analgesic	No effect
Respiratory function	Mu_2	Decrease	No effect
Gastrointestinal tract	Mu_2, kappa	Decrease transit	No effect
Psychotomimesis	Kappa	Increase	No effect
Feeding	Mu, kappa	Increase feeding	Decrease feeding
Sedation	Mu, kappa	Increase	No effect
Diuresis	$Kappa_1$	Increase	
Hormone regulation			
Prolactin	Mu_1	Increase release	Decrease release
Growth hormone	Mu_2 and/or delta	Increase release	Decrease release
Neurotransmitter release			
Acetylcholine	Mu_1	Inhibit	
Dopamine	Mu_2, delta	Inhibit	
Isolated organ bioassays			
Guinea pig ileum	Mu_2	Decrease	No effect
Mouse vas deferens	Delta	Decrease	No effect

*The actions listed for antagonists are seen with the antagonist alone. The subtypes responsible for a number of actions attributed to a general family of receptor have not been idenified. All the correlations in this table are based on studies in rats and mice, which occasionally show species differences. Thus, any extensions of these associations to human beings are tentative. Clinical studies do indicate that mu receptors elicit analgesia both spinally and supraspinally, but the subtypes have not been identified. Preliminary work with a synthetic opioid peptide, [D-Ala[2], D-Leu[5]]enkephalin, suggests that intrathecal delta agonists are analgesic in human beings.

Modified from Pasternak GW: Pharmacological mechanisms of opioid analgesics. Clinical Neuropharmacology *16*:3, 1993. From Reisine T, Pasternak G: Opioid analgesics and antagonists. *In* Hardman JG, Limbird LE, Molinoff PB, et al (eds): *Goodman and Gilman's the Pharmacological Basis of Therapeutics,* 9th ed. New York, McGraw-Hill, p 525, 1996.

opioid agonists, antagonists, and agonist-antagonist agents. These classifications are based on their activity (Table 36–3).

Pharmacokinetics

Opioids are generally well absorbed after oral, rectal, or parenteral administration. Nasal, buccal, or respiratory (for heroin and fentanyl) and transdermal absorption (fentanyl) is also readily accomplished for the more lipid-soluble opioids.[1, 15, 16] For some opioids there is variable reduction in bioavailability as a result of first-pass metabolism when absorbed through the gastrointestinal tract. For example, the bioavailability of morphine is reduced to about 25% (in contrast to codeine at 60%) when comparing oral versus parenteral routes of administration.[1]

After absorption, opioids are rapidly cleared from the blood and deposited primarily in kidney, liver, brain, lung, spleen, skeletal muscle, and placental tissue.[16, 17] Metabolism of individual opioids varies; however, they generally undergo hepatic metabolism with some form of conjugation, hydrolysis, oxidation, or dealkylation. Some of the resulting metabolites have been implicated in the activity or recognized toxic side effects of various opioids. Examples of this

Table 36–3. Actions and Selectivities of Opioids at the Various Receptor Classes

		Receptor Types			
Drug	**Activity**	*Mu*	*Delta*	*Kappa₁*	*Kappa₂*
Morphine	Agonist	+ + +		+	+
Methadone	Agonist	+ + +			
Levorphanol	Agonist	+ + +		NA	+ + +
Fentanyl	Agonist	+ + +			
Sufentanil	Agonist	+ + +	+	+	
Butorphanol	Agonist-Antagonist	P	NA	+ + +	NA
Buprenorphine	Agonist-Antagonist	P	NA	– –	NA
Nalorphine	Agonist-Antagonist	– – –		+	+ + +
Pentazocine	Agonist-Antagonist	P		+ +	+
Nalbupine	Agonist-Antagonist	– – –		+ +	+ +
Naloxone	Antagonist	– – –	–	– –	– –
Naltrexone	Antagonist	– – –	–	– – –	– –

Activities of drugs are given at the receptors for which the agent has reasonable affinity. +, agonist; –, antagonist; P, partial agonist; NA, no data available or inadequate. The number of symbols is an indication of potency, the ratio for a given drug denotes selectivity. These values were obtained primarily from animal studies and should be extrapolated to humans with caution.

Modified with permission from Reisine T, Pasternak G: Opioid analgesics and antagonists. *In* Hardman JG, Limbird LE, Molinoff PB, et al (eds): *Goodman and Gilman's the Pharmacological Basis of Therapeutics,* 9th ed. New York, McGraw-Hill, p 524, 1996.

include the metabolism of codeine to morphine,[18] morphine to the more active morphine-6-glucuronide,[1, 16] meperidine to the potentially harmful neurotoxic normeperidine,[19, 20] and propoxyphene to the potentially cardiotoxic norpropoxyphene.[21]

Protein binding and any interaction that alters it also plays a vital role in pharmacodynamics. The range of bound opioid varies from a low of 7% for codeine,[17] to greater than 90% for methadone.[1] Depression in albumin and other serum proteins resulting in decreased binding may produce higher levels of free opioid with possible opioid toxicity. Changes in serum pH (e.g., renal failure) may also alter protein binding of opiates.

Hepatic dysfunction may play a significant role in contributing to opioid toxicity.[22] Cirrhosis or other conditions associated with liver failure result in delayed hepatic metabolism of certain opioids (meperidine,[23] pentazocine,[24] and proxpoxyphene[25]), leading to accumulation and the development of CNS and respiratory depression.

Excretion of opiates occurs primarily via the renal route, with about 90% of the opioid metabolites eventually being excreted in the urine, usually via glomerular filtration. A small amount may end up in the gastrointestinal tract via enterohepatic circulation (e.g., morphine).[16] Renal failure will also lead to toxic effects, accumulated drug, or active metabolites (morphine-6-glucuronide[26] or normeperidine[18]).

Drug interactions may occur at various sites affecting the absorption, metabolism (e.g., induction of hepatic enzymes), and elimination of opioids (competition for renal excretion) contributing to the potentiation or reduction of their effects (Table 36–4). Acceleration of metabolism in the liver, which results from phenytoin ingestion, may result in diminished activity for certain drugs, such as methadone,[22, 27, 28] but may also result in an increase in potentially toxic metabolites (normeperidine).[29] The discontinuation of an interacting drug may play just as important a role as the addition of one in changing the bioavailability and activity of opioids. These interactions may lead to the onset of overdose or withdrawal symptoms.[30]

Ultimately, relative potency and half-life of each opioid are the key factors in the management of patients with opioid toxicity (Table 36–5). Morphine (10 mg given intramuscularly) is generally the standard against which potency comparisons are made. Duration of action and route of administration varies for each drug. These figures are based on therapeutic dosages. Few data are available to demonstrate pharmacokinetics.

CLINICAL MANIFESTATIONS OF OPIATE USE

As noted earlier, the physiologic effects of opioids are actually the result of interaction between the individual agent and multiple receptors. These interactions exert their primary effects on the CNS, the respiratory system, the cardiovascular system, and the gastrointestinal system.[1]

Table 36–4. Drug Interactions Resulting in Alteration in Opioid Activity

Opiate	Drug	Interaction Mechanism	Effect	Reference
Albentanil	Erythromycins	Decreased metabolism	Possible albentanil toxicity	98
Fentanyl	Enflurane	Decreased metabolism	Possible increased narcotic toxicity with bentanyl	99
Fentanyl	Halothane	Decreased metabolism	Possible increased narcotic toxicity with fentanyl	99
Meperidine	Acyclovir	Decreased renal excretion	Possible meperidine toxicity	100
Meperidine	Barbiturates	Increased merperidine metabolites	Increased CNS depression	101
Meperidine and congeners	β-adrenergic blockers	Mechanism not established	Increased narcotic toxicity	102
Meperidine and congeners	Cimetidine	Decreased metabolism	Increased narcotic toxicity	103
Meperidine and congeners	Monoamine oxidase inhibitors	Mechanism not established	Severe encephalopathy with meperidine	104
Meperidine and congeners	Phenothiazines	Toxic metabolite	Increased narcotic toxicity with chlorpromazine or thioridazine	105
Meperidine and congeners	Phenytoin	Increased metabolism	Decreased meperidine effect	106
Methadone	Barbiturates	Increased metabolism	Methadone withdrawal symptoms	107
Methadone	Carbamazepine	Probably increased metabolism	Methadone withdrawal symptoms	108
Methadone	Phenytoin	Increased metabolism	Decreased methadone effect	109
Methadone	Rifampin	Increased metabolism	Methadone withdrawal symptoms	110
Methadone	Fluvoxamine	Decreased methadone metabolism	Increased methadone effect with fluvoxamine	111
Morphine	Cimetidine	Probably decreased metabolism	Severe narcotic toxicity; renal failure may predispose to this	112
Morphine (controlled-release)	Metoclopramide	Probably increased absorption	Oversedation or possibly other toxicity with oral controlled-release	113
Propoxyphene	Monoamine oxidase inhibitors	Mechanism not established	Increased sedation and somnolence with propoxyphene	114

Table 36–5. A Comparison of Opioid Analgesics with Respect to Dosage, Duration of Action, and Some Distinguishing Features*

Nonproprietary Name	Trade Name	Route†	Dose,‡ mg	Duration of Action,§ h	Plasma Half-Life,¶ h	Distinguishing Features**
Morphine		IM, SC	10	4–5	2	See text
		O	60	4–7		
Heroin		IM, SC	5	4–5	0.5	1
(diacetylmorphine)		O	60			
Hydromorphone	Dilaudid	IM, SC	1.3	4–5	2–3	
(dihydromorphenone)		O	7.5	4–5		
Oxymorphone	Numorphan	IM, SC	1	4–6	2–3	
(dihydrohydroxymorphinone)		R	5	4–6		
Levorphanol	Levo-Dromoran	IM, SC	2	4–5	12–16	2
		O	4	4–7		
Methadone	Dolophine	IM	10	4–5	15–40	2
		O	20	4–6		
Meperidine	Demerol, Pethadol	IM, SC	75	3–5	3–4	3
(pethidine)		O	300	4–6		
Fentanyl	Sublimaze	IM	0.1	1–2	3–4	4
Codeine		IM	130	4–6	2–4	5
		O	200	4–6		
		O	10–20††			
Hydrocodone	Hycodan,	O	5–10‡‡	4–5	4	5, 6
(dihydrocodeinone)	others	O	5–10‡‡			
Drocode (dihydrocodeine)	Synalgos-DC, Compal	O	32‡‡	4–5	4	5, 6
Oxycodone	Roxicodone, Percodan,	O	5–10‡‡	4–5	—	
(dihydrohydroxycodeinone)	Percocet					
Propoxyphene	Darvon, others	O	65‡‡	4–6	6–12	5
Buprenorphine	Buprenex	IM	0.4	4–5	5	7
		SL	0.8	5–6		
Pentazocine	Talwin	IM, SC	30–60	4–6	4–5	7, 8, 9
		O	180	4–7		
Nalbuphine	Nubain	IM	10	4–6	2–3	6, 7
Butorphanol	Stadol	IM	2	4–6	2.5–3.5	6, 7

*The doses and durations of action in this table are based in part on Foley KM: The treatment of cancer pain. N Engl J Med *313*:84–85, 1985.

†IM, intramuscular; SC, subcutaneous; O, oral; SL, sublingual; R, rectal.

‡Except where noted, dose is the amount that produces approximately the same analgesic effect as 10 mg of morphine administered intramuscularly or subcutaneously.

§Average duration of action for the first single dose. The duration of action from a dose may vary with chronic dosing.

¶Average terminal half-life of parent molecule: some drugs have active metabolites with different half-lives.

****1,** Manufacture or importation in the United States is illegal. **2,** May exhibit cumulative effects with repeated dosing. **3,** Should be used cautiously with renal compromise due to accumulation of toxic metabolites. **4,** Transdermal preparations are available. **5,** Traditionally used orally primarily for treatment of moderate pain. **6,** Marketed in the United States in combination with additional ingredients. **7,** May produce withdrawal symptoms in individuals who are physically dependent on mu agonists. **8,** May produce marked irritation at injection sites. **9,** May produce psychotomimetic effects at higher doses.

††Oral antitussive dose.

‡‡Doses for moderate pain that are not necessarily equivalent to 10 mg of SC morphine.

From Reisine T, Pasternak G: Opioid analgesics and antagonists. *In* Hardman JG, Limbird LE, Molinoff PB, et al (eds): *Goodman and Gilman's the Pharmacological Basis of Therapeutics,* 9th ed. New York, McGraw-Hill, p 535, 1996.

CNS effects include analgesia via altered pain tolerance, sedation, euphoria, and dysphoria. Nausea and vomiting are secondary to stimulation of the chemoreceptor trigger zone in the medulla. Respiratory depression occurs by direct stimulation of the medullary respiratory center. The diminished sensitivity at this region results in an elevation of pCO_2 with resultant cerebral vasodilation, increased cerebral perfusion pressure, and increased intracranial pressure.

Cardiovascular effects are minimal at therapeutic doses but may include peripheral vasodilation resulting in orthostatic hypotension. histamine release may contribute strongly to the hemodynamic changes. Not uncommonly, transient bradycardia and hypotension secondary to occasional vasovagal episodes may accompany nausea and vomiting.

Gastrointestinal effects result in decreased gastric motility. Increased antral and proximal duodenal muscle tone results in delayed gastric emptying. This may contribute to (along with the primary central mechanism) the observed nausea and vomiting. Increased segmental tone and decreased longitudinal peristaltic contractions in the small intestine and colon may result in the common side effect of constipation. Spasm of the sphincter of Oddi may also occur with certain narcotics, resulting in symptoms characteristic of biliary colic.[1]

Clinical Presentation of Overdose

The most common settings for opioid overdose include IV heroin administration in the addict, accidental overdose in the pediatric population, or intentional overdose in the adult or adolescent patient as part of a suicide attempt or gesture. The rare "body packer," who presents with the leakage or potential leakage of drugs from the packets that are being transported within the gastrointestinal tract, may also be encountered.

Overdoses in addicts generally occur in two possible scenarios. The first is the user who unknowingly or naively uses a more potent grade of opioid. The second is the uninitiated or abstaining user who administers a dose beyond his or her perceived tolerance. In both of these settings, excessive opioid effects are observed and respiratory depression may result. The patient is typically found or presents in an obtunded state with varying degrees of respiratory depression. Diagnosis is usually aided by the presence of miosis and "track marks" (scarring from prior IV administration) or evidence of "skin popping" (scarring from prior subcutaneous [SC] administration). Patients who overdose as a result of "snorting" heroin may be less straightforward given the lack of cutaneous findings. Positive response to the administration of a narcotic antagonist is usually confirmatory. Additional history is usually unavailable.

Pediatric patients often present with overdoses resulting from access to pain medication or methadone from a family member or other individual in the household. Interpretation of clinical manifestations in this situation is critical, as the available history may be limited or nonexistent, particularly in the cases in which illicit drugs are involved.

The suicidal patient may present with a mixed picture resulting from a polysubstance ingestion, frequently accompanied by the co-ingestion of alcohol. History may be more helpful than in the prior scenarios. The patient is frequently accompanied by a family member or friend who confirms history, the patient's medication use, or simply having found pill bottles. Toxic doses of opioids may be difficult to assess in this circumstance, as tolerance, underlying medical conditions, and the addition of other substances all play a role in the manifestation of toxic side effects.

Patients with mild overdoses present with a slight depression in mental status, miosis, and minimal to no compromise in ventilation. More severe overdoses result in the triad of CNS depression (up to and including coma), miosis, and respiratory depression. Effects on respiration usually begin with a decrease in the respiratory rate while the tidal volume is maintained. In severe overdoses, respiratory arrest ensues. Hypoxia due to respiratory depression is the principal cause of most deaths from opioid agents.

Certain opiates, particularly heroin, can cause a fulminant but rapidly reversible form of pulmonary edema. Noncardiogenic pulmonary edema (NCPE) has been described as the most frequent complication of heroin overdose observed to occur in up to 48% of patients who present with heroin overdose in one study.[31] In contrast, a later study reported NCPE was diagnosed in only 2.4% of patients presenting to emergency departments, compared with the approximately 25% of heroin-using patients who were admitted.[32] The wide range may be reflective of numerous factors, including changes in heroin purity and methods of administration. Pneumonia, the next leading complication of heroin overdose (up to 30%),[30] may also play a role in this discrepancy. The actual incidence of NCPE in the general heroin-abusing population would be somewhat difficult to determine. The etiology of heroin-induced NCPE in heroin overdose remains unclear but may include a hypersensitivity reaction, an acute hypoxemia-induced capillary vasoconstriction resulting in increased hydrostatic pressure, or capillary injury secondary to the drug or adulterants.[33] Hypoxemia-induced injury seems to be the leading theory at present.

NCPE is characterized by tachypnea, tachycardia, hypoxia, and rales on auscultation. Pulmonary capillary wedge pressure is typically normal. Laboratory abnormalities include respiratory acidosis, and radiographic evaluation usually demonstrates bilateral patchy infiltrates. Onset may occur from minutes to several hours after heroin use. Prior reviews indicate that onset may be delayed as much as 24 hours after heroin administration,[34] whereas more recent studies report a much earlier onset.[31] Methadone and other opiates have also been linked to NCPE, although its occurrence is uncommon.[35, 36]

Additional complications from opioid overdoses have included seizures, most often attributed to propoxyphene[37, 38] or meperidine[39] overdose. Heroin also appears to be a potential causative agent.[40] The mechanism for opioid-induced seizures is not totally clear; however, at least two distinct causes have been postulated based on therapy with opioid antagonists. Although seizures from heroin, morphine, and propoxyphene overdose have been treated successfully with naloxone, animal studies indicate that naloxone may actually lower seizure threshold in meperidine overdoses. The toxic metabolite normeperidine has been implicated in cases involving meperidine.[28, 41, 42] Additional neurologic effects have included a parkinsonian syndrome believed to be secondary to 1-methyl-4-phenyl-1,2,3,6-tetrahydropyridine (MPTP), a by-product of meperidine synthesis.[43, 44]

Cardiac conduction disturbances have also been noted and are primarily attributed to proxpoxyphene and its metabolites.[45, 46] Manifestations of cardiac toxicity include QRS prolongation, ventricular irritability, and ST-T wave abnormalities. These changes do not appear to be influenced by narcotic antagonists.[47]

DIAGNOSIS

Diagnosis of the opioid overdose should be based primarily on history and clinical presentation. Additional laboratory data are useful in the consideration of other processes or conditions that may be contributing to the patient's symptoms or findings. This is particularly true in the IV drug user who may have additional underlying conditions or complications.

Drug screens are of mixed utility depending on the information being sought and the time frame in which results will be available to guide the clinical management of the patient. Patients with pure opioid ingestions generally have specific toxindromes (e.g., miosis, respiratory depression, CNS depression), which suggest a specific therapy. Situations involving polysubstance administration may be less straightforward, but clinical judgment, general toxicologic principles, and supportive measures are usually employed before receiving results of a toxic screen. Situations in which opioid screens could be beneficial include monitoring of "detox" patients to ensure compliance with abstinence and methadone use, treating a potential "dual-diagnosis" patient in whom treatment would be altered based on the presence of other drugs, and in occupational settings in which the individual's job may involve public safety. To reiterate, the toxic screen is frequently unhelpful and merely confirmatory in the patient who presents with a presumed acute overdose.

Screening techniques must be able to detect parent compounds and their active metabolites in typical serum or urine ranges after administration in the usual manner for the given agent. Urine drug screens can provide a qualitative method to detect many opioids, including propoxyphene, codeine, methadone, meperidine, and morphine. Screens for fentanyl and its derivatives are usually negative. Quantitative data on opiates from serum are not helpful in the routine management of overdoses. The serum drug screen may, however, be helpful in detecting the presence of agents other than opiates that may alter therapy (e.g., acetominophen).

TREATMENT

The initial evaluation and management of opioid overdoses focuses on stabilization. Priorities include assessment and establishment of effective ventilation and oxygenation, followed by ensuring adequate hemodynamic support. Initial support with a bag-valve-mask (BMV) device is appropriate, along with 100% oxygen supplementation. Oral or nasal airway placement may be helpful. Caution is advised with their use, however, given the potential for vomiting and/or aspiration. Suction apparatus should be available for immediate use at the patient's bedside. Ventilatory support can usually be safely provided with a BMV device while awaiting the reversal of respiratory depression by an opioid antagonist. Endotracheal intubation is indicated in severely compromised patients in whom there is a real risk for aspiration or in patients who do not respond satisfactorily to opioid antagonists. Treatment of NCPE will require 100% oxygen therapy with positive end-expiratory pressure (PEEP), if necessary, to reverse hypoxia. Diuretics and digoxin have no role in NCPE. The role of opioid antagonists in the treatment of NCPE is unclear at this time.

The options for opioid antagonists include naloxone, naltrexone, and the more recently approved and longer-acting nalmefene.[48, 49] These pure opiate antagonists bind with great affinity to mu receptors and should be titrated according to the given situation. Naloxone probably remains the drug of choice as the initial reversal agent in a suspected opioid overdose, given its short half-life and ability to titrate for effect. The need for immediate results (usually in the form of increased ventilation) is balanced by the potential unpleasant effects of inducing withdrawal symptoms in the chronic abuser. In the patient who presents with respiratory arrest, however, precipitation of some acute withdrawal symptoms may be unavoidable. To minimize this risk, consider giving the drug in small increments titrated to the response. Conveniently, naloxone can be administered IV,[50] IM, SC, endotracheally,[51] and intralingually.[52]

Naloxone dose is based on the circumstances; it generally ranges from 0.4 to 2.0 mg, IV, in the adult patient. If a patient presents with a depressed mental status and pinpoint pupils, but without respiratory depression, a lower dose of 0.1 to 0.8 mg, IV, is recommended. For respiratory depression or arrest, 2 mg IV, is suggested initially, to be repeated every 2 to 5 minutes (or sooner if the patient is indeed in respiratory arrest), up to 10 mg. Certain opiate overdose scenarios may require repetitive or continuous administration of opiate antagonist. These include cases involving pentazocine, codeine, proxpoxyphene, methadone, and diphenoxylate, and cases in which body packing is suspected. If no response is observed after a total of 10 mg is reached, it is unlikely that narcotics by themselves are playing a significant role in the patient's clinical status.[53]

Until recently, constant infusion of naloxone was suggested for recurrent cardiorespiratory depression. The recommended dose is 0.4 to 0.8 mg/hour, IV (suggested only if an initial bolus has reversed respiratory depression). Another regimen for constant infusion is recommended by Goldfrank and colleagues.[54] Their scheme requires determining the amount of naloxone that will restore respiratory function but will not induce full-blown withdrawal symptoms, usually 0.4 to 4.0 mg. Next, give two-thirds of that dose as an hourly infusion until naloxone can be discontinued. Finally, approximately 20 to 30 minutes after the initial bolus, give another bolus of approximately half the original size.

Nalmefene may provide a simpler and preferable alternative to naloxone infusions, given its longer half-life (4 to 8 hours compared with 1 hour for naloxone).[48] Nalmefene is given as an initial dose of 0.5 mg, IV, to reverse respiratory depression in the adult patient. A repeat dose of 1.0 mg can be given 2 to 5 minutes later if necessary. Nalmefene will undoubtedly have a role in the treatment of acute opioid overdosage given its safety and longer duration of action.[48, 49]

The current recommendation for pediatric dosing of naloxone is 0.1 mg/kg given IV.[55] Prior recommendations of 0.01 mg/kg are probably acceptable for the neonate but are not adequate for the toddler.[56] Toddlers reportedly have the same number of opioid receptors as an adult. It is believed that the response to naloxone may be more dependent on number of receptors than weight.[57] Naloxone has a wide therapeutic index in the pediatric and adult population. No published pediatric dosing reference is available for nalmefene at this writing.

Routine empiric administration of naloxone has been recommended based on utility and safety to all patients presenting with diminished mental status. This practice has been challenged because a great number of individuals do not benefit.[57, 58] Retrospective studies have been performed analyzing clinical criteria in suspected opiate overdoses to predict potential benefit from naloxone. Criteria found to be somewhat useful include diminished respirations (≥12 per minute), pinpoint pupils, and circumstantial evidence of opiate use, such as needle track marks. One or more of these criteria was found to be 92% sensitive and 76% specific in predicting a positive response to the administration of naloxone in the setting of opiate intoxication.[58]

Administration of naloxone to a patient on discharge is not recommended for a number of reasons. Naloxone frequently has a shorter half-life than many of the agents whose actions it is given to reverse. Patients may show recurrence of CNS and respiratory depression within an hour of administration. Second, the patient may attempt to counteract iatrogenic withdrawal symptoms by using a higher dose of opiate to overcome naloxone's effect. Nalmefene has been suggested as an alternative to naloxone in this setting, given its relative safety and prolonged duration of action. Nalmefene may be beneficial in cases in which prolonged action (e.g., in methadone or propoxyphene overdoses), or delayed onset of action (e.g., in pentazocine and diphenoxylate ingestions) may be concerns. Other conditions in which delayed metabolism is a factor, as in hepatic failure, renal failure, or severe overdoses, may benefit from a narcotic antagonist with a longer half-life.[48, 49]

The safety of naloxone has been demonstrated in numerous studies and by a lack of untoward effects despite its nearly universal administration in the "coma cocktail."[59, 80] There have been, however, scattered reports of adverse reactions from naloxone aside from the initiation of withdrawal symptoms.[55] These include hypertension,[61] pulmonary edema,[62–65] seizures,[65] ventricular irritability,[66] and even death.[67] All of these cases were noted in the peri-operative setting. The presence of additional medications, comorbid conditions, and a lack of supporting documentation in certain cases suggest that these complications may not be attributable to naloxone alone.[64] Caution should be exercised in the administration of naloxone to perioperative critical care patients, especially those with underlying acute cardiac conditions, given the possibility of precipitating unfavorable hemodynamics.

Opioid antagonists are often used in the diagnostic evaluation and treatment of patients who present with altered mental status. However, the decision to administer naloxone and the amount to give may be guided by certain historical and clinical criteria and does not need to be administered reflexively to every individual who presents with altered mental status. The drowsy individual who was found with a syringe at his side or has obvious track marks on his extremities is most probably under the influence of heroin. If the patient's respiratory status is adequate and the patient is easily arousable, the administration of naloxone is not necessarily indicated. Ultimately, the patient may receive naloxone and become more awake, uncomfortable, and unpleasant for the duration of the effect of the antagonist, or he or she may simply remain in a stable, somewhat lethargic state, until the heroin wears off. Naloxone will not expedite the rate at which an opioid is cleared; it merely causes temporary reversal of the effects. In summary, for the individual who by history or examination is suffering the effects of mild heroin overdose without respiratory compromise, observation is generally adequate treatment.

In other situations, including the potential for polysubstance abuse or significant trauma, it is more imperative to establish which of the patient's clinical symptoms can be attributed to opioid as opposed to nonopioids or to non–drug-related issues. In such cases, it is wise to begin with smaller doses of naloxone (0.1 to 0.4 mg, IV) to reverse potential opioid effect on the patient's neurologic status, without inducing a full-blown withdrawal syndrome. If no results are obtained with the initial bolus, higher doses can be given, as suggested in the previous section. Nalmefene or continuous infusions of naloxone can be given if sustained results are necessary.

Decontamination is generally reserved for agents taken orally. Opiates cause decreased gastric emptying and pylorospasm. This decrease in gastrointestinal motility suggests that there may be some benefit to gastrointestinal decontamination several hours post ingestion. Factors that affect gastrointestinal decontamination include the agent, route of administration, additional co-ingestants (which may contribute to potential toxicity or affect gastrointestinal motility), absorption or metabolism, and time from ingestion to presentation. Gastric lavage is effective in debulking large amounts of ingestant, but it may also be beneficial with smaller amounts of ingestants due to slowed gastric motility. In the obtunded patient, endotracheal intubation should be performed prior to the placement of orogastric or nasogastric tubes, to protect against aspiration. If the administration of an opioid antagonist meets initially with good results, nasogastric or orogastric tube placement is possible, as long as the patient is under close observation for deterioration that might increase the risk of aspiration.

Activated charcoal and cathartic (e.g., magnesium citrate or sorbitol) should be administered after gastric emptying if bowel sounds are present. The initial dose of activated charcoal is 1.0 g/kg by mouth or per nasogastric tube. Repetitive dosing of activated charcoal may be beneficial in cases in which large amounts of ingestant are suspected (e.g., "mules" or "body packers," discussed later). The use of whole-bowel irrigation has been employed with mixed reviews. Use of polyethylene glycol solution has been credited for successful recovery of heroin packets.[68] However, it was hypothesized to play a role in the deterioration of one patient's condition, in whom heroin was thought to be solubilized as a result of its administration.[69] Gastric emptying by ipecac is not recommended given the potential for rapid deterioration and the risk of aspiration. Forced diuresis, peritoneal dialysis, and hemodialysis have no role in opiate overdoses.

Assessment and treatment should not preclude workup of other medical conditions or trauma that may explain part or all of the patient's clinical presentation. The IV drug user or polysubstance abuser is also at risk for coincident conditions, both infectious and noninfectious. Some diligence and patience is required in the evaluation of these patients. The duration of observation or decision to admit depends on multiple factors, including the agent ingested, coingestants, amount of ingestant, the patient's tolerance to opioids, the clinical presentation, additional co-morbid conditions, and the provider's ability to satisfactorily remove the ingestant.

Opiate-induced seizures may be treated with naloxone except in cases of meperidine overdose. As previously mentioned, meperidine-related seizures may actually be aggravated by the administration of naloxone.[41, 42] Benzodiazepines are safe in this scenario, although they may potentially increase CNS and respiratory depression. The use of benzodiazepines is also reasonable given the possibility of polysubstance use or even underlying seizure disorders.

Disposition

Factors that favor prolonged observation or admission include abuse of agents with long half-lives, higher amounts of ingestant, low tolerance to opioids (as compared to that of the chronic abuser), persistent respiratory or hemodynamic instability, and comorbid conditions. Drugs with longer half-lives may require prolonged observation and/or admission, even if the patient's initial presentation is relatively stable (e.g., methadone, *L*-α-acetylmethadol [LAAM], propoxyphene, diphenoxylate). Although administering an opiate antagonist can have a temporizing effect, the effects of a methadone overdose, for example, will significantly outlast several doses of naloxone and may require a continuous naloxone drip or the use of nalmetene. The delay in onset of significant symptoms for up to 6 hours after ingestion is an added reason for prolonged observation in cases involving methadone and diphenolxylate.

The amount of ingestant may be important, but if gastric decontamination is performed soon after ingestion, and charcoal is rapidly administered, this may not be as crucial a factor. Such decontamination obviously applies only to oral opioids. It is crucial to search for co-ingestants, as synergistic effects (e.g., decreased respiratory drive with benzodiazipine ingestion) and need for additional treatment or decontamination methods might be necessary.

Specific Treatment Issues

Heroin

Heroin is generally bought by the "bag" (25 mg) or quarter gram, with preferences and purity varying from region to region. Purity and adulterants play a considerable role in the outcome and complications of heroin use. There is a wide range of purity (and lack thereof) in the supply of heroin, with the potential for tampering occurring at several levels before it is actually used by the addict. A Denmark study revealed that the average purity of wholesale samples (45%) was only slightly higher than the purity of retail samples (36%).[70] Adulterants may include noscapine, caffeine, procaine, various sugars, phenobarbital, methaqualone, quinine, and paracetamol in combination with caffeine.[70, 72] Heroin base and heroin hydrochloride each accounted for approximately half of the samples during the 1980s. However, in recent years the base form has become predominant.

IV use of heroin remains the preferred route of administration among heroin addicts. The powder is heated in a spoon or bottle cap until it is dissolved. The heroin is passed through cotton or a cigarette filter into a syringe and is then injected IV or SC ("skin popping"). The attempts to extract additional drug by boiling the cotton filters has resulted in a condition known as "cotton fever," the etiology of which remains unclear.[53]

Comparable pharmacokinetics have been observed when comparing smoking to IV routes of heroin administration. Heroin appeared rapidly in blood and peaked 1 to 5 minutes after smoking, similar to that observed following IV administration. The rapid onset of pharmacologic effects, together with the early appearance of heroin and metabolites in blood following smoked heroin, demonstrated the effectiveness of this route of administration. It is evident that the smoking route enables individuals to obtain similar pharmacologic effects as are produced by IV administration of heroin.[71]

A recent study among heroin addicts found that "chasing the dragon" (the term applied to the inhalation of the fumes of pyrolyzed heroin) was preferred in as many as 44% of studied individuals. Fears of HIV and other infectious complications have made the latter method increasingly popular.[72] A summary of potential complications of opiate use are listed (Table 36–6).

Methadone

Methadone presents a significant problem for clinicians by virtue of its pharmacokinetic properties and widespread availability as the most frequently used agent in heroin treatment programs. Methadone is well absorbed when taken orally and has a duration

Table 36–6. Medical Complications of Opiate Use

Infection

Acquired immunodeficiency syndrome (AIDS)
Endocarditis: Suspected in any user with fever of undetermined origin, murmur, pneumonia, embolic phenomena, or positive blood cultures
- Bacterial: Characteristically right-sided; most commonly *Staphylococcus aureus,* generally penicillin- and possibly methicillin-resistant; *Escherichia coli, Pseudomonas,* and enterococci less frequent; prior cardiac disease is rare; slowly progressive; septic emboli to lungs
- Fungal: Most frequent in users with prior cardiac disease; *Candida* most common; mycotic aneurysm

Soft tissue infections
- Abscess, nodules, ulcers: Fever and leukocytosis with no source of infection are common; infections due to pathogenic contaminants and nonsterile injection technique
- Tetanus: Opportunistic infection at compromised lesion site
- Malaria, tuberculosis: Sharing of contaminated paraphernalia
- Bacteremia, sepsis: Staphylococci most common; streptococci; pneumococci; *Salmonella*
- Hepatitis: Hepatitis B most common; assumed to be present in any hospitalized addict; subclinical to lethal disease

Pulmonary

Pneumonia: Patients treated for pneumonia should be observed for 7–10 d after antibiotic therapy is completed to avoid overlooking signs of endocarditis
- Bacterial: Generally staphylococci
- Fungal: *Candida* predominates
- Aspiration: Must be differentiated from pulmonary edema; typically produces increased respiratory rate as opposed to the slowed respiratory rate observed in pulmonary edema with respiratory center depression

Pulmonary edema: "Heroin lung." Most commonly observed in heroin, propoxyphene, and methadone poisoning; presents in combination with respiratory center depression
Embolism: May result as complication of endocarditis, especially of tricuspid and pulmnic valves, and may result in abscess formation or emboli from injected material such as talc, starch, quinine
Atelectasis
Fibrosis, granulomas: Cause not established; perhaps due to opiate diluent deposition; decreased vital capacity, mild-to-moderate decrease in oxygen diffusion capacity across alveolar capillary membrane; may result in pulmonary hypertension and precipitate heart failure; chest x-ray may be normal or reveal bilateral reticular basilar infiltrates, pulmonary artery enlargement, or hilar adenopathy

Dermatologic

"Tracks" and scars are cutaneous evidence of drug abuse; caused by nonsterile injection technique and injection of fibrogenic particulate matter
Abscess, ulcerative: Usually multiple, hyperpigmented, and linear
Cellulitis: Strong or wood-hard tenseness
Lymphangitis
Phlebitis
Sphaceloderma: Gangrene of the skin

Neurologic

Cerebral edema
Transverse myelitis: Acute paraplegia, occasionally persistent; thoracic sensory levels are characteristic; caused by adulterants, transient ischemia, hypersensitivity reaction, or direct opiate effect
Horner's syndrome: from supraclavicular injection
Postanoxia encephalopathy
Polyneuritis
Crush injury

Hepatic

Cirrhosis: Abnormal liver function likely due to infection sequelae, toxic adulterants, and concomitant chronic alcohol ingestion
Alcoholic hepatic disease

Renal

Nephropathy: Glomerulonephritis
Immune complex nephritis

Musculoskeletal

Infectious spondylitis, sacroiliitis: Hematogenous spread from nonsterile injection
Lumbar vertebral osteomyelitis: *Staphylococcus aureus, Pseudomonas aeruginosa, Klebsiella, Enterobacter, Mycobacterium, Serratia marcescens, Candida*
Myositis ossificans: "Drug abuser's elbow"—extraosseous metaplasia injury to brachialis muscle due to poor injection technique with calcification development
Camptodactylia: Irreducible finger flexion and hand edema from injections into fingers and hand veins

Hematologic

Thrombocytopenia: Immunologic mechanisms, quinine-induced
Leukopenia: Bone marrow depression
Anemia: Repetitive blood donations

Laboratory

Hypergammaglobulinemia: Elevated IgM, IgG in 90% of addicts; may lead to false-positive results on many serologic tests; elevated immunoglobulins return to normal levels when street drug use is discontinued
False-positive VDRL
↓ C_3 and total complement

From Hubbell KC: Opiates and narcotics. *In* Haddad LM, Winchester JF (eds): Clinical Management of Poisoning and Drug Overdose. 2nd ed. Philadelphia, WB Saunders, 1990, p 713.

of action of up to 24 hours after administration. Patients presenting with a history or evidence of a significant methadone ingestion usually require admission and/or prolonged observation.

Lomotil

Lomotil, is a combination of diphenoxylate (2.5 mg) and atropine (0.025 mg) used for symptomatic relief of diarrhea by altering gastrointestinal motility. It has a low therapeutic index and exhibits a biphasic picture after ingestions. Atropinic effects or anticholinergic symptoms usually precede opiate toxicity and may include flushing, mydriasis, tachycardia, tachypnea, hyperpyrexia, hypotonia, confusion, and/or hallucinations. Duration of this phase may be 2 to 3 hours. The subsequent phase is characterized by opioid effects and may begin from 2 to 3 hours postingestion up to several (36) hours postingestion.[73] Treatment considerations include adequate decontamination via gastric lavage and activated charcoal, use of naloxone to reverse opiate effects (usually higher doses and for a more prolonged period of time), and admission or prolonged observation (24 hours). An initial improvement between phases may falsely reassure the inexperienced, leading to inappropriate early discharge. Children, especially younger than 2 years, are much more sensitive to the effects of diphenoxylate and should be observed and/or admitted for prolonged observation.[73]

Pentazocine

A mixed narcotic agonist-antagonist, pentazocine is associated with a fairly specific scenario of parenteral abuse when used in combination with the antihistamine tripelennamine (pyribenzamine). This combination, known as "T's and blues," once solubilized and injected, was previously popular among addicts because of its heroin-like "rush" and lower cost.[74] The initial injection results in a brief rush, which dissipates quickly but is potentiated by multiple subsequent doses, producing a euphoric state for several hours.[75, 76] Pentazocine alone apparently results in dysphoria and therefore does not have the same abusive potential as the combination. Complications from both pentazocine or the parenteral combination have included seizures, local abscesses, and skin necrosis. Treatment issues remain similar to those for opiate ingestions, with the possible need for higher-dose naloxone to effect reversal. Pentazocine is now packaged as Talwin NX (a combination of pentazocine and naloxone). Taken IV, the medication induces withdrawal symptoms. The naloxone component is actually inactivated when taken orally, thus avoiding induction of withdrawal symptoms.

Propoxyphene

Overdoses of Darvon and related compounds are characterized by a rapid onset of symptoms (i.e., generally within 30 minutes), ranging from nausea and vomiting to central nervous system depression, seizures, respiratory depression, and cardiovascular collapse.[37, 38] Pulmonary edema[77] and cardiac conduction disturbances have also been noted.[78, 79] Treatment considerations include rapid gastrointestinal decontamination by gastric lavage while ensuring adequate airway protection. The use of ipecac is not recommended given the potential for CNS depression. Naloxone in higher doses and for longer duration is frequently required to reverse the respiratory and CNS depression caused by propoxyphene. Naloxone may be used to treat propoxyphene-induced seizure activity, but there is too little experience to demonstrate its benefit in humans. Animal studies do not reveal any benefit to naloxone in cardiac disturbances associated with proxpoxyphene.[21, 80] Patients frequently require longer observation or admission to the hospital compared to the typical opioid overdose patient.

Fentanyl and Derivatives

Fentanyl (Sublimaze) was first used in the 1960s as a synthetic narcotic in the perioperative setting. Its potency, rapid onset of action, and short duration of action, make it an ideal agent for operative use. A dose of 100 μg of fentanyl is equivalent to approximately 10 mg of morphine sulfate. Numerous potent, illicitly synthesized derivatives have been based on fentanyl. These include α-methyl fentanyl ("China White"), and 3-methyl fentanyl. The latter may be 6000 times more potent than morphine and may represent great addictive and abuse potential.[81] Although fentanyl derivative overdoses appear clinically similar to opioid overdoses, they may be puzzling diagnostically, as toxic screens frequently do not reveal their presence. Toxic effects may be experienced with very small amounts, which current screens may not be sensitive enough to detect. Also, because they are structurally different compounds than opioids, routine screens for opioids may not reveal fentanyl derivatives. Treatment considerations are similar to those for opioids, although these substances generally have markedly shorter half-lives. A number of deaths have been attributed to these agents secondary to marked increased potency compared to heroin.[81, 82]

"Body Stuffers" and "Body Packers"

The ingestion of of opioids in various types of packages for purposes of concealment—either for smuggling or merely to hide drugs when threatened by authorities—can be quite serious when these parcels open or leak.[68, 83] Although there is significant first-pass metabolism on absorption of opioids from the gastrointestinal tract, the quantities involved are usually relatively large, so they can still be quite hazardous.

The individual who conceals a bag of heroin or other contraband is known as a "body stuffer," frequently using various orifices or body cavities to hide his or her stash. Methods include swallowing packaged drug or inserting it rectally or vaginally. The "body packer" usually swallows multiple packages of heroin or other illicit drugs for purposes of transport across borders with the intent to sell or receive compensation for transporting the drug. Rupture or leakage of these packets can be lethal because of the amounts of opioids involved.

Discovery of these individuals is difficult, and treatment of a symptomatic patient may require some suspicion if the history is not obvious. Radiologic examination may provide evidence of the abdominal packages and aid in the diagnosis. Initial treatment is similar to that for other opioid ingestions and includes stabilization, gastric lavage, and administration of activated charcoal to bind any remaining free opioids. As discussed previously, additional treatment may include cathartics and/or whole-bowel irrigation. Surgery has been suggested in cases involving large amounts of retained packages, especially with evidence of leakage of opioids into the gastrointestinal tract.[68, 83]

Opiate Addiction

The triad of tolerance, psychological dependence, and physical dependence define the addicted or drug-dependent personality. Tolerance is the need for increasing quantities of a given agent to provide an equivalent response over time. This is reflected by either an increase in dose or frequency of the specified agent or substitution of a more potent or longer-acting agent. The speed or degree of tolerance may vary from one agent to the next and from one individual to another. Euphoria, CNS depression, and respiratory depression may be affected variably by tolerance. Constipation and miosis remain despite tolerance, to a lesser degree.

Psychological dependence encompasses the prototypical conduct surrounding the drug-abusing culture. Aspects include compulsive drug seeking and drug procurement behavior.

Physical dependence occurs when the organ systems affected by a given agent, in this case opioids, exhibit signs and symptoms upon withdrawal or when an opioid antagonist is introduced. The presence of a withdrawal syndrome on discontinuing an agent confirms the presence of physical dependence. The withdrawal syndromes of most opioids share similarities. Withdrawal from longer-acting opioids generally provides less intense symptoms.

Abstinence Syndromes

Animal studies have provided evidence that the phenomenon of opiate withdrawal is mediated at multiple sites, both centrally and peripherally. Studies utilizing opiate antagonists have confirmed the role of the mu receptor in mediating withdrawal symptoms. The locus ceruleus and the periaqueductal gray matter have been determined to be activating sites for opiate withdrawal.[84] When the addict abruptly stops using opiates (most commonly heroin), there is an increase in circulating norepinephrine, which leads to increased sympathetic discharge. Lesions at the locus ceruleus (resulting in depletion of norepinephrine) can significantly diminish these symptoms. This may provide an explanation for the utility of clonidine in opiate withdrawal, as it acts on central α_2-receptors and thereby diminishes firing at the locus ceruleus. Fluctuation in levels of cyclic adenosine monophosphate (cAMP) has been demonstrated with administration and withdrawal of both opiates and clonidine. The withdrawal state induced by either the administration of naloxone or the discontinuation of opiate generally results in elevated cAMP levels. The administration or continuation of opiates or clonidinene generally leads to a decrease in cAMP levels that correlates with the resolution of any withdrawal symptoms that may have occurred. Chronic opiate use results in a dampened response and the return of cAMP levels to normal. Peripheral receptors have also been implicated in the manifestation of withdrawal symptoms.[84]

Withdrawal is a factor in frequently encountered scenarios, including encounters with patients seeking detoxification, the unanticipated hospitalization or incarceration of a patient who is denied his usual supply of drugs, and the iatrogenic withdrawal that occurs when an opiate antagonist is given for a suspected opiate overdose. Treatment issues surrounding each depend heavily on the setting and supervision available.

Table 36–7. Time Course of Opiate Withdrawal

Agent	Onset of Withdrawal	Peak of Withdrawal	Duration of Withdrawal
Short-acting			
Meperidine	3–6 h	8–12 h	3–5 d
Intermediate-acting			
Morphine, heroin, codeine, hydromorphone, oxycodone	6–8 h	2–4 d	5–10 d
Long-acting			
Methadone	36–72 h	5–8 d	10–15 d

Factors that play a role in opiate withdrawal include the type of opiate (Table 36–7),[85–87] the total dose used, the interval between administrations, the duration of use, and the general health of the individual addict. Objective signs of opiate withdrawal typically include mild hypertension, tachycardia, increased respiratory rate and depth, mydriasis, lacrimation, rhinorrhea, sneezing, piloerection, cold sweats, vomiting, diarrhea, and yawning (Table 36–8).[88] Subjective symptoms include restlessness, insomnia, anxiety, headache, anorexia, feverishness, chills, nausea, abdominal cramps, and muscle spasm and cramps. Although it is uncomfortable, the withdrawal syndrome is not life-threatening.

Pharmacologic Treatment of Opiate Withdrawal

Prior to the availability of methadone, the detoxification of patients with opiate addiction was essentially accomplished by abstinence, so-called "going cold turkey" (a reference to the gooseflesh appearance of the skin from piloerection during withdrawal). Current treatment of the opiate withdrawal syndrome is primarily pharmacologic. Regimens include long acting opioid agents such as methadone or LAAM, centrally active α_2-blocking agents (e.g., clon-

Table 36–8. Signs and Symptoms of Opiate Withdrawal

Early	Intermediate	Late
Yawning	Mydriasis	Involuntary muscle spasm
Lacrimation	Piloerection	Fever
Rhinorrhea	Flushing	Nausea
"Yen sleep"	Diaphoresis	Intestinal discomfort
Perspiration	Tachycardia	Diarrhea
	Twitching	Vomiting
	Tremor	Spontaneous ejaculation or orgasm
	Restlessness	
	Irritability	Increased blood glucose level
	Anorexia	

From Easom JM, Lovejoy FH: Opiates. *In* Haddad LM, Winchester JF: Clinical Management of Poisoning and Drug Overdose. Philadelphia, WB Saunders, p 429, 1983.

idine), anxiolytic agents to blunt certain unpleasant withdrawal symptoms (e.g., benzodiazepines), or a simple tapering scheme if the agent in question was a prescribed medication.

For many years methadone was the primary pharmacologic therapy for opiate withdrawal. Its relatively short onset of action (30 to 60 minutes) and long half-life permit a once- or twice-daily dosing schedule. Suggested methadone withdrawal regimens include the establishment of an initial dose of methadone by titrating up from 5 to 20 mg every 6 hours until withdrawal symptoms are alleviated.[89] The provider should be guided by objective findings rather than subjective symptoms in the initial titration of methadone. The drug is then left at a stable dose for a variable period of time, followed by a period of tapering.

Methadone is typically dosed at 40 to 80 mg, orally, daily, once the patient's condition has been stabilized. The higher dosing range has been associated with a trend toward decreased illicit drug use.[90] The detoxification period may range anywhere from 10 to 180 days (the standard detoxification period is 21 days), during which the dose is gradually tapered, except in cases of chronic maintenance. During this period, an attempt is also made via counseling to deal with the psychosocial aspects of addiction and the factors that lead to the addictive lifestyle. Methadone provides less euphoria than other opioid agents, which makes it an ideal drug for detoxification. Other opioid agents used for detoxification include LAAM and buprenorphine (agonist-antagonist activity).

Clonidine is an α_2-adrenergic agonist that acts by binding to presynaptic receptors and blocking release of norepinephrine. The action of clonidine is based on its ability to block the sympathetic outflow that occurs when an addicted individual abruptly refrains from opiate use. Clonidine has several advantages in the treatment of withdrawal and opiate detoxification.[91–93] Because clonidine is not an opiate, therapy is not simply based on substitution of an opioid agent.

Clonidine is usually started at 0.1 mg, by mouth, followed by an additional 0.1 mg every 30 to 60 minutes, guided by alleviation of symptoms and limited by hypotension.[94] Dosage regimens for clonidine to prevent or treat withdrawal symptoms range from 0.1 mg, by mouth, three times daily up to 1.2 mg each day in divided doses. Clonidine has the added benefit of a relatively rapid onset of action and can be titrated on the basis of alleviation of symptoms. Limitations of clonidine use primarily concern an incidence of hypotension, especially in the dosage range that may be necessary to adequately prevent withdrawal symptoms. Sedation and hypotension are aggravated by concurrent opiate use, an issue that is a significant factor in the choice of outpatient therapy in an unreliable patient population.

An opiate antagonist has also been employed in detoxification and prevention programs in a way similar to the use of Antabuse (disulfiram) in alcohol abuse. Naltrexone, a competitive antagonist at the mu receptor, is the most advantageous of the antagonists used this way, because of its longer half-life compared to that of naloxone. The use of naltrexone in this setting requires highly motivated individuals and good support systems to ensure compliance.[95]

Neonatal Abstinence Syndrome

Neonatal abstinence syndrome (NAS) can be precipitated by many drugs, but it is most typically seen in neonates of opiate-abusing mothers. Time of presentation and signs and symptoms of NAS may be variable depending on the offending agent, its half-life, the last maternal use of the agent, and the severity of the mother's habit. The first evidence of NAS may range from minutes up to 1 to 2 weeks after delivery.[96] Infants born to heroin-abusing mothers generally become symptomatic earlier than those born to mothers using methadone, because of heroin's shorter half-life. Onset of NAS symptoms in neonates born to mothers enrolled in methadone programs ranged from 42% within 24 hours and up to 87% within 72 hours of delivery.[97] Irritability is generally the most prominent symptom of NAS. Other symptoms are listed in Table 36–9.

Treatment of NAS is initially supportive. Pharmacologic therapy is reserved for neonates demonstrating severe symptoms such as seizures, vomiting, diarrhea, or weight loss. Treatment regimens may

Table 36–9. Signs and Symptoms of Neonatal Withdrawal Syndrome

General	CNS	Respiratory	Gastrointestinal
Irritability	Coarse tremors	Rhinorrhea	Salivation
Wakefulness	Seizures (myoclonic)	Stuffy nose	Hiccups
Yawning	Twitching	Sneezing	Disorganized suck
Lacrimation	Hyperactivity	Respiratory distress	Vomiting
Fever	Hypertonicity	Tachypnea	Diarrhea
Diaphoresis	High-pitched cry	Respiratory alkalosis	Weight loss
Rub marks	Hyperreflexia		Failure to gain weight
Skin mottling	Hyperacusis		
Voracious sucking	Photophobia		
Poor sleep pattern	Apneic spells		
Hypothermia	Hypertonicity		

From Levy M, Spino M: Neonatal withdrawal syndrome: Associated drugs and pharmacologic management. Pharmacotherapy *13*:202–211, 1993.

include paregoric, phenobarbital, diazepam, chlorpromazine, diluted opium tincture, and clonidine.

References

1. Reisine T, Pasternak G: Opioid analgesics and antagonists. *In* Hardman JG, Limbird LE, Molinoff PB, et al (eds): Goodman and Gilman's The Pharmacologic Basis of Therapeutics, 9th ed. New York, McGraw-Hill, 1996, pp 521–555.
2. Shook JE, Watkins WD, Canaporesi EM: Differential roles of opioid receptors in respiration, respiratory disease, and opiate-induced respiratory depression. Am Rev Respir Dis *142:*895–909, 1990.
3. Shakespeare W: Romeo and Juliet, Act 2, Scene 3. *In* Black WJ (ed): The Works of William Shakespeare Complete. Black's Reader's Service Company, pp 1076, 1937.
4. Brownstein MJ: A brief history of opiates, opioid peptides, and opioid receptors. Proc Natl Acad Sci *90:*5391–5393, 1993.
5. Inhalants, Hallucinogens and Heroin: National Household Survey on Drug Abuse: Main Findings 1993. Substance Abuse and Mental Health Services Administration. Washington, DC, DHHS publ No. (SMA)95–3020, June 1995, pp 71–74.
6. Preliminary Estimates from the Drug Abuse Warning Network: January–June 1993: Preliminary Estimates of Drug-Related Emergency Room Episodes, advance report No. 6. Washington, DC, DHHS, March 1994.
7. Illicit drug availability: National Drug Control Strategy: Strengthening Communities Response to Drugs and Crime. Washington, DC, Office of National Drug Control Policy, February 1995, pp 46–47.
8. May EL: A half century of medicinal chemistry with major emphasis on pain-relieving drugs and their antagonists. J Med Chem *35:*3587–3594, 1992.
9. Martin W: Pharmacology of opioids. Pharmacol Rev *35:*285–323, 1983.
10. Hughes J, Smith TW, Kosterlitz HW, et al: Identification of two related pentapeptides from the brain with potent opiate agonist activity. Nature (Lond) *258:*577–579, 1975.
11. Thompson JW: Opioid peptides. BMJ *288:*259–261, 1984.
12. Pasternak GW: Multiple morphine and enkephalin receptors and the relief of pain. JAMA *259:*1362–1367, 1988.
13. Pasternak GW: Pharmacological mechanisms of opioid analgesics. Clin Neuropharmacol *16:*1–18, 1993.
14. Poole JC, Jahr JS: Opiate receptors: A review of analgesic properties and pharmacological side effects. J LA State Med Soc *144:*106–108, 1992.
15. Weinberg DS, Inturrisi CE, Reidenberg B, et al: Sublingual absorption of selected opioid analgesics. Clin Pharmacol Ther *44:*335–342, 1988.
16. Boerner U, Abbott S, Roe RL: The metabolism of morphine and heroin in man. Drug Metab Rev *4:*39–73, 1975.
17. Baselt RC, Crivey RH: Morphine, *In* Disposition of Toxic Drugs and Chemicals in Man. 3rd ed. Littleton, MA, Chicago, Year Book Medical Publishers, pp 575–579, 1989.
18. Baselt RC, Crivey RH: Codeine, *In* Disposition of Toxic Drugs and Chemicals in Man. 3rd ed. Littleton, MA, Chicago, Year Book Medical Publishers, pp 214–218, 1989.
19. Kalko RF, Foley KM, Grabinski PY: Central nervous system excitatory effects of meperidine in cancer patients. Ann Neurol *13:*180–185, 1983.
20. Szeto H, Inturrisi CE, Houde R, et al: Accumulation of normeperidine, an active metabolite of meperidine, in patients with renal failure or cancer. Ann Intern Med *86:*738–741, 1977.
21. Nickander R, Smits SE, Steinberg MI: Propoxyphene and norpropoxyphene: Pharmacologic and toxic effects in animals. J Pharmacol Exp Ther *200:*245–253, 1977.
22. Foley KM: Opioids. Neurol Clin *11:*503–522, 1993.
23. Klotz U, McHorse TS, Wilkinson GR, et al: The effect of cirrhosis on the disposition and elimination of meperidine in man. Clin Pharmacol Ther *16:*667–675, 1974.
24. Neal EA, Meffin PJ, Gregory PB: Enhanced bioavailability and decreased clearance of analgesics in patients with cirrhosis. Gastroenterology *77:*96–102, 1979.
25. Giacomini KM, Giacomini JC, Gibson TP, et al: Propoxyphene and norpropoxyphene plasma concentration after oral propoxyphene in cirrhotic patients with and without surgically constructed portacaval shunt. Clin Pharmacol Ther *28:*417–424, 1980.
26. Osborne RJ, Joel SP, Slevin ML: Morphine intoxication in renal failure: The role of morphine-6-glucuronide. BMJ *292:*1548–1549, 1986.
27. Finelli PF: Phenytoin and methadone tolerance. N Engl J Med *294:*227, 1976.
28. Tong TG: Phenytoin-induced methadone withdrawal. Ann Intern Med *94:*349, 1981.
29. Pond SM, Kretschzmar KM: Effect of phenytoin on meperidine clearance and normeperidine formation. Clin Pharmacol Ther *30:*680, 1981.
30. Maurer PM, Bartkowski RR: Drug interactions of clinical significance with opioid analgesics. Drug Saf *8:*30–48, 1993.
31. Duberstein JL, Kaufman DM: A clinical study of an epidemic of heroin intoxication and heroin induced pulmonary edema. Am J Med *51:*704, 1971.
32. Smith DA, Leake L, Loflin JR, et al: Is admission after intravenous heroin overdose necessary? Ann Emerg Med *21:*1326–1330, 1992.
33. Wang ML, Lin JL, Liaw SJ, et al: Heroin lung: Report of two cases: Department of Emergency, Chang Gung Memorial Hospital, Taipei, Taiwan, R.O.C. J Formos Med Assoc *93:*170–172, 1994.
34. Steinberg AD, Karliner J: The clinical spectrum of heroin pulmonary edema. Arch Intern Med *122:*122–127, 1968.
35. Persky VW, Goldfrank LR: Methadone overdoses in a New York City Hospital. J Am Coll Emerg Phys *65:*111, 1976.
36. Kjeldgaard JM, Hahn GW, Heckenlively JR, et al: Methadone-induced pulmonary edema. JAMA *218:*882–883, 1971.
37. Carson DJL, Carson ED: Fatal dextropropoxyphene poisoning in Northern Ireland. Lancet 1:894–897, 1977.
38. Lovejoy FH, Mitchell AA, Goldman PG: The management of propoxyphene poisoning. Pediatr *85:*98–100, 1974.
39. Clark RF, Wei EM, Anderson PO: Meperidine: Therapeutic use and toxicity. J Emerg Med *13:*797–802, 1995.
40. Ng SK, Brust JC, Hauser WA, et al: Illicit drug use and the risk of new-onset seizures. Am J Epidemiol *132:*47–57, 1990.
41. Bonfiglio MF, Mauro VF: Naloxone in the treatment of meperidine-induced seizures. Drug Intell Clin Pharmacother *21:*174–175, 1987.
42. Mauro VF, Bonfiglio MF, Spunt AL: Meperidine-induced seizures in a patient without renal dysfunction or sickle cell anemia. Clin Pharmacol *5:*837–839, 1986.
43. Langston JW, Ballard P, Tetrud JW, et al: Chronic parkinsonism in humans due to a product of meperidine-analog synthesis. Science *219:*979–980, 1983.
44. Lieberman AN, Goldstein M: Reversible parkinsonism related to meperidine. N Engl J Med *312:*509, 1985.
45. Holland DR, Steinberg MI: Electrophysiologic properties of propoxyphene and norpropoxyphene in canine conductive tissue in vitro and in vivo. J Pharmacol Exp Ther *47:*123–133, 1979.
46. Nickander R, Smits SE, Steinberg MI: Propoxyphene and norpropoxyphene: Pharmacologic and toxic effects in animals. J Pharmacol Exp Ther *200:*245–253, 1977.
47. Bogartz LJ, Miller WC: Pulmonary edema associated with propoxyphene intoxication. JAMA *215:*259–262, 1971.
48. Glass PS, Jhaveri RM, Smith LR: Comparison of potency and duration of action of nalmefene and naloxone. Anesth Analg *78:*536–541, 1994.
49. Kaplan JL, Marx JA: Effectiveness and safety of intravenous nalmefene for emergency department patients with suspected narcotic overdose: A pilot study. Ann Emerg Med *22:*187–190, 1993.
50. Martin WR: Naloxone. Ann Intern Med *85:*765, 1976.
51. Greenberg MI: The use of endotracheal medication in cardiac emergencies. Resuscitation *12:*155–165, 1984.
52. Maio RF, Gaukel B, Freeman B: Intralingual naloxone injection for narcotic-induced respiratory depression. Ann Emerg Med *16:*572, 1987.

53. Hubbell KC: Opiates and narcotics. *In* Haddad LM, Winchester JF (eds): Clinical Management of Poisoning and Drug Overdose, 2nd ed. Philadelphia, WB Saunders, 1990, pp 706–717.
54. Goldfrank L, Weisman RS, Errick JK, et al: A dosing nomogram for continuous infusion of intravenous naloxone. Ann Emerg Med *15:*566–570, 1986.
55. Kauffman RE, Banner W Jr, Blumer JL: Naloxone dosage and route of administration for infants and children: Addendum to emergency drug doses for infants and children. Pediatrics *86:*484–485, 1990.
56. Moore RA, Rumack BH, Conner CS, et al: Naloxone: Underdosage after narcotic poisoning. AJDC *134:*156–158, 1980.
57. Doyan S, Roberts JR: Reappraisal of the "coma cocktail." Emerg Med Clin North Am *12:*301–316, 1994.
58. Hoffman JR, Schriger DL, Luo JS: The empiric use of naloxone in patients with altered mental status: A reappraisal. Ann Emerg Med *20:*246–252, 1991.
59. Cohen MR, Cohen RM, Pickar D, et al: High dose naloxone infusions in normals: Dose dependent behavioral, hormonal and physiological response. Arch Gen Psychiatry *40:*613, 1983.
60. Yealy DM, Paris PM, Kaplan RM, et al: The safety of prehospital naloxone administration by paramedics. Ann Emerg Med *19:*902–905, 1990.
61. Azar I, Turndorf H: Severe hypertension and multiple atrial premature contraction following naloxone administration. Anesth Analg *58:*524, 1979.
62. Flacke JW, Flacke WE, William GD: Acute pulmonary edema following naloxone reversal of high dose morphine anesthesia. Anesthesiology *47:*376, 1977.
63. Taff RH: Pulmonary edema following naloxone administration in a patient without heart disease. Anesthesiology *59:*576, 1983.
64. Schwartz JA, Koenigsberg MD: Naloxone-induced pulmonary edema. Ann Emerg Med *16:*1294, 1987.
65. Mariani P: Seizure associated with low dose naloxone. Am J Emerg Med *6:*127, 1989.
66. Michaelis LL, Hickey PR, Clark TA, et al: Ventricular irritability associated with the use of naloxone hydrochloride: Two case reports and laboratory assessment of the effect of the drug on cardiac excitability. Ann Thorac Surg *18:*608–614, 1974.
67. Andree RA: Sudden death following administration of naloxone. Anesth Analg *59:*782, 1980.
68. Betzelos S, Mueller P: Whole bowel irrigation in a heroin body-packer. Vet Hum Toxicol *33:*353, 1991.
69. Utecht MJ, Stone AF, McCarron MM: Heroin body packers. J Emerg Med *11:*33–40, 1993.
70. Kaa E: Impurities, adulterants and diluents of illicit heroin: Changes during a 12-year period. Forensic Sci Int *64:*171–179, 1994.
71. Jenkins AJ, Keenan RM, Henningfield JE, et al: Pharmacokinetics and pharmacodynamics of smoked heroin. J Anal Toxicol *18:*317–330, 1994.
72. Griffiths P, Gossop M, Powis B, et al: Transitions in patterns of heroin administration: A study of heroin chasers and heroin injectors. Addiction *89:*301–309, 1994.
73. Mack RB: Toxic encounters of the dangerous kind. NC Med J *42:*858, 1981.
74. Stahl SM, Kasser IS: Pentazocine overdose. Ann Emerg Med *12:*63–66, 1983.
75. Showalter CV: "T's and blues": Abuse of pentazocine and tripelennamine. JAMA *244:*1224–1225, 1980.
76. Lahmeyer HW, Steingold RG: Medical and psychiatric complications of pentazocine and tripelennamine abuse. J Clin Psychiatry *41:*275, 1980.
77. Bogartz LJ, Miller WC: Pulmonary edema associated with propoxyphene intoxication. JAMA *215:*259, 1971.
78. Gary N, Maher JF, DeMyttenaeree MH, et al: Acute propoxyphene hydrochloride intoxication. Arch Intern Med *121:*453, 1968.
79. McCarthy WH, Keenan RL: Propoxyphene hydrochloride poisoning. JAMA *187:*164, 1964.
80. Holland DR, Steinberg MI: Electrophysiologic properties of propoxyphene and norpropoxyphene in canine conductive tissue in vitro and in vivo. J Pharmacol Exp Ther *47:*123–133, 1979.
81. Martin M, Hecker J, Clark R, et al: China White epidemic: An Eastern United States emergency department experience. Ann Emerg Med *20*:158–164, 1991.
82. Hibbs J, Perper J, Winek CL: An outbreak of designer drug–related deaths in Pennsylvania. JAMA *265:*1011–1013, 1991.
83. McCleave NR: Drug smuggling by body packers: Detection and removal of internally concealed drugs. Med J Aust *159:*750–754, 1993.
84. Koob GF, Maldonado R, Stinus L: Neural substrates of opiate withdrawal. Trends Neurosci *15:*186–191, 1992.
85. Isbell H, White W: Clinical characteristics of addictions. Am J Med *14:*558–565, 1953.
86. Hodding GC, Jann M, Ackerman IP: Drug withdrawal syndromes: A literature review. West J Med *133:*383–391, 1980.
87. Senay EC, Dorus W, Goldberg F, et al: Withdrawal from methadone maintenance: Rate of withdrawal and expectation. Arch Gen Psychiatry *34:*361–367, 1977.
88. Easom JM, Lovejoy FH: Opiates. *In* Haddad LM, Winchester JF: Clinical Management of Poisoning and Drug Overdose. 2nd ed. Philadelphia, WB Saunders, 1983, p 429.
89. Fultz JM, Senay EC: Guidelines for the management of hospitalized narcotics addicts. Ann Intern Med *82:*815–818, 1975.
90. Banys P, Tusel DJ, Sees KL, et al: Low (40 mg) versus high (180 mg) dose methadone in a 180-day heroin detoxification program. J Substance Abuse Treat *11:*225–232, 1994.
91. Gold MS, Pottash AL, Extein I, et al: Clinical utility of clonidine in opiate withdrawal. NIDA Res Monogr *34:*95–100, 1981.
92. Gerra G, Marcato A, Caccavari R, et al: Clonidine and opiate receptor antagonists in the treatment of heroin addiction. J Substance Abuse Treat *12:*35–41, 1995.
93. Gold MS: Opiate addiction and the locus ceruleus: The clinical utility of clonidine, naltrexone, methadone, and buprenorphine. Psychiatr Clin North Am *16:*61–73, 1993.
94. Gold MS, Redmond DE, Kleber HD: Clonidine blocks acute opiate withdrawal symptoms. Lancet *2:*599, 1978.
95. Shufman EN, Porat S, Witztum E, et al: The efficacy of naltrexone in preventing reabuse of heroin after detoxification. Biol Psychiatry *35:*935–945, 1994.
96. Levy M, Spino M: Neonatal withdrawal syndrome: Associated drugs and pharmacologic management. Pharmacotherapy *13:*202–211, 1993.
97. Harper R, Solish G, Purow H, et al: The effect of a methadone treatment program upon pregnant heroin addicts and their newborn infants. Pediatrics *54:*300–305, 1974.
98. Bartkowski RR, McDonnell TE: Prolonged alfentanil effect following erythromycin administration. Anesthesiology *73:*566–568, 1990.
99. Lehmann KA, Weski C, Hunger L, et al: Biotransformation of fentanyl: II. Acute drug interactions in rats and men. Anaesthesist *31:*221–227, 1982.
100. Johnson R, Douglas J, Corey L: Adverse effects with acyclovir and meperidine. Ann Intern Med 103:962–963, 1985.
101. Stambaugh JE, Hemphill DM, Wainer IW, et al: A potentially toxic drug interaction between pethidine (meperidine) and phenobarbitone. Lancet *1:*398–399, 1977.
102. Roerig DL, Kotrly KJ, Ahlf SB, et al: Effect of propranolol on the first pass uptake of fentanyl in the human and rat lung. Anesthesiology *71:*62–68, 1989.
103. Guay DR, Meatherall RC, Chalmers JL, et al: Cimetidine alters pethidine disposition in man. Br J Clin Pharmacol *18:*907–914, 1984.
104. Meyer D, Halfin V: Toxicity secondary to meperidine in patients on monoamine oxidase inhibitors: A case report and critical review. J Clin Psychopharmacol *1:*319–321, 1981.
105. Grothe DR, Ereshefsky L, Jann MW, et al: Clinical implications of the neuroleptic-opioid interaction. Drug Intell Clin Pharmacol *20:*75–77, 1986.
106. Pond SM, Kretschzmar KM: Effect of phenytoin on meperidine clearance and normeperidine formation. Clin Pharmacol Ther *30:*680–686, 1981.

107. Liu SJ, Wang RI: Case report of barbiturate-induced enhancement of methadone metabolism and withdrawal syndrome. Am J Psychiatry *141:*1287–1288, 1984.
108. Bell J, Seres V, Bowron P, et al: The use of serum methadone levels in patients receiving methadone maintenance. Clin Pharmacol Ther *43:*623–629, 1988.
109. Tong TG, Pond SM, Kreek MJ, et al: Phenytoin-induced methadone withdrawal. Ann Intern Med *94:*349–351, 1981.
110. Kreek MJ, Garfield JW, Gutjahr CL, et al: Rifampin-induced methadone withdrawal. N Engl J Med *294:*1104–1106, 1976.
111. Bertschy G, Baumann P, Eap CB, et al: Probable metabolic interaction between methadone and fluvoxamine in addict patients. Ther Drug Monit *16:*42–45, 1994.
112. Fine A, Churchill DN: Potentially lethal interaction of cimetidine and morphine. Can Med Assoc J *124:*1434–1436, 1981.
113. Manara AR, Shelly MP, Quinn K, et al: The effect of metoclopramide on the absorption of oral controlled release morphine. Br J Clin Pharmacol *25:*518–521, 1988.
114. Garbutt JC: Potentiation of propoxyphene by phenelzine. Am J Psychiatry *144:*251–252, 1987.
115. Foley KM: The treatment of cancer pain. N Engl J Med *313:*84–85, 1985.

ACKNOWLEDGMENT

The author wishes to acknowledge the assistance of Drs. Seth Schonwald and John Patrick in preparing this chapter.

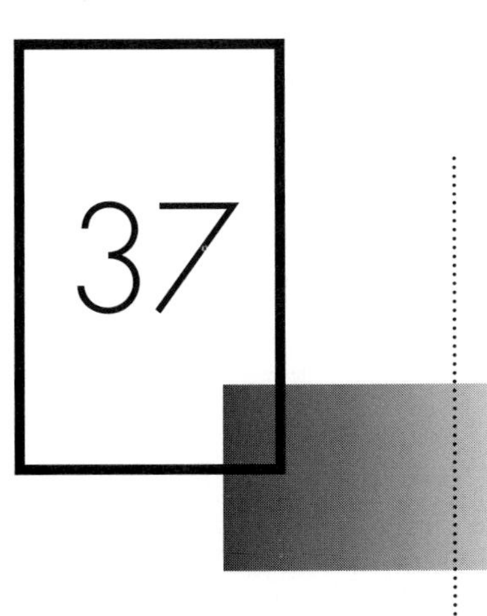

Barbiturates

LESTER M. HADDAD, MD
JAMES F. WINCHESTER, MD

The barbiturates were once the leading cause of death in sedative drug overdose, typified by the tragic death of Marilyn Monroe, allegedly of barbiturates, on August 4, 1962, at age 36 years. The prescription of sleep medications such as secobarbital (Seconal, or "reds"), pentobarbital (Nembutal, or "yellow jackets"), and secobarbital-amobarbital combination (Tuinal or "rainbows") was in vogue during the 1950s and 1960s and accounted for the high incidence of overdose and drug abuse.

Although the barbiturates were largely replaced with the benzodiazepines during the 1970s and 1980s, they are experiencing a resurgence of use. According to data[1] from the Drug Abuse Warning Network (DAWN) of the National Institute on Drug Abuse, barbiturates accounted for 391 deaths in 1993, largely from overdose of phenobarbital, the butalbital-analgesic combination headache medications such as butalbital-aspirin (Fiorinal, Axotal) and butalbital-acetaminophen (Fioricet, Esgic, Bucet, Axocet), and the sleep medications already mentioned. A recent study found short-acting barbiturates the highest odds ratio for death in drug overdose when adjusted for prescription numbers.[2]

PHARMACOLOGY AND PHARMACOKINETICS

Barbituric acid (2,4,6-trioxohexahydropyrimidine) is the parent compound of the barbiturates; barbital was first introduced as a sedative-hypnotic agent in 1903. A general formula with the substituted radicals for the various derivatives of barbituric acid is shown in Table 37–1. In general, agents with long side chains have increased lipid solubility, possess a short duration of action and a high degree of potency, and undergo hepatic degradation. An example is thiopental, an intravenous drug widely used in hospitals for rapid-sequence intubation of patients with status

Table 37–1. Barbiturate Classification

General Formula and Substituted Derivatives

Barbiturate	Trade Name	pK_a	Duration of Action (h)	Plasma Half-Life (h)	R_{5a}	R_{5b}	R_3
Short-Acting Barbiturates							
Ultrashort							
Thiopental	(Pentothal)	7.6	0.3	6–46	Ethyl	1-Methylbutyl	H
Methohexital	(Brevital)	7.9	0.3	?	Allyl	1-Methyl-2-pentynyl	CH_3
Short							
Pentobarbital	(Nembutal)	7.96	3.0	21–42	Ethyl	1-Methylbutyl	H
Secobarbital	(Seconal)	7.90	3.0	20–28	Allyl	1-Methylbutyl	H
Intermediate							
Amobarbital	(Amytal)	7.75	3–6	15–40	Ethyl	Isopentyl	H
Butabarbital	(Butisol)	7.74	3–6	34–42	Ethyl	*sec*-Butyl	H
Long-Acting Barbiturates							
Barbital	(Veronal)	7.74	6–12	48	Ethyl	Ethyl	H
Mephobarbital	(Mebaral)	8.5	6–12	48–52	Ethyl	Phenyl	CH_3
Phenobarbital	(Luminal)	7.24	6–12	48–144	Ethyl	Phenyl	H
Primidone	(Mysoline)	—	6–12	6–22	Ethyl	Phenyl	H

*S= substitution for O= in thiopental, H_2 substitution for O= in primidone.

epilepticus, head injury, cardioversion, and other anesthetic indications. The onset of action of thiopental is within 20 to 30 seconds. In contrast, agents with short side chains have a slower onset and longer duration of action, and they are excreted primarily unchanged by the kidneys. An example is the anticonvulsant phenobarbital.

Most barbiturates in clinical use are given orally. After transit through the stomach, absorption takes place in the small intestine, despite the favorable pH partition occurring in the stomach. Sodium salts are more rapidly absorbed than are free acids. Absorption is more rapid when the barbiturates are diluted with water and slower when food is present in the stomach. In general, the more lipid-soluble the drug, the more highly protein-bound the drug will be.[3] Highly lipid-soluble thiopental is 80% protein bound, but the less lipid-soluble phenobarbital is only 5% protein bound.

Distribution of the highly lipid-soluble barbiturates is into the vascular areas of the brain (gray matter), where maximal uptake occurs within 30 seconds of administration; as a result, sleep is induced within a few minutes. Thirty minutes after intravenous administration, redistribution into the less vascular areas of the brain occurs, and plasma levels of barbiturate may decrease to 10% of peak levels. Thus, *no* correlation exists between the duration of action and the elimination half-life of these drugs, since their activity depends on the rapid vascular distribution phase. For example, patients who are comatose from phenobarbital overdose often begin to awake the following day, even if their blood drug levels have not decreased substantially. The unbound (free) concentrations of barbiturates in the plasma and in the cerebrospinal fluid are equal. Equilibration of barbiturates varies in different tissues and is slowest in the poorly vascular fat tissue. When steady state is reached, the highest concentrations of drug in nonadipose tissue, although less than those in fat, occur in the liver and the kidney.

Nearly all barbiturates undergo hepatic[3] metabolism, although small quantities of the thiobarbiturates (thiopental and thiamylal) are biotransformed in kidney, brain, and other tissues. Some barbiturates have active metabolites. For example, demethylation of mephobarbital yields 15% phenobarbital, whereas primidone is metabolized to phenobarbital and phenylethylmalonamide.[3]

Barbiturates are transformed by oxidation of the side chain radicals to alcohols, ketones, phenols, or carboxylic acids, which appear in the urine as these compounds or as glucuronized conjugates. Desulfuration of thiobarbiturates, opening of the barbituric acid ring, and other processes are also known to occur.[3] The biotransformation process responsible for termination of biologic activity is side-chain oxidation. Phenobarbital also is unique in that it exhibits increased clearance from the gastrointestinal tract by serial administration of activated charcoal.[4]

Barbiturates are filtered by the renal glomerulus in quantities equivalent to those of the unbound fraction in plasma. Highly lipid-soluble barbiturates not only are highly protein-bound but also are poorly filtered; however, they are also readily reabsorbed from the renal tubular lumen. Barbiturates with low lipid-to-water partition coefficients (e.g., barbital, mephobarbital, and phenobarbital) are excreted largely unchanged in the urine.

Alkalization of the urine tends to promote ionization of barbiturates and leads to their enhanced excretion, particularly with phenobarbital. This is because the pK_a of phenobarbital is 7.24. (The pK_a is equivalent to the pH at which the ionized and unionized forms of an acid or base are equal in concentration.) Thus, phenobarbital, a weak organic acid, is 50% non-ionized at pH 7.24, but it is less than 4% non-ionized (or 96% ionized) at pH 7.5. Because only the non-ionized portion is reabsorbed, it follows that attaining an alkaline pH greater than 7.5 causes 96% of phenobarbital to be excreted. In contrast, secobarbital (see Table 37–1), which has a pK_a of 7.9, is 99% non-ionized at pH 7.2 and 98% non-ionized at pH 7.5; thus, alkalization has little effect on the excretion of secobarbital.[3]

The barbiturates have traditionally been classified as ultrashort, short, intermediate, and long acting. However, this classification is somewhat artificial because it is now known that these drugs' elimination half-lives do not correspond to their apparent durations of action. McCarron and co-workers[5] have grouped the barbiturates into the *short-acting barbiturates* (which include the ultrashort-, short-, and intermediate-acting agents) and the *long-acting barbiturates*; this is a useful clinical classification because management differs for long-acting barbiturate overdose.

When given in sedative or hypnotic doses, barbiturates have little effect on skeletal, cardiac, and smooth muscle. However, in acute barbiturate intoxication, muscle inhibitory effects produce serious problems with cardiovascular stability. The desired central nervous system effects of barbiturates range from mild sedation to general anesthesia. In addition, phenobarbital and mephobarbital have selective anticonvulsant activity. Some evidence indicates that barbiturates may have euphoriant activity, and there is equivocal evidence that they may have an effect on anxiety.

Barbiturates have no effect on pain; when given in small doses, they are thought to increase the reaction to painful stimuli and, in certain experimental models, may antagonize the effect of analgesics. In patients with somatic pain, barbiturates may cause paradoxical excitement. Barbiturates decrease the low-frequency electrical activity of the electroencephalogram and increase the low-voltage fast activity (15 to 35 Hz); these findings suggest electrical arousal of the reticular activating substance, although this arousal response is incomplete owing to nonstimulation of the hippocampal component.

The barbiturates decrease sleep latency, increase delta wave activity and fast electroencephalographic activity during sleep, decrease the number of state shifts to stages 0 and 1, and decrease body movement. The pharmacologic basis for activity in the central nervous system most likely is due to the fact that low-dose barbiturates have a γ-aminobutyric acid–like action or enhance the effects of γ-aminobutyric acid activity within the central nervous system. However, barbiturates may also selectively abolish noradrenergic excitation (but not inhibition) in various synapses. During barbiturate-induced anesthesia, oxygen utilization by brain tissue decreases by approximately 50%. This observation has led to the clinical use of high-dose barbiturates for protection against cerebral infarction during cerebral ischemia and head injury.[6–9]

Barbiturates' interaction with γ-aminobutyric acid explains the nonselective inhibition of synaptic responses, such that of the neurogenic drive for respiration is eliminated by a barbiturate dose about threefold greater than that normally used to induce sleep. Similarly, suppression of hypoxic and chemoreceptor drives to respiration is achieved with high doses of barbiturates; the dominant respiratory drive shifts to the carotid and aortic bodies and eventually fails. It is of interest that, unlike the opiates and opioids, the barbiturates suppress the cough reflex only when they are given in doses that depress respiration. The smooth muscle effects, however, are seen particularly in the cardiovascular system. Cardiovascular depression and depression of vascular smooth muscle accompany acute barbiturate poisoning. Both of these effects can be overcome by digitalis and β-adrenergic agonists. The smooth muscle inhibitory effect is also observed in the gastrointestinal tract, where reduction in bowel motility is observed. This effect is reversed on recovery from barbiturate poisoning.

THERAPEUTIC USES OF BARBITURATES

The ultrashort-acting thiopental (pentothal) is an essential in-hospital anesthetic agent used for performing rapid-sequence intubation, such as in status epilepticus, head injury, and cardioversion, and selectively in other conditions for reducing brain edema and metabolism during and after neurosurgery, in near-drowning, in cerebral ischemia, and after resuscitation. Thiopental is also used for short-term sedation in patients (especially children) who must undergo computed tomography or other imaging studies.

The short-acting barbiturates pentobarbital and secobarbital, formerly used as sleep medications and once the most common cause of coma from drug overdose, are uncommonly used therapeutically today.

The intermediate-acting butalbital, in use as a headache medication often in combination with acetaminophen or aspirin, is currently one of the most commonly prescribed barbiturates (Table 37–2).

The long-acting agent phenobarbital, when given orally or parenterally, still has widespread use as an anticonvulsant. The maximum recommended anticonvulsant loading dose of phenobarbital in refractory status epilepticus is up to 20 mg/kg; the mainte-

Table 37–2. Medications Containing Butalbital

Trade Name (Manufacturer)	Butalbital Content (mg)	Acetaminophen Content (mg)	Aspirin Content (mg)	Caffeine Content (mg)	Codeine (mg)
Esgic (Forest)	50	325		40	
Esgic Plus (Forest)	50	500		40	
Fiorinal (Sandoz)	50		325	40	
Fioricet (Sandoz)	50	325		40	
Fiorinal with codeine (Sandoz)	50		325	40	30
Fioricet with codeine (Sandoz)	50	325		40	30
Butisol (Wallace)	15–100				
Axocet (Savage)	50	650			
Axital (Savage)	50		650		
Bucet (UAD)	50	650			
Phrenilin Forte (Carnrick)	50	325			
Sedapap (Mayrand)	50	650			

nance dose in outpatient management of seizure disorder is 45 to 180 mg/d.

TOLERANCE, ABUSE, AND DEPENDENCE

Tolerance to barbiturates is a well-recognized phenomenon.[10] For example, the plasma concentration at which sleep ensues may be lower than that at the time of wakening after a single-dose administration; accordingly, this phenomenon cannot be explained by the induction of hepatic microsomal enzymes. Similarly, with chronic administration, tolerance to increasing doses of barbiturates occurs to the extent that the effective dosage of barbiturate may be increased by as much as sixfold—a phenomenon two- to threefold greater than can be accounted for by enhanced hepatic metabolism. This tolerance to barbiturates also is conferred by other central nervous system depressant drugs, such as meprobamate, glutethimide, methaqualone, and general anesthetics. In addition, cross-tolerance to drugs such as phencyclidine and the benzodiazepines develops; however, no tolerance develops for the muscle-relaxant properties of benzodiazepines.

The effects of the abrupt withdrawal of barbiturates in patients who have been taking them for prolonged periods vary considerably, depending on the degree of tolerance and the duration of abuse before withdrawal. However, discontinuation of barbiturates may result in progressive seizures, delirium, insomnia, tremor, anorexia, and abnormal sleep patterns. In addition, abdominal cramps, nausea, vomiting, and orthostatic hypotension are characteristic of withdrawal, and patients may exhibit purposive behavior patterns. Seizure activity is the most important of all the withdrawal symptoms, and the number of seizures varies from one to the many that characterize status epilepticus. Neither phenytoin nor chlorpromazine prevents seizures; indeed, in this case, barbiturates themselves are indicated for suppression.

DRUG INTERACTIONS

An increased sedative effect is observed when barbiturates are taken in combination with other drugs affecting the central nervous system, in particular alcohol but also antihistamines and other central nervous system depressants. An increased effect of barbiturates is seen during concomitant use of isoniazid, methylphenidate, and monamine oxidase inhibitors. The principal drug interactions observed, however, are the result of the induction of hepatic microsomal enzymes. This process causes an increase in the elimination of dicumarol, digoxin, tetracycline, corticosteroids, oral contraceptives, phenytoin, sulfa drugs, tricyclic antidepressants, hormones such as testosterone, and vitamins D and K. Also, it has been observed that toxic metabolite formation may occur more intensely in patients who have been receiving barbiturates and coingesting other compounds, particularly the hydrocarbon anesthetics, carbon tetrachloride, and acetaminophen. As mentioned, aspirin displaces phenobarbital from its albumin-binding sites, whereas barbiturates displace thyroxine from thyroxine-binding proteins. Barbiturates also decrease the absorption of certain drugs, such as dicumarol and griseofulvin.

Not only is microsomal biotransformation of drugs affected, but the activity of other enzyme systems also is increased; for example, the activity of δ-aminolevulinic acid synthetase is increased, and this increase can precipitate exacerbations of porphyria.

CLINICAL PRESENTATION OF BARBITURATE OVERDOSE

The characteristic signs of barbiturate poisoning are depression of the central nervous and cardiovascular systems.[2, 11, 12] Mild to moderate intoxication resembles that seen with alcohol consumption; with severe intoxication, the patient becomes comatose to a varying degree and may demonstrate progression from stupor to coma, with depression and eventual loss of deep tendon reflexes.[13] The pupils are initially constricted and react to light; however, late in the course of barbiturate poisoning, hypoxic paralytic pupillary dilation may occur. *Persistence of the pupillary light reflex despite the presence of deep coma is a characteristic sign of barbiturate overdose.* As has already been noted, respiration is affected early. Breathing initially may be slow or rapid and shallow, and Cheyne-Stokes respiration may develop. Eventually, depression of respiration and concomitant depression of minute volume and vital capacity occur, with accompanying evidence of hypoxemia and hypercapnia. Blood pressure may decrease precipitously; initially, this is believed to be due to loss of central control of blood pressure at the midbrain level, but cardiac depression and inhibition of vascular smooth muscle tone may contribute. The patient in shock exhibits the classic signs of sweating, a rapid weak pulse, cool and clammy skin, hemoconcentration, and oliguria. Hypothermia is common, and it must be remembered that body temperature must be measured with a rectal thermometer.

Coma from barbiturate overdose has classically been divided into four stages typical of sedative drug overdose (Table 37–3). *Repeated neurologic examinations, with assessment of pupils, eye opening, corneal and gag reflexes, and response to verbal and painful stimuli; checking deep tendon reflexes; and repeated monitoring of vital signs, respiratory status, and oxygen saturation are the best clinical means of assessing both the depth of coma and the clinical status of the patient.*

Bullous skin lesions[14] are reported to occur with an incidence of 6.5%; they occur principally over pressure areas but also between the toes and fingers. At one point, they were thought to be sufficiently characteristic of acute barbiturate intoxication to be considered diagnostic. However, these lesions have also been observed in overdose with methaqualone, meprobamate, glutethimide, opiates, and tricyclic antidepressants.[15]

Early death from barbiturate intoxication is due to cardiorespiratory arrest. Delayed fatalities may occur secondary to circulatory collapse, acute renal failure, aspiration pneumonitis, atelectasis, lung abscess, pulmonary edema, and cerebral edema.[16–18] In addition, in patients who have suffered prolonged hypoxia before admission to an emergency department, permanent brain death may have occurred; in these patients, *all means of eliminating barbiturates from the body should be used before a final diagnosis of brain death is made.* Partial recovery of hypoxic neurologic lesions has been reported in patients surviving severe barbiturate overdose with prolonged coma.[19]

The lethal dose of barbiturates is difficult to establish with any certainty because survival has been reported after ingestion of widely varying doses. However, the potentially fatal dose of phenobarbital is 6 to 10 g, and that of amobarbital, secobarbital, and pentobarbital is 2 to 3 g.[16]

Table 37–3. Stages of Coma in Barbiturate Overdose

Grade	Features
I	Patient is comatose, the patient withdraws from painful stimuli, and the reflexes are intact.
II	Patient is comatose and fails to respond to painful stimuli, but the reflexes are intact and the vital signs are stable.
III	Patient is comatose and fails to respond to painful stimuli, deep tendon reflexes are absent, but vital signs are stable.
IV	Patient is comatose and fails to respond to painful stimui, deep tendon reflexes are absent, and vital signs are unstable with respiratory and cardiovascular depression.

EMERGENCY DEPARTMENT EVALUATION

Acute barbiturate overdose must be differentiated from other forms of coma or central nervous system injury. Information regarding the use or abuse of medications, previous psychiatric history or suicide attempts, or possible exposure to trauma or environmental exposure should be obtained. An accurate history of the type, amount, and time of drug ingestion; the duration of coma; and the possible coingestion of alcohol or other drugs should also be recorded.

Traumatic injury, pressure sores, and bullous lesions on the skin suggest barbiturate overdose. Detection of signs of liver disease such as jaundice, enlargement of the liver, or ascites is important because these conditions necessitate modification of treatment. A physical examination, including a detailed neurologic examination, is essential to proper management. Frequent recording of vital signs is essential; core temperature must be measured because hypothermia[20, 21] is common in barbiturate overdose.

In addition to routine laboratory data, measurements of serum barbiturate, ethanol, acetaminophen, and salicylate levels should be obtained. The therapeutic serum concentration of phenobarbital is 15 to 40 μg/mL; that of the short-acting barbiturates is 6 to 14 μg/mL. However, the plasma barbiturate level is notoriously unreliable. A serum barbiturate level of 1.5 μg/mL may be potentially lethal with concomitant ingestion of alcohol because of synergism. In contrast, tolerance in chronic abuse may enable a patient with a blood level of 40 μg/mL to walk into the emergency department.[22] The use of serial barbiturate levels may be useful in monitoring the efficacy of clinical management.[23]

Cardiac and pulmonary status should be assessed with electrocardiography and cardiac monitoring, chest radiography, and determination of oxygen saturation. Patients in deep coma and those with focal neurologic findings should undergo computed tomography of the head. In patients with fever, a spinal tap may be indicated to rule out meningitis.[23]

EMERGENCY MANAGEMENT

Treatment consists of emergency resuscitation and supportive care, gastric decontamination, and, for phenobarbital and the long-acting barbiturates, an alkaline diuresis and serial administration of activated charcoal.

Establishment of an airway with endotracheal intubation, support of respiration with mechanical ventilation, and maintenance of circulation with fluid resuscitation are essential to the management of the critical patient. Correction of acid-base balance may be indicated. Vasopressors such as dopamine may be necessary for stabilizing the blood pressure. All patients in coma should be administered intravenous naloxone and glucose. Treatment of hypothermia should be initiated in the emergency department.

Following resuscitation, patients should undergo gastric decontamination in the emergency department. Gastric lavage within the first hour of ingestion is indicated; gastric lavage in barbiturate overdose may be worthwhile up to 4 hours after ingestion.[24] The administration of activated charcoal (1 g/kg, or 50 to 100 g) is clearly indicated for barbiturate overdose.[24] Because phenobarbital may cause gastric mass formation, the physician should be aware that endoscopic gastric lavage for removal of such a mass may be indicated.[25]

An alkaline diuresis[22] is indicated for the treatment of phenobarbital and mephobarbital overdose. In patients with no cardiac or renal compromise, alkalization is usually initiated with administration of 1 L of 5% dextrose in water or 5% dextrose in 0.45% sodium chloride solution plus 2 ampoules of sodium bicarbonate (100 mEq, or 1.5 mEq/kg)[22, 23] at a rate necessary to obtain a urine pH of greater than 7.5; if possible, intravenous administration of a 500-mL fluid bolus is followed by infusion at a rate of 150 to 250 mL/h. The general philosophy is that one should carry out fluid-alkaline administration as aggressively as possible without compromising the patient. Renal clearance values for patients with barbiturate overdose may be as high as 17 mL/min with this therapy.

Serial administration of activated charcoal has been shown to increase clearance of phenobarbital and the long-acting barbiturates. In a study of normal volunteers, Neuvonen and Elonen[4] showed that multiple doses of activated charcoal administered 10 hours after ingestion of phenobarbital resulted in a nearly sixfold decrease (from 110 hours to 20 hours) in the elimination half-life of phenobarbital. Treatment of two patients[26] with phenobarbital overdose with multiple doses of activated charcoal resulted in a greater than fourfold reduction in the expected half-life of phenobarbital, as well as a reduction in the duration of coma, which often persists for days in patients who are managed with supportive care only. Further studies[27, 28] confirmed these early reports, which include the successful treatment of a 28-day-old infant.[29] Serial administration of 1 g/kg of activated charcoal every 4 hours is indicated in significant phenobarbital overdose.[24–30]

Supportive care is all that is effective in the conservative management of overdose with ultrashort-, short-, and intermediate-acting barbiturates; alkalization of the urine and serial administration of activated charcoal are ineffective when these agents are ingested in overdose.

Following emergency department evaluation and emergency management, patients who are in critical condition should be transferred to the intensive care unit for critical and often multidisciplinary care.

Hemodialysis and charcoal or resin hemoperfusion are both quite effective in removing barbiturates from the blood. In fact, hemodialysis was first used in the management of poisoning and drug overdose in response to the dramatic upsurge of barbiturate overdose in the 1950s and 1960s.[31, 32]

Again, the long-acting barbiturates are more readily removed by dialysis owing to their low potential for protein binding. In studies of simultaneous hemodialysis and forced diuresis, hemodialysis has been found to be ninefold more efficient for the removal of long-acting drugs and sixfold more efficient for the removal of short-acting drugs than forced diuresis.[33] It has been shown that hemodialysis removes phenobarbital at a rate of 744 mg/h, butabarbital at a rate of 262 mg/h, and cyclobarbital at 323 mg/h; this again reflects the fact that short-acting barbiturates undergo greater protein-binding and sequestration in adipose tissue.[33] There is no significant advantage conferred by the addition of activated charcoal or lipid to the dialysate to achieve further partitioning of barbiturates across hemodialysis membranes.

Yatzidis and associates[34] were the first to report a reduction of phenobarbital and barbital blood levels with the use of uncoated activated charcoal in two patients and the eventual recovery of both patients. Following this, Chang[35] used albumin collodion–coated activated charcoal for the rapid removal of phenobarbital in a poisoned patient. Using charcoal particles coated with an acrylic hydrogel polymer, Gelfand and associates[36] achieved a phenobarbital removal rate of 640 mg/h in one severely intoxicated patient; the patient recovered completely. Because peritoneal dialysis is relatively ineffective in removing barbiturate, it is not indicated for barbiturate overdose.[37]

Conservative management[5, 22, 23, 38] is the mainstay of therapy for the majority of patients with barbiturate overdose. Hemodialysis or hemoperfusion may be considered, especially in critical patients who are in stage IV coma; patients who are unresponsive to intensive supportive care, such as those who have ingested short-acting barbiturates (according to the McCarron classification); patients who have underlying or concomitant illness, such as those with pulmonary edema, aspiration pneumonitis, or adult respiratory distress syndrome; patients with renal or hepatic failure; or patients with severe electrolyte imbalance. Hemodialysis may be a better choice for those patients with pulmonary edema, renal failure, or severe electrolyte imbalance.[40] *Again, an isoelectric electroencephalogram should not be interpreted as evidence of brain death in barbiturate overdose and treatment must not be withheld, as full recovery can occur.*

Psychiatric referral is necessary for any patient who recovers from a suicide attempt as soon as he or she is awake and alert.

References

1. DAWN (Drug Abuse Warning Network): 1993 Annual Medical Examiner Data. Washington, DC, Department of Health and Human Services Publication No. 95-3019, p 21, 1995.
2. Buckley NA, White IM, Dawson AH, et al: Correlations between prescriptions and drugs taken in self-poisoning. Med J Aust *162*:194–197, 1995.
3. Harvey SC: Hypnotics and sedatives. *In* Hardman JG, Limbird LE, Molinoff PB, et al (eds): Goodman and Gilman's The Pharmacologic Basis of Therapeutics. 9th ed. New York, Macmillan Publishing Co., pp 373–380, 471–472, 1996.
4. Neuvonen PJ, Elonen E: Effect of activated charcoal on absorption and elimination of phenobarbitone, carbamazepine and phenylbutazone in man. Eur J Clin Pharmacol *17*:51–57, 1980.
5. McCarron MM, Schulze BW, Walberg CB, et al: Short-acting barbiturate overdosage. JAMA *248*:55–61, 1982.
6. Eisenberg HM, Frankowski RF, Contant CF, et al: High-dose barbiturate control of elevated intracranial pressure in patients with severe head injury. J Neurosurg *69*:15, 1988.
7. Bohn DJ, Biggar WD, Smith CR, et al: Influence of hypothermia, barbiturate therapy, and intracranial pressure monitoring on morbidity and mortality rates after near-drowning. Crit Care Med *14*:529, 1986.
8. Wilberger JE, Cantella D: High-dose barbiturates for intracranial pressure control. New Horiz *3*:469–473, 1995.
9. Miller SM, Cottrell JE, Turndorf H, Ransohoff J: Cerebral protection by barbiturates and loop diuretics in head trauma: possible modes of action. Bull N Y Acad Med *56*:305, 1980.
10. Jaffe JH: Drug addiction and drug abuse. In Gilman AG, Goodman LS, Gilman A (eds): The Pharmacologic Basis of Therapeutics. 6th ed. New York, MacMillan Publishing Co., p 535, 1980.
11. Robinson RR, Gunnells JC, Clapp JR: Treatment of acute barbiturate intoxication. Mod Treatment *8*:561–579, 1971.
12. Winchester JF: Barbiturates. *In* Haddad LM, Winchester JF (eds): Clinical Management of Poisoning and Drug Overdose. 2nd ed. Philadelphia, W.B. Saunders Co., pp 718–730, 1990.
13. Reed CE, Driggs MF, Foote CC: Acute barbiturate intoxication: a study of 300 cases based on a physiologic system of classification of severity of the intoxication. Ann Intern Med *37*:290, 1952.
14. Beveridge AW, Lawson AAH: Occurrence of bullous lesions in acute barbiturate intoxication. BMJ *1*:835, 1965.
15. Matthew H: Drug overdose. Medicine (Medical Education International Ltd) *4*:273, 1972.
16. Goodman JM, Bischel MD, Wagers PW, Barbour BM: Barbiturate intoxication: morbidity and mortality. West J Med *124*:179, 1976.
17. Greenblatt DJ, Allen MD, Harmatz JS, et al: Overdosage with pentobarbital and secobarbital: Assessment of factors related to outcome. J Clin Pharmacol *19*:758, 1979.
18. Afifi AA, Sacks ST, Liu VY, et al: Accumulative prognostic index for patients with barbiturate, glutethimide, and meprobamate intoxication. N Engl J Med *285*:1447, 1971.
19. Cohan SL: Brain death. *In* Haddad LM, Winchester JF (eds): Clinical Management of Poisoning and Drug Overdose. 2nd ed. Philadelphia, W.B. Saunders Co., pp 239–246, 1990.
20. Meredith TJ, Dawling S: Sedative overdose. *In* Haddad LM, Shannon MW, Winchester JF (eds): Clinical Management of Poisoning and Drug Overdose. 3rd ed. Philadelphia, W.B. Saunders Co., pp 581–608, 1998.
21. Linton AL, Ledingham IM: Severe hypothermia with barbiturate intoxication. Lancet *1*:24, 1966.
22. Haddad LM, Robinson RR, Gunnells JC, Clapp JR: Barbiturate overdose. *In* Tintinalli J (ed): Emergency Medicine: A Comprehensive Study Guide. New York, McGraw-Hill Book Co., pp 276–278, 1985.
23. McCarron MM: Barbiturate poisoning. *In* Harwood-Nuss A, Linden CH, Luten RC, et al (eds): The Clinical Practice of Emergency Medicine. Philadelphia, J.B. Lippincott Co., pp 471–474, 1991.
24. Matthew H, Lawson AAH: Acute barbiturate poisoning: A review of two years' experience. Q J Med *35*:539, 1966.
25. Johanson WG: Massive phenobarbital ingestion with survival. JAMA *202*:1106, 1967.
26. Goldberg MJ, Berlinger WG: Treatment of phenobarbital overdose with activated charcoal. JAMA *247*:2400–2401, 1982.
27. Berg MJ, Berlinger WG, Goldberg MJ, et al: Acceleration of the body clearance of phenobarbital by oral activated charcoal. N Engl J Med *307*:642–644, 1982.
28. Pond SM, Olson KR, Osterloh JD, Tong TG: Randomized study of the treatment of phenobarbital overdose with repeated doses of activated charcoal. JAMA *251*:3104–3108, 1984.
29. Amitai Y, Degani Y: Treatment of phenobarbital poisoning with multiple dose activated charcoal in an infant. J Emerg Med *8*:449–450, 1990.
30. Modi NB, Veng-Pedersen P, Wurster DE, et al: Phenobarbital removal characteristics of three brands of activated charcoals: A systems analysis approach. Pharm Res *11*:318–323, 1994.
31. Shreiner GE: The role of hemodialysis (artificial kidney) in acute poisoning. Arch Intern Med *102*:896, 1958.
32. Setter JG, Maher JF, Shreiner GE: Barbiturate intoxication: Evaluation of therapy including dialysis in a large series selectively referred because of severity. Arch Intern Med *117*:224, 1966.
33. Kennedy AC, Lindsay RM, Briggs JD, et al: Successful treatment of three cases of very severe barbiturate poisoning. Lancet *1*:955, 1969.
34. Yatzidis H, Oreopoulos D, Triantaphyllidis D, et al: Treatment of severe barbiturate poisoning. Lancet *2*:216, 1965.
35. Chang TMS: Hemoperfusion alone and in series with hemofiltration or dialysis for uremia, poisoning, and liver failure. Kidney Int *10*:S305, 1976.
36. Gelfand MC, Winchester JF, Knepshield JH, et al: Treatment of severe drug overdose with charcoal hemoperfusion. Trans Am Soc Artif Intern Organs *23*:599, 1977.
37. Winchester JF, Gelfand MC, Knepshield JH, Shreiner GE: Dialysis and hemoperfusion of poisons and drugs: update. Trans Am Soc Artif Intern Organs *23*:762, 1977.
38. Haddad LM: Acute poisoning. *In* Bennett JC, Plum F (eds): Cecil Textbook of Medicine. 20th ed. Philadelphia, W.B. Saunders Co., pp 503–510, 1996.
39. Samtleben W, Gurland HJ, Lysaght MJ, Winchester JF: Plasma exchange and hemoperfusion. *In* Jacobs C, Kjellstrand CM, Koch KM, Winchester JF (eds): Replacement of Renal Function by Dialysis. Boston, Kluwer Academic Publishers, pp 472–500, 1996.
40. Winchester JF: Active methods for detoxification: Oral sorbents, forced diuresis, hemoperfusion and hemodialysis. *In* Haddad LM, Winchester JF (eds): Clinical Management of Poisoning and Drug Overdose. 2nd ed. Philadelphia, W.B. Saunders Co., pp 148–167, 1990.

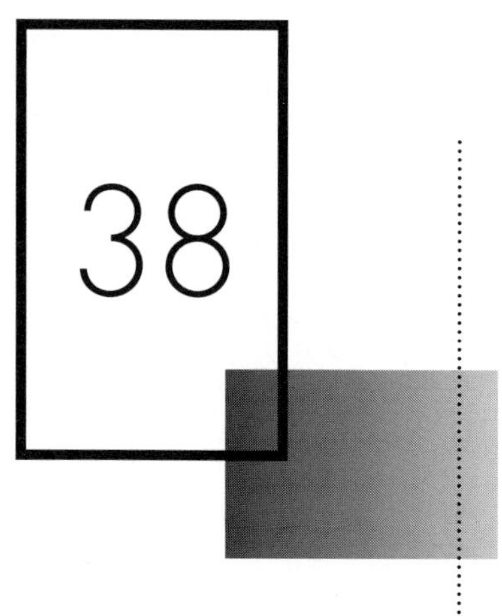

Marijuana

BILLY MARTIN, PhD
STEPHEN SZARA, MD, DSc

The sudden emergence of marijuana as a major drug of abuse in the late 1960s has had a lasting impact on the dynamics of substance abuse. Marijuana continues to be by far the most extensively used illicit drug. As such, it has received much attention ranging from concerns that its acute and chronic use poses a health hazard to consideration of its potential as a therapeutic agent. Despite a wealth of anecdotal information, innumerable clinical studies, and extensive animal experimentation, marijuana use remains a highly controversial and much-debated topic. The views include advocates who proclaim marijuana to be a highly effective therapeutic agent with little potential for producing adverse health effects. Conversely, others consider marijuana to be a highly dangeous substance with no therapeutic potential. The objectives of this chapter are to review the patterns of marijuana use, summarize the health consequences of acute and chronic exposure to marijuana, and discuss the medical uses of marijuana. The discussion also includes some of the issues that contribute to the controversial nature of marijuana. Finally, the progress that has been made in the past decade in terms of identifying the brain mechanisms by which marijuana produces its behavioral effects are reviewed. The purpose of this chapter is to provide the most accurate available data on the potential health problems of marijuana use so that clinicians can recognize medical and psychologic difficulties arising from the widespread use of this drug.

EPIDEMIOLOGY

The most comprehensive evaluation of drug use is conducted through an ongoing national research and reporting program entitled The Monitoring the Future Study, in which secondary school students, college students, and young adults are surveyed annually about the types of drugs used and the frequency of use.[1] This study has consistently shown that alcohol is the most frequently used substance in all subgroups, and marijuana is the most frequently used illicit substance. High school seniors have been closely monitored since 1975. Prevalence is measured in terms of lifetime (used at least once), annual (used at least once during the past year), 30 days (used at least once during the past 30 days), and daily (used at least 20 times during the past 30 days). The prevalence of marijuana use peaked during the late 1970s, when more than 60% of high school seniors reported having smoked marijuana at least once in their lifetime. More importantly, 10% of these studends were smoking marijuana on a daily basis. Since that time, marijuana use continually declined to its lowest levels, in 1991, when more than a third of seniors reported lifetime use and approximately 2% reported daily use. However, a steady rebound in use has been noted during the past 3 years, and approximately 40% of seniors report lifetime use, 31% annual use, and 3.6% daily use. The survey was expanded in 1991 to include 8th- and 10th-grade students. The patterns of use are very similar to that of seniors in that a continual increase has occurred since 1992. Lifetime uses for 8th and 10th graders were 16.7% and 30.4%, respectively, in 1994. Marijuana is also widely used by young adults, although use tends to decline with age. For example, annual use by 20-year-olds is nearly 30%, whereas it is approximately 20% for 30-year-olds. As these statistics suggest, the use of this substance is so prevalent that clinicians should have at least a basic understanding of marijuana's effects and probably should include careful questioning on drug use when taking a history of patients in the youth and young adult age groups.

The most common form of marijuana use in the

United States is in cigarettes. Generally, smoke is inhaled deeply and held in the lungs for 15 to 30 seconds; this represents a very efficient and rapid way to "get high." Smokers easily can control their level of intoxication, because effective brain levels of the active ingredients are rapidly achieved. The oral route is the second most common means of intoxication. Generally, marijuana is baked inside cookies or brownies and ingested. In this mode, the effects after ingestion do not start immediately, as with inhalation. Peak brain levels are reached approximately 2 hours after ingestion; the effects, however, last longer. The user, in this mode of administration, cannot control the level of intoxication, and for some this is rather disconcerting. For example, oral users have periods of being too high and feeling anxious, interspersed with periods of not being high enough and feeling depressed or tired. The intravenous route has been reported in the literature, although primarily in research subjects. Some illicit intravenous use has been reported, and subjects "shoot" crude marijuana plant extracts, but this remains an extremely unusual practice.

BOTANY AND CHEMISTRY

Cannabis sativa has been used for centuries not only for its psychoactive resin but also for hemp fiber and rope. The cannabinoid Δ^9-tetrahydrocannabinol (THC) is the principal psychoactive constituent in the plant. In addition, the plant contains more than 400 other chemicals, including several other cannabinoids, which produce little if any psychoactive effects. The only other cannabinoid with known behavioral effects is cannabinol, which is approximately 10 times less potent than THC. The highest concentration of THC is found in the leaves and the flowering tops of the plant. The term *marijuana* generally refers to tobacco-like preparations of the leaves and flowers. Depending on cultivation techniques, the THC content in marijuana can range from 0.4% to 20%, but the average THC content in confiscated marijuana in the United States has remained steady at approximately 3% for the past 10 years. Hashish, the resin extracted from the tops of the flowering plants, sometimes has a THC concentration exceeding 10%. Hash oil is an extract of cannabis that can provide a THC concentration of 20% or higher. A typical marijuana cigarette contains 500 to 1000 mg of plant material and on average (3% THC content) 15 to 30 mg of THC.

PHARMACOKINETICS

THC is readily absorbed when marijuana is smoked. Although oral ingestion of marijuana produces similar pharmacologic effects, THC is absorbed somewhat more slowly and erratically than by smoking. THC is metabolized in humans first to hydroxylated metabolites, followed by conversion to carboxylic acids. The metabolites are subsequently excreted as conjugates. Although the metabolite 11-hydroxy-Δ^9-THC produces psychotomimetic activity, it is formed in only small amounts when marijuana is smoked. Appoximately 15% and 50% of THC is excreted in urine and feces, respectively, over several days.[2] The primary metabolite excreted in urine is conjugated 11-*nor*-9-carboxy-Δ^9-THC. Pharmacologic effects are produced rapidly and generally peak within 30 minutes of the onset of smoking. Impairment of various performance measures related to driving skills has been demonstrated immediately after marijuana use for as long as 24 hours thereafter. Behavioral and physiologic effects generally return to baseline levels 4 to 6 hours after smoking.

Two general pharmacokinetic issues have attracted considerable attention. The first is whether blood or urine levels of THC can be used to assess the degree of intoxication. It is well recognized that blood concentrations of THC peak before behavioral effects.[3] One interpretation of this time discordance between blood concentrations of THC and effects is that no meaningful relationships exists between blood concentrations and effects.[4, 5] Fortunately, the technology for measuring THC and metabolites in biologic fluids and tissues has improved, along with an understanding of underlying principles governing distribution of lipophilic substances, such as THC, in mammalian systems. Once equilibrium between brain and blood concentrations is established (approximately 45 minutes after use), a linear relationship between blood concentrations and pharmacologic effects appears. Mathematic models that have been introduced are useful in interpretation of the relationship of THC and metabolite concentrations in blood to drug-induced effects and for estimation of time elapsed since marijuana use.[6] Because no reliable model has yet been put into practice for determining degree of impairment, blood and urine levels of THC and metabolites should be used only for determining whether or not an individual has used marijuana. This point brings us to the second issue, which deals with urine testing. The typical means of detecting marijuana use is through measurement of the primary THC metabolite 11-*nor*-Δ^9-THC carboxylic acid in urine using an immunoassay screen. The most frequently asked questions pertain to reliability and sensitivity of these tests. When the results from the initial screen are confirmed by gas chromatography/mass spectrometry, the results are extremely reliable. As for sensitivity, the immunoassay kits have different cutoff limits such as 20, 50, and 100 ng/mL of urine. Some marijuana users are interested in the length of time that urinary metabolites can be detected after last use. In addition to assay sensitivity, individual metabolism and amount of material that was smoked are important variables. Although the length of time for detection varies greatly, monitoring acute marijuana use with a 50-ng/mL cutoff may provide a narrow window of detection of as little as 1 to 2 days or with a lower cutoff as long as a week or more.[7]

INTERPRETATION OF ANIMAL AND HUMAN STUDIES

Before discussing the health implications of marijuana use, it is important to consider some of the factors that complicate interpretation of the existing data. Much of the earlier literature is based on uncontrolled clinical studies of individuals who smoked marijuana or products derived from marijuana. In most of these studies, there was little characterization of the plant material, and comparison among different studies thus was highly problematic. Most of these studies were not only uncontrolled but were retrospective. A major advance occurred with the identification and synthesis of THC.[8] A few years later, the National Institute of Mental Health contracted for large-scale production of THC for distribution to the research community. With the availability of a chemically well-defined active principle, scientific research began in earnest to assess the health consequences of marijuana use and to determine the neurochemical mechanisms responsible for these effects. It must be borne in mind, however, that clinical studies with THC do not elucidate all of the potential harmful effects of marijuana.

The ambiguity of our knowledge may be attributed to a number of other factors. It has been difficult either to prove or disprove health hazards in humans by extrapolation of data from animal studies. The doses used in animals are sometimes much larger than the average amount of drug consumed by humans, and species differences make the extrapolation difficult. On the other hand, higher doses in animals can be justified on the basis that animals are less sensitive to THC than are humans because of pharmacokinetic differences. Marijuana is still used by young persons in the best of health, frequently on an intermittent rather than regular basis, and this fact may lead to an underestimation of the potential impact it has on health. Finally, marijuana is often used in combination with tobacco and alcohol, among licit drugs, as well as various illicit drugs. This fact makes any conclusion from uncontrolled clinical observation less then conclusive. In recognition of these difficulties, research has been conducted with more appropriate doses of the drug in animal studies. The patient population has been more carefully selected in clinical studies, using appropriate control groups whenever feasible, so that the conclusions drawn from these data are more reliable.

ACUTE EFFECTS OF MARIJUANA

Almost all the effects of a single exposure to marijuana can be predicted by dose. As noted, an average marijuana cigarette can contain from 15 to 30 mg of THC. The delivery of THC via smoke is dependent on many factors, such as pyrolysis during smoking, efficiency of smoking, and so on. Ohlsson and colleagues[9] reported that heavy marijuana users smoked more efficiently (23% to 27% bioavailability) than light smokers (10% to 14% bioavailability). If we assume 20% bioavailability, a smoker receives a dose of approximately 3 to 6 mg of THC. This calculation allows for a reasonable comparison of studies conducted with marijuana and THC. The effects that are produced by a single administration of THC or marijuana exposure are for the most part unequivocal.

Acute Cardiovascular Effects

It has been well established that sinus tachycardia is produced by administration of THC or smoking marijuana. This tachycardia is easily reproducible, is clearly related to dose of THC, and occurs with lower doses of THC. Marijuana may produce orthostatic hypotension at higher doses. Electrocardiographic changes in intoxicated individuals have shown nonspecific ST-T changes as well as occasional premature ventricular contractions. The electrocardiographic changes, however, have not been easily reproduced and seem to be subject dependent. These cardiovascular effects are not likely to have serious consequences in young, healthy adults. The effects on patients who have pre-existent angina pectoris can be harmful because the exercise performance in these individuals was reported to be significantly decreased after administration of marijuana. The increase in heart rate, blood pressure changes, and apparent increase in myocardial oxygen demand certainly can add to patients' already compromised cardiovascular problems. The mechanism of action for the cardiovascular effects has been shown to be caused primarily by stimulation of the autonomic nervous system with involvement of both the parasympathetic and sympathetic pathways. No long-term cardiovascular effects have been described to date.

Respiratory Effects

Because inhalation of marijuana is the prevalent mode of administration in the United States today, the effects on the respiratory tract are of major concern. Marijuana smoke, as is true of tobacco smoke, has a high content of particulate matter, or tar. When the smoke is inhaled deeply into the lungs, it appears to have effects at both the anatomic and cellular levels. Although these effects may occur after a single smoking session, the primary effects occur after repetitive administration. What has been demonstrated after acute inhalation of marijuana is bronchodilatation in both normal and asthmatic patients. Additionally, after one-time administration by inhalation, clinicians may note rhinitis, pharyngitis, and hoarseness. These symptoms, however, generally occur along with acute bronchitis-laryngitis after chronic use.

Psychologic and Neurologic Effects

Marijuana's effects on central nervous system functions such as behavior, cognition, perception, and performance are extremely important issues. It is important to understand the mind-altering qualities of this substance that have made it such a popular recreational drug in our society. It is also important to recognize and understand the drug's effects on cognition and performance in intoxicated individuals, particularly in social settings or situations requiring accurate psychomotor functioning—that is, on the job, in the classroom, and on the highways.

In the acute state, it appears that the mood-altering effects of marijuana are in fact dose dependent. Individuals who consume low to moderate quantities generally report a feeling of well-being or euphoria, a dreamlike state, a state of pleasant relaxation, an alteration of time and space perception, and a heightening of their senses—for example, better olfaction, clearer perception of music, and so on. Smoking a large quantity of marijuana can produce a range of effects including mild anxiety, paranoid behavior, acute psychosis, problems in dealing with reality, and obsessional thought content characterized by delusions, hallucinations, illusions, and bizarre behavior. These adverse effects are also sometimes reported to occur in inexperienced users.

Cognitive functioning, such as speaking, problem solving, and memory recall, can be affected by marijuana use. It appears that these cognitive changes are related not only to the dose of the drug but also to the complexity of the tasks or the problem to be solved as well as the individual's familiarity with the given tasks.[10] Marijuana users, while intoxicated, frequently have problems with frequency of speech and organization of thought. Marijuana has been shown to interfere with short-term memory, and this dysfunction is thought to be a major cause of poor cognitive performance during marijuana intoxication. In addition, it appears that material and facts learned while intoxicated are less well recalled than is the same material learned in a nondrugged state. This may of course have significant impact on the performance of students or individuals in work or job-training situations.

Complex Motor Functions

Complex motor functions of individuals are also impaired while in the intoxicated state.[10] Society as well as practicing clinicians may experience far-reaching consequences of marijuana's effect on the important tasks of driving automobiles and flying airplanes. Numerous attempts have been made to assess the impact of marijuana on driving performance, particularly with regard to traffic accidents. Several studies have examined cannabinoid levels in accident victims, including epidemiologic studies, to suggest a link between traffic accidents and marijuana use.[11] Of most importance is that some of the performance parameters continue to be impaired even several hours after a marijuana user no longer feels high. This motor performance impairment is additionally augmented by the common combination of marijuana with alcohol. Practicing clinicians who may encounter individuals who have altered behavior and have been involved in motor vehicle accidents are thus faced with a tremendous challenge. These clinicians must consider whether the behavior is secondary to the trauma itself or to alcohol use, but given the prevalence of the use of marijuana today in our society, they must also consider marijuana intoxication as another potential factor in a patient's altered state. Despite evidence that marijuana interferes with driving performance in the laboratory as well as on the highway, establishing marijuana as the primary cause of traffic accidents has been complicated by confounding variables, such as combined use of marijuana with alcohol.[12] Arguments have also been forwarded that marijuana users are better capable of compensating for impairment, in contrast to those under the influence of alcohol.[12]

Diagnosis and Treatment of Acute Intoxication

The clinical features of acute intoxication with marijuana, either administered orally or after smoking, are nondescript. The signs of hyperemia of the conjunctivae, irritation of mucous membranes of the throat and nose, and tachycardia, coupled with apparent trouble with short-term memory and its effects on continuity of conversation, fluency of speech, and performance of complex tasks, could be the only clues to marijuana use. As stated, acute panic and anxiety reactions as well as an acute toxic psychosis with hallucinations, delusions, illusions, and agitation are primarily observed in inexperienced individuals or in those who take too large a dose. These adverse reactions can generally be managed with a quiet, supportive, and protective environment; reassurance; and, if needed, mild sedation with drugs such as the benzodiazepines. The symptoms of these episodes generally subside within hours. In patients who have a genotype for schizophrenia, even a modest dose of marijuana sometimes can produce a schizophrenic type of psychosis that may be difficult to distinguish from an acute toxic psychosis. In these individuals, the usual drug and support therapies for schizophrenia are needed.

In general, because the clinical presentation of acute marijuana intoxication is so subtle and its use so prevalent, clinicians should suspect marijuana use when confronted with individuals who seem to have problems with cognitive functions such as thinking, speaking, and attention span and have difficulty with complex tasks such as driving. Although urine screening can verify marijuana use, these tests are not practical in the acute clinical intoxication because interpretation is hampered by poor correlation between blood levels and clinical effects. In addition, prolonged elimination of the drug makes determination of the exact time of use difficult.

LONG-TERM EFFECTS

As noted, the effects of marijuana in humans after repetitive or chronic use are most controversial. Attempts at creating a research design investigating the drug's effects on human subjects reveal the reasons for so much controversy and contradiction. The approach used in the majority of long-term studies first identified chronic users and then measured physiologic and psychologic parameters for comparison with non–marijuana-smoking subjects. Obviously, unless gross changes occurred, subtle changes would not be noted or subject to researcher interpretation.

Chronic Pulmonary Effects

Because marijuana is typically smoked, its possible adverse effects on the lungs and pulmonary function have long been of concern. If the public health experience with tobacco smoking can be considered a precedent for pulmonary consequences of chronic inhalation of tar-containing material, we could expect the development of pathology such as emphysema or cancer of the lungs of the user population. Thus far, no large-scale epidemiologic studies such as that with tobacco have been carried out to allow a conclusion to be drawn about the relationship between smoking marijuana and the incidence of lung cancer. It may well be that the American experience has been too brief for this to be a measurable outcome. Nevertheless, there is good reason for concern about the possibility that pulmonary cancer might result from extended use for several decades. Several reports have noted a higher-than-expected incidence of squamous cell carcinoma of the tongue, larynx, and lungs in young adults.[13, 14] Like tobacco smoke residuals, so-called tar cannabis residuals, when applied to the skin of experimental animals, have been shown to be tumor producing. Analysis of marijuana smoke also has revealed large amounts of cancer-producing hydrocarbons. For example, benzopyrene, a known cancer-producing chemical found in tobacco smoke, has been reported to be 70% more abundant in marijuana smoke than in tobacco.[15]

Taskin and his colleagues[16–18] conducted studies of lung function in marijuana-only smokers, marijuana-plus-tobacco smokers, tobacco-only smokers, and nonsmokers. A subset of these individuals were studied longitudinally for changes in lung function, evidence of respiratory disease, and precancerous signs. Light microscopy showed two or more histopathologic changes in the bronchial epithelium of all smokers, regardless of the substance smoked. Squamous metaplasia was observed in all subjects smoking both marijuana and tobacco, a prevalence that was significantly different from that in any of the other groups of subjects. Hyperplasia of basal and goblet cells and cellular disorganization were more prevalent in the marijuana users than in the respective control subjects.

Several clinical studies of human users have reported such symptoms as laryngitis, cough, hoarseness, bronchitis, and cellular change in chronic marijuana smokers; these symptoms resemble symptoms found in heavy tobacco smokers. Although studies of small numbers of long-term cannabis users in Jamaica,[19] Greece,[20] and Costa Rica[21] found no evidence of lung pathology, this may have been because traditional users in those countries do not deeply inhale cannabis smoke and retain it in their lungs as do American users. In the Tashkin studies mentioned earlier, results of the initial testing of participants indicated that daily smoking of marijuana was associated with physiologic and symptomatic evidence of large airways disease, whereas regular tobacco smoking affected mainly the smaller airways and the alveolated regions of the lungs.[18] In follow-up testing, after a 2- to 3-year hiatus, the researchers succeeded in re-examining approximately half of their original cohort. Most of the re-examined participants remained in their original smoking category. When only those participants who did not change their smoking status were considered, chronic respiratory symptoms remained significantly more prevalent among continuing smokers of marijuana or tobacco or both than among nonsmokers. Although the frequency of reported symptoms tended to decline slightly among the smokers of marijuana or tobacco alone, respiratory symptom prevalence tended to increase among those who smoked both marijuana and tobacco. Analysis of lung function data in the retested subjects who retained their original smoking status indicated continuing or worsening abnormality in measures of small airways function and diffusing capacity in tobacco smokers, including those who also smoked marijuana, and an increasingly high frequency of abnormalities in tests of large airways function among smokers of marijuana alone or with tobacco. These results support previous findings from analysis of cross-sectional data[17] of a negative impact of tobacco (but not marijuana alone), mainly on small airways and alveolar function, and of marijuana (but not tobacco) predominantly on large airways function. Thus, the longitudinal data suggest additive effects of marijuana plus tobacco, at least with respect to symptom prevalence, that was not apparent from the cross-sectional findings alone.

In summary, the total body of clinical and experimental evidence appears to indicate that relatively young, habitual, heavy marijuana smokers have a high prevalence of pulmonary symptoms associated with abnormal airway appearance and histologic alterations, irrespective of concomitant tobacco smoking. Because marijuana users also often smoke tobacco and the combination appears to place an additive burden on the pulmonary system, the long-term consequences of this practice deserve additional attention.

Reproductive Effects

Effects on reproduction were attributed to marijuana as early as the first cannabis commission's scientific report, that of the Indian Hemp Drugs Commission of 1894. In animal studies, cannabinoids have been reported to reduce levels of luteinizing hormone releasing hormone, luteinizing hormone, prolactin, and testosterone.[22] As for human studies, some have found changes in sex hormone levels after heavy marijuana use[23]; others found no changes in levels of testosterone, luteinizing hormone, follicle-stimulating hormone, prolactin, and cortisol in men and women.[24] One possible explanation for this discrepancy in experimental findings is that after one smokes marijuana, the temporarily depressed levels of testosterone may rapidly return to normal levels. Depending on the time schedule in which sampling is carried out, the effects may be missed. It is important to note that even when testosterone decreases have been found, the levels have been within normal limits.[25] Whether persistent long-term use of marijuana might result in consistently depressed levels of serum testosterone remains to be established.

An increased incidence of gynecomastia and elevated estrogen levels have been clinically noted in a subset of men engaging in chronic abuse of marijuana; a cause-and-effect relationship has not yet been scientifically established.

Two studies of the semen of male long-term users have found abnormalities in count, motility, and structural characteristics of the sperm examined.[26, 27] In one of these experiments, the semen of 16 healthy young men smoking marijuana under controlled conditions was studied. The levels of use consisted of 8 to 20 joints per day, an amount considered to be very high. Decreases in sperm count and motility were found, as was evidence of structural spermatozoal abnormalities. A second study, of Greek long-term users, also found structural abnormalities in sperm that were associated with heavy use.[27] Although the clinical implications of these findings are still unresolved, decreased fertility might well result, especially in men with already marginal fertility. In the more controlled laboratory study, an apparent gradual return to normal function occurred when marijuana use was discontinued.[26] To date, no published reports have related abnormal offspring to the father's marijuana use. Whether or not alterations in reproductive function might have greater significance for a developing child or adolescent is not known, although a concern is that younger users may be more vulnerable during pubescence.

It was suggested that marijuana abuse during the time of established hormonal cycles may induce human females to become anovulatory and produce delayed and smaller surges in estrogen and progesterone.[28] Data on female monkeys did not corroborate alterations in progesterone, however, although treatment for 1 year suggested a shortened luteal phase and either decreased or had no effect on serum levels of estradiol and progesterone.[28] Rat data suggest that THC is neither proestrogenic nor antiestrogenic with respect to increased uterine macromolecular uptake within 6 hours of estrogen administration. In terms of hyperplasia and hypertrophy after estrogen administration, however, THC was modestly proestrogenic in the progesterone-treated uterus but was antiestrogenic in the presence of estradiol. However, these estrogen agonistic/antagonistic effects of THC did not adversely affect the process of implantation and decidualization.[29] THC can prevent estradiol-induced increase in pituitary weight but has no effect on either the uterine or oviduct weight response.[30]

Mendelson and Mello[31] closely monitored a group of female marijuana users, and they failed to find alterations in the cyclic nature of sex hormones and the cycle itself. In summary, no definitive evidence shows that marijuana use alters sexual function in either males or females to such an extent that reproduction is compromised. However, a comprehensive longitutidal study has not been conducted with sufficient power to detect subtle differences in reproduction rate. Additionally, tolerance to these hormonal changes was shown to develop on continuing administration of THC, and the effects seem to be reversible when cannabis use is discontinued. These aspects further complicate attempts to confirm cannabinoid effects on reproduction.

Pregnancy and Fetal Development

The consequences of adminstration of THC in pregnant laboratory animals has been reviewed.[22] Exposure to high doses of THC resulted in an increase in the number of stillbirths and a decrease in litter size. Reports have also described malformations in the offspring, but they occurred only when the dams received very high doses of THC during the initial stages of organogenesis. No malformations were found when THC was administered after the period of organogenesis. Therefore, it has been difficult to demonstrate tetratogenic effects of cannabinoids with treatment regimens that do not affect nutrition. Abel pointed out that many studies conducted with high doses of THC more likely reflect maternal toxicity rather than direct effects on embryonic and fetal development.[32] Hutchings and colleagues conducted carefully controlled rat studies in which food intake was adjusted and cross-fostering was performed. They reported that THC produced relatively few adverse effects on the offspring.[33] During the postnatal period, somatic growth and brain protein synthesis were reduced; however, these effects were transitory in that these THC-exposed animals caught up to the control animals by the time of weaning.

The effects of maternal marijuana use on the fetal development and the outcome of pregnancy in humans are difficult to study, because these effects are complicated by such variables as nutrition; use of alcohol, tobacco, and other drugs; and socioeconomic status, all of which affect fetal health. In order to determine marijuana's effect, these variables must be equalized or controlled. Large numbers of mother/child pairs are necessary if infrequent disorders are to be identified.

Numerous studies have examined the influence of marijuana exposure on birth weight, and only approximately a third have reported a reduction in weight.[34] It has been suggested that lifestyle likely has an important role in the influence of marijuana on birth weight. Three studies have examined samples of sufficient size to control adequately for confounding effects. Hingston and associates[35] studied 1690 mother/child pairs, Gibson and co-workers[36] sampled 7301 births, and the largest study to date, by Linn and colleagues,[37] involved 12,716 mothers and their newborn babies. The general conclusions from these studies were that marijuana users were more likely than nonusers to have had an unplanned pregnancy, premature labor, and abruptio placentae, and their children were more likely to have lower birth weight and congenital features compatible with fetal alcohol syndrome or some other major malformation. Marijuana use was a better predictor of fetal alcohol syndrome than alcohol use in these studies. The investigators note that the same women who smoke tobacco and marijuana frequently drink alcohol and abuse other drugs. Therefore, some of the adverse effects on fetal development attributed to maternal drinking or smoking may be due to an interaction with marijuana and other psychoactive substances. When a number of these toxic substances are consumed together, their toxic effects on a fetus may be additive.

The long-term consequences of prenatal marijuana exposure have not been fully elucidated. The effects are at most very subtle, and few neurobehavioral consequences are observed up to 3 years of age.[38, 39] Some alterations in language skills are observed at 2 years of age, and verbal ability and memory were different between marijuana-exposed and nonexposed 4-year-olds. However, these differences were not observed in 5- and 6-year-olds. Older children may have altered cognitive ability, but these findings are not definitive.

Immune System

The effects of cannabinoids on all components of the immune system has been studied in humans, monkeys, and rodents using both *in vivo* and *in vitro* approaches. Rat alveolar macrophages were only moderately affected after 30 days of exposure to marijuana smoke, with changes in morphology, superoxide production, and oxygen consumption.[40] Human pulmonary alveolar macrophages obtained from marijuana smokers also displayed a suppression of superoxide production.[41] Macrophages from monkeys exposed to marijuana smoke for as long as 1 year had altered morphology, including an increase in the number of vacuoles, as well as changes in protein expression.[42] Phagocytic and spreading ability of macrophages is also adversely affected in cultures prepared from mice[43] and humans.[44] Interleukin-1 bioactivity and release were increased,[45] and antiviral factor production was suppressed.[46] Because tumor necrosis factor levels have been reported either to increase[45] or decrease,[47] depending on the type of cell culture, the effect of cannabinoids on cytokine levels is probably modulatory.

The effects of cannabinoids on the humoral immunity (production of B-lymphocytes) and cell-mediated immunity (T-lymphocyte production) are inconsistent. Conflicting study results were generated in the 1970s; cannabinoids either suppressed leukocyte numbers and functions or did not affect lymphocytes. These studies were often performed with human patients without controlling lifestyle factors. In monkey studies conducted during the same period, blood cell mitogen responses and serum IgG and IgM levels were reduced in monkeys continually administered THC for 6 months.[48] In another study, rhesus monkeys treated with THC for 3 weeks had elevated neutrophil levels; lymphocytes were not affected.[49] A more recent study reported that in human outpatient marijuana smokers, the T-cell CD4-to-CD8 ratio increased.[50] However, Dax and colleagues demonstrated that in institutionalized patients receiving small amounts of marijuana for 3 weeks, white blood cell and subset lymphocyte counts and killer cell activity were unaffected.[51] When the amount of THC and length of exposure time increased, IgG levels decreased; IgD levels increased, and IgA and IgM levels were unaffected.[52] Marijuana smoking appears to produce moderate disturbances in lymphocyte activity in humans and monkeys *in vivo*. Exposure to high doses of THC suppresses leukocyte migration and lymphoproliferation.

Several studies have suggested that cannabinoids decrease host resistance to infection. Cannabinoids enhanced mortality due to *Listeria monocytogenes* and herpes simplex type II virus.[53] Subsequent animal studies confirmed that cannabinoids decreased antibacterial activity of the host immune system.[54]

The evidence just cited clearly demonstrates that cannabinoids are capable of altering immune function. Additionally, a unique subpopulation of cannabinoid receptors is confined to the immune system (discussed later). The clinical relevance of these findings is uncertain, however. Although it seems reasonable to conclude that marijuana exposure could contribute to immunosuppression in humans, particularly in compromised individuals, direct evidence demonstrating deleterious effects in humans is lacking.

Psychopathology

The most common adverse psychologic reaction to marijuana use is an exaggeration of the more usual marijuana response in which an individual loses perspective (i.e., the realization that what she or he is experiencing is a transient drug-induced distortion of reality) and becomes acutely anxious. This reaction appears to be more common in relatively inexperienced users, although unexpectedly higher doses of the drug (e.g., a more potent variety of marijuana) can cause such a response even in more experienced users. The symptoms generally respond to authoritative assurance and diminish in a few hours as the immediate effects of acute intoxication recede. An acute syndrome associated with cannabis intoxication, including such features as clouding of mental processes, disorientation, confusion, and marked memory impairment, has been reported.[55] Other cannabinoid-induced symptoms may include severe panic and anxiety states, paranoia, depression, personality changes, confusional states, and psychoses, which are indistinguishable from classic psychiatric syndromes unless the drug-induced etiology is known. These symptoms do not routinely occur after use of marijuana, however. The correct diagnosis often cannot and is not made by physicians and psychiatrists unless they keep in mind this possibility and actively pursue verification by asking direct questions and following up with accurate blood and urine testing.[56]

Tolerance and Dependence

Tolerance to cannabis—that is, a diminished physiologic and psychologic response to repeated drug exposure—is now well substantiated. Tolerance development originally was suspected because experienced users in other countries were able to use quantities of the drug that would have been toxic to United States users, who were accustomed to smaller amounts. Carefully conducted studies with known doses of marijuana or THC leave little question that tolerance develops with prolonged use.[57] These data are also consistent with animals studies demonstrating development of profound tolerance to THC and related analogues after long-term exposure.[58]

The term *marijuana dependence* often has been used in an imprecise way, with meanings ranging from a vague desire to continue use, if marijuana is available, to the manifestation of physical withdrawal symptoms after discontinuance. The clinical diagnosis of marijuana dependence was recently changed to reflect the continued drug use in individuals who are unable to quit. If *dependence* is defined as experiencing definite physical symptoms (such as irritability, restlessness, sleep disturbance, nausea, and diarrhea) after withdrawal of the drug, experimental evidence indicates that such symptoms can occur under conditions of extremely heavy administration on a research ward. At first, this appeared as a theoretic curiosity, but clinical reports now indicate that it can also happen in real life.[59, 60] It has been estimated that 100,000 individuals in the United States alone seek medical attention for marijuana dependence.

It is possible that the physical manifestations of dependence are not readily apparent because withdrawal is protacted but subtle owing to sequestration of THC in the body. Animal studies have also provided mixed results when researchers attempt to define a withdrawal syndrome for THC.[61] One valuable tool in clearly demonstrating dependence is the use of an antagonist to precipitate withdrawal in continually treated animals. The recent discovery of the cannabinoid antagonist SR 141716A by Rinaldi-Carmona and associates[62] provided the first opportunity to conduct such studies with cannabinoids. Administration of the cannabinoid antagonist to rats treated continually with THC resulted in a profound withdrawal syndrome[63, 64] resembling naloxone-precipitated withdrawal in morphine-dependent rats. These studies unequivocally demonstrate that cannabinoids are capable of producing dependence, and the findings are consistent with the observations that chronic heavy marijuana users have difficulty giving up marijuana.

Prevention and Treatment

No prevention model can be cited as being successful on a broad scale. In fact, marijuana use among young individuals has continuously increased during the 1990s, as discussed at the beginning of this chapter. This rebound in marijuana use has been attributed to changes in attitude about the consequences of marijuana use, increasing references to marijuana in the entertainment industry, aggressive pro-marijuana campaigns by advocates, and so on. It is obviously much easier to speculate on the causes for increased use than to identify effective means for preventing use.

No pharmacologic methods are effective for intervening in chronic marijuana use. The standard approach is psychotherapy similar to that of a 12-step Alcoholics Anonymous model, which is often quite helpful for adolescent marijuana users and alcoholics. This approach, coupled with urine monitoring, can be effective in terminating marijuana use; however, relapse is common, as it is with most other drugs of abuse. It is unlikely that the newly developed cannabinoid antagonist will be useful as a treatment modality. Although antagonists are theoretically useful for treatment because they prevent the pleasurable effects of the drugs, most addicts refuse to undergo antagonist treatment for this very reason.

EFFECTS OF MARIJUANA IN COMBINATION WITH ALCOHOL AND OTHER DRUGS

Because marijuana is so commonly used with alcohol and other drugs, the combined effects of these drugs have potentially important implications. Given the extremely wide range of possible doses and interactions, it is not surprising that our present knowledge is still quite limited, even in terms of the most common combinations of alcohol and marijuana. Some of the potential dangers to the outcome of pregnancy by a woman's use of both marijuana and alcohol were alluded to earlier.

Few human studies have investigated the interactive effects of marijuana with drugs other than alcohol; however, limited evidence suggests that such interactions may be significant. Cocaine and marijuana are also coabused, although the reasons are not completely clear, given their opposing pharmacologic properties. A general impression is that marijuana potentiates cocaine's subjective effects. Lukas and colleagues reported that coabuse of intranasal cocaine and marijuana smoke enhanced the tachycardia observed with marijuana alone.[65] The duration of the effects of marijuana and cocaine was unaltered when both drugs were given together. However, marijuana pretreatment reduced the time required for the onset of cocaine effects and decreased the duration of negative cocaine effects. Moreover, marijuana pretreatment increased cocaine levels almost twofold. The researchers concluded that marijuana-induced dilation attenuated the vasoconstrictive properties of cocaine and thereby enhanced the absorption of the latter.

It was reported long ago that marijuana is sometimes adulterated with phencyclidine and that severe toxic reactions may result.[66] Doty and associates[67] reported that combinations of phencyclidine and THC produced either additive or supra-addictive effects in disrupting the behavior of animals responding for food. Combinations of ethanol and THC were also additive in this paradigm. Long-term marijuana use may also affect the persistence of barbiturates in the body; simultaneous use of marijuana and amphetamines may increase the intensity and duration of a subjective high.

It stands to reason that the most likely combination of polydrug use would involve ethanol and marijuana because they are the most heavily used substances. Several studies have reported that concomitant marijuana and ethanol use produces either additive or supra-additive effects on psychomotor performance.[68, 69] Lukas and co-workers, however, reported that marijuana attenuates the plasma ethanol levels, with a resultant decrease in the duration of subjective effects for both agents.[70]

THERAPEUTIC ASPECTS

The modern phase of therapeutic use of cannabis began about 140 years ago, when O'Shaughnessy reported on its effectiveness as an analgesic and anticonvulsant.[71] At about the same time, others described marijuana's use in the treatment of psychiatric illnesses and some favorable results in promoting sleep and enhancing appetite without causing physical addiction. It was also tried as a treatment for opium addiction, chronic alcoholism, delirium tremens, and a wide variety of painful disorders. The drawbacks that historically accompanied therapeutic trials of cannabis centered on the highly variable content of THC, its loss of potency while standing on pharmacy shelves, and its variable gastrointestinal absorption. Therefore, when aspirin, barbiturates, and other synthetic analgesics and sedatives became available, the medical use of extracted *Cannabis indica* faded. The Marijuana Tax Act of 1937 was the final blow that eliminated it from medical practice. In the past decades, however, not only has THC been synthesized but also researchers now have available standardized cigarettes and capsules with specific concentrations of the drug. These advances, plus public and scientific interest in the nature of marijuana's effects on humans, have generated renewed activity in researching the therapeutic potential of this substance. Early clinical trials suggested that marijuana may have some beneficial effects in several disorders. Some of the more noteworthy uses include reduction of intraocular pressure, nausea, and vomiting; stimulation of bronchodilation; and attenuation of the AIDS wasting syndrome. The medical community has not enthusiastically endorsed marijuana for medical purposes, however, because of its variability and modest therapeutic effectiveness, the adverse health consequences of administering smoke, other undesirable side effects, and the adequacy of already marketed drugs. However, some efforts have been made to use THC and synthetic derivatives for treatment of several disease states. Those advocating the use of marijuana for medicinal purposes argue that THC is delivered more effectively in smoke, that marijuana is less expensive than THC, and that marijuana produces few if any harmful effects.

Antiemetic Effect

THC and some of its synthetic analogues such as nabilone, levonantradol, and nabitan have been tested in mostly open clinical trials for antiemetic potency on cancer patients receiving chemotherapy and found to be effective in alleviating the invariable side effects of nausea and vomiting.[72] In several controlled studies, THC was found to be at least as useful as prochlorperazine, in standard use, for controlling these symptoms in patients with cancer. Side effects of THC itself can still be a problem, but evidence of its efficacy for this treatment indication led the Food and Drug Administration to make THC capsules legally available for prescription under the trade name Marinol.[41] Because of its high abuse liability, however, THC is controlled as schedule II drug under the Controlled Substances Act, and prescriptions are limited to the amount necessary for a single cycle of chemotherapy (i.e., a few days).

Anticonvulsant Effect

Marijuana's therapeutic potential as an anticonvulsant has sparked interest ever since a study in the 1940s showed that five retarded children whose seizures were poorly controlled on conventional anticonvulsant medication showed improvement after the use of cannabis.[73] However, extensive animal studies have shown that THC is capable of producing both convulsant and anticonvulsant effects. The discovery that cannabidiol, a natural component of marijuana with practically no marijuana-like psychoactivity, exhibited anticonvulsant activity in animals generated considerable attention.[74] Interest waned, however, when it failed to demonstrate sufficient efficacy for clinical use.

Analgesia

Little definitive evidence has showed that marijuana is effective in controlling either acute or chronic pain. However, several controlled studies have been conducted with THC. Regelson and his colleagues reported that THC failed to ameliorate pain in patients with cancer and did not decrease their need for pain medication.[75] On the other hand, Noyes and co-workers demonstrated that orally administered THC was comparable to codeine in analgesic potency, although it produced considerable side effects in the effective dose range.[76] THC is highly effective in almost all animal analgesic assays and has a potency comparable to that of morphine.[77] In addition, numerous analogues have been synthesized and are as much as several hundredfold more potent than THC.[78] The endogenous cannabinoid ligand anandamide (described later) also has analgesic properties.[79] However, the inability to develop a cannabinoid devoid of behavioral effects represents the primary limitation of cannabinoid analgesics. Cannabinoids are quite effective when administered intrathecally to laboratory animals, and this route may provide a means of producing analgesia with minimal behavioral effects.[80] Additionally, cannabinoids have been shown to potentiate the analgesic effects of morphine when both are administered intrathecally.[81]

Glaucoma

The ability of marijuana, THC, and its synthetic derivatives to lower intraocular pressure in patients suffering from glaucoma has received much attention.[82] Although some variability is found among the results of studies, most reveal that smoking marijuana lowers intraocular pressure to a significant degree. The need for smoking marijuana or for systemic administration of synthetic cannabinoids for beneficial effects has tempered the enthusiasm for their use for managing glaucoma. One report describes a topical preparation of marijuana that is effective for glaucoma and is marketed as Canasol in Jamaica.[83] However, no present evidence shows that marijuana or THC is more effective than other agents in controlling glaucoma.

MECHANISM OF ACTION

Cannabinoids produce a complexity of pharmacologic and behavioral effects that most likely involve numerous neurochemical mechanisms. Although researchers devoted several decades to unraveling the actions of the very lipophilic cannabinoids on the brain, in only the past 7 to 10 years has significant progress been made. Definitive evidence now shows that THC acts on unique receptors in the brain to produce most of its effects. The earliest indications of cannabinoid receptors arose for structure-activity relationships.[78] Enantioselectivity has been demonstrated for THC as well as numerous derivatives. Equally important is the finding that subtle changes in the THC structure can have a profound influence on activity. Two significant substances that were developed from these structure-activity relationship studies were the highly potent agonists and structurally diverse analogues with THC-like properties.

The first direct evidence for a cannabinoid receptor was made possible by the synthesis and radiolabeling of the potent bicyclic cannabinoid CP-55,940,[84] which led to the identification of a receptor in rat brain membranes.[85] Analysis of the data revealed a single binding site that possessed saturable and reversible binding. This receptor exhibits high selectivity for cannabinoids in that a vast array of other centrally acting compounds fail to interact with this site.[86] It appears that this receptor is responsible for most of THC's effects on the brain. In an extensive study, Compton and associates demonstrated a high correlation between binding affinities for a large number of cannabinoids and potency in various pharmacologic assays, including production of antinociception, catalepsy, hypothermia, and depression of spontaneous locomotor activity in mice; drug discrimination in rats; and psychotomimetic activity in humans.[87]

According to autoradiograpic studies, the distribution of the cannabinoid receptor is heterogeneous in several mammalian species, conserved, and neuronally located.[88–90] The densest binding occurs in the basal ganglia (substantia nigra pars reticulata, globus pallidus, endopeduncular nucleus, and lateral caudate putamen) and the molecular layer of the cerebellum. Binding in these regions explains cannabinoid alteration in motor function. THC disrupts short-term memory in humans, and this finding is consistent with intermediate levels of receptors in the pyramidal cell layers of the hippocampus, the dentate gyrus, and layers I and VI of the cortex. Cannabinoid effects on memory and cognition are consistent with receptor localization in the hippocampus and cortex. The hippocampus stores memory and codes sensory information. The presence of cannabinoid receptors in regions associated with mediating brain reward (ventromedial striatum and nucleus accumbens) suggests an association with dopamine neurons.[91] Sparse levels were detected in the brain stem, hypothalamus, corpus callosum, and the deep cerebellum nuclei. Low levels of receptors in brain stem areas controlling cardiovascular and respiratory functions are also consistent with the lack of lethality of marijuana. Binding has also been found in the B-lymphocyte–enriched areas, including the marginal zone of the spleen, the nodular corona of Peyer's patches, and the cortex of the lymph nodes.[92]

Unfortunately, binding studies such as those described earlier do not provide definitive evidence for a receptor. Unequivocal evidence was provided when the cannabinoid receptor was cloned.[93] It was found to be a member of a large family of receptors that are coupled to G proteins, which serve as very common second messengers for most neurotransmitter receptors. The human cannabinoid receptor was subsequently cloned and found to have almost identical homology to the rat receptor.[94] A distinct peripheral cannabinoid receptor, designated CB_2, has been identified in macrophages in the marginal zone of the spleen.[95] The role of this receptor in the spleen remains unknown. The discovery of a second receptor raises the possibility that other receptors with unique functional roles may exist.

The discovery of the receptor led to the search for endogenous cannabinoids. Devane and colleagues isolated a substance from porcine brain that competed for cannabinoid receptor binding and, like THC, inhibited electrically stimulated contractions in the murine vas deferens.[96] Anandamide produced similar pharmacologic effects to THC, such as antinociception, catalepsy, hypomotility, and hypothermia,[97] and inhibited adenylate cyclase[98] and N-type calcium channels.[99] A comparison between anandamide and THC revealed that anandamide was 4- to 20-fold less potent and had a shorter duration of action than THC.[100] Neuronal tissue has the ability to both synthesize and degrade anandamide. Deutsch and Chin[101] showed that anandamide was rapidly taken up by neuroblastoma and glioma cells and degraded by a cytosolic amidase. Degradation also occurred in tissues from the brain, heart, kidneys, and lungs. Synthesis was achieved by incubating arachidonate with ethanolamide. The enzyme inhibitor phenymethylsulfonyl fluoride prevented degradation but not synthesis of anandamide. On the other hand, another group found that phenylmethylsulfonyl fluoride did inhibit synthesis in bovine brain.[102] Other investigators have questioned the condensation synthetic pathway by providing evidence that anandamide formation occurs through phosphodiesterase-mediated cleavage of a novel phospholipid precursor, *N*-arachidonoyl-phosphatidylethanolamine.[103] The synthesis of anandamide has also been proposed to occur via a novel eisosanoid pathway that is coenzyme A and adenosine triphosphate independent.[104]

The discovery of the cannabinoid antagonist SR 141716A by Rinaldi-Carmona and colleagues[62] provides a means for delineating receptor- and non–receptor-mediated events. These investigators demonstrated that this antagonist has high affinity for the CB_1 receptor and antagonizes cannabinoid-induced inhibition of adenylate cyclase and smooth muscle contractions. Others have shown that it also antagonizes cannabinoid drug discrimination in rats.[105]

Based on the discoveries during the past decade, one can postulate that a cannabinoid neurochemical system does exist. The function of this system and its interaction with other neurochemical systems remains unclear. It is well known that cannabinoids exert many of their actions by influencing several traditional neurotransmitter systems, as presented in other reviews.[106–108] The results of numerous studies suggest that several neurotransmitters and neuromodulators have a role in the neuropharmacology of cannabinoids. These substances include acetylcholine, dopamine, γ-aminobutyric acid (GABA), histamine, 5-hydroxytryptamine, norepinephrine, opioid peptides, and prostaglandins. The basis for some of the effects of cannabinoids are studied by determining the interaction between cannabinoids and drugs that bind to other receptor types or drugs that alter the synthesis, storage, release, or metabolism of transmitters and modulators.[107] Cannabinoids have been shown to enhance the formation of norepinephrine, dopamine, and 5-hydroxytryptamine. Cannabinoids also stimulated the release of dopamine from rat corpus striatum, nucleus accumbens, and medial prefrontal cortex. GABA turnover is enhanced by cannabinoids. The most commonly studied effects of cannabinoids include hypothermia, antinociception, and changes in locomotor activity. Results of drug interaction studies of catalepsy and depression of spontaneous locomotor activity suggest that these effects are mediated by acetylcholine's acting at muscarinic and nicotinic receptors, GABA's acting at $GABA_A$ and $GABA_B$ receptors, and prostaglandin Es (PGEs). The extrapyramidal system probably has a role in catalepsy, because intrapallidal administration of 11-OH-Δ^8-THC produced this behavior.[109] Hypothermia in rats and mice may be mediated by dopamine, norepinephrine, 5-hydroxytryptamine, GABA, histamine, and opioid peptides. Evidence also suggests that alteration in thermoregulation involves the hypothalamus[110] and brain stem.[111] Results of hypothermia studies are often inconsistent; thus, definite conclusions cannot be drawn about the neuronal pathway involved in cannabinoid-induced antinociception.[107] Several endogenous compounds serve to inhibit nociception (norepinephrine, 5-hydroxytryptamine, acetylcholine, GABA, opioid peptides, PGE_1, and PGD_2), and some of these compounds interact with cannabinoids to produce antinociception. Data support the involvement of PGE_1, and some experiments support the involvement of catecholamines, 5-hydroxytryptamine, and opioid peptides. Interpretation of the actions of cannabinoids on neurotransmitter systems is often difficult, because evidence shows that cannabinoids both inhibit and stimulate neuronal uptake.

The establishment of a cannabinoid receptor and

an endogenous ligand with biosynthetic and degradative pathways suggests the possible presence of a distinct neurochemical system. Future research is needed to establish the physiologic role of this system in the central nervous system.

References

1. Johnston LD, O'Malley PM, Bachman JG (eds): National Survey Results on Drug Use from the Monitoring the Future Study, 1975–1995. Washington, DC, US Department of Health and Human Services, 1995.
2. Wall ME, Sadler BM, Brine D, et al: Metabolism, disposition, and kinetics of Δ^9-tetrahydrocannabinol in men and women. Clin Pharmacol Ther *34:*352–363, 1983.
3. Huestis MA, Sampson AH, Holicky BJ, et al: Characterization of the absorption phase of marijuana smoking. Clin Pharmacol Ther *52:*31–41, 1992.
4. Mason AP, McBay AJ: Cannabis: Pharmacology and interpretation of effects. J Forensic Sci *30:*615–631, 1985.
5. McBay A: Drug concentrations and traffic safety. Adv Alcohol Subst Abuse *2:*51–59, 1986.
6. Huestis MA, Henningfield JE, Cone EJ: Blood cannabinoids. II. Models for the prediction of time of marijuana exposure from plasma concentrations of Δ^9-tetrahydrocannabinol (THC) and 11-nor-9-carboxy-Δ^9-tetrahydrocannabinol (THCCOOH). J Anal Toxicol *16:*283–290, 1992.
7. Huestis MA, Mitchell JM, Cone EJ: Detection times of marijuana metabolites in urine by immunoassay and gc-ms. J Anal Toxicol *19:*443–449, 1995.
8. Gaoni Y, Mechoulam R: Isolation, structure, and partial synthesis of an active constituent of hashish. J Am Chem Soc *86:*1646–1647, 1964.
9. Ohlsson A, Agurell S, Londgren J, et al: Pharmacokinetics studies of delta-1-tetra hydrocannabinol in man. *In* Barnett G, Chiang C (eds): Pharmacokinetics and Pharmacodynamics of Psychoactive Drugs. Biomedical Publications, Foster City, CA, pp 75–92, 1985.
10. Chait LD, Pierri J: Effects of smoked marijuana on human performance: A critical review. *In* Murphy L, Bartke A (eds): Marijuana/Cannabinoids: Neurobiology and Neurophysiology. Boca Raton, FL, CRC Press, pp 387–423, 1992.
11. Hall W, Solowij N, Lemon J (eds): The Health and Psychological Consequences of Cannabis Use. Canberra, Australian Government Printing Service, 1994.
12. Robbe HWJ (ed): Influence of Marijuana on Driving. Maastricht, Institute for Human Psychopharmacology, University of Limburg, 1994.
13. Taylor FM: Marijuana as a potential respiratory tract carcinogen: A retrospective analysis of a community hospital population. South Med J *81:*1213–1216, 1988.
14. Donald PJ: Marijuana and upper aerodigestive tract malignancy in young patients. *In* Nahas GG, Latour C (eds): Cannabis: Physiopathology, Epidemiology, Detection. Boca Raton, FL, CRC Press, pp 165–183, 1993.
15. Peterson RC (ed): Marijuana Research Findings: 1980. Washington, DC, US Government Printing Office, 1980.
16. Gong H, Fligiel S, Tashkin DP, Barbers RG: Tracheobronchial changes in habitual, heavy smokers of marijuana with and without tobacco. Am Rev Respir Dis *136:*142–149, 1987.
17. Tashkin DP, Calvarese BM, Simmons MS, Shapiro BJ: Respiratory status of seventy-four habitual marijuana smokers. Chest *78:*699–706, 1980.
18. Tashkin DP, Coulson AH, Clark VA, et al: Respiratory symptoms and lung function in habitual heavy smokers of marijuana alone, smokers of marijuana and tobacco, smokers of tobacco alone, and nonsmokers. Am Rev Respir Dis *135:*209–216, 1987.
19. Rubin V, Comitas L (eds): Ganja in Jamica. The Effects of Marijuana, New York, Anchor/Doubleday, 1976.
20. Stefanis C, Dornbush R, Fink M (eds): Hashish: Studies of Long-Term Use. New York, Raven Press, 1977.
21. Carter WE (ed): Cannabis in Costa Rica/A Study of Chronic Marijuana Use. Philadelphia, Institute for the Study of Human Issues, 1980.
22. Wenger T, Croix D, Tramu G, Leonardelli J: Effects of Δ^9-tetrahydrocannabinol on pregnancy, puberty, and the neuroendocrine system. *In* Murphy L, Bartke A (eds): Marijuana/Cannabinoids: Neurobiology and Neurophysiology. Boca Raton, FL, CRC Press, pp 539–560, 1992.
23. Kolodny R, Leasin P, Tora G, et al: Depression of plasma testosterone with acute marihuana administration. *In* Braude MC, Szara S (eds): The Pharmacology of Marihuana. New York, Raven Press, pp 217–225, 1976.
24. Block R, Farinpour R, Schlechte J: Effects of chronic marijuana use on testosterone, luteinizing hormone, follicle stimulating hormone, prolactin and cortisol in men and women. Drug Alcohol Depend *28:*121–128, 1991.
25. Hollister LE: Health aspects of cannabis. Pharmacol Rev *38:*1–20, 1986.
26. Hembree W, Nahas GG, Zeidenberg P, Huang HFS: Changes in human spermatozoa associated with high dose marihuana smoking. *In* Nahas GG, Paton WDM (eds): Marihuana: Biological Effects. New York, Pergamon Press, pp 429–439, 1979.
27. Issidorides MR: Observations in chronic hashish users: Nuclear aberrations in blood and sperm and abnormal acrosomes in spermatozoa. *In* Nahas GG, Paton WDM (eds): Marihuana: Biological Effects. New York, Pergamon Press, pp 377–388, 1979.
28. Rosenkrantz H: Cannabis components and responses of neuroendocrine-reproductive targets: An overview. *In* Paton W, Nahas GG (eds): Marihuana '84: Proceedings of the Oxford Symposium on Cannabis. Oxford, UK, IRL Press, pp 457–505, 1985.
29. Paria BC, Kapur S, Dey SK: Effects of 9-ene-tetrahydrocannabinol on uterine estrogenicity in the mouse. J Steroid Biochem Mol Biol *42:*713–719, 1992.
30. Murphy LL, Rodriguez de Fonseca F, Steger RW: Δ^9-tetrahydrocannabinol antagonism of the anterior pituitary response to estradiol in immature female rats. Steroids *56:*97–102, 1991.
31. Mendelson JH, Mello NK: Effects of marijuana on neuroendocrine hormones in human males and females. *In* Braude MC, Ludford JP (eds): Marijuana Effects on the Endocrine and Reproductive Systems. Washington, DC, US Government Printing Office, pp 97–114, 1984.
32. Abel EL: Effects of prenatal exposure to cannabinoids. *In* Pinkert TM (ed): Current Research on the Consequences of Maternal Drug Abuse. Washington, D.C., U.S. Govt. Printing Office, pp 20–35, 1985.
33. Hutchings DE, Morgan B, Brake SC, et al: Δ^9-tetrahydrocannabinol during pregnancy in the rat: I. Differential effects on maternal nutrition, embryotoxicity, and growth in the offspring. Neurotoxicol Teratol *9:*39–43, 1987.
34. Fried PA, O'Connell CM: A comparison of the effects of prenatal exposure to tobacco, alcohol, cannabis and caffeine on birth size and subsequent growth. Neurotoxicol Teratol *9:*79–85, 1987.
35. Hingston R, Zuckerman B, Frank DS, et al: Effects on fetal development of maternal marijuana use during pregnancy. *In* Harvey DJ (ed): Marijuana '84: Proceedings of the Oxford Symposium on Marijuana. Oxford, IRL Press, p 539, 1984.
36. Gibson GT, Baghurst PA, Colley DP: Maternal alcohol, tobacco and cannabis consumption and the outcome of pregnancy. Aust N Z J Obstet Gynaecol *23:*15–19, 1983.
37. Linn S, Schoenbaum SC, Monson RR, et al: The association of marijuana use with outcome of pregnancy. Am J Public Health *73:*1161–1164, 1983.
38. Fried PA, O'Connell CM, Watkinson B: 60- and 72-month follow-up of children prenatally exposed to marijuana, cigarettes, and alcohol: Cognitive and language assessment. J Dev Behav Pediatr *13:*383–391, 1992.
39. Day N, Richardson G, Goldschmidt L, et al: Effect of prenatal marijuana exposure on the cognitive development of offspring at age three. Neurotoxicol Teratol *16:*169–175, 1994.
40. Davies P, Somberger GC, Huber GL: Effects of experimental

marijuana and tobacco smoke inhalation on alveolar macrophages. Lab Invest *41:*220–223, 1979.
41. Sherman MP, Roth MD, Gong H, Tashkin DP: Marijuana smoking, pulmonary function, and lung macrophage oxidant release. Pharmacol Biochem Behav *40:*663–669, 1991.
42. Cabral GA, Stinnett AL, Bailey J, et al: Chronic marijuana smoke alters alveolar macrophage morphology and protein expression. Pharmacol Biochem Behav *40:*643–649, 1991.
43. Lopez-Cepero M, Friedman M, Klein T, Friedman H: Tetrahydrocannabinol induced suppression of macrophages spreading and phagocytic activity *in vivo.* J Leukocyte Biol *39:*679–686, 1986.
44. Spector S, Lancz G: Suppression of human macrophage function *in vitro* by Δ^9-tetrahydrocannabinol. J Leukocyte Biol *50:*423–426, 1991.
45. Shivers SC, Newton C, Friedman H, Klein TW: Δ^9-Tetrahydrocannabinol (THC) modulates IL-1 bioactivity in human monocyte/macrophae cell lines. Life Sci *54:*1281–1289, 1994.
46. Cabral GA, Vasquez R: Δ^9-Tetrahydrocannabinol suppresses macrophage extrinsic antiherpes virus activity. Proc Soc Exp Biol Med *199:*255–263, 1992.
47. Fischer-Stenger K, Pettit DAD, Cabral GA: Δ^9-Tetrahydrocannabinol inhibition of tumor necrosis factor-α: Suppression of post-translational events. J Pharmacol Exp Ther *267:*1558–1565, 1993.
48. Daul CB, Health RG: The effect of chronic marihuana usage on the immunological status of rhesus monkeys. Life Sci *17:*875–882, 1975.
49. Silverman AY, Darnell BJ, Montiel MM, et al: Response of rhesus monkey lymphocytes to short-term administration of THC. Life Sci *30:*107–115, 1982.
50. Wallace JM, Tashkin DP, Oishi JS, Barbers RG: Peripheral blood lymphocyte subpopulations and mitogen responsiveness in tobacco and marijuana smokers. J Psychoactive Drugs *20:*9–14, 1988.
51. Dax EM, Pilotte NS, Adler WH, et al: The effects of 9-ene-tetrahydrocannabinol on hormone release and immune function. J Steroid Biochem *34:*263–270, 1989.
52. Nahas GG, Ossweman EF: Altered serum immunoglobulin concentration in chronic marijuana smokers. *In* Friedman H, Spector S, Klein TW (eds): Drug of Abuse, Immunity, and Immunodeficiency. New York, Plenum Press, pp 25–32, 1991.
53. Morahan PS, Klykken PC, Smith SH, et al: Effects of cannabinoids on host resistance to *Listeria monocytogenes* and herpes simplex virus. Infect Immun *23:*670–674, 1979.
54. Ashfaq MK, Watson ES, ElSohly HN: The effect of subacute marijuana smoke inhalation on experimentally induced dermonecrosis by *S. aureus* infection. Immunopharmacol Immunotoxicol *9:*319–331, 1987.
55. Myer RE: The state of evidence. *In* Tinklenberg JR (ed): Marihuana and Health Hazards: Methodological Issues in Current Research. New York, Academic Press, pp 133–152, 1975.
56. Estroff TW, Gold MS: Psychiatric presentation of marijuana abuse. Psychiatr Ann *16:*221–224, 1986.
57. Jones RT, Benowitz N: The 30-day trip—clinical studies of cannabis tolerance and dependence. *In* Braude MC, Szara S (eds): Pharmacology of Marihuana. New York, Raven Press, pp 627–642, 1976.
58. Fan F, Compton DR, Ward S, et al: Development of cross-tolerance between Δ^9-THC, CP 55,940 and WIN 55,212. J Pharmacol Exp Ther *271:*1383–1390, 1994.
59. Weller RA, Halikas JA: Objective criteria for the diagnosis of marijuana abuse. J Nerv Ment Dis *168:*98–103, 1980.
60. Tennant FS: The clinical syndrome of marijuana dependence. Psychiatr Ann *16:*225–234, 1986.
61. Compton DR, Dewey WL, Martin BR: Cannabis dependence and tolerance production. *In* Erickson CK, Javors MA, Morgan WW (eds): Addiction Potential of Abused Drugs and Drug Classes. Binghampton, NY, Hayworth Press, pp 129–147, 1990.
62. Rinaldi-Carmona M, Barth F, Héaulme M, et al: SR141716A, a potent and selective antagonist of the brain cannabinoid receptor. FEBS Lett *350:*240–244, 1994.
63. Tsou K, Patrick S, Walker JM: Physical withdrawal in rats tolerant to D9-tetrahydrocannabinol precipitated by a cannabinoid receptor antagonist. Eur J Pharmacol *280:*R13–R15, 1995.
64. Aceto M, Scates S, Lowe J, Martin B: Cannabinoid precipitated withdrawal by the selective cannabinoid receptor antagonist, sr 141716A. Eur J Pharmacol *282:*R1–R2, 1995.
65. Lukas S, Sholar M, Kouri E, et al: Marihuana smoking increases plasma cocaine levels and subjective reports of euphoria in male volunteers. Pharmacol Biochem Behav *48:*715–721, 1994.
66. McCabe OL: Psychedelic drug crises: Toxicity and therapeutics. J Psychedelic Drugs *9:*107–114, 1977.
67. Doty P, Dykstra LA, Picker MJ: Δ^9-Tetrahydrocannabinol interactions with phencyclidine and ethanol: Effects on accuracy and rate of responding. Pharmacol Biochem Behav *43:*61–70, 1992.
68. Bird KD, Boleyn T, Chesher GB, et al: Intercannabinoid and cannabinoid-ethanol interactions and their effects on human performance. Psychopharmacology *71:*181–188, 1980.
69. Sutton L: The effects of alcohol, marijuana and their combination on driving ability. J Stud Alcohol *44:*438–445, 1983.
70. Lukas SE, Benedikt R, Mendelson JH, et al: Marihuana attenuates the rise in plasma ethanol levels in human subjects. Neuropsychopharmogy *7:*77–81, 1992.
71. O'Shaughnessy WB: On the preparation of Indian hemp and gunjah. Trans Med Phys Soc Bombay *8:*421–461, 1842.
72. Razdan RK: Structure-activity relationships in cannabinoids. Pharmacol Rev *38:*75–149, 1986.
73. Davis JA, Ramsey HD: Antiepileptic action of amrijuana active substance. Fed Proc *8:*284, 1949.
74. Karler R, Turkanis SA: The cannabinoids as potential antiepileptics. J Clin Pharmacol *21:*417S–448S, 1981.
75. Regelson W, Butler JR, Schulz J, et al: Δ9-Tetrahydrocannabinol as an effective antidepressant and appetite-stimulating agent in advanced cancer patients. *In* Braude MC, Szara S (eds): The Pharmacology of Marihuana. New York, Raven Press, pp 763–776, 1976.
76. Noyes JR, Brunk SF, Avery DH, Canter A: The analgesic properties of Δ^9-tetrahydrocannabinol and codeine. Clin Pharmacol Ther *18:*84–89, 1975.
77. Martin BR: Characterization of the antinociceptive activity of intravenously administered Δ^9-tetrahydrocannabinol in mice. *In* Harvey DJ (ed): Marihuana '84, Proceedings of the Oxford Symposium on Cannabis. Oxford, UK, IRL Press, pp 685–692, 1985.
78. Martin BR, Thomas BF, Razdan RK: Structural requirements for cannabinoid receptor probes. *In* Pertwee RG (ed): Cannabinoid Receptors. New York, Academic Press, pp 36–85, 1995.
79. Adams IB, Ryan W, Singer M, et al: Evaluation of cannabinoid receptor binding and *in vivo* activities for anandamide analogs. J Pharmacol Exp Ther *273:*1172–1181, 1995.
80. Smith PB, Martin BR, Welch SP: Nor-binaltorphimine pretreatment specifically inhibits Δ^9-THC induced antinociception in mice without altering the behavioral effects. *In* Harris LS (ed): Problems of Drug Dependence 1992: Proceedings of the 54th Annual Scientific Meeting. Washington, DC, US Government Printing Office, p 148, 1992.
81. Welch SP, Stevens DL: Antinociceptive activity of intrathecally administered cannabinoids alone, and in combination with morphine, in mice. J Pharmacol Exp Ther *262:*10–18, 1992.
82. Adler MW, Geller EB: Ocular effects of cannabinoids. *In* Mechoulam R (ed): Cannabinoids as Therapeutic Agents. Boca Raton, FL, CRC Press, pp 51–70, 1986.
83. West ME, Homi J: Cannabis as a medicine. Br J Anaesth *76:*167, 1996.
84. Melvin LS, Johnson MR: Structure-activity relationships of tricyclic and nonclassical bicyclic cannabinoids. *In* Rapaka RS, Makriyannis A (ed): Structure-Activity Relationships of the Cannabinoids. Washington, DC, US Government Printing Office, pp 31–47, 1987.
85. Devane WA, Dysarz FA, Johnson MR, et al: Determination and characterization of a cannabinoid receptor in rat brain. Mol Pharmacol *34:*605–613, 1988.

86. Howlett AC, Evans DM, Houston DB: The cannabinoid receptor. *In* Murphy L, Bartke A (eds): Marijuana/Cannabinoids: Neurobiology and Neurophysiology. Boca Raton, FL, CRC Press, pp 35–72, 1992.
87. Compton DR, Rice KC, De Costa BR, et al: Cannabinoid structure-activity relationships: Correlation of receptor binding and *in vivo* activities. J Pharmacol Exp Ther *265:*218–226, 1993.
88. Herkenham M, Lynn AB, Johnson MR, et al: Characterization and localization of cannabinoid receptors in rat brain: A quantitative *in vitro* autoradiographic study. J Neurosci *11:*563–583, 1991.
89. Herkenham M, Lynn AB, DeCosta BR, Richfield EK: Neuronal localization of cannabinoid receptors in the basal ganglia of the rat. Brain Res *547:*267–274, 1991.
90. Herkenham M: Cannabinoid receptor localization in brain. Neurosci Facts *3:*53–54, 1992.
91. Gardner EL, Lowinson JH: Marijuana's interaction with brain reward systems—update 1991. Pharmacol Biochem Behav *40:*571–580, 1991.
92. Lynn A, Herkenham M: Localization of cannabinoid receptors and nonsaturable high-density cannabinoid binding sites in peripheral tissues of the rat: Implications for receptor-mediated immune modulation by cannabinoids. J Pharmacol Exp Ther *268:*1612–1623, 1994.
93. Matsuda L: Cloning of the cannabinoid receptor gene. Neurosci Facts *3:*53, 1992.
94. Gérard CM, Mollereau C, Vassart G, Parmentier M: Molecular cloning of a human cannabinoid receptor which is also expressed in testis. Biochem J *279:*129–134, 1991.
95. Munro S, Thomas KL, Abu-Shaar M: Molecular characterization of a peripheral receptor for cannabinoids. Nature *365:*61–64, 1993.
96. Devane WA, Hanus L, Breuer A, et al: Isolation and structure of a brain constituent that binds to the cannabinoid receptor. Science *258:*1946–1949, 1992.
97. Fride E, Mechoulam R: Pharmacological activity of the cannabinoid receptor agonist anandamide, a brain constituent. Eur J Pharmacol *231:*313–314, 1993.
98. Felder CC, Briley EM, Axelrod J, et al: Anandamide, an endogenous cannabimimetic eicosanoid, binds to the cloned human cannabinoid receptor and stimulates receptor-mediated signal transduction. Proc Natl Acad Sci U S A *90:*7656–7660, 1993.
99. Mackie K, Devane W, Hille B: Anandamide, an endogenous cannabinoid, inhibits calcium currents as a partial agonist in N18 neuroblastoma cells. Mol Pharmacol *44:*498–503, 1993.
100. Smith PB, Compton DR, Welch SP, et al: The pharmacological activity of anandamide, a putative endogenous cannabinoid, in mice. J Pharmacol Exp Ther *270:*219–227, 1994.
101. Deutsch DG, Chin SA: Enzymatic synthesis and degradation of anandamide, a cannabinoid receptor agonist. Biochem Pharmacol *46:*791–796, 1993.
102. Devane W, Axelrod J: Characterization of the enzymatic synthesis of anandamide: Properties and distribution in the brain. Neuropsychopharmacology *10:*146S–146S, 1994.
103. Di Marzo V, Fontana A, Cadas H, et al: Formation and inactivation of endogenous cannabinoid anandamide in central neurons. Nature *372:*686–691, 1994.
104. Kruszka K, Gross R: The ATP-and CoA-independent synthesis of arachidonoylethanolamide. J Biol Chem *269:*14345–14348, 1994.
105. Wiley J, Barrett R, Lowe J, et al: Discriminative stimulus effects of CP 55,940 and structurally dissimilar cannabinoids in rats. Neuropharmacology *34:*669–676, 1995.
106. Dewey WL: Cannabinoid pharmacology. Pharmacol Rev *38:*151–178, 1986.
107. Pertwee R: *In vivo* interactions between psychotropic cannabinoids and other drugs involving central and peripheral neurochemical mediators. *In* Murphy L, Bartke A (eds): Marihuana/Cannabinoids: Neurobiology and Neurophysiology. Boca Raton, FL, CRC Press, pp 165–218, 1992.
108. Pertwee RG: The central neuropharmacology of psychotropic cannabinoids. *In* Balfour DJK (ed): Psychotropic Drugs of Abuse. New York, Pergamon Press, p 355, 1990.
109. Pertwee RG, Wickens AP: Enhancement by chlordiazepoxide of catalepsy induced in rats by intravenous or intrapallidal injections of enantiomeric cannabinoids. Neuropharmacology *30:*237–244, 1991.
110. Fitton AG, Pertwee RG: Changes in body temperature and oxygen consumption rate of conscious mice produced by intrahypothalamic and intracerebroventricular injections of Δ^9-tetrahydrocannabinol. Br J Pharmacol *75:*409–414, 1982.
111. Hosko MJ, Schmeling WT, Hardman HF: Evidence for a caudal brainstem site of action for cannabinoid-induced hypothermia. Res Bull *6:*251–258, 1981.

39

Cocaine

TIMOTHY E. ALBERTSON, MD, PHD
GREGORY P. MARELICH, MD
R. STEVEN THARRATT, MD

Cocaine continues to be a significant drug of abuse in the United States, as well as in many other parts of the world. It is frequently associated with drug-related emergency department (ED) and intensive care unit admissions. The presence of cocaine is frequently identified in the reckless or impaired driver[1] and in the general trauma patient.[2, 3] Although the central nervous and cardiovascular systems are most commonly affected by cocaine, the drug can have toxic manifestations in nearly every organ system. Because of the prevalence and medical significance of cocaine toxicity, health care providers must be knowledgeable of and alert for cocaine toxicity.

COCAINE HISTORY

Cocaine is an alkaloid derived from the leaves of the species *Erythroxylon coca*. The first recorded medicinal uses were by Spanish physicians in 1596.[4] Cocaine was first isolated from coca leaves in 1859 by Albert Nieman, a graduate student at the University of Göttingen.[5] By 1863, Angelo Mariani marketed a wine in France that was fortified with about 6 mg per ounce of the cocaine alkaloid extract.[5] In the United States, the Parke-Davis Company was selling a fluid extract containing 0.5 mg/mL of a crude cocaine by 1880.[5] By 1884, Sigmund Freud had proposed that cocaine be used for the treatment of depression, cachexia, and asthma and as a local anesthetic.[6] That same year, cocaine was also first used in eye surgery, a field revolutionized by the discovery of this drug. Also in 1884, William Steward Halsted, the father of modern American surgery, first used cocaine in regional nerve blocks. Unfortunately, Halsted, like Freud, became heavily dependent on cocaine.[6] In 1885, John Styth Pemberton registered the cocaine-containing “French Wine Cola” in the United States; later, he renamed the product “Coca-Cola.”[5]

By 1893, fatalities from the use of cocaine had been reported. In 1895, a series of six fatalities were reported in *Lancet*.[5, 7] In 1909, over 10 tons of cocaine were imported into the United States without legal restraint. Multiple over-the-counter medical products and elixirs containing various amounts of cocaine were created. A product for nasal application called “Dr. Tucker’s Asthma Specific” contained 420 mg of cocaine per ounce.[5] The passage of the Harrison Narcotics Act of 1914 finally banned nonprescription use of cocaine-containing products. Subsequently, a significant reduction in the use of cocaine in the United States occurred. Cocaine was gradually replaced by amphetamine in the 1950s as the most prevalent stimulant of abuse, but this trend reversed in the 1970s.[6, 8] The Controlled Substances Act of 1970 prohibited the manufacture, distribution, and possession of cocaine in the United States, except for increasingly limited medical uses.[6] By the 1980s, chunks of an alkaloidal cocaine called “crack” (for the cracking-like noise it makes when heated) had become widely available.

As a result of the large-scale, illegal importation and distribution of cocaine, a 15-fold increase in cocaine toxicity–related ED visits was noted between 1976 and 1986.[8] A corresponding increase in cocaine-related deaths also was seen, with some reports indicating that as many as 5 of every 1000 deaths in the United States are associated with cocaine abuse.[8, 9] In 1985, it was estimated that 30 million people in the United States had used cocaine.[4] An estimated 3 to 5 million people in the United States reported using cocaine regularly.[4] A 1987 survey of primary care physicians found that 37% had seen at least one patient with cocaine-related toxicity within a month of the survey. Approximately 11% of Americans older than 12 years of age have used cocaine, with 7% of adults between 18 and 34 years of age having used it within the previous year. Despite a significant overall reduction in the current number of users of cocaine to 1.6 million between 1985 and 1990, no similar decline was found during the same period in the nearly 500,000 people regularly using free base ("crack") cocaine.[10]

Crack cocaine (cocaine alkaloid or base) has a lower melting point than the hydrochloride form (80 to 90°C, versus 180°C). Its increased volatility and stability during pyrolysis allow for an inhalation route of abuse.[6] Crack cocaine's popularity among abusers was first noted in the early 1980s and is likely owing to its ease of production and its rapid and intense drug effect. It is not surprising that smoking cocaine base has become the most common means of self-administration of cocaine in patients presenting to EDs.[11]

PHARMACOLOGIC MECHANISMS

The stimulant cocaine (benzoylmethylecgonine, $C_{17}H_{21}NO_4$) has complex and multiple pharmacologic mechanisms of action. It is a weak base with a pKa of 8.6.[12] It has a volume of distribution of 2 to 3 L/kg.[12] Central and peripheral nervous system blockade of the reuptake of and possible stimulation of presynaptic release of catecholamines, including norepinephrine and dopamine, and the blockade of serotonin reuptake are major actions of cocaine. The predominance of catecholamine reuptake blockade contributes to postsynaptic nervous system stimulation. Reuptake inhibition also leads to metabolism and eventual depletion of catecholamines and serotonin. Cocaine also causes marked local anesthetic effects from the blockade of membrane sodium channels.[8, 12] In addition, cocaine may inhibit potassium channels and sodium-calcium exchange mechanisms in some cellular membranes.[13]

Cocaine has excellent oral absorption, with oral bioavailability of the drug being 30% to 40% for both cocaine hydrochloride (crystalline salt) and its cocaine base. Reasonable nasal absorption of the hydrochloride form is observed. With the advent of crack cocaine's popularity, inhalation use of the drug has increased. Although constriction of nasal vessels inhibits further nasal absorption, it can produce prolonged duration of action and may reduce the risk of high exposure levels and associated toxicity.[12] Although the route of administration does not change the drug's pharmacodynamics, the inhalation route produces a more rapid increase in plasma and brain cocaine levels and more intense euphoria than the nasal and oral routes and has cardiovascular effects similar to those produced by an equivalent intravenous dose of cocaine.[14] When cocaine is taken nasally or by the oral route, attainment of peak levels occurs at 30 to 120 minutes.[12] Self-administration utilizing the intravenous route is often seen, commonly when cocaine is used in combination with other agents. Although arterial levels are higher, peak venous levels of 200 to 600 mg/mL are seen with typical doses (0.2 to 2 mg/kg), depending on the route. Peak venous cocaine levels of several thousand nanograms per milliliter have been reported in intoxicated patients.[12]

About 35% to 45% of cocaine is rapidly metabolized by both enzymatic and nonenzymatic hydrolysis to benzoylecgonine. Another 32% to 49% of cocaine is metabolized to ecgonine methyl ester by enzymatic hydrolysis with hepatic and nonhepatic esterases. A small amount of the benzoylecgonine is metabolized on to ecgonine in a 24-hour period. Although these metabolites tend not to be very active, a small percentage of cocaine, particularly after toxic exposure, undergoes hepatic microsomal oxidative metabolism to norcocaine, a potentially active metabolite, and then to *N*-hydroxynorcocaine, a metabolite potentially toxic to the liver.[12] Endogenous (genetic) loss or induced (e.g., by organophosphate pesticide exposure) loss of cholinesterase activity in a patient may result in a delay in metabolism of cocaine and may increase the toxic risk of a given exposure. Blood or plasma samples must be frozen, or fluoride or cholinesterase inhibitors must be added to samples to prevent cocaine from being hydrolyzed to ecgonine methyl ester by serum cholinesterases.

The serum half-life of cocaine is approximately 30 to 80 minutes. The fact that only 1% to 9% of cocaine appears in the urine unchanged (dependent on urine pH) makes the analysis of the major cocaine metabolites benzoylecgonine and ecgonine more useful for diagnostic and forensic purposes. Benzoylecgonine and ecgonine have serum half-lives of approximately 4 to 6 hours and 3 to 4 hours, respectively. Analysis of both blood and urine for these metabolites can be routinely performed. An enzyme-linked immunoassay directed against benzoylecgonine is useful for the rapid screening of samples for cocaine and its metabolites. Gas chromatography followed by mass spectroscopy represents one of the most sensitive and specific assays available for identifying cocaine and its metabolites.

Intravenous use of cocaine alone or in combination with heroin or with benzodiazepines or other sedative hypnotics is commonly seen. The intravenous use of heroin in combination with cocaine is called "speedballing." The combined use of cocaine and narcotics is estimated to be associated with 12% to 15% of toxic cocaine episodes managed in EDs in the United States.[11] The combined use of ethanol and cocaine appears to facilitate the formation of cocaethylene.[15] This potent cocaine metabolite has a half-life of approximately 2 hours. Animal studies and human epidemiologic studies suggest that cocaethylene is more toxic to the brain and heart than is cocaine or its usual metabolites.[13] The risk of sudden death is 21.5-fold greater with the combined use of ethanol and cocaine than with cocaine use alone. The concomitant use of drugs can increase overall toxicity and can further obscure specific cocaine-induced toxicity.

CLINICAL TOXICITIES AND SPECIFIC MANAGEMENT

Cocaine is capable of inducing toxicities in each organ system. Both acute and chronic abnormalities have been reported with cocaine exposures. Studies have not established the exact prevalence or incidence of the toxicities, which are summarized in Table 39–1.

Cardiovascular

Cocaine use and abuse are frequently associated with cardiovascular toxicity. Acceleration of underlying hypertension and coronary artery disease is thought to occur with chronic cocaine use. Cardiovascular complications of cocaine have been reviewed in detail.[16] Significant cardiac cellular defects have been demonstrated. Indirect, β-adrenergic receptor stimulation by cocaine increases myocardial cell calcium influx and increases free intracellular calcium levels. α-Adrenergic receptor stimulation by cocaine has been shown to activate phospholipase C, which increases inositol triphosphate levels. In turn, the inositol triphosphates initiate a cascade of intracellular second messengers.[16] These two mechanisms have been postulated to cause acute as well as chronic cocaine cardiac toxicity.

Chest pain is a frequent presenting complaint of patients who have used cocaine. Chest pain is responsible for approximately 16% of cocaine admissions to EDs.[2, 17–19] The incidence of cocaine-induced cardiac ischemia resulting in chest pain is unknown. It is believed that much of the cocaine-induced chest pain is noncardiac in origin. However, acute myocardial infarction is the most frequently reported cardiac consequence of cocaine abuse.

Several mechanisms may lead to cocaine-induced myocardial infarction. These include *in situ* coronary artery thrombosis formation, increased myocardial oxygen demand in the setting of limited myocardial oxygen supply, coronary artery vasoconstriction, left ventricular hypertrophy, and accelerated atherosclerosis.[16, 20] Coronary artery spasm leading to myocardial infarction in cocaine users has been widely reported.[17] Patients with cocaine-associated myocardial infarctions are typically young (mean age, 38 years), nonwhite (72%) tobacco smokers (91%) who have a history of cocaine use within the past 24 hours (88%).[17] Angiographic studies of these patients have demonstrated both atherosclerotic and normal coronary arteries.

A number of clinical reports have described cardiomyopathy and myocarditis as consequences of cocaine abuse. It is hypothesized that repeated exposures to cocaine-induced elevations of catecholamine levels may be responsible for myocarditis, the forma-

Table 39–1. Major Noninfectious Medical Complications Associated with Cocaine Use

Cardiac	
Chest pain	+ + +
Myocardial infarction	+ + +
Arrhythmias	+ +
Cardiomyopathy	+ +
Myocarditis	+
Hypertension	+ + +
Sudden death	+ +
Psychiatric	
Anxiety	+ +
Depression	+ +
Paranoia	+ +
Delirium	+ +
Psychosis	+ +
Suicide	+ + +
Obstetric	
Low birth weight	+
Placental abruption	+
Respiratory	
Barotrauma	+ +
Pneumothorax	
Pneumopericardium	
Pneumomediastinum	
Subcutaneous emphysema	
Pulmonary hemorrhage/infarct	+
Diffuse alveolar hemorrhage	+
Pulmonary edema	+ + +
Exacerbation of asthma	+ +
Eosinophilic lung disease	+
Recurrent transient pulmonary infiltrates with peripheral eosinophilia	+
Chronic diffuse interstitial pneumonia with mild fibrosis	+
Sudden infant death syndrome (SIDS)	+
Pulmonary hypertension	+
"Crack lung" with transient pulmonary infiltrates	+ +
Nasal septum perforation/aspiration	+
Bronchiolitis obliterans organizing pneumonia	+
Airway burns/tracheal stenosis	+
Sinusitis	+
Epiglottitis	+
Bronchitis	+ +
Pulmonary cellulose granulomas in lung	+
Panlobar emphysema	+
Foreign body aspiration/needle	+
Alveolar accumulation of carbonaceous material	+ +
Central nervous system respiratory stimulant effect	+ +
Neurogenic Pulmonary Edema	+ + +
Respiratory depression—overdose/post-ictal	+ + +
Abnormal hypoxic response in infants of cocaine-abusing mother	+
Neurologic	
Headaches	+ +
Strokes	+ +
Seizures	+ + +
Cerebral infarcts	+ +
Cerebral hemorrhage	+ +
Cerebral vasculitis	+
Gastrointestinal, Renal, and Other	
Renal failure	+
Rhabdomyolysis	+ +
Hyperthermia	+
Disseminated vasculitis	+
Bowel ischemia/colitis	+ +
Thrombocytopenia/platelet aggregation	+
Hepatitis	+

Estimated frequency and magnitude of events: +, rarely reported; + +, commonly reported; + + +, frequently seen with chronic use or overdose.

tion of myocardial contraction bands, and the development of cardiomyopathy. Immune-mediated or hypersensitivity-generated toxicity from cocaine may also have a role in the development of cardiomyopathy or myocarditis. In addition, it has been postulated that contaminants, including heavy metals such as manganese, have a role in the development of cocaine-associated cardiomyopathy.[16]

Because of cocaine's local anesthetic properties and its effects on catecholamines, it is not surprising that cardiac ventricular arrhythmias are common in patients who abuse cocaine. Several mechanisms have been proposed to explain the cardiac arrhythmias seen with cocaine use. These include direct alteration of myocardial automaticity, autonomic dysregulation by enhanced adrenergic neural stimulation, induction of myocardial tissue ischemia, induction of ischemic electrical disturbances, and potential re-entrant arrhythmias.[16] The severe metabolic acidosis and hypoxemia that often accompany acute cocaine overdose increase the risk of ventricular arrhythmias.

Acute aortic rupture and papillary muscle rupture have been associated with cocaine use in otherwise healthy patients. Endocarditis is a frequent complication of intravenous drug use and thus is seen in the patient abusing intravenous cocaine.

Because of the relatively short half-life of cocaine and its metabolites, supportive care with minimal pharmacologic intervention usually is adequate for most patients with acute cocaine-related cardiovascular toxicity. Hypertension usually responds to sedation alone. If treatment for hypertension is needed, nitroprusside or a calcium channel blocker such as nifedipine can be administered. Malignant cardiac arrhythmias should be treated immediately by correction of hypoxemic, metabolic, and electrolyte abnormalities. The careful use of antiarrhythmics such as lidocaine or short-acting β-adrenergic blockers such as esmolol is indicated. Although lidocaine has been found as an adulterant in street cocaine and even though cocaine has a local anesthetic effect itself, the clinician should not be discouraged from using lidocaine in cocaine-intoxicated patients with severe cardiac arrhythmias. Routine use of β-adrenergic blockers in patients with minimal cardiovascular symptoms should be discouraged because of the effects of unopposed α-adrenergic mechanisms, which can include cocaine-induced coronary artery spasm. The use of agents such as labetolol that have some α-adrenergic in addition to primarily β-adrenergic blocking effects may have theoretic advantages. However, the use of labetolol has not been shown in animal or human studies to be preferable to pure β-blockade in the treatment of cocaine-induced tachycardias and arrhythmias.

Patients with cocaine toxicity frequently present with palpitations and supraventricular tachycardia. Treatment of the patient with no evidence of coronary artery disease includes observation, sedation, generally with benzodiazepines, and the occasional judicious use of labetolol or the short-acting β-adrenergic blocker esmolol for heart rate control.

Cocaine-induced cardiac ischemia has been treated in several reported cases with β-adrenergic blockers or calcium channel blockers as well as with nitrates. According to a review of the treatment of cocaine-associated myocardial ischemia, the use of β-blockers or labetalol in the initial management is not recommended.[20] The use of calcium channel blockers or the α-blocker phentolamine is considered second-line therapy in cocaine-induced coronary ischemia.[20] The need for rapid reperfusion with thrombolytic therapy or angioplasty has been advocated if medical management does not terminate continued myocardial ischemia.[20] A clinical trial has evaluated thrombolytic therapy for cocaine-induced myocardial infarctions. Although thrombolytics appeared to be safe, their efficacy was not examined.[21] The increased risk of cerebrovascular hemorrhage with cocaine-induced toxicity requires that the use of thrombolytics in this patient population be carried out with extreme care.[20] As mentioned earlier, the use of lidocaine has theoretic disadvantages, and some animal data indicate that its use carries a potential risk in cocaine-induced ventricular arrhythmias associated with myocardial ischemia. In review of the use of lidocaine in 29 patients with cocaine-associated myocardial infarctions, no enhanced cocaine toxicity was seen.[22] Ventricular arrhythmias observed immediately after exposure to large doses of cocaine may be treated with sodium bicarbonate because this agent has been shown to reverse cocaine-induced QRS complex prolongation.[20]

Intravascular volume replacement, diuretics, cardiotonic and inotropic agents, and careful vasopressor support have all been utilized in cocaine-induced cardiomyopathy with congestive heart failure. Monitoring of central venous or pulmonary artery wedge pressure may be necessary for titration of these agents. Short-term use of intra-aortic balloon pumps also has been reported to augment cardiac function during transient myocardial dysfunction. General supportive care is important in maintaining cardiomuscular function during cocaine-induced cardiac toxicities. Discontinuation of cocaine use appears to be the most prudent way of reversing or limiting the progression of cocaine-induced chronic cardiomyopathy.

Central Nervous System

It is not surprising that the central nervous system is particularly susceptible to the toxic effects of cocaine, since it is the euphoric effects of cocaine that have drawn so many to its illicit use. Neurologic complaints have ranged in incidence from 17% to 42% in various series of patients with cocaine-related medical problems necessitating ED treatment in the United States.[2, 18, 19] Altered mental status, dizziness, headaches, paresthesias, tremors, seizures, strokes, transient ischemic attacks, and coma represent the majority of these neurologic complaints.

Seizures are a very common manifestation of cocaine toxicity and have been reported in as many as 9% of patients presenting to EDs with cocaine toxicity.[18] Drug-induced seizures are frequently caused by stimulants. Cocaine-induced seizures accounted for the increase in all drug-induced seizure cases from 4% in 1981 to 23% in 1988.[23] Human and animal data suggest that cocaine-induced seizures are typically generalized seizures and are single events without long-lasting neurologic consequences.[24] The majority of cocaine-related seizures are associated with intravenous injection or inhalation of cocaine alkaloid. Pascual-Leone and colleagues have found that when habitual cocaine abuse was associated with seizures, computed tomography frequently showed diffuse brain atrophy; also, diffuse slowing was often found on electroencephalography.[24] Multiple or focal seizures are often associated with acute intracerebral complications (e.g., hemorrhage) or with the toxic manifestations of other medications.[24] Recurrent generalized seizures have been reported in children after mucosal application of the topical anesthetic tetracaine-adrenalin-cocaine. Seizures may be a major determinant of cocaine lethality.[25] This justifies aggressive immediate treatment of sustained cocaine-induced seizures with the correction of seizure-related metabolic acidosis and hypoxemia. Persistent seizures presumed to be caused by cocaine indicate the need for further diagnostic workup that includes computed tomography and possibly lumbar puncture. Aggressive supportive care is often associated with improved cardiac function in the critically ill patient with cocaine toxicity.[25]

Dystonic reactions, cerebral vasculitis, headaches, toxic encephalopathies, transient ischemic events, choreoathetoid movements, and migraine-like events have all been reported with acute and chronic use of cocaine.[26, 27] As would be expected, cerebral hemorrhage, cerebral infarction, and cerebral vasculitis are associated with significant mortality and morbidity among cocaine users. Kaku and Lowenstein reported that 34% of patients between the ages of 15 and 44 years with a diagnosis of ischemic or hemorrhagic stroke had associated drug abuse; cocaine and amphetamine use accounted for the largest percentage of these cases.[28] Psychologic dependence and a cocaine withdrawal or abstinence syndrome have been reported.[12] The *cocaine abstinence syndrome* has been described as having three phases.[12] The first phase is a "crash" that lasts up to 4 days and is characterized by dysphoria, depression, irritability, anxiety, and insomnia followed by hypersomnolence, exhaustion, and drug craving. The second phase lasts from 1 to 10 weeks and is characterized by anergia, anxiety, listlessness, and drug craving. The third phase, which has been called the "extinction phase," may last indefinitely and is associated with normalization of mood and actions but also episodic drug craving that is often triggered by environmental cues.[12] Acute psychiatric disturbances, including agitation, anxiety, depression, psychosis, paranoia, and suicidal ideation have been reported in clinical series evaluating the neurologic toxicity of cocaine abuse.[29] The neurologic complications of cocaine toxicity are responsible for significant morbidity and mortality and have been reviewed in detail.[30]

Treatment for the neurologic complications of cocaine abuse is primarily supportive. Subarachnoid hemorrhage and intracerebral bleeding may require neurosurgical intervention. These hemorrhages may be associated with an underlying cerebral saccular aneurysm or vascular malformation. Ischemic cerebrovascular accidents and transient ischemic attacks are treated symptomatically. Aspirin, heparin, and thrombolytics may be used empirically in acute ischemic strokes associated with cocaine use, but their role has not been formally addressed in the literature. Migraine-like headaches produced by cocaine have been reported to improve with ergotamine treatment. However, there is theoretical concern about the use of another vasospastic agent such as ergotamine in view of the vasospastic side effects of cocaine itself. The use of serotonergic agents such as sumatriptan for cocaine-induced migraine headaches has not been reported.

The use of diazepam and other anticonvulsants, which work through a γ-aminobutyric acid–related mechanism, has been effective in terminating and controlling seizure activity caused by cocaine. Phenytoin, phenobarbital, and pentobarbital may also be useful. Mechanical ventilation for correction of hypoxemia and acidemia may be required in the patient with cocaine-induced seizures.

Sedation with benzodiazepines or butyrophenones such as droperidol or haloperidol can be particularly effective in managing the agitated patient with cocaine toxicity. Use of benzodiazepines (e.g., diazepam) as therapy adjunctive to butyrophenone treatment (e.g., with haloperidol) in the management of acute psychotic agitation is well established and allows reduced dosing of butyrophenones. This combination can lower the risk of extrapyramidal side effects and the theoretic reduction in seizure threshold reported with the use of neuroleptic agents.

Pulmonary

A wide range of pulmonary complications have been reported to occur with cocaine exposure and have been reviewed.[31] Cocaine-induced pulmonary disturbances are often the presenting complaint in EDs and commonly result in intensive care unit admissions. Primary respiratory depression or reduced respiratory drive has been associated with toxic cocaine exposures. This has occurred both in conjunction with and independent of cardiac arrhythmias and seizure-induced cardiovascular collapse.

Cocaine smoking is associated with significant barotrauma manifested by pneumothorax, pneumomediastinum, pneumopericardium, and the presence of subcutaneous air. The self-application of a Valsalva maneuver by cocaine smokers seeking enhancement of euphoric effects (to increase positive airway or intrapleural pressures) may be a significant cause of this barotrauma. High positive airway pressures can also be generated by an "assistant" who blows back into the cocaine pipe being used. Thermal injury from smoking cocaine may also contribute to the development of barotrauma.

Particularly troublesome are the frequent reports of noncardiogenic pulmonary edema associated with cocaine use.[31] Although pulmonary edema has been postulated to occur secondary to acute or chronic heart failure, a vast majority of cases appear to be caused by a noncardiogenic "capillary leak" syndrome. Both neurogenic and non-neurogenic mechanisms for the cocaine-induced noncardiogenic pulmonary edema can be postulated. Treatment for noncardiogenic pulmonary edema is supportive in nature and is similar to that for treating adult respiratory distress syndrome. This includes the use of positive-pressure ventilation, supplemental oxygen, and either positive end-expiratory pressure of the lengthening of inspiratory time intervals to increase the functional residual capacity.

Exacerbation of reversible airway diseases, including asthma, has been reported in association with the use of cocaine. These exacerbations may be the consequences of heat or of exposure to the impurities in cocaine, since its catecholamine effects would not be expected to produce airway bronchospasm.[31, 32]

Dyspnea is the presenting complaint of patients with cocaine-induced toxicity, occurring in 3% to 22% of cases in various series.[2, 18, 19] Hemoptysis, bronchitis, and expectoration of carbonaceous sputum are frequent complaints of cocaine users in the ED. An increased incidence of pulmonary hypertension, pulmonary infarction, pulmonary hemorrhage, and pulmonary foreign body granulomas have been reported in cocaine users. Bronchiolitis obliterans and bronchiolitis obliterans with organizing pneumonia (BOOP) associated with fever and dyspnea may also occur.[31, 33] Loss of a functional alveolocapillary interface as measured by a reduction in carbon monoxide diffusion capacity has been observed in studies of frequent cocaine users.[31] The interpretation of this finding is complicated by other pulmonary exposures to tobacco and marijuana in the population studied.

A specific syndrome of "crack lung" associated with the smoking of cocaine has been defined and comprises chest pain, hemoptysis, and diffuse alveolar infiltrates.[34] Again, whether these manifestations of pulmonary toxicities are related to cocaine exposure itself, to the inhalation of superheated adulterants, or to the exposure to combustion products is unknown.

The treatment of pulmonary problems associated with cocaine use is primarily supportive. Supplemental oxygen, bronchodilator therapy, and mechanical support may be necessary in cocaine-induced bronchospasm. Mechanical ventilation with supplemental oxygen is often needed for patients with cocaine-induced pulmonary edema. Empiric treatment with corticosteroids for bronchiolitis obliterans with organizing pneumonia and eosinophilic pulmonary syndromes has been reported.[31] Chest tube placement is needed in patients with symptomatic pneumothoraces. Avoidance of further cocaine exposure and supportive care is advised for all patients with cocaine-associated pulmonary toxicities.

Hyperthermia

Cocaine-induced hyperthermia has been reported with and in the absence of seizure activity.[35, 36] It has been postulated that cocaine can produce a primary disturbance of thermoregulation.[36] In addition, hyperthermia has been associated with a specific cocaine toxidrome. This toxidrome includes seizures, rhabdomyolysis, renal failure, and shock.[35, 36] Rectal temperatures as high as 40 to 45.6°C (104 to 114.1°F) have been reported.[36] Muscle biopsy and clinical observations have suggested a similarity to the dopamine receptor antagonist–induced neuroleptic malignant syndrome.[36] Supportive care and aggressive cooling attempts have been advocated.[36] Therapy directed toward the rapid lowering of temperatures to prevent cell death, such as the use of a cooling blanket, convection evaporation, cool air ventilation, and gastric lavage with iced saline are indicated. Sedation and paralysis may be useful for reducing muscle activity thought to be a significant cause of the hyperthermia.[36]

Rhabdomyolysis and Renal Failure

As noted earlier, an association between cocaine intoxication and acute rhabdomyolysis has been made.[35, 37] Approximately one third of patients with cocaine-associated rhabdomyolysis develop acute renal failure. Presence of profound hypotension, hyperpyrexia, and marked elevation of serum creatine kinase levels (e.g., 28,000 units/L) at admission was found useful in predicting renal failure.[35] Some cocaine-induced rhabdomyolysis was predicted by the presence of seizures, coma, hypotension, arrhythmia, or cardiac arrest. In one series, six of seven patients who developed cocaine-induced rhabdomyolysis, disseminated intravascular coagulation, and renal failure died.[35] Because of the frequency of chest pain with cocaine use, the possibility exists that cocaine-induced rhabdomyolysis may be mistaken for myocardial ischemia.

Treatment of cocaine-induced rhabdomyolysis and renal failure is generally limited to supportive care. Correction of hypotension and volume depletion, termination of seizure activity, careful monitoring of electrolytes, aggressive efforts to ensure urine flow, and the prevention of myoglobin precipitation in the kidneys with exogenous bicarbonate (to alkalize the urine) are the principles of early supportive care for this disorder. Hemodialysis may be needed for acute renal failure resulting from significant rhabdomyolysis.

Head and Neck

Although rarely life threatening, head and neck complications of cocaine toxicity are not uncommon. An ophthalmologic condition called "crack eye" has been described; it is characterized by pain, photophobia, lacrimation, chemosis, and hyperemia in association with corneal epithelial defects. In addition, microbial keratitis may complicate the syndrome of "crack eye," leading to potential long-term corneal alterations.[38]

Chronic sinusitis as result of cocaine abuse, including osteolytic sinusitis and secondary bilateral optic nerve involvement, has been described.[39] Midline granuloma and loss of olfaction have also been reported with cocaine use. Acute epiglottitis has followed crack cocaine inhalation. Whether this epiglottitis is a direct effect of cocaine or is induced by the inhalation of hot gases is not known. Cocaine-induced dental erosions and gingival necrosis have been noted.[40] A perforated nasal septum is commonly noted with chronic nasal inhalation of cocaine. At least one case of the pulmonary aspiration of a fragment of nasal septum has been reported.[31] Symptomatic care is the sole treatment necessary for most head, neck, and ophthalmologic complications of cocaine abuse.

Gastrointestinal

Ingestion of large amounts of cocaine have been associated with small and large bowel perforation, ischemia, and necrosis.[41, 42] Acute pyloric and gastrointestinal perforations have been reported after prolonged crack cocaine smoking.[42] The intense vasoconstriction from stimulation of α-adrenergic receptors in the mesenteric vasculature is believed to contribute to focal tissue ischemia and perforation. Patients who have ingested packets of cocaine in the illicit smuggling of the drug (so-called "mules" or "body packers") have presented with mechanical bowel obstructions requiring surgical intervention.[43] Although surgical treatment may be needed, conservative management with whole-bowel irrigation or observation of asymptomatic "body packers" has been advocated.[43] Endoscopy may be helpful in the removal of cocaine packets still in the stomach or proximal small bowel. Activated charcoal in the gastrointestinal tract helps bind cocaine that leaks out of the packets. Radiologic imaging studies such as abdominal flat plates or computed tomography of the abdomen are useful in making the diagnosis of the cause of partial or complete bowel obstruction.

Pregnancy and Urologic Effects

Significant alteration in menstrual cycle function, including amenorrhea and infertility, have been noted with cocaine abuse.[44] If the female cocaine user becomes pregnant, increased risk of placental abruption exists.[45] Premature rupture of membranes, spontaneous abortion, pregnancy-induced hypertension, precipitate delivery, or fetal death have been suggested but not proved to be associated with cocaine use.[45] Congenital urinary tract anomalies may be associated with maternal cocaine use.[45] Abnormal ventilatory patterns and increased incidence of sudden infant death syndrome have been reported with maternal cocaine use.[46, 47] Other neurobehavioral abnormalities in the neonate, including tremulousness and an increased startle reflex ("crack baby" behavior), have been noted with maternal cocaine use.[45, 47] The duration and long-term implications of these neurobehavioral abnormalities await clarification.

Several cases of impotence and priapism from acute cocaine use have been reported. Intranasal, intraurethral, and topical application (to the glans penis) of cocaine have all been reported to cause priapism.[47] In these patients, bladder outlet obstruction needs to be relieved with bladder catheterization, if possible. Aspiration, irrigation, and in most cases, surgical intervention have been needed to relieve the priapism.

Hepatic

Approximately 90% of cocaine is biotransformed by hydrolytic reactions of one or both of the ester linkages and the rest by oxidative processes.[48] Both chemical reactions and enzymatic esterases (e.g., serum pseudocholinesterase) rapidly hydrolyze cocaine to yield ecgonine methylester, ecgonine, benzoylecgonine, and benzoic acid.[48] Oxidative processes centered around the tropane nitrogen are responsible for about 10% of cocaine metabolism, using the cytochrome P-450 enzyme system within the liver.[48] This minor pathway appears to be responsible for hepatic toxicity. It produces norcocaine, norcocaine nitroxide, hydrogen peroxide, and superoxide radicals.[48] These products are thought to reduce hepatocyte nicotinamide-adenine dinucleotide phosphate (NADPH) and glutathione levels.[48]

The formation of lipid peroxidation and the resultant superoxide or hydroxyl radical injury are believed to lead to the intrinsic hepatotoxicity seen with cocaine abuse.[48] Agents that deplete NADPH and intracellular glutathione (e.g., acetaminophen) can enhance the risk of cocaine hepatotoxicity. Human cocaine hepatotoxicity is seen most frequently as necrosis in zone 3 of the liver that corresponds to the cytochrome P-450 distribution.[48] Although many case reports of cocaine-induced hepatotoxicity exist and hepatocyte tissue cultures confirm intrinsic toxicity, the clinical incidence of cocaine hepatotoxicity is unknown, but probably is low. Why hepatitis from cocaine toxicity is infrequent also is unknown, but the determination of the exact incidence is complicated by the high prevalence of viral and alcohol-induced liver disease in this patient population.

Table 39–2. Cocaine Toxicity and Treatment Decision Algorithm

Suspected Cocaine Toxicity

↓ ↓ ↓

Mild Cocaine Toxicity

↓

Psychologic support
Decontamination of oral ingestions/administration of activated charcoal
Observe

Severe Cocaine Toxicity

↓

Immediate Supportive Care

Airway control
Oxygenation
Vascular access

↓

Decontaminate/Antagonists

In oral exposures, administer activated charcoal
Consider whole-bowel lavage with polyethylene glycol solutions for "body packers"
Consider empiric dextrose, thiamine, and naloxone
Avoid using benzodiazepine antagonists (e.g., flumazenil)

↓

Terminate Seizures

Benzodiazepines (e.g., diazepam, lorazepam)
Barbiturates (e.g., pentobarbital, phenobarbital)

↓

Correct Immediate Metabolic, Oxygenation, and Electrolyte Abnormalities

↓

Correct Local Tissue Ischemia, Improve Perfusion

↓

Local α-Adrenergic Blockers for Cocaine (e.g., phenoxybenzamine, phentolamine)

↓

Treat Hyperthermia

Evaluate for Other Agents

↓

Initiate specific treatment for additional agents
Consider interactions with cocaine
Monitor for early and late toxicities of other agents

↓

Second-Level Evaluations to Check for Persistent Abnormalities

↓ ↓ ↓

Persistent Hypotension

Intravascular volume resuscitation
Acute cardiopulmonary support
Central hemodynamic monitoring

Ventricular Arrhythmia

Antiarrhythmics (e.g., lidocaine)
Electrolyte correction
Acid-base correction

Renal Failure

Hemodialysis
Intravascular volume

Hypertension

Sedation (e.g., diazepam)
Calcium channel blockers (e.g., nifedipine, nicardipine)
β-Adrenergic blockers (e.g., esmolol)
Nitroprusside

Coronary Artery Ischemia

Antiplatelet agents (e.g., aspirin)
Calcium channel blockers (e.g., nifedipine, diltiazem, nicardipine)
α-Adrenergic blockers (e.g., phentolamine)
β-Adrenergic blockers (e.g., esmolol, metoprolol) may be contraindicated (see text)
Nitrates (e.g., nitroglycerin)
Thrombolytics (e.g., streptokinase, tissue plasminogen activator)
Sedation (e.g., diazepam)

CNS Abnormalities

Seizures
Strokes
Bleeds
Terminate seizures

Pulmonary Edema/Respiratory Failure

Ventilator
Oxygen
PEEP
Electrolyte Abnormalities
Correct hypokalemia (e.g., potassium chloride)
Correct hypocalcemia (e.g., calcium gluconate)

Rhabdomyolysis

Alkalinize urine (e.g., IV bicarbonate)
Calcium replacement (e.g., calcium gluconate)
Intravascular volume

Supportive Care

Psychologic and pharmacologic support for cocaine abstinence and long-term recovery

CNS, central nervous system; PEEP, positive end-expiratory pressure; IV, intravenous.

Hematologic

The association of disseminated intravascular coagulation, rhabdomyolysis, and renal failure was earlier noted.[35] Severe destructive thrombocytopenia unrelated to retroviral infection has been reported in a small series of both intravenous and inhalation cocaine users.[49] Cocaine-associated thrombocytopenia with a clinical course similar to that of immunopathic thrombocytopenic purpura has been noted, with five of six patients apparently responding to corticosteroids. The sixth patient had a partial response to corticosteroids and a complete response to splenectomy.[49] Whether this thrombocytopenia reflects a direct or an indirect immunologic stimulus from cocaine or a contaminant is not known. In addition, increased platelet aggregation is believed to contribute to thrombocytopenia in some cocaine users. Nontraumatic splenic hematomas have also been reported in cocaine abusers.

Endocrine

Thyroid function tests in heavy users of cocaine were found not to be different from normal values. Persistent hyperprolactinemia leading in some cases to galactorrhea may occur in chronic cocaine abusers. Higher peak and trough levels of prolactin-releasing factor have also been reported in male cocaine users with hyperprolactinemia.[44] Prolactin levels remained elevated for 4 weeks in men and women during hospitalization for cocaine withdrawal. The persistent elevation of prolactin was attributed to cocaine-induced derangement in dopaminergic neural regulatory systems. In this same study, levels of plasma luteinizing hormone, testosterone, and cortisol were found to be within the normal range. The clinical importance of these findings is unclear, but they explain the impotence and gynecomastia reported in men who chronically abuse cocaine.

GENERAL PRINCIPLES OF TREATMENT

Table 39–2 outlines an algorithm for the general approach to patients with suspected cocaine toxicity. Prospective human studies evaluating different treatment options for such patients are lacking. Recommendations are instead based on the results of animal studies and small series of human poisonings with cocaine. General supportive care for ingestions includes decontamination of the gastrointestinal tract with activated charcoal and, possibly, gastric lavage. Control of seizures and body temperature remain important aspects of supportive therapy in these patients. Specific measures for each complication have been outlined throughout this chapter. Abdominal imaging studies, including plain films and computed tomography, are useful in diagnosing cocaine "body stuffers" and "body packers." ("Body stuffers" have ingested cocaine in packets not specifically prepared for gut transit, whereas "body packers" have ingested sealed packets that can withstand gut transit.) Both "stuffers" and "packers" can be followed with serial abdominal imaging studies to confirm passage of all cocaine. Whole-bowel irrigation, endoscopy, surgery, cathartics, and repeat doses of activated charcoal have been used to reduce cocaine exposure in these patients. Referral for psychiatric care, for appropriate serologic testing for viral hepatitis and HIV, and for evaluation for complications attendant to intravenous drug abuse should be considered.

CONCLUSION

Since its re-emergence as a cause of death in the 1970s, the incidence of cocaine-associated deaths has remained high, with as many as 26.7% of all deaths in New York City between 1990 and 1992 having been associated with the presence of cocaine or a cocaine metabolite in the blood or urine.[50] In Tennessee in 1993, over 25% of reckless drivers that did not smell of alcohol were found to be intoxicated with cocaine alone or with cocaine in combination with marijuana.[1] Both related trauma and direct toxicity contribute to the high rate of cocaine-associated deaths.[3]

Acute and chronic cocaine toxicity represents a major challenge to the clinician. The ability of cocaine to cause significant multiple-organ system dysfunction contributes to this challenge. Preventive care and new carefully tested approaches to therapy can help reduce the incidence and improve the outcome of patients with this modern affliction.

References

1. Brookoff D, Cook CS, Williams C, Man CS: Testing reckless drivers for cocaine and marijuana. N Engl J Med *331*:518–522, 1994.
2. Rich JA, Singer DE: Cocaine-related symptoms in patients presenting to an urban emergency department. Ann Emerg Med *20*:616–621, 1991.
3. Loiselle JM, Baker MD, Templeton JM, et al: Substance abuse in adolescent trauma. Ann Emerg Med *22*:1530–1534, 1993.
4. Cregler L, Mark H: Medical complications of cocaine abuse. N Engl J Med *315*:1495–1500, 1986.
5. Karch S: The history of cocaine toxicity. Hum Pathol *20*:1037–1039, 1989.
6. Warner E: Cocaine abuse. Ann Intern Med *119*:226–235, 1993.
7. Garland O: Fatal acute poisoning by cocaine. Lancet *2*:1104–1105, 1895.
8. Gawin F, Ellinwood EH: Cocaine and other stimulants actions, abuse, and treatments. N Engl J Med *318*:1173–1182, 1988.
9. Mittleman RE, Wefli CV: Death caused by recreational cocaine use. JAMA *252*:1889–1893, 1984.
10. National survey shows continuing decline in use of illicit drugs; cocaine use drops dramatically. Hosp Comm Psychiatry *42*:1078, 1991.
11. Colliver J, Kopstein A: Trends in cocaine abuse reflected in emergency room episodes reported to DAWN. Public Health Rep *106*:59–68, 1991.

12. Benowitz N: Clinical pharmacology and toxicology of cocaine. Pharmacol Toxicol *72*:3–12, 1993.
13. Henning R, Wilson L, et al: Cocaine plus ethanol is more cardiotoxic than cocaine or ethanol alone. Crit Care Med *22*:1896–1906, 1994.
14. Perez-Reyes M, Di Guiseppi S, et al: Free-base cocaine smoking. Clin Pharmacol Ther *32*:459–465, 1982.
15. Rose JS: Cocaethylene: A current understanding of the active metabolite of cocaine and ethanol. Am J Emerg Med *12*:489–490, 1994.
16. Mouhaffel AH, Madu EC, et al: Cardiovascular complication of cocaine. Chest *107*:1426–1434, 1995.
17. Hollander JE, Hoffman RS, et al: Cocaine-associated myocardial infarction mortality and complications. Arch Intern Med *155*:1081–1086, 1995.
18. Derlet RW, Albertson TE: Emergency department presentation of cocaine intoxication. Ann Emerg Med *18*:182–186, 1989.
19. Brody SL, Slovis CM, Wrenn KD: Cocaine-related medical problems: Consecutive series of 233 patients. Am J Med *88*:325–331, 1990.
20. Hollander JE: The management of cocaine-associated myocardial ischemia. N Engl J Med *333*:1267–1271, 1995.
21. Hollander JE, Burstein JL, et al: Cocaine-associated myocardial infarction: Clinical safety of thrombolytic therapy. Chest *107*:1237–1241, 1995.
22. Shih RD, Hollander JE, et al: Clinical safety of lidocaine in patients with cocaine-associated myocardial infarction. Ann Emerg Med *26*:702–706, 1995.
23. Olson KR, Kearney TE, et al: Seizures associated with poisoning and drug overdose. Am J Emerg Med *11*:565–568, 1993.
24. Pascual-Leone A, Dhuna A, Altafullah IM, Anderson DC: Cocaine-induced seizures. Neurology *40*:404–407, 1990.
25. Johsson S, O'Meara M, Young JB: Acute cocaine poisoning: Importance of treating seizures and acidosis. Am J Med *75*:1061–1064, 1983.
26. Kaye BR, Fainstat M: Cerebral vasculitis associated with cocaine abuse. JAMA *258*:2104–2106, 1987.
27. Daras M, Koppel BS, Atos-Radzion E: Cocaine-induced choreoathetoid movements ('crack dancing'). Neurology *44*:751–752, 1994.
28. Kaku DA, Lowenstein DH: Emergence of recreational drug abuse as a major risk factor for stroke in young adults. Ann Intern Med *113*:821–827, 1990.
29. Lowenstein DH, Massa SM, et al: Acute neurologic and psychiatric implications associated with cocaine abuse. Am J Med *83*:841–846, 1987.
30. Spivey WH, Euerle B: Neurologic complications of cocaine abuse. Ann Emerg Med *19*:1422–1428, 1990.
31. Albertson TE, Walby WF, Derlet RW: Stimulant-induced pulmonary toxicty. Chest *108*:1140–1149, 1995.
32. Shannon M: Clinical toxicity of cocaine adulterants. Ann Emerg Med *17*:1243–1247, 1988.
33. Patel RC, Dutta D, Schonfeld SA: Free-base cocaine use associated with bronchiolitis obliterans organizing pneumonia. Ann Intern Med *107*:186–187, 1987.
34. Forrester JM, Steele AW, Waldron JA, Parsons PE: Crack lung: An acute pulmonary syndrome with a spectrum of clinical and histopathologic findings. Am Rev Respir Dis *142*:462–467, 1990.
35. Roth D, Alarcon FJ, et al: Acute rhabdomyolysis with cocaine intoxication. N Engl J Med *319*:673–377, 1988.
36. Callaway CW, Clark RF: Hyperthermia in psychostimulant overdose. Ann Emerg Med *24*:68–76, 1994.
37. Merigian KS, Roberts JR: Cocaine intoxication: hyperpyrexia, rhabdomyolysis and acute renal failure. Clin Toxicol *25*:135–148, 1987.
38. Strominger MB, Sachs R, Hersh PS: Microbial keratitis with crack cocaine. Arch Ophthalmol *108*:1672, 1990.
39. Newman NM, DiLoreto DA, et al: Bilateral optic neuropathy and osteolytic sinusitis complications of cocaine abuse. JAMA *259*:72–74, 1988.
40. Quart AM, Butkus-Small C, Klein RS: The cocaine connection users imperil their gingiva. J Am Dent Assoc *122*:85–87, 1991.
41. Yang RD, Han MW, McCarthy JH: Ischemic colitis in a crack abuser. Dig Dis Sci *36*:238–240, 1991.
42. Cheng CLY, Suesko V: Acute pyloric perforation after prolonged crack smoking. Ann Emerg Med *23*:126–128, 1994.
43. Caruana DS, Weinbach B, Goerg D, Gardner LB: Cocaine-packet ingestion. Ann Intern Med *100*:73–74, 1984.
44. Mendelson JH, Mello NK, et al: Cocaine effects on pulsatile secretion of anterior pituitary, gonadal, and adrenal hormones. J Clin Endocrinol Metab *69*:1256–1260, 1989.
45. Slutsker L: Risks associated with cocaine use during pregnancy. Obstet Gynecol *79*:778–789, 1992.
46. Durand DJ, Espinoza AM, Nickerson BG: Association between prenatal cocaine exposure and sudden infant death syndrome. J Pediatr *117*:909–911, 1990.
47. Fiorrelli RL, Manfrey SJ, Belikoff LH, Finkelstein LH: Priapism associated with intranasal cocaine abuse. J Urol *143*:584–585, 1990.
48. Kloss MW, Rosen GM, Rauckman EJ: Cocaine-mediated hepatotoxicity: A critical review. Biochem Pharmacol *33*:169–173, 1984.
49. Leissinger CA: Severe thrombocytopenia associated with cocaine use. Ann Intern Med *112*:708–710, 1990.
50. Marzuk PM, Tardiff K, Leon AC, et al: Fatal injuries after cocaine use as a leading cause of death among young adults in New York City. N Engl J Med *332*:1753–1757, 1995.

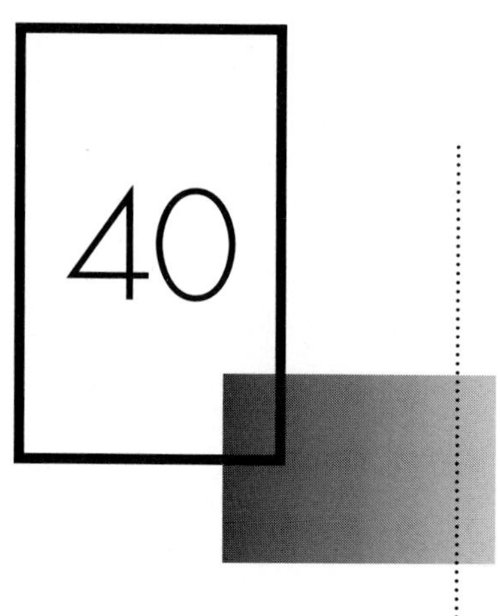

40

Phencyclidine

ROBERT O. WRIGHT, MD
ALAN D. WOOLF, MD, MPH

Phencyclidine (PCP), formerly used as a preinduction anesthetic and as an animal tranquilizer, has no current licit medical indications, although it is still used illegally as a hallucinogenic. PCP is a tertiary amine with a three-ring structure (Fig. 40–1) and is a stable, soluble, white crystalline solid at room temperature. Ketamine, a dissociative anesthetic agent commonly used in pediatrics, is a structural analogue of PCP. Both drugs are classified as arylcyclohexylamines and produce a complicated clinical picture of stimulation, depression, and analgesia. PCP is a common drug of abuse and is also known as "PeaCe pill," "hog," "angel dust," and "elephant" or "horse tranquilizer." PCP was originally marketed in the late 1950s by Parke Davis Pharmaceutical Company as a sedative and surgical anesthetic.[1] Under the trade name Sernyl, PCP was touted as an anesthetic agent free of objectionable cardiorespiratory depression. However, after surgery many patients developed extreme agitation and dysphoric effects, and the drug was subsequently removed from the market. In 1967, PCP returned as Sernylan and was marketed as a veterinary tranquilizer, prompting the street names with allusions to animals.

PCP first emerged as a hallucinogenic in the late 1960s but did not become popular until the 1970s. Its popularity resulted in part from its easy synthesis using relatively inexpensive constituents. Frequently, drug dealers would misrepresent the drug as a more exotic, expensive hallucinogen such as mescaline, psilocybin, or tetrahydrocannabinol.[2, 3] In addition, PCP is often added as an adulterant to

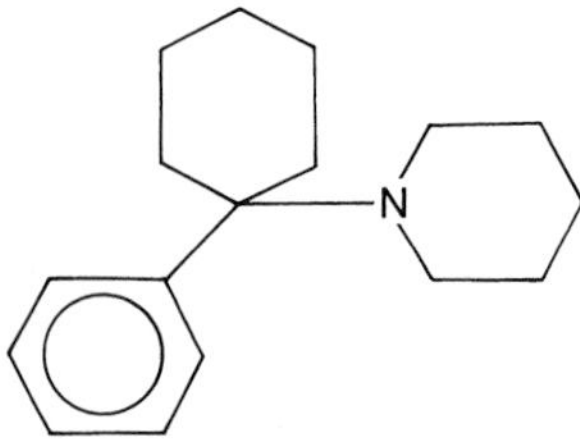

Cl
O
H
N
CH_3
Ketamine

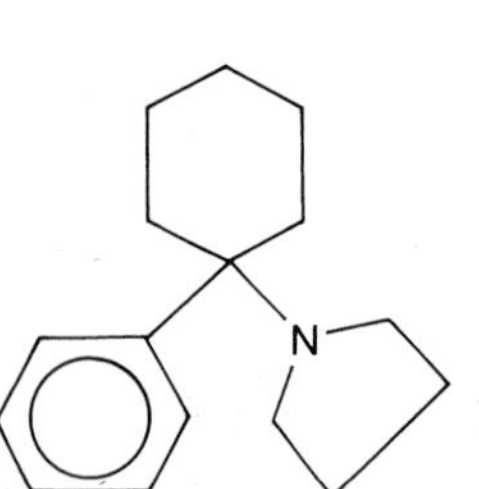

N≡C
N
PCC

Figure 40–1. Phencyclidine (PCP) and several of its psychoactive analogues.

marijuana or cocaine without the knowledge of the user.[2, 4] PCP was classified as a Schedule I agent in 1978, and the sale of its chemical precursor (piperidine) was restricted. Nonetheless, PCP was found in 1% of toxic screens run between 1984 and 1987 by the laboratory of one university hospital.[5] In addition, so-called designer drugs, unregulated synthetic analogues of PCP, have also been used as substitutes by street users.[6, 7] Until recently, the sale of "designer" arylcyclohexylamines was not restricted by law. These drugs are structurally similar to the parent compound with the addition of an aliphatic or aromatic amine, ketone, or halide. Although they may be sufficiently different from PCP so as to escape detection on a routine toxicologic screen of blood or urine, these agents may be more toxic than PCP itself.[8] PCP has more than 60 psychoactive analogues, among which ketamine is the only one legally manufactured for human use. Ketamine has also been used illicitly for its PCP-like effects, and thefts from veterinary facilities have been reported.

EPIDEMIOLOGY

In 1994, there were 343 exposures of PCP reported to the American Association of Poison Control Centers.[9] Forty-three percent of the affected individuals were younger than age 20. Three deaths were reported. The 1993 Monitoring the Future Study reported an annual prevalence rate of PCP use of 1.4% among high school seniors.[10] This prevalence rate has plateaued since 1991 and is down from a peak annual prevalence rate of 7% in 1979. However, PCP is still popular in the inner city; and in 1994, police officials reported an increase in PCP use in both Los Angeles and Washington, DC.

PCP is sold on the street in a variety of forms and is the most versatile of the substances of abuse. It is available as powder, tablets, liquid, leaf mixture, crystals, or capsules and can be snorted, smoked, injected (intravenously or subcutaneously), or ingested. Studies have shown that the typical PCP user is a polydrug user who rarely takes PCP alone, and the average starting age of a PCP user is 14 years.[5, 11] A typical PCP-laced marijuana cigarette contains between 1 and 10 mg of drug. The average dose in tablet form is 5 mg and varies from 1 to 6 mg. The most common route of exposure is smoking, which accounts for about 70% of usage.[12] Passive smoke exposure has led to clinical toxicity in pediatric cases.[5] PCP has been discovered in up to 24% of street marijuana samples and in the hair samples of 19% of patients admitted to one psychiatric facility.[13]

PHARMACOLOGY

PCP is a weak, alkaline salt, soluble in both water and ethanol and is rapidly absorbed after ingestion or inhalation or when it is administered intravenously, subcutaneously, or per rectum.[14] It has a two-ringed molecular structure differing from piperidine by an alkyl side group (see Fig. 40–1). Absorption is minimal in the stomach but occurs rapidly in the upper small intestine.[15] Onset of effect occurs in 30 to 60 minutes when it is ingested and in 2 to 5 minutes when smoked.[16, 17] Acute symptoms and signs of toxicity usually last 4 to 6 hours and generally resolve completely by 24 to 48 hours.[1] The terminal phase serum half-life of PCP is 21 to 24 hours.[14] Up to 50% of PCP present in a cigarette may be converted by pyrolysis to the less potent product phenylcyclohexane; thus, higher doses may be tolerated in inhalational exposures. When ingested, sedation and loss of inhibition are produced at doses between 1 and 5 mg, while only 0.25 mg intravenously is required to produce sedation in an adult. At oral doses between 5 and 10 mg, toxic psychoses and violent behavior may occur. Oral doses greater than 10 mg may produce a schizophreniform reaction; however, the relationship between dose and clinical effects is not completely reliable.[16, 17]

PCP is a highly lipophilic weak base ($pK_a = 8.6$) and thus is widely distributed into the tissues. It has an unusual enterogastric circulation, such that significant amounts of drug are actively secreted into the stomach and then reabsorbed in the small intestine.[20] The concentration of PCP in the stomach may be up to 50 times higher than that in the serum. PCP levels are highest in adipose tissue. The concentration of drug within the brain may be up to 9 times higher than that in the plasma.[15] The slightly acidic nature of cerebrospinal fluid induces ion-trapping of the weak base PCP, and cerebrospinal fluid levels may be 4 times as high as plasma levels. This may account for some of the prolonged neurologic effects of the drug. The apparent volume of distribution of PCP is 6.2 L/kg, and the drug is 78% bound to plasma proteins. The large volume of distribution and the lipophilic nature of this chemical are responsible for its persistence and long duration of action. More than 90% of patients will have positive urine metabolites for 7 days postexposure. Chronic PCP users (about 1% of patients) may still be positive for urine metabolites 4 weeks post exposure.[19]

PCP is metabolized mainly in the liver. Oxidative hydroxylation to the inactive monohydroxypiperidine is followed by glucuronidation to a more water-soluble, conjugated derivative that is then excreted in the urine as the major form of metabolism.[6] Significant first-pass liver metabolism also occurs when the drug is ingested orally, as opposed to being smoked or injected. Approximately 10% of drug is excreted unchanged in the urine.

Considerable effort has been devoted to identifying the site at which PCP mediates its psychomimetic effects. Both an oral PCP dose of 5 mg and an intravenous dose of 0.1 mg/kg would be expected to produce serum PCP concentrations between 0.01 and 0.10 μmol/L. Given this small dose range, the target site must have a high affinity for PCP.[23] Initial theories centered around PCP's interaction with a number of receptors and neurotransmitters including γ-

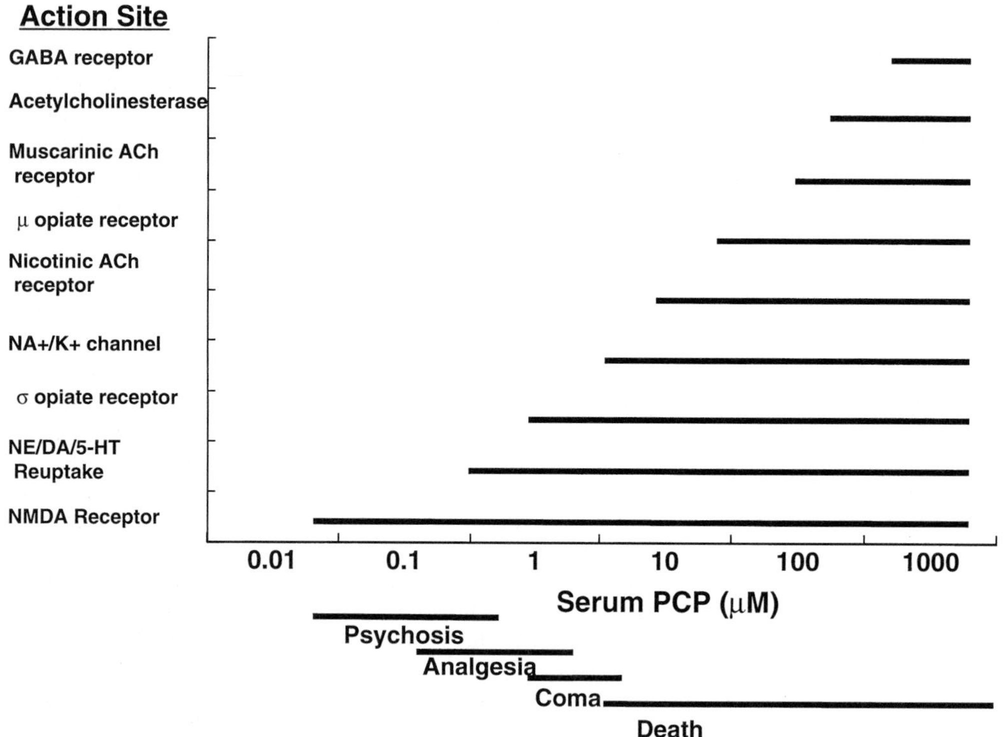

Figure 40–2. PCP receptor interactions and clinical effects. The vertical axis lists endogenous action sites for PCP. The horizontal axis represents PCP concentration. The black lines above the horizontal axis indicate the concentrations at which interactions with PCP would occur. The black lines below the horizontal axis are the clinical effects corresponding with drug concentrations. NMDA, *N*-methyl-D-aspartate; NE/DA/5-HT, norepinephrine, dopamine, and 5-hydroxytryptophan; Na^+/K^+, sodium/potassium; ACh, acetylcholine; GABA, γ-aminobutyric acid. (Adapted from Javitt DC, Zukin SR: Recent advances in the phencyclidine model of schizophrenia. Am J Psychiatry *148*:1301–1308, 1991.)

aminobutyric acid (GABA). However, these interactions occurred at serum levels of approximately 100 μmol/L, a concentration that would be almost uniformly lethal. Hence, direct inhibition of GABAnergic neurons is unlikely to be the principal site of PCP action. Subsequently, PCP had been reported to interact with a large number of receptor and target sites; however, most of these interactions like those with GABA receptors occur at concentrations unlikely to be reached clinically.[23, 24] Interactions with neuronal membrane–associated potassium and sodium channels occur only at concentrations associated with coma (2 to 3 μmol). Interactions with nicotinic cholinergic receptors, muscarinic cholinergic receptors, and μ opiate receptors all occur at serum concentrations that are unobtainable clinically.[18] Only three action sites for PCP have been identified that interact at serum or tissue concentrations seen clinically. These sites, in decreasing order of affinity, include the *N*-methyl-D-aspartate (NMDA) protein complex, the neuronal dopamine/norepinephrine/serotonin reuptake complex, and the σ opiate receptor complex. Figure 40–2 summarizes the previously described receptor interactions with PCP within the context of pharmacologic versus clinical effects.

The NMDA complex is regulated by excitatory amino acid neurotransmitters such as glutamate, glycine, and aspartate. Excitatory amino acids act as neurotransmitters and also play a role in the development of the cytoarchitecture of the central nervous system.[25] A critical level of excitatory amino acids is required for normal neurologic development. NMDA receptors have been located in the hippocampus, neocortex, basal ganglia, and limbic system. A PCP binding site within the L-type calcium channel of the NMDA receptor has been described that has a submicromolar affinity for PCP.[21] Thus, PCP would interact with this receptor at physiologic concentrations. PCP acts as a noncompetitive antagonist to NMDA receptors, inhibiting neurotransmitter release.[22, 23, 26] PCP inhibits calcium flux across the L-type channel by binding to the receptor at a site independent of glutamate or glycine (Fig. 40–3).

The role of the PCP/NMDA receptor complex in mediating the neurobehavioral effects of PCP is supported by *in vivo* animal studies. Stereotypical, dysfunctional behaviors can be induced by PCP and ketamine as well as by several designer drug analogues

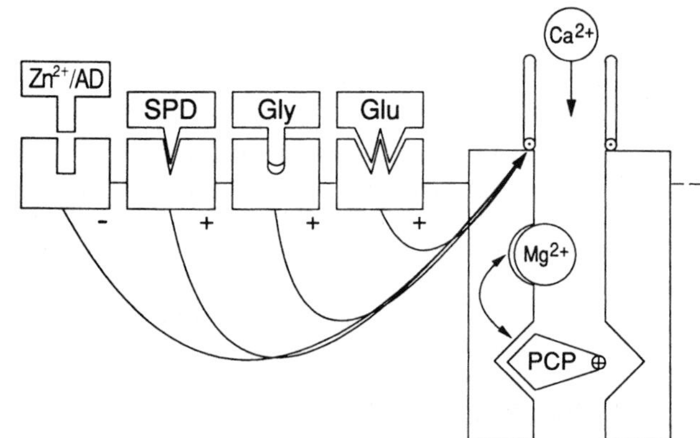

Figure 40–3. Schematic model of NMDA receptor functioning. AD, tricyclic antidepressants; SPD, spermidine; GLY, glycine; GLU, glutamate. (From Javitt DC, Zukin SR: Recent advances in the phencyclidine model of schizophrenia. Am J Psychiatry *148*:1301–1308, 1991.)

of PCP, which have also been demonstrated to bind at the PCP/NMDA binding site.[27–29] The potency of these stimulus effects corresponds to the potency of PCP binding to NMDA receptors. In addition, dopamine antagonists, such as haloperidol, do not inhibit these effects, suggesting that the effects are not mediated by dopaminergic pathways. A wide variety of serotonergic, adrenergic, GABAnergic agents, and opiate agonists also fail to induce or inhibit these PCP stimulus effects in animal models, suggesting that interaction with the NMDA receptor may be responsible.

Calcium channel blockers such as nimodipine and diltiazem have been shown to potentiate the stimulus effects of PCP in animals, presumably by synergistic blockade of the NMDA calcium channel.[30] Verapamil, conversely, has been shown to reverse PCP toxicity in animal models. Verapamil, however, is unique to calcium channel blockers in that it binds directly to the PCP receptor site within the NMDA complex displacing PCP.[30] Other calcium channel blockers bind at sites independent of the PCP receptor. Flunarizine, an experimental calcium channel blocker, also binds directly to the PCP receptor site and has better central nervous system penetration than verapamil. Some animal studies have suggested that verapamil or flunarizine may be potential antidotes for PCP overdose, but this hypothesis requires further investigation.

A second PCP binding site on the neuronal dopamine/norepinephrine/serotonin reuptake complex has also been identified and may modulate the dopaminergic and catecholinergic effects of PCP.[31] PCP has been demonstrated to inhibit dopamine, serotonin, and norepinephrine reuptake at physiologic concentrations (although these concentrations are 5 to 10 times greater than those required for NMDA receptor antagonism). Dopamine, acting at D_2 receptors, inhibits both cholinergic and GABAnergic receptors. In addition, glutamate by means of NMDA receptors, stimulates GABAnergic outflow so that inhibition of NMDA receptors also indirectly inhibits GABA receptor stimulation.[23] Thus, it appears that PCP may act by different synergistic mechanisms to modulate indirectly both GABA-like and dopamine-like effects. In addition, the inhibition of catecholamine reuptake may account for the sympathomimetic effects of PCP.

Lastly, PCP has been demonstrated to have σ opiate receptor agonist action, which could contribute in part to its analgesic and sedative properties.[32] This receptor action is of relatively low affinity, occurring at concentrations generally associated with coma, and may only be significant in severe overdose. MK-801, a selective PCP-NMDA receptor ligand, also induces sedation independent of opiate receptors.[23] Thus, PCP's inhibition of NMDA receptors may play the major role in the development of coma. Activation of σ opiate receptors has been shown to have an inhibitory effect on cholinergic neuron stimulation.[32] This effect may play a role in the anticholinergic properties of PCP and act synergistically with the aforementioned dopaminergic inhibition of cholinergic receptors.

PCP also has specific binding to σ opiate receptors within lymphocytes. *In vitro* studies have suggested that both humoral and cellular immune function is depressed when immunocytes are exposed to PCP.[33] The clinical implications of such findings are unclear.

THERAPEUTIC EFFECTS

At present there are no therapeutic indications for PCP. However, several properties of the drug show promise in the treatment of hypoxic/ischemic brain injury. Acute ischemic injury may lead to the uninhibited firing of NMDA receptor neurons. This intense stimulation in turn may lead to cell death of both the NMDA afferent mediated neuron and the efferent neuron to which it transmits.[34] As an antagonist to NMDA receptors, PCP has been postulated to provide a protective effect in acute hypoxemic/ischemic brain injury; and, indeed, some animal studies have confirmed this.[35, 36] Rats given PCP before temporary carotid and vertebral artery occlusion had decreased spike-wave activity on electroencephalogram versus controls, suggesting less seizure activity. The paradoxical anticonvulsant properties of PCP in low doses (as opposed to the epileptogenic effect of high dose PCP) have been demonstrated in several different animal models. Transient, reversible vacuolation of rat neurons has also been demonstrated after PCP administration, raising questions regarding its safety in ischemic hypoxemic brain injury.[34] Therefore, the potential beneficial effects of PCP in the management of patients with ischemic brain injury require further study before being applied to the clinical setting.

CLINICAL PRESENTATION

PCP has a wide variety of potential clinical effects, some of which are unpredictable but are generally dose related. Table 40–1 shows the most common symptoms and signs manifested by 1000 patients treated for PCP poisoning. Violent behavior, rotatory nystagmus, hypertension, and anesthesia and analgesia are the most characteristic signs of intoxication.[12, 37, 38] Depending on the dose, PCP will produce disorientation, depersonalization, dissociative thought, or a catatonic trancelike state. Drug users can experience a "high" from PCP, with feelings of euphoria, omnipotence, tremendous strength, sociability, and sexual prowess.[39] It is these effects that maintain the psychological dependence on PCP.

At lower doses (less than 10 mg) PCP may cause ataxia, slurred speech, sweating, and muscle rigidity. Neurologic manifestations may range from a blank, dissociative stare to violent hostility. Drug users may be irrational, perseverating, or otherwise uncommunicative. Nystagmus, which may be vertical, horizontal, or rotatory, is present in more than 50% of

Table 40–1. Clinical Findings in 1000 Cases of PCP Toxicity

Finding	%
Hallmarks	
Nystagmus	57.4
Hypertension	57.0
Sensorium	
Alert and oriented	45.9
Acute brain syndrome	36.9
Unconscious	10.6
Lethargy/stupor	6.6
Anticholinergic Signs	
Pupils > 4 mm	6.2
Urinary retention	2.4
Abnormal Vital Signs	
Tachycardia	30.0
Hypothermia	6.4
Apnea/respiratory arrest	2.8
Hyperthermia	2.6
Cardiac arrest	0.3
Motor Signs	
Generalized rigidity	5.2
Grand mal seizures	3.1
Localized dystonia	2.4
Facial grimacing	1.7
Athetosis	1.3
Cholinergic Signs	
Diaphoresis	3.9
Bronchospasm	2.1
Pupils < 1 mm	2.1
Hypersalivation	1.7
Bronchorrhea	0.6
Behavior	
Violent	35.4
Agitated	34.0
Bizarre	28.8
Hallucinating	18.5
Mute/staring	11.7
Nudism	3.3
No effects	3.5

Adapted from McCarron M, et al: Acute phencyclidine intoxication: Incidence of clinical findings in 1000 cases. Ann Emerg Med *10*:232–242, 1981.)

patients. The pupils may be either midsize or miotic and reactive. Reflexes are generally hyperactive. Muscle rigidity, catalepsy, opisthotonus, dystonic reactions, myoclonus, athetosis, and ataxia are sometimes noted.[12] As the dose increases, varying degrees of anesthesia occur and even coma may ensue. Generalized seizures can occur with large overdoses. Unlike those under the effects of hallucinogens, persons taking PCP are unaware that the drug is responsible for their delusional state. Patients report feeling exhilarated with tremendous strength, and it may take several attendants in the emergency department to restrain them. In addition, PCP causes a dissociative state as well as sensory anesthesia; patients are often seemingly unaware of injuries, such as lacerations, contusions, or even fractures.[38] Aggressive hostile behaviors may lead to homicidal, suicidal, or self-mutilatory acts. Patients under the influence of PCP have been known to walk into traffic, jump from buildings, or enucleate their own eye.[40] Patients who have taken more than 10 mg are usually comatose. Coma can last for hours or for many days if the overdose is severe. A characteristic of PCP-induced coma is the unresponsive patient whose eyes remain open.

Prominent psychiatric effects of PCP include the aforementioned violent, aggressive behavior. Mania and marked dysphoria are also common manifestations. Some patients may present with catatonia; visual and auditory hallucinations may also occur.[12] The most common cause of death related to PCP poisoning is the aggressive, violent, psychiatric effect of the drug that causes the patient to take life-threatening risks or attempt suicide.[41] Other causes of death include respiratory depression or arrest, hypertension, intracerebral hemorrhage, and seizures.[41, 42]

Patients recovering from PCP exposure may undergo an emergence reaction consisting of prolonged psychosis, bizarre behavior, or depression that may last for days to weeks. Prolonged psychosis is more commonly seen in chronic users and is a poor prognostic sign. Evidence exists linking chronic PCP abuse and the development of schizophrenia, but cause and effect is unclear.[43] Depression during the emergence phase may also stimulate further drug use.

Cardiovascular effects include hypertension (both systolic and diastolic) and tachycardia.[47] PCP has also been shown to be a direct cardiac depressant and may induce arrhythmias. It may act directly on blood vessels inducing vasospasm.[44] Severe hypertension may be associated with cerebral hemorrhage.[45]

Ventilation is usually maintained except in cases of severe overdose. Respiratory depression, hypoventilation, and apnea can occur in massive overdoses or in cases with respiratory depressant coingestants. Both pharyngeal and laryngeal reflexes are hyperactive, and the risk of laryngospasm and airway obstruction exists in PCP overdose. The sympathomimetic effects may also cause bronchorrhea, further complicating airway management.

A temperature greater than 38.8°C (101.8°F) was found in 2.6% of 1000 patients in one series of PCP ingestions.[12] Although isometric muscle contraction may account in part for the hyperthermia response, centrally mediated hypothalamic disturbances may also be involved. Elevated levels of uric acid, alanine transaminase, and aspartate transaminase may be due to rhabdomyolysis and occur in approximately 25% of ingestions. No elevations of serum bilirubin occurred in this series of 1000 cases, suggesting that the elevated transaminase levels were due to muscle damage.[12] Rhabdomyolysis with myoglobinuria and acute renal failure may complicate the dystonic muscle contractions seen with PCP poisoning.[46] Rhabdomyolysis may occur in the absence of seizures. Submassive liver failure associated with PCP-induced malignant hyperthermia has been described.[48] Approximately one in five patients will be hypoglycemic.

Psychological dependence for PCP, in the absence

of clear physiologic symptoms, has been well described.[49] Whether physiologic dependence (tolerance or withdrawal) occurs has been more controversial. Anecdotal reports of as much as a fourfold tolerance to PCP after repeated use have been published. Animal models have also demonstrated a twofold to fourfold tolerance to PCP's behavioral effects as well.[49, 50] Evidence for withdrawal also exists. Rhesus monkeys who self-administered PCP chronically for over a month developed oculomotor hyperactivity, tremor, diarrhea, and piloerection within 8 hours of drug cessation.[49] Other studies have demonstrated that administration of PCP temporarily reverses withdrawal symptoms, providing more evidence of its addicting properties. Rawson and colleagues studied 68 long-term PCP abusers and described a syndrome of depression, anxiety, irritability, restlessness, anergia, sleep disturbance, and disturbed thoughts after 1 day of abstinence.[51] These studies suggest that a physiologic dependence on PCP can develop in chronic users.

Long-term neuropsychiatric effects of chronic PCP abuse have been described. Chronic PCP abuse predominantly affects the brain's ability to perform integrated higher-order functions. Findings include difficulty with flexibility of thinking, incidental memory loss, and the inability to formulate simple and complex abstractions. Impairment in fine motor function has also been reported.

DIAGNOSIS

PCP poisoning is suspected based on clinical presentation and can be confirmed by laboratory testing. The profile of a patient presenting with typical PCP poisoning is a violent, aggressive, intoxicated adolescent or young adult male with nystagmus and hypertension. Confirmation of PCP intoxication can be made by several qualitative assays. Quantitative serum and urine levels of PCP do not correlate well with symptomatology and are of little use clinically. Several chromatographic tests are available for the rapid qualitative analysis of PCP.[52] Paper and silica gel thin-layer chromatography are inexpensive, rapid screens for PCP. High-performance liquid chromatography or gas chromatography–mass spectrophotometry can be used to quantitate the drug. Radioimmunoassay and enzyme-multilinked immunoassay provide better specificity and sensitivity. Because PCP is lipophilic and may be detected in urine for up to 1 to 4 weeks, urine is the preferred specimen for detection. A routine toxicologic screen of blood and urine by a commercial laboratory may not include an assay for PCP, and clinicians may be required to request it specifically.

Other laboratory tests recommended in PCP poisoning include serum electrolytes, blood urea nitrogen, creatinine, creatine phosphokinase, and glucose. Given the association with rhabdomyolysis, clinicians should be vigilant for electrolyte disturbances, metabolic acidosis, and renal failure.

TREATMENT

Initial management of the patient demonstrating severe clinical toxicity from suspected PCP use includes assessment and management of the airway, breathing, and circulation. Gastric lavage or induced emesis is not indicated in PCP ingestion when the route of exposure is nasal or inhalational (smoking) or if more than 1 hour has passed since the time of ingestion. PCP may hyperstimulate airway musculature, and care should be taken to prevent laryngospasm during passage of a nasogastric tube or during intubation.

Because PCP is actively secreted into the stomach, multiple doses of activated charcoal may be of benefit in binding free PCP. Continuous gastric suctioning has also been recommended for evacuating PCP secreted in the stomach by means of this enterogastric recirculation. Close monitoring for electrolyte imbalance is recommended if this modality is employed, because continuous suction may also remove significant amounts of potassium, hydrogen, and other essential ions.

The mildly intoxicated patient requires only supportive care. This patient should be observed in a quiet darkened environment. Auditory, tactile, or visual stimuli should be kept to a minimum to avoid provoking violent outbursts. Continuous observation is necessary to prevent patients from injuring themselves or others. "Talking down" patients, a technique of verbal reassurance and continuous contact, commonly used in lysergic acid diethylamide (LSD) or mescaline overdose, is generally not efficacious in the PCP-intoxicated patient and may even provoke hostile behavior. Patients taking small oral doses of PCP (less than 10 mg) should recover in 4 to 8 hours. Those who have been exposed to larger doses of PCP may take days to recover. Because of the high risk of rhabdomyolysis resulting from increased muscle tone, physical restraints should be avoided. The combative, aggressive patient may, however, require chemical sedation. Lorazepam, 0.1 mg/kg, or haloperidol, 5 to 10 mg, intramuscularly, may be useful in the management of such patients. In addition, haloperidol has been shown to improve substantially PCP-induced schizophreniform symptoms such as hallucinations, delusions, and disorganized thinking. This is consistent with the known clinical efficacy of neuroleptics in controlling psychotic symptoms of diverse etiology.[53] As a cautionary note, phenothiazines may provoke an anticholinergic reaction or lower seizure threshold. However, clinically reported complications from haloperidol sedation are rare.

In the more seriously intoxicated patient, life-threatening complications may arise. Seizures should be managed with lorazepam, diazepam, or phenytoin administered intravenously. Severe hypertension can be treated with sublingual nifedipine, intravenous diazoxide, or nitroprusside.

Renal failure secondary to rhabdomyolysis occurs in up to 1% of patients.[12] Management of this disorder should include maintaining brisk urinary flow and strict monitoring of serum electrolytes and renal function. Diuretics, such as mannitol or furosemide, may aid in maintaining urinary flow. Urinary alkalinization is a mainstay of rhabdomyolysis management but interferes with the urinary elimination of PCP, a weak base. Thus, use of alkalinization is controversial in PCP-induced rhabdomyolysis. Also, whereas it theoretically enhances elimination, urinary acidification is contraindicated in PCP poisoning, because it may produce further precipitation of myoglobin and calcium and thus worsen rhabdomyolysis.

Severe muscle rigidity, hyperthermia, and status epilepticus may require neuromuscular blockade and mechanical ventilation. Malignant hyperthermia has been described from PCP, and standard treatment with dantrolene and core cooling techniques should be employed when this is encountered. Because the volume of distribution of PCP is high, hemodialysis is not considered an efficient method of enhancing elimination of PCP. However, hemodialysis may be of benefit in rhabdomyolysis-induced renal failure.

Various antidotes for PCP intoxication are being studied. GABA transferase inhibitors, which increase central nervous system levels of the inhibitory neurotransmitter GABA, have also been shown to partially decrease PCP-induced motor activity in mice.[54] Given the discovery of PCP-specific NMDA receptor sites, much of the research has focused here. Verapamil and flunarizine, which displace PCP from its binding site within the L-type calcium channel of the NMDA receptor, have been reported to reverse PCP-induced discriminative behaviors in rats.[32] In addition, verapamil has been reported to reverse the adverse effects of PCP in case reports, but this requires further study.[55] PCP-specific Fab antibody fragments have been developed, but their use is experimental. Preliminary animal studies have shown Fab fragments to have a high affinity for PCP and can change the distribution of PCP in dogs.[56] Such experimental investigations hold great promise for improving our knowledge as to the pharmacology of PCP, as well as improving our management of the PCP-intoxicated patient.

OTHER HALLUCINOGENICS

Hallucinogenic amphetamines are discussed in Chapter 41. Hallucinogenic designer drugs are discussed in Chapter 42. LSD and natural hallucinogenics are discussed in Chapter 106.

References

1. Pradhan SN: Phencyclidine (PCP): Some human studies. Neurosci Biobehav Rev *8*:493–501, 1984.
2. Lundberg GD, Gupta RC, Montgomery SH: Phencyclidine: Patterns seen in street drug analysis. Clin Toxicol *9*:503–510, 1976.
3. Rainey JM, Crowder MK: Prevalence of phencyclidine in street drug preparations. N Engl J Med *290*:466–467, 1974.
4. Bailey DN: Phencyclidine detection during toxicology testing of a university medical patient population. J Toxicol Clinical Tox *25*:517–526, 1987.
5. Welch MJ, Correa GA: PCP intoxication in young children and infants. Clin Pediatr *19*:510–514, 1980.
6. Burns RS, Lerner SE (eds): Phencyclidine: A symposium. Clin Toxicol *9*:473–600, 1976.
7. Shulgin AT, Maclean DE: Illicit synthesis of phencyclidine and several of its analogs. Clin Toxicol *9*:553–560, 1979.
8. Davis WM, Borne RF, Hackett RB: Piperidinocyclohexanecarbonitrile (PCC) acute toxicity alone and potentiation of the lethality of phencyclidine (PCP). Fed Proc *30*:435–439, 1979.
9. Litovitz TL, Felberg L, Soloway RA, et al: 1994 annual report of the American Association of Poison Control Centers Toxic Exposure Surveillance System. Am J Emerg Med *13*:551–597, 1995.
10. Johnston LD, O'Malley PM, Bachman JG: National Survey Results on Drug Use from Monitoring the Future Survey, 1975–1993. NIH publication No. 93-3597. Bethesda, MD, National Institute on Drug Abuse, 1994.
11. Crider R: Phencyclidine: Changing abuse patterns. NIDA Res Monogr *64*:163–173, 1986.
12. McCarron MM, Schulze BW, Thompson GA, et al: Acute phencyclidine intoxication: Incidence of clinical findings in 1000 cases. Ann Emerg Med *10*:232–242, 1981.
13. Sramek JJ, Baumgartner WA, Tallos JA, et al: Hair analysis for detection of phencyclidine in newly admitted psychiatric patients. Am J Psychiatry *142*:950–953, 1985.
14. Showalter CV, Thornton WE: Clinical pharmacology of phencyclidine toxicity. Am J Psychiatry *134*:1234–1238, 1977.
15. Misra AL, Pontani RB, Bartolmeo J: Persistence of phencyclidine and metabolites in brain and adipose tissue and implications for long-lasting behavioral effects. Res Commun Chem Pathol Pharmacol *24*:431–435, 1979.
16. Cook CE, Brine DR, Quin GD, et al: Phencyclidine and phenylcyclohexane disposition after smoking phencyclidine. Clin Pharmacol Ther *31*:635–641, 1982.
17. Cook CE, Brine DR, Jeffcoat AR, et al: Phencyclidine disposition after intravenous and oral doses. Clin Pharmacol Ther *31*:625–634, 1982.
18. Vincent JP, Cavey D, Kamenka JM, et al: Interaction of phencyclidine with muscarinic and opiate receptors in the central nervous system. Brain Res *152*:176–182, 1978.
19. Simpson GM, Khajawall AM, Alatorre E, Staples FR: Urinary phencyclidine excretion in chronic abusers. J Toxicol Clin Toxicol *19*:1051–1059, 1982.
20. Done AK, Aronow, R, Miceli JN: The pharmacokinetics of phencyclidine in overdosage and its treatment. NIDA Res Monogr *21*:210–217, 1978.
21. Macdonald JF, Bartlett MC, Mody I, et al: The PCP site of the NMDA receptor complex. Adv Exp Med Biol *268*:27–33, 1990.
22. Sircar R, Li CS: PCP/NMDA receptor-channel complex and brain development. Neurotoxicol Teratol *16*:369–373, 1994.
23. Javitt DC, Zukin SR: Recent advances in the phencyclidine model of schizophrenia. Am J Psychiatry *148*:1301–1308, 1991.
24. Vincent JP, Kartalovski P, Geneste JM, Lazdunski M: Interaction of phencyclidine (angel dust) with a specific receptor in rat brain membranes. Proc Natl Acad Sci U S A *76*:4678–4682, 1979.
25. McDonald JW, Johnston MV: Excitatory amino acid neurotoxicity in the developing brain. NIDA Res Monogr 133:185–205, 1993.
26. Johnson KM, Snell LD, Sacaan AI, Jones SM: Pharmacologic regulation of the NMDA receptor-ionophore complex. NIDA Res Monogr 133:14–40, 1993.
27. Willets J, Balster RL: Phencyclidine-like discriminative stimulus properties of MK-801 in rats. Eur J Pharmacol 146:167–169, 1988.
28. Browne RG: Discriminative stimulus properties of PCP mimetics. NIDA Res Monogr 64:134–147, 1986.
29. Shannon HE: Evaluation of phencyclidine analogues on the basis of their discriminitive stimulus properties in the rat. J Pharmacol Exp Ther *216*:543–551, 1981.
30. Popoli P, Peezzola A, Benedetti M, Scotti de Carolis A: Vera-

pamil and flunarizine inhibit phencyclidine induced effects: An EEG and behavioral study in rats. Neuropharmacology *31*:1185–1191, 1992.
31. Akunne HC, Reid AA, Thurkuf A, et al: [3H]1-[2-(2-thienyl) cyclohexyl]piperidine labeled two high-affinity binding sites in human cortex: Further evidence for phencyclidine binding sites associated with the biogenic amine reuptake complex. Synapse *8*:289–300, 1991.
32. Wolfe SA, De Souza EB: Sigma and phencyclidine receptors in the brain-endocrine-immune axis. NIDA Res Monogr 133:95–123, 1993.
33. Khansari N, Whitten HD, Fudenberg HH: Phencyclidine-induced immunodepression. Science *225*:76–78, 1984.
34. Hargreaves RJ, Hill RG, Iverson LL: Neuroprotective NMDA antagonist: The controversy over their potential for adverse effects on cortical neuronal morphology. Acta Neurochir Suppl *60*:15–19, 1994.
35. Barone FC, Price WJ, Jakobsen S, et al: Pharmacological profile of a novel neuronal calcium channel blocker includes cerebral damage and neurological deficits in rat focal ischemia. Pharmacol Biochem Behav *48*:77–85, 1994.
36. Lu Yf, Xing YZ, Pan BS et al: Neuroprotective effects of phencyclidine in acute cerebral ischemia and reperfusion injury of rabbits. Abstract. Chung Kuo Yao Li Hsueh Pao *13*:1218–1222, 1992.
37. Liden CB, Lovejoy FH, Costello CE: Phencyclidine: Nine cases of poisoning. JAMA *234*:513–516, 1975.
38. McCarron MM, Schulze BW, Thompson GA, et al: Acute phencyclidine intoxication: Clinical patterns, complications and treatment. Ann Emerg Med *10*:290–297, 1981.
39. Burns RS, Lerner SE: Perspectives: Acute phencyclidine intoxication. Clin Toxicol *9*:477–501, 1976.
40. Moskovitz RA, Byrd T: Rescuing the angel within: PCP related self enucleation. Psychosomatics *24*:402–403, 1983.
41. Heilig SM, Diller J, Nelson FL: A study of 44 PCP related deaths. Int J Addict *17*:1175–1184, 1982.
42. Kessler GF, Demers LM, Berlin C, Brennan RW: Phencyclidine and fatal status epilepticus. N Engl J Med *291*:979, 1974.
43. Wright HH, Cole EA, Batey SR, Hanna K: Phencyclidine-induced psychosis: Eight-year follow-up of ten cases. South Med J *81*:565–567, 1988.
44. Altura BT, Altura BM: Phencyclidine, lysergic acid diethylamide and mescaline: Cerebral artery spasm and hallucinogenic activity. Science *212*:1051–1052, 1982.
45. Bessen HA: Intracranial hemorrhage associated with phencyclidine abuse. JAMA *248*:585–587, 1982.
46. Patel R, Connor G: A review of thirty cases of rhabdomyolysis-associated acute renal failure among PCP users. J Toxicol Clin Toxicol *23*:547–556, 1986.
47. Eastman JW, Cohen SN: Hypertensive crisis and death associated with phencyclidine poisoning. JAMA *231*:1270–1271, 1975.
48. Armen R, Kanel G, Reynolds T: Phencyclidine-induced malignant hyperthermia causing submassive liver necrosis. Am J Med *77*:167–172, 1984.
49. Balster RL: Clinical implications of behavior pharmacology research on phencyclidine. NIDA Res Monogr *64*:148–162, 1986.
50. Balster RL, Johanson CE, Harris RT, Schuster CR: Phencyclidine self-administration in the rhesus monkey. Pharmacol Biochem Behav *1*:167–172, 1973.
51. Rawson RA, Tennant FS, McCann MA: Characteristics of 68 chronic phencyclidine abusers who sought treatment. Drug Alcohol Depend *8*:223–227, 1981.
52. Goldberger BA, Cone EJ: Confirmatory tests for drugs in the workplace by gas chromatography-mass spectrometry. Am J Chromatogr *674*:73–86, 1994.
53. Castellani S, Giannini, AJ, Boeringa JA, Adams PM: Phencyclidine intoxication: Assessment of possible antidotes. J Toxicol Clin Toxicol *19*:313–319, 1982.
54. Seiler N, Grauffel C: Antagonism of phencyclidine-induced hyperactivity in mice by elevated brain GABA concentrations. Pharmacol Biochem Behav *41*:603–606, 1992.
55. Price WA, Giannini, AJ, Krishen A: Management of PCP intoxication with verapamil. J Toxicol Clin Toxicol *24*:85–87, 1986.
56. Owens SM, Mayersohn M: Phencyclidine-specific Fab fragments alter phencyclidine disposition in dogs. Drug Metab Dispos *14*:52–58, 1985.

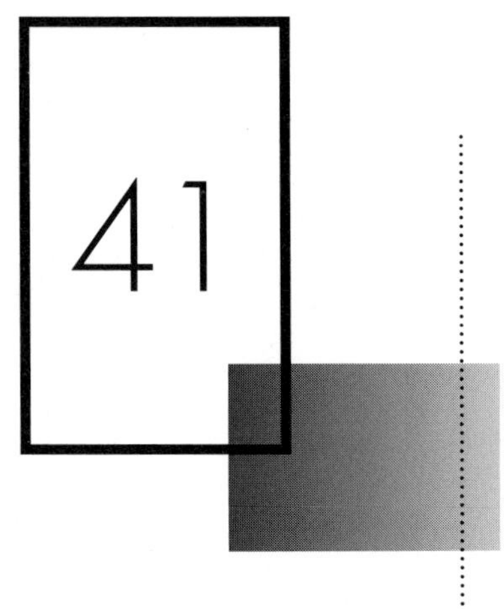

Amphetamines

TIMOTHY E. ALBERTSON, MD, PhD
BRENT E. VAN HOOZEN, MD
ROBLEE P. ALLEN, MD

Amphetamines and related stimulant compounds represent an increasingly important class of recreational drugs of abuse in the United States as well as in many other parts of the world. In some locales, they rival cocaine as a cause of drug-related emergency department (ED) and intensive care unit admissions. Although altered mental status, psychiatric disorders, and cardiovascular symptoms are most commonly encountered with amphetamine use, toxic manifestations in nearly every organ system have been reported (Table 41–1).

HISTORY

The amphetamine-like compounds have a long medical history. Related phenylisopropylamines including the alkaloids ephedrine, obtained from *Ephedra mahuang,* and norpseudoephedrine, or cathine, obtained from *Catha edulis,* have been respectively used for more than 5000 years in China and 600 years in East Africa.[1]

Although racemic β-phenylisopropylamine was first synthesized in 1887, initial investigations into the pharmacology of amphetamine derived from the basic phenylethylamine structure (Fig. 41–1) were not reported until 1930 by Piness.[2, 3] Early medicinal uses of amphetamine included the treatment of rhinitis and asthma.[1] The Smith, Kline and French Pharmaceutical Company introduced the Benzedrine Nasal Inhaler in the United States in 1932. Each inhaler contained 250 mg of synthetic racemic amphetamine base with menthol and various other aromatics.[4] Abuse of amphetamines was quickly noted and increased with a 1936 report claiming enhanced intellectual performance with its use.[4, 5] Because of reports of medical complications, amphetamines became prescription drugs in the United States in 1938; however, inhalers initially remained available without prescription. Limited use and abuse of amphetamine and related compounds continued until World War II, when they were extensively used by the Allies and the Axis powers as stimulants in combat.

The psychologically addicting characteristics were first realized when amphetamine abuse became epidemic in several countries including Japan and Sweden after World War II.[6] The 1950s and 1960s brought widespread abuse of amphetamines to the United States. Abuse was initially limited to using amphetamines as an anorectic or as a stimulant agent in an attempt to improve intellectual and physical performance or to combat fatigue.[7] A second pattern of abuse later emerged, with more recreational use of amphetamines. These abusers used amphetamines to attempt to achieve a euphoric state.[7] In addition to oral use, nasal and intravenous routes were popularized at this time.

Large amounts of amphetamines were legally produced in the United States; production peaked in 1965, with more than 10 billion pills (10,000 kg) manufactured.[7] At that time, much of this amphetamine was diverted from legitimate pharmaceutical sales, mainly for the treatment of obesity, to illicit street use. Additional amphetamine-like compounds that have emerged have limited proven medical uses and varying abuse potential (Table 41–2). Compounds such as methamphetamine, propylhexedrine, aminorex fumarate, fenfluramine, and methylphenidate (Ritalin) are only some of these agents. After the passage of the Controlled Substances Act of 1970, manufacture and distribution of amphetamines were better regulated in the United States, and legal production was markedly reduced.[7]

Table 41–1. Major Signs, Symptoms, and Noninfectious Medical Complications Associated with Use of Amphetamines and Related Compounds

Cardiac		*Neurologic*	
Chest pain	+ + +	Headaches	+
Myocardial infarction	+	Seizures	+ +
Palpitations	+ +	Cerebral infarcts/strokes	+ +
Arrhythmias	+ +	Cerebral vasculitis	+ +
Cardiomyopathy	+	Cerebral edema	+
Myocarditis	+	Mydriasis	+ +
Hypertension	+ +	Cerebral hemorrhage	+ +
Sudden death	+	Subarachnoid	+ +
Psychiatric		Intraventricular	+ + +
		Intracerebral	+ +
Anxiety	+ + +	*Respiratory*	
Depression	+ +		
Paranoia	+ +	Pulmonary edema	+
Delirium/ hallucinations	+ + +	Dyspnea	+ +
		Bronchitis	+
Psychosis	+ + +	Pulmonary hypertension	+
Suicide	+ +	Hemoptysis	+
Aggressive behavior	+ +	Pleuritic chest pain	+ +
Euphoria/ hyperactivity	+ +	Asthma exacerbations	+
		Pulmonary granuloma	+
Irritability	+ +	*Other*	
		Hyperpyrexia	+ +
		Renal failure	+
		Ischemic colitis	+
		Obstetric complications	+ +
		Anorexia/weight loss	+ + +
		Rhabdomyolysis	+ +
		Nausea/vomiting	+
		Disseminated vasculitis	+

Estimated frequency of events: +, reported rare case; + +, commonly reported; + + +, frequently seen or reported with chronic use or overdose.

With reduced amounts of diverted pharmaceutical-grade amphetamines such as D-amphetamine (Dexedrine), large-scale illegal manufacture and illegal importation of amphetamines began. Methamphetamine was found to be synthesized easily in crude street laboratories from readily available precursors such as L-ephedrine.[6] Methamphetamine has provided illicit street users with equal if not longer stimulant and euphoric action than that of D-amphetamine. During the past 20 years, various "designer" illicit amphetamines have enjoyed popularity on the street (see Table 41–2). Additional hallucinogenic properties are gained by methoxyl group substitutions on the phenyl ring, especially at the 3,4 position (see Fig. 41–1). These have included agents such as 3,4-methylenedioxymethamphetamine (MDMA), 3,4-methylenedioxyamphetamine (MDA), and 2,5-dimethoxy-4-methylamphetamine (DOM). These agents have had intermittent popularity on the streets of various communities.

Colorful names have been used to refer to methamphetamines on the street, including "meth," "speed," "crystal," and "crank." Studies in the late 1980s established the illicit manufacture of methamphetamine to be a 3 billion dollar per year industry localized primarily in Hawaii, California, Oregon, and Texas.[1] By the early 1990s, the crude techniques had given way to illicit manufacturers who were able to synthesize very pure methamphetamine. A 99% to 100% pure form of methamphetamine called "ice," because of its purity, has increased volatility when heated. Inhaling these volatile vapors, or "smoking meth," provides the same "rush" as intravenous use of methamphetamine. Increasing use has been noted in many western states, and nearly epidemic use is reported in some parts of Hawaii and California.

Death associated with amphetamine use has been frequently reported the past 25 years to the present.[8–10] These deaths are often associated with assault, suicide, or homicide.[8, 9] Cocaine was involved in one fifth and methamphetamine in about one eighth of all homicides in San Diego County in 1987.[11] By 1989, methamphetamine accounted for 60% of illicit drug seizures by San Diego County law enforcement agencies and 40% of all drug rehabilitation referrals in the area.[12] A large university teaching hospital in San Diego found an increase in the detection of amphetamine compounds on toxicology screens, from 3% to 10% of all tests during a 7- to 8-year period.[13] Predominantly men (56%) between the ages of 21 and 30 (61%) years had positive results.[13] Between 1986 and 1988, a 1.7-fold increase in ED visits for methamphetamine abuse was reported nationwide.[12] Abuse of methcathinone, a cathinone-methamphetamine analogue easily made as an oxidative product of ephedrine, has been widely reported in Russia and most recently in the midwestern United States. Although the heaviest illicit use of methamphetamine and other amphetamine compounds still appears to be more regionally located than does use of cocaine, the use is widespread enough for all practitioners to be aware of the toxicology of these compounds.

Table 41–2. Amphetamines and Related Compounds

Aminorex fumarate
Amphetamine
Benzphetamine
4-Bromo-2,5-methoxyphenylethylamine (2-CB/MFT)
Cathinone (khat)
Cinnamedrine
Desoxyephedrine
Dextroamphetamine
Diethylpropion
4-Bromo-2,5-dimethoxyamphetamine (DOB)
4-Methyl-2,5-dimethoxyamphetamine (DOM/STP)
Fenfluramine
Mescaline (3,4,5-trimethoxyphenylethylamine)
3,4-Methylenedioxyamphetamine (MDA)
3,4-Methylenedioxyethamphetamine (MDEA)
3,4-Methylenedioxymethamphetamine (MDMA)
Methamphetamine
Methcathinone
Methylphenidate
Methoxyamphetamine (PMA)
Pemoline
Phendimetrazine
Phenmetrazine
Phentermine
Phenylephrine
Phenylethylamine
Phenylpropanolamine
Propylhexadrine
Pseudoephedrine

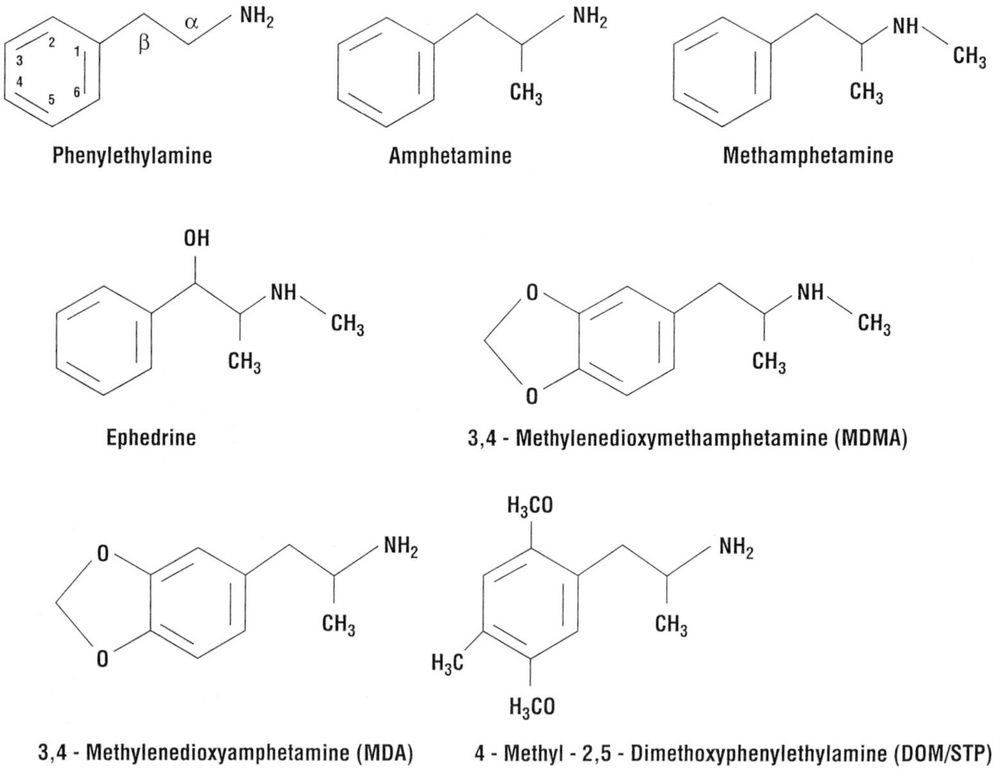

Figure 41–1. The chemical structures of several amphetamine-like compounds are shown. The basic phenylethylamine structure is labeled. Both α and β side chain positions and the phenyl ring itself can be modified to alter the pharmacologic effects of these related compounds.

PHARMACOLOGIC MECHANISMS

The amphetamines have complicated and diverse pharmacologic mechanisms. They have been shown to work primarily (as indirect sympathomimetics) by affecting the release of catecholamines at the neuronal presynaptic terminal.[1, 2, 7] Amphetamines and related compounds work indirectly to cause neuronal stimulation by increasing postsynaptic catecholamines. This is accomplished by blocking the presynaptic uptake transport activity from the synaptic cleft, by blocking presynaptic vesicular storage, and by reducing cytoplastic destruction of catecholamines by inhibiting mitochondrial monoamine oxidase.[1, 2, 7] Together these activities increase the rate of postsynaptic receptor stimulation. Both central and peripheral norepinephrine and dopamine neurotransmitters are affected. Some amphetamine-related compounds (e.g., ephedrine) are thought also to have the ability to directly stimulate sympathetic receptors (direct sympathominetics), but this is probably not a major mechanism of action for most of these compounds.[7] Amphetamines lack the local anesthetic effects on cardiac and nervous tissue that occur with cocaine use. The catecholamine toxicity of amphetamines is similar qualitatively to that of cocaine.

Increased norepinephrine postsynaptically causes sympathetic nervous system stimulation. This results in bronchodilation and increased heart rate, cardiac output, pupil size, and blood pressure, all of which are noted in the fight-or-flight response.[1] The central nervous system effects of amphetamine appear to be mediated primarily by dopaminergic alterations, which affect changes in mood, excitation, motor movements, and appetite.[1] Some evidence suggests that repeated high-dose amphetamine exposures in both adults and in fetuses/neonates may result in long-lasting destruction or depletion of central dopamine neurons.[1] Further alteration in mood, psychotic behavior, and aggressiveness may be the result of central nervous system serotonin release or reuptake blockade.[2] The extent to which serotonin neurotransmission alterations function in the clinical manifestations of amphetamine toxicity remains controversial.[1, 2, 7]

PHARMACOKINETICS

The amphetamines are weak bases with pK_a values around 8.8 to 10.4. For example, amphetamine has a pK_a of 9.9.[7, 14] Amphetamines are easily absorbed across most biologic membranes including gut, airway, nasopharynx, muscle, and vagina. Peak plasma concentrations occur in minutes by the intravenous route, in about 30 minutes by the intramuscular or topical nasal routes, and within 2 to 3 hours after ingestion.[7] Tissue redistribution is extensive, and the high lipid solubility of the amphetamines leads to increased concentrations relative to serum in the liver, kidneys, and lungs. This results in large volumes of distribution ranging from 3 to 6 L/kg for amphetamine, phentermine, and phenylephrine and 12 to 33 L/kg for fenfluramine and methylphenidate.[7]

Cerebrospinal fluid levels are about 80% of plasma levels at steady state. Therapeutic levels of amphetamine itself range between 30 and 40 ng/mL (0.030 to 0.040 mg/L), and death has been associated with average levels of 8600 (range, 500 to 41,000) ng/mL in the blood.[7, 14] Wide variations in doses and blood levels are reported to cause toxicity. This is in part related to the tolerance to amphetamines that can develop. The serum half-lives of various amphetamine-related compounds are urine pH dependent and range between 7 and 34 hours.[14] The more acidic the urine, the shorter the half-life because of reduced renal reabsorption of ionized urinary amphetamines. This leads to increased renal clearance of the iodized amphetamines.

Both active and inactive metabolites exist. Metabolism that results in aromatic hydroxylation, aliphatic hydroxylation, and *n*-dealkylation of amphetamines can give rise to active metabolites such as the potent hallucinogen *p*-hydroxyamphetamine.[7] Other metabolic pathways, including deamination and subsequent side chain oxidation, produce inactive amphetamine derivatives.[7] Glucuronide and glycine conjugation pathways result in urine excretion of metabolites.[14] As much as 30% of amphetamine is excreted in the urine unchanged, whereas between 86% and 97% of ephedrine, pseudoephedrine, and phenylpropanolamine is excreted unchanged.[7, 14]

The use of concomitant drugs such as the opiates (i.e., speedballing) can increase overall toxicity of amphetamines. However, major alterations of the metabolic pathways of amphetamine have not been postulated as an explanation for this increased toxicity.[14] Simultaneous use of methamphetamine and ethanol has been shown to have more psychologic and cardiac effects than use of methamphetamine alone. This response is also presumed to be pharmacodynamic in nature rather than a result of any specific pharmacokinetic interaction.[15]

CLINICAL TOXICITIES AND SPECIFIC MANAGEMENT

The amphetamines are capable of being toxic to each organ system. Both acute and chronic and direct and indirect abnormalities have been reported with the use of amphetamines. The exact prevalence and incidence of the toxicities summarized in Table 41–1 have not been determined and probably vary with route, dose, and length of exposure to each of the amphetamine-related agents.

Central Nervous System

The central nervous system is the target organ for the pharmacologic effects of most amphetamine-related compounds. As such, significant central nervous system toxicity can result from use of amphetamines. With the resurgence of amphetamines as drugs of abuse in the 1960s, it was quickly recognized that the initial sensation of extreme physical and mental powers following amphetamine use could rapidly deteriorate with high doses or chronic moderate doses to recurrent affective lability, confusion, and hallucinations.[16, 17] In a series of 127 amphetamine-toxic patients presenting to an ED, 57% were found to have altered mental status.[18] Agitation, suicidal ideation, hallucinations, delusions, confusion, and despondent affect were the most common major signs and symptoms noted. The presenting manifestations of headaches affected 4%, seizures 3%, and paresthesias 2%.[18] An additional 10% were found to be unresponsive.[18]

Tolerance to the autonomic effects of amphetamine has been reported for body temperature, blood pressure, heart rate, and respirations. In addition, the anorectic effects of amphetamines have also been shown to exhibit tolerance.[19] In contrast, the motor stimulant and stereotypic behavior effects of amphetamine have been shown to display progressive enhancement with repeated intermittent administrations.[19] This has been termed *behavioral sensitization* or *reverse tolerance.*

Researchers have postulated that the acute paranoid delusional psychosis associated with amphetamine use may produce a lasting psychosis similar to schizophrenia that persists long after elimination of the amphetamine through behavioral sensitization.[20] Whether this represents emergence of an underlying psychiatric disorder or simply a lowering of the threshold for drug-induced psychosis is not known.[21, 22] When challenged with large doses of intravenous methamphetamine, patients dependent on amphetamine developed drug-induced psychosis.[22] This same dose of methamphetamine failed to produce drug-induced psychosis in nonamphetamine users.[22] Drug-induced psychotic states have been reported with the abuse of most of the stimulant amphetamine-related compounds, including cathinone, pemoline, and phenmetrazine.[23–25] Psychosis is common with derivatives of amphetamine that are hallucinogens, such as mescaline, DOM, MDA, *p*-methoxyamphetamine, and MDMA.[24] Although tolerance to the hallucinogenic properties of these agents has been noted, prolonged psychotic reactions are also well documented.[24] Acute severe hallucinations with bizarre and risky behavior due to the use of agents such as MDA, MDMA, and 3,4-methylenedioxyethamphetamine have resulted in traumatic deaths.[26] Mild to moderate amphetamine-induced agitated behavior and psychosis can be treated with benzodiazepines (e.g., diazepam or lorazepam), but severe symptoms should be treated with high-potency antipsychotic agents (e.g., haloperidol, droperidol, or thiothixene).[7, 18, 27] Minimizing sensory stimuli with low doses of benzodiazepines in combination with low doses of antipsychotic agents has been a useful approach to amphetamine-induced psychosis.

In addition to behavioral effects including agitation, hallucinations, and psychosis, amphetamine use has been associated with several other neurologic toxicities. The chorea of patients with Huntington's disease has been exacerbated by use of amphetamines.[28] The dopaminergic receptor blocker haloperidol was shown to inhibit the amphetamine-induced exacerbation of the choreoathetoid movements.[28] Choreoathetoid movement disorders have also been seen with acute and chronic amphetamine exposures in patients who do not have Huntington's disease.[29, 30] Treatment of acute amphetamine-induced choreoathetoid movement disorders has included supportive care, gastrointestinal decontamination with activated charcoal, and the use of haloperidol.[29]

Seizures have been reported with severe intoxications of amphetamine and related compounds.[18, 31–33] The seizures have been isolated or associated with hyperpyrexia, coma, metabolic acidosis, and shock. Intravenous benzodiazepines (e.g., diazepam, lorazepam), phenytoin, and barbiturates (e.g., pentobarbital, amobarbital) have been used to terminate amphetamine-induced seizures.[7, 32]

Intracerebral hemorrhage has been associated with the use of amphetamines and related compounds. Amphetamine-related cerebral hemorrhage has occurred in patients with arteriovenous malformations[34] and drug-induced cerebral vasculitis.[35–38] Both oral and intravenous amphetamine exposures have resulted in cases of cerebral vasculitis.[35–38] Traditional approaches to intracerebral hemorrhage have focused on supportive care, correcting the hypotension, use of corticosteroids, and use of antifibrinolytic agents such as ε-aminocaproic acid.[35–38] Treatment directed at the vasculitis in these cases has included use of dexamethasone and cyclophosphamide therapy.[35, 36] The efficacy of these agents in the treatment of amphetamine-associated vasculitis is unknown.

Ischemic strokes have been reported with amphetamine compounds taken orally, intravenously, and by inhalation.[39] Supportive care and hypervolemic hemodilutional therapy using albumin or 10% dextran 40 has been advocated after angiographic demonstration of cerebral artery spasm and occlusion.[39] Elective extracranial/intracranial bypass was performed in at least one case of amphetamine-associated occlusive stroke, but its efficacy is unproven.[39] A recent case of transient cortical blindness in an infant exposed to methamphetamine has been reported.[40] The blindness resolved within 12 hours without specific therapy. It was postulated that this represented a manifestation of amphetamine-induced cerebral vasospasm.[40] The central nervous system is the main target of the pharmacologic actions of the amphetamines and is also the most frequent organ system to manifest amphetamine-induced toxicity.

Cardiovascular

In a retrospective study of patients with amphetamine toxicity presenting to an ED, hypertension and tachycardia were commonly encountered. The same study found that patients complained of chest pain 9% and palpitations 3% of the time.[18] Direct pharmacologic effects of the amphetamines most likely account for the frequently encountered hypertension and the tachycardia. Hypertension and agitated behavior associated with amphetamine use are initially approached by minimizing stimulus or sensory inputs and by using sedating agents. If more specific treatment is needed, the use of intravenous nitroprusside or oral or intravenous calcium channel blockers (e.g., nifedipine or nicardipine) may be indicated. β-Blockers should not be used in the treatment of amphetamine-induced hypertension without concomitant α blockade, because unopposed α blockade can produce intense vasospasm and paradoxical hypertension.

Ectopic ventricular beats as well as supraventricular and ventricular tachyarrhythmias have been reported with amphetamine use. Direct catecholamine effects and ischemic effects secondary to coronary vasospasm generated by amphetamine use are probably responsible for the arrhythmias.[41] Although not normally studied, short-acting β-adrenergic receptor blockers (e.g., esmolol), calcium channel blockers (e.g., verapamil, diltiazam), or lidocaine can be used in treating these arrhythmias. Correction of hypoxia and electrolyte abnormalities is also required.

Myocardial infarctions associated with amphetamine use are thought to be secondary to direct cardiac toxicity (myocarditis), vasospasm, and thrombus formation.[41, 42] In addition to treatment with nitrates and analgesics, at least one report describes the use of thrombolytics in treating amphetamine-induced myocardial infarctions.[42] Profound hypotension, bradycardia, and metabolic acidosis have occurred with massive amphetamine overdoses. The treatment includes aggressive hemodynamic support with intravascular volume replacement and vasopressor agents (e.g., norepinephrine or phenylephrine). Direct-acting catecholamines (norepinephrine or phenylephrine rather than dopamine) are preferred because massive overdoses may result in a relative catecholamine-depleted state.

Both acute and chronic cardiomyopathy have been associated with amphetamine use. This is thought to be secondary to direct amphetamine toxicity and indirect hypertension. Treatment has included avoidance of amphetamines, the use of diuretics and digoxin, and afterload reduction (e.g., nitroprusside acutely and angiotensin-converting enzyme inhibitors such as captopril for long-term use).[43] Intravenous use of amphetamines has been associated with bacterial endocarditis, which can lead to abnormal cardiac valves, dilated cardiomyopathy, and the formation of mycotic aneurysms. Acute aortic dissection, necrotizing angiitis, and both visceral and cerebral aneurysms have also been reported to occur in amphetamine users.[44]

Arterial or tissue-extravasated amphetamine quickly leads to tissue ischemia. Immediate intra-arterial or local tissue injection of α-adrenergic blocking agents such as phentolamine or phenoxybenzamine is indicated to reverse the local vasopressor effects of amphetamines. General supportive or symptomatic care is most important to maintain the cardiac system during acute amphetamine toxicity.

Pulmonary

Respiratory symptoms including chest pain and dyspnea have been presenting complaints of amphetamine-toxic patients presenting to an ED.[18] The actual incidence of respiratory toxicity with amphetamines is not known. The incidence and types of toxicity may vary, depending on the amphetamine compound and the route of exposure. One review examined pulmonary effects of exposure to amphetamine-related compounds.[45] Although the amphetamines are often snorted, inhaled, and smoked, the literature has not noted an association with barotrauma. Cocaine, on the other hand, which has similar routes of administration, has in frequent case reports been associated with barotrauma.[45]

Despite increased use of inhaled or smoked methamphetamine, no extensive reports of exacerbation of reactive airway disease have been noted. One death due to asthma has been reported with the use of the hallucinogenic amphetamine MDMA.[26] Two small case series have noted obstructive spirometric findings associated with 20% to 60% reductions in carbon monoxide diffusion capacity after intravenous methylphenidate use.[45] These patients showed variable responses to β-adrenergic agonist bronchodilators (e.g., albuterol). These same patients were noted to have panlobular emphysema. Foreign particle embolization from intravenous dosing of the methylphenidate was postulated as the cause rather than a direct drug effect.[45]

Case reports describe acute noncardiogenic pulmonary edema associated with amphetamine toxicity.[45] At least one mortality with pulmonary edema has been related to the use of MDMA.[26] Whether this represents a direct amphetamine toxicity leading to leaky pulmonary capillaries or is a result of indirect neurogenic (e.g., seizures) or cardiovascular (e.g., shock, hydrostatic leak) consequences has not been determined. Although reports of noncardiogenic pulmonary edema with cocaine abuse appear more frequently in the literature than do those of amphetamine abuse, a mechanism for it also has not been determined and may be similar.[45]

The literature has for some time described amphetamine use associated with pulmonary hypertension. Intravenous users of amphetamines obtained from nasal inhalers available until the 1960s were noted to have pulmonary artery foreign body granulomas and muscle hypertrophy.[4, 45] Long-term inhalation of methamphetamine and propylhexedrine has also been associated with marked pulmonary hypertension in at least one case.[45] Proposed mechanisms have included direct toxic endothelial injury caused by the drugs or their contaminants, recurrent hypoxic insults, direct spasm in genetically determined sensitive hosts, vasculitis, and dysregulation of the mediators of vascular tone such as nitric oxide. The amphetamine-like anorectic agents fenfluramine and aminorex fumarate have also been associated with several European reports of pulmonary hypertension.[45] No specific therapy has been advocated for these cases of pulmonary hypertension, other than further avoidance of stimulants and supportive care, including supplemental oxygen for hypoxic patients.

Because the incidence of smoking methamphetamine has increased, it will not be surprising to see future reports of pulmonary toxicities similar to these reported with the use of the stimulant crack cocaine. These would include hemoptysis, alveolar hemorrhage, and alveolar accumulation of carbonaceous material associated with cough, bronchitis, sinusitis, and thermal epiglottitis.[45] Basic airway management and supportive care are the only approaches to these complications. In severe cases of amphetamine-induced pulmonary edema, aggressive mechanical ventilatory support with the addition of positive end-expiratory pressure and high levels of inspired oxygen flow are often required.

Systemic Toxicity

Severe systemic toxicity has been reported with overdoses of amphetamine-related compounds. A pattern of fulminant hyperthermia, convulsions, disseminated intravascular coagulation, hepatocellular damage, rhabdomyolysis, acute renal failure, arrhythmias, and refractory hypotension has been reported with use of MDMA.[31]

Hyperthermia, shock, pulmonary edema, rhabdomyolysis, acute renal failure, and disseminated intravascular coagulation have been encountered with use of the designer amphetamines, as well as with the use of phenmetrazine and methamphetamine.[31, 33, 46] Aggressive cardiopulmonary support, large amounts of intravascular volume replacement, electrolyte replacement, temperature control measures, and extracorporeal hemodialysis are needed to overcome the amphetamine toxicity in these patients.[31, 46] It appears that this combination of systemic toxicity from amphetamines predicts a poor outcome.

Hepatotoxicity with hepatocellular damage has also occurred with use of this compound and other amphetamines. Postulated mechanisms for the hepatotoxicity include direct toxic effects, lipid peroxidation, necrotizing angiitis, contaminants, hypotension, and genetic variations in metabolism, which create toxic intermediates. Treatment consists of supportive care and avoidance of amphetamines. At least one liver transplant has been attempted in these patients.[31]

In addition to the severe systemic toxicities described earlier, reversible ischemic colitis induced by methamphetamine abuse has been reported. Abdominal pain was the presenting complaint in 4% of amphetamine-toxic patients presenting to an ED.[18] The exact incidence of ischemic bowel and hemorrhagic colitis in abusers of amphetamines is unknown. Diagnostic efforts to rule out necrotic bowel

Table 41–3. Amphetamine and Related Compound Toxicity and Treatment and Decision Algorithm

Suspected Amphetamine Toxicity

↓

Mild Amphetamine Toxicity

↓

Evaluate
Decontamination of oral ingestions/activated charcoal
Observe
Psychologic support/environmental control
Health care maintenance
HIV testing
Hepatitis screening, etc.

Severe Amphetamine Toxicity

↓

Immediate Supportive Care

Airway control
Oxygenation
Vascular access
Appropriate monitoring

↓

Decontaminate/Antagonists

Oral ingestion/activated charcoal
Consider empirical 50% dextrose, thiamine, naloxone
Avoid benzodiazepine antagonists

↓

Terminate Seizures

Benzodiazepines (e.g., diazepam, lorazepam)
Barbiturates (e.g., pentobarbital, phenobarbital)

↓

Control Severe Psychotic Agitation

Minimize sensory stimulation
Benzodiazepines (e.g, diazepam, lorazepam)
Butyrophenones (e.g., droperidol, haloperidol)
Protect from aggressive or self-destructive behavior

↓

Correct Immediate Metabolic, Oxygenation, and Electrolyte Abnormalities

Avoid acidification of the urine

↓

Local α-Blockers for Exuded or Intra-Arterial Amphetamines (e.g., Phenoxybenzamine, Phentolamine)

↓

Treat Hyperthermia

Passive/active cooling measure

↓

Treat Arrhythmias

Antiarrhythmic (e.g., lidocaine)
Supraventricular arrhythmias (e.g., esmolol)
Electrolyte correction
Acid-base/oxygenation correction

↓

Second-Level Evaluations to Check for Persistent Abnormalities

↓

Persistent Hypotension

Intravascular volume resuscitation
Acute cardiopulmonary support
Central hemodynamic monitoring

Pulmonary Edema/Respiratory Failure

Ventilator
Oxygen
Positive end-expiratory pressure

Rhabdomyolysis

Alkalize urine (e.g., intravenous bicarbonate)
Calcium replacement (e.g., calcium gluconate)
Intravascular volume

Renal Failure/Rhabdomyolysis/Renal Ischemia

Hemodialysis
Intravascular volume

Supportive Care

Observation/monitoring
Psychologic and pharmacologic support for amphetamine abstinence and long-term recovery
Health maintenance/education (e.g., HIV and hepatitis testing)

Coronary Artery Ischemia

Calcium channel blockers (e.g., nifedipine, diltiazem)
β-Blockers (e.g., esmolol, metoprolol)
Nitrates (e.g., nitroglycerin)

Hypertension

Sedation (e.g., diazepam, haloperidol)
Calcium channel blockers (e.g., nifedipine, nicardipine)
β-Blockers (e.g., esmolol)
Nitroprusside

Electrolyte Abnormalities

Correct hypokalemia (e.g., potassium chloride)
Correct hypocalcemia (e.g., calcium gluconate)
Correct hypoglycemia (e.g., dextrose as D_{50})

Central Nervous System Abnormality

Seizures
Strokes
Bleeds
Vasculitis
Agitation

Evaluate for Other Agents

↓

Initiate specific treatment for additional agents
Consider interactions with amphetamine
Monitor for early and late toxicities of other agents

would be prudent in amphetamine-associated cases of persistent abdominal pain, particularly with bloody stools.

Obstetric and Prenatal

Gestational exposure to amphetamines has been postulated but not proved to have lasting effects on neonates.[47] After illicit amphetamine exposure, infants have had hypoglycemia, sweating, poor feeding, poor visual tracking, and seizures.[47] As with cocaine exposure, fetal amphetamine exposure was associated with intrauterine growth retardation, decreased head circumference, preterm delivery with fetal distress, anemia, and placental abruption in one study.[47] An amphetamine withdrawal pattern similar to that of cocaine withdrawal was noted in these infants. This pattern consisted of abnormal sleep patterns, tremors, hypertonia, high-pitched cry, poor feeding, vomiting, sneezing, frantic sucking, and tachycardia.[48] Although long-term behavioral and neurologic follow-up of these infants is not yet available, early reports suggest that chaotic lifestyles with minor neurologic abnormalities continue for these infants after discharge from the hospital.[47] Other studies have reported reduced birth weight with methamphetamine exposure relative to normal populations but no increase in other adverse outcomes.[48] Reports have suggested that pregnant women exposed to amphetamines are at increased risk of serious obstetric complications, including intracranial hemorrhage, seizures, and amniotic fluid embolism.[48] No specific therapy has been identified for neonates or pregnant women heavily exposed to amphetamines. Identification of at-risk women during their prenatal care would give an opportunity to educate. Unfortunately, many pregnant women using amphetamines do not seek prenatal care and may be unable or unwilling to reduce their gestational exposures.

GENERAL PRINCIPLES OF TREATMENT

An algorithm for the general approach to a suspected amphetamine-toxic patient is outlined in Table 41–3. No prospective human trials have evaluated different treatment options. Most recommendations are based on animal studies or case reports of humans. For example, the efficacy of activated charcoal in treating oral methamphetamine exposure has been clearly demonstrated in a study in mice but lacks human trials.[49] Original recommendations to acidify the urine in amphetamine overdoses were based on a single case.[50] The risks of systemic acidification and the potential problems for the kidneys when rhabdomyolysis is present have prevented this recommendation from being widely adopted until controlled trials have demonstrated improved patient outcomes. Clinicians must be aware of the problem of contaminants in addition to the direct toxic effects of amphetamines. A cluster of at least 14 cases of acute lead poisonings were found in intravenous methamphetamine users in Oregon in 1988. Amphetamine products manufactured in clandestine laboratories may be grossly contaminated with a number of toxic heavy metals and chemicals. In addition, we have noticed a cluster of 30 cases of acute botulism poisoning associated with illicit amphetamine drug use.

General supportive care, decontamination of the gastrointestinal tract for ingestions, and control of behavior, seizures, arrhythmias, and temperature remain the mainstay of therapy for amphetamine-poisoned patients. Dialysis and hemoperfusion have no role in amphetamine overdose. Specific measures when available for each complication associated with amphetamine use have been outlined in this chapter. Once the acute toxic amphetamine symptoms have passed, treating physicians should consider referring patients for rehabilitation or psychiatric care to break up the destructive drug abuse pattern. Infectious diseases should also be considered. These patients should be evaluated for complications attendant to intravenous drug abuse such as bacterial endocarditis, viral hepatitis, and human immunodeficiency virus.

CONCLUSION

Although not as widespread as cocaine abuse, amphetamine abuse and toxicity account for significant morbidity, mortality, and ED and intensive care unit admissions in many communities. The impact of amphetamine toxicity is amplified by its association with violent crime and trauma. The various compounds that make up the amphetamines challenge the laboratory and clinical toxicologist. The ability of the various amphetamine-related compounds to cause significant behavioral and multiple organ system dysfunction contributes to the clinical challenge. Further trials that evaluate proposed treatment approaches for amphetamine-toxic patients are needed. Community education and prevention approaches can reduce the incidence of this increasing problem.

References

1. Cho AK: Ice: A new dosage form of an old drug. Science *249*:631–634, 1990.
2. Gawin F, Ellinwood EH: Cocaine and other stimulants: Actions, abuse, and treatments. N Engl J Med *318*:1173–1182, 1988.
3. Piness G, Miller H, Alles GA: Clinical observations on phenylaminoethanol sulfate. JAMA *94*:790–791, 1930.
4. Anderson R, Reed W, Hillis L: History, epidemiology, and medical complications of nasal inhaler abuse. J Toxicol Clin Toxicol *19*:95–107, 1982.
5. Myerson A: Effect of benzedrine sulphate on mood in normal and in neurotic persons. Arch Neurol Psychiatry *36*:816–822, 1936.
6. Derlet R, Heischober B: Methamphetamine: Stimulant of the 1990's? West J Med *153*:625–628, 1990.

7. Linden C, Kulig K, Rumack B: Amphetamines. Top Emerg Med *7*:18–31, 1985.
8. Ellinwood E: Assault and homicide associated with amphetamine abuse. Am J Psychiatry *127*:1170–1175, 1971.
9. Kalant H, Kalant D: Death in amphetamine users: Causes and rates. Can Med Assoc J *112*:299–304, 1993.
10. Katsumata S, Sato K, Kashiwade H, et al: Sudden death due to internal use of methamphetamine. Forensic Sci Int *62*:209–215, 1993.
11. Bailey D, Shaw R: Cocaine- and methamphetamine-related deaths in San Diego County (1987): Homicides and accidental overdoses. J Forensic Sci *34*:407–422, 1989.
12. Beebe D, Walley E: Smokable methamphetamine ('Ice'): An old drug in a different form. Am Fam Physician *51*:449–453, 1995.
13. Bailey D: Amphetamine detection during toxicology screening of a university medical center patient population. Clin Toxicol *25*:399–409, 1987.
14. Baselt R, Cravey R: Amphetamine. *In* Baselt R, Cravey R (eds): Disposition of Toxic Drugs and Chemicals in Man. 4th ed. Foster City, CA, Chemical Toxicology Institute, pp 44–47, 1995.
15. Medelson J, Jones RT, Upton R, Jacob P: Methamphetamine and ethanol interactions in humans. Clin Pharmacol Ther *57*:559–568, 1995.
16. Kramer J, Fischman V, Littlefield D: Amphetamine abuse pattern and effects of high doses taken intravenously. JAMA *201*:89–93, 1967.
17. Smith D, Fischer C: An analysis of 310 cases of acute high-dose methamphetamine toxicity in Haight-Ashbury. Clin Toxicol *3*:117–124, 1970.
18. Derlet R, Rice P, Horowitz B, Lord R: Amphetamine toxicity: Experience with 127 cases. J Emerg Med *7*:157–161, 1989.
19. Robinson T, Becker J: Enduring changes in brain and behavior produced by chronic amphetamine administration: A review and evaluation of animal models of amphetamine psychosis. Brain Res Rev *11*:157–198, 1986.
20. Sato M: A lasting vulnerability to psychosis in patients with previous methamphetamine psychosis. Ann NY Acad Sci *654*:160–170, 1992.
21. Ellinwood E: Amphetamine psychosis: I. Description of the individual and process. J Nerv Ment Dis *144*:273–283, 1967.
22. Bell D: The experimental reproduction of amphetamine psychosis. Arch Gen Psychiatry *29*:35–40, 1973.
23. Polchert S, Morse R: Pemoline abuse. JAMA *254*:946–947, 1985.
24. Castellani S, Petrie W, Ellinwood E: Drug-induced psychosis: Neurobiological mechanisms. *In* Alterman AI (ed): Substance Abuse and Psychopathology. New York, Plenum Press, pp 173–210, 1985.
25. Schecter M, Glennon R: Cathinone, cocaine and methamphetamine: Similarity of behavioral effects. Pharmacol Biochem Behav *22*:913–916, 1985.
26. Dowling G, McDonough E, Bost R: "Eve" and "ecstasy": A report of five deaths associated with the use of MDEA and MDMA. JAMA *257*:1615–1617, 1987.
27. Dubin W, Weiss K, Dirn J: Pharmacotherapy of psychiatric emergencies. J Clin Psychopharmacol *6*:210–222, 1986.
28. Klawans H, Weiner W: The pharmacology of choreatic movement disorders. Prog Neurobiol *6*:49–80, 1976.
29. Rhee K, Albertson T, Douglas J: Choreoathetoid disorders associated with amphetamine-like drugs. Am J Emerg Med *6*:131–133, 1988.
30. Lundh H, Tunving K: An extrapyramidal choreiform syndrome caused by amphetamine addiction. J Neurol Neurosurg Psychiatry *44*:728–730, 1981.
31. Henry J, Jeffreys K, Dawling S: Toxicity and deaths from 3,4-methylenedioxymethamphetamine ("ecstasy"). Lancet *340*: 384–387, 1992.
32. Simpson D, Rumack B: Methylenedioxyamphetamine clinical description of overdose, death, and review of pharmacology. Arch Intern Med *141*:1507–1509, 1987.
33. Chan P, Chen J, Lee M, Deng J: Fatal and nonfatal methamphetamine intoxication in the intensive care unit. Clin Toxicol *32*:147–155, 1994.
34. Lukes S: Intracerebral hemorrhage from an arteriovenous malformation after amphetamine injection. Arch Neurol *40*:60–61, 1983.
35. Salanova V, Taubner R: Intracerebral haemorrhage and vasculitis secondary to amphetamine use. Postgraduate Med J *60*:429–430, 1984.
36. Matick H, Anderson D, Brumlik J: Cerebral vasculitis associated with oral amphetamine overdose. Arch Neurol *40*:253–254, 1983.
37. Hughes J, McCabe M, Evans R: Intracranial haemorrhage associated with ingestion of 'Ecstasy.' Arch Emerg Med *10*:372–374, 1993.
38. Conci F, D'Angelo V, Tampier D, Vecchi G: Intracerebral hemorrhage and angiographic beading following amphetamine abuse. Ital J Neurol Sci *9*:77–81, 1981.
39. Rothrock J, Rubenstein R, Legden P: Ischemic stroke associated with methamphetamine inhalation. Neurology *38*:589–592, 1988.
40. Gospe S: Transient cortical blindness in an infant exposed to methamphetamine. Ann Emerg Med *26*:380–382, 1995.
41. Bashour T: Acute myocardial infarction resulting from amphetamine abuse: A spasm-thrombus interplay? Am Heart J *128*:1237–1239, 1994.
42. Furst S, Fallon S, Reznik G, Shah P: Myocardial infarction after inhalation of methamphetamine. N Engl J Med *323*:1147–1148, 1990.
43. Hong R, Matsuyama E, Nur K: Cardiomyopathy associated with the smoking of crystal methamphetamine. JAMA *265*:1152–1154, 1991.
44. Davis G, Swalwell C: Acute aortic dissections and ruptured berry aneurysms associated with methamphetamine abuse. J Forensic Sci *39*:1481–1485.
45. Albertson T, Walby W, Derlet R: Stimulant-induced pulmonary toxicity. Chest *108*:1140–1149, 1995.
46. Kendrick W, Hall A, Knochel J: Rhabdomyolysis and shock after intravenous amphetamine administration. Ann Intern Med *86*:381–387, 1977.
47. Dixon S: Effects of transplacental exposure to cocaine and methamphetamine on the neonate. West J Med *150*:436–442, 1989.
48. Catanzarite V, Stein D: "Crystal" and pregnancy methamphetamine-associated maternal deaths. West J Med *162*:454–457, 1995.
49. McKinney P, Tomaszewski C, Phillips S, et al: Methamphetamine toxicity prevented by activated charcoal in a mouse model. Ann Emerg Med *24*:220–223, 1994.
50. Gary N, Saidi P: Methamphetamine intoxication: A speedy new treatment. Am J Med *64*:537–540, 1978.

42

Designer Drugs

PATRICK E. McKINNEY, MD

INTERESTING MEDICAL HISTORY

Designer drug is a term that originated in the early 1980s to describe compounds that were synthesized by street chemists that resembled various parent drugs of abuse with minor structural modifications.[1] These drugs were temporarily exempt from control by the Drug Enforcement Administration (DEA) because of structural differences from their parent compounds. At that time, these drugs were not illegal, because until new drugs were formally scheduled by the DEA, existing laws did not apply to them. Because of this loophole in drug regulations, minor modifications of drugs such as phencyclidine (PCP), fentanyl, meperidine, mescaline, and amphetamine yielded compounds that had pharmacologic activity similar to that of the parent drug, but were legal to manufacture, possess, and use. The synthesis of many of these compounds is relatively uncomplicated and inexpensive; therefore, the lure of potentially large profit margins and the continued popularity of many of these substances makes the designer drug phenomenon unlikely to be short-lived.

The designer drug loophole was largely closed by the Controlled Substances Analogue Enforcement Act of 1986; however, the term *designer drug* continues to be used to refer to this diverse group of drugs.[2] Currently, *designer drug* refers to analogues in several classes of drugs of abuse, including opioids, amphetamines, hallucinogens, arylhexylamines, and methaqualone derivatives. Although these compounds might logically be discussed individually in conjunction with related compounds, convention and historical factors make their discussion appropriate here.

Contrary to popular belief, most designer drugs are not novel compounds originally developed and synthesized by street chemists; rather, they are drugs that have been synthesized and studied in the past by researchers and pharmaceutical companies, usually as part of the study of a series of related compounds. The description of the synthetic process and pharmacologic activity of these compounds is often found in the scientific literature. However, many of these substances have never been formally tested for safety, efficacy, and side effects, and their pharmacokinetics and pharmacodynamics may be poorly characterized, if studied at all. Therefore, their use by a potentially large population of substance abusers continues to be a matter of concern. The manufacture of these substances often occurs in conditions that are unsanitary, in which chemical reactions may be poorly monitored, and in which substitutions for unavailable reagents may be made. This has led to the presence of contaminants with potentially significant toxicity, such as the contamination of a synthetic meperidine analogue with 1-methyl-4-phenyl-1,2,3,6-tetrahydropyridine (MPTP), which resulted in cases of drug-induced parkinsonism in the 1980s.[3]

EPIDEMIOLOGY

The incidence and prevalence of designer drug use is difficult to estimate. Statistics collected by the American Association of Poison Control Centers do not specifically reflect designer drug use but rather include them in a miscellaneous subcategory under their parent compound. In addition, many of these substances are difficult to detect using standard urine or blood toxicologic screens, making their identification difficult. A random and anonymous poll conducted at Stanford University reported in 1987 indicated that of the 369 subjects interviewed, 149 (39%) indicated that they had used 3,4-methylenedioxymethamphetamine (MDMA), a substituted amphetamine, at least once.[4] A similar study conducted at Tulane University in 1990 showed that 24.3% of the 1,264 respondents indicated using MDMA at least once, up from 15.5% in 1986.[5] The popular press has noted the widespread phenomenon of MDMA use, especially at "rave parties," large dance gatherings where MDMA is often found.[6]

The use of designer opioids does not currently seem as widespread as the use of MDMA. From 1979 through the mid-1980s, more than 100 deaths from fentanyl analogues were noted in California.[1] A few deaths were also noted in other western states. Then in 1988, a new outbreak was seen in Allegheny County, Pennsylvania.[7] These outbreaks appear to have been limited, but the possibility of recurrence at any time or place remains.

Reports of morbidity in the form of drug-induced parkinsonism from the use of meperidine analogue methylphenylpropionoxypiperidine (MPPP) contaminated with MPTP appear to be limited to a small series of patients in California in the mid-1970s to the mid-1980s.[8] New cases have not surfaced since then, but it is estimated that a large population of currently asymptomatic opioid users injected this drug in doses insufficient to cause parkinsonism acutely, but a risk for development of symptoms in the future is possible.[9]

PHARMACOLOGY

Chemical Identification and Structure

Structural Relationship with Other Compounds

Designer drugs currently available in the United States can be included in four major categories. The first group, the phenylethylamines, are structurally related to both amphetamine and mescaline. The second, synthetic opioids, include fentanyl derivatives and meperidine analogues. The third, arylhexylamine derivatives, include structural modifications of phencyclidine. The last includes modifications of methaqualone.

Phenylethylamines. Phenylethylamine is the core chemical structure for endogenous catecholamines (Fig. 42–1). Modifications of the basic structure of phenylethylamine result in therapeutic agents including ephedrine, phenylpropanolamine, and amphetamine as well as drugs of abuse, including mescaline and MDMA. Because of structural similarity to both amphetamine and mescaline, phenylethylamines are referred to in various fashions including substituted amphetamines, hallucinogenic amphetamines, and amphetamine or mescaline derivatives. Use of the term *phenylethylamine* avoids some of the implications of the other terms that would tend to lump this class of compounds either as sympathomimetics or hallucinogens. Chemical modifications of various sites of the phenylethylamine molecule modify sympathetic activity as well as psychoactive properties, producing a spectrum of compounds that are not easily categorized based on their physiologic properties. In overdose, however, the compounds tend to produce similar symptoms of sympathomimetic excess.

Mescaline is the prototypical phenylethylamine with psychoactive properties. Mescaline is a component of peyote with prominent hallucinogenic properties, first synthesized in 1918.[10] Many subsequent analogues have been produced, but only a fraction of these have been widely used as substances of abuse. Representative analogues are shown in Figure 42–1. One of the first recreationally available mescaline analogues was 4-methyl-2,5-dimethoxyamphetamine (DOM). First reported in 1967, DOM, also known as STP (for serenity, tranquility, and peace), had a low therapeutic index, and its popularity was short-lived.[11] Para-methoxyamphetamine (PMA) appeared in the 1970s and is produced when a methoxy group is added to the 4 carbon of the benzene ring. It was noted for both marked sympathomimetic and hallucinogenic properties.[12] 4-Bromo-2,5-dimethoxyamphetamine (DOB) is produced when a methyl group in the ring structure of DOM is replaced with bromine. The resulting compound has at least 100 times the psychoactive properties of mescaline and a duration of action of 24 to 36 hours.[13] Compounds known as 2-CD and 2-CB are produced when the methyl group is removed from the α carbon of DOM and DOB, respectively, and may be up to 20 times as potent as mescaline. Introduction of a methyl group α to the nitrogen of mescaline yields 2,4,5-trimethoxyamphetamine, a compound with a duration of action of 8 to 10 hours in therapeutic doses.[14] A derivative of a European diet pill aminorex (removed from the market because it caused pulmonary hypertension) is known as U-4-E-Uh (2-amino-5-phenyl-2-oxazoline.[15] Most of these phenylethylamine derivatives are not currently widely available, and currently reports of use and toxicity are uncommon.

The most widely recognized and currently abused additions to this series are 3,4-methylenedioxyamphetamine (MDA), 3,4-methylenedioxymethamphetamine (MDMA), and 3,4-methylenedioxyethamphetamine (MDEA). MDA appeared as a recreational drug in 1967; however, sympathomimetic effects limited its popularity.[15] Currently, the most popular phenylethylamine derivatives include MDMA and MDEA. The legal classification of these compounds is controversial. The DEA has classified these as schedule 1 substances, arguing that as hallucinogenic amphetamines they have no therapeutic role. Some clinicians and researchers argue that MDMA and MDEA are not classically hallucinogenic in usual doses, but that they in fact comprise a new therapeutic group, the entactogens.[16] Largely anecdotal data suggest that these compounds do not cause classic hallucinations, but rather reduce negative feelings and break down barriers of communication, allowing psychotherapeutic breakthroughs.[17] The physical form of MDMA and MDA is often a white powder, usually in a gelatin capsule or tablet. Analysis of

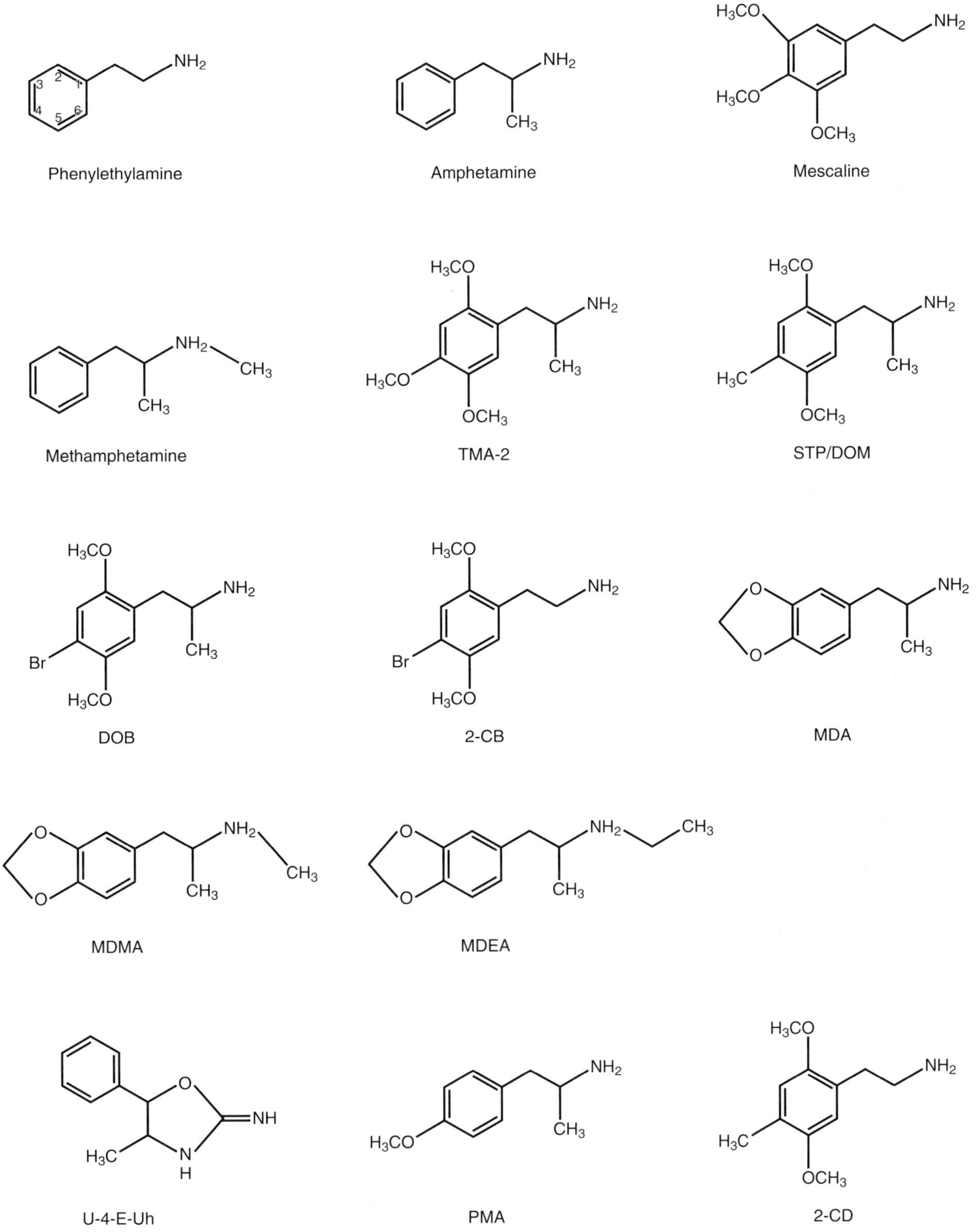

Phenylethylamine   Amphetamine   Mescaline

Methamphetamine   TMA-2   STP/DOM

DOB   2-CB   MDA

MDMA   MDEA

U-4-E-Uh   PMA   2-CD

Figure 42–1. Phenylethylamine and derivatives.

samples submitted anonymously for verification showed that 58% of samples alleged to contain MDMA actually contained that substance, and another 24% contained MDMA plus another substance, usually MDA.[18] Another 16% of samples alleged to be MDMA contained an analogue, usually MDA. Only 2% of samples were found to contain no psychoactive substance.

Synthetic Opioids. Synthetic opioids include two groups: fentanyl and meperidine derivatives. Fentanyl derivatives first surfaced in late 1979 in Orange County, California.[1] Several overdose deaths occurred that clinically resembled opioid overdoses; however, toxicologic analysis of biologic fluids and samples of the abused substance detected no known drug. The substance was finally identified as a fentanyl derivative, first incorrectly as 3-methylfentanyl and then correctly as α-methylfentanyl[1] (Fig. 42–2). A variety of fentanyl derivatives later appeared on the street, ranging in potency from α-methyl acetylfentanyl (10 times as potent as morphine) to 3-methylfentanyl (up to 6000 times as potent as morphine for the *cis* isomer). Street samples containing fentanyl analogues vary in appearance. The actual content of fentanyl derivative is very low, usually less than 1% of the total sample, so the appearance is dependent on the substances that are mixed with the drug. Descriptions of confiscated drug samples have ranged from pure white to brown with textures ranging from powdery to coarse and cake-like.[1] Fentanyls may appear in all the forms that heroin does, and the two cannot be easily distinguished.

Attempts at production of meperidine derivatives were associated with one of the most notorious episodes associated with designer drugs. A chemist of illicit drugs, in an attempt to produce the meperidine analogue MPPP, inadvertently made a product contaminated with MPTP (1-methyl-4-phenyl-1,2,3,6-tetrahydropyridine), which led to his developing parkinsonism.[3] MPTP is metabolized to MPP^+, which is toxic to nigrostriatal neurons.[19] Reappearance of this contaminant in batches of "synthetic heroin" produced in California in the 1980s led to a small outbreak of drug-induced parkinsonism[8] (Fig. 42–3).

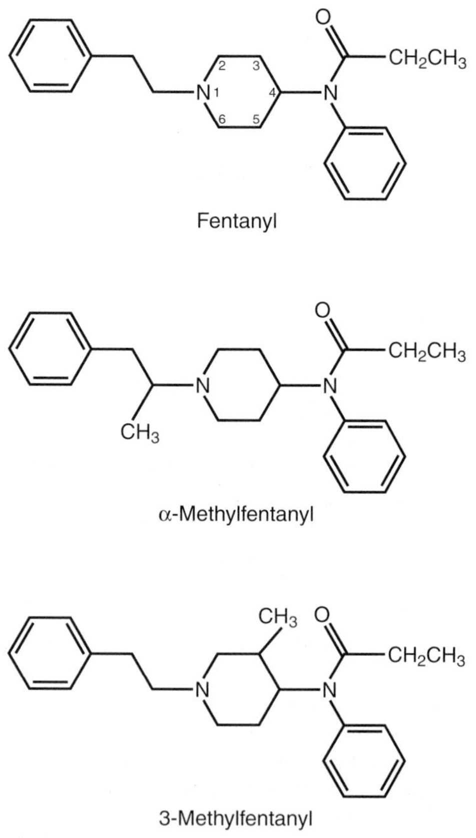

Fentanyl

α-Methylfentanyl

3-Methylfentanyl

Figure 42–2. Fentanyl and analogues.

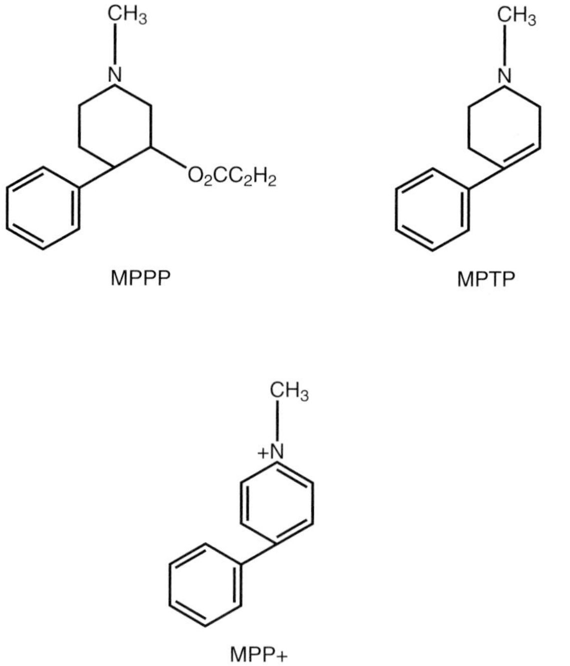

MPPP

MPTP

MPP+

Figure 42–3. 1-Methyl-4-phenyl-1,2,3,6-tetrahydropyridine (MPTP) and metabolites.

Arylhexylamines. Phencyclidine (PCP) is an arylhexylamine. PCP and its analogue ketamine are the most commonly used and abused members of this class. The synthesis of PCP and its analogues is relatively uncomplicated, yielding the potential for future problems with these substances. An intermediate in the synthesis, piperidinocyclohexanecarbonitrile (PCC) has appeared on the street as well as several analogues including TCP (a thiophene analogue of PCP) and PCE (an *N*-ethyl analogue of PCP).[20] Phenylcyclohexylpyrolidine (PHP) has clinical effects similar to those of PCP, but pyrrolidine instead of piperidine is required for its synthesis[21] (Fig. 42–4).

Methaqualone Derivatives. Methaqualone use has subsided in the United States since the 1970s; however, illicit synthesis of methaqualone and two derivatives available in Europe, mecloqualone and nitromethaqualone, has been reported.[22]

Pharmacokinetics (Including Drug Interactions)

Phenylethylamines. MDMA is readily absorbed. Onset of action is 20 to 60 minutes after oral ingestion.[23, 24] Duration of drug effect is usually 4 to 6 hours, although it can be prolonged in overdose. The apparent volume of distribution (V_d) and protein binding are unknown. The elimination half-life ranges from 73.8 to 100.2 minutes in rats.[25] MDMA is metabolized in the liver, in part to MDA, an active metabolite. Renal elimination of unchanged drug can

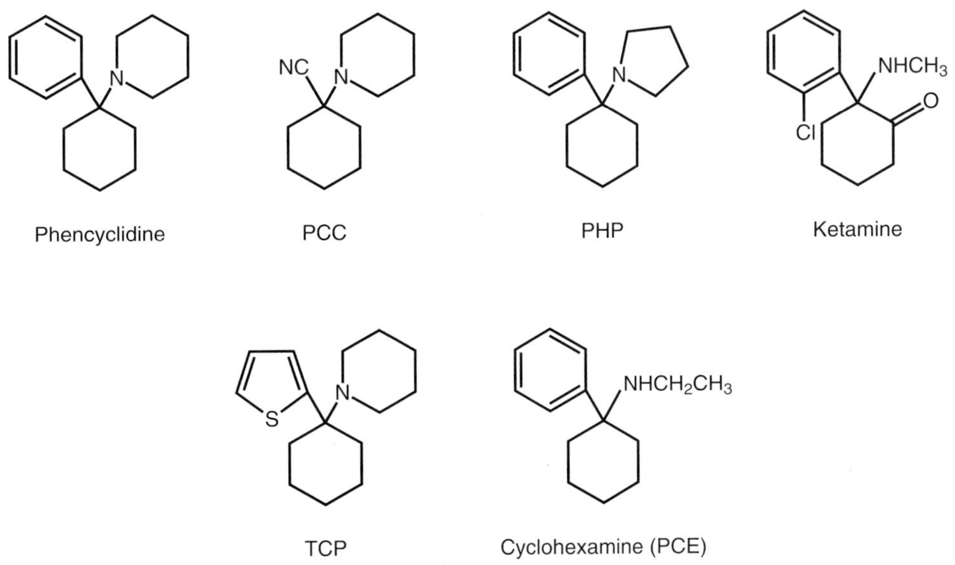

Figure 42–4. Phencyclidine and analogues.

account for up to 65% of an ingested dose within 24 hours.[26] DOM produces effects within 1 to 2 hours of ingestion of doses ranging from 2 to 14 mg. Twenty per cent of an ingested dose appears unchanged in the urine within 24 hours.[10]

An apparent adverse drug interaction may occur when MDMA is co-ingested with monoamine oxidase (MAO) inhibitors. A 50-year-old man experienced mental status changes, hypertension, diaphoresis, and hypertonicity after ingestion of MDMA and phenelzine.[27] It is presumed that MDMA facilitated the release of catecholamines and phenelzine inhibited catecholamine inactivation, although other enzyme inhibition or synergistic amphetamine-like activity is possible as well. Similar interactions with other phenylethylamines might be expected.

Synthetic Opioids. Fentanyl derivatives are very lipophilic and reach maximal brain concentrations within minutes. The apparent volume of distribution of fentanyl has been estimated at 60 to 300 L, with terminal half-life ranging from 1.5 to 6 hours.[28] Fentanyl is primarily cleared by metabolism by the liver and other tissues, with 10% of the drug being cleared renally. Protein binding of fentanyl and legally available analogues ranges from 80% to 95%. Fentanyl analogues are so potent that dermal or inadvertent inhalational exposure may be of concern. Pharmacokinetic parameters for illegal fentanyl analogues are not known.

Arylhexylamines. Phencyclidine is rapidly absorbed both orally and by inhalation. The apparent volume of distribution is 6.2 ± 0.3 L/kg.[29] Protein binding is 50% to 60%.[30] It is metabolized in the liver by oxidative hydroxylation to monohydroxy metabolites.[31] Approximately 10% is excreted unchanged in the urine; however, this is dependent on urine pH, with urinary excretion increasing 100-fold in acidic urine.[32] Elimination half-life is estimated to be 17.6 hours, increasing in overdose. Human pharmacokinetic data regarding PCP analogues are sparse; however, the plasma decay curves of PCP and analogues *N*-ethyl-phenylcyclohexylpyrrolidine (PCE), phenylcyclohexylamine (PCA), phenylcyclohexylpyrrolidine (PCPY), and phenylcyclodiethylamine (PCDE) were noted to be very similar in rats.[33]

Methaqualone. Methaqualone is 70% to 90% protein-bound. The volume of distribution ranges from 2.4 to 6.4 L/kg. It is extensively metabolized in the liver, and numerous metabolites are excreted in the urine and, to a lesser extent, in the bile. The elimination half-life ranges from 33 to 40 hours after therapeutic doses and is prolonged in overdose. The kinetic and metabolic parameters for methaqualone designer analogues are not well described.

Pharmacodynamics/Mechanisms of Action and Toxicity

Phenylethylamines. MDMA produces a mixture of sympathomimetic and psychedelic effects, which appear to be mediated by central nervous system monoamines. In vitro studies indicate that MDMA causes a calcium-independent release of brain monoamines and inhibits their inactivation.[34] Serotonin is primarily affected, dopamine is affected to a lesser extent. In vivo models demonstrate an initial release of serotonin followed by a depletion that is dependent on both dose and duration.[35] In addition, a reduction is seen in tryptophan hydroxylase activity and in the number of serotonin uptake sites that may be persistent.[35] These changes in neurotransmitter concentrations are accompanied by a disappearance of serotonergic axons, suggesting they are related to axonal damage. These neurodegenerative changes are consistent over a range of species from rats to nonhuman primates. Evidence indicates that the serotonergic system in rats is able to recover within 6 to 12 months;[36] however, in some circumstances in nonhuman primates, the damage may be permanent.[37] Studies on MDMA-mediated neurotoxicity have proposed two possible explanations: (1) the generation of a neurotoxic metabolite of MDMA or (2) serotonergic neuron toxicity caused by MDMA-induced elevated CNS concentrations of dopamine.[35] The potential clinical significance of MDMA or related compound serotonin neurotoxicity remains to be demonstrated.

Synthetic Opioids. Meperidine analogues can produce toxicity by interaction at the opioid receptors; however, the major concern has not been opioid toxicity, rather it has been the development of parkinsonism in a number of users of "synthetic heroin" or "China White." This street product has appeared at least twice, first in the late 1970s and second in the early 1980s. In an attempt to produce a meperidine congener, MPPP, an unwanted by-product was unknowingly introduced. This contaminant, MPTP, is metabolized by monoamine oxidase B in the brain to MPP^+. MPP^+ is bound to nearby neuromelatonin in the substantia nigra, where it is released over time.[38] Thought to interrupt mitochondrial respiration, MPP^+ then causes selective death of dopaminergic neurons in the substantia nigra, leading to the rapid development of a presumably permanent parkinsonian state.[39] Subjects who used the MPTP-contaminated product but were asymptomatic have been shown to have abnormal positron emission tomographic studies, in the nigrostriatal area.[39] This suggests that this population may be at risk for the development of parkinsonian syndrome as neurons in the substantia are depleted, which occurs normally with aging.

Fentanyl analogues also act at opioid receptors to cause analgesia, euphoria, CNS depression, and, most significantly, respiratory depression. The depth and duration of symptoms is dependent on tolerance of the user as well as the potency of the specific analogue. Fentanyl itself is approximately 200 times as potent as morphine.[40] The two most common fentanyl analogues, α-methylfentanyl and 3-methylfentanyl, are reported to be 200 and 6000 times as potent as morphine, respectively.

Arylhexylamines. The mechanism of action of phencyclidine and related arylhexylamines is not clear and may involve several mechanisms. These related compounds are usually classified as dissociative anesthetics, meaning that they somehow interfere with the association pathways linking the cerebral cortex with deeper structures.[41] In vitro studies indicate inhibition of norepinephrine, dopamine, and serotonin uptake.[42] PCP is generally described as having central and peripheral anticholinergic activity;[43] however, its structure as well as some case reports suggest cholinergic activity as well.[44] Phencyclidine and related compounds can bind to the opioid σ receptor site. The function of this receptor is unknown. Phencyclidine also blocks the *N*-methyl-D-aspartate excitatory amino acid receptor. The relative role of these effects on clinical toxicity has not been defined. As a result of their multiple mechanisms of action, arylhexylamines have stimulant, depressant, hallucinogenic, and anesthetic activity.

Methaqualone. Methaqualone is a central nervous system depressant that depresses spinal reflexes at higher doses. It also inhibits platelet aggregation and prolongs both the prothrombin time and the partial thromboplastin time. Few data are available regarding the effects and clinical presentation of methaqualone analogues, but it is assumed that toxic effects will be similar to those of methaqualone.

CLINICAL PRESENTATION

Pathophysiology

Phenylethylamines. Phenylethylamines act on the peripheral and central nervous system by α- and β-adrenergic stimulation. These compounds may also have varying degrees of serotonergic and dopaminergic activity, depending on structural similarity to mescaline.

Cardiovascular effects generally reflect sympathetic stimulation. Systolic and diastolic hypertension can be seen. Pulse can be variably affected. Tachycardia can be seen; however, if α-adrenergic effects predominate, hypertension with reflex bradycardia can occur.

Central nervous system effects may be secondary to both sympathetic stimulation and altered perception. Therapeutic or recreational doses may induce feelings of warmth and are purported to promote communication and empathy. Higher doses may induce hallucinations, agitation, delirium, hyperreflexia, or rigidity. Seizures may occur and can reflect either direct CNS stimulation or hypertension-induced cerebrovascular hemorrhage.

Sympathetic stimulation may induce a state of hyperthermia and agitated delirium.[45, 46] Direct sympathetic stimulation and increased metabolic heat production may be the primary pathophysiologic event; however, in many cases, increased muscular activity may be contributory as well. Hyperthermia due to use of MDMA at "rave parties" has been hypothesized to be due to a combination of MDMA use, increased muscular heat production due to dancing, and inadequate fluid intake.[47]

Synthetic Opioids. Synthetic opioids act through stimulation of opioid receptors. Five main receptors have been identified, including mu, kappa, delta, sigma, and epsilon. Mu receptors mediate respiratory depression, alterations in gastrointestinal motility, and decreased blood pressure and bradycardia. Mu, delta, and kappa receptors mediate analgesia.

The primary respiratory effect is respiratory depression. Respiratory rate may be normal in the presence of decreased tidal volume. Respiratory depression may be due to central decrease in respiratory drive as well as to decreased sensitivity to hypoxic and hypercarbic stimuli. Recurrence of respiratory depression after clinical recovery has been reported after fentanyl analgesia.[48] It is thought that this may be due to enteral secretion of parenterally administered drug and subsequent reabsorption. It is unknown if this phenomenon may occur after intoxication with fentanyl analogues.

Noncardiogenic pulmonary edema has been reported after use of several opioids by a variety of routes including intravenous, oral, and inhalational. The source of this pulmonary edema is unknown, but it may include hypoxia-induced pulmonary hypertension with capillary leak, hypersensitivity to opioids, direct toxic effect by the drug on the alveolus, a central neurogenic response, and, last, response to the histamine released by some opioids.

Central nervous system effects include euphoria and drowsiness to coma. Seizures have been reported after fentanyl use as well as following large doses of meperidine. It is unknown whether MPPP, a meperidine congener, is associated with seizures.

Arylhexylamines. Arylhexylamines were originally marketed as dissociative anesthetics, meaning that the perception of pain was somehow separated from its occurrence. The combination of anesthesia with altered judgment and bizarre and sometimes violent behavior can lead to significant injury to both the user and others.

Sympathomimetic effects may cause tachycardia and hypertension. Although these cardiovascular effects are common, clinically significant hypertension and dysrhythmias other than sinus tachycardia appear to be uncommon.

Central nervous system effects appear to range from mild agitation to coma. Confusion, hallucinations, disorientation, and bizarre and violent behavior may be seen. Motor abnormalities may include a variety of movement disorders such as opisthotonus and choreoathetosis. Nystagmus is commonly reported but is variably present, and it may be horizontal, vertical, or rotary.

Methaqualone. Methaqualone was primarily used for its sedative-hypnotic properties, but it also possesses antihistaminic, anticonvulsant, local anesthetic, antitussive, and antispasmodic properties.

Sedative-hypnotic properties are the primary drug effect, but agitation and restlessness are occasionally seen. Excessive dreaming and sleep-walking may occur. Hypertonicity, hyperreflexia, myoclonus, and seizures may occur with overdose.

Cardiorespiratory depression may occur, but it is thought to be less severe than that seen with barbiturates. Hypotension has rarely been seen, but it may be secondary to decreased systemic vascular resistance and decreased contractility.

Clinical Manifestations

Phenylethylamines. Most of the existing data regarding the pathophysiology of phenylethylamines examine the properties of MDMA. Although data for some of the lesser used phenylethylamines are sparse, some generalizations can probably be made from experience with MDMA. Data regarding the clinical presentation of MDMA intoxication and toxic effects come from uncontrolled case reports describing side effects and toxicity, either in the psychotherapeutic setting or after recreational use. No large series or controlled trials are currently available.

Hayner and McKinney divide adverse reactions to MDMA into three classes: acute reactions at therapeutic doses, overdose reactions, and residual effects.[23] Acute reactions at therapeutic doses include tachycardia, tremor, tight jaw muscles, bruxism, nausea, headache, and sweating. Less commonly, numbness and tingling of the extremities, hallucinations, ataxia, blurry vision, and nystagmus were reported. Mydriasis, hyperreflexia, and gait instability have also been reported.[24] Tachycardia has been documented in healthy volunteers,[24] and ventricular dysrhythmias have occurred after allegedly therapeutic ingestions.[45] Four of 21 healthy volunteers who ingested MDMA in doses ranging from 0.8 to 1.9 mg/lb[24] experienced a diastolic blood pressure greater than 100 mm Hg without obvious sequelae. Cerebrovascular accidents have been reported with MDMA.[47] It is presumed that intravascular hemorrhage is secondary to hypertension, possible in the presence of existing intracerebral vascular malformations; however, it is possible that the neurologic events may be associated with amphetamine-like vasculitis. Users also report a variety of emotional and cognitive effects. Euphoria, increased energy, decreased appetite, positive changes in attitude or feelings, expanded mental perspective, and heightened sensual arousal have been noted.[17] Although MDMA is often referred to as the "love drug," its effect on sexual function is often detrimental. Alterations in female sexual function appear to be inconsistent, whereas the majority of men may experience decreased ability to attain and maintain erection and to ejaculate.[49] Although most of the psychological effects of MDMA are generally described as positive, and relate to the perception of improved insight and interpersonal communication, undesirable emotional symptoms, such as anxiety, nervousness, and depression, have been reported as well. Difficulty with cognition (multiplication) and judgment has been noted in volunteers.[24]

Overdose reactions consist of symptoms of sympathetic excess similar to those seen with amphetamine toxicity: tachycardia, dysrhythmias, hypertension progressing to hypotension, hyperthermia, muscular rigidity, disseminated intravascular coagulation, rhabdomyolysis, and renal failure.[23, 46, 47] This clinical scenario has been described after ingestion of presumed therapeutic doses as well as overdose. These signs and symptoms of toxicity have been associated with the use of MDMA at "rave" parties.[47] Rave parties are typically mass gatherings of young people where dance music is played and MDMA is often found. It has been postulated that vigorous dancing coupled with inadequate fluid intake may predispose an MDMA user to hyperthermic crisis and collapse.[47]

The third category of reactions was attributable to residual effects. Mild residual reactions such as exhaustion, fatigue, depression, nausea, numbness, and flashbacks were described as were more significant symptoms, such as anxiety attacks, persistent insomnia, rage reactions, and psychosis. These residual symptoms persisted for hours to 2 weeks.[23] Other authors have described a variety of psychiatric effects, primarily panic disorder, psychosis, flashbacks, and depression, which may be delayed in onset and may persist for months.[50–52] Some cases resemble amphetamine psychosis, some resemble lysergic acid diethlyamide (LSD) psychosis and flashbacks, and others are difficult to distinguish from case-matched psychotic controls.[50] These cases appear to vary with respect to duration of symptoms and response to various psychotherapeutic agents, including haloperidol, amitriptyline, and fluoxetine. Because serotonin is implicated in several psychiatric disorders including depression, psychosis, anxiety, panic, and eating disorders, it is hypothesized that MDMA disruption of serotonin homeostasis may be responsible for these symptoms.

Cases of hepatitis have been reported after single doses as well as after chronic use of MDMA.[47, 53] Hepatitis usually resolves, but some cases have gone on to liver transplantation or death.[53] Aplastic anemia with recovery has been reported.[54] MDMA also modulates immune function in vitro but the clinical correlates of this finding are uncertain.[55] Few data are available regarding the effect of phenylethylamines in pregnancy; however, DOM was found to cause significant uterine and umbilical artery vasoconstriction and evidence of fetal distress in a sheep model.[56] Diffuse vascular spasm responding to tolazoline hydrochloride and nitroprusside has also been reported after ingestion of a related derivative, DOB.[57]

The long-term potential adverse effect of MDMA that causes the most concern is the possibility of central nervous system serotonergic neuron dysfunction or damage, which may or may not be permanent. As of yet, the clinical correlation of serotonergic dysfunction is uncertain, but it has been implicated in the adverse effects of MDMA on mood, sleep, and emotional and psychiatric state.

Synthetic Opioids. The syndrome of MPTP toxicity has been divided into acute intoxication and chronic effects. In the acute stage, users first experience a burning at the injection site. This is followed by a heroin-like euphoria, accompanied by disorientation, illusions or visual hallucinations, and jerking of the extremities. It is unknown if users develop other classic signs of opioid intoxication, such as miosis and hypoventilation. After several days, users may then develop signs of parkinsonism. Although there is some variation in symptoms, patients have presented with bradykinesia, rigidity, tremor, an expressionless face, and virtually all the motor manifestations of Parkinson's disease. It is interesting to note that the initial cases were often misdiagnosed as psychiatric illnesses, such as conversion disorder or catatonia, before the correct diagnosis was made.[8] The onset of symptoms is abrupt and dramatic; some patients progress within weeks to symptoms that are usually not seen until after 9 to 14 years of progression with the idiopathic form of Parkinson's disease.[8] Unlike the classic form of Parkinson's disease, autonomic nervous system changes are not seen, Lewy bodies are not found on microscopic analysis of the brain, and severe dementia does not appear to develop. Mild decreases in performance on tests assessing intelligence and frontal lobe function have been described, but thus far, no cases of dementia have been reported.[58]

Intoxication from fentanyl derivatives resembles narcotic overdose. Users unintentionally overdose due to the high potency of these drugs, and reports have told of addicts found dead with the needle still in their arm.[59] Patients may present with varying degrees of opioid intoxication including central nervous system depression, miosis, hypoventilation, and cardiopulmonary failure. Routine toxicologic analysis of urine, blood, or drug specimens will be negative unless special assays for fentanyl are used. Fentanyl and its analogues are not structurally related to other opioids and are thus not detected on standard assays. Therefore, patients who are clinically diagnosed with opioid intoxication but have a negative toxicologic screen test result for opioids should be suspected of fentanyl or fentanyl derivative use.

Arylhexylamines. Clinical data regarding presentation of non-PCP arylhexylamines are sparse, but they generally reflect reported cases of PCP toxicity. The primary findings of patients intoxicated with PCP presenting to health care facilities include mental status or behavioral changes and nystagmus.[44] In some series, 54.1% of patients had altered sensorium and 35.4% were described as violent.[44] Nystagmus is commonly present (57% to 85%) and may be vertical, horizontal, or rotary.[44, 60] Other findings may include tachycardia, hypertension, seizures, cholinergic signs, anticholinergic signs, and alterations in body temperature. Rhabdomyolysis with or without renal failure may occur. It is uncertain whether this is secondary to increased muscular activity or to a direct toxic effect of the drug or to a combination of factors. Two deaths reported from PCE (cyclohexamine or "rocket fuel") occurred in circumstances similar to PCP deaths.[61] Other potential sources of toxicity include the presence of unwanted contaminants or reaction intermediates. 1-Piperidinocyclohexanecarbonitrile (PCC) has been described as a PCP contaminant and decomposes on heating to release hydrogen cyanide.[62]

Methaqualone. Methaqualone intoxication is usually accompanied by lethargy and ataxia. Increasing CNS depression to coma may be seen. In contrast to most other sedative hypnotics, muscular hyperactivity may be seen. Nitromethaqualone is estimated to be 10 times as potent as mecloqualone or methaqualone.[15]

DIAGNOSIS

Phenylethylamines. The diagnosis of phenylethylamine use or intoxication should be primarily based on the recognition of the clinical symptoms of sympathetic excess or hallucinations. Urine toxicology screening may suggest phenylethylamine use. Commercially available immunoassays including radioimmunoassay, enzyme-multiplied immunoassay technique, and fluorescence polarization immunoassay for amphetamines, have been demonstrated to have cross-reactivity to methamphetamine, MDMA, MDA, and MDEA.[63]

Synthetic Opioids. It is assumed that a large population of heroin users was exposed to MPTP-contaminated products but have not yet developed motor symptoms. It is possible that these people may have partially depleted a portion of their nigrostriatal dopaminergic neuron pool, but not enough to become symptomatic. Because of the normal loss of dopaminergic neurons with age, this population may be at risk for the development of premature Parkinson's syndrome.[38] Acute exposure to MPTP should be suspected whenever parkinsonian symptoms appear in young patients, and a history for intravenous drug use should be elicited. MPTP exposure can also be seen in chemical workers and there is some concern that exposure to structurally similar herbicides may also induce parkinsonism.[64] Laboratory confirmation of MPPP or MPTP exposure is not routinely available. Cerebrospinal fluid from patients with MPTP-induced parkinsonism has been shown to contain lower concentrations of the norepinephrine metabolite 3-methoxy-4-hydroxyphenylethylene glycol when adjusted for plasma concentrations than has cerebrospinal fluid from patients with idiopathic Parkinson's disease.[65] The clinical significance of this finding is uncertain.

The diagnosis of fentanyl or fentanyl derivative use should be considered if a patient presents with a clinical opioid intoxication and responds to an opioid antagonist, but has a urine or blood toxicology screen result that is negative for opioids. Confirmation of fentanyl use is difficult and assays are not widely available, but fentanyl derivatives can be detected by radioimmunoassay (RIA), gas chromatography, and infrared, mass, and nuclear magnetic resonance spectroscopy.[66] Use should also be suspected if the patient identifies the drug as "China White" or "synthetic heroin," although these names may also refer to heroin or other opioids. Fentanyl derivatives cannot be differentiated from heroin based on appearance.

Arylhexylamines. The diagnosis of PCP analogue intoxication may be made by the presence of signs and symptoms of PCP intoxication. Confirmation by laboratory analysis is dependent on the specific analogue involved as well as the laboratory methodology. Using Roche PCP RIA assay, some cross-reactivity was seen for PHP and TCP. Little or no cross-reactivity was noted for PCE, phencyclohexylamine, and ketamine.[67]

Methaqualone. Methaqualone analogues mecloqualone and nitromethaqualone demonstrate some degree of cross-reactivity with methaqualone using the Roche RIA.[68]

TREATMENT

Immediate Supportive Measures and Any Specific Early Interventions

Phenylethylamines. Initial treatment of toxicity from phenylethylamine derivatives should be directed toward assessment and stabilization of the airway, breathing, circulation, and temperature. Agitation and combativeness may make the initial evaluation and treatment of these patients difficult. Rapid control of the situation is essential, as significant hyperthermia or other vital sign or laboratory abnormalities may require emergent therapy. Diazepam or a similar benzodiazepine and haloperidol have both been recommended for agitation.[69, 70] Physical restraint of the patient may also be necessary. Intravenous access should be obtained in all cases of significant vital sign abnormalities or mental status changes. Patients should be placed on a cardiac monitor and oxygen administered as needed. Endotracheal intubation should be performed if hypoventilation is present or if airway protective reflexes are impaired.

Hyperthermia should be treated aggressively. Initial control of agitation must be obtained in these circumstances to prevent further heat generation. Vigorous use of benzodiazepines or butyrophenones should be followed by cooling with mist and fans. If this is not successful, consider intubation and chemical paralysis to reduce muscular thermogenesis. Acetaminophen, acetylsalicylate and cooled blankets probably have little value in these circumstances. The role of dantrolene in this circumstance is unclear. In cases of significant temperature elevation, core temperature should be monitored with a continuous rectal or bladder probe, if available.

Seizures should be treated with a benzodiazepine. If seizure activity persists, phenobarbital should be added, with airway protection as needed. The role of phenytoin in toxin-induced seizures is probably minor. Continued seizure activity that is unresponsive to benzodiazepines and barbiturates, especially if it is contributing to significant hyperthermia, should be treated with chemical paralysis followed by electroencephalographic monitoring and consideration for general anesthesia. Consideration should be given to the possibility of an intracranial hemorrhage and a computed tomographic scan of the head should be done if clinically indicated by focal neurologic defects or persistent nonfocal findings, such as coma.

Phenylethylamines may cause a variety of dysrhythmias. Sinus tachycardia alone without hemodynamic compromise does not usually require treatment. Sinus tachycardia with hypertension may respond to a β-blocking agent, but caution should be used when using a β-adrenergic blocking agent alone, because of the concern of unopposed α-adrenergic stimulation and worsening hypertension. An α-adrenergic blocking agent or a combination of an α-

adrenergic blocking agent, such as phentolamine, with a β-adrenergic blocking agent would be a rational choice in such cases. Likewise, titratable agents such as nitroprusside or nitroglycerin have been recommended for significant hypertension. Oral nifedipine has also been empirically recommended; however, it may not be a good choice if activated charcoal has been given or its administration is anticipated.

Ventricular tachyarrythmias should be treated by standard ACLS measures. Propranolol or other β-blocking agents, such as esmolol, may be of value in these cases.

Hypotension, if present, should first be treated with normal saline or lactated Ringer's solution. Hypotension unresponsive to crystalloid infusion will require the use of vasopressor agents.

Vasospasm has been reported with phenylethylamine use. Local vasospasm may be treated with vasodilators such as nitroprusside or α-adrenergic blocking agents such as phentolamine. These agents may be administered by venous infusion or by local arterial infusion to the affected area. Vasospasm may be recurrent and require prolonged therapy.[57]

Rhabdomyolysis, if present, should be treated with adequate hydration and maintenance of urine output. Most clinicians recommend urinary alkalinization to prevent renal myoglobin deposition. To alkalinize the urine, 88 to 132 mEq/L of sodium bicarbonate can be added to 1 L of 5% dextrose in water, with potassium, 20 to 40 mEq/L, added as needed. The rate can be adjusted to maintain adequate urine flow and a urine pH of 7.5.

Synthetic Opioids. Intoxication from opioid derivatives usually presents as respiratory depression, decreased level of consciousness, and miosis. Patients with suspected opioid intoxication should have airway, breathing, and circulation assessed and stabilized. Oxygenation and ventilation may be assisted with supplemental oxygenation and bag-valve-mask respirations if a trial of naloxone can be accomplished in a timely fashion. Endotracheal intubation may be required for ventilation and airway protection if naloxone cannot be administered in a timely fashion or if the response to naloxone is incomplete. Naloxone should be administered in initial doses of 0.4 to 2 mg up to 10 mg, preferably by the intravenous route, although it may be given intramuscularly, sublingually, or endotracheally if necessary. Hypotension should first be treated with intravenous crystalloid bolus infusion. If hypotension is unresponsive to intravenous fluids, dopamine or norepinephrine may be used. Hypothermia, if present, should be treated by rewarming. Patients who are significantly symptomatic on presentation may develop delayed pulmonary edema. The incidence of this finding after designer opioid intoxication is unknown.

The presentation of young patients with parkinsonian symptoms should prompt inquiry regarding intravenous opioid use. No acute therapy has been determined as clinically beneficial in preventing the development of symptoms, but the possibility of other potential victims presents a public health issue. In experimental models, the prior administration of MAO-β inhibitors prevents the development of parkinsonian symptoms, but the clinical significance of this finding remains untested.[71] Once parkinsonian symptoms have become established, patients have responded to carbidopa-levodopa and bromocriptine or lisuride.[8] Amantidine and anticholinergic agents, such as benztropine and trihexyphenidyl, appear to have little benefit in these patients.

Arylhexylamines. Patients intoxicated with arylhexylamines will require initial stabilization, similar to those intoxicated by phenylethylamines. Seizures, hypertension, hyperthermia, and rhabdomyolysis should be treated as discussed previously. Hypertension appears to be short-lived in many cases and may respond to sedation.[44] Chemical restraint may be necessary, and butyrophenones and benzodiazepines appear to be rational choices.[72]

Methaqualone. Treatment of patients intoxicated by methaqualone or methaqualone derivatives is largely supportive. Aspiration pneumonia and pulmonary edema should be suspected and treated accordingly. Bleeding complications, such as gastrointestinal hemorrhage and retinal bleeding, should be monitored. Platelets or fresh frozen plasma should be considered for uncontrolled hemorrhage with abnormal coagulation parameters.

Decontamination and Prevention of Systemic Absorption

Decontamination after ingestion of designer drugs should follow generally accepted principles. Ipecac should not be used, because all of these substances have the potential to cause rapid deterioration of level of consciousness and seizures. Gastric lavage may be indicated after exposures that are deemed potentially serious, provided it can be accomplished within a reasonable time period. Endotracheal intubation may be indicated before lavage if airway protective reflexes are compromised or if hypoventilation is present. Although the adsorption of many designer drugs to activated charcoal is largely untested, their physicochemical characteristics suggest that all would be well adsorbed. Activated charcoal, 50 to 100 g, should be administered orally by nasogastric or orogastric tube to most patients. Pharmocokinetic parameters do not suggest a role for multiple doses of activated charcoal in enhancing clearance of drug that has already been absorbed; however, repeat doses should be considered in massive ingestions.

Antidotes

No specific antidotes are available for designer drug toxicity from agents with sympathomimetic characteristics. Opioid intoxication should respond to opioid antagonists, including naloxone or nalmefene. Naloxone doses up to 10 mg may be required if potent agents or massive doses are suspected. The role of nalmefene in the management of these cases is unclear. If naloxone is used, resedation should be watched for, both in the cases of shorter-acting fentanyls and the meperidine analogues.

In some animal models, the preadministration of MAO-β inhibitors has been found to prevent the dopaminergic toxicity of MPTP by inhibiting bioactivation to MPP^+; however, the clinical implications of this finding are uncertain.[71]

Elimination Enhancement

The enhanced renal elimination of phenylethylamines and arylhexylamines in acidic urine pH is mentioned only to be condemned. Renal excretion of PCP may be enhanced by 50% when the urine pH decreases from 7.4 to 6.1.[32] The elimination half-life of amphetamine is 8 to 10.5 hours when urine is acidic and 16 to 31 hours when urine is alkaline. The role of urinary pH and renal excretion of phenylethylamine and arylhexylamine derivatives has not been evaluated. However, intoxication from either of these classes of drugs may be accompanied by rhabdomyolysis and the risk of precipitating renal failure due to the precipitation of myoglobin in acidic urine is felt to outweigh any potential benefit from increased drug clearance. Hemodialysis or hemoperfusion play no role in increasing drug clearance in designer drug toxicity.

Disposition

Patients who have mild symptoms, such as tachycardia or anxiety, from any designer drug overdose should be observed until symptoms resolve. The effects of phenylethylamines and arylhexylamines on judgment have been described, but their duration is unknown. Patients with persistent tachycardia, hypertension or significant arrythymias, seizures, or hyperthermia should be admitted to the hospital. Patients who experience significant hypoventilation from opioid ingestion may be at risk for development of delayed pulmonary edema. Although the incidence of this finding is probably small, hospitalization of these patients for 24 hours of observation may be considered.

References

1. Henderson GL: Designer drugs: Past history and future prospects. J Forensic Sci *33:*569–575, 1988.
2. US Congress: CSA (Controlled Substance Analogue) Enforcement Act (21 provision USC 813–CSA) Defn: 21 USC 802 32A. Public Law 99–570, 99th Congress, Oct. 27, 1986.
3. Davis GC, Williams AC, Markey SP, et al: Chronic parkinsonism secondary to intravenous injection of meperidine analogues. Psychiatry Res 1:249–254, 1979.
4. Peroutka SJ: Incidence of recreational use of 3,4-methylene dimethoxymethamphetamine (MDMAA, "ecstasy") on an undergraduate campus. N Engl J Med *317:*1542, 1987.
5. Cuomo MJ, Dyment PG, Gammino VM: Increasing use of "ecstasy" (MDMA) and other hallucinogens on a college campus. J Am Coll Health *42:*271–274, 1994.
6. Randall T: Ectasy-fueled "rave" parties become dance of death for English youths. JAMA *268:*1505, 1992.
7. Hibbs J, Perper J, Winek CL: An outbreak of designer drug-related deaths in Pennsylvania. JAMA *265:*1011, 1991
8. Ballard PA, Tetrud JW, Langston JW: Permanent human parkinsonism due to 1-methyl-4-phenyl-1,2,3,6-tetrahydropyridine (MPTP): Seven cases. Neurology *35:*949–956, 1985.
9. Appler WD: The federal response to designer drugs: A new approach to a new program. J Clin Psychopharmacol *5:*350, 1985.
10. Shulgin AT: Chemistry of phenylethylamines related to mescaline. J Psychedelic Drugs *11:*41, 1979.
11. Snyder SH, Faillace L, Hollister L: 2,5-Dimethoxy-4-methyl-amphetamine (STP): A new hallucinogenic drug. Science *158:*669, 1967.
12. Cimbura G: PMA deaths in Ontario. Can Med Assoc J *110:*1263, 1974.
13. Shulgin AT: Profiles of psychedelic drugs: DOB. J Psychoactive Drugs *13:*99, 1981.
14. Shulgin AT: Profiles of psychedelic drugs: TMA–2, *8:*169, 1976.
15. Buchanan JF, Brown CR: Designer drugs, a problem in clinical toxicology. Med Toxicol *3:*1–17, 1988.
16. Nichols DE: Differences between the mechanism of action of MDMA, MBDB and the classic hallucinogens: Identification of a new therapeutic class: Entactogens. J Psychoactive Drugs *18:*305, 1986.
17. Greer G, Tolbert R: Subjective reports of the effects of MDMA in a clinical setting. J Psychoactive Drugs *18:*319, 1986.
18. Renfroe CL: MDMA on the street: Analysis Anonymous. J Psychoactive Drugs *18:*363, 1986.
19. Langston JW, Irwin I, Langston E, et al: 1-Methyl-4-phenyl-pyridinium ion (MPP+): Identification of a metabolite of MPTP, a toxin selective to the substantia nigra. Neurosci Lett *48:*87–92, 1984.
20. Shulgin AT, Mac Lean DE: Illicit synthesis of phencyclidine (PCP) and several of its analogs. Clin Toxicol *9:*553–560, 1976.
21. Budd RD: PHP, a new drug of abuse. N Engl J Med *303:*588, 1980.
22. Daenens P, Van Boven M: The identification of quinazolinones on the illicit market. J Forensic Sci *21:*552–563, 1976.
23. Hayner GN, McKinney H: MDMA the dark side of ecstasy. J Psychoactive Drugs *18:*341, 1986.
24. Downing J: The psychological and physiological effects of MDMA on normal volunteers. J Psychoactive Drugs *18:*335, 1986.
25. Cho AK, Hiramatsu M, Distefano EW, et al: Stereochemical differences in the metabolism of 3,4-methylene dioxymethamphetamine in vivo and in vitro: A pharmacokinetic analysis. Drug Metab Dispos *18:*686, 1990.
26. Verehey K, Alrazi JJ, Jaffee JH: The complications of "ecstasy" (MDMA). J Am Vet Med Assoc *259:*1649, 1988.
27. Smilkstein ML, Smolinske SC, Rumack BH: A case of MAO inhibitor/MDMA interaction: Agony after ecstasy. Clin Toxicol *25:*147, 1987.
28. Mather LE: Clinical pharmacokinetics of fentanyl and its newer derivatives. Clin Pharmacokinet *8:*422–446, 1983.
29. Cook EC, Perez-Reyes M, Jeffcoat BR, et al: Phencyclidine disposition in humans after small doses of radiolabeled drug. Fed Proc *42:*2566, 1983.
30. Giles HG, Corrigall WA, Khouw V, et al: Plasma protein binding of phencyclidine. Clin Pharmacol Ther *31:*77, 1982.
31. Syracuse CD, Kuhnert BR, Golden NL, et al: Measurement of the amino acid metabolite of phencyclidine by selected ion monitoring. Biomed Environ Mass Spectrometry *13:*113, 1986.
32. Reyes-Perez M, DiGiuseppi S, Brine D, et al: Urine pH and phencyclidine excretion. Clin Pharmacol Ther *32:*635, 1982.
33. Cho AK, Hiramatsu M, Schmitz DA, et al: Pharmacokinetic and pharmacodynamic properties of some phencyclidine analogs in rats. Pharmacol Biochem Behav *39:*947–953, 1991.
34. Steele TD, McCann UD, Ricuarte GA: 3,4-Methylene dioxymethamphetamine (MDMA, "ecstasy"): Pharmacology and toxicology in animals and humans. Addiction *89:*539, 1994.
35. McKenna DJ, Peroutka SJ: Neurochemistry and neurotoxicity

of 3,4-methylene dioxymethamphetamine (MDMA, "ecstasy"). J Neurochem *54:*14, 1990.
36. Scanzello CR, Hatzidimitriou G, Martello AL, et al: Serotonergic recovery after (+/−)3,4,3,4–methylene dioxymethamphetamine injury: Observations in rats. J Pharmacol Exp Ther *264:*1484, 1993.
37. Ricuarte GA, Martello AL, Katz JL, et al: Lasting effects of *(1)*-3,4-methylene dioxymethamphetamine (MDMA) on central serotonergic neurons in nonhuman primates: Neurochemical observations. J Pharmacol Exp Ther *261:*616, 1992.
38. D'Amato RJ, Lipman ZP, Snyder SH: Selectivity of the parkinsonian neurotoxin MPTP: Toxic metabolite MPP+ binds to neuromelanin. Science *231:*987–989, 1986.
39. Heikkila RE, Nicklas WJ: Studies on the mechanism of the dopaminergic neurotoxicity of 1-methyl-4-phenyl-1,2,3,6-tetrahydrapyridine (MPTP). Bioanal Syst Curr Separations *7:*52, 1986.
40. Gardocki JF, Yelnosky J: A study of some of the pharmacologic actions of fentanyl citrate. Toxicol Appl Pharmacol *6:*48, 1964.
41. Pender JW: Dissociative anesthesia. JAMA *215:*1126, 1971.
42. Smith RC, Meltzer HY, Arora RC, et al: Effects of phencyclidine and (^{3}H) serotonin preparations from rat brain. Biochem Pharmacol *26:*1435, 1977.
43. Paster Z, Maayani S, Weinstein H, et al: Cholinolytic action of phencyclidine derivatives. Eur J Pharmacol *25:*270, 1974.
44. McCarron MM, Schulze BW, Thompson GA, et al: Acute phencyclidine intoxication: Incidence of clinical findings in 1000 cases. Ann Emerg Med 10:237–241, 1981.
45. Dowling GP, McDonough ET, Bost RO: "Eve" and "ecstasy:" A report of five deaths associated with the use of MDEA and MDMA. JAMA *257:*1615, 1987.
46. Brown C, Osterloh J: Multiple severe complications from recreational ingestion of MDMA ("ecstasy"). JAMA *258:*780, 1987.
47. Henry JA, Jeffreys KJ, Dawling S: Toxicity and deaths from 3,4-methylene dioxymethamphetamine ("ecstasy"). Lancet *340:*384, 1992.
48. Adams AP, Pybus DA: Delayed respiratory depression after use of fentanyl during anesthesia. BMJ *1:*278, 1978.
49. Buffum J, Moser C: MDMA and human sexual function. J Psychoactive Drugs *18:*355, 1986.
50. McGuire PK, Cope H, Fahy TA: Diversity of psychopathology associated with the use of 3,4–methylene dioxymethamphetamine ("ecstasy"). Br J Psychiatry *165:*391, 1994.
51. McCann UD, Ricaurte GA: Lasting neuropsychiatric sequelae of (±)methylenedioxymethamphetamine ("ecstasy") in recreational users. J Clin Psychopharmacol *11:*302, 1991.
52. Creighton FJ, Black DL, Hyde CE: "Ecstasy" psychosis and flashbacks. Br J Psychiatry *159:*713, 1991.
53. Dykhuizen RS, Brunt PW, Atkinson P, et al: Ecstasy induced hepatitis mimicking viral hepatitis. Gut *36:*939, 1995.
54. Marsh CW, Abboudi ZH, Gibson FM, et al: Aplastic anemia following exposure to 3,4-methylene dioxymethamphetamine ("ecstasy"). Br J Hematol *88:*281, 1994.
55. House RV, Thomas PT, Bhargava HN: Selective modulation of immune function resulting from in vitro exposure to methylenedioxymethamphetamine (ecstasy), Toxicology *96:*59, 1995.
56. Zhang L, Dyer DC, Hembrough FB, et al: Effect of R(−)2,5-dimethoxy-4-methylamphetamine on uterine and umbilical blood flow in conscious pregnant sheep. Eur J Pharmacol *199:*179, 1991.
57. Bowen JS, Davis GB, Kearney TE, et al: Diffuse vascular spasm associated with 4-bromo-2,5-dimethoxyamphetamine ingestion. JAMA *249:*1147, 1983.
58. Stern Y, Langston JW: Intellectual changes in patients with MPTP-induced parkinsonism. Neurology *35:*1506, 1985.
59. Martin M, Hecker R, Clark R, et al: China White epidemic: An eastern United States emergency department experience. Ann Emerg Med *20:*158, 1991.
60. Barton CH, Sterling ML, Vaziri ND: Phencyclidine intoxication: Clinical experience in 27 cases confirmed by urine assay. Ann Emerg Med *10:*243–246, 1981.
61. Smialek JE, Monforte JR, Gault R, et al: Cyclohexamine ("rocket fuel")—phencyclidine's potent analog. J Anal Toxicol *3:*209, 1979.
62. Soine WII, Vincek WC, Agee DT: Phencyclidine contaminant generates cyanide. N Engl J Med *301:*438, 1979.
63. Ruangyuttikarn W, Moody DE: Comparison of three commercial amphetamine immunoassays for detection of methamphetamine, methylenedioxyamphetamine, methylenedioxymethamphetamine and methylenedioxyethylamphetamine. J Anal Toxicol *12:*229, 1988.
64. Bocchetta A, Corsini GU: Parkinson's disease and pesticides. Lancet 2:1163, 1986.
65. Burns RS, LeWitt PA, Ebert MH, et al: The clinical syndrome of striatal dopamine deficiency: Parkinsonism induced by 1-methyl-4-phenyl-1,2,3,6-tetrahydropyridine (MPTP). N Engl J Med *312:*1418–1421, 1985.
66. Cooper D, Jacob M, Allen A: Identification of fentanyl derivatives. J Forensic Sci *31:*511, 1986.
67. Budd RD: Phencyclidine (PCP)-structure versus reactivity. Clin Toxicol *18:*1033–1041, 1981.
68. Budd RD: Methaqualone RIA structure versus reactivity. Clin Toxicol *16:*209, 1980.
69. Derlet RW, Albertson TE, Rice P: Protection against D-amphetamine toxicity. Am J Emerg Med *8:*105, 1990.
70. Solursh LP, Clement WR: Use of diazepam in hallucinogenic drug crises. JAMA *205:*98, 1968.
71. Langston JW, Irwin I, Langston EB: Pargyline prevents MPTP-induced Parkinsonism in primates. Science *225:*1480, 1984.
72. Castellani S, Giannini AJ, Boeringa JA, et al: Phencyclidine intoxication: Assessment of possible antidotes. J Toxicol Clin Toxicol *19:*313, 1982.

43

Sedatives

SHEILA DAWLING, PhD
TIMOTHY J. MEREDITH, MD

Sedative-hypnotic drugs are employed therapeutically to produce drowsiness and to promote sleep. As a group they are structurally diverse, comprising the barbiturates, the benzodiazepines, carbamates, glutethimide, methyprylon, methaqualone, and the chlorinated compounds chlormethiazole, chloral hydrate, chlormezanone, and ethchlorvynol. Two newer and apparently safer sedatives, zolpidem and zopiclone, form part of this group. In addition to sedative-hypnotic properties, some of these drugs possess anesthetic, anxiolytic, muscle relaxant, anticonflict, antihistamine, antitussive, and other properties. Many other drugs have sedative or central nervous system (CNS) depressant properties in overdose, but these have not been included in this chapter because they are dealt with elsewhere in this book on the basis of their major therapeutic indications. Accidental or deliberate self-poisoning with sedative-hypnotic drugs accounts for up to 30% of deaths from drug overdose in many developed countries and is a frequent cause of inquiries made to poison control centers and, of course, of attendances at emergency departments.

HISTORY AND USAGE

Chloral hydrate was first synthesized in 1832 and became a popular sedative after its introduction into clinical practice by Liebreich in 1869. Early reports of toxicity (Borntnager reviewed 44 deaths in 1890, identifying cardiovascular, respiratory, and central nervous system [CNS] depressant effects) and the introduction of the barbiturates led to a decline in its use in the early decades of the 20th century. Sedative action is produced almost exclusively by the main metabolite trichloroethanol. Because of its unpleasant taste, liquid formulation, and propensity to cause gastric irritation, choral hydrate was often given rectally. Subsequently, triclofos (monosodium trichloroethyl phosphate) and dichloralphenazone (chloral hydrate–phenazone ester) also enjoyed popularity owing to their more pleasant tastes and solid formulation, although now chloral betaine has largely replaced both these preparations. Oral preparations are prescribed for short-term sedative use and as surgical premedicants, which produce fewer hangover effects than the barbiturates. Larger doses produce anesthesia, when use is typically restricted to young children and the elderly, because chloral hydrate is thought to induce less paradoxical excitement than the barbiturates. Although chloral hydrate is used as a recreational drug in combination with ethanol (the well-known "Mickey Finn" and "knock-out drops"), it has never been considered a significant social or clinical problem.

The *barbiturates* were used extensively as sedatives and hypnotics in the 1950s and 1960s. By the early 1970s, however, barbiturate poisoning was the leading cause of drug-induced fatalities in many countries, particularly in Europe. The wide availability of barbiturates as prescription drugs, together with concern over their ability to produce psychological and physical dependence, led to prescription restrictions in Europe and legal regulations governing their possession and supply.

After a marked decline in the incidence of barbiturate poisoning in many countries, usage of barbiturates appears to be on the rise. The desired effects of barbiturate administration may range from mild sedation to general anesthesia. Thiopental and methohexital, in particular, have found widespread use in emergency anesthesia, and thiopental and pentobarbital in high doses have been shown to be protective in reducing the extent of infarction from cerebral ischemia after head injury, and they are also beneficial at more modest doses during hepatic coma. In addition, phenobarbital and mephobarbital have selective anticonvulsant activity. Thus the barbiturates remain an important class of drugs.

Since the introduction of the first benzodiazepine (chlordiazepoxide [Librium]) in 1960, the *benzodiazepines* have enjoyed a meteoric rise in popularity and currently dominate drug treatment of sleep disorders and anxiety states. Their extraordinary acceptance in clinical medicine represented a response to medical and public demand for safe and effective sedative and anxiolytic agents, with minimal side effects. Heralded initially as the nonaddictive substitute for barbiturates, the pendulum of approval swung dramatically against them in the mid 1980s, as the potential for dependence at therapeutic doses became appreciated.[1] Limitations on prescription size and duration were introduced in response to these concerns, but benzodiazepines remain the single most commonly prescribed group of drugs in the western world, with a vast spectrum of therapeutic indications.[2] Other uses of benzodiazepines include surgical premedication, provision of retrograde amnesia for conscious surgical procedures, anxiolysis, and as anticonvulsants and muscle relaxants. More than 30 benzodiazepines are marketed worldwide, and 15 preparations are approved for use in the United States. In the United States and United Kingdom, benzodiazepines are available by prescription only, but in some countries in Latin America they can be obtained freely and constitute a major abuse problem.

Glutethimide is related structurally to phenobarbital and was introduced in 1954 as a nonaddictive barbiturate-substitute. Although initially popular, it soon became apparent that glutethimide intoxication was more difficult to manage than that resulting from the barbiturates, with prolonged and cyclical coma, cerebral and pulmonary edema, convulsions, and sudden apnea. In the past decade reports have increased of the abuse of a glutethimide-codeine combination (packs or loads). *Methyprylon* also has structural similarity to the barbiturates and was introduced as a nonbarbiturate hypnotic in the mid 1950s. It causes less CNS depression than the barbiturates, but it is used infrequently and its mechanisms of action and toxicity are not well documented.

Ethchlorvynol was introduced in 1955 as a sedative-hypnotic with a more rapid onset and shorter duration of action than the barbiturates. It was envisaged that its use would be less problematic because it did not induce hepatic microsomal oxidation. However, during the period 1976 through 1977 the Drug Abuse Warning Network (DAWN) estimated that some 5000 emergency department visits and 310 deaths could be attributed to this drug. The drug is an aromatic viscous liquid at room temperature and is therefore only available in a gelatin capsule formulation, which increases its potential for abuse by intravenous injection. Ethchlorvynol was subsequently withdrawn in the United Kingdom and, although it continues to be prescribed in the United States, it has only small pockets of popularity.

Methaqualone was introduced in 1956 as a safe, nonaddictive, nonbarbiturate sedative with low abuse potential. It was initially synthesized as part of a program in India investigating antimalarial drugs. The drug later became available in a combination preparation (Mandrax), containing 250 mg of methaqualone with 25 mg of diphenhydramine, marketed aggressively in 1965 in response to calls for safe sedatives in the aftermath of thalidomide. However, as with glutethimide and ethchlorvynol, it soon became apparent that these claims were erroneous; and it was widely abused with ethanol ("luding out") and produced both physical and psychologic dependence. After restriction by classifying it as a Schedule II drug under the US Controlled Substances Act 1973, and then reclassification under Schedule I in 1984, methaqualone was completely withdrawn from both the United Kingdom and United States markets. Analytical surveys of illicitly manufactured heroin have shown that up to 13% has been adulterated with methaqualone, and it is widely manufactured and supplied on the black market. Methaqualone also has anticonvulsant, antitussive, and weak antihistaminic actions. *Mecloqualone* is a hypnotic that is related structurally to methaqualone and was first synthesized in 1960 and is marketed legally in some parts of Europe. Because it has no legitimate use in the United States, it is, however, placed under Schedule I by the Food and Drug Administration (FDA) and has been manufactured and distributed clandestinely in the United States for some years.

Meprobamate, the prototype of the carbamates, was synthesized in 1950 and introduced into medical practice in 1955 as the first of the modern centrally acting tranquilizers lacking the peripheral autonomic side effects of the phenothiazines. Initially, case reports indicated serious problems in overdose (due to hypotension and depressed myocardial contractility and to bezoar formation in the stomach) and an addiction potential similar to the existing sedative-hypnotics. More recent data are less supportive of this perception. The drug additionally has anticonvulsant and muscle relaxant properties. *Carisoprodol* was synthesized in 1959, and, although used primarily as a skeletal muscle relaxant, it is included in this chapter as a significant proportion of an ingested dose is metabolized to meprobamate, and carisoprodol therefore shares a toxicity profile with this compound. Meprobamate was virtually eliminated from use after reports of its high abuse potential, and in the United States is a FDA Schedule IV drug. Although meprobamate is available in more than a dozen formulations and is prescribed in a number of European countries, often in combination preparations (with, for example, ethoheptazine, aspirin, or trihexyphenidyl), it is not a first-line drug. Carisoprodol is not legally restricted in the United States and can be purchased through veterinary mail order catalogs. Its resurgence as a drug of abuse in recent years has therefore caused concern. Two other carbamate derivatives, *ethinamate* and *methocarbamol,* were synthesized in 1953 and 1956, respectively, and are still used occasionally for their sedative or muscle relaxant properties.

The therapeutic properties of *chlormethiazole* were first investigated in 1957, and in Europe it is used frequently as a sedative-hypnotic and anticonvulsant agent. It is used intravenously in the management of status epilepticus, particularly in patients refractory to benzodiazepines or barbiturates, and in toxemia of pregnancy. Its structural similarity with thiamine and its pharmacologic profile make it ideally suited to the management of acute ethanol withdrawal, including alcoholic psychosis and severe, life-threatening delirium tremens. Chlormethiazole is also used orally in the treatment of ethanol addiction, where its synergistic effects with ethanol can result in significant toxicity. Chlormethiazole has more recently been shown to have neuroprotective action, both prophylactically during prolonged cardiac surgery and in the first few hours after a stroke.

Carbromal is a monoureide derivative used as a mild, short-acting sedative; and although it is commonly considered to be obsolete, its continued availability in combination with pentobarbital (Carbrital, 130 mg carbromal plus 49 mg pentobarbital) occasionally results in serious poisoning. In Europe, the drug is available in a number of popular nonprescription formulations (Obral, for example, is carbromal with phenobarbital and diphenhydramine). Also included in this chapter is a discussion of *chlormezanone*, a mild sedative with muscle relaxant properties first described in 1958 that is used, often in combination with non-narcotic analgesics, for the treatment of painful muscular spasm due to degenerative skeletal disease. This compound is only rarely implicated as a cause of serious toxicity.

The search for safer, more rapidly acting and rapidly cleared sedatives with low abuse potential has given rise to two new series of compounds. *Zopiclone* is the first of the cyclopyrrolone hypnotics, released in European countries from 1987 onward. The drug has a broad spectrum of pharmacologic activity, with anticonvulsant, muscle relaxant, anticonflict, and antiaggressive properties. Thus far, however, its use has been restricted to sedative indications. *Zolpidem* (Ambien), a novel short-acting hypnotic agent first launched in Europe in 1988, is the first example of a new series of imidazopyridine derivatives. It has a narrow spectrum of clinical effects, with no appreciable anxiolytic, muscle relaxant, or anticonflict properties at therapeutic doses. It is believed that the potential for tolerance, dependence, and withdrawal with these drugs is relatively low.

STRUCTURE AND ACTIVITY

Barbituric acid (2,4,6-trioxo-hexa-hydro-pyrimidine), the condensation product of malonic acid and urea, was first prepared in 1864 and forms the barbiturate nucleus, which is itself devoid of CNS activity. Substitution of the two hydrogen atoms at position 5 with alkyl, alkenyl, or aryl groups produces compounds with CNS activity, of which the diethyl derivative barbital was introduced first in 1903. Clinically significant consequences arise from the marked differences in lipid solubility among the individual members of the barbiturate group of drugs. Replacement of the oxygen at position 2 with sulfur confers more lipid solubility on the molecule, giving rise to the thiobarbiturates, of which thiopental and methohexital are important in emergency anesthesia. Methyl substitution at position 1 also increases lipid solubility, which accelerates compartmental transfer of drug, thus shortening its duration of action and increasing its potency, although paradoxically it prolongs the plasma elimination half-life and can prolong CNS activity if longer-acting metabolites are formed. Less lipid-soluble barbiturates generally have a slower onset and longer duration of action owing to their slow transfer into and out of the CNS (see Chapter 37 on Barbiturates for further discussion).

The benzodiazepines also share a common structure, all having a six-membered benzene ring attached to a seven-membered diazepine ring substituted at the 5-position. The substitution of different functional groups produces derivatives with varying degrees of sedative, hypnotic, anxiolytic, amnestic, anticonflict, muscle relaxant, and anticonvulsant properties and with differences in onset and duration of action. Differences in pharmacodynamics and physiochemical properties are also thought to contribute to the marked variation in tolerance and addiction potential among the benzodiazepines. Structurally, they are usually divided into 1,4-benzodiazepines and the imidazo- and the triazolo-benzodiazepines. Clobazam is the sole representative of the 1,5-benzodiazepines; and although not available in the United States, it is prescribed in Europe, where it is used almost exclusively as an adjunct anticonvulsant. Midazolam is a comparatively short-acting imidazo-benzodiazepine that has found widespread use in anesthesia as a premedicant, induction, and maintenance agent. Its use for conscious sedation in minor surgical procedures such as bronchoscopy, cardiac catheterization, and orthopedic and dental procedures is now common. Alprazolam also has significant antidepressant activity (see Chapter 44 on benzodiazepines for further discussion).

Some of the nonbarbiturate sedative-hypnotic drugs have structures that resemble the barbiturates in many respects (Figure 43–1). The compounds concerned were introduced in the mid 1950s and share many of the pharmacologic and toxicologic properties of the barbiturates. Glutethimide (2-ethyl-2-phenyl-glutarimide) is a piperidinedione, with similar hypnotic action to the barbiturates, but is devoid of anticonvulsant, antitussive, or analgesic action. Methaqualone (2-methyl-3-o-tolylquinazolin-4[3H]-one) is a highly lipid-soluble drug with a rapid onset of action. It has anticonvulsant, antitussive, and weak antihistaminic activities. Mecloqualone is similar in structure and differs only by the substitution of a chloro group for the methyl group on the benzene

Trichloroethanol

Ethchlorvynol

Chlormethiazole

Glutethimide

Methyprylon

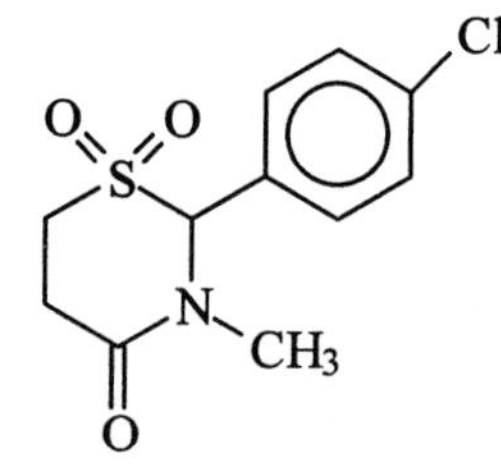

Chlormezanone

Methaqualone R = CH_3
Mecloqualone R = Cl

Meprobamate R = H
Carisoprodol R = C_3H_7

Methocarbamol

Ethinamate

Carbromal

Zopiclone

Zolpidem

Figure 43–1. Structures of nonbarbiturate and nonbenzodiazepine sedative-hypnotics.

ring but has a similar pharmacologic profile. Methyprylon (3,3-diethyl-5-methylpiperidine-2,4-dione) like glutethimide is a piperidinedione derivative and therefore bears a structural resemblance to barbital.

Four compounds with one or more carbamate functional groups are used as skeletal muscle relaxants and sedative-hypnotics. Apart from their functional group they have little other structural similarity. These are carisoprodol (2-methyl-2-propyltrimethylene carbamate isopropyl carbamate), meprobamate (2-methyl-2-propyltrimethylene dicarbamate), ethinamate (1-ethynylcyclohexyl carbamate), and methocarbamol (2-hydroxy-3-[2-methoxyphenoxy]-propyl carbamate). Carbromal, N-(2-bromo-2-ethylbutyryl)-urea, shares some structural similarities with the carbamates and is metabolized in part to bromide, which was once used as a sedative. Their structures are shown in Figure 43–1.

2,2,2-Trichloroethanol is the active metabolite of four prodrugs: chloral hydrate (2,2,2-trichloroethne-1,1-diol), triclofos (trichloroethanol monophosphate sodium), chloral betaine (a complex of chloral hydrate and betaine), and dichloralphenazone (a complex of chloral hydrate and phenazone or antipyrine). The latter two compounds produce rapid-onset sedation by hydrolysis in the gut to chloral hydrate. Chloral hydrate is then rapidly reduced to trichloroethanol in the blood. Chlormethiazole (5-[2-chloroethyl]-4-methythiazole) is structurally unrelated and is a highly metabolized lipid-soluble drug that rarely causes serious complications when taken alone in overdose but that is synergistically toxic with ethanol.

Ethchlorvynol (1-chloro-3-ethylpent-1-en-4-yn-3-ol) is a chlorinated tertiary acetylenic carbinol, with properties similar to those of chloral hydrate, with which it shares some structural similarities (see Fig. 43–1). Ethchlorvynol is a mild nonbarbiturate sedative-hypnotic with anticonvulsant activity. Its onset of action is rapid (15 to 30 minutes), with a short duration of action of about 5 hours. In terms of abuse potential, it offers no advantages over the barbiturates; unlike the barbiturates, it does not induce cytochrome P-450 enzymes or uridine diphosphate (UDP) glucuronosyl transferase, so the potential for pharmacokinetic interaction with concomitant medications is much more limited.

Chlormezanone is a substituted metathiazone (2[4-chlorophenyl]-3-methylperhydro-1,3-thiazin-4-one 1,1-dione), with actions similar to meprobamate, so it is primarily sedative in action (see Fig. 43–1). Chlormezanone is used in treatment of mild neurotic states characterized by anxiety and tension. There is some evidence that it has skeletal muscle-relaxing effects, but this is not proven. Chlormezanone is often used (sometimes in combination with acetaminophen) for treatment of painful musculoskeletal disorders.

Two newer-generation sedatives included in this chapter are zopiclone and zolpidem (see Fig. 43–1). Zopiclone {6-(5-chloro-2-pyridyl)-5-[(4-methyl-1-piperazinyl)carbonyloxy]-6,7-dihydro(5H)-pyrrolo (3,4-b) pyrazine-7-one} is the first of the cyclopyrrolones, with marked sedative properties in addition to anticonvulsant and anxiolytic properties. Suriclone, which is structurally similar, is also under investigation and appears to have a different spectrum of pharmacologic activity. Zolpidem {*N,N*,6-trimethyl-2-(4-methylphenyl)imidazo[1,2-a]pyridine-3-acetamide} is a new sedative of the imidazopyrine class with some muscle relaxant properties. Alpidem, which differs from zolpidem by substitution of phenolic chlorides for methyl groups and propyl substituents on the side chain terminal nitrogen for methyl (which makes it even more lipid-soluble), is also under investigation and appears to have anxiolytic activity and to be devoid of sedative and muscle relaxant actions.[3]

MECHANISM OF PHARMACOLOGIC ACTION

Investigation of the molecular action of the sedatives has been stimulated by the search for nonaddictive sedative-hypnotic agents, and for nonsedating anxiolytics and anticonvulsants. The mechanism of hypnotic action is thought to be at the level of the $GABA_A$ receptor complex in the central nervous system.[4, 5] GABA (γ-aminobutyric acid) is the principal inhibitory neurotransmitter in the CNS, and the benzodiazepine $GABA_A$ receptor is shown in Figure 43–2. On binding at postsynaptic $GABA_A$ receptors, GABA becomes coupled to a transducer (G protein) that elicits an effector sequence resulting in the opening of chloride ion channels. The resulting chloride ion influx hyperpolarizes neurons and stabilizes their resting membrane potential, thereby dampening neuronal excitability.

The benzodiazepine receptor is a complex entity functioning only in concert with the $GABA_A$ receptor. Occupation of the benzodiazepine binding site results in allosteric modulation of the proximal GABA recognition site, such that the effector sequence of the GABA–chloride ion channel becomes more efficiently coupled to the transducer. This promotes an increased frequency of opening of the chloride channel in response to a given GABA stimulus. The $GABA_A$ receptor/chloride channel complex also contains separate and nonoverlapping binding sites for a number of other drugs, the occupation of which allosterically enhances or reduces GABA transmission, giving significant potential for drug interactions to occur at the pharmacologic level, distinct from pharmacokinetic interactions.

The $GABA_A$ receptor is composed of five protein subunits, of which at present six α-, four β-, three γ-, one δ-, and two ρ-subunits have been characterized. Individual $GABA_A$ receptors comprise different combinations of subunits, allowing for perhaps several hundred unique combinations. These confer individual and distinctive electrophysiologic and pharmacologic properties on the receptor, which are reflected in the affinity of binding with individual ligands, and the extent and direction of the ensuing

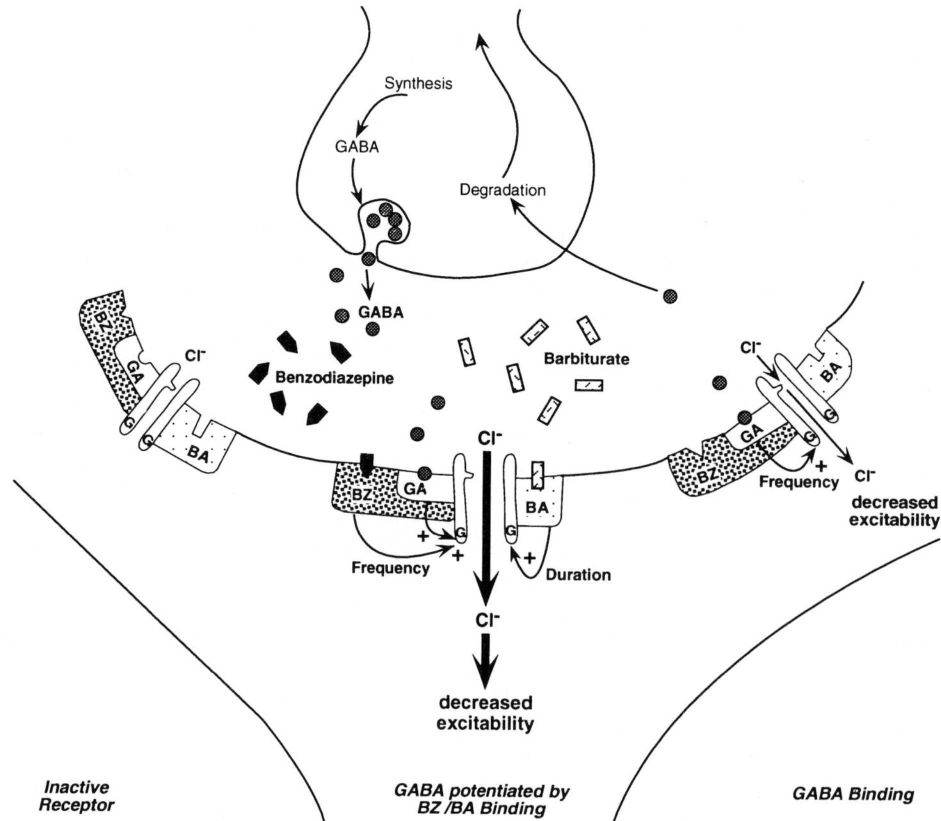

Figure 43–2. The benzodiazepine $GABA_A$ chloride channel receptor. The diagram shows receptors under three different conditions: left, resting state; right, opening with increased frequency due to GABA binding; middle, opening with increased frequency and duration due to binding by GABA, benzodiazepines, and barbiturates.

On binding at postsynaptic $GABA_A$ receptors, GABA becomes coupled to a transducer (G protein), which elicits an effector sequence resulting in the opening of chloride ion channels. The resulting chloride ion influx hyperpolarizes neurons and stabilizes their resting membrane potential, thereby dampening neuronal excitability.

The benzodiazepine receptor is a complex entity functioning only in concert with the $GABA_A$ receptor. Occupation of the benzodiazepine binding site results in allosteric modulation of the proximal GABA recognition site, such that the effector sequence of the GABA-chloride ion channel becomes more efficiently coupled to the transducer. This promotes an increased frequency of opening of the chloride channel in response to a given GABA stimulus.

Once bound to the receptor, the ligand may elicit several different types of response. An agonist, once bound to the receptor, forms a strong complex with the transducer and produces maximal effect. Partial agonists are unable to elicit the same maximal response as a full agonist, possibly because they form only weak complexes with the transducer. In the presence of an agonist, a partial agonist can attenuate the agonist's maximal response. An inverse agonist produces the opposite effect on binding to that produced by an agonist, attenuating the GABA response rather than potentiating it. When an antagonist binds to a receptor, activation does not occur, and binding can be either competitive (the response can be normalized by increasing the concentration of the agonist) or irreversible (blocking the ability to bind the transducer).

Barbiturates also exert their pharmacologic action at the $GABA_A$ receptor/chloride channel complex, but in a slightly different manner to that of the benzodiazepines. Instead of increasing the frequency of opening of chloride channels, they increase chloride ion influx by prolonging the duration of the opening at each given GABA stimulus. (BZ, benzodiazepine binding site; GA, GABA binding site; BA, barbiturate binding site; G, G protein; Cl^-, chloride ion.)

modulation. Only the α-, β-, and γ-subunits are thought to be important for benzodiazepine activity, with the α-subunit being the main determinant of binding selectivity. Once bound to the receptor, the ligand may elicit several different types of response. An agonist, once bound to the receptor, forms a strong complex with the transducer and produces maximal effect. Partial agonists are unable to elicit the same maximal response as a full agonist, possibly because they form only weak complexes with the transducer. In the presence of an agonist, a partial agonist can attenuate the agonist's maximal response. An inverse agonist produces the opposite effect on binding to that produced by an agonist, attenuating GABA response rather than potentiating it. When an antagonist binds to a receptor, activation does not occur, and binding can be either competitive (the response can be normalized by increasing the concentration of the agonist) or irreversible (blocking the ability to bind the transducer). With the benzodiazepines, partial agonists give fewer side effects because their full receptor occupancy is capable of promoting only anticonvulsant or anxiolytic action. They do not produce sufficient activity to elicit sedative-hypnotic or muscle relaxant effects, which require high receptor occupancy by a full agonist.

The ability of some benzodiazepines to bind specifically and with high affinity in some brain regions but not in others has led to the detection of two types of central benzodiazepine receptors. Type I and II benzodiazepine receptors have different α subunits: type I receptors have α_1 subunits and type II have α_2 and α_3 subunits. Alpha$_4$ and α_6 subunits are thought to be important for inverse agonist binding. The β-subunit, however, is not important for benzodiazepine binding but is a requirement for GABA action. The γ_1-subunit preferentially binds agonist ligands, whereas γ_2 has binding preference for antagonists such as flumazenil and is modulated by ethanol. Type I benzodiazepine receptors have wide distribution throughout the brain and are highly concentrated in the cerebellum. These are thought to produce anxiolytic effects at low occupancy or at higher occupancy by compounds with low intrinsic affinity, whereas higher occupancy by ligands with greater intrinsic affinity produces sedative and amnestic effects. Alpidem and zolpidem, the newly introduced imidazopyridines, and the benzodiazepine quazepam have high specificity for these sites. The second central benzodiazepine receptor, type II, is enriched in a few areas of the brain, the hippocampus, striatum, and spinal cord, and it is thought that this receptor is more closely associated with muscle relaxant properties and the development of tolerance and dependence. Thus, depending on the population of receptors with which they interact, some ligands exhibit different actions and may, for example, be agonists when bound to one type of receptor but only partial agonists at another.

Barbiturates also exert their pharmacologic action at the GABA$_A$ receptor–chloride channel complex but in a slightly different manner to the benzodiazepines. Instead of increasing the frequency of opening of chloride channels, they increase chloride ion influx by prolonging the duration of the opening at each given GABA stimulus. However, the barbiturates have far more CNS depressant effect than the benzodiazepines because at higher doses they increase chloride conductance directly by binding with the receptor, without the requirement for GABA. Barbiturate binding has also been found to enhance the binding of benzodiazepines and other GABA agonists and vice versa, thus producing their potentiating (supra-additive) effects. Paradoxically, this effect does not appear to be mediated by an increased flux of chloride ions as might be expected on the basis of their individual modes of action but may be moderated by a compensatory desensitization or adaptation to prolonged exposure to GABA. Barbiturate binding also inhibits receptor binding of antagonists and inverse agonists. In addition, barbiturates are thought to modulate the effects of glycine, another inhibitory CNS neurotransmitter located proximal to the GABA$_A$ receptor complex.

Chlormethiazole also acts at the GABA$_A$ receptor complex, but its spectrum of effects and resistance to flumazenil suggest that it acts at a different locus from the barbiturates and benzodiazepines, independent of the γ-subunit. It potentiates the action of both GABA and of glycine. Chlormethiazole is thought to prolong the opening of chloride channels as do the barbiturates, and preliminary evidence suggests that this effect may be more important at the low concentrations required for sedation than at higher anticonvulsant concentrations. Chlormethiazole does, however, antagonize barbiturate and benzodiazepine interactions, and therefore must share a common site of action even though its nature has not been fully elucidated. Glycine potentiation is thought to be important for the treatment of status epilepticus in patients refractory to benzodiazepines or barbiturates. Inhibition of glycine receptors causes convulsions, and it is these receptors that are thought to mediate the anticonvulsant effect of phenobarbital and propofol. At higher doses, chlormethiazole activates the GABA$_A$ receptor directly and with greater potency than the barbiturates.[6]

The sedative action of trichloroethanol is also thought to be mediated by the GABA$_A$ receptor, because its actions can be inhibited by GABA antagonists. GABA agonists have been found to prolong and to increase the amplitude of the effects of trichloroethanol in a dose-dependent manner, but only at low concentrations. Trichloroethanol potentiates the response to GABA, but in contrast to the barbiturates and benzodiazepines, it is not itself potentiated by GABA, neither is it potentiated by pentobarbital. Trichloroethanol can, however, activate GABA$_A$ receptors directly, and it also blocks N-methy-D-aspartate (NMDA) receptors by inhibition of the ion current through altered gating, rather than by affecting channel conductance, ion permeability, or regulatory sites.[7]

The anesthetic action of barbiturates such as pentobarbital and thiopental is considered to be mediated by direct stimulation of GABA$_A$ receptors in the absence of GABA, and these effects cannot therefore be blocked by antagonists. Anesthesia has also been suggested to be produced as a result of the very high lipid solubility of these drugs, enabling them to enter the cell membrane lipid bilayer to expand the membrane structure, to alter the flux of electrolytes (decreased sodium influx and increased potassium efflux). Barbiturates have also been shown to block central glutamate receptors, the main excitatory neurotransmitter pathway in the CNS. Activation of the NMDA receptor complex by glutamate depolarizes neurons by triggering an increase in membrane sodium conductance. Repeated use of barbiturates produces a compensatory increase in the number of glutamate receptors, and their presence contributes to the hyperexcitability seen in individuals experiencing withdrawal from these drugs. Both chlormethiazole and thiopental (Pentothal) have been shown to have neuroprotective action by their ability to lower the basal metabolic rate and to extend the tolerable ischemic time and have been used for this purpose in status epilepticus, cardiac bypass surgery, raised intracranial pressure after accidental injury, and stroke. Studies have suggested that this action of chlormethiazole results from its ability to stimulate directly the GABA receptor. Brain GABA concentrations are greatly reduced in animal models of cerebral injury, and it is thought that chlormethiazole somehow "replaces" brain GABA. Because the barbiturates (but only at high doses) also share this property, thiopental may also act in this way. However, the associated cardiovascular depression and prolonged duration of clearance associated with these high doses of thiopental has curtailed its use to some extent in favor of other agents such as etomidate.[8] Their inhibitory action at the NMDA receptor may also be contributory; and although the mechanism is not clear, it has been suggested that cell death results from excessive activation of these receptors and subsequent increases in intracytosolic calcium concentrations.[9]

The actions of the new, nonbenzodiazepine sedatives, zolpidem and zopiclone, also appear to be mediated by the $GABA_A$ receptor complex, but by differing mechanisms. Zolpidem has high affinity and selectivity for type I central benzodiazepine receptors that confers a narrow spectrum of clinical activity and characteristic regional distribution within the CNS. Thus, zolpidem has no appreciable anxiolytic, muscle relaxant, or anticonflict properties unless the doses given are 10 to 20 times those required to produce sedation; and it appears to have fewer adverse effects, especially with respect to residual sedation, and potential for rebound insomnia and respiratory depression. These actions are antagonized by flumazenil, and the binding of zolpidem is enhanced in the presence of GABA. The potential for tolerance, dependence, and withdrawal is also much less than with the benzodiazepine sedatives.[10]

Zopiclone is thought to act through $GABA_A$ receptors, but at a site distinct from, but closely related to, the benzodiazepine binding site. However, unlike the benzodiazepines, zopiclone binding is not modulated by GABA. It has been suggested that binding may occur at the same site as the benzodiazepines, but that a different conformational change is induced. The allosteric modification of the complex by benzodiazepines is sensitive to the effects of GABA and chloride, whereas the zopiclone modification is not. An alternative suggestion is that zopiclone binds to the flumazenil binding site because zopiclone is able to displace flumazenil from its GABA binding site but, unlike the benzodiazepines, this displacement is of a noncompetitive rather than a competitive nature. Zopiclone displays high-affinity binding only for central benzodiazepine receptors and does not bind appreciably to those at peripheral sites. There is also negligible binding to other types of neuroreceptors. Zopiclone does not appear to have specificity for type I or type II benzodiazepine receptors, which again suggests that the γ_2 subunit (flumazenil binding site) may be involved in its action. Consequently, the drug has a broad spectrum of pharmacologic activity similar to the benzodiazepines, with sedative-hypnotic, anticonvulsant, muscle relaxant, antiaggressive, and anticonflict properties. Thus far, however, zopiclone has been used almost exclusively as a sedative-hypnotic.[11]

Relatively little is known about the precise mode of action of the other sedative drugs, although chlormezanone is believed to exert its muscle relaxant activity by inhibiting polysynaptic reflex pathways in subcortical spinal centers.

PHARMACODYNAMICS, PHARMACOKINETICS, AND METABOLISM

The intermittent type of clinical effect that is desirable in hypnotic treatment differs fundamentally from many other types of drug therapy where a constant effect is required. Thus, for insomnia, sleep should ideally be achieved rapidly, drug effects should be restricted to the duration of the night, and residual effects should be absent during the daytime. This is particularly important, because although sedatives are often used in the hospital setting, by far the largest amounts are taken by patients who are required to maintain an otherwise normal lifestyle and who need to be alert and able to perform manual and intellectual functions during the daytime. Additionally, there should be no accumulation of drug or active metabolites despite being given on a daily basis. These factors taken together directed early investigators toward designing sedative-hypnotic drugs that had rapid rates of absorption, distribution, and elimination.

Many attempts have been made to understand the complex relationship between the pharmacokinetics and pharmacodynamics of sedative-hypnotic drugs (Table 43–1). *Pharmacokinetics* is the application of mathematical models to describe the time course of drug concentrations in various body fluids, whereas *pharmacodynamics* describes the time course and intensity of drug effects. Originally, evaluation of the kinetics of a particular drug was made in terms of its plasma distribution and elimination characteristics. However, drugs with long plasma elimination half-lives were sometimes found, paradoxically, to have short durations of clinical action. It is now recognized that it is the kinetics of a drug at its site of action (i.e., at the receptor level within the CNS) that is the most important determinant of success as a sedative-hypnotic agent. This can be difficult to measure directly and may require indirect measurements (e.g., plasma drug concentrations) coupled to computer simulations based on available knowledge of the drug's physicochemical properties.

The onset of action for drugs taken orally is obviously controlled by the pharmacokinetic parameters that determine speed of absorption from the gastrointestinal tract, although in practice the speed with which they enter the CNS once absorbed appears to play an equally important role. However, for drugs administered intravenously, and to a lesser extent those given by other nonoral routes, the latter is the major determinant of the speed of onset of therapeutic action. For example, thiopental given intravenously is effective within 20 seconds compared with

Table 43–1. Pharmacokinetics and Physicochemical Properties of the Sedatives

Drug Name	Plasma Half-Life (h)	Distribution Volume (L/kg)	Protein Binding (%)	pK_a	Partition Coefficient
Thiopental	6–46	1.4–6.7	72–86	7.6	
Pentobarbital	20–30	0.5–1.0	65	7.9	1.9
Phenobarbital	48–144	0.5–0.6	50	7.2	1.4
Diazepam	20–80	0.5–2.5	96–98	3.3	2.5
Lorazepam	10–24	1–2	88–92	1.3/11.5	1.9
Midazolam	3–8	0.8–2	95	6.2	1.5
Chloral hydrate	4 min			10.0	0.6
(trichloroethanol)	6–10	0.6	35–40		3.5
Ethchlorvynol	19–32	2–3	62		
Chlormethiazole	3–8–17*	4–12	60–70	3.2	
Glutethimide	5–20	3	47–59	9.2	
Methyprylon	4–20–50*	0.6–1.5	38	12.0	
Chlormezanone†	20–35		50		
Methaqualone	20–50–75*	6	75–95*	2.5	
Carisoprodol	1–2	1.0	41–67		
Meprobamate	6–17	0.7	14–24		0.7
Methocarbamol†	1–2	0.3–0.6	46–50		
Ethinamate	2				
Carbromal	7–15		40		1.7
Zopiclone	3.5–7	1.5	45		
Zolpidem	1–3	0.5	92	6.2	2.42

*Dose-dependent kinetics or protein binding, saturable in overdose.
†Unstable in neutral or alkaline solution.

20 minutes for phenobarbital. The physicochemical properties that influence the rate and extent of drug entry into the CNS are plasma and tissue protein binding, lipid solubility (usually expressed as the octanol/water partition coefficient), and the ionization constant (pK_a). Drug is delivered to the blood-brain barrier by arterioles originating from the carotid arteries. After crossing the arachnoid membranes, the drug enters the extracellular spaces of the brain, which are in equilibrium with cerebrospinal fluid (CSF) in the lateral and fourth ventricles and in the subarachnoid spaces. Drug can then enter the brain cells without further impediment and interact with its receptors. The duration of action of an individual drug is a function of the receptor occupancy (i.e., both the affinity of the drug for the receptor and the individual drug's elimination rate from the CNS). High-affinity binding causes drug to be retained in the CSF, and lower-affinity binding results in more rapid efflux. If receptor affinity were equal for all drugs, then the most lipophilic, least protein bound, and least ionized at physiologic pH would have the shortest duration of action in the CNS because they are most rapidly and extensively redistributed. However, they also tend to have the longest plasma half-lives because they remain in clinically "irrelevant" peripheral storage compartments (fat, muscle) for prolonged periods of time. Ironically, the very characteristic that makes a drug a good sedative-hypnotic is the very one that contributes to its potential for life-threatening toxicity in overdose, namely, a rapid onset of action through high and uninhibited transfer into the CSF. Drugs that are less lipophilic have shorter plasma half-lives, but redistribution from the CNS to the peripheral compartment is more limited and occurs more slowly.

Although the physicochemical properties may regulate the rate and extent of entry of a drug into the CSF, they bear little relationship to the affinity with which a drug binds subsequently to its receptors. Thus, for example, a single dose of lorazepam, which is of relatively low lipophilicity with a short plasma half-life (10 to 24 hours), gives longer seizure control than a single dose of highly lipophilic diazepam, which has a much longer plasma elimination half-life (20 to 80 hours); lorazepam also displays a twofold to threefold higher receptor affinity. These differences become less marked during long-term treatment because of accumulation of diazepam and its active metabolites and by modulation of receptor sensitivity or density. These issues are discussed more fully, in relation to the benzodiazepines in particular, in recent review articles[12, 13] and are represented schematically in Figure 43–3.

The pharmacodynamics of sedative-hypnotic drug action are further complicated by other pharmacokinetic considerations. For example, there are interindividual differences in pharmacokinetics arising from genetic predisposition to fast or slow metabolism, from the effects of age, and from coadministration of drugs or exposure to chemicals. The size of the dose administered and the route of its administration are known to alter pharmacokinetics, because these influence both the rate of metabolism and the metabolic products formed by either first-pass or other metabolism. In turn, these alterations in pharmacokinetics affect the pharmacodynamics, because the acquisition of tolerance of receptors to sedative-hypnotics is also important in defining the concentration-effect relationship. In the acute phase, tolerance is also affected by the route of administration, because the more slowly a drug is delivered the greater the potential for tolerance to the effects.

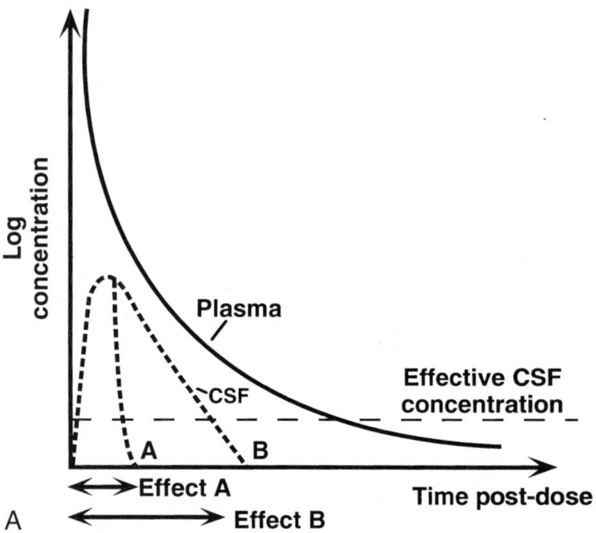

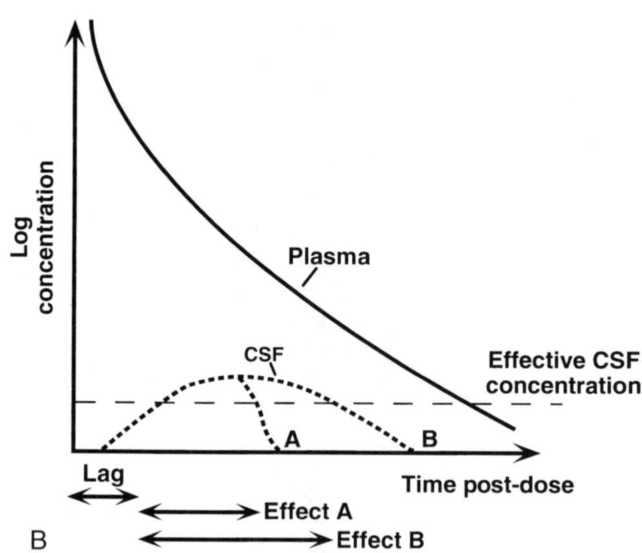

Figure 43–3. Effect of lipophilicity on drug concentration profile in plasma and cerebrospinal fluid (CSF), and duration of action. Concentration with time after dose in plasma and CSF for two hypothetical drugs given intravenously. CSF concentrations are shown for situations of both low *(A)* and high *(B)* affinity binding to receptors, together with the duration and lag time to onset of action. *Solid line,* plasma concentration; *short dashes,* CSF concentration; *long dashes,* effective CSF concentration.

A, Highly lipophilic drug. Plasma concentration shows rapid decline due to extensive tissue distribution, followed by slower terminal half-life due to requirement for extensive metabolism. There is rapid transfer from the plasma compartment to the CSF, resulting in a short lag time to onset of action. A is readily released from receptors and declines quickly to give a shorter duration of action than B, which is strongly bound to receptors and released only slowly.

B, Water-soluble drug. Plasma concentration shows slower decline due to relatively poor tissue distribution, followed by relatively quicker terminal half-life due to limited requirement for metabolism. There is slower transfer from the plasma compartment to the CSF, resulting in a long lag time to onset of action. A is readily released from receptors and declines quickly to give a shorter duration of action than B, which is strongly bound to receptors and released only slowly.

In attempting to define the pharmacokinetic-pharmacodynamic effect relationship for sedative drugs, consideration should also be given to the affinity, specificity, and selectivity of the drugs for their receptors in addition to the mere physical presence of the drugs at the site of action. This concept was addressed in the previous section of this chapter, when it was noted that differences in affinity and selectivity for receptor subtypes conferred characteristic profiles of pharmaceutical activity on the individual sedative-hypnotic drugs.

Barbiturates are most often given orally, except for their use in anesthesia or as anticonvulsants in emergency situations when they are given intravenously. Their metabolism and pharmacokinetics are discussed in Chapter 37. It is worth noting that although the recovery from the anesthetic dose of an ultra-short-acting barbiturate may take place within several hours as a result of rapid transfer out of the CSF, the sedative-hypnotic effects of the drug may persist for much longer (e.g., with thiopental); and this in turn correlates with their long plasma elimination half-lives due to slow tissue redistribution.[14] Absorption of barbiturates is primarily from the small intestine because solutions of barbiturate salts are alkaline. The sodium salts of barbiturates are more rapidly absorbed than the free base formulations. Because the onset of action is dependent on the speed of uptake into the CNS, lipid-soluble barbiturates induce sleep more quickly. Thus, whereas thiopental anesthesia may be achieved in less than 1 minute, there may be a lag time of up to 20 minutes after intravenous phenobarbital. Initial plasma barbiturate concentrations rapidly decline within 30 minutes to some 10% of their maximal concentration after intravenous dosing because of distribution into the tissues. Distribution volumes are between 0.6 and 2.6 L/kg. Lipid-soluble members are more highly protein bound (e.g., thiopental 80%, but phenobarbital only 50%). Excretion of unchanged barbiturate by the kidney contributes significantly to the overall elimination of the less water-soluble, less extensively protein-bound members of the group (barbital and metharbital, 60% to 90%; phenobarbital, 25% to 40%; and aprobarbital, 7% to 18%). Alkalinization of the urine also increases renal excretion of those barbiturates with an acidic/neutral pK_a, owing to an increased production of ionized species, and this has been exploited in the treatment of phenobarbital intoxication ($pK_a = 7.2$). However, most barbiturates are metabolized in the liver. Although most of the metabolic products are to all intents and purposes inactive after therapeutic doses, the hydroxylated metabolites of amylobarbital and secobarbital (about one third of the activity of the parent compound) are thought to contribute to cyclical coma after overdose. Oxidation of the radicals at the 5-position produces more polar and pharmacologically less active compounds: alcohols, ketones, phenols, or carboxylic acids. These are excreted unchanged and as highly polar glucuronide conjugates. N-hydroxylation, N-dealkylation, desulfuration, and ring opening are also known to occur, but, in contrast, N-demethylation of mephobarbital and metharbital yields the active compounds phenobarbital and barbital, respectively, whereas desulfuration of thiopental produces the active compound pentobarbital. Plasma elimination half-lives vary enormously among the group and range from as little as 1 to 2 hours for methohexital to up to 100 hours for phenobarbital.

Benzodiazepines given in the emergency situation for control of convulsions are administered intravenously. As a premedicant or for conscious sedation the intravenous or oral route is usually employed, and more recently midazolam has been administered by nebulizer. Poor water solubility at physiologic pH has limited the widespread availability of suitable injectable preparations of benzodiazepines. However, because the benzodiazepines are so lipophilic, they are able to reach and penetrate the blood-brain barrier quickly by passive diffusion to interact with their receptors within the CNS. In contrast to the barbiturates, therefore, the onset of clinical effect of the individual benzodiazepines is rapid and varies little after intravenous administration. The absorption profile of benzodiazepines after intramuscular injection is erratic and bioavailability variable, and for this reason this route is not popular. Most benzodiazepines are taken for anxiety or night-time sedation, and can be taken orally. Oral or sublingual absorption of benzodiazepines is often rapid and almost complete, dependent on the formulation, with peak plasma concentrations occurring within 30 minutes to 3 hours of administration for the majority of drugs.

Being highly lipophilic drugs, the benzodiazepines require extensive metabolism by one or both of two major pathways to furnish water-soluble products for renal excretion. The first pathway is hepatic oxidative deamination or nitroreduction, which is subject to large interindividual variation. The second pathway is also mainly hepatic and involves conjugation with glucuronic acid and sulfate but is less subject to variability. Some benzodiazepines are eliminated almost exclusively by conjugation; and in general for the 1,4-benzodiazepines, the half-life is more rapid where this mechanism predominates (e.g., lorazepam, oxazepam, and temazepam). The imidazobenzodiazepines have extremely rapid elimination kinetics, but this is through a hepatic oxidation pathway. First-pass metabolism may account for a significant proportion of an oral dose, giving bioavailabilities of 30% to 70%. Many of the metabolites are, however, pharmacologically active, and consequently some drugs (e.g., flurazepam, adinazolam, and chlordiazepoxide) have much longer durations of action from those expected from the pharmacokinetic characteristics of the parent drug alone. A number of different benzodiazepines share common metabolic pathways, of which the most frequently encountered metabolite is desmethyldiazepam, which arises from clorazepate, diazepam, prazepam, halazepam, pinazepam, medazepam, and ketazolam. Because oxazepam is a metabolite of desmethyldiazepam, this is also frequently detected in biologic specimens. Benzodiazepine metabolism is decreased in gross hepatic failure, but because of the large interindividual variability within the population and the large therapeutic index of the benzodiazepines, this usually has little clinical significance. Relatively minor changes are seen in chronic renal failure because elimination is principally hepatic. However, when glucuronide conjugate formation and urinary excretion are the principal routes of elimination, accumulation does occur.[15]

Plasma protein binding of benzodiazepines is generally high (above 85%) but does vary widely among this group of drugs, from 98% for diazepam to only 40% to 70% for bromazepam. When CSF concentrations of benzodiazepines have been measured, these have correlated well with circulating unbound plasma concentrations. Binding is predominantly to plasma albumin and is therefore decreased in renal failure, although for some drugs (e.g., temazepam) significant binding to free fatty acids is clinically important because the changes in fatty acid concentration and therefore in binding that occur postprandially are thought to contribute to observed secondary peaks in plasma drug concentrations. Accumulation of benzodiazepines in the plasma is expected to occur on once-daily dosing when the plasma half-life exceeds 16.7 hours (see Chapter 44 for further discussion).

Glutethimide absorption from the gut is highly variable and erratic. The onset of action is rapid (within 20 minutes), and its duration of action is similar to that of the intermediate-acting barbiturates. Peak plasma concentrations after single therapeutic oral doses occur within 1 to 6 hours and lie in the range of 3 to 7 mg/L. Glutethimide is then rapidly and extensively distributed in tissues with a distribution volume of 2.7 L/kg; plasma protein binding is 47% to 59%. CSF glutethimide concentrations of about one third of those measured in plasma collected simultaneously have been reported. Glutethimide is metabolized extensively, with only about 0.05% of an oral dose being excreted unchanged in the urine. Supplied as a racemate, there is stereospecific hydroxylation of the d-form at the 4-position of the glutarimide ring, and this 4-hydroxy glutethimide is the major metabolite seen in plasma. Stereospecific hydroxylation of both the *d*- and the *l*-form at the ethyl side chain yields both diastereo-isomers of 1′-hydroxyethylglutethimide. The majority of metabolites are conjugated, and these forms of 4-hydroxy and 1′-hydroxyethyl constitute the bulk of the urinary excretion products, representing about 60% of an administered dose. A variety of minor metabolic products are also formed including phenols, γ-butyrolactone and dihydroxy-metabolites of which a dihydrodiol has been identified. *In vitro* investigations have shown 4-hydroxyglutethimide, the 2-phenylglutarimide, and the butyrolactone metabolites to have significant pharmacologic activity when compared with the parent compound. Peak plasma concentrations of 4-hydroxyglutethimide are attained at about 24 hours after oral dosing and lie in the range of 4 to 6 mg/L. Concentrations decline in parallel with the parent compound. A similar pattern is seen after overdose with glutethimide, but whether this metabolite contributes to the toxic effects of the drug in overdose remains a matter of some debate.[16]

Methaqualone is a highly lipid-soluble acidic/neutral drug that is rapidly absorbed after oral administration, with peak plasma concentrations occurring 1 to 2 hours later, which after a therapeutic dose are in the range of 1 to 4 mg/L, declining to 1 mg/L by 5 hours. The plasma elimination half-life is between 20 and 50 hours. The distribution volume is relatively large at 6 L/kg, reflecting its lipid solubility; and reported concentrations in the CSF are some 18% of those seen in serum. Seventy-five to 95% is protein bound to albumin, and the binding has been shown to be concentration dependent. Methaqualone is extensively metabolized in the liver by hydroxylation with at least 12 different hydroxylated metabolites having been identified, together with the N-oxide and conjugated forms of these. The enzyme(s) responsible for methaqualone hydroxylation have not been identified but do not co-segregate with debrisoquine hydroxylase. The N-oxide (6.6% of the dose) and the 4′, 2′, and 3′ hydroxy metabolite conjugates form the major urinary excretion products (10.3%, 4.7%, and 3.5% of an ingested dose, respectively), with less than 1% of the dose being excreted in unchanged form. 6-Hydroxymethaqualone was detected for up to 4 weeks in the urine of a patient after the ingestion of a single therapeutic dose. On a repeated once-daily sedative dosage schedule there is initially some accumulation of methaqualone, but concentrations soon return to single-dose levels because of autoinduction of metabolism (although high concentrations may be found in the plasma of individuals addicted to methaqualone). Significant concentrations of the 2-hydroxy metabolite have been reported in overdose, with concentrations exceeding those of methaqualone by up to 50%. This metabolite is believed to be a more potent CNS depressant than the parent compound.[17]

Methyprylon is moderately quickly absorbed from the gastrointestinal tract, with peak plasma concentrations occurring at 1 to 2 hours after administration of a therapeutic dose and concentrations typically of the order of 3 to 10 mg/L. The distribution volume is modest at 0.6 to 1.5 L/kg, and the extent of protein binding is not known. The plasma elimination half-life is 7 to 11 hours. Methyprylon is metabolized extensively by dehydrogenation and oxidation to a number of more polar compounds, with only 3% of the dose being excreted unchanged in the urine. At least one of these metabolites, 5-methylpyrithyldione (methylpersedon), is known to have hypnotic activity, and this is excreted in a similar quantity to the parent compound. This compound is metabolized by hydroxylation of the 5-methyl group and further oxidized to a carboxylic acid. Both these metabolites are conjugated. It is thought likely that 6-oxomethyprylon is also active. Some 60% of the dose is excreted in the urine as metabolites, with 20% being lost in the feces, but the precise pattern of elimination has not been elucidated fully.[18] After a methyprylon overdose, with a peak plasma concentration of 66 mg/L, measurement of 5-methylpyrithyldione showed a maximal plasma concentration of 17 mg/L at 13 hours after admission, with a half-life of 8 hours.[19] After therapeutic doses, however, only small amounts of this metabolite are seen in plasma, although it is likely to accumulate to amounts equal to that of methyprylon itself on repeated dosing.

The sedative-hypnotic *trichloroethanol* is usually administered as one of several prodrugs: chloral hydrate, triclofos, dichloralphenazone, or chloral betaine. Chloral hydrate is rapidly absorbed from the gastrointestinal tract, with an onset of action within 30 minutes. It is widely distributed throughout the body and is rapidly and almost completely metabolized by alcohol dehydrogenase in the liver and also by erythrocytes, with a half-life of only 4 minutes. After therapeutic doses, peak serum trichloroethanol concentrations are typically about 8 mg/L and are achieved within 1 hour. Trichloroethanol is further oxidized (by alcohol dehydrogenase and an aldehyde dehydrogenase), with a half-life of 6 to 10 hours to the inactive metabolite trichloroacetic acid. Both trichloroethanol and trichloroacetic acid are glucuronide conjugated, the former producing urochloralic acid. Plasma concentrations of trichloroethanol glucuronide slightly exceed those of trichloroethanol, but the elimination rate is similar. The urinary excretion pattern after chloral hydrate administration is 0.7% and 28% of the dose as trichloroethanol and its urochloralic acid, respectively, and the remainder as trichloroacetic acid. The plasma elimination half-life of trichloroacetic acid is 3 to 4 days, and concentrations as high as 100 mg/L have been found; and although not an active metabolite, it is highly protein bound (85% to 95%), which is thought to have implications for interactions with other acidic drugs (see later). In neonates and infants up to 2 years of age, unchanged chloral hydrate is detected in the blood for several hours after administration and may contribute to its pharmacologic action. The half-life of trichloroethanol approaches that of adults by the age of 2 years, but in term and preterm neonates is significantly prolonged at 28 and 40 hours, respectively. Furthermore, concentrations of trichloroacetic acid do not begin to fall until 6 days after administration. This probably reflects an inability to conjugate to glucuronic acid, particularly in the face of competition by bilirubin. The bioavailability of chloral hydrate given rectally is dependent on the vehicle of administration. Hydrophobic vehicles such as polyethylene glycol produce higher trichloroethanol concentrations than if a lipophilic vehicle is used. The pharmacokinetic parameters obtained for trichloroethanol and metabolites after administration of triclofos are not dissimilar to those of chloral hydrate. Triclofos is hydrolyzed to trichloroethanol in the blood at a rate about half that for chloral hydrate. Both chloral betaine and dichloralphenazone are readily degraded in aqueous solution in the gastrointestinal tract to chloral hydrate.[20]

Ethchlorvynol is a highly lipophilic drug, and absorption after oral administration is rapid, with peak plasma concentrations occurring at about 1 hour, which after therapeutic doses typically lie in the range of 1 to 5 mg/L. In keeping with its lipid solubility, the onset of action is rapid (within 15 to 30 minutes), and it has a short duration of action (3 to 5 hours). Tissue distribution is rapid and extensive, with a distribution volume of 2 to 4 L/kg. In comparison to its activity profile, it has a fairly long plasma elimination half-life owing to slow release of the drug from tissues. Early estimates that put the plasma half-life at about 6 hours were almost certainly flawed by inadequately specific or sensitive analytical techniques, and the later estimates of 14 to 32 hours are probably more accurate. In keeping with this, accumulation of drug occurs on repeated dosing, with steady-state plasma ethchlorvynol concentrations of up to 37 mg/L being reported in chronic heavy users. The protein binding of ethchlorvynol is 50% to 60%. The metabolism of ethchlorvynol has not been investigated systematically. Only a fraction (less than 2%) of the dose is excreted unchanged or as conjugates in the urine, and it was therefore proposed that being a volatile compound some excretion must occur through the lungs. However, it was subsequently shown that extensive metabolism occurs by reduction of the unsaturated bond, by hydroxylation to produce several diols, and by conjugation with glucuronic acid and sulfate. The major metabolic product is thought to be the ethynyl 3,4-diol, which together with its conjugated metabolite may constitute up to 40% of an administered dose. Ethchlorvynol metabolism is unaffected by hepatic failure, but the evidence for increased accumulation of drug or metabolites in renal failure is confounded by inadequate specificity of the laboratory analysis.[21] There is some evidence for saturable metabolism after overdose, but again this may be an analytical artifact.

Chlormethiazole, which is used extensively outside the United States, is rapidly absorbed after ingestion, with peak plasma drug concentrations being seen at about 0.5 to 1 hour after a therapeutic dose, typically 0.1 to 0.5 mg/L. The linctus formulation produces a more rapid peak, which is double the value found after ingestion of the capsule formulation. The oral bioavailability is low (10% to 20%) and variable, owing to extensive first-pass metabolism with a high hepatic extraction ratio. The distribution volume is 4 to 12 L/kg, and protein binding is 60% to 70%. Chlormethiazole is extensively metabolized, with less than 1% of a dose excreted unchanged in the urine over 36 hours. The identification of the precise route of metabolism has been difficult, although the identified metabolites are formed by side-chain dechlorination and oxidation at the 1- and 2-positions to produce alcohols, and further oxidation at the 2-position furnishes a carboxylic acid and carbolactone. However, they account for only some 16% of an administered dose and are excreted in free and conjugated forms. The two major urinary metabolites, 4-methylthiazole-5-acetic acid (12% to 14%) and 5-(1-hydroxyethyl)-4-methylthiazole (2% to 3%), are seen in plasma, often at concentrations exceeding that of the parent drug. The pharmacologic activity of these and any other possible metabolites is thought unlikely. The plasma elimination half-life is 3 to 8 hours, with a significant increase (6 to 11 hours) in the elderly and in those with impaired hepatic function (4 to 14 hours). In cirrhosis, the oral bioavailability is increased about 10-fold due to impaired first-pass metabolism and portal shunting, although because systemic clearance is reduced by only 30% the data also suggest saturation of chlormethiazole metabolism.[22] Accumulation of chlormethiazole is not expected at normal therapeutic doses.

Chlormezanone decomposes in aqueous neutral solution to *p*-chlorobenzaldehyde, with a half-life of 48 hours, and is far more labile in both acidic or alkaline media and in strongly concentrated solutions. The drug was therefore believed to be hydrolyzed extensively in the stomach to this pharmacologically active hydrolysis product, which in turn constituted the principal plasma component. Derivation of reliable serum drug concentration data has been hampered by this instability, and it is believed that many analytical techniques that involve an extraction under anything other than neutral conditions probably detect the hydrolysis product rather than the unchanged drug. However, because the decomposition is quantitative and the standards are subject to identical handling, the use of data derived in this manner is acceptable, because it is now known that the amount of degradation product present in the blood is minimal. Absorption after oral administration is moderately quick, and peak serum chlormezanone concentrations are attained at 2 to 3 hours after therapeutic dosing and are in the range of 2.5 to 3.5 mg/L. Larger doses result in an earlier peak, within 1 to 2 hours. Protein binding is about 50%, and the half-life is estimated at 20 to 35 hours, suggesting accumulation on repeated dosing by a factor of 5, something that is observed in practice. The kinetics do not appear significantly altered in the elderly, and there is no evidence for slower elimination after overdose. Therapeutic effect is believed to be optimized at concentrations of 10 to 14 mg/L, with increasingly troublesome adverse effects above 20 mg/L. Unchanged chlormezanone is not detected in the urine, and the urinary excretion products comprise the hydrolysis product (1.3% of the dose), together with further metabolic products *p*-chlorobenzaldehyde (0.5% of the dose), *p*-chlorobenzoic acid (6.5%), *p*-chlorohippuric acid (29%), and *p*-chlorobenzoyl-*N*-methylamide (3.8%).[23]

Meprobamate is rapidly absorbed from the gastrointestinal tract, with peak plasma concentrations occurring within 1 to 2 hours, in the range of 5 to 9 mg/L. The distribution volume is 0.7 L/kg, and the plasma protein binding is relatively low at only 14% to 24%. The plasma elimination half-life is 6 to 17 hours, and repeated administration may therefore cause accumulation in a few individuals, although autoinduction of hydroxylation may compensate. Metabolism is by oxidation of the propyl side chain to hydroxymeprobamate, which is inactive, and by N-glucuronidation of this and the parent compound. Some 5% of the dose is eliminated unchanged in the urine, 10% as hydroxymeprobamate and 65% as the N-glucuronide.[24]

Carisoprodol metabolism was not studied systematically until the recent resurgence of interest in this compound as it became more widely sought as a drug of abuse. Carisoprodol is rapidly absorbed after oral therapeutic dosing, with peak plasma concentrations attained within 0.5 to 1 hour of 2.5 to 3.5 mg/L. The distribution volume is about 1 L/kg, and the plasma protein binding is 41% to 67%. Carisoprodol is rapidly metabolized by N-dealkylation to meprobamate and by oxidation to hydroxymeprobamate and hydroxycarisoprodol, with a plasma half-life of only 1 to 2 hours. Less than 1% of an oral dose is excreted unchanged in the urine. After therapeutic doses, plasma meprobamate concentrations exceed those of carisoprodol within 2.5 hours. This metabolic pathway has been shown to cosegregate with mephenytoin polymorphism but not with debrisoquine, and approximately 5% of persons will have a prolonged half-life of the order of 8 hours.[25]

Ethinamate is quickly absorbed from the gastrointestinal tract, with peak serum concentrations being observed at 0.5 to 1 hour after therapeutic dosing, typically in the range of 8 to 10 mg/L. The distribution volume and protein binding are not known. The drug is metabolized by oxidation of the cyclohexyl ring to 4-hyroxyethinamate, and this is largely glucuronide conjugated and accounts for about 40% of an administered dose in 24 hours. Small amounts of the 2- and 3-hydroxylated metabolites are also formed and conjugated.[26]

Methocarbamol is unstable in neutral/alkaline media and is readily hydrolyzed, mainly through the formation of its isomer 3-(2-methoxyphenoxy)-propanediol 2-carbamate, to guaiphenesin, an antitussive drug in its own right. Peak plasma methocarbamol concentrations occur at 0.5 to 2 hours after therapeutic oral dosing and lie in the region of 20 to 40 mg/L. The distribution volume is small, at 0.3 to 0.6 L/kg, and plasma protein binding is 46% to 50%. Methocarbamol is extensively and rapidly metabolized, with less than 1% of a dose excreted unchanged in the urine. The plasma half-life of methocarbamol is 1 to 2 hours. The major metabolites are not active and are formed by O-demethylation and phenolic oxidation. These are excreted as glucuronide conjugates, accounting for almost an entire dose over a period of 3 days. No alteration in kinetics in renal failure has been observed.[27]

Carbromal is a mild short-acting sedative, taken in doses of up to 1000 mg. It is also available as a tablet and elixir of 130 mg with 49 mg of pentobarbital and in combinations with phenobarbital and diphenhydramine. Peak serum concentrations are observed at 30 minutes after oral administration, which are typically in the region of 6 mg/L, rapidly declining to 1 mg/L by 9 hours with a half-life of 7 to 15 hours. Carbromal is metabolized by hydrolysis to bromoethylbutyramide (carbromide), which is further metabolized by oxidation of the ethyl group to 2-bromo-2-ethyl-3-hydroxybutyramide. This active metabolite has been found to reach peak serum concentrations of 3 mg/L at 2 hours and to decline with a slower half-life than the parent drug. Debromination of carbromal also occurs, with the formation of 2-ethylbutyrylurea and release of bromide ion. In one study, serum concentrations of bromide reached 12.8 mg/L by 9 hours at which time they were still rising. Carbromal, carbromide, and bromide are all thought to contribute to the sedative effect, and both carbromal and carbromide have been shown to have negative inotropic actions at concentrations occurring after overdose.[28] After 10 days of chronic treatment, serum bromide concentrations of 100 mg/L have been measured.

Zolpidem has a rapid onset of action, with peak serum concentrations occurring at 30 minutes to 1 hour after ingestion. Oral bioavailability is some 70%, indicating significant first-pass metabolism. The main metabolic pathway is by oxidation of the phenolic methyl group, furnishing the major carboxylic acid metabolite (50% urinary metabolite). Lesser metabolites are formed by oxidation of methyl groups on the imidazopyridine and substituted amide moieties and by imidazopyridine hydroxylation. None has appreciable pharmacologic activity, and less than 1% of a therapeutic dose is excreted unchanged in the urine. In keeping with its clinical profile, distribution into and out of the CNS is rapid; and, because of its low lipophilicity, zolpidem has a distribution volume of 0.5 L/kg. Plasma protein binding is about 92%, which increases in renal and hepatic insufficiency, although this does not appear to translate into altered kinetics in renal failure. The elimination half-life is 1 to 3 hours, with typical therapeutic serum concentrations of 0.05 to 0.2 mg/L.[3, 29]

Zopiclone is rapidly absorbed after oral administration. Peak plasma concentrations occur within 1 hour after therapeutic dosing, typically being between 0.06 and 0.07 mg/L. Oral bioavailability is about 80%, with little drug (less than 20%) being lost to first-pass metabolism. Zopiclone distribution is rapid and extensive, with a distribution volume of about 1.5 L/kg. Plasma protein binding is relatively low at about 45%, predominantly to albumin. Zopiclone is extensively metabolized, mainly by hepatic oxidation, with less than 5% of the dose excreted unchanged in the urine. Oxidative decarboxylation accounts for 50% of the dose, and further metabolism from this pathway subsequently produces many inactive metabolites. Piperazinyl side-chain oxidation produces a less-active N-oxide metabolite, with a plasma half-life similar to that of the parent compound. This accounts for some 11% of an administered dose of zopiclone. The N-desmethyl piperazine metabolite is not active and accounts for 15% of an administered dose. Zopiclone has a short plasma half-life of 3.5 to 7 hours, increasing slightly with age. In hepatic disease, the time to attain peak plasma concentrations is delayed (to about 3.5 hours), and bioavailability increases to almost 100% due to impaired oxidative metabolism. In these patients, zopiclone plasma half-life is doubled and correlates negatively with the albumin concentration in individual patients. In patients with renal failure, the half-life of zopiclone shows a smaller increase than in hepatic disease, and, again, the time to peak plasma concentration is increased.[29, 30]

PHARMACOKINETICS IN OVERDOSE

From the data available, there appear to be few differences between the pharmacokinetics of sedatives taken in overdose as opposed to therapeutic doses. Three drugs, though, demonstrate evidence of saturation kinetics, which has important clinical consequences. In overdose, the half-life of elimination of chlormethiazole may increase from a normal value of 3 to 8 hours to 4 to 17 hours.[31] This phenomenon is particularly important to remember if the drug is given therapeutically by continuous intravenous infusion for alcohol withdrawal or control of seizures, because, after some hours, respiratory arrest can occur at an infusion rate initially tolerated without respiratory depression. Methyprylon also exhibits saturation kinetics at plasma concentrations above 30 mg/L, with the half-life increasing from 7 to 11 hours to as long as 50 hours.[19] The protein binding of methaqualone is reduced in overdose, and there is some evidence of saturable metabolism, which may prolong elimination half-life from 20 to 50 hours to about 75 hours. This occurs only after massive overdose (plasma methaqualone concentrations above 100 mg/L) and is not, therefore, usually of importance after moderate to severe overdose.[32] Finally, rebound coma may occur in poisoning due to glutethimide, which has been attributed to enterohepatic recirculation (for which there is no evidence).[33] Nevertheless, after overdose, relapse into coma is paralleled by increase in serum concentrations of glutethimide and its active metabolites.

DRUG INTERACTIONS

The principal drug interactions occur either by pharmacodynamic interactions at receptors or by pharmacokinetic effects. The latter can be subdivided into interactions within the gastrointestinal tract, interactions with drug-protein binding sites, and inhibition or induction of drug metabolizing enzymes.

Absorption

The only pharmacokinetic interactions reported are with zopiclone and are those associated with drugs known to alter gastric emptying. Erythromycin has been found to increase the speed and extent of absorption, increasing bioavailability by 80%. Concurrent metoclopramide administration also increased plasma zopiclone concentrations, whereas atropine, which delays gastric emptying, has been found to decrease zopiclone concentrations. In both the studies concerned, subjects experienced significant alterations in the onset and degree of sedation produced, consistent with the changes in kinetics observed.

Pharmacodynamic Interactions

Pharmacodynamic interactions occur at the level of the drug receptors in the CNS, and can be expected for this group of drugs because they have been shown to exert at least some of their clinical effects by allosteric modification at a common receptor-complex (see earlier). The effects of sedative-hypnotic drugs are enhanced by the coadministration of other sedatives or drugs with CNS depressant properties, such as ethanol or tricyclic antidepressants. In many instances, this appears to be little more than an additive effect rather than a synergistic one. Long-term use of sedative-hypnotics leads to the development of receptor tolerance; and there is also a significant amount of cross-tolerance to the sedative effects of other sedatives, but not to their muscle relaxant properties.

Protein Binding

The trichloroethanol metabolite trichloroacetic acid is 65% to 95% bound (concentration-dependent) to plasma albumin and has been shown to displace other highly bound acidic drugs such as coumarins and warfarin and to increase their metabolism, although in practice only a small clinical effect has been demonstrated. However, the extremely high concentrations and slow clearance of trichloroacetic acid seen in neonates may be an important impediment to bilirubin metabolism, owing to competition not only for binding sites on albumin but also for glucuronidation by an inadequately developed UDP glucuronosyl transferase system, and presents a real danger of kernicterus. Barbiturates bind predominantly to plasma albumin (ranging from 25% for barbital to 85% for thiopental). Protein-binding displacements can be an important mechanism of interaction, with some acidic drugs such as aspirin and phenylbutazone that display saturable or dose-dependent binding at therapeutic concentrations. Alterations in protein binding can lead to significant clinical effects if the distribution (particularly that into the CSF for the sedatives) is altered or if lowered drug binding results in unusually high drug concentrations becoming available for metabolism. This latter phenomenon may increase dosage requirements but is distinguished from the enzyme induction effect noted later in that it is usually specific for one particular drug rather than for a wide range of drugs.

Metabolic Induction

Induction of the capacity of metabolic enzymes occurs by gradual de novo synthesis of enzyme material rather than by increasing the capacity (maximal velocity) of existing enzymes and is therefore usually accompanied by an increase in liver mass. Effects therefore develop gradually over a number of days or weeks. Similarly, return to normality is also a gradual process. Unlike enzyme inhibition, induction invariably involves many different enzyme systems simultaneously, and therefore has the potential to affect the metabolism of many different drugs and pathways. The traditional sedatives and hypnotics are well known for their ability to induce hepatic enzyme systems. The barbiturates, glutethimide, methaqualone, methyprylon, meprobamate, carisoprodol, carbromal, and ethinamate are all known enzyme inducers, although there are large differences in the capacities of the individual drugs to induce. Differences reported range from 1.2 times normal activity for hexobarbital and butobarbital up to 2.5 times for methaqualone. They have been shown to induce enzyme production of a wide range of cytochrome P-450 oxidative isoenzymes, some esterases (not cholinesterase), and UDP glucuronosyl transferase, the enzyme responsible for formation of highly water-soluble glucuronide conjugates. Because induction is nonselective there is also often induction of the metabolism of the inducing drug (autoinduction), leading to an increased dosage requirement, aside from any increase that may be required through receptor tolerance as discussed in the preceding section.

When enzymes are induced, an increased dose is required to maintain effective concentrations, and this can usually be dealt with quite easily. However, enzyme induction becomes clinically significant if the induced drug has a narrow therapeutic index or if the consequences of undertreatment carry a significant risk. Adjustment of dosages of other medications can be more difficult on withdrawal of the inducer because there is a rebound decrease in metabolism and possible toxicity ensuing if the drug has a low therapeutic index. Hepatic enzyme induction can also have serious consequences when the enhanced metabolism of other drugs is detrimental, for example, if it is converted to one or more toxic metabolites. Acetaminophen is frequently ingested in overdose, and the production of the hepatotoxic metabolite NAPQI is known to be increased by enzyme inducers such as phenobarbital and phenytoin. Therefore, it has become common practice in patients with acetaminophen overdose known to have received treatment with barbiturates or the other enzyme-inducing sedatives to adjust the treatment line downward by up to 50% of its normal value (see Chapter 49 on acetaminophen). In other instances, barbiturate-induced enzyme induction can be used to advantage, such as in the treatment of icteric infants with phenobarbital to induce the poorly developed UDP glucuronosyl transferase–mediated conjugation of bilirubin.

Metabolic inhibition differs from induction in that the effects are usually limited to one enzyme or group of related enzymes. The time course of the effect is often almost instantaneous, usually increases in keeping with the offending drug concentration, and declines in parallel with the elimination kinetics of the drug. The effect can be quite dramatic and potentially serious as toxic concentrations of drugs accumulate. However, with the sedatives these are extremely rare events. The interaction that occurs with the concomitant ingestion of ethanol with chloral hydrate or chlormethiazole arises primarily by enzyme inhibition, which results from their shared metabolic pathway with alcohol dehydrogenase. Both also have a pharmacodynamic interaction at the receptor level; and although this is probably no more than additive in the case of chloral hydrate, there is significant potentiation with chlormethiazole leading to a higher morbidity and mortality at relatively modest plasma concentrations.[34] Plasma trichloroethanol concentrations peak earlier, are significantly higher, and persist so for about 6 hours after coadministration of chloral hydrate and ethanol, or with chloral hydrate pretreatment, and the extent of the rise correlates with the plasma trichloroethanol concentration present at the time of ethanol ingestion. Correspondingly lower metabolite concentrations in blood and urine are found without changes in the plasma elimination rates. Similarly, blood ethanol concentrations are slightly raised in the presence of trichloroethanol and lower acetaldehyde concentrations are seen, once again without an alteration in the elimination rate of ethanol. Although various mechanisms have been suggested, these observations are entirely consistent with increased systemic availability through competitive inhibition of alcohol dehydrogenase on first-pass metabolism, which is to be expected because alcohol dehydrogenase is known to be saturated at typically encountered (>20 mg/dL) ethanol concentrations. As the drugs become distributed, the portal blood and liver concentrations decline and, thereafter, the metabolism of both compounds proceeds at the usual rate. Similar observations have been made with chlormethiazole; and because chlormethiazole is used in the treatment of alcohol withdrawal, the possibility of such an interaction is all the more likely.

Benzodiazepines as a group have little or no propensity to augment or to inhibit the activity of most of the common groups of drugs by metabolic effects, nor is their metabolism subject to interaction, with the exception of cimetidine. Because of their high therapeutic index, when interactions do occur, the associated 30% rise or fall in plasma concentration is clinically insignificant when compared with the normal level of intersubject variability in metabolism. This ease of use in combination therapies is one reason for the popularity of the benzodiazepines over the barbiturates. However, significant interactions are those that occur at the pharmacologic level, in the presence of ethanol and other CNS depressant drugs. These effects are for the most part additive only and can therefore be predicted and are not usually problematic.

There are no data on clinically significant interactions resulting from the use or abuse of chlormezanone, ethchlorvynol, or zolpidem.

TOLERANCE, ADDICTION, ABUSE, DEPENDENCE, AND WITHDRAWAL

Many of the sedatives and hypnotics discussed in this chapter have been associated with some form of abuse, tolerance, dependence, addiction, or withdrawal; and for the most part the symptoms and signs and treatment of withdrawal are similar irrespective of causative agent and can be treated symptomatically and supportively. There are, however, some important differences and complications arising from the individual drugs that are noteworthy. Distinction is made between the tolerance and dependence that occurs as a result of the normal therapeutic use of the drugs and the addiction that results from abuse, often by a route of administration not employed therapeutically.

Tolerance in itself can be fairly benign and is sometimes beneficial in terms of patient compliance, particularly for the sedative component of a drug given for another clinical indication. Tolerance on repeated dosing to the sedative effects of the barbiturates, benzodiazepines, and other sedative-hypnotic drugs is well recognized, and the demonstration of cross-tolerance between the benzodiazepines and barbiturates, and between ethanol and some of the sedatives, implicates the $GABA_A$ receptor/chloride ion channel complex or the closely associated glycine or glutamate receptors as the locus for this effect. For drugs that induce metabolic enzymes, tolerance can be explained partly by increased drug clearance, but the magnitude of tolerance (often a fivefold or sixfold increase in effective barbiturate dose) is far in excess of any possible consequence of induced metabolism. Evidence of tolerance at the GABA receptor comes from the demonstration of attenuated GABA responses to barbiturates or benzodiazepines, without changes in receptor density or in responses to GABA or GABA agonists. These data suggest a less effective transducer coupling at the benzodiazepine receptor in tolerant animals, but without an effect on the adjacent GABA binding site. Barbiturates and some other sedatives also block the response of the major excitatory neurotransmitter pathway in the CNS (NMDA receptor complex) to glutamate. Repeated use of barbiturates produces a compensatory increase in glutamate receptors, and their presence may contribute to the hyperexcitability that is characteristic of withdrawal from these drugs.

Controversy continues over whether the long-term use of benzodiazepines constitutes a medically sanctioned and potentially dangerous form of addiction.[35] Anxious patients with no premorbid substance or alcohol abuse problems who take benzodiazepines only rarely increase their intake or use them for non–medically intended purposes, so *addiction* is a misleading term. There is, however, good evidence for tolerance and dependence. Accommodating changes in receptor sensitivity occur with chronic use, and the consequences of this become realized when the drug is stopped. Withdrawal quite clearly does occur with benzodiazepines (reported incidence varies between 15% and 45%), although the severity and duration are often underestimated. Acceptance of this has prompted a dramatic reduction in prescriptions and, in particular a move away from the long-term use of benzodiazepines.

True withdrawal symptoms are distinct from a return to the morbid condition being treated or simply the reversal or alleviation of symptoms of drug treatment. By definition, they must occur in a defined spatial relationship in both onset and duration in relation to the drug's pharmacokinetics, and mitigation must be achieved by reintroduction of the drug. Recently, attention has been focused on defining the pharmacodynamic and pharmacokinetic characteristics that predispose a sedative to precipitate a withdrawal syndrome. Because it is the continued exposure of the receptors to an effective concentration that promotes tolerance and therefore subsequent withdrawal, those drugs that have a long residence time in the CSF have a particular propensity to do so. Residence time is determined partly by the affinity with which the drug binds to the receptors and partly by its rate of elimination from the body. Thus, higher potency drugs that bind with strong affinity to receptors have a longer duration of action than those that dissociate readily from receptors and which are then transferred out of the CSF. Slow metabolism or the production of significant active metabolites leads to a long duration of action, and their accumulation on repeated dosing predisposes to receptor modulation and hence to withdrawal. In any event, the degree and severity of the symptoms are related to the dose and duration of use.

Addiction and *abuse* are terms used to denote drug use that results in physical, psychologic, economic, legal, or social harm to the user or to others affected by their behavior. Implicit is the notion of escalating dosage and of ingestion to seek euphoric effects. Predisposition to abuse drugs can be ascribed to a number of different characteristics and circumstances. Some drugs clearly have more potential than others to be abused. Although this can be difficult to quantify, it is, however, possible to define the pharmacodynamic properties that predispose a drug to abuse by considering the aspirations of the abuser, for example, to achieve a rapid and sustainable "high" with limited undesirable effects. Speed of onset of action correlates with lipid solubility and to some extent with absorption. High-affinity receptor binding increases the duration of action, as does slow metabolic clearance (which again is related to lipid solubility).

Specificity and selectivity of receptor binding confers a narrow spectrum of clinical activity and can limit unwanted actions or side effects, hence the appeal of the high-potency benzodiazepines and that of the "short-acting" barbiturates.

Data on the pattern of drug abuse can be obtained from several sources: analysis of confiscated seizure materials, reports of prevalence of drugs in persons apprehended for traffic violations, medical examiner forensic reports on drug-related fatalities, and calls to poison information centers. All have their drawbacks, and none gives a true picture, but they do highlight trends and changes in patterns. Patterns of abuse can be influenced by changes in legal restrictions or may simply indicate the unavailability of a preferred drug. For example, barbiturates were widely abused in the 1960s and 1970s, but the Campaign Against the Use of Barbiturates (CURB) in the United Kingdom in 1975 and worldwide scheduling of these drugs led to a dramatic decline not just in abuse but also in their contribution to overdose statistics.

Barbiturates and benzodiazepines are rarely abused on their own but are more often used to potentiate and prolong the effects of heroin, methadone, and alcohol or to attenuate the withdrawal effects of stimulants such as cocaine. As each new nonbarbiturate hypnotic was released onto the market it was claimed not to share the barbiturates' propensity for addiction and withdrawal, although it in fact transpired that many were abused directly for their euphoric effects. Glutethimide and methaqualone are notorious examples, and these together with methyprylon, meprobamate, carisoprodol, ethchlorvynol, and trichloroethanol have all had periods of considerable usage and resultant morbidity and mortality. Methaqualone abuse was widespread, initially on its own but later as a combination pharmaceutical with diphenhydramine (Mandrax) and in an illicit capsule preparation with a benzodiazepine. Glutethimide abuse enjoyed a resurgence in the mid to late 1980s, being abused together with codeine (as "sets," "hits," or "loads," usually consisting of 1 g of glutethimide plus 240 mg of codeine, often compounded with aspirin, acetaminophen, phenacetin, or caffeine). Its popularity stemmed from its ability to produce heroin-like euphoria of longer duration for a fraction of the cost, with guaranteed pharmaceutical quality and strength. More recent trends in sedative abuse have seen widespread abuse of benzodiazepines, particularly of flunitrazepam, by nasal insufflation, in which the alteration in absorption profile and metabolite patterns arising from this route of administration confer favorable abuse characteristics. Intravenous injection of benzodiazepines is also common among narcotic addicts. After intravenous injection of temazepam, there have been many reports of abscess and thrombosis and of tissue necrosis necessitating amputation of digits and limbs in a number of cases.[36] Toxicity is due to microparticles of precipitated temazepam rather than to the vehicle itself,[37] and the ensuing rhabdomyolysis can lead to renal failure. These problems have led to changes in the formulation of temazepam capsules over the years. Initial attempts in 1989 to deter abuse by injection by replacing the liquid capsule filling with a gel were ineffective and in 1995 this, together with expanding oral abuse of temazepam, led to its scheduling in the United Kingdom as a Class I restricted drug under the Misuse of Drugs Act. The last few years has seen a resurgence in abuse of carisoprodol (Soma), which is rapidly metabolized to meprobamate, a drug that was virtually eliminated from use after realization of its high abuse potential and its placement under the FDA Schedule IV. Although meprobamate is available in more than a dozen formulations prescribed in Europe, often in combination preparations (with, for example, ethoheptazine, aspirin, or trihexyphenidyl), it is not a first-line drug. Carisoprodol is not restricted legally in the United States and can be purchased through veterinary mail order catalogs. Its resurgence as a drug of abuse in recent years is causing concern.

Clinical Features and Treatment

In contrast to opioid withdrawal, withdrawal from barbiturates and the traditional nonbarbiturate hypnotics can present life-threatening emergencies. On discontinuation, signs and symptoms progress over a 3-day period and include seizures, delirium, insomnia, tremor, anorexia, and abnormal sleep patterns. Abdominal cramps, nausea, vomiting, and orthostatic hypotension are characteristic milder features, and persons may exhibit purposive behavior patterns. Clinical features of withdrawal usually resolve within 10 to 14 days. Control of seizures may not be fully achieved with phenytoin or chlormethiazole, and readministration of barbiturates may be indicated in severe cases. Phenothiazines may also be useful for treatment of psychotic symptoms in this context, but their epileptogenic properties make the routine use of phenothiazines questionable. Substitution of the long-acting phenobarbital for shorter-acting barbiturates at the commencement of reduction of drug dosage sometimes gives easier control.

Benzodiazepines also cause withdrawal when medication is abruptly terminated, but this carries an insignificant mortality compared with withdrawal from the traditional sedative-hypnotics. Symptoms include anxiety, dysphoria, insomnia, concentration disturbance, panic reactions, tinnitus, hyperacusia, sweating, palpitations, anorexia, metallic taste, headache, tremor, depersonalization, derealization, and tremor. Mild symptoms appear within 1 to 3 days, peak at 5 to 9 days, and decline over 3 to 4 weeks, with mild residual effects lasting up to several months. Substituting the offending medication with the longer-acting diazepam has been used as a means of achieving gradual dosage reduction. Propranolol and clonidine have been used in treatment with equivocal results, and more recently carbamazepine has been suggested as being potentially useful.

The newer-generation sedative-hypnotics zopiclone and zolpidem seem markedly less prone to induce tolerance and withdrawal. The current literature contains a single case report of physical dependence to zopiclone on a dose some 10 times the maximum recommended. Grand mal convulsions were documented on abrupt withdrawal of this drug on three separate occasions, but there were confounding factors of concurrently prescribed trimipramine and promazine and of ethanol abuse.[38]

Neonatal Sedative-Hypnotic Toxicity and Withdrawal Syndromes

Drug withdrawal in the newborn is most commonly attributed today to maternal opiate or cocaine ingestion. However, maternal use of sedative-hypnotics is well known to produce withdrawal in the neonate, although the features are somewhat different. The symptoms of neonatal barbiturate withdrawal most commonly observed are overactivity, restlessness, tremors, hyperreflexia, persistent hypotonus, voracious appetite with vomiting, sneezing and hiccups, hyperphagia, and vasomotor instability. The treatment calls for the use of CNS depressant drugs or benzodiazepines rather than a phenothiazine, as is often used for neonatal opiate withdrawal. Because of the relatively slow elimination of barbiturates, withdrawal symptoms are typically not noticed until 2 to 3 days after birth and may occur as late as 14 days.[39] In a case report of maternal glutethimide abuse,[40] the fetus was restless if the drug was withheld and settled on drug administration, suggesting intrauterine withdrawal. The infant was tremulous at 8 hours after delivery and was initially treated with chlorpromazine, which was tapered off by the 10th day post partum. Striking features included incessant crying accompanied by an anxious, wide-eyed, alert look. On day 10, the child developed fever, severe diarrhea, dehydration, tachypnea, irritability, hypertonicity, and diaphoresis. Symptoms subsided with the administration of morphine, and methadone and paregoric (camphorated tincture of opium) maintenance was instituted. Weaning from these drugs was difficult and not achieved until day 45. There are also reports of neonatal withdrawal from ethchlorvynol,[41] which were successfully treated with phenobarbital. Symptoms of lethargy with episodes of extreme jitteriness, irritability, and behavior suggesting hunger appeared 1 day after birth, lasting for 4 days and in the absence of hypoglycemia.

Benzodiazepines also cause dependence and withdrawal in the neonate. Again, symptoms include hypertonicity, irritability, tremors, hyperreflexia, tachypnea, and weight loss. Feeding is vigorous, and there is frequent vomiting, which can lead to dehydration if not treated. Because of the slow elimination of these compounds, symptoms of withdrawal may not occur until 2 to 6 days after delivery.

Drug toxicity in neonates has also arisen from the maternal administration of sedative-hypnotics during labor and delivery. After administration of a single therapeutic dose of amobarbital intramuscularly before delivery, amobarbital concentrations were found to be similar in maternal and neonatal blood at the time of delivery but with the elimination half-life 2 to 3 times longer in the neonate (mean, 16 and 39 hours, respectively).[42] Glutethimide also crosses the placenta, with similar concentrations found in maternal and fetal blood when given as a single dose before delivery.[43] Chlormethiazole given by intravenous infusion to treat severe pre-eclamptic toxemia and eclampsia has resulted in hypotonia (of 24 to 36 hours' duration), hypoventilation, and even apnea in newborns. However, analytical data regarding plasma drug concentrations have not been reported.[44]

Laboratory analysis may be helpful in some instances, such as a drug screen on urine from identified high-risk infants shortly after birth. With opiates and amphetamines, the infant urine concentrations are often below detectable limits when symptoms appear. However, with the barbiturates, the 1,4-benzodiazepines, and the other older sedative-hypnotics (excluding the imidazo-benzodiazepines, zolpidem, and zopiclone), the combination of assay sensitivity and relatively slow elimination make detection of these drugs or their metabolites possible for several days post delivery. Drug analysis in meconium and infant hair is becoming increasingly popular, particularly for detection of maternal cocaine use, but these tests are expensive and the potential gain from detection of sedatives is questionable, because by comparison with cocaine the long-term effects from uterine sedative-hypnotic exposure are negligible.

Benzodiazepine Psychoses

Benzodiazepines may rarely cause aberrant or paradoxical effects, which usually occur after the first or first few doses have been administered. These occur most frequently in patients with overt or latent psychoses and organic brain syndrome or in the elderly. The anxiolytic benzodiazepines have been noted to unmask bizarre, uninhibited behavior in some patients, as well as hostility, rage, paranoia, and depression. After short-term use of the short-acting imidazo-benzodiazepine triazolam, there have been reports of visual, auditory, and tactile hallucinations that vanish on reality testing, and although the patient may be aware of the situation, he or she nonetheless feels compelled to react. The symptoms are not responsive to chlorpromazine. Patients have also experienced severe discomfort of the legs, similar to that found in psychotropic-induced akathisia. There is disorientation and reference to familiar persons, and the episode is typically followed by confusion and anterograde amnesia. Longer-term triazolam use has also been associated with an increase in daytime anxiety, weight loss, development of paranoid ideas, and personality changes.[45] Five cases of psychotic reaction similar to triazolam-induced psychosis have so far appeared in the literature attributable to the first (four cases) and third (one case) dose of zolpidem.[46] The fact that both zolpidem and triazolam have exceptionally high affinity for type I benzodiazepine receptors may help elucidate the underlying mechanism for this phenomenon.

Midazolam is a high-affinity benzodiazepine receptor agonist, and recent data suggest that it may also have the ability to cause psychosis. The intravenous formulation of midazolam has been used extensively in the United States and the United Kingdom where single doses are given for conscious sedation during minor surgical procedures. The drug is also given for longer-term maintenance of sedation during assisted ventilation. However, in some parts of Europe midazolam is available as an oral preparation for nighttime sedation in doses of 7.5 to 15 mg. Some patients who have had their sleep disturbed have been able to perform complex activities (such as driving a motor vehicle) or to talk freely to other persons and seem to be awake and attentive. However, next morning they have had complete amnesia for the episode. No other psychotropic drugs or ethanol was involved.[47]

EPIDEMIOLOGY AND INCIDENCE OF POISONING DUE TO SEDATIVES

The incidence of particular types of drug intoxication reflects trends in prescription patterns as well as patterns of drug abuse. Prescription patterns may change because certain drugs fall out of favor because of perceived side effects, because newly marketed preparations represent genuine advances in therapy, or because of attempts to reduce abuse of certain classes of drug.[48] On occasion, drugs may become subject to new legal constraints, for example, because of their abuse potential, and this has certainly been true of some sedative drugs in the United States and elsewhere. Other factors may also play a part in changing prescription patterns, such as the unwillingness of insurance carriers to provide reimbursement for proprietary formulations whose cost is greater than that of perceived generic equivalents. For all these reasons, the pattern of poisoning due to sedatives has changed over the years in the United States and in other countries. Sedatives, nonetheless, have accounted and continue to account for a significant proportion of deaths and hospital admissions from poisoning worldwide.[49, 50]

Once common, serious intoxication and death from *barbiturate* overdose still occurs occasionally in the United States and other developed countries.[50–55] As a result of their wide availability, *benzodiazepines* are commonly ingested in overdose and are found in a fourth to more than one third of poisoning admissions to hospital.[50–52] Official statistics suggest that over 1500 deaths occurred over a 10-year period in the United Kingdom as a result of poisoning due to benzodiazepine compounds, usually in the elderly and often in combination with alcohol. However, these data are based on returns made by Her Majesty's Coroners and, in many cases, the toxicologic diagnosis is based on circumstantial or limited analytical data rather than on comprehensive analytical evidence. Because benzodiazepines are widely available, it is not surprising that they are implicated circumstantially in fatal overdoses, and these data are therefore widely regarded as representing a gross overestimate of the true situation. More reliable estimates come from, for example, the study of Finkle and co-workers,[56] who reviewed 1239 deaths involving diazepam, only two of which could reasonably be attributed to diazepam alone. Similarly, of 1662 suspicious deaths reported in Cuyahoga, Ohio, benzodiazepines were detected in 6.6% of cases, although death was not thought to be due to the direct toxic effects of benzodiazepines in any of them except for one case involving a combination of flurazepam and alcohol.[57] However, fatal self-poisonings with diazepam and temazepam alone have been reported, as well as in cases where temazepam was taken in conjunction with quantities of other drugs that in themselves would not otherwise have caused death. On the other hand, there is good evidence that substantial quantities of a benzodiazepine may be ingested without a fatal consequence.

As indicated earlier, nonfatal poisoning with benzodiazepines occurs commonly in most developed countries where benzodiazepine usage is frequent. In a surveillance study of hospitalizations due to poisoning in Finland in the period 1987 to 1988, benzodiazepines accounted for 19% (2200 cases) of all admissions. Similarly, benzodiazepines were associated with 17.8% of 1212 cases of acute poisoning admitted in 1980 to hospitals in Oslo, Norway. In Australia, there has been a fall in numbers in recent years according to studies undertaken in 1976 through 1979, 1980 through 1982, and 1987 through 1993, with the figures attributable to benzodiazepines being 34.9%, 34.5%, and 26.2%, respectively.[53] The figure for elsewhere in Australia was found to be 39.5% of 325 cases in 1985 through 1986,[53] and 31% (of intensive care unit admissions) in 1986 through 1991.[50] In the United Kingdom, figures from a 12-week survey of six accident and emergency departments in 1994 showed that benzodiazepines accounted for only 15% of cases.[55]

Data are fewer on the incidence of other types of sedative poisoning, principally because denominator data are not available. A review of ethchlorvynol intoxications over a 14-year period (1975–1988) in San Diego[58] revealed 89 cases in toto (51 nonfatal and 38 fatal), but the denominator and annual incidence of poisoning are not known. All the fatalities occurred outside a hospital. In a series of 701 patients admitted to Massachusetts General Hospital in the period 1962 through 1975 because of accidental or deliberate overdosage with a psychotherapeutic drug, 63 (9%) had taken glutethimide.[59] During the mid to late 1980s, there was a series of reports of deaths due to glutethimide taken in combination with codeine (and often also with aspirin, phenacetin, and caffeine) (so-called loads or hits, also known as sets, threes, eights, or four doors). To judge from the serum concentrations of glutethimide and codeine measured in these fatal cases, the two drugs appear to exhibit synergistic toxicity in overdose. Methaqualone abuse and poisoning were seen commonly in the late 1960s and early 1970s, both in the United States where it was marketed as Quaalude, and in the United Kingdom and Canada, where it was most commonly encountered in the context of a proprietary formulation, Mandrax, containing methaqualone and diphenhydramine. Widespread abuse and poisoning incidents were also seen in other countries. In the first 6 months of 1966, Mandrax accounted for 5% of admissions to the Poisoning Treatment Centre at the Edinburgh Royal Infirmary in Scotland, and the proportion had increased to 10% by the last 6 months of 1967. Methaqualone was found in the urine of 3% to 4% of 7000 US Air Force Personnel serving in Germany in 1973. A review from Sweden of self-poisoned patients admitted to intensive care in the period 1972 through 1976 showed a fall in admissions due to methaqualone that exceeded that observed in barbiturate poisoning. A resurgence in methaqualone-related deaths was noted in the United States in the late 1970s.

PATHOPHYSIOLOGY AND CLINICAL MANIFESTATIONS

In overdose, the *barbiturates* act as CNS depressants, causing a fall in the level of consciousness and central respiratory and cardiovascular depression that is dose dependent. Clinical relapse is not uncommonly observed shortly after the beginning of apparent clinical recovery possibly owing to further drug absorption. The presenting clinical features of barbiturate toxicity therefore include depression of the level of consciousness, ranging from drowsiness to deep coma, depressed rate and depth of respiration, and hypotension. Hypothermia results from loss of peripheral vascular tone and accompanying vasodilatation. Bullous cutaneous lesions may also be observed.

Benzodiazepines also act as CNS depressants and may cause peripheral vasodilatation, although in both instances the severity is far less than that which is seen with barbiturates. The degree of sedation and severity of poisoning appears to vary with different benzodiazepine preparations,[60] but this is more of an epidemiologic observation than one that is applicable to an individual patient. Clinical features of toxicity include drowsiness, dizziness, confusion, coma, ataxia, dysarthria, nystagmus (the cerebellar syndrome), hallucinations, and bullous skin lesions. Mild hypotension is not uncommon; but even when substantial quantities of a benzodiazepine have been ingested, mechanical ventilation is required only rarely, although the depressant effects of other drugs or alcohol ingested at the same time may precipitate respiratory failure, particularly in an elderly person or one with chronic airways obstruction. Exceptionally, this may also occur in a young otherwise healthy individual, although the period of assisted ventilation required is usually short and may sometimes be averted with the use of flumazenil (see Treatment). Rarely, coma may persist for 2 or 3 days or, exceptionally, for 10 days. Coma may also be cyclical.

The clinical features of *glutethimide* poisoning are similar to those of barbiturate poisoning, although there are some important differences. First, glutethimide has anticholinergic properties, which can result in fixed dilated pupils, decreased salivary and bronchial secretions, reduced intestinal motility, and urinary retention. Second, the coma observed in glutethimide poisoning may be cyclical, and the observed fluctuations in the level of consciousness appear to correlate in some cases with changes in the plasma concentration of the parent drug. This may be due to release of glutethimide from lipid stores or enterohepatic circulation of the parent drug (or active metabolites). The role of the active metabolite, 4-hydroxyglutethimide, in the prolongation of glutethimide-induced coma remains controversial.[61, 62] Whereas the plasma concentration of this metabolite may be only 50% to 60% of the peak glutethimide concentration after a single therapeutic dose within 24 hours, after overdose it may rise to or exceed the initial measured glutethimide concentration during this time frame. The time-concentration curve for 4-hydroxyglutethimide plateaus because of continued formation; and although the elimination half-life of the metabolite is similar to that of the parent compound, in the days after an overdose (day 2 onward), the concentration of the metabolite may be as much as 10 times that of the parent compound.[59]

Methaqualone poisoning can result in clinical features indistinguishable from those caused by other sedatives, although hypotension and respiratory depression may be less evident than the presence of coma. In evaluating historical reports of methaqualone poisoning, it is important to distinguish between pure methaqualone poisoning and methaqualone ingested concomitantly with diphenhydramine (as Mandrax). In the latter instance, additional features of intoxication may develop, including ophthalmoplegias, hyperreflexia, peripheral sensorimotor neuropathy, prolonged coagulation times, thrombocytopenia, and nonspecific electrocardiographic abnormalities. However, pure methaqualone poisoning may also be complicated by pupillary dilatation, hyperreflexia, hypertonia, muscle twitching, clonus, muscle rigidity, seizure activity, and tachycardia. Respiratory complications observed may include aspiration pneumonitis, noncardiogenic pulmonary edema (which may be unilateral), and adult respiratory distress syndrome. There is some evidence that methaqualone alone may inhibit platelet aggregation. Bleeding problems have more commonly been reported after ingestion of methaqualone and diphenhydramine in combination (Mandrax), although retinal hemorrhage associated with thrombocytopenia has been reported after pure methaqualone overdosage.

The clinical features of poisoning due to *chloral hydrate* are similar to those of barbiturate poisoning, although some additional features may be present. These may include a retrosternal burning sensation after ingestion owing to irritation of the gastric and esophageal mucosae (hemorrhagic gastritis, gastric necrosis, enteritis, and esophageal stricture formation have been reported as rare complications of chloral hydrate poisoning). In addition, chloral hydrate may cause unifocal and multifocal ventricular ectopic beats, bigeminy, and ventricular tachydysrhythmias (ventricular tachycardia, torsades de pointes, ventricular fibrillation) in the absence of pre-existing heart disease. Supraventricular ectopic beats may also be observed. The rapid response of these dysrhythmias to β-adrenergic blockade suggests that chloral hydrate or a metabolite of chloral hydrate sensitizes the myocardium to circulating catecholamines rather than automaticity being directly affected.

The clinical features of toxicity due to *meprobamate* and *carisoprodol* (which can be regarded as a meprobamate prodrug in this context) are similar to those of barbiturate poisoning, and the same is true of ethinamate and methocarbamol, although overdose with these latter agents is now seen only uncommonly. *Methyprylon* overdose results in a similar clinical picture, with depression of the level of consciousness, respiratory depression, and hypotension being the most prominent features of intoxication.

Carbromal has been an uncommon cause of poisoning in the United States, although it was encountered frequently in overdose in Germany in the late 1960s and early 1970s. The clinical features of carbromal toxicity include coma, respiratory depression, and hypotension (due in part to a negative inotropic effect of the drug), but reports in the literature from German physicians suggest that hypothermia, adult respiratory distress syndrome, and disseminated intravascular coagulation occurred with unusual frequency. Tachydysrhythmias, hepatocellular necrosis, renal failure, and pancreatitis have all been reported as complications of carbromal poisoning. The contribution made by the presence of inorganic bromide ion to the clinical features of carbromal toxicity is not known.

The toxicity of *ethchlorvynol* is similar to that of the barbiturates, although coma is often prolonged and there are a few other minor differences. Ethchlorvynol is a pungent volatile aromatic compound, and its distinctive odor can be detected on the breath of patients with overdose. Bailey and Shaw[58] have reported what is probably the largest case series of nonfatal ethchlorvynol poisonings. The most common findings in the 51 reported cases were a depressed level of consciousness (37), dysarthria (18), tachycardia (18), nystagmus (13), and hyporeflexia (12). Hypotension and respiratory depression occurred uncommonly (eight cases and one case, respectively). Some of the observed clinical features may reflect the presence of coingested drugs, which were present in 80% of cases. Teehan and colleagues[63] reviewed the findings in six cases of severe ethchlorvynol poisoning. The patients typically presented in deep coma, which was prolonged (mean duration, 119 hours; range, 10.5 to 288 hours) with hypothermia, marked respiratory depression, hypotension, and relative bradycardia. Complications included pneumonia, cardiorespiratory arrest, and peripheral neuropathy (usually pressure-induced associated with prolonged coma before hospital admission). Pressure necrosis and blisters similar to those observed in barbiturate poisoning have also been reported, as has pancytopenia. The mortality from ethchlorvynol poisoning appears to be low.

Ethchlorvynol is sometimes abused intravenously, and noncardiogenic pulmonary edema is then a common complication that may develop within minutes of injection.[64] Patients develop cough and dyspnea and expectorate pulmonary edema fluid. Hypoxemia, hypocapnia, and respiratory alkalosis are universally present, and radiographic examination typically reveals bilateral interstitial/alveolar infiltrates with a normal-sized heart. Animal models have been used to investigate the pathogenesis of ethchlorvynol-induced noncardiogenic pulmonary edema.[65–68] The phenomenon is accompanied by an increase in pulmonary artery pressure mediated by cyclooxygenase products and can be blocked by prior administration of nonsteroidal anti-inflammatory agents. Hypoxia occurs universally and persists for hours. Ethchlorvynol also appears to have a direct effect on alveolar capillary membrane permeability, which is not blocked by nonsteroidal anti-inflammatory agents.

Chlormezanone poisoning has been reported only uncommonly, except from France, and may be associated with confusion, dizziness, drowsiness, ataxia, a modest depression in the level of consciousness, and mild hypotension. Respiratory depression does not appear to be a prominent or common feature of chlormezanone intoxication. One case of hepatocellular necrosis has been reported after chlormezanone overdose,[69] and a few deaths have also been recorded.[70]

Chlormethiazole is a sedative drug used infrequently in the United States where chlormethiazole poisoning is seen only rarely, in contrast to the situation in other countries where this drug is more widely used. Chlormethiazole given by intravenous infusion has been used in the treatment of alcohol withdrawal and in the management of eclampsia. Chlormethiazole poisoning is similar to that induced by barbiturates,[31, 34] with deep coma, respiratory depression, hypotension, and hypothermia being characteristic features. Chlormethiazole also causes increased salivation, which may compromise respiratory function in the presence of an unprotected airway. Nasal irritation and congestion, sneezing, eye irritation, and facial flushing may also occur. Bullous eruptions of the type seen in barbiturate poisoning have also been reported. The toxicity of chlormethiazole is enhanced by coingestion of ethanol, and the two agents appear to be synergistically toxic. Death typically results from respiratory depression. In part, this may be because alcohol increases the bioavailability of chlormethiazole, probably by impairing first-pass hepatic metabolism.

Bioavailability is also greatly increased in patients with cirrhosis of the liver.[22] Fatal respiratory depression and severe cerebral hypoxic damage after respiratory arrest have been observed after the administration of chlormethiazole by intravenous infusion for the treatment of alcohol withdrawal.[71] This is because the half-life of elimination of the drug increases from 3 to 8 hours to the order of 17 hours after prolonged infusion,[72] resulting in increasing concentrations of the drug if a constant infusion rate is maintained.

Despite the frequency with which the newer sedatives *zolpidem* and *zopiclone* are now prescribed there is a relative paucity of information about their effects in overdose. The first reported zolpidem overdose[73] presented as profound but short-lived coma, pinpoint pupils, respiratory depression, and acidosis, mimicking opioid toxicity. The patient, however, did not respond to naloxone, but all signs cleared rapidly after the administration of flumazenil. Repeated dosing with flumazenil was required. Analytical data collected over a short period did not show evidence of a prolonged elimination half-life in overdose. Interpretation of the clinical findings was, however, complicated by coingestion of a phenothiazine, prothipendyl, together with a significant amount of alcohol. The patient made a full recovery by 6 hours after ingestion but suffered anterograde amnesia. A zolpidem-related death was reported by Tracqui and colleagues,[74] with a blood zolpidem concentration of 3.9 mg/L and a potentially fatal concentration of a phenothiazine, acepromazine. This case, and that reported by Lheureux and colleagues[73] involving another phenothiazine, prothipendyl, suggests that enhanced toxicity may occur when zolpidem is ingested in overdose with a phenothiazine. This supposition is supported by the demonstration of prolongation of chlorpromazine elimination by therapeutic doses of zolpidem.[73, 75]

A larger series of 344 cases of intentional overdose with zolpidem has been reported, but in these cases ingestion of zolpidem was not confirmed analytically.[76] Two thirds of the patients were intoxicated, but this could only be attributed to zolpidem in 105 patients. Half of the total number of the patients had coingested other drugs, principally benzodiazepines, antidepressants, neuroleptics, anticonvulsants, lithium, and alcohol. Drowsiness was the most common clinical feature (89 of 344), with coma being observed in 4 patients, vomiting in 7 patients, and respiratory failure in 1 patient. Patients with electrocardiographic abnormalities had all allegedly taken tricyclic antidepressants, and in 2 patients who presented with acidosis, salicylates, and ethylene glycol had reportedly been ingested. Rapid remission was observed in 91% of patients. There were 11 fatalities (6%), none of which could be attributed to zolpidem.

Royer-Morrot and colleagues[77] reported a patient who ingested 300 mg of zopiclone. The only symptom noted was sleepiness. The patient underwent gastric lavage and was given flumazenil, apparently with a good result. The initial plasma zopiclone concentration at 4.5 hours after ingestion was 1.6 mg/L (about 25 times the normal therapeutic concentration), and the elimination half-life of the drug was 3.5 hours. Ahmad and colleagues[78] reported a patient on multiple psychotropic drug therapy (chlorpromazine, amitriptyline, trifluoperazine, procyclidine, and zopiclone) who presented deeply comatose but breathing spontaneously. The patient was stable from a cardiovascular standpoint but was noted to have loss of doll's eye movements. He responded immediately to flumazenil, admitted to having ingested a pure zopiclone overdose, and then relapsed into coma. An intravenous infusion of flumazenil was required to maintain a satisfactory level of consciousness. A urine screen for benzodiazepines was negative. Regouby and colleagues[79] reported a previously healthy young adult who experienced somnolence and first-degree heart block after ingesting 127.5 mg of zopiclone. Treatment consisted of gastric lavage and oral administration of activated charcoal. After 36 hours, the electrocardiographic abnormality returned to normal, and he made an uneventful recovery. He was also taking alprazolam, ciprofibrate, and mianserin therapeutically but claimed not to have taken these drugs in excess of the prescription.

A young adult found dead no more than 6 hours after ingesting a zopiclone overdose (maximum dose, 420 mg) while under the influence of alcohol was described by Pounder and Davies.[80] The blood zopiclone concentration was 1.2 mg/L, and the blood ethanol concentration 153 mg/dL. The cause of death was given as aspiration of vomit. In a survey of five fatalities implicating zopiclone,[81] fatal concentrations of coingested drugs were present in three patients (trichloroethanol in one patient, dothiepin and procyclidine in another, and amylobarbital in the other). Blood zopiclone concentrations were 0.62, 1.16, and 1.7 mg/L, respectively. One patient died of a non–drug-related cause 24 hours after the ingestion of a single 7.5-mg tablet, and no zopiclone was detected in the blood. The fifth patient had a blood zopiclone concentration of 0.4 mg/L and had also ingested a therapeutic amount of temazepam. The cause of death in this case was given as zopiclone overdose.

DIAGNOSIS

There are no true pathognomonic features of sedative drug overdoses that allow one to identify a particular sedative as being the cause of a particular overdose on clinical grounds. The diagnosis therefore rests on circumstantial evidence; the presence of coma, respiratory depression, and hypotension of differing degrees, and of analytical detection and quantitation of the drugs in question. There may be a few pointers toward particular drugs, but they have limited predictive values. Carbromal is radiodense because it contains bromide, and tablets may be observed on an abdominal radiograph. Coma due to benzodiazepines and zopiclone reverses with the administration of flumazenil in sufficient dosage, but it is arguable as to whether a benzodiazepine antagonist should be used solely for diagnostic purposes, and this practice should be avoided.

TREATMENT

The mainstay of treatment for all types of sedative drug overdose is *supportive care* directed particularly at the cardiovascular and respiratory systems. Respiratory depression due to sedative drug overdose should be managed conventionally, and assisted ventilation is commonly necessary. Hypotension should first be treated with volume replacement, utilizing measurement of central venous pressures (or, exceptionally, pulmonary artery wedge pressures) as necessary. If there is an element of myocardial depression, as may be the case in severe barbiturate and nonbarbiturate sedative drug poisoning, then inotropic agents may be required. There are no good studies of the relative effectiveness of inotropes in this context, and the agents used will depend on the experience of the physician concerned. The authors of this chapter have almost invariably obtained good results with a combination of dobutamine (5 to 20 μg/kg per min) and low-dose dopamine (2 to 3 μg/kg per min). Observation of critically ill patients in an intensive care unit with monitoring of vital signs, telemetry, oxygen saturation, laboratory parameters, and, where appropriate, drug concentrations[104] (Tables 43–1 and 43–2) may be necessary for life support.

There is a specific antidote, flumazenil, that does have a role, although a limited one, in the management of certain types of sedative drug overdose. Flumazenil, a 1,4-imidazodiazepine, is a highly effective specific competitive benzodiazepine antagonist acting at the $GABA_A$ chloride channel receptor. It has a short half-life (about 60 minutes) and a duration of action of 2 to 3 hours. A response usually occurs in patients with benzodiazepine overdose after administration of less than 5 mg in divided doses, but repeated doses may be required if sedation recurs, and an infusion of 0.5 mg/h may be necessary to counter prolonged sedation. The role of flumazenil as a "blanket" treatment for suspected benzodiazepine overdose is, however, controversial.[82–85] Several studies (including those of Hofer and Scollo-Lavizzari,[86] O'Sullivan & Wade,[87] and Knudsen and associates[88]) have investigated the efficacy of flumazenil in the management of sedative intoxication. Flumazenil was found to be highly effective in rapidly reversing coma due to pure benzodiazepine overdose or mitigating the benzodiazepine component of a "mixed" overdose. Other studies, for example that of Höjer and colleagues,[89] have resulted in advocacy for the use of flumazenil in pure and mixed benzodiazepine overdoses because it produces a 30% to 40% reduction in the requirement for invasive procedures (such as gastric lavage, intubation, urinary catheterization, assisted ventilation, and computed tomography of the brain), and many patients are able to give clinically significant information about the drugs ingested. However, adverse effects resulting from the use of flumazenil include agitation, vomiting, dizziness, headache, and injection site pain. On balance, therefore, it is probably better to avoid the routine use of flumazenil in patients with benzodiazepine overdose except in those unusual circumstances when a short period of intubation and assisted ventilation might otherwise be avoided. Although flumazenil is a specific benzodiazepine antagonist, there is evidence that some of the respiratory depressant effects of benzodiazepines may be controlled by a receptor that is not affected by flumazenil.[90, 91]

Additionally, flumazenil reverses the sedative component of toxicity induced by some other drugs whose sedative action is thought to be mediated through the benzodiazepine receptor, for example, chloral hydrate[92] and reversal of the sedative effects of ethanol is sometimes dramatic although it occurs very inconsistently.[93] In mixed overdoses, however, the reversal of benzodiazepine-induced CNS depression can "unmask" the toxic effects of other drugs present. *For example, convulsions have resulted when tricyclic antidepressants had been ingested concomitantly,*[94] *and ventricular tachycardia has been reported in the presence of chloral hydrate.*[80, 91, 95] Flumazenil administration precipitated complete heart block in a patient who ingested atenolol, nifedipine, paracetamol, and temazepam in overdose,[96] and a fatality has been reported after a dothiepin and benzodiazepine overdose.[93] On balance therefore, the conservative use of flumazenil for known pure benzodiazepine overdose is perhaps the safest course of action (see Chapter 44 for further discussion).

Zopiclone also acts at the $GABA_A$/chloride channel complex, and there is evidence from two case reports[77, 78] that flumazenil reverses the pharmacologic effects of zopiclone. *Zolpidem* also acts at the $GABA_A$/chloride channel complex, and there is evidence from animal[97] and human[98] volunteer studies, and from a case report,[73] that flumazenil reverses the pharmacologic effects of zolpidem. The use of this antidote should therefore be considered as a means of reversing respiratory depression induced by either zolpidem or zopiclone, particularly if intubation or assisted ventilation is otherwise indicated.

The ventricular tachydysrhythmias that may complicate *chloral hydrate* overdose do not respond to conventional antiarrhythmic agents such as lidocaine or phenytoin, whereas β-adrenergic blocking drugs have been found to be highly effective[99–101] once hypoxemia and hypokalemia have been corrected. Ideally, in these patients the potassium concentration should be maintained at 4.5 to 4.7 mEq/L as an antidysrhythmic measure. The dose of propranolol required to correct ventricular dysrhythmias is typically of the order of 1 to 2 mg by slow intravenous injection followed by 1 to 2 mg/h, as necessary, to

Table 43–2. Therapeutic and Toxic Plasma Concentrations of Sedative-Hypnotic Drugs in Man*

Drug Name (Significant Active Metabolite)	Therapeutic Below† (mg/L)	Severe Toxicity Above† (mg/L)	Typical Therapeutic Dose Range (mg)
Ultra-Short-Acting Barbiturates			
Methohexital	5	20	50–120
Thiopental (plus pentobarbital)	15/200‡	20	100–200
Short-Acting Barbiturates			
Hexobarbital	5	8	250–500
Pentobarbital	10	100	100–200
Secobarbital	5	40	100–200
Intermediate-Acting Barbiturates			
Allobarbital	15	50	100–200
Amobarbital	5	40	30–200
Aprobarbital	10	40	50–150
Butabarbital	5	30	30–100
Butalbital	5	30	150–400
Butobarbital	10	100	100–200
Cyclobarbital	2	10	100–400
Heptabarbital	2	8	150–400
Vinylbarbitone	2	10	100–200
Long-Acting Barbiturates			
Barbital	15	50	300–600
Mephobarbital (plus phenobarbital)	30	100	90–600
Metharbital (plus barbital)	30	100	100–300
Phenobarbital	30	100	45–180
Primidone (excluding phenobarbital)	12	100	200–1000
Benzodiazepines			
Adinazolam (plus desmethyladinazolam)	0.5	Not known	10–90
Alprazolam	0.02	0.2	0.75–4
Bromazepam	0.2	2	6–20
Chlordiazepoxide (plus metabolites)	1.5	5	15–100
Clobazam (plus desmethylclobazam)	1.5	10	20–80
Clonazepam	0.1	0.5	1.5–20
Clorazepate (as desmethyldiazepam)	1.5	5	15–30
Diazepam (plus desmethyldiazepam)	1.5	5	5–30
Flunitrazepam	0.05	2	1–2
Flurazepam (plus desalkylflurazepam)	0.2	2	15–30
Ketazolam (as desmethyldiazepam)	1.5	5	15–60
Loprazolam	0.02	0.2	1–2
Lorazepam	0.2	2	2–6
Lormetazepam	0.2	1	0.5–2
Midazolam	0.3	2	2.5–7.5
Nitrazepam	0.2	2	5–20
Oxazepam	1	5	30–100
Prazepam (as desmethyldiazepam)	1.5	5	30–120
Quazepam (plus desalkylflurazepam)	0.2	2	20–60
Temazepam	0.5	10	15–60
Tetrazepam	0.5	5	25–150
Triazolam	0.02	0.2	0.5–1.5
Other Sedative-Hypnotics			
Carbromal	5	25	200–1000
(bromoethylbutyramide)	5	15	
(bromide)	100	800	
Carisoprodol (plus meprobamate)	10	80	500–1500
Chlormethiazole	2	20	200–1000
Chlormezanone	8	50	300–800
Ethchlorvynol	10	100	200–500
Ethinamate	10	100	500–1000
Glutethimide	4	30	150–400
Meprobamate	10	80	400–2000
Methaqualone	4	20	150–400
Methocarbamol	25	300	4000–6000
Methyprylon	10	50	200–400
Trichloroethanol (from chloral hydrate, triclofos, dichloralphenazone and chloral betaine)	10	50	250–1000
Zolpidem	0.1	2	10–30
Zopiclone	0.7	Not known	3.75–7.5

*These concentrations are for guidance only. There is a large interindividual difference in drug response; tolerance, coingested drugs, premorbid conditions and complications may affect outcome significantly.

†Concentrations are in plasma or serum in mg/L unless otherwise stated.

‡When given in anesthetic doses during assisted ventilation for cerebral protection.

maintain a heart rate of 80 to 100 beats per minute. Metoprolol, 5 mg by slow intravenous injection, has also been used successfully.[99]

Certain of the sedatives do lend themselves to enhanced elimination, and exceptional measures may be indicated to enhance drug removal. Phenobarbital has a small volume of distribution and an acid pK_a, and as such it is amenable to enhanced elimination by either repeat-dose activated charcoal or alkaline diuresis (see Chapter 37). Urinary alkalinization, however, is not indicated for sedative drugs with neutral or basic pK_a values. There is a report of two patients with meprobamate poisoning in whom the use of repeat-dose activated charcoal was associated with elimination half-lives of approximately 4.5 hours compared with usual values of 7 to 17 hours.[102] Further experience of the utility of this approach is awaited.

In the past, hemoperfusion was employed as a means of removing barbiturate and nonbarbiturate sedatives, with the exception of chlormethiazole, principally to shorten the duration of coma in the belief this would reduce the incidence and severity of complications associated with prolonged intubation and assisted ventilation. Intensive supportive care of poisoned patients is now more commonplace than it was 20 years ago when hemoperfusion was in vogue, and this method of elimination is now no longer used in the routine management of patients. The same considerations also apply to hemodialysis; shortening of the duration of coma is rarely indicated because of the high standards of intensive supportive care that prevail in most hospitals; and in those in whom enhanced elimination would be desirable because of cardiovascular instability, hemodialysis is rarely practicable because of the additional risks involved. In the past, however, hemodialysis has been effective in removing barbiturates, carbromal, chloral hydrate, ethchlorvynol, glutethimide, meprobamate, methaqualone, and methyprylon. Although dialysis has been advocated for the treatment of benzodiazepine poisoning, its utility is doubtful from both pharmacokinetic and practical considerations, and its use for this purpose cannot be recommended. Hemodialysis has been shown not to be effective in removing zopiclone.[103]

The principal and most serious complications that may arise in sedative drug overdose are adult respiratory distress syndrome and acute renal failure. These often arise in the context of prolonged coma before arrival at a hospital and are complicated by pulmonary aspiration, hypoxemia, hypotension, and hypothermia. Their management in the context of sedative drug poisoning is no different from that when they occur in other settings of multiple organ failure.

DISPOSITION

Serious overdose with sedative drugs is complicated by coma, respiratory depression, and hypotension; and patients with one or more of these complications usually require management in an intensive care setting. After recovery of a patient from a deliberate self-ingestion of a sedative drug in overdose, the attending physician will wish to consider obtaining a psychiatric consultation for the patient before discharge. Uncomplicated sedative drug overdose is not usually accompanied by long-term physical sequelae.

References

1. Ashton H: Benzodiazepine withdrawal: An unfinished story. BMJ *288*:1135–1140, 1984.
2. Shader RI, Greenblatt DJ, Balter MB: Appropriate use and regulatory control of benzodiazepines. J Clin Pharmacol *31*:781–784, 1991.
3. Durand A, Thénot JP, Bianchetti G, Morselli PL: Comparative pharmacokinetic profile of two imidazopyridine drugs: Zolpidem and alpidem. Drug Metab Rev *24*:239–266, 1992.
4. Siehart W: Pharmacology of benzodiazepine receptors: An update. J Psychiatr Neurosci *19*:24–29, 1994.
5. Sanger DJ, Benavides J, Perrault G, et al: Recent developments in the behavioural pharmacology of the benzodiazepine (omega) receptors: Evidence for the functional significance of receptor subtypes. Neurosci Biobehav Rev *18*: 255–372, 1994.
6. Hales TG, Lambert JL: Modulation of $GABA_A$ and glycine receptors by chlormethiazole. Eur J Pharmacol *210*:239–246, 1992.
7. Peoples RW, Weight FF: Trichloroethanol potentiation of γ-aminobutyric acid–activated chloride current in mouse hippocampal neurones. Br J Pharmacol *113*:555–563, 1994.
8. Batjer HH: Cerebral protective effects of etomidate: Experimental data and clinical aspects. Cerebrovasc Brain Metab Rev *5*:17–32, 1993.
9. Green AR, Cross AJ: The neuroprotective actions of chlormethiazole. Prog Neurobiol *44*:463–484, 1994.
10. Depoortere H, Zivkovic B, Lloyd KG, et al: Zolpidem, a novel nonbenzodiazepine hypnotic: I. Neuropharmacological and behavioural effects. J Pharmacol Exp Ther *237*:649–658, 1986.
11. Trifiletti RR, Snyder SS: Anxiolytic cyclopyrrolones Zopiclone and Suriclone bind to a novel site linked allosterically to benzodiazepine receptors. Mol Pharmacol *26*:458–469, 1984.
12. Colburn WA, Jack ML: Relationships between CSF drug concentrations, receptor binding characteristics, and pharmacokinetic and pharmacodynamic properties of selected 1,4-substituted benzodiazepines. Clin Pharmacokinet *13*:179–190, 1987.
13. Laurijssens BE, Greenblatt DJ: Pharmacokinetic-pharmacodynamic relationships for benzodiazepines. Clin Pharmacokinet *30*:52–76, 1996.
14. Breimer DD: Clinical pharmacokinetics of hypnotics. Clin Pharmacokinet *2*:93–109, 1977.
15. Bauer TM, Ritz R, Haberthur C, et al: Prolonged sedation due to accumulation of conjugated metabolites of midazolam. Lancet *436*:145–147, 1995.
16. Kennedy KA, Fisher LJ: Quantitative and stereochemical aspects of glutethimide metabolism in humans. Drug Metab Dispos *7*:319–324, 1979.
17. Oram M, Wilson K, Burnett D, et al: Metabolic oxidation of methaqualone in extensive and poor metabolizers of debrisoquine. Eur J Clin Pharmacol *23*:147–150, 1982.
18. Gwilt PR, Pankaskie MC, Thornburg JE, et al: Pharmacokinetics of methyprylon following a single oral dose. J Pharm Sci *74*:1001–1003, 1985.
19. Contos DA, Dixon KF, Guthrie RM, et al: Nonlinear elimination of methyprylon (Noludar) in an overdose patient: Correlation of clinical effects with plasma concentration. J Pharm Sci *80*:768–771, 1991.
20. Sellers EM, Lang M, Koch-Weser J, et al: Interaction of

chloral hydrate and ethanol in man: I. Metabolism. Clin Pharmacol Ther *13*:37–49, 1971.

21. Dawborn JK, Turner A, Pattison G: Ethchlorvynol as a sedative in patients with renal failure. Med J Aust *2*:702–704, 1972.
22. Pentikäinen PJ, Neuvonen PJ, Jostell K-G: Pharmacokinetics of chlormethiazole in healthy volunteers and patients with cirrhosis of the liver. Eur J Clin Pharmacol *17*:275–284, 1980.
23. Köppel C, Kristinsson J, Wagemann A, et al: Chlormezanone plasma and blood levels in patients after single and repeated oral doses and after suicidal drug overdose. Eur J Drug Metab Pharmacokinet *16*:43–47, 1991.
24. Meyer MC, Melikian AP, Straughn AB: Relative bioavailability of meprobamate tablets in humans. J Pharm Sci *67*:1290–1293, 1978.
25. Olsen H, Koppang E, Alvan G, Mørland J: Carisoprodol elimination in humans. Ther Drug Monit *16*:337–340, 1994.
26. Kleber JW, Bechtol LD, Brunson MK, Chernish SM: GLC determination of ethinamate and its hydroxy derivative in biological fluids. J Pharm Sci *66*:992–994, 1977.
27. Florist AA, Judy RW: Comparative pharmacokinetics of chlorphenesin carbamate and methocarbamol in man. J Pharm Sci 60:1686–1688, 1971.
28. Strubelt O: Cardiotoxicity of bromoethylbutyramide (Carbromide). Arch Toxicol *40*:151–154, 1978.
29. Dawling S, Meredith TJ: Second generation anxiolytics and hypnotics. *In* Vale JA, Proudfoot AT, Meredith TJ (eds): The Oxford Textbook of Clinical Toxicology. Oxford, Oxford University Press (in press).
30. Goa KL, Heel RC: Zopiclone: A review of its pharmacodynamic and pharmacokinetic properties and therapeutic efficacy as an hypnotic. Drugs *32*:48–65, 1986.
31. Illingworth RN, Stewart MJ, Jarvie DR: Severe poisoning with chlormethiazole. BMJ *2*:902–903, 1979.
32. Proudfoot AT, Noble J, Nimmo J, et al: Peritoneal dialysis and haemodialysis in methaqualone (Mandrax) poisoning. Scot Med J *13*:232–239, 1968.
33. Decker WJ, Thompson HL, Arneson LA: Glutethimide rebound. Lancet *1*:778–779, 1970.
34. Houston A, Essex EG, Wiseman HM, Flanagan RJ: Acute chlormethiazole poisoning in patients notified to the Poisons Unit, Guy's Hospital, 1978–1981. Human Toxicol *2*:361–369, 1983.
35. Roy-Byrne PP, Hommer D: Benzodiazepine withdrawal: Overview and implications for the treatment of anxiety. JAMA 1988:*84*:1041–1052, 1988.
36. Fox R, Beeching NJ, Morrison C, et al: Misuse of temazepam. BMJ *305*:253, 1992.
37. Launchbury AP, Drake J, Seager H: Misuse of temazepam. BMJ *305*:252–253, 1992.
38. Aranko K, Henriksson M, Hublin C, Seppäläinen AM: Misuse of zopiclone and convulsions during withdrawal. Pharmacopsychiatry *24*:138–140, 1991.
39. Desmond DM, Schwanecke RP, Wilson GS, et al: Maternal barbiturate utilization and neonatal withdrawal symptomatology. J Pediatr *80*:190–197, 1972.
40. Reveri M, Pyati SP, Pildes RS: Neonatal withdrawal symptoms associated with glutethimide (Doriden) addiction in the mother during pregnancy. Clin Pediatr *16*:424–425, 1977.
41. Rumack BH, Walravens PA: Neonatal withdrawal following maternal ingestion of ethchlorvynol (Placidyl). Paediatrics *52*:714–716, 1973.
42. Krauer B, Draffan GH, Williams FM, et al: Elimination kinetics of amobarbital in mothers and their newborn infants. Clin Pharmacol Ther *14*:442–447, 1973.
43. Curry SH, Riddall D, Gordon JS, et al: Disposition of glutethimide in man. Clin Pharmacol Ther *12*:849–857, 1971.
44. Johnson RA: Adverse neonatal reaction to maternal administration of intravenous chlormethiazole and diazoxide. BMJ *1*:943, 1976.
45. Oswald I: Triazolam syndrome 10 years on. Lancet *2*:451–452, 1989.
46. Pies RW: Dose-related sensory distortions with zolpidem. J Clin Psychiatry *56*:35–36, 1995.
47. Häcki M: Amnestische Episoden nach einahme des hypnotikums Midazolam, Wirkung oder Nebenwirkung? Schweiz Med Wochenschr *116*:42–44, 1986.
48. Buckley NA, Whyte IA, Dawson AH, et al: Correlation between prescriptions and drugs taken in self-poisoning. Med J Aust *162*:194–197, 1995.
49. Meredith TJ, Vale JA: Epidemiology of analgesic overdose in England and Wales. Hum Toxicol *3*:61S–74S, 1984.
50. Henderson A, Wright M, Pond SM: Experience with 732 acute overdose patients admitted to an intensive care unit over six years. Med J Aust *158*:28–30, 1993.
51. Arieff AJ, Friedmann EA: Coma following non-narcotic drug overdose: Management of 208 adult patients. Am J Med Sci *266*:405, 1973.
52. Fuller GN, Rea AJ, Payne JF, Lant AF: Parasuicide in central London 1984–1988. J R Soc Med *82*:653–656, 1989.
53. Buckley NA, Whyte IA, Dawson AH, et al: Self-poisoning in Newcastle, 1987–1992. Med J Aust *162*:190–193, 1995.
54. McGrath J: A survey of deliberate self-poisoning. Med J Aust *150*:317–324, 1989.
55. Thomas SHL, Bevan L, Bhattacharyya S, et al: Presentation of poisoned patients to accident and emergency departments in the North of England. Hum Exp Toxicol *15*:466–470, 1996.
56. Finkle BS, McCloskey KL, Goodman LS: Diazepam and drug-associated deaths. JAMA *242*:429–434, 1979.
57. Kelly RC, Kent L, Sunshine I, Balter MB: Association of benzodiazepines with death in a major metropolitan area. J Anal Toxicol *6*:91–96, 1982.
58. Bailey DN, Shaw RF: Ethchlorvynol ingestion in San Diego county: A 14-year review of cases with blood concentration and findings. J Anal Toxicol *14*:348–352, 1990.
59. Greenblatt DJ, Allen MD, Harmatz JS, et al: Correlates of outcome following acute glutethimide overdosage. J Forens Sci *24*:76–86, 1979.
60. Buckley NA, Dawson AH, Whyte IM, O'Connell DL: Relative toxicity of benzodiazepines in overdose. BMJ *310*:219–221, 1995.
61. Hansen AR, Kennedy KA, Ambre JJ, Fischer LJ: Glutethimide poisoning: A metabolite contributes to morbidity and mortality. N Engl J Med *292*:250–252, 1975.
62. Curry SH, Hubbard JM, Gerkin R, et al: Lack of correlation between plasma 4-hydroxyglutethimide and severity of coma in acute glutethimide poisoning: A case report and brief review of the literature. Med Toxicol *2*:309–316, 1987.
63. Teehan BP, Maher JF, Carey JJH, et al: Acute ethchlorvynol (Placidyl) intoxication. Ann Intern Med *72*:875–882, 1970.
64. Reed CR, Glauser FL: Drug-induced noncardiogenic pulmonary edema. Chest *100*:1120–1124, 1991.
65. Glauser FL, Smith WR, Caldwell A, et al: Ethchlorvynol (Placidyl)-induced pulmonary edema. Ann Intern Med *84*:46–48, 1976.
66. Fischer P, Glauser FL, Millen JE, et al: The effects of ethchlorvynol on pulmonary alveolar membrane permeability. Am Rev Respir Med *116*:901–906, 1977.
67. Yagi K, Baudendistel LJ, Dahms TE: Ibuprofen reduces ethchlorvynol lung injury: Possible role of blood flow distribution. J Appl Physiol *72*:1156–1165, 1992.
68. Zanaboni PB, Bradley JD, Webster RO, Dahms TE: Cyclooxygenase inhibitors prevent ethchlorvynol-induced injury in rat and rabbit lungs. J Appl Physiol *71*:43–49, 1991.
69. Sheu B-S, Lin C-Y, Chen K-W, et al: Severe hepatocellular damage induced by chlormezanone overdose. Am J Gastroenterol *90*:833–835, 1995.
70. Köppel C, Kristinsson J, Wagemann A, et al: Chlormezanone plasma and blood levels in patients after single and repeated oral doses and after suicidal drug overdose. Eur J Drug Metab Pharmacokinet *16*:43–47, 1991.
71. McInnes GT: Chlormethiazole and alcohol: A lethal cocktail. BMJ *294*:592, 1987.
72. Robson DJ, Blow C, Gaines P, et al: Accumulation of chlormethiazole during intravenous infusion. Intensive Care Med *10*:315–316, 1984.
73. Lheureux P, Debailleul G, De Witte O, Askenasi R: Zolpidem intoxication mimicking narcotic overdose: Response to flumazenil. Hum Exp Toxicol *9*:105–107, 1990.

74. Tracqui A, Kintz P, Mangin P: A fatality involving two unusual compounds—zolpidem and acepromazine. Am J Forens Med Pathol *14*:309–312, 1993.
75. Desager JP, Hulhoven R, Harvengt C, et al: Possible interactions between zolpidem, a new sleep inducer, and chlorpromazine, a phenothiazine neuroleptic. Psychopharmacology *96*:63–66, 1988.
76. Garnier R, Guerault E, Muzard D, et al: Acute zolpidem poisoning—analysis of 344 cases. Clin Toxicol *32*:391–404, 1994.
77. Royer-Morrot MJ, Bauer PH, Royer RJ: Determination of zopiclone in plasma using column liquid chromatography with ultra-violet detection. J Chromatogr *581*:297–299, 1992.
78. Ahmad Z, Herepath M, Ebden P: Diagnostic utility of flumazenil in coma with suspected poisoning. BMJ *302*:292, 1991.
79. Regouby Y, Delomez G, Tisserant A: First-degree heart block caused by voluntary zopiclone poisoning. Therapie *45*:162, 1990.
80. Pounder DJ, Davies JI: Zopiclone poisoning: Tissue distribution and potential for postmortem diffusion. Forensic Sci Int *65*:177–183, 1994.
81. Boniface PJ, Martin IC, Nolan SL, To Tan S: Development of a method for the determination of zopiclone in whole blood. J Chromatogr *584*:199–206, 1992.
82. Ashton CH: Benzodiazepine overdose: Are specific antagonists useful? BMJ *290*:805–806, 1985.
83. Amrein R, Leishman B, Bentzinger C, Roncari G: Flumazenil in benzodiazepine antagonism: Actions and clinical use in intoxications and anaesthesiology. Med Toxicol *2*:411–419, 1987.
84. Hoffman EJ, Warren EW: Flumazenil: A benzodiazepine antagonist. Clin Pharm *12*:641–656, 1993.
85. Sugarman JM, Paul RI: Flumazenil: A review. Pediatr Emerg Care *10*:37–43, 1994.
86. Hofer P, Scollo-Lavizzari G: Benzodiazepine antagonist RO 15-1788 in self-poisoning: Diagnostic and therapeutic use. Arch Intern Med *145*:663–664, 1985.
87. O'Sullivan GF, Wade DN: Flumazenil in the management of acute drug overdosage with benzodiazepines and other drugs. Clin Pharmacol Ther *42*:254–259, 1987.
88. Knudsen L, Lonka L, Sorensen BH, et al: Benzodiazepine intoxication treated with flumazenil (Anexate, RO 15-1788). Anaesthesia *43*:274–276, 1988.
89. Höjer J, Baehrendtz S, Matell G, Gustafsson LL: Diagnostic utility of flumazenil in coma with suspected poisoning: A double blind, randomised controlled study. BMJ *301*:1308–1311, 1990.
90. Mora CT, Torjman M, White PF: Effects of diazepam and flumazenil on sedation and hypnotic ventilatory response. Anaesth Analg *68*:473–478, 1989.
91. Gross JB, Weller RS, Conard P: Flumazenil antagonism of midazolam induced ventilatory depression. Anaesthesiology *75*:179–185, 1991.
92. Donovan KL, Fisher DJ: Reversal of chloral hydrate overdose with flumazenil. BMJ *298*:1253, 1989.
93. Lheureux P, Askenasi R: Efficacy of flumazenil in acute alcohol intoxication: Double blind placebo controlled evaluation. Hum Exp Toxicol *10*:235–239, 1991.
94. Burr W, Sandham P, Judd A: Death after flumazenil. BMJ *298*:1713, 1989.
95. Short TG, Maling T, Galletly DC: Ventricular arrhythmia precipitated by flumazenil. BMJ *296*:1070–1071, 1988.
96. Herd B, Clark F: Complete heart block after flumazenil. Hum Exp Toxicol *10*:289, 1991.
97. Depoortere H, Zivkovic B, Lloyd KG, et al: Zolpidem, a novel nonbenzodiazepine hypnotic: I Neuropharmacological and behavioural effects. J Pharmacol Exp Ther *237*:649–658, 1986.
98. Patat A, Naef MM, van Gessel E, et al: Flumazenil antagonizes the central effects of zolpidem, an imidazopyridine hypnotic. Clin Pharmacol Ther *56*:430–436, 1994.
99. Singh K, Erickson T, Amitai Y, Hryhorczuk D: Chloral hydrate toxicity from oral and intravenous administration. J Toxicol Clin Toxicol *34*:101–106, 1996.
100. Graham SR, Day RO, Lee R, Fulde GWO: Overdose with chloral hydrate: A pharmacological and therapeutic review. Med J Aust *149*:686–688, 1988.
101. Brown AM, Cade JF: Cardiac arrhythmias after chloral hydrate overdose. Med J Aust *1*:28–29, 1980.
102. Hassan E. Treatment of meprobamate overdose with repeated oral doses of activated charcoal. Ann Emerg Med *15*:73–76, 1986.
103. Marc-Aurele J, Caille G, Bourgoin J: Comparison of zopiclone pharmacokinetics in patients with impaired renal function and normal subjects: Effect of hemodialysis. Sleep *10*(Suppl 1):22–26, 1987.
104. Dawling S, Volans G: Poisons. *In* Noe DA, Rock RC (eds): Laboratory Medicine: The Selection and Interpretation of Clinical Laboratory Studies. Baltimore, Williams & Wilkins, pp 580–617, 1994.

44

Benzodiazepines

SUSAN E. FARRELL, MD
JAMES R. ROBERTS, MD

The first commercially marketed benzodiazepine was accidentally synthesized in 1955 by Roche Laboratories in Nutley, New Jersey, but the scope of its pharmacologic properties and its clinical applications were not appreciated until 1957.[1] That drug, chlordiazepoxide (Librium), was noted to possess clinically effective sedative, hypnotic, and anticonvulsant properties. When it became available in 1960, it ushered in an era of widespread benzodiazepine use that persists today. Diazepam, perhaps the best known and most commercially successful of all the benzodiazepines, was synthesized in 1959 and marketed as Valium in 1963. Since that time, more than 3000 benzodiazepines have been developed, over 120 have been tested for biologic activity, and approximately 50 different benzodiazepines are currently marketed worldwide. Thirteen benzodiazepines are approved for use in the United States (Table 44–1).

Benzodiazepines have various sedative, hypnotic, amnestic, anxiolytic, anticonvulsant, and muscle relaxant properties. Current evidence indicates that all benzodiazepines are effective for the treatment of anxiety and insomnia. However, individual drugs are approved by the Food and Drug Administration and marketed for specific indications on the basis of their clinical and pharmacologic characteristics. For example, alprazolam may have significant antidepressant activity in addition to its sedative properties. Benzodiazepines such as alprazolam and particularly clonazepam have gained use in the treatment of social phobias and panic disorders,[2] and clonazepam and lorazepam may be effective in place of or in combination with a neuroleptic and lithium for the treatment of acute mania in bipolar disorder.[3] Reports also describe the efficacy of benzodiazepines for the initial treatment of catatonia[4] and neuroleptic-induced dystonias.[5] In addition, short-acting benzodiazepines such as temazepam and triazolam have found new uses in the prevention and treatment of jet lag.[6] Their action is presumed to be through the readjustment of sleep patterns and body temperature, and they shorten the time to resynchronize activity rhythms when used in conjunction with regular exercise. In the past several years, certain benzodiazepines have also been reported to be of benefit in the treatment of pain syndromes,[7] by both decreasing situational anxiety in acute pain and relieving anxiety and muscle tension related to some chronic musculoskeletal pain syndromes. Finally, benzodiazepines are also finding greater use in the treatment of patients with cancer, for the relief of anticipatory anxiety and nausea, insomnia, chemotherapy-induced emesis, neuralgias, and psychiatric disorders secondary to use of high-dose steroids.[8] Although not currently in clinical use, one benzodiazepine derivative, R016-0521, has been found to inhibit cholesterol absorption in human studies of hypercholesterolemia.[9]

Since their introduction, the benzodiazepines have enjoyed a meteoric rise in popularity and have largely replaced other sedative-hypnotics. Their extraordinary acceptance in clinical medicine has been based on their safety, efficacy, minimal side effects, relatively low addiction potential, and the medical and public demand for sedative and anxiolytic agents. It is no surprise, therefore, that benzodiazepines are the most widely prescribed class of psychoactive drugs in current therapeutic use in the world. It is estimated that at least 15% of the adult population in the western world ingests a benzodiazepine at least once a year. In 1979, the United States National Household survey revealed that 11% of the adult population in the United States had taken an anxiolytic on one or more occasions in the previous year.[10] Since that time, the annual prevalence of use of benzodiazepine anxiolytics has declined from 13% in

Table 44–1. Benzodiazepines Available in the United States

Generic Name	Trade Name	Year of Introduction	Recommended Adult Dose*	Available Dosage Forms	FDA-Approved Indications	Rate of Oral Absorption
Alprazolam	Xanax	1981	Oral: 0.75–4 mg/d divided t.i.d.	0.25, 0.5, 1 mg tablets	Anxiety Anxious depression	Intermediate
Chlordiazepoxide	Librium	1960	Oral: 15–100 mg/d divided t.i.d. to q.i.d.	5, 10, 25 mg tablets or capsules	Alcohol withdrawal Anxiety Preoperative sedation	Intermediate
Clonazepam	Klonopin	1974	Oral: 7.5–20 mg/d divided t.i.d.	0.5, 1, 2 mg tablets	Seizure disorder	Intermediate
Clorazepate	Tranxene	1972	Oral: 7.5–60 mg/d divided qd to q.i.d.	2.75, 7.5, 15 mg capsules	Anxiety Alcohol withdrawal	Rapid
Diazepam	Valium	1963	Oral: 6–40 mg/d divided qd to q.i.d. IV: 0.1 mg/kg per dose	2, 5, 10 mg tablets	Anxiety/insomnia Alcohol withdrawal Muscle spasm/ seizures Preoperative sedation	Rapid
Flurazepam	Dalmane	1970	Oral: 15–30 mg/ d h.s.	15, 30 mg capsules	Insomnia	Rapid
Halazepam	Paxipam	1981	Oral: 80–160 mg/d divided t.i.d. to q.i.d.	20, 40 mg capsules	Anxiety	Intermediate to slow
Lorazepam	Ativan	1977	Oral: 1–10 mg/d divided b.i.d. to t.i.d. IM: 0.5 mg/kg IV: 0.05 mg/kg	0.5, 1, 2 mg tablets	Anxiety/insomnia Anxious depression Preoperative sedation	Intermediate
Midazolam	Versed	1986	Oral: not available IM: 0.07–0.08 mg/kg IV: Begin 1–2.5 mg, titrate to effect		Preoperative sedation Anesthesia induction Conscious sedation	Rapid†
Oxazepam	Serax	1963	Oral: 30–120 mg/d divided t.i.d. to q.i.d.	10, 15, 30 mg capsules 15 mg tablets	Anxiety Alcohol withdrawal Anxious depression	Slow
Prazepam	Centrax	1977	Oral: 20–60 mg/ d divided b.i.d.	5, 10 mg capsules 10 mg tablets	Anxiety	Ultraslow
Temazepam	Restoril	1981	Oral: 15–30 mg q h.s.	15, 30 mg capsules	Insomnia	Slow
Triazolam	Halcion	1983	Oral: 0.125–0.5 mg q h.s.	0.125, 0.25, 0.5 mg capsules	Insomnia	Intermediate

IV, intravenously.
*Maximum dose not established.
†Oral form of midazolam is not yet commercially available.

1981 to 8.3% in 1990.[11] This decline has largely been attributed to widespread negative publicity and concern about their potential misuse, abuse, and long-term side effects. Regardless of this decline, in 1990 in the United States, one in four users had been regularly taking benzodiazepines for 1 year or longer.

Because of their widespread availability, benzodiazepines are also among the most frequently misused drugs. Many investigators, however, emphasize that dependence and abuse by the general population are largely overstated by the media and are minor compared with alcohol, cocaine, or opiate abuse. As a class, benzodiazepines are not powerful euphoriants and are therefore not frequently abused primarily. Secondary drug abuse is common, however, usually in the form of self-medication to decrease the adverse side effects of stimulants or hallucinogens, to ameliorate the unpleasant symptoms of withdrawal from more highly addictive substances, or to substitute for the drug of primary dependence when it is not available.

Studies show that benzodiazepines are increasingly used by intravenous drug abusers. The United States Treatment Outcome prospective study reported that 73% of heroin abusers also used benzodiazepines on their entry into treatment.[12] This combination of intravenous drug use and benzodiazepine abuse has been correlated with increased incidence of needle sharing, polydrug use, psychosocial dysfunction, depression, anxiety, and poor health.[12] In addition, their availability in the general population has been accompanied by an increased incidence of overdose of the benzodiazepines, particularly diazepam.

In an attempt to limit such widespread availability and the incidence of misuse and abuse, various laws regulating the prescribing of benzodiazepines have been enacted. The resultant effects have become a source of some controversy in the past 5 years. On January 1, 1989, the state of New York enacted a regulation that required prescriptions for benzodiazepines to be written in triplicate, with mandatory reporting of prescriptions to the New York State Department of Health. The purpose of the regulation was to decrease improper prescribing practices in an attempt to restrict overall use of benzodiazepines and to help eliminate fraud and illegal misdirection of the drugs. Mcnutt and colleagues reported the effect of this regulation on an elderly population during the ensuing year.[13] The number of patients using benzodiazepines was reduced by 33%, and the number of prescriptions written was reduced by 45%. However, these changes were accompanied by an increase in number of prescriptions for other miscellaneous anxiolytics, including meprobamate, chloral hydrate, and antidepressants. Schwartz and Blank[14, 15] also reported on the effects of this regulation, noting a decrease of benzodiazepine prescriptions by about 2 million, accompanied by the aforementioned increase in other anxiolytics. According to a 1991 Gallup poll of 200 physicians in New York, approximately 50% had decreased their prescribing of this class of drugs. Schwartz also noted that during the first 3 months after enactment, approximately 50% of patient visits to an urban psychiatric emergency department and clinic were related to the new law, as either a recurrence of previously controlled symptoms or acute withdrawal secondary to inavailability of benzodiazepines. Of note are the statistics of increased sales of distilled spirits during the first 4 months after the law was implemented. Similar findings have been reported in European studies,[16] noting the increase in prescriptions for alternative psychoactive drugs, as the prescribing of benzodiazepines declines. These studies have been followed by reports assessing various strategies for cutting benzodiazepine use in general practice[17] and the resultant reduction in use of outpatient medical and mental health facilities by patients who have been successfully detoxified from benzodiazepines.

In summary, although benzodiazepines are remarkably safe compared with older sedative-hypnotics, their slim yet possible potential for addiction and abuse is still a matter of medical and legal controversy.

STRUCTURE

The benzodiazepines are organic bases (Figs. 44–1 and 44–2). All benzodiazepines share a structure composed of the benzene ring fused to a seven-membered diazepine ring. All of the important benzodiazepines have a 5-aryl substituent and various substitutions at the R1 and R4 positions of the diazepine ring. The aryl ring at position R5 confers greater potency of the molecule. Specific benzodiazepine agonists are formed by varying the substitutions at the R1, R2, R3, R4, R7, and R2′ positions. Substitutions at the R5 and R4 positions are structural features of the benzodiazepine antagonist flumazenil. Despite the myriad benzodiazepine compounds available, all derivatives can be expected to have similar qualitative pharmacologic and clinical effects when adjusted for differences in potency. However, various compounds have significant differences in onset and duration of action and metabolism, and these differences theoretically make them more suitable for certain indications.

PHARMACOKINETICS

Absorption

Although some benzodiazepines form water-soluble salts at acidic pH, at physiologic pH all are moderately to highly lipid-soluble molecules that are rapidly and completely absorbed from the proximal small bowel (Table 44–2). Significant differences in lipid solubility affect the rate of gastrointestinal (GI) absorption and subsequent distribution. Highly lipophilic benzodiazepines (diazepam, flurazepam, midazolam) are rapidly absorbed, and less lipophilic compounds (oxazepam, temazepam) are more slowly absorbed.

The parent forms of two benzodiazepines, clorazepate and prazepam, do not reach the systemic circulation in clinically significant amounts. The active metabolite is formed in the GI tract or liver before systemic absorption and appears in the serum as desmethyldiazepam. Desmethyldiazepam is rapidly formed from clorazepate after acid hydrolysis within the stomach. However, this metabolic conversion may be prevented by the presence of antacids in the stomach.[18] Prazepam is slowly converted to desmethyldiazepam after first-pass metabolism in the liver.

The rate of oral absorption may be influenced by several factors other than lipid solubility. Absorption is enhanced by taking the drugs on an empty stomach or by coingestion of alcohol[19] and is slowed by coadministration of food or aluminum- or magnesium hydroxide–containing antacids. The presence of antacids during ingestion impairs the rate but not the extent of absorption.[18] Absorption also may be altered by manipulating the pharmaceutical preparation, such as slow-release diazepam (Valium CR). The "lag time" between ingestion and appearance in the systemic circulation is secondary to dissolution in the

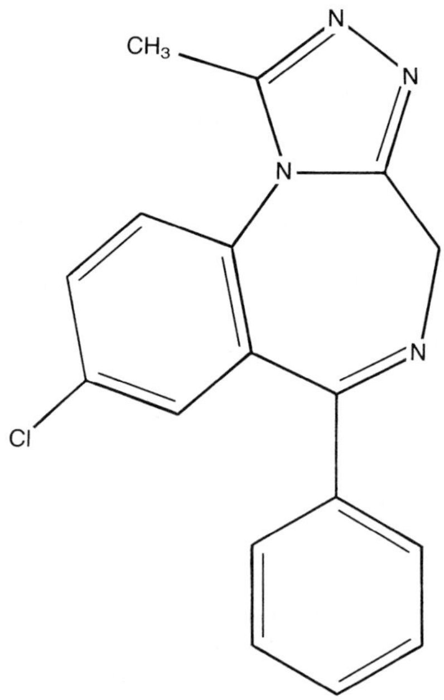

alprazolam (Xanax)

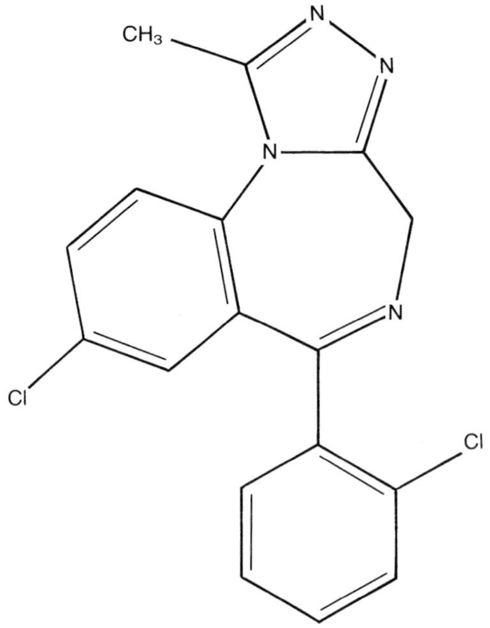

triazolam (Halcion)

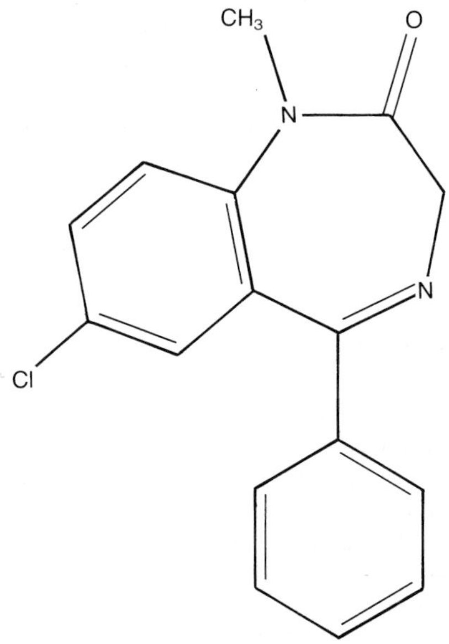

diazepam (Valium)

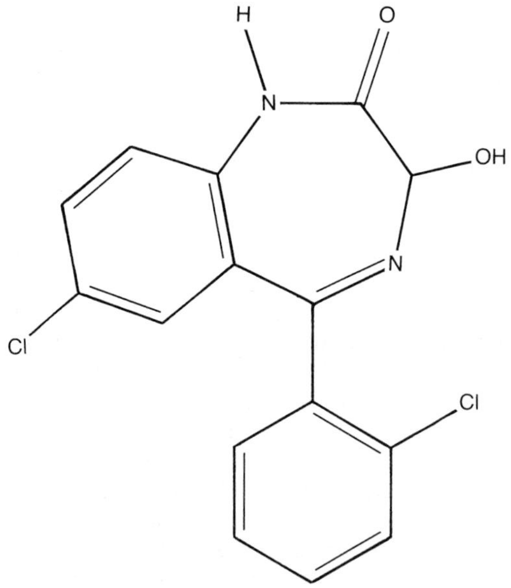

lorazepam (Ativan)

Figure 44–1. The four most prescribed benzodiazepines in the United States.

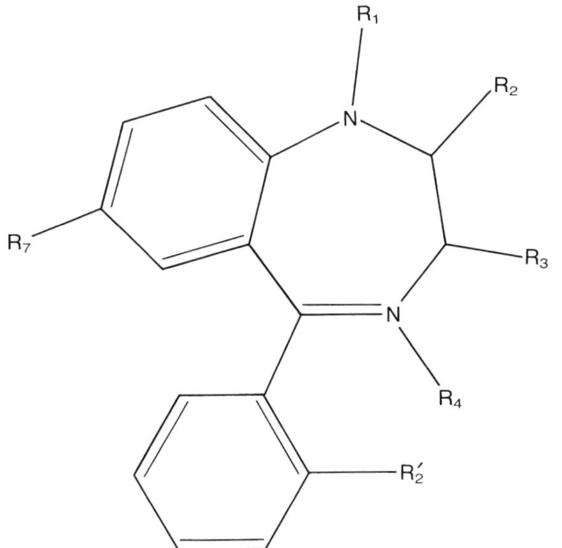

Figure 44–2. The general chemical structure of benzodiazepines.

stomach, passage to the small bowel, absorption from the GI tract, and passage from the portal to systemic circulation. Depending on the drug preparation and the presence of coingestants, this time is approximately 10 to 20 minutes. In general, the time to maximal serum concentration (T_{max}) is inversely proportional to the maximal serum concentration (C_{max}) and may be influenced by the aforementioned factors.[20]

Benzodiazepine absorption from intramuscular injection is variable. Lorazepam and midazolam are the only benzodiazepines adequately absorbed after intramuscular administration. Chlordiazepoxide absorption is particularly slow and erratic, and plasma concentration may not peak for 6 to 12 hours. Diazepam is inconsistently absorbed after intramuscular administration. Serum levels of both chlordiazepoxide and diazepam are more rapidly achieved by the oral route than by intramuscular administration.

After absorption, benzodiazepines are more than 70% protein bound, but the degree of protein binding varies significantly. Protein binding is greatest with diazepam (99%) and least with alprazolam (70%). Only unbound drug is available to cross the blood-brain barrier and interact at central nervous system (CNS) receptors. Drug concentrations in the cerebrospinal fluid are generally 2% to 4% of plasma levels, or roughly parallel to the concentration of free drug in the plasma. Increased protein binding decreases the concentration of free drug in equilibrium with sites of action and elimination. Hypoalbuminemia increases the concentration of active drug and may increase clinical effects. There is little or no glomerular filtration of protein-bound benzodiazepines.

After GI absorption or intravenous administration, benzodiazepines are rapidly distributed to highly perfused organs, particularly the CNS. All benzodiazepines are widely distributed, and tissue concentrations within the brain, liver, and spleen typically exceed that of the serum. The volume of distribution of various benzodiazepines ranges from 0.3 to 5.5 L/kg. Benzodiazepines are lipophilic and quickly penetrate the blood-brain barrier via passive diffusion to reach their sites of action within the CNS. Because penetration into the CNS is rapid, the onset of clinical effects is limited more by the rate of systemic absorption of individual compounds than by their rate of distribution.

Pharmacologically, the serum and CNS are termed the *central compartment* of drug distribution. After initial distribution within this compartment, benzodiazepines are slowly redistributed to more poorly perfused sites (such as adipose tissue and muscle), collectively termed the *peripheral compartment.* Therefore, highly lipid-soluble benzodiazepines distribute more quickly and have a more rapid CNS effect. They then undergo more rapid and extensive redistribution and, thus, termination of that effect.

Duration of Action

Benzodiazepine activity is terminated by at least three mechanisms. Two of these are pharmacokinetic, and the third involves a functional change of the benzodiazepine receptor. The rate of redistribution of drug from the central compartment (CNS) to the peripheral compartment is the most important determinant of duration of clinical effect. The second mechanism responsible for the duration of action is hepatic metabolism and renal excretion. The third mechanism is *acute tolerance* or *acute adaptation,* terms used to describe the clinical observation that

Table 44–2. Absorption Rates of Orally Administered Benzodiazepines

	Time of Peak Plasma Concentration
Rapid	<1.2 h
Desmethyldiazepam (from clorazepate [Tranxene])	
Diazepam (Valium)	
Flurazepam (Dalmane)	
Midazolam* (Versed)	
Intermediate	1.2–2.0 h
Alprazolam (Xanax)	
Chlordiazepoxide (Librium)	
Clonazepam (Klonopin)	
Halazepam (Paxipam)	
Lorazepam (Ativan)	
Triazolam (Halcion)	
Slow	2.0–3.0 h
Oxazepam (Serax)	
Temazepam (Restoril)	
Ultraslow	>3.0
Desmethyldiazepam (from prazepam [Centrax])	
Diazepam CR (slow release)	

*Oral form of midazolam not yet commercially available.

benzodiazepine receptors appear to become less sensitive to drug effects with continued exposure.

Redistribution

It may seem paradoxical that a drug's measured plasma half-life does not predict its duration of action, but such is the case with benzodiazepines. The duration of action of benzodiazepines is a function of the CNS elimination half-life. During single-dose administration, the most lipophilic benzodiazepines have the shortest duration of action in the CNS because they are rapidly and extensively redistributed. They have the longest calculated plasma half-lives after redistribution because they remain in clinically inactive peripheral storage compartments (fat, muscle) for prolonged periods. Drugs that are less lipophilic have shorter plasma half-lives yet a longer duration of action, because redistribution from the CNS to the peripheral compartment is more limited and occurs more slowly. The rapid egress of highly lipid-soluble benzodiazepines from the central compartment results in a shorter duration of action than their respective plasma half-lives might suggest. This is illustrated by comparing the clinical anticonvulsant activity of lorazepam and diazepam. Lorazepam (half-life, 10 to 20 hours), a drug of relatively low lipophilicity, has more prolonged antiseizure activity than the highly lipophilic diazepam (half-life, 20 to 70 hours). The benzodiazepine midazolam is extremely lipophilic and is rapidly biotransformed by the liver. It has an extremely short duration of action because both redistribution and metabolism contribute significantly to the termination of clinical effects and plasma clearance (Table 44–3).

During prolonged administration or repeated dosing, the plasma half-life is a more reliable predictor of response to the highly lipophilic agents. Repeated doses of the lipid-soluble benzodiazepines cause the eventual saturation of peripheral fat stores during redistribution. As they become saturated, the concentration gradient from plasma to peripheral lipid compartment decreases, thus increasing the drug concentration and duration of action at the CNS receptor site. In addition, the lipid stores act as a depot for leaching out of the drug and its active metabolites, further prolonging the persistence of drug plasma concentrations.[18] In general, the longer the elimination half-life, the greater the accumulation after multiple doses, the longer the "washout" after termination of multiple-dose therapy, and the less likely the occurrence of rebound side effects.[20]

Table 44–3. Classification of Benzodiazepines According to Plasma Half-Life

Short	
Flurazepam (Dalmane)	1–4 h
Midazolam (Versed)	2–5 h
Triazolam (Halcion)	2–6 h
Intermediate	
Alprazolam (Xanax)	6–20 h
Chlordiazepoxide (Librium)	5–20 h
Halazepam (Paxipam)	10–20 h
Lorazepam (Ativan)	10–20 h
Oxazepam (Serax)	5–15 h
Temazepam (Restoril)	5–20 h
Long	
Clonazepam (Klonopin)	20–30 h
Diazepam (Valium)	20–70 h
Very Long	
Clorazepate† (Tranxene)	30–200 h
Desalkylflurazepam*	45–300 h
Desmethyldiazepam*	30–200 h
Prazepam† (Centrax)	30–200 h

*Active metabolite of primary benzodiazepine compounds.
†Prodrug or drug precursor that does not reach the system circulation in clinically significant amounts. Compounds are metabolized in the gastrointestinal tract or liver before systemic absorption and appear in the serum as desmethyldiazepam.

Metabolism

Hepatic biotransformation via oxidation or conjugation accounts for virtually all benzodiazepine metabolism and clearance in humans (Fig. 44–3). Hepatic metabolism can be divided into two phases: Phase I metabolism consists of oxidative pathways, either aliphatic hydroxylation by the cytochrome P-450 enzyme system or *N*-dealkylation. Phase I biotransformation produces pharmacologically active metabolites or intermediates. Phase II metabolism consists of hepatic conjugation of hydroxyl and amino groups to form inactive glucuronides, sulfates, and acetylated compounds that are rapidly excreted in the urine. Hepatic metabolism differs among benzodiazepines, and compounds may undergo both phase I and phase II metabolism (diazepam, chlordiazepoxide, flurazepam, halazepam, clorazepate, prazepam, triazolam, alprazolam, midazolam, and clonazepam) or only phase II metabolism (lorazepam, oxazepam, and temazepam).

Phase I oxidation is termed a *susceptible pathway* because the rate of activity may be altered by several factors. Phase I metabolism is inhibited or decreased by increasing age, pre-existing liver disease (including cirrhosis or hepatitis), or coadministration of estrogens, isoniazid, disulfiram, phenytoin, alcohol, or cimetidine. Phase I metabolism is stimulated or induced by cigarette smoking or by long-term administration of substances that induce the cytochrome P-450 system, such as phenobarbital and alcohol. Benzodiazepines are very weak inducers of hepatic microsomal systems and do not significantly alter their own metabolism. Phase II conjugation is considered a *non-susceptible pathway* because those factors that alter benzodiazepine oxidation usually have little or no effect on conjugation.

Studies of benzodiazepines that undergo strictly phase II metabolism reveal various pharmacokinetic data in patients with cirrhosis.[18, 20] In general, however, dose adjustment is not usually necessary for

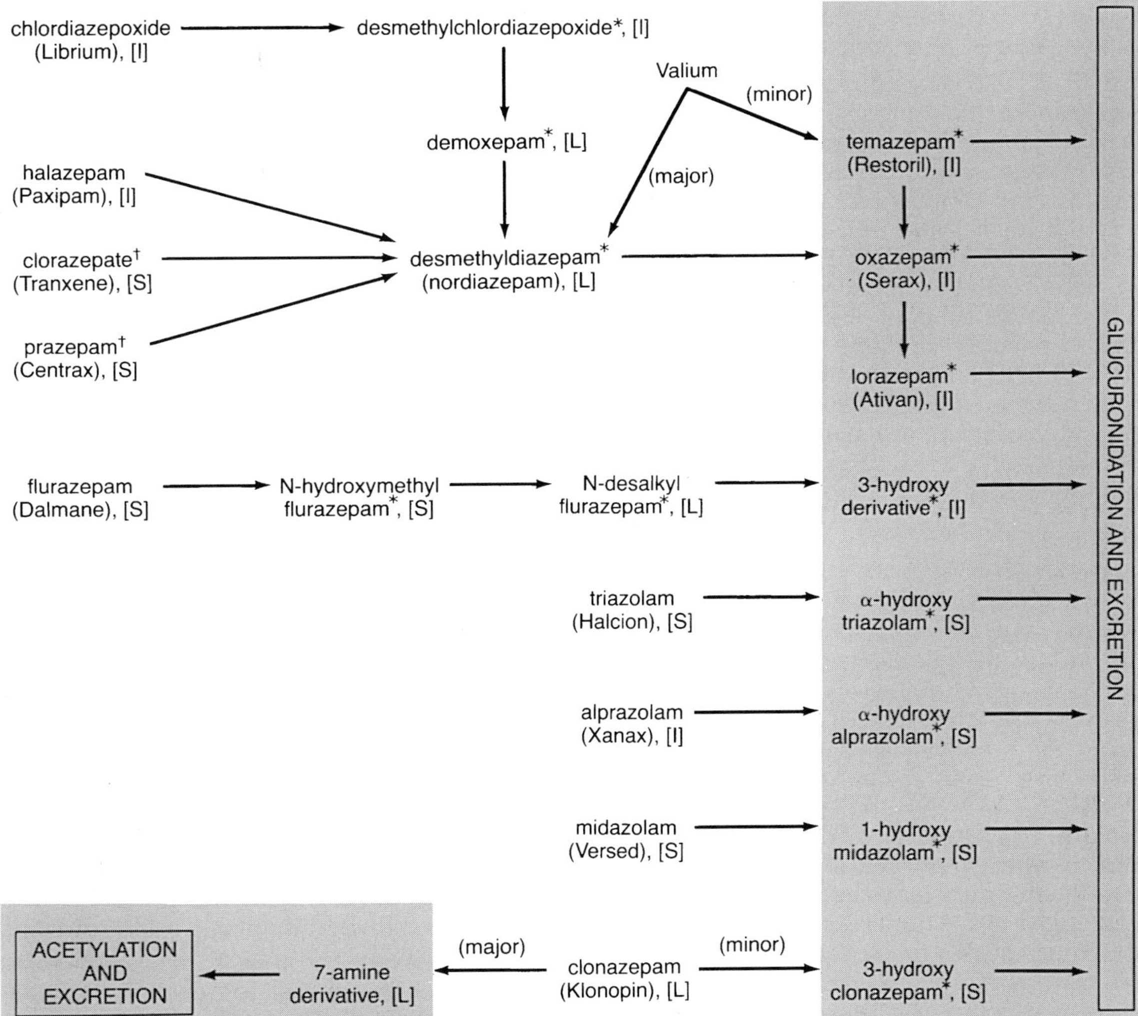

Figure 44–3. Major metabolic pathways of benzodiazepines approved for use in the United States. [S], conversion half-life of less than 6 hours; [I], conversion half-life of 6 to 20 hours; [L], conversion half-life of greater than 20 hours; *, active metabolite; †, prodrug or drug precursor, which does not reach the systemic circulation in clinically significant amounts. Shaded areas denote processes that proceed via phase II metabolism.

those agents that are biotransformed by glucuronidation alone (temazepam, lorazepam, oxazepam). Conversely, agents that undergo multiple biotransformation reactions via the P-450 system (diazepam, chlordiazepoxide) may accumulate in cirrhotic patients secondary to increased volumes of distribution, decreased protein binding, prolonged half-life, and decreased clearance.[18] Because the therapeutic indices of all benzodiazepines are very large, it is unclear whether the effects of higher blood concentrations resulting from decreased metabolism are clinically significant. In one study, Kroboth and colleagues demonstrated no significant difference in psychomotor function in cirrhotic patients after single doses of adinazolam but concluded that there is potential for accumulation after multiple doses.[101]

Similarly, elderly patients with decreased capacity for hepatic oxidative metabolism, hypoalbuminemia, and diminished glomerular filtration rate are at risk for complications secondary to benzodiazepine accumulation. In these subgroups of patients, short-acting, nonaccumulating agents that undergo few hepatic manipulations and have few active metabolites would be the benzodiazepines of choice.

Several benzodiazepines are biotransformed to active metabolites that contribute to their pharmacologic activity. In some cases, the metabolites possess half-lives that far exceed those of the parent compound. In such instances, persistent clinical effects are more likely a consequence of the metabolic products than of the parent compound itself. The activity of the metabolite depends on its blood concentration, its lipophilicity, and its affinity for the benzodiazepine receptor. Flurazepam has a plasma metabolic half-life of 1 to 4 hours, but its pharmacologically active metabolite, desalkylflurazepam, has a serum half-life of 45 to 300 hours. The primary metabolite of diazepam, desmethyldiazepam, is also pharmacologically active, and its half-life exceeds that of diazepam.

Excretion

Elimination of benzodiazepine metabolites occurs via renal clearance. In patients with decreased renal blood flow or decreased glomerular filtration rate, this process is diminished. Certain drugs may also inhibit this process. Golden and colleagues studied the effect of probenecid on renal tubule secretion of *N*-desmethyladinazolam (NDMAD), the active metabolite of adinazolam, a triazolobenzodiazepine.[102] Probenecid inhibits tubular secretion of organic bases, and in this study probenecid decreased renal clearance of NDMAD and increased maximal plasma concentrations of both NDMAD and adinazolam. The effect was a decrease in psychomotor skill performance in healthy volunteers, presumed to be secondary to accumulation of the active metabolite.

Tolerance

Tolerance develops rapidly to the sedative effects of benzodiazepines. It has been reported for nearly all of the effects of benzodiazepines, although the effect on anxiolytic properties is limited. Several studies have been performed to evaluate the mechanism of tolerance. Some researchers mention the presence of a "reverse hysteresis loop" for certain benzodiazepines.[18] During the short term, these drugs seem to cause less mental impairment over the course of hours, although plasma concentrations remain unchanged or even increase. Whether this is a matter of pharmacodynamics and redistribution or a change in central receptor kinetics and adaptation is unclear. During long-term therapy, there may be an actual down-regulation of the γ-aminobutyric acid (GABA) receptors, where benzodiazepines have their effect. This has been hypothesized to occur as a result of a change in the number of receptors or a change in receptor affinity.

The effect of tolerance at the receptor level has been studied in mouse models by Miller.[21] Mice that received doses of lorazepam to maintain a constant brain and plasma drug concentration developed behavioral tolerance within 1 week. After 1 week, benzodiazepine-receptor binding and $GABA_A$ function were decreased in various areas of the cerebral cortex, consistent with down-regulation of the receptors. Four days after discontinuation of lorazepam, drug concentrations in the brain and plasma were undetectable. This finding was accompanied by an increase in motor activity, receptor binding, and function, consistent with up-regulation. These findings were duplicated with alprazolam and clonazepam. In further studies, the researchers again induced tolerance to the effects of lorazepam in mice. Fourteen days after the initiation of drug therapy, levels of mRNA for subunits of the $GABA_A$/benzodiazepine receptor were markedly decreased in the cortex, and these diminished levels persisted, consistent with decreased receptor synthesis during chronic benzodiazepine administration.

In other studies of tolerance and its prevention, Miller and Koff were able to attenuate the tolerance effects of chronic lorazepam in mice.[22] By concomitant administration of a benzodiazepine antagonist with lorazepam, they limited behavioral tolerance and reversed lorazepam-induced neurochemical effects of down-regulation of the $GABA_A$ receptor in some areas of the brain.

The incidence of tolerance is unclear. In one retrospective study of 191 patients receiving long-term benzodiazepine therapy, 92% had had no increase in their dose of benzodiazepine for a mean of 5.6 years.[23] However, the development of tolerance to these medications may limit their utility as sedatives, anticonvulsants, and anxiolytics. Interventions to prevent or reduce tolerance are under study and consist of intermittent dosing, tapering schedules, use of benzodiazepine antagonists, or coadministration of anticonvulsants.[22]

MECHANISM OF ACTION

Benzodiazepines produce their sedative, hypnotic, anxiolytic, and anticonvulsant effects through their ability to potentiate the activity of GABA. GABA is the major inhibitory neurotransmitter in the CNS; it is involved in sleep induction and in control of neuronal excitation and epileptic potentials, anxiety, memory, and hypnosis. GABA is found in highest concentrations in the basal ganglia, hippocampus, cerebellum, hypothalamus, and substantia gelatinosa of the dorsal horn of the spinal cord.[24] GABA acts at two receptors: $GABA_A$, which is also the site of most benzodiazepine action, and $GABA_B$, which is presynaptically involved in autofeedback and postsynaptically involved in control of spasticity in the dorsal horns of the spinal cord.

When GABA binds to the $GABA_A$ receptor, it causes an influx of chloride through a ligand-gated ion channel that is part of the receptor complex in the neuronal membrane (Fig. 44–4). This influx of chloride hyperpolarizes the cell and thus inhibits its excitation. It is at this receptor complex that benzodiazepines exert their effect. The binding of benzodiazepines to their site on the receptor complex facilitates the binding of GABA on its site and increases the frequency of chloride channel opening, thus increasing the hyperpolarized state of the cell. In this way, benzodiazepines potentiate the inhibitory effect of GABA.

Benzodiazepine receptors have been categorized on the basis of their location in the CNS, their relationship to the $GABA_A$ receptor, and their pharmacologic effects. Type I receptors are located throughout the brain, especially in the cerebellum, and are involved in anxiolytic effects. Type II receptors have been found in the cerebral cortex, hippocampus, and spinal cord and may be responsible for sedative and hypnotic effects. Research has also identified a *peripheral benzodiazepine receptor,* named for its location on the outer membrane of mitochondria. These peripheral receptors are found in almost all tissue types but especially in steroid-producing cells, such as the adrenal cortical and glial cells, and in the anterior pituitary. The action of some benzodiazepines at these mitochondrial benzodiazepine receptors is believed to effect the production of steroids, particularly "neurosteroids" in the CNS, which subsequently modulate the action of GABA on the $GABA_A$ receptor.[25]

A tremendous amount of research elucidated the exact structure of the GABA/benzodiazepine receptor complex and facilitated the understanding of various benzodiazepine agonists' mechanisms of action.[24, 26–31] Several GABA receptor subunits have been identified. At present, it has been determined that there are six α, three β, two γ, one δ, and two ρ variants.[24] It is the combination of these various subunits that confers sensitivity and specificity to individual benzodiazepine drugs. The resultant receptor heterogeneity throughout the CNS accounts for the varied responses to benzodiazepines, depending on the drug dose and location of its action. In general, the GABA/benzodiazepine receptor complex is composed of five or fewer subunits. The most abundant receptor subunits are $\alpha 1$, $\alpha 2$, $\beta 1$, $\beta 3$, and $\gamma 1$.[27] The major naturally occurring subunit composition is $\alpha 1\beta 2\gamma 2$, but the theoretical number of possible variant receptors is greater than 5000.[26]

It appears that benzodiazepines bind at the interface of the α and γ subunits that form the benzodiazepine pharmacophore. GABA binds at the β subunit. When benzodiazepines bind at their site of action, they induce a conformational change that may be relayed through the γ subunit to the β subunit, to alter its affinity for GABA and potentiate GABA's effects on the anion channel. The α subunit is responsible for the specific benzodiazepine pharmacology, the affinity for the ligand, and its intrinsic potency. For example, $\alpha 1$ subunits are commonly found in type I receptors, and α 2, 3, and 5 are found in type II. The particular α subunit may be responsible for whether a benzodiazepine has sedative or anxiolytic effects in different areas of the brain, at different concentrations. Finally, scientists have demonstrated that single amino acid alterations in the structure of subunits can intrinsically change their sensitivity or specificity for certain benzodiazepine ligands.[28, 30, 31]

In summary, the variability of a benzodiazepine's pharmacologic profile depends on the heterogeneity of the $GABA_A$ receptor structure, the intrinsic efficacy of the drug at various receptors, and the ability of some benzodiazepines to act on mitochondrial benzodiazepine receptors, producing neurosteroids that modulate GABA effects.[29]

The discovery of specific benzodiazepine receptors in the CNS has led to a search for naturally occurring benzodiazepine-like substances that also bind there, as well as research into their function or dysfunction in psychiatric disease. In 1986, a substance that interacts with the benzodiazepine receptor was purified from bovine brain and later identified as *N*-desmethyldiazepam. Since that time, benzodiazepine-like molecules, *endozepines,* have been purified from bovine, rat, and human brain tissue, at highest concentrations in the limbic system. A similar substance, identified as diazepam, has been quantified in human breast milk retrieved from women who were not taking exogenous benzodiazepines.[32] The source of these substances (food sources, bacterial modification of precursors in the GI tract, or endogenous formation) is controversial. However, their discovery, after the discovery of the high-affinity benzodiazepine receptor, has led to research into the role of the $GABA_A$/benzodiazepine receptor and endogenous benzodiazepine-like ligands in panic disorder,[33] anxiety,[34] memory and learning,[35] and hepatic encephalopathy.[36, 37] Similarly, the possible interaction of endogenous benzodiazepines with other hormones, such as thyroid hormone,[38] and the implications of this interaction on neuropsychiatric disease is being studied. The therapeutic mechanism of action of synthesized benzodiazepines or their antagonists may be better understood in the years to come, as disease states that are related to an imbalance in normal regulation of endogenous benzodiazepine-like substances are elucidated.

DRUG INTERACTION

As a group, the benzodiazepines' most significant drug interactions occur in the presence of alcohol or other CNS depressants and account for the ability of benzodiazepines to enhance the sedation produced by these substances. Not surprisingly, many of these interactions take place at the level of the $GABA_A$ receptor, where many sedative-hypnotics and depressants also bind. Barbiturates bind to a site on the complex apart from the benzodiazepine binding site. They enhance the action of GABA by prolonging the open phase of the ion channel, allowing greater chloride influx into the cell. Pentobarbital also has the ability to increase the affinity of the GABA and benzodiazepine receptors for their individual ligands. Other anesthetics and sedatives are also able to enhance GABA's effects at the receptor, including propofol, some general anesthetics, and sedatives such as meprobamate. Exogenous steroids also bind to the receptor complex, modulating GABA's effects and adding further evidence for the possible role of endogenous neurosteroids. Even ethanol is capable of binding to the GABA receptor complex, enhancing the ability of chloride to enter the cell. The expected CNS effects would be greater CNS depression and diminished psychomotor skills when these drugs are used in combination.

Just as endogenous benzodiazepine agonists have been discovered, so also have antagonists that have the ability to inhibit GABA's effects at the receptor been isolated. Drugs that exhibit similar inhibitory effects would be expected to diminish the sedative or anxiolytic effects of benzodiazepines. These include some antibiotics at high doses. Methylxanthines, particularly theophylline, have been reported to reverse

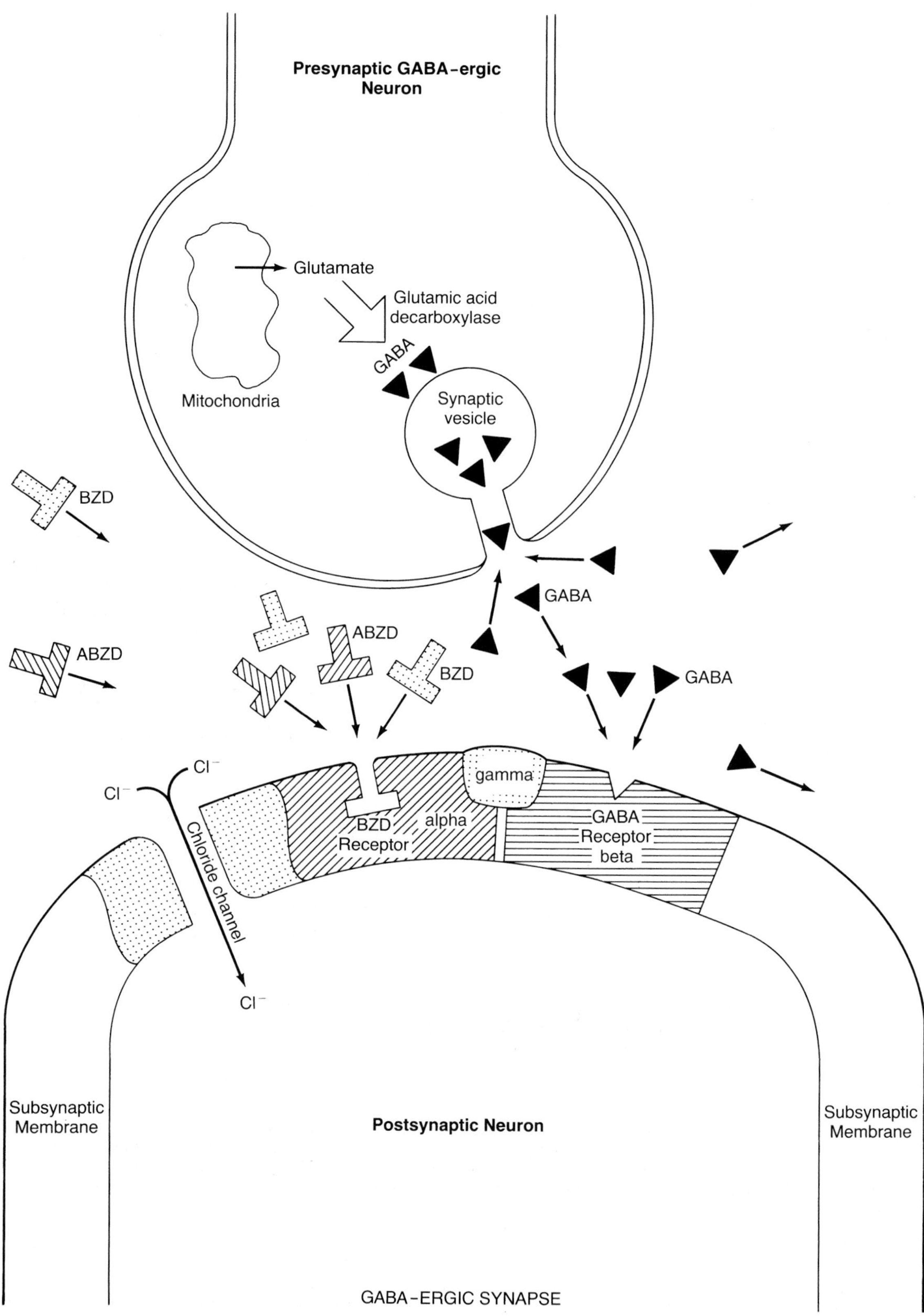

Figure 44–4 *See legend on opposite page*

benzodiazepine-induced sedation. In addition to their activity at the benzodiazepine receptor, benzodiazepines also inhibit the uptake of adenosine, an inhibitory neurotransmitter in the CNS. Reversal of their sedative effect may be related to the adenosine receptor–blocking activity of theophylline. This interaction has been studied therapeutically in the field of anesthesiology and critical care.

BENZODIAZEPINES IN ELDERLY PATIENTS

Rates of benzodiazepine use increase with age, and elderly patients thus account for a disproportionately large percentage of benzodiazepine prescriptions. In one report, it was estimated that more than 10% of elderly patients receive one or more benzodiazepine prescriptions per year. In the United States, the elderly receive more than 35% of the hypnotic prescriptions, and most of these are for benzodiazepines.[13] In addition, the elderly are more likely to be long-term users of these agents. These facts, in combination with age-related differences in sedative effects, place this population of patients at greater risk for the adverse side effects related to benzodiazepine use—namely, excess sedation, falls, and memory impairment.

Even after detoxification from benzodiazepines, impairment of learning and short-term memory has been shown to persist in elderly patients, as compared with younger patients detoxified from ethanol. Research into the neurochemical effects of benzodiazepines in the elderly has been scant and does not shed much light on the reasons for their increased susceptibility. Positron emission tomography (PET) has been used to demonstrate age-related decreases in various neurotransmitter receptors in the human brain; yet in one study using PET, no significant change in benzodiazepine-binding potentials could be shown in older study participants. This result was consistent throughout all examined brain regions. The researchers hypothesized that elderly patients' increased sensitivity to benzodiazepines is not simply secondary to a change in receptor number or affinity. They suggested an age-related change in the coupling between receptor binding and subsequent cellular function. To date, no satisfactory explanation has been offered for elderly patients' sensitivity to benzodiazepines at the CNS level.

Some of the differences in clinical response may be attributed to the changes in benzodiazepine pharmacokinetics noted with aging. As mentioned previously, aging is associated with an increased volume of distribution, an increased plasma half-life, and decreased hepatic clearance of some benzodiazepines, particularly diazepam and chlordiazepoxide.

If excess sedation, confusion, agitation, or other signs of cognitive impairment develop in an elderly patient taking benzodiazepines, it is prudent to discontinue the drug immediately pending further clinical investigation. Larson reported that benzodiazepines, particularly the long-acting ones such as diazepam, were the most common drugs associated with cognitive impairment in elderly people, often producing confusion, forgetfulness, slowing of the thought processes, and loss of the ability to care for oneself.[103] This occurred even if the drugs had been well tolerated for years. Benzodiazepines may also cause increased morbidity in patients with dementia due to other causes, such as Alzheimer's disease. The benzodiazepine effect is often overlooked by family and physicians and wrongly attributed to senility or a worsening of the underlying process.

TOXICITY OF BENZODIAZEPINES

Clinical Toxicity and Untoward Reactions

Therapeutic doses of benzodiazepines cause various degrees of sedation, drowsiness, lightheadedness, lethargy, and lassitude in virtually all patients, especially when therapy is initiated. Dysarthria, ataxia, motor incoordination, impairment of cognition, and amnesia may also be noted. Uncommonly, fatigue, headache, blurred vision, vertigo, nausea and vomiting, diarrhea, arthralgias, chest pain, and incontinence may occur. The frequency and severity of side effects appear to increase with age.

Figure 44–4. Benzodiazepine receptors and the GABAergic synapse. CNS neurotransmission occurs via a complex circuitry consisting of multiple connections, pathways, feedback mechanisms, and inhibitory/disinhibitory neurons, all under the control of neurotransmitters and neuroinhibitors. The body's most important neuroinhibitor, γ-aminobutyric acid (GABA), is synthesized in nerve endings of presynaptic GABAergic neurons from glutamate, under the influence of the enzyme glutamic acid decarboxylase. GABA is stored in synaptic vesicles located in presynaptic nerve endings and is released into the synapse to function as a neuroinhibitor. GABA activity is terminated by diffusion out of the synapse or reuptake into presynaptic nerve endings.

Specific GABA receptors have been identified on the subsynaptic membrane of postsynaptic neurons. GABA receptors are adjacent to and coupled with chloride ion channels in such a way that activation of a GABA receptor "opens" the associated channel, increasing chloride ion influx. The end result is hyperpolarization of the cell membrane and decreased neuronal excitability. The activity of GABA or its functional relationship to GABA receptors may be related to GABA modulin, an endogenous peptide located in synaptic membranes.

The benzodiazepine receptor is located on a subunit of the benzodiazepine-GABA pharmacophore, spatially adjacent to the GABA receptor. Binding of benzodiazepines to the benzodiazepine receptor subunit induces a change in the receptor complex, which facilitates GABA binding to the GABA receptor subunit, increasing the frequency of chloride ion channel opening. Benzodiazepine antagonists competitively block specific benzodiazepine receptor sites and either block the benzodiazepine binding or displace already bound drug, thereby offsetting any benzodiazepine-enhanced GABAergic transmission. GABA, γ-aminobutyric acid; BZD, benzodiazepine; ABZD, benzodiazepine antagonist.

Some differences in side effect profiles are noted between short- and long-acting benzodiazepines.[39] Long-acting benzodiazepines, such as diazepam and flurazepam, have a greater incidence of residual sedation and daytime drowsiness, may be associated with greater risks of falls in the elderly, and may cause greater respiratory depression in patients with pulmonary compromise. In addition, long- and intermediate-acting benzodiazepines are considered to have reinforcing properties that may lead to their persistent use and potential for abuse.[39] The hypnotic effect of long-acting benzodiazepines may not be fully achieved on the first night of administration, as compared with short-acting agents. However, short-acting benzodiazepines, such as triazolam and temezepam, which induce adequate nighttime sedation after only one dose, are more commonly associated with daytime anxiety and rebound insomnia on discontinuation. In fact, as little as one night of triazolam administration has been reported to induce rebound insomnia.[40] In general, rebound insomnia and benzodiazepine-induced amnesia are dose-related symptoms.

Benzodiazepines may rarely cause aberrant or paradoxical effects. These reactions occur most frequently in patients with overt or latent psychoses and organic brain syndrome and in elderly patients. The anxiolytic benzodiazepines have been reported to unmask bizarre, uninhibited behavior in some patients, as well as hostility, rage, paranoia, and depression.

In the late 1970s and 1980s, case reports of adverse reactions occurring in response to triazolam appeared in the media. These reactions consisted of psychosis, delirium, coma, and complete, transient global amnesia. These reports prompted the banning of triazolam in some European countries and a reassessment of its use in the United States. In 1992, Rothschild published a review of the medical literature pertaining to adverse reactions to triazolam as compared with other benzodiazepines.[104] He found that dysinhibition or dyscontrol reactions can occur with various benzodiazepines, are quite rare, and are usually related to the patient's pre-existing expectations of its occurrence and their pretreatment level of aggression and hostility. Anterograde amnesia occurs with administration of all benzodiazepines, affects the recall of events, but does not affect a patient's normal functional behavior. Delirium and withdrawal reactions are also associated with all of the benzodiazepines and, as with dysinhibition and amnesia, are dose related and more likely to occur in elderly users.

As research into the neurochemical effects of benzodiazepines reveals more information, the possibility of subtle or delayed brain toxicity is being considered. It appears that benzodiazepines may interact with GABA in certain areas of the brain to affect cognitive function and memory acquisition. The reversibility of these effects is unclear. In one study of long-term benzodiazepine users who were detoxified from benzodiazepines and remained benzodiazepine free for 6 months, some cognitive defects persisted for those 6 months. These investigators found that in the postwithdrawal period there was no evidence of recovery in verbal memory or learning, visuosymbolic, psychomotor, or conceptual tracking abilities in patients. In addition, their delayed recall was significantly impaired. Six months after withdrawal, mild recovery of cognitive deficits was found, but patients were still significantly deficient compared with controls.

In a related study, infants born to mothers who used benzodiazepines throughout their pregnancies were observed to 18 months of age. The researchers noted consistently lower general development scores in the benzodiazepine-exposed infants, especially in terms of personal-social behavior, eye-hand coordination, and performance at 10 and 18 month of age. Any confounding contribution of the infants' mother's psychiatric conditions to these findings could not be assessed.

In an animal model, fetal exposure to benzodiazepines alters function and stressor-induced responsiveness of the $GABA_A$ receptor in the brains of the exposed adult animals. It is hypothesized that the GABA receptor has a developmental role in integrated stress responses and may also induce developmental changes in other neural systems. Research is ongoing into the effect of prenatal exposure to benzodiazepines on the development of both the neurologic and immunologic systems. Central $GABA_A$ receptors and "peripheral" benzodiazepine receptors may interact with exogenous benzodiazepines in a way that adversely affects fetal development of these systems.

$GABA_A$ receptors appear to be involved in memory acquisition in animals. The long-term effects of benzodiazepines on the $GABA_A$ receptor and GABA physiology are not known. Any benzodiazepine-induced neurochemical or physiologic changes in the amygdala, hippocampus, or frontal lobe may not be quickly or easily reversed.

When given alone, benzodiazepines are relatively benign. They may depress the respiratory and cardiovascular systems indirectly through CNS depression. Uncommon side effects noted to occur after intravenous administration of benzodiazepines include respiratory arrest, cardiac arrest, hypotension, and phlebitis at the site of injection. Cardiorespiratory toxicity is probably secondary to rapid administration of too large a dose for the particular individual. Life-threatening adverse reactions occur with a frequency of 1.7% with intravenous diazepam and may be related in part to the use of propylene glycol as a parenteral vehicle in the formulation. Midazolam has been associated with respiratory depression and fatal cardiorespiratory arrest when administered intravenously for conscious sedation. Patients at particular risk for severe adverse reactions include elderly people, those patients with severe pulmonary or cardiac disease, and patients who have received other cardiorespiratory depressant medications.

Other side effects, such as coronary vasodilatation

and neuromuscular blockade, can occur after the intake of extremely large doses but rarely become clinically significant. Hematologic, renal, and hepatic toxicity have been noted, as well as acute rhabdomyolysis, anaphylaxis, dermatitis, and acute respiratory distress syndrome, but such adverse reactions are unusual and actually may be related to factors other than benzodiazepine overdose. Finally, postoperative exposure to benzodiazepines has been reported to increase the risk of delirium during recovery of surgical patients. Benzodiazepine withdrawal has been reported to be associated with tinnitus and absence seizures.

Early animal data suggested that benzodiazepine use may influence the risk of selected cancers. However, no association between the use of these drugs and the incidence of cancers, including breast, large bowel, malignant melanoma, lung, or endometrium, has been documented.

TOXICITY IN OVERDOSE

One of the most remarkable properties of benzodiazepines is their relative safety after overdose. In contrast to the sedative-hypnotic drugs of the past, such as barbiturates, chloral hydrate, meprobamate, glutethimide, and ethchlorvynol, benzodiazepines have a high therapeutic index. Deaths attributable to benzodiazepines taken alone are extremely rare.[1, 41, 42] When they do occur, deaths are almost always due to benzodiazepines taken in combination with other drugs. When the popularity and widespread use and misuse of benzodiazepines are considered, the paucity of documented fatalities secondary to benzodiazepines alone is a remarkable tribute to their safety.

CNS depression is common in benzodiazepine overdose. Patients usually become acutely drowsy, stuporous, and ataxic or may present in low-grade coma without focal neurologic abnormalities. Patients can generally be aroused from this state with verbal or painful stimulation. Profound coma, significant hypotension, respiratory depression, or hypothermia is extremely uncommon in oral overdose unless other drugs have also been ingested. For example, of the 38 patients with pure benzodiazepine overdose reported by Jatlow and colleagues, 16 were awake and none were more symptomatic than grade 0 coma (asleep but arousable).[43] No patient required hospitalization despite blood levels considered to be in the toxic range (1 to 9 μg/mL). Although cases of prolonged deep coma, prolonged cyclic coma, and benzodiazepine overdose presenting with focal neurologic signs[44] have been reported, such clinical scenarios are unusual. Most overdosed patients become easily arousable or awaken within 12 to 36 hours, secondary to drug redistribution and the development of acute tolerance. The duration of coma in elderly patients may be prolonged. Beyond their transient CNS depression and possible complications secondary to prolonged coma, pulmonary aspiration, or other indirect effects, benzodiazepines are not known to cause any specific injury or long-term toxicity to organ systems.

Although the recovery to consciousness is relatively rapid after benzodiazepine overdose, it is typical for overdosed patients to be dizzy, depressed, and apathetic for an extended period. Clinically, patients are noted to have CNS depression with hypotonia, motor retardation, slowed voluntary movements, and decreased reaction times.

Numerous clinical studies testify to the safety of benzodiazepine overdose. In a study by Finkle and associates of 1239 cases of diazepam-associated deaths, only 2 (0.2%) were possibly attributed to diazepam alone.[19] The investigators concluded that the toxicity of diazepam was low and that its role in fatal overdoses was minimal. A study conducted by Busto and colleagues evaluated 1071 patients with drug overdose who presented to an emergency department in Toronto.[41] They noted that the effects of benzodiazepine overdose were usually mild, requiring only supportive therapy. The patients were rarely unconscious on presentation and were only infrequently admitted to the hospital. Greenblatt and associates studied 773 admissions for drug overdose to Massachusetts General Hospital; 99 involved benzodiazepines, either alone or in combination with other agents.[42] Of the 12 admissions that were due to benzodiazepines alone, only one patient reached stage III coma (minimal response to painful stimuli), and one patient suffered significant cardiac or respiratory depression. In a study of 93 cases of diazepam overdose, Jatlow and associates found that patients required only supportive therapy, and no patient who ingested benzodiazepines alone required hospital admission.[43] Numerous other case reports also attest to benzodiazepines' minimal toxicity, even in massive overdose.[45, 46] In the rare fatal cases of benzodiazepines ingested alone,[47] newer, short-acting benzodiazepines (triazolam, alprazolam, temazepam) have been involved.

Coingestions

The toxicity of benzodiazepines may be significantly enhanced when they are taken in combination with other agents. The study by Greenblatt and associates demonstrated that coingestion of benzodiazepines with any other drug, including ethanol, analgesics, other sedative-hypnotics, tricyclic antidepressants, phenothiazines, or barbiturates, substantially increased the potential for serious toxicity.[42] The combination of benzodiazepines and barbiturates was noted to be particularly dangerous, and 50% of patients studied required mechanical ventilation. Ethanol, identified as a coingestant in 38% of benzodiazepine overdoses in one study,[19] enhances CNS toxicity of these agents directly because of its depressant characteristics and by increasing benzodiazepine absorption and decreasing phase I metabolism.[48] Case reports, clinical studies, and subject reviews have suggested that synergistic toxicity exists between benzodiazepines and tricyclic antidepressants,[49] cimetidine, phenothiazines, narcotics,[19] antihistamines, barbiturates, and alcohol.[19, 48, 50] Understanding of agents' effects at the GABA/benzodiazepine receptor makes some of this synergism predictable.

LABORATORY TESTING AND ANALYSIS

Plasma concentrations of benzodiazepines have been shown to correlate very poorly with the severity of toxic effects, the degree of CNS depression, or final outcome. Quantitative plasma measurements are not available in most hospitals, and they provide no significant therapeutic direction to the treating physician.[41, 43, 45, 50] A lethal dose has not been established for any benzodiazepine.

Blood concentrations and clinical effects of diazepam have been studied in some detail. Daily 10-mg doses of diazepam usually produce serum levels of less than 1μg/mL. Long-term daily doses of 150 to 200 mg/d produce levels of 5 to 6 μg/mL. Therapeutic levels range between 0.5 and 2.0 μg/mL but vary widely. When measured for academic or forensic purposes, diazepam levels commonly reach 2 to 5 μg/mL in overdose cases but may reach 10 to 15 μg/mL. Diazepam levels of 5 to 20 μg/mL are generally regarded as toxic, but many patients with serum concentrations in this range manifest only minimal clinical effects. No reliable or interpretable data exist regarding therapeutic or toxic levels for most newer benzodiazepines.

Quantitative measurement of serum benzodiazepine levels (parent compound and metabolite) may be useful to differentiate acute from chronic ingestions or may be of value in medicolegal or forensic situations. For example, diazepam's principal metabolite, desmethyldiazepam, has a half-life that exceeds that of diazepam. In acute ingestion, the level of diazepam should exceed that of desmethyldiazepam; with long-term ingestion, concentrations of desmethyldiazepam should exceed that of diazepam. Although some research toxicology laboratories have the capability to measure these levels, application of this measurement is not useful in the management of acute overdose.

The use of qualitative urine screening to ascertain the presence or absence of parent benzodiazepines or their metabolites may provide rapid, useful information in the evaluation of patients with an unknown cause of CNS depression. Although thin-layer chromatography is used most frequently for general toxicology screening,[51] its ability to detect benzodiazepines or their metabolites in urine is poor. Most laboratories perform initial screens for benzodiazepines with diagnostic immunoassay tests that identify the presence of benzodiazepines or benzodiazepine metabolites in the urine. When a positive result is obtained with a screening immunoassay study, laboratories should perform confirmatory tests with gas or high-pressure liquid chromatography or mass spectrometry.

Various immunoassay tests are available and are standardized against the detection of a particular single benzodiazepine compound (usually oxazepam). Other structurally similar benzodiazepines are subsequently detected through immunologic cross-reactivity with the compound that is used as a standard in the screening test. The sensitivities for detection of an individual benzodiazepine may differ significantly. For example, the enzyme-multiplied immunoassay technique (EMIT) screen is known to cross-react with chlordiazepoxide, clonazepam, demoxepam, desalkylfurazepam, desmethyldiazepam, flurazepam, lorazepam, oxazepam, prazepam, and temazepam.[52] However, this assay has not been consistently demonstrated to detect several of these compounds unless they are found in extremely high concentrations. Triazolobenzodiazepine derivatives, such as alprazolam or triazolam,[53] may be particularly difficult to detect in small (but clinically significant) ingestions because they possess poor immunologic cross-reactivity with oxazepam since they are administered and excreted in very small quantities. The radioimmunoassay screening test Abuscreen identifies alprazolam, chlordiazepoxide, demoxepam, clorazepate, diazepam, temazepam, desmethyldiazepam, desalkylflurazepam, halazepam, lorazepam, midazolam, and prazepam but does not detect clonazepam or flurazepam.[54] The latest commercially available immunoassay, based on the technique of fluorescence polarization (Abbott Diagnostics, Chicago) offers detection capabilities similar to that of radioimmunoassay with somewhat improved detection of the triazolobenzodiazepines.

One study evaluated six screening tests' ability to detect various benzodiazepines in urine. Screening results were compared with negative chemical ionization–gas chromatography/mass spectrometry.[55] Tests were used to evaluate 231 urine samples. All of the screening tests resulted in some false negatives in 3 to 11 samples. The metabolites most commonly involved in the falsely negative results were lorazepam and 7-aminoclonazepam. None of the screens were able to detect α-hydroxytriazolam or α-hydroxyalprazolam.

The concentration of benzodiazepine metabolites in urine can vary by orders of magnitude, secondary to the individual drug, dose, and time of collection relative to dosing. It is important to recognize that laboratory detection of benzodiazepines depends on the particular toxicologic screen used. Some commonly used screens may indicate negative results despite a clinically significant benzodiazepine ingestion.

In this era of drug screening for legal and management decisions in the workplace, it is important to be aware of the screening technologies in use, as well as their implications. One report has shown the ability to detect benzodiazepines in human hair by radioimmunoassay.[56] However, this mode of screening also revealed false negatives. In addition, reports have described false-positive screening results for benzodiazepines in the urine of patients using a new nonsteroidal anti-inflammatory agent, oxaprozin.[57] Oxaprozin is metabolized via microsomal oxidation and glucuronidation. Its urinary metabolite is probably responsible for these results, which have been noted via radioimmunoassay and fluorescence polarization immunoassay. Thin-layer chromatography and gas chromatography/mass spectometry should be able to identify oxaprozin's metabolite accurately. Similar false-positive results have been noted in the cases of etodolac, naproxen sodium, fenoprofen calcium, and tolmetin sodium.[57]

TERATOGENICITY AND BREAST EXCRETION

Benzodiazepines readily cross the placenta and may accumulate in the fetus, with levels that exceed the maternal serum concentration. Several animal studies have suggested that occasional congenital malformations may occur and the incidence of fetal loss may increase when benzodiazepines are used during pregnancy. A possible association between the development of fetal oral clefts in humans and diazepam use in the first trimester of pregnancy had been suggested by several studies in the early 1970s,[58, 59] but a larger well-controlled study performed in 1983 failed to support this association.[60] Regardless, a syndrome referred to as *benzodiazepine embryopathy* was reported in the 1980s to consist of growth retardation, dysmorphic features, and CNS dysfunction, occurring after exposure to oxazepam.[18] The most recent study on this subject monitored 80 pregnancies during which heavy benzodiazepine use was documented. Of the 64 surviving infants, 6 had diagnoses consistent with teratogenic abnormalities. The study was confounded by the concomitant use of other drugs and alcohol in the mothers. Human fetal exposure to benzodiazepines in combination with valproic acid has been postulated to cause an amplification of valproate-induced congenital malformations; however, the number of cases is very small.

High doses of benzodiazepines taken immediately before or during labor may produce the characteristics of floppy baby syndrome in newborn infants, including lethargy, poor feeding, hypothermia, hypotonia, apnea, and low Apgar scores. The occurrence of floppy baby syndrome is associated with the persistence of long-acting benzodiazepine metabolites in the serum of the neonate.[61, 62] The incidence appears to be decreased when benzodiazepines that are metabolized by only phase II metabolism are administered.[63]

Benzodiazepines and their metabolites are excreted in breast milk in clinically significant amounts[64] and may sedate a nursing neonate. This can result in poor feeding, lethargy, and failure to thrive. Because the metabolic capability of neonates is immature,[65] the benzodiazepines metabolized by phase I pathways may persist for extended periods. Breast-feeding should be avoided if benzodiazepines are to be administered to lactating women.

DEPENDENCE AND THE WITHDRAWAL SYNDROME

Physiologic addiction, characterized by somatic withdrawal symptoms after cessation of therapy, occurs with benzodiazepines.[66–71] The incidence of benzodiazepine dependence varies. In one report from the United Kingdom, 15% of long-term users had experienced withdrawal symptoms and as many as 200,000 people were estimated to be dependent on benzodiazepines.[10] In another community survey of 13,000 patients in the United Kingdom, only 0.5% of patients had been taking benzodiazepines for longer than 1 year. Thirty-three per cent of those had experienced withdrawal symptoms.[72]

Physiologic dependence implies the need for escalation of the drug dose in order to achieve the same pharmacologic effect and the presence of withdrawal symptoms on drug discontinuation. Clinically, the benzodiazepine withdrawal syndrome is similar to barbiturate or alcohol withdrawal; however, benzodiazepine withdrawal occurs less frequently and is usually less severe.

The mechanism of dependence probably involves down-regulation of $GABA_A$ and benzodiazepine receptors in the limbic system.[10] This may occur as a result of effects on the gene expression of receptors, as previously mentioned. Other hypotheses of benzodiazepine dependence suggest an increase in receptor sensitivity to inverse agonists, diminishing the agonist effect of a particular dose of benzodiazepine.

Risk factors for dependence include use of high-potency benzodiazepines, such as lorazepam and alprazolam. Prolonged duration of use has been reported to increase the incidence of dependence. However, some studies report the development of dependence and withdrawal symptoms after only 2 weeks of use. Other factors that may affect the development of physiologic dependence include the drug's half-life, the magnitude of the dose, and the patient's previous drug use, age, and personality.[11] Physiologic dependence can occur even after doses administered in the therapeutic range.

High-dose and low-dose benzodiazepine dependence states with their subsequent withdrawal syndromes have been identified. High-dose dependence is similar to that classically encountered with barbiturate and other sedative-hypnotics and can occur within 1 month if two to four times the maximum daily recommended dose is administered. The intensity of withdrawal is dose and time related and tends to be severe yet short lived.

Low-dose dependence can occur after therapeutic doses are given for prolonged periods. Withdrawal symptoms are less severe but may last for weeks. The validity of the low-dose withdrawal syndrome is somewhat controversial, however, because many individuals take benzodiazepines continually for years without any signs of overt withdrawal when the drug is abruptly discontinued. Some experts believe that the incidence and severity of benzodiazepine withdrawal have been overestimated. Rickels estimated the incidence to be as low as 1% to 3% after long-acting benzodiazepine use for up to 1 year and 5% to 10% after termination of short, rapidly acting drugs that have been administered for as long as 1 year.[73]

The onset and severity of symptoms vary with the type of benzodiazepine used. Withdrawal symptoms from long-acting benzodiazepines such as diazepam are typically evident between 3 and 7 days after termination of therapy. Symptoms may persist for as long as several months.[68, 74]

Complete elimination of a benzodiazepine is not required to produce overt withdrawal, and symptoms may occur after a rapid reduction in dose. It is speculated that the serum or tissue levels in persons taking benzodiazepines with long half-lives or long-acting metabolites decrease more slowly, thereby minimizing the severity of withdrawal symptoms. With long-term use of short-acting benzodiazepines, withdrawal symptoms can occur less than 24 hours after termination of therapy, and the symptoms are usually more severe than those associated with withdrawal from benzodiazepines with longer half-lives.[67, 69, 75, 76] Because of this fact, patients who experience abrupt withdrawal from a short-acting agent may be more likely to resume benzodiazepine use to avoid uncomfortable symptoms of withdrawal.[11]

Symptoms of Withdrawal

Because most patients undergoing long-term benzodiazepine therapy have underlying psychiatric disturbances, it may be difficult to distinguish withdrawal symptoms from rebound or recurrence of the underlying psychiatric illness. Unsuspected concurrent withdrawal from alcohol or other sedative-hypnotics may exacerbate the symptoms of benzodiazepine withdrawal. Benzodiazepine withdrawal is characterized by increased anxiety and apprehension, agitation, insomnia, tremors, nightmares, photophobia, headache, myalgias, and a heightened sensorium (hyperacusis). More severe and less common symptoms include nausea and vomiting, diaphoresis, hyperpyrexia, palpitations, vertigo, and psychosis.[68, 77, 78] Seizures rarely have been reported and may occur as late as 2 weeks after cessation of therapy.[79] Death secondary to benzodiazepine withdrawal has been documented.[80]

Treatment of Withdrawal

The treatment of withdrawal includes administration of long-acting benzodiazepines or occasionally barbiturates, followed by a gradual tapering of dose, preferably for a period of at least 4 weeks.[69, 81] A gradual reduction in dose is recommended whenever benzodiazepines are electively discontinued by patients who have had long-term therapy. Most clinicians prefer to discontinue the short-acting benzodiazepines and replace them with equivalent doses of diazepam. Withdrawal may then be prevented or minimized by decreasing the daily dose by an equivalent of 0.5 to 2.5 mg of diazepam or a maximum of one quarter of the daily dose every 1 to 2 weeks. Individual sensitivity is quite varied, however, and it is best to titrate the dose and rate of reduction to the patient's symptoms. Clonidine,[82, 83] propranolol,[84, 85] and tricyclic antidepressants[74] also have been used successfully as adjunctive therapy to decrease some of the somatic symptoms of benzodiazepine withdrawal. Other alternative anxiolytics used in treatment include buspirone and some antipsychotics.[10] Withdrawal can usually be accomplished on an outpatient basis in compliant and motivated patients.

Fetal Dependence

Women who take benzodiazepines during pregnancy may cause intrauterine benzodiazepine dependence in their fetus and benzodiazepine withdrawal in their neonate. The syndrome resembles neonatal narcotic withdrawal; symptoms include hypertonicity, irritability, tremors, hyperreflexia, tachypnea, and weight loss. Although these infants may feed vigorously, they frequently vomit.[86] Symptoms usually begin 2 to 6 days after delivery but may be delayed for as long as 10 days because of decreased benzodiazepine clearance in the neonate. The withdrawal syndrome in neonates is usually treated with phenobarbital.

DIAGNOSIS OF BENZODIAZEPINE OVERDOSE

Patients with a pure benzodiazepine overdose display mild to moderate sedation, often with dysarthria and ataxia, without serious neurologic, cardiovascular, or respiratory impairment. The diagnosis is usually based entirely on history or laboratory results because there are no diagnostic clinical features or specific toxidromes. Clinical clues that suggest an alternative diagnosis or a concomitant ingestion include hyperreflexia or clonus, cardiovascular instability, and respiratory depression requiring assisted ventilation. Associated trauma, underlying medical disorders, or concomitant ingestion of other drugs may make the clinical diagnosis of benzodiazepine overdose quite difficult. In obtaining the history or analyzing any toxicologic laboratory data, particular attention should be paid to the possible ingestion of any compounds that may potentiate the toxicity of benzodiazepines. It is emphasized that significant ingestions of the newer benzodiazepines may escape the detection of an unsophisticated toxicology laboratory. It should also be emphasized that quantitative serum levels of specific benzodiazepines have no utility in the setting of acute overdose. They do not correlate with symptoms and are of no benefit in the evaluation and treatment of these patients.

TREATMENT

Current therapy for benzodiazepine overdose is conservative and supportive. Coingestion of other toxic substances, concurrent trauma, or other underlying medical conditions may significantly alter the diagnostic and therapeutic approach. One should always be cognizant of conditions that may mimic a benzodiazepine ingestion, such as head trauma, ethanol intoxication, hypoglycemia, carbon monoxide poisoning, or cerebrovascular accident.

Very few patients with a pure benzodiazepine overdose require treatment beyond activated charcoal and observation. Minimally symptomatic patients or those with ingestions more than 2 hours before evaluation can safely be observed and closely monitored. Patients who do not have complications and who are able to ambulate without ataxia after treatment and 4 to 6 hours of observation can be discharged after appropriate psychiatric consultation. In instances of respiratory depression or cardiovascular compromise, airway protection and mechanical ventilation may be instituted. Circulatory support should consist of administration of intravenous crystalloid fluids and, rarely, vasopressors.

There are no practical ways to enhance benzodiazepine elimination significantly. Forced diuresis is of no proven value. Hemoperfusion, hemodialysis, and peritoneal dialysis are relatively ineffective in removing clinically significant amounts of benzodiazepines from the serum because of extensive protein binding. The potential toxicity of benzodiazepine overdose is not sufficient to warrant the use of such aggressive intervention.

BENZODIAZEPINE ANTAGONISTS

Flumazenil is the benzodiazepine antagonist currently available in the United States. It has been available in Europe under the trade name of Anexate since 1987. Flumazenil is a 1,4-imidazobenzodiazepine, a derivative of the antibiotic anthramycin[87] (Fig. 44–5). It contains a diazepine ring that binds the benzodiazepine receptor, where it competitively displaces benzodiazepines from the receptor and reverses their sedative and anxiolytic effects.

In oral dosage form, this antagonist has low bioavailability secondary to significant first-pass metabolism in the liver. It has a volume of distribution of 1.1 L/kg, is 40% to 50% protein bound, and is highly lipid soluble.[87] Flumazenil has a distribution half-life of 5 minutes and rapidly crosses the blood-brain barrier to reverse benzodiazepine-induced sedation within 1 to 2 minutes after intravenous administration.

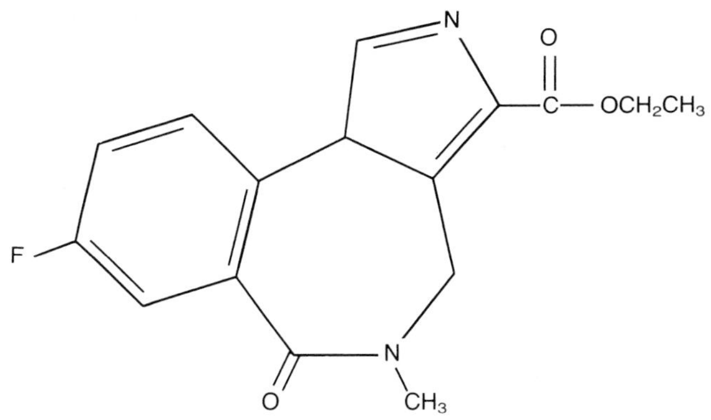

Figure 44–5. The chemical structure of flumazenil (Ro 15-1788), a specific benzodiazepine antagonist.

In studies performed to date, flumazenil has been noted to reverse rapidly and completely the sedative, anxiolytic, anticonvulsant, ataxic, anesthetic, and muscle relaxant effects of benzodiazepines in animals and humans.[88] It also has been shown to restore an encephalogram to the baseline waking state in patients who have previously been administered benzodiazepines,[89] and it has been demonstrated to be an effective antidote in cases of benzodiazepine overdose.[90] In studies of coma secondary to use of benzodiazepines,[91, 92] patients responded dramatically in 1 to 5 minutes after the administration of flumazenil. Incomplete or partial antagonism of benzodiazepine-induced sedation has been reported[92] but may be secondary to coingestion of other sedative-hypnotics or concomitant medical causes of depressed consciousness. In addition, residual memory deficits of events preceding reversal may persist.

The mean half-life of flumazenil is 57 minutes, and thus resedation after administration may occur within 1 to 2 hours. Repeat dosing may be required to maintain an intact mental status. It is hepatically metabolized by conjugation to glucuronide, and the metabolite is renally excreted. The dose is 0.5 to 5 mg in adults and 0.005 mg/kg to 0.01 mg/kg in children. A continuous infusion of 0.1 mg/kg per hour has been used in children.[93]

Flumazenil acts as an antagonist, removing both agonists (benzodiazepines) and inverse agonists from the benzodiazepine receptor–binding site. At high doses, it is reported to have agonist-like anticonvulsant activity. However, it is also reported to have weak inverse agonist properties.[94] This property of benzodiazepine reversal has been used to reverse sedation in selected cases of hepatic encephalopathy, which many believe may be caused by an excess of endogenous benzodiazepines in these patients.[95] Anecdotal reports also describe partial reversal of ethanol- and tegretol-induced depression in consciousness.

The most common side effects of flumazenil administered to normal volunteers are dizziness, facial erythema, anxiety, and headache. Symptoms are mild and disappear within several minutes. Flumazenil has been shown to increase intracranial pressure in head-injured patients with elevated intracranial pressure. Reports also describe ventricular dysrhythmias on administration.[93] Flumazenil has been noted to precipitate convulsions in epileptic patients taking benzodiazepines for seizure control and in patients with coingestion of drugs that lower the seizure threshold.[96]

In 1992, Spivey analyzed 43 reported cases of seizures that occurred after administration of flumazenil in doses of 0.2 to 10 mg.[97] Forty-seven per cent of these cases were in patients who experienced drug-induced seizures that were being suppressed by coingestion of a benzodiazepine. Ninety per cent of these patients had ingested cyclic antidepressants. Two of those developed status epilepticus and died. The other patients who developed seizures after receiving flumazenil had taken benzodiazepines for treatment of a known seizure disorder (16%), had medically induced seizures that were being suppressed by benzodiazepines (12%), received benzodiazepines for conscious sedation (5%), or had acute withdrawal from long-term use of benzodiazepines after flumazenil administration (7%). Treatment for seizures temporally related to flumazenil antagonism of a benzodiazepine included benzodiazepines, barbiturates, phenytoin, and chlormethiazole.

As mentioned, flumazenil has the potential to precipitate withdrawal symptoms in benzodiazepine-dependent individuals.[98] In animal studies, the severity of withdrawal depends on the specific benzodiazepine used, the dose and duration of treatment, and the dose of flumazenil administered.[99] Withdrawal symptoms are usually more severe with flumazenil than when benzodiazepines are simply discontinued.

Controversy exists over the role of flumazenil in patients who present with overdose and altered mental status. In an editorial that reviewed American Association of Poison Control Center data during the 8 years before flumazenil introduction and after its introduction in 1992, no change was noted in the overall morbidity or mortality associated with benzodiazepine overdose.[100]

Although the potential toxicity of benzodiazepines is relatively low and aggressive therapy for pure overdose is rarely required, flumazenil offers several important potential uses in clinical medicine. The antagonist can help to confirm a suspected diagnosis of benzodiazepine overdose. Flumazenil may reverse overdose of zolpidem and zopiclone, and may be indicated for respiratory depression, particularly if intubation and mechanical ventilation would otherwise be indicated (see Chapter 43). Flumazenil may be useful postoperatively to reverse the effects of preoperative sedation or to reverse an inadvertent overdose when benzodiazepines are used for conscious sedation in outpatients. Despite its potential usefulness, flumazenil should not become a "routine" antidote in the treatment of coma secondary to overdose. Patients should be assessed for evidence of ingestion or exposure to epileptogenic agents, cyclic antidepressants in particular. The presence of an anticholinergic toxidrome, abnormal vital signs such as tachycardia, or myoclonic jerking precludes the use of flumazenil. In addition, if a patient's history provides information about long-term benzodiazepine use and possible dependence or benzodiazepine use for anticonvulsant properties, flumazenil should be avoided.

References

1. Greenblatt DJ, Shader RI: Drug therapy. Benzodiazepines. N Engl J Med *291*:1011–1015, 1974.
2. Johnson MR, Lydiard RB, Ballenger JC: Panic disorder. Pathophysiology and drug treatment. Drugs *49*:328–344, 1995.
3. Practice guidelines for the treatment of patients with bipolar disorder. Am J Psychiatry *151*:1–36, 1994.
4. Ungvari GS, Leung CM, Wong MK, Lau J: Benzodiazepines in the treatment of catatonic syndrome. Acta Psychiatr Scand *89*:285–288, 1994.
5. Rosebush PI, Mazurek MF: Do benzodiazepines modify the incidence of neuroloptic-induced dystonia? Letter. Am J Psychiatry *150*:528, 1993.
6. Redfern P, Minors D, Waterhouse J: Circadian rhythms, jet lag, and chronobiotics: An overview. Chronobiol Int *11*:253–265, 1994.
7. Dellemijn PLI, Fields HL: Do benzodiazepines have a role in chronic pain management? Pain *57*:137–152, 1994.
8. Greenberg DB: Strategic use of benzodiazepines in cancer patients. Oncology *5*:83–88, 1991.
9. Kesaniemi YA, Miettinen TA: Inhibition of cholesterol absorption by neomycin, benzodiazepine derivatives and ketoconazole. Eur J Clin Pharmacol *40*(Suppl 1):S65–67, 1991.
10. Livingston MG: Benzodiazepine dependence. Br J Hosp Med *51*:281–286, 1994.
11. Woods JH, Winger G: Current benzodiazepine issues. Psychopharmacology *118*:107–115, 1995.
12. Darke S: Benzodiazepine use among injecting drug users: Problems and implications. Addiction *89*:379–382, 1994.
13. McNutt LA, Coles FB, McAuliffe T, et al: Impact of regulation on benzodiazepine prescribing to a low income elderly population, New York State. J Clin Epidemiol *47*:613–625, 1994.
14. Schwartz HI, Blank K: Regulation of benzodiazepine prescribing practices: Clinical implications. Gen Hosp Psychiatry *13*:219–224, 1991.
15. Schwartz HI: Negative clinical consequences of triplicate prescription regulation of benzodiazepines. N Y State J Med *91*(Suppl 11):9S–12S, 1991.
16. Linden M, Gothe H: Benzodiazepine substitution in medical practice. Analysis of pharmacoepidemiologic data based on expert interviews. Pharmacopsychiatry *26*:107–113, 1993.
17. Cormack MA, Sweeney KG, Hughes-Jones H, Foot GA: Evaluation of an easy, cost-effective strategy for cutting benzodiazepine use in general practice. Br J Gen Pract *44*:5–8, 1994.
18. Bailey L, Ward M, Musa MN: Clinical pharmacokinetics of benzodiazepines. J Clin Pharmacol *34*:804–811, 1994.
19. Finkle BS, McCloskey KL, Goodman LS: Diazepam and drug-associated deaths: A survey in the United States and Canada. JAMA *242*:429–434, 1979.
20. Greenblatt DJ: Benzodiazepine hypnotics: Sorting the pharmacokinetic facts. J Clin Psychiatry *52*(Suppl 9):4–10, 1991.
21. Miller LG: Chronic benzodiazepine administration: From the patient to the gene. J Clin Pharmacol *31*:492–495, 1991.
22. Miller LG, Koff JM: Interaction of central and peripheral benzodiazepine sites in benzodiazepine tolerance and discontinuation. Prog Neuropsychopharmacol Biol Psychiatry *18*:847–857, 1994.
23. Logan KE, Lawrie SM: Long term use of hypnotics and anxiolytics. Letter. BMJ *309*:27–28, 1994.
24. Goodchild CS: GABA receptors and benzodiazepines. Br J Anaesth *71*:127–133, 1993.
25. Whitehouse BJ: Benzodiazepines and steroidogenesis. J Endocrinol *134*:1–3, 1992.

26. Luddens H, Wisden W: Function and pharmacology of multiple GABAa receptor subunits. Trends Pharmacol Sci *12*:49–51, 1991.
27. Fraser DD, Mudrick-Donnon LA, Macvicar BA: Astrocytic GABA receptors. Glia *11*:83–93, 1994.
28. Korpi ER, Seeburg PH: Natural mutation of GABAa receptor alpha6 subunit alters benzodiazepine affinity but not allosteric GABA effects. Eur J Pharmacol Mol Pharmacol Sect *247*:23–27, 1993.
29. Giusti P, Romeo E, Auta J, Guidotti A: Structural variety of GABAa receptors and specificity of benzodiazepines pharmacological profiles. Adv Biochem Psychopharmacol *47*:163–177, 1992.
30. Luddens H, Seeburg PH, Korpi ER: Impact of beta and gamma variants on ligand-binding properties of gamma-aminobutyric acid type A receptors. Mol Pharmacol *45*:810–814, 1994.
31. Mihic SJ, Sanna E, Whiting PJ, Harris RA: Pharmacology of recombinant GABAa receptors. Adv Biochem Psychopharmacol *48*:17–40, 1995.
32. Dencker SJ, Johansson G, Milsom I: Quantification of naturally occurring benzodiazepine-like substances in human breast milk. Psychopharmacology *107*:69–72, 1992.
33. Nutt DJ, Smith CF, Bennett R, Jackson HC: Investigations on the "set-point" theory of benzodiazepine receptor function. Adv Biochem Psychopharmacol *47*:419–429, 1992.
34. Malizia AL, Coupland NJ, Nutt DJ: Benzodiazepine receptor function in anxiety disorders. Adv Biochem Psychopharmacol *48*:115–133, 1995.
35. Izquierdo I, Medina JH: GABAa receptor modulation of memory: The role of endogenous benzodiazepines. Trends Pharmacol Sci *12*:260–265, 1991.
36. Rothstein JD: Benzodiazepine-receptor ligands and hepatic encephalopathy: A causal relationship? Hepatology *19*:248–250, 1994.
37. Mullen KD: Benzodiazepine compounds and hepatic encephalopathy. N Engl J Med *325*:509–511, 1991.
38. Kragie L: Neuropsychiatric implications of thyroid hormone and benzodiazepine interactions. Endocr Res *19*:1–32, 1993.
39. Mendelson WB: Clinical distinctions between long-acting and short-acting benzodiazepines. J Clin Psychiatry *53* (Suppl): 4–7, 1992.
40. Roth T, Roehrs TA: A review of the safety profiles of benzodiazepine hypnotics. J Clin Psychiatry *52*(Suppl):38–41, 1991.
41. Busto U, Kaplan HL, Sellers EM: Benzodiazepine-associated emergencies in Toronto. Am J Psychiatry *137*:224–227, 1980.
42. Greenblatt DJ, Allen MD, Noel BJ, et al: Acute overdosage with benzodiazepine derivatives. Clin Pharmacol Ther *21*:497–514, 1977.
43. Jatlow P, Dobular K, Bailey D: Serum diazepam concentrations in overdose: Their significance. Am J Clin Pathol *72*:571–579, 1979.
44. Deleu D, Keyser J: Flunitrazepam intoxication simulating a structural brainstem lesion. J Neurol Neurosurg Psychiatry *50*:236–237, 1987.
45. Allen-Divoll M, Greenblatt DJ, Lacasse Y: Pharmacokinetic study of lorazepam overdosage. Am J Psychiatry *137*:1414–1415, 1980.
46. McCormick SR, Nielsen J, Jatlow PI: Alprazolam overdose: Clinical findings and serum concentrations in two cases. J Clin Psychiatry *46*:247–248, 1985.
47. Martin CD, Chan SC: Distribution of temazepam in body fluids and tissues in lethal overdose. J Anal Toxicol *10*:77–78, 1986.
48. Sellers EM, Busto U: Benzodiazepines and ethanol: Assessment of the effects and consequences of psychotropic drug interactions. J Clin Pharmacol *22*:249–262, 1982.
49. Goethe JW, Edelman SL: Chlordiazepoxide toxicity in limbitrol overdose. Am J Psychiatry *142*:774, 1985.
50. Bailey DN: Blood concentrations and clinical findings following overdose of chlordiazepoxide alone and chlordiazepoxide plus ethanol. Clin Toxicol *22*:433–446, 1984.
51. Kellermann AL, Fihn SD, LoGerto JP, et al: Impact of drug screening in suspected overdose. Ann Emerg Med *16*:1206–1216, 1987.
52. Package insert, EMIT. Urine Immunoassay. Sylva Company, Palo Alto, CA, August 1985.
53. Fraser AD: Urinary screening for alprazolam, triazolam and their metabolites with the EMIT®d.a.u.™ benzodiazepine metabolite assay. J Anal Toxicol *11*:263–266, 1987.
54. Pachage insert, Abuscreen-Radioimmunoassay for benzodiazepines. Roche Diagnostic Systems, Nutley, NJ, July 1987.
55. Fitzgerald RL, Rexin DA, Herold DA: Detecting benzodiazepines: Immunoassays compared with negative chemical ionization gas chromatography/mass spectrometry. Clin Chem *40*:373–380, 1994.
56. Sramek JJ, Baumgartner WA, Ahrens TN, et al: Detection of benzodiazepines in human hair by radioimmunoassay. Ann Pharmacother *26*:469–472, 1992.
57. Pulini M: False-positive benzodiazepine urine test due to oxaproxin. Letter. JAMA *273*:1905–1906, 1995.
58. Saxen I: Associations between oral clefts and drugs taken during pregnancy. Int J Epidemiol *4*:37, 1975.
59. Safra MJ, Oakley GP: Valium: An oral cleft teratogen. Cleft Palate J *13*:198, 1976.
60. Rosenberg L, Mitchell AA, Parsels JL, et al: Lack of relation of oral clefts to diazepam use during pregnancy. N Engl J Med *309*:1281, 1983.
61. Spreight ANP: Floppy-infant syndrome and maternal diazepam and/or nitrazepam. Lancet *2*:878, 1977.
62. Whitelaw AGL, Cummings AJ, McFadyen IR: Effect of maternal lorazepam on the neonate. Br Med J *282*:1106–1108, 1981.
63. Drury KAD: Floppy-infant syndrome: Is oxazepam the answer? Lancet *2*:1126, 1977.
64. Cole AP, Hailey DM: Diazepam and active metabolites in breast milk and their transfer to the neonate. Arch Dis Child *50*:741–742, 1975.
65. Kaplan SA: Pharmacokinetics of the benzodiazepines. *In* Priest RG, Vianna Filho U, Amrein R, Skreta M (eds): Benzodiazepines Today and Tomorrow. Lancaster, MTP Press, 1980.
66. Ashton H: Benzodiazepine withdrawal: An unfinished story. BMJ *288*:1135–1140, 1984.
67. Owen RT, Tyler P: Benzodiazepine dependence: A review of the evidence. Drugs *25*:385–398, 1983.
68. Petursson H, Lader MH: Withdrawal from long-term benzodiazepine treatment. BMJ *283*:643–645, 1981.
69. Busto U, Sellers EM, Naranjo CA: Withdrawal reaction after long-term therapeutic use of benzodiazepines. N Engl J Med *315*:854–859, 1986.
70. Power KG, Jeffom DWA, Simpson RJ, et al: Controlled study of withdrawal symptoms and rebound anxiety after six week course of diazepam for generalised anxiety. BMJ *290*:1246–1248, 1985.
71. Marks J: The benzodiazepines—use and abuse. Arzneimittelforschung *30*:898–901, 1980.
72. Wright N, Caplan R, Payne S: Community survey of long term daytime use of benzodiazepines. BMJ *309*:27–28, 1994.
73. Rickels K: Benzodiazepines in the treatment of anxiety: The North American experience. *In* Costa E (ed): The Benzodiazepines: From Molecular Biology to Clinical Practice. New York, Raven Press, 1983.
74. Higgitt AC, Lader MH, Fonagy P: Clinical management of benzodiazepine dependence. BMJ *291*:688–690, 1985.
75. Noyes R, Clancy J, Coryell WH, et al: A withdrawal syndrome after abrupt discontinuation of alprazolam. Am J Psychiatry *142*:114–116, 1985.
76. Tyrer PJ: Benzodiazepines on trial. BMJ *288*:1101–1102, 1984.
77. Drury WM: Benzodiazepines—a challenge to rational prescribing. J R Coll Gen Pract *35*:86–88, 1985.
78. Lader M, Petursson H: Long-term effects of benzodiazepines. Neuropharmacology *22*:527–533, 1983.
79. Breier A, Charney DS, Nelson JC: Seizures induced by abrupt discontinuation of alprazolam. Am J Psychiatry *141*:1606–1607, 1984.
80. Relkin R: Death following withdrawal of diazepam. N Y State J Med *66*:1770–1772, 1966.
81. Murphy SM, Owen RT, Tyrer PJ: Withdrawal symptoms

after six weeks' treatment with diazepam. Lancet *2*:1389, 1984.
82. Vinogradov S, Reiss AL, Csernansky JG: Clonidine therapy in withdrawal from high dose alprazolam treatment. Letter. Am J Psychiatry *143*:1188, 1986.
83. Keshavan MS, Crammer JL: Clonidine in benzodiazepine withdrawal. Lancet *1*:1325–1326, 1985.
84. Tyrer P, Rutherford D, Juggett A: Benzodiazepine withdrawal symptoms and propranolol. Lancet *1*:520–522, 1981.
85. Gauche WG: Propranolol for the treatment of diazepam withdrawal symptoms. Letter. S Afr Med J *66*:870, 1984.
86. Smith DE, Wesson DR: Benzodiazepine dependency syndromes. *In* Smith DE, Wesson DR (eds): The Benzodiazepines: Current Standards for Medical Practice. Lancaster, MTP Press, 1985.
87. Longmire AW, Seger DL: Topics in clinical pharmacology: Flumazenil, a benzodiazepine antagonist. Am J Med Sci *306*:49–52, 1993.
88. Darragh A, Lambe R, Scully M, et al: Investigation in man of the efficacy of a benzodiazepine antagonist, Ro15-1788. Lancet *2*:8–10, 1981.
89. Laurian S, Gailard M, Le PK, et al: Effects of a benzodiazepine antagonist on the diazepam-induced electrical brain activity modifications. Neuropsychobiology *11*:55–58, 1984.
90. Hofer P, Scollo-Lavizzari G: Benzodiazepine antagonist Ro 15-1788 in self-poisoning: Diagnostic and therapeutic use. Arch Intern Med *145*:663–664, 1985.
91. Scollo-Lavizzari G: First clinical investigation of the benzodiazepine antagonist Ro 15-1788 in comatose patients. Eur Neurol *22*:7–11, 1983.
92. Chern CH, Chern TL, Hu SC, et al: Complete and partial response to flumazenil in patients with suspected benzodiazepine overdose. Letter. Am J Emerg Med *13*:372–375, 1995.
93. Sugarman JM, Paul RI: Flumazenil: A review. Pediatr Emerg Care *10*:37–43, 1994.
94. Philip BK: Drug reversal: Benzodiazepine receptors and antagonists. J Clin Anesth *5*(Suppl 1):46S–51S, 1993.
95. Hoffman EJ, Warren EW: Flumazenil: A benzodiazepine antagonist. Clin Pharm *12*:641–656, 1993.
96. Haverkos GP, DiSalvo RP, Imhoff TE: Fatal seizures after flumazenil administration in a patient with mixed overdose. Ann Pharmacother *28*:1347–1349, 1994.
97. Spivey WH: Flumazenil and seizures: Analysis of 43 cases. Clin Ther *14*:292–305, 1992.
98. Cumin R, Bonetti EP, Scherchlicht R, et al: Use of the specific benzodiazepine antagonist, Ro 15-1788, in studies of physiological dependence on benzodiazepines. Experientia *38*:833–834, 1982.
99. Intravenous flumazenil (Ro 15-1788): Investigational drug brochure. Hoffmann-La Roche, Nutley, NJ, March 1987.
100. Krenzelok EP: Judicious use of flumazenil. Clin Pharm *12*:691–692, 1993.
101. Kroboth PD, Maxwell RA, Fleishaker JC, et al: Comparison of adinazolam pharmacokinetics and effects in healthy and cirrhotic subjects. J Clin Pharmacol *31*:580–586, 1991.
102. Golden PL, Warner PE, Fleishaker JC, et al: Effects of probenecid on the pharmacokinetics and pharmacodynamics of adinazolam in humans. Clin Pharmacol Ther *56*:133–141, 1994.
103. Larson EB, Kukill WA, Buchner D, Reifler BV: Adverse drug reactions associated with cognitive impairment in elderly persons. Ann Intern Med *107*:169–173, 1987.
104. Rothschild AJ: Disinhibition, amnestic reactions, and other adverse reactions secondary to triazolam: A review of the literature. J Clin Psychiatry *53*(suppl):69–79, 1992.

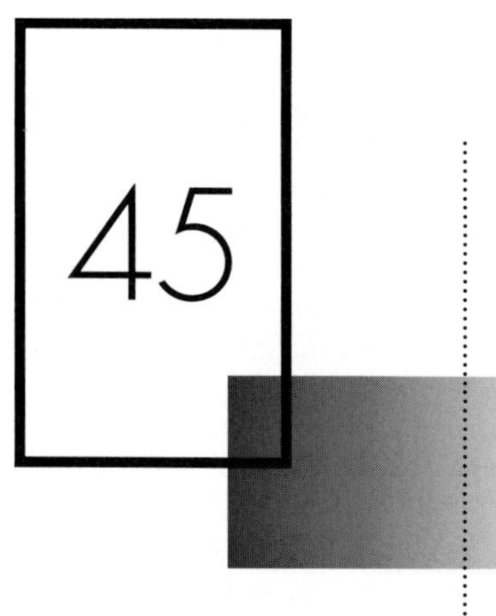

The Antipsychotic Drugs

MICHAEL BURNS, MD

The antipsychotic agents, also called *major tranquilizers* and *neuroleptics,* have been used to treat schizophrenia and other types of psychoses since the discovery of chlorpromazine in 1952. The term *antipsychotic* is somewhat of a misnomer because these agents are often used for purposes other than treating psychoses; they are also used as sedatives and preanesthetics and as treatment for the manic phase of bipolar disorder, agitated behavior, drug-induced hallucinations, nausea and vomiting, migraine and tension headaches, hiccups, and various extrapyramidal movement disorders (e.g., tics, chorea, hemiballismus). The term *major tranquilizer* is misleading because these agents are not simple seda-

Table 45–1. Antipsychotic Agents

Structural Class	Generic Name (Trade Name)	Affinity of Antipsychotic Agent for Dopamine D_2 Receptor (Potency)*	Daily Dose Range (mg)
Phenothiazines	Chlorpromazine (Thorazine)	5.3	25–2000
Aliphatic	Cyamemazine (Tercian)	—	200–300
	Triflupromazine (Vesprin)	—	5–90 (parenteral only)
	Promethazine (Phenergan)†	—	25–150
	Trimeprazine (Temaril)‡	—	2.5–10
	Promazine (Sparine)†	—	50–1000
Piperazine	Fluphenazine (Prolixin)	125	0.5–25
	Perphenazine (Trilafon)	71	4–64
	Prochlorperazine (Compazine)	14	10–150
	Trifluoperazine (Stelazine)	38	2–40
	Thiethylperazine (Torecan)†		10–30
Piperidine	Mesoridazine (Serentil)	5.3	50–400
	Thioridazine (Mellaril)	3.8	30–800
Butyrophenone	Haloperidol (Haldol)	25	1–30
Thioxanthene	Droperidol (Inapsine)	—	2.5–30 (parenteral only)
	Chlorprothixene (Taractan)	13	30–600
	Thiothixene (Navane)	222	6–60
	Zuclopenthixol (Clopixol)	—	20–150
Dihydroindolone	Molindone (Moban)	0.83	15–225
Dibenzoxazepine	Loxapine (Loxitane)	1.4	20–200
	Clozapine (Clozaril)	0.56	100–900
	Olanzapine (Zyprexa)	5.0	5–15
Diphenylbutylpiperidine	Pimozide (Orap)	12.5	1–20
Benzisoxazole	Risperidone (Risperdal)	74.1	1–10
Benzamides	Sulpiride§	0.71	100–3200
	Remoxipride§	0.10	150–600
	Raclopride§	16.7	5–8

*A higher numeric value indicates greater binding and greater antagonism at dopamine D_2 receptor. Binding affinity (potency) at dopamine D_2 receptor correlates with daily dose range.
†Antiemetic only.
‡Antipruritic only.
§Not available for clinical use in the United States.
Adapted from Black JL, Richelson E, Richardson JW: Antipsychotic agents: A clinical update. Mayo Clin Proc *60*:777–789, 1985.

tives. Until recently, the term *neuroleptic* was synonymous with and preferred to *antipsychotic* because all traditional antipsychotics produce extrapyramidal side effects (EPS). The introduction of agents that produce minimal EPS, or atypical antipsychotics (e.g., clozapine, risperidone), has allowed separation of antipsychotic from neuroleptic effects and prevents the ready interchange of terms.

Toxicity of the antipsychotic drugs results from unintentional or intentional overdose or from adverse reactions following therapeutic administration. Because of a large toxic-to-therapeutic ratio, fatalities rarely occur. Death is usually a consequence of polydrug overdose or ingestion of the agents thioridazine or mesoridazine. In 1995, 11,577 antipsychotic agent exposures were reported to the American Association of Poison Control Centers; 355 (3%) of these resulted in major toxicity and 25 (0.2%) in death.[1] Despite the rarity of fatality due to antipsychotic agents, these drugs are commonly used and have a wide range of adverse effects. An understanding of the pharmacology, nature of adverse effects, and appropriate interventions for antipsychotic agent poisoning is thus needed.

STRUCTURE AND CLASSIFICATION

The antipsychotic agents have traditionally been classified according to structure. Using such a scheme, eight different classes are currently available for clinical use. They include phenothiazine, butyrophenone, thioxanthene, indolic derivative (dihydroindolone), dibenzoxazepine, diphenylbutylpiperidine, benzisoxazole, and benzamide (Table 45–1). The phenothiazine class is further subdivided into three groups (aliphatic, piperidine, and piperazine) on the basis of respective side chain substitution at position 10 on the central ring (Fig. 45–1). The piperazine group agents are the least sedating and least likely to cause hypotension but are the most potent (smallest antipsychotic dose) and most likely to cause EPS.

A more clinically useful method of antipsychotic agent classification is obtained not by structure but by relative receptor-binding profiles (Table 45–2).

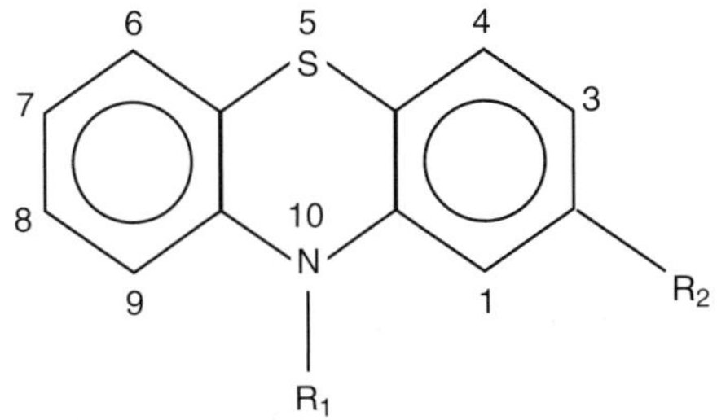

Figure 45–1. Phenothiazine structure.

Table 45–2. Relative Neuroreceptor Affinities for Antipsychotics*

Antipsychotic Agent	Receptor				
	Histamine H_1	*α-Adrenergic*	*M_1 Muscarinic*	*Serotonergic 5-HT_2*	*D_2/M_1 (EPS Risk)*
Typical Agents					
Chlorpromazine	2.1	7.3	0.27	0.94	3.8
Fluphenazine	0.038	0.088	0.00042	0.02	2358
Perphenazine	0.18	0.14	0.00093	—	1050
Prochlorperazine	0.37	0.30	0.0039	0.06	253
Trifluoperazine	0.042	0.11	0.013	0.79	78
Haloperidol	0.0021	0.66	0.00017	0.08	5952
Thiothixene	0.075	0.041	0.00016	—	6529
Molindone	0.00097	0.048	0.00031	0.10	3192
Loxapine	14	2.5	0.16	—	6.4
Pimozide	<0.0008	0.20	0.008	0.73	125
Atypical Agents					
Mesoridazine	10	9.5	0.28	—	3.8
Thioridazine	1.6	5.2	1.4	0.73	0.68
Clozapine	64	20	15	11.2	0.07
Olanzapine	2.8	1.1	4	2.8	0.02
Risperidone	1.12	1.50	—	6.75	—
Remoxipride	<0.02	0.03	0.03	0.04	33

*Relative neuroreceptor affinity = neuroreceptor affinity at receptor X/dopamine D_2 receptor affinity.
A higher numeric value indicates greater blockade of a given receptor when a dopamine receptor-blocking dose is given.
A higher 5-HT_2 relative neuroreceptor affinity (5-HT_2/D_2) and higher D_2/M_1 ratio confers a lower EPS risk.
Adapted from Black JL, Richelson E: Antipsychotic drugs: Prediction of side-effect profile based on neuroreceptor data derived from human brain tissue. Mayo Clin Proc *62*:369, 1987.

Neuroreceptor binding affinity is unique for each agent and allows fairly reliable prediction of adverse effects in both therapeutic and overdose situations.[2, 3] Clinical toxicity of antipsychotics results from exaggerated pharmacologic activity.

PHARMACOLOGY

Antipsychotic agents block D_2-subtype dopamine receptors in nigrostriatal (basal ganglia), tuberoinfundibular (hypothalamus to pituitary), mesocortical, and mesolimbic pathways of the brain. These agents additionally antagonize dopamine receptors in the medulla oblongata and anterior hypothalamus. Antipsychotic efficacy is mediated by a drug's ability to block mesocortical and mesolimbic D_2 receptors. A strong correlation has been noted between D_2 receptor affinity and potency in terms of daily dose of antipsychotic agents (see Table 45–1).[2] The likelihood of developing EPS (i.e., acute dystonia, parkinsonism, akathisia) correlates with nigrostriatal D_2 receptor potency relative to mesolimbic and mesocortical D_2 potency. For typical antipsychotics, basal ganglia D_2 blockade occurs in the same dose range necessary for limbic D_2 blockade, and thus high EPS liability is created.[2] Some atypical agents (e.g., sulpiride, remoxipride, raclopride) are believed to have low EPS liability owing to apparent physiologic selectivity at limbic over nigrostriatal pathways.[4]

D_2 receptor blockade in the pituitary (tuberoinfundibular pathway) causes sustained elevated prolactin secretion, which may result in galactorrhea, gynecomastia, menstrual changes, and sexual dysfunction. Dopamine receptor antagonism in the area postrema (chemoreceptor trigger zone) of the medulla oblongata is primarily responsible for antiemetic activity.

Regulation of core body temperature involves dopamine. Antipsychotic-induced D_2 receptor blockade in the anterior hypothalamus (preoptic area) may alter core temperature set-point, block thermosensitive neuronal inputs, or inhibit centrally mediated thermoregulatory responses. Hypothermia or hyperthermia may result. Body temperature response depends on the ambient temperature, the species involved, the receptor profile of the agent used, and a host of other factors. Chlorpromazine and haloperidol administration to rabbits produces hypothermia at normal and lower ambient temperatures but hyperthermia at elevated ambient temperature.[5] Decreased tolerance to heat and fatal heat stroke have been described in patients taking phenothiazines.[6] Antipsychotic agents have been successfully used to treat hyperthermia associated with use of cocaine and amphetamine.[7, 8]

The ratio of other neuroreceptor-binding affinities to D_2 receptor–binding affinity (relative binding affinities) predicts each drug's likelihood of producing those receptor-mediated effects at clinically effective antipsychotic (D_2-blocking) doses and in overdose (see Table 45–2). Antipsychotics bind to the α_1-adrenergic receptor with variable affinities. Relative potency correlates directly with the ability to cause orthostatic hypotension, reflex tachycardia, and miosis. Relative α_2-adrenergic binding is low for all antipsychotic agents except for clozapine, which has equivalent D_2 and α_2-adrenergic binding affinities. The clinical effect of α_2-adrenergic blockade is unclear. Histamine H_1 receptor antagonism correlates with antipsychotic-induced sedation and hypotension. Antipsychotics bind to and antagonize the muscarinic M_1 acetylcholine receptor. Relative potency correlates directly with the ability to induce anticholinergic stigmata (sedation, delirium, hallucinations, mydriasis, blurred vision, tachycardia, hyperthermia, cutaneous flushing, dry mouth and skin, urinary retention, and ileus) and inversely with the incidence of EPS. EPS occur when dopaminergic activity decreases in relation to cholinergic activity in the basal ganglia.[2, 9] Agents with high dopaminergic potency in relation to cholinergic potency (e.g., piperazine phenothiazines, thioxanthenes, butyrophenones, pimozide, and molindone) have a higher likelihood of inducing EPS. Agents with high relative cholinergic antagonism (e.g., aliphatic and piperidine phenothiazines, clozapine, olanzapine) have a low likelihood of inducing EPS (Fig. 45–2).

Atypia of an antipsychotic agent is not determined by any single or common pharmacologic receptor profile but is unique for each atypical agent. Clozapine, the prototypic atypical antipsychotic, has relatively weak D_2 receptor affinity, binds α_2-adrenergic and D_1 receptors with equal affinity to D_2 receptors, and binds D_4, muscarinic M_1, and serotonin 5-HT_{2A} receptors more avidly than D_2 receptors.[10] All of these pharmacologic actions may be partly responsible for clozapine's low propensity to induce EPS. Olanzapine is a novel antipsychotic agent with a receptor-binding profile similar to that of clozapine. Serotonin antagonism is now considered an important mechanism in both antipsychotic action and low EPS liability. The serotonin-dopamine antagonist concept contends that antipsychotics that are more potent at 5-HT_{2A} receptors than at D_2 receptors (e.g., clozapine, olanzapine, risperidone, thioridazine) have a low EPS liability.[11] Serotonergic fibers normally inhibit dopamine release in the nigrostriatal pathway.[11] Thus, blockade at 5-HT_{2A} receptors increases dopamine release in the striatum, offsets D_2 blockade, and lessens the likelihood of EPS (Fig. 45–3). 5-HT_{2A} antagonism correlates with antipsychotic efficacy. Thus, drugs with high 5-HT_{2A} antagonism in relation to D_2 antagonism can be given in smaller clinically effective antipsychotic doses, which have less risk of causing EPS development (less D_2 antagonism in the striatum). Newer drugs (e.g., risperidone) achieve antipsychotic efficacy for a majority of patients at doses that are less than the EPS threshold.[12]

Phenothiazine antipsychotics have local anesthetic or quinidine-like (antiarrhythmic and myocardial depressant) effects and frequently produce electrocardiogram (ECG) changes in therapeutic and overdose situations. The most cardioactive agents are thioridazine and mesoridazine. Thioridazine, mesori-

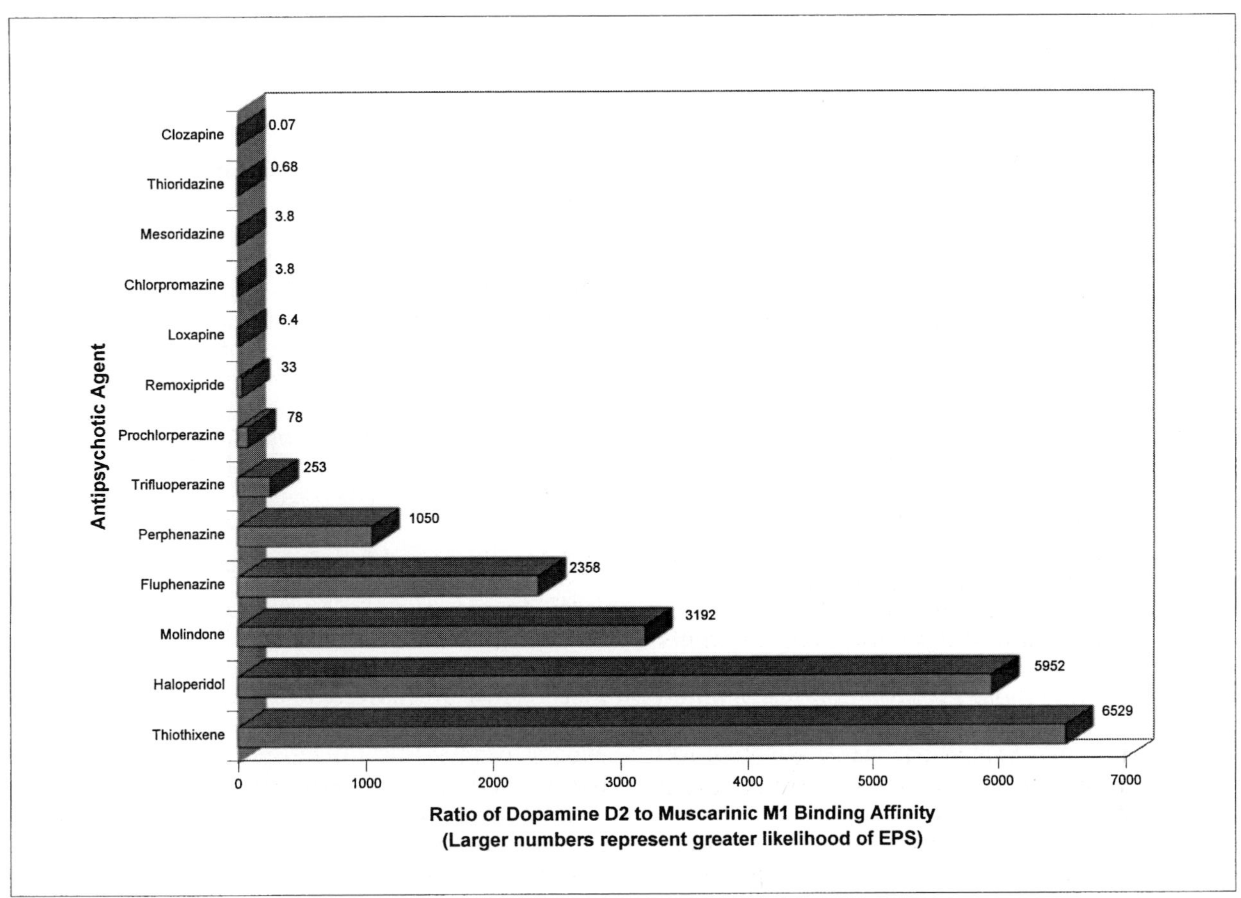

Figure 45–2. Theoretical likelihood of developing extrapyramidal side effects (EPS) with antipsychotic drugs.

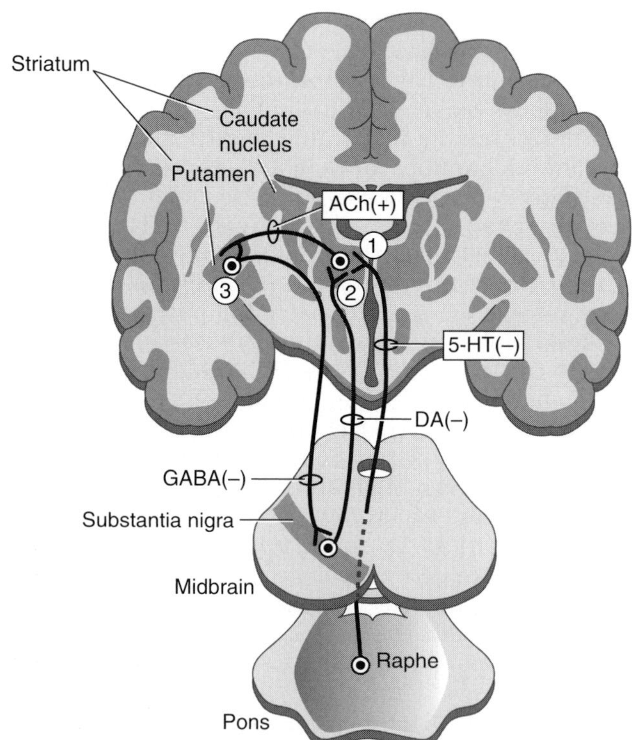

Figure 45–3. Schematic diagram of the nigrostriatal pathway. 1, presynaptic 5-HT_{2A} heteroreceptors; 2, postsynaptic D_2 receptors; 3, postsynaptic M_1 receptors. (Adapted from Cookson J: The development of new drugs for the treatment of schizophrenia. Br J Hosp Med *38*:544, 1987.)

dazine, and pimozide have added properties of calcium channel blockade, which may contribute to their dose-related ECG changes and cardiotoxicity in overdose.[13, 14] Electrophysiologic effects include a depressed rate of phase 0 depolarization, depressed amplitude and duration of phase 2, and prolongation of phase 3 repolarization.

PHARMACOKINETICS

Most chemical classes of antipsychotics have similar pharmacokinetics. They are well absorbed after oral administration, but bioavailability is unpredictable (range 10% to 70%) owing to interindividual variability, intestinal metabolism, and substantial first-pass hepatic clearance. Plasma concentrations peak 2 to 4 hours after therapeutic oral dosing and ½ to 1 hour after immediate-release intramuscular (IM) injections. After oral (PO) overdose, a larger amount of drug is available for absorption. Drug absorption should occur more rapidly (first-order kinetics), but more time is required for complete absorption. The result is more rapid onset of clinical effects but delayed peak serum concentrations and a longer duration of clinical effects. Erratic absorption may occur after ingestion of agents with greater anticholinergic effects.

Drug bioavailability is increased 4- to 10-fold after IM administration.[15] Slow-release or depot IM injections (e.g., fluphenazine and haloperidol decanoate) are created by esterifying the hydroxyl group of an antipsychotic with a long-chain fatty acid and dissolving it in a sesame oil vehicle. After IM administration, peak serum levels occur within 24 hours.[15]

Most antipsychotics are highly bound to plasma proteins (75% to 99%) and are extensively distributed to body tissue (i.e., brain) owing to high lipophilicity. Volumes of distribution are large and range from 10 to 40 L/kg. Neuroleptics readily cross the placenta and enter the fetal circulation.[16] They are also found in breast milk. Antipsychotics are slowly, extensively, and variably eliminated by hepatic metabolism. Urinary excretion of unchanged drug accounts for approximately 1% of the ingested dose. Extensive hepatic metabolism and large volumes of distribution result in long elimination half-lives (usual range, 10 to 40 hours). Molindone and pimozide are exceptions, having elimination half-lives of 1.5 and 50 to 200 hours, respectively.[17] Depot antipsychotics have an apparent elimination half-life of 3 weeks owing to slow tissue absorption.[15] Many hepatic metabolites are pharmacologically active and could be expected to extend the parent drug's effects after therapeutic or toxic dosing. Metabolites are variably excreted in the urine and stool after conjugation and enterohepatic circulation, respectively.

The benzamides are more hydrophilic compounds than other antipsychotics, and thus their pharmacokinetic profile is substantially altered. Elimination half-lives range from 2 to 14 hours, and 10% to 80% of the parent drug is excreted unchanged in the urine.[17]

TOXICOLOGY OF ANTIPSYCHOTIC DRUGS

Adverse Effects

Adverse effects (unintentional side effects that occur during therapeutic use) of antipsychotic agents may be idiosyncratic or dose related, may occur early or late during the course of therapy, and are often a result of receptor antagonism. Toxicity is commonly manifested in the cardiovascular system and central nervous system (CNS).

Extrapyramidal Syndromes

EPS are a group of sustained movement disorders that occur in as many as 90% of patients receiving these drugs and are a common reason why patients discontinue antipsychotic therapy.[18] EPS are a result of basal ganglia dopamine D_2 receptor blockade and consist of four main drug-induced syndromes. These can be divided into reversible syndromes that occur within days to weeks of the onset of antipsychotic therapy (acute dystonia, parkinsonism, and akathisia) and a potentially irreversible syndrome that occurs after months to years of therapy (tardive dyskinesia [TD]).

Acute dystonic reactions (dyskinesias) consist of intermittent spasmodic or sustained involuntary contractions of muscles in the face, neck, trunk, and occasionally extremities. Resulting clinical manifestations include facial grimacing, trismus, blepharospasm, oculogyric crisis, tongue protrusion, buccolingual crisis, retrocollis, torticollis, opisthotonos, abnormal postures and gait, and respiratory difficulty. Acute dystonia (AD), although distressing to patients, is uncommonly life threatening. Rare pharyngeal and laryngeal muscle spasm may produce respiratory distress and asphyxia. AD usually occurs soon after initiation of antipsychotic therapy or after an increase in dose. About 50% occurs within 48 hours and 90% within the first 5 days of treatment.[9, 19] Peak incidence occurs when antipsychotic levels are declining in the serum. In one study of pediatric patients, AD occurred 5 to 50 hours (mean 23 hours) after the first therapeutic dose and 1 to 20 hours (mean 5 hours) after single accidental ingestion of phenothiazines.[20] Incidence rates of AD vary greatly, depending on the agent given. Incidence rates of 0.6%, 3.5%, 8.3%, 16%, and 25% have been reported for thioridazine, chlorpromazine, thiothixene, haloperidol, and IM fluphenazine decanoate, respectively.[19] Risk factors for development of AD include use of antipsychotic drugs with high dopamine D_2, low muscarinic M_1, and low serotonergic 5-HT_{2A} binding affinities; use of depot preparations; male gender; young age (range, 5 to 45 years old); and a family history of AD or recent history of cocaine or alcohol use.[9, 19, 21] AD is an idiosyncratic reaction and is not more likely to occur after an acute overdose.

The pathophysiology of AD is not fully elucidated but involves disruption of dopaminergic–cholinergic–γ-aminobutyric acid (GABA) balance in the basal ganglia. Normally, dopamine is excitatory whereas GABA and acetylcholine act as inhibitory modulators of movement.[22] Serotonin may also have an inhibitory role (see Fig. 45–3).[11] Nigrostriatal dopamine neurons tonically inhibit cholinergic striatal interneurons and are inhibited by striatonigral GABA neurons and (probably) presynaptic serotonin heteroreceptors. Acute antipsychotic administration blocks postsynaptic dopamine D_2 receptors, and the result is increased acetylcholine release. Disruption of the dopaminergic-cholinergic balance in favor of cholinergic excess may underlie AD pathophysiology.[9] Paradoxically, AD may instead be due to enhanced dopamine release onto supersensitive postsynaptic receptors. Acute administration of antipsychotics provokes increased dopamine synthesis and release from nigrostriatal neurons and postsynaptic receptor supersensitivity. These are compensatory attempts to overcome postsynaptic dopamine D_2 receptor blockade. As brain concentrations of the drug decline hours to days after a dose, a state of dopamine excess develops and heightened muscular activity (dystonia) results.[23, 24]

Akathisia is a condition of subjective unease and motor restlessness that occurs within hours to days of initiation or increase of antipsychotic drug dosing. Akathisia is a dose-related complication that occurs at any age. It occurs more commonly in women and with the use of high-potency agents. About 20% of patients taking antipsychotics develop akathisia, usually within the first 3 months of treatment.[3] Akathisia may be a result of dopamine D_2 blockade in mesocortical pathways.[24]

Parkinsonism (akinesia) is a reversible syndrome of muscle rigidity, bradykinesia, and tremor that occurs in 13% of patients who take antipsychotic agents, usually within the first 2 to 3 months of therapy.[3] Drug-induced parkinsonism occurs in all age groups but more commonly in the elderly, in women, and with high-potency agents. Parkinsonism may also develop as a late-onset EPS and persist for years despite discontinuation of drug.[3] The rabbit syndrome is an uncommon reversible late-onset EPS characterized by perioral lip tremor. It is considered a variant of parkinsonism. Drug-induced parkinsonism is a result of nigrostriatal postsynaptic dopamine D_2 receptor blockade. A state of relative dopaminergic depletion and cholinergic excess is created.[24]

TD is a hyperkinetic late-onset EPS that typically occurs after 2 years of antipsychotic therapy and only rarely before 6 months.[25] It is characterized by involuntary and repetitive movements of orofacial structures and, occasionally, the trunk and arms. These movements include chewing; tongue protrusion; lip smacking, sucking, and pursing; facial grimacing; grunting; rapid eye blinking; and occasionally choreoathetosis of the trunk and limbs. TD is associated with all antipsychotic agents (except clozapine), can occur in children, and develops in 27% to 35% of patients on long-term antipsychotic therapy.[26] TD occurs more commonly in women older than 50 years and is frequently elicited in patients who have their drug discontinued or dose lowered after years of therapy.[3] TD is believed to result from supersensitivity and increased numbers of dopamine receptors in the nigrostriatal system as a compensatory response to prolonged receptor blockade by the antipsychotic agent. A state of dopaminergic excess and cholinergic underactivity is created.[3, 24]

Neuroleptic Malignant Syndrome

Neuroleptic malignant syndrome (NMS) is a rare, life-threatening idiosyncratic adverse reaction to antipsychotic agents. It usually occurs early in the course of treatment or soon after a change in dose but may appear at any time during therapy. NMS has been associated with all antipsychotic agents, but most reported cases have been secondary to the high-potency agents haloperidol and fluphenazine (particularly depot preparations). Reported incidence rates range from 0.02% to 12.2%, but prospective studies and pooled data from the literature report incidences of 0.07% to 0.2%.[27–29] NMS is not a result of overdose and usually occurs with antipsychotic serum levels in the therapeutic range. Potential risk factors for development of NMS include rapid initiation of antipsychotic therapy, use of high-potency agents and depot preparations, dehydration, severe patient agitation or catatonia, diagnosis of organic brain disease or affective disorder, preceding history of NMS, and concomitant use of predisposing drugs—namely lithium, anticholinergic agents, and antiparkinsonian agents. NMS occurs more commonly in men (2:1 ratio), with a mean age of 40 years.[30] NMS typically develops over a period of 24 to 72 hours and is variably characterized by hyperthermia (temperature ≥ 38°C), muscle rigidity (usually lead pipe), altered consciousness, autonomic dysfunction (dysrhythmias, urinary incontinence, diaphoresis, sialorrhea, tachycardia, hypertension or hypotension), elevated creatine phosphokinase levels (> three times normal), other signs of EPS, dyspnea, tachypnea, hypoxemia, dysphagia, and leukocytosis (white blood cell count > 12,000/mm^3). NMS may be a distinct entity or it may occur at the extreme end of a spectrum of EPS. Regardless, NMS is a heterogeneous syndrome with various signs, symptoms, degrees of severity, and laboratory abnormalities.[30] Fever, muscle rigidity, autonomic disturbances, and altered mental status occur in 95% to 100% of patients, elevated levels of creatine phosphokinase in 50% to 100%, elevated white blood cell count in 70% to 98%, and respiratory distress in 31% of patients.[27, 31] Abnormal laboratory findings may include elevated levels of hepatic transaminases, metabolic acidosis, myoglobinuria, renal failure, and decreased serum iron levels. No confirmatory laboratory tests exist for NMS, and diagnosis is based on a high level of suspicion in the appropriate clinical situation. Several researchers have proposed standardized but flexible criteria to assist NMS diagnosis.[27, 30] The presence of fever and muscle rigidity is usually required for diagnosis. Most cases of NMS seem to follow a sequence of development. Mental status changes or rigidity precedes autonomic dysfunction and hyperthermia in 82.3% of cases.[32] Thus, early recognition of confusion, catatonia, or worsening EPS may facilitate prompt treatment and halt progression to the fulminant syndrome.

Diagnosis of NMS should not be made before other etiologies, principally CNS infection, are ruled out. The differential diagnosis of NMS includes infection (e.g., meningoencephalitis), heat stroke, intracranial hemorrhage, thyrotoxicosis, pheochromocytoma, tetanus, strychnine poisoning, central anticholinergic syndrome, serotonin syndrome, monoamine oxidase inhibitor overdose or adverse drug interaction, lithium overdose, sympathomimetic intoxication (e.g., cocaine, designer amphetamines), alcohol or sedative-hypnotic withdrawal, malignant hyperthermia, and lethal catatonia. The mean duration of NMS ranges from 6.8 to 10.6 days,[27, 33, 34] and the clinical course is nearly twice as long in patients who have received IM depot preparations.[27] NMS was initially characterized as malignant because of its sometimes fatal outcome. Mortality rate, once estimated to range from 20% to 30%, is now estimated to range from 5% to 11.6%.[27, 34, 35] Death is usually secondary to respiratory failure (e.g., aspiration pneumonia, hypoventilation), cardiovascular collapse, myoglobinuric renal failure, arrhythmias, thromboembolism (e.g., pulmonary embolism), and disseminated intravascular coagulation.[27, 36] Renal failure is associated with a 50% mortality rate.[27] Seizures and pulmonary edema uncommonly complicate NMS.

The pathophysiology of NMS is unclear but may involve a functional dopamine deficiency state induced by antipsychotic dopamine receptor blockade. Blockade of dopaminergic receptors in the substantia nigra and hypothalamus results in rigidity and altered thermoregulation, respectively. Fever is the result of increased heat production from muscle rigidity, impaired heat dissipation, and possibly a higher set-point of core temperature in the hypothalamus. The pathophysiology of NMS may involve iron. Iron is a positive modulator of dopamine receptor activity, and low serum iron levels in NMS may lead to a decreased number of dopamine receptors in the brain.[37]

NMS should not be confused with malignant hyperthermia, a different clinical entity. Malignant hyperthermia is a rare genetically transmitted abnormality of skeletal muscle calcium metabolism. After a patient is exposed to certain anesthetic agents (e.g., succinylcholine, halothane) or stress, enhanced release and impaired reuptake of calcium result from muscle cell sarcoplasmic reticulum. The result is excessive excitation-contraction coupling and a syndrome of muscle rigidity and fever that may appear clinically similar to NMS.

Seizures

Seizures are uncommon side effects of antipsychotic drugs; they typically occur at higher therapeutic doses in susceptible patients and after overdose. All antipsychotic agents lower the seizure threshold, but to variable degrees.[38] The mechanism of seizure production remains obscure. Antipsychotics produce dose-related electroencephalographic (EEG) changes.[39, 40] The type and degree of EEG change vary depending on the neuroleptic. Risk factors for seizures include organic brain disease, epilepsy, a history of electroconvulsive therapy, abnormal EEG results, drug-associated seizures, polypharmacy, large drug doses, initiation of antipsychotic therapy, rapid dose titration, and use of certain antipsychotic agents. Seizures are more likely to occur with chlorpromazine, clozapine, and loxapine and less likely to occur with thioridazine, molindone, pimozide, fluphenazine, and haloperidol. Seizures have been reported in 1.2% of patients taking phenothiazines and 2.4% of patients taking clozapine.[38, 40] The probability of having a seizure with chlorpromazine and clozapine is dose dependent. A 0.5% incidence of seizures has been reported with low to moderate doses of chlorpromazine (30 to 900 mg/day) and 9% incidence with daily doses greater than 1 g.[40] A seizure rate of 1.8% has been reported with moderate doses of clozapine (300 to 600 mg/day), whereas those taking greater than 600 mg/day had an incidence of 14%.[39]

Cardiovascular Toxicity

Cardiovascular toxicity may occur during therapeutic dosing and after overdose of antipsychotic drugs. Effects are dose related and reversible. Hypotension (typically postural) and electrophysiologic changes are the usual toxic manifestations. Hypotension results from α_1-adrenergic blockade (direct vasodilation), central vasomotor reflex depression, and direct myocardial depression. Tachycardia may occur as a vasomotor reflex to hypotension or anticholinergic drug effects. Many antipsychotics (e.g., phenothiazines) exert a quinidine-like action on the myocardium and may impair cardiac conduction and depress myocardial contractility.

ECG changes include prolongation of the PR, QRS, and QT intervals, rightward shift of the terminal QRS vector, T wave abnormalities (widening, flattening, notching, and inversion), depressed ST segments, and increased U wave amplitude. QT prolongation is the earliest ECG change produced, and it reflects a disturbance in ventricular repolarization.[41] Atrioventricular, bundle branch, fascicular, and intraventricular blocks and supraventricular and ventricular arrhythmias all have been described with antipsychotics, particularly after overdose. Torsades de pointes ventricular tachycardia has been reported after high therapeutic doses and overdose of thioridazine, mesoridazine, and haloperidol. Cardiotoxicity is more common in thioridazine and mesoridazine overdose than with other antipsychotic agents.[42] Sudden death has been described in otherwise healthy patients receiving antipsychotic drugs. This may be the result of sudden ventricular tachyarrhythmias.

Miscellaneous Adverse Effects

Agranulocytosis (granulocyte count $< 500/mm^3$) is a serious idiosyncratic side effect of clozapine and phenothiazine therapy. It is rare (0.1 to 1.0/1000 persons) with phenothiazines and usually occurs in the first 12 weeks of therapy. The reported frequency is higher with clozapine (0.6% to 2.0%), and onset usually is within the first 18 weeks of therapy.[43] Mortality rates range from 30% to 85% once agranulocytosis occurs.[43] The risk of clozapine-associated agranulocytosis is minimized by regular white blood cell count monitoring, which is mandated by the Federal Drug Administration. Monitoring allows rapid detection and drug discontinuation. A mortality rate of 4% has been reported with intensive monitoring. If fever or infection develops in patients taking clozapine or phenothiazines, a complete blood count should be performed. Agranulocytosis has not been reported after acute overdose of phenothiazines or clozapine.

Priapism, allergic dermatitis, photosensitivity, cholestatic jaundice, and pigmentation of the skin, cornea, and lens have been described with phenothiazine use.

Drug Interactions

Several drugs may interact with antipsychotic agents to produce synergistic toxic effects or enhanced toxicity from either drug individually. The combination of antipsychotic agents with other CNS depressants (e.g., antihistamines, cyclic antidepressants, sedative-hypnotics, opiates, ethanol) produces enhanced CNS and respiratory depression. Enhanced anticholinergic effects may occur with concurrent use of tricyclic antidepressants (TCAs), certain skeletal muscle relaxants, antihistamines, and antiparkinsonian agents. The combination of thioridazine and mesoridazine with type IA antiarrhythmic agents or TCAs enhances cardiotoxicity. Hypotension may be potentiated when certain antipsychotic agents are combined with antihypertensive agents (e.g., prazosin). Enhanced neurotoxicity may occur when lithium or TCAs are combined with antipsychotics. TCAs and antipsychotics decrease the metabolism of each other and may potentiate toxicity of each other. Some antipsychotics decrease hepatic phenytoin metabolism and may induce toxic serum levels. Carbamazepine and clozapine may result in synergistic granulocytopenia. Drugs that alter hepatic metabolic capabilities may potentiate or inhibit antipsychotic metabolism. Clinicians should be aware of common drug interactions.

Overdose

Pure antipsychotic overdose is rarely fatal. Ingested doses that produce acute toxicity and lethality are highly variable. Many patients have survived ingestions larger than those reported to be lethal in others. Although the ingested dose may vary, seriously poisoned patients invariably demonstrate CNS and cardiovascular toxicity. Peak toxicity usually occurs within 2 to 6 hours after overdose, but delayed onset and peak toxicity are possible after ingestion of drugs that slow gut motility (e.g., anticholinergic drugs). Toxic effects are similar in adults and children.

CNS effects range from lethargy, slurred speech, ataxia, and confusion in mild intoxication to mild coma with respiratory depression in moderate intoxication to deep coma with apnea and loss of brain stem and deep tendon reflexes in severe intoxication. Paradoxical agitation and delirium may occur in mixed overdoses and those due to thioridazine, mesoridazine, olanzapine, and clozapine (central anticholinergic stigmata). CNS depression is usually manifested within 1 to 2 hours after ingestion. Respiratory depression requiring endotracheal intubation is uncommon but occurs with greater frequency in children, with mixed overdoses, and with sedating antipsychotics (e.g., aliphatic and piperidine phenothiazines, clozapine). Apnea and sudden infant death syndrome have been associated with use of antipsychotics. Seizures are uncommon in overdose but occur with greater frequency after loxapine and clozapine ingestions. Generalized major motor seizures typically occur. A seizure incidence of 60% has been reported after loxapine overdose.[44] Loxapine-associated seizures may be recurrent and can result in rhabdomyolysis, myoglobinuria, and acute renal failure.[44] Loxapine and clozapine have tricyclic structures similar to those of classic TCAs, and this may account for their enhanced neurotoxicity.

Mild hypothermia and, less commonly, hyperthermia have occurred in patients taking an antipsychotic overdose. α-Adrenergic vasodilation at high ambient temperature, seizures, and loss of sweating capabilities (anticholinergic syndrome) increase the likelihood of drug-induced hyperthermia. α-Adrenergic vasodilation at low ambient temperature, hypotension, coma, and loss of shivering capabilities increase the likelihood of drug-induced hypothermia. Peripheral anticholinergic stigmata (dry flushed skin, dry mucous membranes, hyperthermia, tachycardia, urinary retention, decreased bowel sounds) may follow ingestion of aliphatic and piperidine phenothiazines, clozapine, and olanzapine. Miosis or mydriasis may occur in overdose. Miosis is more likely to occur in seriously poisoned patients and has been described in 75% of adults and 72% of children after pure phenothiazine overdose.[45, 46]

Serious cardiovascular toxicity is uncommon after antipsychotic overdose unless piperidine phenothiazines have been ingested. Cardiovascular effects include hypotension, rare hypertension, sinus tachycardia, rare sinus bradycardia, conduction abnormalities (atrioventricular block, bundle branch block, intraventricular conduction delay), and arrhythmias (supraventricular tachycardia, premature ventricular contractions, ventricular tachycardia, ventricular fibrillation, and torsades de pointes). ECG abnormalities or obvious cardiotoxicity should be evident within several hours of overdose. Newer agents are not without cardiotoxicity. Prolonged QRS and QT intervals and hypotension have been described after risperidone overdose, and ventricular tachycardia has occurred after remoxipride overdose.[47–49] Acute pulmonary edema has been described anecdotally with perphenazine and chlorpromazine overdose and rapid haloperidol neuroleptization.[50, 51]

Diagnosis

Diagnosis of antipsychotic agent poisoning is based on history of ingestion, suggestive physical examination findings (miosis, variable CNS and respiratory depression, hypotension, sinus tachycardia, acute dystonia), typical ECG changes (QT prolongation), and adjunctive laboratory testing (radiographs, colorimetric urine tests, toxicologic screening). Abdominal radiographs may be obtained because phenothiazines and butyrophenones are radiopaque. Lack of radiographic visualization, however, does not rule out a significant ingestion. The Forrest, ferric chloride, and Phenistix colorimetric urine tests may be used to screen for phenothiazines. These tests do not detect nonphenothiazine antipsychotics, and negative color reactions do not rule out phenothiazine ingestion. Comprehensive screening of urine can be used to qualitatively confirm ingestion of many antipsychotics. Results of qualitative urine screens, however, are often negative, particularly in young children who present with AD more than 24 hours after ingesting a single antipsychotic tablet. Quantitative drug levels do not correlate well with clinical toxicity and are not helpful in treating patients. Antipsychotic agent toxicity may mimic and must be differentiated from toxicity resulting from sedative-hypnotics, opiates, anticonvulsants, alcohols, anticholinergic agents, and antihistamines. Mesoridazine and thioridazine toxicity may mimic that due to tricyclic antidepressants and type IA antiarrhythmic agents. CNS infection, cerebrovascular accident, and head trauma must be considered in the differential diagnosis of antipsychotic agent poisoning. The list of drugs producing dystonic reactions is extensive (Table 45–3) but may be useful in identifying etiologies other than phenothiazine exposure.

MANAGEMENT

Overdose

General

Treatment for antipsychotic agent poisoning is mainly supportive. Patients with significant CNS or respiratory depression should have their airway protected, breathing assisted, and cardiovascular support provided as necessary. All patients should have continuous cardiac monitoring, an intravenous (IV) line established, and ECG performed. Administer supplemental oxygen and parenteral thiamine, dextrose (or rapid fingerstick glucose determination), and naloxone to patients with an altered mental status. Semi-comatose patients should be placed in the left lateral, head-down position to lessen the risk of aspiration. Frequent vital signs and neurologic evaluations are necessary. Arterial blood gas analysis and continuous pulse oximetry are helpful for those patients with significant CNS and respiratory depression. Routine laboratory analysis should include a complete blood count and measurement of electrolytes, blood urea nitrogen/creatinine, and glucose levels. For patients with seizures or hyperthermia, laboratory evaluation should additionally include a urinalysis and serum creatinine phosphokinase, calcium, and magnesium determinations.

Seizures

Seizures should be treated with benzodiazepines (i.e., diazepam or lorazepam) and, if necessary, barbiturates (i.e., phenobarbital). Phenytoin is not a useful anticonvulsant in the setting of drug-associated seizures and is not recommended. Refractory seizures, such as with loxapine, may require induction of thiopental or pentobarbital coma or neuromuscular paralysis with continuous EEG monitoring. Obtain a fingerstick glucose level, monitor temperature frequently, and perform creatine phosphokinase analysis on all patients who have seizures.

Table 45–3. Drugs Reported to Have Caused Acute Dystonic Reactions

Generic Name	Brand Name	Generic Name	Brand Name
Well Documented		*Poorly Documented*	
Chlorpromazine	Thorazine	Alfentanil	Alfenta
Chlorprothixene	Taractan	Benztropine	Cogentin
Fluphenazine*	Prolixin	Bethanechol	Urecholine
Haloperidol	Haldol	Bromocriptine	Parlodel
Loxapine	Loxitane	Bupropion	Wellbutrin
Mesoridazine	Serentil	Buspirone†	BuSpar
Metoclopramide	Reglan	Carbamazepine†	Tegretol
Perphenazine*	Trilafon	Cholinesterase inhibitor insecticides	—
Prochlorperazine	Compazine	Cocaine	—
Promazine	Sparine	Copper	—
Promethazine	Phenergan	Cyanide	—
Thiethylperazine	Torecan	Erythromycin ethylsuccinate	EES
Thioridazine	Mellaril	Etoposide	VePesid
Thiothixene	Navane	Midazolam	Versed
Trifluoperazine*	Stelazine	Nifedipine	Procardia, Adalat
Less Well Documented		Phenobarbital	Luminal
Amitriptyline	Elavil	Sertraline	Zoloft
Amoxapine	Asendin	Trazodone†	Desyrel
Azatadine	Optimine	Verapamil†	Calan, Isoptin
Cimetidine	Tagamet	Antihistamines and decongestants	
Diazepam	Valium	Chlorpheniramine and phenylpropanolamine†	
Diphenhydramine	Benadryl	Pheniramine and phenylephrine†	
Doxepin	Sinequan		
Etomidate	Amidate		
Fluoxetine	Prozac		
Imipramine	Tofranil		
Ketamine	Ketalar		
Methohexital	Brevital		
Phenelzine	Nardil		
Phenytoin‡	Dilantin		
Thiopental	Pentothal		
Tranylcypromine	Parnate		

*Piperazine side chain phenothiazines.
†Symptoms were of latent onset (tardive dyskinesias).
‡Symptoms develop at toxic serum concentrations.
Adapted from McCormick MA, Manoguerra AS: Dystonic reactions. *In* Harwood-Nuss AL, Linden CH, Luten RC, et al (eds): The Clinical Practice of Emergency Medicine, ed 2. Philadelphia, Lippincott-Raven, 1996, p 1320.

Cardiovascular

Hypotension is treated initially with Trendelenburg's position and crystalloid boluses (10 to 40 mL/kg normal saline or Ringer's lactate solution). α-Adrenergic agonists (e.g., norepinephrine, phenylephrine) are first-line agents for treating refractory hypotension, particularly in those patients who have been poisoned by antipsychotics and who have significant α-adrenergic blockade. Epinephrine, a mixed α- and β-adrenergic agonist, may cause unopposed β-adrenergic stimulation and worsen hypotension. Dopamine, an indirect-acting agent, may be ineffective owing to presynaptic depleted norepinephrine stores or its stimulation of β-adrenergic receptors. Hemodynamic monitoring with a pulmonary artery catheter may be helpful for patients on pressors.

Arrhythmias should be treated according to advanced cardiac life support guidelines, with some exceptions. Types IA, IC (e.g., propafenone), II (β-blockers) and possibly III (e.g., amiodarone, bretylium) agents should be avoided in patients with conduction delays and ventricular arrhythmias. Their use may potentiate such cardiotoxicity. Sodium bicarbonate (1 to 2 mEq/kg IV bolus) may be effective and is recommended for patients with wide QRS complexes. Lidocaine is a safe and appropriate therapeutic agent for treating ventricular arrhythmias. Torsades de pointes ventricular tachycardia should be treated in the standard fashion (IV magnesium, chemical [IV isoproterenol] or electric overdrive pacing, and correction of hypoxemia and electrolyte disturbances).

Anticholinergic Syndrome

Physostigmine antidotal therapy may be used safely and effectively in poisoned patients who have peripheral or central anticholinergic stigmata and who are without cardiac conduction abnormalities on ECG. Physostigmine is sometimes helpful as a diagnostic aid and is particularly useful in the treatment of patients with anticholinergic-related hyperthermia, severe hallucinations, and agitated delirium unresponsive to benzodiazepines and requiring physical restraint. Physostigmine is given slowly IV (1 to 2 mg in adults and 0.02 mg/kg in children) over 3 to 5 minutes. Complete resolution of anticholinergic stigmata after initial physostigmine administration should not alter patient disposition. The clinical duration of action of physostigmine (20 to 90 minutes) is short compared with that of antipsychotic agents.

Thus, prolonged observation and potential physostigmine redosing are needed.

Decontamination/Enhanced Elimination

Gastrointestinal decontamination should be performed as rapidly as possible after stabilization of a patient. Activated charcoal (1 g/kg PO) with a cathartic is the preferred method for the majority of patients. Gastric lavage should not be routinely used for patients with an antipsychotic agent overdose when the risk of death is very low. Gastric lavage has not been definitively shown to improve clinical outcome and may cause significant morbidity.[52] It may benefit comatose patients who have ingested thioridazine or mesoridazine and who present within 1 hour after ingestion. Activated charcoal administration should follow gastric lavage if performed. Syrup of ipecac has no role in the emergency department management of patients with antipsychotic overdose. Administration of activated charcoal is still recommended for patients who present many hours after overdose because of decreased gastrointestinal motility that may be associated with antipsychotic toxicity. Multidose activated charcoal has no proven benefit in antipsychotic overdose. Because of extensive tissue and protein binding by antipsychotic agents, hemoperfusion, hemodialysis, and forced diuresis are not effective in overdose management. Urinary alkalization is beneficial in the setting of associated rhabdomyolysis to prevent myoglobinuric renal failure.

Disposition

Most patients with a pure antipsychotic overdose do not require hospitalization. Asymptomatic patients should be observed and monitored for 4 to 6 hours after reported overdose before they are medically safe for psychiatric disposition or discharge. Mildly symptomatic patients (i.e., lethargy, slurred speech, ataxia) should be observed until signs and symptoms have improved or resolved. Patients with arrhythmias, ECG abnormalities, prolonged hypotension, seizures, anticholinergic syndrome, or persistent CNS depression require hospital admission, typically to an intensive care unit.

Acute Dystonia

Treatment of AD may rarely require supplemental oxygen and airway protection for those with pharyngeal or laryngeal spasm. The usual treatment is rapid parenteral administration of the anticholinergic agent diphenhydramine (1 mg/kg IV or IM) or benztropine (1 to 2 mg IV or IM in adults or 0.02 to 0.05 mg/kg IV or IM). Some recommend diazepam (0.1 mg/kg slow IV push). AD usually resolves within 10 minutes of IV drug administration, but repeat dosing may be necessary for its complete resolution. AD also responds to use of biperiden (1 to 2 mg IM or IV in adults), trihexyphenidyl (2 mg PO twice a day), and amantadine (100 to 200 mg PO twice a day). However, these agents are more commonly given concomitantly with chronic antipsychotic therapy to prevent dystonia. Outpatient oral therapy is necessary for 48 to 72 hours after initial parenteral treatment of AD.[53] Benztropine (1 to 2 mg PO twice a day) or diphenhydramine (1 mg/kg PO three times a day) is commonly used, but other anticholinergics are acceptable. Benztropine offers less frequent dosing and less sedation but is associated with greater risk of anticholinergic side effects. Its use in children younger than 3 years is contraindicated owing to atropine-like side effects. Those who develop AD yet necessitate continued neuroleptic treatment may have the dose of neuroleptic decreased, continue anticholinergic drug therapy indefinitely, or be switched to an alternative antipsychotic agent with less EPS liability.

Akathisia

Akathisia is often mistaken for worsening psychosis. This mistake may prompt increased dosing of the antipsychotic agent and result in worsening agitation and restlessness. No treatment for akathisia is uniformly effective, but benefit may be obtained from reduction of neuroleptic dose, administration of the β-blocker propranolol (10 mg PO three times per day), clonidine therapy (0.1 mg PO three times per day), anticholinergic agents (e.g., benztropine, diphenhydramine, trihexyphenidyl), benzodiazepines (e.g., diazepam), or changing to an antipsychotic with less dopaminergic-blocking activity (e.g., thioridazine, clozapine).[3]

Parkinsonism

Treatment options for antipsychotic-induced parkinsonism include agents that enhance dopaminergic tone, such as amantadine, and agents that diminish cholinergic activity, such as benztropine, biperiden, trihexyphenidyl, and diphenhydramine.[3] Doses are similar to those used to treat adverse drug reactions. Symptoms may also improve with reduction of drug dose or change to an antipsychotic with less dopaminergic-blocking activity.

Tardive Dyskinesia

Once TD develops, it is difficult to treat and may be irreversible. No treatment for TD is uniformly effective, but many variably successful therapies have been reported. They include cholinergic agents (e.g., deanol, physostigmine, choline, and lecithin), GABA agonists (e.g., valproate, baclofen, benzodiazepines), dopamine agonists (e.g., levodopa/carbidopa [Sinemet], pergolide, bromocriptine), dopamine-depleting agents (e.g., reserpine, tetrabenazine, α-methyldopa), discontinuation of neuroleptic therapy, and switching to an antipsychotic with minimal TD liability (e.g., clozapine).[3, 54] Shortsighted but effective treatment for TD is to administer higher doses of antipsychotic agents, which temporarily relieve symptoms but further enhance receptor dysfunction. The best treatment for TD is to minimize its risk of development.[3, 55] Neuroleptic agents should be used in the lowest effective antipsychotic doses, and periodic re-evaluation of their need and adjustment of doses should be performed.[55] Anticholinergic agents exacerbate TD; thus, their long-term use with neuroleptics is discouraged. Drug-free intervals or "holidays" were once advocated but are no longer recommended. Because TD may be a progressively irreversible disorder, early detection and prompt neuroleptic withdrawal increase the likelihood of complete recovery.[54]

Neuroleptic Malignant Syndrome

Successful treatment of NMS requires prompt recognition, withdrawal of neuroleptic and NMS-potentiating drugs (e.g., anticholinergics, lithium), exclusion of sepsis and other medical conditions, and institution of intensive supportive care and specific pharmacotherapies. Head computed tomography and lumbar puncture are necessary to preclude other diagnostic possibilities. Empirical antibiotic administration is prudent because of possible concurrent infection and initial difficulty in differentiating NMS from systemic infection. Supportive care includes provision of adequate ventilation and oxygenation, rehydration, temperature reduction, and treatment of metabolic, renal, and cardiopulmonary complications. Prophylactic intubation should be considered for patients with excessive sialorrhea, swallowing dysfunction, coma, significant hypoxemia and acidosis, and rigidity with severe hyperthermia. The role of specific pharmacotherapy in NMS treatment is controversial, because most data on individual agent efficacy come from retrospective studies and case reports. Selection bias, the lack of standardized drug-dosing protocols, and the self-limited course of NMS make it difficult to establish the relative efficacy of specific therapy compared with supportive care alone. The possibility of a prospective controlled study is unlikely owing to the rare incidence of NMS. Specific treatment measures include nondepolarizing neuromuscular paralysis, electroconvulsive therapy, and administration of dantrolene, benzodiazepines, bromocriptine, amantadine, levodopa/carbidopa, nifedipine, and nitroprusside. All have been anecdotally reported to be effective in the management of NMS. Antimuscarinic therapy for NMS is discouraged; it is ineffective and may worsen hyperthermia.

Dantrolene, a congener of phenytoin, inhibits ionized calcium release from the sarcoplasmic reticulum and thus causes direct muscle relaxation. It is used mainly to treat NMS-associated hyperthermia and rigidity. It is given PO or by IV infusion four times daily (0.8 to 2.5 mg/kg per dose, up to 10 mg/kg per day). Bromocriptine, amantadine, and levodopa/carbidopa are dopamine agonists that are given to overcome neuroleptic-induced dopaminergic blockade, which may underlie the pathophysiology of NMS. Dopamine agonists are given alone or in conjunction with dantrolene or other muscle relaxants. Bromocriptine, a dopamine receptor agonist, is given PO three times daily (2.5 to 10 mg/dose). Amantadine, which enhances presynaptic dopamine release, is given PO two times daily (100 to 200 mg/dose). Levodopa/carbidopa, which increases presynaptic dopamine stores, is given PO three to four times daily (25/250 mg dose). In one retrospective analysis of 67 cases of NMS, dantrolene or bromocriptine reduced mean times to improvement and complete resolution as compared with supportive care alone.[33] Mean response time to clinical improvement was 1.0 day for bromocriptine, 1.7 days for dantrolene, and 6.8 days for supportive care alone. Mean time to complete resolution was 9.0 days for dantrolene, 9.8 days for bromocriptine, and 15.8 days for supportive care alone. A prospective nonrandomized study of 20 patients with NMS, however, demonstrated a more prolonged illness and greater complication rates with bromocriptine or dantrolene treatment as compared with supportive care alone.[33] The mean duration of illness was 9.9 days for patients receiving bromocriptine/dantrolene versus 6.8 days for patients receiving supportive care. In retrospective analyses, dopamine agonists (e.g., bromocriptine) have been reported to reduce NMS mortality rates significantly, from 21% to 9.2%.[27, 56] The combination of dantrolene with bromocriptine does not offer additional advantage over either drug alone.[56]

Prompt reduction of NMS-associated muscle rigidity and hyperthermia can be expected to minimize the risk of rhabdomyolysis, renal failure, pneumonia, respiratory failure, disseminated intravascular coagulation, and cardiovascular collapse. These complications are responsible for most NMS-associated deaths, and thus their prevention is paramount. Although hypothalamic thermoregulatory dysfunction may have a causal role in NMS-associated fever, thermogenesis is ultimately due to tonic skeletal muscle contraction.[36, 57] Rapid peripheral muscle relaxation is the goal. Dantrolene has a mean response time of 1.7 days, according to the most favorable analyses.[34] Rigidity and temperature reduction with dantrolene often takes longer, occurs erratically, and is incomplete.[57–59] Dantrolene is also a potentially hepatotoxic drug. It makes intuitive sense to use nondepolarizing neuromuscular paralysis (e.g., pancuronium) to achieve rapid, predictable, and effective resolution of rigidity and fever in those patients who are significantly ill (temperature ≥ 104°F). Pancuronium administration was rapidly successful in controlling rigidity and fever in case reports of two patients, one of whom had failed to respond to dantrolene therapy.[59, 60] A reasonable first approach to rigidity and fever management in NMS includes

IV benzodiazepines (diazepam 0.1 to 0.4 mg/kg IV), antipyretics, evaporative cooling, ice packs, and cooled IV fluids. If rigidity persists and temperature is 104°F or greater, timely neuromuscular paralysis and adjunctive dopamine agonist therapy (e.g., bromocriptine) are recommended. The best approach is to tailor pharmacotherapies to presenting symptoms. The level of intervention depends on the severity of illness.

References

1. Litovitz TL, Felberg L, White S, et al: 1995 Annual report of the American Association of Poison Control Centers Toxic Exposure Surveillance System. Am J Emerg Med *14*:487, 1996.
2. Richelson E: Neuroleptic affinities for human brain receptors and their use in predicting adverse effects. J Clin Psychiatry *45*:331, 1984.
3. Black JL, Richelson E, Richardson JW: Antipsychotic agents: A clinical update. Mayo Clin Proc *60*:777, 1985.
4. Silverstone T: Clinically relevant differences between antipsychotic compounds. Acta Psychiatr Scand *82*(Suppl 358):88, 1990.
5. Lin MT: Effects of dopaminergic antagonist and agonist on thermoregulation in rabbits. J Physiol *293*:217, 1979.
6. Zelman S, Guillan R: Heatstroke in phenothiazine treated patients: A report of three fatalities. Am J Psychiatry *126*:1787, 1970.
7. Catravas JD, Waters IW: Acute cocaine intoxication in the conscious dog: Studies on the mechanism of lethality. J Pharmacol Exp Ther *217*:350, 1981.
8. Espelin DE, Done AK: Amphetamine poisoning: Effectiveness of chlorpromazine. N Engl J Med *278*:1361, 1968.
9. Rupniak NMJ, Jenner P, Marsden CD: Acute dystonia induced by neuroleptic drugs. Psychopharmacology *88*:403, 1986.
10. Meltzer HY: An overview of the mechanism of action of clozapine. J Clin Psychiatry *55*(Suppl B):47, 1994.
11. Huttunen M: The evolution of the seratonin-dopamine antagonist concept. J Clin Psychopharmacol *15*(Suppl 1):4S, 1995.
12. Casey DE: Serotonergic and dopaminergic aspects of neuroleptic-induced extrapyramidal syndromes in nonhuman primates. Psychopharmacology *112*:S55, 1993.
13. Gould RJ, Murphy KMM, Reynolds IJ, et al: Antischizophrenic drugs of the diphenybutylpiperidine type act as calcium channel antagonists. Proc Natl Acad Sci U S A *86*:5122, 1983.
14. Gould RJ, Murphy KMM, Reynolds IJ, et al: Calcium channel blockade: Possible explanation for thioridazine's peripheral side effects. Am J Psychiatry *141*:352, 1984.
15. Javaid JI: Clinical pharmacokinetics of antipsychotics. J Clin Pharmacol *34*:286, 1994.
16. Lipton MA, DiMascio A, Killam KP: Psychotropic drugs in pregnancy. *In* Goldberg HL, DiMascio A (eds): Psychopharmacology: A Generation of Progress. New York, Raven Press, pp 1047–1055, 1978.
17. Dahl SG: Pharmacokinetics of antipsychotic drugs in man. Acta Psychiatr Scand *82*(Suppl 358):37, 1990.
18. Casey DE, Keepers GA: Neuroleptic side effects: Acute extrapyramidal syndromes and tardive dyskinesia. *In* Casey DE, Christensen AV (eds): Psychopharmacology: Current Trends. New York, Springer-Verlag, pp 74–83, 1988.
19. Swett C: Drug-induced dystonia. Am J Psychiatry *132*:532, 1975.
20. Gupta JM, Lovejoy FH: Acute phenothiazine toxicity in childhood: A five-year survey. Pediatrics *39*:771, 1967.
21. Hegarty AM, Lipton RB, Merriam AE, et al: Cocaine as a risk factor for acute dystonic reactions. Neurology *41*:1670, 1991.
22. Young AB, Albion RL, Penney JB: Neuropharmacology of basal ganglia function: Relationship to pathophysiology of movement disorders. *In* Grossman AR, Sambrook MA (eds): Neural Mechanisms in Disorders of Movement. London, Libbey, pp 17–27, 1989.
23. Kolbe H, Clow A, Jenner P, et al: Neuroleptic-induced acute dystonic reactions may be due to enhanced dopamine release on to supersensitive postsynaptic receptors. Neurology *31*:434, 1981.
24. Marsden CD, Jenner P: The pathophysiology of extrapyramidal side-effects of neuroleptic drugs. Psychol Med *10*:55, 1980.
25. Kobayashi RM: Drug therapy of tardive dyskinesia. N Engl J Med *296*:257, 1977.
26. Yassa R, Ananth J, Cordozo S, et al: Tardive dyskinesia in an outpatient population: Prevalence and predisposing factors. Can J Psychiatry *28*:391, 1983.
27. Caroff SN, Mann SC: Neuroleptic malignant syndrome. Med Clin North Am *77*:185, 1993.
28. Kellam AMP: The neuroleptic malignant syndrome, so-called: A survey of the world literature. Br J Psychiatry *150*:752, 1987.
29. Gelenberg AJ, Bellinghausen B, Wojcik JD, et al: A prospective survey of neuroleptic syndrome in a short-term psychiatric hospital. Am J Psychiatry *145*:517, 1988.
30. Nierenberg D, Disch M, Manheimer E, et al: Facilitating prompt diagnosis and treatment of the neuroleptic malignant syndrome. Clin Pharmacol Ther *50*:580, 1991.
31. Heiman-Patterson TD: Neuroleptic malignant syndrome and malignant hyperthermia. Med Clin North Am *77*:477, 1993.
32. Velamoor VR, Swamy GN, Parmar RS, et al: Management of suspected neuroleptic malignant syndrome. Can J Psychiatry *40*:545, 1995.
33. Rosebush PI, Stewart T, Mazurek MF: The treatment of neuroleptic malignant syndrome. Are dantrolene and bromocriptine useful adjuncts to supportive care? Br J Psychiatry *159*:709, 1991.
34. Rosenberg MR, Green M: Neuroleptic malignant syndrome: Review of response to therapy. Arch Intern Med *149*:1927, 1989.
35. Shalev A, Hermesh H, Munitz H: Mortality from neuroleptic malignant syndrome. J Clin Psychiatry *50*:18, 1989.
36. Guze BH, Baxter, LR: Neuroleptic malignant syndrome. N Engl J Med *313*:163, 1985.
37. Rosebush PI, Mazurak MF: Serum iron and neuroleptic malignant syndrome. Lancet *338*:149, 1991.
38. Marks RC, Luchins DJ: Antipsychotic medications and seizures. Psychiatr Med *9*:37, 1991.
39. Cold JA, Wells BG, Froemming JH: Seizure activity associated with antipsychotic therapy. DICP *24*:601, 1990.
40. Logothetis J: Spontaneous epileptic seizures and electroencephalographic changes in the course of phenothiazine therapy. Neurology *17*:869, 1967.
41. Elkayam U, Frishman W: Cardiovascular effects of phenothiazines. Am Heart J *100*:397, 1980.
42. Buckley NA, Whyte IM, Dawson AH: Cardiotoxicity more common in thioridazine overdose than with other neuroleptics. Clin Toxicol *33*:199, 1995.
43. Safferman A, Lieberman JA, Kane JM, et al: Update on the clinical efficacy and side effects of clozapine. Schizophr Bull *17*:247, 1991.
44. Peterson CD: Seizures induced by acute loxapine overdose. Am J Psychiatry *138*:1089, 1981.
45. Barry D, Meyskens FL, Becker CE: Phenothiazine poisoning: A review of 48 cases. Calif Med *118*:1, 1973.
46. Mitchell AA, Lovejoy FH, Goldman P: Drug ingestions associated with miosis in comatose children. J Pediatr *89*:303, 1976.
47. Brown K, Levy H, Brenner C, et al: Overdose of risperidone. Ann Emerg Med *22*:1908, 1993.
48. Acri AA, Henretig FM: The effects of risperidone (Risperdal-Janssen) in overdose. J Toxicol Clin Toxicol *33*:521, 1995.
49. Palatnick W, Meatherall R, Tenenbein M: Ventricular tachycardia associated with remoxipride overdose. J Toxicol Clin Toxicol *33*:492, 1995.
50. Li C, Gefter WB: Acute pulmonary edema induced by overdosage of phenothiazines. Chest *101*:102, 1992.
51. Mahutte CK, Nakasato SK, Light RW: Haloperidol and sudden death due to pulmonary edema. Arch Intern Med *142*: 1951, 1982.

52. Linden CH: General considerations in the evaluation and treatment of poisoning. *In* Rippe JM, Irwin RS, Alpert JS, Fink MP (eds): Intensive Care Medicine. 2nd ed. Boston, Little, Brown & Co., pp 1093–1114, 1991.
53. Corre K, Neimann J, Bessen H: Extended therapy for acute dystonic reactions. Ann Emerg Med *13*:194, 1984.
54. Klawans HL, Goetz CG, Perlik S: Tardive dyskinesia: Review and update. Am J Psychiatry *137*:900, 1980.
55. Casey DE: Neuroleptic-induced acute extrapyramidal syndromes and dyskinesia. Psychiatr Clin North Am *16*:589, 1993.
56. Sakkas P, Davis JM, Hua J, et al: Pharmacotherapy of neuroleptic malignant syndrome. Psychiatr Ann *21*:157, 1991.
57. May DC, Morris SW, Stewart RM, et al: Neuroleptic malignant syndrome: Response to dantrolene sodium. Ann Intern Med *98*:183, 1983.
58. Levenson JL: Neuroleptic malignant syndrome. Am J Psychiatry *142*:1137, 1985.
59. Sangal R, Dimitrijevic R: Neuroleptic malignant syndrome: Successful treatment with pancuronium. JAMA *254*:2795, 1985.
60. Mahmoodian S: Neuroleptic malignant syndrome. WV Med J *82*:435, 1986.

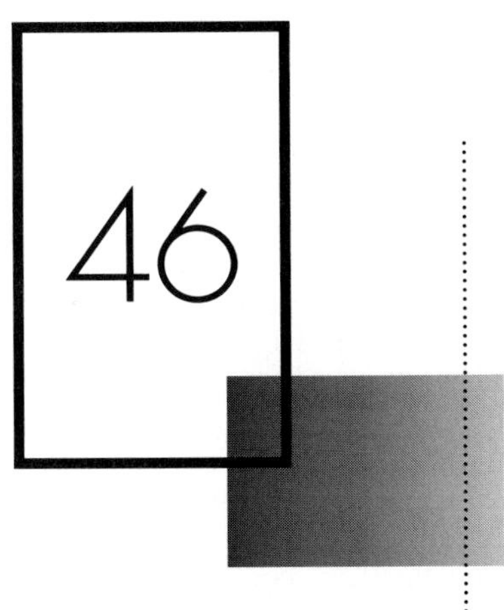

Anticholinergics and Antihistamines

MARK A. KIRK, MD

Anticholinergic drugs and plants have a distinct place in world history. Marc Anthony's military troops were neutralized and defeated after ingesting hallucinogenic anticholinergic plants. In 1676, a witness wrote of British soldiers' antics after they consumed salad containing *Datura stramonium.* His account is a vivid description of anticholinergic poisoning[1]:

"... some of them eat plentiful of it [James-town weed], the Effect of which was a very pleasant Comedy; for they turn'd natural Fools upon it for several Days: One would blow up a Feather in the Air: another wou'd dart Straws at it with much Fury; and another stark naked was sitting up in a Corner, like a Monkey, grinning and making Mows at them; a Fourth would fondly kiss, and paw his Companions, and snear in their faces ... and after Eleven Days return'd to themselves again, not remembring any thing that had pass'd."

In the world of crime, scopolamine has been "truth serum" and "knockout drops" for great detective novels. In the real world, it has produced temporary psychosis so that victims could be robbed. Analgesia for broken bones and cure for the common cold are only a few of the historical uses of anticholinergic drugs. These drugs continue to contribute to modern medicine.

Today, many classes of prescription and over-the-counter medications have anticholinergic properties. Anticholinergic effects are the therapeutic effects for some medications but produce only side effects and adverse drug reactions for others. In addition to medications, a number of plants and mushrooms contain anticholinergic alkaloids. Some are ingested deliberately for their mind-altering effects. Antihistamines are a diverse group of medications, most with potent anticholinergic effects and numerous other pharmacologic activities.

The clinical syndrome of anticholinergic poisoning is one of the most common and most easily recognized. Identifying the signs and symptoms of this syndrome is a basic skill for assessing a poisoned patient.

PHARMACOLOGY

Anticholinergics

Acetylcholine is a neurotransmitter found in various neuroeffector junctions (e.g., secretory glands) and synaptic sites.[2] It is a neurotransmitter in the cerebral cortex and lower centers, such as the reticular activating system and the postganglionic parasympathetic nervous system (muscarinic sites), and in the skeletal muscle motor end plate, spinal cord, and autonomic ganglia (nicotinic sites).[3] Muscarinic receptors are transmembrane proteins that interact with G proteins.[3] Acetylcholine binds to and activates muscarinic receptors, and the result is stimulation or inhibition of cellular function. Nicotinic receptors are cation channels in postsynaptic membranes responsible for skeletal muscle contraction. Acetylcholine is inactivated when metabolized at the synaptic cleft by the enzyme acetylcholinesterase.

Anticholinergic drugs block acetylcholine's action by competitively inhibiting its muscarinic receptor sites. The receptor sites in different organs are not equally sensitive to antimuscarinic effects.[2] Small doses of anticholinergic drugs decrease secretions of the sweat, bronchial, and salivary glands. With increasing doses, the sphincter muscle of the iris (mydriasis) and the ciliary muscle of the lens are paralyzed (cycloplegia). At the same dose, anticholinergic drugs block the vagal effects on the heart, and heart rate is thus increased. Even larger doses cause bladder atony and decreased gastrointestinal motility. These classic peripheral anticholinergic effects are caused by blocking postganglionic cholinergic nerves and predominate in most cases of acute poisoning.[4] Cholinergic neurons are spread widely through the cerebral cortex and subcortical areas.[3] Because of this ubiquitous distribution, they likely have a role in regulation and modulation of other neurotransmitters.[5] Central cholinergic pathways are important to memory, wake-sleep cycle, alertness, and orientation and for fine-tuning motor movements. The *central anticholinergic syndrome* refers to an acute psychosis or delirium resulting from inhibition of central cholinergic transmission. The degree of central anticholinergic activity is related to a medication's ability to cross the blood-brain barrier.

The autonomic ganglia are affected to a much smaller degree, and the nicotinic receptors at the motor end plates are unaffected by drugs that block muscarinic sites.

Antihistamines

Histamine is a mediator of the allergic response, a regulator of gastric acid secretion, and a central nervous system (CNS) neurotransmitter.[6] Three distinct receptors have been identified (H_1, H_2, H_3). Stimulation of H_1 receptors constricts bronchioles, dilates peripheral vasculature, and increases vascular permeability. H_2 receptors are primarily regulators of gastric acid secretion. In the CNS, histamine (H_1 and H_2) modulates activities such as arousal, thermoregulation, and neuroendocrine and vegetative functions that are controlled by the neocortex, hypothalamus, and hippocampus.[7] H_3 receptors are presynaptic regulators of synthesis and release of histamine into the synapse.

The antihistamines are reversible competitive inhibitors of H_1 receptors.[6, 7] This group of drugs can be divided into several classes: ethanolamines (diphenhydramine), ethylenediamines (pyrilamine), alkylamines (chlorpheniramine), piperazines (hydroxyzine), phenothiazines (promethazine), and piperidines (terfenadine and astemizole). Except for the piperidines, all classes readily cross the blood-brain barrier. Antihistamines are presented in this chapter because they possess antimuscarinic effects. In overdoses, their effects are clinically indistinguishable from those of other anticholinergic drugs and respond to physostigmine administration. In addition, antihistamines alter cortical neurons and block sodium channels. These effects cause CNS symptoms and cardiac conduction abnormalities.[8, 9] Promethazine and other phenothiazines have α-adrenergic blocking effects causing hypotension. The piperidines block the outward reuptake potassium rectifier current, and cardiac dysrhythmias result. Some H_1 antagonists such as cyproheptadine affect serotonin receptors.[10]

SYMPTOMS AND SIGNS OF ANTICHOLINERGIC TOXICITY

The diagnosis of the anticholinergic syndrome can easily be made at the bedside in most cases. The most commonly seen effects of anticholinergic poisoning can be divided into peripheral and central toxicity (Table 46–1). Peripheral manifestations are classic for the anticholinergic syndrome. Dry mucous membranes and hot, dry, flushed skin are a result of inhibition of secretions from the salivary glands, bronchioles, and sweat glands. Vasodilation occurs in peripheral blood vessels, especially those of the face. Body temperature rises because of altered CNS regulation and inability to sweat. The pupils are markedly dilated, and vision is blurred. Sinus tachycardia is one of the earliest and most reliable signs of muscarinic receptor blockade.[11] The urinary bladder may be palpable owing to urinary retention, and bowel sounds are hypoactive or absent. Altered peristalsis may result in prolonged symptoms secondary to reduced drug absorption.

Anticholinergic delirium, or the central anticholinergic syndrome, usually occurs in combination with peripheral signs of poisoning. This cause of delirium may be misdiagnosed because the physician does not look for the associated peripheral signs. The presen-

Table 46–1. Symptoms/Signs of Anticholinergic Toxicity

Peripheral (Muscarinic Blockade)
Tachycardia
Dry, flushed skin
Dry mucous membranes
Dilated pupils
Hyperpyrexia
Urinary retention
Decreased bowel sounds
Hypertension
Hypotension (late finding)
Central Anticholinergic Syndrome
Confusion
Disorientation
Loss of short-term memory
Ataxia
Psychomotor agitation
Picking and grasping movements
Extrapyramidal reactions
Visual/auditory hallucinations
Frank psychosis
Coma
Seizures
Respiratory failure
Cardiovascular collapse

tation is characteristically that of an acutely developing organic brain syndrome with disorientation, agitation, impairment of short-term memory, nonsensical or incoherent speech, meaningless motor activity such as repetitive picking at bed clothes or grabbing at nonexistent objects, removal of clothing, and visual hallucinations.[12–17]

In overdose, both central and peripheral anticholinergic signs are commonly present. Indeed, the famous mnemonic well describes the anticholinergic syndrome: *Mad as a hatter, red as a beet, dry as a bone, blind as a bat, and hot as a hare.*

The central anticholinergic syndrome may occasionally occur without evidence of peripheral signs.[18–21] This seems more likely to occur in the elderly and those with underlying organic brain syndrome.[16] It has been encountered even when therapeutic doses of anticholinergic drugs have been administered.[16, 18] Anticholinergic delirium is frequently misdiagnosed as dementia or psychotic depression in elderly patients.[18, 20] Anticholinergic-poisoned children have initially been misdiagnosed with varicella encephalitis.[22, 23]

Because of patients' extreme degree of disorientation, a history of ingestion is frequently impossible to obtain. For this reason, a thorough physical examination for common peripheral anticholinergic findings is of vital importance. All medications available to the patient should be inspected. Any history obtainable from friends or relatives about abuse of drugs or hallucinogenic plants (particularly jimsonweed and mushrooms) may be of value. A history of recent travel and the use of scopolamine patches should be sought. The diagnosis of acute poisoning in an acutely psychotic patient can be made only if it is thought of, and the presence of classic peripheral anticholinergic findings is frequently the key. In a mixed ingestion, the physical findings may be variable and the clinical picture may thus be confused.

As with many other ingestions, a toxicology screen has limited value. Agents producing anticholinergic toxicity may not be part of a routine screen, and a significantly toxic patient and a negative toxicologic screen may thus result.[24] Quantitative levels of many anticholinergic agents are usually unobtainable or do not correlate well with symptoms. It takes time to obtain results from a toxicologic screen; therefore, the tests are useful for confirmation of the presence of a drug and not as a tool for determining treatment. Treatment should be based on information obtained from the clinical evaluation.

Anticholinergic poisoning is included on every list of toxin-induced seizures. Despite this, seizures are not a frequent manifestation of anticholinergic poisoning. Seizures have infrequently been reported in jimsonweed abusers and atropine-poisoned infants. The mechanism of anticholinergic-induced seizures remains unclear. The majority of seizures related to anticholinergic toxicity seem to be associated with medications having other toxic manifestations. Seizures have been reported with antihistamine, cyclic antidepressant, phenothiazine, and carbamazepine poisonings. Interestingly, researchers have suggested that histamine may have a role as a natural anticonvulsant. Positron emission tomography has demonstrated H_1 receptors' coalescence around epileptogenic foci in brain possibly, and this may inhibit generalization of epileptic discharges in the brain.[25] Antihistamines increase electroencephalographic abnormalities and are suspected to produce seizures in epileptic patients. Phenothiazines are a class of antihistamines that has long been thought to decrease the seizure threshold. Doxepin and other cyclic antidepressants are potent histamine blockers that frequently cause seizures when taken in serious overdoses. In addition, seizure activity from some medications with anticholinergic activity is due to interactions at γ-aminobutyric acid (GABA) receptors (cyclic antidepressants) and adenosine receptors (carbamazepine).

Anticholinergic-induced seizures are usually short lived and require no specific therapy. However, large overdoses of diphenhydramine, pyrilamine, hydroxyzine, orphenadrine, cyclic antidepressants, and carbamazepine have caused prolonged or repeated seizures.

Sinus tachycardia is the most common arrhythmia in anticholinergic poisoning. Some medications with anticholinergic properties cause life-threatening cardiac arrhythmias by mechanisms other than muscarinic blockade. Medications with anticholinergic effects and the potential to cause quinidine-like conduction abnormalities include cyclic antidepressants, phenothiazines, diphenhydramine, chlorpheniramine, orphenadrine, pyrilamine, and class IA antiarrhythmics.[9] These drugs have sodium channel–blocking properties that not only slow conduction but also decrease myocardial contractility. Phenothiazines are also potassium channel efflux blockers that prolong QT interval and cause ventricular dysrhythmias.

Rhabdomyolysis is a complication of anticholinergic poisoning.[26] Drug-induced rhabdomyolysis from anticholinergic poisoning is due to excess energy use or inadequate oxygen and nutrient delivery to the muscle, which causes myocyte breakdown. Patients at risk are those with prolonged seizures, coma, compartment syndrome, hyperthermia, or severe agitation requiring restraint.

Polydrug poisoning from a single medication is possible because many over-the-counter products contain a combination of anticholinergic, antihistamine, and analgesic medications. In particular, poisoning by acetaminophen should be ruled out when an anticholinergic syndrome is recognized.

AGENTS THAT PRODUCE THE ANTICHOLINERGIC SYNDROME

Both pharmaceutical agents and plants may cause significant anticholinergic toxicity (Table 46–2). For many medications, such as the gastrointestinal antispasmodics or the local mydriatics, the anticholinergic properties are considered the desired therapeutic responses to the drug. Hence, many of the primary pharmacologic effects are not considered toxic. The desired therapeutic effects of many other medications, such as antipsychotics and antiparkinsonian drugs, are not related to peripheral anticholinergic symptoms. Thus, mydriasis, constipation, tachycardia, and dry mouth are frequently considered manifestations of toxicity.

Combining medications with anticholinergic properties produces synergistic effects.[14–16, 27] For example, antiparkinsonian medications, when given in combination with phenothiazines to prevent the occurrence of undesirable extrapyramidal reactions, greatly increase the incidence of toxic confusional states.[28] Small changes in the dose of either drug may precipitate the central anticholinergic syndrome in a previously unaffected individual.[29] Additive effects may be common because so many medications, including over-the-counter products, have anticholinergic properties. For example, the combined use of oral diphenhydramine with topical application of Caladryl lotion (calamine lotion and diphenhydramine) has produced central anticholinergic toxicity in children.[22, 30, 31]

An unusual form of toxicity involves the use of transdermal scopolamine patches.[32] Several cases of the central anticholinergic syndrome have been reported in adults and children using the patches for treatment of motion sickness. Accidental instillation of the drug into the eyes has occurred after manipulation of the patch. This has resulted in a unilateral fixed dilated pupil or bilateral fixed dilated pupils without focal neurologic changes.[33, 34] An additional method of systemic anticholinergic toxicity involves the absorption of ophthalmologic agents or nasal decongestants through the conjunctiva, nasal mucosa, or gastrointestinal tract.[35–37]

Table 46–2. Examples of Agents with Anticholinergic Properties

Plants and Mushrooms	
Atropa belladonna	Deadly nightshade
Datura stramomium	Jimsonweed
Mandrigora officinarum	Mandrake
Hyoscyamine niger	Henbane
Amanita muscaria	Fly agaric
Amanita pantherina	Panther
Belladonna Alkaloids and Related Synthetic Compounds	
Atropine	
Scopolamine	
Glycopyrrolate (Robinul)	
Antispasmodics	
Clidinium bromide (Librax)	
Dicyclomine (Bentyl)	
Propantheline bromide (Pro-Banthīne)	
Methantheline bromide (Banthīne)	
Flavoxate (Urispas)	
Oxybutynin (Ditropan)	
Antiparkinsonism Medications	
Benztropine mesylate (Cogentin)	
Biperiden (Akineton)	
Trihexyphenidyl (Artane)	
Local Mydriatics	
Cyclopentolate (Cyclogyl)	
Homatropine (Isopto Homatropine)	
Tropicamide (Mydriacyl)	
Antihistamines	
Brompheniramine (Dimetane)	
Chlorpheniramine (Ornade, Chlor-Trimeton)	
Cyclizine (Marezine)	
Dimenhydrinate (Dramamine)	
Diphenhydramine (Benadryl, Caladryl)	
Hydroxyzine (Atarax)	
Meclizine (Antivert)	
Antipsychotics	
Chlorpromazine (Thorazine)	
Prochlorperazine (Compazine)	
Thiothixene (Navane)	
Thioridazine (Mellaril)	
Trifluoperazine (Stelazine)	
Perphenazine (Trilafon)	
Over-the-Counter Sleep Aids	
Diphenhydramine (Benadryl)	
Doxylamine (Unisom)	
Cyclic Antidepressants	
Amitriptyline (Elavil)	
Amoxapine (Asendin)	
Clomipramine (Anafranil)	
Imipramine (Tofranil)	
Others	
Amantadine (Symmetrel)	
Ipratropium (Atrovent)	
Cyproheptadine (Periactin)	

Scopolamine eye drops have allegedly been used deliberately to disorient subsequent victims of theft.[38] The victim is often found naked, disoriented, hallucinating, and amnestic to the events before hospitalization. Scopolamine was believed to have been placed in a beverage ingested by the victim.[24] Many toxicologic laboratories do not routinely screen for scopolamine; therefore, these patients had negative results of toxicologic screens.

Both anticholinergic pharmaceuticals and plants may be abused. Central anticholinergic effects of intentional ingestion may produce euphoria and hallucinogenic effects.[39] It has been proposed that a physiologic dependence and the development of withdrawal symptoms exist when the agent is withheld.[39] Among the most frequently reported anticholinergic drugs abused are the antiparkinsonian agents trihexyphenidyl and benztropine mesylate.[40] These drugs have potent dopamine reuptake inhibition. The resulting dopamine excess is a proposed mechanism for craving of many abused drugs.[40, 41] Drug seekers may feign extrapyramidal symptoms to receive additional anticholinergic agents.[39, 42–45]

Many types of plants contain alkaloids that cause anticholinergic symptoms in humans. Most of these are found in the family Solanaceae, which includes the genera *Atropa, Datura, Hyoscyamus, Lycium,* and *Solanum.* The principal alkaloids found in these plants include solanine, atropine (a racemic mixture of D- and L-hyoscyamine, of which only the levorotatory isomer is pharmacologically active), and scopolamine (L-hyoscine). The mushrooms *Amanita muscaria* and *A. pantherina* have anticholinergic as well as cholinergic activity. Anticholinergic effects can be severe but are rarely the prominent finding with poisoning by these mushrooms.[46] The alkaloid content of each species and each plant varies greatly and depends on such parameters as the time of year, the available moisture, and the temperature. For this reason, it is very difficult to determine predicted toxicity in relation to the amount and the origin of the plant material. Recreational abusers of anticholinergic mushrooms and *D. stramonium* (jimsonweed) are unable to titrate the dose of ingested substance because of this tremendous biologic variability and therefore are prone to severe anticholinergic poisoning.

DIFFERENTIAL DIAGNOSIS OF ANTICHOLINERGIC POISONING

The constellation of symptoms that identify the anticholinergic syndrome can be mimicked, in part, by many other toxins and medical conditions (see Table 46–3). Distinguishing it from adrenergic excess (sympathomimetic poisoning, thyrotoxicosis, or pheochromocytoma) can be difficult. The pupillary, cardiovascular, and CNS effects of sympathomimetic poisons are similar to those produced by anticholinergic poisoning. Sweating frequently accompanies adrenergic stimulation, whereas dry skin and mucous membranes are characteristic of anticholinergic poisoning. Paranoid hallucinations and violent behavior often accompany adrenergic-induced hallucinations, whereas anticholinergic poisoning causes mumbling speech, picking at sheets, and disorientation. The anticholinergic syndrome also has similarities to autonomic dysfunction due to ethanol or sedative-hypnotic withdrawal, serotonin syndrome, neuroleptic malignant syndrome, or disulfiram reaction. Chronic salicylate poisoning can appear similar to anticholinergic poisoning because patients often present with altered mental status, tachycardia, and fever. Medical conditions can also mimic the anticholinergic syndrome. Hypoxia or hypoglycemia causes delirium, agitation, or CNS depression. Dry, hot skin and altered sensorium due to heat stroke, dehydration, or sepsis can be mistaken for anticholinergic toxicity. Central anticholinergic effects in the absence of peripheral signs can be similar to those caused by some hallucinogenic substances, steroid-induced psychosis, vascular or infectious CNS disease, sepsis, or psychiatric illnesses.

Table 46–3. Toxins and Medical Conditions Easily Confused with the Anticholinergic Syndrome

Toxins
Adrenergic poisons
Cocaine
Amphetamines
Phencyclidine
Phenylpropanolamine
Methylphenidate
Theophylline
Caffeine
Autonomic dysfunction
Withdrawal from ethanol or benzodiazepines
Serotonin syndrome
Neuroleptic malignant syndrome
Disulfiram reactions
Salicylate poisoning
Medical Conditions
Hypoxia
Hypoglycemia
Adrenergic excess
Thyrotoxicosis
Pheochromocytoma
Heat stroke
Dehydration
Sepsis
Central Anticholinergic Syndrome Without Peripheral Signs
Hallucinogens
Steroid-induced psychosis
Cerebral vasculitis
Central nervous system infection
Sepsis
Psychiatric illnesses

TREATMENT OF ANTICHOLINERGIC TOXICITY

General Management

The majority of patients poisoned by anticholinergic agents are adequately treated with supportive care and observation.

Anticholinergics inhibit gastrointestinal motility and can cause prolonged, erratic, or delayed drug absorption. After a large overdose of benztropine, a patient demonstrated erratic absorption and repeated worsening of anticholinergic symptoms over 9 days.[47] Because of slowed gastrointestinal absorption, gastric emptying procedures may be useful even when patients present many hours after an ingestion. Administration of charcoal is effective for preventing further drug absorption. Repeated doses of activated charcoal may have a key role in preventing continued absorption, although the development of ileus limits its use.

Treatment of Agitation

Anticholinergic-induced delirium ranges from mild confusion to severe agitation and possibly violence. Controlling agitation is necessary for adequate patient assessment and to prevent rhabdomyolysis, hyperthermia, and physical trauma. Physical or chemical restraints are indicated for treating severe agitation. Administration of haloperidol is frequently recommended for the control of agitated patients. Benzodiazepines are an alternative to haloperidol. They effectively calm a patient and act centrally to diminish hyperdynamic cardiovascular effects of adrenergic or anticholinergic agents. Benzodiazepines are preferable to haloperidol when agitation does not pose a considerable safety risk to the patient or staff. When anticholinergic toxicity is certain, physostigmine is an alternative to haloperidol or benzodiazepines.

Treatment of Seizures

Although mechanisms are not entirely understood, it is known that many toxins alter GABA inhibition, glutamate stimulation, or adenosine modulation at CNS synapses and thus cause toxin-induced seizures. Based on these mechanisms, enhancing CNS neuronal inhibition at GABA receptors with benzodiazepines or barbiturates seems most logical for treating toxin-induced seizures. The mechanism of anticholinergic-induced seizures is unclear. Case reports suggest that physostigmine stops seizures, but clinical experience is limited and no proof of its efficacy for seizure control exists.[48, 49] Therefore, anticholinergic-induced seizures should be treated with benzodiazepines and barbiturates. Reserve physostigmine for refractory seizures.

Treatment of Rhabdomyolysis

Agitation and excessive neuronal stimulation increase the risk of rhabdomyolysis. Controlling agitation and seizures is important to prevent rhabdomyolysis. Measuring creatine phosphokinase and urine myoglobin levels is the key to recognizing those at risk of developing acute renal failure. Ensuring adequate urine output with intravenous fluids, alkalization of the urine, and intravenous mannitol are basic strategies for preventing acute tubular necrosis.[26]

Treatment of Cardiovascular Toxicity

Sinus tachycardia is the most common toxic cardiovascular effect from anticholinergic poisoning but rarely requires intervention. A large number of drugs with anticholinergic effects cause QRS prolongation and dysrhythmias by blocking sodium channels.[50–52] Intravenous sodium bicarbonate improves impaired conduction from sodium blockers such as cyclic antidepressants and diphenhydramine. Rarely, myocardial pump failure occurs with large overdoses. Case reports show that refractory shock develops despite aggressive medical intervention. Patients with such profound cardiovascular toxicity have been successfully rescucitated after cardiac bypass or intra-aortic balloon pump procedures.[53]

Antidote Therapy

The major controversy surrounding the treatment of the anticholinergic syndrome concerns the use of physostigmine. Physostigmine, a naturally occurring alkaloid obtained from the West African vine *Physostigma venenosum,* is a reversible cholinesterase inhibitor.[2] After a single dose of physostigmine, the action of acetylcholine is potentiated at the postganglionic parasympathetic and the central cholinergic neuroreceptors, and the action of anticholinergic agents is reversed. Physostigmine crosses the blood-brain barrier and is capable of reversing coma and delirium and may be beneficial for seizures.[54–58] Peripherally, physostigmine may reverse the tachycardia, mydriasis, ileus, and urinary retention that occur secondary to muscarine blockade.

Physostigmine alters CNS neurotransmitters by still poorly understood mechanisms. Interestingly, toxic effects of drugs without anticholinergic activity have responded to physostigmine administration.[58] In years past, physostigmine was part of a "coma cocktail" administered to a large number of patients. The large published clinical experience from that era demonstrates its relatively safe use.[59]

One must be cautious, however, about the indiscriminate use of physostigmine, which may precipitate seizures, cholinergic crisis, or bradyarrhythmias and asystole. In a clinical series, 2 of 21 patients receiving physostigmine had seizures after administration, and 2 developed cholinergic symptoms (hypersalivation in one patient, bradycardia and hypotension in the other). The investigator concluded that because patients with anticholinergic symptoms usually fare well with supportive therapy alone, physostigmine has "little part to play in routine management."[60] In one series of 26 patients receiving intravenous physostigmine, 3 (12%) suffered seizures thought to be secondary to this medication (although

17 had ingested a tricyclic antidepressant), and one had bradycardia.[61] One case report describes a patient poisoned by *D. stramonium* (jimsonweed), who developed atrial fibrillation and a short run of ventricular tachycardia 45 minutes after administration of physostigmine.[62] In an additional case report, an 85-year-old man developed ventricular ectopy 30 minutes after receiving 1 mg of physostigmine.[63] Therefore, there is little question that physostigmine can be dangerous if given inappropriately (that is, in the absence of severe anticholinergic findings) or too quickly.

Physostigmine is no longer indicated in the treatment of cyclic antidepressant poisoning, and evidence suggests that it may be dangerous.[61, 64–66] A series of 41 patients taking intentional overdoses of maprotiline showed that 6 of 7 patients treated with physostigmine developed seizures.[65] The investigators concluded that the use of physostigmine should be abandoned in overdoses of maprotiline and other cyclic antidepressants. Similar case reports of two patients ingesting tricyclic antidepressants suggest that physostigmine was responsible for the ultimate development of asystole in two complicated resuscitative efforts.[66] The potential risks associated with physostigmine are greater than the benefits gained from its use in cyclic antidepressant toxicity.

The indications for the use of physostigmine in cases of anticholinergic poisoning should be restricted to

- Pronounced hallucinations and agitation in which patients may be dangerous to themselves or others
- Narrow complex supraventricular arrhythmias clearly resulting in hemodynamic instability (hypotension, myocardial ischemia, or congestive heart failure) when other attempts to control heart rate have failed or are believed to be too risky in a particular patient
- Intractable seizures

The relative contraindications to the use of physostigmine include asthma, gangrene, ischemic heart disease, peripheral vascular disease, and mechanical obstruction of the gastrointestinal or urogenital tract.[2, 67]

The suggested doses of physostigmine are as follows:

- For children: A dose of 0.02 mg/kg.
- For adults: 1 to 2 mg slowly intravenously; may be repeated every 10 minutes until cessation of the life-threatening condition. Schneck has recommended an intravenous infusion of 2 mg in 100 mL of normal saline infused over 10 minutes to avoid adverse effects from too rapid administration.[5]

The duration of action is 20 to 60 minutes, and recurrence of anticholinergic symptoms may require repeated doses. Adverse effects are more likely after repeated doses. Cholinergic excess due to physostigmine use is often not life threatening. It has been suggested that atropine be available and be given in half the dose of physostigmine should severe cholinergic toxicity develop.[55] The use of glycopyrrolate, a pure peripheral anticholinergic agent, has been proposed as an alternative treatment to the cholinergic toxicity of physostigmine.

Whenever physostigmine is used, it should (1) be given very slowly (over 5 to 10 minutes) intravenously; (2) not be given merely to "wake the patient up"; (3) be used only in a setting where advanced life support is available; (4) be used only when central and peripheral anticholinergic findings are present; (5) be used only in the absence of cardiac conduction abnormalities suggesting sodium channel blockade; and (6) always be preceded and followed by proper supportive care.

SPECIAL CONSIDERATIONS FOR ANTIHISTAMINE TOXICITY

Nonsedating Piperidine Antihistamines

Antihistamines sedate many people at therapeutic doses. Researchers developed and released terfenadine, a nonsedating H_1 blocker, in 1990. Shortly after its release, clinicians began reporting cases of prolonged QT and torsades de pointes in patients taking terfenadine. The pharmacologically active agent at the H_1 receptor is the hepatic metabolite terfenadine carboxylate.[10] The cardiac toxic effects are due to impaired hepatic metabolism and accumulation of the parent compound. Terfenadine inhibits the potassium rectifier current and thus slows repolarization.[68] This is manifested clinically as prolongation of the QT interval and torsades de pointes. Agents shown to inhibit P-450 metabolism of terfenadine include erythromycin, clarithromycin, ketoconazole, and grapefruit juice. Overdoses and underlying liver disease in the absence of P-450 inhibitors can cause cardiac toxic effects.

Terfenadine, astemizole, and loratadine are currently marketed in the United States nonsedating piperidine antihistamines. In therapeutic doses, their lack of CNS effects is secondary to an inability to cross the blood-brain barrier.[10] Limited experience has been had with acute poisoning by these medications, although astemizole overdoses have resulted in CNS sedation and seizures. All three have been reported to cause significant cardiovascular effects in overdoses.

Histamine$_2$ Receptor Blockers

The H_2 blockers used to treat peptic acid diseases are cimetidine, ranitidine, famotidine, and nizatidine. They are selective and do not block H_1 receptors or have antimuscarinic activity. Blocking central H_2

receptors alters neurotransmitter function and causes delirium, confusion, agitation, and seizures. Mental confusion while taking these medications follows rising blood levels after acute deterioration of renal and hepatic function.[69] Only cimetidine causes significant inhibition of hepatic microsomal mixed-function oxidases that may impair metabolism of other drugs.

Acute overdose of the specific H_2 receptor antagonists typically causes only minor toxic effects such as drowsiness and mild bradycardia.[70] More serious effects such as hypotension or bradycardia are likely to occur with intravenous overdoses and not with ingestion of the drug. Other effects rarely reported include hypersensitivity hepatitis, bone marrow suppression, and renal failure with long-term therapeutic doses.

DISPOSITION

Many factors must be considered for disposition of anticholinergic-poisoned patients. Patients with altered mental status, severe agitation, cardiac dysrhythmias, seizures, or hyperthermia require close observation and possible intervention in a critical care setting. A patient needing large amounts of benzodiazepines for controlling agitation or invasive interventions such as mechanical ventilation requires intensive care.

Decisions to discharge a patient must take into consideration resolution or absence of symptoms, the duration of physostigmine's effects in relation to the toxin's, anticipated complications such as aspiration pneumonitis or rhabdomyolysis, and the potential for delayed or prolonged toxin absorption. In most cases, discharge is safe when symptoms have been absent after 6 to 8 hours of observation or mild symptoms have resolved and ileus or significant coingestants are not present. No patient should be discharged without suicide assessment, substance abuse counseling, or poison prevention counseling.

SUMMARY

Anticholinergic poisoning is common and should be included in the differential diagnosis of any patient with an altered mental status. Evaluation of the vital signs and finding physical signs associated with the anticholinergic syndrome are often the clues to the diagnosis. The majority of patients with anticholinergic poisoning have a good outcome with simple observation and meticulous attention to supportive care. It is important to emphasize that physostigmine must be used cautiously. Treatment with physostigmine should be limited to severe cases.

References

1. Labianca DA, Reeves WJ. Scopolamine: A potent chemical weapon. J Chem Educ *61*:678, 1984.
2. Brown JH, Taylor P: Muscarinic receptor agonists and antagonists. *In* Hardman JG, Limbird LE (eds): Goodman and Gilman's The Pharmacological Basis of Therapeutics, 9th ed. New York, McGraw-Hill, pp 141–161, 1996.
3. Taylor P, Brown JH: Acetylcholine. *In* Siegel GJ (ed): Basic Neurochemistry: Molecular, Cellular, and Medical Aspects. 4th ed. New York, Raven Press, pp 203–231, 1989.
4. Cuello AC, Sofroniew MV: The anatomy of the CNS cholinergic neurons. Trends Neurosci *7*:74, 1984.
5. Schneck HJ, Rupreht J: Central anticholinergic syndrome in anesthesia and intensive care. Acta Anaesthesiol Belg *40*:219, 1989.
6. Bobe KS, Serafin WE: Histamine, bradykinin and their antagonists. *In* Hardman JG, Limbird LE (eds): Goodman and Gilman's The Pharmacological Basis of Therapeutics, 9th ed. New York, McGraw-Hill, pp 581–600, 1996.
7. Green JP: Histamine and serotonin. *In* Siegel GJ (ed): Basic Neurochemistry: Molecular, Cellular, and Medical Aspects. 4th ed. New York, Raven Press, pp 253–269, 1989.
8. Sastry BS, Phillis JW: Depression of rat cerebral cortical neurons by H_1 and H_2 histamine receptor agonists. Eur J Pharmacol *38*:269, 1976.
9. Clark RF, Vance MV: Massive diphenhydramine poisoning resulting in a wide-complex tachycardia: Successful treatment with sodium bicarbonate. Ann Emerg Med *21*:318, 1992.
10. Simons FE, Simons KJ: The pharmacology and use of H_1-receptor-antagonist drugs. N Engl J Med *330*:1663, 1994.
11. Greenblatt DJ, Shader RI: Anticholinergics. N Engl J Med *288*:1215, 1973.
12. Gowdy JM: Stramonium intoxication: Review of symptomatology in 212 cases. JAMA *221*:585, 1972.
13. Perry PJ, Wilding DC, Juhl RP: Anticholinergic psychosis. Am J Hosp Pharm *35*:725, 1978.
14. Hall RC, Fox J, Stickney SK, et al: Anticholinergic delirium: Etiology, presentation, diagnosis and management. J Psychedelic Drugs *10*:237, 1978.
15. Hall RC, Feinsilver DL, Holt RE: Anticholinergic psychosis: Differential diagnosis and management. Psychosomatics *22*:581, 1981.
16. Hvizdos AJ, Bennett JA, Wells BG, et al: Anticholinergic psychosis in a patient receiving usual doses of haloperidol, desipramine and benztropine. Clin Pharm *2*:174, 1983.
17. Fisher CM: Visual hallucinations on eye closure associated with atropine toxicity. A neurological analysis and comparison with other visual hallucinations. Can J Neurol Sci *18*:18, 1991.
18. Johnson AL, Hollister LE, Berger PA: The anticholinergic intoxication syndrome: Diagnosis and treatment. J Clin Psychiatry *42*:313, 1981.
19. Klein-Schwartz W, Oderda GM: Jimson weed intoxication in adolescents and young adults. Am J Dis Child *138*:737, 1984.
20. Moreau A, Jones BD, Banno V: Chronic central anticholinergic toxicity in manic depressive illness mimicking dementia. Can J Psychiatry *31*:339, 1986.
21. Richmond M, Seger D: Central anticholinergic syndrome in a child: A case report. J Emerg Med *3*:453, 1985.
22. Woodward GA, Baldassano RN: Topical diphenhydramine toxicity in a five year old with varicella. Pediatr Emerg Care *4*:18, 1988.
23. Filloux F: Toxic encephalopathy caused by topically applied diphenhydramine. J Pediatr *108*:1018, 1986.
24. Goldfrank L, Flomenbaum N, Lewin N, et al: Anticholinergic poisoning. Clin Toxicol *19*:17, 1982.
25. Tuomisto L, Tacke U: Is histamine an anticonvulsive inhibitory transmitter? Neuropharmacology *25*:955, 1986.
26. Curry SC, Chang D, Conner D: Drug- and toxin-induced rhabdomyolysis. Ann Emerg Med *18*:1068, 1989.
27. Hvizdos AJ, Bennett JA, Wells BG, et al: Anticholinergic psychosis in a patient receiving usual doses of haloperidol, desipramine, and benztropine. Clin Pharm *2*:174, 1983.
28. Cole J: Atropine-like delirium and anticholinergic substances. Am J Psychiatry *128*:898, 1972.
29. Forrester PA: An anticholinergic effect of general anaesthetics on cerebrocortical neurones. Br J Pharmacol *55*:275, 1975.
30. Reilly JF, Weisse ME: Topically induced diphenhydramine toxicity. J Emerg Med *8*:59, 1990.

31. Filloux F: Toxic encephalopathy caused by topically applied diphenhydramine. J Pediatr *108*:1018, 1986.
32. Wilkinson JA: Side effects of transdermal scopolamine. J Emerg Med *5*:389, 1987.
33. Price BH: Anisocoria from scopolamine patches. JAMA *253*:1561, 1985.
34. Patterson JH, Ives T, Greganti MA: Transient bilateral pupillary dilation from scopolamine discs. Drug Intell Clin Pharm *20*:986, 1986.
35. Adler AG, McElwain GE, Merli GJ, et al: Systemic effects of eye drops. Arch Intern Med *142*:2293, 1982.
36. Reid D, Fulton JD: Tachycardia precipitated by topical homatropine. BMJ *299*:795, 1989.
37. Fitzgerald DA, Hanson RM, West C: Seizures associated with 1% cyclopentolate eyedrops. J Paediatr Child Health *26*:106, 1990.
38. Brizer DA, Manning DW: Delirium induced by poisoning with anticholinergic agents. Am J Psychiatry *139*:1343, 1982.
39. Dilsaver SC: Antimuscarinic agents as substances of abuse: A review. J Clin Psychopharmacol *8*:14, 1988.
40. Smith JM: Abuse of the antiparkinson drugs: A review of the literature. J Clin Psychiatry *41*:351, 1980.
41. Modell JG, Tandon R, Beresford TP: Dopaminergic activity of the antimuscarinic antiparkinsonian agents. J Clin Psychopharmacol *9*:347, 1989.
42. Land W, Pinsky D, Salzman C: Abuse and misuse of anticholinergic medications. Hosp Community Psychiatry *42*:580, 1991.
43. MacVicar K: Abuse of antiparkinsonian drugs by psychiatric patients. Am J Psychiatry *134*:809, 1977.
44. Pullen GP, Best NR, Maguire J: Anticholinergic drug abuse: A common problem. BMJ *289*:612, 1984.
45. Crawshaw JA, Mullen PA: A study of benzhexol abuse. Br J Psychiatry *145*:300, 1984.
46. Benjamin MB: Mushroom poisoning in infants and children: The *Amanita pantherina/muscaria* group. Clin Toxicol *30*:13, 1992.
47. Fahy P, Arnold P, Curry SC, et al: Serial serum drug concentrations and prolonged anticholinergic toxicity after benztropine (Cogentin) overdose. Am J Emerg Med *7*:199, 1989.
48. Magera BE, Betlach CJ, Sweatt AP, et al: Hydroxyzine intoxication in a 13-month-old child. Pediatrics *67*:280, 1981.
49. Gillick JS: Atropine toxicity in a neonate. Br J Anaesth *46*:793, 1974.
50. Danze LK, Langdorf MI: Reversal of orphenadrine-induced ventricular tachycardia with physostigmine. J Emerg Med *9*:453, 1991.
51. Lindsay CA, Williams GD, Levin DL: Fatal adult respiratory distress syndrome after diphenhydramine toxicity in a child: A case report. Crit Care Med *23*:777, 1995.
52. Farrell M, Heinrichs M, Tilelli JA: Response of life threatening dimenhydrinate intoxication to sodium bicarbonate administration. Clin Toxicol *29*:527, 1991.
53. Freedberg RS, Friedman GR, Palu RN, et al: Cardiogenic shock due to antihistamine overdose: Reversal with intra-aortic balloon counterpulsation. JAMA *257*:660, 1987.
54. Granacher RP, Baldessarini RJ, Messner E: Physostigmine treatment of delirium induced by anticholinergics. Am Fam Physician *13*:99, 1976.
55. Rumack BH: Anticholinergic poisoning: Treatment with physostigmine. Pediatrics *52*:449, 1973.
56. Burks JS, Walker JE, Rumack BH, et al: Tricyclic antidepressant poisoning. Reversal of coma, choreoathetosis, and myoclonus by physostigmine. JAMA *230*:1405, 1974.
57. Duvoisin RC, Katz R: Reversal of central anticholinergic syndrome in man by physostigmine. JAMA *206*:1963, 1968.
58. Nattel S, Bayne L, Ruedy J: Physostigmine in coma due to drug overdose. Clin Pharmacol Ther *25*:96, 1979.
59. Manoguerra AS, Ruiz E: Physostigmine treatment of anticholinergic poisoning. JACEP *5*:125, 1976.
60. Newton RW: Physostigmine salicylate in the treatment of cyclic antidepressant overdosage. JAMA *231*:941, 1975.
61. Walker WE, Levy RC, Henenson IB: Physostigmine—its use and abuse. J Am Coll Emerg Phys *5*:335, 1976.
62. Levy R: Arrhythmias following physostigmine administration in Jimson weed poisoning. J Am Coll Emerg Physicians *6*:107, 1977.
63. Dysken MW, Janowsky DS: Dose-related physostigmine induced ventricular arrhythmia: Case report. J Clin Psychiatry *46*:446, 1985.
64. Munoz RA, Kuplic JB: Large overdoses of tricyclic antidepressants treated with physostigmine salicylate. Psychosomatics *16*:77, 1975.
65. Knudsen K, Heath A: Effects of self poisoning with maprotiline. BMJ *288*:601, 1984.
66. Pentel P, Peterson CD: Asystole complicating physostigmine treatment of tricyclic antidepressant overdose. Ann Emerg Med *9*:588, 1980.
67. Nilsson E, Meretoja OA, Neuvonen P: Hemodynamic responses to physostigmine in patients with a drug overdose. Anesth Analg *62*:885, 1983.
68. Berul CI, Morad M: Regulation of potassium channels by nonsedating antihistamines. Circulation *91*:2220, 1995.
69. Schentag JJ: Cimetidine-associated mental confusion: Further studies in 36 severely ill patients. Ther Drug Monit *2*:133, 1980.
70. Krenzelok EP, Litovitz T, Lippold KP: Cimetidine toxicity: An assessment of 881 cases. Ann Emerg Med *16*:1217, 1987.

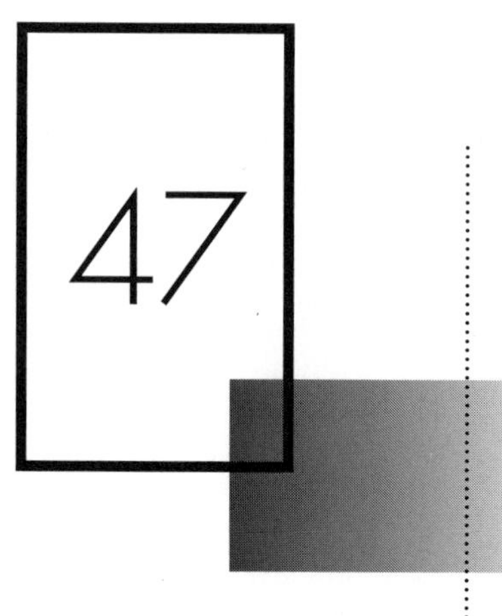

Oral Hypoglycemic Agents

LINDSAY MURRAY, MB, BS

In the majority of patients with non–insulin-dependent diabetes mellitus (NIDDM), an oral hypoglycemic agent is required to achieve the therapeutic ideal of normoglycemia. As a consequence of the prevalence of NIDDM, oral hypoglycemic agents are widely prescribed and are estimated to account for 1% of all prescriptions in the United States.[1]

Oral hypoglycemic agents belong to two groups: the sulfonylureas and the biguanides. Those agents that are available in the United States are listed in Table 47–1.

Subsequent to the discovery of the hypoglycemic action of sulfonamide compounds in the 1940s, a number of sulfonylurea compounds, including tolbutamide, acetohexamide, tolazamide, and chlorpropamide, were developed and introduced into clinical practice specifically for use as hypoglycemic agents. In the 1980s, two significantly more potent agents, glyburide and glipizide, became available. Currently, chlorpropamide, glyburide, and glipizide account for the majority of prescriptions of oral hypoglycemic agents.

Phenformin, a biguanide, was widely used as a hypoglycemic agent until its withdrawal from the market in the United States and Europe in the 1970s because of an association with lactic acidosis.[2] Metformin, another biguanide, is now available in the United States and has been widely prescribed elsewhere for many years.

Table 47–1. Oral Hypoglycemic Agents

Sulfonylureas	*Biguanide*
Tolbutamide	Metformin
Acetohexamide	
Tolazamide	
Chlorpropamide	
Glipizide	
Glyburide	

PHARMACOLOGY

Sulfonylureas

The sulfonylureas are *p*-substituted arylsulfonamides closely related in structure to the sulfonamides and the thiazide diuretics. The different side chains result in varying potency and duration of action, the details of which are shown in Table 47–2. All agents in this group are extensively bound to plasma proteins and can be displaced by other drugs. All are, for the most part, metabolized in the liver to inactive or less active metabolites (with the exception of acetohexamide whose metabolites are more active) with residual quantities of the parent drug and its metabolites being eliminated in the urine. The major mechanism of action of the sulfonylureas is thought to be stimulation of endogenous insulin secretion by pancreatic beta cells. Some extrapancreatic mechanisms may also operate,[3] but they are ineffective *in vivo* without functioning beta cells.[1]

Sulfonylureas are generally well tolerated with less than 2% of patients discontinuing therapy because of side effects.[1] Hematologic (hemolytic anemia, bone marrow aplasia) and dermatologic side effects (rashes, pruritus, erythema nodosum, erythema multiforme, exfoliative dermatitis) are rare and usually occur during the first 6 weeks of therapy. Their incidence (less than 0.1%) is similar with all agents. Gastrointestinal disturbances, including nausea, vomiting, abnormal results of liver function

Table 47–2. Comparison of Sulfonylureas

	Relative Potency	Elimination Half-Life (h)	Duration of Hypoglycemic Action (h)	Therapeutic Dose Range (mg)	Dose Frequency (doses/d)	Frequency of Severe Hypoglycemia (%)
Tolbutamide	1	3–28	6–10	500–3000	2–3	3
Acetohexamide	2.5	1–2	12–18	250–1500	2	4
Tolazamide	5	4–7	16–24	100–1000	1–2	4
Chlorpropamide	6	24–48	24–72	100–500	1	9
Glipizide	100	1–5	16–24	2.5–40	1–2	6
Glyburide	150	1.5–3	18–24	1.25–20	1–2	7

From Gerich JE: Oral hypoglycemic agents. N Engl J Med *321*:1231–1245, 1989. Adapted, by permission, from *The New England Journal of Medicine.*

tests, and cholestasis, occur with a frequency of 1% to 3%. Weight gain is common in patients who achieve improved glycemic control and is probably the result of reduced caloric loss associated with the diminution in glycosuria.[4] Chlorpropamide is unique among the sulfonylureas in being associated with disulfiram-type reactions and the syndrome of inappropriate antidiuretic hormone secretion.[5] The most common severe complication of sulfonylurea therapy is hypoglycemia, an extension of its therapeutic effect. The frequency of clinically significant hypoglycemic reactions is related to the potency and duration of action of the agent used, as shown in Table 47–2.[6] Risk factors for sulfonylurea-induced hypoglycemia include age older than 60, impaired renal function, poor nutrition, and multidrug therapy. Alcohol, sulfonamides, trimethoprim, salicylates, nonsteroidal anti-inflammatory agents, and β-blockers may potentiate the hypoglycemic activity of these agents.[6]

Biguanides

Biguanides contain two guanidine molecules linked together with the elimination of an amino group. Metformin is the only biguanide available in the United States, having been introduced in 1995.

The pharmacokinetics of metformin differ markedly from those of the sulfonylureas. The drug is not significantly bound to plasma proteins, does not undergo biotransformation, and is eliminated in the urine by both glomerular filtration and tubular secretion. The plasma elimination half-life is estimated at 1.5 to 4.9 hours in subjects with normal renal function.[7] Metformin is used either as a single agent or in combination with a sulfonylurea or insulin in the management of NIDDM. The biguanides reduce fasting blood glucose levels and insulin concentrations by improving insulin sensitivity, thus enhancing peripheral insulin-mediated glucose uptake and decreasing hepatic glucose output. The biguanides are better described as antihyperglycemic agents, in contrast to the sulfonylureas, which are correctly described as hypoglycemic agents.

The most common side effects associated with metformin at therapeutic doses are gastrointestinal and include anorexia, nausea, abdominal discomfort, and diarrhea. These symptoms occur in 5% to 20% of patients initially commenced on metformin but rarely persist. Lactic acidosis is associated with metformin, but the incidence is significantly less than that associated with phenformin. When this complication occurs at therapeutic doses it is usually in the context of it having been prescribed in patients for whom the drug is contraindicated (Table 47–3). It appears that a critical blood level of biguanide, as yet undefined, is required to produce the metabolic abnormalities that in turn lead to lactic acidosis.[8] The listed contraindications, especially impaired renal function, are likely to result in impaired elimination and excessive blood levels of metformin, thus increasing the likelihood of the critical blood level being achieved.

CLINICAL PRESENTATION OF OVERDOSE

Sulfonylurea-Induced Hypoglycemia

The chief effect of overdose of any of the sulfonylurea agents, whether occurring in the diabetic or the nondiabetic individual, is hypoglycemia. Although hypoglycemia has been defined in absolute terms as a plasma glucose concentration of less than 2.78 mmol/L (50 mg/dL),[9] it is perhaps more usefully defined in functional terms as a depressed concentration of blood or plasma glucose producing evidence of a physiologic counter-regulatory hormone response or evidence of neurologic dysfunction. As the plasma

Table 47–3. Contraindications to Metformin Therapy

Renal impairment: plasma creatinine > 1.5 mg/dL (132 μmol/L) for men, > 1.4 mg/dL (124 μmol/L) for women
Cardiac or respiratory failure of sufficient magnitude to cause central hypoxia or reduced peripheral perfusion
Past history of lactic acidosis
Severe infection that could lead to decreased tissue perfusion
Liver disease demonstrated by abnormal results of liver function tests
Alcohol abuse with binge drinking sufficient to cause acute hepatotoxicity

From Bailey CJ, Turner RC: Metformin. N Engl J Med *334*:574–579, 1996. Adapted, by permission, from *The New England Journal of Medicine.*

glucose concentration decreases to about 4 mmol/L, there is an increase in the secretion of counterregulatory hormones (glucagon, epinephrine, growth hormone, cortisol) and activation of the autonomic nervous system. If the plasma glucose concentration reaches 3.2 mmol/L, this increase in autonomic activity is normally of a sufficient magnitude as to result in symptoms. This response may be modified in those with diabetic autonomic neuropathy or on β-blocker therapy. Glucose is the principal energy substrate for the brain. The brain does not produce glucose and can only store a few minutes supply; therefore, it is extremely sensitive to hypoglycemia. Concentrations of circulating glucose below 3 mmol/L impair cerebral function, and more severe and prolonged hypoglycemia can cause convulsions, permanent neurologic damage, or death.[10]

The onset of symptomatic hypoglycemia after sulfonylurea overdose occurs at a variable time interval depending on the size of the ingestion and the particular agent involved. It usually occurs within 6 hours of ingestion but may be delayed for up to 16 hours after ingestion of small doses by young children.[11] After deliberate or accidental overdose, the patient may thus present during an asymptomatic phase, before the onset of hypoglycemia.

The symptoms and signs of sulfonylurea-induced hypoglycemia are the same as for those associated with hypoglycemia of other causes and include those of the autonomic response to hypoglycemia and those directly associated with the consequences of neuroglycopenia as listed in Table 47–4.

Neurologic dysfunction may not respond immediately to correction of hypoglycemia in the patient who presents late after a period of prolonged and severe hypoglycemia.

Biguanide-Induced Lactic Acidosis

Hypoglycemia virtually never occurs in association with therapeutic or near-therapeutic doses of biguanides. It has been reported in association with biguanide overdose but appears to be much less severe than sulfonylurea-induced hypoglycemia and is easily managed with dextrose administration of relatively short duration. Of much greater concern is the development of biguanide-associated lactic acidosis, a condition associated with significant morbidity and mortality.

Table 47–4. Signs and Symptoms of Hypoglycemia

Associated with Autonomic Response	Associated with Neuroglycopenia
Sweating	Behavioral disturbance
Tachycardia	Irritability
Pallor	Weakness
Tremor	Confusion
Palpitations	Coma
Piloerection	Seizures
Anxiety	Focal neurologic deficits
Hypertension	
Hunger	
Nausea	

Lactic acidosis is defined as a metabolic acidosis due to accumulation of lactic acid in the blood in excess of 5 mmol/L with an accompanying blood pH of less than 7.25.[12] Biguanide-associated lactic acidosis is classified as a type B lactic acidosis and thought to be multifactorial in origin. The postulated mechanisms include an increase in lactate production, especially in the gastrointestinal mucosa cells, and reduced hepatic uptake and metabolism of lactate secondary to increased intrahepatocyte lactate concentration and reduced intrahepatocyte pH.[8] The incidence of lactic acidosis during metformin therapy is extremely low, estimated at 0.6 per 1000 patient-years in a Swedish study.[13] In this study, all patients who developed lactic acidosis in connection with metformin therapy displayed impaired renal function at the time the diagnosis of acidosis was made.

Relatively few case reports of metformin overdose have been published. However, it is likely that an ingestion sufficient to result in excessive serum concentrations of metformin for a prolonged period of time would produce a clinical picture similar to that after accumulation of the drug in association with impaired renal function. Severe lactic acidosis associated with cardiovascular collapse occurred in an adult diabetic within 10 hours of ingesting 24.5 g of metformin together with a barbiturate. Death ensued at 45 hours after ingestion despite the institution of aggressive intensive care.[14] It is not known what dose is necessary to precipitate lactic acidosis in an individual with normal renal function.

Patients with biguanide-associated lactic acidosis present with relatively nonspecific symptoms and signs such as (in decreasing frequency of occurrence) vomiting, somnolence, nausea, epigastric pain, anorexia, hyperpnea, lethargy, diarrhea, and thirst.[15] Coma, hypothermia, and cardiovascular collapse may develop as the intoxication progresses.

DIAGNOSIS

Sulfonylurea-Induced Hypoglycemia

The diagnosis of hypoglycemia should be entertained in any patient presenting with an alteration in mental status and should be rapidly excluded or confirmed on the basis of a bedside test for blood glucose concentration. When this cannot be done rapidly or when the result is equivocal, an intravenous bolus dose of 50 mL of 50% dextrose should be administered empirically. A clinical response to this intervention confirms the diagnosis of hypoglycemia. A lack of response does not exclude the diagnosis because prolonged severe hypoglycemia can result in permanent neurologic deficits that will not respond to correction of hypoglycemia. If a diagnosis of hypoglycemia is made, the patient's history usually establishes whether sulfonylurea toxicity or overdose is a likely cause. If the history does not establish the diagnosis, other causes of hypoglycemia should be considered (Table 47–5). Specific drug levels are rarely necessary to make the diagnosis, but when no explanation for hypoglycemia is apparent, estimation of plasma insulin, C-peptide, proinsulin, and sulfonylurea concentrations may be necessary to confirm a diagnosis of sulfonylurea toxicity and to avoid missing the diagnosis of accidental, factitious, or felonious sulfonylurea or insulin poisoning.

Biguanide-Induced Lactic Acidosis

This diagnosis should be suspected in any patient on metformin who develops symptoms or in any patient who becomes unwell after a deliberate overdose of metformin (or other biguanide). The hallmark of biguanide-associated lactic acidosis is severe acidosis without evidence of hypotension or hypoxia. The diagnosis is confirmed by documentation of an anion-gap metabolic acidosis and an elevated serum lactate level (>5 mmol/L).

TREATMENT

Sulfonylurea Overdose

A patient usually presents with symptoms and signs of hypoglycemia, which is a medical emergency mandating urgent attention. Less commonly, after overdose of a hypoglycemic agent, the patient may present while still euglycemic, in which case an appropriate strategy for monitoring needs to be devised.

The patient presenting with hypoglycemic coma, seizures, or marked behavioral disturbance after sulfonylurea overdose requires immediate institution of appropriate supportive care, including establishment of an airway, administration of supplemental oxygen, control of seizures, institution of measures to protect against further injury, institution of cardiac monitoring, and establishment of intravenous access. As soon as practicable, concentrated intravenous dextrose (50% solution) should be administered as a bolus dose. Administration of intravenous dextrose is indicated in any patient with altered mental status, unusual behavior, or seizures if an accurate blood glucose determination cannot be rapidly attained. Because focal neurologic deficits are a relatively rare manifestation and because hyperglycemia may exacerbate ischemic cerebral injury,[16] every effort should be made to determine rapidly the blood glucose concentration before empirical intravenous administration of dextrose to patients presenting with a focal neurologic deficit.

Once the patient's condition is stabilized, consideration should be given to gastric decontamination with oral activated charcoal in those instances when presentation occurs within several hours of ingestion. Activated charcoal has been demonstrated to bind effectively chlorpropamide, tolbutamide, tolazamide, glibenclamide, and glypizide *in vitro*[17] and tolbutamide and chlorpropamide *in vivo*.[18, 19] Theoretically, standard therapeutic doses of activated charcoal are likely to be most effective after overdose with the second-generation agents such as glibenclamide and glypizide because the adsorptive charcoal is less likely to be saturated by the smaller doses of these agents.

Once hypoglycemia has been corrected by administration of concentrated intravenous dextrose solution, an infusion of 10% dextrose in water should be begun and blood glucose concentrations determined on a frequent basis (at least hourly). The rate and concentration of the dextrose infusion will need to be adjusted to maintain euglycemia. Depending on the severity of the overdose, the glucose requirement may be quite high. If concentrations of 20% dextrose or greater are used, the infusion should be given through a central venous catheter to avoid damage to peripheral veins.

A number of other drugs have been used as adjuncts in the management of sulfonylurea-induced hypoglycemia. Glucagon may be useful to produce a temporary elevation in blood glucose level in the prehospital setting or when difficulty obtaining intravenous access is encountered. It is only effective when adequate glycogen stores exist and needs to be followed by parenteral administration of dextrose. As such, it has little role in the hospital management of sulfonylurea overdose. Diazoxide effectively inhibits insulin secretion and has been used successfully in the management of refractory sulfonylurea-induced hypoglycemia.[20, 21] This situation may be more likely to occur when sulfonylurea overdose occurs in nondiabetic individuals and is associated with very high plasma insulin levels. Octreotide, a long-acting synthetic analogue of somatostatin, is a potent inhibitor of secretion of insulin, glucagon, and growth hormone. It has been reported to inhibit effectively excessive insulin secretion and significantly reduce dextrose requirements after sulfonylurea overdose[22, 23] and may have a role in the management of severe, refractory sulfonylurea-induced hypoglycemia. Doses of 50 μg of octreotide subcutaneously every 12 hours

Table 47–5. Differential Diagnosis of Hypoglycemia

Nontoxic	Toxic
Pancreatic	Drug
Insulinoma	Insulin
Pancreatitis	Sulfonylurea
Extrapancreatic neoplasms	Biguanide
Post-gastrectomy	Propranolol
Sepsis	Ethanol
Prolonged carbohydrate deprivation	Salicylate
Inborn errors of metabolism	Quinine
Severe hepatic, renal, or cardiac disease	Disopyramide
Endocrine	Pentamidine
Pituitary insufficiency	Nondrug
Adrenocortical insufficiency	Mushrooms
Hypothyroidism	Akee fruit

effectively suppressed endogenous insulin secretion after tolbutamide overdose in a nondiabetic individual without significant adverse effects.[22]

The vast majority of cases of sulfonylurea overdose are adequately managed with dextrose supplementation, and attempts at enhanced elimination are not indicated. Alkalinization of the urine has been demonstrated to enhance the excretion of chlorpropamide (a weak acid, pK_a 4.8), reducing its elimination half-life from 49 to 13 hours.[18] Charcoal hemoperfusion has been used effectively to enhance elimination of chlorpropamide after overdose by a man with chronic renal failure.[24] Repeat-dose activated charcoal is ineffective in enhancing elimination of chlorpropamide but has not been investigated for other sulfonylureas.[18]

Metformin Overdose

Biguanide-induced lactic acidosis is associated with a very high mortality, approximately 50% even if aggressive therapy is instituted.[15] If initiation of treatment is delayed until after the onset of hemodynamic collapse, mortality is even higher.

Initial management should focus on stabilization of the airway, breathing, and circulation. Adequate and early volume expansion is essential. Hypoglycemia, although rarely profound, should be corrected with intravenous administration of dextrose.

The administration of intravenous bicarbonate in lactic acidosis is controversial and may in fact be detrimental by resulting in paradoxical acidification of the intracellular and cerebrospinal fluid; increased hemoglobin affinity for oxygen leading to impaired oxygen delivery to the tissues; hypernatremia and volume overload; and increased cellular membrane permeability to biguanides, resulting in further increases in cellular lactate production.[25] Bicarbonate has not been shown to have any clinical benefit in patients with circulatory insufficiency from either biguanide-associated or other forms of lactic acidosis.[26, 27]

Bicarbonate hemodialysis has been reported to increase dramatically the survival rate in metformin-induced lactic acidosis. Lalau and associates[28] report five cases of patients with severe metformin-induced lactic acidosis whose clinical status and metabolic abnormalities rapidly responded to bicarbonate hemodialysis despite incomplete removal of metformin as determined by serum sampling. All had acute renal failure, and three were in cardiovascular collapse at the time of presentation.

DISPOSITION

Because sulfonylurea-induced hypoglycemia is invariably prolonged, all patients require admission to a hospital for ongoing monitoring of blood glucose concentrations and intravenous administration of dextrose. Because the onset of hypoglycemia after sulfonylurea overdose may be delayed up to 16 hours, all patients with deliberate overdose or children with suspected ingestion must be admitted for monitoring of blood glucose concentrations, at least hourly, for 24 hours. The ingestion of even one tablet of chlorpropamide, glipizide, or glibenclamide is capable of producing significant hypoglycemia in children younger than 4 years of age.[11] A patient is ready for medical discharge when maintenance of an adequate blood glucose concentration without parenteral supplementation has been demonstrated. This may be 3 to 4 days from the time of admission. Appropriate psychiatric evaluation in cases of deliberate self-overdose should take place before final discharge. When the overdose was accidental or a therapeutic error, appropriate educational intervention should occur before discharge.

Evidence of lactic acidosis associated with biguanide therapy or after biguanide overdose mandates hospital admission. Lactic acidosis is unlikely to develop in individuals with normal renal function after relatively small ingestions of metformin, but, because a dose-response relationship has not been well characterized, all patients with metformin overdose should be observed for 6 hours. If there is no evidence of acidosis or hypoglycemia and the patient remains asymptomatic at that time, he or she may be discharged after appropriate psychiatric evaluation and educational intervention.

References

1. Gerich JE: Oral hypoglycemic agents. N Engl J Med *321*:1231–1245, 1989.
2. William RH, Palmer JP: Farewell to phenformin for treating diabetes mellitus. Ann Intern Med *83*:567, 1975.
3. Beck-Neilsen H, Hother-Neilsen O, Pedersen O: Mechanism of action of sulfonylureas with special reference to the extrapancreatic effect: An overview. Diabet Med *5*:613–620, 1988.
4. Welle S, Nair KS, Lockwood D: Effect of sulfonylurea and insulin on energy expenditure in type II diabetes mellitus. J Clin Endocrinol Metab *6*:593–597, 1988.
5. Berger W: Incidence of severe side effects during therapy with sulfonylureas and biguanides. Horm Metab Res *17*(Suppl 15):111–115, 1985.
6. Seltzer HS: Drug-induced hypoglycemia: A review of 1418 cases. Endocrinol Metab Clin North Am *18*:163–183, 1989.
7. Bailey CJ, Turner RC: Metformin. N Engl J Med *334*:574–579, 1996.
8. Gan SC, Barr J, Arieff AI, Pear RG: Biguanide-associated lactic acidosis: Case report and review of the literature. Arch Intern Med *152*:2333–2336, 1992.
9. Field JB: Hypoglycemia: Definition, clinical presentations, classification, and laboratory tests. Endocrin Metabol Clin North Am *18*:27–43, 1989.
10. Gerich JE: Control of glycaemia. Ballieres Clin Endocrinol Metabol *7*:551–586, 1993.
11. Quadrani DA, Spiller HA, Widder P: Five year retrospective evaluation of sulfonylurea ingestion in children. J Toxicol Clin Toxicol *34*:267–270, 1996.
12. Arieff AI: Pathogenesis of lactic acidosis. Diabet Metab Rev *5*:637–649, 1989.
13. Wilholm BE, Myrhed M: Metformin-associated lactic acidosis in Sweden 1977–1991. Eur J Clin Pharmacol *44*:589–591, 1993.
14. Bismuth C, Gaultier M, Conso F, et al: Acidose lactique indu-

ite par l'ingestion excessive de metformine. Nouv Presse Med *5*:26, 1976.
15. Luft D, Schmülling RM, Eggstein M: Lactic acidosis in biguanide-treated diabetics: A review of 330 cases. Diabetologia *14*:75–87, 1978.
16. Browning RG, Olson DW, Stueven HA, Mateer JR: 50% Dextrose: Antidote or toxin? Ann Emerg Med *19*:683–687, 1990.
17. Kannisto H, Neuvonen PJ: Adsorption of sulfonylureas onto activated charcoal. J Pharmacol Sci *73*:253–256, 1984.
18. Neuvonen PJ, Karkhainen S: Effects of charcoal, sodium bicarbonate and ammonia chloride on chlorpropamide kinetics. Clin Pharmacol Ther *33*:386–393, 1983.
19. Neuvonen PJ, Kannisto H, Hirvisalo EL: Effect of activated charcoal on absorption of tolbutamide and valproate in man. Eur J Clin Pharmacol *24*:243–246, 1983.
20. Johnson SF, Schad DS, Peake GT: Chlorpropamide-induced hypoglycemia: Successful treatment with diazoxide. Am J Med *63*:799–804, 1977.
21. Palatnick W, Meatherall RC, Tenenbein M: Clinical spectrum of sulfonylurea overdose and experience with diazoxide. Arch Int Med *151*:1859–1862, 1991.
22. Krentz AJ, Boyle PJ, Justice KM, et al: Successful treatment of severe refractory sulfonylurea-induced hypoglycemia with octreotide. Diabetes Care *16*:184–186, 1993.
23. Boyle PJ, Justice K, Krentz AJ, et al: Octreotide reverses hyperinsulinemia and prevents hypoglycemia induced by sulfonylurea overdoses. J Clin Endocrinol Metab *76*:752–756, 1993.
24. Ludwig SM, McKenzie J, Faiman C: Chlorpropamide overdose in renal failure: Management with charcoal hemoperfusion. Am J Kidney Dis *10*:457–460, 1987.
25. Arieff AJ: Indications for use of bicarbonate in patients with metabolic acidosis. Br J Anaesth *67*:165–177, 1991.
26. Fulop M, Hoberman HD: Phenformin-associated metabolic acidosis. Diabetes *25*:292–296, 1976.
27. Cooper JD, Walley KR, Wiggs BR, Russell JA: Bicarbonate does not improve hemodynamics in critically ill patients who have lactic acidosis. Ann Intern Med *112*:492–498, 1990.
28. Lalau JD, Westeel PF, Debussche X, et al: Bicarbonate haemodialysis: An adequate treatment for lactic acidosis in diabetics treated by metformin. Intensive Care Med *13*:383–387, 1987.

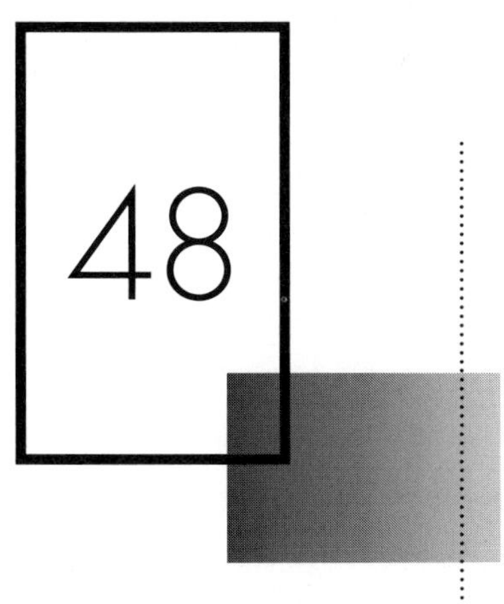

48 Anticonvulsants

DONNA L. SEGER, MD

ANTIEPILEPTIC DRUG ACTIONS

Phenytoin, carbamazepine, and sodium valproate inhibit the voltage-dependent sodium current that is responsible for the action potential in brain neurons. Inhibition of the current is termed *use dependent* because the sodium channel must be opened for the drug to work. Therefore, these drugs have little or no effect on single action potentials, but when a neuron fires repetitively, the latter action potentials are blocked. Each of these anticonvulsants may have other actions as well.[1]

Phenytoin

In addition to sodium channel blockade, phenytoin can inhibit calcium channels and stimulate the sodium/potassium–adenosine triphosphatase pump. Although prescribed primarily for seizure control, phenytoin is also administered for trigeminal neuralgia and behavior disorders.[2, 3]

Preparation and Dosage

Phenytoin may be administered by oral, intravenous, or intraosseous routes. Intramuscular administration is not recommended because absorption is slow and erratic owing to crystallization at the injection site.

Phenytoin sodium (Dilantin) is available in the United States as 30-mg and 100-mg capsules as well as an oral suspension. A sterile solution is available for intravenous administration (see section on intravenous administration).[2]

The maintenance oral dose is 3 to 5 mg/kg per day for adults and 4 to 7 mg/kg per day in divided doses for children. Although prolonged half-life and slow absorption allow single daily dosing, large oral doses cause fluctuations in plasma phenytoin concentrations owing to gastric intolerance and variable product bioavailability (tablets are better absorbed than capsules, increasing dose decreases proportion absorbed).[2]

If phenytoin administration is initiated with standard oral maintenance doses of 300 to 400 mg/d, therapeutic serum concentrations will be approached in 3 to 4 days. Steady state will be attained by 7 to 10 days. Oral "loading" with 15 to 18 mg/kg will yield therapeutic serum concentrations in 8 to 30 hours.[4, 5]

Table 48–1. Phenytoin: Drug Interactions

Drugs That Increase Phenytoin Concentration	
Amiodarone	Imipramine
Chloramphenicol	Isoniazid
Chlorpromazine	Phenothiazines
Cimetidine	Phenylbutazone
Co-trimoxazole	Salicylates
Diazepam	Sulfisoxazole
Dicumarol	Sulfonamides
Disulfiram	Valproate
Drugs That Decrease Phenytoin Concentration	
Antacid	
Calcium	
Carbamazepine	
Diazepam	
Ethanol (↑ or ↓)	
Folic acid	
Phenobarbital (↑ or ↓)	

Pharmacokinetics

Phenytoin has a pK_a of 8.3. Therefore, the solid capsule dissolves while the salt precipitates in the acidic medium of the stomach. Absorption of oral phenytoin is slow, variable, and occasionally incomplete.[2, 6] Phenytoin is 90% bound to plasma protein, has a volume of distribution of 0.6 to 0.7 L/kg (5 to 6 L/kg for unbound phenytoin), and is highly lipid soluble. It freely diffuses into all tissues (including the central nervous system) and is firmly tissue bound.[7]

Ninety-five per cent of the drug is metabolized by the hepatic microsomal enzyme system. The major metabolite, a parahydroxyphenyl derivative, is inactive. Although interindividual variation in metabolism exists, the average therapeutic half-life is 20 to 30 hours. The metabolites are conjugated with glucuronide and excreted in the bile and, subsequently, the urine. Only 5% of the parent drug is excreted unchanged in the urine.[4]

The metabolism of phenytoin is dose dependent. At therapeutic serum concentrations, phenytoin elimination follows first-order (exponential) kinetics (the rate of drug metabolism increases as the concentration of the drug increases). In the upper therapeutic and toxic ranges, the hydroxylation reaction reaches maximum velocity and phenytoin elimination changes from first-order to zero-order kinetics (the rate of phenytoin metabolism remains constant despite increased drug concentration). As phenytoin accumulates, serum phenytoin half-life and time to reach steady state increase disproportionately. Therefore, a small increase in dose may result in a toxic serum phenytoin concentration 2 to 3 weeks after the increased dosage. Supratherapeutic serum phenytoin concentrations decrease slowly until the serum concentration approaches the therapeutic range and elimination again follows first-order kinetics.[3, 4]

Serum Concentrations

Therapeutic serum concentrations of 10 to 20 mg/L equate with a free phenytoin concentration of 1.0 to 2.0 mg/L.[8] Toxic effects occur when free phenytoin concentrations are greater than 5 mg/L. Free phenytoin may be increased by impairment of protein binding caused by drugs that displace phenytoin from serum proteins (Table 48–1) and conditions that decrease serum albumin concentrations (e.g., hepatic dysfunction, chronic renal failure, uremia, age [elderly and neonates] and late pregnancy). In these settings, the total plasma concentration may not reflect the relative increase in unbound phenytoin that may cause phenytoin toxicity.[3, 8] Although serum concentrations do not correlate well with symptoms, a progression of symptoms correlates with increasing serum concentration (Table 48–2).

Side Effects of Chronic Therapy

Side effects occur in 45% of patients receiving maintenance phenytoin therapy and are usually associated with serum concentrations of greater than 15 mg/L. Commonly occurring side effects are listed in Table 48–3.[3] The most serious side effect is a hypersensitivity syndrome (phenytoin syndrome) manifested by fever, rash, lymphadenopathy, hepati-

Table 48–2. Phenytoin Serum Concentrations and Symptoms of Toxicity

Phenytoin Serum Concentrations (mg/mL)	Signs and Symptoms
20	Nystagmus on lateral gaze (spontaneous, horizontal)
30	Nystagmus (vertical) Ataxia Slurred speech Drowsiness
40	Mentation (confusion, disorientation) Lethargy, hyperactivity, mania Coma Respiratory depression
50	Paradoxical seizures

Table 48–3. Phenytoin: Side Effects

Gingival hyperplasia*
Rash
Thyroid function inhibition
Hirsutism
Hypertrichosis
Carbohydrate intolerance
Folic acid deficiency*
Benign intracranial hypertension
Peripheral neuropathy
Osteomalacia
Altered vitamin D metabolism (↑ alkaline phosphatase)
Acne
Lupus-like syndrome
Stevens-Johnson syndrome
↑ Liver function tests

*Dose related.

tis, and eosinophilia. Death occurs secondary to hepatic failure. Phenytoin should be discontinued if patients manifest signs of this syndrome. The drug should not be reinstituted.[9, 10]

Although serum liver enzyme activity may increase after phenytoin ingestion, discontinuation of the drug may not be necessary. When phenytoin and valproate are administered simultaneously, hepatotoxicity may result from protein displacement and enzyme inhibition, causing a rise in serum phenytoin concentrations. It is important to distinguish this mild hepatic dysfunction from hypersensitivity-induced fulminant hepatic failure.[11]

Toxicity During Therapeutic Ingestion

Symptoms of coexisting disease as well as the onset of toxicity with a previously tolerated dose frequently delay the diagnosis of phenytoin toxicity. Signs and symptoms are primarily cerebellar (nystagmus, ataxia, and drowsiness) but may not correlate well with serum concentrations. Cerebellar signs occur at lower serum concentrations than basal ganglia signs (movement disorders). Because phenytoin is usually discontinued when cerebellar signs occur, concentrations in the basal ganglia that would cause movement disorders are seldom attained.[12, 13] Movement disorders most frequently occur when serum concentrations are greater than 20 mg/L, are self-limited, and resolve when serum concentrations are in the therapeutic range. Other manifestations of toxicity (such as behavior change and poor school performance) must also be considered (Table 48–4). Treatment is supportive. The drug should be withdrawn and reinstituted when the patient is asymptomatic and serum concentrations have fallen to within the therapeutic range.

The extent to which phenytoin can produce chronic cerebellar abnormalities is controversial. Animals with chronic phenytoin intoxication demonstrate lesions in the cerebellum, primarily the Purkinje cells. Computed tomography has demonstrated cerebellar atrophy and loss of cerebellar tissue after phenytoin therapy. Seizures also cause cerebellar degeneration and atrophy, which is unable to be differentiated from atrophy caused by phenytoin. Despite anatomic evidence of atrophy, patients with phenytoin-induced cerebellar symptoms demonstrate almost complete symptomatic recovery. There is one report of cerebellar atrophy after acute phenytoin intoxication, but it is very rare.[13–15]

Overdose

Limited phenytoin solubility (dissolution rate decreases with increasing dose) and decreased intestinal motility prolong absorption. Peak serum concentrations may not occur for 3 to 12 hours after ingestion and have occurred as late as 4 days after ingestion.[2, 16]

Symptoms occur 1 to 2 hours after phenytoin ingestion. Manifestations of cerebellar dysfunction (nystagmus, ataxia, and drowsiness) are the classic clinical features of an acute ingestion. Paradoxical seizures may occur if the serum phenytoin concentration is greater than 50 mg/L. If the patient arrives within an hour, gastrointestinal absorption may be minimized by gastrointestinal decontamination. Current evidence does not support the administration of multiple-dose activated charcoal. Treatment is supportive. Hospital admission is indicated in symptomatic cases until ataxia or other debilitating symptoms resolve. Cardiac monitoring is not required. Repeat serum phenytoin concentrations should be obtained to ensure decreasing serum concentrations. Metabolic abnormalities rarely occur as a result of phenytoin toxicity. Because of prolonged elimination half-life, recovery may take several days.[16, 17]

Forced diuresis, modification of urine pH, hemodialysis, charcoal hemoperfusion, exchange transfusion, peritoneal dialysis, and plasmapheresis are ineffective.[18] Fortunately, life-threatening toxicity rarely occurs after overdose.

Intravenous Administration

Because of phenytoin's lack of solubility and stability in unbuffered aqueous solutions, the US Food and

Table 48–4. Signs and Symptoms of Phenytoin Toxicity After Chronic Ingestion

Behavorial changes
↑ Frequency of seizures
Gastrointestinal symptoms
Hypotonia
Pupillary dilatation
Incontinence
Psychosis
Transient hemiparesis
Extrapyramidal signs
Dystonia
Tremor
Tongue protrusion
Lip smacking
Head nodding
Fish mouthing
Facial grimace
Movement disorders

Drug Administration (FDA) recommends intravenous phenytoin administration by manual infusion at a rate less than 50 mg/min. This method has many disadvantages, which include medical staff time (frequently physician time), pain at the infusion site, and a variable drug delivery rate that is an important factor in causing cardiovascular depression. Clinical studies have demonstrated that phenytoin can be safely administered in intravenous solution at a controlled rate.[19–21]

Phenytoin sodium injection preparation is a mixture of 40% propylene glycol and 10% ethanol. The solution is adjusted to a pH of 12 with sodium hydroxide to maintain phenytoin solubility.

Solubility, pH, and crystallization must be considered when placing phenytoin sodium in solution. If the pH is less than 11.7, phenytoin sodium becomes phenytoin acid, hydrolyzes, and precipitates. The pH of normal saline (9.81 to 10.81) makes it the best (most alkaline as compared with dextrose or lactated Ringer's solution) diluent. Propylene glycol is required to solubulize phenytoin. A further consideration is the phenytoin concentration, because the administration of a solution with high phenytoin concentration is associated with increased incidence of cardiovascular complications.[22]

Phenytoin maintains solubility in normal saline at a concentration of 6 to 10 mg/L. Crystallization occurs within an hour even with this concentration, but the degree of crystallization is not harmful. The solution should be made immediately before use and infused within an hour. There is no appreciable difference in delivered phenytoin concentrations when using filtered versus unfiltered infusions.[20, 21]

Administration Guidelines. Rapid attainment of therapeutic serum phenytoin levels is required to treat status epilepticus. An intravenous loading dose of phenytoin is the only method of administration that will produce therapeutic steady state rapidly. Some anticonvulsant activity begins within 3 to 5 minutes after intravenous infusion. Distribution to the brain is rapid, and brain concentrations exceed plasma concentrations 20 minutes after an intravenous loading dose. If the pretreatment serum concentration of phenytoin is zero, an intravenous loading dose of 15 to 18 mg/kg will produce serum concentrations within the therapeutic range lasting 12 to 24 hours in most adult patients. If serum concentration is known, administration of each 100 mg of intravenous phenytoin will increase serum concentration 1.2 mg/L.[23]

Cardiac monitoring is necessary during intravenous phenytoin administration owing to potential adverse cardiovascular effects (hypotension, arrhythmias, bradycardia, apnea, peripheral vasodilatation, myocardial depression). These may be secondary to the rate of administration, the propylene glycol solvent, patient age, pre-existing medical illness, or a combination of these factors. Fatalities have been attributed to the administration of intravenous phenytoin; these have been reported either in elderly patients with a history of heart disease or when administered doses exceeded the recommended rate and concentration (most were administered by manual intravenous infusion).[24, 25] Both concentration and infusion rate must be considered because hypotension and bradycardia occurred in young persons when phenytoin was administered in solutions with high phenytoin concentrations at generally accepted rates (35 to 40 mg/min).[22]

Phenytoin diluted in normal saline to a concentration of 4 to 10 mg of phenytoin in each milliliter of normal saline can be safely administered intravenously at a rate of 50 mg/min in patients younger than 50 years of age.[19–21] If the patient is 50 years or older, 4 mg phenytoin per milliliter of normal saline (e.g., 1 g of phenytoin in 250 mL of normal saline) should be administered no faster than 25 mg/min. Intravenous piggyback delivery should be monitored by a constant infusion pump. Patients should be placed on a cardiac monitor and vital signs recorded frequently. If systemic side effects occur during infusion, the drug should be discontinued. Patients with the following conditions should not receive phenytoin: marked bradycardia, second- or third-degree atrioventricular conduction block, active severe arteriosclerotic heart disease, hypotension, and seizures due to electrolyte abnormalities or hypoglycemia.[19–21]

The highly alkaline solvent in which phenytoin is dissolved may cause burning and aching of the arm at or near the infusion site. If the rate is slowed, or the concentration is decreased, the sensation resolves. Soft tissue or vascular injury has occurred after intravenous administration. An alkaline solution infused into a small vein may exceed the buffering capacity of the blood, causing a local reaction. The majority of cases reported have occurred in elderly women with cardiovascular disease. To minimize the risk of injury in the elderly, phenytoin infusions should be diluted in normal saline, the catheter should be 20 gauge or larger, and the administration rate should not be greater than 25 mg/min.[26]

When more than 1 g of phenytoin is administered intravenously, ataxia, dizziness, and confusion may occur. This clinical picture is not caused by high drug concentration or rapid rate of administration but appears to be related to the total dose administered.[21]

Intraosseous Administration

Intraosseous administration of phenytoin has been reported in a child in whom emergency vascular access failed. Absorption from bone was rapid, and pharmacokinetics appeared to approximate intravenous administration.[27]

Conclusion

Supportive therapy is appropriate for phenytoin toxicity resulting from either an acute overdose or chronic therapeutic ingestion. Toxicity due to intravenous phenytoin is related to phenytoin concentration and rate of delivery. Intravenous administration of phenytoin as a constant infusion is safe and effective.

Carbamazepine

Carbamazepine (CBMZ) was introduced into the United States in 1960 for pain control of trigeminal neuralgia.[1] CBMZ is now the preferred anticonvulsant in children, owing to relative freedom from cosmetic, behavioral, and cognitive side effects. Other indications include manic-depressive illness unresponsive to lithium, phantom limb pain, and postherpetic neuralgia.

Preparations and Dosage

CBMZ (Tegretol) is available as 100- and 200-mg tablets for oral administration. A suspension is also available that contains 100 mg/5 mL.[28]

Pharmacokinetics

CBMZ is an iminostilbene derivative that is chemically and structurally similar to imipramine yet shares few of its pharmacologic properties.[29] CBMZ is absorbed slowly and erratically after oral administration. Peak serum concentrations occur in 4 to 8 hours after ingestion but may be delayed 24 hours. The drug is 75% protein bound and has a volume of distribution of 0.79 to 1.19 L/kg. CBMZ is hepatically metabolized to a 10,11-epoxide, which is as active as the parent compound and which has a half-life of 10 to 20 hours. In adults, the epoxide metabolite is present in blood at a concentration of 10% to 15% of the parent compound, whereas in children the ratio is 20%.[29] The epoxide may be responsible for the neurotoxicity of the drug,[30] and an increased ratio of the epoxide to parent compound may explain neurotoxicity at therapeutic serum CBMZ concentrations. Because CBMZ induces its own metabolism, the half-life of the drug after a single dose (31 to 35 hours) is much longer than the half-life of the drug at steady state (10 to 20 hours). This autoinduction process takes about 4 weeks.[31] CBMZ elimination follows first-order kinetics. The epoxide is metabolized to inactive compounds, which are excreted in the urine. Only 3% of the parent compound is excreted unchanged in the urine. Fifteen percent of the drug is recovered unchanged from feces with evidence of enterohepatic circulation.

Side Effects of Chronic Therapy

Side effects occur in up to 25% of patients receiving CBMZ (Table 48–5). A mild transient leukopenia may occur in 10% of patients during their first month of treatment but usually resolves despite continued drug administration. Persistent leukopenia resolves after discontinuation of the drug. This mild leukopenia appears to be unrelated to aplastic anemia, which occurs in approximately 1 in 575,000 patients who are treated with CMBZ.[32] Recommendations for hematologic monitoring are varied and range from weekly to every 2 months.

Serum liver enzyme activity increases in approximately 10% of patients taking CBMZ. In the asymptomatic patient, mild elevation of serum liver enzyme activity does not require discontinuation of the drug.[33] Drug interactions are listed in Table 48–6.

Table 48–5. Carbamazepine: Adverse Side Effects

↑ Liver function tests (5–10%)
Cardiac conduction disturbance*
Anorexia
Weight loss
Diarrhea
Hyponatremia
Hypersensitivity reactions
Aplastic anemia*
Neurologic side effects†
Drowsiness (40%)
Ataxia (20%)
Slurred speech
Tremor
Asterixis
Dystonic reactions
Diplopia

*See text.
†More common in patients with pre-existing side effects.

Carbamazepine and the Heart

Cardiac conduction disturbances occur in elderly patients on long-term, or after initiation of, CBMZ therapy and do not appear to be dose related. CBMZ-induced clinically significant bradycardia (including complete heart block) may be a result of a defective conduction system or a sick sinus syndrome in older patients.[34–37] The bradycardia may cause symptoms mistakenly diagnosed as seizures. All patients 50 years of age and older should have an electrocardiogram performed before the initiation of CBMZ therapy. If the pattern of seizures changes, cardiac evaluation should be performed.

Animal experiments demonstrate prolonged atrioventricular conduction and membrane depressant effect in higher doses.[38] Clinically insignificant electrocardiographic abnormalities have been noted (primarily first-degree heart block),[39, 40] Unfortunately, many of the case reports of CBMZ overdose do not include electrocardiographic assessment.

Table 48–6. Carbamazepine: Drug Interactions

Drug → ↓ CBMZ	*Drug → ↑ CBMZ*
Phenobarbital	Propoxyphene
Phenytoin	Erythromycin
Primidone	Cimetidine
Valproic acid (↑ or ↓)	Diltiazem
	Verapamil
	Isoniazid
	Troleandomycin

CBMZ → ↓ Drug
Warfarin
Valproate
Haloperidol
Theophylline
Clonazepam
Phenytoin (↑, ↓, =)

Overdose

Ingestion of a toxic amount of CBMZ usually causes a depressed sensorium, nystagmus, ataxia, and mydriasis. Abnormal deep tendon reflexes with hypertonicity and clonus as well as movement disorders may also occur. Seizures occur more frequently in patients with a seizure disorder and are thought to result from CBMZ-epoxide neurotoxicity. Hypokalemia, hyponatremia, hyperglycemia, and transient elevation of serum liver enzyme activity may be present after overdose. Heart block has been reported in two children after overdose.[41, 42] Although cardiac arrhythmias and QRS widening may occur in conjunction with seizures, cardiac arrhythmias are rarely seen in an uncomplicated CBMZ overdose.[43] Although serum CBMZ concentrations greater than 170 μmol/L (40 mg/L) are indicative of severe intoxication, lower serum concentrations are not prognostic of a benign clinical course. The seriousness of toxicity should be judged by clinical status, not serum CBMZ concentration.[41, 42]

Late relapses and a cyclic clinical course occasionally seen after CBMZ overdose are explained by delayed absorption secondary to anticholinergic properties and low water solubility. Peak serum concentrations may not occur until 72 hours after ingestion.[43] Half-life may be up to 39 hours after overdose, even in patients chronically ingesting CBMZ, suggesting the prolongation is due to delayed absorption.[44] Although gastric emptying beyond 1 hour after ingestion does not alter outcome, prolonged absorption must be a special consideration in this overdose. If gastric emptying is performed, subsequent administration of multiple doses of activated charcoal will decrease the half-life and increase elimination of CBMZ. Recommendations include administration of 100 g of activated charcoal followed by 50 g every 4 hours until clinical recovery.[45–49] Although charcoal hemoperfusion may decrease the half-life of both CBMZ and the epoxide,[48] the efficacy of charcoal hemoperfusion has not been compared with the administration of multiple doses of activated charcoal. Hemodialysis and forced diuresis are of no benefit.

Owing to structural similarities between tricyclic antidepressants and CBMZ, physostigmine has been administered to patients with CBMZ toxicity. However, dystonic reactions are the only toxic effect that has resolved with physostigmine administration. Cardiac arrhythmias and decreased sensorium are not affected by administration of physostigmine. Its use is not recommended.[49]

Valproate

Valproate (VPA) was first prescribed for the treatment of absence seizures in 1978 and is currently prescribed for the treatment of all types of seizures.[3] When VPA is discontinued after chronic administration, the anticonvulsant effect continues after plasma drug concentrations are no longer measurable. Long-lived active metabolites or adaptive changes in neuronal function may be important facets of VPA's action.[3]

Preparations and Dosage

VPA (Depakene) is available in the United States as 250-mg capsules and as a syrup containing 250 mg/5 mL of sodium valproate. Usual daily doses are 1000 to 2000 mg in adults and 15 to 60 mg/kg in children. Depakote contains equal proportions of VPA and sodium valproate.[50]

Pharmacokinetics

VPA is rapidly and completely absorbed after oral administration. Peak serum concentrations occur 15 minutes to 2 hours, 1 to 2 hours, and 3 to 8 hours after ingestion of syrup, capsules, and enteric-coated tablets, respectively.[50, 51] The drug is 90% bound to plasma proteins and has a small volume of distribution (0.13 to 0.23 L/kg). Anticonvulsant activity of the many metabolites is negligible. The half-life of VPA is 8 to 14 hours but may be up to 42 hours after overdose. Elimination kinetics of the parent compound appear to be first order in overdose. Elimination kinetic data of the metabolites is still undetermined.[52] Less than 3% of the drug is excreted unchanged in the urine and feces.

Serum Concentration and Laboratory Analysis

Serum concentration does not correlate well with either seizure control or toxicity. Therapeutic serum concentrations of VPA lie between 50 and 100 μg/mL. Because cognitive function is impaired as the dose increases, the lowest dose possible should be used. Once a response occurs, there is no therapeutic gain in achieving higher serum concentrations. Incidence of adverse side effects increases at concentrations greater than 120 μg/mL.[53]

The enzyme-multilinked immunoassay will yield higher values of serum VPA than will gas-liquid chromatography. Serum levels must therefore be monitored by the same analytic method. Free VPA concentration is no more useful than total VPA concentration in achieving optimal seizure control.[51]

VPA is eliminated partly as ketone bodies and may cause a false-positive test result for ketones in the urine. VPA may also decrease serum values of total thyroxine.[50]

Side Effects of Chronic Therapy

Side effects of chronic therapy are listed in Table 48–7.[54] Serum liver enzyme activity increases in up to 60% of patients with therapeutic VPA serum concentrations, with serum bilirubin increasing as VPA concentrations increase. Dose reduction or discontinuation of the drug results in normalization of the serum liver enzyme concentration.[55]

Table 48–7. Valproate: Adverse Side Effects

Gastrointestinal (15%)	Central nervous system*
Anorexia	Sedation
Nausea	Ataxia
Diarrhea	Tremor
Abdominal	
Pancreatitis†	

*Abated by decreasing dose.
†Fatal cases reported.

The most serious side effect is hepatotoxicity and, rarely, hepatic failure. VPA may cause either intrinsic hepatotoxicity (reversible, reproducible, and dose dependent) or idiosyncratic hepatotoxicity (unpredictable, not dose dependent, long latent period). Fatal hepatic failure, histologically evident as microvesicular steatosis, occurs in 1 in 20,000 patients.[56] Children younger than 3 years of age who are receiving multiple antiepileptic agents and with additional medical problems are at highest risk.[57] Lack of clinical signs of hypersensitivity (fever, rash, and eosinophilia) suggests that hepatic failure is an idiosyncratic reaction. Children in their first 6 months of VPA administration, who present with unexplained symptoms of lethargy, vomiting, or general deterioration, should be assessed for hepatotoxicity. An increase in serum ammonia may also cause somnolence, lethargy, and coma.[58] Asymptomatic hyperammonemia without hepatic damage occurs in 20% of patients taking this drug. Routine monitoring of liver function does not predict which patients will develop hepatotoxicity.

The hematologic side effect most commonly reported is thrombocytopenia, which is usually transient despite continuing the drug. Although rare, VPA may induce widespread bone marrow toxicity.[59]

Drug Interactions

VPA inhibits several hepatic metabolic pathways, which alters drug metabolism of coingested drugs (Table 48–8).

Overdose

Central nervous system (CNS) toxicity, from drowsiness to coma, is the most frequent sign after overdose. Onset and progression of CNS depression is rapid. Respiratory distress has been reported, although it is difficult to discern if aspiration is the main factor or if VPA has a direct toxic effect on lung tissue. Although the cause of the multiple metabolic abnormalities that occur is unknown, inhibition of fatty acid oxidation, fatty acid synthesis, pyruvate oxidation, urea synthesis, and gluconeogenesis have been demonstrated in rat hepatocytes.[60] Hypoglycemia, hypocalcemia, hypernatremia, hypophosphatemia, and metabolic acidosis may be life threatening and persist for days. Leukopenia and thrombocytopenia may occur. Thrombocytopenia may be severe enough to require platelet transfusion. Cerebral edema, occurring days after the overdose, has been reported in severe cases. Although the mechanism of delayed-onset cerebral edema is unknown, it may be related to active metabolites that are present in high concentrations in regions of the brain. Although elevation of serum ammonia and hepatic enzymes may occur, hepatic injury appears to be minimal after overdose. Serum liver enzyme elevations are not indicative of the severity of overdose and return to normal within 2 weeks. Fatalities are rare. Serum drug concentrations do not correlate with the severity of the poisoning. Drowsiness has been the only manifestation of serum concentrations as high as 100 mg/L.[51, 61]

High concentrations of VPA may cause abnormal metabolism. Decreased β-oxidation metabolites have been reported after overdose. Because hypocarnitinemia, which inhibits β-oxidation, has been reported after long-term VPA therapy, L-carnitine has been administered in an attempt to increase VPA metabolism by β-oxidation, which is the primary pathway with therapeutic VPA concentrations. Clinical relevance is unknown.[62]

Supportive care is the primary treatment for this overdose. Gastrointestinal decontamination should be considered in the comatose patient or in the patient who presents within 1 hour of ingestion. Both *in vitro* studies and case reports have demonstrated naloxone reversal of VPA-induced CNS depression (probably due to naloxone antagonism of the VPA-induced γ-aminobutyric acid [GABA] elevation). High doses of naloxone should be administered if CNS depression is present. Extracorporeal detoxification has not been shown to alter outcome.[63]

Table 48–8. Valproate: Drug Interactions

Drug → ↓ VPA Concentration
Carbamazepine
Phenobarbital
Phenytoin
VPA → ↓ Drug Concentration
Phenobarbital
VPA → ↑ or ↓ Phenytoin Concentration

PRENATAL ANTICONVULSANT EXPOSURE

Serious malformations occur in 3% of children of epileptic women as compared with 2% of children of nonepileptic women. Risk increases with increase in number of concurrently ingested antiepiletic drugs: 3% with one drug (same incidence in offspring of women with untreated epilepsy) and up to 4% with four drugs. A syndrome of facial dimorphism, cleft lip and palate, cardiac defects, digital hypoplasia, and nail dysplasia occurs not only with phenytoin but with CBMZ and VPA as well. Incidence of fetal neural tube defects is increased by 1% to 2% with VPA and 0.5% to 1% with CBMZ. Phenytoin and

CBMZ, which are enzyme inducers, can cause a transient deficiency in vitamin K–dependent clotting factors in the newborn. Women taking these drugs should receive vitamin K_1 during their last weeks of pregnancy. Their newborns should receive 1 mg of vitamin K_1 intramuscularly at birth.[64, 65]

NEWER ANTICONVULSANTS

Felbamate

Felbamate is a lipophilic, water-insoluble, stable neutral compound that was approved by the FDA in 1993. It is a third-line drug and is administered with other anticonvulsants and as monotherapy for intractable epilepsy. Its mechanism of action is unknown. The pharmacokinetic profile of this drug is incomplete. Felbamate has a mean half-life of 20 hours; 50% of the drug is excreted unchanged in the urine. The primary side effects are insomnia and nausea.[66, 67]

The FDA and Carter Wallace issued a warning regarding 10 cases of felbamate-induced aplastic anemia in October 1994. To date, 33 cases of aplastic anemia, of which 8 were fatal, have been reported. Sixteen cases of hepatic failure have also been reported. Many patients choose to take the drug with its known risk profile owing to its efficacy in the treatment of refractory seizures.[68]

Eighteen cases of felbamate overdose have been reported to its manufacturer. When ingested alone, doses of 36 to 40 g caused only tachycardia and drowsiness. Fatalities have been reported when felbamate was ingested with other drugs (personal communication, Carter Wallace, 1995).

Gabapentin

Gabapentin is structurally related to the inhibitory neurotransmitter GABA, although its antiepileptic activity appear to be unrelated to any effects on the GABA system. The mechanism of action is unknown.[69]

The drug is water-soluble, is not bound to plasma proteins, and is not metabolized but is excreted unchanged by the kidney. Its half-life is 5 to 7 hours. Gabapentin pharmacokinetics are influenced by renal function, with renal clearance decreasing with increasing age. The drug is effectively removed from plasma by hemodialysis.

Gabapentin has no known drug-drug interactions. Gabapentin causes only minor adverse effects (sedation, diplopia, dizziness, slurred speech, and sedation) in overdose.[70] Treatment is supportive.

Lamotrigine

Lamotrigine has been approved for the adjunctive treatment of partial seizures in adult patients and in children older than 12 years of age. The drug is structurally unrelated to other anticonvulsants. It is minimally soluble in water and is rapidly and completely absorbed. Lamotrigine undergoes hepatic metabolism and is eliminated primarily as the glucuronide conjugate. Its half-life is 24 to 30 hours. The most significant adverse effect during therapy is rash. An advantage is the lack of induction or inhibition of metabolism of other drugs. One report of an overdose of lamotrigine revealed QRS widening that was not of hemodynamic significance.[71, 72]

References

1. Dichter MA: Old and new mechanisms of antiepileptic drug actions. Epilepsy Res Suppl *10*:9–17, 1993.
2. Rall T, Schlerfer L: Drugs effective in the therapy of the epilepsies. *In* Gilman AG, Goodman LS, Rall TD, (eds): Goodman and Gilman's The Pharmacological Basis of Therapeutics. New York, Macmillan Publishing Co., pp 436–444, 1990.
3. Brodie M, Dichter M: Antiepileptic drugs. N Engl J Med *334*:168–175, 1996.
4. Tozer T, Winter M: Phenytoin. *In* Evans W, Schentag J, Jusko W (eds): Applied Pharmacokinetics. Vancouver, BC, Applied Therapeutics, pp 275–314, 1992.
5. Osborn H, Zisfein J, Sparano R: Single-dose oral phenytoin loading. Ann Emerg Med *155*:407–412, 1987.
6. Jung D, Powell R, Watson P, Paerrier D: Effect of dose on phenytoin absorption. Clin Pharmacol Ther *28*:479–485, 1985.
7. Hvidberg EF, Dan M: Clinical pharmacokinetics of anticonvulsants. Clin Pharmacokinet *1*:161–188, 1976.
8. The use of free phenytoin levels in adverting phenytoin toxicity. Letter to the editor. NY State J Med *90*:39–41, 1990.
9. Aaron J, Bank S, Ackert G: Diphenylhydantoin-induced hepatotoxicity. Am J Gastroenterol *80*:200–202, 1985.
10. Flowers F, Araujo O, Hanm K: Phenytoin hypersensitivity syndrome. J Emerg Med *5*:103–108, 1987.
11. Palm R, Selsith C, Alvan G: Phenytoin intoxication as the first symptom of fatal liver damage induced by sodium valproate. Br J Clin Pharmacol *17*:597–598, 1984.
12. Kooker J, Sumi S: Movement disorder as a manifestation of diphenylhydantoin intoxication. Neurology *24*:68–71, 1974.
13. Kokenge R, Henn K, McDowell F: Neurological sequelae following Dilantin overdose in a patient and in experimental animals. Neurology *15*:823–829, 1964.
14. Masur H, Elger CE, Ludolph AC, Glanski M: Cerebellar atrophy following acute intoxication with phenytoin. Neurology *39*:432–433, 1989.
15. McLain L, Martin T, Allen J: Cerebellar degeneration due to chronic phenytoin therapy. Ann Neurol 7:18–23, 1980.
16. Chaikin P, Adir J: Unusual absorption profile of phenytoin in a massive overdose case. J Clin Pharmacol *27*:70–73, 1987.
17. Wyte CD, Berk WA: Severe oral phenytoin overdose does not cause cardiovascular morbidity. Ann Emerg Med *20*:508–512, 1991.
18. Czajka P, Anderson W, Christoph R, Banner W: A pharmacokinetics evaluation of peritoneal dialysis for phenytoin intoxication. J Clin Pharmacol *20*:565–569, 1980.
19. Donovan P, Cline D: Phenytoin administration by constant intravenous infusion: Selective rates of administration. Ann Emerg Med *20*:139–142, 1991.
20. Earnest M, Marx J, Druey L: Complications of intravenous phenytoin for acute treatment of seizures. JAMA *249*:762–765, 1983.
21. Carducci B, Hedges J, Beal J, et al: Emergency phenytoin loading by constant intravenous infusion. Ann Emerg Med *13*:1027–1031, 1984.
22. Barron S: Cardiac arrhythmias after small IV dose of phenytoin. N Engl J Med *295*:678, 1976.
23. Wilder JB, Ramsay, RE, Willmore L, et al: Efficacy of intravenous phenytoin in the treatment of status epilepticus: Kinetics

of central nervous system penetration. Ann Neuro *1*:511–518, 1977.

24. York R, Coleridge S: Cardiopulmonary arrest following intravenous phenytoin loading. Am J Emerg Med *6*:255–259, 1988.
25. Zoneraich S, Zoneraich O, Siegel J: Sudden death following intravenous sodium diphenylhydantoin. Am Heart J *92*:375–377, 1976.
26. Spengler R, Arrowsmith J, Kilarski D, et al: Severe soft-tissue injury following intravenous infusion of phenytoin. Arch Intern Med *148*:1329–1333, 1988.
27. Walsh-Kelly C, Berens R, Glaeser P, Losek J: Intraosseous infusion of phenytoin. Am J Emerg Med *4*:523–524, 1986.
28. Rall T, Schlerfer L: Drugs effective in the therapy of the epilepsies. *In* Gilman AG, Goodman LS, Rall TD, et al (eds): Goodman and Gilman's The Pharmacological Basis of Therapeutics. New York, Macmillan Publishing Co., pp 447–448, 1990.
29. Garnett W, Carson S, Pellock J, et al: Carbamazepine and carbamazepine epoxide carbamazepine plasma levels in children following chronic dosing with Tegretol suspension and tablets. Neurology *37*(Suppl 1): 93–94, 1987.
30. Pellock J: Carbamazepine side effects in children and adults. Epilepsia *28*(Suppl 3): 564–570, 1987.
31. Levy RH, Dreifuss FE, Mattson RG, et al (eds): Antiepileptic Drugs. 3rd ed. New York, Raven Press, 1989.
32. O'Connor CP, Schraeder PL, Kurland AH, O'Connor WH: Evaluation of the mechanisms of antiepileptic drug-related leukopenia. Epilepsia *35*:149–154, 1994.
33. Seetharam MN, Pellock JM: Risk benefit assessment of carbamazepine in children. Drug Saf *6*:148–158, 1991.
34. Steiner C, Wit AL, Weis MD, Damato AN: The antiarrhythmic actions of carbamazepine. J Pharm Exp Ther *172*:323–335, 1970.
35. Kenneback G, Bergfeldt L, Vallin H, et al: Electrophysiologic effects and clinical hazards of carbamazepine treatment for neurologic disorders in patients with abnormalities of the cardiac conduction system. Am Heart J *5*:1421–1429, 1981.
36. Puletti M, Iani C, Curione M, et al: Carbamazepine and the heart. Ann Neurol *29*:575–576, 1991.
37. Beerman B, Edhag O: Side effects of drugs. BMJ *2*:171–172, 1978.
38. Seymour JF: Carbamazepine overdose. Drug Saf *8*:81–88, 1993.
39. Apfelbaum J, Caravati EM, Kerns WP, et al: Cardiovascular effects of carbamazepine toxicity. Ann Emerg Med *25*:631–635, 1995.
40. Heart block secondary to erythromycin-induced carbamazepine toxicity. Pediatrics *80*:951–953, 1987.
41. Spiller HA, Krenzelok EP, Cookson E: Carbamazepine overdose: A prospective study of serum levels and toxicity. Clin Toxicol *28*:445–458, 1990
42. Hojer J, Malmlund HO, Berg A: Clinical features in 28 consecutive cases of laboratory confirmed massive poisoning with carbamazepine alone. Clin Toxicol *31*:449–458, 1993.
43. Sethna M, Solomon G, Cedarbaum J, Kutt H: Successful treatment of massive carbamazepine overdose. Epilepsia *30*:71–73, 1989.
44. Boldy D, Heath A, Ruddock S, et al: Activated charcoal for carbamazepine poisoning. Lancet *1*:1027, 1987.
45. Neuvonen PJ, Elonen E: Effect of activated charcoal on absorption and elimination of phenobarbitone, carbamazepine and phenylbutazone in man. Eur J Clin Pharmacol *17*:51–57, 1980.
46. Watson S, Baker RC, Carolan P, et al: Carbamazepine overdose: The effects of multiple dose activated charcoal. Clin Toxicol *30*:39–48, 1992.
47. Stremski E, Brady W, Prasad K, Hennes H: Pediatric carbamazepine intoxication. Ann Emerg Med *25*:624–630, 1995.
48. Groot G, Van Heijst A, Maes R: Charcoal hemoperfusion in the treatment of two cases of acute CBMZ poisoning. Clin Toxicol *4*:349–362, 1984.
49. Sullivan J, Rumack B, Peterson R: Acute carbamazepine toxicity resulting from overdose. Neurology *31*:21–24, 1981.
50. Rall T, Schlerfer L: Drugs effective in the therapy of the epilepsies. *In* Gilman AG, Goodman LS, Rall TD, et al (eds): Goodman and Gilman's The Pharmacological Basis of Therapeutics. New York, Macmillan Publishing Co., pp 450–453, 1985.
51. Dupuis R, Lichtman S, Pollack G. Acute valproic acid overdose. Drug Saf *5*:65–71, 1990.
52. Andersen GO, Ritland S: Life-threatening intoxication with sodium valproate. Clin Toxicol *33*:279–284, 1995.
53. Schmidt D: Adverse effects of valproate. Epilepsia *25*(Suppl 1):544–549, 1984.
54. Binek J, Hany A, Heer M: Valproic acid–induced pancreatitis. J Clin Gastroenterol *13*:690–693, 1991.
55. Ralnaike R, Schapel G, Purdie G, et al: Hyperammonaemia and hepatotoxicity during chronic valproate therapy: Enhancement by combination with other antiepileptic drugs. Br J Clin Pharmacol *22*:100–103, 1986.
56. Dreifuss FE, Santilli N, Langer DH, et al: Valproic acid hepatic fatalities: A retrospective review. Neurology *37*:379–385, 1987.
57. Dreifuss FE, Langer DH, Moline KA, Maxwell JE: Valproic acid hepatic fatalities: US experience since 1984. Neurology *39*:201–207, 1989.
58. Patsalos PN, Wilson SJ, Popovik M, et al: The prevalence of valproic acid–associated hyperammonaemia in patients with intractable epilepsy. J Epilepsy *6*:228–232, 1993.
59. Glanick D, Suner T, Finley JL: Severe hematologic toxicity of valproic acid. Am J Pediatr Hematol Oncol *12*:80–85, 1990.
60. Turnbull DM, Dick DJ, Wilson L, et al: Valproate causes metabolic disturbance in normal man. J Neurol Neurosurg Psychiatry *49*:405–410, 1986.
61. Wason S, Savitt D: Acute valproic acid toxicity at therapeutic concentrations. Clin Pediatr *24*:466–467, 1985.
62. Ishikura H, Matsuo N, Matsubara M, et al: Valproic acid overdose and L-carnitine therapy. J Anal Toxicol *20*:55–58, 1996.
63. Alberto G, Erickson T, Popiel R, et al: Central nervous system manifestations of a valproic acid overdose responsive to naloxone. Ann Emerg Med *18*:889–891, 1989.
64. Nakane Y, Okuma T, Takahashi R, et al: Multi-institutional study on the teratogenicity and fetal toxicity of antiepileptic drugs: A report of a collaborative study group in Japan. Epilepsia *21*:663–680, 1980.
65. Yerby MS, Leppik I. Epilepsy and the outcomes of pregnancy. J Epilepsy *3*:193–199, 1990.
66. Graves NM: Felbamate. Ann Pharmacother *27*:1078–1081, 1993.
67. Leppik IE: Felbamate. Epilepsia *36*(Suppl 2):S66–S72, 1995.
68. Pennell PB, Ogaily MS, Macdonald RL: Aplastic anemia in a patient receiving felbamate for complex partial seizures. Neurology *45*:456–460, 1995.
69. Andrews CO, Fischer JH: Gabapentin: A new agent for the management of epilepsy. Ann Pharmacother *28*:1188–1196, 1994.
70. Fischer JH, Barr AN, Rogers SL, et al: Lack of serious toxicity following gabapentin overdose. Neurology *44*:982, 1994.
71. Messenheimer JA: Lamotrigine. Epilepsia *36*(Suppl 2):S87–S94, 1995.
72. Buckley NA, Whyte IM, Dawson AH: Self-poisoning with lamotrigine. Lancet *342*:1552–1553, 1993.

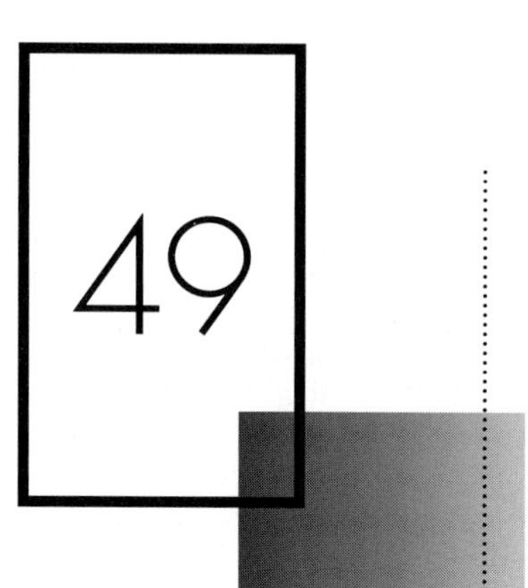

SECTION C

ANALGESICS

Acetaminophen

HOLLY PERRY, MD
MICHAEL W. SHANNON, MD, MPH

IDENTIFICATION AND HISTORY

Acetaminophen is the most widely used analgesic/antipyretic in the world today, partly because of its excellent safety profile. Acetaminophen (also known as paracetamol, *N*-acetyl-*p*-aminophenol, and APAP) was first used in 1893 but did not gain popularity until 1949, when its relationship to another widely used analgesic, phenacetin, was appreciated. Acetaminophen was made available without a prescription in the United States in 1955. Acetaminophen is currently available either singly or in combination with other pharmaceuticals in more than 100 preparations.

Acetaminophen is a member of the family of coal tar analgesics, which also includes acetanilid and phenacetin. Once very popular, acetanilid and phenacetin were found to have serious adverse reactions when continually used, including renal papillary necrosis, hemolysis, and methemoglobinemia. Although acetaminophen is a metabolite of both phenacetin and acetanilid, it does not share the renal or hematologic toxicity of its precursors. Its primary toxicity is hepatic, and it is toxic only when taken in overdose quantities.

EPIDEMIOLOGY

Toxicity due to acetaminophen overdose was not recognized until 1966, when the first case was reported in the British literature.[1, 2] Since that time, morbidity and mortality from acetaminophen overdose have continued to climb steadily. Acetaminophen currently is one of the most frequent causes of poisoning due to a pharmaceutical agent worldwide. It was one of the most common overdoses reported to the American Association of Poison Control Centers Toxic Exposures Surveillance System (AAPCC-TESS) in 1994.[3] One hundred thirty-five deaths attributed to acetaminophen overdose were reported to the AAPCC-TESS in 1994, more deaths than from any other pharmaceutical agent. Acetaminophen-induced hepatic failure is the most common cause of hepatic failure necessitating liver transplant in Great Britain and is the second most common reason for liver transplantation in the United States.[4]

PHARMACOKINETICS AND TOXICOKINETICS

The kinetics and metabolism of acetaminophen are well understood. Absorption of acetaminophen tablets is rapid and usually complete by 1 hour after a therapeutic dose, with slightly faster absorption of the liquid preparations.[5] After ingestion of excessive doses of standard-release preparations, absorption is delayed but invariably is complete within 4 hours. Theoretically, acetaminophen absorption could be delayed by coingestion of agents that reduce gastric emptying. However, only three reported cases of a peak level occurred later than 4 hours after overdose; propoxyphene was a coingestant in all three cases.[6–8] A concern is that the extended-release acetaminophen preparation that was marketed in 1995 might have absorption that extends beyond 4 hours; in one reported case, the plasma acetaminophen level did not peak until 16 hours after overdose.[9]

Acetaminophen has noncomplex, noncumulative log linear kinetics of the first-order type. This means that acetaminophen is metabolized—in the absence of liver damage—at a steady rate (such that the level declines over time in a predictable fashion).

(Salicylates, in contrast, have cumulative kinetics of the zero-order type, and when metabolic capacity is exceeded, elimination is predominantly dependent on urine flow and urine pH.) Acetaminophen has a half-life of 2.5 to 4 hours; the half-life may be prolonged in cases of liver damage. Protein binding of acetaminophen is about 10%, and its volume of distribution is approximately 0.9 L/kg.[5]

Metabolism is the basis of toxicity. Acetaminophen is a rare example of drug toxification rather than detoxification by the liver; other examples include methanol and ethylene glycol. Approximately 2% is excreted unchanged in the urine.[10] More than 90% of acetaminophen is metabolized by either sulfation or glucuronidation, and the remainder is metabolized by the cytochrome P-450 mixed-function oxidase system (Fig. 49–1)[10]; the mixed-function oxidase system is distributed throughout the body, but the majority is in the hepatocytes. The metabolism of acetaminophen is age dependent, with a larger proportion of acetaminophen undergoing sulfation in infants and children.[11] This difference diminishes with age and essentially resolves by age 12. Neither unchanged acetaminophen nor the glucuronide or sulfate conjugates are toxic. However, the metabolite that is elaborated by the mixed-function oxidase system is toxic.[12–14] This metabolite, *N*-acetyl-*p*-benzoquinoneimine (NAPQI), is very short lived, with a half-life of nanoseconds. It attaches to the hepatic cell membrane and injures the lipid bilayer if not neutralized

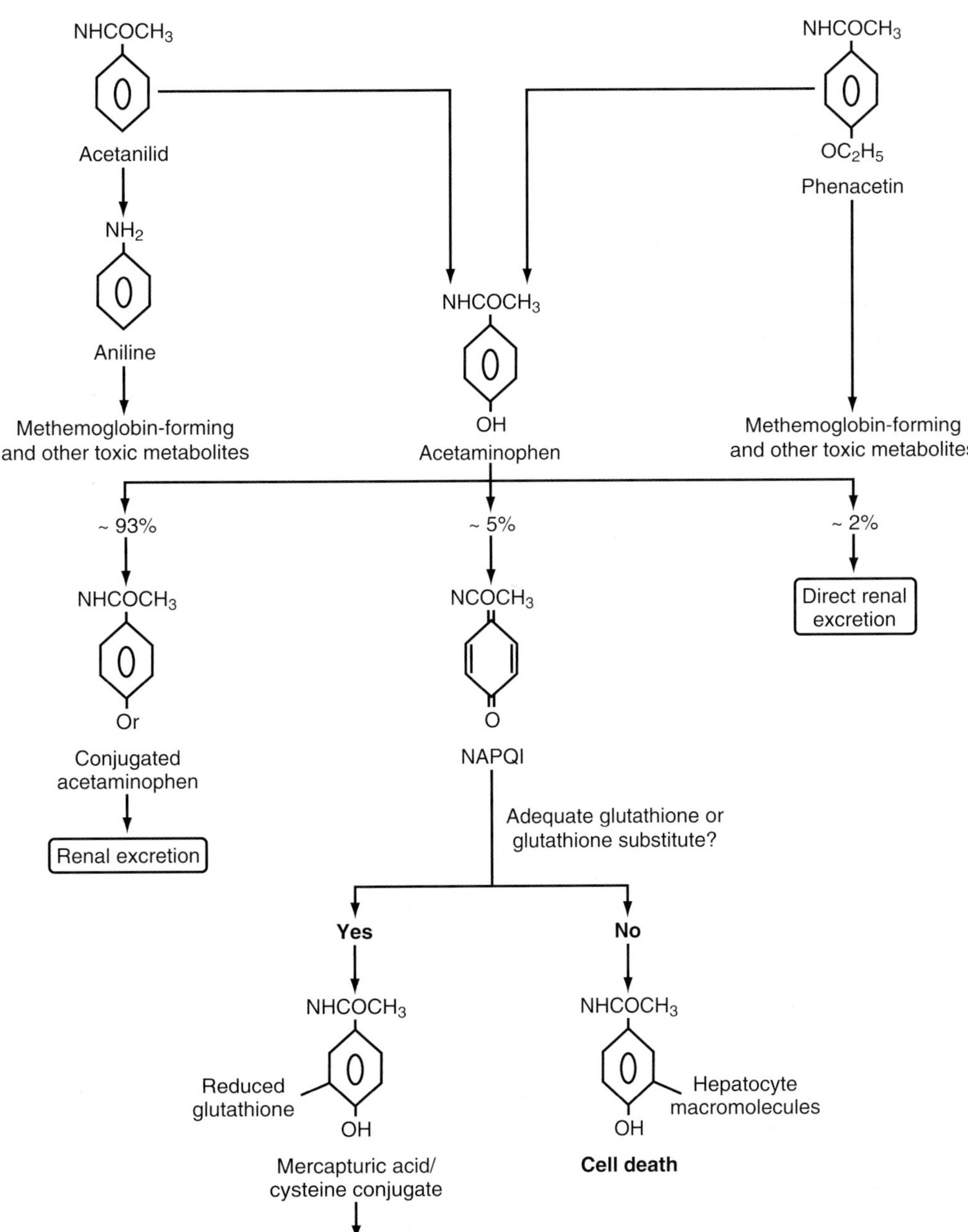

Figure 49–1. Metabolism of acetaminophen and other coal tar analgesics. R, glucuronide or sulfate; NAPQI, *N*-acetyl-*p*-benzoquinoneimine.

by an antioxidant. Hepatic glutathione appears to be the primary antioxidant that conjugates and neutralizes NAPQI.[10, 15–17]

At therapeutic doses, acetaminophen is a very safe drug with essentially no side effects. However, when hepatic glutathione stores have been depleted to less than 70% of normal values, such as after an acetaminophen overdose, NAPQI is not detoxified by glutathione but instead binds to hepatocytes, and arylation and cell death result.

MODULATORS OF TOXICITY

Acetaminophen toxicity results from an imbalance between hepatic glutathione stores and the amount of NAPQI formed by the hepatic mixed-function oxidase system, which is made up of several families of enzymes. Theoretically, any compound that affects the mixed-function oxidase system, specifically either the cyp2E1 or cyp1A2 enzymes, would be anticipated to affect the amount of NAPQI produced and thus to have an impact on the likelihood of developing hepatotoxicity after an acetaminophen overdose. The cyp2E1 enzyme is responsible for most NAPQI formation from acetaminophen, and the cyp1A2 enzyme produces a lesser amount. Probable inducers for cyp2E1 include ethanol, isoniazid, rifampin, phenytoin, and carbamazepine; probable inducers for cyp1A2 include cigarette smoke and charcoal-broiled foods.[18] Indeed, clinical series have demonstrated that patients who are continually ingesting substances that induce cyp2E1 such as anticonvulsants[19] and those who chronically abuse alcohol have poorer outcomes than the general population after acetaminophen overdose.[20–23] Several case reports describe patients' taking antituberculosis medications and subsequently developing hepatotoxicity after both acute single overdose and long-term excessive intake of acetaminophen.[24, 25] Patients with depleted glutathione stores, such as those with anorexia nervosa, may also be at higher risk for development of hepatotoxicity after an acetaminophen overdose.

Age may also be a potential modulator of toxicity. Children younger than 5 years appear to be more resistant to the toxic effects of acetaminophen. Very few deaths have been reported, and the incidence of hepatotoxcity is much lower than that observed in the general population.[26, 27] It is unclear why young children might be more resistant to large ingestions of acetaminophen, but a number of possibilities have been suggested, including early decontamination due to spontaneous or induced emesis, differences in the activity of the mixed-function oxidase system, increased glutathione stores, or a briefer delay before the antidote is administered. The amount of acetaminophen metabolized by the mixed-function oxidase system is difficult to ascertain because it is technically impractical to measure the glutathione-NAPQI complex. Inferences can be drawn from metabolic data for other drugs, such as phenytoin, which use the mixed-function oxidase system; kinetic analyses have shown the mixed-function oxidase systems to have greater activity in young children. Thus, young children would be expected to elaborate more NAPQI and be more susceptible to acetaminophen, which is opposite the clinical observation. Yet another possible explanation is that the lower incidence of severe hepatotoxicity is an effect of early treatment: most toddlers would be expected to present promptly to a health care provider after an accidental ingestion and thus receive treatment earlier than their adult counterparts. The largest reported series of young children with acetaminophen overdose did not address treatment delay.[26] One study that did investigate the role of treatment delay in children found that none who were younger than 6 years (n = 5) and who had acetaminophen levels in the probable or high toxicity range developed severe hepatotoxicity despite an average treatment delay of more than 15 hours.[27] Perhaps the lower incidence of severe hepatotoxicity is due to intrinsic differences in young children's ability to detoxify NAPQI, although there are no clear data to demonstrate this.

CLINICAL MANIFESTATIONS

The minimal single acute toxic dose is 7.5 g for an adult or 150 mg/kg for a child. Symptoms and laboratory abnormalities are predictable after an acetaminophen overdose and have traditionally been divided into four phases (Table 49–1). Symptoms may initially be minimal, although patients who are severely poisoned generally have nausea, vomiting, and occasionally lethargy. These symptoms tend to resolve by 12 to 18 hours and possibly reflect direct effects of the parent compound (because resolution occurs with declining acetaminophen levels). Evidence of hepatic injury as reflected by elevations in aspartate aminotransferase (AST) and alanine ami-

Table 49–1. Phases of Acetaminophen Poisoning

Phase
Phase I (0.5–24 h)
Anorexia, nausea, and vomiting are frequently present.
Malaise and diaphoresis may be present.
Transaminases may be elevated.
Patients may appear normal.
Phase II (24–72 h)
Anorexia, nausea, and vomiting become less pronounced.
Right upper quadrant pain may be present.
Transaminase levels continue to increase.
Bilirubin level may be elevated.
Prothrombin time may be prolonged.
Renal function may deteriorate.
Phase III (72–96 h)
Characterized by the sequelae of hepatic necrosis: jaundice, coagulation defects, renal failure, and hepatic encephalopathy.
Liver biopsy reveals centrilobular necrosis.
Death due to multiorgan failure may result.
Phase IV (4–14 d)
If patients survive, complete resolution of hepatic dysfunction occurs and the liver heals without evidence of fibrosis.

notransferase (ALT) may appear as early as 8 hours after overdose, and more than half of all patients with liver injury develop some elevation in transaminase levels within 24 hours after overdose.[28] (In patients who recover, transaminase levels peak between 48 and 72 hours, with peak values as high as 50,000 IU/L). Transaminases gradually return to normal levels during the ensuing 2 weeks. Patients who develop an elevation of AST or ALT level greater than 1000 IU/L commonly demonstrate other evidence of liver dysfunction by 24 to 72 hours after overdose, including elevations in prothrombin time and bilirubin. Patients who ultimately die or require liver transplantation progress to demonstrate the sequelae of hepatic necrosis, including jaundice, coagulation defects, hepatorenal syndrome, and hepatic encephalopathy. Death results from multiorgan failure and generally occurs 72 to 96 hours after overdose.

The liver is the primary target for toxicity after acetaminophen overdose because the hepatocytes elaborate NAPQI. Because NAPQI has such a short life span, it can damage only cells that elaborate it. The histopathologic signs following acetaminophen overdose are characteristic: centrilobular necrosis (which is where NAPQI is elaborated) with periportal sparing.

Organ systems other than the liver are rarely affected immediately after acute overdose. Multiorgan failure may occur several days after acetaminophen poisoning but only in the setting of severe hepatotoxicity. The mechanism of acute injury to other organs besides the liver is unclear. Isolated case reports describe acute nephrotoxicity[29–31] and altered mental status.[32] Elevation of pancreatic enzyme levels has been reported in as many as 22% of unselected cases.[33, 34] The clinical importance of these laboratory abnormalities is unknown. Although acetaminophen is a metabolite of phenacetin, it does not have the capacity to regenerate phenacetin, and consequently, neither the papillary necrosis nor the methemoglobinemia characteristic of phenacetin toxicity is observed in human beings with acetaminophen toxicity.

All outcome studies have defined severe hepatotoxicity due to acetaminophen overdose as either AST or ALT level greater than 1000 IU/L. Approximately 3.5% of patients who develop severe hepatotoxicity eventually suffer fulminant hepatic failure,[33] and slightly fewer than half of patients with fulminant hepatic failure die or require liver transplantation.[35] Death is most frequently caused by cerebral edema or sepsis. There are several early indicators of decreased survival for patients with fulminant hepatic failure: arterial pH less than 7.30,[35] peak prothrombin time greater than 100 seconds in combination with a serum creatinine level greater than 3.4 mg/dL, and a prothrombin time continuing to rise on day 4 after overdose.[36] In the subset of patients who develop severe hepatotoxicity, initial acetaminophen level and treatment with *N-acetylcysteine (NAC)* have no value for predicting which of those patients will progress to fulminant hepatic failure. Similarly, peak AST and ALT values have no prognostic significance. In one large study of patients who died of acetaminophen overdose, mean peak AST level was less than 3000 IU/L.[35] Patients who do not die have complete recovery of their liver with no evidence of scarring within 30 days.[37]

PREDICTION OF HEPATOXICITY

The natural history of cases treated with supportive care alone was known to be related to plasma acetaminophen concentration as a function of time since ingestion. The outcome measure chosen was elevation in the serum levels of transaminases, with severe hepatotoxicity being defined as either AST or ALT level greater than 1000 IU/L. Transaminases were chosen as a measure of liver injury because of ease of standardization and accessibility. Sixty per cent of patients with plasma acetaminophen concentration above a line connecting the points where plasma acetaminophen concentration is 200 μg/mL 4 hours after overdose to the point where plasma acetaminophen concentration is 100 μg/mL 8 hours after overdose developed severe hepatotoxicty. This percentage increased to 90% in patients with plasma acetaminophen concentration above a line connecting the points where plasma acetaminophen concentration is 300 μg/mL 4 hours after overdose to a point where plasma acetaminophen concentration 150 μg/mL 8 hours after overdose.[38]

Before antidotal therapy with NAC was evaluated in a national study in the United States, a treatment nomogram was devised by Rumack and colleagues using the foregoing data (Fig. 49–2). According to this nomogram, which remains a treatment standard, three levels of risk for development of severe hepatotoxicity following acetaminophen overdose are delineated: possible, probable, and high. Patients are at high risk if the 4-hour (or equivalent) plasma acetaminophen concentration is 300 μg/mL and at probable risk if the 4-hour (or equivalent) plasma acetaminophen concentration is 200 μg/mL. A third level was added to the nomogram to give a 25% margin of safety to allow for variations in measurement of acetaminophen levels among laboratories as well as uncertainty in time of ingestion.[39] The earliest time after ingestion that can be plotted on the nomogram is 4 hours, because this is when absorption of acetaminophen is complete and acetaminophen levels peak; levels obtained sooner than 4 hours after ingestion are uninterpretable. Acetaminophen levels obtained later than 20 hours after the overdose may be difficult to interpret if they are nondetectable. The lower limit of detection of acetaminophen for many laboratories is 10 μg/mL, which represents a toxic concentration if obtained more than 20 hours after acetaminophen overdose.

ANTIDOTE THERAPY

Several drugs have been evaluated as antidotes for acetaminophen overdose, including cysteamine,

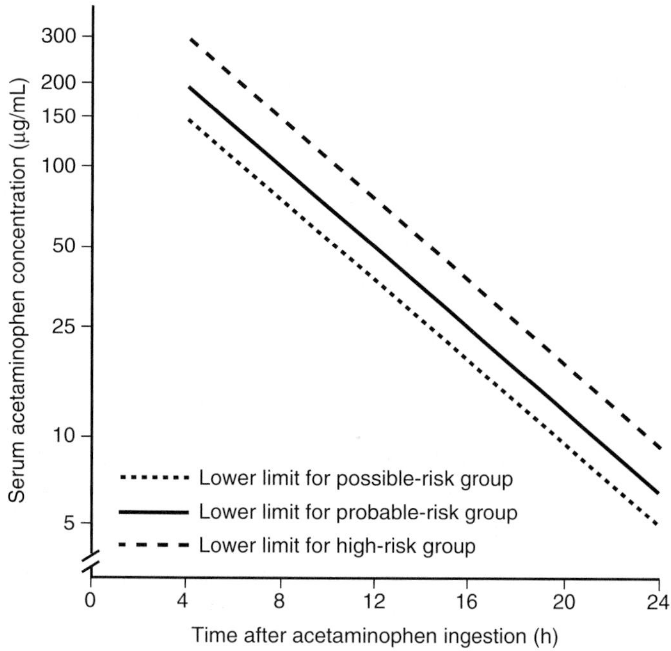

Figure 49–2. Acetaminophen (APAP) overdose treatment nomogram. Adapted from Smilkstein MJ, Knapp GL, Kully KW, et al: Efficacy of oral *N*-acetylcysteine in the treatment of acetaminophen overdose: Analysis of the National Multicenter Study (1976 to 1985). N Engl J Med *319*:1557, 1988.

methionine, and NAC. Each of these antidotes can serve as either a glutathione precursor or substitute. Glutathione itself has not been studied because it does not penetrate cell membranes. Cysteamine, although effective, has unacceptable adverse effects including nausea, vomiting, drowsiness, and cardiotoxicity.[40] Methionine, although safe, has not been very effective. In contrast, NAC is both safe and effective. In addition to serving as a glutathione substitute, NAC is thought to act as an antidote by enhancing glutathione synthesis and increasing the amount of acetaminophen that is metabolized by sulfation.[15] Other compounds such as cimetidine[41, 42] and 4-methylpyrazole,[43] which block the mixed-function oxidase system, have also been postulated to ameliorate the toxic effects of acetaminophen overdose, although no extensive clinical trials using these drugs have been conducted to date. Three different NAC protocols are currently in use worldwide. In the United Kingdom, Canada, Australia, and other countries, NAC is administered continuously for 20 hours by intravenous (IV) infusion. This regimen consists of a loading dose of 150 mg/kg over 15 minutes, followed by 50 mg/kg over the next 4 hours, followed by 100 mg/kg over the next 20 hours (total dose of 300 mg/kg). *In the United States, the only Food and Drug Administration–approved protocol is 72 hours of oral NAC, which consists of a 140 mg/kg loading dose followed by 17 maintenance doses of 70 mg/kg (total dose of 1330 mg/kg).* Although the 72-hour oral NAC regimen is effective, therapy is complicated by the frequent incidence of emesis; this has a negative impact on the usefulness of NAC as an oral antidote. Therefore, an IV regimen of NAC that is as efficacious as the oral regimen is being sought. In the United States, an on-going clinical trial of IV NAC is currently being conducted. The protocol is based on a modification of the oral regimen: a 140 mg/kg loading dose followed by 12 maintenance doses of 70 mg/kg (total dose of 980 mg/kg).

The results of clinical trials of these regimens are compared in Table 49–2.[38, 44, 45] Both the 20-hour IV protocol and the 72-hour oral protocol are efficacious when treatment is begun early, but the 72-hour oral protocol is clearly superior to the 20-hour IV protocol when patients present more than 15 hours after an overdose. The protocol of 72 hours of oral NAC is effective when used within the 24 hours after overdose, although its efficacy is a function of treatment delay. It is most effective when administered within the first 8 hours after acetaminophen overdose, but its effectiveness decreases incrementally every hour thereafter. Patients who are at probable risk for de-

Table 49–2. Comparison of Incidence of Hepatotoxicity After Treatment with Either Oral or Intravenous *N*-Acetylcysteine

Treatment Delay	20-h IV	72-h Oral	52-h IV
Probable Risk			
0–10 h	1/62 (1.6) [0–9%]	32/527 (6.1) [4–8%]	5/50 (10) [3–22%]
10–24 h	20/38 (52.6) [36–69%]	247/935 (26.4) [24–30%]	23/85 (27.1) [18–38%]
High Risk			
0–10 h	1/33 (3) [0–16%]	17/206 (8.3) [5–13%]	1/24 (4.2) [0–21%]
10–24 h	18/27 (67) [46–83%]	199/578 (34.4) [30–37%]	16/50 (32) [19–47%]
16–24 h	9/11 (82) [48–98%]	116/283 (41) [35–47%]	11/19 (57.9) [34–80%]

Values given are number of cases, percent (in parentheses), and 95% confidence intervals (in brackets) with AST or ALT of more than 1000 IU/L.

Adapted from Smilkstein MJ, Bronstein AC, Linden C, et al: Acetaminophen overdose: A 48-hour intravenous *N*-acetylcysteine treatment protocol. Ann Emerg Med *20*:1058, 1991.

veloping hepatotoxicity have a 6.1% incidence of hepatotoxicity if treatment is begun with oral NAC within 10 hours after ingestion; this incidence increases to 26.4% if treatment is initiated between 10 and 24 hours after ingestion. For patients at high risk for developing hepatotoxity, the incidence is 8.3% if treatment with oral NAC is initiated within 10 hours after overdose, 34.4% if treatment is initiated between 10 and 24 hours after overdose, and 41% if treatment is initiated between 16 and 24 hours. The 52-hour IV protocol appears to be equivalent to the 72-hour oral protocol.

Treatment with either the oral or IV forms of NAC is associated with some adverse effects. The incidence of nausea and vomiting associated with the administration of oral NAC is high, but the incidence of anaphylactoid reactions is only 2% to 3%.[45, 46] In contrast, IV infusion of NAC has been associated with a 3% to 14% rate of adverse reactions including erythema at the injection site, diffuse urticaria, bronchospasm, fever, and, rarely, anaphylaxis and death.[45, 47, 48] Anaphylactoid reactions typically respond to administration of antihistamines.[46, 48]

TREATMENT

Acetaminophen intoxication by itself does not typically produce cardiorespiratory compromise unless the patient presents late and is in severe hepatic failure. A patient's airway, breathing, and circulation should always be evaluated first, however, and stabilized if necessary. Decontamination should then be performed. Gastric lavage for an isolated acetaminophen overdose is rarely necessary. One dose of activated charcoal should be given if a patient presents less than 4 to 6 hours after ingestion. Thereafter, the only indication for activated charcoal is coingestion of another toxin. Although activated charcoal does adsorb NAC and reduce its peak serum levels by as much as 29%,[49] the loading dose of NAC does not need to be increased because the amount adsorbed is not considered clinically important.[50, 51] Past guidelines for gastrointestinal decontamination after acetaminophen overdose recommended that activated charcoal be lavaged from the stomach before administration of NAC, that NAC be alternated with activated charcoal, or that the loading dose of NAC be increased. None of these interventions is necessary.

Laboratory evaluation on arrival at a health care facility should include an acetaminophen level obtained 4 or more hours after ingestion, baseline AST level, ALT level, bilirubin level, prothrombin time, creatinine level, pregnancy test for women of childbearing age, and toxicologic screen as appropriate. Aspirin is a frequent coingestant, and a salicylate level should therefore be determined in every patient who presents with an acetaminophen overdose. Consideration should be given to obtaining amylase and lipase determinations, particularly in patients with protracted emesis.

Perhaps the most crucial piece of information required for making appropriate management decisions about a patient who has ingested a single overdose of acetaminophen is *time elapsed since ingestion* (Fig. 49–3). For a patient who has ingested a potentially toxic amount of acetaminophen and presents later than 8 hours after the overdose or in circumstances in which an acetaminophen determination is not available within 8 hours after the overdose, a loading dose of NAC should be administered immediately. If the acetaminophen level is found to be in the nontoxic range, further doses of NAC are unnecessary. Otherwise, a complete course of NAC should be given. For nonpregnant patients who present less than 8 hours after overdose, the decision to initiate NAC therapy may be delayed until an acetaminophen level is available and it is known whether or not the patient has a toxic level. A dose of activated charcoal should be given to these patients on presentation while awaiting the acetaminophen level. A pregnant woman should be administered a loading dose of NAC as soon as possible regardless of time since overdose, for reasons discussed later.

Acetaminophen level should be plotted on the nomogram as a function of time after ingestion. Patients who present within 24 hours of an acute single overdose and have an acetaminophen level above the possible toxicity line should be treated with NAC. The lines denoting probable and high toxicity are not used to make treatment decisions but rather may be used to estimate a patient's risk for development of severe hepatotoxicity.

The oral preparation of NAC (Mucomyst) is available as a 20% solution and should be diluted to a 5% solution with either fruit juice or a carbonated beverage. A loading dose of 140 mg/kg should be administered, followed every 4 hours by 17 maintenance doses of 70 mg/kg. If a patient vomits within 1 hour of receiving NAC, that dose must be repeated. As an example, a 50-kg patient requires (50 × 140) 7000 mg, or 7 g, of NAC or 35 mL of 20% Mucomyst as a loading dose.

Aggressive antiemetic therapy is critical to successful treatment when the oral preparation of NAC is used because emesis of the antidote prevents effective therapy. Acetaminophen overdose by itself is associated with emesis, and NAC, which is foul smelling, only adds to the nausea and vomiting that may already be present. For a patient with emesis, although the usual dose is 10 mg (IV) we recommend metoclopramide (Reglan) at an initial dose up to 25 mg IV with additional doses if needed to a maximum of 1 mg/kg. Consideration should be given to coadministration of diphenhydramine (Benadryl) (25 mg IV) in order to decrease the risk of metoclopramide-induced dystonic reaction, which occurs most frequently in younger patients. If emesis persists, ondansetron (0.15 mg/kg IV) or droperidol (2 to 5 mg IV for adults; 0.15 mg/kg for children) may be useful adjuncts (Table 49–3). If emesis is still persistent, a nasogastric or duodenal tube should be inserted and the NAC dripped in over 30 minutes. If emesis continues despite aggressive antiemetic therapy, the pa-

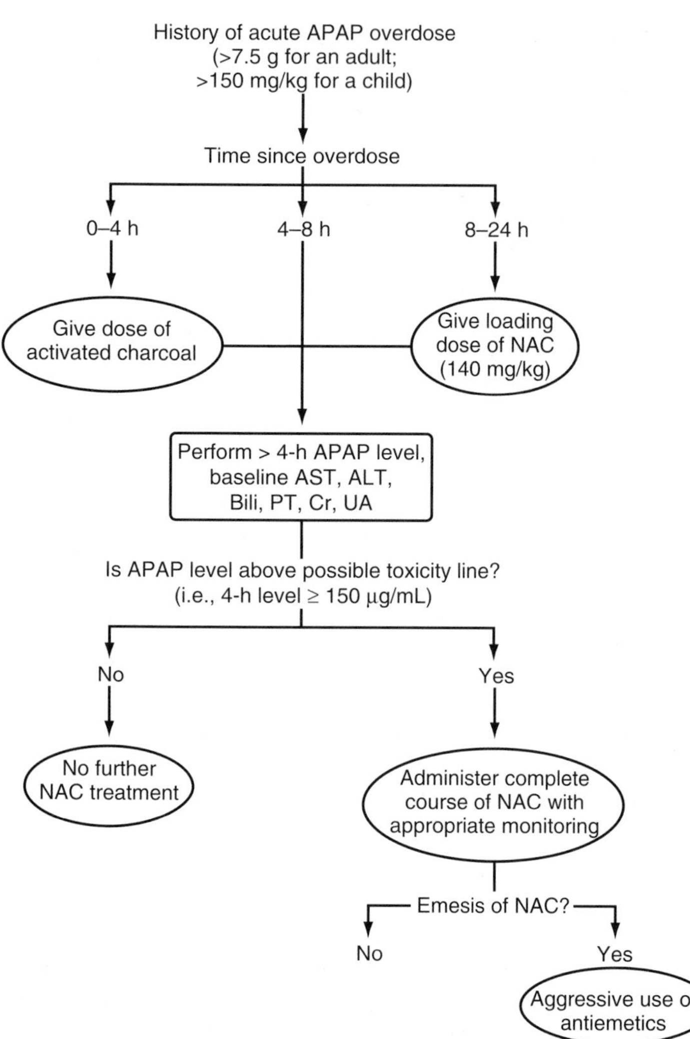

Figure 49–3. Management of acute acetaminophen overdose. NAC, *N*-acetylcysteine; AST, aspartate aminotransferase; ALT, alanine aminotransferase; Bili, bilirubin; PT, prothrombin time; Cr, creatinine; UA, urinalysis.

tient should be transferred to a center that has an IV preparation of NAC available. If this is not feasible, consideration should be given to IV administration of the oral form of NAC through a 25 μ millipore filter, which removes pyrogens and other contaminants. Although substantial experience has been gained with this, it is *not* routinely recommended and should only be done as a last resort; there is a high rate of anaphylaxis when the oral form of NAC is administered IV.

Table 49–3. Administration of Oral *N*-Acetylcysteine After Acetaminophen Overdose

How Supplied	
As 10% (10 g/100 mL) or 20% (20 g/100 mL) solution	
Dosing	
Loading	140 mg/kg
Maintenance	70 mg/kg every 4 h for 17 doses
Administration	
Dilute each dose with carbonated beverage or fruit juice to make a 5% solution.	
Repeat dose if patient vomits within 1 h of administration.	
Aggressive antiemetic therapy may be indicated.	
Antiemetics	
Metoclopramide: 0.5–1.0 mg/kg IV	
Droperidol: 2–5 mg IV (adult); 0.15 mg/kg IV (pediatric)	
Ondansetron: 0.15 mg/kg	

Monitoring in the hospital should include at least daily measurements of AST, ALT, bilirubin, blood urea nitrogen, creatinine, and prothrombin time, as well as urinalysis. Acetaminophen elimination half-life was previously thought to be the most reliable early guide to prognosis: A half-life exceeding 4 hours was almost always (16 of 17) associated with hepatotoxicity, and a half-life of less than 4 hours was practically never (12 of 13) associated with hepatotoxicity.[52] However, the correlation between acetaminophen half-life and development of hepatotoxicity has subsequently been demonstrated to have a low positive predictive value, and thus half-life determination is not helpful.[53] Furthermore, delaying treatment with NAC while awaiting determination of acetaminophen half-life is detrimental to patients who should receive NAC based on a single toxic acetaminophen level. Because acetaminophen itself is not toxic and will continue to be metabolized unless a patient has severe liver damage, no information is gained from serial acetaminophen determinations. It is important to recognize that NAC has no effect on the elimination of acetaminophen from the serum; declining acetaminophen concentrations are not evidence of the efficacy of NAC. Only patients who have ingested an extended-release acetaminophen preparation or who are being considered for an abbreviated course of NAC therapy (discussed later) should receive serial acetaminophen determinations.

SPECIAL CIRCUMSTANCES IN MANAGEMENT

Pregnancy

Acetaminophen is the preferred analgesic/antipyretic for use during pregnancy because it is safe at therapeutic doses; there is no evidence that it is teratogenic.[54] However, there is potential for fetal toxicity after maternal overdose. Animal studies have shown that both acetaminophen[55] and NAC[56] freely cross the placenta. The fetal liver is capable of elaborating NAPQI by 14 weeks' gestation.[57] Little has been published about acetaminophen overdose in pregnancy, but overdose has been reported to result in fetal morbidity[58] and mortality.[59] *Treatment delay is significantly correlated with fetal wastage.* Therefore, it is recommended that any pregnant woman who has ingested a potentially toxic amount of acetaminophen receive a loading dose of NAC on presentation, regardless of time after ingestion. If the acetaminophen level is then found to be in the nontoxic range, further doses of NAC are unnecessary.

Acute Acetaminophen Overdose in Chronic Alcoholics

Several studies have demonstrated that patients who chronically abuse alcohol are more likely to develop hepatotoxicity after an acute acetaminophen overdose[20–22] and, having developed hepatotoxicity, have a higher mortality than the general population.[23] In contrast, Rumack and co-workers found no association between alcohol use and hepatotoxicity; however, only 11 patients in this series met criteria for chronic alcohol use.[39] Most toxicologists agree that patients who chronically ingest ethanol are at higher risk for development of hepatotoxicity than the general population after acetaminophen overdose. Some toxicologists have even recommended that the treatment line on the Rumack nomogram be lowered to a 4-hour or equivalent acetaminophen concentration of 100 μg/mL in the setting of an acute acetaminophen overdose in a chronically alcoholic patient.[60] The increased susceptibility of these patients to acetaminophen overdose is perhaps due to both lower than average glutathione stores as well as increased production of NAPQI due to induction of the cyp2E1 system.

Long-Term Acetaminophen Overdose

Four grams of acetaminophen for an adult and 90 mg/kg for a child are the maximum recommended daily doses of acetaminophen. Ingestion of larger quantities constitutes chronic excess, which may result in hepatotoxicity; a few case reports describe even smaller doses resulting in hepatotoxicity in adults. Young children who have received as little as 150 mg/kg per day have developed hepatotoxicity.[61, 62] Chronic acetaminophen excess is usually a therapeutic misadventure. Common scenarios include increased daily intake because patients believe it is safe, use of combination products such as acetaminophen and codeine along with acetaminophen, or the substitution of pediatric with adult suppositories in a young child. The incidence of hepatotoxicity after chronic excess is unknown. Certain populations appear to be at risk, however, including patients who are fasting or who have ingested alcohol in the preceding 5 days.[63] Additionally, numerous cases of hepatotoxicity have occurred in alcoholic patients after long-term acetaminophen excess, although the apparent frequency may in part be due to ascertainment bias.[64] Indeed, Benson and co-workers showed that alcoholic patients who were given 4 g/day of acetaminophen for 14 days did not develop hepatotoxicity.[65]

The basis of certain patients' sensitivity to long-term acetaminophen excess is not well understood. Fasting is known to decrease the amount of acetaminophen that undergoes glucuronidation; this may increase metabolism by the cyp2E1 system, which would result in elaboration of more NAPQI. Similarly, because ethanol use induces cyp2E1, NAPQI production may be increased in patients who ingest alcohol. Continual alcohol use may also result in glutathione depletion. Finally, patients who chronically abuse alcohol may be at a higher risk because abnormal transaminase values may be wrongly attributed to alcoholic hepatitis instead of acetaminophen toxicity. Chronically alcoholic patients frequently have abnormal transaminase levels; knowledge of the pattern of enzyme abnormalities is important to make an accurate diagnosis of the etiology of hepatitis in patients who continually abuse alcohol. In alcoholic hepatitis, AST level is less than 300 IU/L, ALT level is normal or marginally increased, and AST value is usually greater than twice the ALT. In contrast, chronic excess of acetaminophen in a chronically alcoholic patient leads to an elevation of AST greater than 300 IU/L, although the proportion between AST and ALT remains the same.[63, 66]

For patients who present with a history of chronic acetaminophen excess, with or without a history of long-term ethanol use, a modified treatment approach is necessary. On presentation to the health care facility, baseline values of acetaminophen, AST, ALT, bilirubin, and prothrombin time should be obtained and a loading dose of NAC given pending the results. The nomogram cannot be used to determine which patients may benefit from treatment. In fact, no studies have been performed to prove that NAC provides benefit in the setting of long-term excess. However, it seems prudent to continue NAC if a plasma acetaminophen concentration is detectable or if either the AST or ALT value is abnormal.

Late Treatment of Acute Overdose

NAC, when given early (i.e., < 24 hours after ingestion when the oral protocol is used < 15 hours when the 20-hour IV protocol is used), is beneficial in all patients with a potentially toxic plasma acetaminophen level. Additionally, late administration of NAC is beneficial to patients with fulminant hepatic failure. Although late NAC use does not change the biochemical markers of liver function such as prothrombin time, it has been shown to improve survival and decrease the incidence of cerebral edema as well as the incidence of hypotension requiring inotropic support.[67, 68] In a prospective randomized study,[68] survival was improved from 20% for patients who received intensive liver care only as compared with 48% for patients who received late NAC treatment. Groups were well matched for age, sex, and time to presentation to a health care facility. Administration of NAC was continued until recovery from encephalopathy occurred or death ensued. Unlike methionine, NAC use is safe in patients with encephalopathy. The mechanism for the salutary effect of NAC is not completely understood but may in part be due to improvement of tissue oxygenation.[69]

Extended-Release Tylenol

Tylenol-ER is a new, unique formulation of acetaminophen released in 1995. It is a caplet consisting of 325 mg of immediate-release acetaminophen on one side and 325 mg in a matrix formulation designed for slow release on the other. At therapeutic doses, the manufacturer's *in vitro* studies have shown that 88% of the product is released within 3 hours and 95% within 5 hours. The figures are similar when 10-fold the therapeutic dose is ingested.[70] However, other investigators have shown a decreased rate of dissolution with increasing number of tablets.[71, 72] Therefore, because this formulation potentially changes the absorption kinetics *in vivo* and because experience to date is limited, plasma acetaminophen levels must be interpreted cautiously using the Rumack nomogram. One approach is to measure at least three serial plasma acetaminophen levels, with the first at least 4 hours after overdose and the following measurements at 2-hour intervals. Unequivocally, the full course of NAC should be given if any level is above the treatment nomogram line. NAC therapy should be considered if the second level is greater than the first level or if any level is more than half of the potentially toxic level on the nomogram. The factor of one half is conservative. It is derived from a prospective, randomized, double-blind crossover comparison study of volunteers ingesting 75 mg/kg of acetaminophen. This study showed that peak acetaminophen levels after a dose of Tylenol-ER were 57% of that after an immediate-release Tylenol preparation.[73] Management of any overdose involving Tylenol-ER should be discussed with a consulting toxicologist or poison control center.

NEW DIRECTIONS

Abbreviated Therapy

An increasingly popular view is that 72 hours of oral NAC is longer treatment than many patients require. Therefore, clinicians have begun to administer NAC for only 24 hours (a loading dose of 140 mg/kg and six maintenance doses of 70 mg/kg; total, 560 mg/kg) for selected patients. Two groups of patients appear to be ideal candidates for abbreviated therapy. The first group of patients who should be considered for abbreviated therapy are those with a history of long-term acetaminophen overdose who have transaminases less than 1000 IU/L and a nondetectable acetaminophen level. In the setting of acute overdose, the ideal patient to be considered for abbreviated therapy is otherwise healthy, has no history of chronic alcohol use, and is treated successfully with NAC within 8 hours of overdose. The patient should be re-evaluated after 24 hours of treatment; if the acetaminophen concentration is nondetectable and the transaminase levels are normal, NAC may be discontinued. The major concern with abbreviated therapy is that a minority of patients may not have abnormal transaminase values within 28 hours of ingestion and NAC would be prematurely terminated in these patients, before evidence of liver injury is manifested. Published clinical experience with abbreviated NAC therapy is sparse,[74] and a prospective trial with clinical follow-up is necessary before this approach can be endorsed. Therefore, unless a specific recommendation is made by a consulting toxicologist, the full course of NAC should be considered the standard of care.

Intravenous Therapy

The protocol of 52 hours of IV NAC appears to be as effective as the 72-hour course of oral NAC in reducing hepatotoxicity. Additionally, it has the advantage of assured delivery of treatment to patients who are vomiting. The IV form of NAC is safe, although it has a higher incidence of anaphylactoid reactions than does the oral form. Only a limited number of centers in the United States currently have access to the IV form of NAC on the basis of investigational drug status. It is hoped that the IV form will gain Food and Drug Administration approval in the near future.

SUMMARY

Acetaminophen, although safe when taken at therapeutic doses, is hepatotoxic when taken as an acute single overdose or in continual excess. It is an important cause of morbidity and mortality worldwide.

Toxicity of acetaminophen is a result of its metabolism. Neither the parent compound nor the major metabolites are toxic. However, NAPQI, which is a minor metabolite elaborated by the mixed-function oxidase, is toxic when hepatic glutathione stores have been depleted.

Patients who have ingested overdose quantities of acetaminophen can be effectively treated with NAC. Treatment with NAC is beneficial for all patients with a massive single overdose when begun less than 24 hours after overdose but is most effective if started within 8 hours, and effectiveness declines incrementally for each hour after 8 hours. The Rumack nomogram is a reliable guide for determining which patients require antidote therapy after an acute overdose. The nomogram is not useful for patients who have continually ingested excessive amounts, and its usefulness after an overdose of the extended-release preparation of acetaminophen is untested.

References

1. Davidson DGD, Eastham WN: Acute liver necrosis following overdose of paracetamol. BMJ *2*:497, 1966.
2. Thomson JS, Prescott LF: Liver damage and impaired glucose tolerance after paracetamol overdosage. BMJ *2*:506, 1966.
3. Litovitz TL, Felberg L, Soloway RA, et al: 1994 Annual report of the American Association of Poison Control Centers Toxic Exposure Surveillance System. Am J Emerg Med *13*:551, 1995.
4. Lee WM: Acute liver failure. Am J Med *96*(Suppl 1A):1A, 1994.
5. Forrest JAH, Clements JA, Prescott LF: Clinical pharmacokinetics of paracetamol. Clin Pharmacokinet *7*:93, 1982.
6. Augenstein WL, Kulig KW, Rumack BH: Delayed rise in serum drug levels in overdose patients despite multiple dose charcoal and after charcoal stools. Vet Hum Toxicol *29*:491, 1987.
7. Bartle WR, Paradiso FL, Derry JE, et al: Delayed acetaminophen toxicity despite *N*-acetylcysteine use. Drug Intell Clin Pharmacol *23*:509, 1989.
8. Tighe TV, Walter FG: Delayed toxic acetaminophen level after initial four hour non-toxic level. Clin Toxicol *32*:431, 1994.
9. Bizovi K, Keys N, Rivas J, et al: Tylenol ER, late rise in APAP level after overdose. Abstract. J Toxicol Clin Toxicol *33*:510, 1995.
10. Mitchel JR, Thorgiersson SS, Potter WZ, et al: Acetaminophen-induced hepatic injury: Protective role of glutathione in man and rationale for therapy. Clin Pharmacol Ther *16*:676, 1974.
11. Miller RP, Roberts RJ, Fischer LJ: Acetaminophen kinetics in neonates, children, and adults. Clin Pharmacol Ther *19*:284, 1976.
12. Mitchell JR, Jollow DJ, Gillette JR, et al: Drug metabolism as a cause of drug toxicity. Drug Metab Dispos *1*:418, 1973.
13. Potter WZ, Davis DC, Mitchell, et al: Acetaminophen-induced hepatic necrosis. III. Cytochrome P-450-mediated covalent binding *in vitro*. J Pharmacol Exp Ther *187*:203, 1973.
14. Corcoran GB, Mitchell JR, Vaishnav YN, et al: Evidence that acetaminophen and *N*-hydroxyacetaminophen form a common arylating intermediate, *N*-acetyl-*p*-benzoquinoneimine. Mol Pharmacol *18*:536, 1980.
15. Miners JO, Drew R, Birkett DJ: Mechanism of action of paracetomol protective agents in mice *in vivo*. Biochem Pharmacol *33*:2995, 1984.
16. Corcoran GB, Todd EL, Racz WJ, et al: Effects of *N*-acetylcysteine on the disposition and metabolism of acetaminophen in mice. J Pharmacol Exp Ther *232*:857, 1985.
17. Buckpitt AR, Rollins DE, Mitchell JR: Varying effects of sulfhydryl nucleophiles on acetaminophen oxidation and sulfhydryl adduct formation. Biochem Pharmacol *28*:2941, 1979.
18. Watkins PB: Drug metabolism by cytochromes P450 in the liver and small bowel. Gastroenterol Clin North Am *21*:511, 1992.
19. Bray GP, Harrison PM, O'Grady JG, et al: Long-term anticonvulsant therapy worsens outcome in paracetamol-induced fulminant hepatic failure. Hum Exp Toxicol *11*:26, 1992.
20. Brotodihardjo AE, Batey RG, Farrell GC, et al: Hepatotoxicity from paracetamol self-poisoning in western Sydney: A continuing challenge. Med J Aust *157*:382, 1992.
21. Wright N, Prescott LF: Potentiation by previous drug therapy of hepatotoxicity following paracetamol overdosage. Scot Med J *18*:56, 1973.
22. Scott CR, Stewart MF: Cysteamine treatment in paracetamol overdose. Lancet *1*:452, 1975.
23. Bray GP, Mowat CM, Muir DF, et al: The effect of chronic alcohol intake on prognosis and outcome in paracetamol overdose. Hum Exp Toxicol *10*:435, 1991.
24. Nolan CM, Sandblom RE, Thummel KE, et al: Hepatotoxicity associated with acetaminophen usage in patients receiving multiple drug therapy for tuberculosis. Chest *105*:408, 1994.
25. Crippen JS: Acetaminophen hepatotoxicity: Potentiation by isoniazid. Am J Gastroenterol *88*:590, 1993.
26. Rumack BH: Acetaminophen overdose in young children. Treatment and effects of alcohol and other additional ingestants in 417 cases. Am J Dis Child *138*:428, 1984.
27. Peterson RG, Rumack BH: Age as a variable in acetaminophen overdose. Arch Intern Med *141*:390, 1981.
28. Singer AJ, Carracio TR, Mofenson HC: The temporal profile of increased transaminase levels in patients with acetaminophen-induced liver dysfunction. Ann Emerg Med *26*:49, 1995.
29. Curry RW, Robinson D, Sughrue MJ: Acute renal failure after acetaminophen ingestion. JAMA *247*:1012, 1982.
30. Kher K, Makker S: Acute renal failure due to acetaminophen ingestion without concurrent hepatotoxicty. Letter. Am J Med *82*:1280, 1987.
31. Campbell NR, Bayliss B: Renal impairment associated with an acute paracetamol overdose in the absence of hepatotoxicity. Postgrad Med J *68*:116, 1992.
32. Flanagan RJ, Mant TGK: Coma and metabolic acidosis early in severe acute paracetamol poisoning. Hum Toxicol *5*:179, 1986.
33. Hamlyn AN, James O, Douglas AP: The spectrum of paracetamol (acetaminophen) overdose: Clinical and epidemiological studies. Postgrad Med J *54*:400, 1978.
34. Mofenson HC, Caraccio TR, Nawaz H, et al: Acetaminophen induced pancreatitis. Clin Toxicol *29*:223, 1991.
35. O'Grady JG, Alexander GJM, Hayllar KM, et al: Early indicators of prognosis in fulminant hepatic failure. Gastroenterology *97*:439, 1989.
36. Harrison PM, O'Grady JG, Keays RT, et al: Serial prothrombin time as a prognostic indicator in paracetamol induced fulminant hepatic failure. BMJ *301*:964, 1990.
37. Hamlyn AN, Douglas AP, James OFW, et al: Liver structure and function in survivors of acetaminophen poisoning. Am J Dig Dis *22*:605, 1977.
38. Prescott LF, Illingworth RN, Critchley JA, et al: Intravenous *N*-acetylcysteine: The treatment of choice for paracetamol poisoning. BMJ *2*:1097, 1979.
39. Rumack BH, Peterson RC, Koch GG, et al: Acetaminophen overdose: 662 cases with evaluation of oral acetylcysteine treatment. Arch Intern Med *141*:380, 1981.

40. Prescott LF: Paracetamol overdose: Pharmacological considerations and clinical management. Drugs *25*:290, 1983.
41. Rolband GC, Marcaurd SP: Cimetidine in the treatment of acetaminophen overdose. Clin Gastroenterol *13*:79, 1991.
42. Burkhart KK, Janco N, Kulig K, et al: Cimetidine as adjunctive treatment for acetaminophen overdose. Hum Exp Toxicol *14*:299, 1995.
43. Brennan RJ, Mankes RF, Lefevre R, et al: 4-Methylpyrazole blocks acetaminophen hepatotoxicity in the rat. Ann Emerg Med *23*:487, 1994.
44. Smilkstein MJ, Knapp GL, Kulig KW, et al: Efficacy of oral *N*-acetylcysteine in the treatment of acetaminophen overdose: Analysis of the National Multicenter Study (1976 to 1985). N Engl J Med *319*:1557, 1988.
45. Smilkstein MJ, Bronstein AC, Linden C, et al: Acetaminophen overdose: A 48-hour intravenous *N*-acetylcysteine treatment protocol. Ann Emerg Med *20*:1058, 1991.
46. Tenenbein M: Hypersensitivity-like reactions to *N*-acetylcysteine. Vet Hum Toxicol *26*(Suppl 2):3, 1984.
47. Miller LF, Rumack BH: Clinical safety of high oral doses of acetylcysteine. Semin Oncol *10*(Suppl 1):76, 1983.
48. Chan TYK, Critchley JAJH: Adverse reactions to intravenous *N*-acetylcysteine in Chinese patients with paracetamol (acetaminophen) poisoning. Hum Exp Toxicol *13*:542, 1994.
49. Ekins BR, Ford DC, Thompson MIB, et al: The effect of activated charcoal on *N*-acetylcysteine absorption in normal subjects. Am J Emerg Med *5*:483, 1987.
50. Smilkstein MJ: A new loading dose for *N*-acetylcysteine? The answer is NO. Ann Emerg Med *24*:538, 1994.
51. Spiller HA, Krenzelok EP, Grande GA, et al: A prospective evaluation of the effect of activated charcoal before oral *N*-acetylcysteine in acetaminophen overdose. Ann Emerg Med *23*:519, 1994.
52. Prescott LF, Roscoe P, Wright N, et al: Plasma-paracetamol half-life and hepatic necrosis in patients with paracetamol overdosage. Lancet *1*:519, 1971.
53. Smilkstein MJ, Rumack BH: Elimination half-life ($T_{1/2}$) as a predictor of acetaminophen-induced hepatotoxicity. Abstract. Vet Hum Toxicol *36*:337, 1994.
54. McElhatton PR, Sullivan FM, Volans GN, et al: Paracetamol poisoning in pregnancy: An analysis of the outcomes of cases referred to the teratology information service of the national poisons information service. Hum Exp Toxicol *9*:147, 1990.
55. Wang LH, Rudolph AM, Benet LZ: Pharmacokinetic studies of the disposition of acetaminophen in the sheep maternal-placental-fetal unit. J Pharmacol Exp Ther *238*:198, 1986.
56. Ansai N, Kimura T, Chida S, et al: Studies on the metabolic fate of *N*-acetyl-L-cysteine in rats and dogs. Pharmacometrics *26*:249, 1983.
57. Yaffe SJ, Rane A, Sjoqvist F, et al: The presence of a monooxygenase system in human fetal liver microsomes. Life Sci *9*:1189, 1970.
58. Kurzel RB: Can acetaminophen excess result in maternal and fetal toxicity? South Med J *83*:953, 1990.
59. Riggs BS, Bronstein AC, Kulig K, et al: Acute acetaminophen overdose during pregnancy. Obstet Gynecol *74*:247, 1989.
60. Vale JA, Proudfoot AT: Paracetamol (acetaminophen) poisoning. Lancet *346*:547, 1995.
61. Henretig FM, Selbst SM, Forrest C, et al: Repeated acetaminophen overdosing causing hepatotoxicity in children. Clin Pediatr *28*:525, 1989.
62. Florén C, Thesleff P, Nilsson Å: Severe liver damage caused by therapeutic doses of acetaminophen. Acta Med Scand *222*:285, 1987.
63. Whitcomb DC, Block GD: Association of acetaminophen hepatotoxicity with fasting and ethanol use. JAMA *272*:1845, 1994.
64. Seeff LB, Cuccherini BA, Zimmerman HJ, et al: Acetaminophen hepatotoxicity in alcoholics: A therapeutic misadventure. Ann Intern Med *104*:399, 1986.
65. Benson GD: Acetaminophen in chronic liver disease. Clin Pharmacol Ther *33*:95, 1983.
66. Kumar S, Rex DK: Failure of physicians to recognize acetaminophen hepatotoxicity in chronic alcoholics. Arch Intern Med *151*:1189, 1991.
67. Harrison PM, Keays R, Bray GP, et al: Improved outcome of paracetamol-induced hepatic failure by late administration of acetylcysteine. Lancet *335*:1572, 1990.
68. Keays R, Harrison PM, Wendon JA, et al: Intravenous acetylcysteine in paracetamol induced fulminant hepatic failure: A prospective controlled trial. BMJ *303*:1026, 1991.
69. Harrison PM, Wendon JA, Gimson AES, et al: Improvement by acetylcysteine of hemodynamics and oxygen transport in fulminant hepatic failure. N Engl J Med *324*:1852, 1991.
70. Temple AR, Mrazik TJ: More on extended-release acetaminophen. N Engl J Med *333*:1508, 1995.
71. Vraa EP, Watson WA, Neau SH: Dissolution of Tylenol dosage formulations under overdose conditions. Abstract. J Toxicol Clin Toxicol *33*:510, 1995.
72. Stork CM, Rees S, Howland MA, et al: Pharmacokinetics of extended relief (ER) vs regular release (RR) Tylenol (APAP) in a simulated human overdose model. Abstract. J Toxicol Clin Toxicol *33*:511, 1995.
73. Douglas DR, Smilkstein MJ, Sholar JB: Overdose with "extended-relief" acetaminophen: Is a new approach necessary? Abstract. Acad Emerg Med *2*:397, 1995.
74. Woo OF, Anderson IB, Kim SY, et al: Shorter duration of *N*-acetylcysteine (NAC) for acute acetaminophen poisoning. Abstract. J Toxicol Clin Toxicol *33*:508, 1995.

50

Salicylate Toxicity

EDWARD P. KRENZELOK, PharmD
FERGUS KERR, MB, BS, MPH
A.T. PROUDFOOT, BSc

Salicylates have a long history of use. Hippocrates, Galen, and medieval herbalists relied on salicylate-containing botanicals for their palliative properties. The medicinal properties of willow bark (*Salix alba vulgaris*) have been appreciated by native peoples for centuries. In the mid-19th century, the active ingredient of willow bark, salicylic acid, was isolated and shortly thereafter was synthesized from phenol. It gained widespread use in extemporaneously compounded pharmaceuticals as a pain reliever, anti-inflammatory, and antipyretic. In the latter portion of the 19th century, the Bayer company in Germany developed a salicylic acid derivative, aspirin (or acetylsalicylic acid), for commercial use. Aspirin and its chemically related analogues, all known as salicylates, have since been prescribed widely by the medical profession and have become a staple pharmaceutical for nonprescription use by the public. Few if any pharmaceuticals in the history of therapeutics can rival the scale on which they were consumed until recent years. Since the 1960s, the development of alternatives to salicylates, such as acetaminophen and ibuprofen, has resulted in diminished use of salicylates. However, the ubiquitous nature of salicylates has resulted in the problem of both acute and chronic poisoning.

SALICYLATES AND SALICYLATE ANALOGUES

Aspirin is the most common salicylate, but there are dozens of different salicylate analogues in pharmaceutical preparations, including sodium salicylate, methyl salicylate, bismuth subsalicylate, and salicylic acid. As systemic pharmaceuticals, the salicylates are available in all of the common dosage formulations—tablets, enteric-coated tablets, capsules, suppositories, powder papers, liquids, and effervescent tablets. Methyl salicylate is commonly found in liniments, lotions, creams, and ointments for the treatment of minor musculoskeletal complaints. Methyl salicylate is also known as oil of wintergreen and is used to flavor confectioneries. Bismuth subsalicylate is used in a popular antidiarrheal agent, and most do not recognize it as a possible source of salicylate poisoning (especially when other salicylates are ingested concomitantly). Salicylic acid is present in corn and wart removers. However, the most common use of salicylates is as an oral analgesic, antipyretic, and anti-inflammatory. For this application, salicylates are ingested as the sole pharmaceutical or in combination with synergistic pain relievers, such as opioids.

Although salicylates have enjoyed a prosperous history and have benefited countless individuals, they are now secondary products for the treatment of pain, fever, and inflammation. The development of acetaminophen in the 1960s and of ibuprofen in the 1970s as well as the association of salicylates with the development of Reye's syndrome in the 1980s has greatly changed the pattern of salicylate usage. Salicylate-related poisonings and fatalities still occur, but not as frequently.

EPIDEMIOLOGY OF SALICYLATE POISONING

To paraphrase Paracelsus: *"The only thing which differentiates a poison from a remedy is the dose."* Salicylates exemplify this dictum, and a variant of the epidemiologic model best portrays how salicylate poisoning occurs:

Poison + potential victim
+ conducive environment = poisoning

Exposure to excessive amounts of salicylate results in salicylate poisoning, commonly referred to as *salicylism*. According to the epidemiologic model, salicylate poisoning can be accidental or intentional. For example, a curious 2-year-old child (victim) may ingest aspirin tablets (poison) that were inadvertently left within the child's reach (conducive environment), the result of which is a poisoning incident. Or an elderly individual may self-medicate with excessive doses or have a physical ailment that predisposes him or her to greater sensitivity to salicylate accumulation. Conversely, intentional poisonings occur when an individual chooses salicylate overdose as a means of self-harm due to external stresses or endogenous psychological imbalance. Both acute and chronic toxicity can occur as consequences of accidental and intentional overdose.

A review of salicylate exposures reported to the American Association of Poison Control Centers Toxic Exposure Surveillance System (AAPCC TESS) for the 10-year period of 1985 through 1994 reveals that 30.5% of all salicylate exposures occurred in children younger than 6 years (Fig. 50–1). Although a significant number of exposures occurred in this pediatric age group, only four fatalities related to accidental overdose were reported—only 0.006% of the cases! However, 392 fatalities occurred among the remainder of those with salicylate exposures, and both the mean and median age of those with fatal outcomes was 47 years. It is apparent from these data that salicylate exposures are rarely fatal in those most vulnerable to poisoning—children younger than 6 years. Furthermore, intentional overdose or therapeutic misadventure account for the high morbidity and mortality in adolescents and adults.

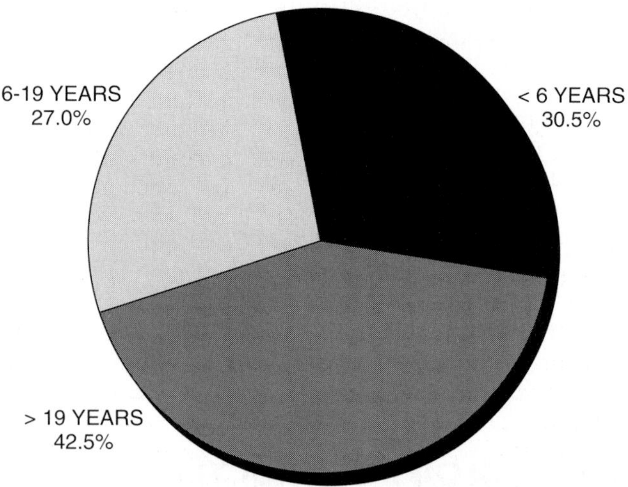

Figure 50–1. Age distribution: accidental and intentional salicylate exposures, 1985 through 1994. Mean age, 47.6 years; median age, 47.7 years. (From the yearly publication of the Toxic Exposure Surveillance System [TESS] of the American Association of Poison Control Centers [AAPCC] as published in the September issues of the Am J Emerg Med, vol 3, 1985, to vol 13, 1994.)

Based on poison center data (AAPCC TESS, 1985 through 1994), the number of salicylate-related poisonings in children younger than 6 years has been declining steadily over the 10-year period. This is especially noteworthy since the number of pediatric salicylate exposures decreased by 30% (8,183 in 1985 versus 5,799 in 1994) while the number of exposures reported to poison centers more than doubled (900,513 in 1985 versus 1,926,438 in 1994). Therefore, relative to all poisoning exposures, the incidence of reported exposures has dropped dramatically. A number of factors may account for this trend. Most important, the enactment of the 1970 Poison Prevention Packaging Act mandated the use of child-resistant closures on aspirin-containing products. Additionally, the enticingly flavored children's aspirin tablets were restricted to 81 mg/tablet and 36 tablets per bottle, thereby limiting the amount taken by children in accidental ingestions. In conjunction with the possible association between Reye's syndrome and the use of aspirin to treat viral diseases in children, the number of annual fatalities due to aspirin in children younger than 5 years dropped from 46 in 1972 to 0 in 1992 (Fig. 50–2). The introduction of alternatives to aspirin-containing products such as acetaminophen and ibuprofen, which have a considerably higher therapeutic index, have contributed to the decreased number of fatalities by decreasing the availability of salicylates.

SALICYLATE TOXICOKINETICS

It took approximately 100 years to elucidate the pharmacokinetics of salicylates. However, this chapter addresses salicylate toxicity and not the therapeutic aspects of salicylate use; therefore, it is more appropriate to refer to the disposition of salicylates as toxicokinetics. Although the toxicokinetics of salicylates are a reflection of research conducted in volunteers who ingested only modest amounts of salicylates, they are representative of the overdose situation. Characterization of the toxicokinetics of salicylate overdose is essential to understanding the genesis of salicylism and its management.

Absorption

Most cases of salicylate poisoning involve the ingestion of a product that contains aspirin. Ingested salicylates are absorbed passively in the non-ionized form from the stomach.[1] Major absorption occurs in the jejunum and elsewhere throughout the small intestine.[2] Absorption is a first-order process that is fairly rapid but dependent on a number of influential variables.[1] For example, the presence of food may impair absorption by retarding gastric emptying. Enteric-coated products are resistant to the acid envi-

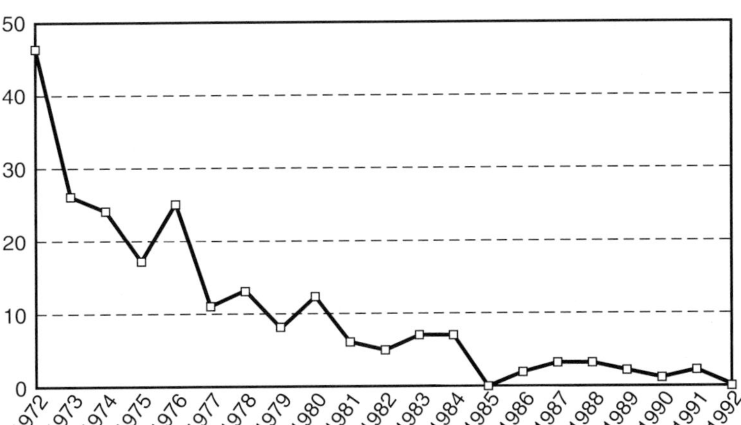

Figure 50–2. Aspirin-related fatalities in children younger than 5 years, 1972 through 1992. (From National Center for Health Statistics: Unpublished data.)

ronment of the stomach, which delays tablet dissolution until it resides in the more alkaline environment of the distal intestines. Alkaline-buffered aspirin tablets have more rapid dissolution, resulting in greater bioavailability. Purportedly, overdosage of salicylates produces pylorospasm, delaying gastric emptying and subsequent absorption. Although it is not a common phenomenon, salicylates have the potential to form gastric concretions or bezoars, which retard the otherwise rapid absorption and result in slow, continuous absorption that simulates the action of a sustained-release pharmaceutical. Overdoses involving multiple poisons that retard gastric emptying and intestinal motility, such as poisons with anticholinergic or opioid properties, have the capacity to slow salicylate absorption. Coexistent pathophysiology such as hypotension or decreased splanchnic circulation may also impede the absorption of salicylates. Liquid forms of salicylate, such as methyl salicylate, are more bioavailable and are not subject to the rate-limiting process of dissolution; therefore, the absorption of liquid products may be more rapid and not retarded by physical or pathophysiologic factors.

Biliary secretion of salicylate is minimal.[3] Therefore, increased reabsorption secondary to enterohepatic circulation is not an important consideration.

Dermal absorption of salicylates is a reported but rarely encountered source of salicylism.[4, 5] Salicylate-containing liniments and topical rubefacients are unlikely to represent a notable risk because their use is usually limited to the nonprescription treatment of minor musculoskeletal discomfort. However, chronic use of highly concentrated products applied to large surface areas of compromised skin may create a condition that allows sufficient salicylate absorption with resultant toxicity.

Chronic excessive use of salicylate suppositories has the potential to produce toxicity. However, it is rarely a cause of acute salicylism. The intentional use of a salicylate enema that contained 700 aspirin tablets produced profound salicylism.[6]

The natural source of salicylates (e.g., willow bark, herbal products) or its pharmaceutical formulation, in conjunction with other variables, affects salicylate absorption. Once absorption and metabolic conversion to salicylic acid occur, the other disposition toxicokinetics are unaffected.

Distribution

Salicylates are distributed throughout body fluids and tissues. The low apparent volume of distribution (V_d) (V_d = 0.16 – 0.35 L/kg) in salicylate overdose victims suggests that salicylate remains largely in the central compartment.[7] This and the low molecular weight and water solubility of salicylates are important factors that favor the effectiveness of hemodialysis in the treatment of severely poisoned patients.

In therapeutic doses salicylates are significantly bound to proteins—possibly as high as 80% to 90%. Albumin is the major protein that is responsible for the extensive protein binding.[2, 8] The degree of protein binding is a function of both the concentration of salicylic acid and the amount of albumin. As protein binding sites become saturated in overdose patients, the amount of free non–protein-bound salicylic acid increases and creates a climate for more significant toxicity. Furthermore, any condition that depletes albumin and other proteins (e.g., liver disease), predisposes the patient to a disproportionate risk of severe salicylism at a given plasma concentration. Larger amounts of salicylate are bioavailable to tissues, the result of which may be greater poisoning of cellular metabolism. As a consequence of reduced protein binding and greater tissue concentrations, the apparent V_d increases in the overdose patient.

Under conditions that favor normal acid-base status, salicylates are highly ionized, which reduces their diffusion across the blood-brain barrier and into the central nervous system (CNS). Patients with salicylate toxic effects may develop metabolic acidosis, which increases the fraction of non-ionized salicylate and results in greater CNS penetration and elevated cerebrospinal fluid (CSF) concentrations. High CSF concentrations are associated with CNS toxicity and greater morbidity.

Salicylates cross the placenta, and sufficient overdosage poses a significant risk to the fetus. In consistent fashion, salicylates are also found in breast milk, but this presents a threat to the infant only when the mother is taking large doses on a daily basis. Infants, whose ability to metabolize and eliminate salicylates and their metabolites is immature, are especially prone to toxic effects under these conditions.

Metabolism and Excretion

The initial metabolic step involves the hydrolysis of the salicylate salt or aspirin to the pharmacologically and toxicologically active chemical, salicylic acid. This is a first-order process with a half-life of 15 to 20 minutes.[9] Salicylic acid undergoes further biotransformation and elimination via first-order processes[10, 11] involving the following:

1. Glucuronide formation → salicyl acyl glucuronide
2. Oxidation → gentisic acid
3. Microsomal oxidation or glycine conjugation → gentisuric acid
4. Salicylic acid → elimination via the urine

Normally, these are minor metabolic pathways. In overdosage they assume more significance, but not enough to compensate for the severely compromised major metabolic pathways.

The major metabolic pathways become saturated rapidly when more than a single therapeutic dose is ingested. Biotransformation converts from a dose-dependent first-order process (rate proportional to the dose) to a zero-order process, which means that a fixed amount of salicylic acid is metabolized per unit of time—regardless of the dose. This is referred to as Michaelis-Menten kinetics. The metabolism results in the slow formation of two major metabolites:

1. Oxidation → salicyluric acid
2. Glucuronide formation → salicyl phenolic glucuronide

Because salicyluric acid and salicyl phenolic glucuronide formation is a saturable process, the biotransformation of salicylic acid proceeds more slowly and creates more opportunity for toxicity to occur.[10, 11] Awareness of the accumulation kinetics of salicylic acid is essential to understanding the long half-life of salicylates in the overdose situation and the subsequent long duration of toxic manifestations. For the same reasons, the well-intentioned Done nomogram is not applicable in the determination of patient prognosis and the management of either acute or chronic salicylism,[12] because Done considered that salicylates followed a first-order elimination process and developed the nomogram accordingly.[13]

The toxicokinetics of salicylic acid account for the prolonged elimination half-life, which approximates 20 to 30 hours. This results in a very slow decline in the plasma salicylate concentration. In contrast to the slow reduction in salicylic acid concentrations, acetylsalicylic acid concentrations decline very rapidly, with a half-life of 15 to 20 minutes, as acetylsalicylic acid is hydrolyzed to salicylic acid.

Kinetics in Children

Neonates absorb salicylate as rapidly as any other age group, but they metabolize it more slowly than those with mature hepatic function. Renal elimination is slower in children, and they have reduced albumin concentrations, which increase plasma salicylate concentrations. The V_d increases in proportion to the dose, suggesting that children may have higher tissue concentrations than is inferred by the plasma concentration.

Kinetics in the Elderly

Salicylate toxicokinetics in the elderly have not been well defined. However, the same accumulation kinetics apparent in younger adults applies to the elderly. Furthermore, the elderly may be at a greater risk in the overdose situation due to underlying pathophysiology that would impair the metabolism or excretion of the salicylates.

CLINICAL FEATURES AND PATHOPHYSIOLOGY

Salicylate poisoning results mostly from either unintentional overdose in the pediatric age group or intentional, suicidal overdose in the adult and adolescent population. Further, therapeutically induced poisoning can occur at any age. Intoxication is typically acute; however chronic salicylism is well recognized.

Acute poisoning with salicylates results in a diverse array of features. Almost invariably these include hyperventilation, hyperpyrexia, tinnitus, nausea and vomiting, dehydration, and central nervous system involvement, which ranges from confusion to coma and seizures. More uncommon clinical features may include bleeding, pulmonary edema, acute renal failure, and anaphylaxis (Table 50–1).

Chronic salicylate poisoning can present as a diagnostic dilemma, with an insidious course and nonspecific clinical findings. (This category of poisoning is discussed in more detail at the end of the chapter.)

The mechanisms by which salicylates exert their toxic effects are complex and not fully understood. However, they include direct respiratory center stim-

Table 50–1. Clinical Findings in Salicylism

Nausea and vomiting	Coma
Dehydration	Tinnitus
Tachypnea	Pulmonary edema
Hyperthermia	Acute renal failure
Confusion	

ulation, uncoupling of oxidative phosphorylation, inhibition of the tricarboxylic acid (TCA) cycle, inhibition of amino acid metabolism, stimulation of glyconeogenesis and lipid metabolism, and increased tissue glycolysis. In addition, interference with hemostatic mechanisms occurs. Together these features contribute to the total picture of salicylate poisoning (Table 50–2).

Acid-Base Disturbance

Acid-base disturbance is one of the most common manifestations of salicylate toxicity. Respiratory alkalosis and a high anion gap metabolic acidosis may occur singly or together. Generally, an initial respiratory alkalosis will be present. However, metabolic acidosis may supervene in sensitive or severely poisoned patients. The co-ingestion of other drugs may influence acid-base balance. For example, Gabow and colleagues found that 40% of the patients in their series who ingested other drugs had a normal anion gap metabolic acidosis.[14] The severity of acidosis increases with decreasing age, with increasing severity of intoxication, and in chronic poisonings as compared with acute single ingestions.[15] In children younger than 4 years, the metabolic component is usually more prominent, and these patients invariably demonstrate metabolic acidosis.[16] In contrast, older children and adults tend to have a predominating respiratory component.[17] In a review of 97 adult patients with high salicylate levels, Chapman and Proudfoot[18] recorded four categories of acid-base disturbance in patients, with mixed respiratory alkalosis and metabolic acidosis or respiratory alkalosis alone predominating in 61% and 19% of patients, respectively. The arterial hydrogen ion concentration (H+), rather than the class of acid-base disturbance, was of greater value in determining clinical severity and mortality.[15] The concomitant ingestion of respiratory depressant drugs may manifest as a mixed or isolated respiratory acidosis.[14]

Table 50–2. Mechanisms and Manifestations in Salicylate Poisoning

Mechanism	Manifestation
Respiratory center stimulation	Respiratory alkalosis Renal HCO_3 elimination increased Increased insensible fluid loss
Oxidative-phosphorylation uncoupling	Metabolic acidosis Increased heat production and fluid loss Hypoglycemia
Inhibition of tricarboxylic acid cycle	Metabolic acidosis
Inhibition of amino acid metabolism	Metabolic acidosis
Stimulation of glyconeogenesis	Hyperglycemia
Stimulation of lipid metabolism	Metabolic acidosis
Increased pulmonary capillary permeability	Pulmonary edema

It is commonly held that in adult salicylate poisoning a dominant metabolic acidosis follows an initial respiratory alkalosis. The latter phase may be very brief.[16] Adults may develop severe acidemia within as little as 3 to 4 hours of a massive aspirin overdose.

The underlying pathophysiology of the acid-base disturbances in salicylate intoxication is complex and has not been fully elucidated. Salicylates have been shown to directly stimulate the central respiratory center.[19, 20] Respiratory alkalosis occurs as a result of hyperventilation, with an increase in depth and rate of respiration. As a result, partial pressure of carbon dioxide in arterial blood ($Paco_2$) is low, plasma pH is increased, and serum bicarbonate (HCO_3^-) level is elevated. As a compensatory measure, HCO_3^- is then vigorously excreted in the urine. Some animal data also suggest a role for peripheral arterial chemoreceptors in the development of hyperventilation.[21]

Metabolic acidosis occurs following an inhibition of the TCA cycle enzymes and of mitochondrial oxidative phosphorylation.[22, 23] The uncoupling of oxidative phosphorylation reduces the production of cellular adenosine triphosphate (ATP) and hence increases the production of pyruvic and lactic acid. Bartels and Lund-Jacobsen cast doubt on the significance of excessive lactate production due to salicylate-induced uncoupling of oxidative phosphorylation. Instead they postulated that observed elevations in lactate may be due to decreased hepatic elimination of lactate.[24] TCA cycle inhibition, specifically of α-ketoglutaric dehydrogenase and succinic acid dehydrogenase, also increases pyruvic and lactic acid levels. Two other mechanisms contribute to the development of acidemia. The first is an increased lipid metabolism, producing the ketone bodies (hydroxybutyric acid, acetoacetic acid, and acetone). The second is inhibition of aminotransferases, producing increased levels of circulating amino acids.[25]

Both salicylate in the CSF and acidemia are powerful stimuli to respiration, and the latter facilitates the former.[26] Together they may be expected to enhance hyperventilation in comparison to ventilation in patients with normal or low arterial H+. Chapman and Proudfoot, however, found that the mean $Paco_2$ was higher in fatal cases (in which acidemia was also present in most), than in survivors (most of whom had normal or low arterial H+).[18] This failure to hyperventilate appropriately in response to an acid stimulus may be a factor in the development of acidemia in these patients.[18]

A final contributing factor to the development of acidosis is the depletion of buffering capacity as a result of increased renal loss of HCO_3^- through the compensatory mechanisms that are a consequence of the initial respiratory alkalosis.[27]

Fluid and Electrolyte Abnormalities

Fluid and electrolyte aberrations are not uncommon in salicylate poisoning and are the result of many factors. Increased insensible losses of water occur as a result of increased metabolism, heat production, and respiratory rate. Water and sodium are lost through increased sweating. Further fluid loss may occur as a result of decreased fluid intake and/or vomiting. Water losses may reach 4 to 6 L/m^2.[15] With increased HCO_3^- excretion at the kidney in the early alkalotic stage, there is concomitant loss of sodium and potassium as the body attempts to conserve hydrogen ions. Severe potassium depletion may produce a paradoxically acid urine while the kidney attempts to conserve potassium over H^+.[15] Robin and colleagues[28] reported on six severely poisoned patients who presented with hypokalemia manifesting as a low serum potassium concentration, ECG changes, and neuromuscular abnormalities.[28] All patients demonstrated respiratory alkalosis. It was postulated that the hypokalemia resulted from a subsequent shift of potassium into the cells and excessive renal loss. In a similar way, forced alkaline diuresis may also lead to significant hypokalemia.[29] In both of these situations, patients responded to potassium supplementation. Hypocalcemia may also complicate attempts to alkalinize the urine.[30] Conversely, transient hypercalcemia has been reported after overdose with soluble aspirin, possibly due to the calcium content of the tablet.[31] Hypernatremia is common, presumably resulting from dehydration. Hyponatremia is less common, but it does occur and may be associated with inappropriate fluid retention.[32]

As indicated previously, fluid loss may occur in salicylate-poisoned patients to the point of causing clinically significant dehydration. This dehydration may account for the observation that urine output lags behind the rate of fluid administration in the process of forcing diuresis. Temple and colleagues[32] reported on two children who demonstrated fluid retention and oliguria despite adequate hydration. It was postulated that this resulted from an inappropriate secretion of antidiuretic hormone.

Pulmonary Edema

Pulmonary edema is an uncommon but well-recognized complication of acute salicylate intoxication; it was first reported in 1950. It is thought to represent the most common cause of significant morbidity in chronic salicylate intoxication.[33] In the 1970s, the noncardiogenic origin of the edema was suspected by Zitnik and colleagues following pulmonary artery catheterization that showed a normal pulmonary artery wedge pressure, and by Bowers and others in studies on sheep.[34, 35] Since that time, a number of studies have suggested an increase in pulmonary capillary permeability as the underlying pathologic process. Three prominent theories[36] postulate explanations: First, aspirin is known to inhibit release of prostacyclin, a chemical that acts to reduce capillary permeability. Second, mild cerebral edema may result in a catecholamine surge, leading to elevated pulmonary vascular pressures. And third, the effect of salicylates on platelet-vessel interaction may result in increased permeability.

Radiologic studies in salicylate intoxication indicate that pulmonary edema occurs in about 35% of patients older than 30 years.[36] Chronic ingestion of the drug, smoking, the presence of metabolic acidosis, and/or neurologic features on admission were major risk factors for its development. In the same study by Walters and co-workers,[36] none of the patients younger than 16 years developed pulmonary edema, whereas Fisher and associates[37] demonstrated development of this complication in 2 of 20 children.

Central Nervous System Abnormalities

CNS toxicity is an important indicator of severe salicylate toxicity. Coma is rare; patients are often agitated, confused, and restless before unconsciousness occurs. In children younger than 5 years, in whom acidemia is the usual acid-base disturbance, these neurologic features are more common.[16, 38]

Adults show CNS toxicity less often, but when they do, it is also associated with acidemia.[14, 18] The severity of CNS manifestations appears to have a direct relationship to brain salicylate levels.[26] Hill demonstrated in rats that the presence of acidemia facilitates the shift of salicylate from the extracellular fluid into the intracellular space, especially in the brain.[26] As the negative logarithm of the ionization constant K_1 $(pKa)_1$ of 3.0 for salicylic acid suggests, as the pH of the blood decreases, a higher percentage of the compound will be found in the non-ionized form. This results in enhanced lipid solubility and, hence, an increased ability to cross cell membranes and the blood-brain barrier. Some patients with significant CNS effects have had alkalemia, but in these cases the plasma salicylate levels have been very high.

Cerebral edema has been reported, but it is uncommon. Hypernatremia and fluid retention or overload may contribute to its development. Convulsions are also documented in severe cases. Some animal studies indicate that they may result from hyperventilation or reduced brain glucose levels, which paradoxically can occur despite normoglycemia.

Concomitant ingestion of CNS depressants, such as alcohol and benzodiazepines, encourages the development of acidosis by reducing the central drive to hyperventilate in response to acidemia.[14]

Metabolic Derangement

The principal metabolic derangements in salicylate poisoning are changes in glucose metabolism, which may produce either hypoglycemia or hyperglycemia. An increased demand for glucose results from an increased metabolism. This, in turn, mobilizes glycogen and fat stores via increased hepatic glycogenolysis and lipid metabolism. Initially, patients may present with a short-lived, or in some cases persistent, hyperglycemia, which may be of high enough magnitude to produce glucosuria.[15, 17] This is thought to be a response to a failure of the tissues to utilize glucose adequately. Eventually, glucose stores are exhausted and hypoglycemia may occur. Contributing to the development of hypoglycemia is an enhanced insulin secretion,[39] which may be due to inhibition of prostaglandin synthesis.[40] The fact that brain hypoglycemia has been demonstrated in animals in the presence of a normal blood glucose level is important.[41]

Hyperpyrexia

Hyperpyrexia is more common in children than in adults.[18] It may result from the increased heat production that occurs following the uncoupling of oxidative phosphorylation. Additionally, toxic levels of salicylate impair the efficiency of the body's cooling mechanisms, and this is compounded by the presence of dehydration.[15] Hyperpyrexia is very uncommon in acute adult salicylate poisoning, and its presence is indicative of a poor prognosis.[18] Other causes of an elevated temperature should also be considered (e.g., infection or concomitant drug ingestion).

Hematologic Abnormalities

Decreased prothrombin formation; decreased production of factors II, V, VII, and X; increased capillary fragility; decreased platelet adhesiveness; and thrombocytopenia have all been demonstrated in salicylate intoxication.[42] Rarely do any of these changes become clinically significant. On occasion, transient petechial rashes may be observed over the face and neck. Significant hemorrhagic complications are, however, very uncommon in salicylate poisoning.

Gastrointestinal and Hepatic Abnormalities

As discussed previously, gastrointestinal bleeding is rare in salicylate-poisoned patients. Gastric perforation has been reported after an acute overdosage; one such reported case occurred following the overdose with enteric-coated aspirin.[43] Nausea and vomiting are by far the most common and consistent gastrointestinal tract findings in these patients.

Direct hepatotoxicity, histologically similar to Reye's syndrome on biopsy, may occur. The presence of larger fatty droplets and a lack of mitochondrial changes differentiate salicylate poisoning from Reye's syndrome.[44, 45]

Renal Abnormalities

Kimberly and Plotz have reported reduced creatinine clearance, elevated urea level, and an increased variety of cells within the urine as adverse effects of aspirin.[46] This acute renal impairment may be either a result of direct nephrotoxicity or the effect of a reduction in renal blood flow. Typically, it is thought that salicylates acutely inhibit prostaglandin synthesis, resulting in vasoconstriction and reduced renal blood flow and glomerular filtration.[47] The resultant oliguria is exacerbated by the presence of dehydration. Pre-existing renal disease may predispose patients to the development of renal impairment.

Other Findings

Tinnitus is well known with salicylate intoxication, and it frequently precedes the onset of deafness. Both effects are reversible. Mongan and co-workers[48] reported tinnitus beginning at levels from 20 to 45 mg/dL. It has been postulated that salicylates increase intralabyrinthine pressure; however, Ramsden and colleagues[49] suggest that salicylates cause their effect by acting at the hair cell–neural interface, causing a transient metabolic blockade.

Ralston and colleagues[50] report a case of a 13-month-old boy with mild to moderate salicylate intoxication who experienced bradyarrhythmias and global myocardial dysfunction, which they could not attribute to acidosis, hypoxia, ischemia, or metabolic or electrolyte abnormalities.

Fatal *in utero* salicylism has been reported following an aspirin overdose in an 8-months' pregnant primigravida.[51]

A number of investigators have reported on multiple-system organ failure following salicylate overdose, sometimes associated with rhabdomyolysis.[52, 53] Vadas and colleagues[53] demonstrated increased phospholipase A_2 concentrations and postulated that this may result from an aspirin-induced intestinal permeability to endotoxin and that these elevated phospholipase A_2 levels may play a role in the development of multiple system organ failure.

DIAGNOSIS

Clinical Aspects

Following an acute overdose of salicylate, the diagnosis is often straightforward. In the pediatric age group, a history of witnessed ingestion or of recent ingestion is usually forthcoming. Adults with salicylate overdose may be more circumspect, but these patients are seldom comatose and commonly admit to their actions. In cases in which CNS depressant drugs have also been ingested, the history is more difficult, and a greater reliance should be placed on physical findings. *The presence of hyperventilation, diaphoresis, tinnitus, and an acid-base abnormality should point to salicylate poisoning.* In severe cases, the presence of an altered state of consciousness may prevent the disclosure of salicylate ingestion and erroneously lead to an involved neuropsychiatric evaluation, delaying the diagnosis and potentially increasing morbidity. Chronic salicylism often presents as a neuropsychiatric problem. Other potential misdiagnoses include diabetic ketoacidosis, alcoholic ketoacidosis, and other causes of high anion gap acidemia.

Laboratory Data

Plasma Salicylate Concentrations

The patient's clinical presentation is usually pathognomonic of salicylism, but a plasma salicylate level is essential in the diagnosis and management of salicylate-poisoned patients. A concentration greater than 30 mg/dL is usually associated with toxicity. Chronic therapeutic plasma concentrations in rheumatoid arthritis sufferers range from 10 to 30 mg/dL. A single level drawn too early may not be representative. Therefore, repeated levels at 2 to 3 hourly intervals should be obtained until a downward trend is established. It is important not to rely on a single level because of the possibility of prolonged or delayed absorption following the ingestion of sustained-release products, enteric-coated tablets, or the formation of a pharmacologic bezoar. Concentrations should be interpreted in conjunction with the patient's overall clinical and acid-base status. The presence of significant acidemia may imply a more serious intoxication, because higher concentrations of non-ionized salicylate can penetrate into the CNS.

Several methods are available to determine plasma salicylate concentrations.[54] The most common is the colorimetric technique, which utilizes the reaction between salicylate and the ferric ion and gives an estimate of the total plasma salicylate concentration. High-performance liquid chromatography and gas chromatography are able to distinguish acetylsalicylic acid (aspirin) from salicylic acid, something the colorimetric test is unable to differentiate. Colorimetric testing is, however, easy and fast. So-called "routine" toxicologic screening for salicylate poisoning has a low positive yield.[55] Spot tests performed in the emergency department have little prognostic value and are fraught with problems due to misinterpretation by inexperienced individuals.

Other Useful Tests

Electrolytes should be analyzed and an anion gap calculated. Glucose, creatinine, blood urea nitrogen (BUN), and arterial blood gas assays are also indicated. Complete blood cell count, coagulation profile, serum calcium level, and liver function tests are appropriate in moderate to severe poisonings. A chest x-ray should be performed if pulmonary edema is suggested on examination or if arterial blood gases demonstrate a widened arterial-alveolar gradient.[37]

Assessing Severity

Assessing the severity of an acute salicylate overdose can be done on the basis of three main parameters. First, from the history, an estimate can be made of the amount ingested, and from this, a prediction of the clinical severity can be made.[17] Generally, ingestions of less than 150 mg/kg follow a benign course, with salicylate toxicity being unlikely.[56] With ingestions above 150 mg/kg, toxicity is dose-dependent, and categories have traditionally been broken into mild (150 to 300 mg/kg), moderate (300 to 500 mg/kg), and severe (>500 mg/kg).[17] These categories are not absolute and should be interpreted in conjunction with the patient's clinical condition.

Second, by evaluating the clinical state of the patient, an approximate severity classification can be made.[17] Early in the course of an acute salicylate overdose, symptoms and signs may be mild and subtle; hence, it is important to evaluate these patients on a regular basis, rather than relying on a single initial assessment as an indicator of severity. Traditionally, cases of mild poisoning are said to be characterized by tachypnea, with lethargy on occasion. Moderate toxicity is characterized by more prominent tachypnea and neurologic disturbances. Finally, severe poisoning is represented by coma or near-coma, possibly with convulsions. It is vital to remember, however, that salicylate poisoning is a dynamic process, and regular assessments and management appraisals are required. It is unwise to strictly categorize such patients.

Finally, an assessment of severity can be attempted from the plasma salicylate level. In 1960, Done studied 38 patients (29 of whom were children) who presented following an acute aspirin overdose.[13] Based on their clinical symptoms and signs and their plasma levels, he created a nomogram that plots salicylate levels at differing times in an attempt to estimate the degree of intoxication (asymptomatic, mild, moderate, or severe) and, hence, to predict expected symptoms. Measurements made before 6 hours were considered misleading because the drug may be incompletely absorbed. In practice, plasma salicylate concentrations do not correlate well with features of acute toxicity, especially in patients who are assessed clinically as being moderately or severely intoxicated.[12] The nomogram has been demonstrated to be unrepresentative of toxicity.[12] More specifically, the nomogram is not useful in the following circumstances: when salicylate ingestion occurs over a prolonged period (chronic ingestion), when a sustained-release preparation or oil of wintergreen has been ingested, in the presence of renal insufficiency, when the time of ingestion is unknown, and when a patient has acidemia.[57] Furthermore, the nomogram is based on the misconception that salicylates are eliminated via first-order toxicokinetics.[13] For all of these limitations, many toxicologists do not now rely on the nomogram to determine severity but instead rely on the combination of the amount ingested (if known), the clinical symptoms and signs, and the plasma salicylate concentration.

The concentration of salicylate in the CSF reflects the concentration of unbound drug in the plasma, and studies in children and animals have shown that the severity of intoxication is closely related to the CSF salicylate concentrations. These, in turn, are related to the total plasma concentration and the H+. High H+ reduces ionization and thereby facilitates the shift of salicylate into the cells. However, CSF levels are not used routinely to assess the magnitude of salicylism.

MANAGEMENT

Initial Treatment

As with all poisoned patients, initial management should be directed toward establishing and maintaining an adequate airway, then maximizing cardiovascular and respiratory support. Intravenous access should be gained in all patients and supplemental oxygen applied when appropriate. During this initial process, the history-taker should attempt to ascertain the amount and type of salicylate ingested and the time of ingestion. Laboratory investigations at this time may include arterial blood gas measurements; plasma salicylate, electrolyte, and blood glucose levels; and renal function tests.

Gut Decontamination

In recent years, the role of syrup of ipecac has been significantly curtailed, such that its use is predominantly restricted to the treatment of children in the home setting if it can be given within 30 to 60 minutes of the ingestion. Gastric lavage has also been the focus of considerable attention. Some limited evidence has indicated that salicylates in toxic amounts may delay gastric emptying. Some investigators have used this as the rationale for extending the time interval in which gastric lavage may be of benefit. Up to 12 hours postingestion has been suggested; however, contemporary practices allow the sole and expeditious use of oral activated charcoal in most acute salicylate overdoses.[58] Although their occurrence is uncommon, pharmacologic bezoars may form after very large overdoses. Their presence, as indicated by sustained or rising salicylate concentrations, may necessitate gastric lavage or even endoscopic procedures to break up the concretions if evidence shows continued gut absorption. Comatose patients who undergo gastric lavage should also undergo endotracheal intubation.

Activated charcoal is effective in reducing the gut absorption of salicylates.[10, 59] An initial oral bolus of 50 g or 1 g/kg should be administered as soon as possible. Subsequent doses should be administered at 2- to 6-hour intervals if evidence indicates that continued absorption is occurring. The mythical dose of activated charcoal in a ratio of 10:1 (charcoal-to-salicylate) is impractical, as overdosage of 50 g would necessitate administration of 500 g of activated charcoal! Conceptually, as enteric-coated salicylates dissolve in the distal gastrointestinal tract, activated charcoal should be effective. However, whole-bowel irrigation may be a more effective means of eliminating enteric-coated products. Kirshenbaum and coworkers[60] have also studied the effectiveness of whole-bowel irrigation, compared with that of single-dose activated charcoal with sorbitol, in preventing salicylate absorption following the ingestion of enteric-coated aspirin in volunteers.[60] They concluded that whole-bowel irrigation was more effective in reducing absorption. Generally, the use of whole-bowel irrigation in the prevention of salicylate absorption has not been fully elucidated, and it cannot be recommended routinely in the management of most salicylate overdoses.

Multi-Dose Activated Charcoal

The use of multi-dose activated charcoal has also been investigated in the role of enhancing the elimination of salicylate, once the drug is absorbed, via "gastrointestinal dialysis."[61–63] Hillman and Prescott[61] demonstrated that multi-dose activated charcoal was effective in enhancing the elimination in patients with mild to moderate toxicity; however, most subsequent studies have failed to demonstrate this finding.[62, 63] Multiple doses of activated charcoal should not be used as a means of enhancing elimination, only as an intervention to prevent the ongoing absorption of salicylates.

Correction of Acid-Base, Fluid, and Electrolyte Disturbances

It is absolutely essential that careful attention be paid to the fluid balance status of the patient. Fluid therapy should be based on the clinical need for rehydration, renal function, and risks of inducing pulmonary edema. Patients may initially require fluid resuscitation in the presence of dehyration.[17]

A hypotonic solution such as half-normal saline is generally appropriate. As hypoglycemia has been implicated in the pathophysiology of CNS injury in salicylate-poisoned patients, glucose should be added (50 to 100 g/L), despite the presence of normoglycemia or even mild hyperglycemia. The potential benefit of giving glucose supplementation is empirical, and no clinical data are available concerning the real glucose requirements.[57] Ultimately, the aim of fluid replacement is to replace fluid deficits and maintain a urine output of between 100 and 200 mL/hour.

Patients who are seriously poisoned by salicylates are at risk of developing pulmonary edema and/or fluid retention through an inappropriate secretion of antidiuretic hormone. In these patients, particularly if at extremes of age, aggressive fluid replacement may be counterproductive. Urine output, renal function, and pulmonary capillary wedge pressure readings will be helpful in assessing these persons. Pulmonary edema in salicylate-poisoned patients is of a noncardiogenic type. Given this, therapy should begin with oxygen; it may progress to continuous positive airway pressure ventilation (CPAP) and finally, perhaps, to intubation with positive end-expiratory pressure ventilation (PEEP). Pulmonary edema improves as salicylate levels fall.[33, 57]

Electrolytes

Hypernatremia is common; hence the recommendation for hypotonic solutions in the initial management phase. Hypokalemia should also be watched for and treated. The presence of a significant acidemia may result in a normal serum potassium level but may mask a true total body potassium deficiency.

Acid-Base Disturbances

As outlined previously, a low serum pH increases the tissue penetration of salicylate and hence increases CNS concentrations. For this reason, acidemia should be corrected using sodium bicarbonate. Hypokalemia should be corrected simultaneously. Alkalemia rarely requires treatment.

Hypoglycemia

All patients should undergo blood glucose analysis. The presence of CNS symptoms or signs of hypoglycemia should be treated with an intravenous bolus of 50% glucose, approximately 1 mL/kg. As described previously, normoglycemia, or even a slightly elevated blood glucose level, may be present with depressed CNS glucose concentrations. In view of this, glucose should be administered with all intravenous fluids.

Other Disturbances

Seizures are not common in salicylate intoxication. Those that occur should be treated along standard lines; diazepam, or a similar benzodiazepine, is the widely accepted drug of first choice. Other causes of seizures should also be considered, including electrolyte abnormalities and hypoglycemia. Hyperpyrexia is more common in children than in adults. The possibilities of other causes should be considered, including infection or other drug ingestion. In cases of severe pyrexia, traditional cooling methods may be needed.

Urinary Alkalinization

Normally salicylate undergoes both glomerular filtration and tubular secretion. In therapeutic doses the metabolic pathways for salicylates become saturated. Renal excretion is therefore very important in the elimination of salicylate in both therapeutic and toxic levels. Only the unbound fraction of salicylate is available for glomerular filtration, but in toxic amounts, this portion increases. Salicylate is also reabsorbed at the proximal convoluted tubules (PCT). The latter process depends on both urine flow rate and urine pH. As explained previously, in an acid environment, salicylate is maximally non-ionized, facilitating transfer across cell membranes and, hence, PCT reabsorption. During periods of high urine output the urinary concentration of salicylate falls, reducing the urine-to-tubular cell concentration gradient; this also theoretically reduces PCT reabsorption. Attempts to apply these fundamental physiologic principles clinically has led to the use of alkalinization of the urine, forced diuresis, or forced alkaline diuresis.

Urinary alkalinization is the administration of sodium bicarbonate alone in an attempt to increase the urine pH to greater than 7.5 while maintaining a normal urine output and avoiding the risks of fluid overload.[64]

In 1982, Prescott and colleagues[64] compared all three methods by studying 44 salicylate-poisoned adults. They concluded that the administration of sodium bicarbonate alone was effective and possibly more effective than either forced diuresis or forced alkaline diuresis. Further, unlike the latter two regimens, fluid retention was not a problem. The large fluid load produced by regimens designed to force a diuresis are usually well-tolerated by young adults with normal renal function; however, even in this age group pulmonary edema and cerebral edema have occurred. The addition of furosemide does reduce the risk of fluid retention, but it may decrease rather than increase renal salicylate elimination.[64] In the study of Prescott and associates, the significant decreases in plasma salicylate levels seen with the group that was treated with forced diuresis and forced alkaline diuresis was greater than expected based on the urinary salicylate excretion. It was felt that this was partly due to hemodilution and that this phenomenon may give a false impression of efficacy.

Generally, urinary alkalinization alone is more effective and probably safer than other regimens in the treatment of mild to moderate salicylate poisoning. Although the indications for urinary alkalinization are not clearly delineated, it is suggested for patients with the presence of clinical features consistent with salicylate poisoning, as seen in those with serum salicylate concentrations of 30 to 60 mg/dL or greater. Hemodialysis may be indicated for patients who are unresponsive to an initial trial of bicarbonate therapy, especially those whose salicylate levels approach 80 to 100 mg/dL, or as clinically indicated. Effective alkalinization of the urine may be very difficult to achieve. One method is through the addition of 100 mEq of sodium bicarbonate to 1000 mL of 5% dextrose in half-normal saline, which is infused at a rate of approximately 200 mL/hour. Unless renal failure is also present, the addition of 20 to 40 mEq of potassium to each 1000 mL of fluid will enhance the ability to alkalinize the urine successfully. Although a number of different methods for alkalinization are available, no specific one has been shown to be better or to result in a greater amount of salicylate elimination.

Significant concerns still exist over the use of sodium bicarbonate in salicylate-poisoned patients; it is important to watch for the worsening of alkalemia in patients with a pre-existing respiratory alkalosis, the development of hypokalemia or hypernatremia, and to a lesser extent, fluid overload and congestive heart failure. The effectiveness of urinary alkalinization in most severe cases of pediatric salicylate poisoning may be in question.[27]

The use of acetazolamide to alkalinize the urine is contraindicated, because it produces metabolic acidosis through renal elimination of sodium bicarbonate, which may worsen salicylism and result in increased tissue penetration of salicylate. Tromethamine is not preferable to the use of sodium bicarbonate when alkalinization is required.

Hemodialysis

Salicylates have a small volume of distribution, approximately 0.2 L/kg, and a low molecular weight. Both of these characteristics enhance the ability to remove salicylate extracorporeally. Further, in toxic states, the plasma protein-binding falls significantly, allowing more free salicylate, and consequently more drug, to be removed.[65] A number of techniques have been tried, including exchange transfusion, peritoneal dialysis, hemoperfusion, and hemodialysis. Although both hemoperfusion and hemodialysis remove similar amounts of salicylate, hemodialysis is considered the best choice, particularly because of its availability and because it allows concurrent correction of fluid, electrolyte, and acid-base abnormalities, which hemoperfusion does not. Hemoperfusion also traps platelets and usually requires higher heparin doses, both of which may theoretically compound the anticoagulant effect of salicylate.[66]

Clinical and laboratory parameters are used as indicators for the need to hemodialyze salicylate-poisoned patients. Little information exists on which to base this decision, and in each case an individual assessment is best. The sole reliance on the plasma salicylate level is not advised. *Generally, as levels approach 80 to 100 mg/dL in an acute overdose, serious consideration should be given to using hemodialysis to enhance the elimination of salicylate.* Further clinical indications for hemodialysis include the presence of volume overload or renal failure, in which cases the administration of fluid or sodium bicarbonate would not be recommended. Furthermore, hemodialysis is recommended in the presence of deterioration despite supportive care and evidence of organ injury (e.g., altered level of consciousness, pulmonary edema, and uncontrolled acid-base disturbances). Early consultation with a nephrologist is prudent to avoid any possible bureaucratic delays in commencing dialysis. Once begun, the endpoint of dialysis is typically considered to be a return to nontoxic salicylate levels, clinical improvement, and correction of major acid-base abnormalities.

CHRONIC SALICYLATE INTOXICATION

Chronic salicylate intoxication is a difficult diagnosis in the pediatric and adult population, and its presentation is often delayed. Chronic salicylate poisoning in children is usually more serious than acute poisoning, and it may manifest with hyperventilation, acidosis, dehydration, electrolyte abnormalities, and an altered level of consciousness.[38] The adult group, especially the elderly, are more likely to have a pre-existing medical problem for which salicylate has been a therapeutic measure—particularly degenerative joint disease and cardiovascular disease.[33] This age group presents with similar symptoms and signs as those of the pediatric age group, but they may also describe nausea and tinnitus or decreased auditory acuity. In chronic toxicity, acid-base disturbances generally consist of metabolic acidosis, which tends to be more severe.[15] Further, pulmonary edema is a more common finding in chronic than in acute intoxication, as are neurologic abnormalities.[33, 36] In their study of 73 consecutive adult salicylate poisonings, Anderson and associates[33] found that 60% of patients had a prolonged neurologic evaluation before salicylate poisoning was diagnosed, with the delay to diagnosis ranging from 6 to 72 hours.[33] Infection is another common misdiagnosis in patients with chronic intoxication because of the presence of fever. Salicylate toxicity should be considered in patients with unexplained acid-base disturbances, hyperventilation, or confusion.

Severe chronic poisoning occurs at a lower plasma salicylate level than does acute intoxication. Clinical features correlate poorly with levels. The Done nomogram is of no use. Supportive measures and the use of urinary alkalinization are the same as for acute toxicity. Given that absorption has already occurred in most patients, the use of activated charcoal in this group is probably of no benefit. Finally, the threshold to institute extracorporeal techniques to enhance salicylate removal is much lower than in the acutely poisoned patients. The presence of significant acidosis, confusion, or pulmonary edema has been used as evidence for the need to begin hemodialysis. Data are not available on which to suggest an exact plasma salicylate concentration that signals a need for hemodialysis. However, it is usually significantly lower than in acute intoxication and varies considerably from patient to patient. Overall, clinical considerations should predominate in the decision process with respect to chronic salicylism.

References

1. Rowland M, Riegelman S, Harris PA, et al: Absorption kinetics of aspirin in man following oral administration of an aqueous solution. J Pharm Sci *61*:379–385, 1972.
2. Needs CJ, Brooks PM: Clinical pharmacokinetics of salicylates. Clin Pharmacokinet *10*:164–177, 1985.
3. Brune K, Nuernberg A, Schneider HT: Biliary elimination of

aspirin after oral and intravenous administration in patients. *In* Variability in Response to Anti-rheumatic Drugs. Basel, Birkhauser Verlag, pp 51–57, 1993.
4. Davies MG, Briffa DV, Greaves MW: Systemic toxicity from topically applied salicylic acid. Br Med J *1*:661, 1979.
5. Brubacher JR, Hoffman RS: Salicylism from topical salicylates: Review of the literature. Clin Toxicol *34*:431–436, 1996.
6. Watson JE, Tagupa ET: Suicide attempt by means of aspirin enema. Ann Pharmacother *28*:467–468, 1994.
7. Levy G, Yaffe SJ: Relationship between dose and apparent volume of distribution of salicylate in children. Pediatrics *54*:713–717, 1974.
8. Kwong TC: Salicylate measurement: Clinical usefulness and methodology. CRC Crit Rev Clin Lab Sci *25*:137–159, 1987.
9. Rowland M, Riegelman S: Pharmacokinetics of acetylsalicylic acid and salicylic acid after intravenous administration in man. J Pharm Sci *57*:717–720, 1968.
10. Levy G, Tsuchiya T: Salicylate accumulation kinetics in man. N Engl J Med *287*:430–432, 1972.
11. Levy G, Tsuchiya T, Amsel LP: Limited capacity for salicyl phenolic glucuronide formation and its effect on the kinetics of salicylate elimination in man. Clin Pharmacol Ther *13*:258–268, 1972.
12. Dugandzic RM, Tierney MG, Dickinson GE, et al: Evaluation of the validity of the Done nomogram in the management of acute salicylate intoxication. Ann Emerg Med *18*:1186–1190, 1989.
13. Done AK: Salicylate intoxication: Significance of measurements of salicylate in blood in cases of acute ingestion. Pediatrics *26*:800–807, 1960.
14. Gabow PA, Anderson RJ, Potts DE, et al: Acid-base disturbances in the salicylate-intoxicated adult. Arch Intern Med *138*:1481–1484, 1978.
15. Temple AR: Pathophysiology of aspirin overdosage toxicity, with implications for management. Pediatrics *62*:873–876, 1978.
16. Winters RW, White JS, Hughes MC, et al: Disturbances of acid-base equilibrium in salicylate intoxication. Pediatrics 23:260–285, 1959.
17. Temple AR: Acute and chronic effects of aspirin toxicity and their treatment. Arch Intern Med *141*:364–369, 1981.
18. Chapman BC, Proudfoot AT: Adult salicylate poisoning: Deaths and outcome in patients with high plasma salicylate concentrations. Q J Med *72*:699–707, 1989.
19. Tenney SM, Miller RM: The respiratory and circulatory actions of salicylate. Am J Med *19*:498–508, 1965.
20. Cameron IR, Semple SJR: The central respiratory stimulation action of salicylates. Clin Sci *35*:391–401, 1968.
21. McQueen DS, Ritchie IM, Birrell GJ: Arterial chemoreceptor involvement in salicylate-induced hyperventilation in rats. Br J Pharmacol *98*:413–424, 1989.
22. Kaplan EH, Kennedy J, Davis J: Effects of salicylate and other benzoates on oxidative enzymes of the tricarboxylic acid cycle in rat tissue homogenates. Arch Biochem Biophys *51*:47–61, 1954.
23. Miyahara JT, Karler R: Effect of salicylate on oxidative phosphorylation and respiration of mitochondrial fragment. Biochem J *97*:194–198, 1965.
24. Bartels PD, Lund-Jacobsen H: Blood lactate and ketone body concentrations in salicylate intoxication. Hum Toxicol *5*:363–366, 1986.
25. Schwartz R, Landy G, Taller D: Organic acid excretion in salicylate intoxication. J Pediatr *66*:658–666, 1965.
26. Hill JB: Salicylate intoxication. N Engl J Med *288*:1110–1113, 1973.
27. Done AK: Treatment of salicylate poisoning: Review of personal and published experiences. Clin Toxicol *1*:451–467, 1968.
28. Robin ED, Davis RP, Rees SB: Salicylate intoxication with special reference to the development of hypokalemia. Am J Med *26*:869–882, 1959.
29. Lawson AAH, Proudfoot AT, Brown SS, et al: Forced diuresis in the treatment of acute salicylate poisoning in adults. Q J Med *38*:31–48, 1969.
30. Fox GN: Hypocalcemia complicating bicarbonate therapy for salicylate poisoning. West J Med *141*:108–109, 1984.
31. Reid IR: Transient hypercalcemia following overdoses of soluble aspirin tablets. Aust N Z J Med *15*:364, 1985.
32. Temple AR, George DJ, Done AK, et al: Salicylate poisoning complicated by fluid retention. Clin Toxicol *9*:61–68, 1976.
33. Anderson RJ, Potts DE, Gabow PA, et al: Unrecognized adult salicylate intoxication. Ann Intern Med *85*:745–748, 1976.
34. Zitnik RJ, Cooper JA: Pulmonary disease due to antirheumatic agents. Clin Chest Med *11*:139–150, 1990.
35. Bowers RE, Brigham KL, Owen PJ: Salicylate pulmonary edema: The mechanism in sheep and review of the clinical literature. Am Rev Respir Dis *115*:261–268, 1977.
36. Walters JS, Woodring JH, Stelling CB, et al: Salicylate-induced pulmonary edema. Radiology *146*:289–293, 1983.
37. Fisher CJ, Albertson TE, Foulke GE: Salicylate-induced pulmonary edema: Clinical characteristics in children. Am J Emerg Med *3*:33–37, 1985.
38. Gaudreault P, Temple AR, Lovejoy FH: The relative severity of acute versus chronic salicylate poisoning in children: A clinical comparison. Pediatrics *70*:566–569, 1982.
39. Giugliano D, Cozzolino D, Ceriello A: Studies on the mechanism of salicylate-induced increase of insulin secretion in man. Diabet Metab *14*:431–436, 1988.
40. Robertson RP: Eicosanoids as pluripotential modulators of pancreatic islet function. Diabetes *37*:367–370, 1988.
41. Thurston JH, Pollock PG, Warren SK: Reduced brain glucose with normal plasma glucose in salicylate poisoning. J Clin Invest *49*:2139–2145, 1970.
42. Smith MJH: The metabolic bases of the major symptoms in acute salicylate intoxication. Clin Toxicol *1*:387–407, 1968.
43. Farrand RJ, Green JH, Haworth C: Enteric-coated aspirin overdose and gastric perforation. Br Med J *4*:85–86, 1975.
44. Rich RR, Johnson JS: Salicylate hepatotoxicity in patients with juvenile rheumatoid arthritis. Arthritis Rheum *16*:1–9, 1973.
45. Wolfe JD, Metzger AL, Goldstein RC: Aspirin hepatitis. Ann Intern Med *80*:74–76, 1974.
46. Kimberly RP, Plotz PH: Aspirin-induced depression of renal function. N Engl J Med *296*:418–424, 1977.
47. Rupp DJ, Seaton RD, Weigmann TB: Acute polyuric renal failure after aspirin intoxication. Arch Intern Med *143*:1237–1238, 1983.
48. Mongan E, Kelly P, Nils K, et al: Tinnitus as an indication of therapeutic serum salicylate levels. JAMA *226*:142–145, 1973.
49. Ramsden RT, Latif A, O'Malley S: Electrocochleographic changes in acute salicylate overdosage. J Laryngol Otol *99*:1269–1273, 1985.
50. Ralston ME, Pearigen PD, Ponaman ML, et al: Transient myocardial dysfunction in a child with salicylate toxicity. J Emerg Med *5*:657–659, 1995.
51. Rejent TA, Baik S: Fatal in utero salicylism. J Forensic Sci *30*:942–944, 1985.
52. Montgomery H, Porter JC, Bradley RD: Salicylate intoxication causing a severe systemic inflammatory response and rhabdomyolysis. Am J Emerg Med *12*:531–532, 1994.
53. Vadas P, Schouten BD, Stefanski E, et al: Association of hyperphospholipasemia A_2 with multiple system organ dysfunction due to salicylate intoxication. Crit Care Med *21*:1087–1091, 1993.
54. Kwong TC: Salicylate measurement: Clinical usefulness and methodology. CRC Crit Rev Clin Lab Sci *25*:137–159, 1987.
55. Krenzelok EP, Guharoy SL, Johnson DR: Toxicology screening in the emergency department: Ethanol, barbiturates and salicylates. Am J Emerg Med *2*:331–332, 1984.
56. Rumack BH, Hess AJ, Gelman CR (eds): Poisindex System, Vol 89. Englewood, Colo, Micromedex, Inc. (expires 8/31/96).
57. Yip L, Dart RC, Gabow PA: Concepts and controversies in salicylate toxicity. Emerg Med Clin North Am *12*:351–364, 1994.
58. Prescott LF: Clinical features and management of analgesic poisoning. Hum Toxicol *3*:75S–84S, 1984.
59. Filippone GA, Fish SS, Lacoutre PG, et al: Reversible adsorption (desorption) of aspirin from activated charcoal. Arch Intern Med *147*:1390–1392, 1987.
60. Kirshenbaum LA, Mathews SC, Sitar DS: Whole-bowel irrigation versus activated charcoal in sorbitol for the ingestion of modified-release pharmaceuticals. Clin Pharmacol Ther *46*:264–271, 1989.

61. Hillman RJ, Prescott LF: Treatment of salicylate poisoning with repeat oral charcoal. Br Med J *291*:1472, 1985.
62. Kirshenbaum LA, Mathews SC, Sitar DS, et al: Does multi-dose charcoal therapy enhance salicylate excretion? Arch Intern Med *150*:1281–1283, 1990.
63. Johnson D, Eppler J, Giesbrecht E, et al: Effect of multi-dose activated charcoal on the clearance of high-dose intravenous aspirin in a porcine model. Ann Emerg Med *26*:569–574, 1995.
64. Prescott LF, Balali-Mood M, Critchley JA, et al: Diuresis or urinary alkalinisation for salicylate poisoning? Br Med J *285*:1383–1386, 1982.
65. Alvan G, Bergman U, Gustafsson LL: High unbound fraction of salicylate in plasma during intoxication. Br J Clin Pharmacol *11*:625–626, 1981.
66. Jacobsen D, Wiik-Larsen E, Bredesen JE: Haemodialysis or haemoperfusion in severe salicylate poisoning? Hum Toxicol 7:161–163, 1988.

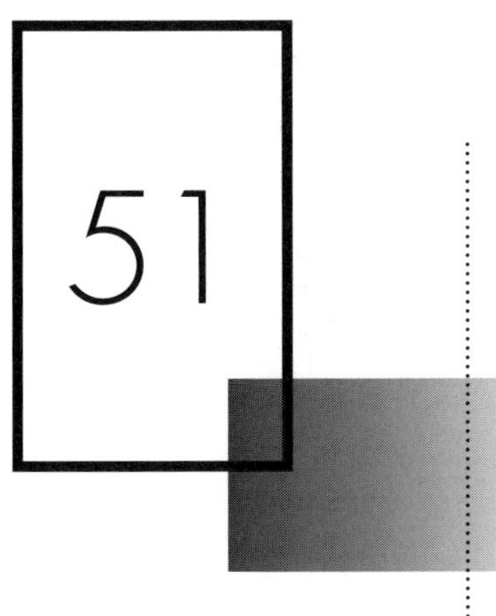

Nonsteroidal Anti-Inflammatory Drugs and Colchicine

J. WARD DONOVAN, MD

Nonsteroidal anti-inflammatory drugs (NSAIDs) were first developed in the late 19th century; they achieved widespread use even before the marketing of acetylsalicylic acid. The first NSAIDs were the pyrazolones, phenazone and amidopyrine; phenylbutazone, of the same class, was not introduced until after World War II. Other NSAIDs were identified in the late 1950s and the 1960s, and they have undergone an explosive increase in use over the past 30 years. Ibuprofen was first introduced into the United States in 1974 and was approved for over-the-counter use in 1984.

The widespread availability of NSAIDs has naturally resulted in a marked increase in the number of overdoses and reported adverse effects. In the 4-year period 1985 through 1988, 55,800 cases of ibuprofen exposure were reported to the American Association of Poison Control Centers (AAPCC), but by 1994, 35,703 ibuprofen exposures and a total of 50,514 NSAID exposures were reported in that year alone.[1, 2] NSAIDs are now the most commonly utilized class of medications in the world, accounting for more than 4% of all prescriptions, with 73 million prescriptions written per year.[3, 4] Piroxicam, with its extended plasma half-life, potency, and safety, has become one of the most widely prescribed NSAIDs in the world.[5]

Despite their extensive use, NSAIDs are among the safest pharmaceuticals in use. Adverse drug reaction frequency is reported as 24.4 per million prescriptions, with fatal adverse reactions of 1.1 per million prescriptions.[6] Symptoms were absent or minor in 93.8% of cases with known outcomes reported to the AAPCC.[2] However, the potential does exist for serious illness and even death, as reflected in the 136 reported serious outcomes and 4 deaths in 1994 in the United States. NSAIDs are now a common cause of renal failure, and at some regional poison treatment centers, mefenamic acid has accounted for the majority of reported drug-induced seizures.[7, 8] Chinese herbal medications have been found to contain NSAIDs, and their use has caused renal failure and aplastic anemia.[9]

NONSTEROIDAL ANTI-INFLAMMATORY DRUGS

Classification and Structure

The NSAIDs are a heterogeneous group of chemicals that share similar therapeutic properties. These acids are classified as subgroups of either of two families: the carboxylic or enolic acids (Table 51–1). Aspirin, a salicylic acid of the carboxylic family, is discussed in Chapter 50.

Pharmacokinetics

The carboxylic acid and enolic acid NSAIDs share similar pharmacokinetics, pharmacodynamic properties, and metabolic pathways. However, there are some clinically significant differences in rates of absorption and elimination and in drug interactions (Table 51–2).[10, 11]

Absorption

Therapeutic oral doses for most NSAIDs are absorbed almost completely, producing peak levels within 1 to 2 hours. Exceptions to this are oxaprozin, mefenamic acid, and diflunisal, which have delays of peak levels up to 3 to 4 hours. The presence of food can delay the absorption of all NSAIDs.[11] In overdose, some delay may take place in achievement of peak serum levels. Five patients in a series of 29 patients with mefenamic acid overdoses had increasing serum levels after admission, which peaked at 8 to 12 hours postingestion.[7]

Table 51–1. Classification of NSAIDs

Class	Trade Name
Carboxylic acids	
Salicylic acids	
Aspirin	
Diflunisal	Dolobid
Phenylacetic acids	
Diclofenac	Voltaren
Carbocyclic and heterocyclic acetic acids	
Indomethacin	Indocin
Sulindac	Clinoril
Tolmetin	Tolectin
Ketorolac	Toradol
Propionic acids	
Ibuprofen	Advil, Nuprin, Motrin
Naproxen	Naproxyn, Anaprox
Flurbiprofen	Ansaid
Fenoprofen	Nalfon
Ketoprofen	Orudis
Oxaprozin	Daypro
Suprofen	Suprol
Fenamic acids	
Mefenamic acid	Ponstel
Meclofenamate	Meclomen
Enolic acids	
Pyrazolones	
Phenylbutazone	Butazolidin
Oxyphenbutazone	Oxalid
Oxicams	
Piroxicam	Feldene

Distribution

The NSAIDs are extensively protein bound (98% to 99%), primarily to albumin. Sulindac and indomethacin have slightly lower degrees of binding, in the range of 90% to 93%.[5, 11] Principally because of their high protein binding, apparent volumes of distribution are low, ranging from 0.10 to 0.36 L/kg.[5, 11] Acute renal insufficiency, liver disease, and hypoalbuminemic states can decrease plasma protein binding and increase volumes of distribution.[11] Plasma protein binding can also decrease when NSAIDs are taken in high doses.

Metabolism

The elimination of NSAIDs is primarily by hepatic biotransformation to metabolites, which are excreted in the urine. The major mechanism is conjugation with glucuronic acid, and in some cases this is preceded by oxidation and hydroxylation.[11] Some NSAIDs undergo significant enterohepatic recirculation, including sulindac, indomethacin, diclofenac, flufenamic acid, ibuprofen, phenylbutazone, and piroxicam.[11] Urinary excretion of unchanged drug is less than 5% for most NSAIDs, but larger amounts of indomethacin, flurbiprofen, tolmetin, and piroxicam are eliminated by this route.[11] Sulindac and nabumetone are metabolized to active metabolites.[10]

The elimination half-lives of NSAIDs vary widely and range from as brief as 1 to 1.5 hours for tolmetin, ketoprofen, and diclofenac to 25 to 50 hours for oxaprozin and piroxicam.[11] The half-lives of many NSAIDs are also prolonged in neonates and patients in renal failure. In overdose, some NSAIDs follow nonlinear kinetics at high serum levels and have prolonged half-lives.[12, 13] Reported half-lives of NSAIDs in overdose are listed in Table 51–2.[7, 11–19]

Drug Interactions

Drug interactions with NSAIDs may be both pharmacokinetic and pharmacodynamic, but the latter is of greatest clinical significance. Significant interactions are primarily effects on the other agents rather than on the NSAID.

The most serious NSAID interactions are with oral anticoagulants, sulfonylurea agents, and methotrexate.[20] The risk of gastrointestinal (GI) bleeding from NSAIDs is enhanced by coumarin-type anticoagulants. NSAID-induced GI bleeding can also be increased by inhibition of NSAID metabolism by the pyrazolones. Methotrexate renal clearance is inhibited by several NSAIDs, and this can result in bone

Table 51–2. Pharmacokinetics of NSAIDs

NSAID (Trade Name)	Absorption T_{max} (h)	Vd (L/kg)	Renal Excretion of Unchanged Drug (%)	Clearance (mL/min)	Elimination $t_{1/2}$ (h) (Therapeutic Dose)	Elimination $t_{1/2}$ (h) (Overdose)
Diclofenac	1–3	0.12–0.17	<1	260	1–2	1.0
Diflunisal	2–3	0.10	3–5	8	8–12	19.4
Etodolac	1.5	0.36	<1	48	7.3	—
Fenoprofen	1–2	0.12	2–5	40–90	3	—
Flurbiprofen	1–2	0.10	20–25	22	3–4	—
Ibuprofen	0.1–1.5	0.11–0.19	1	70	2–2.5	1.5–6
Indomethacin	1–2	0.12	20	70–140	6	3–7
Ketoprofen	0.5–2	0.11	<1	87	1.5	4.4
Ketorolac	1	0.15–0.33	58	32	4–6	
Meclofenamate	0.5–2	—	2–4	190	3	—
Mefenamic acid	2–3	1.3	<6	—	3–4	2–3
Nabumetone	—	—	<5	—	—	—
Naproxen	2	0.10	<1	5	12–15	14
Oxaprozin	3–5	0.14–0.18	<1	2.8	21–25	—
Phenylbutazone	2	0.2	5	2.5	60–72	—
Piroxicam	2	0.12–0.15	10	2.8	38–50	35
Sulindac	1	2	7	105	8	—
Tolmetin	0.5–1	0.10–1.4	17	125	1–1.5	
Zomepirac	1	1.8	0–5	180	4	10

T_{max}, time of maximum concentration; Vd, volume of distribution; $t_{1/2}$, half-life.
Adapted from Verbeeck RK, Blackburn JL, Loewen GR: Clinical pharmacokinetics of non-steroidal anti-inflammatory drugs. Clin Pharmacokinet *8*:302–303, 1983.

marrow toxic effects and renal or hepatic dysfunction. NSAID-drug interactions are summarized in Table 51–3.[20]

Mechanism of Action

The primary mechanism of action of NSAIDs is via inhibition of prostaglandin synthesis. Prostaglandins are derived from phospholipids in cell membranes synthesized from arachidonic acid. This synthesis is mediated by the enzyme cyclo-oxygenase, which is reversibly inhibited by NSAIDs. Thus, NSAIDs block the conversion of arachidonic acid to the various prostaglandins, which are involved in renin release, local vascular tone, regional circulation, water homeostasis, and potassium balance. The prostaglandin pathway and functions are outlined in Figure 51–1.

Prostaglandin E_2 (PGE_2), PGD_2, PGF_2, and prostacyclin (PGI_2) promote salt and water excretion, and the renal vasodilatory action of PGE_2, PGD_2, and prostacyclin enhances this effect. It is thought that PGE_2 and prostacyclin also stimulate renin release.[21] In addition, prostaglandins antagonize the effects of antidiuretic hormone.[22] The net effect of NSAIDs is decreased inhibition of prostaglandins, decreased renal blood flow, and decreased glomerular filtration rate, leading to sodium, potassium, and water retention (Fig. 51–2)

PGE_2 also inhibits lymphocytes and other cells involved in inflammation and allergic response, and this may play a role in the development of interstitial nephritis and hepatotoxic effects in some patients using NSAIDs.[22, 23] This has occurred most with fenoprofen and the carbocyclic and heterocyclic acetic acids.

Other actions of NSAIDs are inhibition of platelet activation and mast cell mediation. The former contributes to prolonged bleeding, and the latter may be involved in NSAID-induced anaphylactic reactions and idiosyncratic hypersensitivity reactions. Also, prostaglandins, particularly prostacyclin, are formed in gastric tissue and exert gastric mucosal protective actions. Inhibition of this action by NSAIDs as well as their direct disruption of the gastric mucosal barrier can cause gastritis and gastrointestinal bleeding.

Table 51–3. Drug Interactions with NSAIDs

Drug	Effect
Anticoagulants	Increase the risk of NSAID-induced GI bleeding; pyrazolones inhibit warfarin metabolism
Sulfonylureas	Metabolism inhibited
Methotrexate	Decreased renal clearance
Digoxin	Decreased renal clearance
Lithium	Decreased renal clearance
Aminoglycosides	Decreased renal clearance
Phenytoin	Displacement of phenytoin from albumin
Antihypertensives, diuretics	Effect antagonized by salt and water retention of NSAIDs
Triamterine	Hyperkalemia; indomethacin combination may precipitate renal failure
Cholestyramine	Binds to and interrupts enterohepatic recirculation of NSAIDs, lowers NSAID levels
Antacids	Reduce absorption of NSAIDs

Range of Toxic Effects

Despite their widespread use, reports of serious acute NSAID overdose have been relatively few. They

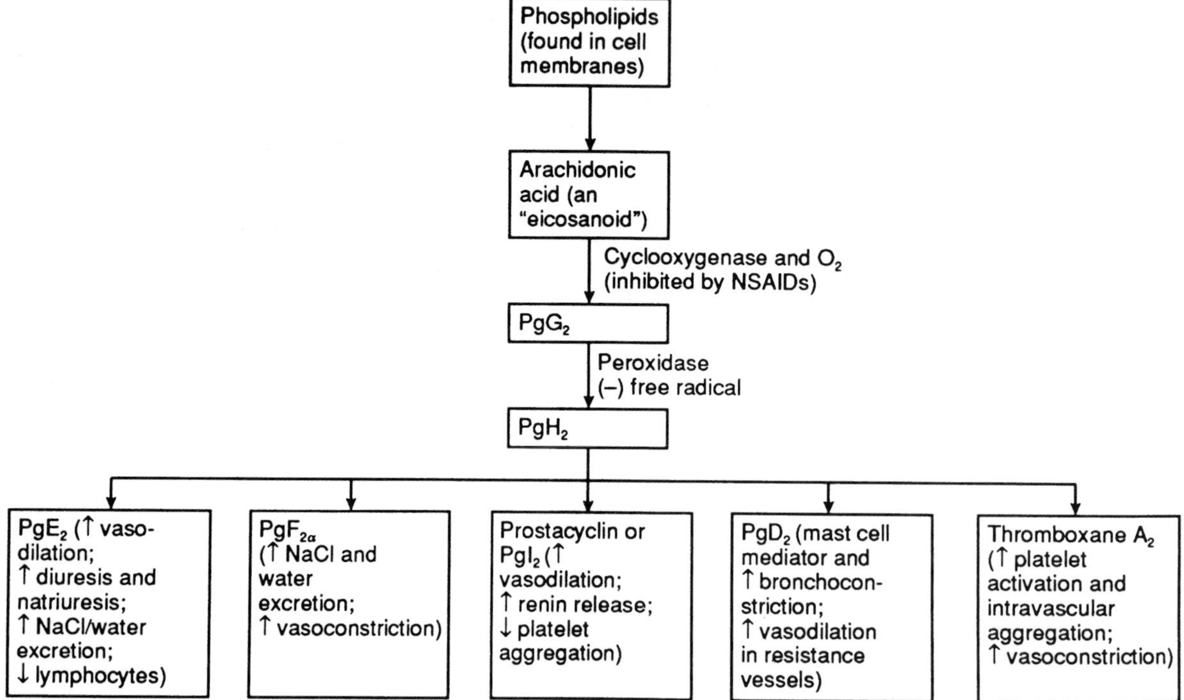

Figure 51–1. Prostaglandin pathway and function.

enjoy a wide therapeutic index, and most overdose cases do not result in serious morbidity and mortality. Nevertheless, severe toxic effects and death can occur with large ingestions.

Chronic NSAID use, particularly in the elderly, causes a greater incidence of toxic and adverse effects. The risk of upper GI tract bleeding is 1.5 to 2.7 times higher in those using NSAIDs than in the general population, with an incidence of 1.0 to 3.3 bleeding events per 1000 users.[24]

The enolic acid NSAIDs are thought to be more toxic in overdose than the carboxylic acids.[5, 12] However, there are multiple exceptions to this, such as the high incidence of serious neurologic effects with mefenamic acid.[7] In chronic use for rheumatoid arthritis, toxicity was consistently greater for indomethacin, tolmetin, meclofenamate, and ketoprofen, whereas the least toxic were the propionic acids ibuprofen and naproxen.[25] Based on case reports, some ranges of toxic doses and serum levels can be established. However, serum quantification for all NSAIDs is neither generally available nor clinically useful.

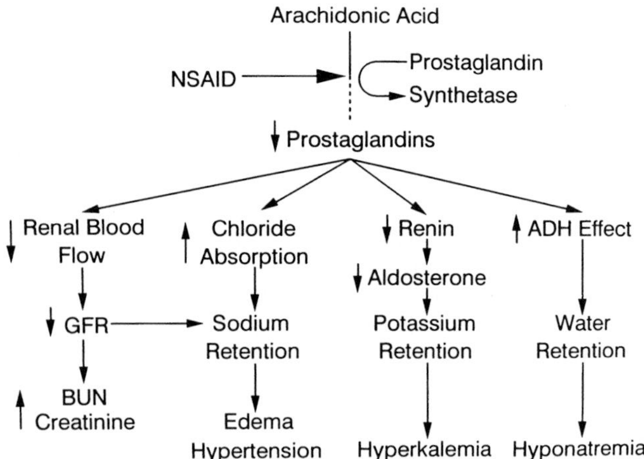

Figure 51–2. The net effect of NSAIDs with prostaglandins. ADH, antidiuretic hormone; GFR, glomerular filtration rate; BUN, blood urea nitrogen.

Ibuprofen

Because of the frequency of its use, considerable data are available on ibuprofen toxicity. In children, doses of less than 100 mg/kg are very unlikely to induce symptoms. In one study, asymptomatic children had a mean ibuprofen dose of 114 mg/kg, but symptoms occurred in those with a mean ingestion of 440 mg/kg.[15, 26] In adults, central nervous system (CNS) symptoms occur only in those who ingest more than 3 g, and renal effects require more than 6 g.[1] Severe symptoms in adults are associated with ingestions of greater than 20 g, although estimated ingestions of up to 60 g have resulted in few or no toxic effects.[1, 26, 27] Complications leading to death have occurred in overdoses of 6.8 g in a child and 24 g in an adult.[15, 26]

As with most overdoses, symptoms correlate better with ibuprofen blood levels than with the history of the ingested amount. In one study, all patients with significant symptoms had plasma ibuprofen levels of greater than 50 μg/mL within 10 hours after ingestion.[1] At 1 to 5 hours postingestion, those with symptoms had a significantly greater mean level (294 μg/mL) than those who were asymptomatic (144 μg/mL).

Renal impairment is associated with levels greater than 280 μg/mL any time within 10 hours postingestion.[16] Multiple organ failure has been reported with levels of 200 to 300 μg/mL at 10 hours postingestion.[27] However, levels up to 725 μg/mL have occurred in asymptomatic patients.[27]

A nomogram of ibuprofen plasma levels versus time postingestion has been constructed to predict the likelihood of toxicity (Fig. 51–3).[1] The nomogram plots a semi-logarithmic line connecting 100 μg/mL at 1 hour and 25 μg/mL at 12 hours postingestion, below which no significant symptoms are expected to occur. However, most ingestions with levels above the line are characterized by only minor symptoms. Considering that symptoms develop within 4 hours of ingestion in most cases, and that ibuprofen levels are usually not readily available, the utility of the nomogram is minimal.[16, 28]

Diflunisal

In children, mild GI symptoms and drowsiness can occur with ingestions of 3.5 g. In adults, only mild symptoms are expected with ingestions of less than 7.5 to 10 g.[12] Serious symptoms can occur with as little as 10 g, although usually more than 15 g is required.[12] Death has been reported with an ingestion of 33 g, but a patient who ingested 29 g survived after a deep coma of 10 hours.[29] The plasma diflunisal level was 500 μg/mL at 16 hours postingestion in a patient with severe symptoms.[12] Levels in fatal cases typically exceed 600 μg/mL.[12] Diflunisal produces false elevations in serum salicylate concentration.

Diclofenac

An acute diclofenac overdose of 1500 mg in a 19-year-old man caused confusion and hypotonia.[14] The

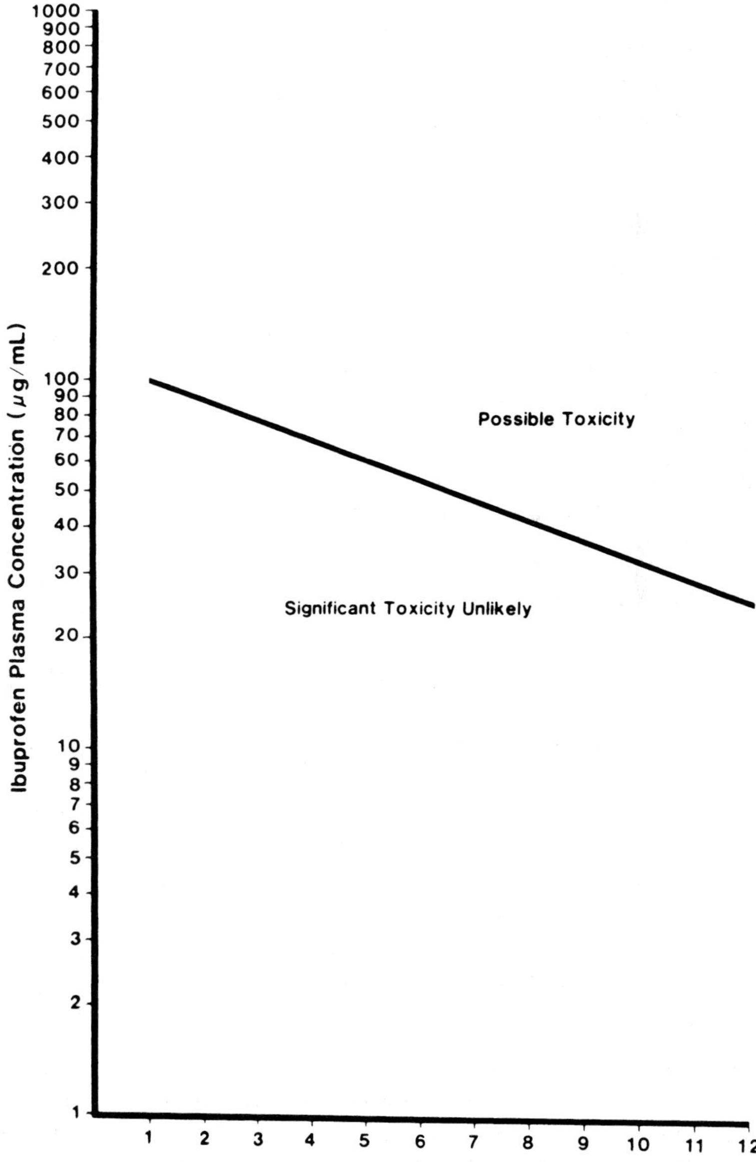

Figure 51–3. Nomogram of ibuprofen plasma levels versus time postingestion, used to predict likelihood of toxicity.

serum level at 7 hours postingestion during the peak toxic effects was 60.1 μg/mL. A 2 g ingestion resulted in renal injury.[30]

Indomethacin

Doses of 75 to 175 mg in children and 175 to 1500 mg in adults have caused only mild CNS or GI symptoms. In a series of 31 indomethacin overdoses in adults, 61% of patients remained asymptomatic and the rest developed only minor GI toxic effects, drowsiness, headache, and tinnitus.[12] Ingestions of 0.5 and 0.9 g caused mild symptoms and plasma levels of 21 and 84 μg/mL, respectively.[17]

Sulindac

Ingestions of 5 to 8 g of sulindac have resulted in mild GI symptoms and brief courses of hematemesis and renal insufficiency.[30] Ingestions of 10 g or more have caused prolonged courses of renal dysfunction.

Naproxen

Ingestions of 3 to 5 g of naproxen have caused mild GI distress and temporary renal insufficiency.[12, 30] Larger overdoses have caused seizures and acidosis.[12, 18]

Flurbiprofen

An ingestion of 3 to 6 g in an adult caused coma and respiratory depression, but it was unknown whether other ingestants were involved.[12]

Fenoprofen

Ingestions of 300 to 3000 mg in children and 2 to 15 g in adults have been reported to cause only mild drowsiness, ataxia, tinnitus, and nausea. However, ingestions of as little as 3.75 g in adults have caused hypotension, tachycardia, and tachypnea.[12] Ingestions of greater than 30 g have resulted in hypotension, coma, and renal failure. A postmortem blood level following death from ingestion of an unknown amount was 711 μg/mL.[12]

Ketoprofen

Overdoses of 2 to 5 g in adults have produced only drowsiness, abdominal pain, and vomiting.[12] Ingestion of an unknown amount in an adolescent resulted in seizures, with a serum level of 1128 μg/mL.[13]

Mefenamic Acid

Seizures can occur with acute overdoses only modestly greater than the recommended maximum daily dose of 1.5 g. A 12-year-old had seizures after a 2.5 g ingestion, and adults can suffer convulsions after doses of less than 5 g.[12] Ingestions of 12 to 15 g have produced status epilepticus, coma, and renal failure.[7, 12]

Seizures have occurred in patients with mefenamic acid plasma levels at or just above the maximum therapeutic level of 10 μg/mL. In one study, plasma concentrations in patients who had convulsions were significantly higher than in those without (73 versus 38 μg/mL).[7] Most patients with seizures have concentrations above a semi-logarithmic line plot connecting 100 μg/mL at 2 hours and 5 μg/mL at 15 hours postingestion.[7] However, seizures can occur with levels well below this line.

Phenylbutazone

Acute phenylbutazone overdoses in children of 1.7 to 3 g result in toxic effects, and death can occur after doses of 2 to 5 g.[12] Severe toxic effects occur in adults after ingestions of 4 to 8 g or more, and death occurs with doses of 14 to 28 g.[8, 12]

Piroxicam

Ingestion of 200 to 400 mg appears to cause only mild symptoms, although 100 mg in a child caused severe multisystem toxicity.[12] Doses of 600 mg in adults have the potential for severe toxicity.

Clinical Effects

Overdoses of NSAIDs result in most cases in minimal or no toxicity. Symptoms that occur are only mild GI or neurologic effects such as abdominal pain, nausea, vomiting, lethargy, confusion, headache, or blurred vision.

In studies of acute overdoses of ibuprofen in adults, about 60% remain asymptomatic, 30% to 40% develop mild to moderate symptoms, and fewer than 3% suffer severe symptoms.[1, 31] Of the symptomatic group, onset is within 4 hours of ingestion and effects are usually of short duration. Severe and even life-threatening toxic effects include acidosis, GI bleeding, dizziness, seizures, coma, respiratory depression, hypotension, and hepatic and renal injury.

The elderly and those with preexisting renal, cardiovascular, or hepatic disease are at particular risk for development of adverse effects with chronic NSAID use. Most organ systems can be involved, but gastrointestinal effects are the most common and account for the majority or deaths from chronic use.

Gastrointestinal

GI effects, primarily nausea, vomiting, diarrhea, and abdominal pain, are common in both overdose and chronic use.[12, 15, 31] The incidence of GI complaints in acute ibuprofen overdose has ranged from 6% to 42%.[26, 27, 32] Peptic ulceration and gastrointestinal hemorrhage are rare in acute overdose; the incidence in chronic use is 1.5%.[7, 31] The associated fluid losses and resultant dehydration cause hypotension, acidosis, and acute renal failure. Acute mild pancreatitis has also been reported after short courses of NSAIDs.[33]

Neurologic

CNS depression is one of the most common effects of NSAID overdose and chronic use.[3, 12, 15] This may range from drowsiness to coma, and it occurred with 30% of ibuprofen overdoses in one series.[32] Coma can occur independent of hypotension, respiratory depression, seizures, or acidosis.[34] Decreased memory and ability to concentrate have been reported with chronic NSAID use, particularly in the elderly taking indomethacin, sulindac, and naproxen.[3]

Seizures occur most commonly after mefenamic overdose, but they have also been reported in overdoses of naproxen, piroxicam, ibuprofen, and ketoprofen.[7, 12, 15, 18] Acute delirium, psychosis, hallucinations, and myoclonus have been described, particularly with indomethacin, sulindac, and mefenamic acid.[3, 7] The mechanism is unexplained, but it is known that indomethacin and sulindac have structural similarities to serotonin.

Aseptic meningitis has occurred rarely with therapeutic NSAID use, usually in patients with systemic lupus erythematosus, but it can occur in otherwise healthy patients.[3] Other neurologic effects include tinnitus, deafness, ataxia, nystagmus, headache, and disorientation.[5, 17]

Metabolic

Metabolic acidosis has been described in adults and children, usually in association with seizures, hypotension, or renal failure.[12, 18, 26, 35] However, metabolic acidosis with increased anion gap has also been reported in the absence of these other effects.[1] The weakly acidic nature of NSAIDs and their metabolites may account for some of this acidosis.[31]

Hyperkalemia is a reported but unusual complication of NSAIDs after therapeutic use and overdose.[22] This can be a result of direct NSAID effect on cellular potassium uptake and delivery to distal renal tubules or of transient renal impairment. Hyponatremia and fluid losses result from both NSAID-induced gastroenteritis and inhibition of prostaglandin-mediated diuresis and natriuresis.

Hematologic

Thrombocytopenia, prolonged prothrombin times, agranulocytosis, and pancytopenia have been reported with acute ibuprofen, piroxicam, naproxen, and etodolac overdoses.[17, 36] Decrease of platelet aggregation and adhesiveness contribute to bleeding disorders and gastrointestinal hemorrhage. With therapeutic use, hematologic effects are uncommon, but they cause a disproportionate number of deaths. Aplastic anemia, agranulocytosis, hemolytic anemia, and thrombocytopenia have been associated with therapeutic use of various NSAIDs.[31, 33, 37]

Hepatic

Hepatotoxicity of both hepatocellular and cholestatic types has occurred with use of all classes of NSAIDs, but it is most common with phenylbutazone and sulindac. The incidence of chronic NSAID-induced hepatic injury is low at 1.1 events per 100,000 prescriptions, and it is seen only rarely in acute overdose.[38] The usual finding is mild elevation of transaminase level, which resolves after discontinuation of the drug. More severe involvement can occur as part of multi-organ involvement. The at-risk populations appear to be the elderly and patients with autoimmune connective tissue diseases, and the mechanism is likely a hypersensitivity reaction.

Renal

Problems associated with chronic use of NSAIDs are now among the most common reasons for hospitalization of patients with renal function abnormalities. It has been estimated that about 1% of those taking NSAIDs on a chronic basis will develop some deterioration of renal function.[22] In acute overdose, renal failure has also been well described in case series and in isolated case reports.[15, 39–41]

Acute renal insufficiency, as a result of alterations in renal blood flow and glomerular filtration rates, is the most common renal complication. Those dependent on prostaglandin-mediated renal regulation are most at risk, including those with volume depletion, congestive heart failure, cirrhosis, hypoalbuminemia, advanced age, and preexisting renal disease.[39] However, renal failure has also been described after acute overdose in healthy individuals and in brief therapeutic use after binge alcohol drinking.[15, 39–41] This may be mediated by increased formation of the leukotrienes, causing renal vasoconstriction and mesangial cell contraction.[40] The renal insufficiency is typically mild; it resolves within 24 to 72 hours and may be oliguric or nonoliguric. The presentation consists of flank pain, elevated blood urea nitrogen (BUN) and creatinine levels, and, in chronic cases, weight gain and hyperkalemia. Urinalysis may show microscopic hematuria and cell casts. In cases associated with other severe manifestations such as coma, acidosis, and hypotension, recovery may be prolonged and require hemodialysis.[35]

Acute interstitial nephritis and the nephrotic syndrome have been reported after short courses of NSAIDs or with chronic use.[9] This syndrome has most often been associated with the acetic and propionic acid derivatives and is a hypersensitivity reaction.[21] Proteinuria is usually, but not always, present. Hemodialysis is required in as many as a third of these cases.[9]

Cardiopulmonary

Hypotension and tachycardia, most likely secondary to volume depletion, occur in fewer than 5% of cases.[15, 32] Congestive heart failure may result from chronic NSAID-induced fluid and salt retention.[31]

Respiratory depression and arrest are unusual-but-reported manifestations of NSAID overdose.[15, 34] Adult respiratory distress syndrome (ARDS) has occurred in the setting of severe multi-organ toxic effects.[35] Bronchospasm may be precipitated by NSAIDs, especially in persons with drug allergies or asthma.[31]

Diagnosis

NSAID toxic effects should be suspected in the case of any overdose that is accompanied by a symptom constellation of gastroenteritis, CNS depression, metabolic acidosis, and renal insufficiency. Ibuprofen (and other NSAIDs) should be included in the differential diagnosis of an increased anion gap acidosis. The clinical appearance with NSAID toxicity can mimic that with salicylate toxicity (acidosis, tachypnea, altered mental status, gastritis) without tinnitus. NSAID toxicity should also be suspected with a history of over-the-counter analgesic ingestion when acetaminophen and salicylates are undetected in the blood.

Laboratory studies for serious overdoses should include assay of electrolytes with anion gap calculation, complete blood count, coagulation studies, and arterial blood gas, BUN, creatinine, and transaminase levels. Renal insufficiency is unlikely to occur if an adult ingests less than 6 g, so renal function tests are not routinely necessary in these cases.[1] In patients at high risk for renal or hepatic complications, baseline renal and liver function tests should be performed prior to initiating NSAID therapy and again in 5 to 7 days.

Routine ibuprofen assays are not particularly useful or predictive of outcomes.[32] However, quantification of ibuprofen levels might be useful to determine if an initially asymptomatic patient will remain so. If the ibuprofen level is in the "significant toxicity unlikely" region (see Fig. 51–3), the patient can safely be discharged from medical care without further observation.[1]

Treatment

Supportive Measures

The therapy of NSAID toxicity is primarily supportive and symptomatic, and there is no antidote. Early correction of any volume depletion is essential to maintain adequate renal blood flow. Hypotension usually responds to fluid replacement, but a short course of vasopressors may be required. Dopamine, in doses of 2 to 5 μg/kg per minute, may be particularly useful in maintaining renal blood flow in patients at high risk of renal insufficiency.[34] Acidosis should resolve with aggressive hydration, but intravenous (IV) administration of sodium bicarbonate, 1 to 2 mEq/kg, may be required if the serum pH is less than 7.1.

The coagulopathies of NSAID overdose rarely warrant specific therapy unless active bleeding is occurring. In such cases, fresh frozen plasma and phytonadione (vitamin K_1), 10 to 20 mg IV, would be appropriate.

Seizures may require immediate therapy with benzodiazepines, such as diazepam, 5 to 10 mg IV (0.2 mg/kg in children). As with most drug-induced seizures, phenytoin is unlikely to be effective, and long-term treatment is usually unnecessary.

Antacids, H_2-receptor antagonists, and/or sucralfate may be considered for reducing any prolonged gastrointestinal effects.[5]

Decontamination

Activated charcoal has been shown to reduce absorption of piroxicam, mefenamic acid, and phenylbutazone, and it is likely to adsorb other NSAIDs as well.[5, 42] Syrup of ipecac and gastric lavage have also been recommended, but effectiveness of these methods has not been studied in NSAID overdose.

Decontamination has been recommended if the amount ingested is more than 10 times the therapeutic dose for adults or 5 times the dose for children.[5] For ibuprofen, decontamination is thought to be unnecessary in children if less than 100 mg/kg is ingested (10 times the therapeutic dose).[15] Although syrup of ipecac has been suggested for child ingestions of ibuprofen of 100 to 400 mg/kg, the symptoms created by ipecac are indistinguishable from ibuprofen toxicity in this dosage range.[5, 15, 32] Because of the rapid absorption of NSAIDs, it is unlikely that decontamination will be of benefit more than 2 to 4 hours postingestion.[5, 11] Patients who have taken overdoses of NSAIDs that carry a high risk of seizures, such as mefenamic acid, or large amounts of other NSAIDs, including more than 400 mg/kg of ibuprofen, should not be given syrup of ipecac.[5, 15]

Elimination Enhancement

Because NSAIDs are greater than 90% protein bound, extensively metabolized, and excreted in essentially unchanged form, it is unlikely that elimination would be enhanced by any method.[5, 11] This has been supported by a lack of efficacy of hemodialysis and hemoperfusion in limited studies.[5, 8] Nevertheless, hemoperfusion has been employed in phenylbutazone overdoses with some limited success.[5] Hemodialysis may be necessary in cases of prolonged or severe renal failure following NSAID overdose.[9, 35]

Multiple doses of activated charcoal have been reported to enhance the elimination of phenylbutazone, indomethacin, and piroxicam by interrupting enterohepatic and/or enteroenteric recirculation.[5, 42] This benefit might also be expected in sulindac, diclofenac, flufenamic acid, and ibuprofen, all of which also undergo some enterohepatic recirculation.[15] However, this therapy would be warranted only in the small number of severely symptomatic patients.

Disposition

Ingestions of greater than 10 times the therapeutic dose of NSAIDs other than ibuprofen in adults, or greater than 5 times in children, probably warrant observation in a medical facility for 4 to 6 hours postingestion.[5, 15] For ibuprofen, ingestions of greater than 300 mg/kg in children and greater than 6 to 20 g in adults warrant observation.[15] Mild symptoms usually resolve quickly and may not necessitate hospitalization. The development of CNS depression, acidosis, seizures, or renal insufficiency should mandate admission and careful monitoring.

COLCHICINE

Colchicine is not an NSAID, but it is included here because of its use as an anti-inflammatory agent in gouty arthritis. It is an alkaloid that can be extracted from two plants of the lily family, *Colchicum autumnale* (autumn crocus, meadow saffron) and *Gloriosa superba* (glory lily).

Colchicum was first recognized as a poison in the 3rd century BC by the Egyptian Dioscorides.[43] In the 6th century AD, Alexander of Trallis first recommended colchicum as a cathartic in the treatment of joint pain.[44] It was advocated as a diuretic in *The New Edinburgh Dispensatory* in 1788 and recommended as specific therapy for gout in medical texts of the early 1800s. It was probably introduced into the United States as therapy for gout by Benjamin Franklin.[43] In 1820, colchicine was isolated from the *C. autumnale* tuber and rapidly gained popularity. It is now used to treat acute gouty arthritis, as prophylaxis for familial Mediterranean fever, and experimentally to study cell division in cytogenetics because of its antimitotic activity.

The infrequency of colchicine use is reflected in the report by the AAPCC of only 125 toxic exposures in 1994, with 4 deaths.[2] Nevertheless, toxic effects may be encountered after accidental, suicidal, or therapeutic use of colchicine tablets. The tubers of the glory lily have also been mistakenly ingested due to their similarity to sweet potatoes. Large volumes of the plants are required to cause toxicity, but the effects are similar to those with tablet ingestion.

Classification and Structure

The alkaloid colchicine has the chemical formula *N*-(5,6,7,9-tetrahydro-1,2,3,10-tetramethoxy-9-oxobenzo[a]heptalen-7-yl) acetamide. The structure is shown in Figure 51–4.[45] Pharmaceutical colchicine is available as 0.5 and 0.6 mg tablets and as a parenteral solution of 0.5 mg/mL. *Colchicum* spp. are cultivated and are popular as houseplants. The species *C. autumnale* has long, tubular purple or white flowers with seeds, and plants emerge from an underground corm or bulb.

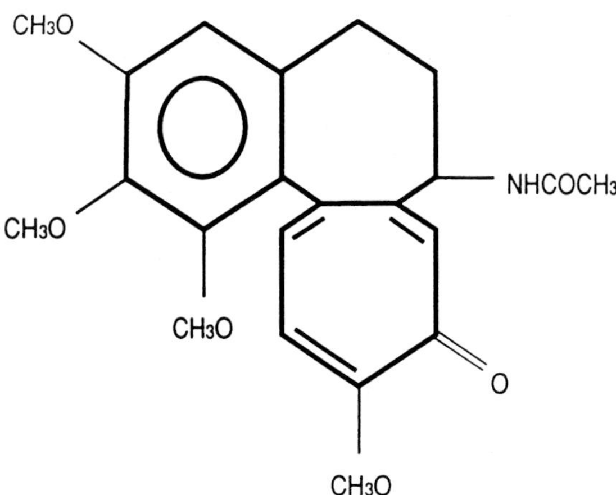

Figure 51–4. Chemical structure of colchicine.

Pharmacokinetics

Colchicine is rapidly absorbed from the GI tract, reaching peak plasma levels within 0.5 to 2 hours.[43] Bioavailability has been estimated to be 25% to 40%.[44] Because higher doses affect jejunal and ileal function, prolonged absorption may occur in toxic doses.[44] However, this was not observed in one study of human poisoning cases.[46]

Approximately 50% of circulating colchicine is bound to plasma proteins. Initial distribution half-lives range from 45 to 90 minutes, and distribution is complete after 3 to 6 hours.[46] The volume of distribution is 2.2 L/kg, but it was reported to be 21 L/kg in patients with toxic effects.[46] A range of 12% to 44% of colchicine is excreted unchanged in the urine with therapeutic doses, similar to the 30% excretion found in overdose. In patients with liver disease, a larger fraction of the drug is excreted unchanged. Metabolism is primarily via deacetylation in the liver, followed by biliary excretion. Significant enterohepatic recirculation occurs, as demonstrated by presence of the parent drug and metabolites in large amounts in bile and intestinal secretions.

The terminal plasma elimination half-life in therapeutic doses has ranged from 9.3 to 31 hours.[44, 46] This is similar to half-lives of 10.6 to 31.7 hours in toxic ingestions.

Drug Interactions

Cimetidine, a cytochrome P-450 inhibitor, causes an increase in colchicine elimination half-life.[44] Likewise, erythromycin has the potential for inhibiting hepatic metabolism of colchicine. Cyclosporine toxicity has resulted with concomitant use of colchicine.

Mechanism of Action and Toxicity

Colchicine binds to intracellular tubulin, a structural protein necessary for motility. This protein binding prevents spindle formation and inhibits cell mitosis. This arrest in cell division in the metaphase affects cells with the highest turnover rate, such as intestinal epithelium, bone marrow, and hair follicles. Its action in gout is to reduce phagocytosis of urate crystals by leukocytes. Colchicine also binds to the terminal portion of tubulin, with inhibition of microtubule function.[47] This may explain some aspects of the multi-organ failure seen in colchicine toxicity, particularly cardiac failure.[48]

Range of Toxic Effects

The usual colchicine dose is 0.5 to 1.0 mg every 2 to 3 hours until relief or GI symptoms occur. Because GI warning symptoms do not occur with IV dosing, the recommended IV dose is half of the equivalent oral dose to a maximum of 4 mg per acute episode.[44] Colchicine is contraindicated in combined hepatorenal disease, with creatinine clearances below 10 mL/min, and in extrahepatic biliary obstruction.[45] Because of reduced elimination, doses should be no larger than 0.6 mg/day if the creatinine clearance is less than 50 mL/min or serum creatinine is greater than 1.6 mg/dL.[49]

Fatalities have occurred with total doses of 8 to 11 mg given therapeutically over several days.[44] Ingestions of 0.5 to 0.8 mg/kg result in severe toxic effects, and doses greater than 0.8 mg/kg or a total of 40 mg are said to almost invariably be fatal.[44] However, severe toxic effects followed by survival have occurred with doses of 50 to 60 mg (>1 mg/kg).[44, 47] Colchicine-containing plants rarely produce severe toxicity due to the low concentrations of toxin. Ten grams of tuber contain about 6 mg of colchicine, and 100 to 125 g of tubers (60 to 95 mg of colchicine) have produced severe toxic effects.[50]

Colchicine plasma levels do not correlate well with level of toxicity and are not clinically useful. Concentrations in acute ingestions accompanied by only GI effects ranged from 11 to 63 ng/mL within 4 hours of exposure.[46] At 27 hours postingestion in a patient with severe hemodynamic instability, the level was 24 ng/mL.[48]

Clinical Presentation

The clinical manifestations of colchicine overdose involve multiple organ systems, including GI, respiratory, hematologic, cardiovascular, renal, and neurologic. Symptoms have been characterized as occurring in three phases after a latent period of 4 to 12 hours.[51] The first phase is characterized by GI symptoms with fluid losses and hypovolemic shock. Life-threatening complications occur during the second stage at 24 to 72 hours. At this time, cardiac insufficiency, arrhythmias, bone marrow depression, renal failure, hepatic injury, respiratory distress, coagulopathies, and neuromuscular involvement are present. This phase can last for 5 to 7 days and is followed by a recovery phase marked by a rebound leukocytosis and alopecia. The duration and features of each phase are outlined in Table 51–4, and details of each involved organ system are described in the following text.

Gastrointestinal

Nausea, vomiting, diarrhea, and burning abdominal pain are the initial symptoms of colchicine toxicity, and they may serve a protective effect by warning of the potential for further toxicity with continued use of the drug. Severe dehydration, hypovolemia, and cardiovascular collapse can result if aggressive treatment is not instituted. GI effects are not prominent after IV use, suggesting a local action of colchicine on gut epithelial cells. Hepatocellular damage and hepatomegaly can also occur, with elevation of transaminase and alkaline phosphatase levels, but fulminant hepatic failure occurs very rarely.[47] Pancreatitis has also been reported.

Cardiovascular

Hypotension occurs due to volume losses, extravasation of fluid into extracellular spaces, and myocardial depression. Development of cardiogenic shock due to a postulated direct myocardial injury is a poor prognostic sign.[52] Colchicine is also thought to impair cardiac conduction, leading to arrhythmias and even late asystole.[51] Marked electrocardiographic (ECG) changes indicative of myocardial injury can occur, with ST- and T-wave changes.[50]

Respiratory

Respiratory distress occurs in about a third of cases and is a result of generalized muscle weakness and ARDS.[45] Colchicine is thought to have a direct toxic effect on the lungs, causing capillary leakage. Prolonged hypotension, sepsis, and multi-organ failure probably also play a major role in this syndrome.

Neurologic

Mental status depression may progress to delirium, seizures, and coma. Peripheral neuropathy, loss of deep tendon reflexes, and ascending paralysis can also occur.[44, 51, 52] Myelin degeneration is thought to be the cause.[45]

Hematologic

The first phase of toxicity includes a peripheral leukocytosis, followed by bone marrow depression in the second phase. Severe leukopenia, thrombocytopenia, and a consumptive coagulopathy peak at 4 to 7 days postingestion.[47] Disseminated intravascular coagulation and sepsis often complicate this phase. Hematologic studies show hypoprothrombinemia, decreased fibrinogen, and increased fibrin split products. At 8 to 10 days postingestion, bone marrow

Table 51–4. Phases of Colchicine Toxicity

Phase	Complication	Treatment
I (0–12 h)	GI symptoms	Gastric lavage to ensure removal of all pills from stomach
	Volume depletion	IV fluid replacement; treatment of shock with use of pressure if needed
	Peripheral leukocytosis	
II (2–7 d)	Respiratory distress, ARDS, hypoxemia	Supplemental oxygen, ET intubation and mechanical ventilation, PEEP
	Cardiovascular shock	Monitor, CVP, Swan-Ganz, fluids, pressors
	Thrombocytopenia, DIC	Replacement therapy with blood products
	Myelosuppression, neutropenia	Blood cultures, treatment with antibiotics
	Hyponatremia, hypocalcemia, hypophosphatemia	Electrolyte replacement
	Metabolic acidosis	Maintain volume status; treatment with HCO_3 if necessary
	Rhabdomyolysis, myoglobinuria, oliguric renal failure	Fluids, diuretics to maintain urine output
III (1–2 wk)	Rebound leukocytosis, alopecia	

recovery is apparent, and a rebound leukocytosis occurs during the recovery phase.

Renal

Renal failure is common in severe colchicine toxicity, probably secondary to hypovolemia, hypoxia, and myoglobinuria.[45] The typical picture is of oliguria responsive to fluids, hematuria, and proteinuria.[50] There is no evidence of direct renal toxicity, although colchicine does concentrate in the kidneys.[46]

Metabolic/Electrolytes

A lactic acid metabolic acidosis is common, again due to hypotension and hypovolemia. This is exacerbated by inhibition of intracellular metabolism and accumulation of organic acids.[51] Hypophosphatemia, hyponatremia, hypocalcemia, and hypomagnesemia occur, primarily due to fluid losses. Hypocalcemia is also thought to be due to direct suppression of bone resorption by colchicine.[44] A direct myopathic effect of colchicine also leads to muscle weakness, necrosis, and rhabdomyolysis.[47]

Alopecia

Scalp hair loss is common and typically occurs during the recovery phase, but it can occur anytime between 6 and 30 days postingestion.[44, 47] Hair growth almost always recovers several weeks after exposure.

Diagnosis

The colchicine toxidrome of gastroenteritis, hypotension, lactic acidosis, and prerenal azotemia could be mistaken for NSAID toxicity. The development later in the course of peripheral neuropathy and alopecia could commonly be mistaken for heavy metal poisoning. Differentiation from both is possible by the presence of severe bone marrow suppression in the second phase of colchicine toxicity.

Laboratory monitoring should include frequent measurements of electrolytes, (including calcium, magnesium, and phosphate), platelets, and creatine kinase; CBC count; prothrombin time; renal and liver function tests; and urinalysis for myoglobinuria. If coagulopathy is suspected, fibrinogen and fibrin split products should be monitored. In severe or persistent hypotension, pulmonary catheter monitoring is warranted. Colchicine measurements are not clinically useful except to establish or confirm the diagnosis.

Treatment

Initial Supportive Measures

Initial therapy must be directed toward aggressive replacement of fluid losses and correction of hypotension with vasopressors, if hemodynamic instability is present. If the latter therapy is necessary, it should be guided by Swan-Ganz catheter placement and measurement of hemodynamic parameters. This is important, given the propensity for myocardial depression, hypovolemia, alterations in systemic vascular resistance, and ARDS. Respiratory deterioration may require endotracheal intubation, mechanical ventilation, and positive end-expiratory pressure.

Transfusions of whole blood, fresh-frozen plasma, vitamin K, and platelets may be necessary to treat coagulopathies. Because of frequent sepsis complicating neutropenia, the use of broad-spectrum antibiotics should be considered in febrile patients.

Decontamination

Gastric emptying is warranted if the patient presents during the latent period prior to the onset of gastroenteritis and a potentially toxic amount (>5 to 10 mg in adults) has been ingested. Adsorption of colchicine by activated charcoal has not been studied but is thought to be effective. Even late decontamination should be performed, because large residual amounts of colchicine have been found in the stomach many hours after ingestion. The known enterohepatic recirculation of colchicine also supports late and repeated doses of activated charcoal, but paralytic ileus may complicate this approach. In such cases, duodenal tube suction could be utilized. Cathartics should not be routinely employed due to the expected onset of spontaneous diarrhea.

Antidotes

Colchicine-specific Fab fragments have been developed and used with success in studies in laboratory animals.[48] The Fab fragments are prepared from the antiserum of goats immunized with colchicine, and their infusion results in reversal of colchicine binding to tubulin. This investigational agent has now also been successfully employed in a case of severe toxicity in a human without any adverse effects.[48] Administration of the Fab fragments resulted in a rapid reversal of life-threatening hemodynamic instability, although bone marrow suppression did not significantly improve. The dose given was 480 mg of colchicine-specific Fab fragments, with half given over 1 hour and the remainder over the ensuing 6 hours.[48] However, this agent remains an investigational antidote and is available only in Europe.

Granulocyte colony-stimulating factor (G-CSF) has been used in colchicine toxicity in an attempt to accelerate production of neutrophils within the bone marrow.[47] In such cases, an accelerated leukocytosis was observed within 1 to 2 days, but at a time when rebound leukocytosis may naturally occur. Because colchicine-induced bone marrow suppression is short-lived, use of G-CSF should be considered only in life-threatening sepsis during the second phase of toxicity.

Enhanced Elimination

As discussed with decontamination, repeated doses of activated charcoal should theoretically enhance colchicine elimination because of its enterohepatic recirculation, but this has not been tested. This treatment would almost certainly be problematic due to the presence of emesis and, possibly, paralytic ileus. With its large volume of distribution, high protein binding, and relatively small fraction of renal excretion, it is unlikely that forced diuresis, hemodialysis, exchange transfusion, or hemoperfusion would be effective.[49]

Disposition

Because of its narrow therapeutic index and latent phase, any patient should be observed for 8 to 12 hours after acute ingestion of colchicine. The onset of GI symptoms or leukocytosis warrants hospital admission until at least the second phase of toxicity has ended.

References

1. Hall AH, Smolinske SC, Stover B, et al: Ibuprofen overdose in adults. J Toxicol Clin Toxicol *30*:23, 1992.
2. Litovitz TL, Felberg AL, Soloway RA, et al: 1994 Annual Report of the American Association of Poison Control Centers Toxic Exposure Surveillance System. Am J Emerg Med *13*:551–597, 1995.
3. Hoppmann RA, Peden JG, Ober SK: Central nervous system side effects of nonsteroidal anti-inflammatory drugs. Arch Intern Med *151*:1309, 1991.
4. Simon LS: Actions and toxicity of nonsteroidal anti-inflammatory drugs. Curr Opin Rheumatol *7*:159, 1995.
5. Vale JA, Meredith TJ: Acute poisoning due to non-steroidal anti-inflammatory drugs. Clinical features and management. Med Toxicol *1*:12, 1986.
6. Boynton CS, Dick CF, Mayor GH: NSAIDs: An overview. J Clin Pharmacol *28*:512, 1988.
7. Balali-Mood M, Proudfoot AT, Critchley JAJH, et al: Mefenamic acid overdosage. Lancet *1*:1354, 1981.
8. Prescott LF, Critchley JAJH, Balali-Mood M: Phenylbutazone overdosage: Abnormal metabolism associated with hepatic and renal damage. Br Med J *281*:1106, 1980.
9. Abt AB, Oh JY, Huntington RA, et al: Chinese herbal medicine induced acute renal failure. Arch Intern Med *155*:211, 1995.
10. Murray MD, Brater DC: Renal toxicity of the nonsteroidal anti-inflammatory drugs. Annu Rev Pharmacol Toxicol *33*:435, 1993.
11. Verbeeck RK, Blackburn JL, Loewen GR: Clinical pharmacokinetics of non-steroidal antiinflammatory drugs. Clin Pharmacokinet *8*:297, 1983.
12. Court H, Volans GN: Poisoning after overdose with non-steroidal and anti-inflammatory drugs. Adverse Drug React Toxicol Rev *3*:1, 1984.
13. Bond GR, Curry SC, Arnold-Capell PA, et al: Generalized seizures and metabolic acidosis after ketoprofen overdose. Vet Hum Toxicol *31*:369, 1989.
14. Netter P, Lambert H, Larcan A, et al: Diclofenac sodium-chlormezanone poisoning. Eur J Clin Pharmacol *26*:535, 1984.
15. Hall AH, Smolinske SC, Conrad FL, et al: Ibuprofen overdose: 126 cases. Ann Emerg Med *15*:1308, 1986.
16. Jenkinson ML, Fitzpatrick R, Streete PJ, et al: The relationship between plasma ibuprofen concentrations and toxicity in acute ibuprofen overdose. Hum Toxicol *7*:319, 1988.
17. Sheehan TMT, Boldy DAR, Vale JA, et al: Indomethacin poisoning. Clin Toxicol *24*:151, 1986.
18. Martinez R, Smith DW, Frankel LR: Severe metabolic acidosis after acute naproxen sodium ingestion. Ann Emerg Med *18*:129, 1989.
19. Backer RC, Kshirsagar VH, Sopher IM: Case report: Zomepirac suicide. J Anal Toxicol *7*:223, 1983.
20. Johnson AG, Seideman P, Day RO: Adverse drug interactions with nonsteroidal anti-inflammatory drugs (NSAIDs): Recognition, management and avoidance. Drug Saf 8:99, 1993.
21. Aronoff GR: Nonsteroidal anti-inflammatory drug induced renal syndromes. J Ky Med Assoc *90*:336, 1992.
22. Whelton A, Hamilton CW: Non-steroidal anti-inflammatory drugs: Effects on kidney function. J Clin Pharmacol *31*:588, 1991.
23. Boelsterli UA, Zimmerman HJ, Kretz-Rommel A: Idiosyncratic liver toxicity of nonsteroidal antiinflammatory drugs: Molecular mechanisms and pathology. Crit Rev Toxicol *25*:207, 1995.
24. Carson JL, Willett LR: Toxicity of nonsteroidal anti-inflammatory drugs: An overview of the epidemiological evidence. Drugs *46*(suppl 1):243, 1993.
25. Fries JF, Williams CA, Bloch DA: The relative toxicity of nonsteroidal antiinflammatory drugs. Arthritis Rheum *34*:1353, 1991.

26. Hall AH, Rumack BH: Treatment of patients with ibuprofen overdose. Ann Emerg Med *17*:185, 1988.
27. Court H, Streete P, Volans GN: Overdose with ibuprofen causing unconsciousness and hypotension. Br Med J *282*:1073, 1981.
29. Upadhyay HP, Gupta SK: Diflunisal (Dolobid) overdose. Br Med J *2*:640, 1978.
30. Kulling PE, Backman EA, Skagius AS: Renal impairment after acute diclofenac, naproxen, and sulindac overdoses. J Toxicol Clin Toxicol *33*:173, 1995.
31. Halpern SM, Fitzpatrick R, Volans GN: Ibuprofen toxicity: A review of adverse reactions and overdose. Adverse Drug React Toxicol Rev *12*:107, 1993.
32. McElwee NE, Veltri JC, Bradford DC, et al: A prospective, population-based study of acute ibuprofen overdose: Complications are rare and routine serum levels not warranted. Ann Emerg Med *19*:657, 1990.
33. Jick SS, Walker AM, Perera DR, et al: Non-steroidal anti-inflammatory drugs and hospital admission for perforated peptic ulcer. Lancet *2*:380, 1987.
34. Bright TP, McNulty CJ: Suspected central nervous system toxicity from inadvertent nonsteroidal antiinflammatory drug overdose. DICP Ann Clin Pharmacother *25*:1066, 1991.
35. Le HT, Bosse GM, Tasi YY: Ibuprofen overdose complicated by renal failure, adult respiratory distress syndrome, and metabolic acidosis. J Toxicol Clin Toxicol *32*:315, 1994.
36. Waugh PK, Keatinge DW: Hypoprothrombinemia in naproxen overdosage. Drug Intell Clin Pharmacol *17*:549, 1983.
37. Inman WHW: Study of fatal bone marrow depression with special reference to phenylbutazone and oxyphenbutazone. Br Med J *1*:1500, 1977.
38. Rodriguez LAG, Williams R, Derby LE, et al: Acute liver injury associated with nonsteroidal anti-inflammatory drugs and the role of risk factors. Arch Intern Med *154*:311, 1994.
39. Wen SF, Parthasarathy R, Iliopoulos O, et al: Acute renal failure following binge drinking and nonsteroidal antiinflammatory drugs. Am J Kidney Dis *20*:281, 1992.
40. Perazella MA, Buller GK: Can ibuprofen cause acute renal failure in a normal individual? A case of acute overdose. Am J Kidney Dis *18*:600, 1991.
41. Kim J, Gazarian M, Verjee Z, et al: Acute renal insufficiency in ibuprofen overdose. Pediatr Emerg Care *11*:107, 1995.
42. Laufen H, Leitold M: The effect of activated charcoal on the bioavailability of piroxicam in man. Int J Clin Pharmacol Ther Toxicol *24*:48, 1986.
43. Mack RB: Achilles and his evil squeeze: Colchicine poisoning. N C Med J *52*:581–583, 1991.
44. Putterman C, Chetrit EB, Caraco Y, et al: Colchicine intoxication: Clinical pharmacology, risk factors, features, and management. Semin Arthritis Rheum *21*:143–155, 1991.
45. Hood RL: Colchicine poisoning. J Emerg Med *12*:171–177, 1992.
46. Rochdi M, Sabouraud A, Baud FJ: Toxicokinetics of colchicine in humans: Analysis of tissue, plasma and urine data in ten cases. Hum Exp Toxicol *11*:510–516, 1992.
47. Folpini A, Furfori P: Colchicine toxicity clinical features and treatment: Massive overdose case report. Clin Toxicol *33*:71–77, 1995.
48. Baud FJ, Sabouraud A, Vicaut E, et al: Brief report: Treatment of severe colchicine overdose with colchicine-specific Fab fragments. N Engl J Med *332*:642–643, 1995.
49. Wallace SL, Singer JZ, Duncan GJ, et al: Renal function predicts colchicine toxicity: Guidelines for the prophylactic use of colchicine in gout. J Rheumatol *18*:264–269, 1991.
50. Mendis S: Colchicine cardiotoxicity following ingestion of *Gloriosa superba* tubers. Postgrad Med J *65*:752–755, 1989.
51. Stapczynski JS, Rothstein RJ, Gaye WA, et al: Colchicine overdose: Report of two cases and review of the literature. Ann Emerg Med *10*:364–369, 1981.
52. De Deyn PP, Cauterick C, Saxena V, et al: Chronic colchicine-induced myopathy and neuropathy. Acta Neurol Belg *95*:29–32, 1995.

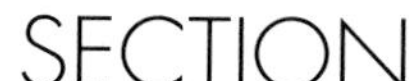

SECTION **D**

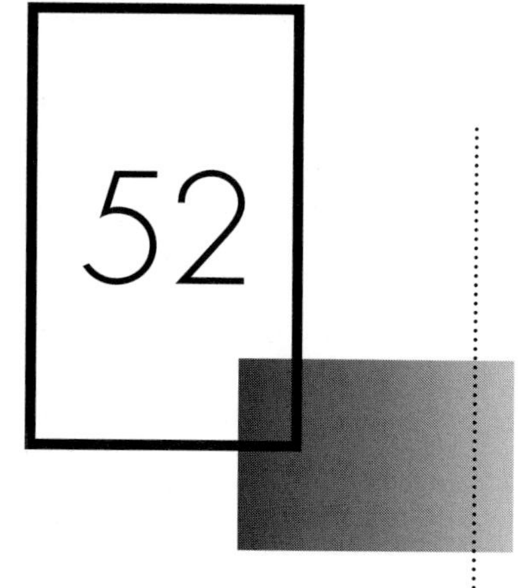

ANTIMICROBIAL AND CHEMOTHERAPEUTIC AGENTS

Antibiotics and Anthelmintics

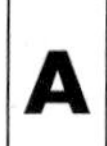

Antibiotics

LESTER M. HADDAD, MD
STEPHEN M. HERMAN, MD

Antibiotics are the most commonly prescribed drugs in primary care. Toxic effects of antibiotics include hypersensitivity reactions and direct drug toxicity. Hypersensitivity reactions to antibiotics are commonplace, and penicillin is the leading cause of death due to anaphylaxis, reported to cause about 400 deaths per year.[1, 2] A study of 120 children in the pediatric age group found β-lactam antibiotics (amoxicillin, cefaclor, and penicillin) to be the most common cause of drug allergy, closely followed by the sulfonamides, then erythromycin and the macrolides.[3] Antibiotics are one of the most common sources of toxic pediatric ingestions, accounting for 39,718 (3.7%) inquiries (up to age 6) to the American Association of Poison Control Centers (AAPCC) in 1995.[4] These pediatric patients drink their sweet-tasting liquid antibiotic and rarely experience clinical symptoms. In fact, of a total of 66,274 cases of human exposures to antimicrobial agents in all age groups reported in 1995 to the AAPCC Toxic Exposure Surveillance System, only one death due solely to antibiotics was reported—from an adverse reaction to rifampin in a 39-year-old patient.[4]

The manifestations of antibiotic toxicity are myriad. Although each antibiotic is associated with a particular toxicity, it is important to remember that each antibiotic may be responsible for an unusual clinical syndrome and it is not until the antibiotic is discontinued and the clinical manifestations resolve that one realizes that the antibiotic was the causative agent. Furthermore, it is not always clear whether the cause of each specific presentation is related to a hypersensitivity reaction or to the direct toxic effect of the antibiotic.

HISTORY

The history of the discovery of penicillin by Alexander Fleming is one of the most famous events in modern medicine. Fleming was a physician and bacteriologist at St. Mary's Medical School in London. After World War I, he began research into effective wound antisepsis. In 1928, while cleaning his bacteriology laboratory, he noticed that an airborne mold had contaminated a culture plate of staphylococci and was inhibiting the growth of staphylococcal colonies around the area of the mold. He discovered the mold was *Penicillium notatum,* which secreted a substance that he called *penicillin.* Fleming published his work in the *British Journal of Experimental Pathology* in 1929.[5] It was not until the beginning of World War II that clinical trials by H. Walter Florey and Ernst Chain at Oxford were begun. World War II propelled the need for and eventual mass manufacture of penicillin. Fleming, Florey, and Chain received the Nobel Prize in 1945 for the discovery of penicillin and its curative effect in infectious disease.

HYPERSENSITIVITY REACTIONS

Hypersensitivity reactions to antibiotics are a result of the interaction between the antibiotic as foreign substance and the components of the immune system.[6] Gell and Coombs have classified four types of immunopathologic reaction.[7] *Type I* reactions involve B-lymphocyte IgE antibody-mediated anaphylaxis, as encountered with penicillin. *Type II* cytotoxic reactions are mediated by IgM or IgG antibodies, which interact with drug antigen adsorbed onto cell membranes. Amoxicillin-induced hemolytic anemia and sulfonamide-induced thrombocytopenia are examples of type II reactions.[8–10] *Type III* or immune complex reactions result from deposition of antigen-IgG or -IgM immune complexes in tissue sites. Penicillin-induced serum sickness and drug fever are examples of type III reactions.[11–12] Cefaclor may induce a serum sickness–like reaction.[13] Finally, delayed hypersensitivity or T-lymphocyte–mediated hypersensitivity reactions are *Type IV* reactions, an example of which is antibiotic-induced contact dermatitis.[14] This chapter reviews the antibiotics that most commonly produce hypersensitivity reactions and then, because of its critical nature, offers a discussion of anaphylaxis and its emergency management.

β-Lactam Antibiotics

The β-lactam antibiotics include five classes: the penicillins, cephalosporins, monobactams, carbapenems, and carbacephems, all of which share a four-membered β-lactam ring.[2, 15]

All types (I to IV) of immunopathologic reactions have occurred with *penicillin.* Penicillin is the most common cause of IgE-mediated (type I) anaphylaxis, which occurs in about 0.01% of patients receiving the drug, with nearly a 10% mortality rate.[1, 15] Commercial skin testing for penicillin allergy is predictive only of IgE reactions to the penicilloyl metabolite, the major determinant in penicillin-induced allergy.[16, 17] Coombs-positive drug-induced hemolytic anemia (type II) of the penicillin type occurs when penicillin acts as a hapten and is directly bound to the red blood cell surface and an antibody directed against the red blood cell–drug complex is formed.[8, 18] This occurs with high-dose penicillin therapy, usually when 10 to 20 million units a day are given for several days. Penicillin-induced serum sickness (type III), occurring after 72 hours, is usually associated with immune complexes formed between the penicilloyl metabolite and IgG and IgM antibodies; these immune complexes deposit in small vessels, particularly in the skin and joints, activating the complement cascade and producing urticaria and joint pain.[19] T-cell delayed hypersensitivity contact dermatitis (type IV) has been known to occur 7 to 14 days after penicillin therapy.

Maculopapular rashes are mediated by idiopathic or unknown pathologic mechanisms and occur more commonly with amoxicillin than with penicillin.[20] The incidence of amoxicillin rashes is markedly increased in patients with Epstein-Barr virus in infectious mononucleosis, cytomegalovirus infections, and acute lymphocytic leukemia, as well as in patients taking allopurinol.[2, 15, 21]

Methicillin is the penicillin that is usually associated with allergic interstitial nephritis, and this may occur in as many as 10% of patients receiving the drug; however, ampicillin has also been implicated.[22] Fortunately, the renal changes are often reversible on withdrawal of the drug.

The *cephalosporins* have a bicyclic structure similar to penicillin, and this accounts for the occasional cross-reactivity in allergic reactions. However, allergic reactions to cephalosporins, with the exception of cefaclor-induced serum sickness, are generally uncommon and considerably less severe than reactions to the penicillins.[15]

Aztreonam (Azactam) is the only *monobactam* antibiotic. It is completely synthetic and has a spectrum of activity against most aerobic gram-negative bacteria. It is poorly immunogenic and has no cross-reactivity with penicillin.[23]

Imipenem (Primaxin) is the only *carbapenem* antibiotic and has a broad range of antimicrobial activity against both gram-positive and aerobic gram-negative activity.[23] Imipenem has a bicyclic ring as penicillin and is cross-reactive with penicillin, as is loracarbef (Lorabid), the only *carbacephem.*[23]

Sulfonamides

The sulfonamides are common causes of antibiotic-induced hypersensitivity reactions, including dermatitis, anaphylaxis, drug fever, hemolytic anemia, systemic vasculitis, and pneumonitis.[24] The clinical manifestations of sulfonamide-induced vasculitis generally result from small vessel vasculitis, with primarily cutaneous manifestations. The process is usually self-limited and subsides on withdrawal of the drug; however, multiple organ involvement, including nephritis, cerebritis, uveitis, hepatitis, and pulmonary involvement, may be encountered and often indicates a poor prognosis.[25, 26] The Stevens-Johnson syndrome has been reported to result from sulfonamide therapy. The most common reaction to trimethoprim-sulfamethoxazole is the type IV cell-mediated delayed hypersensitivity reaction, usually occurring from 7 to 14 days after initiation of therapy, manifesting as pruritic, erythematous, maculopapular lesions often accompanied by fever.[27] The incidence of these skin reactions is especially great in patients with AIDS.[28]

Macrolides

Erythromycin, clarithromycin, and azithromycin in general have low immunogenic potential. The gastric irritation most commonly associated with these antibiotics is due to direct drug toxicity. The cholestatic jaundice following use of erythromycin is probably a manifestation of a hypersensitivity reaction.[29]

Other Antibiotics

Photosensitivity reactions to tetracycline are most likely allergic in nature. Drug allergy is quite uncommon with quinolone therapy.[30] Nitrofurantoin is associated with hypersensitivity pneumonitis and pleural effusions. Urticaria due to vancomycin and polymyxin B use is produced by direct mast cell degranulation and is not mediated by IgE antibody.[19] The thrombocytopenia occurring with use of chloroquine, isoniazid, rifampin, streptomycin, and the sulfonamides is immunologic in origin.[9] As with all of the foregoing antibiotics, *withdrawal of the drug* producing the allergic reaction is key to proper management.

ANAPHYLAXIS

Anaphylaxis was first described in 1902 in France by Portier and Richet[31] when they observed an increased sensitivity instead of immunity on repeat exposure to a particular substance; the term *anaphylaxis* is derived from the Greek *ana,* meaning "backward" and *phylaxis,* or "protection."[1] Anaphylaxis describes the unexpected, immediately occurring, and often catastrophic IgE-mediated response to a sensitizing antigen. Anaphylactic sensitivity is acquired, and prior exposure to the sensitizing agent and a time interval of several weeks are necessary before reintroduction of the sensitizing antigen can evoke an anaphylactic response.[1, 32]

The most common cause of IgE-mediated anaphylaxis is penicillin, followed by β-lactam and other antibiotics; Hymenoptera stings; foods such as peanuts, seafood, and eggs; food additives such as sulfite; intravenous pyelography contrast media; aspirin and other pharmaceuticals; and latex gloves.[1, 32–34] *Anaphylactoid* reactions are clinically similar to anaphylaxis but are triggered independently of IgE antibodies.[1, 32–34] The term *idiopathic anaphylaxis* is used to describe anaphylaxis of unknown cause.[35, 36] Finally, the term *pseudoanaphylaxis* is used to describe the immediate reaction to procaine penicillin injections, the etiology of which is most likely a toxic reaction to procaine.[37] Table 52A–1 lists the antibiotics that are known to precipitate anaphylaxis.

Table 52A–1. Antibiotics That May Produce Anaphylaxis

Penicillin	Amphotericin B
Amoxicillin	Clindamycin
Ampicillin	Lincomycin
Sulfonamides	Ethambutol
Tetracycline	*p*-Aminosalicylic acid
Vancomycin	Chloramphenicol
Cephalosporins	Quinolones
Nitrofurantoin	Other β-lactam antibiotics

Pathophysiology

Haptens are low-molecular-weight substances such as penicillin that in themselves cannot induce an immune response. Penicillin acts as a hapten that binds to endogenous proteins such as serum globulins.[9, 38] On combining with circulating serum globulin, the hapten-protein complex becomes antigenic, causing production of IgE antibodies in certain patients. It is actually the metabolite of penicillin, penicilloyl, that serves as a major determinant and binds as hapten to circulating serum globulin.[14–16] The other metabolites of penicillin, penicilloate and penilloate, and penicillin itself may serve as haptens and are considered minor determinants.[1, 14–16, 29, 39]

Anaphylaxis occurs more commonly after exposure to a parenteral antibiotic.

Combination of circulating hapten-protein antigen with IgE antibody bound to mast cells and basophils causes *cell degranulation* through a calcium-dependent mechanism, as well as release of vasoactive mediators, producing the anaphylactic state (Fig. 52A–1). *Vasoactive mediators include histamine, prostaglandin D_2, leukotrienes C_4 and D_4, platelet-activating factor, and tryptase.*[1, 6, 32, 40] Bradykinin-producing enzymes, as well as neutral proteases, cytokines, and other substances, may also be involved in producing anaphylaxis.[1, 6, 32, 40]

Histamine is secreted by both types of mast cells—mucosal and connective tissue—and by basophils, and it produces arteriolar and venous dilatation and increases vascular permeability.[6, 32, 40] Prostaglandin D_2 is secreted by mast cells only and is a peripheral vasodilator.[32, 40] The leukotrienes are secreted by both mast cells and basophils and constrict coronary and peripheral arterial circulation, increase vascular permeability, and cause bronchoconstriction.[32, 40] Platelet-activating factor is secreted by mast cells only and increases vascular permeability and venous dilatation.[32, 40] The role of mast cell tryptase is unknown, but serum levels peak 60 to 90 minutes after the onset of anaphylaxis and are now used as a clinical marker for anaphylaxis.[40–42]

Clinical Presentation

Anaphylaxis affects the cutaneous, gastrointestinal, respiratory, and cardiovascular systems, which, interestingly enough, contain the largest number of mast cells.[1] Initial manifestations may occur immediately after exposure but generally develop from 10 to 30 minutes after exposure, most often within the first hour. A significant number of patients with anaphylaxis have biphasic or protracted reactions, which may recur several hours after the initial presentation.[43]

Initial symptoms include a feeling of warmth or impending doom, flushing, tachycardia, and pruritus. Urticaria is the most common manifestation of anaphylaxis and may be accompanied by congestion and swelling of the mucous membranes of the eyes, nose,

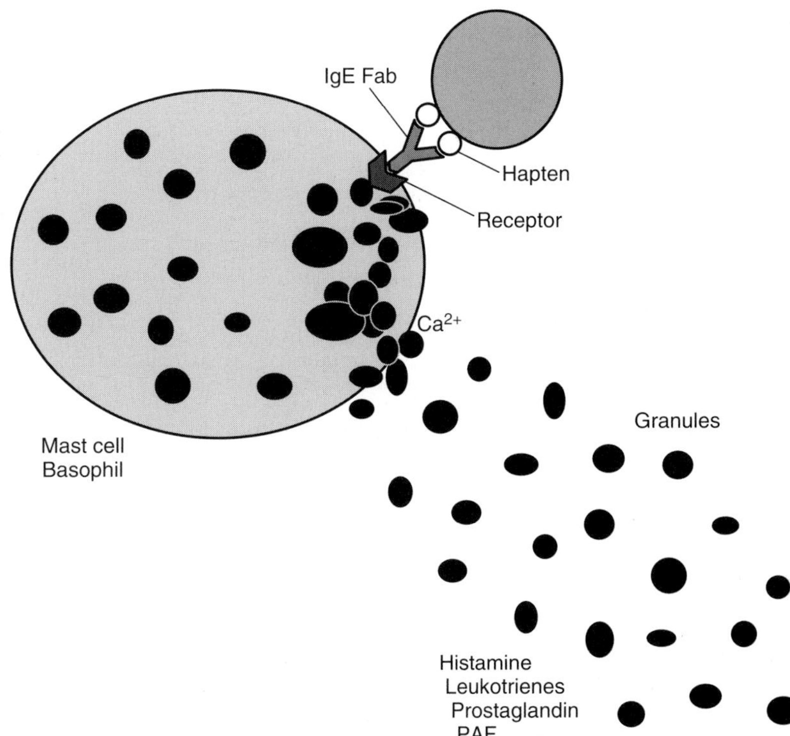

Figure 52A–1. Degranulation of mast cells during anaphylaxis.

mouth, lips, and tongue. Patients may describe a "lump in the throat," which may herald upper airway obstruction due to angioedema of the larynx, epiglottis, and surrounding tissues, producing respiratory stridor and suffocation in untreated cases.

Respiratory involvement further evolves with the development of wheezing, shortness of breath, and tightness in the chest, as with acute asthma. Hypotension frequently develops and may rapidly proceed to cardiac arrest. Seizures, confusion, and loss of consciousness have also been observed, as well as gastrointestinal symptoms such as nausea, vomiting, and abdominal cramps. Table 52A–2 lists clinical findings in anaphylaxis.

Table 52A–2. Primary Clinical Findings in Anaphylaxis

System	Signs	Symptoms
Cutaneous	Flushing, urticaria, angioedema	Pruritus
Cardiovascular	Hypotension, shock, syncope	Weakness
	Cardiac arrhythmia	Palpitations
Pulmonary	Mucous secretions with rhinorrhea and bronchorrhea	Nasal congestion Hoarseness
	Laryngeal edema	Lump in throat Choking
	Wheezing, stridor	Tightness in chest Shortness of breath
	Respiratory arrest	Sense of impending doom
General	Conjunctival edema Diaphoresis	Tearing
	Vomiting and diarrhea	Abdominal cramps

Treatment

Treatment of acute anaphylaxis is a medical emergency and requires immediate attention. *Removing the source of antigen is imperative.* A review of the patient's history to identify possible sources of the reaction or any previous episodes of anaphylaxis may help reveal the cause. For patients who develop anaphylaxis while receiving an intravenous (IV) antibiotic, it is possible to stop the infusion and immediately remove the source of antigen. An IV line of physiologic normal saline should be begun for all patients with anaphylaxis. Maintenance of airway and vital signs and continuous monitoring of cardiac rhythm and pulse oximetry are essential to proper care. Resuscitation with endotracheal intubation and principles of advanced cardiac life support may be necessary in the event of cardiopulmonary arrest. Table 52A–3 outlines treatment measures for the management of acute anaphylaxis.

Epinephrine is the treatment of choice for anaphylaxis.[1, 44–45] Epinephrine counteracts the vasodilation, bronchoconstriction, and other effects of IgE mediator release from mast cells and basophils and may inhibit further mediator release. In patients who have *stable* vital signs and who present with urticaria and early manifestations of anaphylaxis, 0.3 mL of aqueous epinephrine 1:1000 may be administered subcutaneously to an adult or 0.01 mg/kg to a child and repeated every 15 to 30 minutes as necessary. Subcutaneous epinephrine is also quite effective for the treatment of anaphylaxis-induced asthma.

In the event of shock or cardiac arrest, epinephrine

Table 52A–3. Emergency Management of Anaphylaxis

Prevention

Remove the source of antigen!

Epinephrine

Asthma and urticaria (stable blood pressure):
- Epinephrine 0.3 mL 1:1000 (adult) SC, 0.01 mL/kg for a child

Hypotension or cardiac arrest:
- Epinephrine IV 1:10,000 1 mg, 0.1 mL/kg for a child; repeat q 5 min as indicated

Persistent hypotension:
- Epinephrine IV drip
  - 1 mg 1:1000 in normal saline 500 mL (2 μg/mL) begin at 1 μg/min for adults, titrate up to 2–10 μg/min

Patients unresponsive to epinephrine (or who cannot tolerate epinephrine):
- Glucagon, 1 mg IV for adults, 0.5 mg for children; repeat as necessary

Fluid Resuscitation

IV normal saline
- 500–1000 mL IV bolus, then re-evaluate
- Children: 20 mL/kg IV initial bolus

Antihistamines

(H_1) Diphenhydramine, 25–50 mg IV, 1 mg/kg for a child or hydroxyzine, 25–50 mg IV for adults

(H_2) Cimetidine (Tagamet), 300 mg IV for adults, 4 mg/kg for a child

Corticosteroids

Methylprednisolone (Solu-Medrol), 125 mg IV, 1–2 mg/kg for a child

or

Hydrocortisone (Solu-Cortef), 250–500 IV, 4–8 mg/kg up to 250 mg for a child

Additional Treatment as Indicated

Oxygen for patients with cardiac or respiratory symptoms
Nebulized albuterol for asthma
Aminophylline (6 mg/kg IV adult loading dose) for persistent asthma
Dopamine IV for persistent hypotension
Military antishock trousers for persistent hypotension

IV, intravenous(ly).

1:10,000 may be given IV as an initial adult dose of 5 to 10 mL, depending on the clinical situation, and repeated every 5 minutes as indicated, or 0.1 mL/kg for pediatric patients. For persistent or recurrent hypotension, a continuous intravenous drip of epinephrine may be necessary, using the standard advanced cardiac life support protocol. The recommended dose for epinephrine as an IV drip for adults is 1 mg of epinephrine (preferably 1:1000 dilution or 1 mL) to be added to 500 mL of normal saline, to give a concentration of 2 μg/mL. The infusion is begun at 1 μg/min and may be increased up to 2 to 10 μg/min as necessary.[46] Patients should be carefully monitored for potential complications of IV epinephrine, which include cardiac arrhythmias, myocardial ischemia, and accelerated hypertension.

Fluid resuscitation with normal saline and IV vasopressors such as dopamine may also be indicated in patients with shock. IV normal saline is often given as a 500- to 1000-mL bolus for adults or 20 mL/kg for children, followed by reassessment of the patient. For patients who are refractory to the foregoing measures or who may require an alternative to epinephrine, such as patients who are elderly or undergoing β-blocker therapy, 1 mg of IV glucagon, or 0.5 mg in the pediatric age group, may be indicated and repeated as necessary.[47]

Supplemental oxygen is often indicated for patients with cardiac or respiratory symptoms. Patients who develop acute asthma are treated with epinephrine or with albuterol by nebulizer; IV aminophylline may also be indicated for adults at a dose of 6 mg/kg loading dose over 30 minutes, followed by a maintenance dose of 0.5 to 1 mg/kg per hour.

IV antihistamines including H_1 blockers such as diphenhydramine (Benadryl) or hydroxyzine (Atarax), 25 to 50 mg IV (1 mg/kg IV for children), and/or H_2 blockers such as cimetidine (Tagamet), 300 IV for adults (4 mg/kg for children), or famotidine (Pepcid), 20 mg IV for adults, are often administered to provide relief of pruritus and urticaria.[48]

Although intravenous corticosteroids such as methylprednisolone (125 mg IV in an adult or 1 mg/kg in a child) or hydrocortisone (250 to 500 mg in an adult or 4 to 8 mg/kg in a child as an initial loading dose) have no effect on the acute episode, they are often administered and may prevent recurrence of anaphylaxis and delayed bronchospasm; however, in one study of 25 patients, glucocorticoids did *not* reliably suppress biphasic or protracted anaphylaxis.[43]

Biphasic and protracted anaphylaxis occurred in 48% of 25 patients studied by Stark and Sullivan.[43] Antibiotics were the cause of anaphylaxis in 12 of the 25 patients.[43] Biphasic reactions were noted to peak at 4 to 8 hours after the initial stimulus, and the second episode always included the same signs and symptoms as the initial reaction. Protracted anaphylaxis is described as prolonged hypotension after an initial episode. Recurrent and prolonged anaphylaxis in this study were more common in patients who had delayed onset of reactions (> 30 minutes) and in patients who reacted to an oral medication.[43] For this reason, anaphylactic patients who manifest cardiovascular or respiratory signs should be admitted to the hospital for observation.

Prevention

Patients who have a known allergy should be careful to avoid the offending drug. It is important to obtain a history of allergy before prescribing an antibiotic. When there is a question, skin testing for penicillin allergy with the major determinant benzylpenicilloyl polylysine preparation (Pre-Pen) is a far more accurate method of determining penicillin allergy than is the patient's history. Unfortunately, skin testing for the minor determinants of penicillin is not commercially available.[49]

For patients who have a definite history of penicillin allergy or who have positive results of a skin test for penicillin allergy, alternative antibiotics that do not cross-react with penicillin are indicated.[49, 50] In situations in which penicillin remains the drug of choice, such as in patients with syphilis in pregnancy or patients with neurosyphilis, or in situations in which alternative drugs fail or are ineffective or produce unacceptable side effects, as occasionally in *Pseudomonas* sepsis, enterococcal bacterial endocarditis, bacterial meningitis, or staphylococcal osteomyelitis, use of penicillin, piperacillin, ceftazidime, or another β-lactam antibiotic after a desensitization protocol is appropriate.[17, 38, 39, 50]

Patients who experience anaphylaxis should be prescribed EpiPen (or EpiPen Jr.), both of which contain epinephrine in a spring-loaded injectable form for self-administration, with proper instruction in its use.

References

1. Bochner BS, Lichtenstein LM: Anaphylaxis. N Engl J Med *324:*1785–1790, 1991.
2. Boguniewicz M, Leung DYM: Hypersensitivity reactions to antibiotics commonly used in children. Pediatr Infect Dis J *14:*221–231, 1995.
3. Kamada MM, Twarog F, Leung DYM: Multiple antibiotic sensitivity in a pediatric population. Allergy Proc *12:*347–350, 1991.
4. Litovitz TL, Felberg L, White S, Klein-Schwartz W: 1995 Annual Report of the American Association of Poison Control Centers Toxic Exposure Surveillance System. Am J Emerg Med *14:*487–537, 1996.
5. Fleming A: On the antibacterial action of cultures of a penicillium, with special reference to their use in the isolation of B. influenza. Br J Exp Pathol *10:*226–236, 1929.
6. Roitt IM, Brostoff J, Male DK: Immunology. 3rd ed. St. Louis, Mosby–Year Book, 1993.
7. Gell PGH, Coombs RRA: Classification of allergic reactions responsible for clinical hypersensitivity and disease. In Gell PGH, Coombs RRA, Hachmann PJ (eds): Clinical Aspects of Immunology. 3rd ed. Oxford, Blackwell Scientific Publications, pp 761–781, 1975.
8. Garratty G, Petz LD: Drug-induced immune hemolytic anemia. Am J Med *58:*398, 1975.
9. Kerr RO, Cardamone J, Dalmasso AP, Kaplan ME: Two mechanisms of erythrocyte destruction in penicillin-induced hemolytic anemia. N Engl J Med *287:*1322–1325, 1972.
10. Brandwein JM, Keating A: Hematologic consequences of poisoning. *In* Haddad LM, Winchester JF (eds): Clinical Management of Poisoning and Drug Overdose. 3rd ed. Philadelphia, W.B. Saunders Co., pp 296–307, 1990.
11. Erffmeyer JE: Serum sickness. Ann Allergy *56:*105–110, 1986.
12. Mackowiak PH, LeMaistre CF: Drug fever: A critical appraisal of conventional concepts. Ann Intern Med *106:*728–733, 1987.
13. Hebert AA, Sigman ES, Levy ML: Serum-sickness-like reactions from cefaclor in children. J Am Acad Dermatol *25:*805–808, 1991.
14. Reitschel RL: Dermatologic manifestations of antimicrobial adverse reactions with special emphasis on topical exposure. Infect Dis Clin North Am *8:*607–615, 1994.
15. Saxon A: Immediate hypersensitivity reactions to beta-lactam antibiotics. Ann Intern Med *107:*204–215, 1987.
16. Sullivan TJ, Wedner HJ, Shatz GS, et al: Skin testing to detect penicillin allergy. J Allergy Clin Immunol *68:*171–180, 1981.
17. Sullivan TJ: Antigen-specific desensitization of patients allergic to penicillin. J Allergy Clin Immunol *69:*500–508, 1982.
18. Petz LD, Fudenberg HH: Coombs-positive hemolytic anemia caused by penicillin administration. N Engl J Med *274:*171–178, 1966.
19. Huston DR, Bressler RB: Urticaria and angioedema. Med Clin North Am *76:*805–840, 1992.
20. Adcock BB, Rodman DP: Ampicillin-specific rashes. Arch Fam Med *5:*301–304, 1996.
21. Kerns DL, Shira JE, Go S, et al: Ampicillin rash in children: Relationship to penicillin allergy and infectious mononucleosis. Am J Dis Child *125:*187–190, 1973.
22. Maher JF: Clinicopathologic spectrum of drug nephrotoxicity. Adv Intern Med *30:*295–316, 1984.
23. Ennis DM, Cobbs CG: The newer cephalosporins and aztreonam and imipenem. Infect Dis Clin North Am *9:*687–713, 1995.
24. Platt R, Dreis MW, Kennedy DL, Kuritsky JN: Serum sickness-like reactions to amoxicillin, cefaclor, cephalexin, and trimethoprim-sulfamethoxazole. J Infect Dis *158:*474–477, 1988.
25. Somer T, Finegold SM: Vasculitides associated with infections, immunization and antimicrobial drugs. Clin Infect Dis *20:*1010–1036, 1995.
26. Jain KK: Drug-induced cutaneous vasculitis. Adverse Drug React Toxicol Rev *12:*263–276, 1993.
27. Bigby M, Jick S, Jick H, Arndt K: Drug-induced cutaneous reactions: A report from the Boston Collaborative Drug Surveillance Program on 15,438 consecutive patients, 1975 to 1983. JAMA *256:*3358–3363, 1986.
28. Lundstrom TS, Sobel JD: Vancomycin, trimethoprim-sulfamethoxazole, and rifampin. Infect Dis Clin North Am *9:*747–767, 1995.
29. Sullivan D, Csuka ME, Blanchard B: Erythromycin ethylsuccinate hepatotoxicity. JAMA *243:*1074, 1980.
30. Hendershot EF: Fluoroquinolones. Infect Dis Clin North Am *9:*715–730, 1995.
31. Portier P, Richet C: De l'action anaphylactique de certain venins. C R Soc Biol (Paris) *54:*170–172, 1902.
32. Kaplan AP: Anaphylaxis. In Bennett JC, Plum F (eds): Cecil Textbook of Medicine. 10th ed. Philadelphia, W.B. Saunders Co., pp 1417–1420, 1996.
33. Atkinson TP, Kaliner MA: Anaphylaxis. Med Clin North Am *76:*841–855, 1992.
34. Yunginger JW: Anaphylaxis. Ann Allergy *69:*87–96, 1992.
35. Sonin L, Grammer LC, Greenberger PA, Patterson R: Idiopathic anaphylaxis: A clinical summary. Ann Intern Med *99:*634–635, 1983.
36. Stoloff R, Adams SL, Orfan N, et al: Emergency medical recognition and management of idiopathic anaphylaxis. J Emerg Med *10:*693–698, 1992.
37. Galpin JE, Chow AW, Yoshikawa TT, Guze LB: "Pseudoanaphylactic" reactions from inadvertent infusion of procaine penicillin G. Ann Intern Med *81:*358–359, 1974.
38. Weiss ME, Adkinson NF: Immediate hypersensitivity reactions to penicillin and related antibiotics. Clin Allergy *18:*515–540, 1988.
39. Sullivan TJ, Yecies LD, Shatz GS, et al: Desensitization of patients allergic to penicillin using orally-administered beta-lactam antibiotics. J Allergy Clin Immunol *69:*275–282, 1982.
40. Schwartz L, Huff T: Biology of mast cells and basophils. *In* Middleton E, Reed CE, Ellis EF, et al (eds): Allergy–Principles and Practice. 4th ed. St. Louis, C.V. Mosby, pp 135–168, 1993.
41. Tanus T, Mines D, Atkins PC, Levinson AI: Serum tryptase in idiopathic anaphylaxis: A case report and review of the literature, Ann Emerg Med *24:*104–107, 1994.
42. Schwartz LB: Tryptase, a mediator of human mast cells. J Allergy Clin Immunol *86:*594–598, 1990.
43. Stark BJ, Sullivan TJ: Biphasic and protracted anaphylaxis. J Allergy Clin Immunol *78:*76–83, 1986.
44. Barach EM, Nowak RM, Lee TG, Tomlanovich MC: Epinephrine for treatment of anaphylactic shock. JAMA *251:*2118–2122, 1984.
45. Zull DN: Anaphylaxis. *In* Harwood-Nuss AL, Linden CH, Luten RC, et al (eds): Clinical Practice of Emergency Medicine, 2nd ed. Philadelphia, Lippincott-Raven Publishers, pp 929–932, 1996.
46. Cummins RO: Textbook of Advanced Cardiac Life Support. Dallas, American Heart Association, 1994.
47. Zaloga GP, Delacey W, Holmboe E, Chernow B: Glucagon reversal of hypotension in a case of anaphylactoid shock. Ann Intern Med *105:*65–66, 1986.
48. Lieberman P: The use of antihistamines in the prevention and treatment of anaphylaxis and anaphylactoid reactions. J Allergy Clin Immunol *86:*684, 1990.
49. Weiss ME: Drug allergy. Med Clin North Am *76:*857–882, 1992.
50. Segreti J, Trenholme GM, Levin S: Antibiotic therapy in the allergic patient. Med Clin North Am *79:*935–942, 1995.

B Antibiotic Toxicity

MICHAEL W. SHANNON, MD, MPH

In addition to their immunologic effects, antibiotics can produce direct drug toxicity after acute single overdose, soon after therapy is initiated or after several days of use. In many cases, the cause of toxicity is a drug-drug interaction (Table 52B–1). The extensive list of antimicrobials and their adverse effects cannot be discussed entirely in this chapter, and readers are referred to standard pharmacology texts. However, many agents, because of their widespread use or severity of their adverse effects, warrant mention.

ANTIBACTERIALS

Important antibacterials include the penicillins, cephalosporins, sulfonamides, quinolones, aminoglycosides, tetracyclines, macrolides, vancomycin, nitrofurantoin, chloramphenicol, benzyl alcohol, and anti-*Mycobacterium* agents.

The most common adverse effects of penicillins result from immunologic reactions; acute toxicity from the penicillins is rare, and they enjoy a wide margin of safety. Nonetheless, the penicillins can produce direct toxic actions. For example, penicillin G has substantial neurotoxicity (it is used in many animal models to produce seizures). Parenteral administration of large (>20 million units) daily doses is associated with central nervous system (CNS) toxicity that includes lethargy, confusion, or frank seizures. Also, because 20 million units of penicillin G contains 34 mEq of potassium, severe hyperkalemia can result. Finally, injection of procaine penicillin can produce acute neurobehavioral changes (hallucinations, headache, disorientation) or frank seizures.[1] Oral penicillin ingestion has minimal toxicity.[2, 3]

Sulfonamides, although having substantial immunologic toxicity, have little direct toxicity. Most notable of these is hemolysis in glucose-6-phosphate dehydrogenase (G-6-PD) deficient patients and bilirubin displacement from albumin, resulting in a risk of kernicterus in newborn infants given these drugs.[4] CNS system effects, including headache, depression, and hallucinations, may also occur after sulfonamide use. Like penicillins and cephalosporins, sulfonamides have limited toxicity when ingested as an acute single overdose.

Table 52B–1. Antibiotic-Associated Drug Interactions

Agent	Interacting Agent(s)	Clinical Effect	Reference
Antibacterials			
Rifampin	Digitoxin, quinidine, propranolol, verapamil, methadone, cyclosporine, coumadin, theophylline, oral contraceptives, sulfonylurea oral hypoglycemics, phenytoin	↑ Clearance, ↓ Effectiveness	Mandell and Petri[26] Baciewicz et al[27]
Aminoglycosides	Neuromuscular blockers	Prolonged paralysis	Kapusnik-Uner et al[7]
Macrolides	Theophylline, terfenadine, astemizole, carbamazepine, cyclosporine, digoxin, valproate, cisapride	↓ Clearance, prolonged QT syndrome, torsades de pointes	Kapusnik-Uner et al,[7] Ben-Ari et al[10]
Quinolones	Theophylline	↑ Serum [theo]	Brouwers[5]
Chloramphenicol	Phenytoin, coumadin, chlorpropamide	↓ Clearance	Kapusnik-Uner et al[7]
Antivirals			
Saquinavir	Terfenadine Astemizole	Prolonged QT syndrome	Medical Letter[33]
Antifungals			
Ketoconazole	Steroid hormones, terfenadine, astemizole, cisapride, theophylline	↓ Clearance, prolonged QT interval, torsades de pointes	Bennett[37] Honig et al[38]
Fluconazole	Phenytoin, warfarin, cyclosporine	↓ Clearance	Bennett[37]
Antiparasitics			
Quinine	Digoxin Coumadin	↑ Digoxin levels ↓ Anticoagulation	Tracy and Webster[39]
Metronidazole	Ethanol	Disulfiram-like reaction	Sanford et al[48] Waskin et al[49]

Quinolone antibiotics include nalidixic acid, ciprofloxacin, norfloxacin, and ofloxacin. Their major toxic action is inhibition of the cytochrome P-450 isoenzyme CYP1A2, resulting in reduced clearance of drugs, including theophylline and coumadin. Marked reductions in theophylline clearance can result in toxic serum theophylline concentrations.[5] Seizures, which have been reported after the simultaneous use of quinolones and theophylline, may occur despite therapeutic serum theophylline concentrations; these seizures may be the result of both drugs' having an additive effect on the inhibition of γ-aminobutyric acid (GABA) activity.[5]

The aminoglycosides are among the most commonly used antibiotics, owing to their consistent efficacy against gram-negative bacteria. These agents, which include streptomycin, neomycin, kanamycin, gentamicin, amakacin, and tobramycin, are elaborated by different genera of soil actinomycetes, including *Streptomyces* and *Micromonospora.* Aminoglycosides have similar pharmacokinetics that include poor absorption from the gastrointestinal (GI) tract after ingestion, negligible protein binding, and small volumes of distribution. They are eliminated almost exclusively by glomerular filtration and have half-lives of 2 to 4 hours.[6]

The aminoglycosides are associated with several types of toxicity, the best known being nephrotoxicity and ototoxicity. Nephrotoxicity occurs in as many as 26% of patients who receive extended aminoglycoside therapy and produces early manifestations of proteinuria, loss of renal concentrating ability, and the appearance of hyaline or granular casts.[6] Secondary metabolic disturbances include elevated serum creatinine levels and hypokalemia. Unlike ototoxicity, aminoglycoside-induced renal injury has a high likelihood of resolution.

Ototoxicity, although it has occurred after a single dose of tobramycin, most commonly results from prolonged use of aminoglycosides. The appearance of ototoxicity appears to correspond to prolonged elevated concentrations of drug in plasma, which results in accumulation of drug within the endolymph. Also, the half-life of aminoglycosides is as much as six times greater in middle ear fluid than in plasma.[6] Ototoxicity is usually irreversible, corresponding to loss of vestibular and cochlear sensory cells. The earliest sign of ototoxicity is loss of high-frequency hearing (which may be undetectable without audiometric evaluation). Later, low-frequency hearing loss develops. Vestibular toxicity usually appears as labyrinthitis with nausea, vomiting, and vertigo. Ataxia then ensues. Streptomycin and gentamicin are associated primarily with vestibular effects, whereas amikacin, kanamycin, and neomycin are more likely to produce auditory dysfunction. Streptomycin is particularly ototoxic; 20% of patients receiving this drug for 4 weeks develop evidence of vestibular dysfunction.[6]

Aminoglycosides are associated with other neurotoxic consequences. Neuromuscular blockade (a curare-like effect) may appear after use of all aminoglycosides, particularly neomycin. The effect may range from generalized hypotonia to frank apnea. Animal studies suggest that this action results from the combination of aminoglycoside-induced inhibition of acetylcholine release as well as diminished responsiveness of postsynaptic myoneural receptors. The use of aminoglycosides (or the unrelated antibiotic clindamycin) in patients who are receiving skeletal muscle relaxants (e.g., pancuronium) can result in paralysis that continues long after discontinuation of the paralytic.[7] However, the effect is reversible. Other adverse effects of aminoglycosides include visual disturbances and peripheral neuritis (both of which are most common with streptomycin). Treatment of aminoglycoside overdose includes hemodialysis or peritoneal dialysis. However, depending on the specific agent, clearance via extracorporeal techniques may be low, in part because renal elimination relies more on tubular secretion than glomerular filtration, the former being difficult to accelerate.

Tetracyclines include tetracycline, doxycycline, and minocycline. These agents also epitomize broad-spectrum antibiotics, making them useful in a wide range of bacterial infections. Although their side effect profile is relatively low, important adverse effects may result from their long-term use. For example, GI upset is almost universal with tetracyclines. They may also cause severe esophagitis or peptic ulcers. Pancreatitis occurs rarely.[7, 8] Tetracycline-induced hepatitis may develop in those receiving large doses. Tetracyclines may also produce renal disturbances including deterioration of renal function, nephrogenic diabetes insipidus, and a distinct nephropathy manifested by a Fanconi-like syndrome (polyuria, polydipsia, proteinuria, acidosis, and aminoaciduria). The use of outdated tetracycline is associated with the development of pseudotumor cerebri.[9]

Macrolide antibiotics include erythromycin, clarithromycin, troleandomycin, and azithromycin.[7] These agents, derived from the *Streptomyces* actinomycete, are effective against a broad range of bacteria as well as *Chlamydia* and *Mycoplasma* species. Macrolides have pharmacokinetic characteristics such as relatively poor GI absorption and bioavailability, ready distribution across the placenta and into breast milk, and less than 10% renal elimination of unchanged drug. The most important pharmacokinetic difference between these drugs is their metabolism. Troleandomycin, erythromycin, and clarithromycin are potent inhibitors of cytochrome P-450 isoenzymes CYP1A2 and CYP 3A3/4. The clinical consequence of this effect is that these drugs can substantially reduce the clearance of many pharmaceutical agents, including theophylline, the antihistamines terfenadine and astemizole, carbamazepine, cyclosporine, digoxin, cisapride, ergot alkaloids, valproate, and coumadin. Inadvertent intoxication due to these drugs can occur in patients taking macrolides.[10] Prolonged QT syndrome, torsades de pointes, and fatal cardiac arrest have been described after concomitant use of erythromycin or clarithromycin with terfenadine, astemizole, and cisapride. Seizures are often a presenting sign of cardiac disturbances. Interestingly, erythromycin alone can also produce a prolonged QT syndrome after intravenous administration.[11, 12]

Other important toxicities of erythromycin include GI upset and pancreatitis.[13] Hepatic injury may appear in the form of either cholestatic jaundice or frank hepatitis; cholestasis is particularly common after use of erythromycin estolate. Transient auditory disturbances may also occur.

Vancomycin, produced by the actinomycete *Streptococcus orientalis,* is experiencing increased use as the prevalence of penicillin-resistant pneumococcal infection rises.[7] It is also effective against *Staphylococcus epidermidis* infections. Among toxic reactions associated with the use of this agent, the red-man syndrome is best known. This syndrome appears after rapid intravenous infusion of the antibiotic and has manifestations of diffuse flushing with or without urticaria, tachycardia, and hypotension. The facial flushing can be striking and is the basis of the syndrome's name. The red-man syndrome is reversible with supportive measures (discontinuation of the antibiotic and administration of intravenous fluids and diphenhydramine); its appearance does not preclude subsequent use of vancomycin. However, additional infusions should be administered at a considerably slower rate. Acute reversible renal failure also has been associated with excessive administration of vancomycin.[14, 15] Vancomycin is minimally removed by hemodialysis, peritoneal dialysis, and exchange transfusion; however, repeated doses of activated charcoal have been shown to enhance elimination significantly.[15, 16]

Nitrofurantoin is an antibacterial with specificity for the urinary tract. Having a half-life as short as 20 minutes and complete urinary elimination within 8 hours, nitrofurantoin is ideal for the treatment of urinary tract infections.[17] Side effects of this medicine include GI upset (in as many as 30% of patients). A more serious complication is the appearance of acute pulmonary disturbances such as asthma, pulmonary edema, or pneumonia.[18, 19] Acute pulmonary reactions often include fever, tachycardia, tachypnea, rash, and eosinophilia. Treatment consists of drug discontinuation, steroids, and bronchodilator therapy.[19] Complete resolution of acute pulmonary toxicity can generally be expected. A more significant and insidious adverse effect is severe pneumonitis and pulmonary fibrosis; this rare reaction develops after chronic nitrofurantoin use, is usually irreversible, and can be fatal. Treatment of pneumonitis is immediate discontinuation of the drug, plus supportive care.[17] Other toxicities of nitrofurantoin include hepatic injury (both hepatocellular and cholestatic), sensorimotor peripheral neuropathy with stocking-glove paresthesias, and hemolytic anemia, particularly in those with G-6-PD deficiency.[18]

Chloramphenicol, a nitrobenzene-based antibiotic, is derived from *Streptomyces* species. Unlike most antibacterial agents, chloramphenicol is capable of inhibiting protein synthesis in both eukaryotic and bacterial cells. Because of its significant toxicity to mammlian cells, the drug is being used less frequently as safer antibiotics are created.

Chloramphenicol's major toxicity is hematologic.[19] It produces direct, dose-dependent bone marrow depression manifested by reductions in white blood cell, red blood cell, and platelet counts.[20] More well known but extremely rare is an idiosyncratic aplastic anemia. This reaction, which was typically fatal before the advent of bone marrow transplantation, appears to be related to long-term and repeated use of the drug.[20]

In 1959, chloramphenicol use in newborns became associated with a severe illness known as the *gray baby syndrome.*[21] This syndrome occurred in infants, particulary preterm infants, who received chloramphenicol in doses of 100 to 165 mg/kg per day. Characteristically, 4 to 7 days after starting chloramphicol, infants developed vomiting, refusal to suck, irregular respirations, abdominal distention, diarrhea, acidosis, and cyanosis.[7] These early signs were quickly followed by flaccidity, an ashen gray complexion, and hypothermia. At the time of its appearance, mortality in infants was as high as 63%.[20] The etiology of this syndrome remains speculative, although it has largely disappeared. Current theories are that the cause was multifactorial, including impaired chloramphenicol metabolism due to deficient activity of hepatic glucuronyl transferase in the newborn period and reduced renal excretion of the drug or its metabolites. One can also speculate that with its nitrobenzene nucleus, chloramphenicol may have produced methemoglobinemia as well (although this is not documented in case reports of the illness). A similar syndrome may affect adults, having additional features of encephalopathy and cardiomyopathy.

Chloramphenicol is a potent inhibitor of cytochrome P-450 enzymes; the specific isoenzymes involved have not been completely characterized. As a consequence of this inhibition, clearance of drugs including coumadin, phenytoin, and chlorpropamide is reduced.

Treatment of chloramphenicol intoxication is supportive. Exchange transfusion and hemoperfusion have been used to treat both acute overdose and chronic overmedication, although it is unclear whether they significantly enhance drug clearance or alter clinical course.

Another antibacterial of historical importance is benzyl alcohol. Once used as a bacteriostatic agent in multidose vials (e.g., saline), this agent was associated with an epidemic of deaths due to the *gasping baby syndrome,* which occurred in premature newborns. Described in 1982, the gasping baby syndrome consisted of severe metabolic acidosis, encephalopathy, and respiratory depression with gasping.[22–25] The illness was found to result from repeated administration of benzyl alcohol–containing bacteriostatic solutions. The metabolism of this substance produced benzoic acid, among other toxic metabolites. The syndrome, which resulted in as many as 3000 deaths, promptly disappeared when benzyl alcohol was banned from use in nurseries.

The agents that are used for the treatment of mycobacterial infections and that have important clinical toxicity are isoniazid, rifampin, ethambutol, streptomycin, pyrazinamide, and dapsone. The toxicity of isoniazid is discussed in Chapter 53.

Rifampin has a number of uncommon adverse effects, including hepatitis, a flulike illness, and renal injury. Its most important clinical effect is induction of cytochrome P-450 enzymes.[26, 27] As a result, use of rifampin is associated with increased clearance and decreased effectiveness of digitoxin, quinidine, propranolol, verapamil, cyclosporine, methadone, coumadin, theophylline, phenytoin, and sulfonylurea oral hypoglycemics.[26] The clearance of phenytoin can increase by more than 100% in patients who are simultaneously taking rifampin.[27] This effect typically appears in the second week of rifampin use and can persist for as long as a week after rifampin therapy is discontinued.

The most important toxicity of ethambutol is optic neuritis. This dose-related effect may occur in as many as 15% of patients who receive more than 50 mg/kg per day. Visual loss may be unilateral or bilateral and may appear insidiously with initial loss of red-green discrimination. This effect typically resolves after discontinuation of therapy.[26]

Pyrazinamide is a less common antituberculous agent. However, it can produce hepatic injury in as many as 15% of patients; rarely, fulminant hepatic necrosis may occur. The earliest sign of pyrazinamide hepatotoxicity is elevation in serum transaminase values. Although hepatic injury generally resolves after drug discontinuation, progressive hepatic failure occasionally ensues. Other important effects include hyperuricemia (which may result in the precipation of acute gout) and GI upset.

Dapsone is an antibacterial agent that is used in the treatment of leprosy (*Mycobacterium leprae*) as well as *Pneumocystis carinii* pneumonia. The two most important clinical toxicities of dapsone, which may appear after either acute single overdose or long-term administration, are hemolysis (particularly in those with G-6-PD deficiency) and methemoglobinemia.[28] Because of dapsone's enterohepatic recirculation, recurrent methemoglobinemia may occur, requiring repeated methylene blue therapy[29] (see Chapter 13).

ANTIVIRALS (ACYCLOVIR AND RELATED DRUGS, ANTIRETROVIRAL AGENTS, AMANTIDINE)

Although generally safe, acyclovir has a number of important toxicities. The most important of these are renal and central nervous system effects. These may appear after prolonged use as well as after an acute single overdose. Clinical manifestations of nephrotoxicity include flank and abdominal pain and rapid onset of azotemia. This nephrotoxicity is treated with discontinuation of the drug and with intravenous saline hydration. Neurotoxicity may present as altered mental status, delirium, seizures, or dystonia. Adverse drug interactions include marked lethargy in those taking acyclovir in combination with zidovudine, as well as reduced renal clearance of other drugs that are eliminated by renal tubular secretion (e.g., methotrexate).[30] Extracorporeal drug removal techniques (e.g., exchange transfusion and repeated doses of activated charcoal) have proved ineffective in removing acyclovir, despite its low protein binding (15%) and small volume of distribution (0.7 L/kg).[31] However, hemodialysis has been shown to enhance elimination and is considered a very effective therapy for acyclovir overdose.[32]

Structurally related to acyclovir, ganciclovir is active against most herpesviruses but is particularly effective in the treatment of cytomegalovirus (CMV) infections such as retinitis. The toxicity of this agent includes dose-related myelosuppression (manifested by neutropenia and thrombocytopenia); CNS effects including headache, behavioral changes, coma, or seizures; and, less commonly, renal and liver function abnormalities.[30]

Among the antiviral agents, those witnessing the greatest growth are the agents being produced to treat HIV infection. This class includes several agents, such as nucleoside analogues (zidovudine, stavudine, lamivudine, didanosine, and zalcitabine)[30] and a newer group of agents, the protease inhibitors (saquinavir, ritonavir, and indinavir).[33] Toxicity due to these agents is substantial although not life-threatening. The toxicity of zidovudine includes bone marrow suppression, CNS signs including headache or insomnia, a characteristic nail pigmentation, myopathy (skeletal or cardiac), and hepatitis. Severe somnolence may occur with combined use of zidovudine and acyclovir.[30] Didanosine is associated with the distressing adverse effects of peripheral neuropathy and pancreatitis. Paresthesias, numbness, and pain in the lower extremities may be extremely uncomfortable; this effect resolves with discontinuation of therapy. Pancreatitis, which appears in as many as 20% of patients, is more common in those with a prior history of pancreatitis, as well as with concomitant use of intravenous pentamidine. Other adverse effects of didanosine include CNS disturbances, optic neuritis, hepatitis, and cardiomyopathy. Stavudine and lamivudine are also associated with a reversible, dose-related peripheral neuropathy as well as mild hepatitis and pancreatitis. Among the protease inhibitors, side effects include GI upset and inhibition of cytochrome P-450 enzymes. As with the macrolide antibacterials, this can produce decreased elimination of terfenadine and astemizole, resulting in prolonged QT syndrome or torsades de pointes.[33] Side effects are more common with ritonavir and include GI symptoms, paresthesias, and hepatitis. Indinavir has been associated with nephrolithiasis in as many as 5% of patients taking it.

Amantidine was one of the first antiviral agents used clinically. It is an effective treatment for influenza infections and is also used as adjunctive therapy for Parkinson's disease and drug-induced extrapyramidal signs.[34] Pharmacokinetic features of amantadine include a large volume of distribution (7 L/kg), 60% to 70% protein binding, and elimination via excretion of unchanged drug in the urine through the combined mechanisms of glomerular filtration and tubular secretion. The average elimination half-life is 24 hours. Because its elimination is reliant on renal function, the half-life of the drug is prolonged in the elderly and those with renal insufficiency.[30] The toxicity of amantadine affects the CNS; as many as one third of patients develop effects including delirium, hallucinosis, seizures, or coma.[35] Cardiac disturbances such as torsades de pointes can appear after acute overdose or chronic overmedication.[36] Urinary retention may also occur. Fatalities are associated with the ingestion of more than 2 g of amantidine. Treatment of intoxication by this agent involves supportive measures, GI decontamination (in cases of oral overdose), and intravenous hydration sufficient to produce a brisk diuresis. Although urine acidification enhances the elimination of amantidine, it may produce untoward effects (e.g., metabolic acidosis) and is not recommended. Hemodialysis is ineffective for removal of amantidine.

ANTIFUNGALS

Antifungal agents with the most significant clinical toxicity include amphotericin B and the imidazoles/triazoles (ketoconazole, miconazole, fluconazole).

Amphotericin is one of a family of macrolide antibotics unrelated to erythromycin.[37] Because of its relative insolubility, the intravenous solution is prepared with several additives, including the bile salt deoxycholate, lipids, or lecithin.[37] Toxicity after acute amphotericin overdose is generally limited to fever and chills; toxicity after chronic overmedication is more significant.

Amphotericin produces renal toxicity in 80% of patients who receive it. Clinical effects include azotemia, renal tubular acidosis, and urinary losses of potassium and magnesium. Approximately 30% to 35% of patients receiving amphotericin develop hypokalemia sufficient to warrant potassium supplementation. Renal effects are diminished by sodium chloride loading through the liberal administration of intravenous saline. Anemia and encephalopathy may also follow amphotericin use.

Used more commonly for fungal infections are imidazoles (e.g., ketoconazole) and triazoles (e.g., fluconazole). Ketoconazole has direct toxicity that includes GI upset, alopecia, and hepatotoxicity (which can be fatal). However, its most significant adverse effect is inhibition of cytochrome isoenzyme *CYP 3A3/4.* The consequences of this inhibition are endocrinologic abnormalities, resulting from this isoenzyme's role in steroid biosynthesis and metabolism. Ketoconazole may produce menstrual irregularities, gynecomastia, and decreased libido.[37] This enzyme inhibition can also result in life-threatening drug interactions. Ketoconazole used in conjunction with the agents cisapride, terfenadine, and astemizole can produce a prolonged QT syndrome and torsades de pointes; seizures and sudden cardiac death have been reported.[38] Clearance of theophylline, cyclosporine, and coumadin may also be reduced. Finally, ketoconazole has been associated with a disulfiram-like reaction in those drinking ethanol while taking the drug. Fluconazole, a triazole with a spectrum of activity similar to that of ketoconazole, is associated with adverse effects that include rash, abdominal pain, alopecia, hepatitis, and Stevens-Johnson syndrome. Fluconazole is also an inhibitor of cytochrome enzymes but primarily inhibits isoenzyme CYP 2C9/10. This produces decreased clearance of the drugs phenytoin, cyclosporine, coumadin, and sulfonylurea oral hypoglycemics; inadvertent intoxication by these agents can occur with simultaneous use. Unlike ketoconazole, fluconazole appears to have minimal effect on the clearance of theophylline, terfenadine, and astemizole.

Little toxicity is associated with acute ingestion of either agent, and supportive care measures are sufficient in treating acute single overdose. Fluconazole can be removed by hemodialysis, but this therapy is rarely warranted.

ANTIPARASITICS

Important agents in this class include quinine and related drugs, sulfadoxine-pyrimethamine (Fansidar) metronidazole, pentamidine, iodoquinol, benzimidazole, and ivermectin.

Quinine and related drugs are used for the treatment of malaria. Related agents include chloroquine and hydroxychloroquine. Absorbed readily from the GI tract, quinine has a volume of distribution of approximately 1.5 L/kg with an elimination half-life of approximately 11 hours. Therapeutic serum concentrations of drug are 2 to 10 μg/mL.[30] Approximately 10% of drug is excreted in the urine unchanged; elimination is doubled in acidic urine.[39]

The hallmark of quinine overdose is known as *cinchonism.* This syndrome includes features of tinnitus, GI upset, visual disturbances, and hearing impairment. Hearing and vision may be prominently affected; acute single overdose may produce blindness, deafness, or mutism.[28, 40, 41] Other visual disturbances include photophobia, diplopia, narrowed visual fields, and scotomata. These disturbances may be related to spasm of retinal vessels; in overdose, the retina appears pale and ischemic. Other features of cinchonism include abdominal pain, flushing, diaphoresis, and angioedema. Severe hypoglycemia may result from stimulation of pancreatic β-cells.[39] Being a class Ia antiarrhythmic like its stereoisomer quinidine, quinine can produce life-threatening toxicity after acute overdose. Cardiovascular toxicity includes conduction disturbances (e.g., QRS prolongation) and arrhythmias. Seizures are a sign of severe neurotoxicity. The estimated acute fatal dose of quinine is 2 to 8 g.

In addition to cinchonism, chronic quinine use is associated with other toxicities. Blackwater fever is a triad of quinine-associated severe hemolysis, hemoglobinemia, and hemoglobinuria; if untreated, it can result in renal failure and death. It results from a hypersensitivity reaction to quinine during treatment of malaria. Another quinine hypersensitivity reaction is thrombocytopenic purpura, which can appear after chronic ingestion of tonic water ("cocktail purpura").[39]

Treatment of quinine toxicity is largely confined to supportive care. Repeated doses of activated charocal have questionable benefit and are not recommended. Both forced saline diuresis and acid diuresis may produce modest increases in urinary elimination of drug; however, they do not alter the clinical course. Existing data indicate that exchange transfusion, plasmapheresis, hemodialysis, and hemoperfusion all are ineffective in the treatment of quinine intoxication.[42]

Chloroquine is the most commonly used antimalarial. It has a unique pharmacokinetic profile with an enormous volume of distribution (approximately 200 L/kg), low protein binding (50% to 65%), and extremely slow elimination, with a terminal elimination half-life of 200 to 300 hours.[28] As much as 70% of the drug is eliminated in the urine unchanged.

Acute chloroquine ingestion is associated with a dramatic toxicologic syndrome manifested by GI upset that is quickly followed by cardiotoxic effects of hypotension, vasodilatation, electrocardiographic abnormalities (particularly QRS widening), and cardiovascular collapse. These often fatal effects appear after acute ingestions of 5 g or more.[43] A life-saving treatment regimen that has been developed for the treatment of acute chloroquine intoxication includes epinephrine infusion, which begins at a rate of 0.25 μg/kg per minute, rapid-sequence intubation, mechanical ventilation, diazepam 2 mg/kg, and immediate GI decontamination (i.e., gastric lavage followed by activated charcoal.[44–46] Toxicity from chronic overmedication with chloroquine includes GI upset, headache, visual disturbances, ototoxicity, pruritus, and urticaria. Long-term administration of chloroquine may produce torsades de pointes.[36] Chloroquine causes hemolysis in G-6-PD–deficient patients. Rarely, discoloration of the nail beds and mucous membranes may occur.[39] Chloroquine is one of a few drugs that have hypokalemia as a characteristic metabolic complication.[28]

A closely related antimalarial is the aminoquinoline primaquine. Primaquine-associated toxicity includes GI upset, methemoglobinemia, and bone marrow suppression with agranulocytosis.[39] Like chloroquine, this agent can produce hemolysis in patients with G-6-PD deficiency.

Another treatment for malaria is the combination of pyrimethamine-sulfadoxine. Short-term use of this agent has been associated with exfoliative dermatitis. Stevens-Johnson syndrome, and severe hepatic necrosis, often fatal.[39, 47]

Metronidazole is prescribed as both an antiparasitic (e.g., for the treatment of trichomoniasis) and an antibacterial for anaerobic infection (e.g., *Bacteroides, Clostridium,* and *Helicobacter*). The most common adverse effects of metronidazole are headache and a metallic taste in the mouth. GI upset, stomatitis, and pancreatitis also occur frequently.[48] Rarely, neurotoxic effects including dizziness, vertigo, ataxia, and seizures may develop.[39] A peripheral neuropathy has also been associated with its use. Metronidazole produces a disulfiram-like reaction, resulting in abdominal pain, flushing, and severe headache if ethanol is ingested during its use. Acute oral overdose of metronidazole usually does not produce significant toxicity and is treated with supportive care measures only.

Pentamidine is an antiparasitic prescribed for the treatment of *P. carinii* pneumonia; it has received increasing use in the AIDS era. Despite its efficacy, pentamidine is associated with a high rate of side effects (these occurring in as many as 50% of patients[39]). Intravenous administration can produce acute dyspnea, hypotension, and vomiting; these appear to result from histamine release. Other toxic reactions associated with intravenous administration include life-threateining hypoglycemia,[49] rash, azotemia, and hepatitis. Reversible renal dysfunction has occurred in as many as 24% of patients taking the drug.[39] Also, torsades de pointes has been associated with parenteral administration of the drug.[36] Most of these effects have become rarer with increasing use of nebulized pentamidine.

Iodoquinol and clioquinol are prescribed as treatment for amebiasis and other diarrheal illnesses. These drugs are also used topically in the treatment of skin disorders, particularly in children. However, both agents have substantial toxicity. A toxic reaction known as subacute myelo-optic neuropathy results from their use, even after topical application. It presents as an illness that mimics transverse myelitis. Long-term topical administration has also been associated with peripheral neuropathy, optic atrophy, and permanent blindness.[39, 50]

References

1. Mandell GL, Petri WA: Antimicrobial agents: Penicillins, cephalosporins and other beta-lactam antibiotics. *In* Hardman JG, Limbird LE, Molinoff PB, et al (eds): Goodman and Gilman's The Pharmacological Basis of Therapeutics. New York, McGraw-Hill Book Co., pp 1073–1102, 1996.
2. Lascari AD, Amyot K: Fatal hemolysis caused by ceftriaxone. J Pediatr *126:*816–817, 1995.
3. Bernini JC, Mustafa MM, Sutor LJ, Buchanan GR: Fatal hemolysis induced by ceftriaxone in a child with sickle cell anemia. J Pediatr *126:*813–815, 1995.
4. Mandell GL, Petri WA: Antimicrobial agents: Sulfonamides, trimethoprim-sulfamethoxazole, quinolones, and agents for urinary tract infections. *In* Hardman JG, Limbird LE, Molinoff PB, et al (eds): Goodman and Gilman's The Pharmacological Basis of Therapeutics. New York, McGraw-Hill Book Co., pp 1057–1072, 1996.

5. Brouwers JR: Drug interactions with quinolone antibacterials. Drug Saf *7:*268–281, 1992.
6. Chambers HF, Sande MA: Antimicrobial agents: The aminoglycosides. *In* Hardman JG, Limbird LE, Molinoff PB, et al (eds). Goodman and Gilman's The Pharmacological Basis of Therapeutics. New York, McGraw-Hill Book Co., pp 1103–1122, 1996.
7. Kapusnik-Uner JE, Sande MA, Chambers HF: Antimicrobial agents: Tetracyclines, chloramphenicol, erythromycin, and miscellaneous antibacterial agents. *In* Hardman JG, Limbird LE, Molinoff PB, et al: (eds): Goodman and Gilman's The Pharmacological Basis of Therapeutics. New York, McGraw-Hill Book Co., pp 1123–1154, 1996.
8. Shiff A: Doxycycline-induced esophageal ulcers in physicians. JAMA *256:*1893, 1986.
9. Walters BN, Gubbay SS: Tetracycline and benign intracranial hypertension: Report of five cases. BMJ *282:*19–20, 1981.
10. Ben-Ari J, Eisenstein B, Davidovits M, et al: Effect of erythromycin on blood cyclosporine concentrations in kidney transplant patients. J Pediatr *112:*992–993, 1988.
11. Daleau P, Etienne L, Groleau M-F, Turgeon J: Erythromycin blocks the rapid component of the delayed rectifier potassium current and lengthens repolarization of guinea pig ventricular myocytes. Circulation *91:*3010–3016, 1995.
12. Gitler B, Berger LS, Buffa SD: Torsades de pointes induced by erythromycin. Chest *105:*368–372, 1994.
13. Fang C-C, Wang H-P, Lin J-T: Erythromycin-induced acute pancreatitis. Clin Toxicol *34:*93–95, 1996.
14. Tissing W, Umans-Eckenhausen M, vandenAnker J: Vancomycin intoxication in a preterm neonate. Eur J Pediatr *152:*700, 1993.
15. Burkhart KK, Metcalf S, Shurnas E, et al: Exchange transfusion and multidose activated charcoal following vancomycin overdose. Clin Toxicol *30:*285–294, 1992.
16. Kucukguclu S, Tuncok Y, Ozkan H, et al: Multiple-dose activated charcoal in an accidental vancomycin overdose. Clin Toxicol *34:*83–86, 1996.
17. D'Arcy PF: Nitrofurantoin. Drug Intell Clin Pharm *19:*540–547, 1985.
18. Coraggio MJ, Gross TP, Roscelli JD. Nitrofurantoin toxicity in children. Pediatr Infect Dis J *8:*163–166, 1989.
19. Chudnofsky CR, Otten EJ: Acute pulmonary toxicity to nitrofurantoin. J Emerg Med *7:*15–19, 1989.
20. Holt D, Harvey J, Hurley R: Chloramphenicol toxicity. Adverse Drug React Toxicol Rev *12:*83–95, 1993.
21. Sutherland J: Fatal cardiovascular collapse in infants receiving large amounts of chloramphenicol. Am J Dis Child *97:*761–767, 1959.
22. Gershanik J, Boecler B, Ensley H, et al: The gasping syndrome and benzyl alcohol poisoning. N Engl J Med *307:*1384–1388, 1982.
23. Brown WJ, Buist NR, Gipson HTC, et al: Fatal benzyl alcohol poisoning in a neonatal intensive care unit. Lancet *1:*1250, 1982.
24. Newborn Committee on Drugs, American Academy of Pediatrics: Benzyl alcohol: Toxic agent in neonatal units. Pediatrics *73:*356–358, 1983.
25. Benda GI, Hiller HL, Reynolds JW: Benzyl alcohol toxicity: Impact on neurologic handicaps among surviving very low birth weight infants. Pediatrics *77:*507–512, 1986.
26. Mandell GL, Petri WA: Antimicrobial agents: Drugs used in the chemotherapy of tuberculosis and leprosy. *In* Hardman JG, Limbird LE, Molinoff PB, et al (eds): Goodman and Gilman's The Pharmacological Basis of Therapeutics. New York, McGraw-Hill Book Co., pp 1155–1174, 1996.
27. Baciewicz AM, Self TH, Bekemeyer WB: Update on rifampin drug interactions. Arch Intern Med *147:*565–568, 1987.
28. Jaeger A, Sauder P, Kopferschmitt J, Flesch F: Clinical features and management of poisoning due to antimalarial drugs. Med Toxicol *2:*242–273, 1987.
29. Linakis J, Frank C, Shannon M: Recurrent methemoglobinemia in a child after dapsone ingestion. J Emerg Med *7:*477–480, 1989.
30. Hayden FG: Antimicrobial agents: Antiviral agents. *In* Hardman JG, Limbird LE, Molinoff PB, et al (eds): Goodman and Gilman's The Pharmacological Basis of Therapeutics. New York, McGraw-Hill Book Co., pp 1191–1224, 1996.
31. McDonald LK, Tartaglione TA, Mendelman PM, et al: Lack of toxicity in two cases of neonatal acyclovir overdose. Pediatr Infect Dis J *8:*529–532, 1989.
32. Leikin JB, Shicker L, Orlowski J, et al: Hemodialysis removal of acyclovir. Vet Hum Toxicol *37:*233, 1995.
33. New drugs for HIV infection. Med Lett *38:*35–37, 1996.
34. Standaert DG, Young AB: Treatment of central nervous system degenerative disorders. *In* Hardman JG, Limbird LE, Molinoff PB, et al (eds): Goodman and Gilman's The Pharmacological Basis of Therapeutics. New York, McGraw-Hill Book Co., pp 503–519, 1996.
35. Pimentel L, Hughes B: Amantadine toxicity presenting with complex ventricular ectopy and hallucinations. Pediatr Emerg Care *7:*89, 1991.
36. Wharton JM, Demopulos PA, Goldschlager N: Torsade de pointes during administration of pentamidine isethionate. Am J Med *83:*571–575, 1987.
37. Bennett JE: Antimicrobial agents: Antifungal agents. *In* Hardman JG, Limbird LE, Molinoff PB, et al (eds): Goodman and Gilman's The Pharmacological Basis of Therapeutics. New York, McGraw-Hill Book Co., pp 1175–1190, 1996.
38. Honig PK, Wortham DC, Zamani K, et al: Terfenadine-ketoconazole interaction—pharmacokinetic and electrocardiographic consequences. JAMA *269:*1513–1518, 1993.
39. Tracy JW, Webster LT: Chemotherapy of parasitic infections. *In* Hardman JG, Limbird LE, Molinoff PB, et al (eds): Goodman and Gilman's The Pharmacological Basis of Therapeutics. New York, McGraw-Hill Book Co., pp 965–1009, 1996.
40. Schonwald S, Shannon M: Unsuspected quinine intoxication presenting as acute deafness and mutism. Am J Emerg Med *9:*318–320, 1991.
41. Smilkstein M, Kulig KW, Rumack BH: Acute toxic blindness: Unrecognized quinine poisoning. Ann Emerg Med *16:*98–101, 1987.
42. Bateman D, Dyson E: Quinine toxicity. Adverse Drug React Toxicol Rev *4:*215–233, 1986.
43. Kelly JC, Wasserman GS, Bernard WD, et al: Chloroquine poisoning in a child. Ann Emerg Med *19:*47–50, 1990.
44. Riou B, Barriot P, Rimailho A, Baud FJ: Treatment of severe chloroquine poisoning. N Engl J Med *318:*1–6, 1988.
45. Bauer P, Maire B, Weber M, et al: Full recovery after a chlorquine suicide attempt. Clin Toxicol *29:*23–30, 1991.
46. McCarthy VP, Swabe GL: Chloroquine poisoning in a child. Pediatr Emerg Care *12:*207–209, 1996.
47. Zitelli BJ, Alexander J, Taylor S, et al: Fatal hepatic necrosis due to pyrimethamine-sulfadoxine (Fansidar). Ann Intern Med *106:*393–395, 1987.
48. Sanford KA, Mayle JE, Dean HA, Greenbaum DS: Metronidazole-associated pancreatitis. Ann Intern Med *109:*756–757, 1988.
49. Waskin H, Stehr-Green JK, Helmick CG, Sattler FR: Risk factors for hypoglycemia associated with pentamidine therapy for *Pneumocystis* pneumonia. JAMA *260:*345–347, 1988.
50. Committee on Drugs, American Academy of Pediatrics: Clioquinol (iodochlorhydroxyquin, Vioform) and iodoquinol (diiodohydroxyquin): Blindness and neuropathy. Pediatrics *86:*797, 1990.

C Anthelmintics

MAHESH SHRESTHA, MD
CHRISTOPHER KEYES, MD

Infections caused by worms, or helminths, may be the most prevalent of all human infections. It has been estimated that there may be as many worms infecting people as there are people.[1] A thorough review of all the helminths, the clinical syndromes caused, and their diagnoses and treatments are beyond the scope of this chapter. The major organisms are briefly examined, followed by a discussion of the individual chemotherapeutic agents used to treat the infections they cause. Although the mechanisms of action of the anthelmintic medications are poorly understood,[2] they are presented whenever available. A discussion of toxicities of individual agents concludes this chapter.

Helminths are divided into three broad categories: nematodes, trematodes (flatworms, or flukes), and cestodes (tapeworms).

Nematodes include two general categories, intestinal nematodes (roundworms) and tissue nematodes. Intestinal nematodes include the abundant *Ascaris lumbricoides* (giant roundworm), *Trichuris trichiura* (whipworm), and *Enterobius vermicularis* (pinworm), as well as the hookworms *Ancylostoma duodenale* (European hookworm) and *Necatur americanus* (North American hookworm), and *Strongyloides stercoralis.* In the United States, *E. vermicularis,* which causes pruritus ani, is the most common of all helminthic parasites, infecting 42 million people.[3] The prevalence of strongyloidiasis in the southern United States is estimated at 0.4% to 4%. The other helminths are found mainly in tropical areas of the globe, but they are also present in the southeastern United States. It is estimated that 1 billion of the world's population (4.4 million in the United States) are infected with *A. lumbricoides,* 800 million (2.2 million in the United States) with *T. trichiura,* and one fourth of the world's population with hookworm. Hookworm disease was controlled almost in its entirety in the United States during the early part of this century and is uncommon here. The treatment of choice for all of these intestinal nematode infections, except strongyloidiasis, is mebendazole (Vermox), an imidazole. Thiabendazole (Mintezol), a related compound, is currently the treatment of choice for strongyloidiasis. Albendazole is the newest of this group of medications. It achieves greater tissue levels and has a broader spectrum of activity. Pyrantel pamoate can also be used.

Tissue nematodes include *Trichinella spiralis* (the causative agent of trichinosis), *Dracunculus medinensis* (causing skin ulcers through which the worm appears), the three causative agents of filariasis (*Wuchereria bancrofti, Brugia malayi,* and *Brugia timori*), *Loa loa,* and *Onchocerca volvulus.* No completely effective treatment has been found for trichinosis, but use of thiabendazole is recommended within 24 hours for patients known to have ingested trichinous meat. Thiabendazole or metronidazole is recommended for the inflammation of dracunculiasis so that the worms themselves can be physically removed by rolling them on a stick during the course of a week. Filariasis is characterized by acute and chronic lymphatic inflammation eventually resulting in elephantiasis, hydrocele, and chyluria. There is no satisfactory treatment, but administration of diethylcarbamazine reduces the number of microfilaria. Diethylcarbamazine is also effective against *L. loa* and *O. volvulus. L. loa* is characterized by transient subcutaneous swellings (Calabar swellings). *O. volvulus* is the causative agent of river blindness, named for the blackfly that breeds in fast streams, which has caused blindness in whole African villages. The newer drug ivermectin is safer and more effective than diethylcarbamazine for onchocerciasis. Albendazole is the newest of this group of medications (imidazoles) and produces greater tissue levels and a broader spectrum of activity.

Trematodes include the blood flukes, or schistosomes (*Schistosoma mansoni, S. japonicum, S. haematobium,* and *S. mekongi*), which are one of the world's major public health concerns, the liver flukes (*Clonorchis sinensis* and *Fasciola hepatica*); the lung fluke *Paragonimus westermani*; and the intestinal fluke *Fasciolopsis buski.* Praziquantel is the drug of choice for all of these organisms (except *F. hepatica,* for which bithionol is used) and has revolutionized treatment. Metrifonate (Bilarcil) is effective against *S. haematobium,* and oxamniquine is effective against *S. mansoni.*

Cestodes, segmented worms or tapeworms, include the beef tapeworm (*Taenia saginata*), the pork tapeworm (*Taenia solium,* whose eggs cause human cysticercosis), the fish tapeworm (*Diphyllobothrium latum*), the dwarf tapeworm (*Hymenolepis nana*), and *Echinococcus granulosus,* the causative agent of echinococcosis, or hydatid disease. Niclosamide is the usual drug given to eradicate the adult tapeworms, but paromomycin and praziquantel are also effective. For human cysticercosis, praziquantel (with corticosteroids) is the drug of choice, and for hydatid cyst disease, albendazole with surgical removal is effective.

Other helminthic infections include visceral larval migrans (toxocariasis), cutaneous larva migrans (creeping eruption, caused by *Ancylostoma braziliense,* the dog or cat hookworm), and dirofilariasis.

Most patients recover from visceral larva migrans without specific therapy. Thiabendazole has been used along with other agents for severe cases. Thiabendazole administered either orally or topically has also been used successfully for cutaneous larva migrans. *Dirofilaria immitis* is the causative agent of the dog heartworm. In humans, the immature filariae die, causing a local vasculitis in the pulmonary circulation. This may be seen occasionally as a coin lesion on the chest radiograph.

The drugs mentioned earlier are the most common anthelmintics used. Older drugs such as those in the antimony group, pyrantel pamoate, poquil, bephenium hydroxynaphthoate, and hycanthone have special applications and may still be in use, especially in less developed countries and in veterinary medicine. Levamisole, related to mebendazole, and suramin, in use since 1920, have found newer uses as chemotherapeutic agents in the treatment of certain cancers.

In general, the older medications are more toxic to humans than the newer ones. The older medications have reported protean side effects, some of which are worse than the disease being treated. On other occasions, the side effects may be mistaken for progression or complications of the disease itself. It is important to remember that many of the side effects of treatment, such as with praziquantel for cysticercosis or with diethylcarbamazine for onchocerciasis (ivermectin is now used), are due to the large antigenic mass of dying worms released into the blood stream. Similarly, many side effects are really not side effects of the medication because they probably would not occur if uninfected patients were given the same treatment. Pretreatment or concurrent treatment with corticosteroids is used in some cases, and slow progressive therapy is used in others. Medications that are not significantly absorbed (and thus have insignificant systemic toxicity), such as mebendazole, are ideal for susceptible helminths that are limited to the lumen of the gastrointestinal (GI) tract.

In the review that follows, the many agents available are divided into intuitive groups: imidazoles (mebendazole and related compounds), piperazines (diethylcarbamazine and piperazine), drugs identified for schistosomiasis (praziquantel, metrifonate, and others), and other important anthelmintics, such as ivermectin and suramin.

IMIDAZOLES

Mebendazole

Mebendazole is a drug commonly used in the treatment of intestinal nematodal disease, such as ascariasis, trichiuriasis, hookworm (*N. americanus* or *A. duodenale*), and enterobiasis (pinworm). Like the other benzimidazoles, it is thought to selectively and irreversibly block microtubular-dependent glucose uptake by nematodes and cestodes by binding to free β-tublin and inhibiting tublin polymerization.[4] Only 5% to 10% of an orally ingested dose is absorbed from the GI tract. Most of what is absorbed is metabolized in the liver (P-450 system) in a significant first-pass effect. Thus adverse reactions attributable to the medication itself are practically nonexistent, although diarrhea and abdominal pain have been reported. The usual dose used is 100 mg twice daily for 3 days. For pinworm infection, one 100-mg tablet given once is sufficient.

Mebendazole has also been used to treat hydatid disease (echinococcal cysts); a reduction in cyst size has been demonstrated with prolonged treatment. Albendazole, a related imidazole with better absorption, has now replaced mebendazole for this use. Albendazole is given in 4-week cycles of 400 mg, twice daily, separated by 2-week rest periods. At least three cycles are given. When albendazole is given in these higher doses, pyrexia has been noted; it is thought to be due to tissue necrosis of the hydatid cyst.

Another reported side effect of mebendazole is agranulocytosis. In a Russian study, this complication was found in 2 of 75 patients with hydatid cysts treated with 50 mg/kg per day for 30 days, resulting in the death of one patient,[5] Mebendazole has been shown to be teratogenic and embryotoxic in laboratory animals and so is contraindicated in pregnancy and in those younger than 2 years. Cimetidine, by inhibiting the P-450 system, may increase blood levels.

Treatment of poisoning includes decontamination in cases of overdose and is otherwise symptomatic and supportive.

Albendazole

Albendazole is similar to mebendazole but is more completely absorbed from the GI tract. It has a broader spectrum of activity. Its absorption is enhanced by taking it with fatty meals.[6] One of its main uses is in adjunctive treatment with surgery (or single-agent treatment without surgery) in hydatid cyst disease due to echinococci.[7] Mebendazole is probably as effective for most nematodal disease isolated to the lumen of the GI tract. Albendazole appears to be more effective for hookworm.[8] It is also effective against intestinal tapeworms and neurocysticercosis, for which it is an alternative to niclosamide and praziquantel, respectively. In one trial, it was more effective than praziquantel in neurocysticercosis.[9]

Albendazole is rapidly metabolized by the liver into an active metabolite that has a terminal half-life of 8.5 hours. It is given in at least three 4-week cycles separated by 2-week rest periods at a dose of 400 mg twice daily (10 to 14 mg/kg/day) when used for hydatid cyst disease. Side effects are similar to those for mebendazole and usually do not require discontinuation. It, too, has been shown to be teratogenic in animals (rats and rabbits) and is not recommended in pregnancy or in infants younger than 2 years.

Treatment of poisonings is symptomatic and supportive (see also the later discussion of thiabendazole side effects).

Thiabendazole

Thiabendazole, like albendazole, is also rapidly absorbed through the GI tract, metabolized by the hepatic P-450 system, and excreted by the kidneys in the first 24 hours. It is also available for topical application for cutaneous larva migrans. In addition to binding free β-tubulin, it inhibits the helminth-specific fumarate reductase enzyme system. It is the treatment of choice for strongyloidiasis, for which the dosage is 25 mg/kg twice daily (maximum, 3 g/day) for 2 days. In immunocompromised hosts (e.g., HIV-infected patients or those with cancer), a hyperinfection syndrome from *S. stercoralis* can develop. Infective filariform larvae re-enter the host via the lower GI tract or perianal regions in massive numbers. For this, thiabendazole is given at 25 mg/kg twice daily for 2 to 3 weeks.[10]

Thiabendazole has also been used for cutaneous larva migrans (creeping eruption, caused by *A. braziliensis*), visceral larva migrans, and trichinosis (*T. spiralis*), all of which have no proven therapy. Thiabendazole may serve only to decrease the load of growing organisms. It has also been used, at a dose of 25 mg/kg twice daily for 2 days, to treat *D. medinensis* infection (dracontiasis), when it helps to decrease inflammation, allowing slow removal of the helminth by winding it on stick during the course of a week.[11] Metronidazole has also been used for this same purpose.

Numerous adverse reactions have been loosely attributed to thiabendazole. Most reactions are transient and not serious. These include GI effects such as anorexia, nausea, epigastric discomfort, and diarrhea; generalized complaints such as dizziness, drowsiness, weakness, and pruritus; and nervous system complaints such as headaches, tinnitus, and blurred vision. Also reported are hypotension, bradycardia, crystalluria, and malodorous urine. Self-limited abnormalities may be cholestasis, leukopenia, elevated liver transaminase levels, jaundice, and hyperglycemia. Nephrotoxicity has been reported, as well as inhibition of hepatic metabolism of theophylline, which would be expected because both drugs are metabolized by the hepatic P-450 system. Hypersensitivity reactions are also reported and include fever/chills, rashes, angioedema, erythema multiforme, Stevens-Johnson syndrome, and anaphylaxis. Allergy to topically applied medication has also been reported.[12]

Treatment for intoxication with this agent is supportive. Thiabendazole should be avoided by patients with liver and kidney disease. Levels of other hepatic P-450–metabolized medications should be monitored. Because of the possibility of drowsiness due to this drug, heavy machinery should not be operated by patients under treatment. Its safety has not been established in pregnancy or lactation.

Flubendazole

Flubendazole is the parafluoro analogue of mebendazole. Interestingly, it is absorbed better from the GI tract when taken with or after a meal. It is also available in a slow-release parenteral preparation given subcutaneously or intramuscularly, which allows sustained release over 5 days. The usual dosage is 750 mg/wk for onchocerciasis. It is used to treat hookworm, *T. trichiura,* and *A. lumbricoides.* Side effects are vague and mostly abdominal, such as nausea, abdominal pain and rumbling, soft/loose stools, and dyspepsia. Also reported are fatigue and breathlessness. Unlike mebendazole, it has not yet been shown to be teratogenic in laboratory animals. Treatment of poisoning is supportive. If side effects are severe, flubendazole may have to be withdrawn.

Levamisole

Levamisole (Anthelvet, Ripercol, Ketrax) is the more nematocidal L-isomer of tetramisole. Its mechanism of action is thought to be rapid and reversible muscle paralysis of the helminth due to ganglionic stimulation. Like thiabendazole, at high doses, it also inhibits the helminthic fumarate reductase system. It is available as a syrup or tablet, is rapidly absorbed from the GI tract, and is extensively metabolized. Its use is mainly for nematodal disease such as ascariasis, for which it can be given in a single 120- to 150-mg dose.

Today levamisole is used more in combination chemotherapy for cancer (e.g., with 5-fluorouracil in colon cancer) than as an anthelmintic. The doses when used in this manner are different, and more side effects have become evident. Agranulocytosis develops when levamisole is used for a prolonged period.[13] Thrombocytopenia occurring as late as 2 years after its use has been reported.[14] Many skin reactions have been reported, most recently a fixed toxic erythema with pigmentation.[15] Also reported are cases of multifocal inflammatory leukoencephalopathy when used with 5-fluorouracil.[16] In patients taking warfarin, the international normalization ratio has been reported to increase.[17] This may be because of its competitive inhibition of hepatic P-450 system metabolism of warfarin.

Treatment of poisoning is supportive. Severe effects mandate discontinuation of its use.

Niridazole

Niridazole (Ambilhar) is also an imidazole (a substituted nitrothiazole), but it does not have the same uses as the others. It also has the distinction of suppressing cellular immunity and possibly being carcinogenic. Fifty per cent of oral intake is absorbed. It is excreted in the feces and urine after it has been metabolized in the liver. It has a metabolite with a half-life of 40 hours, and this is responsible for the prolonged immune suppression encountered. It causes the urine to become very dark, and patients should be warned about this.

Its main uses are for *S. japonicum* and *S. mansoni* infections, amebiasis, and dracontiasis, in which it may be used like thiabendazole as an anti-inflammatory. It is not as effective against the other species of schistosomes.

Its toxicity includes nervous system problems such as seizures (usually limited to patients with a seizure disorder), subclinical electroencephalographic changes, headaches, dizziness, agitation, insomnia, and hallucinations (usually only in patients with a history of psychosis). In the treatment of schistosomiasis, it is possible that some of the central nervous system effects are due to high drug levels because of hepatic shunting. Other side effects include GI effects such as nausea, vomiting, and abdominal pain. Also reported are rash, slight electrocardiographic abnormalities, and hemolytic anemia in patients with glucose-6-phosphatase deficiency.

Treatment of the toxicity is supportive. It should not be used by patients with a seizure disorder, liver disease, or psychosis.

PIPERAZINES

Piperazine

Piperazine (Antepar, Vermizine) causes paralysis of the helminth and is thought to precipitate expulsion of the helminth from the GI tract. It is orally absorbed and is excreted unchanged in the urine within 24 hours. Its uses include treatment of enterobiasis (pinworm infection), 65 mg/kg per day (maximum 2.5 g) for 7 days; and ascariasis, 75 mg/kg per day (maximum 3.5 g) for 2 days. In cases of intestinal obstruction due to large worm burdens, it is recommended that piperazine syrup be given via nasogastric tube at a dose of 150 mg/kg then 65 mg/kg every 12 hours for 6 doses. It narcotizes the worm in the intestinal or biliary tract, allowing its passage distally.[18]

Side effects are rare but can affect many organ systems. GI symptoms include nausea/vomiting, diarrhea, and abdominal pain. General symptoms include fever, weakness, and rash. Angioneurotic edema has been reported in sensitive patients.[19] Neurologic abnormalities include visual disturbances, seizures and electroencephalographic abnormalities, and cerebellar ataxia, known as "worm wobble."[20] The latter abnormalities are seen mainly in patients with overdoses or with renal failure in which the accumulated levels have become toxic.

Treatment of side effects and toxicities includes discontinuation of treatment and administration of antihistamines if the effects seem to be allergic in nature. Other side effects are treated symptomatically. Piperazine is not recommended for patients with hepatic or renal disturbance or with seizures. Its safety in pregnancy has not been established.

Diethylcarbamazine

Diethylcarbamazine is still in use in many parts of the world. In the United States, it may be found in dog-owning households because it is a treatment for *D. immitis,* the dog heartworm. Ivermectin has become popular for prophylaxsis of this condition (discussed later). It is highly soluble in water and is well absorbed through the GI tract. Its renal clearance is reduced in alkaline urine. It is also available as a lotion for onchocerciasis. In addition to its canine use, it can be used to treat filariasis and *O. volvulus.* In filariasis, like thiabendazole, it may do no more than reduce the number of microfilariae of *W. bancrofti* and *B. malayi* (6 mg/kg daily for 2 weeks). Its effect on adult worms is uncertain, although a higher dose repeated monthly or weekly may be effective.[21] In the treatment of *L. loa,* it eliminates the microfilariae and may also kill the adult worms.

In the treatment of onchocerciasis (and also of filariasis to a lesser degree) with diethylcarbamazine, a severe reaction, probably an immune response to the mass of dying antigenic microfilariae, may develop 16 hours after treatment. It consists of severe pruritus, a fine papular rash, skin edema, fever, tachycardia, headache, swollen lymph nodes, and possibly hypotension. This reaction was first described in 1948 and is called the *Mazzotti reaction.*[22] For this reason, it is recommended that the diethylcarbamazine dose be gradually increased from 50 mg once per day on day 1, to 50 mg three times per day on day 2, to 100 mg three times per day on day 3, to the full 3 mg/kg three times per day on days 4 through 21. Levels of the immune mediator interleukin-6 correlate with the occurrence and severity of clinical symptoms after treatment. Tumor necrosis factors also are elevated in patients with reactions.[23] The Mazzotti reaction can also be used to test whether a rash is caused by *O. volvulus.* This is done by giving a test dose of 50 mg of diethylcarbamazine. If the rash worsens, it probably is due to a reaction against *O. volvulus.* Ivermectin (discussed later) has replaced diethylcarbamazine as the drug of choice in the treatment of onchocerciasis because it is safer and more effective.

Other side effects include changes in the posterior segment of the eye (transient pigment lesions, optic disk leakage, and visual loss).[24] *L. loa* encephalopathy may be aggravated. Pretreatment or concurrent treatment with corticosteroids is helpful. A transient proteinuria, possibly resulting from circulating immune complexes, has also been described in patients.[25]

ANTISCHISTOSOME MEDICATIONS

Praziquantel

The development of praziquantel (Cesol) has been a major advance in the control of schistosomiasis. It also has many other anthelmintic uses. It is readily absorbed through the GI tract and excreted by the kidneys. It can be detected in human breast milk. Its mode of action is not clearly understood. Bioavailability is limited by an extensive first-pass effect through liver metabolism. This is exacerbated by dexamethasone and antiepileptic medication (through P-450 induction), often given concomitantly with praziquantel in patients with neurocysticercosis.[26, 27] Cimetidine, which inhibits P-450 metabolism, lengthens the drug's elimination half-life.[28]

It is effective against all schistosomes as well as most of the other trematodes (flukes).[29] For *S. haematobium* and *S. mansoni,* it is given as a single 40 mg/kg dose, and for *S. japonicum* it is given as 20 mg/kg three times in 1 day. For *C. sinensis,* it is the treatment of choice. Surgery may be necessary for biliary obstruction. *Clonorchis* and intestinal flukes (*F. buski* and *Heterophyes heterophyes*) are treated with a dose of 25 mg/kg three times per day for 1 day. The lung fluke (*Paragonimus*) is treated with 25 mg/kg three times per day for 2 days. The only fluke not responsive to praziquantel is *F. hepatica* (sheep liver), for which bithionol must be used.

In addition to the trematodes, praziquantel is also effective against the cestodes (tapeworms). *T. saginata* (beef tapeworm), *T. solium* (pork tapeworm), and *Diphyllobothrium nana* (fish tapeworm) are treated with 10 mg/kg as a single dose, and *H. nana* (dwarf tapeworm) is treated with 25 mg/kg as a single dose. For human cysticercosis, infection with *T. solium* eggs, treatment is with 50 mg/kg per day in three divided doses for 2 weeks. This is usually given with corticosteroids to avoid the immunologic reaction common with the large antigenic load that is released. It may also have a role in the treatment of *Echinococcus.*

Side effects and toxicity from praziquantel are usually a result of the treatment of the infection rather than of the medication per se. When all inhabitants in an area of high prevalence of *S. mansoni* (61.8%) were treated, 27.2% had side effects (abdominal discomfort, fever, headache), mostly mild, disappearing in 24 hours, correlating with those that were infected.[30]

Toxicity is very rare. Mild toxicity does not require discontinuance of medication. If toxicity is from the rapid killing of worms, corticosteroids may be administered if not already given.

Metrifonate

Metrifonate, also called *trichlorofon,* is an organophosphorus compound that is selective for treatment of *S. haematobium.* It is nonenzymatically transformed into dichlorvos and inhibits plasma cholinesterase activity. It inhibits erythrocyte cholinesterase to a lesser degree. The dose is 7.5 mg/kg (range 5 to 15) every 2 weeks for 6 weeks.

Side effects include those of other cholinergic medications if taken in sufficient quantity. Suicide attempts among patients using metrifonate have been reported. Also reported have been cases of polyneuropathy.[31] Management of toxicity is similar to that with other cholinergic medication.

Oxamniquine

Oxamniquine (Vansil, Mansil) is an antischistosomal quinoline compound selective for *S. mansoni.* Fifty per cent of an oral dose is absorbed; most is excreted in the urine. A metabolite turns the urine dark orange or reddish on the second day. The dosage used varies from 60 mg/kg over 3 days in Egypt or East Africa to a low of 12 mg/kg as a single dose.

Side effects are frequent but usually mild and are likely due to immune reactions to the release antigenic load rather than the medication itself. They include dizziness, headache, vague abdominal pain, nausea, vomiting, and transient increases in results of liver function tests, especially in older patients. In one report, 38% had fever of 38 to 39°C often 24 to 72 hours after completing a 3-day treatment. Six of 40 developed Löffler's syndrome with transient pulmonary infiltrates and eosinophilia.[32] Treatment is supportive.

Hycanthone

Hycanthone (Etronol) has an unknown mechanism of action but is effective against *S. haematobium* and *S. mansoni.* It has good GI absorption and can also be given intramuscularly. It is not sold in the United States.

Side effects are frequent but mild and self-limited. The complaints usually are of GI origin (nausea, vomiting, and abdominal pain) or generalized (weakness, dizziness, headache, and myalgias). Very rarely a serious hepatic necrosis can occur. Hycanthone is mutagenic, carcinogenic, and teratogenic in animals and therefore should not be given to pregnant women until 1 month after delivery, nor to children and young adults. It should also be avoided by patients with liver disease. Treatment is symptomatic and supportive.

Niridazole was discussed earlier in the section on imidazoles.

OTHER ANTHELMINTICS

Other anthelmintics, such as ivermectin and niclosamide, are in common use around the world, and others are of primarily historical importance. Some of the latter are still used in developing countries.

Ivermectin

Ivermectin enjoys widespread use around the world. In the United States, it is used primarily for prophylaxis and treatment of heartworm in dogs. It is often the object of calls to regional poison control centers.

Ivermectin is from a family of chemicals called avermectins. These are macrocyclic lactones from the fermentation broth of *Streptomyces avermitilis.* It is thought to work by opening chloride-sensitive channels. In the free-living nematode *Aenorhabditis elegans,* it binds to a glutamate-gated chloride channel.[33]

It is active primarily in nematodes and is the drug of choice for the treatment of onchocerciasis. It kills the microfilariae of *O. volvulus* but not the adults. Sumarin (discussed later) is the only agent that kills the adults. It is also used to treat *D. immitis* (heartworm) in dogs. For onchocerciasis, it is given in a dose of 150 μg/kg as a single dose. It has been tried in the treatment of lymphatic filariasis (single dose), clearing microfilariae from the blood, but is not active against adult filarial worms in the lymphatic system.[34] It can also be used as an alternative to mebendazole in the treatment of intestinal nematodes.[35]

Adverse reactions are rare and are related to the worm burden rather than the medication itself. In one report, 97% had side effects when ivermectin was used to treat *W. bancrofti.* These consisted of fever, headache, pruritic rash, weakness, myalgias, lymphatic nodules, cough, and elevated alkaline phosphatase levels, all of which subsided in 12 to 72 hours after treatment. Some patients with very dense infection developed serious pulmonary symptoms consisting of cough with production of blood-tinged sputum, shortness of breath, and patchy pneumonitis.[36] Some patients, however, had heavy worm burdens but did not develop side effects. Other reported side effects include facial edema and bullous skin disease.[37] Treatment is symptomatic.

Niclosamide

Niclosamide (Yomesan) is not absorbed through the GI tract and therefore has almost no side effects. It is used to treat cestodes (tapeworms), which include *T. saginata* (beef tapeworm), *T. solium* (pork tapeworm), *D. latum* (fish tapeworm), and *H. nana* (dwarf tapeworm). It is not effective against cysticercosis (eggs of *T. solium*) or *E. granulosus* (hydatid disease), because these require tissue penetration.

Patients occasionally complain of GI symptoms, such as abdominal cramping and nausea. Treatment is supportive and symptomatic.

Sumarin

Sumarin (Antrypol) is an antiparasitic drug that is now used in cancer chemotherapy. It was introduced in 1920 for the treatment of African trypanosomiasis and began to be used in 1947 for the treatment of onchocerciasis. It is the only medication that kills the adult *O. volvulus.* It is not well absorbed orally, and intramuscular injection causes significant local skin irritation; thus, it is given intravenously. Its elimination half-life is 36 to 54 hours. Nearly 100% (99.9%) is protein bound.

It is recommended for onchocerciasis only if the patient has recurrent skin disease after treatment with ivermectin and several courses of diethylcarbamazine or for patients with eye disease. A test dose of 100 mg is first given, and if this is tolerated, 1.0 g is given intravenously each week for 6 weeks. Treatment is stopped if proteinuria or casts appear in the urine or if exfoliative dermatitis develops.

Sumarin toxicity can result in renal and adrenal insufficiency, coagulation factor abnormalities, immune suppression, and polyneuropathy.

Other side effects include a wide variety of skin eruptions,[38] including a lethal toxic epidermal necrolysis,[39] and weakness due to hypophosphatemia, mitochondrial myopathy,[40] or motor axonal polyneuropathy (some with sensory symptoms).[41] Treatment is supportive and symptomatic. The drug should be withdrawn if side effects occur.

Pyrantel Pamoate

Pyrantel pamoate (Combatrin, Antiminth) is a depolarizing neuromuscular blocker. It results in spastic neuromuscular paralysis of the parasite, allowing its expulsion. It is poorly absorbed from the GI tract; 40% is excreted in the feces, and small amounts are detectable in the urine. It is used for enterobiasis (pinworm), ascariasis (giant roundworm), and *N. americanus* (hookworm) infections. The usual dose is 11 mg/kg orally once (maximum 1 g), repeated after 2 weeks.

Because most of an oral ingestion remains in the lumen of the GI tract, the medication itself has very few side effects. Most of the side effects are from the parasitic burden. These include nausea, vomiting, abdominal pain, tenesmus, headache, dizziness, insomnia, drowsiness, fever, rash, and nasal congestion. Liver transaminase levels may become transiently elevated. Use of pyrantel pamoate is contraindicated in pregnancy, in those younger than 1 year, and in patients with liver disease. Treatment is symptomatic and supportive.

Pyrvinium Pamoate

Pyrvinium pamoate (Povan, Vanquin), like pyrantel pamoate, is useful to eliminate certain intestinal parasites because of its minimal absorption from the GI tract. Patients should be warned of changes in stool color, which most often becomes red. It has been largely replaced by mebendazole for the treatment of enterobiasis (oxyuriasis).

It produces minimal side effects, with occasional

nausea, vomiting, and abdominal pain. A photosensitive skin reaction has also been reported. Treatment is symptomatic.

Poquil

Poquil has been used for the treatment of enterobiasis (oxyuriasis) at a dose of 1.5 mg/kg per day for 8 days. Mebendazole treatment is simpler (one dose) and is the agent of choice. Poquil is well tolerated, although occasional nausea and vomiting are reported. It causes a bitter taste in the mouth. Treatment of intoxication is symptomatic and supportive. If vomiting or other effects are severe, it should be discontinued.

Antimony

The trivalent antimonials act by inhibition of phosphofructokinase. They have to be administered intravenously because oral ingestion leads to significant GI irritation. They bind to erythrocytes and thus have slow renal excretion—on the order of weeks to months.

Trivalent antimony has been replaced by other medications for most helminthiasis, but on occasion they are used, mainly for schistosomiasis. *S. japonicum* responds to antimony potassium tartate and antimony sodium dimercaptosuccinate. *S. haematobium* and *S. mansoni* also respond to antimony sodium dimercaptosuccinate. *S. mansoni* also responds to stibophen.

The antimonials have many toxicities. They are contraindicated in hepatic disease, unless it is due to schistosomiasis, because they can cause worsening of liver function. They can rarely cause hepatitis. A host of immunologic reactions can occur, such as an anaphylactoid reaction and anaphylaxis, arthralgias, arthritis, myalgias, headache, fainting, skin rashes, and facial edema. Pulmonary symptoms include pneumonia (especially with tartrates), coughing, dyspnea, and apnea.

More specific side effects include fever, fainting, rashes, and vomiting with use of dimercaptosuccinate; hemolytic anemia, thrombocytopenia, vomiting, and albuminuria with stibophen; and phlebitis, cough, and death due to rapid injection with tartrates. Dimercaptosuccinate is contraindicated in the presence of bacterial infection or herpes (simplex or zoster) infection.

The medication should be withdrawn if the side effects are severe. Treatment is supportive and symptomatic.

Pentavalent antimony is used in the treatment of protozoan infections such as leishmaniasis.

Bephenium Hydroxynaphthoate

Bephenium hydroxynaphthoate is a quaternary ammonium used for the treatment of hookworm (*N. americanus,* 5 g twice per day for 3 days; and *A. duodenale,* 5 g twice per day for 5 days); and also for giant roundworm (*A. lumbricoides*). It has been replaced for the most part by mebendazole but is more effective than tetrachloroethylene.

It has minimal GI absorption. It does have a bitter taste, and this is what usually causes the nausea and vomiting. Treatment is symptomatic.

Bithionol

Bithionol may still be used for human fascioliasis (30 to 50 mg/kg on alternate days for 10 to 15 doses), for which it is the treatment of choice. It may be used for paragonimiasis (30 mg/kg every other day for 20 days), but for the most part treatment of this and other trematode infections has been replaced by praziquantel.

Side effects are skin reactions and GI irritation, which are rarely severe enough to discontinue medication. Treatment is symptomatic.

Paromomycin

Paromomycin (Humatin) can be used to eradicate the cestodes (tapeworms) *T. saginata, T. solium, D. latum,* and *H. nana.* It is given in a dosage of 1 g every 4 hours for 4 days. Treatment with paromomycin has largely been replaced by niclosamide.

References

1. Stoll NR. This wormy world. J Parasitol *33:*1–18, 1947.
2. Liu LX, Weller PF: Antiparasitic drugs. N Engl J Med *334:*1178–1184, 1996.
3. Warren KS: Helminthic diseases endemic in the United States. Am J Trop Med Hyg *23*:723, 1974.
4. Lacey E: Mode of action of benzimidaziles. Parasitol Today *6:*112–115, 1990.
5. Shcherbakov AM, Kozlova TL, Bebris NK: Agranulocytosis—a complication of the chemotherapy of echinococcosis with mebendazole. Med Parazitol (Mosk) 5–6:9–11, 1992.
6. Awadzi K, Hero M, Opoku NO, et al: The chemotherapy of onchocerciasis XVII: A clinical evaluation of albendazole in patients with onchocerciasis; effects of food and pretreatment with ivermectin on drug response and pharmokinetics. Trop Med Parasitol *45:*203–208, 1994.
7. Dickson B: Albendazole for hydatid cysts. Lancet *1:*37, 1984.
8. Albonico M, Smith PG, Hall A, et al: A randomized controlled trial comparing mebendazole and albendazole against *Ascaris, Trichuris* and hookwork infections. Trans R Soc Trop Med Hyg *88:*585–589, 1994.
9. Takayanagui OM, Jardim E: Therapy for neurocysticercosis: Comparison between albendezole and praziquantel. Arch Neurol *49:*290–294, 1992.
10. Grove DI: Treatment of strongyloidiasis with thiobendazole: An analysis of toxicity and effectiveness. Trans R Soc Trop Med Hyg *76:*114–118, 1982.
11. Sastry SC, Jayakumar K, Lakshminarayana V: The treatment of dracontiasis with thiabendazole. J Trop Med Hyg *81:*32, 1978.
12. Mancuso G: Topical thiabendazole allergy. Contact Dermatitis *31:*207, 1994.
13. Renoux G: The general immunopharmacology of levamisole. Drugs *19:*89–90, 1980.

14. Winquist EW, Lassam NJ: Reversible thrombocytopenia with levamisole. Med Pediatr Oncol *24:*262–264, 1995.
15. Clavere P, Bonnafoux-Clavere A, Delrous JL, et al: Fixed pigmented erythema caused by levamisole administration. Ann Dermatol Venereol *121:*238–239, 1994.
16. Enterline DS, Davey NC, Tien RD: Multifocal inflammatory leukoencephalopathy due to treatment with 5-fluorouracil and levamisole. AJR Am J Roentgenol *165:*214–215, 1995.
17. Scarfe MA, Israel MK: Possible drug interaction between warfarin and combination of levamisole and fluorouracil. Ann Pharmacol *28:*264–267, 1994.
18. Swartwelder JC, Miller JH, Sappenfield RW: The use of piperazine for the treatment of human helminthiases. Gastroenterology *33:*87, 1957.
19. Eedy DJ: Angioneurotic oedema following piperazine ingestion in an ethylenediamine-sensitive subject. Contact Dermatitis *28:*48–49, 1993.
20. Conners GP: Piperazine neurotoxicity: Worm wobble revisited. J Emerg Med *13:*341–343, 1995.
21. Ottesen EA: Efficacy of diethylcarbamazine in eradicating infection with lymphatic-dwelling filariae in humans. Rev Infect Dis *7:*341, 1985.
22. Mazzotti L: Posibilidad de utilizar como medio diagnóstico en la onchocercosis las reacciones alérgicas consecutivas a la administratión de Heterozan. Rev Inst Salubr Enferm Trop *9:*235–237, 1948.
23. Turner PF, Rockett KA, Ottesen EA, et al: Interleukin-6 and tumor necrosis factor in the pathogenesis of adverse reactions after treatment of lymphatic filariasis and onchocerciasis. J Infect Dis *169:*1071–1075, 1994.
24. Bird AC, Hall EL, Sheil CH, et al: Changes in visual function and in the posterior segment of the eye during the treatment of onchocerciasis with diethylcarbamazine citrate. Br J Ophthalmol *64:*1191, 1980.
25. Ngu JL, Mate A: Proteinuria associated with diethylcarbamazine. Lancet *1:*710, 1980.
26. Vazquez ML, Jung H, Sotelo J: Plasma levels of praziquantel decrease when dexamethasone is given simultaneously. Neurology *37:*1561–1562, 1987.
27. Bittencourt PR, Garcia CM, Martins R, et al: Phenytoin and carbamazepine decrease and bioavailability of praziquantel. Neurology *42:*492–496, 1992.
28. Duchman WD, Adubofour KO, Biken DS, et al: Cimetidine-induced rise in praziquantel levels in a patient with neurocysticercosis being treated with anti-c. J Infect Dis *169:*689–691, 1994.
29. Day TA, Bennett JL, Pax RA: Praziquantel: The enigmatic antiparasitic. Parisitol Today *8:*342–344, 1992.
30. Boisier P, Ravaoalimalala VA, Serieye J, et al: *Schistosoma mansoni* infection in a hyperendemic region of midwestern Madagascar: Epidemiology, morbidity and secondary effects of praziquantel (French). Arch Inst Pasteur Madagascar *61:*43–48, 1994.
31. Akimor GA, Buchko VM, Kremleva RV: Neurological disorders in trichlorfon poisoning. Klin Med (Mosk) *5:*65, 1975.
32. Higashi GI, Farid Z: Oxamniquine—drug-induced or immune-complex reaction? BMJ *2:*830, 1979.
33. Cully DF, Vassilatis DK, Liu KK, et al: Cloning of an ivermectin-sensitive glutamate-gated chloride channel from *Caenorhabiditis elegans.* Nature *371:*707–711, 1994.
34. Ottesen EA, Vijayasekaran V, Kumaraswami V, et al: A controlled trial of ivermectin and diethylcarbamazine in lymphatic filariasis. N Engl J Med *322:*1113–1117, 1990.
35. Naquira C, Jimenez G, Guerra JG, et al: Ivermectin for human strongyloidiasis and other intestinal helminths. Am J Trop Med Hyg *40:*304–309, 1989.
36. Kar SK, Patnaik S, Kumaraswami V, Murty RS: Side reactions following ivermectin therapy in high density bancroftian microfilaraemics. Acta Trop *55:*21–31, 1993.
37. Burnham GM: Adverse reactions to ivermectin treatment for onchocerciasis. Results of a placebo-controlled, double-blind trial in Malawi. Trans R Soc Trop Med Hyg *87:*313–317, 1993.
38. Lowitt MH, Eisenberg M, Sina B, Kao GF: Cutaneous eruptions from suramin. A clinical and histopathologic study of 60 patients. Arch Dermatol *131:*1147–1153, 1995.
39. Falkson G, Rapoport BL: Lethal toxic epidermal necrolysis during sumarin treatment. Eur J Cancer *28A:*1294, 1992.
40. Rago RP, Miles JM, Sufit RL, et al: Suramin-induced weakness from hypophosphatemia and mitochondrial myopathy. Cancer *73:*1954–1959, 1994.
41. Bitton RJ, Figg WD, Venzon DJ, et al: Pharmacologic variables associated with the development of neurologic toxicity in patients treated with suramin. J Clin Oncol *13:*2223–2229, 1995.

ACKNOWLEDGMENT

The authors wish to thank Donald G. Barceloux, MD, for his thoughtful review and commentary on this chapter.

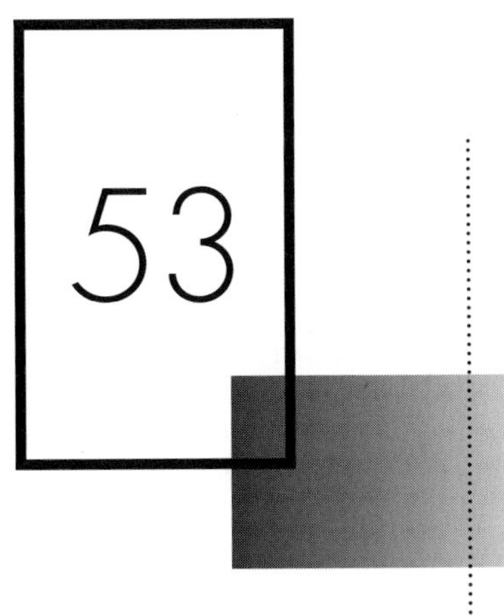

Isoniazid

MICHAEL W. SHANNON, MD, MPH

Isoniazid (INH) was introduced in 1952 and remains the antibiotic most commonly used in the treatment of tuberculosis.[1] Because of an increase in the incidence of tuberculosis, INH has become more widely prescribed.[2–4] With this expanded use has come a greater frequency of INH poisoning.[3, 5] Fortunately, a greater understanding of the biochemical mechanisms underlying its effects has led to the development of effective strategies for the treatment of INH intoxication.[1–3]

PHARMACOLOGY

INH, which contains a pyridine nucleus, is structurally related to the nutrients nicotinic acid (niacin, vitamin B_3), nicotinamide-adenine dinucleotide (NAD), and pyridoxine (vitamin B_6) (Fig. 53–1). INH is also a congener of the monoamine oxidase inhibitor antidepressant isocarboxazid. Its complete name, isonicotinic acid hydrazide, identifies INH as a congener of nicotinic acid.[1] INH has primary pK_a of 1.9.[6]

INH is rapidly absorbed from the gastrointestinal tract (primarily the small intestine), and peak serum concentrations are achieved within 1 to 2 hours.[6] Absorption is delayed by concomitant administrations of antacids.[1] Once absorbed, INH is distributed throughout body water and has an apparent volume of distribution of 0.6 L/kg.[6] INH has negligible binding to plasma proteins.[6]

The primary metabolic pathway for INH is acetylation by the enzyme *N*-acetyltransferase. This enzyme is located in the liver and intestinal mucosa. Acetyltransferase has been identified as a polymorphic enzyme whose pharmacokinetic activity follows Michaelis-Menten (saturable) kinetics. Additionally, the activity of this enzyme is genetically controlled by autosomal dominant inheritance.[6] Phenotypically, slow and fast acetylators are clinically identifiable. The slow acetylation enzyme is found in 50% to 60% of American whites and blacks. Acetylation activity is responsible for a number of the clinical differences observed in slow versus fast acetylators: (1) Slow acetylators have a smaller degree of presystemic clearance (first-pass effect) than fast acetylators, (2) fast acetylators metabolize INH five to six times faster than slow acetylators, and (3) plasma INH concentrations are 30% to 50% lower in fast versus slow acetylators. The elimination half-life of INH in fast acetylators is approximately 70 minutes, compared with a mean of 3 hours in slow acetylators. The primary metabolites after INH biotransformation are acetylisoniazid, isonicotinic acid, and hydrazine.[4, 6, 7] Standard daily doses of INH for antituberculous therapy are 600 mg for adults and 10 to 20 mg/kg for children.[8]

INH and its inactive metabolites are excreted in the urine, and 75% to 95% of a single dose is eliminated within 24 hours. Twenty-seven per cent of INH is excreted unchanged in slow acetylators, in contrast to 11% in fast acetylators.[6] The clearance of INH averages 46 mL/min.[6]

INH has a significant effect on several biochemical pathways (Table 53–1).

INH is an inhibitor of several cytochrome P-450–mediated functions, particularly demethylation, oxidation, and hydroxylation.[9] INH also affects the enzymes involved in the metabolism of the central nervous system (CNS) neurotransmitter γ-aminobutyric acid (GABA). GABA is the primary neurotransmitter at the motor inhibitory neurons of the CNS. GABA levels are regulated by two enzymes, glutamic acid decarboxylase (GAD) and GABA aminotransferase. GAD catalyzes the synthesis of GABA, whereas GABA aminotransferase promotes GABA breakdown. INH is an inhibitor of both enzymes but has a greater inhibitory effect on GAD, leading to reduced GABA levels.[10–12] Reduction in GABA has been di-

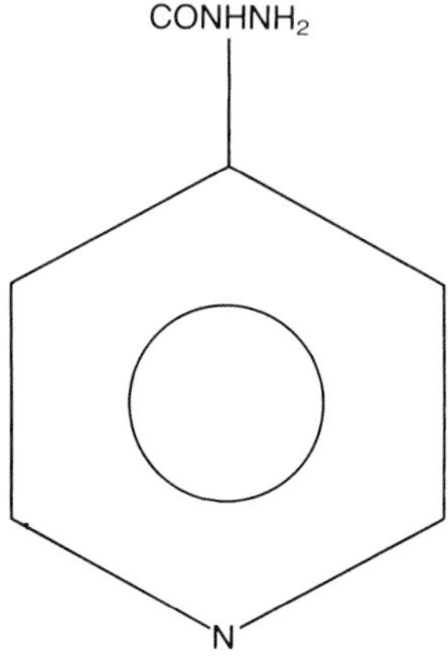

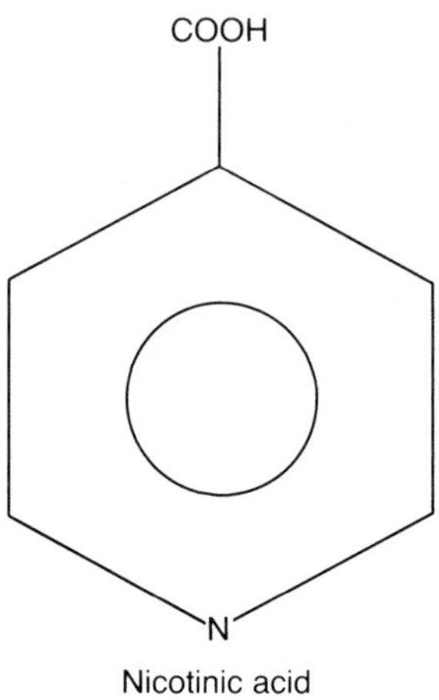

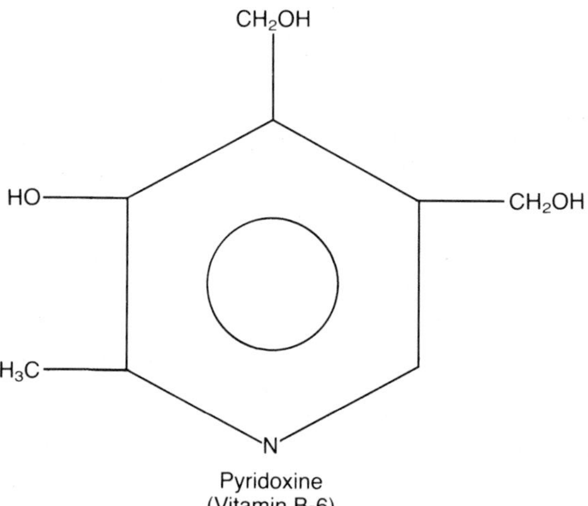

Figure 53–1. Structural relationships of isoniazid.

rectly associated with the development of seizures.[13] Monomethylhydrazine, a constituent of mushrooms of the *Gyromitra* genus, has a similar pharmacologic action.

INH's effect on pyridoxine metabolism is pivotal in the drug's toxicity. Pyridoxine activity is markedly reduced by INH, and pyridoxine depletion ultimately results. At least two mechanisms are responsible for this loss of pyridoxine activity: (1) INH inhibition of the enzyme pydridoxine phosphokinase, which converts pyridoxine to its active form, pyridoxal phosphate,[10, 14, 15] and (2) INH binding to pyridoxal phosphate, which forms an inactive hydrazone complex that is excreted in the urine.[6, 15] Daily urinary excretion of pyridoxine is doubled with INH doses of 3 to 5 mg/kg and is quadrupled with INH doses of 20 mg/kg.[6] The consequences of pyridoxine depletion include impaired activity of pyridoxine-dependent transaminases and decarboxylases (including GAD). Inhibition of these enzymes also leads to a decrease in catecholamine synthesis.

Because of INH's structural similarity to nicotinic acid, it may replace nicotinic acid in the synthesis of NAD, and an inactive compound may form.[6, 15–18]

INH readily crosses the placenta and enters breast milk. No teratogenic or mutagenic effects have been identified with INH use during pregnancy.[6]

CLINICAL TOXICOLOGY

Chronic Intoxication

Because of its many biochemical effects, INH is associated with a myriad of adverse reactions when taken in therapeutic doses. The overall incidence of adverse drug reactions with INH is 5.4%.[1] The most common of these are rash, fever, and abnormal liver function with the appearance of jaundice. INH-induced hepatotoxicity occurs in as many as 10% to 22% of patients, is age dependent, and appears more often in older patients.[1, 6, 19–21] INH hepatotoxicity may result from the generation of hepatotoxic hydrazines.[1, 21] Fulminant hepatitis occurs in an estimated 20.7 per 1000 persons; among these, approximately 5% of cases result in fatality.[22, 23] Liver transplantation may be necessary.[24, 25] Isolated acute pancreatitis has also been associated with INH use.[26] Less commonly, autoimmune phenomena or frank lupus erythematosus occurs. Approximately 25% of those taking INH develop antinuclear antibodies.[27] Autoimmune manifestations may include hemolytic anemia, thrombocytopenia or agranulocytosis, arthritis, vasculitis, and polyserositis.[6, 28]

Peripheral or optic neuritis may also occur with INH use. Optic neuritis generally is manifested as decreased visual acuity (often unilateral).[1, 2, 29] Symptoms of peripheral neuritis include paresthesias in a stocking-glove distribution, which may progress proximally.[2, 30] Although primarily a sensory neuritis, myalgias and weakness may occur.[2] Less commonly, CNS toxicity occurs, with manifestations of dysarthria, ataxia, and psychiatric disturbances.[30, 31] Neurologic complications are usually reversible and may be due to INH inhibition of the neuronal enzyme

Table 53–1. Metabolic Actions of Isoniazid

Biochemical Effect	Clinical Effect	Reference
Enzyme inhibition		
P-450	↓ Clearance of other drugs	10
Monoamine oxidase	Mood elevation	2
	↑ Sensitivity to tyramine	
Glutamate decarboxylase	↓ GABA activity	11, 14, 21
GABA aminotransferase	↑ GABA activity	11
Apotryptophanase	Peripheral neuritis	2
Histaminase	↑ Sensitivity to scombroid	10
Pyridoxine phosphokinase	↓ Conversion of pyridoxine to pyridoxal phosphate	11, 16
Transaminases	↓ Catecholamine synthesis	16
Decarboxylases		
Binding of pyridoxal phosphate	↓ Pyridoxine activity	16
Replacement of nicotinic acid, producing inactive nicotinamide-adenine dinucleotide	Impaired glucose and fatty acid oxidation, metabolic acidosis	16–18, 21

GABA, γ-aminobutyric acid.

apotryptophanase.[2] Coadministration of pyridoxine with INH prevents their occurrence.

INH may precipitate seizures in those with seizure disorder. In patients without a seizure history, an INH dose of 14 mg/kg is associated with a 1% to 3% incidence of seizures.[1, 2] INH doses of 35 to 40 mg/kg uniformly produce seizures.

Significant drug interactions exist with INH.[2, 9] An effect on the anticonvulsant phenytoin has been well described; altered mental status (occasionally coma) has occurred in patients who were simultaneously prescribed INH and phenytoin, associated with the development of toxic serum phenytoin concentrations. Phenytoin toxicity has a frequency of up to 27% and results from INH inhibition of cytochrome P-450 hydroxylases.[1, 9, 19] This decrease in phenytoin clearance tends to occur in the second week of combined treatment.[19] Other drugs whose elimination is reduced by concomitant administration of INH are carbamazepine, valproate,[32] coumarin anticoagulants, and rifampin.[9] Although case reports have suggested a significant adverse interaction between INH and acetaminophen,[33] well-controlled clinical studies have failed to demonstrate a greater risk of hepatotoxicity when these two are taken simultaneously.[34, 35]

INH use also may have a significant effect on diet. Inhibition of the enzyme monoamine oxidase has been associated with an increased sensitivity to tyramine-containing foods; flushing, palpitations, and hypertension all have been reported after such an ingestion. An inhibitory effect on the enzyme histaminase has led to adverse reactions after the ingestion of scombroid fish.[2, 9]

Acute Intoxication

Acute ingestion of more than 1.5 g of INH leads to minor toxicity, whereas ingestion of more than 6 to 10 g is usually fatal without aggressive treatment.[2] *Severe INH toxicity correlates with serum INH concentrations of greater than 30 mg/L.*

Clinical manifestations of INH intoxication may appear as soon as 30 minutes after an ingestion.[2, 36, 37] Early signs and symptoms include nausea, vomiting, slurred speech, dizziness, mydriasis, and tachycardia. A subsequent cascade of biochemical events soon leads to the striking clinical features that characterize INH intoxication—namely, *recurrent seizures, severe metabolic acidosis, and coma.* A proposed mechanism for this sequence is shown in Figure 53–2.

Seizures after INH overdose are episodic and tend to occur at regular intervals; either hyperreflexia or areflexia precedes their onset.[2] Improvement in consciousness may occur between seizures.[16] Once they begin, seizures are difficult to control despite the administration of anticonvulsants.

Severe metabolic acidosis is another prominent feature of INH overdose. Although pH ranges of 6.80 to 7.30 are common, surviving victims may present with a systemic pH as low as 6.49.[36] The etiology of metabolic acidosis appears to be an increase in the generation of lactic acid as a result of the muscular activity of recurrent seizures. Experimental data have demonstrated that paralyzed animals with INH intoxication do not develop severe metabolic acidosis.[14] Other theories of metabolic acidosis have been proposed, however, including (1) the generation of acidic INH metabolites, (2) an increase in keto acids due to enhanced fatty acid oxidation, and (3) the formation of inactive NAD, leading to impairment of both glucose and fatty acid metabolism. The last-named theory has led to the suggestion that nicotinic acid be administered in INH overdose.[6, 15–18, 37]

Coma may be protracted after overdose (lasting more than 24 hours) and may continue after seizures have abated and metabolic acidosis has been corrected. This profound CNS depression has been attributed to CNS catecholamine depletion.[36]

Other clinical effects of acute INH intoxication are severe hypotension, hyperglycemia, acetonuria, abnormal results of liver function tests, and renal failure.[2, 16, 36] INH-induced renal failure is often exacerbated by the myoglobinuria that develops from seizure-induced rhabdomyolysis.[18, 38]

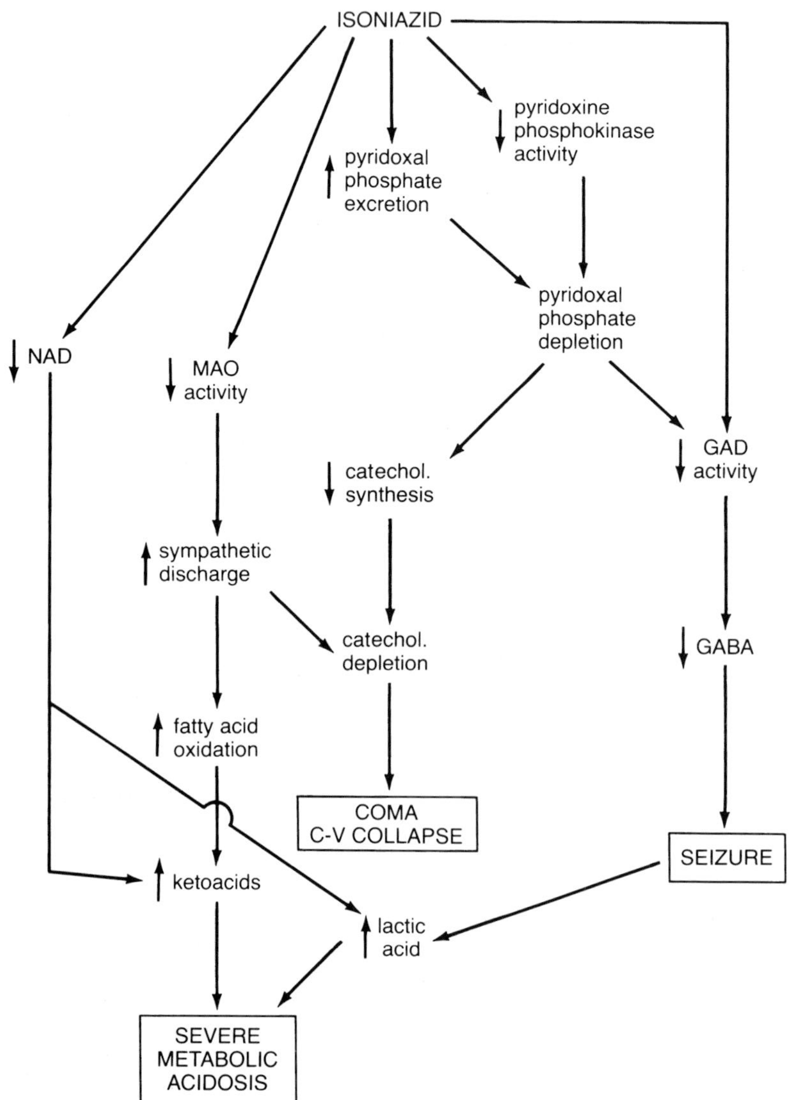

Figure 53–2. Proposed mechanisms of isoniazid toxicity.

DIAGNOSIS

In the absence of a history of overdose, INH overdose may be suspected in patients who present with the characteristic symptom complex. The differential diagnosis of severe metabolic acidosis includes diabetic ketoacidosis and the ingestion of methanol, ethylene glycol, iron, ibuprofen, or salicylates. Of these, only INH overdose has recurrent seizures as its hallmark.

The toxic screen generally does not detect the presence of INH, although serum INH concentrations can be measured if confirmation is required. Other important laboratory tests are an arterial blood gas determination, electrocardiogram, electrolytes measurements, liver function tests, creatine phosphokinase determination, and urinalysis.

MANAGEMENT (Table 53–2)

The initial management of INH intoxication requires stabilization of vital signs with provision of a patent airway, oxygen, cardiovascular support with intravenous fluids, and administration of sodium bicarbonate to treat metabolic acidosis.

If emergency department arrival is within 1 to 2 hours of ingestion, gastrointestinal decontamination with gastric lavage followed by administration of activated charcoal with a cathartic is indicated. Ipecac-induced emesis is contraindicated owing to the potentially rapid onset of seizures. Delayed absorption of INH after an overdose has not been observed, and it is thus suggested that late gastrointestinal decontamination may be ineffective.

Intravenous pyridoxine has been shown to be highly effective for INH intoxication and should be administered to all symptomatic patients.[39] *The milligram dose of pyridoxine should equal the ingested dose of INH.* Pyridoxine (given as pyridoxine hydrochloride) has been shown to terminate seizures, correct metabolic acidosis, and abbreviate the duration of coma.[2, 40] The efficacy of pyridoxine is directly correlated with the administered dose; in one study, recurrent seizures occurred in 60% of patients who

Table 53–2. Summary of Treatment Strategies for Isoniazid Overdose

Supportive Care
Ventilatory support
Vascular access
Fluids, vasopressors

Gastrointestinal Decontamination
Gastric lavage
Activated charcoal
Cathartic

Pharmacologic Treatment
Sodium bicarbonate to correct metabolic acidosis
Benzodiazepines and/or barbiturates as anticonvulsants
Pyridoxine: gram for gram per dose ingested, 5 g (75 mg/kg for children) if isoniazid dose is unknown; may be repeated if necessary

Elimination Enhancement
Forced diuresis
Furosemide
Hemodialysis
? Multiple-dose activated charcoal

received no pyridoxine, 47% of those who received 10% of the ideal pyridoxine dose, and none of the patients who received a full dose of pyridoxine.[40] When the quantity of ingested INH is unknown, a pyridoxine dose of 5 g (75 mg/kg in children) should be administered. Repeated doses of pyridoxine may be required on the basis of the resolution of signs and symptoms. Large doses of pyridoxine (up to 5 g/kg) can be given acutely without adverse effect.[3] Of note, pyridoxine is commonly dispensed in vials of 1 g. A significant INH overdose may deplete local supplies of pyridoxine. Contingency plans should be created for access to pyridoxine in the event of multiple INH exposures within a brief period.[41]

Conventional anticonvulsants remain important in the early treatment of seizures.[42] The benzodiazepines are agents of choice because they have a synergistic effect with pyridoxine as well as inherent GABA agonist activity.[2, 40, 42–44] Prophylactic administration of benzodiazepines has no proven efficacy. Several researchers have recommended against the use of phenytoin in INH overdose because of an apparent lack of efficacy and the potential for phenytoin intoxication.[2, 16] However, impaired phenytoin metabolism has been documented only in those ingesting INH continually, not after acute intoxication. Phenytoin may be an acceptable anticonvulsant, although its efficacy remains in question.[43] Phenobarbital, like the benzodiazepines, is a potent GABA agonist that may be effective in the treatment of seizures. Phenobarbital may worsen CNS depression, however, especially if administered after a benzodiazepine.

Forced diuresis with furosemide or mannitol enhances the elimination of INH.[2, 17] Similarly, hemodialysis and peritoneal dialysis are effective in the treatment of INH intoxication. Seventy-five per cent of an INH dose may be removed within 5 hours by hemodialysis, with clearance rates as high as 120 mL/min.[6] Hemodialysis should be reserved for patients who develop INH-induced renal failure. Interestingly, INH has a small volume of distribution and low protein binding, pharmacokinetic features that are found in drugs (e.g., theophylline, phenobarbital) whose elimination is enhanced by multiple-dose activated charcoal.[45] Therefore, while data are lacking, multiple-dose activated charcoal should be considered as a potential means of elimination enhancement in patients with severe intoxication.

References

1. Mandell GL, Geral L, Petri WA: Isoniazid. *In* Hardman JG, Limbird LE, Molinoff PB, et al (eds): Goodman and Gilman's 9th ed The Pharmacological Basis of Therapeutics. New York, Macmillan, pp 1155–1159, 1996.
2. Holdiness MR: Neurological manifestations and toxicities of the antituberculosis drugs—a review. Med Toxicol *2*:33–51, 1987.
3. Blanchard PD, Yao JDC, McAlpine DE, et al: Isoniazid overdose in the Cambodian population of Olmstead County, Minnesota. JAMA *256*:3131–3133, 1986.
4. Tuberculosis and acquired immunodeficiency syndrome (AIDS). MMWR *36*:785–794, 1987.
5. Shah BR, Santucci K, Sinert R, Steiner P: Acute isoniazid neurotoxicity in an urban hospital. Pediatrics *95*:700–704, 1995.
6. Weber WW, Hein DW: Clinical pharmacokinetics of isoniazid. Clin Pharmacol *4*:401, 1979.
7. Boxenbaum HC, Riegelman S: Pharmacokinetics of isoniazid and some metabolites in man. J Pharmacokinet Biopharm *287*:325, 1976.
8. Drugs for tuberculosis. Med Lett Drugs Ther *37*:67–70, 1995.
9. Baciewicz AW, Self TH: Isoniazid interactions. South Med J *78*:714–718, 1985.
10. Holtz P, Parm D: Pharmacological aspects of vitamin B-6. Pharm Rev *16*:113–178, 1964.
11. Wood JD, Paesker SJ: The effect on GABA metabolism in brain of isonicotinic acid hydrazide and pyridoxine as a function of time after administration. J Neurochem *19*:1527–1537, 1972.
12. Biggs CS, Pearce BR, Fowler LJ, Whitton PS: Effect of isonicotinic acid hydrazide on extracellular amino acids and convulsions in the rat: Reversal of neurochemical and behavioural deficits by sodium valproate. J Neurochem *63*:2197–2201, 1994.
13. Wood JD, Paesker SJ: A correlation between changes in GABA metabolism and isonicotinic acid hydrazide induced seizures. Brain Res *45*:489–498, 1972.
14. Chin L, Sievers ML, Herrier HE, et al: Convulsions as the etiology of lactic acidosis in acute isoniazid toxicity in dogs. Toxicol Appl Pharmacol *49*:377–384, 1949.
15. Mailler J, Robinson A, Percy AKL: Acute isoniazid poisoning in childhood. Am J Dis Child *134*:290–292s, 1980.
16. Orlowski JP, Paganini EP, Pippenger CE: Treatment of a potentially lethal dose of isoniazid ingestion. Ann Emerg Med *17*:73–76, 1988.
17. Pahl MV, Vaziri ND, Ness R, et al: Association of beta-hydroxybutyric acidosis with isoniazid intoxication. Clin Toxicol *22*:167–176, 1984.
18. DiAugustine RP: Formation *in vitro* and *in vivo* of the isonicotinic acid hydrazide analogue of nicotinamide adenine dinucleotide by lung nicotinamide adenine dinucleotide glycohydralase. Mol Pharmacol *12*:291–298, 1976.
19. Miller RR, Porter J, Greenblatt DJ: Clinical importance of the interaction of phenytoin and isoniazid. Chest *75*:356–358, 1979.
20. Byrd RB, Hom BR, Soloman DA, et al: Toxic effects of isoniazid in tuberculosis chemoprophylaxis. JAMA *241*:1239–1241, 1979.
21. Mitchell JR, Zimmerman HJ, Ishak KG, et al: Isoniazid liver

injury: Clinical spectrum, pathology and probable pathogenesis. Ann Intern Med *84*:181–192, 1976.
22. Stewart MF, Freemont AJ, Richardson T: Fatal isoniazid poisoning. Ann Clin Biochem *32*:229–231, 1995.
23. Snider DE, Caras GJ: Isoniazid-associated hepatitis deaths: A review of available information. Am Rev Respir Dis *145*:494–497, 1992.
24. Farrell FJ, Keeffe EB, Man KM, et al: Treatment of hepatic failure secondary to isoniazid hepatitis with liver transplantation. Dig Dis Sci *39*:2255–2259, 1994.
25. Hasagawa T, Reyes J, Nour B, et al: Successful liver transplantation for isoniazid-induced hepatic failure—a case report. Transplantation *57*:1274–1277, 1994.
26. Rabassa AA, Trey G, Shukla U, et al: Isoniazid-induced acute pancreatitis. Ann Intern Med *121*:433–434, 1994.
27. Yung RL, Richardson BC: Drug-induced lupus. Rheum Dis Clin North Am *20*:61–84, 1994.
28. Skaer NL: Medication-induced systemic lupus erythematosus. Clin Ther *14*:496–505, 1992.
29. Gonzalez-Gay MA, Sanchez-Andrade A, Aguero JJ, et al: Optic neuritis following treatment with isoniazid in a hemodialyzed patient. Nephron *63*:360, 1993.
30. Siskind MS, Thienemann D, Kirlin L: Isoniazid-induced neurotoxicity in chronic dialysis patients: Report of three cases and a review of the literature. Nephron *64*:303–306, 1993.
31. Gnam W, Flint A, Goldbloom D: Isoniazid-induced hallucinosis: Response to pyridoxine. Psychosomatics *34*:537–539, 1993.
32. Jonville P, Gauchez AS, Autret E, et al: Interaction between isoniazid and valproate: A case of valproate overdosage. Eur J Clin Pharmacol *40*:197–198, 1991.
33. Crippin JS: Acetaminophen hepatotoxicity: Potentiation by isoniazid. Am J Gastroenterol *88*:590–592, 1993.
34. Epstein MM, Nelson SD, Slattery JT, et al: Inhibition of the metabolism of paracetamol by isoniazid. Br J Clin Pharm *31*:139–142, 1991.
35. Zand R, Nelson SD, Slattery JT, et al: Inhibition and induction of cytochrome P4502E1-catalyzed oxidation by isoniazid in humans. Clin Pharmacol Ther *54*:142–149, 1993.
36. Hankinns DG, Saxena K, Faville RJ, et al: Profound acidosis caused by isoniazid ingestion. Am J Emerg Med *5*:165–166, 1987.
37. Terman DS, Teitelbaum DT: Isoniazid self-poisoning. Neurology *20*:299–304, 1970.
38. Blowey DL, Johnson D, Verjee Z: Isoniazid-associated rhabdomyolysis. Am J Emerg Med *13*:543–544, 1995.
39. Sievers ML, Herrier RN: Treatment of acute isoniazid toxicity. Am J Hosp Pharm *32*:202–206, 1973.
40. Wason S, Lacouture PG, Lovejoy F: Single high-dose pyridoxine treatment for isoniazid overdose. JAMA *246*:1102–1104, 1981.
41. Scharman EJ, Rosencrance JG: Isoniazid toxicity: A survey of pyridoxine availability. Am J Emerg Med *12*:386–388, 1994.
42. Boehnert MT, Lewander WJ, Lacouture PG: Advances in clinical toxicology. Pediatr Clin North Am *32*:193–211, 1985.
43. Chin L, Sievers ML, Laird HE, et al: Potentiation of pyridoxine by depressants and anticonvulsants in the treatment of acute isoniazid intoxication in dogs. Toxicol Appl Pharmacol *58*:504–509, 1981.
44. Chin L, Sievers ML, Laird HE, et al: Evaluation of diazepam and pyridoxine as antidotes to isoniazid intoxication in rats and dogs. Toxicol Appl Pharmacol *45*:713–722, 1978.
45. Levy G: Gastrointestinal clearance of drugs with activated charcoal. N Engl J Med *307*:676–678, 1982.

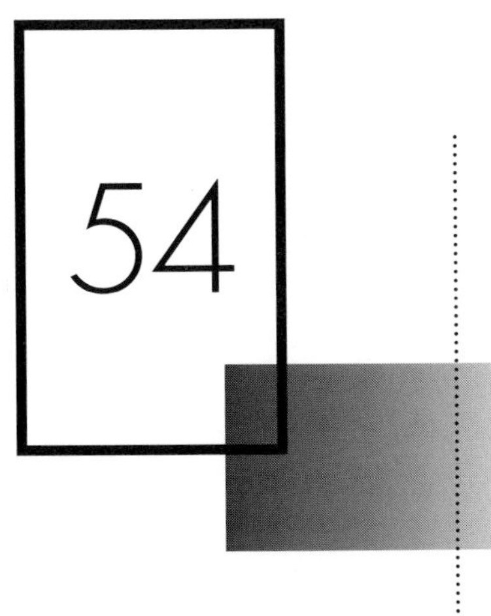

Chemotherapeutic Agents and Transplant Agents

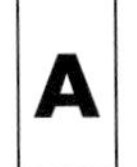

A Chemotherapeutic Agents

JOHN L. MARSHALL, MD
DONELLA NAZZARO, RPH

PRINCIPLES OF CHEMOTHERAPY

The treatment of cancer is undergoing a rapid evolution. Twenty years ago, virtually all antineoplastic agents could be classified as cytotoxins designed to kill dividing cells more readily than resting cells. These agents frequently result in moderate to severe toxicity, with clinical success in a limited range of malignancies. Although these drugs have been effective in curing some patients with Hodgkin's disease, leukemia, testicular cancer, and some childhood malignancies, most clinical benefit has been limited to small increases in survival or tumor shrinkage. As a result, the word *chemotherapy* instantly evoked visions of futile misery, which many patients and physicians maintain today. Efforts of the past decade have resulted in new cytotoxic agents with improved clinical activity, new administration and supportive care techniques that have decreased toxicity, and, most importantly, a better understanding of the molecular mechanisms of cancer, which has allowed for more focused, less toxic agents to make their way to the clinic.

This chapter offers a review of some basic principles of anticancer therapy and pharmacology, the toxicity of the currently available anticancer agents, (Table 54A–1), the many agents used in cancer supportive care, and the specific methods of managing these toxicities when available. This chapter is not intended to be a complete review of the toxicology of chemotherapeutic agents but instead to be a practical guide for clinicians unfamiliar with these agents.

TRADITIONAL AND NOVEL MECHANISMS OF ACTION

In order to gain a better understanding of the range of potential chemotherapy toxicities that might be experienced by a practicing physician, a basic understanding of the molecular chemotherapeutic targets is essential. Today, clinicians are using many new agents, new administration techniques, and new dose schedules to attempt to increase therapeutic efficacy. By understanding the mechanisms of these agents, one is better equipped to predict toxicity patterns. As is increasingly being defined, in order for a cancer cell to become malignant, many cellular changes must occur. Cells must lose their ability to regulate growth, maintain or increase their ability to replicate DNA, lose attachments to neighboring cells, gain the ability to invade through stromal matrix, stimulate neovascularization in order to grow beyond several micrometers in size, and ultimately evade the immune system. Such tumor-promoting cellular errors and changes occur constantly in normal cells, but through various cellular repair or destructive processes, the damaged cell is virtually always either fixed or "scraped" (a process termed *apoptosis*). Backing up these processes, the immune system may recognize a mutated cell as foreign and cause its destruction. It is only those cells that evade cellular repair and destruction processes that become viable cancers with fatal potential. It would seem that such an intricate system would be easy to disrupt, but unfortunately, this has not been the case.

Table 54A–1. Toxicities of Chemotherapeutic Agents

Aldesleukin (Proleukin), IL-2	IV, SC	Fever, chills, hypotension, capillary leak syndrome, dyspnea, sinus tachycardia, eosinophilia, anemia, hepatic, renal, and neurotoxicities
Altretamine (Hexalen), HMM	PO	N/V, diarrhea, abdominal cramping, mental depression, vertigo, BM suppression, peripheral neuropathies
Aminoglutethiamide (Cytadren)	PO	Adrenal insufficiency, rash, N/V, anorexia, headache, fever, myalgia, lethargy, orthostasis
Androgens	PO, IM	N/V, fluid retention, virilization in females, hepatic and renal toxicities
L-Asparaginase (Elspar), PEG-LA	IM, IV	Anaphylactoid reaction, clotting dysfunction, N/V, hepatotoxicity, EEG changes, malaise, confusion
BCG live (TheraCys, Tice BCG)	Intravesical	Hematuria, urinary frequency, dysuria, urinary tract infection, N/V, anorexia, malaise, fever, chills
Bleomycin (Blenoxane, Bleo)	IV, IM, SC	Pneumonitis, pulmonary fibrosis, fever, anaphylaxis, hyperpigmentation, nail changes, alopecia, anorexia
Busulfan (Myleran)	PO	Neutropenia, N/V, hyperpigmentation, anemia, VOD*, seizures*, thrombocytopenia*, pulmonary fibrosis*
Carboplatin (Paraplatin)	IV, IP	BM suppression, N/V, alopecia, electrolyte imbalances, peripheral neuropathy, hepatotoxicity
Carmustine (BiCNU)	IV	Delayed BM suppression, N/V, flushing (face and neck), optic neuritis, renal and hepatic toxicity
Chlorambucil (Leukeran)	PO	BM suppression, N/V, dermatitis, seizures, pulmonary fibrosis, renal and hepatic toxicity
Cisplatin (Platinol)	IV	Severe N/V, hypomagnesemia, BM suppression, anorexia, fatigue, nephrotoxicity, ototoxicity, peripheral neuropathy, visual disturbances
Cladribine (Leustatin), 2-CDA	IV	Lymphopenia, BM suppression, fever, chills, N/V, headache
Corticosteroids	PO, IV	Immunosuppression, GI toxicities, euphoria, insomnia, agitation, psychosis, fluid retention
Cyclophosphamide (Cytoxan), CTX	IV, PO	BM suppression, hemorrhagic cystitis, N/V, alopecia, nasal congestion, SIADH, pulmonary fibrosis, cardiac necrosis*, hepatic dysfunction
Cytarabine ARA-C, (Cytosar)	IV, IT, SC	BM suppression, stomatitis, diarrhea, N/V, flulike symptoms, alopecia, cerebellar toxicity, pancreatitis, conjunctivitis*, urinary retention
Dacarbazine, DTIC	IV	N/V, BM suppression, diarrhea, flulike symptomss, facial flushing, photosensitivity, metallic taste, hepatotoxicity
Dactinomycin (Cosmegen), ACT-D	IV	BM suppression, N/V, alopecia, radiation recall, hepatomegaly, vesicant properties
Daunorubicin (Cerubidine)	IV	BM suppression, mucositis, N/V, diarrhea, alopecia, red urine, vesicant properties, radiation recall, CHF*
Dexrazoxane (Zinecard)	IV	BM suppression, nausea, hepatotoxicity, fever, malaise, phlebitis
Doxorubicin (Adriamycin)	IV	BM suppression, alopecia, stomatitis, red urine, N/V, radiation recall, CHF*, arrhythmias, ECG changes, vesicant properties, venous flare, excessive tearing, conjunctivitis
Estramustine (Emcyt)	PO	N/V, gynecomastia, diarrhea, headache, fever, rash, hypertension, venous thrombosis, thrombocytopenia
Estrogens	PO, IM, IV	N/V, gynecomastia, feminization in males, sodium retention, hypercalcemia
Etoposide (VePesid), VP-16	IV, PO	BM suppression, alopecia, hypotension, headache, fever, N/V, anorexia, anaphylaxis
Floxuridine FUDR	IV, intra-arterial	N/V, mucositis, diarrhea, BM suppression, rash, hepatotoxicity, hiccups, vertigo, lethargy
Fludarabine (Fludara)	IV	BM suppression, N/V, diarrhea, stomatitis, agitation, confusion, visual disturbances, elevated LFTs
5-Fluorouracil, 5-FU	IV	Mucositis, diarrhea, N/V, BM suppression, nail changes, hand-foot syndrome, cerebellar toxicity, excessive lacrimation, cardiac ischemia*
Flutamide (Eulexin)	PO	Gynecomastia, galactorrhea, impotence, N/V, confusion, headache, insomnia, hepatitis
Gemcitabine	IV	BM suppression (thrombocytopenia), rash, fever, N/V
Groserelin (Zoladex)	SC	Sexual dysfunction, hot flashes, gynecomastia, lethargy, tumor flare, bone pain, edema
Hydroxyurea (Hydrea)	PO	BM suppression, anorexia, N/V, stomatitis, rash, facial erythema, dysuria, fever
Idarubicin (Idamycin)	IV	BM suppression, N/V, mucositis, diarrhea, urticaria, vesicant properties, arrhythmias, CHF*, abnormal LFTs
Ifosfamide (Ifex)	IV	BM suppression, hemorrhagic cystitis, N/V, alopecia, mild to severe neurotoxicity, abnormal LFTs, nephrotoxicity
Interferon alfa (Intron, Roferon)	SC, IM	Flulike symptoms, fatigue, nausea, anorexia, diarrhea, weight loss, altered taste, CNS toxicity, erythema, mild BM suppression
Interferon gamma (Actimune)	SC, IM	Flulike symptoms, hypotension, N/V, diarrhea, pulmonary edema, disorientation, BM suppression
Leucovorin (Wellcovorin)	PO, IV, IM	Allergic sensitization

Table 54A–1. Toxicities of Chemotherapeutic Agents *(Continued)*

Leuprolide (Lupron)	IM, SC	Hot flashes, tumor flare, bone pain, dysuria, peripheral edema
Levamisole (Ergamisol)	PO	N/V, diarrhea, rash, disulfiram-like reaction
Lomustine (CeeNU)	PO	Delayed BM suppression, N/V, anorexia, stomatitis, alopecia, hepatic and renal toxicity
Mechlorethamine, nitrogen mustard (Mustargen)	IV	Severe N/V, metallic taste, BM suppression, alopecia, phlebitis, vesicant properties, vertigo, weakness, tinnitus, jaundice, hyperuricemia
Melphalan (Alkeran)	PO, IV	BM suppression, N/V, anorexia, diarrhea, stomatitis, rash, pruritus, pulmonary scarring
Mercaptopurine (Purinethol), 6-MP	PO	BM suppression, GI toxicity, abnormal LFTs, jaundice, hepatic encephalopathy, fever, headache
Mesna (Mesnex)	IV	Altered taste sensation, nausea, diarrhea, headache, fatigue
Methotrexate, MTX	IV, PO, IT, IM	BM suppression, mucositis, GI ulceration, alopecia, N/V, fever, malaise, renal failure, interstitial pneumonitis, hepatotoxicity, photosensitivity
Mitomycin C (Mutamycin)	IV, intravesical	Delayed BM suppression, N/V, alopecia, erythema, vesicant properties, renal toxicity, hemolytic-uremic syndrome, VOD*, lethargy
Mitotane (Lysodren)	PO	N/V, anorexia, adrenal insufficiency, rash, lethargy, vertigo, visual disturbances
Mitoxantrone (Novantrone)	IV	BM suppression, N/V, mucositis, alopecia, phlebitis, blue-green urine, bluish sclera, ECG changes, CHF*
Octreotide (Sandostatin)	SC, IV	Abdominal pain, nausea, pain and/or irritation at injection site
Paclitaxel (Taxol)	IV	BM suppression, hypersensitivity, alopecia, myalgia, bradycardia, fatigue, mucositis, paralytic ileus, peripheral neuropathy, phlebitis
Pentostatin (Nipen), DCF	IV	BM suppression; renal, hepatic, and CNS toxicity; fever; arthralgia; fatigue; rash; N/V
Plicamycin, mithramycin	IV	Hemorrhage, facial flushing, electrolyte imbalance, fever, N/V, renal, hepatic and CNS toxicity
Procarbazine (Matulane)	PO	BM suppression, N/V, rash, xerostomia, myalgia, weakness, confusion, visual disturbances, fever
Progestins (Megace, Provera)	PO, IM	Cushing's syndrome, fluid retention, weight gain, abnormal LFTs, deep vein thrombosis, alopecia
Streptozocin (Zanosar)	IV	N/V, real dysfunction, proteinuria, BM suppression, fever, duodenal ulcer, hypoglycemia, hepatotoxicity
Docetaxel (Taxotere)	IV	BM suppression, hypersensitivity reactions, rash, phlebitis, alopecia, edema
Tamoxifen (Nolvadex)	PO	Hot flashes, N/V, headache, dizziness, rash, peripheral edema, leg cramps, rash, ocular changes
Teniposide (Vumor), VM-26	IV	BM suppression, mucositis, hypotension, N/V, rash, hepatic and biliary toxicity, hypersensitivity
6-Thioguanine (Tabloid), 6-TG	PO	BM suppression, anorexia, stomatitis, hyperuricemia, rash, unsteady gait, renal and hepatic toxicity
Thiotepa	IV, IT	BM suppression, stomatitis, headache, paresthesias, N/V, anorexia, pruritus, dizziness
Trentinoin (Veasnoid)	PO	Headache, dry skin, xerostomia, elevated LFTs, hypertriglyceridemia, leukocytosis, ocular changes, photosensitivity, "retinoic acid syndrome," fetal abnormalities, bone pain
Trimetrexate, TMTX	IV	BM suppression, mucositis, fever, malaise, rash, N/V, anorexia, elevated serum creatine levels, abnormal LFTs
Vinblastine (Velban), VBL	IV	BM suppression, vesicant properties, alopecia, N/V, ileus, constipation, urinary retention, muscular and tumor pain, vocal cord paralysis
Vincristine (Oncovir), VCR	IV	Peripheral and autonomic neuropathies, vesicant properties, bronchospasm, jaw pain, ocular changes, SIADH
Vinorelbine (Navelbine)	IV	BM suppression, N/V, constipation, loss of deep-tendon reflexes, alopecia, vesicant properties, dyspnea, arthralgia

IV, intravenous; SC, subcutaneously; PO, orally; IM, intramuscularly; IT, intrathecally; N/V, nausea and vomiting; BM, bone marrow; EEG, electroencephalogram; GI, gastrointestinal; CHF, congestive heart failure; VOD, veno-occlusive disease; LFTs, liver function tests; ECG, electrocardiogram; SIADH, syndrome of inappropriate secretion of antidiuretic hormone; CNS, central nervous system.

*Seen with high-dose therapy.

The development of anticancer therapy has focused primarily on finding new agents that inhibit, disrupt, or impair the required functions of malignant cells. DNA, RNA, and protein synthesis are the primary targets for most familiar chemotherapeutic agents. The logic behind this is simple: (1) Cancer cells must divide in order to survive; (2) DNA, RNA, and proteins are required for this division; and (3) because most cells in the body are resting and not dividing, cancer cells should be more vulnerable to disruption of DNA, RNA, and protein synthesis than normal cells. The majority of traditional chemotherapeutic agents target the synthesis and repair of these biologic molecules. Although the "logic" for cellular selectivity of the agents is sound, the clinical reality is that many normal tissues in the body are dependent on DNA, RNA, and protein synthesis, and this dependence is linked to much of the toxicity of these agents. In addition, many tumor cells either are already resistant or, under selective pressure, gain resistance to many commonly used agents. The desired effect is thus reversed by increasing the selective toxicity of the normal tissues instead of the malignant cells. Combination chemotherapy, standardly used for many common tumor types, was in fact born from attempts to overcome the multiple mechanisms of resistance that cancer cells develop. Combination chemotherapy has increased the therapeutic efficacy of treatments for many tumors but has not resolved the issue of tumor resistance.[1] Novel cytotoxic agents, high-dose therapy, and agents that directly interfere with resistance mechanisms all are being used clinically to overcome tumor resistance.[2] It is important for clinicians to be aware of these new agents and administration techniques in order to understand more clearly the potential for novel toxicities (Table 54A–2).

Perhaps the most exciting areas of new drug development for the treatment of cancer take advantage of our greater understanding of immunology and tumor-specific mechanisms. Discoveries about the basic molecular mechanisms of immunology and carcinogenesis have yielded novel molecular targets for antineoplastic agent development. Immunotherapy, a clinical concept of the past two to three decades, has found a legitimate role in the treatment of human cancers (e.g., interleukin-2 and α-interferon for renal cell cancer and melanoma). Other immunologically active agents and techniques such as other cytokines and vaccines are being explored, with the hope of generating specific immunoactive cells to recognize and destroy malignant cells. In addition to the expanding number of cytotoxic agents directed toward novel cellular replication targets such as topoisomerases and mitotic spindles, agents are being developed to interfere with tumor-specific molecular processes such as angiogenesis, oncogene expression, cell cycle regulation, and signal transduction pathways. The hope is that these agents will allow for a more tumor-specific effect that would result in a lower toxicity profile and better tolerance. Until these agents find their way to the clinic, most cancer patients will continue to be treated with traditional cytotoxic agents.

INDICATIONS FOR CHEMOTHERAPY

Chemotherapy is offered to patients in essentially four clinical situations: (1) after resection of all gross tumor but when the risk for micrometastatic disease is high (adjuvant); (2) before surgical resection, typically when the tumor is not easily resectable owing to the extent of organ involvment or extension beyond the organ into surrounding structures (neoadjuvant); (3) for patients with metastatic cancer, as palliation; and (4) for patients with cancers that are curable with chemotherapy alone (i.e., lymphoma, leukemia, testicular cancer). Depending on the clinical setting, doses of agents, clinical endpoints, and "acceptable" toxicities vary widely. For example, for a patient receiving chemotherapy for lymphoma, maximum doses are used and greater toxicities are accepted given the curative goal. Neoadjuvant and adjuvant chemotherapy are given with the intent of improving overall survival (over surgery or radiation alone) and are typically given at high doses, which increase the risk of toxicity. The ultimate extension of "aggressive" chemotherapy is high-dose chemotherapy followed by a bone marrow transplant. In such cases, physicians and patients accept potentially fatal toxicity in the hopes of producing long-term disease-free survival or even cures. However, in patients with metastatic, incurable cancers, such as those of the breast, colon, and lung, high toxicity is unacceptable unless clear benefit can be achieved. Therefore, treatment regimens used in a palliative setting are designed to balance effectiveness against quality of life, with dose adjustments to prevent severe toxicity. In clinical decision making, physicians must evaluate and treat patients with these different endpoints in mind while recognizing the different levels of acceptable toxicity for different clinical goals.

PHARMACOLOGY OF CHEMOTHERAPY

Administration

Nearly all chemotherapeutic agents are administered by an intravenous (IV) route, either by bolus, by limited infusion, or by prolonged infusion. Exceptions to this are listed in Table 54A–3. IV administration allows for greater control of peak blood levels (C_{max}) and area under the (drug concentration) curve (AUC) and thus avoids variable oral bioavailability and first-pass metabolism in the liver. This control is critical during administration of chemotherapy, because doses of agents are typically close to or on the steep part of the dose/toxicity curve. Standard doses of chemotherapy are individualized to a patient's body surface area, as calculated from his or her height and weight. Despite attempts at precise control, many abnormalities can alter an agent's pharmacokinetics and therefore its resulting toxicity. The more obvious examples include hepatic and renal dysfunction, but consideration should be given to hypoalbuminemia (leading to altered protein binding), gastrointestinal (GI) abnormalities (for orally administered agents or agents that are activated/excreted through the gut), third-space fluid's acting as a reservoir (methotrexate), and concomitant medicines.

The clinical antitumor activity and subsequent toxicity of many agents depend on the administration dose and schedule. These agents are characterized by different efficacy and toxicity profiles when given by shorter bolus infusions compared with longer infu-

Table 54A–2. Disease Treatments—Drug Regimens and Drugs of Choice

Site of Disease	Treatments	Site of Disease	Treatments
Brain	PCV (procarbazine, CCNU, vincristine) PVP (cisplatin and etoposide) BCNU + XRT	Leukemia ALL (adult)	*Induction:* DVPA (D, daunorubicin; V, vincristine; P, prednisone; A, asparaginase) *Maintenance:* 6-mercaptopurine + methotrexate *Consolidation:* No standard regimen
Breast	CA (AC), CAF (FAC), CMF, VATH Paclitaxel (Taxol); docetaxel (Taxotere) Mitomycin C + vinblastine, 5-FU ± leucovorin, hormonal agents (i.e., tamoxifen, megace) (A, doxorubicin; C, cyclophosphamide; F, 5-FU; M, methotrexate; V, vinblastine; T, thiotepa; H, fluoxymesterone)	ANLL	*Induction:* 7 + 3, 5 + 2 cytarabine + daunorubicin or idarubicin or mitoxantrone *Consolidation:* HiDAC (high-dose araC)
Endocrine Carcinoid	Streptozotocin + 5-FU Octreotide	CLL	CVP, chlorambucil + prednisone, fludarabine, cladribine, pentostatin (C, cyclophosphamide; V, vincristine; P, prednisone)
Thyroid	Doxorubicin ± cisplatin	CML	Busulfan, hydroxyurea, interferon
Gastrointestinal Anal	Mitomycin + 5-FU + XRT Cisplatin + 5-FU + XRT	Hairy cell leukemia	Cladribine, pentostatin, interferon
Colorectal	5-FU + levamisole 5-FU + leucovorin	Lung Non–small cell	Cisplatin or carboplatin + etoposide or paclitaxel or vinorelbine; oral etoposide, cisplatin + vinblastine ± mitomycin
Esophageal	Cisplatin + 5-FU ± XRT		
Gastric	FAM, FAMTX, EAP, FAP, ELF (F, 5-FU; A, doxorubicin; M, mitomycin; MTX, methotrexate; E, etoposide; P, cisplatin; L, leucovorin)	Small cell (Oat cell)	PE, CAV, ACE, CEP, ICE; oral etoposide, paclitaxel (P, cisplatin; E, etoposide; C, cyclophosphamide; A, doxorubicin; V, vincristine; I, ifosfamide + mesna [in ICE, *C* is cisplatin or carboplatin])
Pancreatic	Streptozocin + mitomycin + 5-FU Gemcitabine 5-FU ± leucovorin		
Genitourinary Bladder	CMV, M-VAC, CisCa Intravesical BCG, thiotepa, or mitomycin (C/Cis, cisplatin; M, methotrexate; V, vinblastine; A, doxorubicin; Ca, cyclophosphamide)	Lymphoma Hodgkin's lymphoma	MOPP, ABV, ABVD, MVPP, EVA (M, mechlorethamine; O, vincristine; P, procarbazine; P, prednisone; A, doxorubicin; B, bleomycin; V, vinblastine; D, dacarbazine; E, etoposide [in EVA, *A* is cytarabine])
Prostate	Leuprolide or goserelin ± flutamide Estramustine ± vinblastine, diethylstilbestrol, doxorubicin	Non-Hodgkin's lymphoma	CHOP, ProMACE-CYTABOM, MACOP-B, m-BACOD (C, cyclophosphamide; H/A, doxorubicin; O, vincristine; P/Pro, prednisone; E, etoposide; CYTA, cytarabine; B, bleomycin; M, methotrexate; D, dexamethasone)
Renal	Aldesleukin (IL-2), interferon, deoxyribonucleoside, vinblastine		
Testicular	BEP (PEB), PVB, VIP, paclitaxel (P, cisplatin; E, etoposide; B, bleomycin; V, vinblastine; I, ifosfamide + mesna [in VIP, *V* can also be etoposide]); 5-FU	Melanoma	Tamoxifen + carmustine + cisplatin + dacarbazine, interferon, Aldesleukin (IL-2)
Gynecologic Cervical	BOMP (MOB-PT), BIC (B, bleomycin; O, vincristine; M, mitomycin; P/PT/C, cisplatin; I, ifosofamide + mesna)	Multiple myeloma	VAD, VMCP-VCAP, VMCP-VBAP Melphalan + prednisone, interferon (V, vincristine; A, doxorubicin; D, dexamethasone; M, melphalan; C, cyclophosphamide; P, prednisone; B, carmustine)
Endometrial	PAC (CAP), hormonal agents (i.e., tamoxifen) (P, cisplatin; A, doxorubicin; C, cyclophosphamide)		
Ovarian	Cisplatin or carboplatin + paclitaxel Cyclophosphamide + carboplatin or cisplatin ± doxorubicin Ifosfamide + mesna, melphalan	Sarcoma Osteosarcoma	CyVADic, VAdriaC-XRT Cisplatin + doxorubicin ± ifosfamide or etoposide (Cy/C, cyclophosphamide; V, vincristine; A/Adria, doxorubicin; Dic, dacarbazine)
Head and neck	PF, PFL, carboplatin, methotrexate, paclitaxel (P, cisplatin; F, 5-FU; L, leucovorin); + XRT	Soft tissue	CyADic, CyVADic, MAID, VAC (Cy/C, cyclophosphamide; A, doxorubicin; Dic/D, dacarbazine; V, vincristine; M, mesna; I, ifosfamide [in VAC, *A* is dactinomycin])
Kaposi's sarcoma	Interferon, etoposide Vincristine alt vinblastine Doxil		

XRT, radiation therapy; CCNU, lomustine; BCNU, carmustine; 5-FU, fluorouracil.

Table 54A–3. Oral Chemotherapeutic Agents

Altretamine*	Estrogens	Mercaptopurine*
Aminoglutethimide*	Etoposide	Methotrexate
Androgens	Flutamide*	Mitotane*
Busulfan*	Hydroxyureas*	Procarbazine*
Chlorambucil*	Leucovorin	Progestins
Corticosteroids	Levamisole*	Tamoxifen*
Cyclophosphamide	Lomustine*	6-Thioguanine*
Estramustine*	Melphalan	Tretinoin*

*Available *only* in oral formulation.

sions.[3] Clinically relevant examples of this include the following: The cardiac toxicity of doxorubicin occurs at higher cummulative doses when the agent is administered by continuous infusion compared with bolus.[4] Similarly, 5-fluorouracil (5-FU) has a different toxicity profile and may have increased clinical activity when infused continuously for several weeks compared with the more standard bolus administration. Paclitaxel, initially given as a 24-hour infusion, has been shown to be equally effective but with less associated myelotoxicity when given over 3 hours.[5] These phenomena suggest that peak blood levels are not the only determinant of anticancer activity and toxicity. In prolonged infusions compared with bolus administration, the peak levels are typically lower but cellular exposure as measured by the AUC is increased. The availability and safety of semi-permanent central venous catheters along with these interesting clinical and pharmacokinetic findings have sparked an increased interest in administration of chemotherapy by prolonged infusion.

Maximizing dose intensity may be important to increasing the efficacy of chemotherapeutic agents.[6] Most chemotherapy regimens are given in cycles—that is, the agents are administered at or near maximally tolerated doses over 1 to 5 days, and no further chemotherapy can be given until the patient recovers sufficiently from the toxicities so that another cycle may begin. Cycles range from 3 to 8 weeks, depending on the agents used. To increase the dose intensity of a given regimen, either the dose must be increased or the treatment interval must be shortened. Improved supportive care and the development of agents that speed the recovery of systemic side effects (colony-stimulating factors [CSFs]) have enabled clinicians to increase the dose intensity of many regimens in an attempt to improve clinical outcomes. In doing so, atypical toxicity patterns have emerged (e.g., profound anemia and thrombocytopenia from higher doses of cyclophosphamide given every 2 weeks for breast cancer). Certainly, in the bone marrow transplant setting, a distinct set of toxicities characterize the post-treatment recovery phase but are not observed with the same agents at standard doses.[7] With further changes in treatment schedules will come changes in the toxicity profiles of agents and regimens.

Many chemotherapeutic agents require metabolic conversion or active intracellular transport *in vivo* in order to become activated and reach their cellular target. These include methotrexate, 5-FU, cytosine arabinoside (ara-C), 6-thioguanine (6-TG), 6-mercaptopurine (6-MP), cisplatin, and cyclophosphamide. Fortunately, few other drugs interact or compete with chemotherapy for transport and activation, and thus concerns about interference with an agent's activation are lessened. The inactivation and elimination of these agents are also dependent on metabolic processes, many of which are expressed with wide variability in the population. A good example is the inactivation of 5-FU by dihydropyrimidine dehydrogenase (DPD).[8] This cellular enzyme is the major pathway for inactivation and elimination of 5-FU and is found in highest concentrations in the GI tract and liver. However, the expression of this enzyme varies in the population, from very low to very high. Rarely, patients express only negligible amounts of the enzyme. When such patients are treated with standard doses of 5-FU, they can suffer life-threatening bone marrow suppression and mucositis. Although DPD deficiency can be accurately determined in patients, the incidence of severe DPD deficiency is sufficiently rare not to warrant screening every patient treated with 5-FU. In an attempt to take advantage of our understanding of DPD metabolism of 5-FU, trials using DPD inhibitors to increase the cytotoxic potential of 5-FU are under way.

Unfortunately, there is much about the metabolism of chemotherapy and interpatient variability that we do not understand. Without the ability to make accurate dose calculations for a given individual, standard initial chemotherapy doses have been empirically determined in clinical trials and are subsequently modified or tailored by the prescribing physician. Dose adjustments can be made before each subsequent cycle of treatment on the basis of the toxicities from the previous cycle—in essence, dose finding by trial and error. Individual patients receiving the same agents may experience a wide range of toxicity, and it is not uncommon for toxicities to increase in intensity and character as individual patients receive a higher cumulative dose after a greater number of cycles. A better understanding of interpatient variability in drug metabolism would improve our ability to predict toxicity and to determine individual doses of chemotherapy at the beginning of treatment. In addition, this understanding might uncover pharmacologic methods for protecting normal tissues to improve cancer cell selectivity and lower systemic toxicity. A well-described clinical application of this principle involves methotrexate and leucovorin. Methotrexate requires active transport into the cell through the cellular membrane reduced folate carrier. Leucovorin, a reduced folate, competes with methotrexate for this transport protein and, once inside the cell, provides the molecular end product. Methotrexate's site of action is bypassed. Understanding this system has allowed clinicians to administer extremely high doses of methotrexate that would have otherwise been fatal, followed by a leucovorin "rescue" allowing for recovery. Twenty-four to 48 hours after administration of high-dose methotrexate, leucovorin is administered (IV or orally) every 6 hours until blood levels of methotrexate have declined to less than 5×10^{-8}. Doses of leucovorin are increased when methotrexate levels exceed those outlined in Table 54A–4 at the given time points.

CHEMOTHERAPEUTIC AGENTS

End-Organ Toxicity

Hematologic Toxicity

Hematologic toxicity is the most frequent consequence of cytotoxic chemotherapy administration, and virtually all chemotherapeutic regimens contain one or more agents that cause bone marrow toxicity. Fortunately, bone marrow suppression is nearly always reversible, with recovery within 1 to 4 weeks after treatment, and rarely results in chronic myelosuppression. In many clinical settings in which higher doses of chemotherapy are desired, bone marrow suppression frequently limits the oncologist's ability to escalate doses. In fact, with the progressive dose escalation of certain cytotoxic agents, complete eradication of bone marrow progenitor cells can occur, and permanent bone marrow aplasia and death can ensue. To allow for such high-dose therapy in clinical practice, previously harvested autologous or allogeneic bone marrow may be administered after treatment to rescue patients or to transplant recipients, respectively, and permanent aplasia is thus prevented. Outside of the bone marrow transplant setting, chemotherapy regimens are frequently designed to maximize chemotherapy doses balanced against the degree of anticipated myelosuppression. The reversible nature of hematologic toxicity allows for repeat dosing once the marrow has recovered. It is important to note that there is a limit to the bone marrow reserve, and patients who have received multiple cycles of highly myelotoxic agents may not recover as quickly or as strongly. Although interpatient variability is great, bone marrow reserve limits the number of possible treatments when using many chemotherapy regimens. Life-threatening consequences of myelosuppression include leukopenia with increased risk of infection, thrombocytopenia with increased risk of hemorrhage, and anemia leading to fatigue and cardiopulmonary dysfunction.

Table 54A–4. Leucovorin Rescue After High-Dose Methotrexate Administration

1. Leucovorin should be started 24 h after methotrexate administration.
2. For most regimens, 15 mg/m² of leucovorin intravenously or orally is the initial dose.
3. Methotrexate blood levels should be obtained daily beginning 24 to 48 h after methotrexate administration until level falls below 5×10^{-8} M.
4. Leucovorin doses should be adjusted daily according to the methotrexate levels as outlined below:

Methotrexate Level	*Leucovorin Dose*
$\leq 5 \times 10^{-7}$ M	15 mg/m²
$\leq 1 \times 10^{-6}$ M	100 mg/m²
$\leq 2 \times 10^{-6}$ M	200–1000 mg/m²

Rescue is used routinely for methotrexate doses ≥300 mg/m²

Prehydration and alkalization of the urine before and 24 h after therapy are critical.

Two to 5 days are commonly required to complete leucovorin rescue.

The pathophysiology of bone marrow suppression by cytotoxic chemotherapy is clear. Chemotherapeutic agents damage cells that are actively undergoing cell division. The hematogenous progenitor cells of the bone marrow must constantly divide in order to supply new white bloods cells (WBCs), red blood cells (RBCs), and platelets, which replace the cells lost to normal turnover. This need for constant cell division makes marrow progenitor cells particularly vulnerable to chemotherapeutic agents. After administration of cytotoxic agents, marrow progenitor cell division is disrupted, and production of the mature cells is transiently decreased. After the cytotoxic agent is cleared or inactivated, progenitor cells begin to replace the deficit by forming daughter cells under the stimulus of various cytokines. The three different cell lines are affected and subsequently respond in distinct patterns depending on the dose and combinations of agents used. The differences in the natural life cycle of the three hematologic cell lines result in the differential expression of hematologic toxicity observed after chemotherapy administration.[9] WBCs have a circulating half-life of 7 to 8 hours. Without constant replacement, the WBC supply would quickly become depleted and leukopenia would result. On average, depending on the cytotoxic agent used, division and maturation of neutrophils begin shortly after the clearance of the cytotoxic agent, with adequate recovery in 7 to 10 days. Because platelets survive for 7 to 10 days and RBCs survive for approximately 90 days in the circulation, their nadirs occur with less consistency and predictability. If one monitors closely, a nadir of platelets and RBCs can be detected, but severe thrombocytopenia and anemia, being less common after chemotherapy, rarely are the limiting factors in further treatment. Unlike leukocytes, platelets and RBC transfusions are used to support patients through cytopenic episodes if necessary. Certain chemotherapeutic agents display lineage-specific myelotoxicity, phenomena with unclear mechanisms of action. Examples of lineage selectivity include the neutropenia predominantly caused by paclitaxel, the thrombocytopenia caused by nitrosoureas, and the thrombocytopenia and anemia predominantly caused by platinum analogues. Other agents such as vincristine, bleomycin, and hormonal agents have very little significant clinical effect on the bone marrow.

Leukopenia is the most common and therefore most clinically significant hematologic toxicity of chemotherapy. The absolute neutrophil count (ANC) is the critical quantitative value to calculate when evaluating a patient with neutropenia. It is calculated by adding the percentages of band forms and segmented neutrophils and multiplying this figure by the total WBC count. This gives a total number of WBCs that are capable of fighting bacterial infections. Patients with an absolute neutrophil count of less than 1000 are described as *neutropenic*. Neutropenic patients are vulnerable to bacterial infections because they do not have adequate WBCs to mount an effective immune response.[10] Most patients become neutropenic during chemotherapy, but relatively few develop fever during the neutropenic period. No specific symptoms are suggestive of neutropenia, although patients frequently complain of fatigue. However, should a neutropenic patient develop a fever (typically >38.5°C), the patient is at markedly elevated risk for a potentially fatal septic episode; thus, this is a medical emergency. Fever/neutropenia can occur as a consequence of many treatment regimens, and all physicians should have some familiarity with its management. The management of neutropenic fever has been reviewed elsewhere but can be summarized by the need for a thorough search for a source of infection by careful, directed physical examination (no rectal examinations during neutropenic periods) and blood and urine cultures. Additionally, chest radiographs and other tests as directed by the specific clinical situation are immediately followed by administration of appropriate broad-spectrum antibiotics continued until hematologic recovery. The most common sources for bacterial infections during neutropenic episodes are the gram-negative rods of the mouth and colon.[11] Central venous catheters increasingly are a source of infection and may partially account for the rise in the incidence of gram-positive organisms with neutropenic sepsis. Although less common, viral and fungal infections should be considered, and adequate treatment should be added to the antibiotic regimen if the results of history-taking, physical examination, or laboratory tests are suggestive. The error in fever/neutropenia is using too narrow a diagnostic and therapeutic approach. CSFs have helped reduce the incidence of fever/neutropenia.[12] However, if patients present with fever/neutropenia and currently are not receiving CSFs as prophylaxis, little evidence supports the initiation of CSFs.

The primary role for CSFs is the prevention of fever/neutropenia. Before the development of CSFs, physicians either had to decrease chemotherapy doses or to delay treatments in the presence of severe or prolonged neutropenia. These drugs do not prevent neutropenia but can lessen the depth of the nadir and shorten the length of time a patient is neutropenic. The use of CSFs allows the oncologist to administer dose-intense chemotherapy without delays. The high cost of CSFs has led the American Society of Clinical Oncology (ASCO) to publish guidelines for the appropriate and cost-effective use of these drugs in patients who are not enrolled in clinical trials.[13] In chemotherapy-naive patients, CSFs are indicated when using regimens associated with a 40% or greater risk of developing febrile neutropenia. When using less-myelosuppressive regimens, the use of CSFs is justified in patients with comorbid diseases or other known risk factors such as prior irradiation to the pelvis or other areas containing large amounts of bone marrow. The ASCO guidelines also recommend the use of CSFs after a documented episode of febrile neutropenia in a prior chemotherapy cycle. CSF therapy is initiated 24 to 72 hours after chemotherapy is completed and is continued until the WBC count has recovered to above the normal range. Once the CSF therapy is discontinued, the WBC count declines precipitously. The manufacturers' recommendation of a therapeutic endpoint of an ANC of 10,000 or greater is considered safe and effective. Each of the CSFs differs in its indications, dosing, and toxicity profiles (Table 54A–5).

Thrombocytopenia is the second most common hematologic toxicity caused by chemotherapeutic agents. Agents that most commonly cause thrombocytopenia include the nitrosoureas, thiotepa, and platinum compounds. In addition, thrombocytopenia frequently occurs when other agents are used in higher-dose chemotherapy regimens and bone marrow rescue/transplant regimens. The most severe consequences of thrombocytopenia are GI bleeding, epistaxis, and intracranial bleeding. A platelet count less than 50,000/mm^3 carries an increased risk of hemorrhage, but platelet counts less than 20,000/mm^3 carry significantly higher risk.[14,15] Patients with severe thrombocytopenia and evidence of hemorrhage should be immediately transfused with platelets. In the absence of bleeding, the decision to transfuse platelets for chemotherapy-induced thrombocytopenia should be based on the patient's prior platelet transfusion history, the expected length of the platelet nadir, and any significant comorbid conditions that would increase the risk for hemorrhage.[16] No CSF to stimulate platelet production has been approved to date.

Anemia, a frequent finding in patients with cancer, results from both chemotherapy and the chronic disease itself. Although not particularly limiting in terms of acute chemotherapy administration, clinically significant anemia is increasingly recognized as a subacute or long-term consequence of chemotherapy. Repetitive cycles of high-dose chemotherapy or agents likely to cause anemia can result in a gradual decline in the RBC number, and RBC transfusions are often required. Sudden and severe changes in the RBC count of a patient receiving chemotherapy are unlikely to be secondary to the chemotherapy, however, and alternate explanations such as acute blood loss or hemolysis should be considered (discussed later). Agents associated with anemia include the platinum compounds, paclitaxel, methotrexate, trimetrexate, and high-dose myeloablative therapy. Use of hydoxyurea is associated with a marked peripheral macrocytosis and anemia. The RBC-specific CSF erythropoetin has been approved for use in cancer patients receiving chemotherapy for the prevention of anemia.[17] As with other CSFs, erythropoietin does not reverse anemia acutely and therefore should be

Table 54A–5. Colony-Stimulating Factors

Colony-Stimulating Factor	Generic Name	Trade Name	Dose	Toxicities
G-CSF	Filgrastim	Neupogen	5 μg/kg	Bone pain, exacerbation of pre-existing eczema, elevated LDH and alkaline phosphatase levels
GM-CSF	Sargramostim	Leukine	250 mg/m^2	Fever, malaise, lethargy, headache, bone pain, local irritation of injection sites, elevated LDH and alkaline phosphatase levels, dysonea
Erythropoetin	Epoetin alfa	Procrit Epogen	150–300 units/kg 3 × weekly	Hypertension, headache, arthalgias, nausea, rash

LDH, lactate dehydrogenase.

started in patients at risk for developing anemia or when evidence suggests that the anemia will persist and is not explained by other factors. Erythropoetin should not be used in place of transfusions for acute treatment of severe symptomatic anemia.

The temporal relationship between the chemotherapy administration and the time to hematologic nadirs varies according to the dose, schedule, and agents used.[18] With most agents, the nadir of the WBC count and platelet count occurs 7 to 14 days after chemotherapy administration. The decline in RBC count, as stated earlier, tends to be of a more long-term reduction not showing a marked nadir phenomenon with each cycle. In contrast, agents such as mitomycin C and the nitrosoureas cause delayed nadirs as long as 6 to 8 weeks after administration of the agent. The cause of this is not known.[19] In taking a chemotherapy history, it is useful to determine when a patient is expected to undergo a hematologic nadir as well as the anticipated depth and length of the nadir. All medical decisions about further chemotherapy and dental and surgical procedures would be influenced by this information. This information gives patients the ability to plan their life events and offers some control over what is a very difficult, unpredictable time.

As more patients with cancer have an increased survival after receiving chemotherapy, it has become well recognized that many cytotoxic chemotherapeutic agents and radiation therapy have long-term consequences on the hematologic system. Apart from persistent myelosuppression, it has been noted that alkylating agents, nitrosoureas, and radiation therapy (alone or in combination) given for the treatment of malignancies or other conditions can lead to secondary hematologic malignancies, most typically acute nonlymphoblastic leukemia, which develops from 3 to 10 years after treatment.[20] Although most clinical settings leave few therapeutic alternatives, physicians and patients should be aware of this potential long-term toxicity.

Finally, coagulopathies can occur with use of several chemotherapeutic agents.[21] Fibrinogen levels decrease after use of L-asparginase. Plicamycin is associated with platelet dysfunction. Suramin causes a coagulopathy. Interestingly, increasing cumulative doses of mitomycin C lead to an increased risk of developing hemolytic-uremic syndrome.

Gastrointestinal Toxicity

Nausea/Vomiting

Nausea and vomiting are often the earliest manifestations of the toxic effects caused by chemotherapy drugs and are among the side effects most feared by patients with cancer. Individuals at increased risk for developing nausea and vomiting include (1) younger patients; (2) females, especially those with a history of emesis during pregnancy; (3) patients with a history of motion sickness; (4) nonalcohol drinkers; (5) non drug users (i.e., illicit drugs).[22] The consequences of poorly controlled nausea and vomiting vary from mild physical discomfort to life-threatening physical conditions. As an intangible consequence of nausea and vomiting, decreased treatment efficacy when a patient delays or refuses to continue potentially curative treatment may result in a decrease in overall survival of a given treatment. Second only to the hematologic toxicities, nausea and vomiting are extremely frequent results of chemotherapy. Chemotherapy-induced emesis is due to stimulation of the vomiting center in the reticular formation by the chemoreceptor trigger zone or other afferent signals from the brain, GI tract, and vestibular system.[23] Although chemotherapy is the most frequent cause of nausea and vomiting in a patient receiving treatment, it must be realized that multiple alternate causes of nausea and vomiting such as brain metastasis, structural or functional GI tract abnormalities, or other medicines may have a role. Therefore, one should obtain a complete history to search for other possible explanations for the symptoms. For adequate evaluation of a patient presenting with poorly controlled nausea and vomiting, it is important to know the relative emetogenic potential of chemotherapeutic agents, the time interval between the administration of chemotherapeutic agents and the onset of nausea and vomiting, and the patient's prior history of nausea and vomiting with use of chemotherapeutic agents.

Most chemotherapeutic agents cause only mild or moderate nausea and vomiting. Few agents cause severe, dose-limiting nausea and vomiting. Some agents that frequently cause severe nausea and vomiting include the platinum compounds, dacarbazine, streptozocin, high-dose cytarabine, and nitrogen mustard (Table 54A–6).

Nausea and vomiting are classified into three types: acute, delayed, and anticipatory. The acute phase is the most common and generally begins 1 to 3 hours after receiving chemotherapy, peaks within 6 to 10 hours, and subsides in 12 to 24 hours. When agents such as cisplatin and high-dose doxorubicin are given, however, delayed emesis, occurring 2 to 5 days after the administration of the chemotherapy, is a common complication. Unfortunately, no antiemetic agent has been shown to prevent or control delayed emesis. Delayed nausea and vomiting are usually less severe, peak at 48 to 72 hours, can persist for as long as 5 days, and are difficult to control. Anticipatory nausea and vomiting occur before or very soon after receiving chemotherapy. This type of emesis is often a result of poorly controlled nausea and vomiting during a previous cycle of chemotherapy. Introduction of the selective serotonin antagonists has dramatically improved our ability to treat patients receiving highly emetogenic and high-dose chemotherapy regimens during the acute phase (Table 54A–7). These drugs are less effective in controlling anticipatory and delayed emesis and should not be routinely used in these settings. With their low toxicity profile, these highly effective 5-HT_3 antagonists have gained widespread use.

The primary goal of antiemetic therapy is prevention of nausea and vomiting. When developing an antiemetic regimen for a particular patient, the physician must consider the emetogenic potential for each chemotherapy drug to be administered. Onset and duration of nausea and vomiting vary greatly with each drug. Antiemetic therapy should begin before the chemotherapy treatment and continue for 1 to 5 days, depending on the drugs included in the prescribed regimen. A combination of antiemetic agents often provides the best approach to achieve a complete response (no episodes of vomiting and only mild nausea) to therapy (Table 54A–8).

With appropriate use of antiemetics, alone or in combination, satisfactory control of most acute emesis can be achieved. Failure to treat nausea and vomiting successfully can result in severe dehydration and electrolyte imbalances, which potentially require intensive IV fluids and supportive care. In addition, poor control of emesis increases the risk for developing anticipatory nausea and vomiting, and the result is poor patient compliance and eventually patient withdrawal from treatment.[24] Therefore, aggressive management and understanding of chemotherapy-induced emesis are important to the success of a given chemotherapy treatment.

Mucositis

The epithelial layer of the GI tract consists of a mucosal lining of cells that are constantly being sloughed and replaced through cell division. As with any tissue in the body that undergoes frequent division, the GI tract lining is at risk for toxicities from chemotherapy. The general term for chemotherapy-induced damage to the lining of the GI tract is *mucositis*. Presenting findings include the common abnormalities of sores in the mouth and oropharynx (stomatitis), abdominal pain, and diarrhea (potentially bloody diarrhea). A rare yet severe GI mucosal toxicity is *typhlitis*, the transmural inflammation of the bowel with hematologic seeding of bacteria and subsequent sepsis. Agents that frequently cause mucositis include 5-FU, methotrexate, vinca alkaloids, bleomycin, paclitaxel, high-dose cytarabine, anthracyclines, and dactinomycin. The direct consequences of mucositis include breakdown of the mucosal barrier, which increases the risk for bacterial, fungal (*Candida*), or viral (herpes) infections. Indirectly, the pain and dysphagia associated with mucositis frequently result in poor oral intake and malnutrition. Avoiding dehydration is important in the prevention of more severe consequences. When the combination

Table 54A–6. Emetogenic Potential of Chemotherapy Agents

High (<90%)	Moderately High (60–90%)	Moderate (30–60%)	Moderately Low (10–30%)	Low (<10%)
Cisplatin	Carmustine	Altretamine	Bleomycin	Busulfan
Cytarabine*	Cyclophosphamide	Asparaginase	Cytarabine	Chlorambucil
Dacarbazine	Dactinomycin	Carboplatin	Etoposide	Cladribine
Mechlorethamine	Etoposide*	Daunorubicin	Fludarabine	Hormonal agents
Melphalan*	Ifosphamide	Doxorubicin	Gemcitabine	Paclitaxel
Streptozotocin	Lomustine	5-Fluorouracil	Hydroxyurea	Taxotere
	Methotrexate*	Idarubucin	Melphalan	6-Thioguanine
	Plicamycin	Mitomycin-C	6-Mercaptopurine	Vincristine
	Procarbazine	Vinorelbine	Mitoxantrone	
	Thiotepa*		Pentostatin	
			Teniposide	
			Thiotepa	
			Vinblastine	

*High dose.

Table 54A–7. Antiemetics of Choice

Emetogenic Potential	Primary Antiemetic	Secondary Drugs
Highly emetogenic	Serotonin antagonist	Corticosteroid
	Substituted benzamide (high dose)	Corticosteroid Benzodiazepine and antihistamine
Moderately emetogenic	Serotonin antagonist	Corticosteroid
	Substituted benzamide	Corticosteroid and antihistamine
	Phenothiazine	Corticosteroid
	Butyrophenone	Corticosteroid
	Corticosteroid	Benzodiazepine
	Cannabinoid	Phenothiazine
Mildly emetogenic	Phenothiazine	
	Benzodiazepine	

of poor oral intake and diarrhea results in moderate to severe dehydration, the increased risk of morbidity and mortality is significant. Patients should be aggressively supported to prevent the more serious morbidity. The severity of mucositis tends to increase with increasing chemotherapy doses and can be fatal after administration of high-dose methotrexate or high-dose 5-FU or after bone marrow transplantation. It is important to note that different infusion schedules of the same agents (e.g., 5-FU) are associated with different degrees of mucositis.

Initial management of mucositis depends on the degree of toxicity. Mild mucositis rarely requires more therapy than topical anesthetics. More severe cases may require fluid and electrolyte replacement, topical or systemic pain medication, use of topical or systemic steroids, treatment of any fungal overgrowth, treatment of oral herpes if diagnosed or suspected, and frequent reassessment. The specific management of mucositis after administration of high-dose methotrexate also includes leucovorin rescue if methotrexate levels are elevated. Although moderate to severe mucositis can frequently be managed at home with IV fluids, patients may require more intensive inpatient supportive care.

Recovery from mucositis occurs in 2 to 10 days, the time depending on the severity and the causative agents. Despite efforts to develop agents that prevent or reverse mucositis, no specific treatments have been found. Supportive care is considered the mainstay of therapy. Investigations have shown that vitamin B_6 decreased the intensity and length of mucositis.[25] Oral mucositis has been shown to be alleviated by chewing ice during the administration of the causative agent, but this has not proved helpful once mucositis is established. Studies using CSFs have

Table 54A–8. Antiemetic Therapy

Antiemetic Agent	Dose	Interval	Side Effect
Antihistamines			
Diphenhydramine (Benadryl)	25–50 mg	q 6–8 h	Drowsiness, blurred vision, dry mucous membranes
Benzodiazepines			
Diazepam (Valium)	5–10 mg	q 6 h	Sedation, mild hypotension
Lorazepam (Ativan)	0.5–2 mg	q 4–6 h	
Butyrophenones			
Droperidol (Inapsine)	1–4 mg	q 3–6 h	Extrapyramidal side effects, sedation
Haloperidol (Haldol)	1–5 mg	q 3–6 h	
Cannabinoids			
Dronabinol (Marinol)	2.5–10 mg	q 6–8 h	Hallucinations, euphoria, motor incoordination, dry mouth
Nabilone (Cesamet)	1–2 mg	q 8 h	
Corticosteroids			
Dexamethasone (Decadron)	10–20 mg	q 6 h	Restlessness, mood changes, euphoria
Methylprednisolone (Medrol)	125–250 mg	q 6 h	
Phenothiazines			
Chlorpromazine (Thorazine)	25–50 mg	q 4–6 h	Extrapyramidal side effects, anticholinergic effects, orthostatic hypotension, drowsiness
Perphenazine (Trilafon)	2–4 mg	q 4–6 h	
Prochlorperazine (Compazine)	10–20 mg	q 4–6 h	
Promethazine (Phenergan)	25–50 mg	q 4–6 h	
Thiethylperazine (Torecan)	10 mg	q 4–6 h	
Serotonin antagonists			
Granisetron (Kytril)	IV: 10 μg/kg before chemotherapy only PO: 1 mg bid	q 24 h	Headache, elevated liver function values
Ondansetron (Zofran)	32 mg	q 24 h	
Substituted benzamides			
Metoclopramide (Reglan)	1–3 mg/kg	q 2–6 h	Extrapyramidal side effects, diarrhea, drowsiness, fatigue
Trimethobenzamide (Tigan)	200 mg	q 6 h	

failed to document improvement in mucositis despite early anecdotal evidence of benefit.[26]

Diarrhea

Mild diarrhea occurs after many chemotherapy treatments and is typically characterized by 1 to 2 days of loose stools. Moderate to severe diarrhea, including bloody diarrhea, may follow treatment with 5-FU, ara-C, 6-MP, and a new, yet-to-be-approved class of drugs, the camptothecins. Diarrhea, as with hematologic toxicities, commonly ensues 7 to 10 days after completion of chemotherapy but may occur earlier, depending on the treatment schedule, concomitant medications, and comorbid conditions. The consequences of chronic or persistent diarrhea include decreased energy, poor nutrition, electrolyte abnormalities, significant blood loss, malabsorption, and dehydration. Management of chemotherapy-induced diarrhea includes fluid and electrolyte replacement and other supportive care as indicated. A thorough history taking and physical examination should be performed to rule out other causes of diarrhea in patients with cancer, such as prior or current treatment with antibiotics, use of laxatives, or bowel resections. Depending on severity, binding agents (i.e., Kaopectate) or bowel motility inhibitors (i.e., Lomotil) may be used to slow the diarrhea and fluid loss. Systemic steroids are occasionally used for severe diarrhea from mucositis but with little success. As with other chemotherapy-induced toxicities, care should be taken not to assume that diarrhea is due to chemotherapy unless the history, agents used, and the temporal relationship between the administration of the agent and the onset of the diarrhea are appropriate.

Constipation

Constipation resulting in abdominal pain is a common consequence of certain chemotherapy agents and many supportive care agents used in patients with cancer. The vinca alkaloids lead the list of cytotoxic agents causing constipation, with as many as one third of all patients treated with vincristine. Constipation can be so severe that it results in death.[27] Suramin also has a high rate of associated constipation. Systemic narcotics represent the most common class of constipation-causing agents used in patients with cancer. Patients on long-term or as-needed schedules of systemic narcotics should be advised of this risk and treated prophylactically with laxatives. Serotoninergic antagonists, the new class of antiemetics, are associated with mild to moderate constipation.

HEPATIC TOXICITY

Somewhat surprisingly, chemotherapeutic agents given in standard doses rarely cause clinically significant hepatic toxicity, despite the fact that many agents are processed and cleared through the liver. Hepatic toxicities that are encountered range from mildly elevated results of liver function tests to acute jaundice, chemical hepatitis, hepatic encephalopathy, and hepatic failure. Ara-C, asparaginase, 6-MP, methotrexate, mithramycin, streptozotocin, nitrosoureas, and dacarbazine are commonly associated with hepatic toxicity, but many other agents have also been reported to cause hepatic toxicity.[28] When combination chemotherapy or higher doses of busulfan, carmustine, or carboplatin are used, as in bone marrow transplantation, hepatotoxicity occurs with increased frequency. Veno-occlusive disease, the nonthrombotic obliteration of small intrahepatic veins, is a striking example of severe hepatotoxicity due to chemotherapy. It typically presents 1 to 4 weeks after high-dose combination therapy or transplant.[29] Veno-occlusive disease carries a high mortality rate and requires intensive supportive care. Efforts at improving prevention and treatment of veno-occlusive disease continue. In the bone marrow transplant setting, graft-versus-host disease also may present as hepatic toxicity/failure.[30] Distinguishing between these two entities often requires a liver biopsy. In evaluating patients with abnormal results of liver function tests or symptoms attributable to hepatic toxicity, other possible causes such as progressive cancer, drug interactions, or viral hepatitis should be considered in the differential diagnosis, along with the chemotherapeutic agent. In the presence of abnormal results of liver function tests, dose adjustments should be considered for daunorubicin, doxorubicin, vinblastine, vincristine, procarbazine, etoposide, cyclophosphamide, and methotrexate.[31]

GENITOURINARY SYSTEM

Sexual dysfunction and infertility are the most common genitourinary toxicities of chemotherapeutic agents. As reviewed elsewhere, many chemotherapeutic agents can suppress gonadal function either transiently or permanently.[32] A patient's risk for developing infertility or becoming menopausal increases with increasing age, total dose of chemotherapy administered, and the agents used.[33] The majority of data regarding fertility after chemotherapy come from patients with a long survival after chemotherapy. These data suggest that agents used for Hodgkin's and non-Hodgkin's lymphoma, leukemia, testicular cancer, and breast cancer have a moderate to high risk of causing hormonal dysfunction. In male patients with a high probability of infertility, sperm donation and storage may offer a mechanism to maintain reproductive opportunities. Interestingly, many patients, particularly men, are found to be infertile or have reduced fertility before chemotherapy.[34] Although many believe that this is a result of a paraneoplastic process or hormonal dysfunction secondary to physical debilitation, no clear mechanism has been found. The long-term fertility of patients who are not cured after systemic chemotherapy is not well understood. Although it is assumed that many of the agents used for palliation cause infertility, the advanced stage and clinical course of the disease often result in a low priority given to maintaining fertility.

Beyond the obvious reproductive consequences, chemotherapy can cause premature menopause, leading to increased risks of heart disease, osteoporosis, and decreased libido.[35] Sexual dysfunction and impotence may persist for several months or permanently after completion of chemotherapy. Agents commonly associated with hormone dysfunction include cyclophosphamide, doxorubicin, procarbazine, busulfan, nitrogen mustard, and chlorambucil used alone or in combination. Treatment of breast and prostate cancers typically includes estrogen or testosterone ablative therapy, respectively, but the loss of fertility is a reasonable tradeoff for highly efficacious, low-toxicity therapy. If alterative treatments have a lower risk of hormonal dysfunction but maintain efficacy (e.g., chemotherapy versus radiation for Hodgkin's disease), patients should be made aware of both options. However, it must be remembered that not all agents cause infertility/hormone disruption, and both male and female patients may remain fertile, despite cytotoxic chemotherapy. Patients should therefore use effective contraception during chemotherapeutic treatment. If given during pregnancy, radiation and many agents carry an increased risk of abnormal fetal development and spontaneous miscarriages.[36] Although it is advisable to avoid all chemotherapy during pregnancy, fetal malformations are not inevitable. Decisions about carrying such a pregnancy to term should balance the risk of malformation, the desires of the parents, the need for continuing a potentially teratogenic treatment during pregnancy, and the underlying course and prognosis of the disease itself.

Hemorrhagic cystitis is a potentially severe toxicity most commonly encountered with use of ifosfamide and high doses of cyclophosphamide. Acrolein, a metabolite of ifosfamide and cyclophosphamide, is excreted in the urine and has been implicated as the urotoxic substance, but the exact mechanism by which it damages the urothelium is unknown (see also the later sections on renal toxicity and neurotoxicity). Mesna (sodium 2-mercaptoethane sulfonate), a free radical scavenger that is thought to bind the acrolein compound, is given prophylactically to prevent the development of hemorrhagic cystitis and is frequently used during an acute episode of hemorrhagic cystitis.[37] Other symptomatic treatments include bladder irrigation and IV hydration. The risk of secondary bladder cancers increases after hemorrhagic cystitis, and thus aggressive prevention is justified.

Patients frequently express concern about changes in urine color after chemotherapy. Anthracyclines commonly cause a reddish discoloration of the urine. Mitoxantrone changes urine to blue-green. This is of no clinical significance and should clear within 24 to 48 hours after chemotherapy.

RENAL TOXICITY

When confronting a patient who has cancer and evidence of renal dysfunction either before or after treatment, two things must be kept in mind. First, many chemotherapeutic agents have direct renal toxicity and require specific preventive measures for safe administration. Second, many agents are cleared by the kidneys and thus require either dose adjustment or avoidance in patients with renal insufficiency.[38] Therefore, it is mandatory to evaluate renal function before administration of many agents. Agents most commonly associated with direct renal toxicity include cisplatin, ifosfamide, cyclophosphamide, methotrexate, pentostatin, streptozocin, and suramin. Mitomycin C has been associated with hemolytic-uremic syndrome/thrombotic thrombocytopenic purpura. Agents that require dose modifications in the presence of renal dysfunction include cisplatin, carboplatin, cyclophosphamide, plicamycin, mitomycin C, bleomycin, methotrexate, and streptozotocin.[39]

Cisplatin is the most notorious agent with regard to nephrotoxicity, and some degree of renal insufficiency is evident after every cycle of cisplatin. There is a dose relationship between cisplatin and nephrotoxicity, in that higher single-dose treatments as well as increasing cumulative doses lead to increasing nephrotoxicity.[40] An operational assumption could be that cisplatin damages a certain number of nephrons with each milligram administered, and clinically evident nephrotoxicity results once a particular patient's renal reserve has been depleted. After acute administration of cisplatin, it is not uncommon to observe mild elevations in blood urea nitrogen and creatinine levels for as long as 1 to 2 weeks. However, most commonly, renal function returns to normal after each treatment with cisplatin. Typically, only high cumulative doses result in permanent end-organ damage. Prehydration with a chloride-containing IV solution and adequate diuresis ameliorate much of the nephrotoxicity of cisplatin use. If proper hydration techniques are used, it is extremely uncommon for cisplatin to cause acute renal failure. In the presence of pre-existing mild to moderate renal insufficiency, the dose of cisplatin must be either reduced or completely avoided. The cisplatin analogue carboplatin can be used in renal insufficiency, with doses adjusted according to a patient's creatinine clearance, weight, and age. Carboplatin is not renal toxic but is cleared by the kidneys, and doses must be reduced in the presence of impaired renal function. Newer analogues are being developed, and it is hoped that these will retain the clinical activity but lessen the nephrotoxicity.[41]

In standard doses, methotrexate is not normally toxic to the kidneys even though 90% of the drug is excreted unchanged through the kidneys. However, when given in high doses, methotrexate may precipitate in the renal tubules and can cause acute renal failure.[42] Prehydration with an IV fluid containing sodium bicarbonate to alkalize the urine to a pH exceeding 7 can ameliorate this problem. This alkalization (with or without diuresis) prevents methotrexate precipitation within the tubules. High-dose methotrexate administration should be avoided in patients with pre-existing renal insufficiency (see the section on leucovorin rescue of methotrexate).

The alkylating agents ifosfamide and cyclophosphamide are directly toxic to the kidneys. Ifosfamide is known to cause a Fanconi-like syndrome, and cyclophosphamide has been associated with the syndrome of inappropriate antidiuretic hormone (SIADH) secretion. These toxicities typically occur soon after administration of the agent, may worsen with increasing doses, and appear to be reversible with appropriate supportive care. A particularly challenging pairing of toxicities is simultaneous hemorrhagic cystitis and SIADH due to use of cyclophosphamide. Faced with this rare scenario, the clinician must balance the need for IV fluids against the need to limit free water intake.

The tumor lysis syndrome can result in multiple end-organ toxicities, but the kidneys are the focus. For tumor lysis to occur, a patient must have a large volume of tumor that is likely to respond rapidly to chemotherapy, and the result is synchronous death of large numbers of cells. Cell death results in rapid extrusion of intracellular contents into the extracellular compartment, and the capacity of clearance mechanisms is overwhelmed. Common clinical settings for tumor lysis include lymphoma, leukemia, and rarely solid tumors such as germ cell and small cell tumors. Nephrotoxicity results from the rapid rise in the extracellular uric acid levels, which allow for crystallization within the renal tubules and subsequent renal dysfunction.[43] Precautions against the tumor lysis syndrome should be taken in all patients at risk, especially those who have evidence of renal insufficiency, hyperuricemia, hypercalcemia, or hyperphosphatemia before beginning treatment. Allopurinol, aggressive hydration with an alkaline solution to achieve urine pH greater than 7, and aggressive monitoring of chemistry and electrolyte values are essential. Tumor lysis syndrome may result in the need for dialysis after chemotherapy.

PULMONARY TOXICITY

Nearly 40 antineoplastic agents currently in use today have associated pulmonary toxicity.[44] Fortunately, from a practical point of view, pulmonary toxicity is not a common complication of chemotherapy, for when it does occur, it can be chronic, severe, and life threatening. Agents that are commonly associated with pulmonary toxicity include bleomycin, mitomycin, carmustine, cytarabine, interleukin-2, and methotrexate. Toxicities can include hypersensitivity reactions, pulmonary hypertension, thromboembolism, enhanced pulmonary capillary permeability, veno-occlusive disease, anaphylaxis, bronchiolitis obliterans, pleural effusion, chest pain, and adult respiratory distress syndrome.[45] Therefore, virtually any pathologic finding within the chest could be attributed to chemotherapy. Chemotherapy-induced pulmonary toxicity is frequently a diagnosis of exclusion, and other sources for pulmonary pathology must be ruled out.

Bleomycin is the agent most commonly associated with pulmonary toxicity. Bleomycin concentrates in the lungs and skin and has a direct action on the pulmonary capillary endothelium and type II pneumocytes.[46] The damage that is inflicted on the lungs is through the production of free radicals, which overcome the protective effects of reducing agents such as glutathione. The initial injury acutely follows the administration of the chemotherapy, which is then followed by a more chronic toxicity from lymphocytic and plasma cell infiltration, an infiltration of fibroblasts, and subsequent deposition of collagen and fibrosis. The incidence of reported pulmonary toxicity has a wide range, with most studies describing bleomycin toxicities in 3% to 5% of patients treated. The risk factors for bleomycin toxicity include age over 70, cumulative dose greater than 400 units, prior or subsequent radiotherapy of the chest, exposure to high oxygen concentrations at any time after treatment, renal dysfunction, bolus administration, and, interestingly, the condition of non-Hodgkin's lymphoma.[47] Common clinical features of bleomycin toxicity include dyspnea and pulmonary infiltrates. Pleural friction rubs are occasionally heard. Gallium scanning and computed tomography of the thorax may be of use. Radiographic abnormalities may rarely be limited to one lung. Bronchoalveolar lavage or pulmonary biopsy may be of use in the diagnosis. The typical pathologic findings for bleomycin toxicity as well as most chemotherapy-induced pulmonary toxicity are diffuse alveolar damage, cellular infiltrates, capillary leak, and fibrosis. Once pulmonary toxicity is diagnosed, the treatment of bleomycin-induced lung disease consists of systemic corticosteroids. Approximately half of patients have resolution of their radiographic abnormalities within 9 months of completing therapy, but many patients have persistent symptoms and pathologic changes causing a great potential for high morbidity and mortality.[48]

The nitrosoureas, namely bis-chloroethyl-nitrosourea (BCNU), are associated with severe pulmonary toxicity. The overall incidence may be as high as 30% to 50% in patients who have received a cumulative dose of 1500 mg/m^2 or greater.[49] Although less common, pulmonary toxicities occur after a single high dose of BCNU, such as in the bone marrow transplantation setting. This acute pulmonary toxicity generally develops 12 to 100 days after bone marrow transplantation. Chronic pulmonary toxicity due to standard-dose BCNU has been reported as late as 8 months after discontinuing use of the agent. Younger patients and those with pre-existing pulmonary disease are at increased risk for developing pulmonary toxicity. Clinically, pulmonary toxicity can range from mild shortness of breath to frank adult respiratory distress syndrome. Systemic steroids have failed to prevent nitrosourea-induced pulmonary toxicity or reverse its natural course once diagnosed.[50]

Cyclophosphamide rarely causes pulmonary toxicity, but when it occurs it can be severe. The onset of symptoms begins as early as 2 weeks after the start of therapy and as late as several years after termination of therapy. As with other agents, higher doses of cyclophosphamide increase the risk of developing toxicity, which pathologically includes alveolar hemorrhage and fibrin deposition. Radiation and increasing doses of cyclophosphamide have been reported to have a synergistic role in causing pulmonary toxicity[51] (Table 54A–9).

The pulmonary toxicities of methotrexate display a distinct pattern compared with other cytotoxic agents. This pattern includes capillary leak, pulmonary edema, interstitial pneumonitis with diffuse aveolar damage, hypersensitivity reactions, and noncaseating granulomatous reactions.[52] Although not rare, methotrexate toxicity affects slightly fewer than 1% of patients receiving the agent. Patients can develop pulmonary toxicity after oral, IV, or intrathecal administration. Methotrexate lung toxicity may develop as late as 5 years after administration of the agent and may occur in patients already receiving corticosteroids.[53] The onset of clinical findings ranges from acute shortness of breath, secondary to pulmonary edema, to a more gradual onset of symptoms secondary to progressive interstitial fibrosis. Use of high-dose methotrexate has been associated with chemical pleuritis. Radiographic features of methotrexate toxicity in the lungs are somewhat unique in that the typical presentation is parenchymal infiltrates or pleural effusions. Differential diagnoses includes chronic pneumonia, sarcoidosis, and adenopathy secondary to recurrent tumor. Corticosteroids may speed resolution of the pneumonitis, but no intervention may be necessary, because recovery frequently occurs within days, even if methotrexate is continued.

Radiation therapy of the lung parenchyma can result in acute and chronic pulmonary toxicities. Clinically relevant radiation pneumonitis occurs in as many as 15% of patients irradiated. The risk is much higher and the toxicity more severe when administered to patients who have had prior radiation, patients treated before or concurrently with chemotherapeutic agents (particularly doxorubicin, bleomycin, busulfan, and mitomycin C), and to patients undergoing a steroid taper.[54] The high incidence of severe morbidity and mortality due to adult respiratory distress syndrome in patients receiving concurrent doxorubicin and radiation is such that this practice is rarely if ever done. It is unclear if the pulmonary toxicity following use of radiation and doxorubicin shares common mechanisms with the severe skin reaction of "radiation recall" seen with the same combination. Dyspnea, the primary presenting symptom of radiation pneumonitis, begins a few months after completion of therapy. The total lung damage is in proportion to the amount of lung tissue radiated, which is the prime motivation for minimizing radiation port sizes by using three-dimensional port designs.[55] Corticosteroids and supportive care are the cornerstones of treatment.

Table 54A–9. Chemotherapeutic Agents That Interact Synergistically with Radiation Therapy

Anthracyclines (doxorubicin)
5-Fluorouracil
Paclitaxel
Platinum compounds
Bleomycin
Cyclophosphamide
Methotrexate

CARDIAC TOXICITY

Cardiac toxicity is a relatively uncommon phenomenon following chemotherapy administration. Although many agents have been associated with cardiac toxicity (bleomycin, cyclophosphamide, ifosphamide, paclitaxel, vincristine, hormonal agents, and immunotherapies, among others), relatively few actually cause clinically relevant cardiac abnormalities.[56] Doxorubicin and the other intercalating agents are the cause of most chemotherapy-induced cardiac damage. Although the acute effects of doxorubicin may result in tachyarrhythmias during administration, the more common abnormality of myocardial damage occurs with long-term dosing. When patients receive more than 450 mg/m^2 of doxorubicin given by bolus administration, the incidence of congestive heart failure shows a steady, predictable rise. The precise pathogenesis of doxorubicin-induced cardiomyopathy is unclear, and multiple hypotheses have been put forward.[57] Although congestive heart failure is more prominent at doses exceeding 450 mg/m^2, congestive heart failure can occur at doses lower than the 450 mg/m^2 cutoff. Therefore, doxorubicin may have an etiologic role in patients presenting with congestive heart failure at any point in their treatment. Clinical evaluations can include radionuclide ventriculography or other functional cardiac imaging, but the definitive diagnosis is made only with an endomyocardial biopsy. Dexrazoxane, a cardioprotective agent, has been approved for use in women with metastatic breast cancer who have received a cumulative doxorubicin dose of 300 mg/m^2. Dexrazoxane is indicated for reducing the incidence and severity of cardiomyopathy associated with doxorubicin administration and may allow for the administration of higher cumulative doses of doxorubicin.[58] However, no agent is capable of reversing the cardiac damage due to doxorubicin. Management should include careful cardiac monitoring, both radiographically and pathologically, to avoid cardiac toxicity. If congestive heart failure occurs, management is the same as for other causes of congestive heart failure. Analogues of doxorubicin have been developed with the hope of finding agents with lower cardiac toxicity. Idarubicin, an agent that is frequently used in the treatment of leukemia, may have less cardiac toxicity than doxorubicin. Mitoxantrone, structurally similar to anthracyclines, has a similar clinical activity and appears to cause less cardiotoxicity. With both these agents, however, congestive heart failure occurs and patients should be monitored closely.

Paclitaxel, a new agent licensed for the treatment of breast cancer, ovarian cancer, and lung cancer, was found to have frequent association with bradyarrhythmias and tachyarrhythmias during the acute administration of the drug. After extensive clinical evaluation with inpatient and outpatient monitoring, it was determined that these arrhythmias were of little clinical significance.[59] Cases of more prolonged and severe arrhythmias have occurred, however, and should be a consideration when evaluating a patient during the administration of paclitaxel. Taxotere, the semi-synthetic agent likely to be approved for use in breast cancer, reportedly has a lower associated incidence of arrhythmias than paclitaxel.

5-FU causes a distinctive cardiac toxicity that typically presents as angina associated with nonspecific ST-T wave changes, arrhythmias, global myocardial dysfunction, and rarely myocardial infarct, cardiac failure, and sudden death.[60] Although cardiac ischemia can occur with any infusion schedule of 5-FU, it most frequently occurs during a prolonged infusion of high-dose 5-FU. It has been reported to occur 3 to 18 hours after treatment. The overall incidence is measured at 1.6%, with an increased incidence in patients with prior ischemic cardiomyopathy. The mechanism for cardiac ischemia (which rarely results in permanent myocardial damage) is uncertain. If a patient complains of angina, the infusion should be stopped, an electrocardiogram should be obtained (diffuse ST segment changes are common), and treatment should include nitrates if pain or electrocardiographic changes persist. Frequent response to nitrates suggests a coronary spastic etiology, but this has not been proved.

Radiation can cause damage to all portions of the heart. The pericardium, myocardium, valves, conduction system, and vessels are at risk after moderate- to high-dose radiation to the heart. Inflammation and fibrosis are the major pathologic findings, occurring 1 to 10 years after treatment. There is no prevention or treatment, but cardiac assessment should be considered to detect early signs of vascular or valvular disease and to allow for early surgical intervention when appropriate.

NEUROTOXICITY OF CHEMOTHERAPEUTIC AGENTS

Neurotoxicity is a frequent complication of many commonly used chemotherapy agents (e.g., cisplatin, carboplatin, paclitaxel, methotrexate, cytarabine, fludarabine, the vinca alkaloids, ifosfamide, suramin, interleukin-2, and interferon) and is often a clinical symptom forcing either a reduction or cessation of the causative agent.[61] Damage to the nervous system may be acute and reversible or chronic and irreversible. All portions of the nervous system are at risk for damage due to chemotherapeutic agents.

The most common acute central nervous system toxicity caused by chemotherapy and supportive care drugs is altered mental status. Patients with cancer suffer from many medical conditions and take many medicines that may result in altered mental status. Several chemotherapy agents such as high-dose cytarabine, fludarabine, procarbazine, interferon, and ifosfamide carry independent risks for mental status changes. Ifosfamide neurotoxicity in particular can be quite an unpleasant experience for patients and medical staff because the mental status changes frequently include vivid, horrid hallucinations.[62] Although of unproven benefit, maintaining a patient's serum albumin level above 3.0 g/dE may prevent or treat this particular toxicity. The cause of this toxicity is not entirely clear. Frank encephalopathy can follow both IV and intrathecal administration of methotrexate and cytarabine; high-dose etoposide, nitrogen mustard, carmustine, and procarbazine; and standard doses of mitotane, L-asparaginase, and the vinca alkaloids.[63]

Peripheral neuropathy, the most common chronic neurotoxicity, results from use of the vinca alkaloids, paclitaxel, and cisplatin. The incidence of this toxicity increases with increasing cumulative doses. The severity can range from mild tingling to marked motor and sensory dysfunction leading to inability to ambulate. Cranial nerves are not necessarily spared. Loss of deep tendon reflexes is a useful early clinical finding. Although much of the peripheral neuropathy may reverse after cessation of the agent, it is not uncommon for some level of chronic neuropathy to persist throughout a patient's life. These neuropathies are often quite painful and difficult to treat with conventional analgesics. No agent has been proved to reverse neuropathies, but adding a tricyclic antidepressant or an antiseizure drug to the patient's pain regimen is often effective in relieving the neuropathic pain. Few successes have occurred in the prevention of chemotherapy-induced neurotoxicity.

Cerebellar ataxia can result from use of high-dose cytarabine and 5-FU. Typically, the ataxia occurs acutely during the infusions or within the first few days of treatment and may be reversible after cessation of the agent. Complete resolution may often take weeks to months. The ataxia of cytarabine tends to be more severe, less reversible, and associated with a wide range of other severe neurotoxicities.

Not surprisingly, neurotoxicity is more common with intrathecal chemotherapy. Methotrexate is the most frequently used agent. It may acutely cause a chemical meningitis, fever, headache and nuchal rigidity, and cerebrospinal fluid leukocytosis. Resolution is typically spontaneous within hours after the injection. On a more continual treatment schedule, progressive leukoencephalopathy may also result from intrathecal administration of methotrexate. The risk of developing leukoencephalopathy increases with increasing total dose of methotrexate as well as concurrent radiotherapy.[64] Although less commonly used, intrathecal cytarabine is associated with a high incidence of central neurotoxicity similar to that caused by methotrexate.

Radiation may also result in both acute and chronic central nervous system damage. In the chronic setting, memory loss and mild cognitive dysfunction are frequent results of radiotherapy 1 to 4 years after its completion.[65] The increased recognition of this phenomenon has led to reduced use of prophylactic cranial irradiation in clinical settings where it has not been proved to be of benefit.

Corticosteroids are widely used in oncology and often at high doses over long-term courses. The most common neurotoxicity associated with corticosteroid use is proximal myopathy, but mood alterations, insomnia, tremor, and depression all are side effects of steroid use. In patients who have been on long-term steroid therapy and whose dose is being tapered or discontinued, one must be cognizant of potential steroid withdrawal symptoms such as depression, anorexia, muscle aches, joint pains, and, most severe, addisonian crisis.

The following is a brief summary of other chemotherapy-induced neurotoxicites. Cranial nerve damage can occur with use of agents such as cisplatin, which affects the auditory system, and high-dose cytarabine, 5-FU, and chlorambucil, which cause damage to the eyes and ocular structures. The risk of auditory damage by cisplatin increases with increased cumulative doses and is rarely reversible. The combination of 5-FU and levamisole used in the adjuvant treatment of colorectal cancers has been associated with cerebral demyelination.[66] Arthralgias and myalgias are frequently encountered with use of paclitaxel, cytarabine, and dacarbazine. Headache is a prominent toxicity of the new agent topotecan. Autonomic neuropathies primarily occur with use of the vinca alkaloids. The most common clinical manifestation of an autonomic neuropathy in patients with cancer is an ileus, which is often severe and slow to resolve.

DERMATOLOGIC TOXICITIES

As with use of any pharmaceutical agent, chemotherapy has a wide range of associated dermatologic toxicities. Because the cells of the epidermis, hair, nails, and mucosal surfaces are rapidly dividing, they are particularly vulnerable to cytotoxic agents. Therefore, alopecia, pigmentation changes, and nail disorders are common with chemotherapy. These toxicities are among the most disturbing to patients despite the rarity of significant, long-lasting physical consequences. For many patients, if it were not for alopecia, there would be no public evidence of their condition and they could maintain the privacy of their diagnosis. The psychologic consequences of these toxicities must be respected. One should be aware that not all chemotherapy causes these abnormalities, and when appropriate, other explanations should be considered. Alopecia, hyperpigmentation, and nail disorders are almost always reversible on cessation of the chemotherapeutic agent.

Chemotherapeutic agents are relatively uncommon causes of cutaneous hypersensitivity reactions. A complete history and medication list should be obtained from any patient presenting with such a reaction, because patients with cancer are frequently taking multiple medicines likely to cause a dermatologic reaction. L-Asparaginase is the agent most commonly associated with urticaria and hypersensitivity reactions. Other associated agents include doxorubicin, busulfan, bleomycin, aminoglutethimide, methotrexate, mitotane, and procarbazine.[67] Immunotherapies including interleukin-2 and interferon commonly cause transient erythema and pruritus, which should not be considered allergic reactions.

Both therapeutic and passive radiation can enhance the toxicity of many chemotherapeutic agents. The skin reactions of patients receiving both radiation and chemotherapy are typically increased, found almost exclusively within the radiation port. Any reaction distant from the port is unlikely to be caused by combination therapy, and other causes should be sought. Radiation recall is a dramatic, inflammatory skin reaction localized to the prior radiation port in a patient who received radiation at some point in the past and is now receiving chemotherapy (doxorubicin and dactinomycin are most common).[68] Patients and physicians frequently forget the sun as a source of radiation, but 5-FU, methotrexate, 6-TG, vinblastine, and dacarbazine all can cause photosensitivity. Treatment for all skin reactions include discontinuation of the offending agent if possible and symptomatic care. Systemic or topical steroids and skin grafting are of little benefit in severe cases.

Acroerythema (palmar-plantar acrodysesthesia syndrome) can be caused by a number of chemotherapeutic agents including cytarabine, cyclophosphamide, doxorubicin, 6-MP, 5-FU, methotrexate, hydroxyurea, and mitotane. Erythema multiforme, liver disease, and long-term estrogen therapy must be considered in the differential diagnosis. Treatment of this usually entails symptomatic treatment with cool compresses and analgesics. Acroerythema typically reverses within 2 to 5 days after cessation of chemotherapy.

5-FU is known to inflame pre-existing actinic keratoses. In fact, 5-FU is frequently used as a topical treatment for actinic keratoses.[69] Other agents reported to do this include doxorubicin, dactinomycin, cisplatin, and vincristine. The inflammatory reaction may be mistaken for an allergic reaction or dermatitis and is not an indication to discontinue therapy.

Extravasation is the leakage of a fluid from a vein into the surrounding soft tissue. Chemotherapy extravasation during infusion can result in serious soft tissue damage.[70] Many chemotherapy agents are nonulcerogenic, whereas others are classified as vesicants or irritants (Table 54A–10). Irritants may cause discomfort but do not cause necrosis. It is important to recognize extravasation early, discontinue

Table 54A–10. Vesicant Chemotherapeutic Agents

Dactinomycin	Carmustine
Daunorubicin	Cisplatin
Doxorubicin	Dacarbazine
Idarubicin	Etoposide
Mechlorethamine	Fluorouracil
Mitomycin C	Floxuridine
Vinblastine	Mitoxantrone
Vincristine	Paclitaxel
Vinorelbine	Plicamycin
	Teniposide

Table 54A–11. Vesicant Chemotherapeutic Agents

Drug	Treatment
Cisplatin Mechlorethamine	Isotonic sodium thiosulfite injected into the site.
Mitomycin C	Dimethyl sulfoxide (DMSO) 50–99% applied topically every 6 hours × 14 days.
Doxorubicin Daunorubicin Idarubicin	Ice or cold compresses immediately and repeat every 6 hours for 24 to 48 hours. DMSO applied topically as above. Elevate the extremity.
Vinblastine Vincristine Vinorelbine	Warm compresses immediately and repeat at least four times in the first 24 hours. Inject 150 U hyaluronidase into site.
Etoposide Teniposide	Warm compresses immediately and repeat at least 4 times in the first 24 hours. Inject 150 U hyaluronidase into site.

the therapy if extravasation is recognized during the infusion, and consider antidotes when appropriate. The extent of tissue damage incurred varies with the chemical and irritant properties of the specific drug, its concentration, and the duration of exposure to the tissue. The mechanism for the damage and the treatment of the injury vary according to the agent in question.

When an extravasation occurs, the first symptom often is a sensation of pain or burning during or after infusion. Erythema and swelling may occur. Prompt recognition and treatment of an extravasation are essential to minimize tissue destruction. In some cases of delayed extravasation, however, symptoms or injuries have developed days or weeks after administration of chemotherapy. Initial treatments are varied and controversial and often lack scientific basis. After extravasation of a potent vesicant (e.g., doxorubicin), ulcers can develop over a period of hours or days, and the extent and depth of tissue damage may not be evident for weeks. As a necrotic lesion develops, the risk for more serious complications increases. With decreased blood flow, healing is impaired and significant pain can interfere with the functional use of the affected hand or arm. Surgical débridement with skin grafting may be necessary to treat severe cases.

The local treatments for extravasations include injection of specific antidotes, altering temperature of the skin with the application of ice or heat, adjusting the pH of the exposed tissue, topical application of antioxidants, and systemic administration of glucocorticoids, antihistamines, and lidocaine[71] (Table 54A–11). Many of these treatments are anecdotal and have not been proved to be of clinical benefit. Standard practice for all drugs except vinca alkaloids and epipodophyllotoxins is immediate application of ice and repeated applications during the first 24 to 48 hours, with elevation of the extremity. All treatment should be initiated immediately, because delayed treatment in most cases is ineffective.

PAIN

The cause of pain in patients with cancer is often multifactorial. Pain can be a side effect of the prescribed treatment but more frequently is caused by the underlying disease. Nearly 75% of patients with advanced cancer experience pain. Forty to 50% of those patients report their pain as moderate or severe. Cancer pain is usually chronic and is frequently very debilitating for patients. Effective pain management can have a significant impact on a patient's quality of life. The World Health Organization has developed a "pain ladder" as a rational approach to the treatment of chronic pain. Mild pain is treated with acetaminophen or nonsteroidal anti-inflammatory drugs (NSAIDs). For moderate pain, a weak opiate is combined with a non-narcotic drug such as acetaminophen with codeine or oxycodone. A strong opiate is recommended for unresponsive or severe pain, and morphine is the drug of choice. Adjuvant drugs may be added to the pain regimen to treat specific types of pain. NSAIDs are effective for bone pain, and tricyclic antidepressants can alleviate neuropathic pain.

The side effects of pain therapy are well documented and should be anticipated. NSAIDs and aspirin-containing products cause GI irritation and alter platelet function. Opiates can cause sedation, nausea, vomiting, constipation, itching, and respiratory depression. Constipation is the one toxicity that is always expected and should be treated prophylactically with stool softeners and laxatives. In most cases, patients develop a tolerance to the nausea, vomiting, and sedation. Antiemetics can be useful for patients experiencing nausea or vomiting when narcotic therapy is initiated. If sedation remains problematic, the addition of methylphenidate or dextroamphetamine to the pain regimen is an option. Respiratory depression is a risk when prescribing narcotics for opioid-naive patients but is seldom an issue with opiate-tolerant patients and is uncommon with oral narcotics.

References

1. Morrow CS, Cowan K: Drug resistance and cancer. Adv Exp Med Biol *330*:287, 1993.
2. Goldstein LJ: Clinical reversal of drug resistance. Curr Probl Cancer *19*:65, 1995.

3. Dela Flor-Weiss E, Uziely B, Muggia FM: Protracted drug infusions in cancer treatment: An appraisal of 5-fluorouracil, doxorubicin, and platinums. Ann Oncol *4*:723, 1993.
4. de Valeriola D: Dose optimization of anthracyclines. Anticancer Res *14*:2307, 1994.
5. Arbuck SG, Canetta R, Onetto N, Christian MC: Current dosage and schedule issues in the development of paclitaxel (Taxol). Semin Oncol *20*:31, 1993.
6. Livingston RB: Dose intensity and high dose therapy. Two different concepts. Cancer *74*:1177, 1994.
7. van der Wall E, Beijnen JH, Rodenhuis S: High-dose chemotherapy regimens for solid tumors. Cancer Treat Rev *21*:105, 1995.
8. Milano G, Etienne MC: Dihydropyrimidine dehydrogenase (DPD) and clinical pharmacology of 5-fluorouracil (review). Anticancer Res *14*:2295, 1994.
9. Creaven PJ, Mihich E: The clinical toxicity of anticancer drugs and its prediction. Semin Oncol *4*:147, 1977.
10. Lee JW, Pizzo PA: Management of the cancer patient with fever and prolonged neutropenia. Hematol Oncol Clin North Am *7*:937, 1993.
11. Klastersky J: Febrile neutropenia. Curr Opin Oncol *5*:625, 1993.
12. Roilides E, Pizzo PA: Perspectives on the use of cytokines in the management of infectious complications of cancer. Clin Infect Dis *17*(Suppl 2):385, 1993.
13. Vose JM, Armitage JO: Clinical applications of hematopoetic growth factors. J Clin Oncol *13*:1023, 1995.
14. Bishop JF: Platelet support and the use of cytokines. Stem Cells *12*:370, 1994.
15. Bock M, Heim MU, Salat C, et al: Thrombocyte transfusion. Indications, side effects and problems. Fortschr Med *111*:332, 1993.
16. Goldberg GL, Gibbon DG, Smith HO, et al: Clinical impact of chemotherapy-induced thrombocytopenia in patients with gynecologic cancer. J Clin Oncol *12*:2317, 1994.
17. Markham A, Bryson HM: Epoetin alfa. A review of its pharmacodynamic and pharmacokinetic properties and therapeutic use in nonrenal applications. Drugs *49*:232, 1995.
18. Chabner BA, Myers CE, Coleman CN, et al: The clinical pharmacology of antineoplastic agents. N Engl J Med *292*:1107, 1975.
19. Wasserman TH, Slavic M, Carter SK: Clinical comparison of the nitrosureas. Cancer *36*:1258, 1975.
20. Boffetta P, Kaldor JM: Secondary malignancies following cancer chemotherapy. Acta Oncol *33*:591, 1994.
21. Hoagland HC: Hematologic complications of cancer chemotherapy. *In* Perry MC (ed): The Chemotherapy Source Book. Baltimore, Williams & Wilkins, pp 498–507, 1992.
22. Gralla RJ: Current issues in the management of nausea and vomiting. Ann Oncol *4*(Suppl):3, 1993.
23. Cubeddu LX: Mechanisms by which cancer chemotherapeutic drugs induce emesis. Semin Oncol *19*(Suppl):2, 1992.
24. Bilgrami S, Fallon BG: Chemotherapy-induced nausea and vomiting. Easing patients' fear and discomfort with effective antiemetic regimens. Postgrad Med *94*:55, 1993.
25. Lopez I, Goudou C, Ribrag V, et al: Treatment of mucositis with vitamin E during administration of neutropenic antineoplastic agents. Ann Med Interne (Paris) *145*:405, 1994.
26. Gordon B, Spadinger A, Hodges E, et al: effect of granulocyte-macrophage colony-stimulating factor on oral mucositis after hematopoeitic stem-cell transplantation. J Clin Oncol *12*:1917, 1994.
27. Cappell MS, Simon T: Colonic toxicity of administered medications and chemicals. Am J Gastroenterol *88*:1684, 1994.
28. Perry MC: Hepatotoxicity of chemotherapeutic agents. *In* Perry MC (ed): The Chemotherapy Source Book. Baltimore, Williams & Wilkins, pp 635–647, 1992.
29. Bearman SI, Anderson GL, Mori M, et al: Venoocclusive disease of the liver: Development of a model for predicting fatal outcome after marrow transplantation. J Clin Oncol *11*:1729, 1993.
30. Vogelsang GB, Morris LE: Prevention and management of graft-versus-host disease. Practical recommendations. Drugs *45*:668, 1993.
31. Koren G, Beatty K, Seto A, et al: The effects of impaired liver function on the elimination of antineoplastic agents. Ann Pharmacother *26*:363, 1992.
32. Chapman RM: Gonadal injury resulting from chemotherapy. Am J Intern Med *4*:149, 1983.
33. Goldman S, Johnson FL: Effects of chemotherapy and irradiation on the gonads. Endocrinol Metab Clin North Am *22*:617, 1993.
34. Chapman RM, Sutcliffe SB, Malpas JS: Male gonadal dysfunction in Hodgkin's disease. JAMA *245*:1323, 1981.
35. Valagussa P, Moliterni A, Zambetti M, et al: Long-term sequelae from adjuvant chemotherapy. Recent Results Cancer Res *127*:247, 1993.
36. Mulvihill JJ, McKeen EA, Rosner F, et al: Pregnancy outcome in cancer patients. Cancer *60*:1143, 1987.
37. Vose JM, Reed EC, Pippert GC, et al: Mesna compared with continuous bladder irrigation as uroprotection during high-dose chemotherapy and transplantation: A randomized trial. J Clin Oncol *11*:1306, 1993.
38. Kintzel PE, Dorr RT: Anticancer drug renal toxicity and elimination: dosing guidelines for altered renal function. Cancer Treat Rev *21*:33, 1995.
39. Vogelzang NJ: Nephrotoxicity from chemotherapy: Prevention and management. Oncology *5*:97, 1991.
40. Anand AJ, Bashey B: Newer insights into cisplatin nephrotoxicity. Ann Pharmacother *27*:1519, 1993.
41. Cornelison TL, Reed E: Nephrotoxicity and hydration management for cisplatin, carboplatin, and ormaplatin. Gynecol Oncol *50*:147, 1993.
42. Patterson WP, Reams GP: Renal and electrolyte abnormalities due to chemotherapy. *In* Perry MC (ed): The Chemotherapy Source Book. Baltimore, Williams & Wilkins, pp 648–665, 1992.
43. Jones DP, Mahmoud H, Chesney RW: Tumor lysis syndrome: Pathogenesis and management. Pediatr Nephrol *9*:206, 1995.
44. Kreisman H, Wolkove N: Pulmonary toxicity of antineoplastic therapy. *In* Perry MC (ed): The Chemotherapy Source Book. Baltimore, Williams & Wilkins, pp 598–619, 1992.
45. McDonald S, Rubin P, Philips TL, et al: Injury to the lung from cancer therapy: Clinical syndromes, measurable endpoints, and potential scoring systems. Int J Radiat Oncol Biol Phys *31*:1187, 1995.
46. Comis RL: Bleomycin pulmonary toxicity: Current status and future directions. Semin Oncol *19*(Suppl):64, 1992.
47. Bauer KA, Skarin A, Balikian JP, et al: Pulmonary complications with combination chemotherapy programs containing bleomycin. Am J Med *74*:557, 1983.
48. Cooper AD, White AD, Matthay RA: State of the art drug-induced pulmonary disease. Am Rev Respir Dis *133*:321, 1986.
49. Aronin PA, Mahaley MS, Rudnick SA, et al: Prediction of pulmonary toxicity in patients with malignant gliomas: An assessment of risk factors. N Engl J Med *303*:183, 1980.
50. Kalaycioglu M, Kavuru M, Tuason L, et al: Empiric prednisone therapy for pulmonary toxicity reaction after high-dose chemotherapy containing carmustine (BCNU). Chest *107*:482, 1995.
51. Trask CWL, Joannides T, Harper PG, et al: Radiation-induced lung fibrosis after treatment of small cell carcinoma of the lung with very high dose cyclophosphamide. Cancer *55*:57, 1985.
52. Hand SH, Smith JK, Chaudhary BA: Methotrexate pneumonitis: A case report and summary of the literature. J Med Assoc Ga *78*:625, 1989.
53. Bedrossian CWM, Miller WC, Luna MA: Methotrexate-induced diffuse interstitial pulmonary fibrosis. South Med J *72*:313, 1979.
54. Morgan GW, Breit SN: Radiation and the lung: A reevaluation of the mechanisms mediating pulmonary injury. Int J Radiat Oncol Biol Phys *31*:361, 1995.
55. Choi NC, Kanarek DJ: Toxicity of thoracic radiotherapy on pulmonary function in lung cancer. Lung Cancer *10*(Suppl):219, 1994.
56. de Forni M, Armand JP: Cardiotoxicity of chemotherapy. Curr Opin Oncol *6*:340, 1994.
57. Olson RD, Mushlin PS: Doxorubicin cardiotoxicity: Analysis of prevailing hypotheses. FASEB J *4*:3076, 1990.

58. Seifert CF, Nesser ME, Thompson DF: Dexrazoxane in the prevention of doxorubicin-induced cardiotoxicity. Ann Pharmacother *28*:1063, 1994.
59. Biadi O, Mengozzi G, Gherarducci G, et al: Evaluation of taxol cardiotoxicity in metastatic breast cancer. Ann N Y Acad Sci *698*:403, 1993.
60. Anand AJ: Fluorouracil cardiotoxicity. Ann Pharmacother *28*:374, 1994.
61. MacDonald DR: Neurologic complications of chemotherapy. Neurol Clin *9*:955, 1991.
62. Di Maggio JR, Brown R, Baile WF, et al: Hallucinations and ifosfamide-induced neurotoxicity. Cancer *73*:1509, 1994.
63. MacDonald DR: Neurotoxicity of chemotherapeutic agents. *In* Perry MC (ed): The Chemotherapy Source Book. Baltimore, Williams & Wilkins, pp 666–679, 1992.
64. Bleyer WA, Griffin TW: White matter necrosis, mineralizing microangiopathy, and intellectual abilities in survivors of childhood leukemia: Associations with central nervous system irradiation and methotrexate therapy. *In* Gilbert HA, Kagan AR (eds): Radiation Damage to the Central Nervous System. New York, Raven Press, pp 155–174, 1980.
65. Dropcho EJ: Central nervous system injury by therapeutic irradiation. Neurol Clin *9*:968, 1991.
66. Fassas AB, Gattani AM, Morgello S: Cerebral demyelination with 5-fluorouracil and levamisole. Cancer Invest *12*:379, 1994.
67. De Spain JD: Dermatologic toxicity of chemotherapy. Semin Oncol *19*:501, 1992.
68. Donaldson SS, Glick JM, Wilbur JR: Adriamycin activating a recall phenomenon after radiation therapy. Ann Intern Med *81*:407, 1974.
69. Leo S, Tatulli C, Taveri R, et al: Dermatologic toxicity from chemotherapy containing 5-fluorouracil. J Chemother *6*:423, 1994.
70. Tsavaris NB, Karagiaouris P, Tzannou I, et al: Conservative approach to the treatment of chemotherapy-induced extravasation. J Dermatol Surg Oncol *16*:519, 1990.
71. Dorr RT: Antidotes to vesicant chemotherapy extravasations. Blood Rev *4*:41, 1990.

B Transplant Agents

DAVID J. COHEN, MD, PHD
MARY H. BRANTON, MD
BOON S. OOI, MD

The use of pharmacologic agents to suppress the host immune response is the mainstay of clinical transplantation. Since the first kidney transplant in the 1950s, the dosing of immunosuppressive drugs has been considerably refined to minimize toxicity while maintaining graft function. In this chapter, the effects of transplant immunosuppression overdose and the clinical management of such overdosage are the major focus. Agents discussed are limited to those used specifically to maintain allograft function. Agents with immunosuppressive activity (i.e., antineoplastic agents) not commonly used in long-term transplant management are not included. For the purposes of this discussion, overdosage is defined as an acute ingestion, either accidental or intentional, that results in toxic supratherapeutic tissue and blood drug levels. Immunosuppressive agents used in transplantation have many toxic effects, both acutely and in the long term. It is important to distinguish the known complications of immunosuppressive therapy from the sequelae of acute overdose. Toward this goal, the common toxicities encountered with these agents are discussed with the effects of poisoning.

The major transplant immunosuppressive agents in use today that clinicians are likely to encounter are the steroid preparations (prednisone or methylprednisolone), azathioprine, and cyclosporine. Newer agents such as FK-506 (tacrolimus), mycophenolate, and rapamycin currently are in limited use, and no data on or clinical experiences with overdosage of these drugs have yet been accumulated. Antibody preparations such as OKT3 (monoclonal) and ALG (polyclonal) are important in the induction of transplant immunosuppression and the treatment of acute rejection; however, overdosage has not been reported for these drugs. As an example, the cytokine release syndrome associated with OKT3 cannot be described as an overdose-related toxicity, because it can occur with the first dose of only 5 mg. It is important to recognize that during the initial trials of many of these agents, doses used were substantially higher than those in use today. The titration between transplant function and dysfunction versus overimmunosuppression or underimmunosuppression is highly empirical, requiring close monitoring of the patient's and the graft's condition. The adverse reactions noted during the early trials of an immunosuppressive transplant agent with large dosing may mimic the toxicity caused by acute overdose. In general, it should be noted that overdosing or poisoning with transplant agents is uncommon. Patients with transplants are carefully instructed in the use of these drugs, and the patients themselves are screened before transplantation for emotional stability and the absence of psychiatric disorders that would predispose them to ingestion of drug overdose.

Each transplant agent of interest is discussed individually with respect to its mechanism of action, dosing, generally encountered adverse reactions, and experience with overdosage and poisoning. The relevant literature is cited, including overdose case reports of interest. Finally, clinical guidelines for overdose management are provided, along with the relevant citations.

REVIEW OF SPECIFIC TRANSPLANT AGENTS

Corticosteroids

Mechanism of Action. Steroid preparations have been central to pharmacologic immunosuppression for transplantation for almost 40 years. Although corticosteroids are able to suppress immune responses, these drugs have diffuse effects on the body because most tissues have glucocorticoid receptors.[1] The mechanism of corticosteroid immunosuppression has been difficult to define on a molecular basis. Steroids have been postulated to interfere with T-cell activation by blocking macrophage or T-cell cytokine elaboration. It is now known that corticosteroids increase the transcriptional activation of inhibitor at kappa β alpha (IKBA), a potent inhibitor of the transcriptional activator NFKB (nuclear factor of kappa light-chain gene enhancer in B cells).[2] NFKB is also essential for T-cell activation of cytokine genes such as interleukin-2. (IL-2).[1]

Toxicity, Overdosage, and Treatment. Clinically, the most commonly used corticosteroid preparations are prednisolone, prednisone (the 11-keto metabolite of prednisolone), and methylprednisolone. In vivo, prednisolone has the most active immunosuppressive activity; methylprednisolone is the preparation most commonly used for intravenous use. The toxicity of chronic corticosteroid use is protean, including hypertension, diabetes, cataract formation, bone demineralization, cushingoid facies and habitus, hyperlipidemia, decreased wound healing, increased susceptibility to infection, and emotional lability.[3] However, acute overdosage, even in massive quantities, does not result in significant clinical problems. Toxicity generally is not encountered with corticosteroid preparations when used for less than 3 weeks, even with substantial doses. Toxicity must be distinguished from overimmunosuppression (i.e., increased susceptibility to serious infection), occasionally noted during the treatment of acute rejection with very large, repeated doses of intravenous steroids (pulse therapy). With the advent of OKT3 monoclonal antibody for the treatment of steroid-refractory acute rejection, the use of repeated pulse steroid therapy has diminished.[3]

Azathioprine

Mechanism of Action. Azathioprine has been used as an immunosuppressant in organ transplantation since the 1960s. It is an imidazole derivative of 6-mercaptopurine, a purine analogue that inhibits purine nucleotide synthesis as well as RNA synthesis. Azathioprine is a myelosuppressant, and much of its toxicity is related to this effect. Leukopenia, thrombocytopenia, and macrocytic anemia are common hematologic findings with chronic use of the drug.[3]

Toxicity, Overdosage, and Treatment. In 1974, Carney and colleagues reported a patient with a massive overdose of azathioprine.[4] A cadaveric renal transplant recipient was taking 150 mg of azathioprine and 50 mg of prednisone daily 3 weeks after transplantation. The recipient developed symptoms of rejection (weight gain and increase in serum creatinine level) and was told to take 1 g of prednisone (200 5-mg tablets) and continue with the 150 mg of azathioprine. The patient mistakenly ingested 150 50-mg tablets of azathioprine, a total of 7500 mg, in addition to the 1 g of prednisone. The patient reported nausea, vomiting, and diarrhea at 6 and 8 hours and was subsequently hospitalized. During the 1-week hospitalization, the patient remained asymptomatic. Minor elevations in the serum levels of glutamic-oxaloacetic transaminase, glutamic-pyruvic transaminase, and bilirubin were observed. Leukopenia was identified but was mild; no thrombocytopenia was observed. No specific therapy for the overdose was prescribed. Azathioprine was restarted, and the transplant continued to function well. The researchers stated that the patient likely absorbed most of the drug because intestinal mucosal absorption is complete, based on studies originally performed with ^{35}S-6-mercaptopurine,[5] by the 6- to 8-hour onset of symptoms reported by the patient. The usual dosing of azathioprine is 1 to 5 mg/kg per day for humans undergoing solid organ transplantation; animal studies have shown median lethality (LD_{50}) doses of 2500 mg/kg for mice and 400 mg/kg for rats.[6] Death usually occurs within 7 days, with the histologic finding of agranulocytosis in the spleen and marrow. This patient ingested approximately 100 mg/kg in a single dose and had only minor myelosuppression and somatic toxicity. No significant hepatic toxicity was observed, despite the known ability of azathioprine to cause hepatic injury.[7, 8]

In summary, although the clinical experience with acute overdosage of azathioprine is limited, it is clear that serious toxicity and death have not been encountered, even with a dose up to 20 times the upper limit of the usual prescription. Supportive care is indicated, as well as discontinuation of the drug until hematologic and hepatic parameters have stabilized.

Cyclosporine

Mechanism of Action. Cyclosporine, a cyclic polypeptide isolated from fungi, has immunosuppressive properties.[9] Cylcosporine binds to cyclophilin in the cytoplasm.[9] The complex of cyclosporin and its binding protein, cyclophilin, have the effect of blocking IL-2 transcription in T-cells by blocking the function of calcineurin, an enzyme that activates nuclear factor of activated T-cells (NF-AT).[3] NF-AT is a major transcriptional activator/regulator of the IL-2 gene complex. By blocking IL-2, a growth hormone necessary for immune activation of T-cells, cyclosporine mediates its immunosuppressive effect.[3] Cyclosporine has nonimmunosuppressive effects as well. It can inhibit various ATP-dependent cellular export proteins,[10] which may account for its ability to inhibit cellular multidrug resistance. Cyclosporine has been shown to bind to renal P-glycoprotein and block excretion of renal substrates that bind to P-glycoprotein, a possible mechanism for its significant renal toxicity.[11]

Cyclosporine Pharmacokinetics

Cyclosporine is lipophilic, is insoluble in water, and has a wide range of bioavailability when taken orally. In the setting of organ transplantation, doses as great as 15 mg/kg routinely are used.[9] In other settings, such as treatment of autoimmune disorders or as an inhibitor of the multiple drug resistance enzyme, doses of 4 to 8 mg/kg are common. Patients with satisfactory long-term transplant function (>6 months) are generally maintained on dosages of 1 to 4 mg/kg per day.[9] A new formulation of cyclosporine microemulsion (Neoral) has superior bioavailability characteristics, resulting in increased predictability of serum levels and significantly decreased patient-to-patient variability.[12] Cyclosporine is metabolized via the hepatic microsomal P-450 system.[9] Drugs that inhibit P-450 increase cyclosporine levels, and drugs that induce P-450 decrease cyclosporine levels.[9] The parent drug has an elimination half-life of 8 hours, but P-450 breakdown yields at least 15 metabolites, some of which may have immunosuppressive or toxic potential.[9] Cyclosporine is excreted in the bile, and renal elimination is minimal.[3] Owing to the paucity of renal excretion, cyclosporine dosing is not adjusted for renal dysfunction, nor is it eliminated by dialysis.[3] Various assays are available to monitor cyclosporine blood levels, with various degrees of specificity for the parent compound and its metabolites, as well as variations in compartment measured (i.e., whole blood, plasma, or erythrocytes).[3]

Toxicity, Overdosage, and Treatment. Cyclosporine has been shown to be a nephrotoxin in both the acute and chronic settings.[3] Cyclosporine is also toxic to organs other than the kidneys.[13] Because cyclosporine is a potent inducer of endothelin, constriction of vascular beds, particularly renal, is a commonly encountered clinical problem that may be manifested by renal insufficiency.[3] The effects of cyclosporine on the vascular endothelium rarely may include a thrombotic microangiopathy due to direct endothelial toxicity.[3] Cyclosporine hepatotoxicity, which is manifested as transaminase and bilirubin elevations, likely related to inhibition of bile secretion pathways, is another common toxicity.[3]

Cyclosporine overdose has been documented in various settings, both accidental and intentional. A review by Arellano and colleagues[14] describes the experience with cyclosporine overdose in a series of 27 patients with oral (20) or intravenous (7) drug overdose. This, the largest series of reported cyclosporine overdosage, comes from the Drug Monitoring Center at Sandoz Pharmaceuticals. The investigators reported four cases of intentional cyclosporine overdose, and the remaining were accidental as a result of either dosing errors or errors in drug prescription. The degree of dosing ranged from 30 to 400 mg/kg, which is at least twice the highest current recommended dose for immunosuppression. The largest total dose recorded was 10 g. The adult population surveyed had no serious adverse reactions to cyclosporine overdose. The most common signs and symptoms reported included hypertension, tachycardia, nausea and vomiting, and mild drowsiness. Serious symptoms did occur in the pediatric population—oliguric renal failure, metabolic acidosis, and respiratory depression. In one premature neonate who received 178 mg/kg of cyclosporine, death resulted in the setting of metabolic acidosis and oliguric renal failure. One adult patient was reported to have taken a total of 25 g of cyclosporine during an 8-day period and to have experienced gingivitis, gastric discomfort, and burning sensations in the mouth, feet, and face.

Despite measured blood peak concentrations of up to 6700 μ/L, overall the symptoms reported are surprisingly minor. In general, acute toxicity in adults was confined to hepatic enzyme elevation, transient hypertension, and mild changes in renal function (in a minority of patients). Blood levels were noted to be extremely variable in this study because the time of measurement was variable from patient to patient and because the technique used to measure cyclosporine levels varies among laboratories.

These data obtained by Arellano and colleagues[14] provide clear distinction between oral and parenteral overdosing in terms of severity of toxicity, as well as a distinction between the adult and pediatric population (particularly infant and neonate) in terms of degree of morbidity and mortality. Parenteral overdose (including intramuscular) resulted in one death and several cases of oliguria in the pediatric and neonate group. However, it should be noted that in adults, even parenteral overdosage (30 mg/kg) did not result in symptoms more serious than abdominal pain and increased bilirubin levels. The erratic bioavailability of the orally administered drug likely accounts for the wide variations in peak drug levels as well as the general lack of significant symptoms.

The investigators in this Sandoz[14] study point out that cyclosporine overdosing does not appear to be a significant clinical hazard, except for the already vulnerable neonatal population.

Treatment options for oral overdose should be stratified as follows. Adult patients with normal renal function generally require only clinical monitoring and serial evaluations of renal function. Adult patients with impaired renal function may benefit from gastric lavage and induced emesis. It was shown that emesis and lavage were useful up to 6 hours after ingestion. Although reports have described the use of activated charcoal in cyclosporine overdoses,[15, 16] its true efficacy is controversial. Cyclosporine's relatively large molecular weight (1.2 kd), limited oral bioavailability (30% absorption from the intestinal tract), and potentially large volume of distribution (up to 13.8 L/kg)[14] are characteristics that minimize the utility of activated charcoal. The Sandoz group did not recommend routine use of oral charcoal for treatment of oral overdose. However, in 1992, Anderson and Primack[16] reported an accidental cyclosporine overdose (170 mg/kg) in a 4½-year-old renal transplant recipient treated with ipecac and activated charcoal. The researchers pointed out that liquid cyclosporine preparations contain 12.5% alcohol, which contributed to their patient's intoxicated presentation. Rapid elimination of the drug by emesis and activated charcoal was advocated by these investigators. Their patient required only clinical monitoring after emesis and administration of activated charcoal and suffered no toxicity (including absence of laboratory abnormalities) from the drug. Furthermore, it should be noted that at the time of this writing, no experience is reported with oral overdosage of the cyclosporine microemulsion Neoral. Oral bioavailability is significantly improved with this microemulsion,[12] although molecular weight and volume of distribution are not altered. Future experience and studies are needed to address the true value of activated charcoal in the treatment of cyclosporine microemulsion overdose. In 1997, it seems reasonable to recommend induced emesis and, in the absence of contraindication, the possible use of activated charcoal for the treatment of oral cyclosporine overdose.

Treatment options for parenteral overdose are defined by the limited clinical experience with this entity. However, it appears that the neonatal population, premature in particular, is also at greater risk for serious manifestations of cyclosporine toxicity. Total blood exchange has been used in the setting of neonatal cyclosporine overdosage;[14] however, because of tissue compartmental sequestration (hepatic and renal), it does not appear that this would be a particularly effective method for rapid cyclosporine removal. The Sandoz group noted that the only fatality in the series was a premature neonate[14] who developed renal failure and did receive total blood exchange. Because of the limited experience with total blood transfusion and the limitations due to tissue distribution of the drug, total blood exchange does not have an important role in the management of parenteral cyclosporine overdose, even in the neonatal population most at risk for serious complications. The most appropriate course in neonates who develop metabolic acidosis and renal failure is discontinuation of the drug and clinical monitoring with supportive care.

Adult patients with parenteral cyclosporine overdose require little treatment beyond discontinuation of the drug and supportive care.[14] Renal failure and severe metabolic acidosis were not reported in the Sandoz study among this patient population. The use of plasmapheresis in the treatment of parenteral cyclosporine overdose has been reported.[17] However, the utility of plasmapheresis in this setting would seem to be limited, because cyclosporine is more than 50% cellular bound (not available for plasmapheresis) and has a very large volume of distribution.[14] Both these characteristics severely limit the amount of drug removable by plasmapheresis. The Sandoz group stated that this technique could not be recommended for the treatment of cyclosporine overdose.[14]

Blood level monitoring of cyclosporine in the setting of overdose was not shown to be of particular value in the Sandoz series.[14] The only utility of monitoring blood levels arises when the decision to restart the drug must be made. Based on the results of their series, Arellano and colleagues[14] state that no evidence suggests that blood levels are a useful guide to initiate therapy because there is no significant correlation between blood levels and the toxicity of overdose.

Multiple Agent Overdose

In 1993, Zylber-Katz and associates reported on a 60-year-old renal transplant recipient who had taken an overdose of several transplant agents.[18] The patient's clinical course after transplant was complicated by depression and noncompliance. The patient was treated with imipramine and alprazolam for depression, in addition to his immunosuppressive regimen consisting of cyclosporine, azathioprine, and prednisone. The patient was found unconscious 24 hours after ingesting various medications including his immunosuppressives. It was estimated that the patient could have taken as much as 10 g of cyclosporine, 125 mg of prednisone, and 500 mg of azathioprine, in addition to alcohol, benzodiazepines, and tricyclics. The patient was treated with a benzodiazepine antagonist and activated charcoal. No gastric lavage was performed owing to the time elapsed since ingestion. The patient improved with supportive care, and no toxic manifestations due to cyclosporine were observed; the patient's renal function was stable at baseline, and no other laboratory abnormalities were noted. Although blood cyclosporine levels were measured by various methods (CsA-T, CsA-Sp, and TCA), no correlation was found between clinical toxicity (none observed) and peak cyclosporine concentrations. The tricyclic antidepressant cardiotoxicity was managed by conservative means. Unfortunately, after recovering from the multiple-drug overdose, the patient succeeded at committing suicide by jumping from the hospital's eighth floor.

CONCLUSIONS

Although the total experience with the common agents used for transplant immunosuppression (prednisone, azathioprine, and cyclosporine) is relatively small, sufficient clinical experience is available to state that the overall hazard associated with overdose is minimal. Only the neonatal pediatric population appears to be at significant risk for serious toxicity from cyclosporine, and even in these cases it would appear that supportive care alone is indicated. At this time, no benefit is found for attempting to monitor blood cyclosporine levels as a correlate of toxicity. For the currently used agents described in this chapter, the major source of important toxicity is derived from chronic exposure rather than acute overdose. Certainly, time and the introduction of new transplant immunosuppressive agents on a widespread basis may demand a revised approach to the current experience and practice.

References

1. Carpenter CB: Immunosuppression in organ transplantation. N Engl J Med *322:*1224, 1990.
2. Scheinman RI, Cogswell PC, Lofquist AK, Baldwin AS Jr: Role of transcriptional activation of I kappa B alpha in mediation of immunosuppression by glucocorticoids. Science *270:*283, 1995.
3. Danovitch GM: Immunosuppressive medications and protocols for kidney transplantation. *In* Danovitch GM (ed): Handbook of Kidney Transplantation. Boston, Little, Brown & Co., pp 67–103, 1992.
4. Carney DM, Zukoski CF, Ogden DA: Massive azathioprine overdose. Case report and review of the literature. Am J Med *56:*133, 1974.
5. Elion GB: Biochemistry and pharmacology of purine analogues. Fed Proc *26:*918, 1967.
6. Elion GB, Callahan S, Bieber S, et al: A summary of investigations with 6-(1-methyl-4-nitro-5-imidazolyl)-thiopurine (B.W. 57-332). Cancer Chemother Rep *14:*93, 1961.
7. Gross R: Hepatotoxicity of 6-mercaptopurine and azathioprine. Letter; comment. Mayo Clin Proc *69:*498, 1994.
8. Lawson DH, Lovatt GE, Gurton CS, Hennings RC: Adverse effects of azathioprine. Adverse Drug React Acute Poisoning Rev *3:*161, 1984.
9. Kahan BD: Cyclosporine. N Engl J Med *321:*1725, 1989.
10. Bohme M, Jedlitschky G, Leier I, et al: ATP-dependent export pumps and their inhibition by cyclosporins. Adv Enzyme Regul *34:*371, 1994.
11. Charuk JH, Wong PY, Reithmeier RA: Differential interaction of human renal P-glycoprotein with various metabolites and analogues of cyclosporin A. Am J Physiol *269:*F31, 1995.
12. Keown PA: New options in pharmacologic immunosuppression. Lit Scan Transplantation *11:*1, 1995.
13. Rush DN: Cyclosporine toxicity to organs other than the kidney. Clin Biochem *24:*101, 1991.
14. Arellano F, Monka C, Krupp PF: Acute cyclosporin overdose. A review of present clinical experience [published erratum appears in Drug Saf *6:*338, 1991]. Drug Saf *6:*266, 1991.
15. Honcharik N, Anthone S: Activated charcoal in acute cyclosporin overdose. Lancet *1:*1051, 1985.
16. Anderson AB, Primack W: Treatment of a child with acute cyclosporine overdose Letter. Pediatr Nephrol *6:*222, 1992.
17. Kokado Y, Takahara S, Ishibashi M, Sonoda T: An acute overdose of cyclosporine. Transplantation *47:*1096, 1989.
18. Zylber-Katz E, Putterman C, Caraco Y: Multiple drug overdose in a kidney transplant patient. Ther Drug Monit *16:*327, 1994.

SECTION **E**

HEAVY METALS AND INORGANIC AGENTS

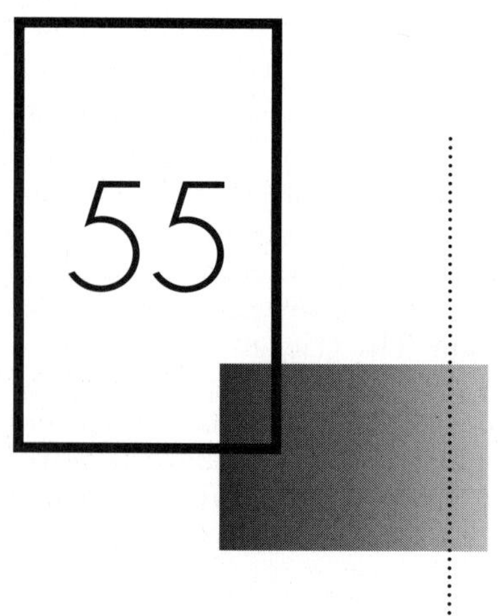

Mercury

BRIAN A. BATES, MD

Mercury, a heavy metal, exists in the environment in three major forms: organic, inorganic, and elemental.[1] As with most toxic heavy metals, human poisonings have been associated with mercury for centuries. In the 1800s, there were many reports in which chronic occupational exposure to elemental mercury fumes caused a dementia-like syndrome among hat felters. This central nervous system toxicity led to the coining of the phrase "mad as a hatter."[1–4] The approved use of mercury-containing medicinals in the form of antisyphilitic agents, diuretics, cathartics, topical salves, teething compounds, and diaper powders has, fortunately, been eliminated in the United States. However, historically, these compounds were responsible for numerous outbreaks of mercurialism. The most widely known outbreaks were in children exposed to products containing calomel (mercurous chloride). In the 1940s and 1950s, it became known that these products caused *acrodynia,* or so-called "pink disease." The manifestations of acrodynia include pain and erythema of the palms and soles, irritability, insomnia, anorexia, diaphoresis, photophobia, and skin rash.[5] Human exposure to methyl mercury, the most common environmental form of organic mercury, has resulted in massive environmental disasters. One such massive exposure occurred in the 1950s in Japan, in which the effluent from an industrial plant contaminated Minamata Bay. The consumption of methyl mercury–contaminated seafood by area residents resulted in more than 1000 deaths.[6] Other mass exposures have been associated with grain contaminated with ethyl and methyl mercury.[7, 8] In addition, almost every year, attempts at the home to extract gold or silver from metals by heating, and the vacuuming of accidentally spilled elemental mercury have resulted in acute inhalation exposure to vaporized elemental mercury.[9–12]

Sources of mercury are numerous. Mercury exists in the earth's crust and is released into the environment by erosion, volcanic eruptions, and the natural degassing of rock. Non-natural means of production include mining, smelting, and the combustion of fossil fuels. Mercury is produced directly by industry through the mining of mercuric sulfide (HgS), or cinnabar, which is the major ore from which mercury is extracted. Independent of the initial source (natural or industrial), mercury undergoes extensive transformation once it is released into the environment.[13] For example, aquatic microorganisms can methylate inorganic mercury, and as a result methyl mercury accumulates in sea animals. Consumption of seafood contaminated with methyl mercury is the major source of nonoccupational mercury exposure in humans. In addition, metallic (elemental) mercury can be oxidized to divalent inorganic mercury under the correct environmental conditions. Conversely, inorganic mercury is often converted back to its elemental form by *in vivo* reduction reactions.[1, 13]

Mercury is used in the production of chloralkali (caustic soda), batteries and measuring devices (thermometers, barometers, and sphygmomanometers), and it is used as a fungicide in the agricultural industry and as an antimildew agent in paint. Although indoor latex paints manufactured after 1990 cannot lawfully contain mercury, those mercury-containing products manufactured prior to August 20, 1990 may still be sold.[14] Mercury also is used in dental amalgams and in various medicinal and antiseptic agents.[13] Table 55–1 lists many sources and uses of mercury.

The occupational and environmental use of mercurial agents is regulated, and guidelines exist to limit exposure to these products. The Environmental Protection Agency includes mercury on its list of hazardous air pollutants and regulates its emission from industrial plants. Also, threshold limit values (TLVs), permissible exposure limits (PELs), and short-term exposure limits (STELs) have been established for various forms of mercury.[13]

PHARMACOLOGY

The chemical symbol for mercury, Hg, is derived from the Greek word *hydrargyros,* meaning "water silver."[13] This description is appropriate because mercury is the only metal that is liquid at room temperature. The three forms of mercury (organic, inorganic, and elemental) have different biologic and toxicologic properties. In general, however, mercury forms covalent bonds to sulfide groups; thus, it interferes with the function of sulfhydryl enzymes, disrupting many important metabolic cellular functions.[15]

Elemental Mercury

Elemental mercury (Hg^{0+}) is liquid at room temperature. Commonly known as *quicksilver* or *hy-*

Table 55–1. Mercury-Containing Products and Other Sources of Mercury

Elemental	Inorganic	Organic
Barometers	Antisyphilitic agents	Antiseptics
Batteries	Acetaldehyde production	Bactericidal agents
Bronzing	Chemical laboratory workers	Embalming agents
Calibration instruments	Cosmetics	Farming industry
Chloralkali production	Disinfectants	Fungicides
Dental amalgams	Explosives	Germicidal agents
Electroplating	Embalming preparations	Insecticidal products
Fingerprinting products	Fur hat processing	Laundry/diaper products
Fluorescent, mercury lamps	Ink manufacturing	Paper manufacturing
Infrared detectors	Mercury vapor lamps	Pathology/histology products
Jewelry industry	Mirror silvering	Seed preservatives
Manometers	Perfume industry	Wood preservatives
Neon lamps	Photography	
Paints	Spermicidal jellies	
Paper pulp production	Tattooing inks	
Photography	Taxidermy products	
Silver and gold production	Vinyl chloride production	
Semiconductor cells	Wood preservatives	
Thermometers		

drargyrum, elemental mercury vaporizes easily at room temperature, and this enables it to be inhaled. Consequently, the lung is the major target organ of toxicity during acute exposure. Elemental mercury is lipid soluble and, once inhaled, easily passes through the alveoli into the bloodstream and red blood cells. Once absorbed, most of the elemental mercury is oxidized to the inorganic divalent or mercuric form (Hg^{2+}) through the action of catalase enzymes. Consequently, after intense inhalation exposures, signs and symptoms of subacute or chronic inorganic mercurialism predominate.[16] Although nonexcreted elemental mercury can accumulate to some degree in the kidney, it does not usually produce renal damage. The mercuric ion is not lipid soluble and does not readily cross the blood-brain barrier; however, a small but potentially significant amount of nonoxidized elemental mercury persists and readily penetrates into the central nervous system, where significant toxicity does occur. Most of the circulating mercuric ion is excreted in feces, urine, and to a small degree, saliva. Elemental mercury is not absorbed well by an intact gastrointestinal tract. As a result, ingested forms of elemental mercury, such as those found in thermometers, are generally nontoxic.[1, 13]

Inorganic Mercury

Historically, inorganic forms of mercury present in topical medicines, cathartic agents, and diuretics were important sources of human poisonings; however, most of these agents have been banned in the United States. Of interest, mercury-containing creams and soaps (used for skin-lightening in dark-skinned individuals), although banned in the United States, continue to be manufactured and distributed in some European countries and have been discovered in areas in which their use is banned.[17] Currently, the occupational inhalation of elemental mercury with *in vivo* conversion to inorganic mercury is probably the most common source of inorganic mercury poisoning.[18] Inorganic mercury exists primarily as a salt of divalent (mercuric) and monovalent (mercurous) forms. The bichloride ($HgCl_2$) form of inorganic mercury, *corrosive sublimate,* is one of the most common of these salts, and as its name suggests, it is directly toxic to the mucosa.[15] This corrosive property constitutes the major initial toxicity associated with acute exposure to inorganic mercury. Unlike elemental mercury, inorganic mercury is absorbed by the gastrointestinal tract (approximately 2% to 15% of the ingested dose) and accumulates in the kidney, causing renal cell damage.[1] Cutaneous absorption of inorganic mercurials also occurs, and chronic exposure to topical inorganic mercurials can lead to significant toxicity.

Once inorganic mercury is absorbed, a small majority remains in the plasma (red blood cell-to-plasma ratio, 1:2.5) and is transported by plasma proteins, accumulating in the kidney. Inorganic mercury is filtered at the glomerulus, undergoing tubular secretion and reabsorption before it is ultimately eliminated.[1, 15] However, because renal excretion is inefficient, the mercury continues to accumulate unless the metal binds to a chelating agent. Although inorganic mercury's lipid solubility is poor, chronic exposure gradually results in accumulation of the mercuric ions in the cerebellar and cerebral cortices of the brain, causing central nervous system disease.[19] Mercuric ions do not readily cross the placenta, and fetotoxicity, if it occurs, is rare.[15]

Organic Mercury

Organic mercurials are used extensively in agriculture as fungicides and seed dressings. Organic mercury exists in three major forms: aryl (phenylmercuric acetate), long-chain, and short-chain alkyl (methyl and ethyl) compounds. Absorption, distribution, and elimination of the two classes differ, as does their mode of toxicity. The aryl and long-chain organic mercurials, once absorbed, are rapidly converted to inorganic forms, and their toxicity is similar to that of inorganic mercury. On the other hand, the alkyl mercurials, methyl and ethyl mercury, are quite stable after absorption, with only a small amount of the parent compound being converted to the mercuric form. Organic methyl mercury is the most widely distributed and toxic form of organic mercury in the environment and is responsible for most of the mass toxic exposures. Short-chain organic mercurials, like methyl and ethyl mercury, are readily absorbed by the gastrointestinal tract (90% to 95%) and rapidly penetrate red blood cells; this results in a large red blood cell–to–plasma ratio. Because of its lipid solubility, alkyl organic mercury is distributed throughout the entire body, accumulating in the brain, kidney, liver, hair, and skin. Organic mercury avidly binds to and inactivates sulfhydryl-group enzymes.[1, 15] Even though the alkyl organic mercurials are widely distributed, their toxic effects are primarily evident in the brain. Methyl mercury also readily passes through the placenta and is of major concern in pregnant women because of its profound fetotoxicity.[6] Methyl mercury is acetylated or conjugated to cysteine or glutathione in the liver and is then excreted in the bile. The *N*-acetyl-homocysteine-methyl mercury metabolite undergoes enterohepatic recirculation and is ultimately excreted in the feces (approximately 90%) and in the urine.[20]

CLINICAL PRESENTATION

The manner in which patients present with mercury poisoning depends on the form of mercury, the duration of exposure, the intensity of the exposure, and certain conditions of the patient. Acute toxicity is usually seen after inhalation exposure to elemental mercury and ingestion of inorganic mercurial compounds. Exposure to organic mercury generally causes signs and symptoms of chronic toxicity.

Elemental Mercury

Exposure to high concentrations of vaporized elemental mercury can cause acute pulmonary symptoms. Initial symptoms consist of fever, chills, shortness of breath, and a metallic taste in the mouth—all signs and symptoms of metal fume fever. Other symptoms include stomatitis, lethargy, confusion, vomiting, and colitis. These clinical findings usually abate within 1 week; however, in some instances, they worsen and progress to pulmonary edema, respiratory failure, and death.[9–11] Young children are particularly susceptible to the acute pulmonary effects of elemental mercury vapor. Following exposure, usually from the melting of metals or vacuuming of elemental mercury in the home, the child may develop severe pulmonary disease, including alveolar dilatation, interstitial emphysema, and pneumatocele, pneumothorax, and pneumomediastinum formation. Small airway obstruction from cellular desquamation may occur, and pulmonary fibrosis, granuloma formation, and respiratory failure often ensue.[10, 11]

Elemental mercury–containing dental amalgams are another potential source of exposure. If appropriate guidelines for use and handling are not followed, dental workers may be exposed to toxic amounts of aerosolized elemental mercury.[21] The effects of vaporized dental amalgam fillings within patients' mouths is a subject of controversy. Although chewing does result in the release of elemental mercury vapor, and urinary mercury levels of patients with mercury fillings is slightly higher than those in people without mercury fillings, to date no scientifically rigorous studies have identified clinical evidence of associated disease.[22]

Ingestion of elemental mercury is usually of no concern because of its poor gastrointestinal absorption. However, if gastrointestinal function or anatomy is abnormal (e.g., in patients with fistulous tracts or decreased gut motility), elemental mercury may be absorbed into the blood stream or may leak into the peritoneal space.[23] The common scenario of a child's swallowing or having a small amount of elemental mercury from a broken thermometer in the rectum is of no concern unless direct trauma from the broken glass is evident.

After intentional intravenous injection (usually in the form of a suicide attempt), elemental mercury can embolize to the lungs, causing signs and symptoms of acute pulmonary embolus, including shortness of breath, dyspnea, chest pain, hypoxemia, and death.[24] In addition, elemental mercury may be transformed to its inorganic form and subsequently lead to renal disease. Accidentally or intentionally injected inorganic mercury may be gradually absorbed, resulting in systemic symptoms unless the mercury is surgically removed.[25]

Intense acute or chronic exposure to elemental mercury fumes causes cutaneous and central nervous system dysfunction. The classic description is a triad of tremor, gingivitis, and erethism. *Erethism* is a constellation of findings that includes insomnia, shyness, memory loss, emotional lability, anorexia, and depression. Oral signs of toxicity include gingivitis, stomatitis, and loose dentition. Additional findings may include headaches, visual disturbances (constricted or tunnel vision), peripheral neuropathy with sensory or motor abnormalities (or both), anosmia, and ataxia.[2, 4, 18] Unless specifically gleaned from a thorough medical and occupational history, chronic mercurialism may be misdiagnosed as Parkinsonism, depression, or Alzheimer's disease. Inhalation exposures have also been diagnosed as pheochromocytoma and toxic shock syndrome.[26, 27]

Inorganic Mercury

The major route of poisoning by inorganic mercury is oral. Acute signs and symptoms of poisoning are related to the direct caustic effects of inorganic mercurial salts. Initial signs and symptoms depend to some degree on the concentration and type of the inorganic mercury salt, with mercuric forms being more toxic than mercurous forms.[28] At high concentrations, symptoms are usually immediate and include pain, vomiting, and hematemesis. Necrosis of any portion of the gastrointestinal tract may occur with subsequent luminal pooling of body fluids, hypovolemia, electrolyte imbalance, acute tubular necrosis, and death. In those who survive the acute phase of toxicity, renal failure may develop. Home accidents involving stool preservatives (mercuric chloride 4.5%) are not uncommon and should be considered in patients presenting with signs of corrosive gastrointestinal injury.[29, 30] The accidental ingestion of disk batteries, many of which contain mercury, is relatively common in pediatric patients. Although these batteries have the potential to break apart and spill inorganic mercury into the gut, complications are usually related to local corrosive injury; systemic absorption of mercury following ingestion of button batteries with subsequent clinical signs of mercurialism is very rare.[31]

Chronic inorganic mercury poisoning typically results from prolonged inhalation exposure to elemental mercury in an occupational setting.[18] Historically, the topical application of inorganic mercurial salves and the chronic ingestion of diuretics or cathartics were common sources of inorganic mercury poisoning, causing renal failure, dementia, and acrodynia. *Acrodynia,* which means "painful extremities" and is also known as "pink disease," presents as erythema and edema of the hands and feet, skin rash, diaphoresis, tachycardia, hypertension, photophobia, irritability, and decreased proximal muscle tone.[32] In addition, subtle neuropsychiatric disturbances have been reported in patients chronically exposed to inorganic mercury.[33] In the 1940s and 1950s, numerous cases of pediatric acrodynia were finally found to be caused by exposure to mercurous chloride.[5] Fortunately, owing to federal regulations limiting or banning many inorganic mercurial compounds, chronic poisoning is now rare outside the occupational setting. However, newer cases continue to be seen and have been associated with exposures to broken mercury-containing light bulbs and spilled elemental mercury.[12, 34, 35] Of importance, acrodynia does not develop in everyone exposed to mercurial compounds; consequently, its presence often is a marker for a more widespread problem. In 1980, three cases of acrodynia led to the discovery of up to 12,000 infants exposed to a phenylmercuric fungicide used by a commercial diaper service.[36]

Organic Mercury

Organic mercury exposure is usually in the form of ingestion of contaminated food products, even though inhalation and dermal exposure may cause toxicity. Poisonings by the long-chain and the aryl organic compounds have similar characteristics of chronic inorganic mercury toxicity. Depending on the amount ingested, symptoms of short-chain alkyl organic mercurial poisoning begin days to weeks after ingestion. This delay occurs primarily because organic mercury targets enzymes, and the depletion of important enzymes must take place before clinical signs develop. The major signs and symptoms of alkyl mercury poisoning are neurologic, consisting of visual field constriction, ataxia, paresthesia, neurasthenia, hearing loss, dysarthria, mental deterioration, muscle tremor, movement disorders, and even death.[15] Dermal exposure to these products may induce burns or cause dermatitis. Ingestion of methyl mercury rarely, if ever, causes gastrointestinal symptoms; however, the ingestion of ethyl mercury can induce vomiting, cramping, and diarrhea. Organic mercurials have been reported to cause thrombocytopenia and agranulocytosis.[1, 6] Symptoms of acute and chronic exposures to organic mercury are similar, with the central nervous system abnormalities predominating. Pathologic and magnetic resonance imaging findings include damage to the cerebral cortex, specifically the visual cortex (calcarine region), the motor and sensory centers (pre- and postcentral cortex), and the auditory center (temporal cortex); and to the cerebellar cortex. Destruction and demyelination of the sensory nerve fibers and dorsal roots of the peripheral nervous system also occur.[37]

Organic mercurials are extremely toxic to the fetus. Although all forms of mercury can cross the placenta, organic mercury passes through most readily. Maternal exposure can lead to spontaneous abortion or severe mental retardation of the child, with global developmental delay, cerebellar ataxia, tremor, nystagmus, dysmetria, limb deformities, and seizure disorders.[6]

DIAGNOSIS

Acute intoxication from exposure to a mercurial compound can usually be diagnosed on the basis of a thorough patient history. However, because inorganic mercury ingestions mimic those of many other caustic or irritant products, identification of ingested compounds should be vigorously sought after suicide attempts by patients who present with signs and symptoms of caustic ingestion. Acute inhalation exposures to elemental mercury may not be discovered unless an environmental history is obtained, particularly if the only symptomatic patient is a child.

The diagnosis of chronic or subacute mercury poisoning may be more difficult. Because the major target organs of toxicity include the central nervous system, the kidneys, and skin and mucous membranes, any patient with an altered mental status and renal failure, with or without cutaneous findings, should be evaluated for mercury intoxication. The constellation of findings of acrodynia should also alert the physician to the possibility of exposure to mercurial compounds. Probably the most important tool in the diagnosis of chronic mercury poisoning is a very thorough occupational and environmental history.

If mercury poisoning is suspected, confirmatory laboratory evaluation is usually necessary, particularly following chronic exposures. Measurement of urine mercury levels is generally considered the best method for determining whether exposure to inorganic or elemental mercury has occurred and whether chelation therapy is effective. Concentrations of mercury in urine greater than 20 to 25 μg/L should be considered elevated. Although no absolute correlation exists between urinary mercury concentrations and symptoms, levels greater than 150 μg/L have been associated with nonspecific symptoms after chronic exposure to mercury vapors; levels greater than 300 μg/L are usually associated with overt symptoms. Urine levels are helpful in confirming exposure to elemental and inorganic mercury. However, because organic mercury is poorly excreted in urine, organic mercurial exposure should not be ruled out on the basis of results of urinary mercury determination.

Blood (not serum) mercury levels in the normal population are usually less than 5 μg/L. Mercury levels in the blood may accurately reflect inorganic mercury exposure if they are obtained soon after exposure. However, because of redistribution to other body tissues, these levels may become less accurate as time from exposure becomes more remote. Following methyl mercury exposure, however, blood levels may remain elevated and are relatively accurate in determining the body's burden of organic mercury.[15]

Mercury accumulates in hair, and levels in hair can be used to document exposure. However, hair is easily contaminated by environmental mercury; therefore, measurement values may be inaccurate following aerosol or other extraneous exposures.

Thus, hair analysis should never be used alone for confirmation of exposure to mercury.[1]

For ingested, intravenous, or subcutaneous exposures to elemental mercury, radiographs should be obtained to document the presence and the efficacy of removal of these compounds, if necessary. X-ray fluorescence techniques have been used for estimating body burdens of mercury. However, these techniques remain experimental and are currently not routinely used.[38]

TREATMENT

Initial treatment of the mercury-poisoned patient is the same as that for any intoxicated patient. Assessment and management of the patient's *a*irway, *b*reathing, and *c*irculation (ABCs) are of primary importance. Initial decontamination should include the removal of contaminated clothing, and copious flushing of contaminated skin and eyes. All patient's with signs of acute mercurialism should undergo continuous cardiac monitoring and pulse oximetry.

Acute inhalation exposure to elemental mercury may cause, as discussed earlier, symptoms of metal fume fever, pneumonitis, and respiratory failure. Humidified supplemental oxygen should be provided; endotracheal intubation may be necessary for those with signs of respiratory failure. There are no known aerosolized antidotes for acute inhalation exposures; therefore, respiratory support is the mainstay of treatment. Infants with severe respiratory compromise after inhalation of elemental mercury have survived with vigorous respiratory support, including the use of high-frequency ventilation when conventional mechanical ventilation has failed.[11] Patients with acute inhalation exposures to mercury may develop systemic poisoning once transformation of elemental mercury to inorganic mercury has occurred; thus, they may require chelation therapy (see later).

Ingestion of caustic inorganic mercury requires rapid assessment and treatment to prevent circulatory collapse. Rapid vascular access should be established, and vigorous replacement of fluid losses should be instituted. Caustic injury to the oropharyngeal mucosa may cause severe local edema, and endotracheal intubation or tracheostomy may be required to prevent obstruction of the airway. Decontamination procedures should be instituted early to prevent further corrosive injury and systemic absorption. The induction of emesis is, as with any caustic ingestion, contraindicated. The role of antiemetics has not been specifically studied, but their use may be of benefit. Gastric lavage is indicated for the ingestion of mercurial compounds unless gastric or esophageal perforation is expected. Anecdotal evidence indicates that lavage with milk or egg whites may help bind mercurial compounds; thus, their use should be considered, especially since there is no evidence that these materials cause harm. If perforation is suspected or radiopaque objects remain present, direct endoscopic removal should be considered. Activated charcoal does not appreciably bind to metallic compounds. However, some evidence indicates that some binding may occur; therefore, it should be administered unless perforation is suspected.[23] Finally, whole-bowel irrigation with polyethylene glycol may be administered until the rectal effluent is clear and the radiopaque material is absent. Extracorporeal methods of mercury removal are not recommended; however, hemodialysis may be necessary if renal failure ensues.

Initial laboratory tests should include serum chemistry assessments and a complete blood count. Type and crossmatch of blood should be performed if exposure to caustic inorganic mercury is suspected. Because elemental mercury is radiopaque, appropriate radiographs should be obtained. Blood and urine should be obtained for appropriate evaluation for the presence of mercury (see diagnosis) and other toxins, as indicated.

Following initial management, chelation therapy should be instituted if systemic absorption is expected, if the patient is symptomatic, or if elevated mercury levels in the blood or urine are discovered. Effective chelating agents include dimercaprol (British antilewisite [BAL]), D-penicillamine (PCN), and 2,3-dimercaptosuccinic acid (DMSA). Each of these agents contains thiol groups, which are thought to compete with mercury for endogenous sulfhydryl groups.[15]

After the acute ingestion of caustic inorganic mercury, chelation is best limited to the use of BAL. BAL is administered intramuscularly at a dose of 2.5–5 mg/kg every 4 to 12 hours. Common side effects of BAL include transient hypertension, tachycardia, pain at the injection site, nausea and vomiting, headache, and diaphoresis. Hemolysis may be induced if the patient is glucose-6-phosphate dehydrogenase–deficient. BAL should not be used for the treatment of alkyl organic mercury poisoning because it may actually worsen neurotoxicity.[39]

If the patient is able to tolerate oral medications, PCN or DMSA may be used instead of or in addition to BAL. PCN forms a complex with mercury that is excreted in the urine. Therefore, it should not be used if the patient has renal failure. It is administered four times a day at 250 mg per dose (20 to 30 mg/kg for children). One- to 2-week courses of PCN therapy are given until the 24-hour urine mercury level is within an acceptable range. Side effects of PCN therapy include gastrointestinal upset, rash, leukopenia, thrombocytopenia, proteinuria, and hematuria. PCN should not be administered if mercury remains present in the gastrointestinal tract because of the potential for increased absorption of mercury.[15, 23]

DMSA is an oral, water-soluble congener of BAL. Its use in mercury-poisoned patients is increasing, and it seems to be more effective than PCN at increasing urinary mercury levels in chronically exposed patients. DMSA has a better side effect profile than do PCN and BAL; its adverse effects are usually limited to mild transient elevations in hepatic transaminase levels and mild gastrointestinal upset.

Table 55–2. Clinical Characteristics of Mercury Exposure

	Elemental	**Inorganic**	**Organic**
Major Route of Exposure	Inhalation	Inhalation (chronic), oral, dermal	Oral
Clinical Effects			
CNS	Tremor	Erethism, tremor	Minamata disease
Pulmonary	+ + +	−	−
GI	+	+ + +	+
Renal	+	+ + +	+
Acrodynia	+	+	−
Treatment	BAL, DMSA	BAL, DMSA	DMSA

BAL, British antilewisite; DMSA, 2,3,-dimercaptosuccinic acid; +, present; −, absent.

DMSA is administered at a dose of 10 mg/kg three times per day for the first 5 days of treatment, and two times per day for the next 14 days. Repeated administrations may be necessary, with a 2-week interval between treatments.[40] Table 55–2 summarizes the clinical effects and treatment for the three forms of mercury poisoning.

References

1. Goyer RA: Toxic effects of metals. *In* Amdur MO, Doull J, Klaassen CD (eds): Casarett and Doull's Toxicology: The Basic Science of Poisons. 4th ed. New York, Pergamon Press, pp 646–650, 1991.
2. Bucknell M, Hunter D, Milton R, Perry KM: Chronic mercury poisoning: 1946 classic article. Br J Ind Med *50*:97, 1993.
3. Hamilton A: Exploring the dangerous trades. J Ind Hyg *4*:219, 1992.
4. Neal PA, Jones RR: Chronic mercurialism in the hatter's fur cutting industry. JAMA *110*:337, 1938.
5. Warkany J, Hubbard DM: Acrodynia and mercury. J Pediatr *42*:365, 1953.
6. Harada M: Minamata disease: Methylmercury poisoning in Japan caused by environmental pollution. Crit Rev Toxicol *25*:1, 1995.
7. Clarkson TW, Amin-Zaki L, Al-Tikriti SK: An outbreak of methylmercury poisoning due to consumption of contaminated grain. Fed Proc *35*:2395, 1976.
8. Bakir F, Damluji SF, Amin-Zaki, L, et al: Methyl mercury poisoning in Iraq. Science *181*:230, 1973.
9. Zelman M, Camfield P, Moss M, et al: Toxicity from vacuumed mercury: A household hazard. Clin Pediatr *30*:121, 1991.
10. Rowens B, Guerrero-Betancourt D, Gottlieb CA, et al: Respiratory failure and death following acute inhalation of mercury vapor. Chest *99*:185, 1991.
11. Moromisato DY, Anas NG, Goodman G: Mercury inhalation poisoning and acute lung in a child: Use of high-frequency oscillatory ventilation. Chest *105*:613, 1994.
12. Schwartz J, Snider T, Montiel MM: Toxicity of a family from vacuumed mercury. Am J Emerg Med *10*:258, 1992.
13. Campbell D, Gonzales M, Sullivan JB: *In* Sullivan JB Jr, Krieger GR (eds): Hazardous Materials Toxicology: Clinical Principles of Environmental Health. Baltimore, Williams & Wilkins, pp 824–833, 1992.
14. Agocs MM, Etzel RA, Parrish RG, et al: Mercury exposure from interior latex paint. N Engl J Med *323*:1096, 1990.
15. Klaassen CD: Heavy metals and heavy-metal antagonists. *In* Gilman AG, Rall TW, Nies AS, Taylor P (eds): Goodman & Gilman's The Pharmacological Basis of Therapeutics. 8th ed. New York, Pergamon Press, pp 1598–1602, 1990.
16. Magos L, Halbach S, Clarkson TW: Role of catalase in the oxidation of mercury vapor. Biochem Pharmacol *27*:1373, 1978.
17. World Health Organization: Environmental Health Criteria 118. Inorganic Mercury—Sources of Human Environmental Exposure. Chapter 3. Geneva, World Health Organization, 1991.
18. Bluhm RE, Bobbitt RG, Welch LW, et al: Elemental mercury vapour toxicity, treatment, and prognosis after acute, intensive exposure in chloralkali plant workers: Part I. History, neuropsychological findings and chelator effects. Hum Exp Toxicol *11*:201, 1992.
19. Williamson AM, Teo RK, Sanderson J: Occupational mercury exposure and its consequences for behaviour. Int Arch Occup Environ Health 50:273, 1982.
20. Graef JW: Mercury. I. Clin Toxicol Rev *2*:(7), 1980.
21. Pohl L, Bergman M: The dentist's exposure to elemental mercury vapor during clinical work with amalgam. Acta Odontol Scand *53*:44, 1995.
22. Eti S, Weisman R, Hoffman R, Reidenberg MM: Slight renal effect of mercury from amalgam fillings. Pharmacol Toxicol *76*:47, 1995.
23. Sue YJ: Mercury. *In* Goldfrank LR, Flomenbaum NE, Lewin NA, et al (eds): Goldfrank's Toxicologic Emergencies. 5th ed. Norwalk, Appleton & Lange, pp 1051–1062, 1994.
24. Anderson WJ: Intravenous mercury: A three-year follow-up. Ulster Med J *62*:180, 1993.
25. Cole JK, Holbrook JL: Focal mercury toxicity: A case report. J Hand Surg *19*:602, 1994.
26. Henningsson C, Hoffmann S, McGonigle L, Winter JSD: Acute mercury poisoning (acrodynia) mimicking pheochromocytoma in an adolescent. J Pediatr *122*:252, 1993.
27. Mohan SB, Tamilarasan A, Buhl M: Inhalational mercury poisoning masquerading as toxic shock syndrome. Anaesth Intensive Care *22*:305, 1994.
28. Gosselin RE, Smith RP, Hodge HC: Mercury. *In* Gosselin RE, Smith RP, Hodge HC (eds): Clinical Toxicology of Commercial Products. 5th ed. Baltimore, Williams & Wilkins, pp 262–275, 1984.
29. Seidel J: Acute mercury poisoning after polyvinyl alcohol preservative ingestion. Pediatrics *66*:132, 1980.
30. Wang RY, Henry GC, Fine J, et al: Mercuric chloride poisonings from stool fixative ingestion. Vet Hum Toxicol *34*:341, 1992.
31. Litovitz T, Schmitz BF: Ingestion of cylindrical and button batteries: An analysis of 2382 cases. Pediatrics *89*:747, 1992.
32. Matherson DS, Clarkson TW, Gelfand EW: Mercury toxicity (acrodynia) induced by long term injection of gammaglobulin. J Pediatr *97*:153, 1980.
33. Andersen A, Ellingsen DG, Morland T, Kjuus H: A neurological and neurophysiological study of chloralkali workers previously exposed to mercury vapour. Acta Neurol Scand *88*:427, 1993.
34. Tunnessen WW, McMahon KJ, Baser M: Acrodynia: Exposure to mercury from fluorescent light bulbs. Pediatrics *79*:786, 1987.
35. Foulds DM, Copeland KC, Franks RC: Mercury poisoning and acrodynia. Am J Dis Child *141*:124, 1987.
36. Clarkson TW: Mercury: An element of mystery. N Engl J Med *323*:1137, 1990.
37. Korogi Y, Takahashi M, Shinzato J, Okajima T: MR findings in seven patients with organic mercury poisoning (Minamata disease). Am J Neuroradiol *15*:1575, 1994.
38. Borjesson J, Barregard L, Sallsten G, et al: *In vivo* XRF analysis of mercury: The relation between concentrations in the kidney and the urine. Phys Med Biol *40*:413, 1995.
39. Howland MA: Antidotes in depth: dimercaprol (BAL). *In* Goldfrank LR, Flomenbaum NE, Lewin NA, et al (eds): Goldfrank's Toxicologic Emergencies. 5th ed. Norwalk, Appleton & Lange, pp 1026–1027, 1994.
40. Graziano JH: Antidotes in depth: 2,3-Dimercaptosuccinic acid (DMSA, Succimer). *In* Goldfrank LR, Flomenbaum NE, Lewin NA, et al (eds): Goldfrank's Toxicologic Emergencies. 5th ed. Norwalk, Appleton & Lange 1045–1047, 1994.

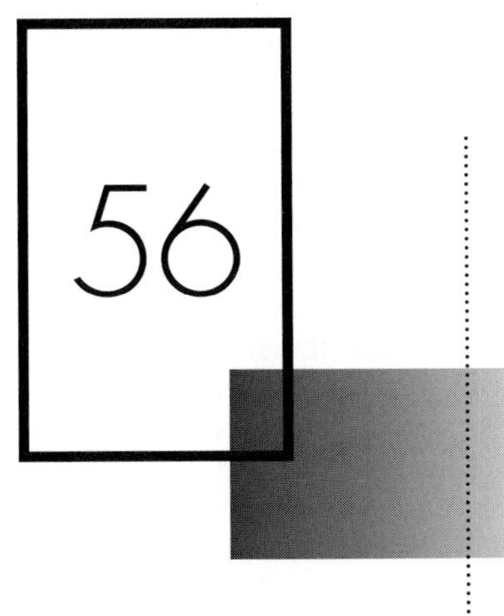

Iron

ERICA L. LIEBELT, MD

Acute iron poisoning continues to be a common and potentially lethal toxicologic problem, especially in the pediatric population. In 1993 and 1994 there were over 40,000 reported exposures to iron-containing products in the United States. These exposures were primarily unintentional ingestions in children younger than 6 years of age, and the majority resulted in either minor or no adverse outcomes. However, iron continues to be a leading cause of unintentional poisoning deaths among children who ingest pharmaceutical preparations. Many factors account for this high incidence of exposures and deaths. First, iron-containing compounds such as multivitamins with iron or iron tablets are readily available and widely used in households as nutritional supplements during childhood and adulthood, particularly during pregnancy. Second, many iron preparations are brightly colored, are sugar coated, and look like candy, making them attractive to curious young children. Finally, parents and the general public do not recognize the potential toxicity of a product that is regarded as healthy. Legislation has been proposed to mandate safer packaging of iron products in an effort to decrease the number of serious exposures. Currently, products containing more than 250 mg of elemental iron per bottle are required to be packaged in child-resistant containers. The Food and Drug Administration (FDA) has proposed that packages of capsules and tablets containing iron be labeled with warnings not to leave the packages open or within reach of children. The FDA has also proposed that any product with 30 mg or more of iron per pill or capsule be packaged in individual doses such as "blister packs."

IRON FORMULATIONS

Three major categories of iron preparations are available, each with varying potential for toxicity based on their content of elemental iron (Table 56–1). Children's chewable multivitamins have a low concentration of elemental iron (10 to 18 mg per tablet packaged in bottles of 60 to 100 tablets) and are rarely associated with serious toxicity. Nonprescription iron products (adult multivitamins with iron and iron supplements) and prescription iron supplements (i.e., prenatal vitamins) contain substantially higher concentrations of iron in the form of ferrous salts. The toxicity of iron results from the amount of elemental iron ingested, which, in turn, depends on the type of iron preparation. Ferrous fumarate contains 33% elemental iron; ferrous sulfate, 20%; and ferrous gluconate, 12%. These iron products are responsible for the moderate and serious toxicity and fatal outcomes that are reported with exposures.

When determining the potential dose of iron ingested, it is important to calculate the amount of *elemental iron* present in the iron preparation by multiplying the milligram amount of the preparation times the percent elemental iron in that preparation. For example, each 325-mg tablet of ferrous sulfate contains 20% (65 mg) elemental iron. Thus, if a 12-kg child ingests fifteen 325-mg ferrous sulfate tablets, the dose ingested is

$$\frac{15 \text{ tablets} \times 65 \text{ mg}}{12 \text{ kg body weight}} = 81 \text{ mg/kg of elemental iron.}$$

PHARMACOKINETICS AND METABOLISM OF IRON

The average healthy adult body contains 3 to 5 g of iron, of which 70% is present in the ferrous state (Fe^{2+}) in hemoglobin and myoglobin and 25% occurs in the ferric state (Fe^{3+}) in the form of ferritin and stored as hemosiderin. The remainder is found attached to transferrin or in heme and flavin en-

Table 56–1. Elemental Iron Content of Common Iron-Containing Products

Product	Total Elemental Iron per Dosage Unit (mg/tablet)
Iron Supplements	
Ferrous Sulfate	
Feosol Capsules (250 mg)	50 mg
Feosol Elixir	44 mg/5 mL
Feosol Tablets (325 mg)	65 mg
Slow Fe Tablets	50 mg
Feo-Grad-500 Tablets (525 mg)	105 mg
Ferrous Fumarate	
Ferancee Chewable Tablets	104 mg
Natalins Rx Tablets	60 mg
Stuartinic Tablets	100 mg
Nephro-Fer Tablets	106.5 mg
Ferrous Gluconate	
Mission Prenatal	39 mg
Ferralet	37 mg
Fergon (320 mg)	36 mg
Adult Multivitamins with Iron	
Centrum Multivitamins	18 mg
Geritol Complete Tablets	18 mg
Theragram Stress Formula High Potency	27 mg
Multivitamins with Iron	
One-A-Day plus Iron	18 mg
Children's Multivitamins with Iron	
Bugs Bunny Plus Iron Chewable Vitamins	15 mg
Centrum Jr. Children's Chewable Vitamins + Iron	18 mg
Flintstones + Iron Children's Chewable Multivitamins	15 mg
Poly-Vi-Sol Vitamins with Iron, Drops	10 mg/1.0 mL
Poly-Vi-Sol Chewable Vitamins with Iron	12 mg
Sesame Street Plus Iron Multivitamins	10 mg

zymes. Dietary iron is absorbed in the ferrous form in the duodenum and upper jejunum. A transferrin-like protein facilitates the energy-dependent carrier-mediated transport across intestinal mucosal cells. This mucosal receptor-dependent process acts as a limiting barrier for normal iron absorption, thus regulating iron balance. Free iron is toxic to many cellular processes; however, the body has many protective mechanisms to prevent this toxicity. Once absorbed, iron is either stored within ferritin or prepared for release to transferrin, an iron-binding protein carrier. The constant sloughing of intestinal cells provides the main mechanism of physiologic iron excretion.

Plasma iron is bound to transferrin in the ferric state with 30% to 40% of the iron-binding sites usually saturated. Transferrin is a protein carrier that transports either dietary or storage iron that is entering the plasma for redistribution and utilization. Total iron-binding capacity (TIBC) is a measurement of the total amount of iron that transferrin can bind and normally exceeds serum iron concentration by twofold to threefold.

The majority of iron is transported to the reticuloendothelial system and hepatocytes, where it is stored within the protein ferritin after ferrous ions are oxidized to the ferric state and complexed with apoferritin. With increasing iron storage, some of the ferritin is transformed into hemosiderin. The small percentage of iron not stored as ferritin is incorporated into iron-containing enzymes or proteins such as hemoglobin and cytochrome enzymes. Humans can eliminate only a small fixed amount of iron per day (1 mg in adult males and 1 to 2 mg in adult females) primarily through exfoliation of gastrointestinal mucosal cells or menstrual blood loss, which can increase up to only 2 mg/d when excess iron accumulation occurs.

CLINICAL TOXICOLOGY

It is evident from the description of normal iron metabolism that the body is poorly equipped to handle excessive amounts of iron. Regulation of iron absorption does not occur in the presence of excessive iron ingestions; rather, iron continues to be absorbed passively down a concentration gradient.[1] Intestinal mucosal injury produced by excess iron disrupts the mucosal barrier, further promoting iron absorption. In acute iron poisoning, iron absorption can occur along the entire length of the small and large intestine rather than just the duodenum and upper jejunum. Furthermore, the normal protective mechanisms (transport and storage proteins) become saturated, resulting in more free circulating iron, the agent responsible for cellular toxicity. Excess free iron catalyzes redox reactions, producing secondary toxicity with lipid peroxidation and free radical formation. Iron has effects on the gastrointestinal and cardiovascular systems as well as on the central nervous system.[2, 3]

Gastrointestinal Tract

Iron has direct corrosive effects on the gastrointestinal mucosa, resulting in ulceration, edema, bleeding, venous thrombosis, infarction, and perforation.[4] Deposition of iron can be demonstrated histologically in mucosal collagen and basement membranes as well as vascular tissues supplying the small intestine. These effects can lead to severe fluid losses both by direct hemorrhage and the "third spacing" of fluids, both contributing to systemic hypovolemia. The severity of these local corrosive effects depends on the quantity of elemental iron ingested, the concentration of iron in the preparation, the duration of its contact with the mucosa, and the amount of mucosal protection provided by food in the stomach at the time of ingestion; greatest mucosal damage occurs on an empty stomach. Gastric scarring may follow severe iron ingestion, resulting in stenosis of the gastric outlet and small bowel.[5]

Cardiovascular System

Multiple cardiovascular manifestations of iron excess are evident on the heart and blood vessels.[3, 6–8] Both free iron and ferritin (whose release is stimulated by free iron) are potent vasodilators that can cause hypotension as a result of venodilation. Iron also directly injures blood vessels, resulting in postarteriolar dilation and decreased venous tone. Capillary membrane permeability increases from direct toxic effects of iron, resulting in diffusion of fluids from the vascular compartment into the interstitium, exacerbating hypovolemia and hypotension. Cardiac output is ultimately decreased as a result of decreased filling pressures from fluid losses, of decreased systemic vascular resistance, and probably from metabolic acidosis and its depression of myocardial contractility. Iron infiltrates myocardial cells and produces fatty degeneration, which can produce a cardiomyopathy.

Liver

Circulating free iron accumulates initially in the Kupffer cells of the reticuloendothelial system and then in the hepatocytes, localizing in the mitochondria, where its toxicity is exerted. The liver is probably the organ most susceptible to injury because it is the first organ to receive portal blood containing toxic amounts of iron; the liver also has the greatest capacity to sequester iron that is not bound to transferrin.[9] Histopathologically, the demonstrated effects of excess iron in the liver include cloudy swelling of the hepatocytes, portal iron deposition, fatty metamorphosis, and massive periportal necrosis.[10] Hepatocellular toxicity is manifested by elevated bilirubin concentrations 3 to 4 days after ingestion, hypoglycemia, hyperammonemia, coagulation defects, and, ultimately, encephalopathy. Acute hepatic failure is rare except in massive iron overdoses.

Hematopoietic System

Several mechanisms are responsible for the coagulation disturbances often noted with iron intoxication. Free iron inhibits the thrombin-induced conversion of fibrinogen to fibrin, resulting in a direct and early effect on coagulation that precedes liver dysfunction.[11] The bleeding from this iron-induced coagulopathy may contribute to the early gastrointestinal blood loss. In addition, experimental iron poisoning has been associated with decreased thrombin production, thrombocytopenia, hypoprothrombinemia, and synthetic disturbances at several stages in the coagulation cascade.[12] In the later stages of iron poisoning, impaired synthesis of clotting factors occurs as a result of hepatotoxicity.

Metabolic Acidosis

The metabolic acidosis of acute iron poisoning can be explained by a number of different mechanisms. Lactic acidosis may result from hypovolemia, hypotension, and anemia, producing tissue hypoperfusion that causes increased anaerobic metabolism. Iron also disrupts oxidative phosphorylation through interference of the electron transport system, promoting anaerobic metabolism.[13, 14] Lipid peroxidation, catalyzed by ferrous ions, alters the membrane permeability of the mitochondria, allowing greater intramitochondrial accumulation of iron. The *in situ* conversion of iron from the ferrous to ferric state releases hydrogen ions that contribute to the metabolic acidosis. Finally, iron directly inhibits enzymatic processes of the Krebs cycle, with the resultant accumulation of organic acids. Thus, metabolic acidosis is multifactorial in etiology and must be aggressively managed from all aspects.

Central Nervous System

Neurologic manifestations from iron toxicity are probably a result of the systemic manifestations of hypoperfusion, metabolic acidosis, hepatic toxicity, and coagulopathy. Iron can produce cerebral edema by an unknown mechanism that manifests itself as lethargy, coma, and seizures.

CLINICAL PRESENTATION

The clinical presentation of acute iron toxicity has traditionally been divided into four stages, which were first described in 1964.[15] Progression of signs and symptoms may occur rapidly depending on the severity of the ingestion; thus, this clinical staging should be determined primarily by the patient's clinical manifestations and not solely by the time since the ingestion.

Stage I (30 Minutes to 6 Hours After Ingestion)

This stage is characterized by the acute gastrointestinal effects of iron toxicity—nausea, abdominal pain, vomiting, and diarrhea. Local corrosive effects of iron to the stomach and intestinal tract may result in hematemesis, hematochezia, and melena. The vomitus and stools may also be dark gray, green, or black owing to the presence of disintegrating iron tablets. Vomiting is the most sensitive indicator of serious ingestions. Most patients with mild to moderate iron toxicity do not progress beyond this stage, with symptoms resolving within 6 to 8 hours. In severe ingestions, cardiovascular toxicity may also appear at this stage as pallor, tachycardia, and hypotension. Central nervous system toxicity may include lethargy and coma. The presence of shock and lethargy on initial presentation are poor prognostic signs. If no gastrointestinal symptoms develop within 6 hours of a presumed iron ingestion, it is unlikely that iron toxicity will develop.

Stage II (6 to 24 Hours After Ingestion)

This second phase of iron poisoning is sometimes referred to as the latent or quiescent period and is characterized by a transient resolution of gastrointestinal symptoms and cardiovascular instability (if adequate fluid resuscitation has been performed in the initial stage). The abatement of symptoms is presumed to occur as circulating free iron is redistributed into the reticuloendothelial system. Some patients may be prematurely discharged from a health care facility despite potentially life-threatening ingestions because of the false reassurance of clinical improvement. This phase may be transient or not appear at all in those with severe iron ingestions.

Stage III (12 to 48 Hours After Ingestion)

Life-threatening systemic symptoms predominate during this stage. Fortunately, only a small percentage of patients with iron ingestions progress to this phase. Some patients with severe ingestions will progress to this phase of multisystem failure without experiencing a quiescent phase. Recurrence of gastrointestinal hemorrhage, hematemesis, melena, and bowel perforation may be seen. Acute circulatory shock characterized by tachycardia, tachypnea, pallor, hypotension, and cyanosis may recur. Metabolic acidosis and coagulopathy are present. However, the hallmark of this phase is progressive pulmonary dysfunction with a radiologic appearance of adult-type respiratory distress syndrome or shock lung. The etiology is multifactorial—iron generation of free radicals that disrupt alveolar membranes in addition to the hypotension and metabolic acidosis. Hepatic, renal, and neurologic dysfunction all may occur during this time. Death from iron toxicity is common in this phase; thus, aggressive supportive treatment in addition to antidotal treatment is mandatory for survival.

Stage IV (4 to 6 Weeks After Ingestion)

Patients with severe poisoning who survive as well as those who do not develop systemic toxicity may go on to have gastric outlet obstruction or pyloric stenosis as a result of gastrointestinal scarring. Vomiting is the presenting symptom of these late sequelae.

Serum iron concentrations less than 300 μg/dL (4 to 6 hours after ingestion) are associated with little to no toxicity, concentrations greater than 500 μg/dL are associated with definite serious toxicity, and concentrations greater than 1000 μg/dL have resulted in death. Iron concentrations between 300 and 500 μg/dL may be associated with mild, moderate, or no toxicity. Such concentrations must be used in conjunction with the patient's history and symptom-complex to assess toxicity and the need for further intervention.

EVALUATION AND DIAGNOSIS

The relative infrequency of deaths associated with the large number of iron exposures suggests that a wide range of clinical toxicity exists in iron poisoning. Evaluation, diagnosis, and subsequent management of the patient requires a knowledge of the pathophysiology and clinical presentation as well as the factors that can guide in predicting the severity of toxicity. Acute iron poisoning is a clinical diagnosis. It is unlikely that a patient who does not have clinical signs and symptoms within 6 hours of reported ingestion will develop iron toxicity. There are many ancillary diagnostic tests that can help to confirm the diagnosis, although none of these should be used independently to determine disposition and treatment. It is important to accurately interpret and understand the limitations of these diagnostic tests in assessing a patient with suspected or known iron poisoning.

History

An important component of the history is the type of iron formulation and amount of elemental iron ingested because the likelihood of iron toxicity can be predicted based on this information. Ingestions of children's multivitamins with iron tablets are rarely associated with significant clinical toxicity and have never been reported to cause death. The content of elemental iron is relatively small (10 to 18 mg/tablet), and thus an enormous number of pills must be ingested for toxicity to occur. On the other hand, pure iron preparations that contain ferrous salts (found in prenatal vitamins and nonprescription iron supplements) contain significantly more elemental iron per tablet. Very few tablets can produce toxicity when accidentally ingested by a small child.

Determining the estimated amount of elemental iron ingested on a milligram per kilogram basis can help predict iron toxicity, thereby directing the triage and management of patients with unintentional ingestions. The reliability of estimating the number of tablets ingested depends on an accurate history, which may not always be possible in every scenario, assuming the worst case scenario in estimating total number of pills available. The minimum toxic dose and the lethal dose of iron are not well established. Ingestions of less than 20 mg/kg of elemental iron have little risk for toxicity and require no specific treatment, although ingestion of 20 mg/kg in an adult human volunteer study resulted in nausea, malaise, and diarrhea in all six subjects.[16] Ingestions of greater than 60 mg/kg can be associated with serious toxicity and require immediate referral to a health care facility for evaluation. Death from iron toxicity has been reported with a wide range of doses—60 to 300 mg/kg. Ingestions of 20 to 60 mg/kg may or may not produce symptoms of serious toxicity and require other historical factors in making a decision regarding triage and referral. In a retrospective study of iron ingestions in children, 28% of 380 children who ingested 40 to 60 mg/kg of iron had symptoms of vomiting, diarrhea, and abdominal pain that resolved.[17] A retrospective review of 199 acute iron exposures revealed that only a small percentage of patients who ingested between 40 and 60 mg/kg of iron developed clinical symptoms (vomiting, diarrhea, abdominal pain) and no one developed serious toxicity.[18] No patient in this study who ingested between 20 and 60 mg/kg of elemental iron had a serum iron level of more than 385 μg/dL, and no one developed serious manifestations. Adult and adolescent overdoses should be considered as intentional and require immediate referral regardless of the dose assessment.

Physical Examination

Careful assessment of vital signs, mental status, and hemodynamic status is imperative and should be performed repeatedly in the first several hours after presentation. Serial abdominal examinations and Hemoccult testing of stool for occult blood should also be included.

Abdominal Radiographs

Because certain iron-containing preparations are radiopaque, an abdominal radiograph can be useful in confirming an iron ingestion and in determining the quantity and location of undissolved iron tablets in the intestinal tract. However, the radiopacity of these tablets depends on the type of formulation and content of elemental iron. Thus, many liquid iron preparations and chewable vitamins with iron (which have low concentrations of iron) are not visible.[19] Also, the usefulness of the radiograph in determining the presence of iron pills may be limited if it is obtained more than 2 hours after the ingestion because the iron preparations may have dissolved and may not appear radiopaque despite their remaining in the gastrointestinal tract. Thus, negative radiographs, especially 2 or more hours after ingestion, do not exclude iron overdose. Serial abdominal radiographs may be useful in determining the efficacy of gastrointestinal decontamination.

Serum Iron Concentration

Serum iron concentrations cannot always be correlated with the severity or the clinical stage of iron intoxication because it is the intracellular iron, not the free circulating iron in the blood, that is responsible for systemic toxicity. The serum iron concentration is useful in confirming an ingestion and may be useful in predicting serious toxicity only if blood samples are drawn at the appropriate time. The most valuable time to assess potential toxicity with an iron concentration is 4 to 6 hours after ingestion, because this time reflects the peak absorption for most preparations with the exception of slow-release iron. A serum iron measured after this time may be "normal" and inappropriately interpreted as "nontoxic" in the presence of a potentially toxic ingestion because of the intracellular distribution of iron. If the time of the ingestion is unknown, serial iron concentrations should be obtained to determine the peak iron concentration.

Iron concentrations are occasionally difficult to obtain on an emergency basis at many health care facilities. Thus, many studies have attempted to identify clinical symptoms and other laboratory data that would predict toxic iron concentrations. Invariably these studies have been limited by their retrospective design and have not resulted in consistent identifiers. In one study, a white blood cell count greater than 15,000/mm^3 or a serum glucose concentration greater than 150 mg/dL had a high positive predictive value identifying the child with an iron concentration of more than 300 μg/dL.[20] Both parameters had very low specificity; thus, their absence did not exclude a high iron concentration. Vomiting was the most sensitive indicator for an iron concentration greater than 300 μg/dL. A subsequent study concluded that neither white blood cell count nor glucose concentration was accurate in identifying significant iron toxicity.[21] In a retrospective study of 92 children with iron poisoning, a serum iron concentration exceeding 500 μg/dL was associated with one single variable—coma.[22] Concurrent coma, radiopacities on abdominal radiographs, leukocytosis, and an elevated anion gap had a positive predictive value of 100%, and the absence of all of the variables had a negative predictive value of 95% for a serum iron concentration over 500 μg/dL. These studies highlight the importance of inability to use a single laboratory test to predict iron toxicity.

A serum iron concentration should be obtained from every patient who has a history of ingesting more than 60 mg/kg elemental iron as well as anyone with significant clinical symptoms or an intentional overdose. Serial iron concentrations may be necessary if the time of ingestion is unknown. Serum iron concentrations may be falsely low in the presence of deferoxamine (DFO) because this chelator interferes with the standard colorimetric and radioimmunoassay methods for iron measurement.[23] When a patient is receiving DFO therapy, iron concentrations should be measured by atomic absorption spectrophotometry.

Total Iron-Binding Capacity

In the past, a serum iron concentration that exceeded the TIBC was considered an indication for chelation therapy and was believed to be a necessary laboratory test in the evaluation of the patient with iron poisoning. This was based on the assumption that the binding of iron to plasma proteins prevents any toxicity—when a serum iron concentration is less than the TIBC, there is little risk for toxicity. However, clinical experience has shown this maxim is untrue. No data have shown that iron toxicity only occurs when the serum iron concentration exceeds the TIBC. Also, TIBC measurements may be unreliable in the presence of excess serum iron or deferoxamine.[24] An *in vitro* study demonstrated that adding iron to pooled serum resulted in an artifactual rise in the TIBC.[25] This same study showed that TIBC determinations varied substantially among different laboratories. Another study demonstrated that even though the TIBC increased and remained above the serum iron concentration in patients with iron ingestions, symptoms of iron toxicity still occurred.[16] Because of the unreliability of the measured TIBC, this measurement is neither a useful nor a clinically indicated laboratory test in the evaluation of iron poisoning.

Other Laboratory Tests

Other laboratory studies that should be obtained in a patient with a significant iron ingestion include an arterial blood gas analysis; complete blood cell count; electrolyte, blood urea nitrogen, creatinine, glucose, and coagulation studies; serum transaminase determinations; and blood sampling for type and crossmatch.

MANAGEMENT

Gastric decontamination, laboratory studies, and an abdominal radiograph are indicated when the amount of elemental iron ingested exceeds 60 mg/kg or an unknown amount of pure iron supplement is ingested. For those unintentional ingestions of between 40 and 60 mg/kg of elemental iron, the reliability of the history, reliability of the caretaker, and presence of clinical symptoms should dictate whether further diagnostic studies are necessary after home decontamination. Unintentional ingestions of less than 20 mg/kg of elemental iron require observation only (Fig. 56–1). Initial management should focus on ensuring an adequate airway, ventilation, and circulation. Hypovolemia should be aggressively managed with isotonic fluid.

Gastrointestinal Decontamination

Of major importance in limiting the severity of iron poisoning is preventing its absorption by removing as much as possible from the gastrointestinal tract. Decisions regarding the optimal method for gastrointestinal decontamination in iron ingestions are complicated by many issues. Many patients have already vomited, reducing the need for further gastric evacuation. This issue is addressed by obtaining an abdominal radiograph. Second, although ipecac-induced emesis may be beneficial in evacuating residual iron pills, vomiting may mimic the early phase of iron poisoning, limiting the usefulness of this sensitive clinical indicator. Third, many adult iron preparations are too large to be removed from the holes in a gastric lavage tube, limiting the value of lavage in this setting. Finally, iron is not adsorbed by charcoal, increasing the overall importance of gastric evacuation efforts.

Syrup of ipecac is indicated for home use in children with unintentional ingestions of 20 to 60 mg/kg of elemental iron unless there are contraindications to its use (e.g., lethargy, concomitant ingestants). These children require close follow-up to identify the development of serious toxicity. Children who ingest 40 to 60 mg/kg should receive ipecac and then be referred to a health care facility for further evaluation. Gastric lavage with a large-bore orogastric tube may be indicated for intentional overdoses of iron and unintentional ingestions of more than 60 mg/kg of iron in those who have not vomited or who have visible pills in the stomach on abdominal radiograph. There are no studies comparing the efficacy of ipecac versus gastric lavage in removing iron preparations; however, it logically follows that their effectiveness is comparable, being greatest if performed immediately after the ingestion. Normal saline is recommended as the lavage fluid. After emesis or lavage, a repeat abdominal radiograph should be obtained to assess the efficacy of gastric evacuation and determine whether further decontamination measures are necessary.

The use of complexing agents in lavage fluid is an interesting historical issue in iron poisoning. Sodium bicarbonate and phosphate solutions have been utilized on the theoretical assumption that insoluble ferrous salts will be formed in the stomach, limiting iron's systemic absorption.[26] However, multiple human and *in vitro* studies have failed to demonstrate benefits from these solutions. Moreover, toxicity from administration of phosphate solutions, hyperphosphatemia, hypocalcemia, and hypernatremia contraindicates their use.[27] Complexing iron in the gastrointestinal tract using oral DFO as a lavage fluid has also been advocated. Although some human and animal studies have suggested benefit from enterally administered DFO, others have shown it does not

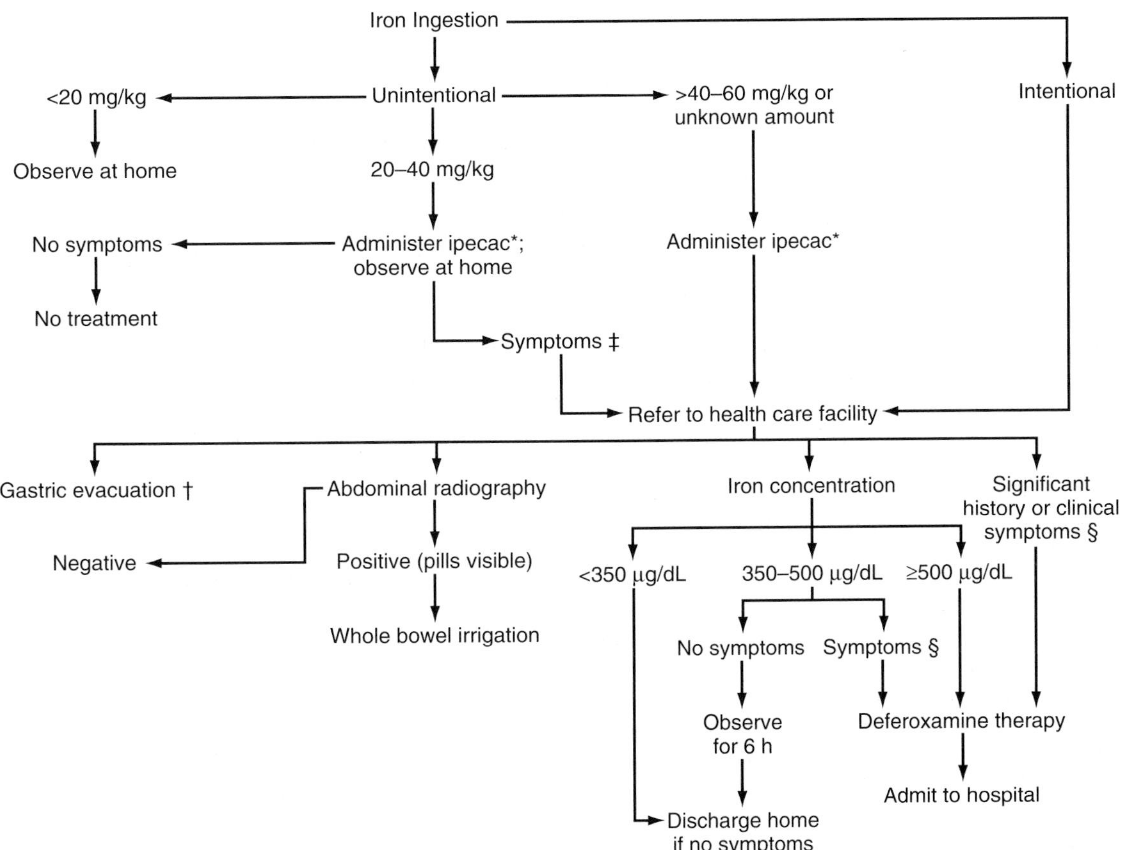

Figure 56–1. Management of the patient with iron ingestion. *, if no spontaneous vomiting; †, see text regarding indications for ipecac or gastric lavage; ‡, persistent vomiting, lethargy, abdominal pain, diarrhea; §, persistent vomiting, lethargy, coma, hypotension, metabolic acidosis.

substantially reduce the amount of iron available for absorption.[13, 28, 29] Furthermore, some investigators have suggested that the iron-DFO complex ferrioxamine can be absorbed and contribute to increases in serum iron concentrations; there is potential toxicity from the ferrioxamine compound as well.[30] From a clinical standpoint, oral DFO is impractical because of the large volumes required in overdose to have any appreciable effect (100 mg of DFO will bind only 8 or 9 mg of iron). Thus, no agent has proven advantage over normal saline; these alternatives are therefore not recommended.

Other measures to decrease the gastrointestinal absorption of iron have been studied. Animal studies have demonstrated a marked reduction of iron absorption after administration of oral magnesium hydroxide preparations such as milk of magnesia, in a dose five times the amount of elemental iron ingested.[31] In addition, this solution may also provide a protective effect against the local corrosive effects of iron in the stomach and intestine. No human studies using magnesium hydroxide have been published. The use of an oral charcoal/DFO mixture has been shown in preliminary experimental studies to effectively decrease the amount of gastrointestinal iron absorption.[32] Further studies are needed with this combination before it can be routinely recommended for gastrointestinal decontamination.

If iron tablets persist in the gastrointestinal tract despite vomiting or gastric lavage and serum iron concentrations continue to rise, whole-bowel irrigation with a polyethylene glycol electrolyte solution such as Colyte or GoLYTELY should be initiated. Whole-bowel irrigation is an effective method of gastrointestinal decontamination, decreasing the passage time of iron through the gastrointestinal tract and thereby reducing the time available for absorption.[33] Given the fact that iron preparations may not be completely removed by emesis or lavage as well as the fact that iron is poorly adsorbed to charcoal, whole-bowel irrigation is theoretically the most effective means of gastrointestinal decontamination. Polyethylene glycol solutions should be administered at a rate of 2 L/h in adolescents and adults, 1 L/h in children, and 500 mL/h in toddlers until the rectal effluent is clear.

Iron tablets may become embedded in the gastric wall, forming bezoars or pseudoconcentrations that are resistant to normal methods of decontamination. In such cases, endoscopy or surgical gastrotomy may be indicated in patients whose iron concentrations are persistently rising.[34] Aggressive decontamination measures in combination with supportive care and appropriate chelation therapy should obviate the need for the surgical removal of iron tablets except in rare circumstances.

Chelation

Deferoxamine is a relatively selective chelator of iron produced by the organism *Streptomyces pilosus* and is the antidote of choice for serious iron poisonings. Guidelines for DFO's use, route of administration, duration of therapy, and dosing are not clear-cut, although general recommendations can be gleaned from clinical experience and several studies (Table 56–2).[29, 30, 35]

DFO combines with iron to form the iron-DFO complex known as ferrioxamine, which is then excreted through the kidneys. Ferrioxamine gives urine the classically described "vin rose" color, which actually is orange to reddish brown. DFO has a volume of distribution of 0.6 L/kg and a half-life of 10 to 30 minutes and is rapidly metabolized in the liver to inactive products. It binds iron in a 1:1 molar ratio with 100 mg of DFO binding 9 mg of iron. Ferrioxamine has a volume of distribution of 0.2 L/kg. DFO binds circulating free iron in the ferric state. DFO also chelates ferric iron from ferritin and hemosiderin. DFO does not bind iron present in hemoglobin, myoglobin, transferrin, or cytochromes. However, there are other mechanisms that are probably responsible for DFO's protective effect; because it has a volume of distribution of 0.6 L/kg (indicating intracellular diffusion), it likely binds both cytosolic and intramitochondrial iron, preventing mitochondrial injury.

Indications for DFO chelation therapy are (1) peak serum iron concentration greater than or equal to 500 μg/dL; (2) significant clinical toxicity (i.e., mental status changes, metabolic acidosis, cardiovascular instability); and (3) patients with history of significant ingestions and abdominal radiographs that demonstrate significant number of pills despite attempts at gastrointestinal decontamination. Patients with peak iron concentrations between 350 and 500 μg/dL must be evaluated for chelation therapy on an individual basis; the presence of significant clinical symptoms mandates treatment.

Table 56–2. Guidelines for Deferoxamine Administration, Dosing, and Termination

Indications for Deferoxamine Chelation Therapy

1. Peak serum iron concentration ≥500 μg/dL
2. Significant clinical symptomatology—lethargy, coma, hypovolemia, metabolic acidosis, coagulopathy
3. Abdominal radiograph demonstrating significant number of pills despite attempts at gastrointestinal decontamination
4. Peak serum iron concentration between 350 and 500 μg/dL *and* the presence of persistent clinical symptoms (persistent vomiting, diarrhea, severe abdominal pain)

*Criteria for Termination of Deferoxamine Therapy**

1. Resolution of clinical signs and symptoms of systemic iron poisoning
2. Serum iron concentration below 150 μg/dL
3. Absence of radiopaque pills (if initially present)
4. Return of normal urine color if vin rose–colored urine present initially

Dosing of Deferoxamine

1. Continuous intravenous infusion starting at 15 mg/kg per h
2. May titrate dose according to severity of clinical symptomatology and development of hypotension (maximum infusion rate 30 mg/kg per h)
3. Ensure adequate intravascular volume

*All four criteria should be present before discontinuing deferoxamine

In the past, a positive DFO challenge test has been proposed as an indication for chelation therapy, particularly in settings where iron concentration levels are not readily obtainable. This test was performed by administering an intramuscular dose of DFO and then observing urine for the vin rose color. The ability to detect this urine color change is subjective, is qualitative, and requires prechelation urine samples for comparison. Several studies had found this urine color change to be an insensitive marker for the presence of significantly elevated serum iron concentrations or serious iron poisoning.[18, 36] Thus, the absence of vin rose urine does not rule out severe iron toxicity. The DFO challenge test is therefore no longer recommended as a guide to determine the need for further chelation therapy.

Although DFO can be administered intravenously, intramuscularly, or subcutaneously, the preferred method for treatment of acute iron intoxication is a continuous intravenous infusion. Because of DFO's short half-life, the benefits of constant exposure to both the free circulating iron and the labile iron pool, this route is more advantageous. Intravenous administration of DFO has also been shown to be more efficient in removing iron than intramuscular administration.

DFO should be administered at a starting rate of 15 mg/kg per hour. There has been considerable debate about the maximum dose of DFO that should be administered. This results from concerns about DFO-induced hypotension and about its possible relationship to the development of adult respiratory distress syndrome.[37] Although the package insert states that the maximum dose should be 6 g/d, there have been numerous cases in which doses up to 35 to 45 mg/kg per hour or 16 to 20 g/d were administered to seriously ill patients without complications.[38] The limiting factor in DFO use is development of hypotension; dosing should be titrated according to patient response and the development of side effects. With severe intoxication, blood pressure support with fluid and vasopressors may be necessary to give high-dose DFO. Dosing of DFO is based on the amount of "free iron"; theoretically then, higher doses should be administered in the first 24 hours. Some investigators have recommended intermittent boluses of DFO or an initial "loading dose" followed by a reduced infusion rate.[39] Adequate hydration before and during DFO therapy is necessary because acute administration of DFO may lower glomerular filtration rate.[40]

Duration of DFO therapy is variable, and published guidelines for discontinuing DFO therapy are vague, occasionally being misleading or unsupported by scientific data. Rational criteria for termination of DFO are (1) resolution of clinical signs and symptoms of systemic iron poisoning; (2) serum iron concentration below 150 μg/dL; (3) disappearance of radiopaque iron pills on repeat abdominal radiographs; and (4) return of normal urine color if vin rose–colored urine was initially present. Some investigators had advocated use of a urine iron-to-creatinine ratio to determine the endpoint of chelation; however, this measurement needs further clinical validation.[41]

Potential adverse effects from DFO administration in acute iron poisoning are hypotension, rash, and *Yersinia enterocolitica* sepsis. Although the mechanism of hypotension is unknown, it may be caused by histamine release and is related to the rate of DFO infusion. The maximum rate of administration before hypotension develops is reported to be 45 mg/kg per hour; human reports have demonstrated infusion rates up to 35 mg/kg per hour without hypotension.[42] *Yersinia entercolitica* sepsis has been reported in patients receiving DFO therapy.[43, 44] DFO acts as a siderophore, supplying iron to the bacteria and thereby increasing its virulence. Any patient presenting with fever, nausea, diarrhea, or pulmonary symptoms during or after DFO therapy needs an assessment of infection, including blood and stool cultures for this pathogen.

Continuous DFO infusion for greater than 24 hours has been associated with the development of adult respiratory distress syndrome.[37] However, the validity of this association remains controversial, because iron poisoning itself has been reported to cause similar pulmonary sequelae. The mechanism of action for this adverse effect is postulated to be production of free radicals in the lungs after prolonged exposure to DFO. However, iron can also generate free radicals that are capable of producing alveolar damage. The possibility of producing the adult respiratory distress syndrome in a patient with serious iron intoxication should not limit the use of DFO. Aggressive supportive therapy, careful monitoring, and appropriate discontinuation of DFO therapy should prevent this complication.

The same guidelines for DFO administration should be applied to the pregnant patient without concern for adverse fetal effects from the DFO. Animal and human studies had demonstrated that neither toxic amounts of iron nor DFO cross the placenta.[45, 46] Fetal death results from maternal death, not from the effects of iron or DFO on the fetus.

A new oral iron chelator, 1,2-dimethyl-3-hydroxypyrid-4-one (L1, deferiprone) is being investigated for treatment in chronically iron-overloaded patients.[47] Its utility in acute iron poisoning remains to be elucidated.

Elimination Enhancement

Extracorporeal methods for enhancing the elimination of iron have been studied, although their potential effectiveness is quite limited because they only remove free circulating iron and must be initiated before significant intracellular transport of iron has occurred. Exchange transfusion is theoretically useful in removing a larger burden of free and bound iron from the blood, although there are no data to support its routine use.[48] Because the volume of distribution of ferrioxamine is low (0.2 L/kg), hemodialysis is effective in removing it should the patient develop renal failure.[49]

However, the role of hemodialysis in enhancing ferrioxamine removal is limited because the ferrioxamine complex is nontoxic. Continuous arteriovenous hemofiltration has been investigated in experimental iron poisoning for removing ferrioxamine.[50] Further investigations with this technique are needed to better determine its utility in the clinical setting. None of these therapies have been shown to decrease morbidity or mortality of iron intoxication.

References

1. Banner W, Tong TG: Iron poisoning. Pediatr Clin North Am *33*:393–409, 1986.
2. Ryan TP, Aust SD: The role of iron in oxygen-mediated toxicities. CRC Crit Rev Toxicol *22*:119–141, 1992.
3. Whitten CF, Brough AJ: The pathophysiology of acute iron poisoning. Clin Toxicol *4*:585–595, 1971.
4. Tenenbein M, Littman C, Stimpson RE: Gastrointestinal pathology in adult iron overdose. J Toxicol Clin Toxicol *28*:311–320, 1990.
5. Ghandi R, Robarts F: Hourglass stricture of the stomach and pyloric stenosis due to ferrous sulfate poisoning. Br J Surg *49*:613–617, 1962.
6. Vernon DD, Banner W, Dean JM: Hemodynamic effects of experimental iron poisoning. Ann Emerg Med *18*:863–866, 1989.
7. Whitten CF, Chen YC, Gibson GW: Studies in acute iron poisoning: III. The hemodynamic alterations in acute experimental iron poisoning. Pediatr Res *2*:479–485, 1968.
8. Jacobs J, Greene H, Gendel BR: Acute iron intoxication. N Engl J Med *273*:1124–1127, 1965.
9. Gleason WA, de Mello DE, deCastro FJ, et al: Acute hepatic failure in severe iron poisoning. J Pediatr *95*:138–140, 1979.
10. Bonkovsky HL: Iron and the liver. Am J Med Sci 301:32–43, 1991.
11. Tenenbein M, Israels SJ: Early coagulopathy in severe iron poisoning. J Pediatr *113*:695–697, 1988.
12. Rosenmund A, Haeberli A, Straub PW: Blood coagulation and acute iron toxicity. J Lab Clin Med *103*:524–533, 1984.
13. Robotham JL, Lietman PS: Acute iron poisoning: A review. Am J Dis Child *134*:875–879, 1980.
14. Proudfoot AT, Simpson D, Dyson EH: Management of acute iron poisoning. Med Toxicol *1*:83–100, 1986.
15. Covey TJ: Ferrous sulfate poisoning: A review, case summaries, and therapeutic regimen. J Pediatr *64*:218–226, 1964.
16. Burkhart KK, Kulig KW, Hammond KB, et al: The rise in the total iron-binding capacity after iron overdose. Ann Emerg Med *20*:532–535, 1991.
17. Oderda GM, Gorman RL, Rose SR, et al: When is referral to the hospital necessary in acute iron ingestion? Abstract. Vet Hum Toxicol *29*:465, 1987.
18. Klein-Schwartz W, Oderda GM, Gorman RL, et al: Assessment of management guidelines: Acute iron ingestion. Clin Pediatr *29*:316–321, 1990.
19. Everson GW, Oukjhane K, Young LW, et al: Effectiveness of abdominal radiographs in visualizing chewable iron supplements following overdose. Am J Emerg Med *7*:459–463, 1989.
20. Lacouture PG, Wason S, Temple AR, et al: Emergency assessment of severity in iron overdose by clinical and laboratory methods. J Pediatr *99*:89–91, 1981.
21. Knasel AL, Collins-Barrow AL: Applicability of early indicators of iron toxicity. J Natl Med Assoc *78*:1037–1040, 1986.

22. Chyka PA, Butler AY: Assessment of acute iron poisoning by laboratory and clinical observations. Am J Emerg Med *11*:99–103, 1993.
23. Helfer RE, Rodgerson DO: The effect of deferoxamine on the determination of serum iron and iron binding capacity. J Pediatr *68*:804–806, 1966.
24. Bentur Y, St. Louis P, Klein J, Koren G: Misinterpretation of iron-binding capacity in the presence of deferoxamine. J Pediatr *118*:139–142, 1991.
25. Tenenbein M, Yatscoff RW: The total iron-binding capacity in iron poisoning: Is it useful? Am J Dis Child *145*:437–439, 1991.
26. Czajka PA, Konrad JD, Duffy JP: Iron poisoning: An *in vitro* comparison of bicarbonate and phosphate lavage solutions. J Pediatr *98*:491–494, 1981.
27. Geffner ME, Opas LM: Phosphate poisoning complicating treatment for iron ingestion. Am J Dis Child *134*:509–510, 1980.
28. Henretig FM, Karl SR, Weintraub WH: Severe iron poisoning treated with enteral and intravenous deferoxamine. Ann Emerg Med *12*:306–309, 1983.
29. McEnery JT, Greengard J: Treatment of acute iron ingestion with deferoxamine in 20 children. J Pediatr *68*:773–779, 1966.
30. Whitten CF, Chen YC, Gibson GW: Studies in acute iron poisoning: II. Further observations on desferrioxamine in the treatment of acute experimental iron poisoning. Pediatrics *38*:102–110, 1966.
31. Corby DG, McCullen AH, Chadwick EW, Decker WJ: Effect of orally administered magnesium hydroxide in experimental iron intoxication. J Toxicol Clin Toxicol *23*:489–499, 1985–1986.
32. Gomez HF, McClafferty H, Flory D, et al: Prevention of GI iron absorption by an orally administered deferoxamine/charcoal mixture. Abstract. J Toxicol Clin Toxicol *33*:556, 1995.
33. Tenenbein M: Whole bowel irrigation in iron poisoning. J Pediatr *111*:142–145, 1987.
34. Foxford R, Goldfrank L: Gastrotomy—A surgical approach to iron overdose. Ann Emerg Med *14*:1223–1226, 1985.
35. Whitten CF, Gibson GW, Good MH, et al: Studies in acute iron poisoning: I. Desferrioxamine in the treatment of acute iron poisoning: Clinical observations, experimental studies and theoretical considerations. Pediatrics *36*:322–335, 1965.
36. Villalobos D: Reliability of urine color changes after deferoxamine challenge. Abstract. Vet Hum Toxicol *34*:330, 1992.
37. Tenenbein M, Kowalski S, Sienko A, et al: Pulmonary toxic effects of continuous desferrioxamine administration in acute iron poisoning. Lancet *339*:699–701, 1992.
38. Shannon M: Desferrioxamine in acute iron poisoning. Lancet *339*:1601, 1992.
39. Cheney K, Gumbiner C, Benson B, Tenenbein M: Survival after a severe iron poisoning treated with intermittent infusions of deferoxamine. Clin Toxicol *33*:61–66, 1995.
40. Koren G, Bentur Y, Strong D, et al: Acute changes in renal function associated with deferoxamine therapy. Am J Dis Child *143*:1077–1080, 1989.
41. Yatscoff RW, Wayne EA, Tenenbein M: An objective criterion for the cessation of deferoxamine therapy in the acutely iron poisoned patient. Clin Toxicol *29*:1–10, 1991.
42. Bentur Y, McGuigan M, Koren G: Deferoxamine: New toxicities for an old drug. Drug Saf *6*:37–46, 1991.
43. Melby K, Slorhahl S, Gutteberg TJ, Mordbo SA: Septicemia due to *Yersinia enterocolitica* oral doses of iron. BMJ *285*:487–488, 1982.
44. Mofenson HC, Caraccio TR, Sharieff N: Iron sepsis: *Yersinia enterocolitica* septicemia possibly caused by an overdose of iron. N Engl J Med *316*:1092–1093, 1987.
45. Curry SC, Bond GR, Raschke R, et al: An ovine model of maternal iron poisoning in pregnancy. Ann Emerg Med *19*:632–638, 1990.
46. McElhatton PR, Roberts JC, Sullivan FM: The consequences of iron overdose and its treatment with desferrioxamine in pregnancy. Hum Exp Toxicol *10*:251–259, 1991.
47. Kontoghiorghes GJ: New concepts of iron and aluminum chelation therapy with oral L1 (deferiprone) and other chelators: A review. Analyst *120*:845–851, 1995.
48. Movassaghi N, Purugganan GG, Leikin S: Comparison of exchange transfusion and deferoxamine in the treatment of acute iron poisoning. J Pediatr *75*:604–608, 1969.
49. Richardson JR, Sugerman DL, Hulet WH: Extraction of iron by chelation with desferrioxamine and hemodialysis. Clin Res *15*:368, 1967.
50. Banner W, Vernon DD, Ward RM, et al: Continuous arteriovenous hemofiltration in experimental iron intoxication. Crit Care Med *17*:1187–1190, 1989.

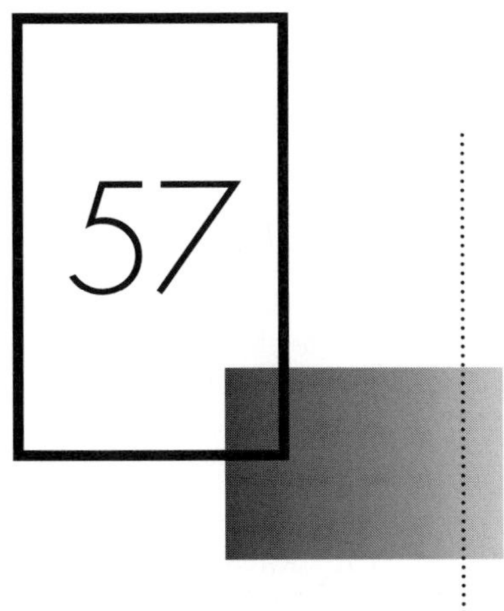

Lead

MICHAEL W. SHANNON, MD, MPH

Lead was previously considered one of the most valuable elements on earth. Because it has a number of highly desirable properties (low melting point, malleability, durability, low cost, ability to augment octane number in gasoline), lead has become ubiquitous in both urban and rural areas. Both industrial and developing nations have found beneficial uses for lead. However, lead is also a potent toxin. In the past century, an explosion of scientific data has demonstrated the toxic effects of lead on the human body. This has been highlighted by the growing body of evidence that even small amounts of lead can have long-standing or permanent sequelae, particularly in young children. Lead poisoning (plumbism) is now considered the most common disease of environmental origin.[1]

This chapter reviews the toxicology of lead poisoning. Because of unique differences in the epidemiology, clinical toxicity, and treatment strategies of lead poisoning in adults versus children, the chapter is later subdivided into lead poisoning among adults and then among children.

HISTORY

Lead has been mined for thousands of years; the earliest recorded lead mine reportedly existed in Turkey in 6500 BC.[2, 3] Evidence of high lead use can be found in the skeletons of ancient Egyptians (reflecting the increased use of lead over time, contemporary skeletons have bone lead concentrations 500 times higher than skeletons from ancient societies).[2, 4] By the Greek Bronze Age, lead was widely used in the manufacture of brass and cosmetics. Also, because lead geologically coexisted with silver, the mining of silver resulted in a marked increase in lead exposure. It is estimated that as long as 2200 years ago, 25,000 tons of lead were produced annually.[2]

The fall of the Roman empire is thought to have resulted from lead intoxication.[3–5] During this era, lead-induced gout was endemic. Romans used lead in their plumbing (the word *plumbing* is derived from the traditional use of lead in water conduits), in their cooking utensils, and in the vessels that concentrated grape juice for wine. Lead was popular in wine because it enhanced the color, wetness, and bouquet. The lead content of wine in the Roman era may have been as high as 15 to 30 mg/L. In fact, well into the 20th century, wines contained added lead. Lead poisoning was described at the same time that the metal became popular. Hippocrates wrote descriptions of lead colic. Similar descriptions have been recorded throughout history by Benjamin Franklin and others.

Large-scale interest in lead poisoning has been attributed to an 1839 publication by Tanquerel des Plances in which he described the clinical course of workers, primarily painters, who developed lead colic.[4] In 1860, corresponding with the industrialization of Europe, epidemiologists described widespread reproductive toxicity in those with lead-related occupations as well as their spouses. These occurrences, which were also being identified in the United States, led in the 20th century to regulations that protected workers from occupational exposure to lead. At an extreme, laws were passed to exclude women from lead-related occupations; the United States Supreme Court has reversed these laws.[4]

The increasing desire to reduce exposure to lead also resulted in legislation to protect not only workers but the public at large from the hazards of lead exposure. Establishment of the Environmental Protection Agency (EPA) and passage of important laws including the Clean Air Act, the Clean Water Act, the Lead Poisoning Prevention Act, and the Housing and Community Development Act (Title X) all have served to dramatically reduce nonoccupational exposure to lead.

EPIDEMIOLOGY

Population Rates

The blood lead level of Americans has been monitored through the periodic conductance of the National Health and Nutrition Examination Survey (NHANES). The results of the most recent study, NHANES III, has revealed that mean blood lead level has declined 80% since the performance of NHANES II (1976 to 1980), from 12.8 μg/dL to a current level of approximately 3 μg/dL.[6,7] Age-specific analyses show that higher levels are found in young children (who have a mean lead level of 4 to 5 μg/dL). In males, however, blood lead levels begin to rise in adolescence, continuing through most of adulthood, reflecting occupational exposure. In both elderly men and women, blood lead levels rise again, representing remobilization of lead that accompanies bone resorption.

No particular blood lead level has clearly defined lead poisoning in adults. In the past, the "reference" or normal range for blood lead in adults was 60 μg/dL. The reference range of lead levels is currently considered to be less than 40 μg/dL. However, many clinicians continue to believe that lead poisoning in adults is defined only by the presence of clinical symptoms, not by any particular blood lead level. The increasing evidence of subclinical effects at low blood levels in adults argues for defining lead intoxication as a blood lead level of greater than 25 μg/dL.

Sources

Lead is ubiquitous and can be found throughout the environment. Exposure to lead therefore usually occurs from a number of sources (Fig. 57–1). Many of these sources are highly age dependent. For example, most (but not all) lead-based occupations expose adults but not children to excess lead. Although lead exposure can occur after a single event—for example, after ingestion of a lead-containing object—it is usually chronic.

Occupational

In adults, the most significant exposures to lead usually occur in the workplace. The list of occupations associated with lead exposure is large (Table 57–1). Occupation-specific tasks including demolition, radiator repair, home remodeling, burning, blasting, firearm instruction (indoor and outdoor), grinding, and sanding all can result in frank lead poisoning.[8–10]

Occupational lead standards were introduced by the Occupational Safety and Health Administration (OSHA) in 1978.[11] Under these guidelines, the permissible exposure limit for lead is 50 μg/m³ for an 8-hour time-weighted average. Employers are responsible for maintaining proper working conditions as well as for environmental and medical monitoring.[11] Workers with blood lead levels of 60 μg/dL or greater must be removed from the workplace; those with blood lead levels of 50 μg/dL or greater on three occasions at 1-month intervals in the prior 3 months must also be removed from work. Those with blood lead levels of 40 μg/dL or greater must undergo medical evaluation.[9] Employers are responsible for paying the salaries of employees who are removed from work for lead-related reasons.[11] Because of the reproduc-

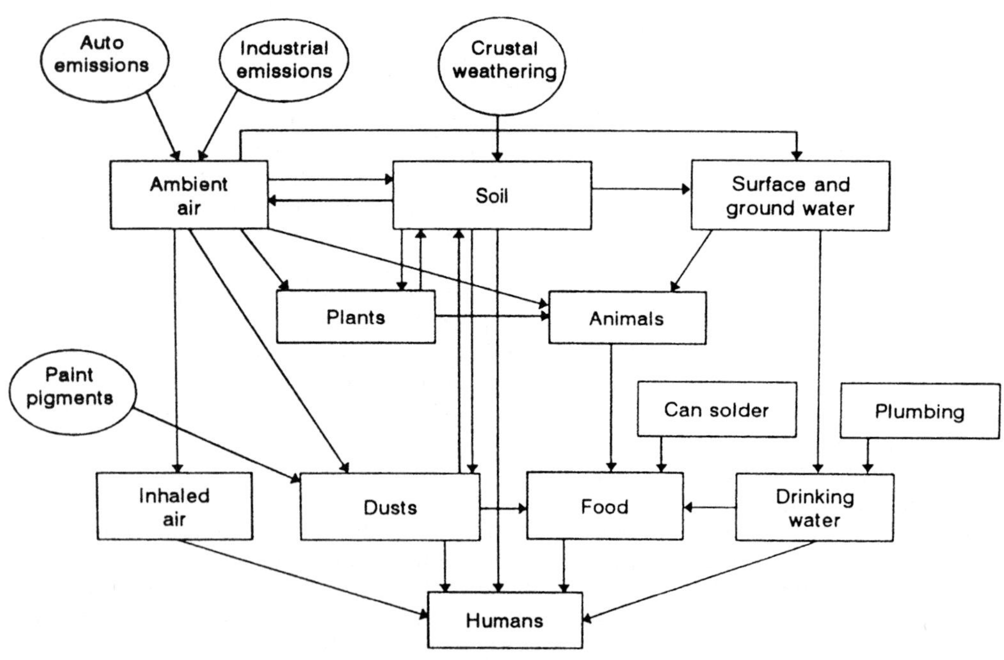

Figure 57–1. Sources and pathways of lead from environment to humans. (From US Environmental Protection Agency: Air Quality Criteria for Lead. EPA-600/08-83/028aF-dF. Research Triangle Park, NC, EPA, 1986.)

Table 57–1. Sites and Industries with Lead Exposure

Lead smelters
Battery manufacturing
Welding and cutting operations
Construction and demolition
Rubber industry
Plastics industry
Printing industry
Firing ranges
Radiator repair
Soldering of lead products
Production of gasoline additives
Zinc smelting
Solid waste combustion
Organic lead production
Copper smelting
Ore crushing and grinding
Frit manufacture
Paint and pigment manufacture

From Kough JP: Lead. *In* Sullivan JB, Krieger GR (eds): Hazardous Materials Toxicology. Baltimore, Williams & Wilkins, pp 834–844, 1992.

tive effects of lead at lower lead levels, recommendations have been made that the permissible blood lead level in workers be reduced to 10 μg/dL.[1]

Lead Paint

Lead has been added to paint for centuries in order to make pigments more vivid, colors more stable, and the paint more durable. For the years that these beneficial properties were exploited, the addition of lead was an industry standard. It is because of its durability under adverse weather conditions that lead-based paint became most popular in the northeastern United States. Interestingly, in Canada, which has even harsher climatic conditions, lead was banned from residential paint early in the 20th century. In the United States, however, lead was added to paint until 1978, when, in an effort to reduce lead exposure, particularly among young children, lead was effectively banned (restricted to a concentration of no more than 0.06%) from use in residential paint. Lead-containing paint is still used in nonresidential settings.[9] As a result of its extensive application, lead paint can be found in more than 50% of American homes and more than 70% of New England homes.

The presence of lead-based paint in homes has led to several problems. First, the natural decay of paint results in both chipping and the creation of lead dust. Also, when lead-containing homes undergo renovation of any type (e.g., scraping, demolition, window or wall removal), lead is released into the environment.[12] Certain types of renovation, particularly paint removal with a heat gun, are extremely hazardous, resulting in the creation of highly toxic lead fumes.[13] Even when homes are undergoing deleading in an effort to reduce lead hazards, improper techniques can result in lead poisoning in all family members.[14] The EPA has established guidelines for safe levels of lead in household dust as follows: maximum lead concentration in uncarpeted floors—100 μg/ft^2, interior window wells—500 μg/ft^2, and window wells—800 μg/ft^2.

Air

Industrial and automobile emissions are historically a major source of lead exposure. Leaded gasoline has released more than 30 million tons of lead into the air.[15] The extent of airborne lead's contribution to lead levels is reflected by the impact of lead's removal from gasoline; when the phaseout began in the 1970s, the mean blood lead of all Americans promptly declined by 35%. The phaseout of leaded gasoline was completed in December 1995. In areas with high concentrations of atmospheric lead, blood lead levels are higher among runners than nonrunners.[16]

Water

Water has become an increasingly important source of lead exposure, especially as the contributions of paint, dust, food, and air diminish. Lead has contaminated bodies of water as it has settled from the atmosphere. The increasing acidity of fresh water, due to acid rain, increases the solubility of waterborne lead. Soft water presents more of a lead hazard than hard water.[17]

Regulation of lead in public water supplies is the responsibility of the EPA. In a 1991 revision of the Clean Water Act, the maximum contaminant level of lead in water, which had been 50 parts per billion (ppb, μg/L), was replaced by an action level of 15 ppb. Under these new regulations, water suppliers must implement measures to reduce the level of lead in water if a significant number of homes are found to have elevated levels of lead.

Plumbing is an important cause of lead contamination in residential water. When public plumbing systems became widespread in the early 20th century, lead pipes served as the primary conduits that directed water from public water sources into the home. In the 1950s, the use of lead pipes declined considerably. However, old public water systems continue to have extensive networks of lead pipe plumbing. Lead pipes have been largely replaced by copper or polyvinylchloride (PVC) pipes.

Unfortunately, the use of lead-based solder for fusing the copper pipe joints was permitted until 1986. Therefore, homes with copper plumbing are assumed to have lead in their water. Because of the continued presence of lead pipes and copper pipes with lead solder joints, many cities in the United States have a high prevalence of lead-contaminated water.

Bottled water, which is under the regulation and oversight of the Food and Drug Administration, must have a lead content of no more than 5 ppb.

Soil

Lead in soil can result either from its natural occurrence or contamination. The latter is responsible for most soil contamination in the United States. For example, studies of soil surrounding lead-emitting industries (e.g., smelters) have revealed soil lead concentrations higher than 60,000 parts per million (ppm, mg/L). In homes, lead contamination of soil occurs as exterior surfaces deteriorate.

Lead in soil results in human exposure through a number of mechanisms. In adults, the most important of these is contamination of home-grown vegetables. Vegetables easily develop surface contamination; less commonly, lead can be incorporated into the flesh of the vegetable. The EPA, in conjunction with the United States Department of Housing and Urban Development, has sought to reduce human exposure to lead through the development of guidelines on safe levels in soil. Under these new standards, a safe concentration of lead in soil is considered to be less than 400 ppm. Soil that contains 400 to 5000 ppm is believed to represent a moderate exposure risk; ground cover (shrubs, grass, or mulch) is recommended. Residential homes that contain soil with lead concentrations greater than 5000 ppm should be fully abated, either through removal of contaminated soil or provision of permanent barriers (e.g., cement paving).

Hobbies

Certain household hobbies can result in lead exposure. These include any work that involves the use of solder (which, when volatilized, produces highly absorbable lead fumes), the manufacture of fishing weights, and various aspects of artisanship. In the latter category, ceramic glazes occasionally contain lead. Although the use of lead glaze has been markedly reduced, it still occurs. Acute lead intoxication has been reported to result from inadvertent ingestion of ceramic glaze among the elderly.[18, 19]

Folk/Alternative Medicines

As discussed in Chapter 97, lead is sometimes found in alternative medicines including Ayurvedic and folk remedies.[20–23] Dolomite, clamshell powder, and other calcium supplements may contain lead, particularly if their source is pulverized bone.[22, 24–26]

Food

Like air, food has been considered an important source of chronic lead exposure. Lead enters the food chain through various avenues. Vegetables, particularly home-grown vegetables that are grown in lead-contaminated soil, can introduce lead into the diet. Storage cans ("tin cans") were previously manufactured with a lead-solder seam.[7] This seam, coming into direct contact with food, could readily release lead, particularly into acidic foods. In some studies the solder seam raised the lead content of food as much as 4000-fold. The use of lead solder for the seam was banned in November 1991.[7] However, its widespread use has left many lead-containing cans still available.[7] Also, cans brought from other areas of the world are likely to contain lead.

Kitchenware can also be a source of lead. Previous reports have identified frank lead poisoning from the use of lead-containing vessels. These include samovars (Asian urns), plates, bowls, cups, pots, and containers made of pewter.[27] Although lead in crystal should not be a source of leachable lead, wine stored in crystal decanters has been reported to have elevated concentrations of lead.[28]

Other

Lead exposure can result from substance abuse. First, the age-old practice of "moonshining"—that is, making illicit ethanol—has long been associated with lead poisoning as a result of using lead-containing vessels such as discarded automobile radiators. Lead poisoning can be caused by sniffing gasoline if leaded gasoline is used (gasoline sniffing is one of the few causes of organic lead exposure). Finally, the synthesis of methamphetamine involves lead acetate. Sporadic reports have described lead intoxication from the injection of lead-contaminated methamphetamine.

Although uncommon, particularly in adults, ingestion of lead-containing foreign bodies can result in significant exposure to lead.

Lead absorption from retained bullets can occur in those with gunshot wounds.[29] However, the kinetics of lead absorption from soft tissue have not been well characterized. For example, in animal models, lead appears to be poorly absorbed from muscle and fat; absorption from pleura and synovial fluid is most efficient.[30] Data from armed conflicts since the Civil War have documented lead absorption.[30] This documentation is complicated by the possibility of mobilization of lead from bone due to complete bed rest with resulting bone resorption.

TOXICOKINETICS

Lead is variably absorbed after ingestion. Its absorption is active, mediated by the same mucosal transport proteins that mediate calcium transport.[31] However, absorption is dependent on several factors including the form of lead, particle size, gastrointestinal (GI) transit time, nutritional status, and chronologic age. Lead absorption is inversely proportional to size; the smaller the particle, the more complete the absorption. This is why exposure to lead dust results in higher lead concentrations than ingestion of an equal amount of lead from a paint chip.

Nutritional status is being increasingly shown to influence the extent of lead absorption. For example, iron deficiency results in increased lead absorption, probably because these atoms use the same transport system, with lead substituting for iron.[31] The prevalence of lead intoxication in childhood results, in part, from the relatively high incidence of iron deficiency in this population. Similarly, calcium deficiency is associated with increased lead absorption. High intake of fat and inadequate intake of calories have also been associated with enhanced lead absorption. Lead absorption is increased when the stomach is empty; small frequent meals reduce absorption, probably through lead binding by dietary phytates and other complexing agents.[31] Finally, lead absorption is inversely proportional to chronologic age. As a general rule, 30% to 50% of ingested lead is absorbed from the gut of a child versus no more than 10% in an adult.[9, 31] This may be related to a higher density of intestinal transport proteins during periods of rapid growth.[31] Lead is also readily absorbed after inhalation of dust or fumes. Generally speaking, lead particles must be less than 0.5 μm to be absorbed from the respiratory tract.[32] Although inorganic lead is not absorbed through intact skin, organic lead compounds are.[9]

After absorption, lead is circulated in blood, having a half-life of approximately 30 days in adults.[33] However, half-life is related to the duration of exposure. Those with short-term exposure experience more rapid disappearance of lead from blood than those with long-term exposure.[34] In the blood, 95% of lead is attached to the erythrocyte; thus, it is *blood lead* and not serum lead levels that are measured. The volume of distribution of lead is unclear but is presumed to be large; only 1% to 5% of the body's lead burden is in the circulation.[1] Lead readily crosses the placenta; fetal blood lead levels are 80% to 100% of maternal values.[9, 35–37]

The distribution kinetics of lead follow a three-compartment model. From blood, lead diffuses into soft tissues (which include the liver, kidneys, bone marrow, and brain). This compartment is the primary site of lead's cellular toxicity. After a period that corresponds to a half-life of 1 to 2 months, lead diffuses from these tissues into bone. In bone, lead is incorporated into the hydroxyapatite lattice.[9] Lead is similarly incorporated into teeth. Once it is a part of bone, lead is presumed to be inert and nontoxic; however, this issue has been revisited as it becomes clear that conditions associated with bone mobilization (e.g., zero gravity, complete bed rest, medications, advancing years, and thyrotoxicosis) can also result in mobilization of lead.[38] Several researchers have described recurrent lead intoxication in children with a prior history of lead intoxication when they suffer conditions producing bone mobilization.[39, 40] Concerns have been expressed that pregnancy, another state of bone resorption, can result in increased lead mobilization with the potential for fetal exposure to excess lead.[41, 42]

Because of lead's incorporation into bone, the majority of lead is retained in the body with very little elimination (in the absence of chelation); only about 30 μg/d is excreted by the kidneys.[9] Therefore, declining blood lead levels in those with lead poisoning not undergoing chelation represent only lead's distribution into soft tissues. In occupational monitoring, urinary lead excretion of less than 50 μg/g of creatinine is within normal limits. Lead's overall half-life is approximately 10,000 days (20 to 30 years).[1, 3, 43]

MECHANISMS OF TOXICITY

The cellular mechanisms of lead's toxicity are multiple and involve many different physiologic actions. Lead is particularly toxic to enzyme systems, particularly zinc-dependent enzymes. The blood lead levels at which adverse health effects occur are variable (Table 59–2).

Organs most sensitive to lead's toxicity are the

Table 57–2. Significant Health Effects of Lead at Lowest Observed Blood Lead (PbB) Levels in Adults

Lowest Observed Effect PbB (μg/dL)	Heme Synthesis and Hematologic Effects	Neurologic Effects	Effects on the Kidneys	Reproductive Function Effects	Cardiovascular Effects
100–120		Encephalopathic signs and symptoms	Chronic nephropathy		
80	Frank anemia				
60		— ↑		Female reproductive effects	
50	Reduced hemoglobin production	Overt subencephalopathic neurologic symptoms ↓		Altered testicular function	
40	Increased urinary ALA and elevated coproporphyrins	Peripheral nerve dysfunction (slowed nerve conduction) ↓	↓ —	↓ —	
30		—			Elevated blood pressure (white males, age 40–59)
25–30	Erythrocyte protoporphyrin elevation in males				
15–20	Erythrocyte protoporphyrin elevation in females				↓ ?
<10	ALA-D inhibition				

ALA, aminolevulinic acid.
Adapted from U.S. Environmental Protection Agency. Air Quality Criteria of Lead. Washington, DC, 1986, vol 1, p 143.

kidneys, hematopoietic system, and nervous system. In the kidneys, lead interferes with the heme-containing hydroxylase enzyme, which converts 25-vitamin D to 1,25-vitamin D, an effect that is reversible.[9, 44] Additionally, a toxic action affects the renal tubules, producing a tubulopathy characterized by selective proteinuria. At blood levels as low as 40 μg/dL, lead produces dense intranuclear inclusion bodies in renal tubules.[1] More advanced stages of lead nephropathy are associated with interstitial fibrosis, as well as tubular atrophy with relative sparing of the glomeruli.[1]

Lead has a high affinity for sulfydryl groups, particularly those of metalloenzymes. Such enzymes include those in the heme synthetic pathway, particularly δ-aminolevulinic acid dehydratase, coproporphyrinogen oxidase, and ferrochelatase.[34] δ-Aminolevulinic acid dehydratase activity is inhibited at blood lead levels as low as 5 μg/dL.[34, 45] This results in accumulation of δ-aminolevulinic acid, a putative neurotoxin.[37, 46] Inhibition of ferrochelatase, which is responsible for incorporating iron into the porphyrin core, leads to elevated levels of erythrocyte protoporphyrin (EP).

Lead also affects neurotransmitter production.[42] This may be related to its ability to inhibit calmodulin, pyruvate kinase, and other enzymes essential to neuronal function. Many of lead's neurotoxic effects appear to result from its inhibition of cellular functions requiring zinc and calcium (which are also divalent cations).[46, 47] Lead interferes with normal calcium metabolism, causing intracellular calcium buildup; it binds to most calcium-activated proteins with 100,000 times the affinity of calcium.[4]

LEAD POISONING IN ADULTS

Clinical Manifestations

Acute lead intoxication in adults is rare but can occur after high-dose respiratory exposure, such as after use of a heating gun, acetylene torching of lead-coated steel, or organic lead exposure (because organic lead penetrates the blood-brain barrier more readily).[9] Acute intoxication can produce encephalopathy, severe GI upset, and renal failure. More commonly, lead intoxication results from long-term exposure.

Nervous system manifestations predominate in lead-poisoned adults. Signs and symptoms include fatigue, irritability, lethargy, insomnia, headache, difficulty concentrating, memory loss, and tremor.[48] Other symptoms include myalgias, vomiting, constipation, and loss of libido.[9] Severe lead intoxication can result in an encephalopathy characterized by depressed consciousness, seizures, and coma, in association with cerebral edema. Life-threatening neurotoxicity usually develops with blood lead levels exceeding 150 μg/dL. Other central nervous system (CNS) effects include a marked disturbance in auditory brain stem evoked potentials.[49, 50]

Lead is also toxic to the peripheral nervous system, producing an axonopathy that results in motor disturbances.[11, 50] The distinctive pattern of lead-induced peripheral neuropathy affects the upper extremities more than the lower extremities, the extensors more than the flexors, and the dominant more than the nondominant arm. Painter's wristdrop is a once-endemic syndrome of upper extremity paresis found in painters who regularly used or removed lead-based paint. The initial segmental demyelination eventually leads to injury of both the axon and cell body.[3] Nerve conduction studies have shown that ulnar nerve conduction is disturbed at lead levels as low as 30 μg/dL.[1, 9, 43, 50]

The kidneys can be considered a second major site for lead's clinical toxicity. After lead poisoning, concentrations of lead are highest in the kidneys, particularly in the proximal tubules. As a result, lead, like cadmium, produces a renal injury characterized by excretion of β_2-microglobulin and *N*-acetylglucosidase.[51, 52] These proteins have been suggested as early markers of subacute lead-induced renal injury. Finally, chronic exposure to lead can result in hypertension; animal models suggest that the etiology of this is disturbance in calcium metabolism as it modulates vascular tone.[3, 52–54]

Lead's effect on the hematopoietic system is one of its most well-defined toxicities and has been used as a measure of its lead-induced physiologic dysfunction. *Basophilic stippling, the precipitation of nuclear material, is a hallmark of severe lead exposure.* In fact, before laboratory techniques were available for measuring blood lead levels, the degree of basophilic stippling served as a diagnostic tool. Lead is also a potent suppressor of heme synthesis, producing anemia once lead levels exceed 50 μg/dL; the anemia can be either normochromic or hypochromic.[1]

Lead's effects on reproduction are profound and multiple. For example, because of lead's diffusibility across the placenta, pregnant women with lead intoxication invariably have lead-poisoned offspring.[36, 37] Also, because pregnancy is a condition associated with bone mobilization, women with a past history of lead poisoning may have elevated lead levels during pregnancy. Other reproductive effects of lead poisoning in women include a higher rate of spontaneous abortion and stillbirth.[3, 4, 34, 37] Lead is one of the few toxins in which paternal exposure is also associated with adverse reproductive outcomes.[1, 43, 55] Lead-poisoned men have decreased sperm counts and a higher number of abnormal sperm; these effects can appear at blood lead levels as low as 40 μg/dL.[9, 11]

Other manifestations of lead intoxication include GI disturbances, mild liver function abnormalities, gingival lead lines (blue discolorations of the gingiva), muscle and joint aches, and gouty arthritis.[3, 9]

Assessment

The diagnostic evaluation of lead intoxication focuses on quantification and identification of those disturbances that can be readily diagnosed. The first important test is measurement of blood lead level. Because of lead's 30-day half-life and large volume of distribution, blood lead level is a relatively poor measure of total body burden; however, because blood is easy to obtain and does provide useful information after recent exposure, blood lead determination remains valuable. Blood lead levels can currently be measured by a number of techniques, including atomic absorption spectrometry, aniodic strip voltammetry, and thermal-ionization mass spectrometry.[4] All of these, when performed with appropriate quality control measures, are extremely accurate.

Because blood lead levels can be a poor representation of body lead burden, better methods of assessing lead exposure are being sought. Because lead is ultimately deposited in bone, with the skeleton serving as the primary *in situ* reservoir, diagnostic tools that measure lead in the skeleton are being developed. One of the most promising of these is x-ray fluorescence (XRF).[4, 56, 57] XRF works by emitting x-rays at bone in order to activate electrons in various shells, a process that produces energy that can be measured. L-line XRF stimulates electrons in the L electron shell, whereas K-line XRF acts only at electrons in the K shell. The latter technique appears to have greater accuracy in assessing total bone lead concentration. Studies are demonstrating that XRF analysis of bone assesses body lead burden far more accurately than does blood lead determination. For example, Hu and colleagues showed that among carpenters with long-term lead exposure, lead burden as assessed by XRF correlated more closely with lead suppression of heme synthesis than did blood lead level.[57] Although promising, XRF has been difficult to develop in children because they have relatively little bone calcification and because lead incorporation into bone appears to occur at less predictable rates. Nonetheless, XRF has the potential to replace blood lead measurement as a method of assessing lead exposure.

EP determination remains an important test in the evaluation of lead exposure. Because it is not only the quantity of lead in blood that one is interested in but also the effect of that lead burden on body function, EP measurement serves to provide information on lead's organ toxicity. EP is easily measured through hematofluorometry.[25] As a general rule, adults with lead poisoning have less EP elevation than children. It is also notable that rises in EP lag behind lead exposure by several days; therefore, if measured shortly after exposure, EP levels may not yet be abnormal.

Other laboratory tests that are useful in the evaluation of lead exposure include abdominal radiographs, renal function tests, complete blood count, and δ-aminolevulinic acid dehydratase activity. Abdominal radiographs are useful only if acute lead ingestion is suspected. Blood urea nitrogen and serum creatinine levels should be measured, and urinalysis should be performed. Although investigators have suggested that *N*-acetylglucosidase can be used as a marker of lead-induced renal injury, the clinical utility of this test has not yet been proved. A complete blood count (CBC) serves to identify either preexisting iron deficiency anemia or lead suppression of hematopoiesis; also, basophilic stippling can be identified on blood smear. δ-Aminolevulinic acid dehydratase activity has been used as a research tool because its activity is sensitive to low-level lead exposure.

Methods of assessing nervous system function after lead intoxication include measurement of auditory brain stem evoked potentials and nerve conduction velocity.[49] Lumbar puncture should not be performed on patients with altered mental status from suspected lead poisoning; because lead encephalopathy is associated with cerebral edema, a lumbar puncture could produce a herniation syndrome.

Treatment

Treatment of adult lead poisoning begins with cessation of further exposure. For those exposed in the workplace, OSHA standards must be implemented (if the business falls under OSHA regulations). Even for nonoccupationally exposed adults (e.g., artisans or family members with lead poisoning due to home renovation), the primary intervention is prevention of further exposure.

Chelation Therapy

Parenteral agents. Chelators are agents that form stable ligands with metal, effecting enhanced renal or biliary excretion of the drug-chelate complex. Chelators have been developed during the past century. However, it has only been since the mid-20th century that chelation therapy has flourished. As a result, more than five lead chelators have been identified.

The most important lead chelator developed is *dimercaprol.* This agent was created in England during World War II after the search for an antidote to the deadly arsenic-containing gas lewisite. The resulting antidote was an arsenic chelator termed *British antilewisite* (BAL). Since its creation, BAL has proved to be one of the most potent heavy metal chelators. In addition to lead, BAL chelates mercury, arsenic, and gold. BAL forms a stable dithiol bond with lead; the resulting complex is eliminated in both bile and urine.

BAL has a significant side effect profile; as many as 50% of those who receive this drug develop an adverse reaction. Part of this results from BAL's required preparation in a peanut oil vehicle; having such an excipient, the drug can only be administered intramuscularly. BAL has oxidant properties that can produce hemolysis in those with glucose-6-phosphate dehydrogenase (G-6-PD) deficiency. Other adverse effects include hypotension, rash, vomiting, and a metallic taste in the mouth.[58] Toxic reactions occur when BAL is administered simultaneously with oral iron supplements.

BAL should be administered to any patient with encephalopathy or a whole blood lead level greater than 100 μg/dL.[9] The dose is 4 to 6 mg/kg per dose (maximum 300 mg per dose). Because of its peanut oil vehicle, BAL should not be administered to patients with a history of peanut allergy.[58]

Another effective lead chelator is calcium disodium ethylene diamine tetraacetic acid (CaNa2EDTA, *calcium edetate*). Developed in the 1950s, this chelator became an important intervention in the treatment of childhood lead intoxication. Like BAL, EDTA forms a stable bond with the lead atom. The resulting complex is excreted in urine. EDTA can be administered intravenously or intramuscularly; it is not administered orally, both because this route is less effective and because evidence shows that oral EDTA can enhance GI absorption of ingested lead. EDTA has a short half-life (approximately 65 minutes).[3] As a result, it is ideally administered by continuous intravenous infusion. Alternative administration strategies include intramuscular or intravenous administration two to three times daily.

As with BAL, adverse effects of EDTA limit its use to well-outlined protocols. EDTA chelates nutrients, particularly zinc, in addition to lead. Therefore, in order to avoid zinc deficiency, courses of EDTA are limited to 5 days, followed by at least a 48-hour hiatus for nutritional recovery. EDTA courses are also limited to minimize its nephrotoxicity (manifested by proteinuria, hematuria, or glycosuria).[58] Other limitations of EDTA include its relative ineffectiveness with blood lead levels less than 30 to 40 μg/dL, which narrows its range of utility. The dose of EDTA given to adults is 1 to 2 g daily.

Oral Chelators. A group of oral chelators has been developed to provide the option of outpatient therapy for those with clinically asymptomatic lead intoxication. These include dimercaptosuccinic acid (DMSA) and D-penicillamine. They are discussed in the section on childhood lead poisoning.

Indications

Because adults, compared with children, are considered relatively resistant to the toxic effects of lead, indications for chelation therapy are controversial. In the general practice of occupational medicine, treatment of lead poisoning has been reserved for symptomatic adults, independent of blood lead level. Therefore, chelation therapy is often withheld until blood lead levels exceed 70 μg/dL, the range at which adults typically develop overt signs of lead toxicity. In such patients, hospitalization for EDTA chelation is recommended. Experience with childhood lead poisoning has indicated that EDTA chelation can exacerbate CNS toxicity when it is used as sole therapy in those with blood lead levels greater than 70 to 100 μg/dL; this CNS toxicity probably represents EDTA promotion of lead penetration into the brain. To prevent this, dual therapy with both EDTA and BAL should be considered for adults with blood lead levels greater than 100 μg/dL. BAL can be discontinued once blood lead level has fallen below the range of 70 to 80 μg/dL.

As the toxicity of lead becomes more appreciated, a growing opinion is that in adults, chelation therapy should be provided before overt clinical symptoms appear in order to prevent subclinical toxicity as well as to reduce overall lead burden. Therefore, clinically asymptomatic adults should be considered candidates for chelation therapy even at lead levels of 25 to 40 μg/dL. Pregnant lead-poisoned women, unless their plumbism is severe, should not undergo chelation because of the possibility that the chelating agent might enhance lead movement across the placenta[1] and because of evidence of EDTA teratogenicity.[11]

CHILDHOOD LEAD POISONING

History

The history of concern for childhood lead intoxication is comparatively brief. Childhood lead poisoning was clearly identified in Brisbane, Australia, approximately 100 years ago, when, after extensive epidemiologic investigation, A.J. Turner and J.L. Gibson associated the poisoning of young children with the ingestion of paint in their homes. Through the 20th century, increasing reports worldwide described catastrophic illness in children related to their ingestion of lead paint. Clinical features included basophilic stippling, abdominal pain, irritability, and often coma, seizures, and death. In 1943, Byers and Lord published a seminal article indicating that although childhood lead poisoning had been thought of as an illness that, among survivors, produced no obvious sequelae, many children who survived lead intoxication suffered cognitive disturbances or frank mental retardation. During the next 15 years, additional studies reported that lead poisoning in children could lead to subnormal intelligence, hyperactivity, aggression, and school failure.[4, 59]

In the 1950s and 1960s, many areas of the United States were found to have endemic rates of lead poisoning. These so-called lead belts were synonymous with large inner city slums.[34] Such observations led to public outcries until, in 1959, the United States Public Health Service recommended that blood lead levels of 60 to 80 μg/dL be considered evidence of lead absorption in children; levels below this were not thought to have any clinical effect.[34] In 1970, the Surgeon General reduced this to 40 μg/dL and for the first time shifted the focus from case finding to prevention through mass screening for childhood lead poisoning. Interestingly, the American Academy of Pediatrics, in a move thought to reverse this progress, initially recommended that environmental inspection be performed only after a child had two blood lead levels of 50 μg/dL or greater.[34] Mass screening was facilitated through passage of the 1971 Lead-Based Paint Poisoning Prevention Act.[34] In 1975, the Centers for Disease Control (CDC) began to establish classifications and risk categories for childhood lead poisoning. The blood lead level of concern was reduced to 30 μg/dL in 1975, to 25 μg/dL in 1985, and to 10 μg/dL in 1991. According to the 1991 CDC document, the redefinition of childhood lead intoxication as a blood lead of 10 μg/dL or greater was based on increasing scientific data indicating that toxic effects of lead were demonstrable at this level.[60] The 1991 CDC guidelines also moved from a single definition of lead poisoning to a tiered approach that recommended interventions based on a range of lead levels.[60]

The most important legislative action to prevent lead poisoning in children was the banning of lead from residential paint in 1978. However, with decades of using lead-based paint, the problem of lead poisoning due to exposure to paint continues. Nonetheless, as a result of additional legislation and greater federal oversight through organizations such as the EPA, lead exposure in children has declined dramatically.

Epidemiology

Childhood lead poisoning is now defined as a blood lead level of 10 μg/dL or greater. The new classification of lead poisoning also establishes degrees of lead exposure as a means of prioritizing interventions (Table 57–3).

Data from NHANES III on the epidemiology of childhood lead poisoning indicate that the average lead level of American children is 3 to 4 μg/dL, which is 80% less than mean blood lead levels in 1976. This blood lead level represents "background" exposure, the sum of different environmental sources. An estimated 1.7 million children, or 8.9% of American children, have lead poisoning.[1, 6, 7] Childhood lead intoxication is more prevalent in minority groups and among those living in the Northeast. The peak onset of lead poisoning in children is the second year of life, although *de novo* lead poisoning can appear in later childhood years.[61]

As with exposure to lead in adults, childhood lead exposure can result from many sources, including lead paint or dust, air, soil, water, and food.[4, 34, 60] However, there are significant differences in the etiology of frank lead poisoning according to age. For example, in children, lead paint and dust are the primary source of lead poisoning (in contrast to vocational or avocational exposure in adults). Also, children develop congenital lead intoxication if their mother has lead intoxication.[35, 62]

Lead paint remains the most common cause of frank lead poisoning in children.[60] The singular importance of paint results from several factors: (1) Lead-containing paint chips are relatively sweet. (2) The small size and color of paint chips make them attractive to curious young children. (3) Containing up to 50% lead by weight, paint chips are a high-dose source of lead capable of producing fatal degrees of exposure.[63, 64] (4) Pica, or repeated ingestion of nonfood objects, is most prevalent in early childhood; in infants, hand-to-mouth activity is a completely normal developmental process. (5) Children are more likely to have their hands dirtied by dust from the window well, the floor, or outdoor soil. (6) Household renovation of homes with lead generally results in greater contamination of the environment; this is a particular risk factor for lead poisoning in infancy.[62] (7) Even household deleading can also result in greater exposure to lead if not performed properly. Children who live with an adult who has a lead-related occupation are at greater risk of lead intoxication as a result of dust importation by the adult.[65]

Exposure to lead in water has greater impact on young children because of their relatively small size and the greater proportion of dietary lead absorbed by a child's gut. Lead poisoning from lead-contaminated water has been reported by several researchers.[62, 66, 67] In all of these cases, water was being used to prepare infant formula. Water can become highly

Table 57–3. Interpretation of Blood Lead Test Results and Follow-up Activities: Class of Child Based on Blood Lead Concentration

Class	Blood Lead Concentration (μg/dL)	Comment
I	≤9	A child in class I is not considered to be lead poisoned.
IIA	10–14	Many children (or a large proportion of children) with blood lead levels in this range should trigger communitywide childhood lead poisoning prevention activities. Children in this range may need to be rescreened more frequently.
IIB	15–19	A child in class IIB should receive nutritional and educational interventions and more frequent screening. If the blood lead level persists in this range, environmental investigation and intervention should be done.
III	20–44	A child in class III should receive environmental evaluation and remediation and a medical evaluation. Such a child may need pharmacologic treatment of lead poisoning.
IV	45–69	A child in class IV needs both medical and environmental interventions, including chelation therapy.
V	≥70	A child with class V lead poisoning poses a medical emergency. Medical and environmental management must begin immediately.

From The Centers for Disease Control: Preventing Lead Poisoning in Children. Atlanta, CDC, 1991, p 3.

contaminated if warmed or boiled in a vessel that contains lead.[66]

Although soil has not been clearly associated with the development of lead poisoning, it clearly contributes to background lead levels in children. Also, in areas with highly contaminated soil (e.g., homes near smelter), children tend to have higher blood lead levels.[68] In a study of the impact of soil lead abatement on blood lead levels in children, Weitzman and colleagues[124] showed that elimination of lead in soil could effect a reduction in blood lead of approximately 1 μg/dL, an amount insufficient to justify large-scale soil abatement measures.

Other potential causes of lead poisoning in children include administration of folk remedies (e.g., greta, azarcon, or Paylooah), congenital exposure, and ingestion of foreign bodies.[1, 4, 15, 36, 37, 60, 62, 69] A reported case of fatal childhood lead intoxication (blood lead level 283 μg/dL) occurred after a child ingested a lead curtain weight, which was retained in the GI tract for several weeks.[70]

All children do not have equal risk of lead intoxication; rather, it is the unique relationship between the individual child and his or her environment that results in lead exposure. This explains the common phenomenon of one child's developing lead poisoning while living in a house that contains lead although other children in the same environment do not have increased lead exposure. The most important risk factor is generally the oral habits of the child, particularly the presence of pica. Another risk factor for childhood lead poisoning is developmental delay. Children with significant delays—for example, those with autism—are more likely to develop lead poisoning.[60, 71–73] Moreover, the pattern of lead poisoning in these children has atypical features including its appearance at an older age and the tendency for recurrent exposure, despite environmental lead hazard reduction.[73] Finally, for reasons that are not clearly explained, childhood lead poisoning is more prevalent in summer than winter.[34]

Toxicokinetics

The kinetics of lead in children have not been extensively analyzed but are thought, with some exception, to parallel the kinetics in adults.[4] However, certain differences have been well characterized. For example, the extent of lead absorption is greater in children than in adults (30% to 50% versus 10%). Also, nutritional factors have a greater role in the development of childhood plumbism. Inadequate intake of iron, calcium, and total calories, all of which are more prevalent in children, are associated with higher blood lead levels.[31, 74] After its absorption, lead is distributed through soft tissues before its deposition into bone. The half-life of lead in the soft tissues of children may be longer, probably because children have less bone available for lead incorporation. As with adults, the estimated body elimination half-life of lead is 20 years.

Clinical Toxicity

Although the mechanisms of toxicity for lead poisoning in childhood are similar to those in adults, clinical manifestations are different. Also, the lead level at which these toxic manifestations appear is lower in children (Table 57–4). Children, for example, are more susceptible to all of lead's neurotoxic effects.[4]

Lead encephalopathy in children has presenting

Table 57–4. Significant Health Effects of Lead at Lowest Observed Blood Lead (PbB) Levels in Children

Lowest Observed Effect PbB (μg/dL)	Neurologic Effects	Heme Synthesis Effects	Other Effects
10–15 (prenatal and postnatal)	Deficits in neurobehavioral development (Bayley and McCarthy scales); electrophysiologic changes	ALA-D inhibition	Reduced gestational age and weight at birth; reduced size up to age 7–8 years
15–20		Erythrocyte protoporphyrin elevation	Impaired vitamin D metabolism; pyrimidine-5′-nucleotidase inhibition
<25	Lower IQ, slower reaction time (studied cross-sectionally)		
30	Slowed nerve conduction velocity		
40		Reduced hemoglobin; elevated EP and ALA-U	
70	Peripheral neuropathies	Frank anemia	
80–100	Encephalopathy		Colic, other gastrointestinal effects; kidney effects

ALA, aminolevulinic acid; EP, erythrocyte protoporphyrin.

Adapted from Agency for Toxic Substances and Disease Registry: The Nature and Extent of Lead Poisoning in Children in the United States: A Report to Congress, 1988, p IV-21; and U.S. Environmental Protection Agency: Air Quality Criteria of Lead. Washington, DC, 1986, vol 1, p 144.

features that are comparable to the disease in adults.[4] However, encephalopathy appears in children at blood lead levels as low as 50 to 60 μg/dL.[34, 75] Prominent features are irritability, anorexia, abdominal pain, obtundation, and, if untreated, cerebral edema, seizures, and death.[75]

The CNS effects of lead have caused the greatest concern about childhood lead poisoning.[34, 60] Exposure to lead during critical periods of neurodevelopment can produce permanent changes in cerebral architecture. The mechanisms of these changes have been described by Goldstein[76]: During the first 2 years of life, synaptic density and complexity are markedly increased such that by the third year of life, these "arborizations" exceed the normal adult pattern by almost twofold.[76] The enzymes that have an important role in mediating this process, including protein kinase C and calmodulin, are inhibited at very low concentrations of lead because of lead's replacement of calcium in the enzymes' reaction.[47] Another critical factor in normal dendritic arborization is the activity of neural cell adhesions molecules; the actions of these proteins are also impaired by lead. The consequences of lead exposure at this time are both reduced synaptogenesis and imprecise synaptic "pruning."[46, 76, 77] Functional changes including decreased neurotransmitter synthesis also occur after lead exposure.[46, 76, 77] The hippocampus is thought to be the primary anatomic site for these effects, this being an area with a high zinc content.[42] High-level lead exposure can disrupt the integrity of the blood-brain barrier.[34]

The clinical consequences of lead neurotoxicity in childhood are vast. At an extreme, children with severe lead intoxication can be left with profound cognitive disturbances (mental retardation).[59, 78] Estimates from several population-based studies are that children can lose approximately 5 points (95% confidence intervals ranging from 2 to 14) in intelligence quotient (IQ) for every 10 μg/dL elevation in their blood lead level.[11, 15, 79–81] Although a loss of 5 IQ points is arguably insignificant in any child, the potential left shift of the normal distribution of IQ among children would result in greater numbers of children with low IQ and a reduction in the number of children with superior IQ.[32] It is this principle that has, in part, maintained public health momentum to reduce blood lead levels in children to the lowest range possible. Other adverse developmental outcomes in lead-poisoned children include aggression, hyperactivity, school failure, and antisocial behaviors.[82–85] Another relatively common consequence of lead poisoning is the development of a learning disability in which overall IQ is normal by standardized testing but the child demonstrates discrete learning weaknesses such as impairment in memory, auditory processing, and visual-motor integration.[59, 80, 86, 87] These effects, which have been demonstrated in children with blood lead levels as low as 6 μg/dL, can persist into the preadolescent and adolescent years.[82, 84, 88–90] Other researchers have failed to find clear evidence that lead poisoning is causal in learning problems among children with a history of plumbism.[91, 92]

Peripheral neuropathy occurs in children with lead intoxication[93]; children with sickle cell disease may be at higher risk for this complication.[94] Children can develop subclinical peripheral neuropathy at lead levels as low as 30 μg/dL.[93] Hearing is also significantly depressed by low levels of lead exposure (Fig. 57–2).[95–97] Motor disturbances including poorer scores on bilateral coordination, upper limb speed, and dexterity tests may also occur.[98, 99]

Renal toxicity due to childhood lead poisoning includes impairment of vitamin D activation[44]; this appears to be a reversible effect. A 50-year follow-up of lead-poisoned children has shown that they have a sevenfold greater risk of adult hypertension.[53]

Hematopoietic effects of lead poisoning in children include suppression of erythropoiesis with resulting anemia. Children are more sensitive to lead suppression of heme synthesis, as evidenced by their higher EP concentrations. However, the anemia that accompanies lead poisoning is sometimes cause rather than effect, because iron deficiency results in greater lead absorption.[60] Isolated iron deficiency as well as lead intoxication can raise EP levels.

Lead can disturb bone development, leading to the formation of lead lines. These lines represent periods of growth arrest, not lead per se. Lead lines are best identified at the metaphyses of long bones, particularly the distal radius and proximal fibula. These lines generally appear 3 to 6 weeks after a period of significant lead exposure and generally correlate

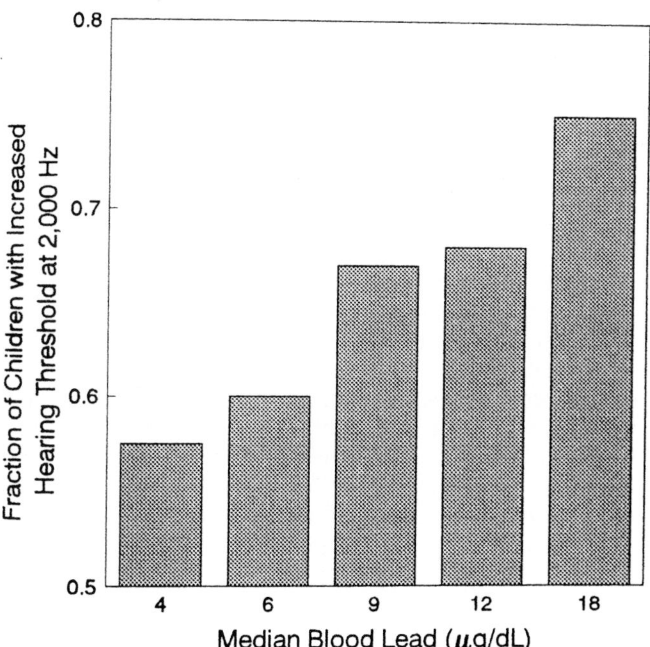

Figure 57–2. Fraction of children with hearing worse than a reference group stratified by quintiles of blood lead concentration, after adjustment for covariates. (From Schwartz J, Otto D: Lead and minor hearing impairment. Arch Environ Health *46*:300–305, 1991.)

with a peak blood lead level of greater than 45 to 50 μg/dL.[100]

Diagnosis

Assessment of children with known or suspected lead intoxication requires a careful physical evaluation that includes investigation of clinically overt signs and symptoms such as irritability and abdominal pain. The laboratory evaluation is an important adjunct. All children with lead intoxication should receive tests for venous blood lead and EP levels, a CBC, measurement of blood urea nitrogen and creatinine, urinalysis, and measures of iron status (serum iron with total iron-binding capacity or serum ferritin). The need for radiographs should be individualized. If recent ingestion of lead-containing material is suspected, an abdominal radiograph should be obtained. Radiographs of the long bones can be useful as an assessment of timing and magnitude of exposure.[60] In children with blood lead level less than 45 to 50 μg/dL, long bone radiographs are usually valueless. As a general rule, long bone films never alter clinical management.

Newer means of assessing lead burden are being explored. For example, the research use of deciduous teeth has the potential to be clinically valuable. Also, XRF in children may ultimately prove to have the same value that is being found in the assessment of adult lead intoxication.[84]

Treatment

Treatment of lead intoxication in children focuses on three components, in the following order of importance: environmental inspection/hazard reduction, nutritional supplementation, and, if necessary, chelation therapy.[60]

Whenever lead poisoning is found, the source must be identified. Unless the source is clearly known, a complete environmental inspection is necessary. This inspection is guided by data obtained from an environmental history. Investigating previous lead tests of the child, the age and condition of the child's housing, recent renovations, water intake, use of kitchenware that may contain lead, time spent elsewhere (including daycare, school, and relatives' homes), occupations of adult family members, oral habits of the child, and siblings or playmates with lead intoxication. The results of the history should guide inspection of areas that may include the home interior and exterior, water, and alternate housing.[60] Inspections for lead are generally performed using either a sodium sulfide test (the reaction between this solution and lead produces gray-black lead sulfide) or XRF. The latter test is best able to detect lead paint that is covered by a nonlead surface. Interior home inspection should include dust wipings, especially when children are younger than 1 year old (more likely to have dust-laden hands because of crawling). Household lead hazards, if found, should be reduced or fully abated (i.e., deleaded). In one study, deleading alone was shown to reduce blood lead levels by as much as 30%.[101] On the other hand, deleading has the potential to result in greater lead exposure if not conducted properly.[14] Therefore, it is important that work be done with minimal environmental contamination, with the family living elsewhere and with final inspection before reoccupancy. Methods of reducing without removing household lead hazards include use of trisodium phosphate detergent, a lead binder on floors and window wells, and application of encapsulants, chemical polymers that effectively (albeit temporarily) cover lead surfaces.

Nutritional supplementation focuses on eliminating iron and calcium deficiency, both of which result in greater absorption of ingested lead.[31, 60] Because there are no consistently accurate measures of iron status in children,[60] iron supplementation should be empirically initiated; iron sulfate elixir or drops can be prescribed in a dose of 3 to 6 mg/kg per day for a period of 4 to 6 weeks. Although evidence in animal models suggests that iron supplementation promotes the elimination of lead from the body, in human subjects, its only proven effect is reduction of further lead absorption.[31] Calcium deficiency is uncommon in children who have a varied diet with regular milk intake. If there is any question about calcium intake, however, the diet should be enhanced with calcium-rich foods (e.g., yogurt, cheese, milk) or calcium supplementation should be prescribed.[31] The combination of environmental abatement and nutritional supplementation is often sufficient to produce prompt reductions in blood lead level. However, the diminution in blood lead level may not be sufficient or may not occur rapidly enough to reduce the risk of multisystem injury. In these cases, chelation therapy is warranted.

Chelation Therapy

Chelation therapy for lead intoxication was initially developed to reduce the mortality associated with childhood lead poisoning. Increasing emphasis is being placed on its use to prevent morbidity as well. Therefore, although the same agents are available for both adults and children with lead intoxication, the greater focus, particularly the development of oral chelators, has been directed to pediatric treatment.

Increasing options in both parenteral and oral chelation therapy have brought into question the indications for hospitalization of lead-poisoned children. Decisions for hospitalization should be individualized. However, the goals of hospitalization are at least threefold: (1) to provide environmental protection so that the child has no further lead exposure, (2) to provide close monitoring for evidence of clinical toxicity, and (3) to provide aggressive chelation therapy.[60] With these principles, hospitalization should be considered for all children who are younger than

6 years and who have a blood lead level exceeding 45 to 55 μg/dL. Children who are hospitalized for lead intoxication should never be returned to the environment in which their lead poisoning occurred unless hazard reduction measures have been completed.

Parenteral Chelating Agents

Parenteral agents for lead intoxication in childhood are BAL and EDTA. However, both of these agents are used in different fashions in the pediatric population. For example, because of the risk of deterioration in CNS status or death when EDTA alone is given to children with severe lead intoxication,[102] therapy with both BAL and EDTA should always be instituted for children with blood lead levels of 70 μg/dL or greater.[58] BAL should be given in a dose of 3 to 5 mg/kg per dose. EDTA is begun approximately 4 hours after the first dose of BAL. BAL is given every 6 to 8 hours until the blood lead level is less than 70 μg/dL. Adverse reactions and cautions are the same in children as in adults, although children appear to have a higher prevalence of febrile reactions.[58] BAL should be used cautiously in those with glucose-6-phosphate dehydrogenase (G-6-PD) deficiency and oral iron therapy must be discontinued. Peanut allergy is a contraindication to the use of BAL.[58]

EDTA is given in a daily dose of 35 to 50 mg/kg per day (1000 to 1500 mg/m^2). Although the agent can be given intramuscularly, intravenous administration is preferred because intramuscular EDTA is extremely painful and because brisk urine output, necessary to prevent EDTA nephrotoxicity, is better achieved with intravenous hydration. Because of EDTA's short half-life, continuous intravenous infusion is preferred; however, administration every 8 to 12 hours is an acceptable alternative.[58] The duration of therapy is 3 to 5 days, depending on the blood lead level.[58] Thereafter, therapy is discontinued. A "rebound" blood lead level measurement should be obtained 2 to 3 days after the EDTA is discontinued for those in whom an immediate second course of EDTA chelation is anticipated. For others, a 2- to 3-week rebound level is obtained. Some degree of rebound, which represents redistribution of lead from soft tissues into blood, always occurs after chelation. Additional courses of EDTA may be necessary, depending on the degree of rebound. It is not uncommon for children with blood lead levels of 60 μg/dL or greater to require two or more courses of EDTA.[58]

Because not every child with lead intoxication has a gratifying response to EDTA chelation, particularly children with blood levels less than 45 μg/dL, the EDTA mobilization test has become a widely used method of identifying children who will benefit from chelation therapy.[103, 104] To perform the test, a child is given a single intravenous or intramuscular dose of EDTA (35 to 50 mg/kg, maximum 1 g), followed by an 8-hour collection of urine, which is analyzed for total lead excretion. A positive mobilization test is considered a ratio of greater than 0.6 between the dose of EDTA administered (in milligrams) versus the quantity of urine excreted (in micrograms). For example, a child who is given 500 mg of EDTA and who excretes 400 μg lead in an 8-hour urine test has a ratio of 0.8 and should receive 3 to 5 days of EDTA therapy. In those with ratios less than 0.6, alternative therapies should be considered. Iron deficiency produces a poor response to the mobilization test[105]; therefore, those with negative results may benefit from a period of iron supplementation followed by a repeat test. Alternatively, oral chelation therapy can be initiated.

The lead mobilization test, although valuable, has shortcomings.[58, 106] First, it is difficult to collect 8 hours' worth of urine in small children in the absence of catheterization, which is traumatic. Spilled or lost urine makes data interpretation difficult if not impossible.[107] The performance of the test is labor intensive and requires an 8- to 10-hour health care visit (or brief hospitalization).[108] Moreover, the chance of a positive mobilization test is inversely related to the blood lead level. As a result, there is little likelihood of a positive mobilization test result in children with blood lead levels less than 25 to 35 μg/dL.[104] Collectively, these factors plus the option of oral chelation therapy have made the mobilization test a less attractive though acceptable option.[58]

Oral Chelating Agents

Numerous oral chelating agents have been used or are in current use for the treatment of lead poisoning. The two most commonly used agents are D-penicillamine and DMSA.

D-Penicillamine was fortuitously discovered in 1953 by Walshe[109] and, because of its copper-chelating ability, was quickly used in the treatment of Wilson's disease. Identification of its efficacy at chelating lead initially resulted in suggestions that penicillamine be used to treat lead-exposed workers without their removal from work.

D-Penicillamine has unique, incompletely understood chelating properties.[102] For example, it does not appear to be capable of forming stable bonds with the lead atom. Nonetheless, it does enhance urinary lead excretion, posssibly by forming a heterocylic ring (sulfur and nitrogen atoms binding the lead).[110] Like BAL, penicillamine is capable of chelating other metals including arsenic and mercury.

The efficacy of D-penicillamine in childhood lead intoxication has been demonstrated in studies by Sachs, Vitale, Marcus, Shannon, and others.[102, 111–115] Data from these studies have shown that penicillamine can reduce blood levels, even in children with low-level lead poisoning (blood lead 20 to 35 μg/dL). Blood lead levels as low as 3 μg/dL can be achieved using this drug.[114] D-Penicillamine can be considered for children with blood lead levels in the range of 25 to 40 μg/dL, especially those who have a negative EDTA mobilization test result.[58]

D-Penicillamine is given in a dose of 10 to 30 mg/kg daily. Its use is initiated after baseline CBC and renal function tests are obtained. Available only in capsules or tablets of 125 and 250 mg, the tablets must usually be crushed or the capsules opened and placed in food or drink. Having an unpleasant odor and taste, penicillamine must often be concealed in juice or food. Because iron may decrease D-penicillamine absorption by as much as 65%, iron supplementation should be discontinued during penicillamine therapy.[110] The agent is given twice a day at home by the parents. During treatment, children must be monitored every 2 to 4 weeks for evidence of adverse effects. Monitoring laboratory tests include CBC, urinalysis, blood lead measurement, and EP determinations. Typical courses of D-penicillamine therapy are 2 to 6 months in length.

Penicillamine has an overall adverse effect rate of 33%, a rate that has led to considerable reluctance to use it. The most common adverse effect is GI upset. More serious effects occur in as many as 10% of children and include rash, platelet and white blood cell count depression, and renal disturbances, manifested by glycosuria, proteinuria, hematuria, or pyuria. The occurrence of any of these adverse effects should prompt discontinuation of therapy (although these adverse effects resolve without discontinuation in 70% of cases[110]). In all reported experience with D-penicillamine use for childhood lead poisoning in otherwise healthy children, these effects have been mild and reversible.

DMSA is an oral chelating agent that was discovered in the 1950s; in 1991, it became the first oral chelating agent ever approved for the treatment of lead intoxication.[110, 116–118] An oral congener of BAL, DMSA has, interestingly, not been approved for adult lead intoxication, in part because of the ever-present risk of its abuse by workers, employers, or physicians.[119]

DMSA has been approved for use in children with blood lead levels exceeding 45 µg/dL. However, studies have demonstrated that its efficacy extends to children with blood lead-levels between 25 and 45 µg/dL[118, 120]; it is therefore a therapeutic option for these patients. Although there is no clearly defined upper limit of lead level for which DMSA can be used, it is prudent to use conventional, dual parenteral therapy (EDTA and BAL) in children with blood lead levels of 70 µg/dL or greater.

DMSA is available in 100-mg capsules. The current treatment protocol is adminstration of 10 mg/kg per dose. For the first 5 days of DMSA therapy, it is given three times daily. For the next 14 days, treatment is twice a day. A complete course of DMSA chelation is therefore 19 days. During therapy, because adverse effects associated with DMSA include rash, white blood cell count depression, and liver function abnormalities, monitoring should include blood lead, EP, white blood cell count, and liver function testing.[58, 110, 113] DMSA, unlike BAL, does not produce hemolysis in those with G-6-PD deficiency. Also, DMSA can be administered concomitantly with iron therapy. Mean reductions in blood lead with DMSA therapy are as great as 70% to 80%.[110, 116, 117] However, in contrast to penicillamine, DMSA discontinuation is followed by large lead rebounds, appearing 2 to 4 weeks after completion of therapy. It is not unusual to experience rebound lead values that approximate the pretreatment value. As a result, multiple courses of DMSA are invariably necessary to produce enduring reductions in blood lead levels. Because lead rebounds can be confused with re-exposure to lead, it is important to monitor EP levels. Lead re-exposure is associated with increases in EP values, but lead rebound is not.

Additional agents that have been used for the treatment of lead intoxication are dimercaptopropanesulfonate and trientine.[121, 122] Neither of these agents has moved beyond the investigational stage.

Indications and Goals for Chelation Therapy

The indications for initiating chelation therapy in children are controversial. For children with blood lead levels of 10 to 20 µg/dL—the majority of lead-poisoned children in the United States—chelation therapy is not recommended, primarily because it is difficult to identify a single source of lead to abate and because for lead levels in this range, the risk of adverse effects from chelation therapy are likely to outweigh the potential benefits.[58, 60] Instead, education, hazard reduction (if lead hazards are found), and nutritional supplementation are provided. For those children with blood lead levels of 20 µg/dL or greater, consultation with a lead specialist is recommended.[60] Among these children, chelation therapy should be considered. The decision to begin therapy should be based on (1) evidence that the blood lead level is not declining despite environmental abatement and nutritional supplementation, (2) the age of the child (evidence strongly suggests that the most neurodevelopmentally vulnerable age is the first 24 months of life[89]), (3) evidence of biochemical disturbances (i.e., an elevated EP level), (4) the assumption that reducing lead burden does reverse some toxicity (e.g., renal and hematopoietic) and may reverse neurodevelopmental disturbances,[46, 123] and (5) the desire to reduce lead burden to prevent its deposition in bone, where recrudescence later in life could occur. In initiating chelation therapy, the goals of treatment must also be established. Although this is also an area of some controversy, it is rational to have a goal of reducing blood lead level to the range of 10 to 15 mg/dL, if not lower. This requires long-term treatment strategies and frequent monitoring.

In children with more serious lead poisoning (blood lead > 30 to 35 µg/dL), formal cognitive or neuropsychologic testing should be performed to identify neurodevelopmental weaknesses and initiate remedial programs as soon as possible. Because these weaknesses are generally not identifiable with gross developmental assessment (e.g., the Denver Developmental Screening Test) and may not be evident in the first few years of life, formal testing is recommended after the ages of 4 to 6 years of age.

Prevention

Prevention of lead poisoning in children has led to both primary and secondary prevention strategies.[60] Primary prevention consists of environmental inspection and abatement before a child develops lead intoxication. Because the cost of identifying and abating all homes (or other sources) with lead is prohibitive, primary prevention efforts have been difficult to implement. However, federal and state legislation that includes lead notification before home renting or purchase is being passed to ensure safe housing. Other primary preventive measures, including lead removal from soil, were attempted in a pilot study by Weitzman and colleagues, with little success.[124]

Prevention has focused primarily on secondary efforts. Under this philosophy, because lead poisoning is asymptomatic in its early phases, the goal is to identify children who have developed lead poisoning, in order to prevent their lead levels from rising further and to protect their siblings and playmates from lead exposure. Secondary prevention forms the basis of routine lead screening in children.[60]

Secondary prevention through screening initially consisted of capillary (fingerstick) measurement of EP levels. This test was used both because EP level rises with lead intoxication and because capillary lead tests are easily contaminated by lead on the fingertip, leading to a high rate of false-positive results. When the definition of lead poisoning was reduced to 10 μg/dL in 1991, EP screening had to be abandoned because EP level generally does not rise when blood lead levels are 10 to 25 μg/dL.[125] Therefore, with a desire to identify all children who have blood lead levels of 10 μg/dL or greater, the current recommendation is to measure blood lead only.[60] Although capillary lead testing can produce false-positive results, making it less useful, it is an acceptable means of screening children if performed properly.[126, 127] Finding children who have elevated EP levels due to iron deficiency is still of benefit, because iron supplementation can be initiated as a primary preventive measure.

Another aspect of secondary prevention has been the call for universal lead screening.[60] Because lead intoxication is present throughout the United States and there are no completely reliable means of case finding, recommendations have been that all children receive periodic lead screening, regardless of where they live or their socioeconomic status. This recommendation has been strongly criticized because it is costly and because, in many areas, its yield is extremely low.[126] Opponents believe that resources devoted to lead screening in areas that have been shown through small-scale screening to have a low incidence of lead poisoning are a financial waste.[128] Targeted screening—that is, screening of children thought to be at risk for lead exposure—is likely to be a more cost-effective strategy. Such screening would include blood lead measurment in siblings and close playmates. Lead poisoning in domestic pets may signal lead intoxication in the child.[129] Other high-risk children include those with developmental delays, those with a history of foreign body ingestion/insertion, and those with a history of physical abuse.[60, 73, 130–132]

References

1. Landrigan PJ, Todd AC: Lead poisoning. West J Med *161:*153–159, 1994.
2. Ericson JE, Shirahata H, Patterson C: Skeletal concentrations of lead in ancient Peruvians. N Engl J Med *300:*946–951, 1979.
3. Ibels LS, Pollock CA: Lead intoxication. Med Toxicol *1:*387–410, 1986.
4. Council NR: Measuring Lead Exposure in Infants, Children and Other Sensitive Populations. Washington, DC, National Academy Press, p 337, 1993.
5. Gilfillan SC: Lead poisoning and the fall of Rome. J Occup Environ Med *7:*53–60, 1965.
6. Brody DJ, Pirkle JL, Kramer RA, et al: Blood lead levels in the US population—Phase 1 of the Third National Health and Nutrition Examination Survey (NHANES III, 1988 to 1991). JAMA *272:*277–283, 1994.
7. Pirkel JL, Brody DJ, Gunter EW, et al: The decline in blood lead levels in the United States—The National Health and Nutrition Examination Surveys (NHANES). JAMA *272:*284–291, 1994.
8. Goldman RH, Baker EL, Hannan M, Kamerow DB: Lead poisoning in automobile radiator mechanics. N Engl J Med *317:*214–218, 1987.
9. Keogh JP: Lead. *In* Sullivan J, Krieger G (eds): Hazardous Materials Toxicology—Clinical Principles of Environmental Health. Baltimore, Williams & Wilkins, pp 834–844, 1992.
10. Tripathi RK, Sherertz PC, Llewellyn GC, Armstrong CW: Lead exposure in outdoor firearm instructors. Am J Public Health *81:*753–755, 1991.
11. Rempel D: The lead-exposed worker. JAMA *262:*532–534, 1989.
12. Schneitzer L, Osborn HH, Bierman A, et al: Lead poisoning in adults from renovation of an older home. Ann Emerg Med *19:*415–420, 1990.
13. Fischbein A, Anderson KE, Sassa S, et al: Lead poisoning from "do-it-yourself" heat guns for removing lead-based paint: Report of two cases. Environ Res *24:*425–431, 1981.
14. Amitai Y, Graef JW, Brown MJ, et al: Hazards of deleading homes of children with lead poisoning. Am J Dis Child *1411:*758–760, 1987.
15. American Academy of Pediatrics Committee on Environmental Health: Lead poisoning: From screening to primary prevention. Pediatrics *92:*176–183, 1993.
16. Orlando P, Perdelli F, Gallelli G, et al: Increased blood lead levels in runners training in urban areas. Arch Environ Health *49:*200–203, 1994.
17. Beattie D, Moore MR, Devenay WT, et al: Environmental lead pollution in an urban soft-water area. BMJ *2:*491–493, 1972.
18. Roberge RJ, Martin TG: Whole bowel irrigation in an acute oral lead intoxication. Am J Emerg Med *10:*577–583, 1992.
19. Vance MV, Curry SC, Bradley JM, et al: Acute lead poisoning in nursing home and psychiatric patients from the ingestion of lead-based ceramic glazes. Arch Intern Med *150:*1085–2092, 1990.
20. Bayly GR, Braithwaite RA, Sheehan TMT, Dyer NH, et al: Lead poisoning from Asian traditional remedies in the West Midlands—report of a series of five cases. Hum Exp Toxicol *14:*24–28, 1995.
21. Bose A, Vashistha K, O'Loughlin BJ: Azarcon por Empacho—another cause of lead toxicity. Pediatrics *42:*106–108, 1983.
22. Markowitz SB, Nunez CM, Klitzman S, et al: Lead poisoning due to Hai Ge Fen—the porphyrin content of individual erythrocytes. JAMA *271:*932–934, 1994.
23. Smitherman J, Harber P: A case of mistaken identity: Herbal

medicine as a cause of lead toxicity. Am J Ind Med *20:*795–798, 1991.
24. Boourgoin BP, Evans DR, Cornett JR, et al: Lead content in 70 brands of dietary calcium supplements. Am J Public Health *83:*1155–1160, 1993.
25. Lamola AA, Joselow M, Yamane T: Zinc protoporphyrin (ZPP): A simple, sensitive, fluorometric screening test for lead poisoning. Clin Chem *21:*93–97, 1975.
26. Miller SA: Lead in calcium supplements. JAMA *257:*1810, 1987.
27. Matte TD, Proops D, Palazuelos E, et al: Acute high-dose lead exposure from beverage contaminated by traditional Mexican pottery. Lancet *344:*1064–1065, 1994.
28. Graziano J, Blum C: Lead exposure from lead crystal. Lancet *337:*141–142, 1991.
29. Lees RE, Scott GD, Miles CG: Subacute lead poisoning from retained lead shot. Can Med Assoc J *138:*130–131, 1988.
30. Magos L: Lead poisoning from retained lead projectiles. A critical review of case reports. Hum Exp Toxicol *13:*735–742, 1994.
31. Sargent JD: The role of nutrition in the prevention of lead poisoning in children. Pediatr Ann *23:*636–642, 1994.
32. Goyer RA: Toxic effects of metals. *In* Amdur MO, Doull J, Klaassen CD (eds): Casarett and Doull's Toxicology—The Basic Science of Poisons. New York, Pergamon Press, 1991.
33. Rabinowitz MB, Wetherill GW, Kopple JD: Kinetic analysis of lead metabolism in healthy humans. J Clin Invest *58:*260–270, 1976.
34. Chisolm JJ Jr, O'Hara DM: Lead Absorption in Children: Management, Clinical and Environmental Aspects. Baltimore-Munich, Urban & Schwarzenberg, p 229, 1982.
35. Ryu JE, Ziegler EE, Fomon S: Maternal lead exposure and blood lead concentration in infancy. J Pediatr *93:*476–478, 1978.
36. Timpo AE, Ain JS, Casalino MB, Yuceoglu AM: Congenital lead intoxication. J Pediatr *94:*765–766, 1979.
37. Wong GP, Ng TL, Martin TR, Farquharson DF: Effects of low-level lead exposure in utero. Obstet Gynecol *47:*285–289, 1992.
38. Goldman RH, White R, Kales SN, Hu H: Lead poisoning from mobilizatioon of bone stores during thyrotoxicosis. Am J Ind Med *25:*417–424, 1994.
39. Shannon M, Landy H, Anast C, Graef J: Recurrent lead poisoning in a child with immobilization osteoporosis. Vet Hum Toxicol *30:*586–588, 1988.
40. Markowitz ME, Weinberger HL: Immobilization-related lead toxicity in previously lead-poisoned children. Pediatrics *86:*455–457, 1990.
41. Mahaffey KR: Biokinetics of lead during pregnancy. Fund Appl Toxicol *16:*15–16, 1991.
42. Silbergeld EK: Lead in bone: Implications for toxicology during pregnancy and lactation. Environ Health Perspect *91:*63–70, 1991.
43. Landrigan PJ: Lead in the modern workplace. Am J Public Health *80:*907–908, 1990.
44. Rosen JF, Chesney RW, Hamstra A, et al: Reduction in 1,25-dihydroxyvitamin D in children with increased lead absorption. N Engl J Med *302:*1128–1130, 1980.
45. Hernberg S, Nikkanen J: Enzyme inhibition by lead under normal urban conditions. Lancet *1:*63–64, 1970.
46. Silbergeld EK: Mechanisms of lead neurotoxicity, or looking beyond the lamppost. FASEB J *6:*3201–3206, 1992.
47. Sandhir R, Gill KD: Lead perturbs calmodulin dependent cyclic AMP metabolism in rat central nervous system. Biochem Mol Biol Int *33:*729–742, 1994.
48. Stollery BT, Broadbent DE, Banks HA, Lee WR: Short term prospective study of cognitive functioning in lead workers. Br J Ind Med *48:*739–749, 1991.
49. Holdstein Y, Pratt H, Goldsher M, et al: Auditory brainstem evoked potentials in asymptomatic lead-exposed subjects. J Laryngol Otol *100:*1031–1036, 1986.
50. Murata K, Araki S, Yokoyama K, et al: Assessment of central, peripheral, and autonomic nervous system functions in lead workers: Neuroelectrophysiological studies. Environ Res *61:*323–336, 1993.
51. Kumar BD, Krishnaswamy K: Detection of occupational lead nephropathy using early renal markers. Clin Toxicol *33:*331–335, 1995.
52. Staessen JA, Lauwerys RR, Buchet J-P, et al: Impairment of renal function with increasing blood lead concentrations in the general populations. N Engl J Med *327:*151–156, 1992.
53. Hu H: A 50-year follow-up of childhood plumbism: Hypertension, renal function and hemoglobin levels among survivors. Am J Dis Child *145:*681–687, 1991.
54. Schwartz J: Lead, blood pressure, and cardiovascular disease in men. Arch Environ Health *50:*31–37, 1995.
55. Levine F, Muenke M: VACTERL association with high prenatal lead exposure: Similarities to animal models of lead teratogenicity. Pediatrics *87:*390–392, 1991.
56. Kosnett MJ, Becker CE, Osterloh J, Kelly TJ, Pasta DJ: Factors influencing bone lead concentration in a suburban community assessed by noninvasive K X-ray fluorescence. JAMA *271:*197–203, 1994.
57. Hu H, Watanabe H, Payton M, et al: The relationship between blood lead and hemoglobin. JAMA *272:*1512–1517, 1994.
58. American Academy of Pediatrics Committee on Drugs: Treatment guidelines for lead exposure in children. Pediatrics *96:*155, 1995.
59. delaBurde B, Choate MS: Does asymptomatic lead exposure in children have latent sequelae? J Pediatr *81:*1088–1091, 1972.
60. Centers for Disease Control and Prevention: Preventing Lead Poisoning in Young Children. Atlanta, US Department of Health and Human Services, p 105, 1991.
61. Brown MJ, DeGiacomo JM, Gallagher G, et al: Lead poisoning in children of different ages. N Engl J Med *323:*135–136, 1990.
62. Shannon M, Graef JW: Lead intoxication in infancy. Pediatrics *89:*87–90, 1992.
63. McElvaine MD, DeUngria EG, Matte TD, et al: Prevalence of radiographic evidence of paint chip ingestion among children with moderate to severe lead poisoning, St. Louis, Missouri, 1989 through 1990. Pediatrics *89:*740–742, 1992.
64. Centers for Disease Control: Fatal pediatric poisoning from leaded paint—Wisconsin 1990. MMWR *40:*193–195, 1991.
65. Baker EL, Folland DS, Taylor TA, et al: Lead poisoning in children of lead workers—house contamination with industrial dust. N Engl J Med *296:*260–261, 1977.
66. Lockitch G, Berry B, Roland E, et al: Seizures in a 10-week-old infant: Lead poisoning from an unexpected source. Can Med Assoc J *145:*1465–1468, 1991.
67. Shannon M, Graef JW: Lead intoxication from lead-contaminated water used to reconstitute infant formula. Clin Pediatr *28:*380–382, 1989.
68. Levallois P, Lavoie M, Goulet L, et al: Blood lead levels in children and pregnant women living near a lead-reclamation plant. Can Med Assoc J *144:*877–885, 1991.
69. Centers for Disease Control: Lead poisoning associated with use of traditional ethnic remedies—California, 1991–1992. MMWR *42:*521–524, 1993.
70. Hugelmeyer CD, Moorhead JC, Horenblas L, Bayer MJ: Fatal lead encephalopathy following foreign body ingestion: Case report. J Emerg Med *6:*397–400, 1988.
71. Accardo P, Whitman B, Calu J, Rolfe U: Autism and plumbism—a possible association. Clin Pediatr *27:*41–44, 1988.
72. Cohen DJ, Johnson WT, Caparulo BK: Pica and elevated blood lead level in autistic and atypical children. Am J Dis Child *130:*47–48, 1976.
73. Shannon MW, Graef JW: Lead intoxication in children with pervasive developmental delays. Clin Toxicol *34:*177–181, 1996.
74. Mahaffey KR: Environmental lead toxicity: Nutrition as a component of intervention. Environ Health Perspect *89:*75–78, 1990.
75. Yaish HM, Niazi GA, Soby AA: Lead poisoning among Saudi children. Ann Saudi Med *13:*395–401, 1993.
76. Goldstein GW: Lead poisoning and brain cell function. Environ Health Perspect *89:*91–94, 1990.
77. Goldstein GW: Neurologic concepts of lead poisoning in children. Pediatr Ann *21:*384–388, 1992.

78. Byers RK, Lord EE: Effects of lead poisoning on mental development. Am J Dis Child *66:*471–494, 1943.
79. Baghurst PA, McMichael AJ, Wigg NR, et al: Environmental exposure to lead and children's intelligence at the age of seven years—the Port Pirie cohort study. N Engl J Med *327:*1279–1284, 1992.
80. Faust D, Brown J: Moderately elevated blood lead levels: Effects on neuropsychologic functioning in children. Pediatrics *80:*623–629, 1987.
81. McMichael AJ, Baghurst PA, Wigg NR, et al: Port Pirie cohort study: Environmental exposure to lead and children's abilities at the age of four years. N Engl J Med *319:*468–475, 1988.
82. Bellinger D, Leviton A, Allred E, Rabinowitz M: Pre- and postnatal lead exposure and behavior problems in school-aged children. Environ Res *66:*12–30, 1994
83. Needleman HL, Schell A, Bellinger D, et al: The long-term effects of exposure to low doses of lead in childhood—an 11-year follow-up report. N Engl J Med *322:*83–88, 1990.
84. Needleman HL, Riess JA, Tobin MJ, et al: Bone lead levels and delinquent behavior. JAMA *275:*363–369, 1996.
85. Sciarillo WG, Alexander G, Farrell KP: Lead exposure and child behavior. Am J Public Health *82:*1356–1360, 1992.
86. Baghurst PA, McMichael AJ, Tong S, et al: Exposure to environmental lead and visual-motor integration at age 7 years: The Port Pirie cohort study. Epidemiology *6:*104–109, 1995.
87. Fergusson DM, Horwood LJ: The effects of lead levels on the growth of word recognition in middle childhood. Int J Epidemiol *22:*891–897, 1993.
88. Bellinger D, Leviton A, Waternaux C, et al: Longitudinal analyses of prenatal and postnatal lead exposure and early cognitive development. N Engl J Med *316:*1037–1043, 1987.
89. Bellinger DC, Stiles KM, Needleman HL: Low-level lead exposure, intelligence and academic achievement: A long-term follow-up study. Pediatrics *90:*855–861, 1992.
90. Needleman HL, Gatsonis CA: Low-level lead exposure and the IQ of children—a meta-analysis of modern studies. JAMA *263:*673–678, 1990.
91. Greene T, Ernhart CB: Dentine lead and intelligence prior to school entry: A statistical sensitivity analysis. J Clin Epidemiol *46:*323–339, 1993.
92. Pocock SJ, Smith M, Baghurst P: Environmental lead and children's intelligence: A systematic review of the epidemiological evidence. BMJ *309:*1189–1197, 1994.
93. Schwartz J, Landrigan PJ, Feldman RG, et al: Threshold effect in lead-induced peripheral neuropathy. J Pediatr *112:*12–17, 1988.
94. Erenberg G, Rinsler SS, Fish BG: Lead neuropathy and sickle cell disease. Pediatrics *54:*438–441, 1974.
95. Schwartz J, Otto D: Lead and minor hearing impairment. Arch Environ Health *46:*300–305, 1987.
96. Schwartz J, Otto D: Blood lead hearing thresholds, and neurobehavioral development in children and youth. Arch Environ Health *42:*153–160, 1987.
97. Schwartz J, Otto D: Blood lead, hearing thresholds, and neurobehavioral development in children and youth. Arch Environ Health *42*:153–160, 1987.
98. Dietrich KN, Berger OG, Succop PA: Lead exposure and the motor developmental status of urban six-year-old children in the Cincinnati prospective study. Pediatrics *91:*301–307, 1993.
99. Needleman HL, Gunnoe C, Leviton A, et al: Deficits in psychologic and classroom performance of children with elevated dentine lead levels. N Engl J Med *300:*689–695, 1979.
100. Blickman JG, Wilkinson RH, Graef JW: The radiologic "lead band" revisited. Am J Radiol *146:*245–247, 1986.
101. Amitai Y, Brown MJ, Graef JW, Cosgrove E: Residential deleading: Effects on the blood lead levels of lead-poisoned children. Pediatrics *88:*893–897, 1991.
102. Chisolm JJ: The use of chelating agents in the treatment of acute and chronic lead intoxication in childhood. J Pediatr *73:*1–38, 1968.
103. Markowitz ME, Rose JF: Assessment of lead stores in children: Validation of an 8-hour CaNa2EDTA provocative test. J Pediatr *104:*337–341, 1984.
104. Markowitz ME, Rosen JF: Need for the lead mobilization test in children with lead poisoning. J Pediatr *119:*305–310, 1991.
105. Markowitz ME, Rosen JF, Bijur PE: Effects of iron deficiency on lead excretion in children with moderate lead intoxication. J Pediatr *116:*360–364, 1990
106. Weitzman M, Glotzer D: Lead poisoning. Pediatr Rev *13:*461–468, 1992.
107. Shannon M, Grace A, Graef J: Use of urinary lead concentration in interpretation of the EDTA mobilization test. Vet Hum Toxicol *31:*140–142, 1989.
108. Kassner J, Shannon M, Graef J: Role of forced diuresis of urinary lead excretion after the ethylenediaminetetraacetic acid mobilization test. J Pediatr *117:*914–916, 1990.
109. Walshe JM: Penicillamine, a new oral therapy for Wilson's disease. Am J Med *21:*487–495, 1956.
110. Liebelt EL, Shannon MW: Oral chelators for childhood lead poisoning. Pediatr Ann *23:*616–626, 1994.
111. Marcus SM: Experience with D-penicillamine in treating lead poisoning. Vet Hum Toxicol *24:*18–20, 1982.
112. Sachs HK, Blanksma LA, Murray EF, O'Connell MJ: Ambulatory treatment of lead poisoning: Report of 1155 cases. Pediatrics *46:*389–396, 1970.
113. Vitale LF, Rosalinas-Bailon A, Folland D, et al: Oral penicillamine therapy for chronic lead poisoning in children. J Pediatr *83:*1041–1045, 1973.
114. Shannon M, Grace A, Graef JW: Use of penicillamine in children with small lead burdens. N Engl J Med *321:*979–980, 1989.
115. Shannon M, Graef J, Lovejoy FH: Efficacy and toxicity of D-penicillamine in low-level lead poisoning. J Pediatr *112:*799–804, 1988.
116. Graziano JH, Lolacono NJ, Meyer P: Dose-response study of oral 2,3-dimercaptosuccinic acid in children with elevated blood lead concentrations. J Pediatr *113:*751–757, 1988.
117. Graziano JH, Lolacono NJ, Moulton T, et al: Controlled study of meso-2,3-dimercaptosuccinic acid for the management of childhood lead intoxication. J Pediatr *120:*133–139, 1992.
118. Liebelt EL, Shannon M, Graef JW: Efficacy of oral meso-2,3 dimercaptosuccinic acid therapy for low-level childhood plumbism. J Pediatr *124:*313–317, 1994.
119. Royce S, Rosenberg J: Chelation therapy in workers with lead exposure. West J Med *158:*372–375, 1993.
120. Besunder JB, Anderson RL, Super DM: Short-term efficacy of oral dimercaptosuccinic acid in children with low to moderate lead intoxication. Pediatrics *96:*683–687, 1995.
121. Chisolm JJ, Thomas DJ: Use of 2,3-dimercaptopropane-1-sulfonate in treatment of lead poisoning in children. J Pharmacol Exp Ther *235:*665–669, 1985.
122. Chisolm JJ: BAL, EDTA, DMSA and DMPS in the treatment of lead poisoning in children. Clin Toxicol *30:*493–504, 1992.
123. Ruff HA, Bijur PE, Markowitz M, et al: Declining blood lead levels and cognitive changes in moderately lead-poisoned children. JAMA *269:*1641–1646, 1993.
124. Weitzman M, Aaschengrau A, Bellinger D, et al: Lead-contaminated soil abatement and urban children's blood lead levels. JAMA *269:*1647–1654, 1993.
125. Rolfe PB, Marcinak JF, Nice AJ, Williams RH: Use of zinc protoporphyrin measured by the Protofluor-Z hematofluormeter in screening children for elevated blood lead levels. Am J Dis Child *147:*66–68, 1993.
126. Gellert GA, Wagner GA, Maxwell RM, et al: Lead poisoning among low-income children in Orange County, California—a need for regionally differentiated policy. JAMA *270:*69–71, 1993.
127. Schlenker TL, Fritz CJ, Mark D, et al: Screening for pediatric lead poisoning—comparability of simultaneously drawn capillary and venous blood samples. JAMA *271:*1346–1348, 1994.
128. Schoen EJ: Lead toxicity in the 21st century: Will we still be treating it? Pediatrics *90:*481–482, 1992.
129. Dowsett R, Shannon M: Childhood plumbism identified after lead poisoning in household pets. N Engl J Med *331:*1661–1662, 1994.
130. Bithoney WG, Vandeven AM, Ryan A: Elevated lead levels in reportedly abused children. J Pediatr *122:*719–720, 1993.
131. Flaherty EG: Risk of lead poisoning in abused and neglected children. Clin Pediatr *34:*128–132, 1995.
132. Wiley JF, Henretig FM, Selbst SM: Blood lead levels in children with foreign bodies. Pediatrics *89:*593–596, 1992.

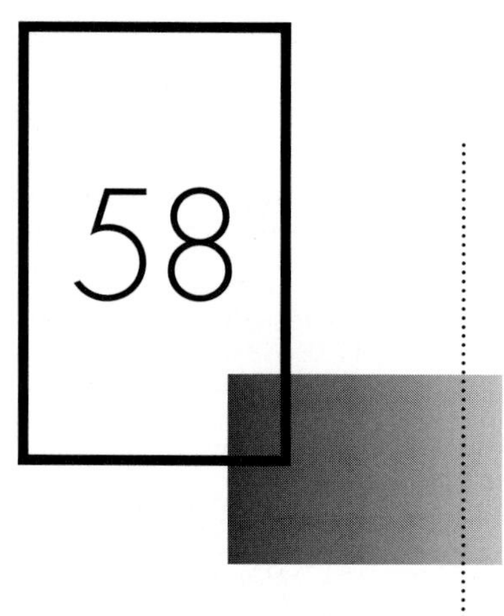

58 Arsenic and Arsine

ALAN H. HALL, MD

ARSENIC

Arsenic is found throughout the earth's crust and is a contaminant in a wide variety of metal ores.[1] Because some arsenical compounds are nearly tasteless and resemble sugar in appearance, they have been used as suicidal and homicidal poisons since the Middle Ages. Cases of this use of arsenic continue to be reported.[2–6] Arsenic has even been injected intravenously in suicide attempts.[7] Also, arsenic compounds were widely used as medicinals in the past.

Arsenic can be extracted in the smelting of copper, gold, lead, and zinc.[1, 8] It is used in metallurgy for hardening alloys of copper and lead, as a dopant in semiconductor production, in the manufacturing of pigments and some types of glass, and in rodenticides, pesticides, and fungicides.[8]

Arsenic compounds occur in various chemical states (a metallic form is not known to exist), including *trivalent* compounds (the most toxic and carcinogenic species), *pentavalent* compounds (species that are less toxic but that may be metabolically converted to trivalent arsenic following systemic absorption),[9, 10] and *organoarsenical* compounds, some of which are commonly called "fish arsenic" and are found in many seafood products. The organoarsenical compounds are generally considered to be nontoxic.[1] This lack of organoarsenical toxicity, however, is not seen with exposure to alkane arsenate herbicides, such as monosodium methane arsenate, which has caused shock as well as liver and kidney impairment following acute ingestion.[6]

In 1994, arsenic exposures represented 741 of 1,926,438 total poison exposures reported to the American Association of Poison Control Centers Toxic Exposure Surveillance System (TESS).[5] Of these, 358 were in children younger than 6 years of age, 91 were in patients aged 6 to 19 years, and 222 were in patients older than 19 years.[5] Of these 741 exposures, 721 were unintentional.

Health care facility evaluation was sought by 111 of these patients. During 1994, no arsenic-related deaths were reported for inclusion in the database. One patient developed major (life-threatening) symptoms, 17 patients developed moderate symptoms, and 93 patients developed minor symptoms; 119 arsenic-exposed patients remained asymptomatic (the outcome was unknown in 511 cases).[5] Single acute small ingestions of sodium arsenate (<5 mL of <3% solutions) found in formerly marketed ant baits did not result in serious toxicity in one study of 149 cases, although urine arsenic levels reported in this study were as high as 5819 μg per 24 hours.[11]

Pathophysiology

Pathophysiologic Mechanisms

The mechanisms of arsenic toxicity are thought to be the inhibition of sulfhydryl group–containing cellular enzymes and the replacement of phosphate molecules in "high-energy" compounds (so-called "arsenolysis").[12, 13] Trivalent arsenic compounds are more potent in inhibiting enzymes, whereas pentavalent compounds are involved in arsenolysis.[13]

Trivalent arsenic compounds are human carcinogens,[1, 8] causing tracheal and bronchogenic carcinomas, hepatic angiosarcomas,[14] and various skin cancers, such as intraepidermal carcinomas (Bowen's disease), squamous cell carcinomas, basal cell carcinomas, and "combined" forms of skin cancer (i.e., more than one type in the same patient).[12, 13, 15, 16] Myelogenous leukemia also may occur.[17] An increased risk of Hodgkin's disease was found in a cohort of arsenic-exposed French gold miners.[18]

Internal cancers also have been associated with

chronic ingestion of arsenical medications (e.g., Fowler's solution) or arsenic-contaminated drinking water.[14, 19, 20] With such exposures, increased risk of developing lung, liver, bladder, and kidney cancers has been found.[14, 19, 20]

Toxicokinetics

Sixty per cent to 90% of soluble arsenic compounds are absorbed from the gastrointestinal tract following ingestion; the percentage of a dose absorbed following inhalation is thought to be within this range.[13] Absorption through intact skin is usually negligible, but rare occupational accidents involving arsenic trichloride and arsenic acid have resulted in systemic poisoning.[13]

In *in vitro* studies and experimental animals, absorbed pentavalent arsenic is converted to the more toxic and carcinogenic trivalent form.[9, 21] In humans, absorbed inorganic pentavalent arsenic is biotransformed to trivalent arsenic. The trivalent arsenic then undergoes methylation to monomethylarsenate and dimethylarsenate, which are less toxic compounds that are excreted in the urine.[10] However, regardless of the magnitude of exposure, some amount of inorganic arsenic is always excreted unchanged in the urine.[22]

Water-soluble arsenic compounds such as organoarsenicals and sodium arsenate are rapidly excreted in the urine following absorption, and measurement of total urinary arsenic excretion shortly after exposure may not accurately reflect potential toxicity.[11] In human volunteers who ingested "fish" organoarsenic, elimination was biphasic, with a first-component half-life ($t_{1/2}$) of 6.9 to 11.0 hours (approximately 50% of the total dose) and a second-component $t_{1/2}$ of 75.7 hours.[10]

Toxic doses for various arsenic compounds have been estimated to be between 1 mg and 10 g. An arsenic trioxide dose of between 9 and 14 mg caused characteristic poisoning in a child[23]; an ingestion of 2150 mg of arsenic oxide did not prove fatal.[4] The potentially fatal human arsenic dose has been estimated to be between 1 and 4 mg/kg.

By 2 to 4 weeks after cessation of exposure, the remaining body burden of arsenic is found mainly in the skin, hair, and nails; lesser amounts are found in teeth and bone.[13] Arsenic is primarily excreted by the kidneys. Because arsenic is cleared rapidly from the blood, blood levels may become unmeasurable at a time when urine levels are still quite elevated.[13]

Clinical Presentation

Acute Exposure

Although most acute arsenic poisonings occur following ingestion, serious toxicity and peripheral neuropathy have rarely occurred following inhalation and dermal exposure.[24] In humans, acute arsenic ingestion characteristically makes an impact on the gastrointestinal tract. Although arsenic is noncorrosive (in contrast to some mercurial compounds), ingestion leads to oral irritation and a sensation of burning in the mouth and throat; this is followed by the development of nausea, vomiting, significant diarrhea, and extensive inflammation and necrosis of the lining of the stomach and intestine, which may lead to perforation.[13] Hemorrhagic gastroenteritis may occur in serious cases. Arsenic causes dilation of blood vessels and damages the vascular lining tissue, resulting in fluid leakage into the interstitial space ("third-spacing"); intravascular volume depletion and severe hypovolemic shock ensue if adequate fluid replacement is not sufficiently rapid.

A garlic-like odor may be noted on the patient's breath. Seizures have been observed in some patients.[25] Muscle twitches and spasms may ensue. Hepatic involvement later becomes evident, with multiple abnormalities in the liver profile. This is followed by kidney involvement and subsequent renal failure. In severe acute arsenic poisonings, multiple organ system failure may develop; rarely, adult respiratory distress syndrome may be seen.[26] Delirium, coma, and death may occur. Rapid onset of respiratory failure and asystole have occurred following ingestion.[27]

Peripheral polyneuropathy and bone marrow depression with anemia, leukopenia, or pancytopenia may be the late sequelae of acute arsenic poisoning.[13] Toxic delirium and encephalopathy may be seen.[28] A variety of electrocardiographic abnormalities demonstrate cardiac irregularities and arrhythmias. Visual disturbances, including "dimness" of vision, photophobia, and conjunctivitis have been described in some cases.[7, 25]

Arsenic crosses the placental barrier, and acute maternal arsenic poisoning during pregnancy has caused intrauterine fetal death.[26, 29] Some forms of arsenic are teratogenic in experimental animals.[30, 31]

Chronic Exposure

Symptomatic arsenic poisoning is not often seen in occupational exposure settings. Attempted homicide and deliberate long-term poisoning for the purpose of maintaining invalidism have resulted in chronic toxicity.[2] Skin pigmentation changes, palmar and plantar hyperkeratoses, gastrointestinal symptoms, anemia, and liver disease are common in chronically exposed persons.[13, 32]

Noncirrhotic portal hypertension with bleeding esophageal varices, splenomegaly, hypersplenism, and typical skin manifestations have been found in patients treated with Fowler's solution for psoriasis.[33] A metallic taste in the mouth and gastrointestinal disturbances may be reported by the patient. Mee's lines (white transverse bands in the nails) may be seen. Bone marrow depression with anemia, leukopenia, or pancytopenia is commonly found in patients with chronic arsenic poisoning.[13, 34]

Gangrene of the feet ("blackfoot disease") has been associated with chronic ingestion of arsenic-contaminated drinking water; Raynaud's phenomenon and acrocyanosis also may occur.[13] Toxic delirium and encephalopathy can be present in persons with chronic arsenic poisoning.[35]

In a group of Swedish copper smelter workers chronically exposed to mainly arsenic trioxide, subclinical nerve injuries were demonstrated by electrodiagnostic testing. These nerve injuries were dependent on long-term arsenic exposure rather than on short-term exposure–related level fluctuations.[36] Peripheral neuropathy is common in persons chronically exposed to arsenic-contaminated drinking water.[13, 32] When exposure is not immediately apparent, patients with arsenical peripheral neuropathy have been misdiagnosed as having Guillain-Barré syndrome.[37] Asymmetric bilateral phrenic neuropathy has been seen in chronic poisoning with arsenic-contaminated opium.[38]

Despite the general lack of a suitable experimental animal model, exposure to certain forms of arsenic either in the workplace or through chronic ingestion of arsenic-contaminated water or arsenical medications has been associated with the development of cancer, particularly that of the skin and lungs.[8, 13] The International Agency for Research on Cancer (IARC) has stated that there is sufficient evidence for arsenic carcinogenicity in humans.[8]

Evaluation and Treatment

Clinical Evaluation

The exposure source may not be determined in up to 50% of arsenic poisoning cases.[13] Especially in cases of homicidal or environmental exposure, the patient may have no idea that arsenic exposure is occurring.

Medical history-taking should address such topics as patients' home heating methods (e.g., patients should be questioned about whether they burn arsenic-treated wood in woodstoves or fireplaces); drinking water source; gardening, farming, or forestry activities (owing to the potential for exposure to arsenical pesticides); use of folk, herbal, or naturopathic medications; location of residence in relation to agricultural or industrial activities (present or past); usual diet; and occupational history.[13] The physician should perform a thorough physical examination, seeking the stigmata described earlier.

Laboratory Evaluation

The best test for confirmation of excessive arsenic exposure is a 24-hour urine collection and analysis, although spot urine measurements may be helpful for emergent diagnosis. When seafood containing fish arsenic has not been recently ingested, urinary excretion of greater than 100 μg per 24 hours is usually abnormal. Also, values less than 50 μg/L are considered normal, whereas those greater than 200 μg/L are abnormal.[13] When seafood is ingested, urinary arsenic levels may transiently increase to 200 to 1700 μg/L.[39] The usual measurement is of total urinary arsenic. When available, laboratory arsenic speciation into organic versus inorganic levels can assist in determining the actual potential for significant toxicity.

Analysis of arsenic in hair or nails is generally not useful in evaluating individual patients. Such testing may be useful to confirm exposure in population or epidemiologic studies.

As arsenic is radiopaque, its presence in the gastrointestinal tract may be determined by abdominal radiography.[40] A negative result, however, does not rule out significant exposure.

Screening and other diagnostic tests can be useful in the evaluation of arsenic-exposed patients.[13] These include a complete blood count with peripheral smear, liver and renal function tests, and urinalysis. Chest radiography and electrocardiography or cardiac monitoring may be useful in some circumstances. Nerve conduction velocity and bone marrow biopsy may be indicated if significant peripheral neuropathy or bone marrow depression is present.

Treatment

The treatment of arsenic poisoning consists of supportive measures and chelation therapy. Although many clinicians prefer to start chelation therapy as soon as possible, fluid loss (and potential blood loss) and direct cardiac toxicity resulting in hypovolemia, cardiogenic shock, or arrhythmias are responsible for fatalities early in the course of acute arsenic poisoning. Continuous electrocardiographic monitoring is required. The clinician must adequately assess volume status by following hourly urine output. Invasive central venous pressure or cardiac output monitoring may be required in severe poisoning cases.

Supportive Measures

Exposed skin and eyes should be copiously flushed with water or normal saline. Patients with inhalation exposure should be moved to fresh air, and supplemental oxygen administered if required.

Following ingestion, gastric lavage is recommended. If the patient is not obtunded or experiencing seizures, whole-bowel irrigation with polyethylene glycol solution may be indicated if abdominal radiography demonstrates the presence of arsenic in the lower bowel.[40] Activated charcoal may not adsorb significant amounts of arsenic,[41] but its use is frequently recommended. Cathartics should be withheld in patients with renal compromise, diarrhea, hemorrhagic gastroenteritis, suspected bowel perforation, or ileus.

Hypotension usually occurs secondary to hypovolemia, and the use of vasopressors should be considered only after fluid replacement efforts have failed to increase the blood pressure to acceptable levels. Transfusion of blood or blood products is indicated only if there is evidence of bleeding or significant hemolysis. Standard antiarrhythmic and anticonvulsant medications can be given if cardiac arrhythmias or seizures are present. If hemolysis occurs, alkalization of the urine with sodium bicarbonate infused in intravenous fluids may protect the kidneys from damage by red blood cell breakdown products.

Chelation Therapy

Chelators that have been used clinically in arsenic poisoning include dimercaprol (British antilewisite; BAL), D-penicillamine, dimercaptosuccinic acid DMSA (Succimer), and dimercaptopropanesulfonic acid (DMPS). One source suggests beginning chelation therapy in asymptomatic patients with urinary arsenic concentrations of 200 μg/L,[42] but another cautions that this may be unnecessary with ingestion of rapidly excreted arsenic compounds such as fish arsenic and sodium arsenate.[11] Chelation is generally ineffective for treating established arsenical peripheral neuropathies and may not prevent their development in all cases.

Dimercaprol is given by deep intramuscular injection at a dose of 3 to 5 mg/kg every 4 to 12 hours until the symptoms resolve or until another chelating agent is substituted. Adverse effects include pain at the injection site, hypertension, tachycardia, anorexia, restlessness, vomiting, excessive salivation, fever, and rarely, seizures. Treatment courses of 5 days each are usual.

D-Penicillamine is given orally at a dose of 25 mg/kg four times daily, up to a total dose of 1 g/d. Although the drug has a number of adverse effects during use in the long-term therapy of other conditions, these effects are seldom seen during metal chelation. Some cross-reactivity with penicillin may occur, and other drugs are best considered for penicillin-allergic patients.

D-Penicillamine has only one arsenic binding site, whereas the other chelators have two sites. Treatment courses of 7 to 10 days each are usual.

Dimercaptosuccinic acid is not currently labeled by the Food and Drug Administration for use in arsenic poisoning, but it has been used successfully in acute poisoning cases.[6] It is usually given in the same doses recommended for childhood lead poisoning: 10 mg/kg per m^2 every 8 hours for 5 days, followed thereafter by the same dose every 12 hours for 14 days. Adverse effects have included transient increases in liver function test results, vesicular eruption on the mucosa, rash, pruritus, nausea, vomiting, diarrhea, drowsiness, paresthesias, sore throat, rhinorrhea, and a sulfurous odor on the breath.

Dimercaptopropanesulfonic acid has been used in Europe at an adult oral dose of 100 mg given three times daily for 3 weeks to 9 months.[43, 44]

The efficacy of and therapeutic endpoints for chelation therapy are usually assessed on the basis of periodic 24-hour urine testing for arsenic. An increase in arsenic excretion with resumption of chelation after a "drug holiday" of 2 days or longer may be an indication for further chelation therapy.

Extracorporeal Elimination Techniques

Hemodialysis is useful for supportive treatment and should be initiated if any degree of renal failure occurs, as the kidneys are the primary route of arsenic excretion. Its use for active extracorporeal removal of absorbed arsenic remains controversial. In one case report, however, hemodialysis seemed to be efficacious and removed arsenic bound to erythrocytes; there was no significant difference in dialysis arsenic clearance when dimercaprol was administered.[45]

Disposition

Arsenic-exposed patients who are asymptomatic should receive basic decontamination and should be observed in a controlled setting for 4 to 6 hours. If the patients remain asymptomatic, they may then be discharged home with instructions to return to the hospital immediately if any symptoms develop.

Patients who are either symptomatic on admission or who develop symptoms during initial observation require hospital admission. Those with vital sign derangements or evidence of significant arsenic poisoning should be admitted to an intensive care unit.

Following complete symptom resolution, patients should have outpatient followup arranged to ensure that renal and liver functions and hematopoiesis have returned to normal and to screen for the possible late development of peripheral neuropathy or encephalopathy.

Until the source of arsenic exposure has been identified by public health officials, it may not be advisable to discharge patients from the hospital, as re-exposure might occur.[13] If the exposure was occupational, the patient should be considered as a possible index case, and the proper authorities should be notified so that a workplace evaluation can be done.

ARSINE

Arsine is a nonirritating, colorless, heavier-than-air gas with an odor of garlic.[8] It is widely used as a dopant gas in the semiconductor industry (it is mixed with gallium to form gallium arsenide), and it may also be generated when acids come into contact with arsenic residues or when water acts on metallic arsenide compounds.[1, 8] Exposures may occur during the refining of metal, the galvanizing of lead, lead plating, and soldering operations.

Pathophysiology

Pathophysiologic Mechanisms

Arsine depletes erythrocyte glutathione stores, resulting in cell membrane instability and rapidly causing massive intravascular hemolytic anemia in the presence of negative results on Coombs' test. Deposition of erythrocyte breakdown products in the renal tubules results in acute renal failure.[1, 8]

Toxicokinetics

Inhalation of an airborne concentration of 250 ppm or greater may cause death within 30 minutes after exposure, whereas more lengthy exposure to 10 to 50 ppm may still cause fatality due to hemolytic anemia.[8] A cumulative effect may occur with long-term exposure to low arsine concentrations.[8] Following arsine absorption, the compound is oxidized to elemental trivalent arsenic and arsenous oxide, compounds known to be human carcinogens.[8]

Clinical Presentation

With the onset of intravascular hemolysis, possible initial symptoms include headache, lightheadedness, malaise, weakness, thirst, muscle cramping, abdominal and flank pain, nausea, vomiting, and occasionally, hypotension. Excretion of dark-red urine frequently develops 4 to 6 hours after exposure; 24 to 48 hours thereafter, what may appear to be jaundice but is actually bronzing of the skin is observed. There may be a latent period of up to 24 hours before symptom onset.[46]

Subsequently, acute renal failure secondary to kidney damage from tubular deposition of erythrocyte breakdown products may develop. Pulmonary edema and congestive heart failure may occasionally occur. Electrocardiographic abnormalities have been noted, and delayed neurologic sequelae such as peripheral polyneuropathy and encephalopathy have been described.

An unusual case of arsine poisoning occurred following chronic exposure to the gas generated by the cleaning of automotive parts contaminated with arsenical herbicides in a mixed acid bath. The patient developed chronic arsenicalism manifested by malaise, nausea, headache, peripheral neuropathies, liver dysfunction, marked leukopenia, and Mee's lines in the fingernails.[47]

Evaluation and Treatment

Clinical Evaluation

The triad of abdominal pain, hematuria, and bronzing of the skin is characteristic of arsine poisoning. A garlic-like odor may be present on the patient's breath. The conjunctivae may be stained a red color.

Laboratory Evaluation

Hyperkalemia is common with massive hemolysis, and vomiting may cause fluid and electrolyte losses; thus, serum electrolyte levels must be monitored. Also, determination of plasma free hemoglobin, hemoglobin, and hematocrit can be used to guide transfusion or exchange transfusion decisions. A Coombs' test may be useful for ruling out other causes of hemolytic anemia.

Dipstick test results are positive for the presence of blood in the urine, but microscopic examination does not reveal intact erythrocytes. Urine output, blood urea nitrogen level, and serum creatinine concentration should be monitored.

Treatment

Transfusion, exchange transfusion, and hemodialysis (for supportive therapy, if renal failure develops) are the treatments of choice for acute arsine poisoning. Exchange transfusion may be considered when plasma free hemoglobin levels are greater than 1.5 g/dL. However, simple transfusion may be an adequate treatment and is much easier to accomplish.

Supportive Measures

Urine alkalization with sodium bicarbonate infused with intravenous fluids, as well as maintenance of a brisk urine flow may help prevent kidney damage caused by red blood cell breakdown products. If hyperkalemia develops, measures must be taken to maintain normal serum potassium levels. Urine output should be monitored, and electrocardiography performed. Chest radiographs should be obtained, and invasive monitoring considered if pulmonary edema or congestive heart failure are suspected.

Chelation Therapy

The place of chelation therapy in acute arsine poisoning, if any, is unclear. An increase in urinary arsenic excretion may be produced in acute arsine poisoning by chelating agents, but dimercaprol administration does not protect against development of hemolysis, even when given soon after exposure.[48] However, in one case of chronic arsine exposure with resultant arsenicalism, administration of D-penicillamine was associated with amelioration of typical arsenic poisoning symptoms.[47]

Extracorporeal Elimination Techniques

Hemodialysis may be required as supportive treatment for patients who develop renal failure secondary to massive hemolysis.

Disposition

Arsine-exposed patients who are asymptomatic should receive basic decontamination and should be observed in a controlled setting for 4 to 6 hours. If they remain asymptomatic, patients may then be discharged home with instructions to return to the hospital immediately if any symptoms or urine discoloration develop.

Patients who are either symptomatic on admission or who develop symptoms during initial observation require hospital admission. Those with vital sign derangements or evidence of hemolysis should be admitted to an intensive care unit.

Following complete symptom resolution, patients should have outpatient followup arranged to ensure that renal function has returned to normal and hematopoiesis is normal, as well as to screen for the possible late development of rare peripheral neuropathy or encephalopathy.

References

1. Gochfeld M: Chemical agents. *In* Brooks S, Gochfeld M, Herzstein J, et al (eds): Environmental Medicine. St. Louis, C.V. Mosby Co., pp 592–614, 1995.
2. Hutton JT, Christians BL, Dippel RL: Arsenic poisoning. N Engl J Med *307*:1080, 1982.
3. Levin-Scherz JK, Patrick JD, Weber FH, Garabedian C: Acute arsenic ingestion. Ann Emerg Med *16*:702, 1987.
4. Fesmire FM, Schauben JL, Roberge RJ: Survival following massive arsenic ingestion. Am J Emerg Med *6*:602, 1988.
5. Litovitz TL, Felberg L, Soloway RA, et al: 1994 Annual Report of the American Association of Poison Control Centers Toxic Exposure Surveillance System. Am J Emerg Med *13*:551, 1995.
6. Shum S, Whitehead J, Vaughn L, et al: Chelation of organoarsenate with dimercaptosuccinic acid. Vet Hum Toxicol *37*:239, 1995.
7. DiNapoli J, Hall AH, Drake R, Rumack BH: Cyanide and arsenic poisoning by intravenous injection. Am J Emerg Med *18*:308, 1989.
8. Hathaway GJ, Proctor NH, Hughes JP, Fischman ML: Arsenic and arsine. *In* Proctor and Hughes' Chemical Hazards of the Workplace. 3rd ed. New York, Van Nostrand Reinhold Co., pp 92–96, 1991.
9. Tsukamoto H, Parker HR, Peoples SA: Metabolism and renal handling of sodium arsenate in dogs. Am J Vet Res *44*:2331, 1983.
10. Johnson LR, Farmer JG: Use of human metabolic studies and urinary arsenic speciation in assessing arsenic exposure. Bull Environ Contam Toxicol *46*:53, 1991.
11. Kingston RL, Hall S, Sioris L: Clinical observations and medical outcome in 149 cases of arsenate ant killer ingestion. Clin Toxicol *31*:581, 1993.
12. Schoolmeester WL, White DR: Arsenic poisoning. South Med J *73*:198, 1980.
13. Agency for Toxic Substances and Disease Registry (ATSDR): ATSDR Case Studies in Environmental Medicine. Atlanta, Agency for Toxic Substances and Disease Registry, 1990.
14. Bates MN, Smith AH, Hopenhayn-Rich C: Arsenic ingestion and internal cancers: A review. Am J Epidemiol *135*:462, 1992.
15. Rees I, Adelman M, Pratilas V: Chronic arsenic poisoning. Anesthesiology *51*:84, 1979.
16. Popper H, Thomas LB, Telles NC, Falk H: Development of hepatic angiosarcoma in man induced by vinylchloride, Thorotrast, or arsenic. Am J Pathol *92*:349, 1978.
17. Kjeldsberg CR, Ward HP: Leukemia in arsenic poisoning. Ann Intern Med *77*:935, 1972.
18. Simonato L, Moulin JJ, Javelaud B, et al: A retrospective mortality study of workers exposed to arsenic in a gold mine and refinery in France. Am J Ind Med *25*:625, 1994.
19. Cuzick J, Sasieni P, Evans S: Ingested arsenic, keratoses, and bladder cancer. Am J Epidemiol *136*:417, 1992.
20. Chiou HY, Hsueh YM, Liaw KF, et al: Incidence of internal cancers and ingested inorganic arsenic: A seven-year followup study in Taiwan. Cancer Res *55*:1296, 1995.
21. Bertolero F, Pozzi G, Sabbioni E, Saffiotti U: Cellular uptake and metabolic reduction of pentavalent to trivalent arsenic as determinants of cytotoxicity and morphological transformation. Carcinogenesis *8*:803, 1987.
22. Hopenhayn-Rich C, Smith AH, Goeden HM: Human studies do not support the methylation threshold hypothesis for the toxicity of inorganic arsenic. Environ Res *60*:161, 1993.
23. Watson WA, Veltri JC, Metcalf TJ: Acute arsenic exposure treated with oral D-penicillamine. Vet Hum Toxicol *23*:164, 1981.
24. Hessl SM, Berman E: Severe peripheral neuropathy after exposure to monosodium methyl arsenate. J Toxicol Clin Toxicol *19*:281, 1982.
25. Peterson RG, Rumack BH: D-Penicillamine therapy of acute arsenic poisoning. J Pediatr *91*:661, 1977.
26. Bolliger CT, van Zijl P, Louw JA: Multiple organ failure with the adult respiratory distress syndrome in homicidal arsenic poisoning. Respiration *59*:57, 1992.
27. Moore DF, O'Callaghan CA, Berlyne G: Acute arsenic poisoning: Absence of polyneuropathy after treatment with 2,3-dimercaptopropanesulphonate (DMPS). J Neurol Neurosurg Psychiatry *57*:1133, 1994.
28. Quatrehomme G, Ricq O, Lapalus P: Acute arsenic intoxication: Forensic and toxicologic aspects (an observation). J Forensic Sci *37*:1163, 1992.
29. Lugo G, Cassady G, Palmisano P: Acute maternal arsenic intoxication with neonatal death. Am J Dis Child *117*:328, 1969.
30. Ferm VH, Saxon A, Smith BM: The teratogenic profile of sodium arsenate in the golden hamster. Arch Environ Health *22*:557, 1971.
31. Morrissey RE, Mottet NK: Arsenic-induced exencephalopathy in the mouse and associated lesions occurring during neurulation. Teratology *28*:399, 1983.
32. Mazumder DN, Das Gupta J, Chakraborty AK, et al: Environmental pollution and chronic arsenicosis in south Calcutta. Bull World Health Organ *70*:481, 1992.
33. Nevens F, Fevery J, van Steenbergen W, et al: Arsenic and non-cirrhotic portal hypertension: A report of eight cases. J Hepatol *11*:80, 1990.
34. Rezuke WN, Anderson C, Pastuszak WT: Arsenic intoxication presenting as a myelodysplastic syndrome: A case report. Am J Hematol *26*:291, 1991.
35. Morton WE, Caron GA: Encephalopathy: An uncommon manifestation of workplace arsenic poisoning? Am J Ind Med *15*:1, 1989.
36. Lagerkvist BJ, Zetterlund B: Assessment of exposure to arsenic among smelter workers: A five-year followup. Am J Ind Med *25*:477, 1994.
37. Goddard MJ, Tanhehco JL, Dau PC: Chronic arsenic poisoning masquerading as Landry-Guillain-Barré syndrome. Electromyogr Clin Neurophysiol *32*:419, 1992.
38. Bansal HK, Haldar N, Dhand UK: Phrenic neuropathy in arsenic poisoning. Chest *100*:878, 1991.
39. Baselt RC, Cravey RH: Arsenic. *In* Baselt RC, Cravey RH (eds): Disposition of Toxic Drugs and Chemicals in Man. 3rd ed. Chicago, Year Book Medical Publishers, 1989.
40. Lee DC, Roberts JR, Kelly JJ: Whole-bowel irrigation as an adjunct in the treatment of radiopaque arsenic. Am J Emerg Med *13*:244, 1995.
41. Al-Mahasneh QM, Rodgers GC, Benz FW: Activated charcoal (AC) as an adsorbent for inorganic arsenic: Study in rats. Vet Hum Toxicol *32*:351, 1990.
42. Kersjes MP, Maurer JR, Trestrail JH: An analysis of arsenic exposures referred to the Blodgett Regional Poison Center. Vet Hum Toxicol *29*:75, 1987.
43. Kew J, Morris C, Aihie A: Arsenic and mercury intoxication due to Indian ethnic remedies. BMJ *306*:506, 1993.
44. Goebel HH, Schmidt PF, Bohl J: Polyneuropathy due to acute arsenic intoxication: Biopsy studies. J Neuropathol Exp Neurol *49*:137, 1990.
45. Mathieu D, Mathieu-Nolf M, Germain-Alonso M, et al: Massive arsenic poisoning: Effect of hemodialysis and dimercaprol on arsenic kinetics. Intensive Care Med *18*:47, 1992.
46. Kleinfeld MJ: Arsine poisoning. J Occup Med *22*:820, 1980.
47. Risk M, Fuortes L: Chronic arsenicalism suspected from arsine exposure: A case report and literature review. Vet Hum Toxicol *33*:590, 1991.
48. Fowler BA, Weissberg JF: Arsine poisoning. N Engl J Med *291*:1171, 1974.

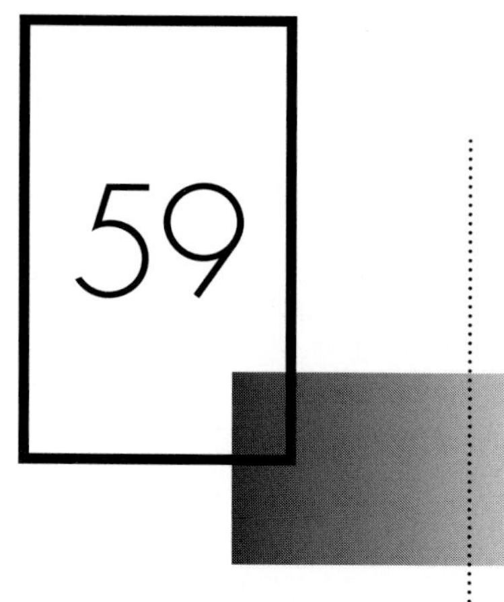

The Toxicology of Other Heavy Metals

MICHAEL W. SHANNON, MD, MPH

SPECIFIC AGENTS

Aluminum

Aluminum is the most abundant metal in the earth's crust. It has no known essential human function. Exposure to aluminum occurs through a number of mechanisms. Contaminated drinking water, aluminum cans, containers, and cooking utensils all are important sources of daily aluminum. Dermal exposure to the metal occurs regularly from aluminum-containing deodorants. There is also general exposure by inhalation of atmospheric aluminum.

The body absorbs less than 1% of an ingested aluminum dose. The body burden of 30 to 40 mg is kept low by renal homeostatic mechanisms. Normal plasma aluminum level is 5 to 10 μg/L. Aluminum is concentrated in the bones and liver.[1] Because excretion of aluminum is primarily renal, aluminum intoxication is a risk in those who have renal insufficiency and are taking aluminum-containing antacids (although elevated plasma aluminum concentrations have been found in those with normal renal function who were taking aluminum antacids).[2] Aluminum toxicity is characterized by encephalopathy, microcytic anemia, and osteomalacia. *Dialysis encephalopathy* is attributed to accumulation of aluminum,[2] as is dialysis osteodystrophy. These illnesses largely disappeared once aluminum was removed from the water used to prepare dialysate.[1]

Two fatalities due to aluminum were reported when a cement containing aluminum-calcium fluorosilicate was used for bone reconstruction after middle ear surgery. In both cases, refractory status epilepticus occurred, and death resulted despite deferoxamine chelation.[3]

Aluminum toxicity is treated with supportive care, diuresis, and, when necessary, with the chelator deferoxamine.

Antimony

Antimony is a silver-gray metal with an atomic weight of 121.8. It belongs to the same periodic table group as arsenic and resembles this heavy metal in its clinical manifestations.[4] Antimony exists primarily in two valence states, Sb^{+3} and Sb^{+5}. Another form of antimony, stibine (antimony hydride, SbH_3), is an extremely toxic gas. Antimony is used in the textile industry, to harden lead, as an alloy with copper or tin, and in glass manufacture. Therefore, occupations including metallurgy, welding, and zinc etching involve use of antimony. Antimony tartrate and sodium stibogluconate are still prescribed as antibiotics for treatment of leishmaniasis and schistosomiasis.

Antimony compounds are rapidly and completely absorbed from the lungs after inhalation. Gastrointestinal (GI) absorption is less efficient, and only 10% to 20% of an oral dose is absorbed. Distribution and organ concentration are dependent on valence form: Pentavalent antimony has no significant binding to blood elements and is concentrated in the heart, liver, and thyroid. In contrast, trivalent antimony is more than 90% bound to red blood cells.[5] Pentavalent antimony is quickly excreted from the body through the kidneys. After a single dose, more than 95% can be recovered in the urine within 24 hours. The elimination half-life of pentavalent antimony is 2 to 4 hours. Trivalent antimony is primarily excreted through the feces as a result of biliary secretion; only about 25% of a dose can be recovered in the urine. With trivalent antimony, the distribution half-life is 30 hours and the terminal half-life is 40 days.[6]

The mechanism of antimony's toxicity is unclear but may be related to its inhibition of thiol-containing enzymes.[4] The manifestations of antimony intoxication are variable, depending on its form and the route of exposure. After ingestion, the most prominent manifestations of antimony intoxication are vomiting, diarrhea, and abdominal pain (cholera stibie). Severe fluid and electrolyte disturbances can quickly ensue. After acute inhalation, both forms of antimony can produce severe respiratory tract irritation; high-concentration exposures can result in pulmonary edema. Other manifestations of acute toxicity include cardiovascular disturbances (QT prolongation and T wave abnormalities) and liver function abnormalities.

Chronic intoxication with antimonials has been associated with a different clinical picture. For example, epistaxis of unclear cause is a common presenting complaint. Occupational exposure produces a pneumoconiosis that resembles silicosis. A cardiomyopathy can develop. *Antimony spots* are distinctive white spots on a pustular base. They appear distinctively on parts of the skin with a high concentration of sweat glands. Death due to either acute or chronic antimony intoxication results from multiorgan failure.

Stibine is an odorless and colorless gas. Similar to arsine gas, it is capable of producing massive intravascular hemolysis, which results in hemoglobinuria and acute renal failure.

Diagnosis is based on urinary measurement for pentavalent antimony exposure and blood measurement for trivalent compound (although urinary trivalent antimony levels have some value). Twenty-four-hour urine collections should be obtained. Laboratory assessment includes evaluation of pulmonary function, a chest radiograph (after inhalation exposure), an electrocardiogram, and liver function tests.

Treatment of antimony exposure begins with aggressive supportive care. Activated charcoal has been recommended after ingestion, although it is doubtful whether a significant degree of adsorption occurs.[4] Fluid and electrolyte values should be closely monitored because of the risk of excessive GI losses. Chelation therapy, if initiated early, appears to improve the clinical course.[4] Agents that have been advocated include dimercaprol (BAL), dimercaptosuccinic acid (DMSA), and dimercaptopropanesulfonic acid (DMPS).[4] Treatment of stibine exposure consists of immediate removal from the toxic site, supportive care, alkalization of the urine, and exchange transfusion.

Barium

Barium is a heavy metal that is best known as a contrast agent for radiographic studies. Because of its density (molecular weight 137), it is a metal that x-rays do not readily penetrate, thus providing a mechanism for visualizing visceral lesions. This particular form of barium, barium sulfate, is insoluble and has no human toxicity when ingested. However, barium is also commonly used as a pesticide (rodenticide or insecticide). Although safer pesticides have permitted the phaseout of barium carbonate for this indication, barium carbonate is still used in other countries, where it continues to pose the hazard of inadvertent food contamination (particularly contamination of flour) and inadvertent clinical toxicity.[7] Other forms of barium are used industrially, including barium hydroxide, barium chlorate, barium chloride, barium fluoride, barium acetate, barium sulfide, and barium hexafluorosilicate. These chemicals are used in the manufacture of matches, explosives, and glass.

Soluble barium compounds are well absorbed after ingestion or inhalation, with peak serum levels occurring within 2 hours. The elimination half-life in serum is approximately 4 days. As much as 93% of an absorbed barium dose is ultimately sequestered in bone rather than eliminated from the body.

The onset of symptoms after barium exposure is rapid. The first signs of exposure are GI and consist of epigastric pain, nausea, vomiting, and watery diarrhea.[7, 8]

Barium intoxication is characterized by a severe, potentially fatal hypokalemia. Serum potassium concentrations of less than 0.8 mEq/L may occur.[7, 8] Either ingestion or inhalation of barium can produce this effect; patients usually have a corresponding hypokalemic paralysis.[8] The cause of this hypokalemia is a shift of potassium into cells, which results from a specific effect on potassium channels. According to current theories, barium salts block potassium channels that permit the normal efflux of potassium. With potassium uptake unaffected, hypokalemia results. Barium has no identified action on the sodium-potassium pump.[9]

The clinical picture of barium ingestion consists of initial GI toxicity followed by the sudden onset of areflexia and motor weakness that involves all extremities. Consciousness is not altered, and anal sphincter tone is typically preserved.[8] Trismus has also been described.[10] The degree of hypokalemia does not correspond to the degree of weakness.[8] Serious electrocardiographic changes may occur, including atrioventricular dissociation or QRS widening; U waves are often present. These can be associated with the development of fatal ventricular fibrillation.[9,11] Other clinical features include bradycardia, ventricular premature beats, rhabdomyolysis, hypophosphatemia, and acute renal failure. The duration of paralysis ranges from 8 hours to 5 days.[8] The estimated lethal dose of barium is 900 mg, although doses of 0.2 to 0.5 mg/kg have resulted in life-threatening toxicity.[8] Children seem to have greater tolerance to barium than adults, and typically develop toxicity that is confined to GI symptoms.[9]

Long-term barium inhalation can produce a benign pneumoconiosis known as *baritosis*.[8] Diagnosis is based on a history of barium exposure. Even in the absence of history, the triad of GI upset, weakness, and profound hypokalemia limits the diagnosis to barium intoxication. Other syndromes of hypokalemia, including those resulting from exposure to β_2-adrenergic agonists, theophylline, and chloroquine, do not have the other clinical signs as a prominent feature. Abrupt paralysis due to toxins including tetrodotoxin and tick paralysis should not be associated with hypokalemia. Important laboratory tests include a complete blood count and measurement of electrolytes, blood urea nitrogen, blood sugar, and serum creatinine, calcium, and phosphorus. Determinations of urinary potassium, arterial blood gas, and muscle enzymes (creatine phosphokinase and aldolase) and liver function tests have also been recommended.[8] An electrocardiogram is essential in order to identify potassium-induced cardiac disturbances. Toxicity can also be identified by measurement of serum barium levels (normal levels, 3 to 29 μg/dL[9]).

Treatment of barium exposure begins with assessment of respiration and circulation. After barium inhalation, intervention begins by transporting the victim to fresh air and giving supplemental oxygen if there is any concern about hypoxia. Because of the possibility of severe skeletal muscle weakness leading to respiratory embarrassment, the need for assisted ventilation should be anticipated. Cardiac disturbances should be treated according to advanced cardiac life support algorithms. For barium ingestions, GI decontamination should be performed. Gastric lavage with the cathartic sodium sulfate or magnesium sulfate precipitates soluble barium compounds as insoluble barium sulfate and theoretically prevents further absorption. Although no data prove efficacy, the absence of significant toxicity from the use of these cathartics argues for their use. Activated charcoal does not adsorb significant amounts of barium and should not be administered.[9] Another decontamination option is whole-bowel irrigation. Decontamination can be guided by abdominal radiographs, which can visualize barium. Potassium supplementation should be provided to those with significant hypokalemia, particularly those with corresponding electrocardiographic disturbances. Potassium doses of up to 400 mEq may be required within the first 24 hours.[9] Because total-body potassium is preserved in barium intoxication, serum potassium levels should be closely monitored during supplementation in order to prevent hyperkalemia, which could occur as clinical toxicity abates; however, animal studies suggest that iatrogenic hyperkalemia is well tolerated after barium-induced hypokalemia.[9] Although researchers have also recommended intravenous administration of magnesium sulfate in order to render circulating barium insoluble, this risks precipitation of barium in renal tubules. Barium can be removed by hemodialysis.[8] However, the indications for this procedure have not been clearly established.

Beryllium

Beryllium is a potent human toxin. Coal combustion has become the principal source of environmental beryllium.[12] However, occupational exposure is the most common source of severe beryllium intoxication.

Beryllium had its first widespread use in the manufacture of fluorescent lights. Shortly after its use for this purpose began in the 1930s, beryllium-related pneumonitis became epidemic. The term *Salem sarcoid* was coined because Salem, Massachusetts, was a major site for fluorescent bulb manufacture and because the pulmonary disease resembled that of sarcoid.[12] Beryllium currently is used primarily in the aerospace and nuclear industries. Toxic forms of beryllium include elemental beryllium, beryllium oxide, beryllium fluoride, and beryllium copper.

Acute Exposure. Beryllium is a respiratory irritant that can cause conjunctivitis, periorbital edema, pharyngitis, tracheobronchitis, and pneumonitis. Dermal exposure can produce a marked dermatitis. However, pulmonary signs are most prominent. Common features include dyspnea, productive cough, chest pain, rales, and cyanosis. Marked infiltrates may be seen on chest radiographs, and hypoxia may occur at rest.[12]

Long-Term Exposure. Berylliosis is a systemic granulomatous disease resulting from long-term exposure.[12] It can appear anytime from a few months to 25 years after regular exposure. Noncaseating granulomas may appear in the liver, spleen, lymph nodes, heart, kidneys, bone, salivary glands, and skin. However, the primary target organ is the lung. Pulmonary manifestations include dyspnea, rales, chest pain, and clubbing. Patients may present with right ventricular heart failure (cor pulmonale). Pulmonary function tests reveal evidence of either restrictive or obstructive lung disease. Chest radiographs characteristically demonstrate diffuse infiltrates and hilar adenopathy. The pulmonary toxicity of beryllium almost certainly represents a type IV immune-mediated hypersensitivity phenomenon.[12] A unique aspect of beryllium's toxicity is its extremely slow elimination from the lungs.[12]

The diagnosis of berylliosis is usually based on a history of beryllium exposure. However, berylliosis can be identical to sarcoidosis in appearance, and an extensive evaluation is required to distinguish the two.

Treatment of berylliosis is largely confined to supportive care. Corticosteroids may improve pulmonary symptoms. Lung transplantation is a potential intervention for progressive respiratory failure.

Bismuth

Bismuth has a molecular weight of 208.9; it is found in the Vb group of elements, with antimony and arsenic. Bismuth is adjacent to lead in molecular weight. Its current use is limited to ingestion for antidiarrheal effects (bismuth subsalicylate [Pepto-Bismol]). Because it is water insoluble, poorly absorbed from the gut, and rapidly excreted in urine, bismuth accumulation rarely occurs despite excess use.[13]

The kinetics of bismuth are not completely understood. Although poorly absorbed, bismuth is measureable in blood after ingestion. Highest concentrations are ultimately found in the kidneys and liver. Bismuth also concentrates in the placenta.[14] Excretion of bismuth, which is primarily renal, is rapid, being complete within 24 hours. Only about 10% of an absorbed dose is found in feces.[14]

The symptoms of bismuth intoxication have been compared with those of lead and mercury intoxication.[14] Early signs are oral and consist of hypersalivation and a characteristic blue discoloration of the gums, resulting from deposition of bismuth sulfide in fibrous tissue.[14] Stomatitis may also occur. Renal injury has been reported and presents either as acute renal failure or Fanconi's syndrome. Hepatic injury and peripheral neuritis have also been reported.[14] Skeletal disturbances, including osteoarthropathy, osteomalacia, and osteoporosis, have been associated with chronic bismuth intoxication; these may result in pathologic fractures.[14]

Encephalopathy has been reported after long-term, high-grade exposure to bismuth salts. Manifestations include altered mental status, ataxia, myoclonus, and distinctively abnormal findings on the electroencephalogram.[13, 14] Outbreaks of bismuth encephalopathy have been reported; between 1973 and 1980, approximately 1000 cases of bismuth intoxication were identified, and 72 of these were fatal.[15] However, Noach and colleagues, in a recent placebo-controlled clinical trial that included electroencephalography, failed to demonstrate neurotoxicity when bismuth was administered.[15]

The diagnosis of bismuth intoxication is made on the basis of history, characteristic clinical features, and laboratory evaluation. Serum bismuth concentrations can be diagnostic; the normal serum bismuth level is less than 50 μg/L.[15]

Supportive care is generally all that is required to treat bismuth toxicity. However, bismuth elimination can be enhanced by administration of BAL.[14]

Other aspects of bismuth intoxication have been well summarized by Winship.[14]

Cadmium

Cadmium is a heavy metal of clinical and historical importance. It is considered one of the most common causes of environmentally associated renal injury. The major sources of cadmium are industrial use and food contamination.[16, 17] Cadmium is also found in cigarettes (1 to 2 μg per cigarette), and thus larger cadmium burdens are found among smokers.[18] Cadmium is used industrially for the fabrication of alloys, for plating of metals, in pigments, and in the manufacture of rechargeable (nickel-cadmium) batteries. Cadmium's high volatility makes it particularly hazardous to welders.[19]

Cadmium is well absorbed after inhalation (up to 50% of an inhaled dose). In contrast, only about 5% of an ingested dose is absorbed.[17, 19] It is notable that GI absorption is enhanced by low intake of calcium, protein, or iron. Cadmium is circulated and stored attached to the metal-carrying protein metallothionein. The main storage organs of cadmium are the liver and the kidneys. The biologic half-life of cadmium in the liver is 5 to 10 years; it is twice that in the kidney. The overall biologic half-life of cadmium is 30 years.[19]

It is because of cadmium's extremely long half-life that progressive accumulation occurs; there is no effective endogenous mechanism for cadmium elimination from the body. Although cadmium's stimulation of metallothionein production reduces its overall toxicity, metallothionein also leads to selective accumulation of cadmium in the kidneys, with injury to this organ.

Acute ingestion of cadmium produces nausea, vomiting, salivation, abdominal pain, and diarrhea. Fatal cases result from cardiovascular collapse. The acute lethal oral dose is estimated at 350 to 8900 mg. Acute inhalation of cadmium oxide fumes as a result of welding, smelting, or soldering can produce a severe, sometimes fatal pneumonitis.[17]

After long-term exposure, the major target organs of cadmium toxicity are the kidneys, where it produces injury manifested by a proximal tubulopathy with excretion of proteins weighing less than 40,000. This includes the circulating proteins β_2-microglobulin, lysozyme, and retinol-binding protein. Cadmium acts by preventing the normal tubular reabsorption of these freely filtered proteins. *N*-acetyl-β-D-glucosaminidase (NAG) is another small-molecular-weight plasma protein whose urinary elimination occurs with cadmium toxicity. Elevated urinary concentrations of NAG are being increasingly promoted as a measure of cadmium-induced proximal tubule disease. However, increased excretion of NAG and other proteins can also occur after exposure to lead, solvents, and other occupational toxins.[20, 21] β_2-Microglobulin excretion is still considered a sensitive indicator of early cadmium-induced renal disease. Larger proteins such as albumin, transferrin, and IgG may also be lost in cadmium nephropathy.[19] Marked excretion of calcium and phosphorus also occurs, leading to osteopenia or nephrolithiasis. Effects on calcium and phosphate homeostasis result in part from cadmium inhibition of vitamin D hydroxylation. Finally, cadmium exposure has been epidemiologically linked with the development of essential hypertension. Renal disturbances may appear more than 10 years after intense cadmium exposure. Other nonrenal clinical effects associated with cadmium intoxication include ulceration of the nasal mucosa, anemia, and hepatitis.[19]

In the latter part of World War II, an epidemic illness in Japan was coined *itai-itai* ("ouch-ouch"). Clinical characteristics were leg and low back pain, chest pain, and difficulty walking. Severe, diffuse osteopenia occurred, resulting in fractures after the slightest trauma; these often produced physical deformities. The disease acquired its name because the victims constantly complained of fracture pain. Proteinuria, glycosuria, and aminoaciduria were also common. Autopsy revealed marked renal tubule atrophy and degeneration. It was notable that the disease was confined to the Jinzu River system, and this distribution suggested water contamination of rice, beans, fish, and other staples by an unknown toxin.[22] The low-protein and low-calcium diet of the victims seemed to contribute to the development of the disease. It was also observed that itai-itai occurred primarily in multiparous women, probably because they were already deficient in calcium and phosphorus. Much of the disease was readily cured by vitamin D supplementation. Cadmium contamination of water was ultimately identified as the cause and traced to industrial discharge from a nearby zinc mine.[19]

The diagnosis of chronic cadmium exposure can be made not only through urinary β_2-microglobulin excretion but also through measurement of cadmium in blood because blood identifies average intake during the past few months. The normal blood cadmium level is less than 5 μg/L. The normal urinary excretion of cadmium is less than 1 μg/g creatinine. Twenty-four-hour urine collections for measurement of cadmium, creatinine, total protein, selective proteins (if available), and amino acids can be diagnostic.

Chelation of cadmium is difficult because of its high affinity for metallothionein. Treatment with BAL has been associated with increased renal accumulation and accelerated renal injury (although an animal study has suggested that BAL has a potential therapeutic role).[23] In the risk-benefit analysis, chelation therapy should not be performed. All treatment is therefore supportive.

Chromium

Chromium is abundant in the earth's crust. It is an essential micronutrient and acts as a cofactor in insulin function.[24] Chromium is widely used in industry for the manufacture of stainless steel and in tanning, photography, and electroplating. Chromium is generally found in one of three valence states: bivalent, trivalent, and hexavalent. Hexavalent compounds include chromic acid, potassium and ammonium dichromate, and chromium trioxide; most of these are extremely corrosive when ingested. Although toxic exposure to chromium most commonly results in the occupational setting, ingestions occasionally occur.

Trivalent chromium is poorly absorbed (< 1%) from the GI tract; however, more than 50% of ingested hexavalent chromium can be absorbed from the gut. Organ accumulation of chromium is extensive and includes the brain, liver, spleen, testes, bone marrow, and reticuloendothelial system. Serum half-life is 15 to 41 hours. Approximately 80% of a chromium dose is readily excreted in the urine. The basis of chromium toxicity is its apparent ability to penetrate cell membranes, where it produces mutagenic events that result in cell death.

Exposure to hexavalent chromium is associated with widespread organ toxicity. Respiratory tract disturbances include acute pulmonary edema (which can appear up to 72 hours after a significant exposure), nasal septal perforation, and diffuse pulmonary inflammation. Dermal exposure to chromium in felt produces eczematous changes referred to as *blackjack disease*, and painless ulcers develop on the hands, periumbilical region, axillae, and forearms ("chromes holes").[11] GI toxicity includes severe hemorrhagic gastroenteritis, with a characteristic yellow-green emesis. Hepatitis, which progresses to fulminant hepatic failure, may result. Renal toxicity includes acute tubular necrosis and glomerulonephritis. Hematologic disturbances are methemoglobinemia, thrombocytopenia, anemia, and intravascular hemolysis. Cardiovascular disturbances can include circulatory collapse and shock, usually secondary to extensive GI corrosion/perforation. Ocular disturbances include corneal opacification, keratitis, and conjunctivitis. As little as 500 mg of ingested chromium can produce life-threatening toxicity; 1 to 2 g is potentially lethal. In a case report by Meert and colleagues, a 2-year-old ingested approximately 1 g of ammonium dichromate crystals. On arrival at the emergency department, he underwent gastric lavage and was given 100 mg of ascorbic acid intravenously. He had no oral lesions. Profuse diarrhea developed in association with coagulopathy, liver function disturbances, obtundation, and respiratory failure. Ascorbic acid was continued, and an exchange transfusion was performed. Nonetheless, 24 hours after ingestion he developed anuria, hypotension, and pulmonary edema. Despite hemodialysis, he had progressive coagulopathy and hepatic failure, resulting in his death. Autopsy was notable for diffuse mucosal erosion as well as injury to the liver, kidneys, adrenal cortex, and brain. The peak plasma chromium concentration was recorded at 4163 μg/L.[25]

Occupational exposure to hexavalent chromium has also been associated with an increased incidence of nasal cancers and bronchial carcinoma. The dietary trivalent form cannot be oxidized to the hexavalent form and has no carcinogenic risk.[24]

Chromium intoxication can be diagnosed through analysis of serum or urine. Normal serum concentrations are 0.3 to 1.0 μg/L. Urinary chromium concentration should be less than 40 μg/L.

Treatment of hexavalent chromium ingestion includes management of hypotension or shock, forced diuresis (which can include administration of furosemide), and aggressive treatment of corrosive GI injury. Ascorbic acid (vitamin C) reacts with hexavalent chromium to form the poorly absorbed trivalent form. Oral doses of 2 to 4 g per gram are recommended if there are no symptoms of severe gastroesophageal injury. The use of *N*-acetylcysteine has also been advocated to maintain chromium in its less toxic trivalent state.[25] Evaluation for intravascular hemolysis, methemoglobinemia, and renal failure should be performed. Forced diuresis is considered an integral part of management.[25]

Treatment of chromium inhalation includes fresh air; the possibility of late pulmonary edema should be considered in decisions about patient disposition. Dermal exposures should be treated by cleansing the skin with copious soap and water; débridement may be required for significant burns. Ocular exposures require copious irrigation and ophthalmology consultation.

Ingestions of chromium supplements appear nontoxic; significant clinical toxicity has not been reported after this ingestion. However, additional ingredients in chromium supplements (e.g., niacin and pyridoxine) have the potential to produce their own toxicity.

Cobalt

Cobalt is an essential trace element that forms the active component of vitamin B_{12} (cyanocobalamin). Cobalt is also found in magnets. Having the unusual property of erythropoiesis stimulation, it has been used in the treatment of select anemias. Normal serum cobalt value is 2 to 17 nmol/L.[26]

Long-term excessive cobalt exposure has been associated with the development of flushing, chest pain, tinnitus, nausea, vomiting, nerve deafness, thyroid hyperplasia, congestive heart failure, and renal disease. Frank hypothyroidism can result. Alopecia is a manifestation of cobalt intoxication found with few other toxins.

Historically, cobalt was responsible for recurring epidemics of cardiomyopathy (beer-drinkers cardiomyopathy), which occurred after cobalt was added to beer to stabilize its foam, a practice not abandoned until the 1970s.[27]

Cobalt intoxication has been successfuly treated with calcium disodium EDTA.[27]

Copper

Copper is an essential micronutrient element; enzymes including catalase, peroxidase, and cytochrome oxidase require copper for their activity. Copper deficiency is associated with microcytic anemia, leukopenia, and pathologic effects on the skeletal, cardiovascular, and nervous systems.

Copper is rapidly absorbed across the stomach and upper part of the small intestines; the extent of copper absorption is regulated by poorly characterized mechanisms. It is then transported both by albumin and by the specific α_2-globulin carrier protein ceruloplasmin. Organs in which copper is concentrated are the liver, kidneys, heart, and brain. Stored copper is bound to metallothionein. The primary route of copper excretion is the feces.[28]

An inherited disease associated with copper excess is Wilson's disease, also referred to as *hepatolenticular degeneration* because of its target pathology. This illness is characterized by accumulation of copper in the viscera and the cornea.

Acquired copper intoxication usually results from acute ingestion. Copper sulfate was once used as an emetic before its toxicity was recognized. Ingestions of copper sulfate produce severe GI upset, blue-green vomitus, hematemesis, hypotension, centrilobular hepatic necrosis, coma, seizures, and death. Hemolytic anemia and methemoglobinemia are also prominent features. Chronic exposure to copper, either occupationally or as a result of excess dietary copper (e.g., from use of copper-containing vessels) is associated with the development of hepatic injury with resulting cirrhosis.[28–31]

The diagnosis of copper intoxication is based on an elevated serum level of copper (normal, 50 to 120 mg/dL).[31] Treatment consists of airway and blood pressure support. Elimination of copper can be enhanced by chelation with either D-penicillamine or BAL.

Gold

Gold is a precious metal with no known essential human function. Exposure to gold can occur from environmental sources including seafood ingestion. Gold is also widely used in industry because of its properties. However, most human exposure to gold results from its medicinal use (chrysotherapy); it is prescribed for treatment of rheumatoid arthritis. Gold-containing pharmaceuticals are aurothioglucose, gold sodium thiomalate, and auranofin.[32]

Gold salts are administered orally or parenterally. When ingested, they are poorly absorbed from the GI tract.[33] Once absorbed, circulating gold is bound primarily to albumin.[32] Interestingly, gold concentrations in synovium are approximately half those in plasma. Gold has a half-life of approximately 7 days. Half-life lengthens after prolonged therapy as a result of avid tissue binding; blood levels are measurable 10 months after treatment is terminated.[33] Elimination is 60% to 90% fecal and 10% to 40% renal.[32]

Despite its beneficial properties, gold has significant clinical toxicity. Many of these effects result from gold-mediated formation of immune complexes. As is typical of immune complex diseases, adverse effects of gold therapy are primarily dermatologic and renal. Dermatitis is the most common side effect of chrysotherapy and may be associated with elevated IgE levels.[30, 33] Mucositis, manifested by stomatitis, tracheitis, gastritis, colitis, glossitis, or vaginitis, is also a common adverse effect. Renal effects, occurring in 5% to 10% of those receiving chrysotherapy, are more serious and consist of proteinuria, frank nephrosis, or immune complex glomerulonephritis. Blood disorders including thrombocytopenia, leukopenia and, rarely, aplastic anemia can occur. Other toxic effects are encephalitis, peripheral neuropathy, hepatitis, and pneumonitis.[32]

Treatment of gold toxicity is primarily symptomatic. Dermatitis and mucositis can be treated with antihistamines and corticosteroids. Corticosteroids can also be used for gold-induced nephrosis. Gold elimination can be enhanced with *N*-acetylcysteine, BAL, and D-penicillamine.[32]

Magnesium

Magnesium is the eighth most abundant element in the earth. It is found in ores such as dolomite and in seawater and is a component of asbestos. Also an essential nutrient, magnesium is necessary for numerous biologic processes including glycolysis and formation of cyclic adenosine monophosphate. More than 300 enzymes are known to be activated by magnesium. Magnesium homeostasis maintains serum magnesium concentrations in a narrow range. Regulation of magnesium levels is performed by the kidneys.

Hypermagnesemia has several causes, the most common being excess ingestion. This can either occur through ingestion of magnesium-containing antacids or excess administration of magnesium cathartic (see Chapter 1). Inhalation of magnesium oxide can produce metal fume fever (MFF). Dermal exposure to magnesium dust or fumes can produce a contact dermatitis. Finally, hypermagnesemia can result when the glomerular filtration rate declines below 30 mL/min and magnesium intake is not reduced.[34]

Acute magnesium toxicity produces central nervous system depression, which includes lethargy and coma, neuromuscular paralysis, hypotonia, and hyporeflexia. Cardiac disturbances consist of prolonged PR, QRS, and QT intervals. Inhalation can also produce pulmonary irritation with frank pulmonary edema.

Diagnosis is made by measuring serum magnesium concentration, although concentrations may not correlate with clinical symptoms. In general, manifestations of toxicity according to serum magnesium concentration are as follows: 3 to 9 mEq/L—vomiting, bradycardia, hypotension, hyporeflexia, lethargy; greater than 10 mEq/L—muscle paralysis, hypoventilation, stupor, cardiac conduction disturbances, ventricular arrhythmias; and greater than 14 mEq/L—cardiac arrest and death.[34]

Treatment begins by terminating exposure. *Calcium administration ameliorates many toxic manifestations.* Forced diuresis enhances the elimination of magnesium ion; hemodialysis is extremely effective at magnesium removal but is rarely necessary in the absence of renal failure.

Manganese

Manganese is an essential nutrent. Several enzymes including decarboxylases, kinases, and transferases are activated by manganese; the enzymes pyruvate carboxylase and superoxide dismutase contain manganese. A daily dietary intake of 2 to 5 mg has been recommended.[24]

Manganese is used in the manufacture of batteries and as an ingredient in paints and varnishes, bleaching agents, laboratory reagents, motor oils, and disinfectants. Manganese is also used for decolorizing glass/ceramics and as a fertilizer for grapes and tobacco.

Occupational and environmental exposures to manganese occur in steel manufacture, in welding, and through the ingestion of contaminated water. Manganese has begun to enter the atmosphere through its addition to methylcyclopentadienyl manganese tricarbonyl (MMT), an antiknock gas additive for unleaded fuels.[34] Of the valence forms of manganese, Mn^{+2} is more toxic than Mn^{+3}.

Manganese can be readily absorbed from the GI tract as well as the lungs. Its absorption is enhanced by iron deficiency and calcium or phosphorus intake. Once absorbed, manganese is transported by a specific β_1-globulin, transmanganin.[34] The primary route of excretion is fecal; less than 6% of a dose appears in the urine.

Chronic manganese intoxication is associated with a distinct clinical picture. Although manganese penetrates the central nervous system poorly, it can eventually lead to illness characterized by neurologic complaints. Once in the brain, the metal is concentrated in the globus pallidus and corpus striatum, where accumulation results in decreased synthesis and ultimate depletion of catecholamines, including dopamine. Initial complaints consist of anorexia, insomnia, and fatigue. A delirium known as *manganese madness* can appear, manifested by inappropriate laughter, hallucinations, and confusion. Victims often report vivid hallucinations and may commit acts of physical violence. This is followed by a marked diminution in spontaneous motor acts, ataxia, slurred speech, limb stiffness, tremor, paresthesias, amnesia, dysphagia, and a metallic taste in the mouth. Difficulties in ambulation produce impaired tandem gait and a loss of associated movements. Other manifestations include masked facies, micrographia, and torticollis. The neurologic syndrome mimics parkinsonism and may improve with levodopa therapy.[35] Other manifestations of chronic manganese intoxication include marked hypocalcemia and reduced spermatogenesis. Birth defects including talipes equinovarus and cleft lip have been reported in association with long-term manganese exposure.[34]

Acute inhalation of manganese oxide can produce either MFF or a distinct manganese pneumonitis.[34] Unlike MFF, manganese pneumonitis is more severe and has sequelae including persistent asthma.

The diagnosis of manganese intoxication should be suspected on the basis of the clinical picture (particularly the appearance of a Parkinson's-like syndrome) and can be confirmed by measurement of manganese in blood. The normal mean whole blood manganese concentration is 3 to 15 μg/L; normal mean serum manganese concentration is 1 to 3 μg/L.

The management of manganese intoxication is dependent on the clinical picture. Treatment of MFF is discussed later. Manganese pneumonitis may require antibiotic and bronchodilator therapy. For symptoms of parkinsonism, therapy with either levodopa or a diet high in tryptophan (a dopamine precursor) may improve motor activity. There are no chelators with an established role in the treatment of manganese toxicity.

Nickel

Nickel exists in three major forms: elemental, inorganic (water soluble and water insoluble), and organic (including nickel carbonyl).[35] Nickel is used for the production of stainless steel, in electroplating, in the manufacture of nickel-cadmium (rechargeable) batteries and magnetic tape, and as a catalyst for the hydrogenation of soaps, fats, and oils. Nickel carbonyl is an extremely toxic gas that is used as a catalyst in the petroleum, plastic, and rubber industries. This gaseous organometal is heavier than air and has a musty odor; its odor threshold is 1 ppm. Readily oxidizing in air, nickel carbonyl is highly explosive.[36] Human exposure to nickel occurs through contamination of water or by dermal contact with nickel-plated jewelry.

Nickel is poorly absorbed (< 1%) from the gut. In the circulation, it is bound to albumin and α_2-microglobulin. Nickel induces metallothionein synthesis.[35, 36]

Long-term exposure to nickel has a number of toxic effects, particularly on the immune system and respiratory tract. Its most characteristic effect is the production of nickel hypersensitivity, which results in allergic contact dermatitis. Rashes that occur in association with the use of nonrusting jewelry most often result from nickel dermatitis.[36] As many as 10% of women and 5% of men may develop nickel dermatitis after contact with nickel-plated jewelry. Other hypersensitivity phenomena occurring after chronic nickel exposure include asthma and conjunctivitis. In addition to asthma, respiratory effects include chronic restrictive lung disease (nickel pneumoconiosis), sinusitis, nasal polyps, and nasal septum perforations.[37, 38] Parenteral injection of nickel-containing medications has been associated with the development of anaphylaxis.[37] Nickel's reactivity and ability to participate in free radical reactions are thought to be the basis of its apparent carcinogenicity.[38]

Nickel carbonyl produces a different profile of toxicity. The potent toxicity of this gas has been compared with that of cyanide gas; exposure to 30 ppm for more than 30 minutes is lethal.[38] Illness may be biphasic. Death can be immediate but is typically delayed for several days. A case report by Kurta and colleagues[39] typifies the clinical course of patients with nickel carbonyl inhalation: A 46-year-old man presented several hours later after a combination dermal/inhalation exposure. At that time, he had tachypnea, fever, sinus tachycardia, and diffuse rales. His initial oxygen tension was 29 mm Hg. A chest radiograph revealed infiltrates consistent with adult-type respiratory distress syndrome. His initial urinary nickel concentration was 172 μg/dL (normal, < 5 μg/dL) with a serum nickel concentration of 14.6 μg/dL (normal, 0.26 to 0.46 μg/dL). He required aggressive treatment of severe respiratory disease with corticosteroids, aminophylline, albuterol, and antibiotics.

Because it is highly lipophilic, nickel carbonyl readily penetrates the central nervous system and produces neurologic toxicity that includes delirium and coma. Other disturbances include hepatic injury, hyperglycemia, glycosuria, mucositis, and dermatitis. Fatalities after acute nickel carbonyl poisoning typically occur 4 to 11 days after exposure and result from respiratory and neurologic toxicity.[39] Chronic nickel carbonyl exposure has been associated with the development of lung cancer.

The diagnosis of nickel intoxication is made by clinical suspicion as well as urine or serum nickel measurement. After nickel exposure, severity can be determined by results of 8-hour urinary elimination: Mild toxicity corresponds to a urinary nickel concentration of less than 100 μg/L, moderate toxicity equals 100 to 500 μg/L, and severe toxicity is associated with urinary concentrations exceeding 500 μg/L. Nickel carbonyl is metabolized by the liver, and liberation of carbon monoxide results; therefore, carboxyhemoglobin concentrations should also be obtained.

Treatment of severe nickel intoxication consists of aggressive cardiorespiratory support. After ingestions, GI decontamination should include activated charcoal administration for organic nickel compounds; ingestion of inorganic or elemental nickel should require only gastric emptying or catharsis. Nickel compounds can be chelated with sodium diethyldithiocarbamate (dithiocarb). This agent substantially reduces morbidity and mortality after nickel carbonyl exposure; however, its efficacy after exposure to elemental nickel is unestablished. Sunderman has suggested that dithiocarb enhances cerebral uptake of elemental nickel and should not be administered.[36] A potential alternative to dithiocarb is the administration of disulfiram (Antabuse), which is metabolized to two molecules of dithiocarb.[39] Because significant amounts of nickel are eliminated in urine, forced diuresis may also be beneficial.

Selenium

Selenium is an essential micronutrient that is chemically similar to sulfur and tellurium. It is an active part of the enzyme glutathione peroxidase, which catalyzes the scavenging of oxygen radicals. Selenium deficiency is associated with a cardiomyopathy known as *Keshan's cardiomyopathy*.[24] The recommended daily allowance of selenium is 50 to 100 μg. Dietary selenium supplements have become popular because of evidence suggesting they are helpful in preventing cancer, cardiovascular disease, cataracts, and arthritis.[40,41] Normal serum selenium concentrations are approximately 100 ng/mL; whole blood selenium measurements are approximately 30% higher than serum measurements.[40]

Selenium is widely used in paints, dyes, semi-conductors, photoelectric cells, fertilizers, and dandruff shampoos. Sheep drench is a common agricultural compound containing sodium selenate. A particularly hazardous form of selenium is gun bluing, which contains selenious acid as well as nitric acid, copper nitrate, and occasionally methanol and other solvents.

Selenium can penetrate the skin, can be inhaled as dust, or can be absorbed after ingestion. Most of a selenium dose is excreted within 2 weeks.[41]

Excess dietary selenium, as described in seleniferous regions of China and the United States,[42] produces fingernail abnormalities, peripheral neuropathy fatigue, muscle spasm, nausea, vomiting, alopecia, and a garlic odor on the breath. The garlic odor of chronic selenium exposure (selenosis) is thought to result from exhalation of selenide.[43,44] Liver function abnormalities, prolonged QT interval, and hypotension, the result of decreased cardiac contractility and reduced systemic vascular resistance, have also been reported after selenosis.[45] Low-grade occupational exposure has been associated with a slightly different clinical picture, which has abdominal pain, chronic diarrhea, alopecia, garlicky breath, and a metallic taste in the mouth as prominent complaints.[40,41] Transverse nail creases, similar to Mees' lines, may occur.[41] Occupational exposures can also produce chemical pneumonitis.[46]

Acute selenium poisoning from ingestion of gun bluing can result in death.[44,47–51] Being highly corrosive, gun bluing produces severe burns of the stomach and esophagus, with initial hypersalivation and vomiting. This is followed by metabolic acidosis, leukocytosis, myocardial depression, hepatitis, renal injury, pulmonary dysfunction (including adult respiratory distress syndrome), and seizures.[44,49] Death has been associated with ingestion of as little as 15 mL of gun bluing.[41]

The diagnosis of chronic selenium exposure is based on clinical suspicion. Alopecia with garlicky breath is pathognomonic. Measurement of urine or blood selenium concentrations can be diagnostic; urinary selenium concentrations of up to 150 μg/L are normal. Treatment of selenium toxicity consists of general supportive measures and appropriate management of corrosive ingestion or toxic inhalation. GI decontamination after gun bluing ingestion is complicated by corrosive injury to the GI tract but should be considered.

Case reports have suggested a beneficial role for forced diuresis and administration of BAL in enhancing selenium elimination.

Silver

Silver was once widely used in medicine to treat syphilis and other conditions. Its pharmacologic use now is restricted to silver nitrate antiseptic. Silver nitrate is also an astrigent, and it remains popular for treatment of burns and granulation tissue and as prophylaxis for ophthalmia neonatorum. When ingested, it can be highly corrosive; doses as small as 3 g can be lethal.[52] Topical application of silver nitrate results in local hyperpigmentation.[52]

Silver exposure also occurs occupationally in the extraction and manufacture of precious metals. It is used in jewelry manufacture and as a component of films, inks, and ceramics. Occupational standards that limit workplace exposure have been created by the Occupational Safety and Health Administration; the permissible exposure limit for silver is 0.01 mg/m^3. Occupational exposure to silver produces irritation of the mucous membranes (eyes, nose, and throat) and respiratory complaints, including cough, wheezing, chest tightness, and epistaxis.[21]

Argyria is an unusual silver-related illness marked by discoloration of the skin, nails, mucous membranes, and organs as a result of silver deposition.[53] The hyperpigmentation, which ranges from pale blue to slate gray, is striking in appearance and pathognomonic for this otherwise asymptomatic disease.[21] Patients have been described as resembling a corpse who has come to life.[53, 54] The most vivid areas of discoloration are sun-exposed skin (e.g., face and hands). The pigmentation has been attributed to deposition of silver and to a silver-induced increase in melanin production. The same blue-gray discoloration can be found throughout the organs on surgery or autopsy. Corneal deposition of silver can result in nyctalopia (disturbed night vision).[21] Argyria can occur after excess exposure to silver by any route (injection, ingestion, or inhalation). Workers in the silver extraction industry are at greatest risk of argyria owing to long-term inhalation. The quantity of silver sufficient to produce argyria is estimated to be 6 g by inhalation and 25 to 50 g by ingestion.[53]

The diagnosis of argyria is readily established by skin biopsy; specimens show silver deposits, particularly in elastic tissue. Normal excretion of silver in unexposed individuals is 1 to 2 μg/L in urine and less than 0.27 μg/100 mL in blood.[21] There is no effective treatment, and the pigmentation of argyria is permanent.

Thallium

Thallium is a heavy metal with a molecular weight between that of mercury and lead. Thallium salts are odorless, colorless, and tasteless. Once used widely in this country as a rodenticide, thallium has been banned from use in the United States since 1965[55]; the World Health Organization has recommended an end to its use worldwide. However, it is still a popular rodenticide. The possibility of importation continues to make thallitoxicosis a possible occurrence in this country. Because it is highly toxic but has characteristics making it easy to conceal, thallium is commonly used as a homicidal agent[56]; Insley and colleagues described three men who developed thallitoxicosis after using what they thought was cocaine but was discovered to be 99% thallium.[57] Thallium is used in the optical, electronic, and chemical research industries as well.[56]

Thallium is rapidly absorbed from the gut after ingestion and by the lungs after inhalation. Once it is absorbed, its distribution is extensive; no significant plasma protein binding occurs. The volume of distribution of thallium is estimated at 20 L/kg. There is significant enterohepatic recycling of the metal. Elimination half-life ranges from 3 to 8 days, although half-lives as long as 15 days have been reported after severe poisoning. Approximately two thirds of a thallium dose is excreted in feces, the remainder in urine. Seventy per cent of a single dose is excreted within a month.[58]

Thallium's toxicity results from its similarity to potassium, an ion with a comparable ionic radius (0.15 versus 0.138 nm).[59] Like potassium, thallium depolarizes excitable membranes and disturbs the function of sodium-potassium adenosine triphosphatase, having a 110-fold greater affinity for this enzyme. Because they have an abundance of sodium-potassium adenosine triphosphatase, mitochondria are particularly susceptible to thallium's effects. Additional toxic effects include interruption of flavin synthesis (flavin adenine dinucleotide and flavin mononucleotide). Thallium's high affinity for thiol groups explains many of its clinical effects, including alopecia and Mees' lines.[59] Severe toxicity occurs with ingestions exceeding 200 mg; the average lethal dose is 1 g in an adult.[55, 60]

The clinical hallmark of thallium intoxication is the triad of gastroenteritis, polyneuropathy, and alopecia. Early manifestations mimic arsenic or antimony intoxication. The immediate phase of intoxication consists of GI effects, which appear within 3 to 4 hours and consist of nausea, vomiting, diarrhea, abdominal pain, and hematochezia. An intermediate phase, appearing within 1 week of exposure, consists of cardiac disturbances: hypertension, tachycardia, and chest pain. At this stage, signs of central and peripheral nervous system disease appear. Central nervous system signs include optic neuritis, ptosis, confusion, seizure, coma, and psychosis. Peripheral neuropathy is more striking. Victims often complain of intense hyperesthesia of the soles, which makes walking difficult. Weakness and ataxia may also occur.[56] Polyneuropathy may be severe enough to produce respiratory failure.[61] At this stage, gingival hyperpigmentation as well as pigmentation of the hair may appear. Severe intractable constipation may develop. The late stage of thallitoxicosis, appearing 2 to 4 weeks after exposure, consists of marked alopecia, a diffuse nonspecific rash, palmar erythema, perioral ulcers, and Aldrich-Mees lines on the fingernails.[55, 57, 58, 61] A "residual" stage, occurring more than 4 weeks after exposure, consists of memory loss, ataxia, tremor, and footdrop. In fatal cases, death generally occurs 10 to 15 days after exposure.[60] Laboratory abnormalities consist of anemia, thrombocytopenia, increased hepatic transaminases, decreased complement, flat or inverted T waves on electrocardiogram, and axonal destruction with demyelination on sural nerve biopsy.[55]

Diagnosis is made on the basis of clinical manifestations and confirmed by measurement of thallium in serum or urine. Serum levels that suggest poisoning are greater than 50 μg/dL. However, because 70% of thallium is bound to the erythrocytes, whole blood measurement is likely to be more accurate.[57] Urinary excretion of greater than 10 to 20 mg/24 hours is considered excessive. Other potential methods for identifying thallium intoxication are electroretinography and electromyography (which demonstrates decreased distal motor units and membrane instability). Thallium may be misdiagnosed as Guillain-Barré syndrome, selenosis, arsenic poisoning, and acute porphyria.[57, 61]

Treatment goals consist of enhancing fecal excretion, enhancing urinary excretion, and, when necessary, extracorporeal elimination. Fecal excretion can be enhanced by early, aggressive GI decontamination. Ferric ferrocyanide (Prussian blue) avidly binds thallium and is considered the adsorbent of choice; however, activated charcoal also effectively binds thallium and should be administered initially. Prussian blue has also been used to interrupt enterohepatic recirculation of thallium; 250 mg/kg daily should be given in four divided doses with a cathartic. Early administration of sodium iodide can form an insoluble thallium-iodine complex that is poorly absorbed.[61] Forced diuresis also has potential benefit; human studies have suggested it increases urinary elimination of thallium twofold to sixfold.[62] Forced diuresis with potassium chloride supplementation has also been advocated; however, exogenous potassium may displace thallium into the serum and thus provide greater opportunity for nervous system penetration.[57] Moreover, Koshy and Lovejoy found that potassium chloride supplementation with forced diuresis had no clear benefit in a thallium overdose.[63] Dithiocarb is a chelating agent that enhances urinary excretion of thallium; however, the resulting chelate is highly lipophilic. It crosses the blood-brain barrier and exacerbates neurologic toxicity and therefore is not recommended. Extracorporeal drug removal techniques including peritoneal dialysis are unlikely to be effective because of thallium's large volume of distribution. If extracorporeal drug removal techniques are considered, hemoperfusion is probably more effective than hemodialysis.[60]

Tin

Tin is a ubiquitous element that may be an essential nutrient.[24, 64] Tin commonly exists in three forms—metallic, inorganic, and organic—with metallic and inorganic being the least toxic.[65] Organotins are used as stabilizers in polymers and as catalysts.

Most tin salts are insoluble, with less than 5% absorbed from the GI tract. Once absorbed, tin is distributed, then deposited in the kidneys, lungs, and bone. Most circulating tin is attached to the erythrocytes.[64]

Among the organotins, the trialkyltins are the most toxic. Being highly lipophilic, they readily penetrate the central nervous system, where they exert their major toxicity.[64, 66] Exposure to organotin has been associated with altered mental status, confusion, and amnesia.[66] Other complaints include headache, tinnitus, deafness, disorientation, syncope, and loss of consciousness; electroencephalographic changes may be associated.[64, 66] Triethyltin, unlike trimethyltin may also produce acute cerebral edema.[64] Long-term tin inhalation can produce a benign pneumoconiosis (stannosis).[65] Illness associated with the use of tin compounds in interior paint have led to its ban in certain states.[65]

Diagnosis can be based on the clinical picture, history, and elevated serum tin levels; in a case of trimethyltin exposure, urinary excretion was 52 μg/dL, compared with a normal urine tin concentration of approximately 0.1 μg/dL.[66]

Treatment is supportive. No chelators have been shown to alter the course of the disease.

Zinc

Zinc is an essential nutrient that is a part of many biologic functions. More than 70 metalloenzymes require zinc for their function, including alcohol dehydrogenase and carbonic anhydrase. There is also a strong reciprocal relationship between zinc and copper metabolism. For example, zinc has been used to treat the copper accumulation associated with Wilson's disease.[29] Like other nutrients, zinc supplements are widely sold; their use can result in toxic manifestations.[67] Severe zinc intoxication has also been described after long-term ingestion of pennies.[67] Finally, excess exposure can occur in the workplace and in those who receive hemodialysis that uses water that has been stored in galvanized tanks.[68]

Acute ingestion of 2 g or more of zinc produces GI irritation and vomiting. Continual excessive zinc intake results in reductions in serum levels of copper (hypocupremia), sideroblastic anemia, and neutropenia.[29, 67] A child with long-term zinc ingestion developed listlessness, anemia, neutropenia, poor weight gain, and sideroblastic anemia, all indicative of copper deficiency.[67] The child had an undetectable serum copper concentration.

The diagnosis of zinc intoxication is confirmed by an elevated serum zinc level (normal, 9.2 to 23 μmol/L).

Treatment of zinc intoxication includes supportive measures and, after ingestion, GI decontamination measures such as administration of activated charcoal. Chelation therapy is very effective for elevated zinc levels; options include ethylenediaminetetraacetic acid, dimercaprol, D-penicillamine, and *N*-acetylcysteine.[69]

METAL FUME FEVER

MFF has been recognized for centuries, although it was not until 1822 that it was characterized by Potissier.[70]

MFF is an occupational disease produced by inhalation of freshly oxidized metal fumes that have a particle size smaller than 0.5 to 1.0 μm.[71] MFF is also referred to as Monday morning fever, the smothers, brass founder's ague, brazier's disease, foundry fever, galvanizer's poisoning, smelter's chills, zinc chills, zinc fume fever, brass chills, and copper fever.[72] Extremely common, MFF is reported more than 1000 times annually.[70] The disease is primarily associated with welding, a task consistently causing the oxidation of metals. Although welding is the occupation most highly associated with the disease, MFF is encountered after soldering, forging, melting, and casting of metal.

MFF is associated with a number of metals, including zinc, copper, magnesium, cadmium, manganese, and antimony (Table 59–1). Zinc, iron, and copper are the most common causes of MFF. Cadmium and tin, although associated with MFF, appear to produce a different, more severe illness that shares some features with MFF.

The clinical syndrome consists of chills, fever, leukocytosis, myalgias, dyspnea, chest pain, nonproductive cough, dry throat, intense thirst, and a metallic taste in the mouth.[72] These symptoms usually appear 4 to 12 hours after an acute exposure. Temperature may be as high as 104°F, accompanied by sinus tachycardia and rales. Chest radiographs may appear normal or may reveal a patchy infiltrate. These findings characteristically appear to be more severe than the patient's clinical picture would suggest. Bronchoalveolar lavage, if performed, may reveal inflammatory cells. Other clinical features include elevated lactate dehydrogenase levels and hypoxia.[70] Tolerance to MFF quickly develops. As a result, exposed workers often complain of illness developing at the beginning of the week, improving by the end of the week, and completely resolving during the weekend before recurring the next work week. The benign clinical course of MFF distinguishes it from acute cadmium or tin pneumonitis.[70]

The cause of MFF is unclear, although it has been attributed to release of endogenous pyrogens or production of antigenic metal proteinates (a theory supported by its clinical similarity to hypersensitivity pneumonitis).[70] Delayed hypersensitivity pneumonitis or allergic reaction has been theorized.[72] Others have proposed that it results from a direct toxic effect on alveolar cells.

Table 59–1. Metals Commonly Associated with Metal Fume Fever

Zinc	Copper
Magnesium	Cadmium
Manganese	Tin
Iron	

MFF is self-limited and resolves within 48 hours. Bed rest and antipyretics are the recommended therapy. Corticosteroids have been recommended for those with interstitial infiltrates on chest radiographs after a history of zinc exposure. A history of exposure to cadmium or tin fumes warrants hospitalization for observation and supportive care. No permanent sequelae of MFF have been identified. Elevated serum zinc levels and increased urinary copper levels have been reported; their significance is unclear.[71,72]

CHELATORS

Exogenous

A growing number of chelating agents have been explored in an attempt to find effective treatment for exposure to toxic metals and minerals. This search has yielded a large number of compounds with a variable profile of safety, efficacy, and toxicity. Table 59–2 summarizes the potential role of a number of available chelators. A complete review of the pharmacology of these agents is beyond the scope of this chapter, and readers are directed to pharmacology texts. Recent symposia by Kosnett and others have attempted to identify the role of chelators in medical toxicology as one evaluates their benefits versus risks.[73]

Table 59–2. Metal Chelators

Chelator	Useful	Possibly Effective	Unlikely to Be Effective	Potentially Detrimental
Edetate calcium disodium	Zinc Cobalt		Chromium Nickel Thallium	Selenium
Dimercaprol (BAL)	Lead Nickel Copper Antimony Bismuth Gold Zinc Arsenic Mercury	Chromium	Thallium	Selenium Cadmium
Dithiocarb (sodium diethyldithiocarbonate)	Nickel carbonyl	Cadmium		Thallium Elemental nickel
D-Penicillamine	Copper Lead Arsenic Mercury Zinc Gold		Nickel	Selenium
Dimercaptosuccinic acid (DMSA)	Antimony Lead Arsenic			
Dimercapto-propane-sulfonic acid (DMPS)	Antimony Lead Mercury			
Deferoxamine	Iron Aluminum			
N-acetylcysteine	Gold Zinc			

Endogenous

A number of endogenous metal-carrying proteins have been identified in humans and lower animals. Many of these, such as albumin, have multiple roles and carry not only metals but xenobiotics. Transferrin, ferritin, ceruloplasmin, and transmanganin, proteins made by the body to carry iron, copper, and manganese, have been well characterized and appear to be extremely narrow in their binding capacity. In forming stable bonds with metals, these agents have been referred to as *endogenous chelators*.

Discovered in 1957, metallothionein is a low-molecular-weight protein (molecular weight, 6600) that appears to be an essential protein transport molecule in humans. Metallothionein has been called a "protein in search of a function" because its exact role has not been fully defined.[74–76]

Thirty per cent of metallothionein is made up of the amino acid cysteine. The high sulfur content permits the formation of several types of stable bonds with metals, including tetrahedral arrangements.[74–76] Metallothionein can be found in every tissue of the body including the intestine, pancreas, brain, thymus, and bone marrow. Although it is primarily found in intracellular sites, it is also secreted into bile, urine, and plasma. The normal rate of metallothionein production is highly variable and is influenced by many nutritional, physiologic, and developmental factors. Zinc has the most profound influence on metallothionein production. For example, metallothionein synthesis decreases with zinc deficiency. Conversely, zinc excess produces a marked increase in metallothionein production. Synthesis of metallothionein can also be induced by exposure to toxic metals including cadmium, mercury, silver, platinum, gold, and bismuth. Cadmium is a particularly potent inducer of synthesis. It is notable that cadmium has many physical properties that are similar to those of zinc. Both exist as divalent cations. Other, nonmetal inducers of metallothionein include estrogen, progesterone, and glucocorticoids. Infection also results in increased hepatic metallothionein levels.[74–76] Very little is known about the degradation of this protein, although its loss is directly related to the metal to which it is attached; in animal models, the half-life of cadmium-, zinc-, and copper-induced metallothioneins is 80, 20, and 17 hours, respectively.[76]

Despite this information, the purpose of metallothionein remains unclear. Some theories suggest that it may be a simple acute phase reactant. As such, its purpose is probably to provide resistance to environmental stress with its production of a metal-sequestering protein. The toxicity of cadmium is clearly reduced by the presence of metallothionein; thus, metallothionein production is an important response to metal intoxication.[30]

Although it has been attractive to use the protective value of metallothionein in cadmium toxicity as evidence that the body manufactures it as an endogenous chelator, in fact, there is no evidence to prove this. Rather, metallothionein most likely represents a metal-carrying protein whose primary function is the transport of essential metal nutrients.[76]

References

1. American Academy of Pediatrics Committee on Nutrition: Aluminum toxicity in infants and children. Pediatrics *78*:1150–1153, 1986.
2. Tsou VM, Young RM, Hart MH, Vanderhoof JA: Elevated plasma aluminum levels in normal infants receiving antacids containing aluminum. Pediatrics *87*:148–151, 1991.
3. Hantson P, Nahieu P, Gersdorff M, et al: Fatal encephalopathy after otoneurosurgery procedure with an aluminum-containing biomaterial. Clin Toxicol *33*:645–648, 1995.
4. Lauwers LF, Roelants A, Rosseel PM, et al: Oral antimony intoxications in man. Crit Care Med *18*:324–326, 1990.
5. Agency for Toxic Substances and Disease Registry: Toxicological Profile for Antimony. US Public Health Service, 1992.
6. Rees PH, Kager PA, Keating MI, Hockmeyer WT: Renal clearance of pentavalent antimony (sodium stibogluconate). Lancet *2*:226–229, 1980.
7. Deng JF, Jan IS, Cheng HS: The essential role of a poison center in handling an outbreak of barium carbonate poisoning. Vet Hum Toxicol *33*:173–175, 1991.
8. Agarwal AK, Ahlawat SK, Gupta S, et al: Hypokalaemic paralysis secondary to acute barium carbonate toxicity. Trop Doct *25*:101–103, 1995.
9. Johnson CH, Van Tassell VJ: Acute barium poisoning with respiratory failure and rhabdomyolysis. Ann Emerg Med *20*:1138–1142, 1991.
10. Gupta S: Barium carbonate, hypokalemic paralysis and trismus. Postgrad Med J *70*:938–939, 1994.
11. Deng J-F, Fleeger AK: An outbreak of chromium ulcer in a manufacturing plant. Vet Hum Toxicol *32*:142, 1990.
12. Kriebel D, Brain JD, Sprince NL, Kazemi H: The pulmonary toxicity of beryllium. Am Rev Respir Dis *137*:464–473, 1988.
13. Mendelowitz PC, Hoffman RS, Weber S: Bismuth absorption and myoclonic encephalopathy during bismuth subsalicylate therapy. Ann Intern Med *112*:140–141, 1990.
14. Winship KA: Toxicity of bismuth salts. Adv Drug React Acute Poisoning Rev *2*:103–121, 1983.
15. Noach LA, Eekhof JL, Bour LJ, et al: Bismuth salts and neurotoxicity. A randomised, single-blind and controlled study. Hum Exp Tox *14*:349–355, 1995.
16. Sherlock JC: Cadmium in foods and the diet. Experientia *40*:152–156, 1984.
17. Hallenbeck WH: Human health effects of exposure to cadmium. Experientia *40*:136–142, 1984.
18. Kowal NE, Johnson DE, Draemer DF, Pahren HR: Normal levels of cadmium in diet, urine, blood, and tissues of inhabitants of the United States. J Toxicol Environ Health *5*:995–1014, 1979.
19. Bernard A, Lauwerys R: Cadmium in human population. Experientia *40*:143–152, 1984.
20. Nogawa K: Biologic indicators of cadmium nephrotoxicity in persons with low-level cadmium exposure. Environ Health Perspect *54*:163–169, 1984.
21. Rosenman KD, Seixas N, Jacobs J: Potential nephrotoxic effects of exposure to silver. Br J Ind Med *44*:267–272, 1987.
22. Ishizaki A: On 'Itai-itai' (ouch-ouch) disease. Asian Med J *14*:421–436, 1971.
23. Cherian MG, Rodgers K: Chelation of cadmium from metallothionein *in vivo* and its excretion in rats repeatedly injected with cadmium chloride. J Pharmacol Exp Ther *222*:699–704, 1982.
24. National Research Council: Recommended Daily Allowances. Washington, DC, National Academy Press, 1989.
25. Meert KL, Ellis J, Aronow R, Perrin E: Acute ammonium dichromate poisoning. Ann Emerg Med *24*:748–750, 1994.
26. Mucklow ES, Griffin SJ, Delves HT, Suchak B: Cobalt poisoning in a 6-year-old. Lancet *335*:981, 1990.
27. Morin Y, Daniel P: Quebec beer-drinkers' cardiomyopathy: Etiological considerations. Can Med Assoc J *97*:926–928, 1967.
28. Walsh FM, Crosson FJ, Bayley M, et al: Acute copper intoxication. Am J Dis Child *131*:149–151, 1977.
29. Botash AS, Nasca J, Dubowy R, et al: Zinc-induced copper deficiency in an infant. Am J Dis Child *146*:709–711, 1992.
30. Ringenberg QS, Doll DC, Patterson WP, et al: Hematologic effects of heavy metal poisoning. South Med J *81*:1132–1139, 1988.
31. Schwartz E, Schmidt E: Refractory shock secondary to copper sulfate ingestion. Ann Emerg Med *15*:952–954, 1986.
32. Insel PA: Analgesic-antipyretic and antiinflammatory agents and drugs employed in the treatment of gout. *In* Hardman JG, Limbird LE, Molinoff PB, et al (eds): Goodman & Gilman's The Pharmacological Basis of Therapeutics. New York, McGraw-Hill, pp 617–657, 1996.
33. Goyer RA: Toxic effects of metals. *In* Klaassen CD (ed): Casarett and Doull's Toxicology—The Basic Science of Poisons. 5th ed. New York, McGraw-Hill, pp 691–736, 1996.
34. Gilmore DA, Bronstein AC: Manganese and magnesium. *In* Sullivan J, Krieger G (eds): Hazardous Materials Toxicology—Clinical Principles of Environmental Health. Baltimore, Williams & Wilkins, 1992.
35. Cook DG, Fahn S, Brait KA: Chronic manganese intoxication. Arch Neurol *30*:59–64, 1974.
36. Leach CN, Sunderman FW: Nickel contamination of human serum albumin solutions. N Engl J Med *313*:1232, 1985.
37. Maibach HI, Menne T: Nickel and the Skin: Immunology and Toxicology. Boca Raton, FL, CRC Press, 1989.
38. Siegers C-P, Sullivan JB: Organometals and reactive metals. *In* Sullivan JB, Krieger GR (eds): Hazardous Materials Toxicology—Clinical Principles of Environmental Health. Baltimore, Williams & Wilkins, pp 928–936, 1992.
39. Kurta DL, Dean BS, Krenzelok EP: Acute nickel carbonyl poisoning. Am J Emerg Med *11*:64–66, 1993.
40. Selenium intoxication—New York. MMWR *33*:157–158, 1984.
41. Alderman LC, Ergin JJ: Hydrogen selenide poisoning: An illustrative case with review of the literature. Arch Environ Health *41*:354–358, 1986.
42. Ruta DA, Haider S: Attempted murder by selenium poisoning. BMJ *299*:316–317, 1989.
43. Clark RF, William SR, Manoguerra A, Turchen S: Acute selenium poisoning resulting from vitamin supplements. Abstract. Clin Toxicol *33*:541, 1995.
44. Lombeck I, Menzel H, Frosch D: Acute selenium poisoning of a 2-year-old child. Eur J Pediatr *146*:308–312, 1987.
45. Civil IDS, McDonald MJA: Acute selenium poisoning: A case report. N Z Med J *87*:354, 1978.
46. Wilson HM: Selenium oxide poisoning. N C Med J *23*:73–75, 1962.
47. Carter RF: Acute selenium poisoning. Med J Aust *1*:525, 1966.
48. Matoba R: An autopsy case of acute selenium (selenious acid) poisoning and selenium levels in human tissues. Forensic Sci Int *31*:87–92, 1986.
49. Nantel AJ: Acute poisoning by selenious acid. Vet Hum Toxicol *27*:531, 1985.
50. Normann SA: Acute selenious acid poisoning. Vet Hum Toxicol *26*:49, 1984.
51. Pentel P: Fatal acute selenium toxicity. J Forensic Sci *30*:556–562, 1985.
52. Rauber A, Bruner B: Ingestion of concentrated silver nitrate: A report of two cases. Vet Hum Toxicol *29*:321–322, 1987.
53. Greene RM, Su WPD: Argyria. Am Family Physician *36*:151–154, 1987.
54. Bryant BL: Argyria resulting from intranasal medication: A clinical and experimental study. Arch Otolaryngol *31*:127–138, 1940.
55. Schwartz JG, Stuckey JH, Kunkel SP, et al: Poisoning from thallium. Tex Med *84*:46–48, 1988.

56. Desenclos J-CA, Wilder MH, Coppenger GW, et al: Thallium poisoning: An outbreak in Florida, 1988. South Med J *85*:1203–1206, 1992.
57. Insley BM, Grufferman S, Ayliffe HE: Thallium poisoning in cocaine abusers. Am J Emerg Med *4*:545–548, 1986.
58. Pai V: Acute thallium poisoning. West Indian Med J *36*:256–258, 1987.
59. Mulkey JP, Oehme FW: A review of thallium toxicity. Vet Hum Toxicol *35*:445–453, 1993.
60. Moeschlin S: Thallium poisoning. Clin Toxicol *17*:133–146, 1980.
61. Vergauwe PL, Knockaert DC, Van Titelboom TJ: Near fatal subacute thallium poisoning necessitating prolonged mechanical ventilation. Am J Emerg Med *8*:548–550, 1990.
62. Pedersen RS, Olesen AS, Freund, LG, et al: Thallium intoxication treated with long-term hemodialysis, forced diuresis, and prussian blue. Acta Med Scand *204*:429–432, 1978.
63. Koshy KM, Lovejoy FH: Thallium ingestion with survival: Ineffectiveness of peritoneal dialysis and KCl diuresis. Clin Toxicol *18*:521–525, 1981.
64. Krigman MR, Silverman AP: General toxicology of tin and its organic compounds. Neurotoxicology *5*:129–140, 1984.
65. Wax PM, Dockstader L: Tributyltin use in interior paints: A continuing health hazard. Clin Toxicol *33*:239–241, 1995.
66. Yanofsky NN, Nieerenberg D, Turco JH: Acute short-term memory loss from trimethyltin exposure. J Emerg Med *9*:137–139, 1991.
67. Broun ER, Greist A, Tricot G, Hoffman R: Excessive zinc ingestion—a reversible cause of sideroblastic anemia and bone marrow depression. JAMA *264*:1441–1443, 1990.
68. Domingo JL, Llobet JM, Paternain JL, Corbella J: Acute zinc intoxication: Comparison of the antidotal efficacy of several chelating agents. Vet Hum Toxicol *30*:224–227, 1988.
69. Fisher D: Zinc. *In* Sullivan JB, Krieger GR (eds): Hazardous Materials Toxicology—Clinical Principles of Environmental Health. Baltimore, Williams & Wilkins, pp 865–868, 1992.
70. Offermann PV, Finley C: Metal fume fever. Ann Emerg Med *21*:872–875, 1992.
71. Vogelmeier C, Konig G, Bencze K, Gruhmann G: Pulmonary involvement in zinc fume fever. Chest *92*:946–948, 1987.
72. Noel NE, Ruthman JC: Elevated serum zinc levels in metal fume fever. Am J Emerg Med *6*:609–610, 1988.
73. Kosnett M: Unanswered questions in metal chelation. Clin Toxicol *30*:529–547, 1992.
74. Bremner I, Beattie JH: Metallothionein and the trace mineral. Ann Rev Nutr *10*:63–83, 1990.
75. Nordberg GF: Modulation of metal toxicity by metallothionein. Biol Trace Elem Res *21*:131–135, 1989.
76. Vallee BL: The function of metallothionein. Neurochem Int *27*:23–33, 1995.

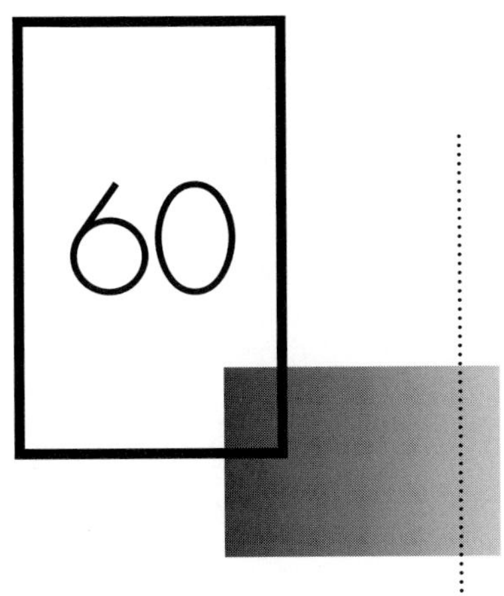

Bromine and Iodine Compounds

MICHAEL W. SHANNON, MD, MPH

The four members of group VIIB of the periodic table—fluorine, chlorine, bromine, and iodine—are collectively known as the *halides*. These nonmetallic elements have many common features. All are strongly electronegative agents with potent oxidizing ability; their ionic forms are known as fluoride, chloride, bromide, and iodide. With the exception of bromine, all are essential for human health. Bromine, although not an essential element, has an important clinical role because of its historic use in the treatment of many illnesses followed by the discovery of its potent toxicity.

This chapter reviews bromine, iodine, and their related compounds. Hydrofluoric acid is discussed in Chapter 61. The fumigants methyl bromide and ethylene dibromide are discussed in Chapter 81.

BROMINE COMPOUNDS

History

Bromide has a molecular weight of 79.9. After it was discovered in 1826, its clinical effects were quickly noted, and by the mid 1800s, bromides were widely prescribed as sedative-hypnotics. By 1857, they were recognized as effective anticonvulsants[1]; before the advent of barbiturate anticonvulsants in the 1920s, bromides were one of the only anticonvulsants available. Bromide salts were also popular as "nerve" remedies, leading to the admonition to "take a bromide," suggested to those who felt anxious. By 1938, more than 200 bromide preparations were in use.[2] Two bromide-containing medications in widespread use until 1975 were Bromo-Seltzer (which was 67% bromide) and Miles Nervine (which contained ammonium bromide and was 82% bromide).[1] Organic bromides, also known as *bromureides*, have been less commonly used. Two such compounds are carbromal and bromisoval.

The bromides are ubiquitous in nature. They can be found in trace amounts in natural soils and waters (e.g., igneous rock contains 0.02 mmol/kg bromide; fresh waters contain 0.05 to 10 μmol/L, and seawater 0.4 to 0.8 mmol/L). Many vegetables contain bromide residues as a result of soil fumigation with methyl dibromide and ethylene dibromide. Bromide exposure therefore occurs in all humans.

The bromide salts are used in photographic chemicals (e.g., activators and developers). They are also found in fire extinguishers and refrigerants, as well as in several medications (Table 60–1). Pharmaceutical bromides can be divided into inorganic bromide salts (NaBr, KBr, NH_4Br, and CaBr) and organic bromides (e.g., brompheniramine). Halothane, a popular inhalation anesthetic, contains significant amounts of bromide; as much as 25% of a halothane dose is metabolized by the liver, and thus bromide is liberated. Its use has been associated with the development of detectable serum bromide levels (which can remain elevated for 9 to 22 days in those with prolonged anesthesia).[3] Ingestions of dextromethorphan, a common over-the-counter cough suppressant, can also result in significant bromide absorption.[4]

Table 60–1. Bromide-Containing Medications

Medication	% Bromide
Acecarbromal	29
Ammonium bromide	80
Bromisovalum	36
Bromodiphenhydramine	24
Carbromal	34
Dextromethorphan hydrobromide	23
Pyridostigmine bromide	31
Brompheniramine maleate	25
Halothane hydrobromide	81
Homatropine methylbromide	29
Neostigmine bromide	38
Bromocriptine	12
Pancuronium bromide	37
Potassium bromide	67
Propantheline bromide	18
Quinine hydrobromide	17
Vecuronium bromide	25
Scopolamine hydrobromide	29

Adapted from Bowers GN, Onoroski M: Hypochloremia and the incidence of bromism in 1990. Clin Chem *36*:1399–1403, 1990; and Rothenberg DM, Berns AS, Barkin R, Glantz RH: Bromide intoxication secondary to pyridostigmine bromide therapy. JAMA *263*:1121–1122, 1990.

Pharmacokinetics

Bromide is well absorbed from the gastrointestinal (GI) tract along a pathway similar to chloride. Its oral bioavailability is approximately 96%, and peak serum concentrations are reached within 2 hours. Bromide has a volume of distribution of 0.35 to 0.48 L/kg.[5] A substantial intracellular concentration of bromide is found in erythrocytes and nerve cells.[6]

Serum bromide concentrations are expressed interchangeably in several units including mEq/L, mg/L, mg/dL, and mmol/L. The interpretation of recorded values is thus subject to considerable confusion. Because of bromide's close relationship with chloride, its serum concentrations are best expressed as mmol/L. Unit relationships are as follows:

$$1 \text{ mg/L} = 1 \text{ mmol/L} = 0.1 \text{ mg/dL} = 0.0125 \text{ mEq/L}$$
$$1 \text{ mEq/L} = 80 \text{ mg/L} = 8 \text{ mg/dL}$$

Common daily intakes of bromide taken to achieve a sedative effect are 3 to 5 g daily. This corresponds to serum concentrations of approximately 50 mmol/L.

Bromide is readily filtered by the glomeruli. Once in the tubular lumen, bromide competes with chloride for reabsorption with tubules having a higher affinity for bromide ion; therefore, chloride is preferentially excreted under typical circumstances. As a result, prolonged administration of bromide results in significant total-body loss of chloride. The elimination half-life of bromide is 7 to 12 days; this half-life is increased with a salt-deficient diet.[1, 5] Average renal bromide clearance is approximately 26 mL/kg per day.

An intimate relationship exists between *in situ* chloride and bromide concentrations; the body maintains the molar sum of chloride and bromide ion at approximately 110 mmol/L.[5]

Bromide readily diffuses across the placenta and accumulates in fetal tissues. It is also secreted into breast milk.

The primary pharmacologic action of bromide is a central nervous system (CNS) membrane-stabilizing effect that results in sedation and an elevated seizure threshold. This effect may result from the disturbance of active and passive transport of chloride across neuronal membranes.

Laboratory Findings

Although total-body chloride is decreased with chronic bromide use, measured serum chloride concentrations may be elevated after bromide intake.[7] Serum chloride concentrations as high as 282 mEq/L have been reported with bromide intoxication.[8] With certain analytic systems such as the PVA-4 ion-selective electrode, measured chloride increases by approximately 2.25 mol for each mole of bromide.[7] The interference ratio for the Ektachem 700 is 3.94 mol/mol of bromide. Bromide interferes with all laboratory methods for chloride determination; other halides may produce the same effect.[9, 10] Three common methods are currently used for serum chloride measurement: ion-selective electrode (ISE), colorimetric, and coulometric.[6] Of these, coulometric analysis is least influenced by bromide whereas ISE is most disturbed (*ISE > colorimetric > coulometric*). Serum chloride concentrations that are elevated by any two of the available testing methods should be considered diagnostic of bromide intoxication. Despite the artifactual chloride elevation that bromide produces, the degree of elevation cannot be used to estimate serum bromide concentration.

Because chloride ion concentration is included in the measurement of the anion gap, the pseudohyperchloremia of bromide intoxication can result in a low anion gap, which can be diagnostic.[10] The anion gap, calculated as (Na − [Cl^- + HCO_3^-]) is normally 12 to 16 mEq/L. Elevated serum bromide concentrations produce an anion gap of less than 10 mEq/L. With high bromide concentrations, negative anion gaps as low as −60 mEq/L can occur. This abnormal anion gap can mask diagnoses that are generally identified by an elevated anion gap. Heckerling reported a case of ethylene glycol poisoning in which an expected elevated anion gap was masked by concomitant ingestion of bromide.[11] Other causes of a low anion gap include hyperlipidemia, hypoalbuminemia, use of polymixin B, and lithium intoxication.[4, 12]

Serum bromide concentrations can be measured by a gold chloride colorimetric procedure as well as by ion-exchange chromatography.[4, 13] Normal "background" bromide concentrations in adults are 3 to 4 mmol/L. Although serum bromide concentrations do not consistently correlate with severity of intoxication, levels of greater than 1000 mmol/L are associated with important clinical toxicity. Serious toxicity occurs when serum concentrations exceed 2000 mmol/L. Serum concentrations of greater than 3000 mg/L may be lethal. Elderly and debilitated patients, especially those on salt-restricted diets or with congestive heart failure, hypertension, or chronic renal failure, manifest toxicity at much lower levels.

Clinical Toxicity

In addition to sedative and anticonvulsant effects, bromide produces a number of neuropsychiatric changes. In retrospective studies, it was found that many patients who were hospitalized in psychiatric institutions in the mid-20th century in fact had bromide intoxication. In one such study, Trump and Hochberg reported that 10% to 20% of patients admitted to a psychiatric hospital had detectable bromide levels and 2% to 10% had clinical signs of bromide intoxication.[2] Case reports have also described evidence of bromide psychosis after prolonged use of pyridostigmine (used to treat myasthenia gravis) and other medications.[12, 14, 15] Widespread use of Bromo-Seltzer and Miles Nervine was once associated with widespread cases of bromide intoxication.[16]

Because bromide salts are extremely irritating to the GI tract and thus can cause a high rate of spontaneous vomiting, acute intoxication is uncommon. The estimated acute oral lethal dose of bromide is 20 to 30 g. Instead, bromide intoxication usually results from long-term overmedication, resulting in the clinical syndrome known as *bromism.*

Bromism is a clinical syndrome that consists of GI, dermatologic, and CNS manifestations (Table 60–2). GI manifestations include nausea, vomiting, a fetid odor on the breath, anorexia, and weight loss.[2] Dermatologic manifestations are found in as many as 30% of those with bromism[2]; *bromoderma* is the name given to the associated skin lesions. The most common lesion is an acneiform eruption on the face. Another frequent finding is an eruption resembling ecthyma, appearing on the lower extremities (nodose bromoderma). Other skin lesions include pemphigus-like, bromide-filled vesicles on the lower extremity, erythema multiforme, pyoderma gangrenosum, and bromoderma tuberosum (tumor-like lesions).

The neurobehavioral signs and symptoms of bromism are prominent. Behavioral disturbances include the appearance of a bromide dementia characterized by delirium, agitation, auditory and visual hallucinations, depression, and schizophrenic and manic-depressive psychosis. Hallucinosis may occur with an otherwise clear consciousness. Neurologic manifestations of bromism include dysarthria, hyporeflexia, and coma. An increased cerebrospinal fluid protein level occurs in 2% to 40% of patients.[26] Low-grade fever may be found in as many as 25% of cases.[2] Papilledema may also be present. Neurologic signs of bromism are slow to resolve and lag behind the decrease in serum bromide concentration because of the slow diffusion of bromide out of the CNS.[6] Among those who present with obtundation or coma, retrograde amnesia may develop. Ocular findings may also be striking in bromide intoxication and may consist of mydriasis, color disturbances, blurred vision, and micropsia or macropsia. Ocular bobbing (opsoclonus) has been described in a patient with

Table 60–2. Clinical Manifestations of Bromism

Behavioral	*Neurologic*	*Laboratory*
Delirium Hallucinations Agitation Amnesia Depression Mania	Dysarthria Hyporeflexia Encephalopathy Fever Papilledema Ataxia Tremor	Pseudohyperchloremia Low or negative anion gap
Gastrointestinal	*Dermatologic*	*Ocular*
Nausea, vomiting Abdominal pain Halitosis Anorexia Weight loss	Facial acneiform eruption Nodose bromoderma Bromide-filled vesicles	Mydriasis Color disturbances Blurred vision Micropsia Ocular bobbing

bromide encephalopathy.[17] Papilledema is occasionally found on funduscopic evaluation.

Bromide ingestions of 9 mg/kg per day have been associated with modest increases in serum thyroxine and triiodothyronine concentrations.[18]

Although most sedative-hypnotics are associated with tolerance, dependence, and a withdrawal syndrome when therapy is abruptly terminated, a bromide withdrawal syndrome has not been clearly described.

Because of its ready diffusion across the placenta, bromide accumulates in the fetus and can produce neonatal bromism. Clinical features of neonatal bromism are CNS depression, hypotonia, and weak suck and cry.[19, 20] CNS manifestations of bromism are thought to be more prominent in neonates because their larger brains (15% of body weight versus 2% of body weight in an adult) are the storage site of a large bromide pool.[20] Bromide also appears to be teratogenic; in a case report, Mangurten and Kaye described a woman who ingested bromides throughout pregnancy and who gave birth to a hypotonic infant with macrocephaly, hypertelorism, and clinodactyly.[19]

Diagnosis

The diagnosis of bromide intoxication is usually suspected on the basis of presenting clinical or laboratory features. Direct laboratory measurement of serum bromide concentrations is used to support the diagnosis. Bromide toxicity can appear with serum levels exceeding 100 mmol/L. Laboratory studies that are most useful in the assessment of patients with known or suspected bromide intoxication include measurements of electrolytes, blood urea nitrogen, and serum creatinine level. A general toxic screen may be indicated to identify other potential causes of altered mental status.

Management

It is unusual for bromide intoxication to result in severe cardiorespiratory embarrassment. Nonetheless, in the treatment of patients with bromide intoxication, assessment of airway, breathing, and circulation remains the foundation of treatment.

Bromide intoxication most commonly occurs after chronic ingestion. In these cases, there is no role for GI decontamination. In the rare case of acute bromide ingestion, immediate management consists of prompt GI decontamination. There are no contraindications to the use of ipecac syrup for gastric emptying; therefore, in an isolated bromide ingestion, discovered promptly, with ipecac immediately available, induced emesis would be appropriate. In the emergency department setting, ingestions within approximately 1 hour of presentation may benefit from gastric lavage. No clear evidence shows that significant amounts of bromide ion are adsorbed to activated charcoal. Organic bromides are thought to be well adsorbed to charcoal, however, and thus the administration of charcoal after organic bromide ingestion is supported.

Intravenous sodium chloride is the most important treatment intervention for bromide intoxication. It causes elimination enhancement through accelerated renal excretion. Because of its competitive action with chloride ion, bromide excretion is significantly enhanced by saline diuresis; half-life reductions to 2 to 3 days have been reported with diuresis alone. Although ammonium chloride was formerly recommended as a means of chloride loading, it is no longer recommended owing to the potential for creating metabolic acidosis. Urinary output should be maintained at 3 to 6 mL/kg per hour. Saline diuresis carries the risk of excess sodium administration; therefore, serum electrolyte values should be monitored closely. Monitoring of chloride therapy is complicated by bromide-induced pseudohyperchloremia. This prevents accurate determinations of serum chloride. Paradoxically, serum chloride concentrations decline during saline diuresis as the degree of bromide interference diminishes.

Administration of diuretics is associated with as much as 30-fold increases in bromide clearance. Both osmotic diuretics such as mannitol and loop diuretics such as furosemide can reduce the bromide elimination half-life to as little as 9 hours. In one case report, the combination of a loop and osmotic diuretic shortened the bromide half-life to less than 2 hours.[21] Intravenous furosemide should be administered in a dose of 1 mg/kg. The therapeutic endpoint of saline diuresis is improvement of symptoms and, if measurable, a serum bromide concentration of less than 1000 mmol/L. Hemodialysis is also highly effective in removing bromide ion; it produces an elimination half-life of 2 hours. Hemodialysis is rarely necessary, however, because of the efficacy of saline and diuretics. Those who are treated with hemodialysis may have a rebound in serum bromide concentration, which represents ion redistribution from intracellular spaces back to the vascular compartment.

Bromates

The bromates ($KBrO_3$, $NaBrO_3$) are distinct from bromide ion. These agents are used widely to bleach flour and produce explosives. Bromates are also found in the "neutralizers" that are part of cold-wave hair permanent kits. Cold-wave kits generally contain two solutions: a thioglycollate waving solution that acts on keratin to make hair more flexible by reducing the disulfide bond of cysteine and a bromate-containing neutralizing solution that reverses the process and stiffens hair by oxidizing the newly formed sulfhydryl groups.[22] Hair neutralizers may contain either 2% potassium bromate or 10% sodium bromate. Reports of intoxication from these agents have appeared since the 1940s. Many cases of adult bromate poisoning occurred in Japan in the 1960s and 1970s when suicide attempts by hairdressers resulted in renal failure, which led to a clinical syndrome known as "hairdresser's anuria."[22, 23] In the most complete review of these episodes, Matsumoto and colleagues described 31 cases of bromate intoxication, almost all in women, more than half of whom were hairdressers.[23] Although use of bromate-containing hair permanent kits has diminished, reports of childhood poisonings continue to appear.[24, 25]

Pharmacology/Pharmacokinetics

Bromates are colorless, odorless, tasteless compounds that are readily absorbed from the GI tract. Once they are absorbed, a fraction of bromate is reduced to bromide, and modestly elevated serum bromide concentrations result. Serum bromate concentrations are not readily measurable, and thus toxic serum bromate concentrations are unknown. Bromates are excreted unchanged in urine.

Potentially lethal doses of potassium bromate are estimated at 200 to 500 mg/kg. Life-threatening toxicity has occurred in children who ingested as little as 2 to 4 oz of potassium bromate solution.[23] Potassium bromate appears to be more toxic than sodium bromate.

Symptoms of bromate intoxication are diverse (Table 60–3). Manifestations appear within 2 hours of ingestion and begin with the GI effects of nausea, vomiting, diarrhea, and abdominal pain. These are thought to result from the formation of irritating hydrobromic acid in the gut. Cardiovascular instability with hypotension may be an early manifestation with severe exposures.

Nephrotoxicity and ototoxicity are the hallmarks of bromate intoxication. Renal injury accounts for the major morbidity and mortality of bromates. Acute renal failure usually appears 1 to 3 days after ingestion and presents as oliguria or frank anuria. Renal failure occurs in 90% to 100% of patients with significant bromate intoxication and is the most common cause of death. In children, bromate-induced acute renal failure typically resolves within 1 to 3 weeks of onset. In adult case series, however, many victims eventually develop chronic renal failure or persistent renal tubular acidosis.[22, 25, 26] Pathologic findings in the kidneys consist of acute tubular necrosis with relative glomerular sparing. Tubular histopathology consists of karyorrhexis, karyolysis, and lymphocytic interstitial infiltrates. Later changes consist of scarring, interstitial fibrosis, and glomerular sclerosis.[22]

Table 60–3. Clinical Manifestations of Bromate Intoxication

Gastrointestinal	*Renal*	*Auditory*
Nausea Vomiting, diarrhea Abdominal pain	Acute renal failure Uremia	Sensorineural hearing loss
Central Nervous System	*Cardiovascular*	
Encephalopathy Seizures	Hypotension	

Bromate ototoxicity can result in permanent sensorineural hearing loss with intact vestibular function. The mechanism of this effect is unclear; it may be related to damage of the stria vascularis with degenerative changes in the outer hair cells of the cochlea.[22] Deafness has been reported in as many as 85% of adults with significant bromate poisoning but is less frequent in children. Tinnitus and decreased hearing may appear as early as 4 to 6 hours after ingestion.[27] Other toxicities of bromate poisoning include encephalopathy, myocarditis, and hepatitis.[22] Encephalopathy is typically manifested as agitation, delirium, seizures, and coma. A peripheral neuropathy with burning in the feet has also been described.[22] Hematologic toxicity of bromate intoxication consists of anemia, which may result from microangiopathy, a clinical picture resembling hemolytic-uremic syndrome.[24]

Management

General management principles (airway, breathing, circulation) apply to unstable patients who present after bromate intoxication. Fluid, acid-base, and electrolyte status should be carefully assessed, with particular attention to hyperkalemia secondary to renal failure. An electrocardiogram should be obtained in all cases of bromate ingestion. Acute renal failure, if present, should be treated with fluid restriction, fluid and electrolyte monitoring, and, if indicated, with hemodialysis or peritoneal dialysis.

GI decontamination should proceed immediately after a bromate ingestion is recognized in order to prevent early onset of toxicity. Gastric lavage with a 2% to 5% solution of sodium bicarbonate should be performed to reduce bromate absorption and prevent hydrobromic acid production. Activated charcoal should be administered because of its potential adsorption to bromate.

Bromate ion can be reduced to less toxic bromide by intravenous administration of sodium thiosulfate. This therapy appears to be highly effective in preventing both ototoxicity and nephrotoxicity, particularly if administered early. One to 5 g of sodium thiosulfate should be administered to adults, 150 to 200 mg/kg to children, over 30 to 60 minutes. Administration of thiosulfate is associated with immediate elevations in serum bromide concentration, which confirm the conversion of bromate to less-toxic bromide.[27]

Early dialysis may remove bromate and thus prevent clinical toxicity. Both hemodialysis and peritoneal dialysis are useful adjuncts to sodium thiosulfate therapy and increase the elimination of both bromate and bromide ion. Dialysis should be strongly considered for patients who present within a few hours of a significant bromate ingestion.[27]

Bromine

Bromine is a reddish-brown gas with high water solubility. In its gaseous phase, bromine produces a dense brown cloud. Because it is heavier than air, bromine gas is found in lower layers of air.[28] Elemental bromine is widely used in industry; its largest use is as an additive to gasoline.[29] Significant occupational exposure is controlled by an Occupational Safety and Health Administration–permissible exposure limit of 1 ppm and a threshold limit value of 0.1 ppm.

Bromine is very irritating to mucous membranes and produces pain and irritation of the upper airways and the eyes. Lacrimation, tearing, coughing, respiratory distress, and headaches all develop after inhalation exposures. High concentrations of bromine can cause inflammatory lesions of the upper airway as well as photophobia and blepharospasm.[28] Other clinical manifestations are dizziness, headache, and nosebleeds. Animal studies have shown that 3-hour exposures to bromine at 3 ppm can result in pulmonary edema.[29] Bromine gas at a concentration of 10 ppm is a severe irritant that cannot be tolerated. Death may occur secondary to bromine pneumonitis, which resembles adult respiratory distress syndrome. Necropsy revealed massive hemorrhagic alveolitis. Direct skin exposure to liquid bromine can result in formation of vesicles and pustules, which develop into deep, painful ulcers with a brown discoloration of skin.[30] The manifestations of bromine exposure parallel those of chlorine exposure.

Exposure to elemental bromine is uncommon but has been reported after occupational or environmental disasters. In one of the most important such exposures, a chemical plant in Geneva, Switzerland, released bromine gas in November 1984, and approximately 25,000 inhabitants were exposed to high concentrations of bromine. Clinical manifestations were extensive (Table 60–4).[28] Many of these symptoms persisted 1 month later, particularly eye and upper airway irritation, headache, and cough.

Table 60–4. Clinical Manifestations Reported After Bromine Gas Exposure in 59 Patients

Symptoms	Number of Patients (%)
Eye irritation	53 (90)
Upper airway irritation	40 (68)
Cough	28 (47)
Expectoration	20 (34)
Headache	27 (46)
Photophobia	7 (12)
Weakness	7 (12)
Nausea	6 (10)
Dizziness	6 (10)
Abdominal pain	4 (7)
Itching	2 (3)
Sweating	2 (3)
Vomiting	2 (3)

From Morabia A, Selleger C, Landry JC, et al: Accidental bromine exposure in an urban population: An acute epidemiological assessment. Int J Epidemiol *17*:148–152, 1988.

Treatment of bromine exposure consists of ventilation and copious irrigation of eyes and skin with water and isotonic saline.[28] Corticosteroids have been administered in cases of severe respiratory distress without clear efficacy.[28] Prophylactic antibiotics are not recommended for bromine pneumonitis because they may promote the selection of resistant organisms.

IODINE COMPOUNDS

Iodine

With a molecular weight of 127, iodine is the heaviest of the halides. Iodine was discovered in 1812. Shortly thereafter, its antiseptic/antimicrobial properties were recognized and it became widely used for infection control. Iodine was subsequently found to be a nutrient necessary for the synthesis of thyroid hormones.

Industrial uses of iodine include the manufacture of organic chemicals, pharmaceuticals such as contrast media for radiographic procedures, antiseptics and germicides, dyes and inks, and catalysts for photography, engraving, and lithography. The threshold limit value for occupational iodine exposure is 0.1 ppm.

Iodine is also an essential micronutrient and is a moiety in the thyroid hormones thyroxine and triiodothyronine. A regular intake of dietary iodine (in the form of iodide) is therefore essential; a daily requirement of 150 μg/day is recommended for adults.

Elemental iodine is used almost exclusively for topical application. Available products are iodine topical solution (which contains approximately 2 g of iodine and 2 g of sodium iodide per 100 mL) and tincture of iodine (which has the same composition as iodine solution but in a 50% alcohol base). Solutions of iodine have a characteristic deep brown color and odor. In aqueous solutions, iodine is present as seven different species: elemental iodine (I_2), hypoiodic acid (HOI), iodine cation ($[H_2OI]^+$), triiodide ion (I_3^-), iodide ion (I^-), hypoiodite ion (OI^-), and iodate ion (IO_3^-).[31] Elemental iodine, hypoiodic acid, and iodine cation are potent germicides, whereas triiodide and hypoiodite ions are relatively weak antiseptics. Topically applied iodide ion has no antimicrobial activity. Although the exact mechanism of its antimicrobial effect remains unclear, iodine compounds may work by (1) reacting with ubiquitous amine groups, (2) oxidizing the sulfhydryl group of cysteine, (3) disrupting protein synthesis, (4) reacting with the phenolic group of tyrosine, or (5) reacting with fatty acid double bonds, thereby disrupting the cell wall lipid bilayer.

Because of its oxidizing ability, iodine compounds can produce false-positive test results for blood when orthotoluidine (Hematest) or guaiac reagents are used. When used as a topical antiseptic, iodine may also produce a false elevation in blood glucose level when measured by certain methods.[32] Iodine can produce a false elevation in chloride level, which can result in pseudohyperchloremia.

Pharmacokinetics

When ingested in its elemental form, iodine must be reduced to iodide in the intestine before its systemic absorption. After absorption, interconversion occurs between iodine and iodide. Both species are readily excreted in urine. As a result, persons with renal failure due to any cause are at greater risk of iodide accumulation, regardless of the iodide form or its method of administration.

Clinical Toxicity

Two per cent iodine has minimal toxicity when applied topically, although it may stain the skin and produce dermal injury (iodine burns). Iodine solutions of greater than 7% are invariably corrosive to skin. Sensitization may occur in susceptible individuals.[31] Tincture of iodine is more irritating than aqueous solution. Occlusive dressing increases the risk of dermal injury after iodine application.

Iodine is strongly irritating to all mucous membranes, including the eyes and respiratory tract. Possessing the characteristics of an acid corrosive, concentrated iodine produces a coagulation necrosis. Eye exposures to iodine result in intense pain and blepharospasm; prolonged occupational exposure to iodine gas can produce brown staining of the corneal epithelium. With severe inhalation exposures, pulmonary edema secondary to iodine pneumonitis may appear in a pattern similar to that of other halide gas exposures (fluorine, bromine, and chlorine).

Ingestion of 2 to 4 g of iodine is potentially fatal, although ingestions of as much as 20 g have been associated with survival. The hallmark of iodine ingestion is corrosion of the GI tract with potential peritonitis, perforation, metabolic acidosis, sepsis, and death. The metabolic acidosis can be profound and has an unclear cause. Any starch-containing food complexes with iodine, and a blue emesis that is considered pathognomonic for iodine ingestion is produced. Significant iodine ingestion also produces a clinical syndrome that includes tachycardia, parotitis, bronchitis, and insomnia.[30]

Management

Victims of iodine ingestion may present with shock secondary to GI injury and possible perforation. These unstable patients must be managed by airway support, aggressive fluid resuscitation, and correction of acid-base disturbances. A surgical evaluation may be necessary for the evaluation and management of possible esophageal or gastric perforation. In the absence of clear signs of perforation, diagnostic esophagoscopy should be performed.

The issue of GI decontamination in patients with iodine ingestion is complex and difficult. Administration of ipecac is absolutely contraindicated owing to the risk of additional corrosive injury to the esophagus. Orogastric lavage with a large-bore lavage tube is also relatively contraindicated because it may worsen any esophageal injury. Although activated charcoal may adsorb small amounts of iodine, dietary complex sugars are more effective in gut decontamination because of their ability both to complex with iodine and to promote its reduction to less-toxic iodide. In a patient who has no signs of significant esophageal or gastric injury, administration of either flour (or some other starch) or milk may be beneficial. However, because significant esophageal or gastric injury may occur and because patients with corrosive ingestions must take nothing by mouth, GI decontamination measures may not be a practical option. Treatment of iodine ingestions also includes oral administration of sodium thiosulfate; 100 mL of a 1% solution can rapidly reduce iodine to iodide and thereby reduce the risk of corrosive injury. Thiosulfate can also be used to remove iodine stains from skin and clothing.[31]

Radioactive Iodine

Exposure to radioactive iodines occurs in three distinct clinical settings. First, ^{131}I is a commonly prescribed treatment for hyperthyroid states. ^{131}I exposure may also occur after nuclear reactor mishaps, which often result in mass exposures. Finally, ^{123}I, a related radioisotope, is used in radiographic imaging to identify thyroid tissue.

Radioactive iodine has a half-life of 8 days. During its decay, it emits both x-rays and β-particles.[33] More than 99% of ^{131}I radioactivity is emitted within 56 days of administration or exposure. Once absorbed from either the respiratory or GI tract, radioactive iodine is rapidly incorporated into the thyroid gland. The destructive β-particles destroy the parenchymal cells of the thyroid with little or no damage to surrounding tissue. The x-rays produced by radioactive thyroid can pass through tissue and be measured by external detection.[33] The cytotoxic actions of ^{131}I are well described: Pyknosis and necrosis of follicular cells are followed by the disappearance of glandular colloid. Fibrosis eventually results. Carefully measured doses of ^{131}I can destroy the thyroid gland completely without identifiable injury to adjacent tissues.[33] ^{123}I has a considerably shorter half-life and is used in the performance of thyroid scans. Because of its rapid incorporation into functioning thyroid tissue, producing "hot" and "cold" areas on imaging, it is a valuable tool in the identification of ectopic thyroid tissue, including metastatic tumors.[33]

^{131}I is available in solution and capsule forms. The administered dose is based on the estimated weight of the thyroid gland; the thyroid weight is used to calculate a dose of isotope necessary to provide 7000 to 10,000 rad per gram of thyroid tissue.[33] Approximate doses are 80 to 150 μCi per gram of thyroid tissue. Within a few weeks of treatment, symptoms of hyperthyroidism resolve unless the dose has been inadequate. Depending on the dose, 50% to 65% of hyperthyroid patients are cured by a single dose of ^{131}I, an additional 20% to 30% by two doses, and the remainder by three or more doses.

The primary clinical toxicity from ^{131}I exposure is the eventual development of hypothyroidism. In the therapeutic setting, even after elaborate dose calculations, a significant percentage of patients have complete destruction of the thyroid gland and eventually develop hypothyroidism. In pregnancy, radioactive iodine can accumulate in fetal thyroid, with the potential for its permanent ablation.

Treatment of radioiodine exposure consists primarily of administration of potassium iodide. Thyroid gland uptake of ^{131}I can be reduced by more than 90% through oral administration of potassium iodide if iodide therapy is initiated immediately after acute exposure. Some benefit from potassium iodide therapy is still possible as late as 12 hours after exposure to ^{131}I. Potassium iodide is administered as a 130-mg oral dose; it is generally recommended when the projected exposure to ^{131}I exceeds 10 to 30 rad (although less conservative recommendations of exposures greater than 50 to 100 rad have been recommended). The treatment interval is typically 7 to 14 days unless exposure is ongoing.

Iodides

Like elemental iodine, iodide has a long history of use as an antimicrobial agent. Within 20 years of iodine's discovery, potassium iodide became used for the treatment of tertiary syphilis.[34] In 1927, the first edition of the *Cecil Textbook of Medicine* recommended potassium iodide for the treatment of 30 diseases.[34] Iodide was recognized as an essential nutrient once the etiology of endemic goiter was discovered. Potassium iodide is now added to table salt in order to prevent goiter (thyroid hyperplasia secondary to iodide deficiency). The iodized salt manufactured in the United States contains 100 μg iodide and 6 mEq potassium per gram.[33] Dairy products and seafood are other major dietary sources of iodide.

Iodide salts remain commonly prescribed for the treatment of hyperthyroidism and sporotrichosis.[33] They are also used as expectorants (in the form of iodinated glycerol) because they are mildly effective in liquefying thick bronchial secretions.[33] Other medications that contain iodide include saturated solution of potassium iodide, Elixophyllin (a theophylline combination product), the antimicrobial agent iodoquinol, the antiarrhythmic amiodarone, and enteric-coated potassium iodide. Iodide salts are also provided as protection from thyroid ablation after unintentional exposure to ^{131}I.

Therapeutic doses of iodide vary widely. Used as an expectorant, as much as 1 g daily is recommended. In the management of hyperthyroid crises, as much as 2 g daily is administered.

Pharmacokinetics

Ingested iodide is readily absorbed from the GI tract. Blood concentrations of iodide are typically low (0.2 to 0.4 μg/dL). Iodide is actively transported into thyroid tissue through a mechanism that is under tight negative feedback.

Elevated iodide concentrations can produce falsely elevated serum chloride measurements (pseudohyperchloremia). As with bromide intoxication, this artifactual elevation is greatest for the ion-selective method of chloride analysis rather than the coulometric measurement. Serum chloride concentrations of 168 mEq/L have been reported after iodide intoxication.[35] A low or negative anion gap may also occur. The silver halide precipitation method of serum chloride measurement is not influenced by iodide elevation.[36]

Clinical Toxicity

Chronic intoxication with iodide is known as *iodism*. This syndrome consists of oral, respiratory, salivary, pulmonary, dermatologic, and GI effects (Table 60–5). Oral effects include a metallic taste and burning in the mouth as well as soreness of the teeth and gums. The occurrence of sialorrhea, coryza, frontal headache, and productive cough simulates sinusitis or a head cold.[33] When severe, bronchorrhea can result in pulmonary edema. Other signs of iodism include salivary gland enlargement (iodide mumps)[37, 38] and skin lesions that resemble those found in bromism (iododerma). Iodism can also produce unexplained fever.

Iodide excess can result in both hypothyroidism and hyperthyroidism. Iodide is a potent inhibitor of

Table 60–5. Clinical Manifestations of Iodism

Oral	*Salivary*	*Dermatologic*
Metallic taste Gingivitis Pharyngitis Laryngitis	Excess salivation Salivary gland enlargement	Acneiform eruption Vesicles Pustules
Nasal	*Pulmonary*	*Gastrointestinal*
Nasal congestion Sneezing "Sinus" headache	Productive cough Pulmonary edema	Bloody diarrhea Anorexia
Thyroid		
Thyroid enlargement Hypothyroidism Cretinism Adenoma Myxedema		
Ocular		
Eye irritation Periorbital edema		

thyroid hormone synthesis (the Wolff-Chaikoff effect).[33] It also inhibits thyroid hormone release. This is the basis of its use in the treatment of hyperthyroid states. It is also the reason why excess iodide intake during pregnancy can result in neonatal hypothyroidism (cretinism).[33] Prolonged use of iodide salts produces thyroid gland hyperplasia, goiter, thyroid adenoma, or severe hypothyroidism. Concomitant use of lithium salts amplifies the hypothyroid effect of iodides. Simultaneous use of potassium iodide and potassium-sparing diuretics can produce hyperkalemia, with associated cardiac arrhythmias or cardiac arrest. Enteric-coated potassium iodide can produce small intestinal injury with associated obstruction, hemorrhage, perforation, and death.

Intravenous administration of iodides has resulted in anaphylactoid reactions with the immediate appearance of angioedema, laryngeal swelling, rash, and fever. A serum sickness–like syndrome can also occur, with arthralgia, lymph gland swelling, arthritis, hematuria, proteinuria, and eosinophilia. Other hypersensitivity manifestations include thrombotic thrombocytopenic purpura and fatal periarteritis nodosa.[33] Hypersensitivity reactions to iodinated contrast agents are idiosyncratic. These are often fatal.

Management

Symptoms of iodism resolve rapidly after discontinuation of iodide. As with bromide, iodide competes with chloride for reabsorption in the proximal tubule; therefore, saline diuresis enhances the renal excretion of iodide and is appropriate in cases of significant iodism. Hemodialysis readily removes iodide ion but should not be necessary in a patient with normal renal function.

Certain manifestations of iodism, particularly salivary gland inflammation and ioderma, may respond to corticosteroid therapy.[39, 40]

Iodophors

Iodophors are substances that have elemental iodine attached to a high-molecular-weight moiety. As a general rule, iodophors enhance the bactericidal activity of iodine. The most common iodophor, povidone-iodine (Betadine), is an iodine molecule linked to polyvinylpyrrolidone. Betadine is used most commonly as a 10% solution (which contains only 0.001% free iodine). Iodophors are found in solutions, ointments, and surgical scrubs. Because iodine is tightly bound to the carrier, iodophors have very low rates of iodine release. These substances are therefore nonirritating after ingestion and generally have low toxicity. However, because they do contain substantial amounts of iodine, iodophors can result in significant iodine absorption, particularly (1) when the integrity of the skin is compromised; (2) in infants, who have greater skin permeability; (3) after mucosal application (e.g., vaginal instillation); and (4) after excessive topical application.[36] Because of iodine diffusion into breast milk, vaginal application of povidone-iodine has been associated with elevated serum iodide levels in a breast-fed infant.[41] Neonates readily absorb iodine from topical povidone-iodine solutions, and their total plasma iodine levels remain elevated for 3 days after a single application. Goiter and hypothyroidism, dermatitis, liver function abnormalities, and neutropenia have also been described after prolonged exposure to povidone-iodine and other iodophors. Serum iodide concentrations can increase 100-fold in those who have iodophors applied to open wounds, burns, or decubitus ulcers, and iodide-related fatalities are reported.[42] In an unusual report, Kurt and colleagues described a 9-week-old infant who received 150 mL of povidone-iodide via a nasogastric tube and died of severe corrosive injury to the GI tract with a blood iodine level of 14,600 μg/dL.[43] Systemic absorption of iodophors has also been associated with the development of a metabolic acidosis. The cause of the acidosis has not been identified, although its etiology may be related to either the acidity of the povidone-iodine solution ($pH < 3$), bicarbonate complexation to iodine, or renal tubular acidosis. Both normal and elevated lactate levels have been described after iodine absorption from iodophors.[36] Other metabolic abnormalities associated with iodine absorption from iodophors include hypernatremia, hyperchloremia, renal insufficiency, and renal tubular acidosis.

Treatment of iodine intoxication resulting from iodophor exposure consists of basic interventions used to treat iodide toxicity. However, because iodophors have very low toxicity unless ingested in massive amounts, no specific intervention is recommended after ingestion. Activated charcoal has a potential role, because iodophors are organic compounds; charcoal should be considered after ingestion of more than 6 to 8 oz of Betadine (or other iodophor). Because of the potential disturbances in thyroid function, thyroid hormone should be monitored for up to 4 weeks after very large ingestions.

Acknowledgments

Lydia Baltarowich, MD, Daniel Carl Postellon, MD, and Regine Aronow, MD, contributed to this chapter in a previous edition.

References

1. Bowers GN, Onoroski M: Hypochloremia and the incidence of bromism in 1990. Clin Chem *36*:1399–1403, 1990.
2. Trump DL, Hochberg MC: Bromide intoxication. Johns Hopkins Med J *138*:119–123, 1976.
3. Meldgaard OT, Cold GE: Serum bromide after general anaesthesia with halothane. Acta Anaesth Scand *23*:513–518, 1979.
4. Ng Y-Y, Lin W-L, Chen T-W, et al: Spurious hyperchloremia and decreased anion gap in a patient with dextromethorphan bromide. Am J Nephrol *12*:268–270, 1992.
5. Rauws AG: Pharmacokinetics of bromide ion—an overview. Food Chem Toxicol *21*:379–382, 1983.
6. Iberti TJ, Patterson BK, Fisher CJ: Prolonged bromide intox-

ication resulting from a gastric bezoar. Arch Intern Med *144*:402–403, 1984.
7. Emancipator K, Kroll MH: Bromide interference: Is less really better? Clin Chem *36*:1470–1473, 1990.
8. Kan K, Satowa S, Takeuchi I, et al: Unusual apparent hyperchloremia induced by long-term abuse of bromide-containing drugs. Int J Clin Pharmacol Ther Toxicol *24*:399–402, 1986.
9. Elin RJ, Arthur RE, Johnson E: Bromide interferes with determination of chloride by each of four methods. Clin Chem *27*:778–779, 1981.
10. Vasuvattakul S, Lertpattanasuwan N, Vareesangthip K, et al: A negative anion gap as a clue to diagnose bromide intoxication. Nephron *69*:311–313, 1995.
11. Heckerling PS: Ethylene glycol poisoning with a normal anion gap due to occult bromide intoxication. Ann Emerg Med *16*:1384–1386, 1987.
12. Rothenberg DM, Berns AS, Barkin R, Glantz RH: Bromide intoxication secondary to pyridostigmine bromide therapy. JAMA *263*:1121–1122, 1990.
13. Miller ME, Cappon CJ: Anion-exchange chromatographic determination of bromide in serum. Clin Chem *30*:781–783, 1984.
14. Jinkins JR, Chaleby K: Acute toxic encephalopathy secondary to bromide sedative ingestion. Neuroradiology *29*:212, 1987.
15. Senecal P-E, Osterloh J: Confusion from pyridostigmine bromide: Was there bromide intoxication? JAMA *264*:454–455, 1990.
16. McDanal CE, Owens D, Bolman WM: Bromide abuse: A continuing problem. Am J Psychiatry *131*:913–915, 1974.
17. Paty DW, Sherr H: Ocular bobbing in bromism. Neurology *22*:526–527, 1971.
18. Sangster B, Blom JL, Sekhuis VM, et al: The influence of sodium bromide in man: A study in human volunteers with special emphasis on the endocrine and the central nervous system. Food Chem Toxicol *21*:409–419, 1983.
19. Mangurten HH, Kaye CI: Neonatal bromism secondary to maternal exposure in a photographic laboratory. J Pediatr *100*:596–598, 1982.
20. Pleasure JR, Blackburn MG: Neonatal bromide intoxication: Prenatal ingestion of a large quantity of bromides with transplacental accumulation in the fetus. Pediatrics *55*:503–506, 1975.
21. Steen PA, Sejersted OM, Hartmann A, Kiil F: Transcellular and intercellular transport of anions in the kidney tubules of dogs. Acta Physiol Scand *113*:239–244, 1981.
22. Kutom A, Bazilinshi NG, Magana L, Dunea G: Bromate intoxication: Hairdressers' anuria. Am J Kidney Dis *15*:84–85, 1990.
23. Matsumoto I, Morizono T, Paparella MM: Hearing loss following potassium bromate: Two case reports. Otolaryngol Head Neck Surg *88*:625–629, 1980.
24. Warshaw BL, Carter MC, Hymes LC, et al: Bromate poisoning from hair permanent preparations. Pediatrics *7*:975–978, 1985.
25. Lue JN, Johnson CE, Edwards DL: Bromate poisoning from ingestion of professional hair-care neutralizer. Clin Pharmacol *7*:66–70, 1988.
26. Kuwahara T, Ikehara Y, Kanatsu K, et al: Two cases of potassium bromate poisoning requiring long-term hemodialysis therapy for irreversible tubular damage. Nephron *37*:278–280, 1984.
27. Lichtenberg R, Zeller WP, Gatson R, Hurley RM: Bromate poisoning. J Pediatr *114*:891–894, 1989.
28. Morabia A, Selleger C, Landry JC, et al: Accidental bromine exposure in an urban population: An acute epidemiological assessment. Int J Epidemiol *17*:148–152, 1988.
29. Broderick A, Schwartz DA: Halogen gases, ammonia, and phosgene. *In* Sullivan JB, Krieger GR (eds): Hazardous Materials Toxicology—Clinical Principles of Environmental Health. Baltimore, Williams & Wilkins, pp 792–793, 1992.
30. Sullivan JB: Cryogenics, oxidizers, reducing agents, and explosives. *In* Sullivan JB, Krieger GR (eds): Hazardous Materials Toxicology—Clinical Principles of Environmental Health. Baltimore, Williams & Wilkins, pp 1192–1201, 1992.
31. American Hospital Formulary Service: Iodine. *In* McEvoy GK (ed): Drug Information 95. Bethesda, MD, American Society of Health-System Pharmacists, pp 2427–2428, 1995.
32. Feingold KR, Sater B, Engle B: Iodine-induced artifacts in home blood glucose measurements. Diabetes Care *6*:317–318, 1983.
33. Haynes RC: Thyroid and antithyroid drugs. *In* Gilman AG, Rall TW, Nies AS, Taylor P (eds): Goodman and Gilman's The Pharmacological Basis of Therapeutics. New York, Pergamon Press, pp 1361–1383, 1990.
34. Beeson PB: Effects of iodides on inflammatory processes. Perspect Biol Med *37*:173–181, 1994.
35. Soldin SJ, Nicholson S, Einhorn A, Koppes S: Serendipitous diagnosis of iodide intoxication. Clin Chem *34*:2391–2392, 1988.
36. Dela Cruz F, Brown DH, Leikin JB: Iodine absorption after topical administration. West J Med *146*:43–45, 1987.
37. Sussman RM, Miller J: Iodide "mumps" after intravenous urography. N Engl J Med *255*:433–434, 1956.
38. Carter JE: Iodide "mumps". N Engl J Med *264*:987–988, 1961.
39. Aquilina JT: Fungating ioderma treated with hydrocortisone. JAMA *158*:727–728, 1955.
40. Waugh WH: Use of cortisone by mouth in the prevention and therapy of severer iodism. Arch Intern Med *93*:299–303, 1954.
41. Postellon DC, Aronow R: Iodine in mother's milk. JAMA *247*:463, 1982.
42. D'Auria J, Lipson S, Garfield JM: Fatal iodine toxicity following surgical debridement of a hip wound: Case report. J Trauma *30*:353–355, 1990.
43. Kurt TL, Morgan ML, Hnilica V: Fatal iatrogenic iodine toxicity in a 9-week old infant. Abstract. Vet Hum Toxicol *34*:333, 1992.

61

Hydrofluoric Acid

MICHAEL W. CARLTON, MD
MICHAEL V. VANCE, MD

In 1670, a crude preparation of hydrofluoric acid (HF) was first used for artistic glass etching. Aqueous HF was first produced in 1771. By 1800, the injurious properties of HF were becoming clear, and Gay-Lussac described the toxicity of HF with delayed onset of symptoms in 1809.[1] During the late 18th and early 19th centuries HF was used to clean sand from castings. Since then, the industrial utility of HF has increased dramatically (Table 61–1). The introduction of HF into commercial products such as rust removers and chrome and wire-wheel cleaners has made clinical exposures to HF commonplace. HF is a weak inorganic acid produced by reacting fluorospar (CaF_2) with sulfuric acid. HF gas is released and is then cooled to the liquid state. Anhydrous HF must be stored at low temperature or under pressure because its boiling point is 19.4°C and it fumes at concentrations in excess of 48%. Industrial uses require concentrations of 1% to 100%. Concentrations in home use products generally range from 1% to 12%, such as in Whink rust stain remover.

HF attacks glass and stoneware, dissolving the silica. It must therefore be stored in plastic, lead, wax, or paraffin paper bottles. Natural rubber, polyvinyl chloride, neoprene, or nitrile handwear must be used to avoid dermal exposure. Hospital-grade latex gloves are insufficient for protection. Human toxicity is usually the result of noncompliance with the manufacturer's safety guidelines and most frequently results in exposure to the extremities. Workplace exposure limits are shown in Table 61–2.

Table 61–1. Industrial Uses of Hydrofluoric Acid

Cleaning sandstone and marble	High octane fuel production
Insecticide	Propellent manufacture
Control fermentation	Byproduct in fertilizer production
Etching and glazing ceramics	Stain remover
Etching microchip wafers	Etching and frosting glassware
Cleaning foundry castings	Electroplating
Removal of trace metals from textiles	Rust removal
	Dye and drug production
	Oil well injecting

PATHOPHYSIOLOGY

With a pK_a of 3.8, HF acid is a relatively weak acid. As do other inorganic acids, HF produces corrosive burns to the skin. Coagulation necrosis limits the penetration of most acids. HF's ability to penetrate intact skin into deeper tissues where the fluoride ion may dissociate and produce further toxicity is unique among inorganic acids. In concentrated solutions or in the presence of dermal necrosis, the ability of HF to reach the deeper tissues is increased.[1]

With concentrated solutions there is immediate pain and injury owing to the dehydrating and corrosive effects of HF. In tissue, free fluoride ion is able to bind calcium and magnesium to form insoluble salts. Profound hypocalcemia and hypomagnesemia may result. The delay in pain and injury that is often characteristic of HF injuries is attributed to the precipitation of calcium fluoride and magnesium fluoride salts in deeper tissues. Hypocalcemia and hypomagnesemia lead to intracellular potassium release. Hyperkalemia leads to neural stimulation, yielding the painful stimuli associated with the deep

Table 61–2. Exposure Limits for Hydrofluoric Acid

Odor threshold	0.03 mg/m^3
Immediately dangerous to life and health	20 ppm
Threshold limit value—ceiling	2.5 mg/m^3 (3 ppm)
Short-term exposure limit	2.5 mg/m^3 (3 ppm)

tissue injury of HF. The lack of early dehydrating and corrosive injury delays presentation and treatment.

CLINICAL PRESENTATION

Toxicity and clinical presentation after exposure to HF depend on the route of exposure, amount and duration of tissue exposed, and the HF concentration. The adequacy of decontamination measures taken also plays a role in toxic presentation. In 1943, the Division of Industrial Hygiene of the National Institutes of Health classified HF exposure solely on the concentration of the agent involved.[2] Solutions with less than 20% HF could produce symptoms that were delayed by up to 24 hours. Agents with concentrations of 20% to 50% produce symptoms within 8 hours of exposure. Compounds with greater than 50% HF produce immediate tissue damage and pain. Although these guidelines remain useful, it must be remembered that even dilute solutions may produce symptoms more rapidly than these guidelines suggest.

Dermal Exposure. The most common route of exposure to HF is dermal. The site of exposure is usually the distal upper extremities, with the hands being involved in over 70% of all injuries. Misuse of HF solutions, damaged or the absence of protective gear, and noncompliance with recommendations are involved in a majority of cases. Although HF is used in many industrial applications, as many as 60% of injuries may occur in the home.[3]

In an animal model of HF exposure, solutions as dilute as 0.01% produced visible lesions in 5 minutes, whereas a 2% solution was corrosive after 1 hour of application and produced elevated serum fluoride levels.[1] Theoretically, the application of 7 mL of 99% HF can bind all of the calcium in a 70-kg man.[4] One fatality was reported after a 2.5% total body surface area burn to the face, mouth, and pharynx. Aspiration and systemic toxicity contributed to the victim's death.[5]

When the solution is dilute, symptomatology and presentation may be delayed by up to 24 hours. Progressive itching, burning, and pain are generally the reason the patient seeks medical attention. There is a predilection for subungual areas. Blanching of the skin or erythema may be present. Blisters may be absent early. A blackish necrotic area appears later. With exposure to concentrated HF solutions the free hydrogen ion concentration produces immediate pain. Coagulation necrosis occurs. The breakdown of the epidermal and dermal barrier increases systemic absorption of the undissociated HF. Systemic toxicity may follow.

Ocular Exposure. Ocular tissues are extremely sensitive to HF. Concentrations as low as 5 mg/L (5 ppm) may produce irritation to the eye.[6] Although the proteinaceous precipitation of coagulation necrosis limits the penetration of other inorganic acids, HF is able to penetrate the ocular tissues and produces severe damage to ocular structures. Lacrimation, pain, and conjunctival injection are early symptoms of HF exposure.[7, 8] Corneal and conjunctival epithelium may be denuded, leading to edema and ischemia. Corneal vascularization and scarring may result. Toxicity may be delayed by up to 4 days after dilute exposures.[9] Global perforation has also been reported.[10]

Inhalational Exposure. HF is an irritant to the mucosa of the upper and lower portions of the respiratory tract. As in ocular tissues, concentrations as low as 5 mg/L (5 ppm) may produce irritation to the nasal mucosa.[6] When HF is present in concentrations greater than 48%, the solution fumes, adding to the volatile airborne fraction. Mucosal edema, bronchospasm, bronchorrhea, wheezing, atelectasis, and airways obstruction may result. A chemical tracheobronchitis or pneumonitis, either of which may be hemorrhagic, and pulmonary edema may follow. Onset of signs and symptoms may be immediate, with death reported in as little as 30 minutes after exposure,[11–13] or they may not appear for several days.[14] Symptoms in survivors may be sustained for greater than 1 year.[14]

Gastrointestinal Exposure. Nausea, vomiting, and abdominal pain are the usual symptoms after HF ingestion. Painful erosions or ulcerations of the mouth, esophagus, and stomach may also occur. Hemorrhagic gastritis without ulceration was reported in one patient in whom death occurred within 90 minutes of ingestion.[15] Autopsy revealed hemorrhagic pulmonary edema and hemorrhagic gastritis without ulceration. Fulminant colitis after an HF enema[16] and perforation of the sigmoid colon secondary to rectal HF exposure[17] occurred in two patients intoxicated with cocaine. Both of these patients self-administered the HF preparation inadvertently and required partial bowel resection.

Systemic Toxicity. Systemic toxicity can follow any route of exposure but is unlikely after one limited to the ocular route. Once HF penetrates the dermal or mucosal barrier the fluoride ion dissociates and binds calcium and magnesium ions. Profound hypocalcemia and hypomagnesemia may result. A serum calcium level as low as 2.2 mg/dL and a serum magnesium level as low as 0.6 mg/dL have been reported.[5] Weakness, respiratory arrest, hypotension, and cardiac arrhythmias may result.[5, 18–22] Hyperkalemia, secondary to systemic fluoride toxicity, leads to cardiac toxicity in animals[23, 24] and humans[23, 25] and may be the most significant factor contributing to death. Hyperphosphatemia, hyponatremia, metabolic acidosis, and death may also occur. The severity of illness is related to the surface area exposed, duration of exposure, and concentration of HF. Renal toxicity has also been reported.[12, 14]

LABORATORY DIAGNOSIS

During assessment for chronic exposure, urine and blood levels may identify persons with excessive exposure, but these levels have no place in the management of acute toxicity. Diagnosis is made on clinical grounds based on history and physical examination. Hypocalcemia, hypomagnesemia, acidemia, and hyperkalemia suggest the presence of HF toxicity in the appropriate setting, and these laboratory values can be useful in guiding therapy.

TREATMENT

Dermal Exposure

Initial management of HF burns after dermal exposure is removal from the source and irrigation with copious amounts of water. All contaminated clothing should be removed. Caution must be used when removing and disposing of contaminated clothing because health care and janitorial workers may become secondarily exposed. Irrigation should last for 15 to 30 minutes. Irrigation is more effective in concentrated exposures because persons affected by low HF concentrations generally have a delayed presentation.

Topical application of various substances including calcium gluconate gel, calcium carbonate paste, benzalkonium chloride magnesium ointments, concentrated aloe gel, and vitamin A and D ointment has been studied after dermal application of HF in animal models.[26, 27] Only calcium gluconate gel proved effective in decreasing the size and severity of skin lesions. Addition of the penetration enhancer dimethyl sulfoxide improved outcome when compared with use of calcium gluconate gel alone in another study.[28] *Topical application of calcium gluconate gel is the first-line emergency department treatment for HF burns after irrigation.*

Subcutaneous injection of calcium gluconate has proven useful in the treatment of HF acid–induced dermal burns.[2, 28–31] With a 25- to 30-gauge needle, 0.5 mL/cm^2 is injected into the subcutaneous space below the injured tissue. This procedure is painful and is seldom used in modern clinical practice. Local and regional anesthesia have been used, but this negates the elimination of pain as the target goal. Calcium chloride should never be used, owing to its irritant effects. Subungual injection may not be effective, and removal of the nail may be required. Subcutaneous and intravenous injection of magnesium sulfate has been shown to be beneficial by several authors, but no advantage of these methods over subcutaneous administration of calcium gluconate has been demonstrated in humans.[32, 33] Severe hand and foot burns are often treated with intra-arterial calcium gluconate.

In cases of moderate to severe toxicity to the hands and feet, intra-arterial infusion of calcium gluconate may be required,[34–37] especially in patients who have persistent pain after irrigation and topical application of calcium gluconate. The choice of artery is based on the location of the burn. If the thumb or index finger is involved, then the radial artery is used. If other portions of the hand are affected, the brachial artery may be used. The posterior tibial or femoral artery may be used when the foot is involved. An arteriogram may be helpful in establishing which artery to use. Ten milliliters of 10% calcium gluconate is added to 40 mL of normal saline or 5% dextrose in water and infused into the appropriate artery over 4 hours. The addition of heparin decreases the incidence of catheter occlusion. If pain does not resolve, then the infusion may be repeated.

Ocular Exposure. After ocular exposure, copious irrigation with tap water, normal saline, or lactated Ringer's solution should be initiated. Contact lenses should be removed before irrigation. Transport of the patient to an emergency department or other site should be delayed until the irrigation is complete. One liter of irrigation solution should be administered over 30 minutes. The pH should be checked and irrigation continued until it is normal. Administration of a topical ophthalmic anesthetic solution may increase compliance with irrigation. Lactated Ringer's solution contains 20 mg/L of calcium chloride. Given the affinity of calcium ion for fluoride, a role for this solution has been suggested.[38] However, various solutions have been used and none has proven more effective than lukewarm tap water or normal saline.[7, 8] Subconjunctival injection of calcium gluconate and calcium chloride was administered to rabbits and resulted in increased toxicity after ocular exposure. Repeated instillation of 1% calcium gluconate eye drops was of benefit in a single case report.[38] All exposed persons should receive ophthalmologic consultation as soon as possible because of the risk of ocular perforation.

Inhalation Exposure. Treatment for inhalational exposure is largely supportive. Given the rapid progression of tracheobronchitis, hemorrhagic pulmonary edema, and death, local emergency medical services should be activated and the patient should be transported to the nearest emergency department. The airway should be maintained, and the patient should be mechanically ventilated if needed. Humidified oxygen should be administered, and aggressive pulmonary toilet should be undertaken. Nebulized calcium gluconate (2.5% to 3%) has been recommended,[39] but there is no evidence that this is effective therapy.[6, 40]

Gastrointestinal Exposure. Immediate dilution of HF with water should be undertaken. Milk has been suggested as a diluent with the possible benefit of its calcium binding some of the ingested fluoride ion. As with all caustic substances, induction of emesis is contraindicated. Activated charcoal plays no role in absorbing small ions such as hydrogen or fluoride. Because of the high mortality associated with systemic toxicity, gastric lavage through a nasogastric tube should be undertaken in all cases when presentation is within 60 to 120 minutes after ingestion in which perforation has not yet occurred. Extreme care must be taken by the health care providers to avoid contact with the irrigating solution that has been removed from the patient's intestinal tract because even dilute HF solutions may cause injury. The augmentation of the irrigating solution with 10% calcium gluconate has a theoretical advantage but has not proven more beneficial than tap water or normal saline alone.[6]

Gastrointestinal bleeding, intestinal perforation, and bowel necrosis are concerns. Endoscopy may be useful in the assessment of the extent of injury. Laparoscopy may also be a useful diagnostic technique. Wounds that appear to be full thickness may require surgical resection. Patients with evidence of intestinal perforation should have prompt surgical evaluation. Calcium carbonate enemas have been used after rectal exposure.[16] Long-term formation of gastric and intestinal strictures may be complicating factors. Close observation and evaluation for signs and symptoms of systemic toxicity is warranted after gastrointestinal exposure.

Systemic Toxicity. All patients with significant exposures should be monitored closely for signs and symptoms of systemic toxicity for 12 to 24 hours. Intravenous access must be established. Continuous cardiac monitoring is necessary to recognize cardiovascular toxicity immediately. Although excision of the affected tissues has been advocated in the past,[41] this mode of treatment has not been shown to have benefit over medical management and should be avoided.

Hypocalcemia and hypomagnesemia should be anticipated. The addition of 20 mL of 10% calcium gluconate to the first liter of fluids has been suggested. Addition of 1 g of magnesium sulfate to this same liter also may be of benefit. Prophylactic use of sodium bicarbonate increased urinary fluoride elimination and improved outcome in one animal study.[42] Treatment of acidosis is important owing to the increased likelihood of cardiac arrhythmia in systemic acidosis.

Cardiac arrhythmias may be secondary to hypocalcemia, hypomagnesemia, hyperkalemia, acidemia, or hypoxia. Hypotension is also a common problem in systemic HF toxicity. Because fluoride binds calcium, treatment with intravenous calcium gluconate or calcium chloride should be the first response to hypotension or cardiac arrhythmia. Administration of calcium chloride may be preferable to giving calcium gluconate because of the former's higher concentration of calcium. However, calcium chloride can cause significant pain and necrosis if infused into a small vein should it infiltrate into the surrounding tissues. Intravenous fluid boluses and vasopressors aid in maintaining blood pressure. Immediate identification of the specific underlying electrolyte abnormality is essential. Large quantities of calcium may be required. In the presence of continued hypocalcemia, the use of antiarrhythmic medications and electrical cardioversion is likely to be futile. Hyperkalemia may require hemodialysis.

References

1. MacKinnon MA: Hydrofluoric acid burns. Dermatol Clin *6*:67–74, 1988.
2. Division of Industrial Hygiene, National Institutes of Health. Hydrofluoric acid burns. Ind Med *12*:634, 1943.
3. El Saadi MS, Hall AH, Hall PK, et al: Hydrofluoric acid dermal exposure. Vet Hum Toxicol *31*:243–247, 1989.
4. Derelanko MJ, Gadsc, Gavigan F, Dunn DB: Acute dermal toxicity of dilute hydrofluoric acid. J Toxicol Cutan Ocular Toxicol *4*:73–85, 1985.
5. Tepperman PB: Fatality due to acute systemic fluoride poisoning following a hydrofluoric acid skin burn. J Occup Med *22*:691–692, 1980.
6. Caravati EM: Acute hydrofluoric acid exposure. Am J Emerg Med *6*:143–150, 1988.
7. McCulley JP, Whiting DW, Petitt MG, Lauber SE: Hydrofluoric acid burns of the eye. J Occup Med *25*:447–450, 1983.
8. Rubinfield RS, Silbert DI, Arentsen JJ, Laibson PR: Ocular hydrofluoric acid burns. Am J Ophthalmol *114*:420–423, 1992.
9. Hatai JK, Weber JN, Doizaki K: Hydrofluoric acid burns of the eye: Report of possible delayed toxicity. J Toxicol Cutan Toxicol *5*:179–184, 1986.
10. Krenzlok EP: Hydrofluoric acid. *In* Sullivan JB, Krieger GR (eds): Hazardous Materials Toxicology. Baltimore: Williams & Wilkins, pp 785–790, 1992.
11. Kleinfeld M: Acute pulmonary edema of chemical origin. Arch Environ Health *10*:942–946, 1965.
12. Watson AA, Oliver JS, Thorpe JW: Accidental death due to inhalation of hydrofluoric acid. Med Sci Law *13*:277–279, 1973.
13. Mayer L, Guelich J: Hydrogen fluoride inhalation and burns. Arch Environ Health *7*:445–447, 1963.
14. Braun J, Stob H, Zober A: Intoxication following the inhalation of hydrogen fluoride. Arch Toxicol *56*:50–54, 1984.
15. Manoguerra AS, Neuman TS: Fatal poisoning from acute hydrofluoric acid poisoning. Am J Emerg Med *4*:362–363, 1986.
16. Cappell MS, Simon T: Fulminant acute colitis following self-administered hydrofluoric acid enema. Am J Gastroenterol *88*:122–126, 1993.
17. Foster DE, Barone JA: Rectal hydrofluoric acid exposure. Clin Pharm *8*:516–518, 1989.
18. Mullett T, Zoeller T, Bingham H: Fatal hydrofluoric acid cutaneous exposure with refractory ventricular fibrillation. J Burn Care Rehabil *8*:216–218, 1987.
19. Mayer TG, Gross PL: Fatal systemic fluorosis due to hydrofluoric acid burns. Ann Emerg Med *14*:149–153, 1985.
20. Chan K, Svancarek WP, Creer M: Fatality due to acute hydrofluoric acid exposure. Clin Toxicol *25*:333–339, 1987.
21. Greco RJ, Hartford CE, Haith LR, Patton ML: Hydrofluoric acid induced hypocalcemia. J Trauma *28*:1593–1596, 1988.
22. Sheridan RL, Ryan CM, Quinby WC Jr, et al: Emergency management of major hydrofluoric acid exposures. Burns *21*:62–64, 1995.
23. Baltazar RF, Mower MM, Reider R: Acute fluoride poisoning leading to fatal hyperkalemia. Chest *78*:660–663, 1980.
24. McIvor ME, Cummings CE, Mower MM: Sudden cardiac death from acute fluoride intoxication: The role of potassium. Ann Emerg Med *16*:777–781, 1987.
25. McIvor ME: Delayed fatal hyperkalemia in a patient with acute fluoride intoxication. Ann Emerg Med *16*:1165–1167, 1987.
26. Bracken WM, Cuppage F, McLaury RL, et al: Comparative effectiveness of topical treatments for hydrofluoric acid burns. J Occup Med *27*:733–739, 1985.
27. Burchard KK, Brent J, Kirk MA, et al: Comparison of topical magnesium and calcium treatment for dermal hydrofluoric acid burns. Ann Emerg Med *24*:9–13, 1994.
28. Seyb ST, Noordhoek L, Botens S, Mani MM: A study to determine the efficacy of treatments for hydrofluoric acid burns. J Burn Care Rehabil *16*:253–257, 1995.
29. Paley S, Seifter J: Treatment of experimental hydrofluoric acid corrosion. Proc Soc Exp Biol Med *46*:190–192, 1941.
30. Dibbell DG, Iverson RE, Jones W, et al: Hydrofluoric acid burns of the hand. J Bone Joint Surg Am *52*:931–936, 1970.
31. Iverson RE, Laub DR, Madison MS: Hydrofluoric acid burns. Plast Reconstr Surg *48*:107–112, 1971.
32. Anderson WJ, Anderson JR: Hydrofluoric acid burns of the hand: Mechanism of injury and treatment. J Hand Surg [Am] *13*:52–57, 1988.

33. Williams JM, Hammad A, Cottington EC, Harchelroad TC: Intravenous magnesium in the treatment of hydrofluoric acid burns in rats. Ann Emerg Med *23*:464–469, 1994.
34. Velyart J: Arterial perfusion for hydrofluoric acid burns. Hum Toxicol *2*:233–238, 1983.
35. Pegg SP, Siu S, Gillett G: Intra-arterial infusion in the treatment of hydrofluoric acid burns. Burns *11*:440–443, 1985.
36. Vance MV, Curry SC, Kunkel DB, et al: Digital hydrofluoric acid burns: Treatment with intra-arterial calcium infusion. Ann Emerg Med *15*:890–896, 1986.
37. Siegel DC, Heard JM: Intra-arterial calcium infusion for hydrofluoric acid burns. Aviat Space Environ Med *63*:206–211, 1992.
38. Bentur Y, Tannenbaum S, Yaffe Y, Halpert M: The role of calcium gluconate in the treatment of hydrofluoric acid eye burn. Ann Emerg Med *22*:1488–1490, 1993.
39. Trevino MA, Herrmann GH, Sprout WL: Treatment of severe hydrofluoric acid exposures. J Occup Med *25*:861–863, 1983.
40. Lee DC, Wiley JF, Snyder JW: Treatment of inhalational exposure to hydrofluoric acid with nebulized calcium gluconate. J Occup Med *35*:470, 1993.
41. Buckingham FM: Surgery: A radical approach to severe hydrofluoric acid burns. J Occup Med *30*:873–874, 1988.
42. Reynolds KE, Whitford GM, Pashley DH: Acute fluoride toxicity: The influence of acid-base status. Toxicol Appl Pharmacol *45*:415–427, 1978.

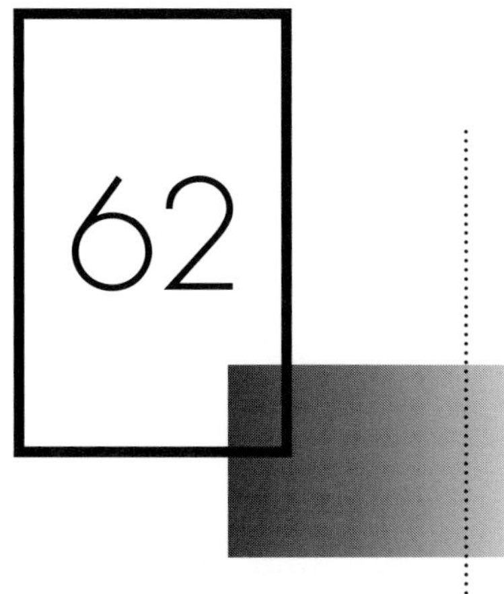

62 Alkali Injury

A Caustics

MICHAEL A. McGUIGAN, MD, MBA

CAUSTIC ALKALI INGESTION

Definitions

Alkali caustics are substances that have an alkaline pH capable of destroying the texture or substance of a tissue. The nine chemicals that are generally considered to be caustic or corrosive alkalis[1] are listed in Table 62A–1. Of these, the caustic alkali most commonly found in household products is sodium hydroxide. The full treatment of patients who have ingested a caustic alkali involves a combination of clinical toxicology, gastroenterology, and surgery. This chapter focuses on the medical toxicology of alkali ingestions and does not address the surgical interventions for esophageal perforation or stricture.

Demographics

Alkali caustics are widely available to the general public. The American Association of Poison Control Centers Toxic Exposure Surveillance System identifies eight categories of alkali products. Table 62A–2 lists these categories and their average relative frequency of exposure and severe outcomes, which are based on reported data from 1990 to 1994.[2–6] The substances most commonly involved in alkali exposures were miscellaneous household cleaners, household wall/floor/tile cleaners, and chemicals. Chemicals and household drain cleaners were the two most

Table 62A–1. Caustic Alkali Chemicals

Ammonia (≥5%)
Calcium carbide
Calcium hydroxide (dry)
Calcium oxide
Sodium hydroxide
Sodium metasilicate
Tetraethylene pentamine
Triethylene tetramine
Trisodium phosphate (dry or concentrated solution)

Table 62A–2. Classes of Alkali Products, Frequency of Exposure, and Outcomes*

Class of Alkali	Exposures† (N = 138,851)	Major (N = 641)	Death (N = 38)
Chemicals	20.1%	29.0%	13.2%
Cleaning substances (household)			
Drain cleaners	10.0%	23.9%	55.3%
Miscellaneous cleaners	24.8%	17.3%	21.0%
Oven cleaner	11.9%	11.2%	5.3%
Rust remover	0.2%	0.2%	0.0%
Toilet bowl cleaner	1.3%	0.0%	0.0%
Wall/floor/tile cleaner	24.1%	4.4%	2.6%
Industrial cleaners	7.7%	14.0%	2.6%

*American Association of Poison Control Centers, 1990 to 1994.
†Total number of exposures for which outcomes were reported.

toxic categories, accounting for 30.1% of exposures but 52.9% of major morbidity and 68.5% of fatalities. Children younger than 6 years and adults older than 19 years each accounted for approximately 45.5% of alkali exposures, with the vast majority of exposures (96.9%) classified as unintentional. These exposures have resulted in no morbidity in 29.4%, minor complaints in 57.2%, moderate effects in 12.7%, major consequences in 0.7%, and death in 0.04% of cases.

Pathophysiology

When caustic alkalis come into contact with tissues, the fatty acids in the cell membranes are saponified and the membranes lose integrity. In addition, the hydroxide ion reacts with collagen and causes it to swell, thicken, and shorten. The result is focal softening and liquefaction of the tissue, often referred to as *liquefactive necrosis.*[7] In clinical toxicology, this type of tissue injury is commonly called an *alkali burn.* Although alkalis may damage the external skin and oropharyngeal and gastric mucosa, most attention has been directed toward esophageal injuries because of the risk of perforation and the long-term complication of esophageal stricture.

The damage caused by caustic alkalis depends on the duration of contact with the tissue and the pH or titratable alkaline reserve of the product. Longer duration of contact is believed to be associated with the ingestion of a large volume of a low-viscosity liquid, a product that is solid or granular, or a liquid formation that has high viscosity. However, the formulation alone has poor predictive value. For example, one retrospective study found that of nine patients who developed an esophageal stricture, none had ingested a granular formulation.[8] A pH greater than 12.5 is associated with a high potential to cause esophageal ulceration.[9] Although a product's titratable alkaline reserve (the number of milliliters of a 0.1-M solution of hydrochloric acid required to titrate 100 mL of a 1% solution of the alkali product to a pH of 8) correlates better than its pH with esophageal erosion,[10] the pH is more practical and readily available.

Table 62A–3 describes the classification of the severity of esophageal burns.[11] Although the injury may initially be severe, esophageal damage progresses over time. The immediate development of an area of erythema signals the beginning of the inflammatory phase, which lasts for 1 to 2 days. Ulceration may be seen within the first 24 hours. The necrotic phase begins 24 to 48 hours after the initial contact, and sloughing of tissue may continue for several days. The risk of esophageal perforation is highest during the necrotic phase. If the esophageal damage has been severe, a constriction phase may start 2 to 3 weeks after the injury. During this period, collagen fibers are deposited and begin to contract and the esophageal lumen begins to narrow. The esophageal wall is weakest between 7 and 21 days after the ingestion.[12] Stricture formation is complete in 4 to 6 weeks.

Patient Management

Initial assessment of a patient who has ingested a caustic should include an evaluation of airway and circulatory status.

History and Physical Examination

Critical elements in the history include the pH of the product and the volume ingested. Determining if the ingestion was accidental (as in a young child) or intentional (as in a suicidal adult) is also important. Alkaline solutions are relatively odorless and tasteless, and ingestion may not cause immediate discomfort.[12]

Clinical manifestations of caustic alkali ingestion include pain, crying, excessive salivation, drooling, dysphagia, vomiting, hematemesis, and respiratory distress (if the larynx is involved). Pain, crying, excessive salivation, and dysphagia tend to be associated with lesions of the buccal mucosa but do not accurately predict lesions elsewhere.[13] Spontaneous vomiting is associated with a higher incidence of more severe esophageal injury.[13] Caustic burns of the facial skin, lips, and oropharyngeal mucosa may appear as white or gray patches with an erythema-

Table 62A–3. Classification of Esophageal Burns

First-degree	Mucosa only Hyperemic edematous mucosa May be superficial sloughing
Second-degree	Destruction of mucosa and submucosa Penetration into muscle layers Exudate is present Erosions and shallow ulcers
Third-degree	Full-thickness injury Possible perforation Deep ulcerations, black coagulum

tous border. Fever, tachypnea, tachycardia, hypotension, and shock may result from extensive tissue injury.

Decontamination

The use of induced emesis, gastric lavage, or activated charcoal is contraindicated, as is administration of a weak acid to neutralize the ingested alkali. Immediate dilution of the ingested alkali with milk or water is intuitively appealing and appears to reduce the acute injury in experimental animals.[14] Although dilution of an alkali with milk or water creates an exothermic reaction,[15] clinical thermal damage has not been reported.

Predicting Esophageal Injury

The utility of presenting symptoms and signs in predicting esophageal injury has been discussed in the literature for nearly 30 years. At present, four general conclusions can be reached: (1) Absence of visible signs of exposure cannot be equated with absence of esophageal lesions.[16–18] (2) The presence of at least two[19] or three[20] symptoms or signs is associated with significant esophageal burns. (3) The severity of the esophageal lesions appears to be related to the severity of the oropharyngeal burns.[13, 21] (4) No single or group of presenting symptoms and signs can identify all patients with potentially serious esophageal burns.[20] Table 62A–4 summarizes the major factors that contribute to the risk of significant esophageal injury.

Investigations

Endoscopy is the only reliable way to establish the severity of esophageal burns and identify high-risk patients who might benefit from pharmacologic or surgical interventions. Only patients at significant risk for second- or third-degree esophageal burns (see Table 62A–4) should undergo endoscopy. Asymptomatic patients with accidental ingestions do not need endoscopy because their esophageal lesions are likely to be minor.[13] If endoscopy is indicated, it should be performed 12 to 24 hours after the ingestion.

Pharmacologic Treatment

The use of corticosteroids and antibiotics to treat alkali-induced esophageal injury has been (and will continue to be) controversial. Although a large number of studies and reports have been published since 1950, the data are difficult to interpret and definitive claims about effectiveness cannot be made.[22] It is clear, however, that not all caustic alkali ingestions should be treated with corticosteroids. If corticosteroids are to be used, patients should be selected on the basis of objective endoscopic assessment of the esophageal lesions. First-degree burns do not need to be treated with corticosteroids because stricture formation does not occur in these cases. Second-degree burns that are extensive or circumferential may benefit from treatment with corticosteroids,[23, 24] although the data supporting this claim are not strong. Third-degree burns are unlikely to benefit from corticosteroid therapy.

Reviews cite lack of proven efficacy and potential complications as reasons for not using corticosteroid therapy.[12, 25] Uncertainties associated with the use of corticosteroids include the lack of consensus on the choice or dose of corticosteroid, the time of initiation of treatment (early may be more efficacious than late treatment), the duration of therapy (2 to 6 weeks), and the therapeutic endpoint (stricture formation or esophageal function).

Pharmacologic therapy other than corticosteroids may be beneficial. Even in a mild caustic ingestion, esophageal dysmotility may occur and esophageal reflux of gastric acid is likely. The use of H_2-blocking agents may help to prevent secondary acid injury to the esophagus.[12] Patients with severe tissue injury who are unable to take adequate oral nutrition for extended periods benefit from appropriate parenteral nutrition.[26]

A number of experimental approaches for the management of caustic-induced esophageal mucosal injury have been investigated (Table 62A–5). No controlled clinical trials have been carried out; therefore, although these therapies are promising, their clinical efficacy is unknown and their use cannot be recommended.

Table 62A–4. Factors Associated with Higher Risk of Esophageal Damage

Product pH >12.5	At least three symptoms
Stridor or dyspnea	Ingestion of a large volume
Intentional ingestion	Severe oropharyngeal burns
Spontaneous vomiting	

Table 62A–5. Experimental Therapy of Caustic Alkali Injury

Lathyrogens
Colchicine[27]
Penicillamine[27]
β-Aminopropionitrile[28]
N-acetylcysteine[29]
Surface Protectors
Sucralfate[30]
Bismuth subsalicylate[31]
Neutralizers
Carbon dioxide inhalation[32]
Hormones
Epidermal growth factor and interferon gamma[33]
Estradiol and progesterone[34]

Outcome

Although corticosteroid treatment may reduce the likelihood of developing esophageal strictures, it does not eliminate the possibility.[22, 24] An average of 24% of patients with documented second- and third-degree esophageal burns treated with corticosteroids developed strictures (range, 10% to 70%).[24]

Patients who develop esophageal strictures are at significantly higher risk than the general population for the development of squamous cell carcinoma.[35, 36] The mean latency period is 41 years after ingestion,[35] and in 84% the carcinomas were located in the area of the tracheal bifurcation.

SUMMARY

Ingestion of a strong alkali product may result in significant esophageal injury. Immediate treatment should consist of dilution with milk or water. Endoscopy is the only way to obtain an objective assessment of the degree of esophageal injury. The use of corticosteroids to treat serious esophageal injuries is controversial but may be beneficial for patients with extensive or circumferential second-degree burns. Periodic examinations later in life are needed to screen for esophageal carcinoma.

References

1. Corrosives—Alkaline. In Poisindex Toxicologic Management. Vol. 85. Denver, Micromedex, 1995.
2. Litovitz TL, Bailey KM, Schmitz BF, et al: 1990 Annual Report of the American Association of Poison Control Centers National Data Collection System. Am J Emerg Med *9:*461, 1991.
3. Litovitz TL, Holm KC, Bailey KM, et al: 1991 Annual Report of the American Association of Poison Control Centers National Data Collection System. Am J Emerg Med *10:*452, 1992.
4. Litovitz TL, Holm KC, Clancy C, et al: 1992 Annual Report of the American Association of Poison Control Centers Toxic Surveillance System. Am J Emerg Med *11:*494, 1993.
5. Litovitz TL, Clark LR, Soloway RA: 1993 Annual Report of the American Association of Poison Control Centers Toxic Exposure Surveillance System. Am J Emerg Med *12:*546, 1994.
6. Litovitz TL, Felberg L, Soloway RA, et al: 1994 Annual Report of the American Association of Poison Control Centers Toxic Exposure Surveillance System. Am J Emerg Med *13:*551, 1995.
7. Scarpelli DG, Iannaccone PM: Cell injury and errors of metabolism. *In* Kissane JM (ed): Anderson's Pathology. 9th ed. Vol. 1. St. Louis, C.V. Mosby Co., pp 1–65, 1990.
8. Ferguson MK, Migliore M, Staszak VM, et al: Early evaluation and therapy for caustic esophageal injury. Am J Surg *157:*116, 1989.
9. Vacura EM, Clinton JE, Ruiz E, et al: Toxicity of alkaline solutions. Ann Emerg Med *9:*118, 1980.
10. Hoffman RS, Howland MA, Kamerow HN, et al: Comparison of titratable acid/alkaline reserve and pH in potentially caustic household products. Clin Toxicol *27:*241, 1989.
11. Holinger P: Management of lesions caused by chemical burns. Ann Otol Rhinol Laryngol *71:*819, 1968.
12. Byrne WJ: Foreign bodies, bezoars, and caustic ingestion. Gastrointest Endosc Clin N Am, *4:*99, 1994.
13. Vergauwen P, Moulin D, Buts JP, et al: Caustic burns of the upper digestive and respiratory tracts. Eur J Pediatr *150:* 700, 1991.
14. Homan CS, Maitra SR, Lane B, et al: Therapeutic effects of water and milk for acute alkali injury of the esophagus. Ann Emerg Med *24:*14, 1994.
15. Rumack BH, Burrington JD: Caustic ingestions: A rational look at diluents. Clin Toxicol *11:*27, 1977.
16. Middelkamp JM, Ferguson TB, Roper CL, et al: The management and problems of caustic burns in children. J Thorac Cardiovasc Surg *57:*341, 1969.
17. Gaudreault P, Parent M, McGuigan MA, et al: Predictability of esophageal injury from signs and symptoms: A study of caustic ingestion in 378 children. Pediatrics *71:*767, 1983.
18. Hawkins DB, Demeter MJ, Barnett TE: Caustic ingestion: Controversies in management: A review of 214 cases. Laryngoscope *90:*98, 1985.
19. Crain EF, Gershel JC, Mezey AP: Caustic ingestions. Symptoms as predictors of esophageal injury. Am J Dis Child *138:*863, 1984.
20. Gorman RL, Kin-Maung-Gyi MT, Klein-Schwartz W, et al: Initial symptoms as predictors of esophageal injury in alkaline corrosive ingestions. Am J Emerg Med *10:*189, 1992.
21. Previtera C, Giusti F, Guglielmi M: Predictive value of visible lesions (cheeks, lips, oropharynx) in suspected caustic ingestion: May endoscopy reasonably be omitted in completely negative pediatric patients? Pediatr Emerg Care *6:*176, 1990.
22. Wason S: The emergency management of caustic ingestions. J Emerg Med *2:*175, 1985.
23. Anderson KD, Rouse TM, Randolph JG: A controlled trial of corticosteroids in children with corrosive injury of the esophagus. N Engl J Med *323:*637, 1990.
24. Howell JM, Dalsey WC, Hartsell FW, et al: Steroids for the treatment of corrosive esophageal injury: A statistical analysis of past studies. Am J Emerg Med *10:*421.
25. Kikendall JW: Caustic ingestion injuries. Gastroenterol Clin N Am *20:*847, 1991.
26. DiCostanzo J, Noirclerc M, Jouglard J, et al: New therapeutic approach to corrosive burns of the upper gastrointestinal tract. Gut *21:*370, 1980.
27. Thompson JN: Corrosive esophageal injuries: II. An investigation of treatment methods and histochemical analysis of esophageal strictures in a new animal model. Laryngoscope *97:*1191, 1987.
28. Madden JW, Davis WM, Butler C, et al: Experimental esophageal lye burns. II. Correcting established strictures with BAPN and bouginage. Ann Surg *178:*277, 1973.
29. Liu AJ, Richardson MA: Effects of *N*-acetylcysteine on experimentally induced esophageal lye injury. Ann Otol Rhinol Laryngol *94:*477, 1985.
30. Reddy AN, Budhraja M: Sucralfate therapy for lye-induced esophagitis. Am J Gastroenterol *83:*71, 1988.
31. Tay HP, Chaparala RC, Harmon JW, et al: Bismuth subsalicylate reduces peptic injury of the oesophagus in rabbits. Gut *31:*11, 1990.
32. Meyers RL, Glenn L, Orlando RC: Protection against alkali injury to rabbit esophagus by CO_2 inhalation. Am J Physiol *264:*G150, 1993.
33. Berthet B, DiCostanzo J, Arnaud C, et al: Influence of epidermal growth factor and interferon g on healing of oesophageal corrosive burns in the rat. Br J Surg *81:*395, 1994.
34. Demirbilek S, Bernay F, Rizalar R, et al: Effects of estradiol and progesterone on the synthesis of collagen in corrosive esophageal burns in rats. J Pediatr Surg *29:*1425, 1994.
35. Appelqvist P: Lye corrosion carcinoma of the esophagus. A review of 63 cases. Cancer *45:*2655, 1980.
36. Hopkins RA, Postlethwait RW: Caustic burns and carcinoma of the esophagus. Ann Surg *194:*146, 1981.

B The Miniature Battery Hazard

TOBY LITOVITZ, MD

In 1995, 1786 disk battery ingestions were reported to the American Association of Poison Control Centers Toxic Exposure Surveillance System. The vast majority of exposure cases involve the ingestion route, and a favorable prognosis can be anticipated in the absence of esophageal lodgment. More serious outcomes are seen when batteries lodge in the esophagus or when they are placed in the ear or nose, especially when diagnosis or removal is delayed.

DESCRIPTION OF THE INGESTION SCENARIO

As in other poisoning cases, children are implicated in the majority of button cell ingestions. Of 2382 cases reviewed,[1] 61.8% involved children under the age of 5 years, with a peak incidence occurring in 1- and 2-year-olds. A second but less profound frequency surge was observed after the age of 60 years. Simultaneous ingestion of multiple button cells was reported in 8.5% of cases, with up to 36 batteries ingested at once. Suicidal intent was evident in only 1.3% of battery ingestions; ingestion to avoid incarceration occurred in 0.4% of cases.

Batteries were most frequently ingested immediately following removal from a product (53%) such as a toy or hearing aid. Batteries that were loose, sitting out, or discarded were involved in 41% of ingestions. Only 5% of ingested batteries were obtained directly from the battery packaging. In a number of incidents, the battery "fell" or "popped" out of a product, either during use or when the product was dropped. Batteries were frequently mistaken for pills (12% of cases), with young or middle-aged adults often reaching into a pocket for an analgesic tablet and ingesting the battery instead. Older patients have described placing medication (e.g., digoxin) in the hearing aid and swallowing the battery, only to note the problem when the hearing aid was malfunctioning. Other recurring ingestion scenarios included patients' use of the mouth as a "third hand" while they were changing the battery in a product or placing the button cell in the mouth for testing (a misconceived testing method, as button cells have relatively low voltages and do not generate the characteristic "buzz" produced by larger batteries). Occasionally, batteries were ingested while still in the product—that is, the entire hearing aid or watch was swallowed.

Hearing aids had long been the single most common intended use of ingested button cells. Of concern is the observation that in nearly one third of cases in which the battery was intended for a hearing aid, the battery was removed by a child from his or her own aid. Industry attempts to provide more secure closures on hearing aid battery compartments have helped to limit this occurrence.

From 1991 through 1993, games and toys temporarily surpassed hearing aids in battery ingestion cases; this led to renewed pleas to the toy industry for more secure closures on battery compartments. The importance of a secure battery compartment was illustrated in 1989 when 2.8 million Ghost Blaster toys were distributed by Hardees restaurants as an advertising premium. These noisemakers were recalled 18 days after the promotion began. Fifty-three children ingested button cells from Ghost Blasters over the 8 weeks following the product's introduction because the battery compartment opened easily, even spontaneously, allowing the button batteries to fall out during use.[2] Other sources of ingested button cells include watches and clocks, calculators, camera equipment, beeping or lighted keychains, remote control devices, thermometers, phones, fishing bobbers, as well as musical, beeping, or lighted jewelry, greeting cards, shoelaces, shoes, clothing, pens, doormats, and story books.

Most ingested batteries are button cells (97.4%). Standard cylindrical cells (AA, AAA, C, and N) are ingested in the remaining cases. Data for the year ending in June 1995 showed a decline in the role of mercuric oxide as the chemical system of ingested button cells as a result of environmental concerns and legislation impacting on the disposal of mercury-containing batteries. These data demonstrated the following distribution of chemical systems for ingested cells: 50.4%, manganese dioxide (compared with 29.6% of cells ingested in 1983 through 1990); 31.1%, zinc/air; 10.6%, silver oxide; 4.5%, mercuric oxide (compared with 24.7% of cells ingested in 1983 through 1990); and 3.4%, lithium. In addition to the positive environmental impact, clinicians have applauded the declining role of mercuric oxide button cells, as these cells evidenced more frequent symptoms and local corrosive effects,[1, 3] presumably from the inherent corrosive properties of mercuric oxide. Federal legislation enacted May 13, 1996 bans the sale of mercuric oxide in button cells in the U.S.

MECHANISM OF BATTERY-INDUCED TISSUE INJURY

Although injury is infrequent following battery ingestion, when it does occur the mechanism is multifactorial, including the following:

1. Leakage of potassium or sodium hydroxide electrolyte from the cell (concentration up to 45%).

Corrosive dissolution of the crimp region surrounding the seal increases the risk of subsequent leakage. Corrosion is accelerated in the acid environment of the stomach. In gastrointestinal fluids with a neutral or slightly alkaline pH, the reaction is slower and causes formation or iron oxides and hydroxides that precipitate along the crimp area and may prevent further can dissolution or disassembly. This theoretic chemical prediction is corroborated by the clinical observation that batteries that arrest in the stomach are more frequently fragmented and more severely corroded than those that arrest in the more distal regions of the gastrointestinal tract.[1]

2. An external current between battery cathode and anode can be generated and may pass through adjacent tissue, causing hydrolysis of tissue fluids and local generation of hydroxides. Bathing a button cell in an electrolyte-rich fluid, such as when otic drops are used in the ear canal in which a battery is lodged, increases the external current and hydroxide formation.
3. Corrosive effects of mercuric oxide may contribute to injury when mercuric oxide cells are implicated. These cells also appear to be more likely to leak or split.
4. Pressure necrosis of an impacted battery on adjacent tissue may occur, as occurs with coin ingestion. Presumably, this is the least important contributing mechanism.

Both the first and second mechanisms (leakage and generation of an external current) produce an alkaline-type injury to surrounding tissue. The relative contribution of each of these mechanisms in an individual patient has not been determined.

The role of heavy metal leakage from button cells in subsequent injury has proved insignificant. Despite the tens of thousands of button cell ingestions that have occurred over the years, symptomatic cases of heavy metal poisoning following battery ingestion have not been reported. The medical literature cites at least four cases of modestly elevated mercury levels following battery ingestion when button cell disassembly occurred in the gastrointestinal tract.[1, 4–6] The patients had no clinical evidence of mercury poisoning. All patients with elevated levels ingested batteries that split (before or after passage) *and* displayed evidence of radiopaque droplets in the gut. Of note, most mercuric oxide batteries that split were 15.6 mm in diameter. The theoretic mercury hazard is minimized by the reduction of the toxic mercuric oxide released from a split button cell to nearly nontoxic elemental mercury. This chemical reaction occurs in the presence of gastric acid and iron dissolved from the corroding steel battery can.[7] In addition, battery discharge results in the reduction of mercuric oxide to elemental mercury. Thus, spent batteries contain mercury predominantly in the less toxic elemental form. Note that, for environmental reasons, mercuric oxide button cells are no longer sold in the United States.

CLINICAL PRESENTATION AND PROGNOSTIC FACTORS

Battery lodgment, whether in the esophagus, nose, or ear canal, is the sole consistent predictor of a severe clinical outcome. Button cells range in diameter from 6.8 mm to 23.0 mm, but 97% of ingested cells are smaller than 15 mm in diameter (7.9 mm and 11.6 mm are the most popular standard sizes). Esophageal lodgment generally follows ingestions of larger cells (20 to 23 mm in diameter), although even these larger cells may pass to the stomach without consequence. Occasionally, esophageal lodgment is reported following the ingestion of batteries with diameters as small as 7.9 to 11.6 mm. Two patients, both younger than the age of 1 year, are known to have experienced a severe outcome following esophageal lodgment of a button cell smaller than 20 mm in diameter. These patients include an 11-month-old infant who developed a tracheoesophageal fistula and esophageal scarring requiring partial surgical resection following ingestion of a 15.6-mm diameter cell,[8] and a 4-month-old infant who developed a tracheoesophageal fistula and required esophageal reconstruction following ingestion of an 11.6-mm diameter battery.[9] Two pediatric fatalities have been reported following battery lodgment in the esophagus, with 24-hour to 4-day delays in diagnosis.[10, 11] More than a dozen cases of severe injury, ranging from esophageal burns occurring within only 4 to 6 hours of ingestion to permanent esophageal injury, have been reported.

Symptoms associated with esophageal lodgment include vomiting, fever, dysphagia, odynophagia, tachypnea, irritability, and refusal of food. Prompt removal of batteries positioned in the esophagus is essential to the prevention of severe consequences, including esophageal stenosis requiring repeated dilatation or surgical repair, tracheoesophageal fistula, tension pneumo- or hemothorax, perforation through the aortic arch or its branches, massive exsanguination, and cardiac arrest. Second-degree esophageal burns have followed battery lodgment in the esophagus for as little as 4 hours. Esophageal rupture has occurred after battery lodgment for only 6 hours.

In contrast, the vast majority of button battery ingestions are associated with a benign clinical outcome[1, 3] and involve the more common 7.9- to 11.6-mm diameter cells. Only 0.08% of cases in the author's series of 2382 ingestion cases[1] demonstrated a severe effect that was either life-threatening or led to long-term disability. In the absence of esophageal lodgment, spontaneous passage through the gastrointestinal tract is the rule. Within 72 hours, 78% of ingested batteries pass spontaneously. Of note, battery passage required more than a week in 4.5% of cases and more than 2 weeks (and up to 596 days) in 1.1% of cases. Delayed transit was a more common finding in patients older than 20 years of age (especially the elderly), and although delayed transit was associated with a higher incidence of gastrointestinal manifestations, it was generally not associated with a severe outcome. When arrested transit was documented radiographically, it is of note that larger cells arrest more proximally (15- to 23-mm batteries arrest in the esophagus or stomach), whereas small cells tend to arrest more distally (7.9-mm cells lodge in the small or large bowel).

At least 83% of all battery ingestors remain entirely asymptomatic. Symptoms are reported in 9.9% of all battery ingestion cases. (The occurrence of symptoms was unknown in 6.8% of cases.) The more common symptoms reported include vomiting (2.4%), abdominal pain (2.0%), discolored or bloody stool (1.7%), fever (1.3%), and diarrhea (1.3%). Rashes are reported in about 1.2% of cases and may be manifestations of nickel hypersensitivity, as many of the ingested button cells are nickel-plated. Dietary nickel is a known factor in nickel dermatitis flare-up in individuals with sensitivity to nickel.[12] In patients with batteries that fragment in the gastrointestinal tract, 42% have symptoms. (Mercuric oxide cells accounted for two thirds of fragmented cells.)

Only a few unusual cases have been reported with severe outcomes, despite successful passage beyond the esophagus. These cases include perforation of a Meckel diverticulum 3 days after ingestion of two hearing aid batteries by a 2.5-year-old boy who presented with vomiting and abdominal pain,[13] and the infrequent occurrence of significant localized mucosal damage of the more distal gastrointestinal tract. Interestingly, these latter cases are more often noted on endoscopic examination and are generally not associated with sequelae.

Batteries placed in the ear or nose that are not promptly removed routinely damage surrounding tissue. Observed injuries include tympanic membrane perforation or destruction, necrosis of the dermis of the external ear canal, destruction of the ossicles, hearing impairment, nasal septal perforation, nasal turbinate destruction, facial nerve paralysis, chondritis, and atrophic rhinitis.[14, 15] Discharge and pain are clinical indicators of battery lodgment in the nose or ear canal. Although these symptoms are manifestations of other more common clinical entities, a thorough examination of the ear or nose is essential for excluding the presence of a foreign body.

PATIENT EVALUATION, MANAGEMENT, AND DISPOSITION

Ipecac administration is ineffective and unsafe. Emetics resulted in battery expulsion in only 2.7% of button cell ingestion cases in which emetics were used. In one case, ipecac caused retrograde movement of a battery from the stomach to the esophagus, with resultant lodgment requiring emergency endoscopic retrieval.[1]

Prompt radiographic determination of the position of an ingested battery is essential. Early symptoms and battery diameter are unreliable indicators of esophageal lodgment. More than one third of patients with batteries in the esophagus are asymptomatic at the time of diagnosis; thus, symptoms are an unreliable predictor of an esophageal position.[1] Furthermore, esophageal lodgment and severe esophageal injury have been reported with cells as small as 11.6 mm.

Surgical removal is rarely indicated. In those infrequent instances when any type of removal is required (e.g., related to esophageal position, failure of a large cell to pass through the pylorus in a young child, or the occurrence of significant symptoms), the endoscopic approach is preferred. However, in the author's series of 2382 ingestions,[1] endoscopy was indicated in only 28% of patients in which it was performed. If the patient requires electrocardiography before a procedure, it should be noted that ingested batteries may interfere with attempts to obtain the electrocardiogram.[16]

Endoscopic retrieval success rates are related to battery location. Endoscopic retrieval from the esophagus is associated with a 90% retrieval rate, compared with rates of 30% to 50% for batteries in the stomach, small bowel, cecum, or colon. A number of alternatives to endoscopic retrieval have been proposed, including the blind insertion of various types of balloon catheters. Blind removal of button batteries lodged in the esophagus should be avoided because (1) the extent of injury cannot be determined, (2) the risk of esophageal perforation may be increased, and (3) tracheal obstruction may ensue when the button cell is pulled back. Several authors have successfully used magnetized nasogastric tubes or magnetized endoscopes for esophageal and gastric removal. Although the author believes that such blind removal is not indicated, if it is employed, then it is worth noting that the success rate is improved by the use of strong, rare-earth magnets rather than iron or steel magnets, as the former is less likely to result in detachment of the battery during the procedure.[3] Endoscopic basket snares and coin-grasping or toothed forceps also have been used to assist retrieval.

Battery lodgment in the nose or ear mandates urgent retrieval. Delays in removal of even 1 to 2 hours or misdiagnosis can lead to very severe outcomes. The use of nasal and otic drops must be avoided, as they bathe the battery in an electrolyte-rich medium, enhancing corrosion, leakage, generation of an external current, and local injury. Battery removal may require patient sedation and direct visualization through an operating microscope. When the button cell is magnetic, a magnetized instrument (even a magnetized screwdriver!)[17] may prove invaluable. Alternatively, a 1-mm 90-degree pick can be positioned beyond a button cell in the ear canal, rotated, and then retracted.

CLINICAL GUIDELINES FOR TREATMENT OF BATTERY INGESTION CASES

1. Obtain a radiograph promptly to determine battery location. Neither battery size nor symptom occurrence can reliably be used to identify every patient with a button cell lodged in the esophagus.

2. Remove batteries lodged in the esophagus emergently. Burns have occurred as early as 4 hours after ingestion, and perforation as soon as 6 hours after ingestion. Removal should be accomplished under direct visualization (i.e., endoscopically).
3. Attempt to identify the battery's diameter and chemical system by determining the imprint code of a duplicate battery, by measuring the battery compartment within the product, or by reviewing instructions and packaging. Once the imprint code is known, the battery system and diameter can be determined by calling the National Button Battery Ingestion Hotline at (202) 625-3333. An accurate assessment of a battery's diameter is difficult to determine reliably on a radiograph.
4. Do not retrieve batteries that have passed beyond the esophagus unless the patient manifests signs or symptoms indicative of significant injury to the gastrointestinal tract (e.g., hematochezia or abdominal pain with tenderness). Minor gastrointestinal symptoms (a few episodes of vomiting or stool discoloration in the absence of evidence of gastrointestinal blood) are *not* indications for battery retrieval. Batteries that have passed beyond the esophagus may also require removal if they are too large to pass spontaneously (see 5.). If the battery is beyond the esophagus and the patient has no signs or symptoms indicative of significant injury to the gastrointestinal tract, the patient can be managed at home, with a regular diet and normal activity to promote gastrointestinal transit. Each stool is checked by the patient or parent to document battery passage.
5. In asymptomatic patients, a repeat radiograph can be obtained 7 to 14 days after ingestion to confirm battery passage. However, it is preferable to confirm such passage by inspection of stools. Obtaining radiographs more frequently (once or twice weekly) should be considered if a 15.6-mm diameter mercuric oxide cell has been ingested owing to the greater likelihood that the battery will split in the gastrointestinal tract. Another clinical situation that generally warrants more frequent radiography is the ingestion of a large diameter cell ($\geq$15 mm) by a child younger than 6 years of age. Despite successful esophageal transit, if these larger cells do not pass through the pylorus within 48 hours, then they are unlikely to pass, and the patients will benefit from endoscopic retrieval. Administration of metoclopramide (to enhance gastric passage) in combination with an H_2-antagonist (to limit corrosive damage and local injury) is often advised for cells which remain in the stomach, although their presumed efficacy remains theoretic. In contrast, pharmacologic interventions (administration of cathartics, metoclopramide, H_2-antagonists) are not advised in more routine cases on the basis of the results of investigations in the dog model, in which they showed no significant effect when transit was uninterrupted.[18] Smaller cells that appear "hung up" in the stomach or bowel do not require removal unless clinical signs or symptoms indicative of gastrointestinal injury are present.
6. Determination of blood and urine mercury levels is indicated only when mercuric oxide cells split in the gastrointestinal tract or when radiopaque droplets are evident in the gut. Chelation therapy is instituted only in the unlikely event that toxic mercury levels or clinical manifestations of mercury poisoning become evident. Mercuric oxide button cells are no longer marketed in the United States.
7. The National Capital Poison Center in Washington, DC has maintained the National Button Battery Ingestion Hotline and Registry since 1982 and has provided telephone consultations and gathered data on more than 5400 battery ingestion cases. For interpretation of the battery imprint code and assistance with patient management, clinicians should report all ingestions and exposures to miniature batteries to the Registry at (202) 625-3333 (call collect). After passage or removal, ingested batteries are mailed to the Poison Center for determination of the extent of corrosion, crimp area dissolution, and pitting.

References

1. Litovitz TL, Schmitz BF: Ingestion of cylindrical and button batteries: An analysis of 2382 cases. Pediatrics *89:*747, 1992.
2. Litovitz TL, Schmitz BF, Soloway RA: Ghost blasting with button batteries. Pediatrics *85:*384, 1990.
3. Thompson N, Lowe-Ponsford F, Mant TGK, Volans GN: Button battery ingestion: A review. Adverse Drug React Acute Poisoning Rev *9:*157, 1990.
4. Kulig K, Rumack CM, Rumack BH, et al: Disk battery ingestion: Elevated urine mercury levels and enema removal of battery fragments. JAMA *249:*2503, 1983.
5. Mofenson HC, Greensher J, Caraccio T, et al: Ingestion of small flat disc batteries. Ann Emerg Med *12:*88, 1983.
6. Mant TGK, Lewis JL, Mattoo TK, et al: Mercury poisoning after disc-battery ingestion. Hum Toxicol *6:*179, 1987.
7. Barber TE, Menke RD: The relationship of ingested iron to the absorption of mercuric oxide. Am J Emerg Med *2:*500, 1984.
8. Maves MD, Carithers JS, Birck HG: Esophageal burns secondary to disc battery ingestion. Ann Otol Rhinol Laryngol *93:*364, 1984.
9. Sigalet D, Lees G: Tracheoesophageal injury secondary to disc battery ingestion. J Pediatr Surg *23:*996, 1988.
10. Blatnik BS, Toohill RJ, Lehman RH: Fatal complications from an alkaline battery foreign body in the esophagus. Ann Otol *86:*611, 1977.
11. Shabino CL, Feinberg AN: Esophageal perforation secondary to alkaline battery ingestion. J Am Coll Emerg Phys *8:*360, 1979.
12. Toxicologic Profile for Nickel. Atlanta, Agency for Toxic Substances and Disease Registry, p 48, 1988.
13. Willis GA, Ho WC: Perforation of Meckel's diverticulum by an alkaline hearing aid battery. Can Med Assoc J *126:*497, 1982.
14. Kavanagh KT, Litovitz T: Miniature battery foreign bodies in auditory and nasal cavities. JAMA *255:*1470, 1986.
15. Skinner DW, Chui P: The hazards of "button sized" batteries as foreign bodies in the nose and ear. J Laryngol Otol *100:*1315, 1986.
16. Proctor MH: Assault by battery. N Engl J Med *316:*554, 1987.
17. Landry GL, Edmonson MB: Attractive method for battery removal. JAMA *256:*3351, 1986.
18. Litovitz T, Butterfield AB, Holloway RR, et al: Button battery ingestion: Assessment of therapeutic modalities and battery discharge state. J Pediatr *105:*868, 1984.

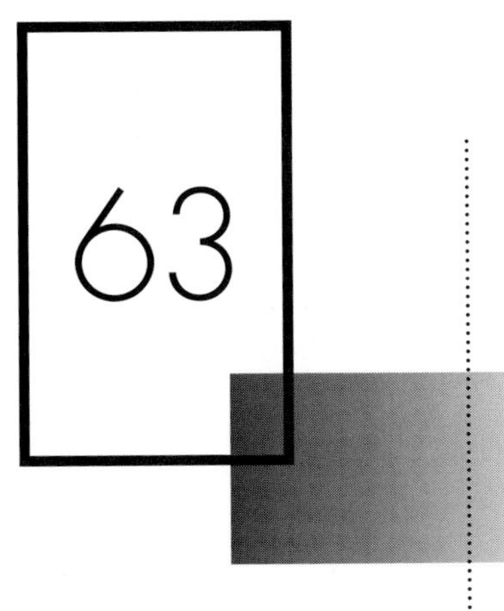

Acids and Antacids

THOMAS MASON, MD
MARSHA FORD, MD

ACIDS

Acids are ubiquitous chemicals in both industry and the home (Table 63–1). The diagnosis and treatment of acid ingestion have been made more difficult because previous studies combined both acid and alkali exposures into a single category as caustic or corrosive agents. We now know that these agents have different effects on biologic systems. Since the first reported case of fatal acid ingestion,[1] mineral acids have continued to be an infrequent yet potentially fatal toxin. The 1994 Annual Report of the American Association of Poison Control Centers (AAPCC) Toxic Exposure Surveillance System[2] (TESS) listed 9386 acid exposures, which accounted for fewer than 1% of all nonpharmaceutical exposures. However, 47% of those patients exposed sought treatment in a medical facility. Hydrochloric acid was the most common acid, accounting for 2772 or 29% of acid exposures, and these exposures resulted in four of the six deaths due to acid exposure.

Table 63–1. Sources of Common Acids

Acetic acid	Permanent wave neutralizers, photography stop bath, disinfectants, hat making, printing, dyeing, rayon manufacturing
Boric acid	Roach powders, water softener, germicide
Carbolic acid	Disinfectants, pharmaceuticals, dyes, plastics manufacturing, preservatives
Formic acid	Airplane glue makers, tanning, deodorizing tablets, plastic menders, fumigants, embalming fluids
Hydrochloric acid (muriatic acid)	Bleaching agents, metal and toilet bowl cleaners, dye and chemical synthesis, metal refining
Oxalic acid	Tanning, blueprint paper, disinfectants, household bleach, iron cleaner, leather, chemical synthesis, antirust polishes
Nitric acid	Engravers, electroplating, metal refiners, fertilizer manufacturing
Phosphoric acid	Metal and toilet bowl cleaner, rustproofing, disinfectants
Sulfuric acid	Automobile batteries, drain cleaners, chemical munitions, fertilizer manufacturing

Pharmacology and Pathophysiology

Acids are hydrogen-containing molecules that dissociate on contact with water to release hydronium ions (H^+). This release produces surface protein desiccation and coagulative necrosis with eschar formation that theoretically limits further acid penetration and additional injury. However, full-thickness burns can occur, including perforation.[3] Concentration, volume, and contact time with tissues all are important predictors of injury potential.[4, 5] For ingestions, the absence of stomach contents and the presence of pylorospasm are also contributors to more severe injury.[4, 6, 7] Acids are eliminated by the body-buffering systems and may form complexes with other ions.

Acid ingestions may result in esophageal lesions, although these are less common than with alkali ingestions.[8, 9] In one series of 34 patients, approximately 50% were found to have second- or third-degree esophageal burns, especially in the distal two thirds.[10] Gastric injuries are more common.[11] This may be because of the magenstrasse fluid flow along the lesser curvature of the stomach to the pylorus, as well as subsequent pylorospasm resulting in acid pooling. Duodenal injury is less common, probably because of this pylorospasm, which was demonstrated radiographically by Testa.[7] However, duodenal injury may occur in as many as one third of patients[11] and is associated with increased mortality.[12]

Clinical Presentation

Patients who ingest mineral acids often present with oropharyngeal pain, dysphagia, chest or epigastric pain, salivation, odynophagia, and vomiting.[9, 11] Oropharyngeal burns may be present, and a swollen, necrotic uvula may be seen, but the absence of these findings does not preclude serious injury to the esophagus or stomach.[9, 13, 14] Aspiration of acid may produce stridor, rales, or rhonchi with potential progression to acute respiratory distress syndrome. Signs of gastrointestinal (GI) hemorrhage or perforation may be seen. Systemic effects include metabolic acidosis, disseminated intravascular coagulation, hyponatremia, and hypotension.[15–17]

Cutaneous mineral acid burns produce similar findings, as in thermal burns including erythema, blistering, or full-thickness skin loss. Tissue damage may be estimated by the duration of contact, quantity, strength, and concentration of the acid.

Mild ocular mineral acid burns may acutely produce conjunctival hyperemia, diffuse chemosis, and mild corneal clouding or epithelial erosions. The stroma may be mildly edematous, and the anterior chamber may have cells and flare. More severe burns caused by strong acids may cause corneal and conjunctival opacification, epithelial sloughing, corneal anesthesia, limbal pallor, and uveitis. Intraocular pressure may rise. Injuries to the limbal area are most severe because this area is most important in revascularization and re-epithelialization.[18]

Diagnosis

Emergent endoscopic examination is required in all mineral acid ingestions.[11, 19, 20] Previous researchers have suggested that early surgical exploration and resection of nonviable tissue should be the primary diagnostic staging procedure.[21] However, unless there is evidence of perforation on clinical examination or radiographic study, emergent endoscopy is recommended to grade the extent of injury. This procedure allows evaluation of the supraglottic structures and upper GI tract. Endoscopic examination should include the esophagus, stomach, and if possible the duodenum. If severe esophageal burns are found, a pediatric endoscope can be passed to view beyond the burns.[22] Gastric necrosis and perforation are a common cause of death, and endoscopic examination of the stomach is essential to determine the need for emergency laparotomy to resect nonviable tissue. Water-soluble radiographic studies may be undertaken if endoscopy cannot be performed. These studies can detect perforation but are inadequate for staging the burn severity.[11] The burns may be staged according to a classification system for acid burns of the upper GI tract established by Zargar and colleagues (Table 63–2).[19]

In cases of ingestion, laboratory studies should include complete blood count, electrolyte determinations, type and crossmatch, renal and liver function tests, coagulation studies, and arterial blood gas measurements. Chest and abdominal radiographs may be obtained if aspiration or GI perforation is suspected. An electrocardiogram should be obtained if the patient's clinical status warrants.

Diagnosis of dermal and ocular lesions depends on finding the clinical manifestations noted earlier in the section on clinical presentation. Ocular slit-lamp examination with topical fluorescein dye can assist in determining the extent of corneal burns.

Treatment

Prehospital workers should beware of contaminating themselves during rescue, and decontamination of skin and ocular exposures should begin at the scene. After the patient is removed from the source and all clothing and other apparel removed, immediate irrigation of cutaneous and ocular exposures with tap water or normal saline should begin.

Treatment of acid ingestion is somewhat controversial. Even the most benign-appearing case requires aggressive patient assessment with particular attention to airway patency, respiratory support, and rapid endoscopic examination.[9] Large-bore intravenous access with crystalloid administration and cardiopulmonary monitoring are indicated. Placement of a nasogastric tube with suction may remove pooled acid from the stomach and theoretically reduce systemic complications.[3, 9, 15] The safety of this procedure has been demonstrated in a small number of patients.[4] Neutralization or diluent therapy cannot be recommended because of concerns related to exothermic neutralization reactions and vomiting with possible aspiration and re-exposure of the esophagus to acid.[4, 9] Pain control with opioids should be compassionate but judicious because this may affect the abdominal examination for perforation.

There is no antidotal therapy for mineral acid exposure. Antibiotics are recommended for documented

Table 63–2. Endoscopic Acid Burn Classification

Grade 0	Normal findings on examination
Grade 1	Edema, hyperemia of mucosa
Grade 2a	Friability, blisters, hemorrhages, erosions, whitish membranes, exudates, superficial ulcerations
Grade 2b	Grade 2a plus deep discrete or circumferential ulceration
Grade 3a	Small scattered areas of multiple ulcerations and areas of necrosis (brown-black or grayish discoloration)
Grade 3b	Extensive necrosis

From Zargar SA, Kochhar R, Mehta S, et al: The role of fiberoptic endoscopy in the management of corrosive ingestion and modified endoscopic classification of burns. Gastroenterol Endosc *37*:165–169, 1991.

infections but otherwise should not be given. No trials have documented the efficacy of corticosteroids in preventing strictures due to mineral acid ingestions, and their use is not recommended.[9, 15, 23] Corticosteroids theoretically may mask signs of visceral perforation and retard wound repair.

Patients with grade 0 or 1 endoscopic lesions may be observed in a regular hospital bed with analgesics, antacids, H_2 blockers, and diet as tolerated. Patients with grade 2 and 3 lesions require intensive care unit admission and nothing-by-mouth status with intravenous hydration and hyperalimentation or feeding jejunostomy as needed.[19, 24] Repeated abdominal examinations for signs of perforation are required. Repeat endoscopy in the following 24 to 48 hours may be helpful in re-evaluation of the burns. Patients with signs of intra-abdominal perforation or necrotic gastric lesions should undergo laparotomy with exploration for perforation and débridement of nonviable tissue.

Endoscopic examination usually reveals healing of grades 0, 1, and 2a lesions in 21 to 28 days; grade 2b lesions in approximately 35 days; and grade 3 lesions in an average of 43 days.[19] Stricture formation, including gastric strictures, can be expected in approximately two thirds of patients with grade 2b or 3 lesions.[19] Strictures may present with dysphagia, weight loss, or vomiting. Gastric outlet obstruction due to pyloric, antral, or duodenal stenosis can occur. Subsequent gastric scarring may result in a small, contracted stomach susceptible to the development of the dumping syndrome or pernicious anemia requiring lifelong vitamin B_{12} replacement. Dilation or surgical repair may be required.[11, 25] Adenocarcinoma and squamous carcinoma of the stomach have been reported as a late complication of acid-induced GI strictures.[26] Patients with these strictures should have lifelong monitoring for this potentially life-threatening complication.

The treatment of cutaneous burns due to mineral acids includes copious irrigation and, if possible, pH monitoring of the tissue. Opioid analgesics are frequently required for pain control. Local wound care is similar to the care of thermal burns, except that blisters should be opened and drained of fluid, which may contain the mineral acid. For minor cutaneous burns, antibiotic ointment to combat possible staphylococcal or streptococcal secondary infection should be applied. For more severe skin exposures, patients may require admission, possibly to a burn intensive care unit. Parenteral antibiotics should be withheld until cultures and documentation of infection can be obtained to prevent the development of resistant organisms. Tetanus immunization should be updated. Surgical consultation may be required, depending on burn severity and cosmetic considerations.

Ocular burns should receive immediate copious irrigation with tap water or normal saline for a minimum of 30 minutes or using at least 2 L of irrigation fluid. Any retained particles should be removed. Analgesics are recommended, and irrigation should be continued until the conjunctival sac pH is between 7.3 and 7.7. This pH should be rechecked 30 minutes after discontinuation of irrigation, and if the pH has declined to less than 7.3, the irrigation procedure should be repeated until the pH remains above 7.3. All but the most minor burns produce uveitis, and cycloplegia with 1% atropine or 0.25% scopolamine is recommended. Phenylephrine is contraindicated because it may worsen perilimbal ischemia. Increased intraocular pressures may be treated with carbonic anhydrase inhibitors such as acetazolamide, 250 mg orally or intravenously every 6 hours, or with ophthalmologic β-blocker topical solutions such as timolol 0.5%, two drops twice a day. Antibiotic ointment and a semi-pressure patch should be applied. Topical steroids are controversial and should be used only in consultation with an ophthalmologist.[18]

ANTACIDS

Antacids accounted for 17,959 exposures reported to the AAPCC TESS in 1994. Of these patients, 484 sought medical attention, and there were no deaths.[2]

Pharmacology and Pathophysiology

Antacids possess acid-buffering ability provided by an anionic base. The most commonly used agents are combined with a metallic cation, usually magnesium (Mg^{2+}), calcium (Ca^{2+}), or aluminum (Al^{3+}), which is ultimately responsible for most antacid toxicity.

Most antacids are incompletely absorbed in the gut and thus have minimal systemic effects in normal doses. Exceptions include sodium bicarbonate and sodium citrate, both of which are highly absorbed and have the potential for causing severe systemic alkalosis. Renal impairment can lead to toxic accumulations of Mg^{2+}, Ca^{2+}, and Al^{3+}. Potential serious drug interactions can occur with use of β-blockers, cimetidine, chloroquine, digoxin, nonsteroidal anti-inflammatory drugs, phenytoin, and quinidine.[27]

Clinical Presentation

Diarrhea, constipation,[28] GI obstruction, and perforation[29, 30] have been associated with chronic overdose or massive acute ingestions of antacids. Other symptoms of antacid overdose are due to the development of systemic alkalosis or elevations in specific cations. Prolonged administration or extreme doses may result in toxic manifestations of the cationic component.[27, 31–34] Hypermagnesemia causes hypotension, dysrhythmias, respiratory depression, central nervous system depression, and potentially death.[31, 34, 35] Fatalities have been reported with sodium bicarbonate overdose, which resulted in congestive heart failure, stomach perforation, and systemic alkalosis.[29] Elevated aluminum levels cause encephalopathy, hypercalcemia, osteodystrophy with pathologic fractures, and anemia in patients with chronic renal failure.[36–38] Hypercalciuria may produce nephrolithiasis and acute renal failure.

Two antacid-related syndromes have been reported. The milk-alkali syndrome may be associated with excessive ingestion of milk or with Ca^{2+}-containing preparations. Features include hypercalcemia, reduced parathyroid hormone secretion, phosphate retention, calcium salt precipitation in the kidneys, renal insufficiency, and metabolic alkalosis.[27] The phosphate depletion syndrome may occur after prolonged therapy with aluminum hydroxide. Hypophosphatemia, hypophosphaturia, hypercalciuria, bone pain, muscle weakness, paresthesias, seizures, and anorexia may occur.[27]

Diagnosis

A patient's history is the most important diagnostic tool, with particular attention paid to chronic overuse of nonprescription preparations. Patients tend to underestimate antacid use, and family and friends may provide a more accurate history. Electrolyte determinations, pH measurement, electrocardiography, and renal function tests should be performed for all symptomatic patients. Specific cation measurements of aluminum, calcium, or magnesium are dictated by the history and clinical presentation.

Treatment

Acute antacid toxicity is unlikely because of poor GI absorption. Thus, gastric decontamination is not indicated unless coingestants are suspected.

Aluminum may be removed by use of deferoxamine and subsequent hemodialysis.[39] Symptomatic hypercalcemia can be treated with fluids and loop diuretics,[40] with mithramycin reserved for severe cases or for patients unresponsive to fluids and diuretics. Symptomatic hypermagnesemia is treated with calcium (which directly displaces Mg^{2+} from cell membranes), fluids, and vasopressors as needed for hypotension. Hemodialysis reduces serum levels of Mg^{2+}, Ca^{2+}, and Al^{3+}. Table 63–3 reviews the treatment of antacid-related cation toxicity.

Disposition

Most acute ingestions are not toxic. Asymptomatic patients with normal results of laboratory studies and electrocardiography can be discharged after several hours of observation. Symptomatic patients should be admitted for intravenous hydration and cardiopulmonary monitoring. The presence of symptoms other than GI most likely represents severe electrolyte or acid-base disturbances, which require more aggressive therapy.

Table 63–3. Therapies for Antacid-Induced Cation Overdose

Cation	Therapy	Dose
Aluminum	Deferoxamine	40–90 mg/kg IM, not to exceed 2 g per injection. IV in severe cases, at 15 mg/kg/h
	Hemodialysis	
Calcium	Normal saline	High volumes to correct hypovolemia
	Furosemide	1–3 mg/kg IV
	Mithramycin	25 μg/kg IV if no response after 24 hours of saline diuresis
	Calcitonin	4 IU/kg SQ or IM q12h increased to 8 IU/kg if inadequate response in 1–2 d; if still inadequate, give maximum dose 8 IU/kg q6h
	Hemodialysis	
Magnesium	Calcium gluconate	10 mL of 10% solution; repeat as needed for respiratory depression or hypotension
	Normal saline	High volumes to correct hypovolemia
	Furosemide	1–3 mg/kg IV
	Hemodialysis	

One or more of the above treatment modalities may be indicated in management of the specific cation overdose, depending on the clinical condition and the response to therapy.[31, 36, 39, 40]

References

1. McLanahan S: Pyloric occlusion following the ingestion of corrosive liquids. JAMA *102*:735–736, 1934.
2. Litovitz TL, Felberg L, Soloway RA, et al: 1994 Annual report of the American Association of Poison Control Centers Toxic Exposure Surveillance System. Am J Emerg Med *13*:551–603, 1995.
3. Fisher RA, Eckhauser ML, Radivoyevitch M: Acid ingestion in an experimental model. Surg Gynecol Obstet *161*:91–99, 1985.
4. Penner GE: Acid ingestion: Toxicology and treatment. Ann Emerg Med *9*:374–379, 1980.
5. Scher LA, Maull KI: Emergency management and sequelae of acid ingestion. JACEP *7*:206–208, 1978.
6. Nicosia JF, Thornton JP, Folk FA, et al: Surgical management of corrosive gastric injuries. Ann Surg *180*:139–143, 1974.
7. Testa GF: Contrileta radiologica e sperimentale alla studio dell lesione esofagee e gastriche nelle causticazioni da alcali. Radiol Med (Torino) *25*:17–24, 1938.
8. Wormald PJ, Wilson DAB: Battery acid burns of the upper gastrointestinal tract. Clin Otolaryngol *18*:112–114, 1993.
9. Ford M: Alkali and acid injuries of the upper gastrointestinal tract. *In* Hoffman RS, Goldfrank LR (eds): Critical Care Toxicology. New York, Churchill Livingstone, pp 225–249, 1991.
10. Hawkins DB, Demeter MJ: Caustic ingestion. Controversies in management: A review of 214 cases. Laryngoscope *90*:98–108, 1980.
11. Zargar SA, Kochhar R, Nagi B, et al: Ingestion of corrosive acids: Spectrum of injury to the upper gastrointestinal tract and natural history. Gastroenterology *97*:702–707, 1989.
12. Jeng LB, Chen H, Chen S, et al: Upper gastrointestinal tract ablation for patients with extensive injury after ingestion of strong acid. Arch Surg *129*:1086–1090, 1994.

13. Gaudreault P, Parent M, McGuigan MA, et al: Predictability of esophageal injury from signs and symptoms: A study of caustic ingestion in 378 children. Pediatrics *71*:767–769, 1983.
14. Previtera C, Giusti F, Guglielmi M: Predictive value of visible lesions (cheeks, lips, oropharynx) in suspected caustic ingestion: May endoscopy reasonably be admitted in completely negative pediatric patients? Pediatr Emerg Med *6*:176–178, 1990.
15. Chodak GW, Passaro E: Acid ingestion: Need for gastric resection. JAMA *239*:225–226, 1978.
16. Jelenko CI, Story J, Ellison RG Jr: Ingestion of mineral acid. South Med J *65*:868–871, 1972.
17. Greif F, Kaplan O: Acid ingestion: Another cause of disseminated intravascular coagulopathy. Crit Care Med *14*:990–991, 1986.
18. Catalano RA: Ocular Emergencies. Philadelphia, WB Saunders, pp 179–190, 1992.
19. Zargar SA, Kochhar R, Mehta S, et al: The role of fiberoptic endoscopy in the management of corrosive ingestion and modified endoscopic classification of burns. Gastroenterol Endosc *37*:165–169, 1991.
20. Gumaste VV, Dave PB: Ingestion of corrosive substances by adults. Am J Gastroenterol *87*:1–5, 1992.
21. Estrera A, Taylor W, Mills LJ, et al: Corrosive burns of the esophagus and stomach: A recommendation for an aggressive surgical approach. Ann Thorac Surg *41*:276–283, 1986.
22. Sugawa C, Lucas CE: Caustic injury of the upper gastrointestinal tract in adults: A clinical and endoscopic study. Surgery *106*:802, 1989.
23. Anderson KD, Rouse TM, Randolph JG: A controlled trial of corticosteroids in children with corrosive injury of the esophagus. N Engl J Med *323*:637–640, 1990.
24. Dilawari JB, Singh S, Rao PN, et al: Corrosive acid ingestion in man—a clinical and endoscopic study. Gut *25*:183–187, 1984.
25. Chong GC, Beahrs OH, Payne WS: Management of corrosive gastritis due to ingested acid. Mayo Clin Proc *49*:861–865, 1974.
26. Eaton H, Tennekoon GE: Squamous carcinoma of the stomach following corrosive acid burns. Br J Surg *59*:382–387, 1972.
27. Walan A: Metabolic side effects of and interactions of antacids. Scand J Gastroenterol *17*(Suppl):63–67, 1982.
28. Strom M: Antacid side effects on bowel habits. Scand J Gastroenterol *17*(Suppl 75):54–55, 1982.
29. Downs NM, Stonebridge PA: Gastric rupture due to excessive sodium bicarbonate ingestion. Scot Med J *34*:535–536, 1989.
30. Brand JM, Greer FR: Hypermagnesemia and intestinal perforation following antacid administration in a premature infant. Pediatrics *85*:121–123, 1990.
31. Smilkstein MJ, Smolinske S, Kulig K, et al: Severe hypermagnesemia due to multiple cathartic therapy. West J Med *148*:208–211, 1988.
32. Hoffman RS, Smilkstein MJ, Rubenstein F: An "amp" by any other name: The hazards of intravenous magnesium dosing. JAMA *261*:557, 1989.
33. Garrelts JC, Watson WA, Holloway KD, et al: Magnesium toxicity secondary to catharsis during management of theophylline poisoning. Am J Emerg Med *7*:34–37, 1989.
34. Fassler CA, Rodriguez M, Badesch DB, et al: Magnesium toxicity as a cause of hypotension and hypoventilation. Occurrence in patients with normal renal function. Arch Intern Med *145*:1604–1606, 1985.
35. Ferdanandus J, Pederson JA, Whang R: Hypermagnesemia as a cause of refractory hypotension, respiratory depression, and coma. Arch Intern Med *141*:669–670, 1981.
36. Wills MR, Savory J: Aluminum poisoning: Dialysis encephalopathy, osteomalacia and anemia. Lancet *2*:29–33, 1983.
37. Alfrey AC: Aluminum intoxication. N Engl J Med *310*:1113–1115, 1984.
38. Cannata JB, Briggs JD, Junor BJR, et al: Effect of acute aluminum overload on calcium and parathyroid hormone metabolism. Lancet *1*:501–503, 1983.
39. Malluche HH, Smith AJ, Abreo KA, et al: The use of deferoxamine in the management of aluminum accumulation in bone in patients with renal failure. N Engl J Med *311*:140–144, 1984.
40. Suki WN, Yium JJ, Von Minden M, et al: Acute treatment of hypercalcemia with furosemide. N Engl J Med *283*:836–840, 1970.

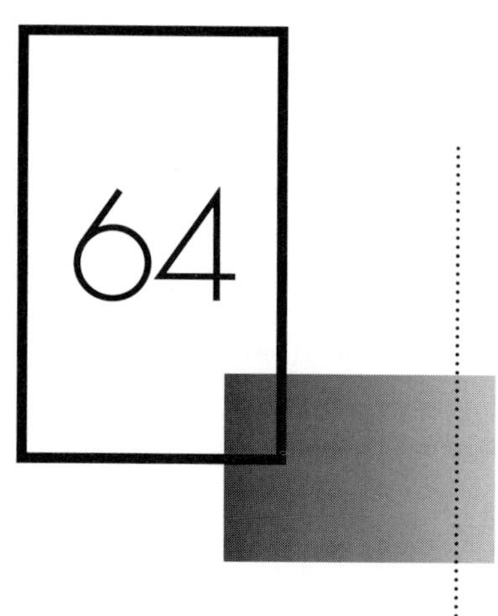

64 Bleach, Soaps, Detergents, and Other Corrosives

MICHAEL A. McGUIGAN, MD, MBA

The ingestion of cleaning products accounts for a large number of calls to poison control centers. This chapter reviews the clinical toxicology of soaps, detergents, bleach, ammonia compounds, and mixed cleaning products. Only those products used in the household are considered. Although similar compounds are used in various industrial settings, they are not discussed in this chapter. The demographic descriptions are based data reported by the American Association of Poison Control Centers (AAPCC) from 1990 to 1994.[1–5] Table 64–1 presents age-related data on exposure to a selected item from each of the five categories of household products. Table 64–2 summarizes reported outcomes of exposures to the same items from the same categories. In each table, personal care soaps were used as an example of "soaps," laundry detergents were used as a representative of "detergents," hypochlorite bleach was used as an example of "bleach," all-purpose ammonia cleaners were used for "ammonia compounds," and household chlorine and chloramine were combined to represent "mixed products."

Table 64–1. Age-Related Exposure Data, 1990–1994

Category	Exposures*	Age		
		<6 y	6–19 y	>19 y†
Soaps	50,301	81.0%	6.0%	13.0%
Detergents	60,871	85.0%	4.4%	10.6%
Bleach	191,718	48.6%	8.9%	42.5%
Ammonia	21,528	52.7%	7.8%	39.5%
Mixed	14,572	3.8%	6.5%	89.7%

*Five-year total number of exposures for which patient age was available.
†For the years 1990 to 1992, these categories were "6–17 y" and ">17 y."

INDIVIDUAL PRODUCT CATEGORIES

Soaps

A *soap* is specifically defined as the salt of a fatty acid that usually results from the reaction of an alkali with natural fats and oils or with fatty acids obtained from animal or vegetable sources. A soap is a surfactant but has the disadvantage of combining with minerals in water to form an insoluble precipitate. The term "soap" is often used to refer to a personal care product; for the purposes of this discussion, such a personal care product is used as an example of a soap.

Tables 64–1 and 64–2 summarize the demographics of exposure to personal care soaps. As might be expected, an average of 81% of these exposures are to children younger than 6 years of age; an additional 13% are to adults. The toxicity of soaps is generally quite low; these exposures resulted in no effects in 57.5%, of patients and caused minor symptoms in 41% of patients.

Exposure to soaps, as well as to other mild irritants, may produce cutaneous, ocular, oral, or gastrointestinal irritation. Ingestion of large amounts of soap may cause spontaneous vomiting (usually within 1 hour) and mild diarrhea. Soap products are

Table 64–2. Outcome Data, 1990–1994

Category	Exposures*	None	Minor	Moderate	Major	Death
Soaps	23,319	57.5%	41.0%	1.5%	0.04%	0.009%
Detergents	36,894	47.3%	49.7%	2.8%	0.1%	0.005%
Bleach	117,551	31.2%	63.4%	5.2%	0.1%	0.006%
Ammonia	13,069	37.6%	56.7%	5.5%	0.2%	0.0%
Mixed	11,122	5.6%	81.1%	13.1%	0.2%	0.02%

*Five-year total number of exposures for which outcome data were available.

not absorbed to any appreciable extent, and systemic toxicity has not been reported following a single ingestion of a soap. However, it has been postulated that hypochloremic alkalosis might occur if vomiting after soap ingestion is protracted. Only two fatalities attributable to soap exposure have been reported by the AAPCC from 1990 to 1994[1, 4]; the cause of one of these was identified as aspiration.[4]

No specific treatment is indicated following a soap ingestion. Dilution with water may provide some symptomatic relief. Rinsing with water is an effective treatment for eye irritation caused by soap exposure.

Detergents

A *detergent* is simply a cleansing agent. However, as commonly used, the term "detergents" refers to synthetic detergents, usually household cleaning products based on nonsoap surfactants that are used for laundering and dishwashing. Household detergents are mixtures of organic and inorganic substances. Composition varies within as well as among product types.[6] The principal organic ingredient is a surfactant. *Surfactants* can be classified according to the electrical charge of the chemical moiety—that is, anionic, cationic, nonionic, or amphoteric. Household detergents generally contain anionic or nonionic surfactants or mixtures of these types. Cationic and amphoteric surfactants are used less frequently in household products. Table 64–3 lists chemical examples of the three most commonly used classes of surfactant. Nonionic surfactants are found in heavy-duty liquid laundry detergents and nonphosphate granular products. Cationic surfactants are frequently used as disinfectants, and they are found in fabric softeners.

The principal inorganic ingredients in most detergents are "builders" such as phosphates, carbonates, silicates, and aluminosilicates. *Builders* help maintain an appropriate washing pH and inactivate calcium and other minerals that interfere with detergency. Low- or nonphosphate laundry detergents have higher concentrations of surfactants and nonphosphate builders. Detergents may also contain small amounts of other functional ingredients, such as soil-redeposition inhibitors, fluorescent whitening agents, fabric softeners, suds-controlling agents, enzymes, bleaches, fragrances, and colorants.

Demographics

Table 64–1 demonstrates that most exposures to detergents occur among young children. Although the number of exposures to detergents increased from 1990 to 1994, the greatest relative increase has been among persons in the 6- to 19-year-old age group; this group accounted for 3.38% of exposures in 1990 compared with 5.89% of exposures in 1994. Table 64–2 shows that 97% of such exposures are associated with benign outcomes. However, it was only in 1993 and 1994 that deaths (one each year) were attributed to laundry detergent exposure. In each case, pulmonary aspiration of a liquid detergent occurred.

Because liquid detergents (especially those for automatic dishwashers) generally have a higher pH (11.8 to 12.7) than their granular counterparts, there is concern that they might be more toxic. However, the volume of liquid automatic dishwasher detergents ingested is often small,[7] and exposures are associated with only minor symptoms.[8] Analysis of the AAPCC data for 1990 to 1994 indicates that there is little difference between the two formulations with regard to the frequencies of outcomes (Table 64–4).

Table 64–3. Chemicals Used in Household Synthetic Detergents

Anionic
Alkyl sodium sulfates
Alkyl sodium sulfonates
Dioctyl sodium sulfosuccinate
Linear alkyl benzene sulfonate (Na^+)
Sodium lauryl sulfate
Tetrapropylene benzene sulfonate (Na^+)
Nonionic
Alkyl ethoxylate
Alkyl phenoxy polyethoxy ethanols
Polyethylene glycol stearate
Cationic
Quaternary Ammonium Compounds
Benzalkonium chloride
Benzethonium chloride
Quaternary Pyridium Germicides
Cetylpyridinium chloride
Quinolinium Compounds
Dequalinium chloride

Table 64–4. Outcomes—Liquid Versus Granular Forms

	Laundry Detergents		Automatic Dishwasher Detergents	
Outcome	*Liquids (N = 9137)*	*Granules (N = 26,872)*	*Liquids (N = 6030)*	*Granules (N = 15,740)*
None	43.76%	48.38%	69.98%	70.82%
Minor	53.42%	48.60%	28.22%	28.30%
Moderate	2.68%	2.91%	1.76%	0.84%
Major	0.11%	0.11%	0.03%	0.02%
Death	0.02%	0.00%	0.00%	0.00%

Clinical Toxicology

The primary clinical toxicity of detergents results from local or topical irritation, with both surfactants and builders contributing to the irritant properties of a given product. Surfactants are of relatively low systemic toxicity but are irritating to mucosal surfaces to different degrees. The relative potency of the different categories of surfactants *CAN* easily be remembered because cationics are more toxic than anionics and nonionics. Concentrated (>10%) quaternary ammonium solutions may be corrosive.[9] Builders contribute significantly to the toxicity of detergents by increasing these products' irritant properties. Simple phosphates are the safest, whereas silicates, carbonates, and complex phosphates (e.g., trisodium phosphate, sodium tripolyphosphate) significantly increase the irritant quality of a product. The relative irritant potency of the various combinations of surfactants and builders is demonstrated in Table 64–5. In all cases, dilute solutions tend to be only irritating, whereas concentrated formulations can be caustic. Clinically, following ingestion, local irritant properties produce burning sensations in the mouth and throat and cause nausea, vomiting, and diarrhea. Spontaneous emesis usually occurs within 1 hour of ingestion. Pulmonary aspiration of either liquid or powdered detergents may cause upper airway irritation that is manifested as cough, stridor, and respiratory distress.[10]

Cationic surfactants may be absorbed and can cause systemic toxicity. Clinical effects attributed to cationic surfactants include hemolysis, restlessness, confusion, convulsions, shock, cyanosis, coma, respiratory paralysis, and muscular weakness.[9] Hemolysis is postulated to be due to the dissolution of red blood cell membranes.[11] The systemic effects of quaternary ammonium compounds may be related to ganglionic blocking effects and to a curare-like action causing paralysis at the neuromuscular junction of striated muscle.[11]

Anionic and nonionic surfactants are not absorbed significantly through the skin. Mild skin irritation may result from contact with undiluted detergents. Occluded dermal application of cationic surfactant powders or concentrated solutions produces varying degrees of dermatitis, including pustular or bullous reactions and dermal necrosis.[12, 13] Varying degrees of conjunctival and corneal irritation may result from accidental ocular exposure to detergents, with products that contain cationic surfactants having greater potential for causing damage.

Table 64–5. Relative Irritant Potency of Detergent Ingredients

	Surfactant Type		
Builder Type	*Cationic*	*Anionic*	*Nonionic*
Silicates	+ + + +	+ +	+ +
Carbonates	+ + + +	+ +	+ +
Complex phosphates	+ + + +	+ +	+ +
Simple phosphates	+ + +	+	+

+ + + +, most irritating; +, least irritating.

Management of Exposure

The ingestion of an anionic or nonionic household detergent is generally not serious. Water or milk may be used to relieve symptoms of irritation. Spontaneous emesis should be anticipated. The use of gastrointestinal decontamination techniques is not indicated. Ingestions of detergents containing cationic surfactants or nonphosphate builders may result in caustic burns, and the patient should be managed accordingly. Standard recommendations for treating ocular exposure to detergents are to rinse the eyes with copious amounts of water for at least 15 minutes and subsequently to perform an ophthalmologic examination if symptoms persist. Areas of dermal irritation should be washed with water; if irritation persists, these areas should be treated with standard topical therapy.

Bleach

The first commercial hypochlorite solution, *Eau de Javel,* was produced about 200 years ago in the French town of Javel.[14] Today, household bleaches contain varying concentrations of sodium peroxide, sodium perborate, or sodium hypochlorite. The most commonly used household bleaches are approximately 3% to 6% solutions of sodium hypochlorite in water; granular bleaches may have higher concentrations. Commercial bleaches contain peroxides or perborates.

The average age distribution of exposures to household hypochlorite bleach from 1990 to 1994 is presented in Table 64–1. The relative distribution of cases among the three age groups did not change much over these years. In another series, the most common route of exposure was shown to be ingestion.[14] The average distribution of outcomes is presented in Table 64–2. A change in the severity of cases reported by poison control centers appears to have occurred between 1990 and 1994. In 1990, 843 cases of "moderate" outcome and 15 cases of "major" outcome were reported, representing 3.8% and 0.07%, respectively, of the total number of cases for which outcomes were available. In 1994, 2080 cases of "moderate" outcome and 39 cases of "major" outcome were reported, representing 8.3% and 0.16%, respectively, of the total number of cases for which outcomes were available. Thus, the severity of the cases reported to poison centers from 1990 to 1994 appears to have increased. From 1990 to 1994, seven deaths have been attributed to household hypochlorite bleach exposure. Of the four fatalities for which case data were published, all involved the inhalation of fumes as a route of exposure.

Clinical Toxicology

Household bleaches are mild to moderate irritants (pH, 10.8 to 11.4) and are generally not associated with any degree of tissue destruction.[14] Following accidental ingestion, the incidence of oropharyngeal, esophageal, and gastrointestinal burns is very low. However, the ingestion of large quantities of bleach (≥5 mL/kg) may be associated with corrosive damage.[15] Although esophageal strictures or perforations were not found in 522 patients,[16, 17] these effects have been reported.[18, 19] Ingestions commonly result in spontaneous emesis. In the stomach, hypochlorite reacts with hydrochloric acid to form hypochlorous acid and chlorine[20]; thus, emesis following hypochlorite bleach ingestion may expose the esophagus to an acid. Reported systemic effects following a large ingestion of bleach have been hypernatremia (Na^+, 169 mmol/L) and hyperchloremic acidosis ($Cl-$, 130 mmol/L, pH 7.25).[20]

External contamination may result in eye or skin irritation. Because of its pH, bleach may cause an alkali-type of burn when it is splashed in the eye. Ocular injury is usually limited to mild superficial erosion of the corneal epithelium and faint haziness of the cornea, both of which resolve spontaneously.[21] If the contact is prolonged, corneal edema and conjunctival hemorrhage may occur. Uncovered dermal application of bleach (2% sodium hypochlorite) causes negligible skin irritation.[22]

Management of Exposure

Forced emesis, gastric lavage, and gastric aspiration are not indicated in a household bleach ingestion. Symptomatic care, including dilution with water or milk, is all that is necessary. Any patient who ingests a large amount of bleach should undergo monitoring of serum electrolytes and plasma pH for 2 hours after the ingestion. Patients who ingest large amounts of bleach or who have significant esophageal or gastric symptoms after vomiting may have acid-induced injuries and should be evaluated for corrosive damage.

Immediate irrigation of the eye with copious amounts of water minimizes the damage caused by bleach. Delays in irrigation may be associated with the development of more significant ocular lesions. Patients who have persistent eye symptoms following irrigation should undergo an ophthalmologic examination for assessment of the damage. Skin contaminated with bleach should be washed thoroughly with mild soap and tepid water. Complications are unlikely.

Ammonia Compounds

Composition and Definition

Aqueous ammonia solutions are alkaline and colorless. Most ammonias for household use are 5% to 10% solutions of ammonia, whereas more concentrated solutions (27% to 30%) are available in pharmacies or are found in industrial settings. So-called "smelling salts" are capsules of aromatic spirits of ammonia and contain a small volume (<0.5 mL) of 15% to 18% ammonia hydroxide in alcohol. This section addresses the hazards associated with exposure to household ammonia compounds. The management of patients with oral or dermal exposure to industrial-strength ammonia is similar to that presented in Chapter 62. Inhalation of ammonia fumes is managed as a respiratory tract irritant.

Demographics

The distribution of ages and outcomes are presented in Tables 64–1 and 64–2. From 1992 to 1994, the number of exposures dropped by about 25%; most of the decrease (65%) was attributable to a reduction in the number of exposures in those older than 19 years of age. Interestingly, as the number of exposures decreased, the number of outcomes classified as "none" and as "minor" decreased, but the number of "moderate" outcomes increased and the number of "major" outcomes did not change.

Clinical Toxicology

The combination ammonia and water forms ammonium hydroxide, which dissociates into ammonium and hydroxyl ions; the latter is responsible for any tissue damage.[23] A 1.0-N aqueous ammonia solution has a pH of 11.6 and causes liquifactive necrosis of tissues; in lower concentrations (e.g., household concentrations), ammonia solutions are tissue irritants. Nausea, vomiting, pain in the mouth and throat, drooling, dysphagia, and swelling of the lips and mucous membranes may occur following ingestion. Although uncommon, caustic-like esophageal burns were reported in 3 adults who ingested 30 mL or more of household ammonia products (3% to 3.6% ammonia, pH 11.5 to 11.8) in suicide attempts.[24]

Oropharyngeal burns have been reported in children who have bitten into aromatic ammonia capsules, but there have been no reports of esophageal burns from this type of exposure.[25]

Ocular contamination with an ammonia solution results in conjunctival hyperemia, lacrimation, photophobia, and a dull-looking cornea. Inhalation of ammonia vapors from household solutions may be mildly irritating to the upper respiratory tract. Bronchospasm, dyspnea, pulmonary edema, and ventilation-perfusion abnormalities have been reported following exposure to concentrated ammonia vapors[26] but not to vapors from household ammonia. Pulmonary aspiration of a household ammonia solution may result in chemical pneumonitis and respiratory distress syndrome.[24] Accidental exposure of the skin to household ammonia may produce minor irritation but is unlikely to result in significant damage.

Management of Exposure

Patients with accidental nonsuicidal ingestions of household ammonia products should be treated symptomatically. Milk or water may be used for dilution, but removal from the stomach is not indicated. No benefit is derived from the use of either activated charcoal or cathartics. Children who bite into a smelling salt capsule should be given milk or water for dilution; endoscopy should be considered for only those children who meet criteria for endoscopy proposed for alkaline corrosive ingestion (see Chapter 62). Similarly, patients who have intentionally ingested household ammonia should be managed as if they had ingested alkaline corrosives. Contaminated eyes should be flushed immediately with copious amounts of running water for at least 15 minutes. Instillation of ointments, including antibiotics, is controversial because of the claim that ointments promote the penetration of ammonium hydroxide.[27] Ophthalmologic examination is appropriate if ocular symptoms and signs persist after flushing. Areas of skin that have accidentally been exposed to household ammonia should be washed with mild soap and water. Removal from further exposure is the appropriate first aid measure. Any respiratory symptoms should be treated symptomatically.

Mixed Chemicals

Composition and Definition

One of the most common mixtures of household products is hypochlorite bleach in combination with either a strong acid or an ammonia solution. Mixing an aqueous solution of hypochlorite with a strong acid results in the release of chlorine gas, whereas combining a solution of hypochlorite with an ammonia solution releases chloramine gas.

Table 64-1 presents the age distribution of persons with exposures to chlorine and chloramine produced by the mixture of household products. Table 64-2 presents the outcome data for exposures to household chlorine or chloramine gas. The percentage of cases reported as having "moderate" outcomes has increased nearly 10-fold, from 2.1% in 1990 to 20.8% in 1994; this suggests an increase in the severity of cases reported to poison control centers.

Clinical Toxicology

Both chlorine gas and chloramine gas are respiratory irritants and are considered together. Inhalation of either chlorine or chloramine gas results in immediate mucous membrane irritation. Chlorine acts by reacting with water to liberate hydrogen chloride and a free oxygen radical.[28]

Although one case of pulmonary edema[29] and two cases of pneumomediastinum secondary to violent coughing[30] have been reported, the vast majority of patients exposed to chlorine or chloramine gas at home seem to have a benign clinical course. A prospective study of exposed patients who contacted a poison control center found that nearly 85% of patients developed coughing and roughly 20% complained of shortness of breath (which usually was related to the coughing); few patients complained of chest pain, wheezing, dizziness, vomiting, ocular irritation, nasal irritation, or abdominal pain.[31]

Management of Exposure

Moving the patient from the contaminated atmosphere to fresh air is the most important first aid measure. Most patients can be managed at home because symptoms usually last for fewer than 6 hours.[31] Patients who have persistent symptoms should be evaluated by a physician for assessment of the degree of airway and alveolar compromise. Treatment is primarily symptomatic and supportive. Inhaled sympathomimetic bronchodilator agents may be beneficial if bronchospasm is significant. The benefits of nebulized sodium bicarbonate in the treatment of respiratory effects and those of systemic corticosteroids for the prevention of noncardiogenic pulmonary edema are still unproven. Patients with significant respiratory compromise should be monitored in a hospital for 24 hours.

References

1. Litovitz TL, Bailey KM, Schmitz BF, et al: 1990 Annual Report of the American Association of Poison Control Centers National Data Collection System. Am J Emerg Med *9*:461, 1991.
2. Litovitz TL, Holm KC, Bailey KM, et al: 1991 Annual Report of the American Association of Poison Control Centers National Data Collection System. Am J Emerg Med *10*:452, 1992.
3. Litovitz TL, Holm KC, Clancy C, et al: 1992 Annual Report of the American Association of Poison Control Centers Toxic Surveillance System. Am J Emerg Med *11*:494, 1993.
4. Litovitz TL, Clark LR, Soloway RA: 1993 Annual Report of

the American Association of Poison Control Centers Toxic Exposure Surveillance System. Am J Emerg Med *12*:546, 1994.

5. Litovitz TL, Felberg L, Soloway RA, et al: 1994 Annual Report of the American Association of Poison Control Centers Toxic Exposure Surveillance System. Am J Emerg Med *13*:551, 1995.
6. Temple AR, Lovejoy Jr FH: Household Cleaning Products and Their Accidental Ingestion: SDA Scientific and Technical Report No. 5R. New York, Soap and Detergent Association, 1980.
7. Sublet VH, Baldwin S, Wilke DL, et al: A survey of automatic dishwashing liquid ingestions: Child-resistant closures limit accidental ingestions. Abstract. Vet Hum Toxicol *30*:375, 1988.
8. Krenzelok EP: Liquid automatic dishwashing detergents: A profile of toxicity. Ann Emerg Med *18*:60, 1989.
9. van Berkel M, de Wolff FA: Survival after acute benzalkonium chloride poisoning. Hum Toxicol *7*:191, 1988.
10. Einhorn A, Horton L, Altieri M, et al: Serious respiratory consequences of detergent ingestions in children. Pediatrics *84*:472, 1989.
11. Gluxhuber C: Toxicological properties of surfactants. Arch Toxicol *32*:245, 1974.
12. Mercer DM: Cetrimide burn in an infant. Postgrad Med J *59*:472, 1983.
13. Wahlberg JE, Wrangs JK, Hietasalo A: Skin irritancy from nonanoic acid. Contact Dermatitis *13*:266, 1985.
14. Racioppi F, Daskaleros PA, Besbelli N, et al: Household bleaches based on sodium hypochlorite: Review of acute toxicology and poison control center experience. Food Chem Toxicol *32*:845, 1994.
15. Jakobsson SW, Rajs J, Jonsson JA, Persson H: Poisoning with sodium hypochlorite solution: Report of a fatal case, supplemented with an experimental and clinico-epidemiology study. Am J Forensic Med Pathol *12*:320, 1991.
16. Pike DG, Peabody Jr JW, Davis EW, et al: A re-evaluation of the dangers of Clorox ingestion. J Pediatr *63*:303, 1963.
17. Landau GD, Saunders WH: The effect of chlorine bleach on the esophagus. Arch Otolaryngol *80*:174, 1964.
18. Strange DC, Finneran JC, Shumacker Jr HB, et al: Corrosive injury of the stomach. Arch Surg *62*:350, 1951.
19. French RJ, Tabb HG, Rutledge LJ: Esophageal stenosis produced by ingestion of bleach: Report of two cases. South Med J *63*:1140, 1970.
20. Ward MJ, Routledge PA: Hypernatraemia and hyperchloraemic acidosis after bleach ingestion. Hum Toxicol *7*:37, 1988.
21. Ingram TA: Response of the human eye to accidental exposure to sodium hypochlorite. J Endodontic *16*:235, 1990.
22. Eun HC, Lee AY, Lee YS: Sodium hypochlorite dermatitis. Contact Dermatitis *11*:45, 1984.
23. Balmes JR: Acute pulmonary injury from hazardous materials. *In* Sullivan Jr JB, Krieger GR (eds): Hazardous Materials Toxicology. Baltimore, Williams & Wilkins, pp 425–432, 1992.
24. Klein J, Olson KR, McKinney HE: Caustic injury from household ammonia. Am J Emerg Med *3*:320, 1985.
25. Wason S, Stephan M, Breide C: Ingestion of aromatic ammonia "smelling salts" capsules. Am J Dis Child *144*:139, 1990.
26. Kocks DJ, Scott D: Ammonia—still a health hazard in the workplace. South Afr Med J *78*:45, 1990.
27. Broderick A, Schwartz DA: Halogen gases, ammonia, and phosgene. *In* Sullivan Jr JB, Krieger GR (eds): Hazardous Materials Toxicology. Baltimore, Williams & Wilkins, pp 791–796, 1992.
28. Adelson L, Kaufman J: Fatal chlorine poisoning: Report of two cases with clinicopathologic correlation. Am J Clin Pathol *56*:430, 1971.
29. Jones FL: Chlorine poisoning from mixing household cleaners. JAMA *222*:1312, 1972.
30. Gapany-Gapanavicius M, Yellin A, Almog S, et al: Pneumomediastinum: A complication of chlorine exposure from mixing household cleaning agents. JAMA *248*:349, 1982.
31. Mrvos R, Dean BS, Krenzelok EP: Home exposures to chlorine/chloramine gas: Review of 216 cases. South Med J *86*:654, 1993.

SECTION F

PESTICIDES

65

The Organophosphates and Other Insecticides

FREDERICK B. CARLTON, JR., MD
WILLIAM M. SIMPSON, JR., MD
LESTER M. HADDAD, MD

The organophosphates are the most commonly used insecticides in the United States as well as in the world. These agents are also potent chemical warfare agents, traditionally known as nerve gas. The organophosphates have been in military arsenals since World War II and most recently achieved international notoriety as the causative agent in the terrorist attack on the Japanese subway March 19, 1995 (March 20 in Japan).[1] They are also the most common cause of insecticide poisoning. The American Association of Poison Control Centers reported 18,650 exposures to organophosphates in 1994, with 4 deaths.[2]

Warfare agents include chemical agents, such as the organophosphate nerve gases, cyanide, arsine, phosgene, nitrogen mustard, and tear gas and other riot control agents; and biologic agents such as aflatoxins, anthrax, and botulism. This chapter includes a discussion of the organophosphate nerve gases sarin, soman, tabun, and VX.

The World Health Organization estimates that approximately 3 million pesticide poisonings occur annually worldwide and cause more than 220,000 deaths.[3] Developing countries such as Sri Lanka and India report alarming rates of toxicity and death.[4]

In addition to the organophosphates, other insecticides include the carbamates, dichlorodiphenyltrichloroethane (DDT) and the organochlorines, the botanic insecticides, and the insect repellents. Approximately 249 million pounds of insecticides are used annually in the United States alone, at a cost of $2.4 billion.

ORGANOPHOSPHATES

The organophosphates have achieved great popularity because of their effectiveness as insecticides and their lack of persistence in the environment. Because of their unstable chemical structure, they disintegrate into harmless radicals within days of application. Because they do not persist in body tissues or the environment, as do DDT and other organochlorines, they have replaced DDT as the insecticide agent of choice.

Although the first organophosphate, tetraethyl pyrophosphate (TEPP), was synthesized in 1854, it was not until World War II that the Germans used TEPP as a substitute for the scarce botanic insecticide nicotine. Because TEPP is water soluble, its absorption is most rapid by either the oral or dermal route, and it is the most toxic of the organophosphate insecticides.

Organophosphate poisoning occurs in various settings. Occupational exposures occur in farm workers involved in the application of these agents and those engaged in their manufacture. Children are accidentally exposed to these agents in the treatment of pets for fleas and other pests. Misuse, whether intentional or unintentional, and suicide attempts account for the remainder of civilian cases. The 1995 terrorist attack on the Tokyo subway involved the nerve gas sarin.

The toxicity of organophosphate compounds varies greatly. The highly toxic group of organophosphates is used primarily for agricultural and military purposes. The organophosphate most suited for agricultural use is parathion, which is the most common cause of human poisoning and fatality.[1, 2] An intermediate group exists, used primarily as an insecticide for animals. Those with low toxicity are available for use by households and on golf courses. Malathion is often found in the garage as a garden spray for roses; its toxicity and absorption are low, and it can be metabolized. Table 65–1 lists some of the better-known commercial compounds and their uses.

Pharmacokinetics and Pharmacodynamics

Organophosphates are a heterogeneous group of compounds that are composed of a phosphoric acid derivative with two organic side chains and an additional side chain that can be a cyanide, thiocyanate, halide, phosphate, phenoxy, thiophenoxy, or carboxylate group.

Most of the organophosphate insecticides are rapidly absorbed by all routes—dermal, respiratory, gastrointestinal (GI), and conjunctival. Organophosphates may be classified as direct or indirect acetylcholinesterase inhibitors. Metabolism, primarily by the hepatic cytochrome P-450 system, is required to activate the indirect inhibitors. Acute effects may be noted almost immediately after exposure to the direct-acting group, such as the nerve gases, although a delay of 2 to 3 hours may be noted after dermal absorption. Parathion is an example of the indirect-acting group, because it first must be converted to paraoxon by substitution of an oxygen for a sulfur to be physiologically active; for this reason, symptoms of parathion intoxication may not begin until 6 to 24 hours after exposure. The organophosphates are generally highly lipid soluble. One drop of VX, soman, or sarin may be lethal.[5]

Pathophysiology

The organophosphates cause a specific biochemical lesion, that of acetylcholinesterase inhibition, thus producing a striking physiologic picture in human poisoning. Acetylcholine is the most important chemical transmitter at synaptic junctions. Acetylcholinesterase breaks down acetylcholine by hydrolysis into its two primary fragments, acetic acid and choline, both of which are essentially inert. This breakdown prevents further neurotransmission at the synapse. The two principal human cholinesterases are true acetylcholinesterase, found primarily in nervous tissue and red blood cells (RBCs), and pseudocholinesterase, found in serum and the liver.

The toxicologic effects of the organophosphates are almost entirely due to the inhibition of acetylcholinesterase in the nervous system, resulting in accumulation of acetylcholine at synapses and the myoneural junction.[6,7] Although organophosphate poisoning is more accurately assessed by measurement of RBC cholinesterase, serum cholinesterase measurements are technically simpler to run and are more readily available in hospitals. Although most organophosphates inhibit both (true) RBC and (pseudo-) serum cholinesterase, the nerve gas VX inhibits RBC but not pseudocholinesterase.[5]

The overabundance of acetylcholine initially excites and then paralyzes transmission in cholinergic synapses, which includes (1) the central nervous system (CNS), (2) the parasympathetic nerve endings

Table 65–1. Examples of Organophosphate Insecticides

Common Name	Product Example	Chemical Name	Estimated Fatal Oral Dose (g/70 kg)
Agricultural Insecticides (high toxicity)			
Tetraethyl pyrophosphate	Miller Kilmite 40	Tetraethyl pyrophosphate	0.05
Phorate	Thimet (American Cyanamid)	*0,0*-Diethyl(*S*-ethylmercaptomethyl) dithiophosphate	
Parathion	Niagara Phoskil Dust	*0,0*-Diethyl-*0*-*p*-nitrophenyl phosphorothioate	0.1
Phosdrin	Mevinphos (Shell)	Dimethyl-0-(1-methyl-2-carbomethoxy-vinyl) phosphate	0.15
Disulfoton	Disyston	Diethyl-*S*-2-ethyl-2-mercaptoethyl phosphorodithioate	0.2
Animal Insecticides (intermediate toxicity)			
Coumaphos	Co-Ral Animal Insecticide	Diethyl-*0*-(3-chloro-4-methyl-7-coumarinyl) phosphorothioate	
Chlorpyrifos (Dursban)	Rid-A-Bug (Kenco)	*0,0*-Diethyl-*0*-(3,5,6-trichloro-2-pyridyl) phosphorothioate	
Trichlorfon	Trichlorfon Pour On (Hess & Clark)	Dimethyl trichlorohydroxyethyl phosphonate	
Ronnel	Korlan Livestock Spray (Dow)	*0,0*-dimethyl-*0*-(2,4,5-trichlorophenyl) phosphorothioate	
Household Use or Golf Course Spray (low toxicity)			
Diazinon	Security Fire Ant Killer (Woolfolk)	Diethyl-*0*-(2-isopropyl-4-methyl-6-pyrimidyl) phosphorothioate	25.0
Malathion	Ortho Malathion 50 Insect Spray	Dimethyl-*S*-(1,2-bis-carboethoxy) ethyl phosphorodithioate	60.0
Vapona (dichlorvos, DDVP)	Shell No-Pest Strip	*0,0*-Dimethyl-*0*-2,2-dichlorovinyl phosphate	
Acephate	Chevron Orthene	*0,S*-Dimethylacetylphosphoramidothioate	

and a few sympathetic nerve endings, such as the sweat glands (muscarinic effects), and (3) the somatic nerves and the ganglionic synapses of autonomic ganglia (nicotinic effects). The signs and symptoms of organophosphate poisoning are thus an expression of these three effects of acetylcholine excess, as outlined in Table 65–2. Thus, parasympathetic stimulation causes miosis, bradycardia, bronchoconstriction, hyperactivity of GI smooth muscle, and secretion of the exocrine glands (salivary, lacrimal, bronchial, and pancreatic). It is interesting to note that stimulation of the autonomic ganglia (nicotinic effects) produces sympathetic stimulation, resulting in tachycardia and mydriasis. Patients with organophosphate poisoning manifest either bradycardia if parasympathetic stimulation prevails or tachycardia if sympathetic stimulation via the ganglia prevails. In our experience, although heart rate is often variable, miosis usually prevails.

Inhibition of the enzyme acetylcholinesterase by organophosphate is initially by ionic bonding, but the enzyme eventually is progressively phosphorylated by covalent bonding, a process that normally takes 24 to 48 hours; this process is called *aging,* and this period is known as the *critical interval,* because during this time administration of antidote is still effective in reversing the process.[6] Once aging is completed, the enzyme cannot be reactivated. Although the aging process generally takes 24 to 48 hours, the nerve gas soman produces such rapid aging that pralidoxime antidotal therapy is often ineffective.[5]

Once complete aging has occurred, enzyme resynthesis is the only means to restore acetylcholinesterase, and it takes weeks to occur. During this time, critically ill patients unresponsive to antidotal therapy require complete pulmonary support until sufficient enzyme resynthesis occurs. Recovery has occurred after weeks of such therapy.[6]

Table 65–2. Clinical Effects of Organophosphate Poisoning (Acetylcholine Excess)

Anatomic Site of Action	Physiologic Effects
Muscarinic Effects	
Sweat glands	Sweating
Pupils	Constricted pupils
Lacrimal glands	Lacrimation
Salivary glands	Excessive salivation
Bronchial tree	Wheezing
Gastrointestinal	Cramps, vomiting, diarrhea, tenesmus
Cardiovascular	Bradycardia, decrease in blood pressure
Ciliary body	Blurred vision
Bladder	Urinary incontinence
Nicotinic Effects	
Striated muscle	Fasciculations, cramps, weakness, twitching, paralysis, respiratory embarrassment, cyanosis, arrest
Sympathetic ganglia	Tachycardia, elevated blood pressure
Central Nervous System Effects	Anxiety, restlessness, ataxia, convulsions, insomnia, coma, absent reflexes, Cheyne-Stokes respirations, respiratory and circulatory depression

Clinical Presentation

The presentation of an organophosphate exposure depends on the specific agent, the quantity, and the route of entry. Initial symptoms may range from mild, as a flulike syndrome, to immediately life threatening. Toxicity typically occurs soon after exposure but may be delayed, depending on the agent and route of entry. The most rapid onset of symptoms occurs with inhalation, and the slowest with dermal exposure. For example, parathion intoxication takes time to be fully manifested, and it is not unusual for a patient to present to the emergency department with symptoms of gastroenteritis, to be sent home, and to return hours later in respiratory distress. In contrast, significant inhalation of the nerve gas sarin can produce respiratory arrest within 5 minutes. Although organophosphate toxicity generally occurs within 4 to 12 hours, full-blown toxicity may not be manifested for 24 hours.[8]

Cholinergic excess produces the signs and symptoms of acute organophosphate exposure. The predominant clinical findings are usually muscarinic, followed by CNS and then nicotinic manifestations (see Table 65–2). GI symptoms and signs are usually seen first after ingestion of organophosphates. Aerosol exposure typically presents with respiratory and ocular complaints. Any constellation of findings may occur with significant exposures, and thus the diagnosis is often difficult to make. In one study,[9] 16 of 20 transfer patients were incorrectly diagnosed as having other conditions. The initial presence of excessive salivation, lacrimation, and weakness during the initial phase is more indicative of organophosphate poisoning. Miosis, a typical muscarinic sign, is not always present, because mydriasis may result from nicotinic stimulation.

CNS effects generally include anxiety, restlessness, coma, and seizures, but chorea, psychosis, depression, and choreoathetosis have been described.[10] Muscle weakness and paralysis develop in severe exposures, and untreated patients die as a result of respiratory arrest.

Pancreatitis with hyperamylasemia and hyperglycemia is an uncommon but definite presentation of organophosphate poisoning.[11, 12] Organophosphates produce an increase in the secretion rate of acinar pancreatic glands because of their cholinergic innervation.

Diagnosis

Organophosphate poisoning is generally diagnosed clinically. The most common presentation is a patient with a characteristic odor (similar to garlic), miosis, increased airway secretions, lacrimation, bradycardia, and GI complaints. A history of exposure is most helpful when present but often is not available. The development of coma, pulmonary edema, ataxia, psychosis, dyspnea or cyanosis, fasciculations, pancreatitis, bradycardia, and weakness and paralysis indicates severe poisoning, and aggressive emergency management must be instituted.

On physical examination, the presence of lacrimation, miosis, fasciculations, and weakness when found are characteristic of organophosphate poisoning and should be managed as such until proved otherwise. When the diagnosis is not evident, a depressed serum or RBC cholinesterase level is helpful. If organophosphate poisoning is suspected, therapy should never be withheld pending confirmation of laboratory values.

Other conditions in which the serum cholinesterase level may be depressed include parenchymal liver disease, including viral hepatitis, cirrhosis, congestion secondary to congestive heart failure, metastatic carcinoma, and reduced levels of serum albumin.[13] Depression of serum cholinesterase level may be a genetic variant in 3% of patients. The serum cholinesterase level is depressed before the RBC cholinesterase level and is a sensitive indicator of exposure to organophosphates.[14] Twenty-five per cent or greater depression of the RBC cholinesterase level is a true indicator of poisoning. RBC cholinesterase levels may take up to 90 to 120 days to return to normal values, whereas serum cholinesterase levels recover in days to weeks.

Treatment

Immediate Supportive Measures. Immediate attention to the airway and adequate oxygenation is essential. Atropine (as later described) should be administered until secretions dry. Frequent suctioning of the airway is usually necessary until the patient is adequately atropinized. Endotracheal intubation is often necessary in severe poisonings because of secretions, decreased level of consciousness, or weakness of the respiratory muscles. Although rapid-sequence intubation is a useful technique for intubation, succinylcholine can produce prolonged apnea in the setting of organophosphate poisoning[15] and should be avoided. If neuromuscular blockade is needed for airway control, a nondepolarizing agent such as *rocuronium* is advisable.

Pulmonary Support. Adequate ventilation is paramount in these patients because respiratory distress is common and is the primary cause of mortality in critical cases. Continuous pulse oximetry, antidote administration, mechanical ventilation, and admission to an intensive care unit are essential to proper management. Cardiac monitoring during atropine administration is indicated. Pressor agents are seldom necessary.

Decontamination. Gastric lavage should be considered with a recent ingestion. Activated charcoal (with sorbitol in adults and older children) should be given, although it lacks efficacy with some organophosphates such as malathion.

After dermal exposure, clothes should be removed immediately and the patient washed with soap and water. A second washing of ethyl alcohol may be advantageous. Remember to remove shoes! Care must be taken to avoid exposure of health care personnel, who should wear protective clothing, including gloves.

Antidotal Therapy: Atropine and Pralidoxime. Administration of both atropine and pralidoxime should be initiated concomitantly with significant organophosphate poisoning. The physiologic antidote for organophosphate poisoning is atropine, which competes with acetylcholine at the synapses and antagonizes both muscarinic and CNS effects. The use of atropine is particularly helpful in drying excessive secretions and improving respiratory status. Atropine has no effect on nicotinic receptors. Therefore, muscle weakness and respiratory depression persist despite adequate atropinization and require pralidoxime for treatment. Atropine should be administered as soon as the diagnosis is suspected, while carefully observing the patient's response. Failure to respond to a trial dose of atropine is virtually diagnostic of organophosphate poisoning. Proper oxygenation and cardiac monitoring are essential during atropine administration.

The initial dose of atropine should be 1 to 2 mg for an adult and 0.05 mg/kg for a child. The preferred route is intravenous, but intramuscular is effective. Treatment must be individualized on the basis of the response to the initial dose. Signs of atropinization include flushing, drying of airway secretions, and pinpoint pupils (if present), which become dilated. Similarly, if the patient originally exhibited bradycardia, an increase in the heart rate to normal or tachycardia suggests an adequate atropine dose.

Repeat doses of atropine may be necessary and are generally given every 15 to 30 minutes until signs of atropinization occur. The repeat dose is 2 mg intravenously for adults and 0.02 to 0.05 mg/kg for children. Intermittent bolus therapy is usually adequate to control muscarinic signs and symptoms, but a continuous intravenous infusion may occasionally be needed for a severely poisoned patient. Signs of excessive atropinization include fever, delirium, and ileus.

Atropine may be required for 24 hours and should be tapered before being discontinued. Prolonged atropine administration and tapered withdrawal are especially warranted in poisoning by the lipid-soluble organophosphates.

Pralidoxime (Protopam, 2-PAM chloride) is a specific antidote for organophosphate toxicity. Pralidoxime can reverse the phosphorylation of acetylcholinesterase and thereby reactivate the enzyme. Pralidoxime may also detoxify the organophosphate molecule and has an anticholinergic effect.[16] Because its efficacy is time dependent and the drug must be given in the first 24- to 48-hour critical interval after exposure, it should be administered as soon as possible in all clinically significant poisonings. Nonetheless, atropine should be given concurrently with oxime therapy to alleviate the acute muscarinic effects.

Because the nerve gas soman causes rapid phosphorylation of acetylcholinesterase, pralidoxime may be ineffective unless given almost immediately after exposure. In addition to undergoing pretreatment with oral pyridostigmine,[17] military personnel in the Gulf War carried autoinjectors containing pralidoxime and atropine in the event of exposure to nerve gas.[5]

The initial dose of pralidoxime is 1 to 2 g for adults and 25 to 50 mg/kg for children, given intravenously for 15 to 30 minutes. The effects are often dramatic, as patients will recover their strength and be able to walk. Pralidoxime is a very safe drug. Its few side effects are more likely to be encountered if it is given rapidly. Known adverse reactions include visual disturbances, confusion, mania, headache, and tachycardia; neuromuscular blockade and weakness are uncommon. Because pralidoxime undergoes renal elimination, it should be administered with caution to patients with renal insufficiency.[16, 18–21] Because of the low toxicity of this agent and its benefit in organophosphate poisoning, an initial dose should virtually always be given in suspected and symptomatic cases. After the initial dose, a continuous intravenous infusion of pralidoxime at 10 to 20 mg/kg per hour up to 500 mg/h has also been effective in the treatment of severe cases of organophosphate poisoning.[20] Although adverse effects with pralidoxime are infrequently encountered, continuous intravenous infusion may further lower their incidence. By providing sustained therapeutic levels of pralidoxime, continuous infusion may be more effective in reactivation of acetylcholinesterase.

Persistent or recurrent symptoms in organophosphate intoxication are generally indicative of inadequate pralidoxime therapy.[8, 22–24] In some countries, obidoxime (Toxogonin) is an alternative oxime.[19]

Complications

Chronic neurologic sequelae[25–30] may occur after heavy organophosphate exposure, such as cognitive impairment, depression, Guillain-Barré syndrome, and peripheral neuropathy.

Prevention

Because of the toxicity of organophosphates, prevention of unintentional exposure is essential. Proper education of all workers involved in the manufacture, transport, or use of these products is imperative. Proper application, labeling, and storage are necessary to avoid either unintentional occupational or domestic exposure.

CARBAMATES

The carbamates are a group of insecticides derived from carbamic acid. They have a broad spectrum of use as agricultural and household garden insecticides. Sevin, Baygon, and Lannate are used most commonly. Table 65–3 lists a group of carbamate insecticides in decreasing order of toxicity. Aldicarb is considered a systemic insecticide because it is taken up from the soil and incorporated into the plant and fruit. Aldicarb was the responsible agent in 1350 cases including 8 deaths due to food poisoning by contaminated watermelons in California during 1985.

The carbamates are *reversible* cholinesterase inhibitors. They cause this effect by reversible carbamoylation of the enzyme cholinesterase, allowing overabundance of acetylcholine, as with organophosphate poisoning. The carbamates are absorbed by all routes, including inhalation, ingestion, and dermal exposure.

The 1994 annual report of the American Association of Poison Control Centers reported 6139 exposures to carbamate insecticides, with 1184 patients treated at a health care facility and no deaths. Also reported were 1022 joint exposures to carbamates and organophosphates, with 225 patients treated at a health care facility and no deaths.[2]

Clinical Presentation: Carbamates Versus Organophosphates

Because both the carbamate insecticides and the organophosphates are cholinesterase inhibitors, both produce the syndrome of cholinergic crisis, as described in the preceding section on organophosphates and outlined in Table 65–2. Contrasting the clinical presentation and diagnostic considerations of the two groups helps in understanding the carbamates.

1. The clinical syndrome is more benign and of much shorter duration with the carbamate insecticides. The carbamate insecticides cause *reversible* in-

Table 65–3. Carbamate Insecticides

Commercial Name	Chemical
Temik	Aldicarb
Matacil	Aminocarb
Vydate	Oxamyl
Isolan	Isolan
Furadan	Carbofuran
Lannate	Methomyl
Zectran	Mexacarbate
Mesurol	Methiocarb
Dimetilan	Dimetilan
Baygon	Propoxur
Sevin	Carbaryl

From Coye MJ, Barnett PJ, Midtling JE, et al: Clinical confirmation of organophosphate poisoning by serial cholinesterase analyses. Arch Intern Med *147*:438, 1987.

hibition, and the carbamoyl-enzyme complex dissociates far more readily than the organophosphate complex, which generally progresses to irreversible inhibition.

2. Unlike the organophosphates, the carbamates poorly penetrate the CNS. Thus, carbamate poisoning resembles organophosphate poisoning with the absence of prominent CNS effects such as convulsions. Convulsions are rare with carbamate insecticides.

3. Serum and RBC cholinesterase values are not reliable in confirming the diagnosis of carbamate poisoning as they are with the organophosphates, because enzyme activity returns to normal within a few hours. A patient may show symptoms in the emergency department 6 hours after exposure, but the cholinesterase levels may have already returned to normal. Thus, one may rely only on clinical judgment when managing the carbamate insecticides.

Treatment

The clinical picture of carbamate poisoning is one of cholinergic crisis (see Table 65–2). Treatment of symptomatic carbamate insecticide poisoning includes establishment of the airway, stabilization of vital signs, removal of poison by gastric lavage if the ingestion is recent, and removal of contaminated clothes and shoes and thorough cleansing of the skin. Use of activated charcoal and cathartics is indicated in the event of ingestion.

Atropine is the drug of choice in the management of carbamate insecticide poisoning. The dosage for adults is 0.5 to 2.0 mg intravenously, repeated generally every 15 to 30 minutes until signs of atropinization appear (dry mouth, flushing, and dilated pupils if pupils were originally pinpoint). Atropine may be necessary for only 6 to 12 hours for the majority of patients. Patients should preferably be well oxygenated with the use of atropine. A child's dosage of atropine is 0.05 mg/kg initially, with repeat dose of 0.02 mg/kg to 0.05 mg/kg (up to the adult dose for teenagers) as necessary at intervals similar to those for adults. The rationale for use of atropine is the same as that for the organophosphate insecticides.

Observation, at least for serious cases, is recommended for at least 24 hours. Milder intoxications that are purely from carbamate exposure do not require such prolonged observation. As with all insecticide poisonings, patients must be observed because of possible exposure to a second insecticide, such as an organophosphate. In one study of 52 patients with insecticide poisoning,[32] the largest group, 34.5%, consisted of mixed organophosphate and carbamate poisoning, with organophosphate alone and carbamate alone each with 13 patients, representing 25% each. Patients must also be observed with respect to possible toxicity from the carrier, which may be methyl alcohol, or a hydrocarbon, which poses the risk of an aspiration pneumonitis.

Pulmonary edema and respiratory failure are uncommon with carbamate poisoning[31, 32] and, as with CNS signs, if present suggest toxicity from a second insecticide, such as an organophosphate. General supportive care is indicated.

Pralidoxime is not indicated for pure carbamate poisoning, because the carbamoyl-enzyme complex is reversible and readily dissociates.[33] The physiologic antidote atropine, which is competitive with acetylcholine at the neuroreceptor site, is all that is necessary until the enzyme acetylcholinesterase is able to dissociate, recover function, and metabolize overabundant acetylcholine.

Early reports stated that pralidoxime reduced the antidotal effect of atropine in the early management of carbamate poisoning, especially with carbaryl. At one time, pralidoxime was not used in the presence of carbamate poisoning. However, pralidoxime has been used in two instances in the presence of carbamate poisoning: (1) when the etiology of the insecticide poisoning was unknown and (2) when a patient suffers from mixed organophosphate and carbamate insecticide toxicity.

The first situation, the unknown insecticide poisoning, is rather common. In fact, common sense tells us that in several cases through the years, patients with carbamate intoxication were administered pralidoxime by well-intentioned emergency physicians who thought they were faced with organophosphate poisoning. We recommend administering pralidoxime to a critically ill patient with possibly mixed carbamate-organophosphate poisoning or unknown insecticide poisoning.

When a physician is faced with a critically ill patient exhibiting signs and symptoms of cholinesterase inhibition, either from an unknown insecticide or from concomitant organophosphate and carbamate exposure, a trial of pralidoxime is clearly warranted.

Recovery from pure carbamate insecticide exposure is generally complete.

ORGANOCHLORINE INSECTICIDES

Once the most important group of insecticides, the organochlorines have been largely banned in the United States and many foreign countries (Table 65–4).

DDT, first introduced in 1942, was the first modern

Table 65–4. Organochlorine Insecticides

Endrin	Heptachlor
Aldrin	Kepone
Endosulfan	Terpene polychlorinates
Dieldrin	Chlordane
Toxaphene	Dicofol (kelthane)
Lindane	Chlorobenzilate
Benzene hexachloride (BHC)	Mirex
DDT	Methoxychlor

From DeBleeker JF, DeReuck JL, Willems JL: Neurologic aspects of organophosphate poisoning. Clin Neurol Neurosurg *94*:93–103, 1992.

pesticide used in the United States.[34] Malaria was brought under control worldwide largely as a result of the efficacy of DDT. Chlordane, another organochlorine, was widely used for termite and roach control. Mirex was used primarily for control of imported red fire ants.

Most organochlorines are stored indefinitely in human tissues (primarily fat). Even persons with only incidental contact with the pesticides can be found to have tissue levels of these chemicals.[34] Studies of Arctic indigenous women who consume moderate amounts of fatty meat (seal and walrus meat and blubber) indicate that they may exceed acceptable daily intake levels for chlordane, toxaphene, dieldrin, and polychlorinated biphenyls 50% of the time.[35]

Heptachlor, chemically related to chlordane, has been associated with malignant tumor development in mice and rats.[36] Blood levels of organochlorines have been shown to be elevated in cohorts of breast cancer victims compared with matched controls.[37] These findings suggest that environmental chemical contamination with organochlorine residues may be an etiologic factor in the development of breast cancer. This and other possible long-term effects of organochlorines in humans are still being debated.

DDT was banned in 1972 in the United States. Heptachlor, kepone, mirex, endrin, aldrin, dieldrin, benzene hexachloride, strobane, chlorobenzilate, and chlordane were later banned by the Environmental Protection Agency. Toxaphene, methoxychlor, and kelthane are still available but for restricted use. Lindane is still used widely and thus is discussed further as a representative of the class.

Lindane

Lindane is the γ isomer of benzene hexachloride. It is widely used as a general garden insecticide; for control of ticks, scabies, and lice; and for extermination of powderpost beetles. It is well absorbed via oral and inhalation routes. It is less well absorbed dermally unless prolonged skin contact or repeated applications occur or the skin is abraded. Lindane is partially metabolized in the liver and directly excreted in the urine, feces, and breast milk.

Lindane interferes with axonal transmission of nerve impulses by disruption of the normal flow of sodium and potassium across the axon membrane. This slowing results in propagation of multiple action potentials for each stimulus.[38] Lindane may also exert toxic effects through release of arachidonic acid in the kidney.[39]

Common clinical presentations include seizures in children exposed repeatedly to lindane for treatment of scabies or lice or more insidious symptoms of apprehension, confusion, dizziness, or coma. Patients may complain of muscle twitching, tremors, or paresthesias. If the compound is ingested, vomiting is often the presenting symptom. Severe overdose may produce death due to respiratory failure. Cough, wheezing, rales, or cyanosis may develop if hydrocarbon (frequently the vehicle) aspiration has occurred.

Hepatic and renal compromise are present only in overwhelming overdose situations (usually ingestion with suicidal intention). Agranulocytosis and aplastic anemia have been reported to be associated with lindane exposure.[40]

Diagnosis of organochlorine toxicity is usually based on history of dermal or inhalation exposure or intentional ingestion. Physical findings are often minimal except for occasional muscle twitching or other signs of CNS hyperexcitability. Respiratory findings may be present owing to aspiration of a petroleum distillate often used as the "inert" ingredient in the preparation.

Treatment is symptomatic and supportive. Laboratory values are of no help in the management of lindane poisoning because lindane is stored in the tissues of the general population. Organochlorines do not affect serum or RBC cholinesterase levels.

Gastric lavage and use of activated charcoal are indicated for ingestion. Decontamination of skin with soap and water should be undertaken for dermal exposure.

Seizures should be controlled with diazepam or lorazepam. Phenobarbital can be used intravenously for uncontrolled seizure activity. Supplemental oxygen, intravenous dextrose, and thiamine should also be given for seizure activity.

Arrhythmias, a result of the myocardial irritant effect of the organochlorines, can be treated with a bolus and continuous infusion of lidocaine (1 mg/kg of body weight bolus followed by 2 to 4 mg/min continuous infusion). Atropine and epinephrine should be avoided in the organochlorine-sensitized myocardium.[41] However, in critically ill patients with unknown insecticide exposure, a trial of atropine and pralidoxime should not be withheld until the etiologic agent is discovered, because use of these agents may be life saving in acute organophosphate poisoning. Rhabdomyolysis, disseminated intravascular coagulation, and lactic acidosis have been reported after lindane ingestions and should be managed with standard specific and supportive therapies. All patients with lindane ingestion or extensive skin contamination should be observed for 6 hours for development of symptoms. Patients who develop CNS depression, irritability, or seizures or who have suspected hydrocarbon aspiration should be admitted for further monitoring and treatment.

BOTANIC INSECTICIDES

The botanic insecticides include nicotine, pyrethrum, and rotenone. The oldest and most widely used agent in this class is pyrethrum. More than 2000 products contain pyrethrum and its related compounds.

The flowers of *Chrysanthemum cineriifolium* are dried and ground to produce pyrethrum, which is actually a composite of six active chemicals known as *pyrethrins.* Synthetic derivatives of these compounds are also widely available and are called *pyrethroids.* Pyrethrum and pyrethroids may be available as dusts or liquids, usually in a hydrocarbon base. Most insecticides containing the pyrethrins have a synergist, piperonyl butoxide, which increases their effectiveness.

Pyrethrum-based insecticides possess little toxicity but can cause nausea, vomiting, diarrhea, hyperexcitability, tremors, incoordination, muscle weakness and paralysis, and respiratory failure. Treatment is supportive. Allergy is a more commonly encountered problem and can include dermatitis, asthma, allergic rhinitis, hypersensitivity pneumonitis, and anaphylaxis.[42] About 50% of patients sensitive to ragweed exhibit cross-reactivity to pyrethrum.

In humans, the compounds produce cutaneous and inhalation allergic reactions. In insects, they prolong nerve sodium currents, resulting in repetitive nerve discharges.[43]

They are well absorbed from the GI tract and minimally absorbed from skin contact. Little is known about inhalation exposures. Pyrethrins and pyrethroids are metabolized in the liver. This rapid inactivation in the liver accounts for their relative lack of systemic toxicity in humans.[44]

Patients report a history of insecticide exposure followed by skin, pulmonary, GI, or neurologic symptoms.

Skin manifestations include erythema and vesiculation. Upper airway irritation and lower airway reactions (cough, wheezing, shortness of breath) can occur, particularly in sensitized patients. Nausea, vomiting, diarrhea, and abdominal cramping can occur with both oral and inhalation exposures. CNS excitation, tremors, incoordination, paralysis, paresthesias, and seizures may result.

The course is usually benign. Most symptoms resolve with symptomatic therapy, although death has occurred secondary to bronchospasm in an asthmatic patient.

No specific laboratory tests are indicated for diagnosis. These compounds do not react with acetylcholinesterase.

Physical findings are nonspecific. History is the primary diagnostic tool. Supportive therapy should be based on signs and symptoms present. Topical vitamin E oil has been reported to relieve paresthesias following skin contact.[45] GI decontamination is not indicated unless the patient has ingested more than 1 g/kg of body weight of pyrethrum or pyrethrin. At smaller doses than this, the risk of hydrocarbon vehicle aspiration outweighs the potential adverse impact of the insecticide.[46]

Atropine and pralidoxime are of no benefit. Follow-up is determined by the patient's symptoms, underlying health problems, and clinical course. Most patients do not require hospitalization.

Rotenone

Rotenone, prepared from the roots of derris, *Lonchocarpus,* and *Tephrosia* plants, is also widely used as a household and horticultural insecticide. It is available in dusts or sprays alone or in combination with other insecticides, frequently pyrethrum. The fresh derris root in Malaya is much more toxic than other sources and has been used for suicides. Rotenone is highly toxic to birds and fish and is often used as a fish poison.

The biochemical mode of action for rotenone in insect and mammalian tissues is the inhibition of the oxidation of reduced nicotinamide-adenine dinucleotide (NAD) ($NADH_2$ to NAD). The consequence of this blockage is that oxidation of substrates via the NAD system, such as glutamate and pyruvate, are blocked by rotenone.[47] Rotenone is rapidly metabolized in the liver. It quickly decomposes on exposure to light and air.

At normal concentrations, rotenone is relatively nontoxic to humans. It causes emesis on ingestion and has low GI absorption. No deaths have been reported in the United States as a result of rotenone ingestion or exposure, but a previously healthy 3-year-old child from Belgium died after ingesting 10 mL of an insecticidal preparation of rotenone.[48] In massive overdose situations, vomiting, respiratory depression, and hypoglycemia have been reported.

History is primary, because there are no typical laboratory or physical findings. Treatment is entirely supportive.

INSECT REPELLENTS

Insect repellents are intended for human use and thus are generally nontoxic with routine use. By topical application or spraying of clothes, they repel mosquitoes, gnats, or other insects. Two insect repellents that may cause clinical poisoning are *N, N*-diethyltoluamide (DEET) and *p*-dichlorobenzene.

DEET

DEET is absorbed through the skin in low concentrations and distributed rapidly, reaching a peak blood concentration 1 hour after application. It is rapidly eliminated, mainly in the urine and to a lesser extent in the feces.

Excessive topical use of this compound has been associated with a toxic encephalopathy, especially in young girls and female infants.[49] Symptoms include lethargy, anxiety, involuntary movements including opisthotonos and athetosis, ataxia, seizures, and coma. The encephalopathy is an idiosyncratic response and may mimic encephalopathy due to any cause. Oral ingestions of 50 mL of insect repellent containing 50% to 90% concentration of DEET have resulted in coma, seizures, and hypotension within 1 hour after ingestion and death in at least two cases.[49] Irritant contact dermatitis,[50] conjunctivitis, and exacerbations of seborrhea and acne have been reported. Anaphylaxis has also occurred. Diagnosis is by history and characteristic physical signs. No characteristic laboratory abnormalities have been noted. A thorough differential diagnosis for encephalopathy must be considered because other causes are far more common than exposure to or ingestion of DEET. Treatment is symptomatic and supportive.

p-Dichlorobenzene

Originally used as a moth repellent and insecticide, *p*-dichlorobenzene is now most commonly used as a deodorizer for bathrooms and diaper and garbage pails. Its use as a moth repellent continues. It is now the least toxic ingredient in mothballs.

Experimental oral and inhalation exposures result in recovery of more than half of the dose in the bile with an enterohepatic circulation and eventual excretion in the urine. After repeated oral and inhalation exposures, dichlorobenzene is found concentrated in fat, but levels quickly decline with cessation of exposure.

Ingestion is common when children eat a part of the deodorant cakes in toilet bowls or diaper pails. It is an irritant to the eyes, nose, and throat, and allergic symptoms have been reported. Massive ingestions produce tremors and hepatic or renal injury.

No characteristic features are noted in terms of physical findings or laboratory abnormalities. Diagnosis is by history of ingestion. Treatment is supportive and symptomatic.

References

1. Okumura T, Takasu N, Ishimatsu S, et al: Report on 640 victims of the Tokyo subway sarin attack. Ann Emerg Med *28*:129–135, 1996.
2. Litovitz TL, Felberg L, Soloway RA, et al: 1994 Annual Report of the American Association of Poison Control Centers Toxic Exposure Surveillance System (TESS). Am J Emerg Med *13*:551–597, 1995.
3. World Health Organization: Public Health Impact of Pesticides Used in Agriculture. Geneva, World Health Organization, 1990.
4. Senanayake N, Petris H: Mortality due to poisoning in a developing agricultural country: Trends over 20 years. Hum Exp Toxicol *14*:437–445, 1995.
5. Hall AH: Warfare Agents. Micromedex, Englewood, CO, 1996.
6. Smith PW: Bulletin: Medical Problems in Aerial Applications. Washington, DC, Office of Aviation Medicine, Federal Aviation Administration, Department of Transportation, 1977.
7. Namba T, Nolte CT, Jackrel J, Grob D: Poisoning due to organophosphate insecticides. Am J Med *50*:475–490, 1971.
8. Haddad LM: Editorial on organophosphate poisoning. J Toxicol Clin Toxicol *30*:331–332, 1992.
9. Zwiener RJ, Ginsburg CM: Organophosphate and carbamate poisoning in infants and children. Pediatrics *81*:121, 1988.
10. Joubert J, Joubert PH, van der Spuy M, van Graan E: Acute organophosphate poisoning presenting with choreoathetosis. Clin Toxicol *22*:187–191, 1984.
11. Dressel TD, Goodale RL, Arneson MA, Borner JW: Pancreatitis as a complication of anticholinesterase insecticide intoxication. Ann Surg *189*:199–204, 1979.
12. Moore PG, James OF: Acute pancreatitis induced by acute organophosphate poisoning. Postgrad Med J *57*:660–662, 1981.
13. Henry JB. Clinical Diagnosis and Management by Laboratory Methods. 19th ed. Philadelphia, W. B. Saunders Co., 1996.
14. Coye MJ, Barnett PJ, Midtling JE, et al: Clinical confirmation of organophosphate poisoning by serial cholinesterase analyses. Arch Intern Med *147*:438, 1987.
15. Perez-Guillermo F, Martinez-Pretel CM, Royo FT, et al: Prolonged suxamethonium-induced neuromuscular blockade associated with organophosphate poisoning. Br J Anaesth *61*:233–236, 1988.
16. Hayes WJ, Laws ER: Handbook of Pesticide Toxicology. San Diego, Academic Press, 1991.
17. Keeler JR, Hurst CJ, Dunn MA: Pyridostigmine used as a nerve agent pretreatment under wartime conditions. JAMA *266*:693–695, 1991.
18. Agarwai SB: Clinical study of 190 patients as a result of acute organophosphorus poisoning. Environ Res *62*:63–70, 1993.
19. Lotti M: Treatment of acute organophosphate poisoning. Med J Aust *154*:51–55, 1991.
20. Farrar H, Wells T, Kearns G: Use of continuous infusion of pralidoxime for treatment of organophosphate poisoning in children. J Pediatr *116*:658–661, 1990.
21. Barden PG, van Eeden SF, Moolman JA, et al: Organophosphate and carbamate poisoning. Arch Intern Med *154*:1433–1444, 1994.
22. Wadia RS, Sadagopan C, Amin RB, Sandesai HV: Neurological manifestations of organophosphorus insecticide poisoning. J Neurol Neurosurg Psychiatry *37*:841–847, 1974.
23. Gadoth N, Fisher A: Late onset of neuromuscular block in organophosphorus poisoning. Ann Intern Med *88*:654, 1978.
24. Tchernilas J: Poisoning with organophosphorus insecticides in Israel. Doctoral thesis. Tel Aviv, University of Tel Aviv Medical School, 1970.
25. Eyer P: Neuropsychopathological changes by organophosphorus compounds—a review. Hum Exp Toxicol *14*:857–864, 1995.
26. Fisher J: Guillain-Barre syndrome following organophosphate poisoning. JAMA *238*:1950, 1977.
27. Rosenstock L, Keifer M, Daniell WE, et al: Chronic central nervous system effects of acute organophosphate pesticide poisoning. Lancet *338*:223–227, 1991.
28. Savage EP, Keefe TJ, Mounce LM, et al: Chronic neurologic sequelae of acute organophosphorus insecticide poisoning. Arch Environ Health *43*:38–45, 1988.
29. DeJager A, van Weerden TW, Houthoff HJ, de Monchy J: Polyneuropathy after massive exposure to parathion. Neurology *31*:603–605, 1981.
30. DeBleeker JF, DeReuck JL, Willems JL: Neurologic aspects of organophosphate poisoning. Clin Neurol Neurosurg *94*:93–103, 1992.
31. Goswami R, Chaudhuri A, Mahashur AA: Study of respiratory failure in organophosphate and carbamate poisoning. Heart Lung *23*:466–472, 1994.
32. Saadeh AM, Al-Ali MK, Farsakh NA: Clinical and sociodemographic features of acute carbamate and organophosphate poisoning: A study of 70 adult patients in North Jordan. Clin Toxicol *34*:45–51, 1996.
33. Arena JM: Poisoning: Toxicology, Symptoms, Treatment. 2nd ed. Springfield, IL, Charles C Thomas, Publisher, 1970.
34. Hayes WJ: Pesticides Studied in Man. Baltimore, Williams & Wilkins, 1982.
35. Kuhnlein HV, Receveur O, Muir DCG, et al: Arctic indigenous women consume greater than acceptable levels of organochlorines. J Nutr *125*:2501–2510, 1995.
36. Murphy SD: Toxic effects of pesticides. *In* Klassen CD, Amdur MO, Doull J (eds): Casarett and Doullis Toxicology. New York, Macmillan, p 548, 1986.
37. Wolff MS, Toniolo PG, Lee EW, et al: Blood levels of organochlorine residues and risk of breast cancer. J Natl Cancer Inst *85*:648–652, 1993.
38. Woo OF: Chlorinated hydrocarbon pesticides. *In* Olson KR (ed): Poisoning and Drug Overdose. Norwalk, CT, Appleton & Lange, pp 117–118, 1990.
39. Senar S, Puente JC, Loper-Aparicio P, et al: Increased intracellular glycerophosphoinositol and arachidonic acid are biochemical markers for lindane toxicity. Cell Signal *6*:915–921, 1994.
40. Gosselin RE, Smith RP, Hodge HC: Clinical Toxicology of

Commercial Products. 5th ed. Baltimore, Williams & Wilkins, pp 239–241, 1984.
41. Morgan DP: Recognition and Management of Pesticide Poisonings. 3rd ed. Washington, DC, Environmental Protection Agency, 1982.
42. Heick HM, Shipman RI, Norman MG: Reye-like syndrome associated with the use of insect repellent. J Pediatr *97*:471, 1980.
43. Paton DL, Walker JS: Pyrethrin poisoning from commercial strength flea and tick spray. Am J Emerg Med *6*:232–234, 1988.
44. Abernathy CO, Casida JE: Pyrethroid insecticides: Esterase cleavage in relation to selective toxicity. Science *179*:1235–1240, 1973.
45. McCord CP: Pyrethrum dermatitis: A record of the occurrence of occupational dermatoses among workers in the pyrethrum industry. JAMA *77*:448–452, 1921.
46. Ford M: Insecticide and pesticides. *In* Viccellio P (ed): Handbook of Medical Toxicology. Boston, Little, Brown & Co., p 311, 1993.
47. Ray DE: Pesticides derived from plants and other organisms. *In* Hayes WJ, Laws ER (eds): Handbook of Pesticide Toxicity. San Diego, Academic Press, p 601, 1991.
48. DeWilde AR, Heyndrickx A, Carton D: A case of fatal rotenone poisoning in a child. J Forensic Sci *31*:1492–1498, 1986.
49. Tenenbein M: Severe toxic reactions and death following the ingestion of diethyltoluamide-containing insect repellents. JAMA *258*:1509–1510, 1987.
50. Amichei B, Lazarov A, Halevy S: Contact dermatitis from diethyltoluamide. Contact Dermatitis *30*:188, 1994.

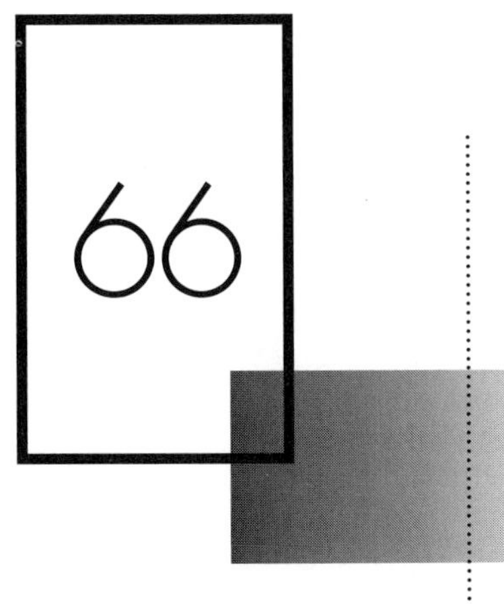

Paraquat and the Bipyridyl Herbicides

JAMES F. WINCHESTER, MD

PARAQUAT

Paraquat (1,1-dimethyl-4,4′-bipyridylium chloride) is the most important of the bipyridyl herbicides, which also include paraquat, diquat, chlormequat, and morfamquat. Difenzoquat, although an herbicide, is a pirazolium compound that may be confused with a bipyridyl. Paraquat (Fig. 66–1) is widely used in agriculture, and it acts as a nonselective herbicide. It can be sprayed from ground level or the air. It is used to desiccate crops such as cotton, allowing a single harvest, and is in turn totally denatured on contact with the earth. Farmers thus can plant seed into the soil directly or with minimal tilling.

Paraquat was introduced as an herbicide in 1962. Early deaths were accidental and resulted from drinking the concentrate from unauthorized containers, but deaths due to suicide soon followed. Legislation in most countries to limit sales and use of the concentrated solution to licensed agricultural workers, as well as replacement of paraquat by diquat to give a paraquat/diquat mixture,[1] reduced the likelihood of accidental exposure but also drew the attention of potential suicide candidates toward the compound.[2] In the 1994 report by the American Association of Poison Control Centers, accidental exposure seems to be increasing, with 175 exposures (164 unintentional); 79 patients reported to a health care facility, and 4 deaths occurred, with a further 13 moderate and 29 minor medical outcomes.[3]

Review of the world literature in 1977 by Harley and associates disclosed approximately 600 deaths due to accidental or intentional ingestion, and 60% of the fatalities were attributed to successful suicides.[4] A report from Mexico has highlighted the involvement of alcohol along with paraquat in the

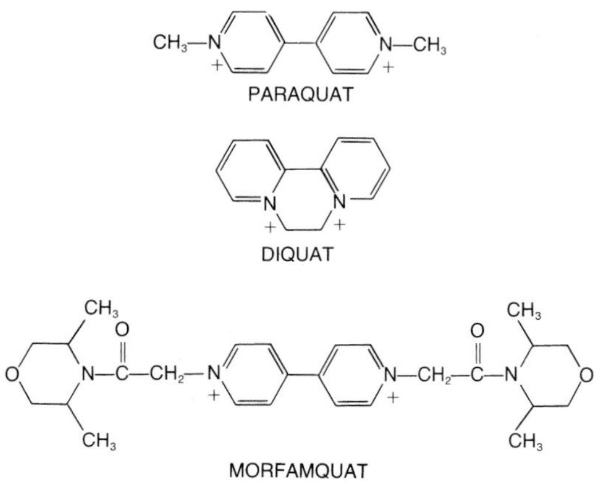

Figure 66–1. Bipyridyl herbicides.

suicide process.[5] Interestingly, heavy alcohol consumption may be protective.[6]

Paraquat Preparations and Toxic Action

Paraquat is available in a liquid concentrate, as granules to be dissolved in water, and as an aerosol. The compound has the following trade names: Cekuquat, Dextron X, Dextrone, Gramoxone, Herbaxon, Herboxone, Pillarxone, Total, and Toxer. Previous substances were esgram, Goldquat, dexuron, Sweep, and Weedol. The concentrates are available for agricultural use as dichloride or dimethyl salts, both of which are water soluble. Paraquat is a parasubstituted quaternary bipyridyl cation. On a weight-to-weight basis, the 29.1% liquid concentrate contains 239.6 g/L of paraquat cations, and the 0.44% aerosol solution contains 0.2% of paraquat cation. Paraquat itself is caustic. The concentrate, in some countries but not in the United States, also may contain a detergent (15% of an aliphatic petroleum solvent) that solubilizes wax on plant leaves and thus allows paraquat to enter cells and exert its phytotoxicity. In some countries, a malodorous agent, a blue dye, and an emetic are added in an attempt to minimize toxicity.[7]

Paraquat exerts its herbicidal activity by interfering with intracellular electron transfer systems, inhibiting reduction of NADP to NADPH during photosynthesis, at which time superoxide, singlet oxygen, and hydroxyl and peroxide radicals are formed.[8] This eventually leads to the destruction of lipid cell membranes by polymerization of unsaturated lipid compounds.[9] Human toxicity is thought to follow a mechanism similar to that in plants, with depletion of the naturally occurring enzyme superoxide dismutase. Recruitment of inflammatory cells then leads to late and irreversible pulmonary fibrosis.[10] Oxidative reactions probably account for the toxicity of the bipyridyls, because the major tissue biochemical features are lipid peroxidation and superoxide and hydroxyl radical formation.[11] These are inextricably linked but by themselves may not account for all of the toxicity. Vitamin E (α-tocopherol), a potent antioxidant, may partially or completely prevent the cytotoxic effects of paraquat in cultured hepatocytes, but in human beings it had no effect on survival.[12] In one study, patients with acute lethal toxicity (discussed later) had no evidence of lipid peroxidation (assessed by serum methylmalondialdehyde determinations), whereas those with subacute toxicity had elevated serum methylmalondialdehyde concentrations compared with controls, which preceded pulmonary fibrosis. Lipid peroxidation may be the consequence of cell damage rather than the cause of it.[10]

Metal ions also may be involved in tissue injury induced by paraquat and its biochemical products. Lipid peroxidation may be enhanced by iron radicals, whereas removal of iron by the chelating agent deferoxamine reduces paraquat toxicity in bacterial preparations or in normal mice as well as in vitamin E–deficient rats.[10, 13] Selenium, a cofactor for glutathione peroxidase, added to the diet induces some protection against paraquat lethality in chicks.[14] Exogenous glutathione also may protect against injury by paraquat, and so may N-acetylcysteine, a donor of glutathione.[15, 16] Sulfite or thiosulfite (redox agents) may also protect against paraquat, by reversing oxidized glutathione, which competes with glutathione for peroxide, hydroxyl, and superoxide radicals.[17] Dimethylthiourea (another free radical scavenger) given to animals poisoned with paraquat actually increases paraquat toxicity, increases plasma concentrations, decreases whole-body clearance, and decreases apparent volume of distribution of paraquat.[18] Vasoactive intestinal peptide, a quencher of oxygen radicals, may also decrease paraquat injury in animals.[19] Little investigation has addressed many of these observations in humans, but some preliminary results are discussed here.

Clinical Exposure and Manifestations of Poisoning

After the first reported death due to the concentrated solution, the rate of accidental poisoning rose to give a mortality rate of 33% to 50%. Most early cases were accidental because of the resemblance of paraquat to root beer or a cola drink, especially when decanted into soft drink bottles left unlabeled. The compound also may resemble dark vinegar, and use as such by one patient led to death.

Studies of paraquat sprayers who have been subjected to heavy exposure have revealed that although skin rashes (particularly on scrotal and intergluteal areas, resulting from paraquat trickling down the back from leaking knapsack sprays), cracked nails, and epistaxis occur, systemic reactions are not observed. Chest roentgenograms, measures of liver and renal function, and diffusion capacity for carbon monoxide are nondiagnostic despite the detection of minute quantities of paraquat in the urine.[20] These studies demonstrate that inhalation and dermal absorption of paraquat are slight if paraquat is used in the recommended way, with proper attention being paid to spray equipment and accurate dilution, protective clothing, and protection of pre-existing skin lesions.

Several experiments have been designed to study absorption of paraquat through the skin. Early experiments in rabbits, using moderate to highly concentrated solutions of paraquat (240 mg cation/kg), demonstrated systemic absorption from occluded dermal sites and fatality from absorption. On the other hand, absorption in mice (from application of 1 mg/kg) is considerably slower than from other pesticides. Of overriding importance, however, is the demonstration *in vitro* that human skin is much less permeable to paraquat than is the skin of some experimental animals, with factors ranging from 40 times (haired rat) to 1460 times (hairless mouse) greater than human skin, with a human skin permeability constant[21, 22] of 0.73 cm/h $\times$ 10^5. Therefore, it is necessary to examine results of *in vivo* skin permeability to paraquat; Wester and associates have demonstrated that only 0.03 μg/cm^2 of a paraquat solution containing 9 μg/cm^2 would be absorbed from intact skin in 24 hours. That this may increase somewhat can be predicted from results of absorption of the closely related chemical diquat; 0.4% of a topical dose is absorbed from an unoccluded site, 1.4% from an occluded site, and 3.8% from an occluded and damaged dermal site.[23] This latter observation is extremely important for making recommendations to spray workers with pre-existing skin lesions and for interpreting published cases of poisoning following dermal exposure.

The published descriptions of cases, in which the skin of patients was believed to be the site of absorption, invariably describe patients with skin ulcers, desquamation, dermal burns, dermatitis, and so on.[24, 25] In many cases, it is impossible to preclude ingestion fully. One patient who had skin abrasions and frequent exposure to concentrate developed an indolent ulcer and progressive (and fatal) respiratory failure.[26] Another died after a single dermal exposure to paraquat concentrate over a large surface area and pre-existing skin lesions; another (with an indolent skin ulcer) died after repeated exposure to 2.8% paraquat and subsequent development of respiratory failure with pathologic features different from the classic picture after paraquat ingestion.[27] In the latter study, hypertrophic pulmonary artery lesions were seen in the patient; in animal experiments, the same lesions developed in the lungs of rats exposed to dermal contact of 8 mg of paraquat at weekly intervals for as long as 9 weeks. Others have mistakenly used paraquat for the treatment of lice or other skin disorders.[28, 29] Putative evidence from these studies suggests that contact exposure to paraquat on the skin might lead to fatal pulmonary disease. Unfortunately, in many of the human fatalities, paraquat identification procedures were not used in lung (or other) tissues. It must therefore be stated that contact exposure (particularly if the skin is not washed immediately after soaking, or if clothing is not changed, or if skin lesions are present) rarely might produce sufficient dermal absorption and subsequent fatal pulmonary lesions. This should prompt identification of paraquat in blood and urine in such exposed patients before instituting therapy. An extensive review of reported cases of purported skin absorption and animal and human experiments supports this view; prolonged exposure to solutions containing more than 5 g/L concentration might lead to fatal poisoning, and exposure to less-concentrated solutions may produce fatalities in patients with pre-existing skin lesions.[30] Subcutaneous injection of paraquat has produced a fatality. Corneal exposure to paraquat can result in ulceration and scarring. Recovery after developing paraquat toxicity from dermal absorption has been reported.[31]

Inhalation of spray is unlikely to cause systemic toxicity because of its low vapor pressure and large spray droplets. Moreover, elegant experiments have been conducted using accurate analytic techniques for the detection of significant exposure to paraquat in respirator filter pads and clothing or dermal contamination in field workers spraying paraquat with low-beam spray machines. These studies have suggested that if paraquat is properly used, a person wearing a short-sleeved and open-necked shirt would be exposed to only 0.06% of the acute dermal LD_{50} dose obtained in male white rats. There is some suggestion that the human pulmonary changes could result from ingestion of smaller amounts of paraquat than in rats; nevertheless, with such low doses, the margin for safety is considerable.[32]

Attention has been directed to possible hazards of inhalation of smoke from paraquat-sprayed marijuana. Poisoning is unlikely, owing first to the low concentration of paraquat used and second to the conversion of paraquat into bipyridines (4,4′-bipyridyl) by smoking marijuana.[33] No cases of paraquat lung have been encountered in heavy users of contaminated marijuana, nor from inhalation of paraquat vapor. In view of its tastelessness in food, paraquat has been implicated in, or later proved to be responsible for, homicidal deaths in the United Kingdom, the United States, and Japan.

The overriding effect of paraquat is the production of pulmonary toxicity, first because paraquat is concentrated by an energy-dependent process in the lung[34] and second because of the free availability of oxygen to form superoxide radicals in the highest oxygen tensions (alveoli) in the body.

Clinical Features

Acute Toxicity

Local Effects. The major acute local effects result from the caustic properties of paraquat, which produce local ulceration of epithelial surfaces. Blistering of the skin and cracking and even loss of the fingernails have been reported. Corneal ulceration has

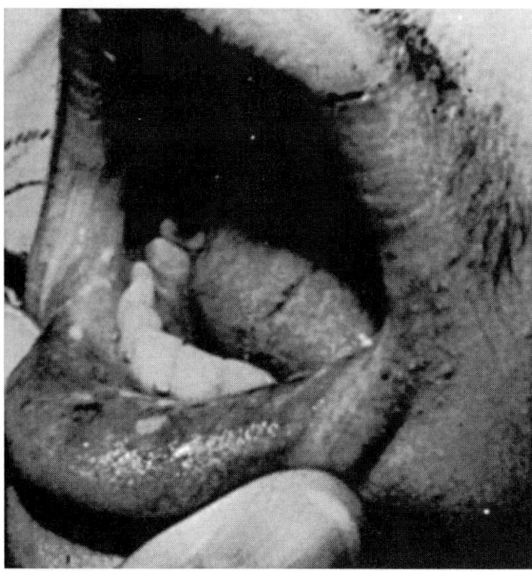

Figure 66–2. Ulceration of the buccal mucosa 24 hours after paraquat ingestion.

been reported after paraquat concentrate was splashed into the eyes.[35] The major local effects, however, are seen in the mouth and esophagus after ingestion of the concentrate. These may include ulcers on the lips (Fig. 66–2) and burning and ulceration of the tongue and pharynx, even to the point of producing a pseudomembrane reminiscent of diphtheria.[36] Esophageal ulceration can proceed to esophageal perforation (Fig. 66–3), with all its attendant problems. All these manifestations become apparent within a few minutes to hours of ingestion, but the initial presenting symptoms may be just a burning sensation in the buccal cavity, with ulceration seen within 1 to 2 days.

Systemic Effects. After massive ingestion (> 30 mg/kg or 50 mL of the paraquat concentrate), patients may have pulmonary edema, cardiac failure, renal failure (which may result within hours of ingestion), hepatic failure, and convulsions caused by central nervous system involvement. After massive ingestion, death may occur within several hours to a few days as a result of multiple organ failure.

Subacute Toxicity

Ingestion of 4 mL/kg or more causes the aforementioned symptoms, with development of renal failure within 24 hours of ingestion in those who have consumed significant quantities; although reversible, this impairs paraquat excretion and increases the likelihood of death. Renal failure may be manifested by proteinuria and oliguria within 2 to 6 days, with renal tubular functional changes that can produce glycosuria, aminoaciduria, and increased fractional excretion of sodium, urate, and phosphate.[37] Paraquat itself may interfere with the Jaffe reaction for the measurement of creatinine.[38] It is imperative that renal function be preserved for as long as possible.

The major effect of paraquat poisoning, however, is pulmonary involvement. Pulmonary edema begins 24 to 48 hours after ingestion and produces the syndrome resembling adult respiratory distress syndrome. It progresses to pulmonary fibrosis over a few days (Fig. 66–4). The respiratory involvement begins with pulmonary hemorrhage and congestion and is followed by intra-alveolar and obliterative fibrosis, which in most cases is irreversible although isolated reports have described full recovery, even with severe pulmonary involvement. Hypoxemia with respiratory distress is the predominant feature, accompanied by severe agitation. A metabolic acidosis often accompanies the respiratory problem and other manifestations of organ involvement. Myocarditis and epicardial hemorrhage may produce electrocardiographic changes with arrhythmias. Paraquat is one of the few poisons that may produce necrosis of the adrenal glands, and this must be borne in mind if a patient becomes hypotensive.

The pulmonary changes depend on the quantity of

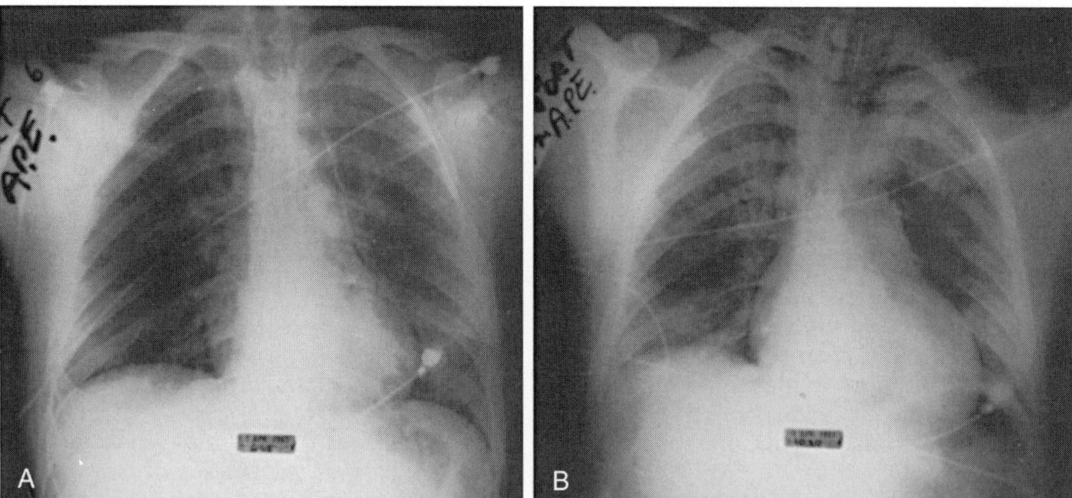

Figure 66–3. Esophageal rupture after fatal paraquat poisoning. Chest radiograph of a man 3 days after ingestion. *A,* Pneumomediastinum (radiolucent shadow left heart border). *B,* Tracking of air into the superior mediastinum 4 hours later.

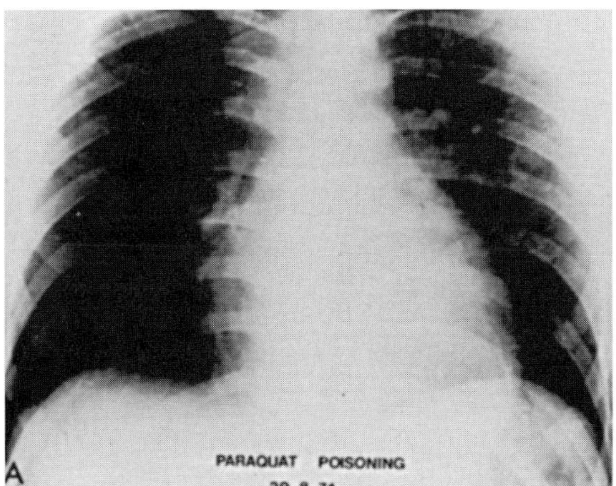

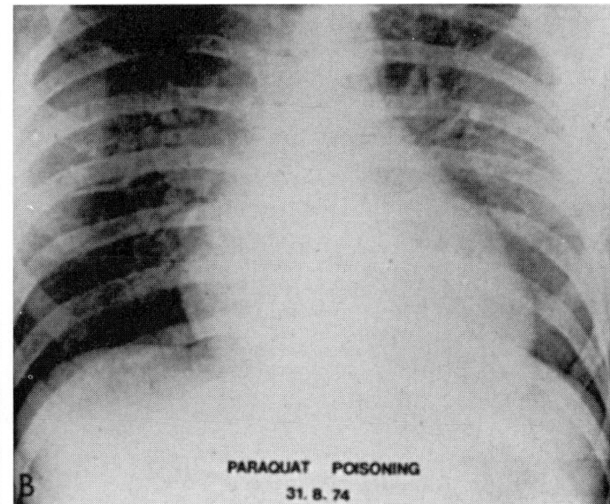

Figure 66–4. Fatal paraquat poisoning. *A,* Radiograph of an 18-year-old man 6 hours after paraquat ingestion. *B,* Evidence of pulmonary fibrosis 3 days later.

paraquat ingested, which is often 20 mL of concentrate (a mouthful, the volume of which may vary from 4.5 mL in a child to 10 to 20 mL in an adult), and initially the lesions in the lung may well be reversible. Radiographic changes in the first week after ingestion are diffuse consolidation, pneumomediastinum with or without pneumothorax, and cardiomegaly with widened superior mediastinum.[39] Pneumomediastinum and subcutaneous emphysema have also been reported.[40] Pulmonary fibrosis develops only in those patients who survive the first few days after ingestion. Although death occurs within 1 to 2 weeks, progressive pulmonary fibrosis and progressive respiratory failure may occur even as long as 6 weeks after ingestion of the agent.

Laboratory Abnormalities

Paraquat Estimation. A simple urine test for paraquat, sensitive only to concentrations of 1 μg/mL or greater (1 ppm), is to add 2 mL of a 1% solution of sodium dithionite in 1 N sodium hydroxide to 10 mL of urine; a blue reaction indicates the presence of paraquat. Gas chromatography and high-pressure liquid chromatography can detect levels of 0.1 to 0.2 with some accuracy.

The introduction of a radioimmunoassay has improved the delectability of paraquat and has given a clearer predictability of survival, because it can detect and measure blood levels well below 0.1 μg/mL.[41] It has been demonstrated that serum levels greater than 0.2 μg/mL at 24 hours and 0.1 μg/mL at 48 hours are usually associated with a fatal outcome[42] (Fig. 66–5*A*). A more detailed analysis of blood concentration data has resulted in probability curves for survival related to time after ingestion and blood concentration of paraquat (Fig. 66–5*B*).[43] The predicted effect of plasma paraquat concentrations on prognosis has been confirmed, extending beyond (Fig. 66–5*C*) the 35-hour period of the original analysis (see Fig. 66–5*A*).[44]

In addition to being detected in urine or blood, paraquat may cause other organ damage. In general, toxicity may be graded by repeated evaluation of pulmonary function. Pulmonary toxicity is manifested by pulmonary hemorrhage, edema, atelectasis, hyaline membranes, interstitial and alveolar fibrosis, and bronchial epithelial proliferation, as well as pleural effusions. Serial measurements of arterial oxygen tension indicate a low arterial oxygen tension (Pa_{O_2}), as well as an increased alveolar oxygen tension gradient ($P_{AO_2} - Pa_{O_2}$), and these should all be monitored in a serial fashion. Additionally, diffusion capacity for carbon monoxide, which should also be measured serially, indicates the severity and progression of the alveolocapillary block that develops when pulmonary fibrosis ensues.[45] One study has suggested that the respiratory index ($RI = P_{AO_2} - Pa_{O_2}/P_{O_2}$) is a simple method to predict survival; in 51 patients with paraquat poisoning, survivors had an RI consistently less than 1.5, and nonsurvivors had an RI equal to or greater than 1.5 at any time point after ingestion[46] (even in late cases in which graphed plasma paraquat/time of ingestion fell outside the predictive graph).[41] $P_{AO_2} - Pa_{O_2}$ is a measure of diffusion capacity for oxygen derived from the following expression:

$$P_{AO_2} - Pa_{O_2} = 713 \times F_{IO_2} - P_{CO_2} - [F_{IO_2} + (1 - F_{IO_2})/R] - P_{O_2}$$

where F_{IO_2} is inspired oxygen concentration (%), P_{CO_2} and P_{O_2} are arterial partial pressures of carbon dioxide and oxygen, respectively (mm Hg); and R is the respiratory quotient assumed to be equal to 0.8.

Treatment

In view of the proposed mechanisms for the production of paraquat toxicity (Fig. 66–6), it is possible at several points to interrupt the pathway for paraquat toxicity (see Fig. 66–6). Management is primarily directed at removing paraquat from the gastrointestinal (GI) tract, increasing its excretion from blood, and, traditionally, adopting measures aimed at preventing pulmonary damage with anti-inflammatory

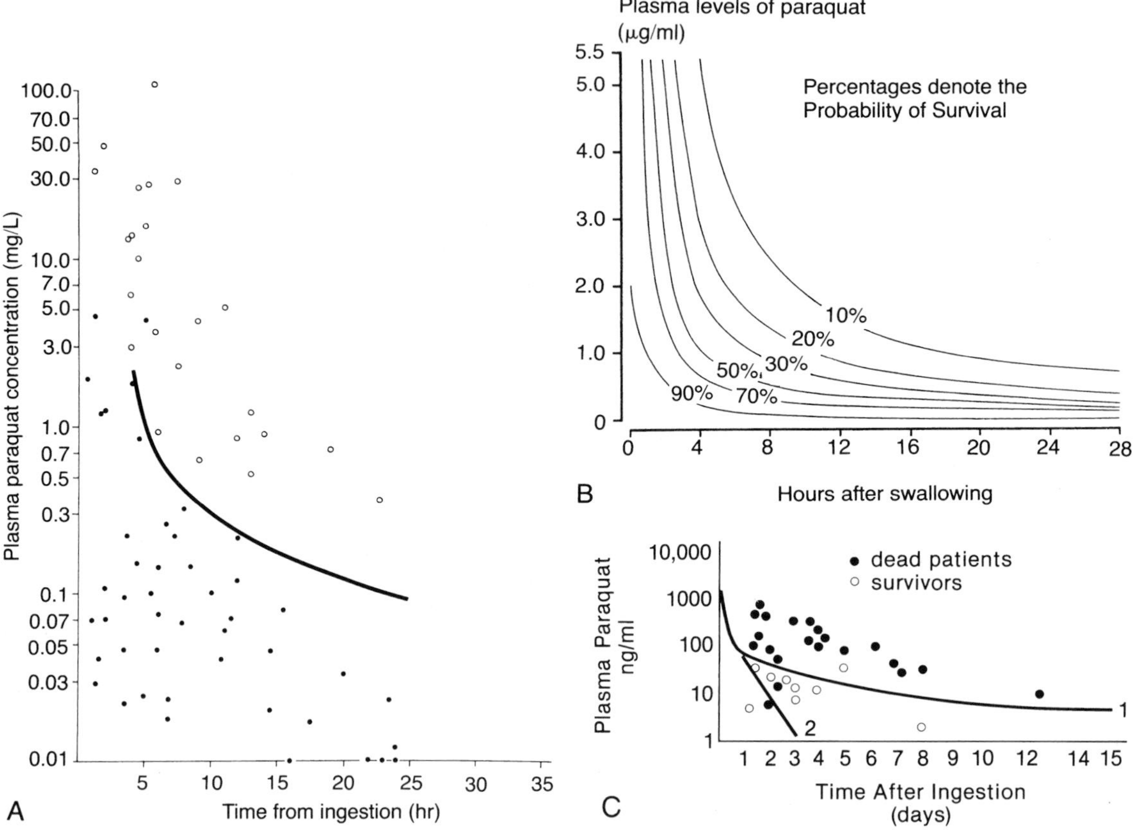

Figure 66–5. Correlation of plasma paraquat concentration and time from ingestion with survival. *A*, Analysis of raw data. *B*, Statistical probability of survival, analyzed from data in *A*. *C*, Probability of survival in late presenters. (*A* from Proudfoot AT, Stewart MS, Levitt T, Widdop B: Paraquat poisoning: Significance of plasma paraquat concentrations. Lancet *2*:330, 1979. *B* from Hart TB, Nevitt A, Whitehead A: A new statistical approach to the prognostic significance of plasma paraquat concentrations. Lancet *2*:1222, 1984. *C* from Schermann JM, Galliott M, Garnier R, Bismuth C: Acute paraquat poisoning: Prognostic significance and therapeutical interest of blood assay. Toxicol Eur Res *3*:141, 1983.)

agents and some newer drugs. Hospitalization is mandatory in all cases suspected (and confirmed by urine or plasma tests) of paraquat poisoning.

Prevention of Absorption from Gastrointestinal Tract

Recommended Treatment. Although removal of paraquat from the intestine has long been a goal of therapy, analysis has now cast doubt on the true efficacy of GI decontamination, because the quantity of paraquat systemically absorbed is not significantly reduced with conventional agents, such as diatomaceous earths and activated charcoals, and other methods.[47] However, current opinion now holds that an attempt be made to restrict the GI absorption using the methods outlined next. Gastric lavage should be performed, using diatomaceous clays in the lavage solution. The diatomaceous earths are bentonite and fuller's earth. Lavage must be performed cautiously in view of the ulceration of the pharynx and the esophagus, with rupture possible in the esophagus, and the recovery of paraquat may be small. Bentonite can be poured only in a 6% to 7.5% suspension and should be given if fuller's earth is not available. On the other hand, fuller's earth can be administered in a 30% suspension, at which it remains pourable, along with magnesium sulfate, to produce catharsis. Three hundred grams of fuller's earth and 50 g of magnesium sulfate are mixed with 1 L of sterile water and autoclaved. After lavage using 250 to 500 mL, a dosage of 250 to 500 mL is given every 2 to 4 hours for 2 or 3 days, or until paraquat cannot be detected in any biologic solution. It must be remembered that omission of magnesium sulfate (or any other cathartic agent) allows the absorption of water from the suspension and produces constipation or even intestinal obstruction. If fuller's earth is not available, activated charcoal may be used. Activated charcoal absorbs paraquat as effectively as bentonite or fuller's earth. Ion-exchange resin (Kayexalate or sodium resonium) has been demonstrated to be an effective absorbent, as have modern high-capacity activated charcoals.

Success with severe human bipyridyl poisoning has been reported with total gut lavage,[48] and animal experimentation using polyethylene glycol solutions has shown a significant decrease in paraquat concentrations compared with control animals.[49] The theoretic risk of paraquat passively accompanying the fluid absorption (0.5 to 1 L) with gut lavage has led some to recommend against gut lavage.[50]

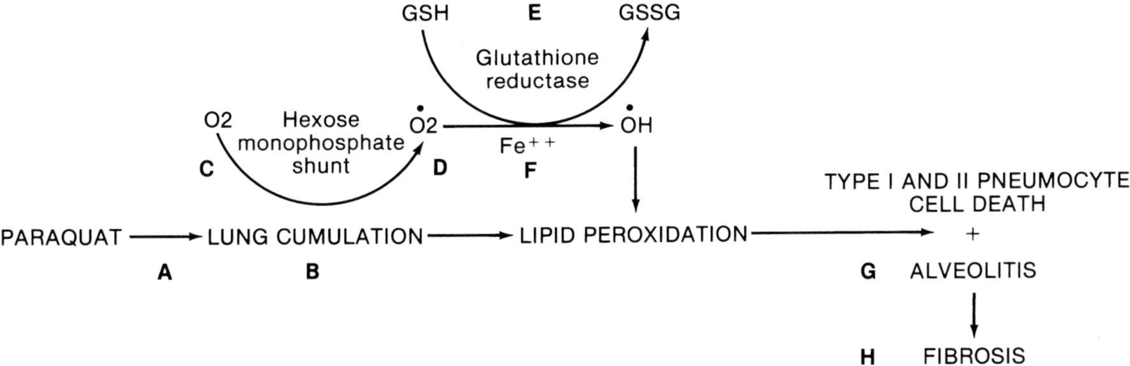

Figure 66–6. Proposed mechanisms of paraquat toxicity and therapy (some therapies of no value—see text). A, Fuller's earth, gastrointestinal decontamination, removal from blood; B, paraquat antibody Fab fragments, D-propranolol; C, low F_{IO_2}, nitric oxide; D, free radical scavengers, antioxidants (vitamin E), superoxide dismutase; E, glutathione, N-acetylcysteine; F, deferoxamine; G, cyclophosphamide, prednisone, radiotherapy; H, antifibrotic agents.

Increasing Excretion from the Blood

A reduction of *p*-aminohippurate clearance (a marker of renal plasma flow) suggests that bipyridyls may themselves cause profound changes in renal hemodynamics as a result of fluid redistribution from the GI tract and that forced diuresis for removal of paraquat will be unsuccessful, because it is not reabsorbed by the tubules. Moreover, the technique is likely to be effective within only the first 24 hours after ingestion, during the period of maximal excretion of urinary paraquat; the onset of renal failure makes this method unlikely to be of any effect. Careful attention must be paid to the maintenance of renal function in the early stages of paraquat poisoning, because ensuing renal failure would allow accumulation of paraquat in other tissues, particularly the lungs.

Both peritoneal dialysis and hemodialysis have been suggested as measures for removing paraquat from blood. Peritoneal dialysis seems to be ineffective and is not recommended, because only small amounts of paraquat are removed. Hemodialysis or hemoperfusion, on the other hand, has been associated with successful outcomes in paraquat-poisoned patients, usually when the paraquat level or ingested dose has been moderate to low. Hemoperfusion offers better clearance of paraquat than hemodialysis (see Chapter 10). On the other hand, others have not had successful outcomes with hemodialysis alone or combined with hemoperfusion or with continuous dialysis therapies (despite maintaining low serum concentrations of paraquat).[51–53]

In animals, charcoal or ion-exchange resin hemoperfusion did reduce plasma concentrations of paraquat.[54] In other animal experiments, hemoperfusion within 12 hours after poisoning with paraquat appeared to reduce the mortality, but its use in severely poisoned humans was not associated with success.[55, 56] However, prolonged hemoperfusion or hemodialysis, with almost continuous treatment periods of up to 2 to 3 weeks after an ingestion, was associated with successful clinical outcomes in two patients in whom the plasma paraquat concentration was kept below the critical level of 0.1 μg/mL and in others in whom the plasma level foretold a moderate to poor prognosis (Fig. 66–7).[57] Paraquat antibodies immobilized on agarose-polyacrolein spheres enclosed in hemoperfusion devices have been shown experimentally to bind paraquat avidly from animal blood passing through the devices.[58] Plasmapheresis has also been advocated, but further studies are needed before its effectiveness is proved.

Summary Statement. The recommended regimen for increased paraquat excretion from the blood at this point is hemoperfusion or hemodialysis when necessary. In an analysis of 42 patients treated by hemoperfusion or hemodialysis, Hampson and Pond drew attention to the fact that there were no survivors after treatment if the plasma paraquat concen-

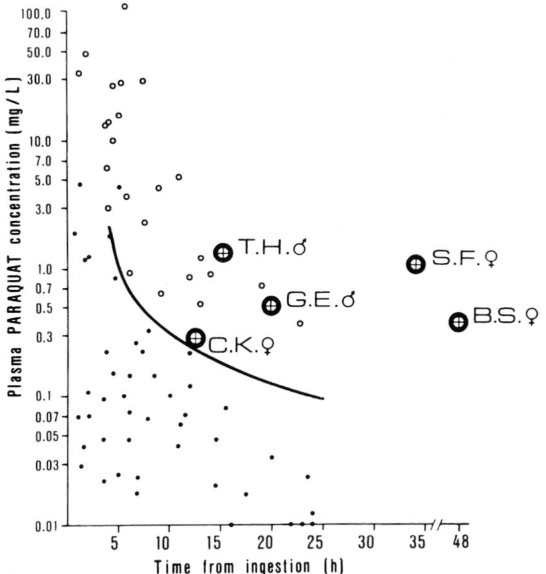

Figure 66–7. Patients (TH, SF, GE, BS, CK) who survived potentially fatal paraquat concentrations after intensive hemoperfusion/hemodialysis. (From Okonek S, Weileman LS, Majdanzic J, et al: Successful treatment of paraquat poisoning. Activated charcoal per os and "continuous" hemoperfusion. J Toxicol Clin Toxicol *19*:807, 1982. Data from Fig. 66–5*A* drawn for comparison.)

tration was greater than 3 mg/L, regardless of time after ingestion.[53] As do others,[59, 60] they suggest that hemoperfusion or hemodialysis is likely to benefit those with a probability of survival of between 20% and 70% (see Fig. 66–5*B*) and within the first 10 to 12 hours after ingestion, because paraquat is rapidly distributed to tissues in the first few hours after ingestion.[61] Ikebuchi and colleagues have devised a discriminant function analysis to predict outcome. D, the toxicologic index, is based on the following formula:

$$D = 1.3114 - 0.1617 \ln T - 0.408 [\ln C \times 1000]$$

where T = hours after ingestion and C is the serum concentration of paraquat (μg/mL). When D was greater than zero, lethality was low; when less than zero, lethality was high.[62]

Prevention of Pulmonary Damage

Paraquat accumulates selectively in lung tissue by an energy-dependent process, and the main efforts of therapeutic intervention have been to prevent this cumulation. The lung changes are similar to the direct toxicity of high alveolar oxygen tension, as observed with lung changes in oxygen toxicity. In addition to the measures previously outlined, prevention of superoxide radical formation may be accomplished by using low-oxygen breathing mixtures with production of therapeutic hypoxemia. It has been shown in animals that paraquat-poisoned rats allowed to breathe normal room air die in far more significant numbers than those allowed to breathe low-oxygen mixtures. Hyperoxia (100% oxygen) enhances the toxicity of paraquat in rats, compared with those breathing room air. Oxygen administration to patients poisoned with paraquat appears to accelerate the lung changes. Use of low F_{IO_2} mixtures requires positive end-expiratory pressure and continuous positive pressure breathing, and it is suggested that an inspired oxygen concentration of greater than 21% should be used only when arterial oxygen pressure declines below 40 mm Hg. Although the value of low inspired oxygen has not been established in humans, putative evidence suggests that this should be used.[63] Other methods of reducing oxygen toxicity, such as cardiopulmonary bypass, also have been proposed, although again, this method has not been proved.

In keeping with the known effects of nitric oxide in adult respiratory distress syndrome, in producing selective pulmonary vasodilatation and improvement in ventilation/perfusion mismatching, a study examined the effect of nitric oxide in paraquat intoxication.[64] A severely respiratory impaired paraquat-poisoned patient with a Pa_{O_2} of 50 mm Hg or less had 25 ppm nitric oxide added to the inspired gases. The patient's Pa_{O_2} increased, and the mean pulmonary artery pressure and right-to-left shunt decreased, with reversal on discontinuing nitric oxide. The patient was maintained for 3 days on nitric oxide therapy but succumbed to massive pleural effusions and died during discontinuation of nitric oxide.[65]

Immunosuppression

Corticosteroids have traditionally been used in addition to these measures, although they have not been proved to be effective. Their role has been brought into question. It has been shown in sheep that methylprednisolone given before or after paraquat exposure reduces the increase in lymph flow and prostacyclin but not thromboxane B_2 accumulation in lymph nor the increase in lung neutrophils induced by the agent alone. Moreover, in rabbits, paraquat pneumonitis was not prevented with prednisone given under carefully controlled conditions. Prostanoids are known suppressors of inflammatory reactions, but injections of prostaglandin E have been shown to increase the early respiratory failure–induced mortality.

Other agents, such as azathioprine, beclomethasone, bleomycin, fluorouracil, and fibrinolytic agents (potassium aminobenzoate) have been used without clear-cut benefit being shown.

A great deal of attention has been paid to the use of radiotherapy in the prevention and treatment of paraquat-induced pulmonary fibrosis, after a case report by Webb and associates[66] described successful reversal of pulmonary damage (in a patient who was not improving on cyclophosphamide and methylprednisolone therapy) after radiotherapy. (The patient ingested 3 g; the plasma paraquat concentration was 80 μg/L at 36 hours.) A further successful outcome was observed in a paraquat-poisoned patient (plasma paraquat concentration of 2.1 mg/L 7.5 hours after ingestion) given an intensive regimen including hemoperfusion and 1125 rad to each lung beginning on day 3. More extensive studies of single-dose radiation at different times after paraquat administration in mice have not confirmed that radiotherapy has any benefit on paraquat-induced pulmonary injury. One patient more intoxicated (the patient ingested 10 to 20 g; the plasma paraquat concentration was 120 μg/L at 36 hours) than that of Webb and colleagues and five others (four in a follow-up series from Webb's group, with toxic paraquat concentrations, and one in Taiwan, for whom no plasma paraquat data were given) failed to respond to radiation and succumbed. D-Propranolol has been used to displace paraquat from lungs in a manner similar to imipramine displacement from isolated perfused rat lungs with chlorpromazine. It has generally been given concomitantly with the enzyme superoxide dismutase, and no clear-cut results have been forthcoming. It is possible that D-propranolol was infused too late in the course of paraquat poisoning, when lung damage had already occurred; similarly, the same situation exists with the enzyme superoxide dismutase.

Cyclophosphamide combined with high-dose dexamethasone has been used. Addo and Poon-King reported a 72% survival in 72 patients treated with no increment in oxygen inhalation, forced diuresis, gut decontamination, and dexamethasone and cyclophosphamide given intravenously.[67] It was subsequently pointed out that of the 25 patients in whom plasma paraquat concentrations were measured, 18 had high concentrations and 12 died; of the 6 survivors, the chance of survival was 30%. Controlled clinical trials would be necessary to confirm these results.[68]

Antioxidant Therapy in Humans

Superoxide dismutase reverses the formation of superoxide radicals and has been used in several clinical studies with both aerosol and intravenous administration, all without benefit.[69] A patient with serious paraquat intoxication was treated with decontamination, hemodialysis, and the combined use of deferoxamine and N-acetylcysteine as antioxidants. The patient survived after developing acute renal failure and liver dysfunction and had demonstrable impaired diffusing capacity of carbon monoxide at the outset and 14 months later.[70]

Lung Transplantation

Lung transplantation has been performed in at least four patients, without success; when blood levels of paraquat were still high, patients developed respiratory failure with lung histology consistent with either rejection or paraquat toxicity. Serial lung transplant in one patient resulted in a successful transplant (the first developed paraquat toxicity), but the patient was ventilator dependent owing to progressive toxic myopathy (a new feature of paraquat toxicity) and eventually died of bronchopneumonia.[71] The patient reported by Kamholz and associates had a successful transplant but died of complications arising from a ruptured bronchial stump.[72]

Immunotherapy

Monoclonal and polyclonal antibodies to paraquat can be manufactured. Plasma paraquat concentrations rise, in test animals compared with controls, after Fab antibody fragment administration, whether given before or after paraquat administration. Specific antibodies have been shown to bind paraquat *in vitro* and to prevent uptake of paraquat into lung slices by pretreatment of the incubation media. However, pretreatment or treatment after exposure to paraquat does not influence displacement of paraquat from lung tissue. Moreover, 100-mg monoclonal antibody pretreatment did not prevent paraquat toxicity in mice after an LD_{10} dose 17 hours later, and the investigators predicted that a 100- to 200-g Fab fragment antibody dose would be required for an adult human, an amount beyond production capabilities.[73] It thus appears that immunotherapy is of limited value in treating paraquat poisoning.

Summary and Conclusions

Ingestion of paraquat concentrate is almost always associated with a fatal outcome, but this should not detract from intensive management of such poisoned patients, because occasional patients, even after massive ingestion with pulmonary involvement, have fully recovered. The mechanisms producing paraquat lung toxicity have been partially elucidated and have given rise to the treatment regimens outlined in this chapter, with the additional measures required to reduce blood levels below those associated with a fatal outcome. In this regard, intensive, almost continuous hemoperfusion or hemodialysis is recommended, especially within the first few hours after ingestion; additionally, lower inspired oxygen therapy should be used. The other immunosuppressive and immunotherapy regimens outlined require further study until their efficacy is demonstrated.

Because of its dramatic nature, paraquat poisoning often arouses press comment on the availability of the agent. As with many chemicals, however, the overriding public health issue is to ensure proper labeling of containers holding paraquat, not to decant it into soft drink bottles, and to make sure that the compound is not likely to arouse children's interest. Moreover, the unauthorized use of small quantities of concentrate by those who take it home from authorized agricultural depots should be strongly discouraged. Only improper use of the paraquat concentrate results in accidental or suicidal poisoning. Poison information on paraquat can be obtained in the United States from National Pesticide Telecommunications Network at 1-800-858-7378 (outside the United States, 806-743-3091) and in the United Kingdom from the International Paraquat/Diquat Poisoning Registry at New Cross Hospital, London, 011-44-171-407-7600.

DIQUAT

Diquat (1,1-ethylene-2,2-bipyridylium), closely related to paraquat, exerts the same activity as an herbicide in photosynthesizing plants. The lungs are most severely damaged in paraquat toxicity, but no histologic evidence of lung damage is noted in animals after diquat administration. Diquat produces more GI disturbances, more renal effects, and less pulmonary toxicity than does paraquat. Diquat appears not to accumulate selectively in any organ, except perhaps the kidneys, in which event subsequent renal failure is more common. Diquat apparently is reduced by a different electron-transferring agent from paraquat or even morfamquat. Fortunately, diquat is usually ingested in a much lower concentration, and it is usually admixed with low concentrations of paraquat. Although it has been stated that lung toxicity with diquat is less than that with paraquat, animal experiments have suggested that in a hyperoxic environment, diquat may well be equal to paraquat in its pulmonary toxicity. It has been suggested that diquat as well as paraquat exerts a greater effect on GI water content, which can produce hemoconcentration and changes in water distribution so that renal failure ensues.[74] For diquat poisoning, the absence of changes in histology at necropsy in animals may be explained by its greater effect on fluid redistribution. Fluid redistribution but also cerebral hemorrhage may be the major determinants of a fatal outcome in diquat poisoning.[75] Full-thickness dermal "burns" have also been reported.[76]

Treatment

Treatment is identical to that for paraquat, with removal of diquat from the GI tract with adsorbent catharsis or gut lavage or both. Hemoperfusion is more effective than hemodialysis for removal of diquat, but because renal failure is of prime concern, it may be necessary to use hemodialysis early in the course of diquat poisoning.

CHLORMEQUAT

Chlormequat is available as an 11.8% solution (Cycocel) for commercial control of peppers, grains, and cereals. It has caused accidental death after ingestion of a mouthful, but toxicity is usually associated with large volumes (>1 L). Toxicity resembles anticholinesterase poisoning, but chlormequat is *NOT* an anticholinesterase and should not be treated as such (i.e., with atropine). It can produce seizures and coma from cerebral edema,[77] but the most striking symptoms are mucosal irritation, with salivation, miosis, and cardiac effects such as bradycardia, ventricular arrhythmias, cardiac arrest, and pulmonary edema.[78] Treatment of seizures with diazepam, avoidance of atropine, and GI decontamination with charcoal are the mainstays of therapy.

MORFAMQUAT

Morfamquat has found less use than the other two bipyridyls, paraquat and diquat, but can produce mammalian toxicity. Studies by Conning and associates showed that rats fed morfamquat developed renal damage, whereas diquat was the only one of the three bipyridyls that produced bilateral cataracts.[79] No human or animal toxicity has been reported with morfamquat. Its use is limited in the United Kingdom, but the general recommendation can be made that treatment should be along the lines proposed for paraquat poisoning.

References

1. Yoshioka T, Sugimoto T, Kinoshita N, et al: Effects of concentration reduction and partial replacement of paraquat by diquat on human toxicity. A clinical survey. Hum Exp Toxicol *11*:241, 1992.
2. Winchester JF: History of paraquat intoxication. *In* Bismuth C, Hall AH (eds): Paraquat Poisoning: Mechanisms, Prevention, Treatment. Series: Drug and Chemical Toxicology. Vol. 10. New York, Marcel Dekker, pp 1–16, 1995.
3. Litovitz TL, Felberg L, Soloway RA, et al: 1994 Annual Report of the American Association of Poison Control Centers Toxic Exposure Surveillance System. Am J Emerg Med *13*:551, 1995.
4. Harley JB, Grinspan S, Root RK: Paraquat suicide in a young woman: Results of therapy directed against the superoxide radical. Yale J Biol Med *50*:481, 1977.
5. Tinoco R, Tinoco R, Parsonnet J, Halperin D: Paraquat poisoning in southern Mexico: A report of 25 cases. Arch Environ Health *48*:78, 1993.
6. Ragoucy-Sengler C, Pileire B, Daijardin JB: Survival from severe paraquat intoxication in heavy drinkers. Lancet *2*:1461, 1991.
7. Onyon LJ, Volans GN: The epidemiology and prevention of paraquat poisoning. Hum Toxicol *6*:19, 1987.
8. Lewis CPL, Nemery B: Pathophysiology and biochemical mechanisms of the pulmonary toxicity of paraquat. *In* Bismuth C, Hall AH (eds): Paraquat Poisoning: Mechanisms, Prevention, Treatment. Series: Drug and Chemical Toxicology. Vol. 10. New York, Marcel Dekker, p 107, 1995.
9. Sandy MS, Moldeus P, Ross D, Smith MT: Role of redox cycling and lipid peroxidation in bipyridyl herbicide cytotoxicity. Studies with a compromised isolated hepatocyte model system. Biochem Pharmacol *35*:3095, 1986.
10. Snider GL: Interstitial pulmonary fibrosis: Which cell is the culprit? Am Rev Respir Dis *127*:535, 1983.
11. Jaeger A, Sauder P, Kopferschmitt J: Mechanisms of paraquat toxicity and therapeutic implications. *In* Bismuth C, Hall AH (eds): Paraquat Poisoning: Mechanisms, Prevention, Treatment. Series: Drug and Chemical Toxicology. Vol. 10. New York, Marcel Dekker, p 141, 1995.
12. Watanabe N, Shiki Y, Morisaki N, et al: Cytotoxic effects of paraquat and inhibition of them by vitamin E. Biochim Biophys Acta *883*:420, 1986.
13. van Asbeck BS, Hillen EC, Boonen HC, et al: Continuous intravenous infusion of deferoxamine reduces mortality by paraquat in vitamin E deficient rats. Am Rev Respir Dis *139*:769, 1989.
14. Mercurio SD, Combs GE Jr: Selenium-dependent glutathione peroxidase inhibitors increase toxicity of prooxidant compounds in chicks. J Nutr *116*:1726, 1986.
15. Hagen TM, Brown LA, Jones DP: Protection against paraquat-induced injury by exogenous GSH in pulmonary alveolar type II cells. Biochem Pharmacol *35*:4537, 1977.
16. Wegener T, Sandhagen B, Chan KW, Saldeen T: *N*-acetylcysteine in paraquat toxicity: Toxicological and histological evaluation in rats. Ups J Med Sci *93*:81, 1988.
17. Yamamoto H: Protection against paraquat-induced toxicity with sulfite or thiosulfite in mice. Toxicology *79*:37, 1993.
18. Fairshter RD, Vaziri ND, Crosby SA, et al: Effect of dimethylthiourea on plasma paraquat concentrations. Toxicology *50*:47, 1988.
19. Pakbaz H, Foda HD, Berisha HI, et al: Paraquat induced lung injury: Prevention by vasoactive peptide and related peptide helodermin. Am J Physiol *265*:L369, 1993.
20. Swan AAB: Exposure of spray operators to paraquat. Br J Ind Med *26*:322, 1969.
21. Grissom RE Jr, Brownie C, Guthrie FE: Dermal absorption of pesticides in mice. Pesticide Biochem Physiol *24*:119, 1985.
22. Scott RC, Walker M, Dugard PH: A comparison of the *in vitro* permeability properties of human and some laboratory animal skins. Int J Cosmet Sci *8*:189, 1986.
23. Wester RC, Maibach HI, Bucks DAW, Aufrere MB: *In vivo* percutaneous absorption of paraquat from hand, leg, and forearm of humans. J Toxicol Environ Health *14*:759, 1984.
24. Fitzgerald GR, Barniville G, Black J, et al: Paraquat poisoning in agricultural workers. Ir Med Assoc J *71*:336, 1978.
25. Garnier R: Paraquat poisoning by inhalation or skin absorption. *In* Bismuth C, Hall AH (eds): Paraquat Poisoning: Mechanisms, Prevention, Treatment. Series: Drug and Chemical Toxicology. Vol. 10. New York, Marcel Dekker, p 211, 1995.
26. Jaros F: Acute percutaneous paraquat absorption. Lancet *1*:275, 1978.
27. Levin PJ, Klaff LJ, Rose AG, Ferguson AD: Pulmonary effects of contact exposure to paraquat: A clinical and experimental study. Thorax *34*:150, 1979.

28. Ongum VL, Owor R, Tonuisange ET: Paraquat (Gramoxone) used as a pediculocide. *In* Bagshawe AE, Maina G, Magela EN (eds): Use and Abuse of Drugs and Chemicals in Tropical Africa. East African Literature Bureau, p 229, 1974.
29. Binns CW: A deadly cure for lice—a case of paraquat poisoning. Papua New Guinea Med J *19*:105, 1976.
30. Smith JG: Paraquat poisoning by skin absorption: A review. Hum Toxicol 7:15, 1988.
31. Papiris SA, Maniati MA, Kyriakidis V, Constanopoulos SH: Pulmonary damage due to paraquat poisoning through skin absorption. Respiration *62*:101, 1995.
32. Hall AH, Becker CE: Occupational health and safety issues in paraquat handling. *In* Bismuth C, Hall AH (eds): Paraquat Poisoning: Mechanisms, Prevention, Treatment. Series: Drug and Chemical Toxicology. Vol. 10. New York, Marcel Dekker, p 249, 1995.
33. Chemistry and toxicology of paraquat-contaminated marijuana. Final report to the National Institutes for Drug Abuse, Washington, D.C., Government Printing Office, June 1978.
34. Rose MS, Smith LL, Wyatt I: Evidence for an energy-dependent accumulation of paraquat into rat lung. Nature *252*:315, 1974.
35. Cant JS, Lewis DRH: Ocular damage due to paraquat and diquat. BMJ *3*:59, 1968.
36. Stephens DS, Walker DH, Schaffner W, et al: Pseudo-diphtheria: Prominent pharyngeal membrane associated with fatal paraquat ingestion. Ann Intern Med *94*:202, 1981.
37. Vaziri ND, Ness RL, Fairshter RD, et al: Nephrotoxicity of paraquat in man. Arch Intern Med *139*:172, 1979.
38. Webb DB, Davies CG: Paraquat poisoning and kidney function tests. Lancet *1*:1424, 1981.
39. Im JG, Lee KS, Han MC, et al: Paraquat poisoning: Findings on chest radiography and CT in 42 patients. Am J Radiol *157*:697, 1991.
40. Chen KW, Wu MH, Huang JJ, Yu CY: Bilateral spontaneous pneumothoraces, pneumopericardium, pneumomediastinum, and subcutaneous emphysema: A rare presentation of paraquat intoxication. Ann Emerg Med *23*:1132, 1994.
41. Levitt T: Determination of paraquat in clinical practice using radioimmunoassay. Proc Anal Div Chem Soc *16*:72, 1979.
42. Proudfoot AT, Stewart MS, Levitt T, Widdop B: Paraquat poisoning: Significance of plasma paraquat concentrations. Lancet *2*:330, 1979.
43. Hart TB, Nevitt A, Whitehead A: A new statistical approach to the prognostic significance of plasma paraquat concentrations. Lancet *2*:1222, 1984.
44. Schermann JM, Galliott M, Garnier R, Bismuth C: Acute paraquat poisoning: Prognostic significance and therapeutical interest of blood assay. Toxicol Eur Res *3*:141, 1983.
45. Cooke NJ, Flenley DC, Matthew IT: Paraquat poisoning: Serial studies of lung function. Q J Med *42*:683, 1973.
46. Suzuki K, Takasu N, Arita S, et al: A new method for predicting the outcome and survival period in paraquat poisoning. Hum Toxicol *8*:31, 1989.
47. Meredith T, Vale JA: Treatment of paraquat poisoning: Gastrointestinal decontamination. *In* Bismuth C, Hall AH (eds): Paraquat Poisoning: Mechanisms, Prevention, Treatment. Series: Drug and Chemical Toxicology. Vol. 10. New York, Marcel Dekker, p 297, 1995.
48. Okonek S, Hofmann A, Hennigsen B: Efficacy of gut lavage, haemodialysis in the therapy of paraquat or diquat intoxication. Arch Toxicol *36*:43, 1976.
49. Mizutani T, Yamashita M, Okubo N, et al: Efficacy of whole bowel irrigation using solutions with or without adsorbent in the removal of paraquat in dogs. Hum Exp Toxicol *11*:495, 1992.
50. Meredith TJ, Vale JA: Treatment of paraquat poisoning in man: Methods to prevent absorption. Hum Toxicol *6*:49, 1987.
51. Mascie-Taylor BH, Thompson J, Davison AM: Haemoperfusion ineffective for paraquat removal in life threatening paraquat poisoning. Lancet *1*:1376, 1983.
52. Van De Vyver FL, Giuliano RA, Paulus J, et al: Hemoperfusion-hemodialysis ineffective for paraquat removal in life-threatening poisoning? J Toxicol Clin Toxicol *23*:117, 1985.
53. Hampson EC, Pond SM: Failure of haemoperfusion and haemodialysis to prevent death in paraquat poisoning. A retrospective review of 42 patients. Med Toxicol Adverse Drug Exp *3*:64, 1988.
54. Maini R, Winchester JF: Removal of paraquat from blood by haemoperfusion over sorbent materials. BMJ *3*:281, 1975.
55. Widdop B, Medd RK, Braithwaite RA, Vale JA: Haemoperfusion in the treatment of paraquat poisoning. Proc Eur Soc Artif Organs *2*:244, 1975.
56. Gelfand MC, Winchester JF, Knepshield JH, et al: Treatment of severe drug overdosage with charcoal hemoperfusion. Trans Am Soc Artif Intern Organs *23*:599, 1977.
57. Okonek S, Weileman LS, Majdanzic J, et al: Successful treatment of paraquat poisoning. Activated charcoal per os and continuous "hemoperfusion." J Toxicol Clin Toxicol *19*:807, 1982.
58. Azhari R, Margel S, Labes A, Haviv Y: Specific removal of paraquat by hemoperfusion through antiparaquat conjugated agarose-polyacrylein microsphere beads. J Biomed Mater Res *21*:25, 1987.
59. Smith LL: Mechanisms of paraquat toxicity in lung and its relevance to treatment. Hum Toxicol *6*:31, 1987.
60. Proudfoot AT, Prescott LF, Jarvie DR: Haemodialysis for paraquat poisoning. Hum Toxicol *6*:69, 1987.
61. Bismuth C, Scherrmann JM, Garnier R, et al: Elimination of paraquat. Hum Toxicol *6*:63, 1987.
62. Ikebuchi J, Proudfoot AT, Matsubara K, et al: Toxicological index of paraquat; a new strategy for assessment of severity of paraquat poisoning in 128 patients. Forensic Sci Int *59*:85, 1993.
63. Chollet A, Muszynzky J, Bismuth C, et al: L'hypooxygenation dans l'intoxication par le paraquat a propos de six cas. Toxicol Eur Res *5*:71, 1983.
64. Rossaint R, Falke KJ, Lopez F, et al: Inhaled nitric oxide for the adult respiratory distress syndrome. N Engl J Med *328*:399, 1993.
65. Koppel C, von Wissmann C, Barckow D, et al: Inhaled nitric oxide in advanced paraquat poisoning. J Toxicol Clin Toxicol *32*:205, 1994.
66. Webb DB, Williams MV, Davies BH, James KW: Resolution after radiotherapy of severe pulmonary damage due to paraquat poisoning. BMJ *288*:1259, 1984.
67. Addo E, Poon-King T: Leucocyte suppression in treatment of 72 patients with paraquat poisoning. Lancet *1*:1117, 1986.
68. Vale JA, Meredith TJ, Buckley BM: Paraquat poisoning. Lancet *1*:1439, 1986.
69. Connolly ME, Davies DS, Draffan GH, et al: Clinical experience with paraquat poisoning. *In* Fletcher K (ed): Clinical Aspects of Paraquat Poisoning. London, Imperial Chemical Industries, p 1, 1975.
70. Lheureux P, Leduc D, Vanbist R, Askenazi R. Survival in a case of massive paraquat ingestion. Chest *107*:285, 1995.
71. Cooper JD, The Toronto Lung Transplant Group: Sequential bilateral lung transplantation for paraquat poisonings case report. J Thorac Cardiovasc Surg *89*:734, 1985.
72. Kamholz S, Veith FJ, Mollenkopf F, et al: Single lung transplant in paraquat intoxication. N Y State J Med *84*:82, 1984.
73. Wright AF, Green TP, Daleyyat P, Smith LL: Monoclonal-antibody does not protect mice from paraquat toxicity. Vet Hum Toxicol *29*(Suppl 2):102, 1987.
74. Crabtree HC, Lock EA, Rose MS: Effects of diquat on the gastrointestinal tract of rats. Toxicol Appl Pharmacol *41*:585, 1973.
75. Vanholder R, Colardyn F, De Rueck J, et al: Diquat intoxication. Report of two cases and review of the literature. Am J Med *76*:1267, 1981.
76. Manoguerra AS: Full thickness skin burns secondary to an unusual exposure to diquat dibromide. J Toxicol Clin Toxicol *28*:107, 1990.
77. von Freislederer A, Besserer K, Mallach HJ: Selbsttotung mit einem als unschadlich geltenden Pflanzenwachstrumsregler. Beitr Gerichtl Med *47*:107, 1989.
78. Winek CL, Wahba WW, Edelstein JM: Sudden death following ingestion of chlormequat. J Anal Toxicol *14*:257, 1990.
79. Conning DM, Fletcher K, Swan AAB: Paraquat and related bipyridyls. Br Med Bull *25*:245, 1969.

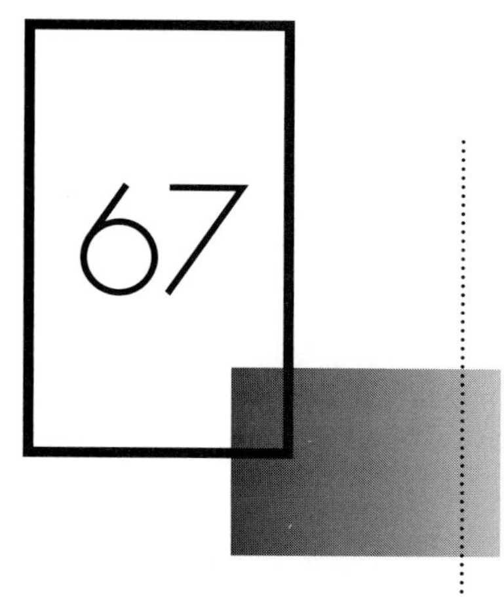

Chlorophenoxy Herbicides and Dioxin Contaminants; Other Herbicides and Fungicides

KENNETH KULIG, M.D.

CHLOROPHENOXY HERBICIDES

Chlorophenoxy herbicides are auxins, or growth regulators, that cause abnormal plant growth that ultimately destroys the plant. They are commonly used for control of broadleaf weeds in cereal crops and pastures.[1] They are all congeners of phenoxyacetic acid; the more common chlorophenoxy herbicides are represented in Figure 67–1. Their notoriety originates primarily from the use of Agent Orange in Vietnam as a defoliant and its alleged health effects on exposed individuals. Agent Orange was an equal mixture of 2,4-dichlorodiphenoxyacetic acid (2,4-D) and 2,4,5-trichlorophenoxyacetic acid (2,4,5-T) in diesel fuel. It was delivered in 55-gallon drums with an orange stripe to distinguish the drums visually from those containing other chemical agents. Most of the alleged adverse health effects of Agent Orange are blamed on the contaminant 2,3,7,8-tetrachlorodibenzo-*p*-dioxin (TCDD, or dioxin).

Chlorophenoxy herbicides as a group include various salts of 2,4-D, 2,4,5-T, 4-chloro-2-methylphenoxyacetic acid (MCPA), 4-methyl, 4-chlorophenoxypropionic acid (MCPP), Dicamba, and Silvex. Many of the products available to consumers contain a mixture of salts in a petroleum distillate solvent. Their toxicity is similar; only minor differences in toxicokinetics distinguish them from one another. Their alleged carcinogenic and neuropathy-inducing potential is of concern but not widely accepted as proven.

The clinical presentation in cases of accidental or intentional chlorophenoxy ingestion may include irritation of the eyes, mucous membranes, and gastrointestinal (GI) tract (vomiting and diarrhea), along with muscle twitching and tenderness, myotonia, rhabdomyolysis, metabolic acidosis, fever, tachycardia, tachypnea, vasodilatation, sweating, seizures, and coma.[2] Abnormal renal and hepatic functions and an elevated creatine phosphokinase level are commonly noted after a massive exposure. Minor electrocardiographic changes have been reported and should be evaluated in cases of excessive exposure. Thrombocytopenia has been rarely reported. Carcinogenicity, teratogenicity, and reproductive abnormalities have been alleged but not confirmed.

Chlorophenoxy herbicides can be measured in plasma and urine by radioimmunoassay[3] and gas liquid chromatography.[4] However, the need for treatment is based on the history of exposure and physical findings rather than on chlorophenoxy levels. Other laboratory parameters that should be monitored after significant exposures include electrocardiogram findings, complete blood count (CBC) results, electro-

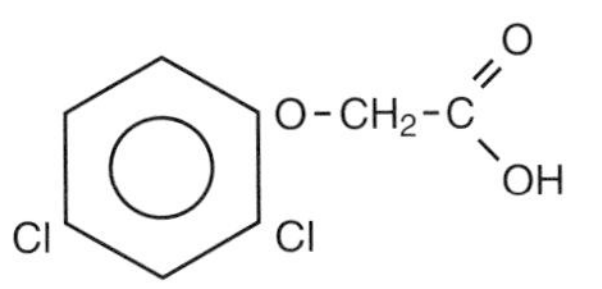

2,4-Dichlorophenoxyacetic acid
(2,4-D)

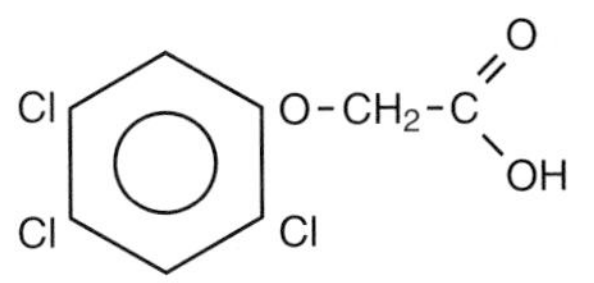

2,4,5-Trichlorophenoxyacetic acid
(2,4,5-T)

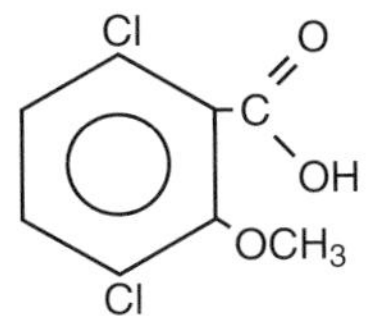

Dicamba

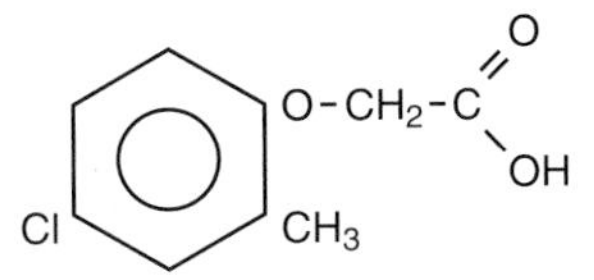

MCPA
2-Methyl-4-chlorophenoxyacetic acid
(2,4,5-T)

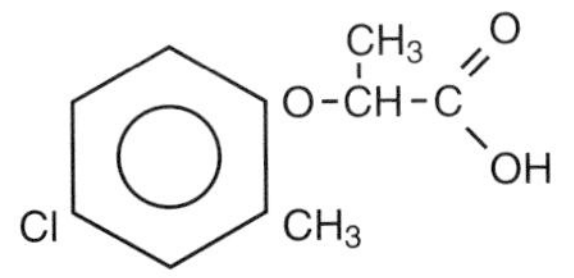

2-(2-Methyl-4-chlorophenoxy)proprionic acid

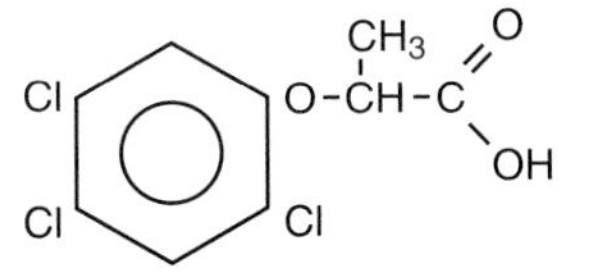

Silvex

Figure 67–1. The most common chlorophenoxy herbicides.

lytes, results of hepatic and renal function studies, serum creatine phosphokinase level, and urine levels of albumin and myoglobin.

Aggressive GI decontamination procedures should be performed after oral exposure to chlorophenoxy compounds. Gastric lavage might be useful if performed very soon after ingestion, followed by administration of 50 to 100 g of activated charcoal in adults (1 g/kg in children). If several hours have elapsed since ingestion, charcoal alone should be administered. After dermal exposure, the skin should be washed thoroughly with soap and water, with attention to easily overlooked areas such as the hair, umbilicus, and nails. Inhalation exposure results primarily in an irritant effect.

Aggressive supportive care consists of protecting the airway, including intubation and mechanical ventilation when needed, and correcting hypotension, arrhythmias, hyperthermia, seizures, and acidosis. Urine output and other parameters indicating the patient's volume status should be monitored until recovery. Although there is no specific antidote, alkaline diuresis has been reported to be of value in enhancing elimination of several chlorophenoxy derivatives.[5, 6]

2,4-Dichlorophenoxyacetic Acid

Studies of human volunteers have demonstrated that 2,4-D is well absorbed from the GI tract[7, 8] but less well absorbed via the dermal route.[9] In a study of six human volunteers who were given a dose of 5 mg/kg orally, 2,4-D was detectable in the plasma in 1 hour and in the urine within 2 hours.[7] The volume of distribution was 10.1 +/− 0.3 L/kg, and more than 75% was excreted unchanged in the urine within 96 hours. A second volunteer study using the same oral dose found the average elimination half-life ($t_{1/2}\beta$) to be 11.7 hours.[8] The $t_{1/2}\beta$ in one patient who ingested an overdose of 2,4-D and Dicamba was 16.7 hours.[10] The mean elimination $t_{1/2}$ in volunteers in one study was 33 hours.[7]

In a patient with disseminated coccidioidomycosis, 2,4-D was given therapeutically in gradually increasing intravenous doses.[11] Although an intravenous dose of 2000 mg (37 mg/kg) produced no side effects, 3600 mg intravenously (66 mg/kg) resulted in coma, muscle twitching, hyporeflexia, and urinary incontinence. At 24 hours after administration, the patient was awake but complained of profound muscle weakness, which resolved 24 hours later.

Several cases of intentional self-poisoning with 2,4-D have been reported. A 76-year-old man who ingested an unknown amount of 2,4-D was found vomiting and combative. Twenty hours later, he was unarousable and had Cheyne-Stokes respirations, myotonia, and guaiac-positive nasogastric aspirate. The patient died 6 days after ingestion.[12]

In another case of suicidal ingestion of 50 g of 2,4-D, the patient was comatose, hypotonic, hyporeflexic, and hypotensive 9 hours after ingestion. Treatment included diuresis and supportive care, but the patient died 12 hours after ingestion.[13]

Iritis has been reported in a worker who rubbed his eyes after moving containers of 2,4-D.[14]

Peripheral neuropathy with painful paresthesias and muscle stiffness has been reported after dermal and inhalation exposure to 2,4-D in a few anecdotal cases.[15–18] Product contaminants and concomitant exposures, however, could not be adequately ruled out as alternative explanations.

Significantly enhanced renal elimination with alkaline diuresis has been reported for several of the chlorophenoxy compounds.[5, 6, 19] Alkaline diuresis can be accomplished by adding 88 to 132 mEq of sodium bicarbonate (1 to 2 adult ampules) per liter of 5% dextrose in water and administering intravenously at a rate to produce adequate urine output (i.e., 2 mL/kg per hour) with a pH of 7.5 or more. One starting point for the maintenance intravenous solution after any volume deficits from vomiting have been corrected might be 200 mL/h for an average-sized adult. Alkalizing the urine may also help to prevent myoglobin deposition in the renal tubules if the patient has chlorophenoxy-induced rhabdomyolysis. Careful monitoring of fluid and electrolyte balance must be performed to prevent the complications of fluid overload such as pulmonary edema.

The Occupational Safety and Health Administration (OSHA) has established a permissible exposure limit of 10 mg/m^3 for 2,4-D, which is the same as the threshold limit value (time-weighted average).

2,4,5-Trichlorophenoxyacetic Acid

Most uses of 2,4,5-T were banned by the United States Environmental Protection Agency (EPA) in 1979,[18] and all remaining uses were subsequently disqualified.[19] TCDD is a byproduct of 2,4,5-T production and is often a contaminant of the final product, a fact largely responsible for the banning of 2,4,5-T.

The acute toxicity is identical to that of 2,4-D, with which it is commonly coingested. Chronic toxicity is alleged to be secondary to TCDD contamination.

The kinetics of 2,4,5-T have been studied in five human volunteers who ingested a single dose of 5 mg/kg. Good absorption from the GI tract was demonstrated, and 88.5 +/− 5.1% of the ingested dose was excreted unchanged in the urine within 96 hours.[20] First-order kinetics were described with a volume of distribution of 0.079 L/kg and a $t_{1/2}\beta$ of 23.1 hours.

A 61-year-old man who ingested 24 g of 2,4-D and 7.5 g of 2,4,5-T in a hydrocarbon solvent was hypertonic, hyperreflexic, hyperthermic, and responsive only to pain by 6 hours after ingestion. By 24 hours after ingestion, he was completely unresponsive to pain. Although he remained unconscious for 4 days, he recovered by 5 days after ingestion. One month later, he had difficulty walking and had evidence of a peripheral neuropathy, which resolved 3 months later.[21]

A 48-year-old man who drank a mixture of equal parts of 2,4-D, 2,4,5-T butyl ester, and inert ingredients was found drowsy and vomiting. By 3 hours after ingestion he was vomiting, diaphoretic, hypotensive, tachycardiac, tachypneic, and responsive only to pain. During 43 hours of hospitalization, the patient developed hyperthermia, oliguria, hemoconcentration, a rising blood urea nitrogen level, and shock unresponsive to pressors.[1]

Dioxin as Contaminant

Dioxins are a group of compounds that are not deliberately manufactured for commercial use but are trace contaminants or products of combustion of other products. One specific compound, 2,3,7,8 (TCDD) (Fig. 67–2), is extremely toxic to some species of laboratory animals, giving it a reputation as one of the most toxic chemicals ever produced, although human toxicity appears to be minimal. This particular compound is often referred to specifically as *dioxin.* It can be a trace contaminant of 2,4,5-T, the antibacterial agent hexachlorophene, or trichlorophenol. It is also created from bleaching wood pulp to make paper, from incineration of wastes containing chlorine such as polyvinyl chloride pipes, and polychlorinated biphenyls from burning coal and diesel fuel, and in nature from volcanoes and forest fires. It is found in the smoke of cigarettes and barbeques. One of the primary sources of human exposure to TCDD is from food, particularly meat, milk, and fish.[22] Consumption of fatty fish such as salmon and herring from the Baltic Sea has been shown to elevate adipose tissue levels of TCDD in humans.[23]

Polychlorodibenzofuran compounds are also contaminants from the same processes but in general are thought to be less toxic than the polychlorodibenzodioxins and are not discussed here.

TCDD is colorless, odorless, and lipid soluble; it accumulates in the food chain, and in fact food accounts for 98% of total adult exposures.[24] United States population means for adipose tissue TCDD have been established from a sample of 865 specimens collected in 1987: 5.38 pg/g (range from below detection limits to 15.1 pg/g).[25] The values increased significantly with age but showed no correlation with sex, race, or geographic location. For comparison, TCDD adipose tissue levels of Vietnam veterans heavily exposed to Agent Orange had a mean value of 41.7 pg/g (SEM 16.8, median 15.4).[26] Blood plasma TCDD levels were also higher in the exposed population than in unexposed controls (46.3 pg/g, SEM 19.1; versus 5.7 g/g, SEM 0.7) in this study. However a similar study investigating serum TCDD levels

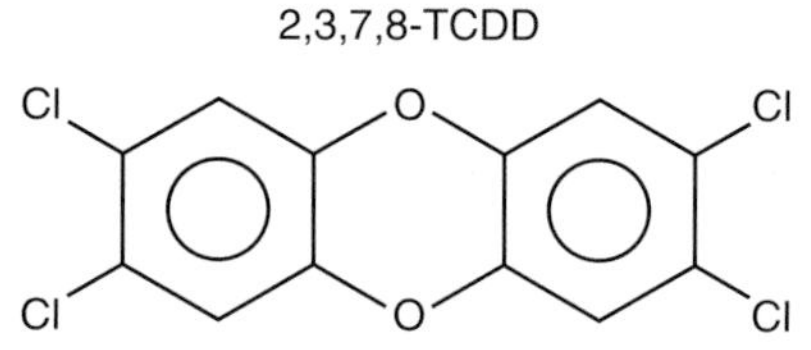

2,3,7,8-TCDD

Figure 67–2. The structure of 2,3,7,8-tetrachlorodibenzo-*p*-dioxin, also referred to as TCDD or dioxin. Hundreds of congeners exist.

showed no difference between exposed veterans and controls.[27] Adipose tissue TCDD levels in residents of Times Beach, Missouri, who were exposed to TCDD from a mixture of materials used to spray the roads showed a mean of 79.7 pg/g, which was higher than that of controls.[28]

The metabolic fate of TCDD in humans is not well defined but is likely to be the formation of oxidation hepatic metabolites, which are conjugated and excreted.[24, 29] The half-life in humans is approximately 7 years. Being lipid soluble, TCDD is excreted in breast milk.

The toxicity of TCDD to animals is well studied. There is a very large difference in species susceptibility to the adverse effects of TCDD, with guinea pigs being the most sensitive. By comparison, hamsters are 5000 to 10,000 times more resistant, and humans even more so. The only proven effects of TCDD on humans are chloracne and transient mild hepatotoxicity.[24] Chemical plant workers with elevated adipose tissue levels of TCDD were found to have no significant elevation of risk for the development of GI or hepatic disease.[30] Residents of Seveso, Italy, with the highest levels of exposure to TCDD from an industrial accident, had minimal elevations of γ-glutamyltransferase and alanine aminotransferase at long-term follow-up without clinical hepatic disease.[31]

In animals, TCDD causes a wasting syndrome not encountered in humans. Soft tissue sarcomas, lymphomas, neuropathy, altered reproductive function, teratogenicity, and various immunotoxic responses are observed in some sensitive animal species. It has been suggested, however, that extrapolation of adverse health effects in animals given the maximum tolerated dose (MTD) of TCDD to lower doses in humans is unreliable. Immune effects in primates at low doses of TCDD are the opposite of those at higher doses.[32] Cancer incidence in some animal models is actually lower than expected at low levels of TCDD exposure; the dose-response curve actually slopes downward at the low doses.[33] The theory for this phenomenon is that TCDD exposure at very low doses stimulates the immune system to eliminate naturally occurring cancers.

Epidemiologic studies of TCDD-exposed workers have demonstrated little if any increased risk for the development of malignancy from the exposure.[34, 35] Similar results have been demonstrated for Vietnam veterans exposed to Agent Orange.[36] Although any increased risk of malignancy may be low (although on occasion statistically significant), these data are likely to be used by both proponents and opponents of the concept that TCDD is a human carcinogen.[37]

Chloracne in humans is characterized by pale yellow cysts located primarily on the face and trunk. Its development does not follow a dose-response model, and therefore its absence does not rule out TCDD exposure.[24] Conversely, even severe chloracne was not associated with other adverse health effects in long-term studies of a population of heavily exposed residents of Seveso, Italy.[38]

No permissible exposure limit or threshold limit value has been established for TCDD. The EPA lists a maximum contaminant level for TCDD in drinking water of 0.05 parts per trillion. The Food and Drug Administration has defined a limit for TCDD in fish of 25 parts per trillion.

Acute human TCDD exposure can be treated only by removal from exposure, skin or GI decontamination, and supportive therapy. Chloracne may respond to topical retinoic acid. Levels of hepatic transaminases, if elevated, should be monitored over time until normal. The need for or utility of long-term medical monitoring of TCDD-exposed persons has not been demonstrated.

4-Chloro-2-Methylphenoxyacetic Acid

Another chlorophenoxy herbicide, MCPA (metaxon) is used to control annual and perennial weeds in cereals, grassland, and turf.[1]

Five volunteers given an oral dose of 15 μg/kg body weight of MCPA had a peak plasma concentration of 0.15 μg/mL at 1 hour. During the first 24 hours, 40% of the dose was excreted in urine. Dermal absorption was demonstrated after 1 g of MCPA emulsion was placed on the skin and washed off after 2 hours. A maximum plasma level of 0.12 μg/mL was reached after 24 hours. Maximal urinary excretion occurred 24 to 48 hours after application, with slow excretion continuing for up to 5 days.[39]

Significant toxicity has been reported after ingestion of MCPA in a suicide attempt. A 61-year-old man ingested a weed killer later identified as MCPA and shortly thereafter developed vomiting, slurred speech, and muscle jerking. By 1.5 hours after ingestion, he was unconscious and had copious oral secretions. Physical examination revealed edema of the tongue and face, coarse rales at the bases of the lungs, small unreactive pupils, hyporeflexia, generalized fibrillary twitching of the skeletal muscles, and clonic spasms of the limbs. Treatment included intubation, gastric lavage, administration of paraldehyde to control abnormal muscle movements, and use of pressors for hypotension. The patient remained unconscious for 72 hours but recovered. Laboratory abnormalities included occult fecal blood for 21 days, elevated transaminase levels, and decreased hemoglobin and platelet counts.[40]

Hypocalcemia complicated the course of one fatal case of ingestion of Herbatox (22.7% MCPA and 9.1% 2,4-D). A 55-year-old woman became confused and aggressive shortly after ingestion and later became unconscious, hypertonic, areflexic, tachycardiac, and hypoxic. Initial treatment included lavage and alkaline diuresis. The hospital course was complicated by hypotension, renal insufficiency, and hypocalcemia requiring calcium infusion. After 15 days, the patient died of multiple organ failure.[41] Two other fatal cases have been described.[42, 43]

2-Methyl,4-Chlorophenoxypropionic Acid

2-Methyl,4-chlorophenoxypropionic acid (MCPP, or mecoprop) has also been involved in cases of human poisoning. Two cases of MCPP ingestion followed a similar clinical course with rapid loss of consciousness, muscle cramps, and hypotension. Laboratory abnormalities included decreased platelets and hemoglobin and elevated creatine phosphokinase and myoglobin levels. One patient also developed acute renal failure secondary to rhabdomyolysis and required hemodialysis. Both recovered.[44]

UREA-SUBSTITUTED HERBICIDES

Urea-substituted herbicides, which are photosynthesis inhibitors, are used mainly for weed control in noncrop areas.[1] Examples of this class of herbicides include chlorimuron, chlorotoluron, diuron, fluometuron, isoproturon, linuron, methabenzthiazuron, metobromuron, monolinuron, monuron, neburon, siduron, tebuthioron, and tetrafluoron.

Diuron is well absorbed from the GI and respiratory systems, but information about dermal absorption is lacking.[1] Diuron undergoes hepatic metabolism, and the majority of metabolites are excreted in the urine.[1] Monuron has also been shown to undergo metabolism via the liver microsomes.[45]

Urea-substituted herbicides have low systemic toxicity based on animal feeding studies. Diuron, for example, had a median lethal dose (LD_{50}) of 1017 mg/kg in normal juvenile rats, an LD_{50} of 437 mg/kg in rats on a low-protein diet, and an LD_{50} of 2390 mg/kg in rats on a high-protein diet.[46]

Cases of human ingestion also generally support the idea that these compounds are of low systemic toxicity. A 39-year-old woman ingested an herbicide containing 56% diuron and 30% amitrole (38 and 20 mg/kg, respectively). She showed no clinical evidence of toxicity, but her urine contained metabolites of diuron.[47]

In another case, however, significant clinical findings did occur after ingestion of an herbicide containing monolinuron. A 63-year-old woman drank 1 cup of Gramonol, containing monolinuron 14% and paraquat 10%. Nine hours after ingestion, the patient was noted to have a cyanotic appearance. At 43 hours after ingestion, she had a 36% methemoglobin level and a 7% sulfhemoglobin level. Hemolysis was also noted. The patient recovered after treatment with 50 mg of methylene blue. Her paraquat level was not in the serious risk category, and her methemoglobinemia was attributed to monolinuron, which is metabolized to aniline.[48] Another similar case with methemoglobinemia, hemolysis, and a nontoxic paraquat level following Gramonol ingestion has also been reported.[49]

Plasma determinations of these herbicides are not clinically useful. Methemoglobin and sulfhemoglobin levels should be measured in patients who have a history of urea-substituted herbicide ingestions and who appear to be cyanotic or are dyspneic.

Treatment should include decontamination and aggressive supportive care. Additionally, methylene blue, 1 to 2 mg/kg per dose, should be given if significant methemoglobinemia is present. If other evidence of severe toxicity is present, other causes should be sought and appropriate treatment given.

ENDOTHALL

Endothall (3,6-bendoxohexahydrophthalic acid) is an herbicide with significant toxicity. The acute oral LD_{50} is 51 mg/kg. It is irritating to the eyes, mucous membranes, GI tract (vomiting and diarrhea), and skin. Seizures, hypotension, respiratory failure, cardiac failure, and death can occur after ingestion.

In one fatal case, a 23-year-old man ingested 40 mL of endothall. He vomited spontaneously six times and complained of abdominal pain on arrival in an emergency department 50 minutes after ingestion. The patient was given a charcoal slurry but vomited again. Six hours after presentation, he complained of dyspnea and abdominal pain. During the next several hours, the patient developed hematemesis, hypotension, acidosis, anuria, disseminated intravascular coagulation, and cardiovascular collapse. Despite aggressive supportive care, the patient expired 12 hours after ingestion. No toxicology studies were reported to exclude the possibility that other toxins were involved.[50] In another fatal case, a 21-year-old man ingested 7 to 8 g (two mouthfuls of a 17.5% solution) and died of multiorgan failure.[51] Postmortem blood endothall level was 10 μg/mL.

Treatment of endothall ingestion should include GI decontamination with activated charcoal and aggressive supportive care.

CARBAMATE HERBICIDES AND FUNGICIDES

Carbamate herbicides and fungicides differ from the carbamate insecticides by a substitution on the nitrogen rather than the oxygen moiety (Fig. 67–3). Unlike the carbamate insecticides, these compounds do not produce inhibition of cholinesterase enzymes or a cholinergic syndrome.[1] Toxicity is unusual.

(Mono)thiocarbamates. This group includes cycloate, molinate, pebulate, diallate, and triallate, which are selective herbicides with generally low mammalian toxicity.[1] Molinate, used to control weeds in rice paddies, was implicated in the illness of eight people who were exposed to contaminated water.[52] After molinate was applied to nearby rice paddies, the well, which was the source of water for four families, developed an odor. Eight people subsequently developed nausea, diarrhea, abdominal pain, fever, weakness, and conjunctivitis, whereas four additional people developed only abdominal pain. Symptoms resolved when the families stopped using

(MONO) THIOCARBAMATES

R O

N — C — S — R″

Ar or R′

THIOCARBAMATE
HERBICIDE

GENERAL CHEMICAL STRUCTURE

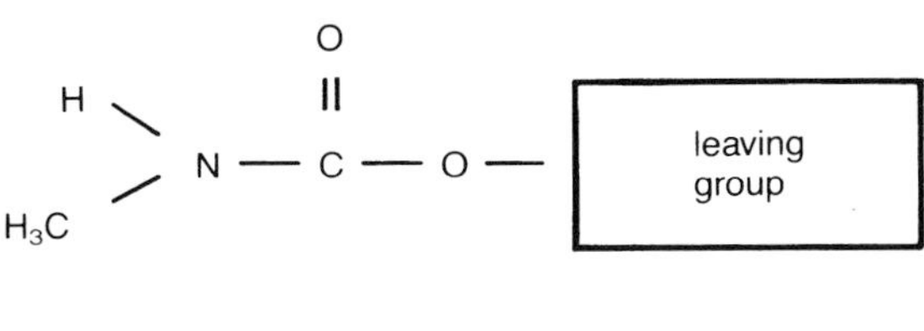

CARBAMATE
INSECTICIDE

Figure 67–3. Structure of carbamate herbicides and cholinesterase-inhibiting carbamate insecticides. (From Morgan DP: Recognition and Management of Pesticide Poisonings. 3rd ed. Washington, DC, US Environmental Protection Agency, 1982.)

the well water. Analysis of the water 15 days later revealed a molinate concentration of 0.006 ppm.

Bisdithiocarbamates. Thiram belongs to the bisdithiocarbamate class and is used as a fungicide. It is structurally similar to disulfiram, and this compound may produce a disulfiram reaction when ethanol is ingested after a significant exposure to thiram. This reaction is characterized by flushing, sweating, headache, weakness, tachycardia, and hypotension.[53–55] One such case resulted in a fatality 4 days after a 10-hour exposure to thiram.[56] Contact dermatitis with a positive patch test result occurred in a man who bowled on a green treated with thiram[57] and in a man who golfed on a course treated with thiram.[58] Allergic contact dermatitis occurred in four patients who were treated in the same hemodialysis unit and who had results of positive skin tests for thiram.[59] The source of the thiram was reportedly from rubber parts of the hemodialysis unit that came into contact with the dialysate. One case of Henoch-Schönlein purpura was reported to have occurred in a 23-year-old man who was exposed to thiram for 1 month while planting seedlings treated with the fungicide. The patient had nausea and signs of eye, skin, and respiratory tract irritation on the job; however, a causal association between thiram exposure and Henoch-Schönlein purpura was not proved.[60]

Metallobisdithiocarbamates. These comprise a class of carbamate fungicides that includes ziram, nabam, and ferbam. The bisdithiocarbamates are named for the metallic component (e.g., ziram for zinc and ferbam for iron). These compounds are moderately irritating to the skin and respiratory mucous membranes after exposure to sprays or dusts. Nausea, vomiting, and diarrhea may result from ingestion. One case of an ingestion of 500 mL of ziram solution of unknown concentration resulted in a fatality a few hours after ingestion. Autopsy revealed only nonspecific findings such as focal necrosis of the mucosa of the small intestine, congestion of the viscera, acute emphysema, focal atelectasis, and desquamation of alveolar and bronchial epithelia.[61]

Ethylene Bisdithiocarbamates. These fungicides are maneb and zineb. These compounds are irritating to the skin and respiratory tract mucosa. Cases of contact dermatitis have been reported.

A case of acute intoxication with maneb and zineb occurred in a 42-year-old man who walked through a field 1 day after it had been sprayed with maneb and zineb.[62] The patient became transiently uncommunicative, nervous, tired, weak, and dizzy. Six days later, he again walked through a recently sprayed field and developed headache, nausea, fatigue, weakness, difficulty undressing, unclear speech, decreased level of consciousness, and tonic-clonic seizures. An electroencephalogram showed diffuse slowing, and results of computed tomography of the brain were normal. The patient was fully recovered 5 days later.

One case of acute renal failure after exposure to maneb has been reported.[63] A 62-year-old man with stomach cancer treated for 2 years with fluorouracil applied maneb to his garden on two occasions 2 days apart. He had worn protective clothing. The day after the second application, he ate corn from the garden without first washing it and afterward washed his hands with water only. That night he had diarrhea followed by hoarseness and muscle weakness. Five days later, he presented with acute renal failure requiring hemodialysis. The patient recovered and later had normal results of a work-up including intravenous pyelography.

Chronic exposure to maneb purportedly produced a complex of symptoms similar to those of chronic manganese toxicity.[64] After two agricultural workers, a 41-year-old woman and a 27-year-old man, developed a parkinsonian syndrome after maneb exposure, a formal study of exposed workers was undertaken. Fifty farm workers with more than 6 months of exposure to maneb were compared with 19 rural workers without exposure. The exposed workers displayed a statistically significant increase in headaches, nervousness, memory problems, fatigue, and muscle rigidity with cogwheeling. However, no significant difference in manganese levels was noted between the two groups.[64]

HEXACHLOROBENZENE

Hexachlorobenzene, an aromatic hydrocarbon fungicide, has been used since 1945 for seed treatment.[3] Kinetic information in humans is unavailable.

The toxicity of hexachlorobenzene in humans was demonstrated by an outbreak of cutaneous porphyria in Turkey that occurred when seed wheat, which had been treated with a fungicide containing hexachlorobenzene, was used instead for human consumption.[65] From 1955 to 1959, approximately 3000 cases of hexachlorobenzene-induced porphyria occurred in southeastern Turkey.[66] Symptoms included hyperpigmentation, hypertrichosis, weight loss, hepatomegaly, and painless arthritis. The most striking finding was blistering and epidermolysis of exposed parts of the skin. Healing was poor and occurred in winter, leaving pigmented scars and contractures. Relapses occurred in the summer with increased sun exposure.[65] Breast-fed infants of affected mothers were noted to develop "pembe yara," or pink sore, and had a mortality rate of 95%.[66] Treatment of seven patients with 1 to 2 g of edetic acid daily for up to 1 year resulted in symptomatic improvement. Chelation also resulted in increased excretion of urine uroporphyrins but no change in the excretion of urine coproporphyrins.[66]

Twenty years after hexachlorobenzene exposure, 32 Turkish patients were studied. Clinically, patients were noted to have small stature, hyperpigmentation, hypertrichosis, pinched faces, arthritis, and scars on the cheeks, arms, and hands. The most striking finding was that of small hands, with sclerodermoid thickening of the skin and an abnormal shape secondary to osteoporosis and almost complete atrophy of the terminal phalanges.[67] A hexachlorobenzene level of 0.7 ppm was detected in breast milk from one porphyric patient; none was detected in milk from four controls. Subcutaneous fat from one porphyric patient had a hexachlorobenzene level of 0.21 ppm. Urine and stool uroporphyrin levels were still elevated in 5 of 29 patients in whom levels were obtained.

GLYPHOSATE-SURFACTANT HERBICIDE (ROUNDUP)

Roundup, a commercial product made by Monsanto, contains 41% glyphosate as the isopropylamine salt and 15% surfactant and water. It has rapidly become one of the most popular herbicides worldwide. Developed as an alternative to paraquat, it is also known as nian-nian-chun in China and Taiwan.

Talbot and colleagues[68] reported 93 cases of Roundup exposure. Although accidental exposure caused no harm after dermal contact with spray in 6 cases, 80 cases with seven deaths were reported from intentional ingestion. GI erosion was the primary site of toxicity, although renal, hepatic, central nervous system, and pulmonary involvement were less frequently noted. The five deaths occurring from Roundup ingestion alone were associated with hypotension unresponsive to intravenous fluids and pressor agents and often pulmonary edema.

References

1. Hayes WJ Jr: Pesticides Studied in Man. Baltimore, Williams & Wilkins, 1982.
2. Morgan DP: Recognition and Management of Pesticide Poisonings. 3rd ed. Washington, DC, US Environmental Protection Agency, 1982.
3. Knopp D, Nuhn P, Dobberkau HJ: Radioimmunology assay for 2,4-dichlorophenoxyacetic acid. Arch Toxicol *58*:27–32, 1985.
4. Rivers JB, Yauger WL, Klemmer HW: Simultaneous gas chromatographic determination of 2,4-D and dicamba in human blood and urine. J Chromatogr *50*:334–337, 1970.
5. Prescott LF, Park J, Darrien I: Treatment of severe 2,4-D and mecoprop intoxication with alkaline diuresis. Br J Clin Pharmacol *7*:111–116, 1979.
6. Flanagan RJ, Meredith TJ, Ruprah M, et al: Alkaline diuresis for acute poisoning with chlorophenoxy herbicides and ioxynil. Lancet *335*:454–458, 1990.
7. Kohli JD, Khanna RN, Gupta BN, et al: Absorption and excretion of 2,4-dichlorophenoxyacetic acid in man. Xenobiotica *4*:97–100, 1974.
8. Sauerhoff MW, Braun WH, Blau GE, et al: The fate of 2,4-dichlorophenoxyacetic add (2,4-D) following oral administration to man. Abstract. Toxicol Appl Pharmacol *37*:136–137, 1976.
9. Feldmann RJ, Maibach HI: Percutaneous penetration of some pesticides and herbicides in man. Toxicol Appl Pharmacol *28*:126–132, 1974.
10. Young JF, Haley TJ: Pharmacokinetic study of a patient intoxicated with 2,4-dichlorophenoxyacetic acid and 2-methoxy-3,6-dichlorobenzoic acid. Toxicology *11*:489–500, 1977.
11. Seabury JH: Toxicity of 2,4-dichlorophenoxyacetic acid for man and dog. Arch Environ Health *7*:202–209, 1963.
12. Dudley AW Jr, Thapar NT: Fatal human ingestion of 2,4-D, a common herbicide. Arch Pathol *94*:270–275, 1972.
13. deLarrard J, Barbaste M: Fatal suicidal poisoning due to 2,4-D. Arch Mal Prof Med Trav Secur Soc *30*:434, 1969.
14. McMillin RB, Samples JR: Iritis after herbicide exposure. Am J Ophthalmol *99*:726–727, 1985.
15. Berkley MC, Magee KR: Neuropathy following exposure to a dimethylamine salt of 2,4-D. Arch Intern Med *111*:351–352, 1963.
16. Goldstein NP, Jones PH, Brown JR: Peripheral neuropathy after exposure to an ester of dichlorophenoxyacetic acid. JAMA *171*:1306–1309, 1959.
17. Wallis WE, Van Poznak A, Plum F: Generalized muscular stiffness, fasciculations, and myokymia of peripheral nerve origin. Arch Neurol *22*:430–439, 1970.
18. Environmental Protection Agency: Rebuttal presumption against registration on 2,4,5-T. Federal Register. April 21, 1978, 43:17116–17157.
19. Baselt RC: Deposition of Toxic Drugs and Chemicals in Man. 2nd ed. Davis, CA, Biomedical Publications, 1982.
20. Gehring PJ, Kramer CG, Schwetz BA, et al: The fate of 2,4,5-trichlorophenoxyacetic acid (2,4,5-T) following oral administration to man. Toxicol Appl Pharmacol *26*:352–361, 1973.
21. O'Reilly JF: Prolonged coma and delayed peripheral neuropathy after ingestion of phenoxyacetic weed killers. Postgrad Med J *60*:76–77, 1984.
22. Schecter A, Startin J, Wright C, et al: Congener-specific levels of dioxins and dibenzofurans in US food and estimated daily dioxin toxic equivalent intake. Environ Health Perspect *102*:962–966, 1994.
23. Svensson BG, Nilsson A, Hansson M, et al: Exposure to dioxins and dibenzofurans through the consumption of fish. N Engl J Med *324*:8–12, 1991.
24. Demers R: Dioxin toxicity. ATSDR case studies in environmental medicine. Washington, DC, US Department of Health and Human Services, 1990.
25. Orban JE, Stanley JS, Schwemberger JG, et al: Dioxins and dibenzofurans in adipose tissue of the general US population and selected subpopulations. Am J Public Health *84*:439–445, 1994.
26. Kahn PC, Gochfeld M, Nygren M: Dioxins and dibenzofurans

in blood and adipose tissue of agent orange–exposed Vietnam veterans and matched controls. JAMA *259*:1661–1667, 1988.
27. Centers for Disease Control: TCDD levels in Vietnam Veterans—CDC Veterans Health Study. JAMA *260*:1249–1254, 1988.
28. Patterson DG, Hoffman RE, Needham LL, et al: 2,3,7,8-Tetrachlorodibenzo-*p*-dioxin levels in adipose tissue of exposed and control persons in Missouri: An interim report. JAMA *256*:2683–2686, 1986.
29. Van den Berg M, De Jongh J, Poiger H, et al: The toxicokinetics and metabolism of polychlorinated dibenzo-*p*-dioxins (PCDDs) and dibenzofurans (PCDFs) and their relevance for toxicity. Crit Rev Toxicol *24*:1–74, 1994.
30. Calvert GM, Hornung RW, Sweeney MH, et al: Hepatic and gastrointestinal effects in an occupational cohort exposed to 2,3,7,8-tetrachlorodibenzo-para-dioxin. JAMA *267*:2209–2214, 1992.
31. Mocarelli P, Marocchi A, Brambilla P, et al: Clinical laboratory manifestations of exposure to dioxin in children. JAMA *256*:2687–2696, 1986.
32. Neubert R, Golor G, Stahlmann R, et al: Polyhalogenated dibenzo-*p*-dioxins and dibenzofurans and the immune system. 4. Effects of multiple-dose treatment with 2,3,7,8-tetrachlorodibenzo-*p*-dioxin (TCDD) on peripheral lymphocyte subpopulations of a non-human primate. Arch Toxicol *66*:250–259, 1992.
33. Stevenson DE, Sielken RL, Bretzlaff RS: Challenges to low-dose linearity in carcinogenesis from interactions among mechanistic components as exemplified by the concept of "invaders" and "defenders." Biol Eff Low Level Exposures Newsl *3*:1–8, 1994.
34. Zober A, Messerer P, Huber P: Thirty-four year mortality follow up of BASF employees exposed to 2,3,7,8-TCDD after the 1953 accident. Int Arch Occup Environ Health *62*:139–157, 1990.
35. Fingerhut MA, Halperin WE, Marlow DA, et al: Cancer mortality in workers exposed to 2,3,7,8-tetrachlorodibenzo-*p*-dioxin. N Engl J Med *324*:212–218, 1991.
36. Watanabe KK, Kang HK: Mortality patterns among Vietnam veterans. J Occup Environ Med *38*:272–278, 1996.
37. Bailar JC III: How dangerous is dioxin? N Engl J Med *324*:260–262, 1991.
38. Caputo R, Moti M, Ermacora E, et al: Cutaneous manifestations of tetrachlorobenzo-*p*-dioxin in children and adolescents. Follow-up 10 years after the Seveso, Italy, accident. J Am Acad Dermatol *19*:812–819, 1988.
39. Kolmodin-Hedman B, Hoglui S, Swensson A, et al: Studies on phenox acid herbicides: II. Oral and dermal uptake and elimination in urine of MCPA in humans. Arch Toxicol *54*:267, 1983.
40. Jones DIR, Knight AG, Smith AJ: Attempted suicide with herbicide containing MCPA. Arch Environ Health *14*:363–366, 1967.
41. Kancir CB, Andersen C, Olesen AS: Marked hypocalcemia in a fatal poisoning with chlorinated phenoxy acid derivatives. J Toxicol *26*:257–264, 1988.
42. Popham RD, Davies DM: A case of MCPA poisoning. BMJ *1*:677–678, 1964.
43. Johnson HRM, Kounmides O: A further case of MCPA poisoning. BMJ *2*:629–630, 1965.
44. Meulenbeit J, Zwaveling JH, Van Zoonen P, et al: Acute MCPP intoxication: Report of two cases. Hum Toxicol *7*:289–292, 1988.
45. Ross D, Farmer PB, Gescher A, et al: The formation and metabolism of *N*-hydroxymethyl compounds—I. The oxidative *N*-demethylation of *N*-dimethyl derivatives of arylamines, aryltriazines, arylformamidines and arylureas including the herbicide monuron. Biochem Pharmacol *31*:3621–3627, 1981.
46. Boyd EM, Krupta V: Protein deficiency diet and diuron toxicity. J Agric Food Chem *18*:1104–1107, 1970.
47. Geldmacher-von Mallinckrodt M, Schussler E: Zu stoffwechsel und toxicitaet von 1-(3,4-dichlorophenyl)-3,3-dimethylharnstoff (Diuron) beim menschen. Arch Toxikol *27*:187–192, 1971.
48. Proudfoot AT: Methaemoglobinaemia due to monolinuron—not paraquat. BMJ *285*:812, 1982.
49. Ng LL, Naik RB, Polak A: Paraquat ingestion with methaemoglobinaemia treated with methylene blue. BMJ *284*:1445–1446, 1982.
50. Day LC: Delayed death by Endothall, an herbicide. Abstract. Vet Hum Toxicol *30*:366, 1988.
51. Allender WJ: Suicidal poisoning by endothall. J Analyt Toxicol *7*:79–82, 1983.
52. Minakawa O, Ishii S, Konno H: Analytical method of residue of molinate, a herbicide in paddy field, and actions of molinate to living bodies. Jpn J Public Health *25*:645–651, 1978.
53. Barnes BA, Fox LE: Screening some thiuram disulfides and related compounds for acute toxicity and Antabuse-like activity. J Am Pharm Assoc *44*:756–759, 1955.
54. Reinl W: Hypersensitivity to alcohol after exposure to the fungicide tetramethylthiuram disulfide (TMTD). Arch Toxikol *22*:12–15, 1966.
55. Krupa A, Pienkowska H, Tarka Z: Acute poisoning with "thiram." Med Wiejsk *6*:29–31, 1971.
56. Marcinkowski T, Manikowski W: Fatal case of intoxication with "Seed Dressing T." Med Pr *24*:91–95, 1973.
57. Gunther DW: Tetramethylthiuramdisulphide (TMTD) and bowls. Med J Aust *1*:1177, 1970.
58. Shelley WB: Golf-course dermatitis due to thiram fungicide: Cross-hazards of alcohol, disulfiram, and rubber. JAMA *188*:415–417, 1964.
59. Penneys NS, Edwards LS, Katsikas JL: Allergic contact sensitivity to thiuram compounds in a hemodialysis unit. Arch Dermatol *112*:811–813, 1976.
60. Duell PB, Morton WE: Henoch-Schönlein purpura following thiram exposure. Arch Intern Med *147*:778–779, 1987.
61. Buklan AI: Acute poisoning with ziram. Sud Med Ekspert *17*:51, 1974.
62. Israeli R, Sculsky M, Tiberin P: Acute intoxication due to exposure to maneb and zineb: A case with behavioral and central nervous system changes. Scand J Work Environ Health *9*:47–51, 1983.
63. Koizumi A, Shiojima S, Orrdva M, et al: Acute renal failure and maneb (manganous ethvienebis [dithiocarbamate]) exposure. JAMA *242*:2583–2585, 1979.
64. Ferraz HB, Bertolucci PHF, Pereira JS, et al: Chronic exposure to the fungicide maneb may produce symptoms and signs of CNS manganese intoxication. Neurology *38*:550–553, 1988.
65. Schmid R: Cutaneous porphyria in Turkey. N Engl J Med *263*:397–398, 1960.
66. Peters HA, Johnson SAM, Cam S, et al: Hexachlorobenzene-induced porphyria: Effect of chelation on the disease, porphyrin and metal metabolism. Am J Med Sci *251*:314–322, 1966.
67. Cripps DJ, Gocmen A, Peters HA: Porphyria turcica: Twenty years after hexachlorobenzene intoxication. Arch Dermatol *116*:46–50, 1980.
68. Talbot RA, Shiaw M, Huang J, et al: Acute poisoning with a glyphosate-surfactant herbicide (Roundup): A review of 93 cases. Hum Exp Toxicol *10*:1–8, 1991.

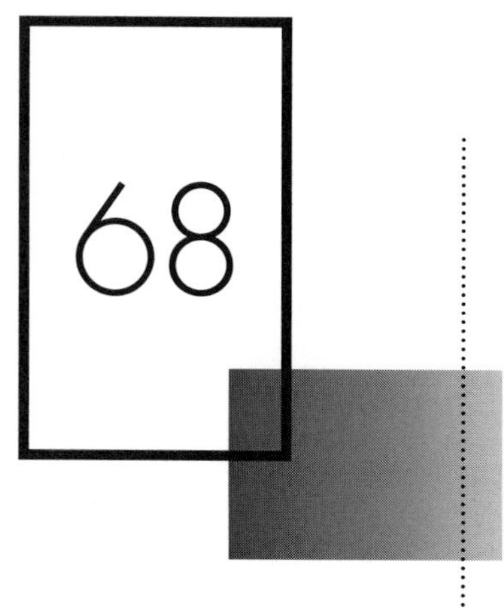

Rodenticides

BROOKS C. METTS, JR., PharmD
N. JOHN STEWART, JR., MD

Competition between humans and lower animals for food and shelter, whether real or imagined, is a constant struggle. In an attempt to gain the ecologic upper hand, humans have endeavored to develop ways to curb rodent populations. The rodenticides encompass a diverse group of chemicals with a wide variety of actions. Whether organic or inorganic, mildly or highly toxic, all of these agents are designed to kill in a cost-effective manner. A problem arises when humans or nontarget animals come into contact with these chemicals. Table 68–1 lists rodenticides by trade name and type of agent.

Rodenticides are designed to kill rodents considered a nuisance, such as rats, mice, gophers, moles, voles, ground squirrels, and prairie dogs. These animals damage crops in the field and foods in storage, host human diseases, bite people, and are capable of causing material damage by gnawing. It makes sense from both an economic and health perspective to attempt to control populations of these animals.[1, 2]

Historically, a wide variety of inorganic and organic compounds have been used as rodenticides. Early rodenticides were agents derived from plant material such as strychnine and red squill or were inorganic chemicals such as arsenic trioxide and thallium. Newer agents tend to be synthetic organic compounds. Regardless of type, virtually all rodenticides are referred to as "rat poisons" by the lay public.

Some substances used as rodenticides proved to be nearly as dangerous to humans and other animals as they are to rodents. Thallium is no longer marketed in the United States because of its toxicity. Efforts have been made to lessen the risk of using rodenticides by restricting the use of some substances and by requiring premarketing studies of potential new products. Still, all rodenticides are toxic if misused.[1]

A number of groups of persons are poisoned by rodenticides. Children are especially at risk. Of 16,478 calls about rodenticides recorded by members of the American Association of Poison Control Centers Toxic Exposure Surveillance System in 1994, 87% involved children younger than 6 years.[3] Other exposures occur in suicide attempts, victims of attempted homicide, exterminators and others putting out rodenticides, intoxicated individuals, psychiatric or mentally impaired patients, and people who accidentally eat rodenticides that are stored in containers normally used for edible products.

The many chemical agents used as rat poisons are listed in Table 68–2. When possible, use only the container label to identify a particular product. Even labeling can be a problem if not read carefully. For example, bromethalin, a neurotoxin, can be confused with bromodiolone or brodifacoum, which are long-acting anticoagulants. It is generally worth the effort to find the container and positively identify the ingredients in order to know what effects might be expected and how to approach treatment.

LONG-ACTING ANTICOAGULANTS (SECOND-GENERATION ANTICOAGULANTS, SUPERWARFARINS)

Description

The long-acting anticoagulants (Table 68–3) are responsible for almost 80% of the human rodenticide exposures reported in the United States.[4] Since their introduction during the mid to late 1970s as a second generation of anticoagulants, these agents have essentially replaced the older warfarin-containing prod-

Table 68–1. Alphabetical List of Rodenticides by Trade Name and Type of Agent*

Trade Name	Active Ingredients	Type of Rodenticide
Acme Mole and Gopher Killer	Zinc phosphide	Phosphides
Anchor Rat and Mouse Bait Packet	Warfarin	Warfarin
Assault Rat Pellets	Bromethalin	Bromethalin
Assault Rat Place Pack	Bromethalin	Bromethalin
Assault Rat WR	Bromethalin	Bromethalin
Bantu	ANTU	ANTU
Bengal Mouse Bait	Chlorophacinone	Long-acting anticoagulant
Black Magic Rat Killer	Pivalyl	Long-acting anticoagulant
Blue Ball Rat Killer	Arsenous oxide	Arsenic
Bromone Mouse Killer	Bromodiolone	Long-acting anticoagulant
Caid	Chlorphacinone	Long-acting anticoagulant
Chopped Poison Peanuts	Strychnine	Strychnine
College Brand Rodenticide	ANTU	ANTU
Compound 1080	Sodium monofluoroacetate	Sodium monofluoroacetate
Compound 1081	Sodium monofluoroacetate	Sodium monofluoroacetate
Contrac	Brodifacoum	Long-acting anticoagulant
D-Con Mouse Prufe (no longer sold)	Warfarin	Warfarin
D-Con Mouse Prufe II	Brodifacoum	Long-acting anticoagulant
Death to Gophers	Strychnine	Strychnine
Deathdiet	Red squill	Red squill
Dipaxin	Diphacinone	Long-acting anticoagulant
Diphacin	Diphacinone	Long-acting anticoagulant
DLP 787 Tracking Powder	Pyriminil	Pyriminil
Dr. Hess Anturat	ANTU	ANTU
Drat	Chlorphacinone	Long-acting anticoagulant
Eagles 7 Final Bite	Diphacinone	Long-acting anticoagulant
El Ray Mouse Bait	Strychnine	Strychnine
Endox	Coumatetral	Long-acting anticoagulant
Endrocide	Coumatetral	Long-acting anticoagulant
Enforcer Rat and Mouse Killer	Chlorophacinone	Long-acting anticoagulant
Enforcer Mouse Kill III	Bromodiolone	Long-acting anticoagulant
Enforcer Rat and Mouse Bars II	Diphacinone	Long-acting anticoagulant
Final Bite	Diphacinone	Long-acting anticoagulant
Finis Rat and Mouse Killer	Diphacinone	Long-acting anticoagulant
Fluorakil 3	Sodium monofluoroacetate	Sodium monofluoroacetate
Fluorakil 100	Sodium monofluoroacetate	Sodium monofluoroacetate
Fluoroacetamide	Sodium monofluoroacetate	Sodium monofluoroacetate
Formula 163 Rat Kill	Diphacinone	Long-acting anticoagulant
Fratol	Sodium monofluoroacetate	Sodium monofluoroacetate
Fussol	Sodium monofluoroacetate	Sodium monofluoroacetate
Gopha Rid	Zinc phosphide	Phosphides
Gopher and Mole Killer Pellets	Zinc phosphide	Phosphides
Gopher Corn	Strychnine	Strychnine
Gopher Getter Bait	Strychnine	Strychnine
Gopher Getter Pills	Strychnine	Strychnine
Gopher Go	Strychnine	Strychnine
Gopher Gone	Diphacinone	Long-acting anticoagulant
Gopher Killer Pellets	Zinc phosphide	Phosphides
Gopher Mix	Strychnine	Strychnine
Gopher Poison Grain Bait	Strychnine	Strychnine
Gopher Probe Mix	Strychnine	Strychnine
Gopher Tabs	Strychnine	Strychnine
Gopher-Rodent Killer	Strychnine	Strychnine
Guardian Rat Bait	Diphacinone	Long-acting anticoagulant
Havoc Rodenticide Bait Pack	Brodifacoum	Long-acting anticoagulant
Hot Shot Sudden Death Mouse Killer	Bromethalin	Bromethalin
Isotrac Tracking Powder	Isovaleryl	Long-acting anticoagulant
Just One Bite Rat and Mouse Bait	Bromodiolone	Long-acting anticoagulant
Kil-Ko Rat Killer	Diphacinone	Long-acting anticoagulant
Kill Kantz	ANTU	ANTU
Klerat	Brodifacoum	Long-acting anticoagulant
Krysid	ANTU	ANTU
Maki Rat and Mouse Meal Bait	Bromodiolone	Long-acting anticoagulant
Maki Rat and Mouse Bait Packs Pellets	Bromodiolone	Long-acting anticoagulant
Megarox	Sodium monofluoroacetate	Sodium monofluoroacetate
Milo Gopher Bait	Strychnine	Strychnine
Miracle Mouse Bait	Strychnine	Strychnine
Mouse-B-Gon, Ortho	Cholecalciferol	Cholecalciferol
Mous-Con No. 2	Zinc phosphide	Phosphides
Mouse Feast	Strychnine	Strychnine
Mouse Maize	Strychnine	Strychnine

Table continued on following page

Table 68–1. Alphabetical List of Rodenticides by Trade Name and Type of Agent* *Continued*

Trade Name	Active Ingredients	Type of Rodenticide
Mouse Nots	Strychnine	Strychnine
Mouse Prufe II	Brodifacoum	Long-acting anticoagulant
Mouse Sault	Strychnine	Strychnine
Mouse Rid	Strychnine	Strychnine
Mr. Rat Guard	Zinc phosphide	Phosphides
Nott's	ANTU	ANTU
Packet Mouse Seed Bait	Strychnine	Strychnine
Patterson Mole Killer	Strychnine	Strychnine
PCQ Rat and Mouse Bait	Diphacinone	Long-acting anticoagulant
Phostoxin Fumigant	Aluminum phosphide	Phosphides
Phosvin	Zinc phosphide	Phosphides
Phosyin	Zinc phosphide	Phosphides
Piper Mouse Bait Packet	Strychnine	Strychnine
Pivalyl	Pindone	Long-acting anticoagulant
Pival	Pindone	Long-acting anticoagulant
Poison Peanut	Strychnine	Strychnine
Prolin	Warfarin	Warfarin
Promar Bait Pellets	Diphacinone	Long-acting anticoagulant
Purina Rat Kill	Pindone	Long-acting anticoagulant
Quick Ravac	Chlorphacinone	Long-acting anticoagulant
Quintox	Cholecalciferol	Cholecalciferol
Ramik Bait Pack	Diphacinone	Long-acting anticoagulant
Ramik Brown	Diphacinone	Long-acting anticoagulant
Ramik Green	Diphacinone	Long-acting anticoagulant
Rampage	Cholecalciferol	Cholecalciferol
Ratangle II	Warfarin	Warfarin
Rat-A-Rest	Bromodiolone	Long-acting anticoagulant
Ratak Bait Pack	Diphenicoum	Long-acting anticoagulant
Rat Bait Meat Bits	Warfarin	Warfarin
Rat Busters	Warfarin	Warfarin
Rat Death Liquid	Sodium arsonite	Arsenic
Rat Doom	Warfarin	Warfarin
Rat Dragon	Warfarin	Warfarin
Rat End	Warfarin	Warfarin
Rat-Fix	Warfarin	Warfarin
Rat Free Rat and Mouse Bait Pack	Bromodiolone	Long-acting anticoagulant
Rat-I-Cide	Warfarin	Warfarin
Raticate	Norbromide	Norbromide
Ratindan	Ratindan	Long-acting anticoagulant
Ratimus	Bromodiolone	Long-acting anticoagulant
Rat Kakes	Warfarin	Warfarin
Rat Kill Formula 163	Diphacinone	Long-acting anticoagulant
Rat Lunches	Strychnine	Strychnine
Ratmort	Warfarin	Warfarin
Rat Nip (Nip-Co)	Red squill	Red squill
Rat Nots	Red squill	Red squill
Rat-O-Cide	Warfarin	Warfarin
Rat-Ola	Diphacinone	Long-acting anticoagulant
Ratorex	Warfarin	Warfarin
Rat Poison (Pearson)	Zinc phosphide	Phosphides
Rat Snak	Arsenic trioxide	Arsenic
Rat Snax	Red squill	Red squill
Rat Squill	Red squill	Red squill
Rattrach	ANTU	ANTU
Rat-tu	ANTU	ANTU
Rat War	Warfarin	Warfarin
Real-Kill Ratex	Bromethalin	Bromethalin
Reardon Mouse Seed	Strychnine	Strychnine
Ro-Dex	Strychnine	Strychnine
Rodentin	Coumatetral	Long-acting anticoagulant
Rodent Kill	Diphacinone	Long-acting anticoagulant
Rodent Pellets	Zinc phosphide	Phosphides
Rodere Paraffinized Rat Bait	Diphacinone	Long-acting anticoagulant
Rodine	Red squill	Red squill
Ropax	Brodifacoum	Long-acting anticoagulant
Rozol	Chlorphacinone	Long-acting anticoagulant
Rumetan	Zinc phosphide	Phosphides
S.L. Cowley & Sons Rat and Mouse Poison	Arsenic trioxide	Arsenic
Shoxin	Norbromide	Norbromide
Sla-Rat	Warfarin	Warfarin
Sodium fluoroacetate	Sodium monofluoroacetate	Sodium monofluoroacetate

Table 68–1. Alphabetical List of Rodenticides by Trade Name and Type of Agent* *Continued*

Trade Name	Active Ingredients	Type of Rodenticide
Sodium monofluoroacetate	Sodium monofluoroacetate	Sodium monofluoroacetate
Stearn's Electric Brand Paste	Phosphorus	Phosphorus
Strike	Warfarin	Warfarin
Super Caid	Bromodiolone	Long-acting anticoagulant
Sweeney's Ready Mixed	Warfarin	Warfarin
Sweeney's Mouse Bait	Warfarin	Warfarin
T&C Gopher Pellets from Sears	Strychnine	Strychnine
Talon	Brodifacoum	Long-acting anticoagulant
Talon G	Brodifacoum	Long-acting anticoagulant
Thro Pac Rat and Mouse Killer Pellets	Diphacinone	Long-acting anticoagulant
Trax-one	Bromodiolone	Long-acting anticoagulant
Tri-Ban	Pindone	Long-acting anticoagulant
Trounce	Bromethalin	Bromethalin
True Grit Tracking Powder	Zinc phosphide	Phosphides
True Grit Gopher Rid	Zinc phosphide	Phosphides
Vacor Rat Bait	Pyriminil	Pyriminil
Vam-o	Warfarin	Warfarin
Vengeance	Bromethalin	Bromethalin
Yancock	Sodium monofluoroacetate	Sodium monofluoroacetate
Zinc-Tox	Zinc phosphide	Phosphides
ZP	Zinc phosphide	Phosphides
ZP AG	Zinc phosphide	Phosphides
ZP Tracking Powder	Zinc phosphide	Phosphides

ANTU, α-naphthyl-thiourea.
*Many trade names sound similar. Package labels should always be checked to verify the type of rodenticide when possible.

ucts. The long-acting agents have the same mechanism of action as warfarin[3]; however, these second-generation substances have two important differences—they are more potent and their half-life is longer. They thus have advantages as rodenticides in that they are effective in single or limited feedings (warfarin requires repeated feeding for 4 to 5 days) and they are effective against animals that are resistant or more tolerant to older anticoagulants.[5] The longer half-life of these agents is significant in cases of human exposure.

The long-acting anticoagulants decrease the activity of the vitamin K–dependent blood-clotting factors (II, VII, IX, X). When clotting factors are sufficiently reduced, bleeding may occur. Signs of bleeding in order of frequency of occurrence include ecchymosis, hematuria, uterine bleeding, melena or hematochezia, epistaxis, hematoma, gingival bleeding, and hematemesis.[6] In humans, a single ingestion of 0.12 mg/kg of brodifacoum has caused anticoagulation lasting 51 days.[7] Others have reported coagulation defects lasting from 45 days to more than 7 months (>210 days).[7–9] A 3-year-old child was found to have elevated levels of brodifacoum and a prolonged prothrombin time (PT) of 40 seconds after exhibiting a tendency to bruising for a week and recent bleeding. The parents had been using D-Con Mouse Prufe II

Table 68–2. Substances Used as Rodenticides

Long-acting anticoagulants	Thallium
Warfarin	Arsenic
Bromethalin	Zinc phosphide
Cholecalciferol	Phosphorus
Pyriminil	α-Naphthyl-thiourea (ANTU)
Sodium monofluoroacetate	Norbromide
Red squill	Barium carbonate
Strychnine	

Table 68–3. Long-Acting Anticoagulant Products

Brodifacoum
Enforcer, Talon, Talon G, Havoc, Ropax, Mouse Prufe II, Ratak, Conrac, Klerat, Enforcer Rat and Mouse Bars II

Bromadiolone
Bromone, Super Caid, Ratimus, Maki, Rat-A-Rest, Just One Bite, Trax-one, Enforcer Mouse Kill III, Rat Free Rat and Mouse Bait Pack

Chlorophacinone
Rozol, Caid, Drat, Quick Ravac, Liphadione, Bengal Mouse Bait, Enforcer Rat and Mouse Killer

Coumatetral
Endox, Racumin 57, Rodentin, Endrocide

Diphacinone
Diphacin, Ramik, Promar, PCQ, Finis, Thro Pac Pellets, Guardian, Kill-Ko, Formula 163, Rat-Ola, Rodere Paraffinized Rat Bait, Ratindan, Dipaxin, Eagles 7 Final Bite, Gopher Gone, Rat Kill Formula 163

Diphenacoum
Ratak

Isovaleryl
Isotrac

Pindone
Purina Rat Kill, Pival, Pivalyl, Tri-Ban

Valone
Black Magic

for 1 month, although the child had not been known to ingest it.

Management

A few pellets or grains ingested by a child are unlikely to cause bleeding, and the child can be monitored at home.[10] Patients who are taking anticoagulants or who have bleeding disorders are at risk with much smaller amounts. Patients with recent large ingestions (>0.1 mg/kg) should have gastric decontamination performed by using syrup of ipecac or gastric lavage. Care must be taken in any patient with a bleeding problem or known prolonged PT because the evacuation procedures can potentially cause harm. Charcoal (1 g/kg) with a suitable cathartic may be used to adsorb the anticoagulant.

Baseline determinations of PT and partial thromboplastin time (PTT) are helpful in those patients suspected of having consumed large amounts. In a review of 110 children who ingested long-acting anticoagulants, only 8 developed a prolonged PT. Unfortunately, prolongation of the PT could not be predicted by the history of the amount ingested. Repeat measurement of PT and PTT at 24 and 48 hours is the only current method for documenting that a significant ingestion has not occurred.[11] If at either time the values are increased, they may continue to rise until there is a risk of bleeding. If the PT or PTT is increased at either 24 or 48 hours, phytonadione (vitamin K_1) should be started before they reach the point where the patient is at risk for hemorrhage. Administer 1 to 5 mg for children and 15 to 20 mg for adults by subcutaneous injection. In critical adult ingestions, a total of 50 to 200 mg of vitamin K_1 can be given by *slow* intravenous infusion; because intravenous vitamin K has caused ventricular fibrillation,[12] no more than 0.5 mg may be given intravenously per minute. Because the half-life of vitamin K is only 1.7 hours, repeat doses of vitamin K may be necessary until the patient is stable. Check the PT and PTT every 4 hours until the patient is stable, and then check every 24 hours. If hemorrhage occurs, use fresh frozen plasma and whole blood to control blood loss and replace clotting factors.

Once patients are stable, they can be switched to oral phytonadione. Very high doses of phytonadione administered for long periods (3 to 7 months or longer) may be required for exposures to the long-acting anticoagulants.[8] Regular monitoring of the PT is essential in these patients. Compliance with treatment can be a problem in patients who intentionally ingest these compounds. Close monitoring as well as psychiatric care is necessary. Phytonadione doses can be tapered as PT values decline toward normal.

WARFARIN-TYPE ANTICOAGULANTS

Description

Although warfarin has now been made obsolete by the second-generation agents, its introduction in the early 1950s revolutionized rodent control. Warfarin proved to be an effective rodenticide and was safer than agents being used at that time. Toxicity requires large amounts as a single exposure or smaller doses for 4 to 6 days.[13] Although a single exposure rarely results in problems, they can occur.

The emergence of rats who were resistant to the effects of warfarin led companies to add an antibiotic, sulfaquinoxaline, to the formulation. This increases effectiveness by reducing vitamin K–producing bacteria in the gut. Although warfarin-containing products (Table 68–4) have largely been replaced by more potent and effective agents, they were still responsible for more than 1300 exposures in 1994.[3]

Warfarin compounds decrease the formation of biologically active vitamin K–dependent blood-clotting factors (II, VII, IX, X). If clotting factors are sufficiently reduced, bleeding occurs.[6] In adults, 5 to 10 mg/d of warfarin produces prothrombin levels about 1.5 to 2.5 times normal. Loading doses of 20 to 60 mg were formerly used to achieve these levels. Ingestions exceeding this amount could cause bleeding.

No reliable studies have correlated rodent bait formulations and prothrombin activity in humans. A 4-oz pack (113 g) of a 0.25% bait contains 28 mg of warfarin. Even if completely absorbed, this is unlikely to produce bleeding in an adult with a single acute exposure. Patients taking anticoagulants are at risk with much smaller amounts. Identification of the product is important because the second-generation anticoagulants are more potent and have longer half-lives.

Management

In children, single-mouthful amounts present no risk and treatment is usually not necessary. Single exposures seldom warrant medical intervention. However, exposures to amounts larger then 0.5 mg/kg or long-term exposures should be evaluated. For recent single exposures, one may prevent absorption by administering syrup of ipecac or performing gastric lavage; follow with activated charcoal and a cathartic to reduce absorption. PT and PTT should be measured and rechecked in 12 to 24 hours. When the PT is two or more times normal, a patient has some risk for bleeding. At this level, phytonadione should

Table 68–4. Products Containing Warfarin*

Hydroxycoumarin (Warfarin) (Wincon)
Kill-Ko, Rat Busters, Rat Kakes, Rat Doom, Rat Dragon, Rat End, Ratmort, Rat-I-Cide, Rat-Ola, D-Con, Sweeney's Mouse Bait, Mouse-Nots, Mouse Prufe, Rat War, Sla-Rat, Vam-O
Warfarin plus Sulfaquinoxalone
Anchor Rat and Mouse Bait Packet, Strike, Sweeney's Ready Mixed Ratangle II, Rat Bait Meat Bits, Rat-Fix, Rat-O-Cide, Ratorex, Final, Eagle 7

*Most warfarin-containing products are no longer manufactured. Check the package carefully for ingredients to be sure of the type of rodenticide.

be given. Administer 1 to 5 mg orally or intramuscularly to children or 10 mg to adults. Vitamin K_1 has a fast turnover rate and has to be given three to five times daily.[14] PT should be measured every 4 hours until stable, then every 24 hours. If hemorrhage occurs, use whole blood or plasma to control blood loss and replace clotting factors.

In patients who are undergoing anticoagulant therapy, emesis and gastric lavage as a decontamination measure to remove bait should be avoided. The risk of inducing gastrointestinal or intracerebral bleeding should always be considered. Activated charcoal is used to adsorb the rat bait formulation. PT should be measured immediately, and phytonadione given if it is significantly prolonged. Because these patients are undergoing anticoagulation for a medical reason, one should maintain the PT at 1.5 to 2 times normal unless future anticoagulation is no longer desired. If desired, heparin may be substituted as an anticoagulant until the PT is stable. In any patient who develops bleeding, monitor the hematocrit closely. Few deaths are reported with warfarin compounds. Therefore, the treatment should not be worse than the problem. When identified early, these patients can be effectively treated.

BROMETHALIN

Available Products

Assault, Vengeance, Trounce, Hot Shot Sudden Death Mouse Killer

Description

Purina Assault is available as green pellets in two sizes: 1/8-inch mouse size, 45 mg per pellet, 22 pellets per gram, 935 pellets per pack; and 3/16-inch rat size, 142 mg per pellet, 7 pellets per gram, 298 pellets per pack. Pellets are packaged in waterproof paper place packs weighing 1.5 oz each and as 1.5-oz prefilled bait stations.[13] Bitrex (denatonium benzoate) has recently been added to bromethalin bait to deter human consumption. This substance does not interfere with its use as a rodenticide but because of its bad taste makes it difficult for humans to consume a toxic dose.

Bromethalin is one of the newer rodenticides, having entered the market in 1985.[15] It is available in pellets of 0.01% concentration as a general-use rodenticide. Bromethalin acts as a neurotoxin. It is metabolized to desmethylbromethalin, which has much more potent neurotoxic activity.[16] The central nervous system (CNS) effects appear to be secondary to the uncoupling of mitochondrial oxidative phosphorylation. A resultant decrease in the production of adenosine triphosphate causes the development of fluid-filled vacuoles between the myelin sheaths covering the central nerves. Increased CNS pressure and pressure on nerve axons result in decreased nerve impulse conduction. Resulting paralysis is followed by eventual death.[14] Bromethalin is a nonselective mammalian poison. All animals, including humans, are vulnerable to its toxic effects. Its effectiveness as a rodenticide is based on smaller rodents' consuming larger quantities per kilogram of body weight than larger animals.[17] No human exposures have been reported. Treatment would be symptomatic and supportive.[17–20]

CHOLECALCIFEROL

Available Products

Rampage, Quintox, Ortho Mouse-B-Gon

Description

A recently marketed rodenticide, cholecalciferol (vitamin D_3) takes advantage of the fact that rodents are extremely sensitive to small percentage changes in the calcium balance in their blood. Cholecalciferol causes hypercalcemia by mobilization of the body stores of calcium primarily found in bone. This hypercalcemic state results in calcification of the organs, blood vessels, and soft tissue. It may also lead to nerve and muscle dysfunction as well as cardiac rhythm disturbances.[21]

Rodenticide baits are a 0.75% concentration of cholecalciferol formulated as pellets or mouse seed. Pellets are available in 30-g packs and in bulk containers. Each pellet contains 0.0577 mg, or 2308 IU of vitamin D. There are 13 pellets per gram (30,000 IU).[22]

There is wide individual variation in the amount of cholecalciferol required to produce hypervitaminosis D in humans. Continued ingestion of 50,000 IU or more per day can cause poisoning. Most reported poisonings are a result of continually taking too much vitamin D.[23] No information is available on acute exposures. However, because of the long elimination half-life (>30 days), a very large single dose might produce the same effects as long-term exposures.

Cholecalciferol (vitamin D) toxicity results in hypercalcemia.[23] When calcium levels rise above 11.5 to 12 mg/dL, symptoms are common. These include confusion, anorexia, headache, fatigue, nausea, vomiting, and diarrhea. Levels exceeding 13 mg/dL may produce seizures and renal insufficiency. Calcification in the kidneys, skin, vessels, lungs, heart, and stomach may occur at this level. In children, one episode of moderately severe hypercalcemia may result in growth retardation. Six months or more may pass before growth resumes.[24]

Management

Several bait pellets or a small amount of the mouse seed should not be toxic, and no treatment is necessary. Larger quantities should be removed from the gastrointestinal (GI) tract before absorption occurs. Charcoal in pulsed doses may be effective. Monitoring serum calcium levels 24 hours after ingestion is indicated because levels may become elevated within 24 to 48 hours after ingestion. Hypercalcemia should be aggressively treated. Institute a low-calcium diet. Forced diuresis using normal saline increases the elimination of calcium. Furosemide is the preferred diuretic. Vitamin D is a fat-soluble vitamin and is not eliminated by diuresis, but the resultant hypercalcemia is effectively treated in this manner. Prednisone, 5 to 15 mg every 6 hours by mouth, is effective in vitamin D intoxication to lower calcium levels. Calcitonin, 4 MRC units/kg intramuscularly every 12 hours, may be necessary. Calcitonin may lower calcium levels by decreasing bone resorption. Lukaszkiewicz and colleagues have shown that phenobarbital and phenytoin are effective in inducing hepatic microsomal enzyme systems in an infant to hasten removal of vitamin D.[25] In severe hypercalcemia (>15 mg/dL), for those patients not responding to other measures, the use of mithramycin should be considered.

PYRIMINIL, PNU

Available Products

Vacor Rat Bait, DLP 787 Tracking Powder

Description

This agent was released in 1975 as a one-feeding (acute-acting), highly toxic rodenticide. Because of the severe toxicity demonstrated by the agent, it was withdrawn as a general-use pesticide in 1979. Although pyriminil has not been available to the public for many years, occasional exposures still occur.

Pyriminil destroys the β-cells of the islets of Langerhans in the pancreas, resulting in inadequate production of insulin. Survivors develop classic diabetes mellitus, and death may result from diabetic ketoacidosis and dysrhythmias. Sensory and motor neuropathies as well as other nervous system dysfunctions are also noted.[26–28] Death has been reported with a dose of 780 mg, and symptoms have been produced with 390 mg (5.6 mg/kg).[28]

The exact mechanism of action of pyriminil is not known, but in animals it seems to act as a niacinamide antagonist interfering with the pentose phosphate pathway. The resulting damage to cellular metabolism, especially in the pancreas, leaves the organism deficient in insulin production.

Management

Recent ingestion should be treated by evacuating the stomach with ipecac or gastric lavage. Administration of activated charcoal and a cathartic are indicated. As an antidote, 500 mg of niacinamide, administered intravenously (slow push) may be effective if given immediately, then 100 to 200 mg every 4 hours for 48 hours.

One should monitor patients' blood and urine glucose levels and check the levels of serum alkaline phosphatase, lactate dehydrogenase, serum glutamic-oxaloacetic transaminase, ketones, electrolytes, and blood urea nitrogen. Diabetic ketoacidosis should be treated with insulin and fluid as necessary. The resulting diabetes may be brittle and difficult to control.

SODIUM MONOFLUOROACETATE

Available Products

Sodium monofluoroacetate, Sodium fluoroacetate, Compound 1080, Fratol, Fluoroacetamide, Compound 1081, Fluorakil 3, Fluorakil 100, Fussol, Megarox, Yancock

Description

Sodium fluoroacetate was developed during World War II as an alternative to imported natural rodenticides.[30] This compound is readily absorbed through the GI tract and respiratory tract, mucous membranes, and broken skin. It is a highly toxic rodenticide. In humans, doses of 0.5 to 2 mg/kg should be considered highly dangerous and 5 mg/kg is estimated to be the lethal dose.[31] Sodium fluoroacetate must first be metabolized to fluorocitrate before toxicity develops. This produces a lag time of up to several hours before symptoms develop. The toxicity may be related to interrupting the Krebs' cycle, thus blocking energy metabolism; however, this mechanism has been challenged.[32] Critical effects are associated with the CNS (seizures and respiratory depression) and heart (tachycardia and ventricular fibrillation).

Fluoroacetamide has essentially the same actions as fluoroacetate but is less toxic.[1] Because it is so highly toxic, sodium monofluoroacetate is restricted to use by licensed exterminators.

After ingestion, effects are delayed. Vomiting is common. Apprehension, auditory hallucinations, and facial paresthesias often precede convulsions. Cardiac effects often follow and may include ectopic beats, tachycardia, ventricular fibrillation, and cardiac failure. Diffuse tubular degeneration of the kidneys has occurred in two cases.[1]

Management

Immediately after ingestion of sodium monofluoroacetate, the stomach should be emptied, followed by administration of activated charcoal. If beyond 30 minutes after exposure or if substantial vomiting has occurred, use of activated charcoal and cathartic alone should be considered. There is not specific therapy for fluoroacetate toxicity. Diazepam or phenobarbital should be used for convulsions. Continuous cardiac monitoring is suggested, along with general supportive care.

RED SQUILL

Available Products

Deathdiet, Rat Snax, Rat Squill, Rat Nip, Rat Not, Rodine

Description

Red squill is a botanic rodenticide derived from the red variety of *Urginea maritima*, or sea onion. Red squill contains two cardiac glycosides, scillaren A and scillaren B.[33]

Red squill is very bitter and has a powerful emetic action; hence, much of the material may be spontaneously removed from the stomach before it is absorbed. The cardiac glycosides produce effects similar to digitalis, and treatment is the same as for digitalis toxicity, including the use of Digibind (see Chapter 85).

STRYCHNINE

Available Products

Ro-Dex, Miracle Mouse Bait, Piper Mouse Bait Packet, Mouse Feast, Mouse Maize, Mouse Nots, Mouse Rid, Mouse Sault, Poison Peanut, Reardon Mouse Seed, El Ray Mouse Bait, Milo Gopher Bait, Gopher Corn, Gopher Getter Pills, Gopher Go, Gopher Mix, T&C Gopher Pellets from Sears, Gopher Poison Grain Bait, Gopher-Rodent Killer, Rat Lunches, Death to Gophers, Patterson Mole Killer, Chopped Poison Peanuts, Packet Mouse Seed Bait

Strychnine

Strychnine is a plant alkaloid found in the seeds of *Strychnos nux-vomica*, a tree native to India. It was introduced into Germany in the 16th century as a poison for rats and other animal pests and is still used today.[34] Although human exposure is now uncommon, 186 exposures were reported in 1994.[3, 35]

Toxic amounts are rapidly absorbed.[36, 37] Some tightness and twitching of facial and neck muscles, or *risus sardonicus*, are often noted initially. Increased reflex excitability is observed. Generalized convulsions may occur within 15 to 30 minutes. Seizures may be clonic at first but rapidly become tonic. All voluntary muscles contract. Respiration is impossible during seizures. Convulsive episodes occur repeatedly, followed by periods of remission. Seizures can be precipitated by sensory stimuli.

Management

The primary goal is prevention or control of convulsions.[34, 35, 37–39] Emptying the stomach with ipecac or lavage is not recommended because strychnine is rapidly absorbed and stimulation can precipitate convulsions. Activated charcoal should be given to reduce absorption if symptoms are minimal or absent; otherwise, administer charcoal after convulsions are controlled. Hayes recommends the use of anticonvulsants as quickly as possible after diagnosis to reduce fear, reflex stimulation, and respiratory paralysis.[1] *Diazepam* may be the most useful drug for this purpose because it antagonizes the convulsions without potentiating postictal depression.[34, 40] Phenobarbital or phenytoin may be used if a patient is not responsive to diazepam. Avoid overstimulating patients. Patients can tolerate manipulation as long as motions are expected and gentle. Morphine should not be used because it causes respiratory depression. Be prepared to intubate and ventilate patients when using any drug that depresses respirations. Monitor patients for metabolic acidosis (lactic acidosis).[40] Death is thought to be a result of hypoxia, and animal studies have shown that artificial ventilation protects from otherwise fatal doses of strychnine.

The prognosis is generally favorable if patients can be supported for the first 24 hours.[37] Convulsions generally decrease within 12 to 24 hours.

THALLIUM

Available Products

No thallium rodenticides are sold in the United States but they are available in Mexico. Exposures still occur in the United States.

Description

Thallium sulfate is a tasteless and odorless powder. It was introduced in the United States in the 1920s as a rodenticide.[41] Thallium is absorbed rapidly from the GI tract. It is also absorbed through the skin and by inhalation.[42] The use of thallium as a pesticide was prohibited in the United States in 1965.[41, 42] Fatalities have resulted from ingestion of 8 mg/kg by adults. The usual lethal dose is 10 to 15 mg/kg.[43]

Ingestion of thallium sulfate often causes nausea and vomiting. For 3 to 4 days (up to 1 week), the only symptom may be constipation. This constipation is usually unresponsive to laxatives.[43] After a latent period, patients develop neurologic pains, usually starting in the lower extremities. During the second week, severe toxic polyneuritis is evident and alopecia begins. Survival may be attended by long-term neuropathies. In chronic thallium poisoning, the primary symptoms are alopecia, peripheral neuropathies, and possibly the development of a toxic psychosis.[42] According to Moeschlin, symptoms essential for diagnosis include dark bands at the roots of hair, retrosternal pain, abdominal cramps, constipation, hysteriform behavior, polyneuritis, tachycardia, hair loss, and lunula strips in the nails.[43] Mees' lines, transverse white lines found on the nails, may also develop. Abnormal results of liver function tests as well as urinalysis results reflecting renal involvement are often found.

Management

Treatment of thallium poisoning is very difficult. Gastric decontamination procedures including lavage and administration of charcoal with a cathartic should be used for any patient presenting with acute ingestion of thallium. Agreement on a treatment protocol is lacking. Forced potassium diuresis can be used. Intravenous fluid support with potassium chloride may be of help. Potassium chloride has been used to displace thallium and increase its excretion by the kidney, using competitive inhibition of reabsorption. Several studies have indicated the benefit of administering potassium to decrease the half-life of thallium. Potassium can decrease the half-life from 30 days to 8 to 10 days.[44–46] The use of hemoperfusion or hemoperfusion alternating with hemodialysis may enhance the elimination of thallium to some degree.[43, 44, 47]

Prussian blue (Berlin blue) is used in Europe to chelate thallium in the gut and stop intestinal reabsorption. This drug is not available in the United States.[42, 44] Activated charcoal also binds thallium in the gut, and multiple-dose charcoal could also be used to reduce reabsorption.[42] Thallium damage to organ systems may be permanent, but patients surviving 4 to 5 weeks usually survive.

ARSENIC

Available Products

Arsenic Trioxide

S.L. Cowley & Sons Rat and Mouse Poison, Rat Snak

Sodium Arsenite

Rat Death Liquid

Arsenious Oxide

Blue Ball Rat Killer

Description

Although more commonly used as a pesticide or herbicide, arsenic finds some limited use as a rodenticide. Arsenites are salts of arsenous acid (from arsenic trioxide). Arsenites are more soluble and have a faster onset of toxicity than other forms of arsenic, thus making them likely choices for rodenticides, herbicides, and pesticides.[1]

For effects and treatment of exposure to arsenic, see Chapter 58.

ALUMINUM PHOSPHIDE, MAGNESIUM PHOSPHIDE, ZINC PHOSPHIDE, AND PHOSPHINE GAS

Available Products

Zinc Phosphide

Acme Mole and Gopher killer, Gopha Rid, Gopher Killer Pellets, Kikrat, Mous-Con, Mr. Rat Guard, Phosvin, Phosyin, Rumetan, True Grit Tracking Powder, True Grit Gopher Rid, Pearson Rat Poison, Zinc-Tox, ZP, ZP Tracking powder, ZP AG

Aluminum Phosphide

Phostoxin

Description

Phosphides are used throughout the world to protect stored grains from rodents and other pests.[48] They are also available as mole and gopher killers. On contact with moisture or acids, phosphides produce phosphine gas, which is thought to be primarily responsible for their toxicity.[48–52]

Phosphine gas is rapidly formed in contact with dilute acids or more slowly in contact with water.[49] It is heavier than air and has an odor that has been described as similar to rotten fish. This odor can be detected at levels of 2 ppm.[48, 53] Unfortunately, odor cannot be relied on as a warning sign or diagnostic aid because toxicity can occur below the level that can be smelled.[53]

Oral exposures to phosphides have become more numerous, and phosphides are now reported to be the most common suicidal agent used in Northern India.[48, 54, 55] Toxic exposures to phosphine gas by inhalation have also been reported.[50, 51, 56]

The lethal dose in humans is not known, but patients ingesting zinc phosphide have died after ingesting as little as 4 to 5 g and have survived ingestion of 25 to 50 g. The threshold limit value for phosphine gas is 0.3 ppm, and the inhalation LD_{50} in rats is 11 ppm over 4 hours.[53]

The exact mechanism of action is unclear, but phosphine has been shown to block cytochrome C oxidase, inhibiting oxidative phosphorylation. This block of the energy-producing process found within cellular mitochondria results in cell death.[48]

Phosphides can cause severe GI irritation. Nausea and vomiting with epigastric pain can ensue within 10 to 15 minutes.[48] Vomiting can be prolonged. Hypotension and shock are common features in serious cases. Myocardial injury results in arrhythmias and conduction disturbances. Patients with moderate to severe cases develop tachypnea, cyanosis, and occasionally adult respiratory distress syndrome. CNS symptoms are not prominent. Shock, early dyspnea, thirst, oliguria, convulsions, and coma have occurred in fatal cases.[49, 50]

Effects that may develop over time include delayed pulmonary edema, metabolic acidosis, hypocalcemic tetany, circulatory collapse, liver damage, bradycardia and electrocardiographic abnormalities, thrombocytopenia, and methemoglobinemia.

The majority of deaths occur approximately 30 hours after ingestion and are probably due to myocardial damage.[53]

Management

Time is critical after ingestion, because vomiting within the first hour may improve the prognosis. If spontaneous vomiting has not occurred, the use of activated charcoal followed by gastric lavage should be considered. Intragastric sodium bicarbonate to increase the stomach pH has been suggested as a means of slowing the release of phosphine gas. The use of 1:1000 potassium permanganate as the lavage solution has also been suggested. This would theoretically oxidize the phosphide to phosphate. However, experimental and clinical evidence supporting this cannot be found. It is important to clear phosphide from the entire GI tract. Charcoal and a cathartic should be left in the stomach after gastric emptying.

Symptomatic patients should be placed on 100% oxygen via a nonrebreathing mask. Treatment is symptomatic and supportive. Patients who are symptomatic should be monitored in an intensive care setting for at least 72 hours. Fluids should be given, and the electrolytes and calcium levels closely monitored. A cardiac monitor should be used because cardiac irregularities are fairly common. Renal and liver functions may need to be checked daily.

The prognosis for patients with severe cardiovascular and pulmonary problems is grave. Those who live for a 3-day period usually recover.

PHOSPHORUS

Available Products

Stearn's Electric Brand Paste

Description

Elemental phosphorus exists in two forms. The red form is insoluble, is not absorbed, and is nontoxic. The yellow (also called white) form is a highly toxic protoplasmic poison and is available as a rat or roach paste.[57] The acute lethal dose has been reported to be approximately 1 mg/kg. Recovery has occurred after ingestions of 1.5 g, and death occurred with exposure to 3 mg in a 2-year-old.

Symptoms have classically been divided into three stages. In stage 1, oral burns, vomiting, stomach pain, garlic-like odor on the breath, and diarrhea may be noted. The feces or vomitus may appear phosphorescent in a darkened room, and hence phosphorus poisoning has been called the *smoking stool syndrome*. Death in stage I has been attributed to ventricular dysrhythmia and cardiovascular collapse. Stage II is a symptom-free period that may last for several weeks. The third stage represents systemic toxicity caused by phosphorus. It affects the GI tract, liver, heart, kidneys, or CNS.[58]

Management

Treatment is directed toward removing and preventing absorption of the phosphorus, as well as symptomatic and supportive care of patients. The extent of the exposure should not be based on the time of onset or seriousness of the initial symptoms. Vomiting is common but should not be interpreted to mean that the stomach is free of phosphorus. Phosphorescent vomitus or stools are diagnostic, but this sign is absent in many cases. Lavage with 1:5000 potassium permanganate or a 2% solution of hydrogen perioxide to oxidize phosphorus to the less harmful phosphate may be useful if begun before onset of symptoms. Mineral oil has been shown in animal studies to decrease the absorption of phosphorus. Administer 200 to 250 after lavage. Digestible oils and fats (e.g., butterfat in milk) should be avoided. Monitor the GI tract, liver, kidneys, heart, and cardiovascular system because these are most commonly affected. Hypoglycemia, hypoprothrombinemia, and clotting abnormalities may be noted with liver damage, and clotting studies should be performed in seriously affected patients. Hypocalcemia has been reported. Early cardiac and CNS disturbances are associated with higher mortality rates.

α-NAPHTHYL-THIOUREA (ANTU)

Available Products

Dr. Hess Anturat, Bantu, Rattrach, Kill Kantz, Krysid, Nott's, Rat-tu, College Brand Rodenticide

Description

ANTU produces pulmonary edema and pulmonary effusion in adult Norway rats. Young Norway rats, roof rats, and most other animals except dogs are resistant to its effects.[1]

Animal studies suggest the lethal dose for humans may be about 4 g/kg. Expected effects following ingestion include vomiting, dyspnea, cyanosis, and pulmonary rales or edema. Fourteen exposures were reported in 1994.

Management

Treatment includes emptying the stomach in large exposures, followed by activated charcoal and a cathartic. Patients should be observed for 72 hours for delayed pulmonary edema. Significant toxicity is not expected for most small ingestions.

NORBROMIDE

Available Products

Shoxin, Raticate

Description

Norbromide is selectively toxic to Norway rats, in whom it acts to produce smooth muscle constriction. Death is a result of intense peripheral vasoconstriction.[59] Other rats, rodents, and animals, including humans, are resistant because they do not have the receptor for this compound in their blood vessels. Human volunteers given 20 to 300 mg had no symptomatic complaints but at the higher doses demonstrated slight decreases in temperature and blood pressure. Lowest values were at 1 hour after ingestion, and values returned to normal by 2 hours.[1]

Management

After large exposures, the stomach should be emptied and activated charcoal given. Treatment, if needed, is symptomatic and supportive.

BARIUM

Available Products

No rodenticides containing barium are sold in the United States.

Description

Barium carbonate is one of several soluble barium salts, including sulfide, chloride, chlorate, and nitrate. All are highly toxic. On the other hand, barium sulfate, an insoluble salt, is harmless and is used in medicine as a radiopaque contrast medium. Rodenticides contain 20% to 25% barium carbonate. The lethal dose is estimated to be 2 g. Acute toxicity may occur with 200 mg.[1]

Barium apparently produces a depolarizing neuromuscular blockade resulting in weakness of striated, cardiac, and smooth muscle. Hypokalemia, often profound, may occur. Symptoms include paresthesias around the mouth; this may spread to the hands and feet. Vomiting and diarrhea with colicky abdominal pain may ensue 1 to 8 hours after ingestion. Tightness in the throat, dysarthria, headache, muscle twitching, general weakness, and paralysis may be noted. Paralysis can range from weakness of one limb to complete paralysis with respiratory failure.[60] Many of the reported cases have resulted from contamination of food. In such cases, the rapidity of onset and absence of eye signs can help rule out botulism.[60]

Management

Treatment should start with emptying the stomach by emesis or lavage unless substantial vomiting has already occurred. Sodium sulfate (30 g in 250 mL of water) should be administered to precipitate the barium as insoluble barium sulfate. Repeat sodium sulfate administration in 1 hour. Monitor patients' fluids and electrolytes. Hypokalemia is common and potassium replacement is often indicated.[61, 62] Observe patients' muscle tone and respiratory status. Mechanical ventilation may be needed in severe cases and can be life saving.

The prognosis is favorable if patients are stabilized and are maintained for 24 hours. Recovery is usually complete.

References

1. Hayes WJ: Pesticides Studied in Man. Baltimore, Williams & Wilkins, 1982.
2. Public Health Study Team: Pest Control and Public Health. Vol 5. Washington, DC, National Academy of Sciences, p 81, 1976.
3. Brekenridge AM, Cholerton S, Hart JAD, et al: A study of the relationship between the pharmacokinetics and the pharmacodynamics of the 4-hydroxycoumarin anticoagulants warfarin, difenacoum and brodifacoum in the rabbit. Br J Pharmacol *84*:81, 1985.
4. Litovitz TL, Feldberg L, Soloway RA, et al: 1994 Annual Report of the American Association of Poison Control Centers Toxic Exposure Surveillance System. Am J Emerg Med *13*:551, 1995.
5. Kaukeinen D: A review of the secondary poisoning hazard potential to wildlife from the use of anticoagulant rodenticides. *In* Proceedings of the 10th Vertebrate Pest Conference, University of California–Davis, p 123, 1982.
6. O'Reilly RA: Anticoagulant, antithrombotic and thrombolytic drugs. *In* Gilman AG, Goodman LA, Rall TW, Murad F: The Pharmacological Basis of Therapeutics. 7th ed. New York, Macmillan, 1985.
7. Jones EC, Growe GH, Naiman SC: Prolonged anticoagulation in rat poisoning. JAMA *252*:3005, 1984.
8. Lipton RA, Klass EM: Human ingestion of a 'superwarfarin' rodenticide resulting in a prolonged anticoagulation effect. JAMA *252*:3004, 1984.
9. Swigar ME, Clemow LP, Saidi P, et al: "Superwarfarin" inges-

tion: A new problem in covert anticoagulant overdose. Gen Hosp Psychiatry *12*:309, 1990.
10. Mack RB: Not all rats have four legs, superwarfarin poisoning. N C Med J *55*:554, 1984.
11. Smolinske SC, Scherger DL, Kearns PS, et al: Superwarfarin poisoning in children: A prospective study. Pediatrics *84*:490, 1989.
12. Lefere JJ, Girot R: Acute cardiovascular collapse during intravenous vitamin K injection. Thromb Haemost *58*:790, 1987.
13. Bjornsson TD, Blaschke TF: Vitamin K_1 disposition and therapy of warfarin overdose. Letter. Lancet *2*:846, 1978.
14. Technical Bulletin: Assault (bromethalin). St. Louis, Purina Mills, 1988.
15. Holmes RW, Love J: Suicide attempt with warfarin, Bishydroxycoumarin-like rodenticide. JAMA *148*:935, 1952.
16. Cherry JT, Gunnoe MD, VanLier RBL: The metabolism of bromethalin and its effects on oxidative phosphorylation and cerebral fluid pressure. Toxicologist *2*:108, 1982.
17. VanLier RBL, Cherry LD: The toxicity and mechanism of toxicity of bromethalin: A new single-feeding rodenticide. Fund Appl Toxicol *11*:664, 1988.
18. Dreikorn BA, O'Doherty OP: The discovery of bromethalin, an acute rodenticide with a unique mode of action. American Chemical Society Symposium Series *255*:45, 1984.
19. Jackson WB, Spaulding SR, VanLier RBL, Dreicorn BA: Bromethalin—a promising new rodenticide. *In* Proceedings of the Material Safety Data Sheet: Bromethalin Concentrate 2%. Indianapolis, Elanco Products Co., 1987.
20. Grant R, Dickerson C: Verbal Communication. St. Louis, Purina Mills, May 1995.
21. Product Information: True Grit Rampage Rat and Mouse Bait. Overland Park, KS, Ceva Laboratories, 1986.
22. Production Information: Quintox Rat and Mouse Bait, Quintox Mouse Seed. Rodent control product and label catalog. Madison, WI, Bell Laboratories, 1985.
23. Paterson CR: Vitamin D poisoning: Survey of causes in 21 patients with hypercalcemia. Lancet *1*:1165, 1980.
24. Haynes RC, Murad F: Agents affecting calcification. *In* Gilman AG, Goodman LS, Rall TW, Murad F: The Pharmacological Basis of Therapeutics. 7th ed. New York, Macillan, 1985.
25. Lukaszkiewicz J, Proszynska K, Lorenc RS: Hepatic microsomal enzyme induction: Treatment of vitamin D poisoning in a 7 month old baby. BMJ *295*:6607, 1987.
26. Prosser PR, Karam JH: Diabetes mellitus following rodenticide ingestion in man. JAMA *239*:1148, 1978.
27. Pont A, Rubino JM, Bishop D, Peal R: Diabetes mellitus and neuropathy following vacor ingestion in man. Arch Intern Med *139*:185, 1979.
28. LeWitt PA: The neurotoxicity of the rat poison vacor. N Engl J Med *301*:73, 1980.
29. LeWitt PA: The rat poison vacor. N Engl J Med *302*:1147, 1980.
30. Egekeze JO, Oehme FW: Sodium monofluoroacetate (SMFA, compound 1080): A literature review. Vet Hum Toxicol *21*:411, 1979.
31. Proctor NH, Hughes JP: Chemical Hazards of the Workplace. Philadelphia, J.B. Lippincott Co., 1978.
32. Kun E: Monofluoroacetic acid (compound 1080), its pharmacology and toxicology. *In* Proceedings of the 10th Vertebrate Pest Conference, University of California–Davis, p 34, 1982.
33. Klaassen CD: Nonmetallic environmental toxicants: Air pollutants, solvents and vapors and pesticides. *In* Gillman AG, Goodman LS, Rall TD, Murad F (eds): The Pharmacological Basis of Therapeutics. 7th ed. New York, Macmillan, 1985.
34. Teitlebaum DT, Ott JE: Acute strychnine intoxication. Clin Toxicol *3*:267, 1970.
35. Edmunds M, Sheehan TMT, Van't-Hoff W: Strychnine poisoning: Clinical and toxicological observations on a non-fatal case. Clin Toxicol *24*:245, 1986.
36. Blain PG, Nightingale S, Stoddart JC: Strychnine poisoning: Abnormal eye movements. J Toxicol Clin Toxicol *19*:215, 1982.
37. Boyd RE, Brennan PT, Deng JF, et al: Strychnine poisoning. Am J Med *74*:507, 1983.
38. Maron BJ, Krupp JR, Tune B: Strychnine poisoning successfully treated with diazepam. J Pediatr *78*:697, 1971.
39. Sgaragli GP, Mannaioni PF: Pharmacokinetic observations on a case of massive strychnine poisoning. Clin Toxicol *6*:533, 1973.
40. Lambert JR, Byrick RJ, Hammeke MD: Management of acute strychnine poisoning. Can Med Assoc J *124*:1268, 1981.
41. Mack RB: Schemes Gang Aft Agley, thallium poisoning. N C Med J *51*:156, 1990.
42. Saddique A, Peterson CD: Thallium poisoning: A review. Vet Hum Toxicol *25*:16, 1983.
43. Moeschlin MD: Thallium poisoning. Clin Toxicol *17*:133, 1980.
44. Nogue S, Mas A, Pares A, et al: Acute thallium poisoning: An evaluation of different forms of treatment. J Toxicol Clin Toxicol *19*:1015, 1982–83.
45. Chamberlain PH, Stavinoha WB, Davis H, et al: Thallium poisoning. Pediatrics *22*:1170, 1958.
46. Reed D, Crawley J, Faro SN, et al: Thallotoxicosis. JAMA *183*:516, 1963.
47. DeBaker W, Zachee P, Verpooten GA, et al: Thallium intoxication treated with combined hemoperfusion-hemodialysis. J Toxicol Clin Toxicol *19*:259, 1982.
48. Gupta S, Ahlawat SK: Aluminum phosphide poisoning–a review. Clin Toxicol *33*:19, 1995.
49. Stephenson JBP: Zinc phosphide poisoning. Arch Environ Health *15*:83, 1967.
50. Wilson R, Lovejoy FH, Jaeger RJ, Landrigan PL: Acute phosphene poisoning aboard a grain freighter. JAMA *244*:148, 1980.
51. Garry VF, Good PF, Manivel C, et al: Investigation of a fatality from nonoccupational aluminum phosphide exposure: Measurement of aluminum in tissue and body fluids as a marker of exposure. J Lab Clin Med *122*:139, 1993.
52. Johnson HD, Voss E: Toxicological studies of zinc phosphide. J Am Pharm Assoc *41*:468, 1952.
53. Rodenberg HD, Chang CC, Watson WA: Zinc phosphide ingestion: A case report and review. Vet Hum Toxicol *31*:559, 1989.
54. Banjaj R, Wasir HS: Epidemic aluminum phosphide poisoning in northern India. Lancet *1*:820, 1988.
55. Jayaraman KS: Death pills from pesticide. Nature *353*:377, 1991.
56. Feldstein A, Heumann M, Barnett M: Fumigant intoxication during transport of grain by railroad. J Occup Med *33*:377, 1991.
57. Simon FA, Pickering LK: Acute yellow phosphorus poisoning. JAMA *235*:1343, 1976.
58. McCarron MM, Trotter AT: Acute yellow phosphorus poisoning from pesticide pastes. Clin Toxicol *18*:693, 1981.
59. Morgan DP: Recognition and Management of Pesticide Poisonings. 3rd ed. Washington, DC, United States Environmental Protection Agency, 1982.
60. Lewi Z, Bar-Khayim Y: Food poisoning from barium carbonate. Lancet *2*:342, 1964.
61. Phelan DM, Hagley SR: Is hypokalemia the cause of paralysis in barium poisoning? BMJ *289*:882, 1984.
62. Bering J: Hypokalemia of barium poisoning. Letter. Lancet *1*:110, 1975.

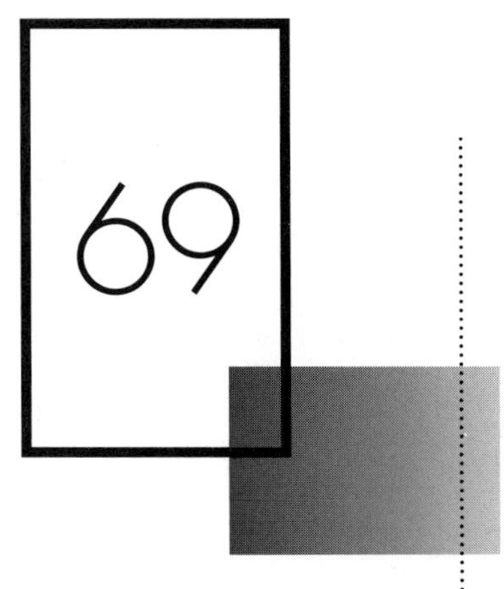

SECTION **G**

INHALATIONAL POISONING AND SOLVENTS

Smoke Inhalation

CHRISTOPHER H. LINDEN, MD

DEFINITIONS

From the perspective of combustion toxicology, smoke is more than just the visible cloud emitted from a material that has been ignited. It is a complex mixture of liquid and solid aerosols, fumes, gases, and vapors resulting from thermal decomposition.[1, 2] Although heat is a prerequisite for smoke production, flame, a zone of gaseous combustion that emits light, is not, and smoke is not always visible.

Thermal decomposition can result from the application of intense heat (pyrolysis) as well as from flaming combustion. Pyrolysis may occur under conditions of relatively low or high oxygen concentrations. Oxidative pyrolysis is commonly referred to as *smoldering*. In most fires, thermal decomposition begins as flaming combustion resulting from the application of an igniting source (e.g., a spark or flame) to a flammable material. As heat is generated and oxygen is consumed, pyrolysis then becomes the dominant process. Of note, more carbon monoxide (CO), a product of incomplete combustion, is evolved during smoldering combustion than during flaming combustion.

HISTORY

Scientific study of combustion toxicology began in 1951, when Zapp, considered to be its founding father, reported that most fire fatalities were caused by smoke inhalation and thermal damage to the respiratory tract rather than by surface burns.[3] This observation has been substantiated by data from many infamous structural fires that occurred in the United States during the 20th century, such as those at the Cleveland Clinic in 1929, the Coconut Grove (Boston) night club in 1942, the Maura County (Tennessee) jail in 1977, the Newport (Kentucky) nightclub in 1978, the Las Vegas MGM Grand and White Plains Stouffers hotels in 1980, and the Las Vegas and Westchase (Houston) Hilton hotels in 1982. In the more recent fires, many victims were discovered in areas were there was no evidence of fire or heat. In some instances, there was also no visible evidence of smoke or soot. These observations emphasize the fact that in enclosed spaces, fatal smoke inhalation can occur without heat, flame, or visible warning.

As early as 1962, differences between the thermal decomposition products of natural and synthetic materials and their toxicities were recognized.[4] However, the fire hazards of now ubiquitous plastics (e.g., polyethylene, polypropylene, polystyrene, polyurethane, polyvinyl chloride, and related polymers), which were introduced during the previous two decades and increasingly used in the construction and furnishing of buildings, were initially minimized by those involved in their manufacture. It was not until after 1972, when the Federal Trade Commission initiated a complaint charging the plastics industry with failing to disclose, misrepresenting, and falsifying evidence, that the combustion toxicity of plastics became public knowledge and serious scientific inquiry commenced.[2] It is now known that plastics are neither nonburning nor self-extinguishing. Compared with natural materials (e.g., cotton, wood, and wool products), plastics spread flame faster, make "flashover" (i.e., the simultaneous ignition of all surfaces of a room or structure, which occurs without the progressive spread of flame when combustible gases are generated) more likely, generate more heat and do so more quickly, generate more and denser visible smoke, and release more toxic and greater amounts of invisible products of thermal decomposition.

In more recent years, the safety of fire retardants has been the focus of study. When added to products (especially plastics), fire retardants make them more difficult to ignite and less likely to propagate flame. Although numerous agents (e.g., antimony oxide; aluminum, boron, bromine, chlorine, molybdenum, and organophosphorus compounds; halogenated polymers) have been developed, a practical but nontoxic fire retardant has yet to be discovered.[1, 2]

COMBUSTION TOXICOLOGY

Thousands of toxic chemicals are known to be generated when materials undergo thermal decomposition. Their identity, amount, and rate of production depend on the nature of the material that is decomposed; the temperature, rate, and mode of decomposition; and the availability of oxygen during decomposition.[5] More than 75 different compounds are released during the thermal decomposition of Douglas fir, and at least 56 are released from polypropylene, 55 from polyethylene, 50 from polyvinyl chloride, and 30 from polystyrene and polyamine.[6–8] Table 69–1 lists the sources and effects of some of the most common and best-characterized products of thermal decomposition that have acute toxicity.[9] It is impossible to predict, however, which toxicants and physical agents will be present at the scene of naturally occurring events with any degree of certainty, because the nature of materials involved and the conditions of thermal degradation are rarely known and may change with time.

Toxic products of thermal decomposition also include a number of carcinogens that represent a potential health hazard to those with chronic exposure to smoke (e.g., blacksmiths, firefighters, foundry workers, and tobacco smokers).[5, 10] All fires generate benzopyrene, the classic chemical initiator of carcinogenesis, as well as hundreds of other polyaromatic hydrocarbons, some of which are known to be promoting agents. Fires involving plastics, especially polyvinyl chloride, can emit acrylonitrile, arsenic, benzene, chromium, and vinyl chloride. Those involving transformers may result in exposure to polychlorinated biphenyls, their polychlorinated dibenzofuran contaminants, and their pyrolysis products (e.g., polychlorinated dibenzofuran, chlorinated biphenylenes, and dioxin). Finally, smoke from wood as well as plastics may contain formaldehyde. All of these products are known or suspected human carcinogens.

An increased incidence of scrotal cancer in chimney sweeps exposed to soot, which is now known to contain polyaromatic hydrocarbons, has long been recognized. Similarly, the increased risk of lung cancer in tobacco smokers is well established. Whether or not those with occupational exposure to smoke are at increased risk for other cancers is extremely controversial.

Table 69–1. Some Acutely Toxic Products of Thermal Decomposition

Agents	Source(s)	Toxic Effect
Chemical Agents		
Acrolein	Acrylics, cellulosics, cotton, polyolefins, polystyrene, paper, wood	Respiratory tract irritation
Aldehydes	Acrylonitrile-butadiene-styrene (ABS), alkyds (polyesters), phenolics, polyalkenes	Respiratory tract irritation
Ammonia	Melamine/phenolic resins, polyamides/polyimides (nylons), silk, wool	Respiratory tract irritation
Carbon monoxide	Incomplete combustion of organic material	Functional anemia, cellular asphyxia
Carbon dioxide	Complete combustion of organic material	Simple asphyxia, narcosis
Carbonyl fluoride	Fluoropolymers (Teflons and related)	Polymer fume fever
Halogen acids (e.g., hydrochloric acid, hydrobromic acid, hydrofluoric acid)	Acrylics, films and resins, fire extinguishers and retardants, vinyls (polyvinyl chloride)	Respiratory tract irritation
Hydrogen Cyanide	Acrylonitriles, melamine resins Polyamides/polyimides (nylons), paper, silk, urethanes, wool	Cellular asphyxia
Isocyanates	Urethanes (foam)	Respiratory tract irritation
Organic acids	Cellulosics, cotton, paper, wood, wool	Respiratory tract irritation
Nitrogen oxides	Cellulosics, paper, petroleum products, wood	Respiratory tract irritation; possible methemoglobinemia
Phosgene	Fire extinguishers and retardants, vinyls (polyvinyl chloride)	Respiratory tract irritation
Styrene	ABS, polystyrene	Respiratory tract irritation
Sulfur oxides	Cellulosics, fur, hair, hides, petroleum products, rubber, wool	Respiratory tract irritation
Unidentified	Aromatic amino and nitroso compounds	Methemoglobinemia
Physical Agents		
Heat/flame	Flaming combustion	Surface burns, laryngotracheitis
Oxygen depletion	Combustion, pyrolysis	Hypoxic asphyxia
Soot	Organic material	Airway obstruction
Steam	Water heated to boiling point	Laryngotracheitis, bronchitis, alveolitis
Trauma	Explosions, falling objects, jumping to safety, structural collapse	Blunt or penetrating injuries

EPIDEMIOLOGY

It is estimated that more than 6000 people die of fire-related injuries each year and that over 80% of the deaths are primarily caused by smoke inhalation rather than surface burns.[1, 2] Some 70% of fatalities result from residential fires. Carelessness with cigarettes, matches, flammable liquids (e.g., fuels and cooking oils), wood stoves, and other heating devices and malfunctioning appliances and heating systems are the underlying causes in most instances. It is also noteworthy that a significant number of fatalities resulting from commercial aircraft crashes are due to smoke inhalation in postcrash fires rather than to injuries sustained on impact.

Eighty per cent of deaths occur within 6 hours of exposure, usually as a result of fulminant pneumonitis. Many victims are unquestionably dead when discovered and do not receive resuscitation attempts. Delayed deaths are primarily due to anoxic brain damage, bacterial pneumonia, and sepsis. Paradoxically, although stricter building codes have made newer structures less likely to catch fire, materials used to make them have become more dangerous when subjected to thermal decomposition. These changes, along with population increases, may account for the fact that despite improvements in medical care, the annual number of fatalities from both surface burns and smoke inhalation is only slightly less than it was 60 years ago.

CLINICAL TOXICOLOGY

CO, heat, and oxygen deficiency are the primary causes of death due to enclosed space fuel fires under experimental conditions.[3] However, the specific toxicants responsible for morbidity and mortality in humans exposed to smoke remain uncertain. Additional causative or contributing factors include cyanide (CN), irritant gases, humidity, particulate matter, carbon dioxide (CO_2), methemoglobinemia, dermal burns, alcohol intoxication, trauma, and underlying cardiovascular or pulmonary disease.

CO is invariably present in smoke, and CO poisoning is thought to be responsible for most prehospital deaths.[11] However, carboxyhemoglobin (COHb) fractions do not always correlate with the severity of inhalation injury,[12–17] and the effects of CO are difficult to separate from those of other causes of asphyxia (discussed later). In one study,[12] 40% of scene fatalities were found to have COHb fractions less than 50%, the fraction generally considered to be evidence of death due to CO poisoning in the forensic literature. Although this definition is disputable, it is clear that in many cases, death cannot be ascribed to CO poisoning alone: In the same study, 20% to 25% had postmortem COHb fractions less than 30% and up to 10% had COHb fractions less than 10%.

In animal studies, the higher the ambient air temperature and humidity, the greater the morbidity and mortality.[18] Exposure to dry air heated to 200°C for 5 minutes or to 125°C for 15 minutes is potentially lethal.[9] Shorter exposures to dry air at temperatures of 350 to 500°C result in tracheitis.[19] Exposure to steam, which has much greater heat capacity, results in bronchitis and pulmonary parenchymal damage in addition to tracheitis at similar temperatures. Respiratory tract injury secondary to heat and humidity is relatively uncommon in human exposures and occurs primarily in those with concomitant surface burns.[20]

Decreased ambient oxygen fractions, which occur as oxygen is progressively consumed during combustion, result in hypoxic asphyxia.[1] At sea level, the normal oxygen fraction is approximately 21%. An acute reduction of the ambient oxygen fraction to 15% to 18% results in dyspnea or exertion; a reduction to 10% to 14% results in dyspnea at rest and impaired mentation; and at fractions of 6% to 8%, loss of consciousness followed by death occurs within 5 to 8 minutes.

Hydrogen cyanide has been implicated as another cause of morbidity and mortality in human smoke inhalation victims. Potentially toxic CN levels have been noted in as many as 30% of survivors and 100% of fatalities, and potentially lethal levels have been reported in as many as 10% of survivors and 70% of fatalities.[17, 21–24] Data are difficult to interpret, however, because the technique and time of blood sampling, storage, and analysis and definitions of potentially toxic and potentially fatal blood CN concentrations vary from study to study. In addition, blood CN levels correlate with both COHb fractions[21, 22] and the severity of inhalation injury,[17, 23, 24] the effects of CN resemble those of other causes of asphyxia, and the effects of CN and CO are probably additive, thus making the contribution of CN difficult to quantify. Finally, the short half-life of CN (approximately 1 hour[21]) suggests that its role in victims who are not dead at the scene is minor.

Irritant gases (see Table 69–1) are corrosive to the mucosal surfaces of the respiratory tract.[9] Ammonia and the halogen acids have high water solubility and tend to dissolve in the moist tissues of the upper airway, where they cause nasopharyngeal, laryngeal, and tracheal inflammation. Other respiratory tract irritants have lower water solubility and travel to the distal respiratory tract, where they cause bronchial, bronchiolar, and alveolar inflammation. Because their concentrations in air and tissues and their effects are difficult to measure directly, the role of irritants in causing morbidity and mortality is based on circumstantial evidence such as clinical manifestations of airway dysfunction and postmortem respiratory tract pathology.

Particulate matter (dust or soot) by itself is relatively inert.[25] Large amounts can cause mechanical airway obstruction. Although this usually occurs at the bronchiolar level (resulting in atelectasis and subsequent pneumonia), in extreme situations (e.g., the Mount Saint Helens volcanic eruption), it can result in upper airway obstruction. More significant, however, is the ability of particulate matter to adsorb toxic gases and liquids and act as vehicle for delivering them to various locations along the respiratory tract. The location at which particulate matter settles depends on its size.[2] Particles smaller than 1 μm reach the alveoli (primarily by diffusion). Those that are 1 to 5 μm settle on tracheal, bronchial, and bronchiolar surfaces (as a result of sedimentation), and those 5 to 30 μm are trapped in the nasopharynx (by inertial impaction). The same is true for aerosolized liquid particles of similar size.

CO_2, along with CO, constitutes most of the gaseous fraction of smoke.[2] CO_2 may result in simple asphyxia by physically displacing oxygen. Increasing blood levels of CO_2 initially stimulate respiration and later cause central nervous system (CNS) depression. As the minute ventilation increases, exposure to smoke increases, resulting in escalating toxicity.

Methemoglobinemia is an infrequently reported complication of smoke inhalation.[26] Whether this is because of infrequent occurrence or infrequent recognition is unclear. The offending toxicants also remain unidentified. Oxides of nitrogen and aromatic amines have been suggested as causes. The effects of methemoglobinemia are similar to those due to other causes of hypoxia, making the relative contribution of this factor to morbidity and mortality difficult to determine. Although COHb fractions are usually also elevated when methemoglobinemia is present, there does not appear to be a direct correlation between the two. Given that the oxygen binding and delivery by hemoglobin are inhibited by both COHb and methemoglobin (MetHb), their combined effects are likely to be additive.

Mortality from smoke inhalation is higher in those with concomitant thermal burns than in those without them.[27] Intoxicating levels of ethanol have been reported in as many as 30% of fatalities, particularly those due to residential fires.[17] By causing impaired mentation and mobility, alcohol may prevent both recognition of and escape from danger. Traumatic injuries due to falling objects, jumping to escape, and structural collapse sometimes contribute to or cause fire-related morbidity and mortality. Underlying cardiovascular disease may increase the risk of cardiac arrhythmias and dysfunction secondary to inhalation injury, toxicants, and emotional and physical stress. It may be a contributing factor in as many as 20% of fatalities.[17] Those with pre-existing pulmonary disease appear to be more susceptible to the respiratory effects of smoke.

PATHOPHYSIOLOGY

Smoke inhalation can be characterized with respect to the mechanism of action of individual toxicants, their physiologic effects, or the course of clinical toxicity after exposure. The pathophysiology of CO poisoning, CN poisoning, and methemoglobinemia is discussed in Chapters 13, 70, and 71. The actions and consequences of exposure to oxygen depletion, particulate matter, and CO_2 are discussed in the previous section.

Heat (hot air and steam) results in thermal burns, and irritant gases cause both thermal and chemical burns. The mucosal surfaces of the eyes and respiratory tract are the target tissues. Effects appear to be mediated by arachidonic acid metabolites (e.g., leukotrienes, prostacyclins, and thromboxanes), cytokines (e.g., platelet-activating factor), free radicals (e.g., superoxide, peroxide, hydroxyl) and activated polymorphonuclear leukocytes.[27] Exposure usually results in tissue inflammation, but ulceration and necrosis can occur in severe cases. Inflammation of the larynx, trachea, bronchi, bronchioles, and alveoli causes edema, bronchospasm, loss of ciliary function, destruction of surfactant, and increased microvascular permeability.[28, 29] Upper and lower airway obstruction, atelectasis, increased shunting (secondary to pulmonary vasoconstriction), loss of lung compliance, and ventilation-perfusion mismatching may ensue.

From a functional perspective, smoke inhalation results in progressive physiologic dysfunction ultimately culminating in death.[30] Regardless of the cause, asphyxia is the underlying mechanism. Asphyxia may be due to inhibition of cellular respiration (e.g., by CO and CN), impaired oxygen transport and delivery (e.g., by COHb and MetHb), central respiratory depression (e.g., by CO, CO_2, and CN), direct or indirect occlusion of air passages (e.g., by the effects of irritant gases, heat, humidity, and soot), or a decreased supply of oxygen (e.g., air rarified by combustion or containing gases that lower the partial pressure of oxygen). There is a direct correlation between the duration of exposure and severity of effects: The longer the exposure, the greater the effect of a given level of exposure. There is also a hyperbolic relationship between the time to effect and the severity of effects and exposure conditions: The greater the exposure, the more rapid and pronounced the effects and vice versa.

Exposure to smoke initially causes incapacitation (cognitive dysfunction) and escape impairment (decreased mobility due to muscle weakness and incoordination). Concomitant inhalation, thermal, and traumatic injuries also limit physical mobility. Impaired vision due to smoke, darkness, and ocular toxicity; physical obstacles such as debris, fire, heat, and slippery surfaces; and underlying conditions such as concurrent alcohol intoxication, extremes of age, disease states, and physical handicaps prolong exposure, resulting in further incapacitation and escape impairment. As the exposure time progresses, physical collapse, loss of consciousness, and death may ensue.

From a temporal standpoint, the clinical course following smoke inhalation can be divided into early, intermediate, and late stages.[31] During the first 36 hours, the systemic effects of CO, CO_2, CN, and MetHb and the airway effects of irritant gases, heat, humidity, and soot predominate. Six hours to 5 days after injury, pulmonary edema may become the most significant clinical problem. This complication is noted in 5% to 30% of hospitalized patients. It can be acute or insidious in onset, progress to fulminant adult respiratory distress syndrome, and is associated with a mortality rate as great as 70%. Pulmonary edema can also occur in patients with extensive cutaneous burns in the absence of significant smoke inhalation. Cerebral edema and the multiple-organ dysfunction syndrome may develop in patients with prolonged or severe hypoxia.

Late manifestations, occurring days to weeks after exposure, include permanent CNS damage (e.g., coma, encephalopathy) due to anoxia, bronchiectasis and subglottic stenosis due to airway injury or its treatment (e.g., endotracheal intubation), and pneumonia and sepsis due to impaired defense mechanisms. Pneumonia is the most common late complication, occurring in 15% to 60% of hospitalized patients.[31] It is usually due to *Staphylococcus aureus* when it occurs early (i.e., within 3 to 4 days of injury) and to gram-negative organisms such as *Enterobacter, Escherichia coli, Klebsiella* and *Pseudomonas* when it occurs later. This complication is associated with a mortality of 50% or higher. Complications associated with prolonged critical illness such as malnutrition, pressure sores, and thromboembolism may also be noted.

Chronic sequelae such as asthma, bronchiolitis obliterans, chronic obstructive pulmonary disease, and pulmonary fibrosis can develop days to years after the original insult.

CLINICAL PRESENTATION

Victims of smoke inhalation usually present with signs and symptoms of respiratory tract injury, systemic toxicity, or both.[31–33] Concomitant surface burns, trauma, and alcohol or drug intoxication may also be noted. Cutaneous burns of more than 15% body surface area, a history of exposure in an enclosed space, an altered level of consciousness, and carbonaceous sputum production are associated with a high incidence of bronchopulmonary injury. Facial and neck burns are associated with a high incidence of both upper and lower respiratory tract injury. It is important to note that respiratory pathology may progressively worsen with time, whereas systemic toxicity is maximal at the time of exposure. Most commonly, smoke inhalation injury causes injury predominantly involving or confined to the lower respiratory tract.

Nonspecific manifestations of airway involvement include cough, dyspnea, tachycardia, tachypnea, and hypoxemia. Some degree of conjunctivitis, lacrimation, pharyngitis, and rhinitis is almost always present. Examination of the nose, mouth, and throat may reveal erythema, edema, or soot. In severe cases, mucosal ulcerations and hemorrhage may be seen. Corneal abrasions are relatively common. Exposure to fire or extreme heat may result in corneal burns or desiccation with superficial sloughing and singed nasal hair. Cyanosis, retractions, and metabolic or respiratory acidosis may occur in severe cases. A decreased ratio of arterial oxygen tension (PO_2) to inspired oxygen fraction (FIO_2) is a sensitive but nonspecific finding that correlates with inhalation injury.

Signs and symptoms of laryngotracheal involvement include drooling, dysphasia, hoarseness, neck pain, retractions, and stridor. Complete obstruction of the upper airway can occur in severe cases. Mucosal edema, erythema, blistering, ulceration, and sloughing; laryngospasm; increased secretions; and soot may be seen on laryngoscopy.[34] Laryngeal, epiglottic, and periglottic edema may be visible on soft tissue neck radiographs. A chest radiograph may reveal tracheal narrowing. A saw-toothed or plateau pattern of the inspiratory curve and an expiratory-inspiratory ratio greater than one may be seen on flow-volume loop measurements.[35]

Complaints and physical findings in patients with lower respiratory tract injury include chest burning or tightness, carbonaceous sputum production, rhonchi, rales, and wheezing. Rales or crackles may be localized (e.g., from atelectasis) or diffuse (e.g., from pneumonitis or pulmonary edema). Fever and leukocytosis may accompany atelectasis and pneumonitis. When they occur within 2 days of exposure, these complications, rather than infection, are the likely cause. In symptomatic patients without auscultatory abnormalities, bedside pulmonary function testing often reveals evidence of obstructive disease such as decreased peak expiratory flow rate, forced expiratory volume in the first second, and forced vital capacity.[36] An increased expiratory-inspiratory ratio on flow-volume loop measurement is even more sensitive in detecting increases in small airway resistance. Formal spirometry may reveal a restrictive pattern due to decreased lung compliance in patients with parenchymal damage. Bronchoscopy may reveal mucosal injury similar to that described earlier.[37, 38] Crusts, casts, and plugs (mucus or soot) may be present. A chest radiograph may reveal peribronchial cuffing (due to airway edema) and patchy or diffuse infiltrates (due to atelectasis, pneumonitis, or pulmonary edema).[39, 40] It may appear normal, however, when obtained soon after exposure.[15, 36] Radionuclide ventilation-perfusion imaging may show segmental delayed washout (retention of gas for more than 90 seconds) in areas of small airway obstruction before abnormalities appear on plain films.[36, 41] Unventilated areas on lung scanning and decreased CO_2 diffusing capacity usually indicate parenchymal injury but can also be seen with severe airway obstruction.

Systemic toxicity resulting from tissue hypoxia and hypercarbia is manifested primarily by CNS and cardiovascular dysfunction. Nausea, vomiting, and diarrhea may also be noted. CNS effects range from agitation, anxiety, confusion, dizziness, and transient loss of consciousness to coma with seizures or abnormal posturing. Headache is a prominent, sensitive, and relatively specific manifestation of CO poisoning. It can, however, be present in CN poisoning and with methemoglobinemia. In comatose patients, a decreased density differential between gray and white matter indicative of cerebral edema may be noted on computed tomography of the head. Cardiovascular manifestations may include dysrhythmias, heart failure, hypotension, and myocardial ischemia or infarction. Patients with underlying cardiovascular disease are especially susceptible to these complications.

Findings that are relatively uncommon yet specific to CO poisoning include retinal hemorrhages and cherry-red skin color. Lack of a color difference between retinal arterioles and venules (i.e., an equally red appearance) has been described in CN poisoning. An elevated plasma lactate concentration (>10 mEq/L) correlates with the presence of high blood CN levels.[21] However, lactic acidosis invariably accompanies severe or prolonged tissue hypoxia or shock regardless of the underlying cause. Cyanosis due to methemoglobinemia usually appears more gray or brown than that due to hypoxia, and blood containing a high MetHb fraction has a milk-chocolate color.

The COHb fraction is elevated in virtually all patients with significant signs and symptoms of either inhalation injury or systemic toxicity. COHb fractions correlate with clinical toxicity only after relatively brief exposures (see Chapter 70). The longer the exposure, the greater the toxicity at a given COHb fraction.[30] CN levels may also be elevated, particularly in patients with significant CNS and cardiovascular dysfunction. Significant methemoglobinemia appears to be rare.

DIAGNOSTIC EVALUATION

The history should include details of exposure, symptoms, condition and treatment before arrival, and past medical history. If details cannot be obtained from the patient, rescuers or other witnesses should be questioned. The nature of the material that generated the smoke (e.g., natural or synthetic); the presence or absence of flame, heat, steam, or explosion; a description of the smoke (e.g., density, color, odor); and the duration of exposure and the time elapsed since exposure should be noted. Of particular importance is whether the exposure occurred indoors or out in the open. The possibility of concomitant drug or alcohol use, trauma, and attempted arson, murder, or suicide should also be explored. How and where a comatose victim was found may provide valuable clues. Firefighters should be asked about mask use, its fit and functioning, and its method of oxygen delivery (e.g., by demand valve or by continuous positive pressure). Exposure to invisible gases may occur when they remove their masks after a fire has been extinguished (e.g., during the clean-up or cool-down period). The duration and intensity of exertion, the type and amount of protective gear, and environmental conditions may suggest the possibility of dehydration and hypothermia or hyperthermia.

The nature of symptoms at the time of exposure or discovery as well as at the time of arrival is important in assessing the severity of an exposure. Altered mental status, collapse, or syncope at the scene suggests CO or CN poisoning. These diagnoses may be overlooked if oxygen is administered in the field or delayed presentation has resulted in clinical improvement by the time of arrival. Cyanosis unresponsive to oxygen, particularly in a patient without respiratory distress, suggests methemoglobinemia. The presence of pre-existing disease must be considered when interpreting clinical events and determining disposition and treatment.

Vital signs should be carefully evaluated. Particular attention should be given to the respiratory rate. Body temperature should be measured as soon as possible for all patients. In critically ill patients (i.e., those at greater risk of having hyperthermia or hypothermia), this vital sign is often not measured until very late in the evaluation. The physical examination should first focus on assessing the patency of the airway and adequacy of respirations. The cardiovascular stability, CNS function (mental status as well as level of consciousness), and skin color and integrity should then be evaluated. A trauma survey should be included in the evaluation of those with a history of trauma or altered mental status. Patients with respiratory symptoms must be frequently reevaluated for signs of upper airway obstruction, hypoxia, and hypercapnea. Those with abnormal vital signs, altered mental status, hypoxemia, hypercapnea, chest pain, or respiratory distress should have continuous cardiac monitoring. Those who are unable to respond verbally or who have eye complaints should have an ophthalmologic examination that includes funduscopy and fluorescein evaluation of the cornea.

Oxygen saturation measured by ear or finger pulse oximetry (Spo_2) should be considered a fifth vital sign and obtained in all patients. The oxygen saturation value measured by this method may be falsely elevated and near normal when COHb and MetHb are present. Hence, unless the history suggests trivial exposure and the patient is asymptomatic and has normal results on physical examination, a COHb fraction should also be measured. Patients who have cyanosis despite normal vital signs and an Spo_2 greater than 90% should have a MetHb fraction measured. In those who are awake and who have mild respiratory symptoms and normal cardiopulmonary findings, venous blood, placed in a heparinized arterial blood gas collection syringe, can be used instead of an arterial sample for measuring COHb and MetHb fractions.[41]

Patients with abnormal mental status, respiratory distress, and abnormal findings on auscultation should be additionally assessed for acid-base disturbances and hypercapnea by formal arterial blood gas analysis. Calculation of the $Po_2/F{\rm IO}_2$ ratio may also be helpful. If COHb and MetHb fractions cannot readily be measured, a decreased oxygen saturation measured directly by co-oximetry in conjunction with a normal Po_2 (and hence normal calculated oxygen saturation) suggests the diagnosis of either CO poisoning or methemoglobinemia. The difference between the calculated and measured oxygen saturation can be used to estimate the fraction of CO or methemoglobin. If metabolic (lactic) acidosis is present, the COHb and MetHb fractions are not elevated, and the Po_2 is normal, CN poisoning should be suspected. Unexplained coma and refractory hypotension also suggest CN poisoning. Although CN levels are not widely or readily measurable and results usually are not known in time to alter therapy, obtaining a blood CN level may retrospectively confirm the diagnosis.

Patients with nonspecific respiratory symptoms should have bedside pulmonary function testing. These tests may reveal evidence of pulmonary pathology despite a normal Spo_2 and normal findings on physical examination. Those who have persistent symptoms and who are otherwise found to be normal should be referred for comprehensive pulmonary function testing.

The evaluation of patients who have upper respiratory tract signs and symptoms and who do not have respiratory distress or other indications for immediate endotracheal intubation is best accomplished by fiberoptic laryngoscopy. Alternatively, soft tissue radiographs of the neck and flow volume loop spirometry can be used to detect upper airway narrowing.

Patients with hypoxemia, respiratory distress, abnormal lung sounds, or altered mental status should have a chest radiograph and electrocardiogram. Those with chest pain, hypertension, palpitations, an abnormal cardiac rhythm, or a history of cardiopulmonary disease should also have an electrocardiogram.[41]

Bronchoscopy can be performed to assess the lower airways. It is more commonly used for therapeutic rather than for diagnostic purposes (discussed later). The possibility of occult alcohol or drug intoxication and trauma should also be considered in those with abnormal mental status or vital signs. Depending on the history and clinical presentation, toxicology testing and computed tomography of the head or abdomen may be indicated. Women who are of childbearing age and who have findings suggestive of significant smoke exposure, particularly those with elevated COHb fractions, should have a pregnancy test.

TREATMENT

In the event that a call for help comes from someone trapped in a burning building and rescue attempts are already in progress, advise the victim to feel the top of any door and the doorknob before opening it. If either is hot, the door should not be opened. If escape is possible but smoke is present, the victim should crawl to safety or stay close to the floor. Stairwells rather than elevators should be used for exiting.

If escape is not possible, then towels and blankets should be used to seal doorways and keep out smoke. If the victim is above the second floor, he or she should be advised to open a window, but only enough to signal rescuers (e.g., by hanging out a sheet) and obtain fresh air. If the room is smoky, placing a wet blanket over one's head and connecting it to the window opening is recommended.

Patients who have escaped and have been or remain symptomatic should be advised to seek immediate medical attention. The mode of transportation recommended depends on the severity of symptoms and a patient's underlying health status. Those who report moderate or severe symptoms, are very young or elderly, or have a history of cardiovascular or pulmonary disease should be advised to call an ambulance.

Prehospital care should begin with the prompt but safe removal of the patient from the smoky environment. Unless emergency medical personnel are equipped with respiratory, eye, and skin protection, rescue is best left to firefighters. Rescuers should never enter potentially hazardous environments without such protection. Basic and advanced cardiac and trauma life support measures should be instituted as necessary. All patients should receive supplemental oxygen. Decontamination measures such as irrigation of the eyes and skin may also be indicated. Blankets should be provided if clothing removal is necessary.

Indications for immediate endotracheal intubation include respiratory distress with signs or symptoms of upper airway obstruction, cyanosis or hypoxia ($Spo_2 < 90\%$ or $Po_2 < 60$ mm Hg) despite maximal oxygen therapy by nonrebreathing mask, respiratory depression (respiratory rate < 12/min or $Pco_2 > 50$ mm Hg), pulmonary edema, altered or depressed mental status, and full-thickness burns of the face or neck.[31, 33, 34] Early endotracheal intubation should also be considered for patients who have less severe injury but who do not improve with treatment. The largest possible endotracheal tube size should be used so that bronchoscopy can be performed if necessary. If hypoxia, respiratory failure, or pulmonary edema is the only problem, continuous positive airway pressure (CPAP or BiPAP) by mask may obviate the need for endotracheal intubation.[42] Blind nasal intubation or use of a fiberoptic laryngoscope or bronchoscope may be helpful in those with constricting perioral or neck burns and airway edema if direct visualization of the larynx is impossible. If the history or physical examination suggests the possibility of head or neck trauma, cervical spine injury precautions should be taken until radiographs preclude this possibility.

After intubation, the airway should be suctioned aggressively to remove secretions and inhaled debris. Oxygen should be humidified to prevent drying of secretions. Positive end-expiratory pressure at 5 to 10 cm of water should be routinely administered to prevent or treat atelectasis.[31] Higher pressures may be necessary for patients who remain hypoxic despite administration of 100% oxygen. Bronchoscopy is also indicated for intubated patients because it allows for more effective and directed removal of bronchial secretions. It may be especially useful in patients with lobar atelectasis or focal infiltrates on chest radiographs. For those with inspissated mucus plugs or bronchial casts, repeated bronchoscopy may be necessary. Although bronchoscopy can be used for the diagnosis of smoke inhalation, the prognostic value of abnormal findings remains controversial.[43] Hence, performing bronchoscopy solely for this purpose is not indicated. Tracheostomy should be reserved for those who require prolonged intubation (3 weeks or more) because it is associated with significant complications and increased mortality.[44] Chest physiotherapy and postural drainage may also be helpful.

Inhaled (aerosolized) racemic epinephrine may be beneficial for patients who have upper airway signs and symptoms but who do not require immediate endotracheal intubation. Such patients must be carefully monitored for deterioration. If laryngoscopy reveals upper airway pathology and the patient fails to improve with treatment, prophylactic intubation should be considered.

Inhaled and parenteral bronchodilators (e.g., β_2-adrenergic agonists) should be administered to patients with wheezing. Incentive spirometry and encouragement of coughing may also be helpful.

Corticosteroids are of potential benefit for laryngeal edema and small airways dysfunction. They may also be useful in the treatment of cerebral edema, irritant-induced bronchiolitis obliterans, and postextubation stridor. However, corticosteroids may increase mortality from infection, particularly in patients with pulmonary parenchymal injury and surface burns.[45] In patients with both airway and parenchymal pathology or burn injury, a single large dose of corticosteroid administered at the time of presentation is recommended. The risks of corticosteroids must be weighed against their benefits when deciding whether or not to continue therapy. Reserving subsequent doses for those with severe upper airway obstruction and refractory wheezing is suggested.

Positive pressure ventilation with positive end-expiratory pressure (PEEP) is the treatment of choice for pulmonary edema.[46] Complications include decreased cardiac output and pulmonary barotrauma. High-frequency ventilation may reduce the incidence of pneumonia and decrease mortality.[47] Arteriovenous or venovenous extracorporeal membrane oxygenation (ECMO) should be considered for patients with hypoxemia refractory to other measures.

Burn victims with concomitant inhalation injury may require more fluids for circulatory support than those without such injury.[47] However, excessive fluid resuscitation may worsen pulmonary dysfunction and should be avoided. Similarly, both fluid restriction and diuretics are ineffective and potentially dangerous, particularly in those with surface burns or shock. Hence, the goal of fluid therapy should be to maintain normal cardiac output. Swan-Ganz catheterization with hemodynamic monitoring may be necessary to optimize such therapy.

Experimental evidence suggests that administration of nonsteroidal anti-inflammatory drugs, inhaled nitric oxide, endotracheal fluorocarbons, and hyperbaric oxygen (HBO) may be beneficial in the treatment of pneumonitis and pulmonary edema. Other anti-inflammatory agents, antioxidants, and free radical scavengers are being investigated. Of the nonsteroidal agents, ibuprofen seems to be the most effective.[48] HBO can also be effective in treating CO poisoning, CN poisoning, cerebral edema, and thermal burns.[49] It should also be considered for patients with refractory hypoxemia. In such patients, however, HBO may not be effective for treating CO or CN poisoning unless a high Po_2 level can be achieved; management of the pulmonary injury may take precedence over transfer for HBO. Indications for its use in these conditions remain controversial.

CO poisoning and methemoglobinemia should generally be treated according to usual guidelines (see Chapters 13 and 70). The treatment of CN poisoning (see Chapter 71) in victims of smoke inhalation is controversial. Although sodium thiosulfate and hydroxycobalamin can be given safely, an effective formulation of hydroxycobalamin is not yet available in the United States, and nitrites, which induce methemoglobinemia, could be harmful in patients with hypoxemia or elevated COHb fractions. Hence, it is recommended that nitrites be reserved for those *in extremis* or those who remain critically ill with persistent coma, seizures, cardiac dysrhythmias, shock, and lactic acidosis despite intubation and 100% oxygen.[50] Because HBO therapy provides enough dissolved oxygen to sustain life in the absence of hemoglobin and obviates concerns over the use of nitrites, it has also been suggested that nitrites be withheld until after HBO therapy has been begun. However, the short half-life of CN and the length of time usually required to arrange for HBO therapy makes it unlikely that nitrites will be necessary or effective in those who survive long enough to receive HBO therapy.

Antibiotic therapy should be reserved for patients with documented infection. Prophylactic use of antibiotics is of no benefit and may foster the development of infection by drug-resistant organisms. The choice of agent should be guided by the results of sputum Gram's stain, culture, and sensitivity.

In patients with fever and leukocytosis persisting or developing more than 2 days after exposure, empirical therapy with an agent effective against *S. aureus* (e.g., cefazolin or nafcillin) as well as gram-negative bacteria including *Pseudomonas* (e.g., gentamicin, cefotaxime, or ticarcillin) can be initiated if laboratory results are not immediately available.

Patients who are asymptomatic on arrival or who become asymptomatic with oxygen therapy alone can be discharged if they have normal findings on physical examination and ancillary testing. Those with mild symptoms and minor abnormalities on evaluation can also be discharged if they are otherwise healthy and their condition is stable. Depending on clinical findings, a 1- to 6-hour period of observation is recommended before discharge. All discharged patients should be instructed to call or return immediately if symptoms develop or recur. Patients who do not meet discharge criteria should be admitted for observation or treatment. Depending on the nature and severity of injury and the presence or absence of pre-existing disease, a floor bed, telemetry unit, or critical care unit may be appropriate. Critically ill patients are best managed at an adult or pediatric tertiary care facility or burn center and should be transferred if such services are not available. Patients with severe CO poisoning are candidates for HBO therapy. However, because HBO treatment centers do not necessarily provide adult or pediatric intensive care or burn services, the nature and severity of other injuries must be considered when deciding if transfer for HBO therapy is appropriate.

References

1. Landrock AH: Handbook of Plastics Flammability and Combustion Toxicology. Park Ridge, NJ, Noyes Publications, 1983.
2. Gad SC, Anderson RC: Combustion Toxicology. Boca Raton, FL, CRC Press, 1990.
3. Zapp JA: The Toxicology of Fire. Medical Division Special Report No. 4. Aberdeen, MD, U.S. Army Chemical Center, 1951.
4. Zapp JA: Toxic and health effects of plastics and resins. Arch Environ Health *4*:335, 1962.
5. Kaplan HL, Grand AF, Hartzell GE: Combustion Toxicology: Principles and Test Methods. Lancaster, PA, Technomic Publishing Co., 1983.
6. Autian J: Toxicologic aspects of flammability and combustion of polymeric materials. J Fire Flam *1*:239, 1970.
7. Packham SC, Hartzell GE: Fundamentals of combustion toxicology in fire hazard assessment. J Test Eval *9*:341, 1981.
8. Mitera J, Michal J: The combustion products of polymeric materials, II: GC - MS analysis of the combustion products of polyethylene, polypropylene, polystyrene, and polyamide. Fire Mater *9*:11, 1985.
9. Terril JB, Montgomery RR, Reinhardt CF: Toxic gases from fires. Science *200*:1343, 1978.
10. Morse LH, Pasternak G, Fujimoto G: Toxic hazards of firefighters. *In* Sullivan JB, Drieger GR (eds): Hazardous Materials Toxicology: Clinical Principles of Environmental Health. Baltimore, Williams & Wilkins, pp 454–550, 1992.
11. Anderson RA, Watson AA: Fire deaths in the Glasgow area II: The role of carbon monoxide. Med Sci Law *21*:288, 1981.
12. Birky MM, Halpin BM, Caplan YH, et al: Fire fatality study. Fire Mater *3*:211, 1979.
13. Zikria BA, Weston GC, Chodoff M, et al: Smoke and carbon monoxide poisoning in fire victims. J Trauma *12*:641, 1972.
14. Zarem HA, Rattenborg CC, Harmel MH: Carbon monoxide toxicity in human fire victims. Arch Surg *107*:851, 1973.
15. Clark WR, Bonaventura M, Myers W: Smoke inhalation and airway management at a regional burn unit: 1975–1983. Part I: Diagnosis and consequences of smoke inhalation. J Burn Care Rehabil *10*:52, 1989.
16. Shusterman D, Alexeff G, Hargis C, et al: Predictors of carbon monoxide and hydrogen cyanide exposure in smoke inhalation patients. Clin Toxicol *34*:61, 1996.
17. Halpin BM, Berl WG: Human fatalities from unwanted fires. Fire J *73*:105, 1979.
18. Stone HH: Respiratory burns: A correlation of clinical and laboratory results. Ann Surg *165*:157, 1967.
19. Moritz AR, Henriques FC, McLean R: The effects of inhaled heat on the air passages and lungs. Am J Pathol *21*:311, 1945.
20. Fein A, Leff A, Hopewell PC: Pathophysiology and management of complications resulting from fire and the inhaled products of combustion. Crit Care Med *8*:94, 1980.
21. Baud FJ, Barriot P, Toffis V, et al: Elevated blood cyanide concentrations in victims of smoke inhalation. N Engl J Med *325*:1761, 1991.
22. Anderson RA, Harland WA: Fire deaths in the Glasgow area III: The role of hydrogen cyanide. Med Sci Law *22*:35, 1982.
23. Birky MM, Clark FB: Inhalation of toxic products from fires. Bull N Y Acad Med *57*:997, 1981.
24. Clark CJ, Campbell D, Reid WH: Blood carboxyhemoglobin and cyanide levels in fire survivors. Lancet *1*:1332, 1981.
25. Zikria BA, Ferrer JM, Floch HF: The chemical factors contributing to pulmonary damage. Surgery *71*:704, 1972.
26. Hoffman RS, Santer D: Methemoglobinemia resulting from smoke inhalation. Vet Hum Toxicol *31*:168, 1989.
27. Traber DI, Linares HA, Herndon DN: The pathophysiology of inhalation injury—a review. Burns *14*:357, 1988.
28. Clark WR, Nieman GF: Smoke inhalation. Burns *14*:473, 1988.
29. Kinsella J: Smoke inhalation: The James Ellsworth Laing prize-winning essay for 1988. Burns *14*:269, 1988.
30. Hartzell GF, Packham SC, Switzer WG: Toxic products from fires. Am Ind Hyg Assoc J *44*:248, 1983.
31. Herndon DN, Thompson PB, Traber DL: Pulmonary injury in burned patients. Crit Care Clin *1*:79, 1985.
32. Mosley S: Inhalation injury: A review of the literature. Heart Lung *17*:3, 1988.
33. Clark WR: Smoke Inhalation: Diagnosis and treatment. World J Surg *16*:24, 1992.
34. Haponik EF, Summer WR: Respiratory complications in burned patients: Diagnosis and management of inhalation injury. J Crit Care *2*:121, 1987.
35. Haponik EF, Munster AM, Wise RA, et al: Upper airway function in burn patients: Correlation of flow volume curves and nasopharyngoscopy. Am Rev Respir Dis *129*:251, 1984.
36. Whitener DR, Whitener LM, Robertson J, et al: Pulmonary function measurements in patients with thermal injury and smoke inhalation. Am Rev Respir Dis *122*:731, 1980.
37. Hunt JL, Agee RN, Pruitt BA: Fiberoptic bronchoscopy in acute inhalation injury. J Trauma *15*:641, 1975.
38. Robinson L, Miller RH: Smoke inhalation injuries. Am J Otolaryngol *7*:375, 1986.
39. Lee MJ, O'Connell DJ: The plain chest radiograph after acute smoke inhalation. Clin Radiol *39*:33, 1988.
40. Peitzman AB, Shires GT, Teixidor S, et al: Smoke inhalation injury: Evaluation of radiographic manifestations and pulmonary dysfunction. J Trauma *29*:1232, 1989.
41. Moylan JA, Wilmore DW, Mouton DE, et al: Early diagnosis of inhalation injury using ^{133}xenon lung scan. Ann Surg *176*:477, 1972.
42. Davies LK, Poulton TJ, Modell JH: Continuous positive airway pressure is beneficial in treatment of smoke inhalation. Crit Care Med *11*:726, 1983.
43. Bingham HG, Gallagher TJ, Powell MD: Early bronchoscopy as a predictor of ventilatory support for burned patients. J Trauma *27*:1286, 1987.
44. Lund T, Goodwin CW, McManus WF, et al: Upper airway sequelae in burn patients requiring endotracheal intubation or tracheostomy. Ann Surg *201*:304, 1985.
45. Robinson NB, Hudson LD, Riem M, et al: Steroid therapy following isolated smoke inhalation injury. J Trauma *22*:876, 1982.
46. Cox CS, Zwischenberger JB, Traber DL, et al: Immediate positive pressure ventilation with positive end expiratory pressure (PEEP) improves survival in ovine smoke inhalation. J Trauma *33*:821, 1992.
47. Pruitt BA, Cioff WG, Shimazu T, et al: Evaluation and management of patients with inhalation injury. J Trauma *30*:563, 1990.
48. Shinozawa Y, Hales C, Jung W, et al: Ibuprofen prevents synthetic smoke-induced pulmonary edema. Am Rev Respir Dis *134*:1145, 1986.
49. Hart GB, Strauss MB, Lennon PA, et al: Treatment of smoke inhalation by hyperbaric oxygen. J Emerg Med *3*:211, 1985.
50. Kulig K: Cyanide antidotes and fire toxicology. N Engl J Med *325*:1801, 1991.

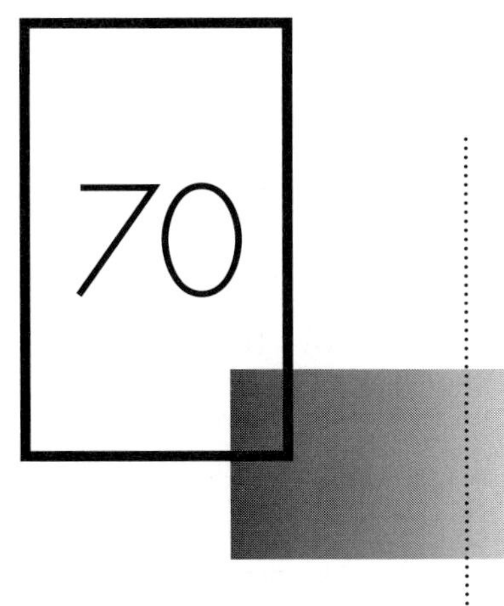

Carbon Monoxide Poisoning

ROBERT BARTLETT, MD

Imagine for a moment that you are in a busy emergency department on a cold winter day. As you make your rounds, you talk with a gentleman complaining of "stress headaches" that are associated with work, then another man who reports a history of chronic angina that is suddenly worse for no apparent reason. You stop to recheck the intoxicated patient who was found passed out in a parked car several hours ago and is still not arousable but has a blood alcohol level of only 200 mg/dL. Later in the day, a family of four returns for the second visit this month complaining of the "flu," which they describe as myalgias, headache, vomiting, and malaise. They mention casually that several other families in the same apartment complex also have the flu. All preceding scenarios are possible presentations for carbon monoxide (CO) poisoning.

Because CO causes the most common form of poisoning in the United States and other industrial countries, it is important to be familiar with this substance. From 1979 to 1988, approximately 56,000 death certificates implicated CO as a primary or contributing cause of death, and thousands more suffered nonlethal consequences of exposure to this pervasive toxin.[1] It is estimated that approximately 10,000 workdays are lost secondary to CO poisoning.[2] Many patients are unwitting victims. Oil and gas home heating can be a common source of CO, but living in a warmer climate does not necessarily change the attack rate. As Figure 70–1 illustrates, the attack rate in Maine is the same as in Florida.

In its pure form, CO is undetectable. It is colorless, odorless, and nonirritating. The specific gravity of CO is 0.97 relative to air, and thus it disperses easily and does not stratify. The gas is produced whenever incomplete oxidation of a carbon-containing compound occurs. Table 70–1 lists many sources for CO; several deserve special mention. For instance, it is a common misconception that propane-powered vehicles produce only carbon dioxide and water. All produce moderate amounts of CO, and because proper maintenance is costly and compliance with maintenance schedules is usually poor, the CO production may be considerably higher than the manufacturer's specifications. This can be further compounded by poor ventilation. The operation of gas-powered equipment outdoors does not guarantee adequate ventilation either, because several case reports have described individuals who suffered from CO poisoning when working close to equipment outdoors. Methylene chloride (dichloromethane) is a very interesting source because it is metabolized to CO. This compound, which can be inhaled or absorbed transdermally, is common in the paint industry and is present commercially in many paint strippers, hydrocarbon solvents, and some spray paints. Once it is absorbed, the CO half-life can be very long owing to ongoing metabolism, and persons thus exposed continue to produce CO for hours. Finally, some CO is always being produced internally through the breakdown of hemoglobin, and carboxyhemoglobin (COHb) levels may be elevated physiologically (4% to 6%) in the setting of hemolytic anemia.

PHARMACOLOGY

Hemoglobin Impairment

The classic theory of CO poisoning was one of "transport hypoxia." In 1895, Haldane first demonstrated that CO combined with hemoglobin to form

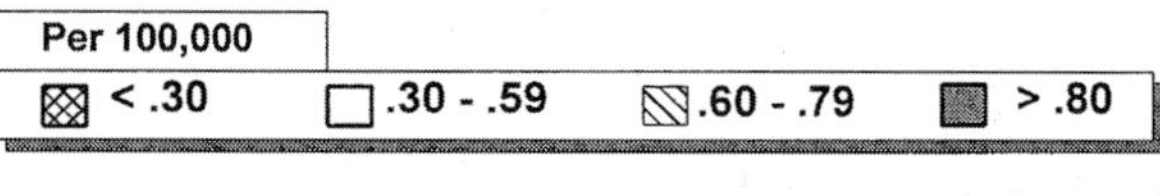

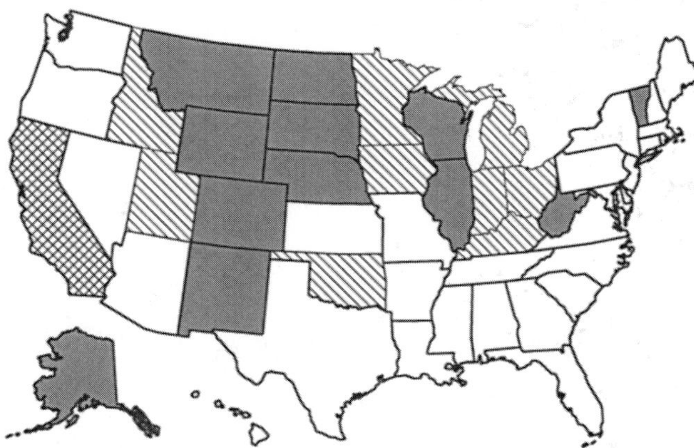

Figure 70–1. Incidence of carbon monoxide-related deaths during a 10-year period. (From Cobb N, Etzel RA: Unintentional carbon monoxide related deaths in the United States, 1979 through 1988. JAMA *266*:659–663, 1991.)

COHb, which had a diminished capacity for oxygen transport. The affinity of CO for hemoglobin oxygen receptor sites is 240 times greater than that of oxygen. The occupation of oxygen transport sites results in tissue hypoxia. Blood normally contains 20 volumes per cent (vol%) of oxygen, and at rest the *average* extraction is approximately 5 vol%. Among organs, the brain and heart extract the greatest volumes of oxygen, 6 vol% and 11 vol%, respectively, and the high demand for oxygen by these organs partially explains why they are so commonly affected.

The molecular structure of hemoglobin is characterized as a tetramer with four oxygen-binding sites. The fixation of CO at any one of these sites increases the oxygen affinity of the remaining sites, thereby interfering with the proper unloading or release of oxygen in the peripheral tissues. This enhanced affinity and impaired unloading of oxygen is referred to as the *Haldane effect* and is demonstrated graphically as a shift to the left of the oxyhemoglobin dissociation curve. To appreciate the clinical significance, consider the following. A healthy person with 14 g of hemoglobin releases on average 5 vol% of oxygen at a tissue partial pressure of oxygen (Po_2) of 40 mm Hg. With only 7 g of hemoglobin (50% of normal), a much lower tissue Po_2 is required (27 mm Hg) to draw 5 vol% of oxygen. Because a patient with a COHb level of 50% has a high-affinity, left-shifted oxygen dissociation curve, a tissue Po_2 of 14 mm Hg is required to draw off 5 vol% of oxygen. Assuming no other compensatory mechanisms, this level of hypoxemia is extremely dangerous, because cells subject to acute hypoxia usually require a minimum oxygen pressure of 20 mm Hg (Fig. 70–2). If the patient has sufficient cardiac reserve, an increased cardiac output can partially compensate for the impaired release of oxygen and improve tissue Po_2.

Table 70–1. Sources of Carbon Monoxide

Propane-powered engines	Kerosene heaters
Natural gas appliances	Hibachi grills
Automobile exhaust	Paint strippers
Portable generators	Spray paints
Gas log fireplaces	

Although the classic theory accounted for some of the clinical phenomena, many clinical observations could not be accounted for using this paradigm. For example, the classic theory of CO poisoning would predict that a patient with 14 g of hemoglobin and a 50% COHb level should have the same functional capacity as a person with only 7 g of hemoglobin. In reality, a patient with 50% COHb is often obtunded or possibly comatose, whereas a patient with an acute anemia and only 7 g of hemoglobin may be alert and may complain only of some weakness. Other mechanisms clearly are at work.

To clarify further the pathophysiology of CO poisoning, Goldbaum and colleagues[54] designed a dog model that compared the outcome of three different groups. Group 1 dogs were allowed to breathe spontaneously 13% CO in room air for 15 minutes and developed COHb levels ranging from 54% to 73% (an average of approximately 65%). All of these animals died within an hour of breathing the CO gas. Group 2 were rendered anemic through venesection, with simultaneous volume replacement using a mixture of lactated Ringer's solution and dextran 70. Their hemoglobin content was reduced by an average of 68% (range, 65 to 73%). All of these animals lived. Group 3 dogs were reduced to the same anemic state as group 2 but were transfused with COHb red blood cells to replenish their red blood cell mass to normal and, producing an average COHb level of 60%, survived. Several inferences can be drawn. First, animals that are spontaneously breathing CO have a higher total body content because of the redistribution of plasma dissolved CO. Second, it would appear that the redistributed "tissue" CO is toxic. Third, the introduction of CO that is already fixed or "chelated" to hemoglobin is relatively nontoxic despite the functional reduction of oxygen-carrying capacity. Fourth, a comparable loss of hemoglobin transport capacity through hemorrhage is not fatal. In summary, this experiment demonstrated that the creation of COHb has a minor role in the pathogenesis of CO poisoning.

Myoglobin Impairment

Chemically, CO has a significant affinity for all iron- or copper-containing proteins and competes with oxygen for the active sites. Representative metalloproteins include myoglobin, cytochrome C oxidase, and cytochrome P-450 oxidase. After hemoglobin, myoglobin is the second most plentiful hemoprotein in the body and functions as a short-term oxygen reservoir. In addition, myoglobin appears to

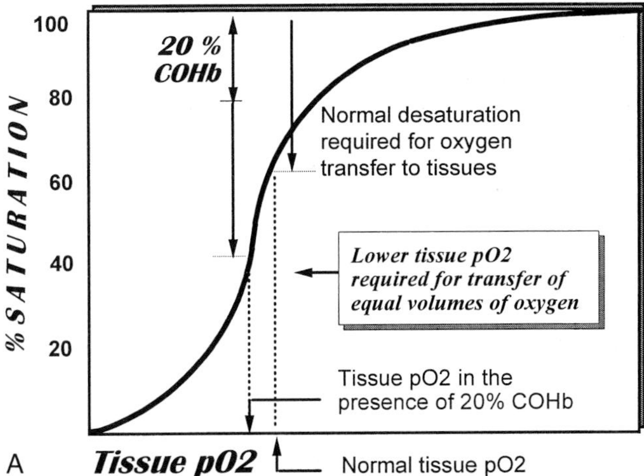

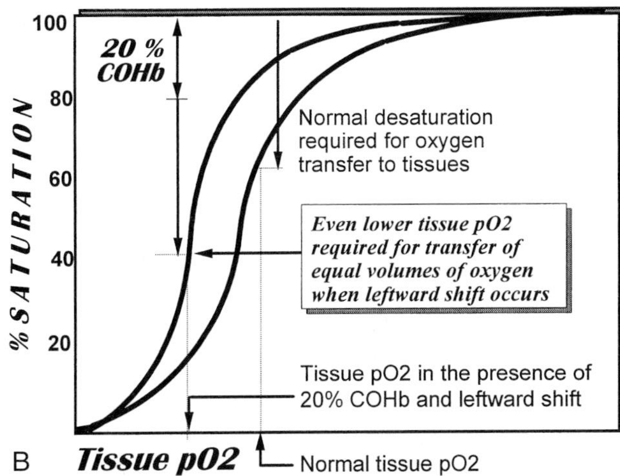

Figure 70–2. *A*, Normal oxygen dissociation curve. Oxygen saturation of hemoglobin governs the final "operating pressure" of oxygen at the tissue level. Carbon monoxide displaces oxygen from hemoglobin, decreasing the maximum oxygen saturation of hemoglobin and forcing the tissue P_{O_2} to a lower level. *B*, Leftward shift of the oxygen dissociation curve. The combined effects of carbon monoxide displacement of oxygen and carbon monoxide-mediated leftward shift of the oxyhemoglobin dissociation curve can force the tissue oxygen pressure to dangerously low levels.

facilitate oxygen transport and diffusion from the blood stream to the mitochondria. For example, the chemical oxidation of myoglobin to metmyoglobin, which cannot bind oxygen, halts oxygen uptake *in vitro* by skeletal muscle strips.[3] Myoglobin's affinity for CO is 40 times greater than that for oxygen, and like hemoglobin, the oxymyoglobin dissociation curve also exhibits a leftward shift when CO is present. Rat heart studies show that this toxic interference with myoglobin-mediated oxygen transport exists regardless of COHb formation.[4] The precipitous reduction in blood pressure that commonly occurs with severe CO poisoning is associated with electrocardiographic evidence of myocardial ischemia and the development of systolic hypotension.[5]

Mitochondrial Impairment

Interference with cellular respiration at the mitochondrial level has been postulated as an additional mechanism, and *in vivo* evidence now shows that CO binds to cytochrome *c* oxidase. Although cytochrome oxidase has an affinity for oxygen that is nine times greater than its affinity for CO, under conditions of hypotension or local hypoxia, CO effectively competes for and occupies the oxygen receptor sites.[6] Perhaps of greater significance is the slow dissociation rate of CO from cytochrome oxidase once binding has occurred. This type of blockade may cause the electron transport chain, proximal to cytochrome oxidase, to become fully reduced. Such a state of "electron congestion" may be associated with electron leakage and the generation of mitochondrial-based fee radicals that occur after CO exposure. Although mitochondrial uptake of CO has been shown experimentally, it does not appear to be directly responsible for the cause of death in fatal cases. Experiments in a bloodless animal model using fluorocarbon solution indicate that survival can occur with very high tissue concentrations of CO.[7]

In addition to cytochrome oxidase blockade, a second mechanism for mitochondrial dysfunction may be related to free radical generation by platelets, in conjunction with the simultaneous release of nitric oxide by platelets. In the presence of free radicals, nitric oxide is converted to peroxynitrite, which has a high affinity for heme proteins such as cytochrome oxidase. Peroxynitrite has been shown to inactivate mitochondrial enzymes and impair electron transport.[8] This platelet-based pathway for mitochondrial dysfunction would also account for the higher survival rate in the bloodless (platelet free) model.

Guanylate Cyclase Impairment

Another hemoprotein affected by CO is guanylate cyclase, which is responsible for the production of cyclic guanosine monophosphate (GMP), a smooth muscle relaxant. It is postulated that CO binding to this enzyme stimulates its activity. After exposure to CO, brain perfusion increases too rapidly to be explained by "hypoxic" mechanisms. CO-induced vascular muscle relaxation appears to be similar to that caused by nitric oxide (NO), although CO is only 1/1000 as potent as NO.[9, 10]

A second mechanism for CO-mediated smooth muscle relaxation is through the displacement of NO from heme-containing proteins in platelets.[11] NO, also known as *endothelial derived relaxation factor*, is a potent smooth muscle relaxant that causes vascular dilatation. NO is a gaseous messenger molecule that has other important biologic functions. Platelets are known producers of NO and contain proteins that normally scavenge excess intraplatelet NO, preventing its diffusion beyond the platelet membrane. Although the displacement of NO from the intraplatelet reservoir may be only a transient phenomenon, it would readily explain the transient nature of the hypotension that occurs with CO-induced syncope.

Clinically, the occurrence of syncope in the setting of CO poisoning is an ominous predictor for serious neurologic sequelae. In monkeys, cerebral white matter lesions correlated better with decreases in blood pressure than with COHb levels, and it has been suggested that an episode of hypotension must coexist for severe neurologic deficits to occur. CO-induced vasodilatation probably works in concert with carboxymyoglobin-induced cardiac ischemia to induce a hypotensive state.[3, 12]

The demonstration that NO was a neuronal messenger led to the suggestion that it might be the first member of a family of gaseous messengers. The chemical similarity of CO to NO hinted that CO might also be a member of this new class of messenger gases, and this appears to be the case. CO is produced by heme oxygenase, the enzyme that metabolizes heme groups to biliverdin and CO. There are two forms of heme oxygenase: an inducible form (type 1) found in the liver and spleen and responsible for breakdown of old blood, and a noninducible form (type 2) which is in significant concentrations in highly discrete areas of the brain.[13–15] The biologic role of CO as a neural messenger is evolving, but it has been established that it has a physiologic function in regulating brain cyclic GMP levels. If this is the case, inhalation of CO, is equivalent to inhaling a neurotransmitter. It may well be that exogenous CO diffuses into neurons where it binds to guanylate cyclase increasing cyclic GMP levels, producing a state of neuronal "overheating" to the detriment of the cell. This phenomenon is likely to be worse in those areas of the brain where NO is the primary regulator of cyclic GMP, because CO can substitute for NO at the regulatory sites. Unlike NO, CO is a more stable gas biologically and persists longer than NO.[16]

Microvascular Impairment—Reperfusion Injury

The histopathology of CO poisoning is strikingly similar to that of postanoxic encephalopathy, or so-called reperfusion injury. Brain reperfusion injury patterns appear to be driven by uncontrolled oxidative damage initiated by oxygen free radicals but sustained by second-generation lipid radicals. Several mechanisms have been postulated for the generation of these radicals.[17] Current evidence suggests that xanthine oxidase activity or possibly leukocyte membrane oxidase activity is responsible for most of the free radical activity associated with CO-mediated lipid peroxidation and brain injury.

Xanthine oxidase generation of free radicals is possible whenever hypoxic or ischemic stress has occurred. During the interval of hypoxia, adenosine dinucleotide triphosphate (ATP) stores are depleted to meet the continuing energy requirements. In the process, ATP is converted to adenosine dinucleotide diphosphate, then to adenosine dinucleotide monophosphate, and then to adenosine as the cell progressively continues to extract molecular energy. Next, adenosine is converted to the purine xanthine. The final disposition of xanthine is the critical step in this cascade of events, which culminates in the generation of a free radical. Normally, most purine metabolism is mediated by xanthine dehydrogenase; however, a protease-mediated conversion of this enzyme into the xanthine oxidase form disposes of xanthine by combining it with oxygen to create uric acid and an oxygen free radical (Fig. 70–3).

Investigations by Thom indicate that the following events lead to the generation of oxygen free radicals after a significant CO exposure: (1) An initial disturbance of endothelial homeostasis occurs and may be due to local hypoxic injury from CO-mediated mitochondrial dysfunction; (2) polymorphonuclear leukocytes are attracted to the site of oxidative endothelial injury; (3) adherent polymorphonuclear leukocytes release a protease that converts xanthine dehydrogenase to xanthine oxidase; and (5) the resulting free radicals perpetuate further injury and continued recruitment of polymorphonuclear leukocytes, resulting in brain lipid peroxidation, which accumulates over time and produces the symptoms of delayed neurologic sequelae.[18]

CLINICAL PRESENTATION

As suggested earlier, CO poisoning has a protean presentation and is notoriously nonspecific. Headache, dizziness, nausea, malaise, and difficulty thinking are common complaints. Abdominal cramps, vomiting, and diarrhea are variations that may occur more commonly in young children. Many factors in-

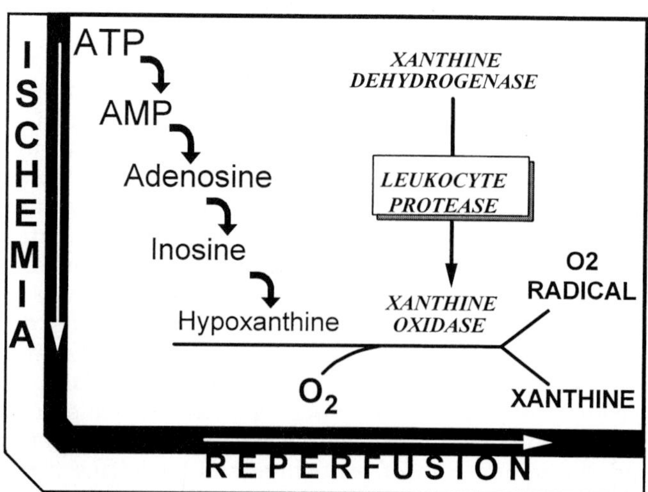

Figure 70–3. Leukocyte-mediated carbon monoxide reperfusion injury pathway following carbon monoxide poisoning has many similarities to proposed mechanisms for traditional ischemic injury. The xanthine oxidase generation of free radicals is probably only one of the several pathways for free radical generation.

Table 70–2. Clinical Grading of Carbon Monoxide Poisoning

Grade	Symptoms	Signs
Mild	Headache Nausea Dizziness	Vomiting
Moderate	Confusion Slow thinking Shortness of breath Blurred vision Weakness	Tachycardia Tachypnea Ataxia Abnormal psychometrics
Severe	Chest pain Palpitations Severe drowsiness Disorientation	Dysrhythmias Electrocardiographic ischemia Hypotension Syncope Lactic acidosis Obtundation Seizures Pulmonary edema Coma Brain changes on computed tomography

fluence the actual presentation, such as the CO concentration, the duration of exposure, the minute ventilation, cardiac output, age, and the presence of cardiac or cerebrovascular disease. Table 70–2 gives a clinical grading system for severity of poisoning.

The earliest symptoms of CO poisoning are headache and dizziness. If a patient has a history of ischemic heart disease, angina may be among the early symptoms. As the poisoning progresses, difficulty with concentration occurs and irritability, weakness, and nausea develop. Physical findings may include mild tachycardia, tachypnea, systolic hypotension, and decreased exercise tolerance. Subtle impairment of cognitive function often occurs, and it can be detected only by neuropsychometric examination. Such cerebral dysfunction is easily missed by a clinician but may be readily apparent to the patient or relatives, especially if the patient has to perform any problem solving.

With more severe poisoning, syncope, seizures, obtundation, generalized muscle rigidity, and coma can occur. The heart, another excessively oxygen-dependent organ, is commonly affected in severe poisoning. Premature ventricular contractions, atrial fibrillation, heart block, ischemic changes on electrocardiography, and myocardial infarction can occur. Transient or persistent hypotension with syncope accompanies myocardial depression and is associated with neurologic complications. In summary, the brain is clearly the principal target organ of CO poisoning. To a much smaller degree, the heart may also be affected, followed by a longer list of complications that affect only severely poisoned patients, in whom the clinical picture is again shaped by neuropsychiatric signs and symptoms. Table 70–3 lists the spectrum of complications that can be associated with CO poisoning.

Neuropathology

The clinical picture of CO poisoning is predominantly one of neurologic and psychiatric manifestations. Almost every known central neurologic syndrome has been reported as a complication of CO poisoning.[19] From the anatomic perspective, the most common lesions occur in the basal ganglia and cerebral gray and white matter. Pathologically, white matter changes range from small multifocal necrotic areas in the commissure and cerebral centrum to extensive zones of necrosis through both hemispheres. Symmetric subcortical demyelination is quite common and probably accounts for delayed neurologic deterioration. Decreased density of the globus pallidus on computed tomography scan of the brain is commonly found in patients with severe neurologic complications and has the best correlation with poor neurologic outcome.[20] As a more sensitive form of imaging, magnetic resonance imaging (MRI) has been advocated as the preferred method of investigation. In sequential MRI studies, a decrease in the extent and signal intensity of white matter lesions accompanied the resolution of clinical symptoms. These observations suggest that the main feature of

Table 70–3. Spectrum of Complications Due to Carbon Monoxide Poisoning

System	Complications
Central nervous system	Impaired cognition, memory dysfunction, vertigo, ataxia, parkinsonism, muscle rigidity, gait disturbance, disorientation, mutism, urinary incontinence, fecal incontinence, cortical blindness, hearing loss, tinnitus, nystagmus, seizures, coma, electroencephalographic abnormalities, cerebral edema, leukoencephalopathy, diabetes insipidus, globus pallidus necrosis
Psychiatric	Personality changes, depression, flattened affect, Tourette's syndrome, anxiety, agitation, poor impulse control
Cardiovascular	Tachycardia, easy fatigue, hypotension, ischemic electrocardiographic changes, arrhythmias, new-onset angina or exacerbation of existing angina, myocardial infarction
Pulmonary	Shortness of breath, pulmonary edema, hemoptysis
Gastrointestinal	Nausea, vomiting, abdominal cramps, diarrhea, gastrointestinal bleeding
Ophthalmologic	Decreased acuity, retrobulbar neuritis, paracentral scotomata, papilledema, flame-shaped retinal hemorrhages
Dermatologic	Erythematous patches, cherry-red skin, bullae, alopecia, sweat gland necrosis
Muscular	Rhabdomyolysis, compartment syndrome
Hematologic	Disseminated intravascular coagulation, thrombotic thrombocytopenic purpura, leukocytosis
Metabolic	Lactic acidosis, hyperglycemia, hypocalcemia, hyperamylasemia (salivary origin)

delayed encephalopathy is a demyelinating process of the cerebral white matter, which for some patients may be reversible.[21] Both computed tomography and MRI are limited studies because they provide only anatomic information as opposed to physiologic information. Newer imaging techniques that can record functional activity in the form of regional cerebral perfusion may be more desirable and more sensitive. Single-photon emission computed tomography (SPECT) has been used as a functional assessment of cerebral perfusion. In SPECT of the brain, a radioisotope (technetium 99m hexamethyl prophyleneamine oxime) that can cross the intact blood-brain barrier and remain fixed long enough to image is administered by intravenous injection. A rotating γ camera is used to produce tomographic images of the radiotracer distribution. Because there usually is an intimate coupling between metabolism and blood flow, SPECT provides a physiologic brain study and may serve as a useful guide to therapy in the near future.[22, 23]

Neurologic Presentations

CO poisoning can produce three different forms of symptoms. Immediately after a CO exposure, the symptoms of *acute intoxication* ensue. These symptoms were detailed earlier. If the CO exposure is stopped, the patient's condition usually improves but may deteriorate 1 to 2 weeks later with new symptoms reminiscent of the acute intoxication. This is the *recurrent symptom syndrome*. Fortunately, a second phase of recovery usually follows this. For other patients, a more severe syndrome of *delayed neuropsychiatric sequelae* may evolve, and some patients may never recover from this.

Recurrent Symptom Syndrome. After an episode of moderate poisoning, patients can have a lucid asymptomatic interval of 1 to 40 days followed by a recurrence of headache, nausea, irritability, confusion, disorientation, apathy, and memory problems. This syndrome may affect 12% to 21% of patients with moderate poisoning. If formally tested with a psychometric examination, these patients have abnormal scores. The average time to onset is 7 days. Without treatment, these patients gradually recover over 40 days on average.

Delayed Neuropsychiatric Sequelae. The syndrome of delayed neuropsychiatric sequelae is a more severe form of secondary deterioration characterized by the appearance of overt signs of neurologic or psychiatric impairment. Neurologic findings include mask face, glabella sign, grasp reflex, dementia, parkinsonism, chorea, apraxia, agnosia, gait disturbance, bradykinesia, mutism, ataxia, nystagmus, tinnitus, hearing loss, partial or complete blindness, and fecal and urinary incontinence. Psychiatric findings include hallucinations, personality changes, impulsiveness, verbal aggressiveness, Tourette's syndrome, and extreme emotional lability. Many of these symptoms are associated with frontal or temporal lobe impairment.

The development of delayed symptoms usually is sudden, with rapid deterioration over only a few days. For many patients, the first symptoms may be disorientation and amnestic confabulation. The onset can be so fast that some patients get lost during their morning errands before family members are even aware of the evolving problem.[19] When the history of a recent CO exposure is overlooked, the constellation of symptoms involving apathy, mutism, and amnesia in conjunction with other bizarre behaviors such as silly smiles, negativism, irrational confabulation, and gait disturbance has led to a false diagnosis of schizophrenia, hysteria, or depression.[19]

In contrast to the recurrent symptom syndrome, only 50% of patients with the syndrome of delayed neuropsychiatric sequelae recover, and as long as 1 year may be required to make a full recovery. This syndrome is frequently associated with a syncopal episode or a period of coma during the initial exposure, followed by a lucid asymptomatic interval. Although loss of consciousness is not an absolute requirement, it is present in 98% of those patients who develop delayed neuropsychiatric sequelae. As seen from a different perspective, approximately 24% of those individuals who lose consciousness develop neurologic problems, half of which are acute and half of which follow a lucid interval and present in a delayed fashion. The true incidence of this syndrome is difficult to determine, but the range reported in the literature is 3% to 40%.

Cardiac Effects

Patients with coronary artery disease can experience exacerbation of anginal symptoms after mild exposures to CO with COHb concentrations less than 10%. The ventricular fibrillation threshold can be affected by a COHb level as low as 9%. If COHb levels rise above 15%, myocardial infarction can occur. A lowered exercise threshold is observed in patients with claudication. Patients without fixed coronary lesions have an increase in coronary blood flow. However, this increased coronary blood flow is inadequate, because lactate production increases, subendocardial flow decreases, and relative subendocardial hypoperfusion supervenes. An increase in platelet adhesiveness has been reported during CO poisoning. The combination of increased platelet activity and relative subendocardial ischemia may account for the case report of a 46-year-old patient who suffered an acute myocardial infarction after CO exposure despite having normal coronary arteries.[24] A report of 18 burn victims with COHb levels exceeding 10% on admission found that 5 (28%) had electrocardiographic changes consistent with myocardial ischemia. Three (17%) of these patients had elevations of creatine kinase–MB levels, consistent with a subendocardial injury.[25] These observations suggest that myocardial damage can result from acute CO poisoning, and appropriate screening is indicated for the detection of such injuries.

Miscellaneous Effects

Severe CO poisoning may be associated with noncardiogenic pulmonary edema due to fluid shifts over increased alveolar-epithelial junctions.[26] Rhabdomyolysis and compartment syndromes have been described but are rare.[27] Oliguric and nonoliguric acute renal failure have been reported. The often cited finding of cherry-red skin is primarily an observation advanced by pathologists at autopsy. In clinical practice, it is rarely seen and varies with the observer and the complexion of the patient. On rare occasions, superficial blisters may develop and may look like second-degree thermal burns. Table 70–2 lists the full spectrum of CO-related effects.

DIAGNOSIS

For fire victims, the possibility of CO poisoning is frequently considered. For the remainder of the general population, the diagnosis is easily missed in the ebb and flow of nonspecific patient complaints. Although headache, dizziness, and nausea are the most common symptoms of CO poisoning, they are encountered commonly in general practice. On occasion, the diagnosis is considered when several individuals from the same occupation or residence present with similar complaints. However, it is easy to dismiss a multiple-case scenario as the simple spread of a viral syndrome. Features that may distinguish CO poisoning from a viral illness include a history of improvement with exposure to fresh air or a change in location and the absence of sore throat, fever, and adenopathy. Three other observations should alert an astute clinician. First is the simultaneous appearance of the illness in many individuals without the typical index case or domino effect. This picture of a group illness may also be misinterpreted as food poisoning whenever CO affects a large group of people with a common food source (e.g., schools or conventions). The second observation pertains to the duration of the illness. Viral syndromes typically run their course in 5 to 7 days. For CO victims, the symptoms persist or continue to recur for as long as a patient continues to be exposed or re-exposed. The third observation is the concurrent illness or death of any family pets, which should alert the physician to an environmental toxin.

In a study investigating the misdiagnosis of CO poisoning, the incidence of misdiagnosis during a 3-year period was 30%. After a campaign for heightened awareness of CO poisoning in the differential diagnosis, the incidence decreased to 5%. Table 70–4 outlines the nature of the misdiagnoses and their relative percentages.[28]

Table 70–4. Common Misdiagnoses for Carbon Monoxide Poisoning

Food poisoning	38%
Psychiatric disease; hysteria, confusion, depression	18%
Heart disease presenting as angina or syncope	13%
Alcohol intoxication or delirium tremens	7%
Acute solvent intoxication	7%
Migraine headache	6%
Ischemic cerebral disease	4%
Cerebral hemorrhage	4%
Cerebral tumor (convulsions)	3%

It is estimated that in winter, the emergency department prevalence of occult CO poisoning among patients with headache or dizziness is 3% to 5%. Certainly it is not practical to screen routinely for COHb on the basis of these complaints alone. Heckerling and colleagues found a COHb screen to be more effective when the physician first inquired about the use of gas stoves, gas heat, or gas hot-water heaters or whether any cohabitants had similar symptoms.[29] Use of this decision rule for obtaining COHb levels eliminates the need for COHb testing in the majority of patients. This decision algorithm for COHb screening correctly identifies patients with COHb levels greater than 10%, with a sensitivity of 75%, and correctly excludes most patients with a lower level (specificity of 74%).

Another historical factor that should be added to Heckerling's rule is the history of an occupational exposure to propane-powered engines. In a study of warehouse workers' headaches, it was determined that CO poisoning should be considered whenever a patient has a history of activity involving propane engines. Crude fuels such as gasoline, kerosene, and coal are commonly associated with CO production, and cleaner fuels such as butane and propane are often thought to undergo complete combustion. A common misconception is that propane-fueled machinery can be safely operated indoors. A study found that propane-powered forklifts maintained within manufacturer's specifications produced sufficient volumes of CO to contaminate even a large warehouse if ventilation was poor.[30] The same researchers noted that the average CO emission from forklifts receiving routine maintenance exceeds current automobile exhaust emission standards and, in fact, corresponds to pre-1968 exhaust emission measurements. CO poisoning from propane engines is most likely to occur when buildings are fully closed, such as during cold winter months or during hot summer months in air-conditioned warehouses. The United States Environmental Protection Agency standards for ambient CO exposures in industrial workplaces are 35 ppm for a 1-hour limit and 9 ppm for an 8-hour limit. An average forklift throttled up to work capacity would produce enough CO to equilibrate to 1 ppm of CO per minute in a large 60,000-m^3 warehouse ($100 \times 60 \times 10$). With a hypothetical ventilation rate of zero, the workplace would exceed Environmental Protection Agency standards for 8-hour exposures in only 9 minutes.

Carboxyhemoglobin Levels

Normal COHb levels range from 0% to 5%. For smokers consuming one pack of cigarettes per day, levels may range from 6% to 10%. Levels are usually determined with a co-oximeter using spectrophotometry to determine the percentage of hemoglobin saturated with CO. Because COHb absorbs light at the same wavelength as oxyhemoglobin, a pulse oximeter shows falsely elevated oxyhemoglobin saturation, and results should be interpreted with caution in the setting of CO poisoning.[31] Anticoagulated blood specimens commonly obtained in conjunction with arterial blood gas are required to measure COHb levels. No substantial difference in COHb values is noted between arterial and venous specimens because of the high affinity of CO for hemoglobin.[32] This point makes it possible for paramedics to draw venous COHb specimens at the scene using heparinized tubes. The use of venous spcimens is also more convenient for COHb measurements in young children. For screening purposes, hand-held CO breath analyzers have been used when patients are capable of holding them. The correlation between breath analyzed values and COHb values is not extraordinarily high (Pearson $r = 0.80$), and breath analysis tends to overestimate rather than underestimate COHb levels. Because false-positive values are more common than false-negative values, it would appear to be quite sensitive but less specific for CO exposure.[33] If this method is used, it is important to know that ethanol, a common cointoxicant, can falsely elevate CO breath levels in the absence of an activated charcoal filter.

The finding of an elevated COHb level is used to confirm the clinical impression of possible CO poisoning. Nevertheless, an elevated COHb value is not a reliable index of the severity of poisoning, nor does it predict the development of the recurrent symptom syndrome or delayed neurologic sequelae. The clinical role of a COHb measurement is simply to determine that CO exposure has occurred. It should not be used to quantitate the severity of poisoning. Many investigators at one time laid out tabular relationships between COHb levels and severity of poisoning. It is now quite clear that the correlation between COHb levels and symptoms is too poor to be of any value.[34] For example, the COHb values in a series of 38 comatose patients, with specimens drawn at the scene, ranged from less than 10% to more than 70%.[35] Eighteen of these patients had COHb levels exceeding 40%, 11 were between 20% and 40%, and 9 were less than 20%. There is no test for the total-body content of CO, and some patients with levels of 30% to 40% may be asymptomatic. Although this is unusual, it illustrates the poor correlation that exists between COHb levels and clinical symptoms.

Neuropsychometric Testing

Given the limited clinical utility of COHb levels to predict or detect severe poisoning, physicians are now moving toward more functional measures of impairment. The development of an abbreviated neuropsychometric battery that could meet the practical requirements of a screening test for subtle cerebral impairment in an emergency setting has provided physicians with a new tool. The test battery can be completed in 20 to 25 minutes and can be administered by a nurse or hyperbaric technician. The tests help detect subtle cerebral dysfunction that could easily be missed with a casual bedside examination. The neuropsychometric screening examination consists of six subtests that help determine various cognitive deficits, including dysgraphia, dysphasia, agnosia, and dyspraxia. The screening battery is composed of the following subtests:

- *Test 1, general orientation*, is used to establish rapport and assess recall of personal facts.
- *Test 2, digit span*, is a test of short-term memory that requires a patient to listen to and recite back a series of digits.
- *Test 3, trail making*, is a timed assessment of temporospacial orientation and visual discrimination based on the patient's ability to connect a pattern of dots.
- *Test 4, digit symbol*, is a timed assessment of temporospacial orientation and visual discrimination and visual-motor coordination in which patients pair numbers with symbols according to a reference key.
- *Test 5, aphasia screen*, is a series of questions that evaluate language and praxic functions.
- *Test 6, block design*, is a timed test of visual-spatial function evaluated by using red and white blocks to construct or reduplicate geometric designs that match the pattern shown in a test booklet.

The screening battery provides a practical cerebral stress test for rapid detection and measurement of subtle neurologic impairment. As the name implies, it is simply a screening test that goes a step beyond the simple "oriented times three" that characterizes most neurologic examinations by non-neurologists. For symptomatic patients who are not obtunded, the examination is used to determine if the poisoning is mild or moderate. It specifically screens for high-level cortical impairment, which would classify a patient as moderately poisoned. Evidence of cortical impairment is regarded as an indication for hyperbaric oxygen (HBO) therapy by most hyperbaric centers.[36] However, a symptomatic patient with normal findings on a neuropsychometric screening examination would be classified as having mild poisoning and would be treated with ambient oxygen. Finally, many hyperbaric units use the examination as an endpoint to therapy and provide repeat HBO treatments until the examination scores normalize or plateau. When using this test, several important qualifiers must be kept in mind:

- The test is not specific for CO. Several investigators have misinterpreted the original work published by Messier and Myers by stating "that it can reliably distinguish between CO poisoned patients and controls 79% of the time." Such statements are misleading and do not take into account that some CO victims may be symptomatic with headaches or dizziness but may still have normal brain function. In other words, their performance scores are expected to be in the control range *because* they have no cortical impairment.

- Screening exams should not be used whenever the clinical impression suggests possible impairment secondary to alcohol, drugs, mental retardation, head injury, or other confounding diseases of the central nervous system.
- The relationship of immediate post-CO-exposure examination scores to the recurrent symptom syndrome or delayed neurologic sequelae is unknown.
- The lower age limit for examination is 15 years.
- A small improvement in scores appears to occur with repetition.
- In Thom's randomized prospective study, patients who were treated with ambient oxygen failed to improve their scores with repetition on the trail-making subtest. This was significantly different from the improved scores noted in the HBO-treated group and normal controls (no CO exposure). The lack of improvement may reflect the presence of subtle CO-induced learning disability when the patients first took the examination after oxygen therapy.

TREATMENT

The antidote for CO poisoning is 100% oxygen, which should be administered by a tight-fitting non-rebreathing mask or an endotracheal tube. Cardiac monitoring and an electrocardiogram are necessary if a patient complains of chest pain, has a history of heart disease, or has an altered mental status. The physician should consider entering the patient into a "rule-out" subendocardial infarction protocol if the patient has a history of any significant chest pain or is severely poisoned. Dysrhythmias should be treated by standard advanced cardiac life support protocols, and hypotension corrected with intravenous normal saline. From a metabolic standpoint, hypoglycemia should be precluded as a cause of an altered mental status or a contributer to it. Patients with moderate or severe poisoning should be checked for acidosis (low serum bicarbonate or an elevated lactate level). Patients suffering from closed-space structural fires with significant metabolic acidosis or elevated lactate levels should also be treated for concomitant cyanide poisoning (see Chapter 71).

The use of 100% oxygen facilitates the dissociation of CO from hemoglobin. The half-life of CO is reduced from 5 hours on room air (range 2 to 7 hours) to approximately 90 minutes on 100% oxygen by conventional nonrebreathing plastic face masks (range, 31 to 150 minutes) to 60 minutes when delivered by a cuffed endotracheal tube. The use of 100% oxygen administered at greater than atmospheric pressure (HBO) can shorten the half-life even further, to 23 minutes (range, 4 to 86 minutes).[35] More importantly, it appears that only HBO can bring about pharmacologic effects that transcend the simple shortening of the COHb half-life. Collectively, these effects prevent CO-mediated oxidative brain injury.

The use of HBO in the management of CO poisoning continues to gain support as the preferred treatment for moderate and severe poisoning. Previous investigations into the utility of HBO suffered from a lack of controls, failure to control for the severity of poisoning, time to treatment, and uncertainty about the correct pressure and number of HBO treatments.* In a retrospective study of severely poisoned patients, Goulon and colleagues demonstrated a reduction in mortality if HBO was administered within 6 hours after discovery of the victim. The mortality was 13.5% if HBO treatment was begun within 6 hours and 30.1% if HBO treatment was delayed for more than 6 hours. In a similar fashion, neurologic morbidity also appeared to be affected by any delays in treatment. The incidence of delayed neurologic sequelae was similar (36%) for those patients treated with 100% normobaric oxygen (ambient pressure) and for those whose treatment with HBO was delayed for more than 6 hours. In contrast, the incidence of delayed neurologic sequelae was only 0.7% among patients treated with HBO within 6 hours after presentation.[37] Experimental animal work by Thom suggests that *time to treatment* is an important variable in preventing leukocyte-mediated oxidative brain injury.[18]

The dosing of oxygen in a hyperbaric unit is prescribed in units of pressure, commonly referred to as atmospheres absolute (ATA). Using this scale, 1 ATA is equal to sea level pressure, or 760 mm Hg. A comparison of outcomes using HBO at different pressures indicates that those studies that used a higher-pressure (2.8 to 3 ATA) protocol had better outcomes than protocols using 2.0 or 2.5 ATA. For example, a prospective study by Raphael and colleagues using 2.0 ATA of oxygen pressure found no significant benefit over conventional ambient oxygen, whereas studies by Myers and associates and Thom and co-workers, which used pressures of 2.8 to 3.0 ATA, did find significant benefit compared with normobaric oxygen.[38–40]

The study by Thom and colleagues deserves special mention, because it was a controlled prospective randomized study in the more commonly encountered form of moderate CO poisoning. The study applied treatment within the first 6 hours of presentation and used the higher pressure of 2.8 ATA. Patients with cardiac instability or loss of consciousness were excluded from the study. The incidence of delayed

*Readers should be aware that it is not possible to have a pressure control group in the "classic" sense because pressurization with an air control drives nitrogen into tissues and introduces the confounding variable of decompression illness from nitrogen off-gasing.

neurologic sequelae was compared between groups treated with 100% oxygen at ambient pressure or HBO. Delayed neurologic sequelae were defined as the development of new symptoms plus deterioration on one or more subtests of a standardized neuropsychologic screening battery. The researchers found delayed neurologic sequelae in 23% of patients treated with ambient-pressure oxygen but none when HBO was used. In the ambient oxygen group, delayed neurologic sequelae occurred 6±1 days after poisoning and persisted for 41±8 days. In this study of moderate poisoning in which the delayed neurologic sequelae manifested as impaired cognition, in distinction to impaired basal ganglia function, all patients recovered. However, from a cost-benefit perspective, the high incidence of delayed neurologic sequelae (23%) and the duration (41 days) suggested that it would be more cost effective to provide a single HBO treatment than to incur the costs for return evaluations, lost work, and reduction in personal performance.

Single Versus Multiple Hyperbaric Oxygen Treatments

In a longitudinal study of 100 consecutive admissions for CO poisoning, the frequency of neuropsychiatric sequelae in patients who received only oxygen at ambient pressure was 63% at discharge and 67% at 1-month follow-up.[41] For those patients receiving one hyperbaric oxygen treatment (2.8 ATA), the frequency was 46% at discharge and 50% at 1-month follow-up. In contrast, the frequency of neuropsychiatric sequelae in patients who had two or more HBO treatments was only 13% at discharge ($P < .005$) and 18% at follow-up ($P < .005$). The frequency of sequelae was significantly greater if HBO was delayed ($P < .005$). However, a prospective randomized study of patients with initial impairment of consciousness compared a single HBO treatment (2.0 ATA) with two HBO treatments and showed a slightly better but insignificant recovery rate for two versus one.[42] Again, important differences between these two studies are the time to treatment and the treatment pressures (2.8 ATA versus 2.0 ATA).

Delayed Hyperbaric Oxygen Treatments

The clinical studies by Goulon and colleagues and Thom and associates suggest that the optimal therapeutic window for CO treatment is within the first 6 hours after exposure. Although delayed HBO treatment is less effective, it should still be considered after suspected or confirmed poisonings in the moderate to severe range. Myers and co-workers described four cases of CO poisoning in which the COHb level was reduced to the normal values using ambient oxygen, without clinical improvement.[43] HBO was subsequently begun, with dramatic improvement or complete resolution of symptoms. More recently, two cases of acute CO poisoning with serious neurologic symptoms and normal COHb levels were reported. Despite the passage of more than 6 hours before instituting HBO, the researchers described complete resolution of symptoms.[44] Myers also reported a series of 10 patients who developed the recurrent symptom syndrome approximately 6 days after recovery from the initial exposure and symptoms. These patients experienced a mild recurrence of symptoms such as headache, nausea, apathy, and dizziness, which in most cases were accompanied by abnormal neuropsychometric findings. After a single HBO treatment, all patients experienced prompt resolution of their recurring symptoms.[39]

Although these case reports are of interest, very limited information describes the use of HBO for subacute or chronic exposures. No animal studies have investigated the effects of delayed HBO after a course of ambient oxygen therapy. It is unclear when the acute effects of CO become translated into chronic brain injury. Also debated is the best treatment for chronic brain injury. Some investigators believe that a low-pressure HBO protocol (1.5 ATA) is more desirable. HBO currently appears to be beneficial for moderate or severe poisoning within the first 24 hours; however, its role for HBO after the first 24 hours is largely undefined.

Carbon Monoxide Poisoning in Pregnancy

Treatment recommendations for CO-poisoned pregnant women must take into consideration the sensitivity of the fetus to CO and the altered kinetics of uptake and elimination of CO from the fetus. Specifically, fetal hemoglobin has a higher affinity for CO than adult hemoglobin, the peak fetal COHb levels are higher than the maternal, the elimination rate of fetal CO is slower, and the oxyhemoglobin dissociation curve for fetal hemoglobin is shifted to the left naturally compared with maternal hemoglobin. Fetal hemoglobin is therefore susceptible to extreme left shifting in the presence of CO (Fig. 70–4). Figuratively speaking, the fetus behaves like a biochemical sponge pulling CO from the maternal circulation, and in some cases a woman is relatively asymptomatic compared with her fetus. In primate studies, a single CO exposure insufficient to cause maternal disease led to intrauterine hypoxia, fetal brain injury, and increased rates of fetal death.[45, 46] In the clinical literature, it is common to find that a woman survives exposures that were fatal to her fetus.[47, 48]

Because of the elimination delay and the known risks of CO to a fetus, HBO should be considered in any pregnant woman who, based on history, is thought to have had a significant or prolonged exposure. Even greater consideration should be given to the use of HBO if the woman is symptomatic, and

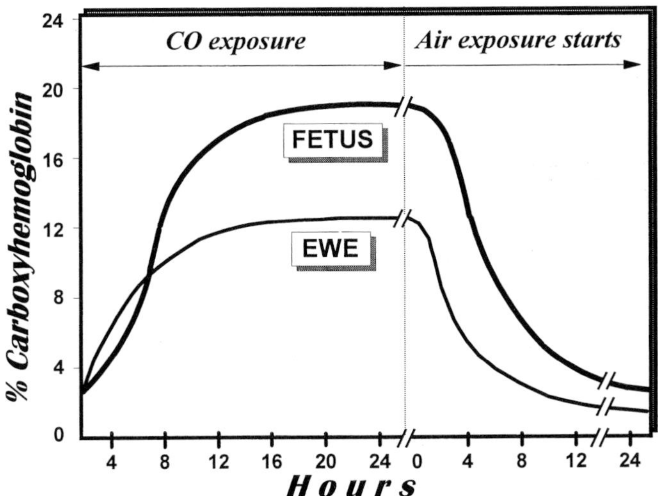

Figure 70–4. Kinetic data from the investigations by Longo and Hill using pregnant sheep exposed to carbon monoxide. The fetus initially lags behind the ewe but will ultimately have higher levels and longer elimination times.

certainly if she has a history of syncope. Theoretic concerns about adverse effects of HBO in pregnancy are no longer warranted. At present, no clear evidence shows that HBO poses any harm when using conventional treatment protocols. Animal studies questioning the use of HBO have used oxygen dosages that *exceed* the normal clinical range and therefore are not relevant. In those animal models assessing the effects of HBO in pregnancy using dosages within the normal clinical range, no deleterious effects were noted. Clinicians in the former Soviet Union have used intermittent HBO to treat more than 700 pregnant women for hypoxemia of various etiologies, such as congenital heart defects, eclampsia or pre-eclampsia, placental insufficiency, anemia, and diabetes, without detrimental effects on the fetus. The Western literature also contains numerous case reports, and one prospective study describes 44 pregnant women who sustained CO poisoning and were treated using HBO, with no reported side effects.[49]

The current recommendations, advanced by Van Hoesen and colleagues for HBO therapy for pregnant patients suffering acute CO poisoning, are the following.[50]

1. Administer HBO if the maternal COHb level exceeds 20% at any time during the exposure.
2. Administer HBO if the patient has suffered or demonstrates any neurologic signs, regardless of the COHb level. In addition, other researchers would consider the presence of any cognitive impairment on psychometric examinations to be a neurologic sign.
3. Administer HBO if signs of fetal distress are present in the form of
   - Fetal tachycardia
   - Beat-to-beat variability
   - Late decelerations
4. If HBO is unavailable, administer 100% oxygen by a tightly fitting mask for five times as long as needed to reduce the maternal COHb to normal (<5%). This recommendation is based on a mathematic model that attempts to predict the elimation COHb rate for the human fetus.[51]
5. If the patient continues to demonstrate neurologic signs or if signs of fetal distress occur within 12 hours after initial treatment, additional HBO may be indicated.

In general, a liberal approach should be taken for the administration of HBO in the setting of pregnancy. A woman should be informed about the increased risk for fetal abnormalities due to CO exposure and told that HBO therapy does not completely eliminate those risks. Pending further investigations, HBO does not appear to pose any substantial risk to the fetus when provided within the customary dose ranges of clinical practice.

How Does Hyperbaric Oxygen Work?

Certainly the most intuitive mechanism of action for hyperbaric therapy is Le Chatelier's principle, which states that the rate of a reaction is proportional to the concentration of the reactants. More simply put, CO dissociates from hemoglobin more rapidly when the concentration of oxygen competing for the binding sites is increased. This concept is also known as the *law of mass action*. As previously discussed, the actual concentration of COHb is not as important as previously thought. CO binding to myoglobin may be deleterious where the heart is concerned, and the rapid dissociation of CO under hyperbaric conditions may be beneficial. The binding of CO to cytochrome oxidase, which interferes with energy production, may also produce free radicals, which have been implicated in the neuropathogenesis of CO. HBO at 3 ATA markedly accelerates the dissociation of CO from cytochrome *c* oxidase, restoring oxidative phosphorylation and perhaps arresting further production of free radicals.[6] Evidence also suggests that HBO may generate hydroperoxyl radicals, which could terminate the self-propagating organic radicals.[52] Finally, substantial evidence shows that leukocytes are involved in the pathogenesis of oxidative injury to the central nervous system. After the initial exposure to CO, an endothelial injury evolves and triggers the adherence of leukocytes to the brain microvasculature. Once attached, the leukocytes amplify local injury by initiating further free radical production. HBO has been shown to prevent leukocyte adherence by interfering with leukocyte β_2 integrin functions, which are responsible for adherence to microvasculature.[53] This aspect of HBO therapy is perhaps the most interesting, because it suggests that much of the physiology of HBO may be related to protein and enzyme alterations rather

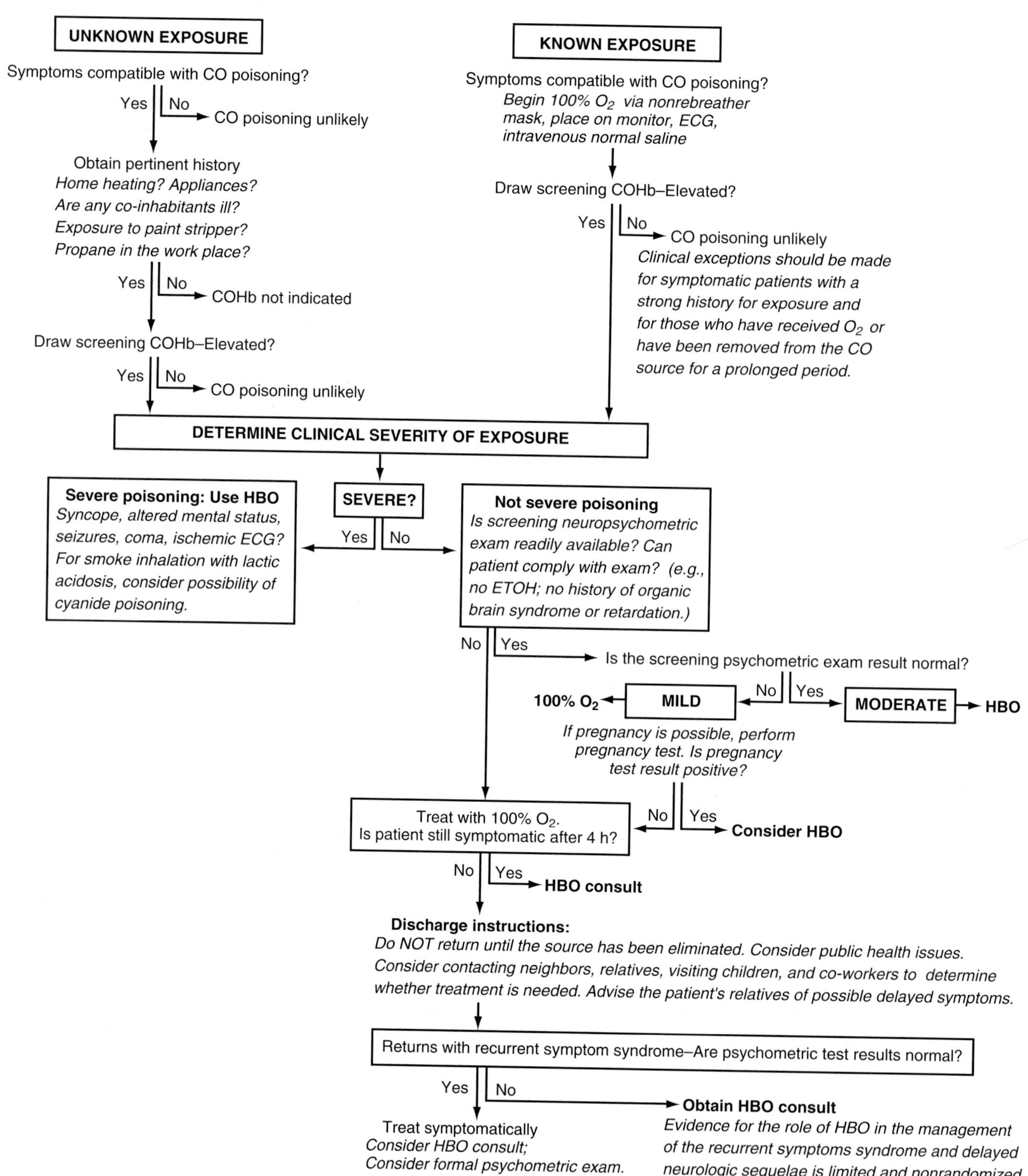

Figure 70–5. Carbon monoxide management algorithm. ECG, electrocardiography; ETOH, ethanol; HBO, hyperbaric oxygenation.

than being simply a function of increased oxygen pressure.

CONCLUSION

To date, more than 3000 articles have been written on the subject of CO poisoning, and yet we still cannot explain physiologically all of the associated clinical phenomena. In the past 5 years, the role of CO in biologic systems has evolved from a toxic substance to a sophisticated neuroregulator. The CO paradigm has shifted from a simple concept of COHb-mediated hypoxia to the more complex understanding that acute cerebral impairment may in effect be an inhalation overdose of "neurotransmitter." In the past, HBO was reserved for only comatose patients. Current evidence suggests a much broader role in the management of moderate poisoning. Likewise, the effect or mechanism for HBO has changed from the role of simple oxygen "flush" to that of a modulator for reperfusion injury. Finally, our approach to the detection and assessment of impaired patients has evolved from the simplistic notion that COHb levels correlate with disease severity to a more practical assessment of cerebral function via psychometric tests. Although assessment of brain performance via psychometric tests is more "functional" than use of COHb levels, these tests are limited by an examiner's skill and a patient's motivation and are subject to confounding factors such as alcohol and stress. In the future, we will probably devise purer forms of assessment that are not subject to psychologic "set" or setting. Such assessments will probably be in the form of imaging true neurophysiologic function via spectamine scanning, positron emission tomography scanning, or some derivative. The evolving story of CO poisoning teaches us that we should be ever flexible in our thinking, avoid the comfortable path of unchallenged ideas, and realize that definitive studies are only the stepping stones of work in progress. Figure 70–5 provides an algorithm that summarizes most of the clinical decision points for the management of CO poisoning.

References

1. Cobb N, Etzel RA: Unintentional carbon monoxide related deaths in the United States, 1979 through 1988. JAMA *266*:659, 1991.
2. Schaplowsky AF, Oglesbay FB, Morrison JH, et al: Carbon monoxide contamination of the living environment: A national survey of home air and children's blood. J Environ Health *36*:569, 1974.
3. Wittenberg BA, Wittenberg JB: Role of myoglobin in the oxygen supply of red skeletal muscle. J Biol Chem *250*:9038, 1975.
4. Chen KC, McGrath JJ: Response of the isolated heart to carbon monoxide and nitrogen anoxia. Toxicol Appl Pharmacol *81*:363, 1985.
5. Ginsberg MD, Myers RE, McDonagh BF: Experimental carbon monoxide encephalopathy in the primate. II. Clinical aspects, neuropathology, and physiologic correlation. Arch Neurol *30*:209, 1974.
6. Brown SD, Piantadosi CA: In vivo binding of carbon monoxide to cytochrome C oxidase in rat brain. J Appl Physiol *68*:604, 1990.
7. Geyer RP: Review of perfluorochemical-type blood substitutes. *In* Proceedings of the 10th International Congress for Nutrition: Symposium on Perfluorochemical Artificial Blood. Igakushobe, Osaka, Japan, p 3, 1976.
8. Radi R, Rodriguez M, Castro L, et al: Inhibition of mitochondrial electron transport by peroxynitrite. Arch Biochem Biophys *308*:89, 1994.
9. Furchgott RF, Jothianandan D: Endothelium-dependent and independent vasodilation involving cyclic GMP: Relaxation induced by nitric oxide, carbon monoxide and light. Blood Vessels *28*:52, 1991.
10. Utz J, Ullrich V: Carbon monoxide relaxes ileal smooth muscle through activation of guanylate cyclase. Biochem Pharmacol *41*:1195, 1991.
11. Thom SR, Ohnishi TS, Ischiropoulos H: Nitric oxide release by platelets inhibits neutrophil B2 integrin function following acute carbon monoxide poisoning. Toxicol Applied Pharmacol *128*:105, 1994.
12. Thom SR: Carbon monoxide-mediated brain lipid peroxidation in the rat. J Appl Physiol *68*:997, 1990.
13. Snyder SH, Bredt DS: Biological roles of nitric oxide. Sci Am *266*:68, 1992.
14. Baringa M: Carbon monoxide: Killer to brain messenger in one step. Science *259*:309, 1993.
15. Marks GS, Brien JF, Nakatsu K, et al: Does carbon monoxide have a physiological function? Trends Pharmacol Sci *12*:185, 1991.
16. Gorman D: Carbon monoxide: From toxic poison to brain messenger. S Pac Underwater Med Soc J *25*:77, 1995.
17. Hallenbeck JM, Dutka AJ: Background review and current concepts of reperfusion injury. Arch Neurol *47*:1245, 1990.
18. Thom SR: Leukocytes in carbon monoxide-mediated brain oxidative injury. Toxicol Appl Pharmacol *123*:234, 1993.
19. Min SK: A brain syndrome associated with delayed neuropsychiatric sequelae following acute carbon monoxide intoxication. Acta Psychiatr Scand *73*:80, 1986.
20. Sawada Y, Ohashi N, Maemura K, et al: Computed tomography as an indication of long-term outcome after acute carbon monoxide poisoning. Lancet *1*:783, 1980.
21. Chang KH, Moon HH, Kim HS, et al: Delayed encephalopathy after acute carbon monoxide intoxication: MR imaging features and distribution of cerebral white matter lesions. Radiology *184*:117, 1992.
22. Choi S, Lee MS: Early hypoperfusion of technetium-99m hexamethylprophylene amine oxime brain single photon emission computed tomography in a patient with carbon monoxide poisoning. Eur Neurol *33*:461, 1993.
23. Van Meter KW, Harch PG, Andrews LC, et al: Should the pressure be off or on in the use of oxygen in the treatment of carbon monoxide-poisoned patients? Ann Emerg Med *24*:283, 1994.
24. Marius-Nunez AL: Myocardial infarction with normal coronary arteries after acute exposure to carbon monoxide. Chest *87*:491, 1990.
25. Williams J, Lewis RW, Kealey GP: Carbon monoxide poisoning and myocardial ischemia in patients with burns. J Burn Care Rehabil *13*:210, 1992.
26. Fein A, Grossman RF, Jones JG, et al: Carbon monoxide effect on alveolar epithelium permeability. Chest *78*:726, 1980.
27. Florkowski CM, Rossi ML, Carey MP, et al: Rhabdomyolysis and acute renal failure following carbon monoxide poisoning: Two case reports with muscle histopathology and enzyme activities. J Toxicol Clin Toxicol *30*:443, 1992.
28. Barret L, Danel V, Faure J: Carbon monoxide poisoning, a diagnosis frequently overlooked. Clin Toxicol *23*:309, 1985.
29. Heckerling PS, Leikin JB, Maturen A: Occult carbon monoxide poisoning: Validation of a prediction model. Am J Med *84*:251, 1988.
30. Fawcett TA, Moon RE, Fracica PJ, et al: Warehouse worker's headache; carbon monoxide poisoning from propane-fueled forklifts. J Occup Med *34*:12, 1992.
31. Buckley RG, Aks SE, Eshom JL, et al: The pulse oximetry gap in carbon monoxide intoxication. Ann Emerg Med *24*:252, 1994.

32. Touger M, Gallagher JE, Tyrell J: Relationship between venous and arterial carboxyhemoglobin levels in patients with suspected carbon monoxide poisoning. Ann Emerg Med *25*:481, 1995.
33. Turnbull TL, Hart RG, Strange GR, et al: Emergency department screening for unsuspected carbon monoxide exposure. Ann Emerg Med *17*:478, 1988.
34. Benignus VA, Muller KE, Malott CM: Dose-effects function for carboxyhemoglobin and behavior. Neurotoxicol Teratol *12*:111, 1990.
35. Myers RAM: Carbon monoxide poisoning: *In* Haddad LM, Winchester JF (eds): Clinical Management of Poisoning and Drug Overdose. 2nd ed. Philadelphia, W. B. Saunders Co., pp 1139–1152.
36. Hampson NB, Dunford RG, Kramer CC, et al: Selection criteria utilized for hyperbaric oxygen treatment of carbon monoxide poisoning. J Emerg Med *13*:227, 1995.
37. Goulon M, Barois A, Rapin M, et al: Carbon monoxide poisoning and acute anoxia due to breathing coal gas and hydrocarbons. Ann Med Interne (Paris) *120*:335, 1969.
38. Raphael JC, Elkharrat D, Jars-Guincestre MC, et al: Trial of normobaric and hyperbaric oxygen for acute carbon monoxide intoxication. Lancet *1*:414, 1989.
39. Myers RAM, Snyder SK, Emhoff TA: Subacute sequelae of carbon monoxide poisoning. Ann Emerg Med *14*:1163, 1985.
40. Thom SR, Taber RL, Mendiguren I, et al: Delayed neurological sequelae following carbon monoxide poisoning. Ann Emerg Med *25*:474, 1995.
41. Gorman DF, Clayton D, Gilligan JE, et al: A longitudinal study of 100 consecutive admissions for carbon monoxide poisoning to the Royal Adelaide Hospital. Anaesth Intensive Care *20*:311, 1992.
42. Raphael JC, Elkharrat D, Jars-Guincestre MC, et al: Trial of normobaric and hyperbaric oxygen for acute carbon monoxide intoxication. Lancet *1*:414, 1989.
43. Myers RAM, Snyder SK, Linberg S, et al: Value of hyperbaric oxygen in suspected carbon monoxide poisoning. JAMA *246*:2478, 1981.
44. Gibson AJ, Davis FM, Ewer T: Delayed hyperbaric oxygen therapy for carbon monoxide intoxication—two case reports. N Z Med J *104*:64, 1991.
45. Ginsburg MD, Myers RE: Fetal brain damage following maternal carbon monoxide intoxication: An experimental study. Acta Obstet Gynecol Scand *53*:309, 1974.
46. Ginsburg MD, Myers RE: Fetal brain injury after maternal carbon monoxide intoxication: Clinical and neuropathologic aspects. Neurology *26*:14, 1976.
47. Caravati EM, Adams CJ, Joyce SM, et al: Fetal toxicity associated with maternal carbon monoxide poisoning. Ann Emerg Med *17*:714, 1988.
48. Koren G, Sharav T, Pastuszak A, et al: A multicenter prospective study of fetal outcome following accidental carbon monoxide poisoning in pregnancy. Reprod Toxicol *5*:397, 1991.
49. Elkharrat D, Raphael JC, Korach JM, et al: Acute carbon monoxide intoxication and hyperbaric oxygen in pregnancy. Intensive Care Med *17*:289, 1991.
50. Van Hoesen KB, Camporesi EM, Moon RE, et al: Should hyperbaric oxygen be used to treat the pregnant patient for carbon monoxide poisoning? A case report and literature review. JAMA *261*:1039, 1989.
51. Hill EP, Hill JR, Power GG, et al: Carbon monoxide exchanges between human fetus and mother: A mathematical model. Am J Physiol *232*:H311, 1977.
52. Thom SR, Elbukin EM: Oxygen-dependent antagonism of lipid peroxidation. Free Radic Biol Med *10*:413, 1991.
53. Thom SR: Functional inhibition of leukocyte B2 integrins by hyperbaric oxygen in carbon monoxide–mediated brain injury in rats. Toxicol Appl Pharmacol *123*:248, 1993.
54. Goldbaum LR, Orellano T, Dergal E: Studies on the relationship between carboxyhemoglobin concentration and toxicity. Aviat Space Environ Med *48*:969, 1977.

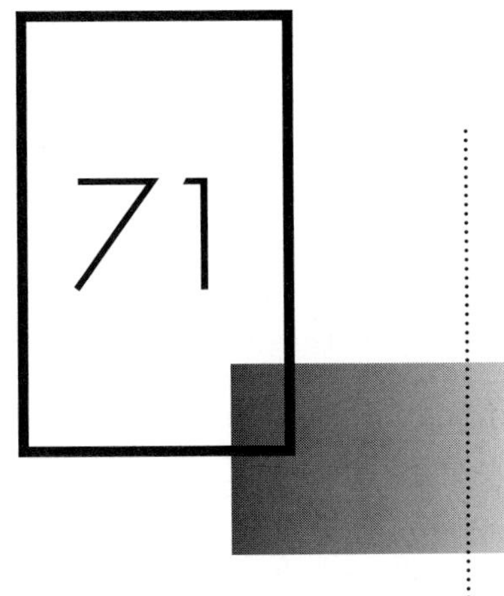

Cyanide and Related Compounds

ALAN H. HALL, MD
BARRY H. RUMACK, MD

HISTORY

Cyanide poisoning may be encountered in a wide variety of settings. Cyanide salts and hydrocyanic acid are used in common industrial processes, such as electroplating, jewelry and metal cleaning, precious metal extraction, laboratory assays, and photographic processes.[1–4] Hydrogen cyanide gas is a fumigant rodenticide.[3] "Coyote getters" (snub-nosed guns blasting sodium cyanide concealed in baits into the mouths of predators) continue to be used in Canada.[5] Criminal tampering by replacement of the ingredients in over-the-counter capsules with cyanide salts has resulted in a number of deaths.[6, 7]

Victims of enclosed-space fire-smoke inhalation may have cyanide toxicity in addition to carbon monoxide poisoning,[8, 9] and cyanide and carbon monoxide have been shown to be synergistic poisons.[10] Nontraumatic deaths in aircraft accidents may be related to inhalation of carbon monoxide and cyanide products of combustion.[11] A number of compounds can liberate cyanide on spontaneous or thermal decomposition, or by chemical reaction with acids or acid fumes (e.g., cyanogen, cyanogen bromide, cyanogen iodide, cyanogen chloride, and calcium cyanide).[1, 3] The use of cyanogen halides and hydrogen cyanide as chemical warfare agents has been considered.[12] At low concentrations, however, the cyanogen halides have primarily lacrimating and pulmonary irritant effects.[3]

Cyanogenic compounds (laetrile, amygdalin from plant sources, nitrile compounds such as acetonitrile or propionitrile, and aliphatic thiocyanates, such as Lethane and Thanate) can release cyanide during metabolism, chemical reaction in the gut, or bacterial degradation following ingestion.[3, 13–16] Severe or fatal cyanide poisoning with a delay in symptom onset of several hours or longer has followed accidental ingestion of acetonitrile from glue-on nail removing compounds.[17, 18]

Sodium nitroprusside releases cyanide during metabolism and can cause elevated blood cyanide levels, and, occasionally, clinical manifestations of cyanide poisoning.[19–21] The frequent lack of correlation between blood cyanide levels and cyanide poisoning symptomatology during nitroprusside administration suggests that the decision of whether to employ antidote therapy must be made more on clinical grounds (e.g., presence of metabolic [lactic] acidosis or of signs and symptoms consistent with cyanide poisoning) than on blood cyanide levels alone. Clinical symptoms in this setting may, however, be due to *thiocyanate* accumulation.[22]

Isocyanates (e.g., methyl isocyanate, toluene diisocyanate) do not release cyanide after absorption and do not cause cyanide poisoning, being primarily irritant and sensitizing agents.[3]

Chronic exposure to low levels of cyanide has been postulated to cause retrobulbar optic atrophy (in heavy smokers) and ataxic peripheral neuropathy (tropical ataxic neuropathy), as well as *konzo* (spastic upper motor neuron paraparesis) in persons who consume large amounts of improperly prepared cyanogenic cassava.[23, 24] Development of neuropathies seems to require both chronic low-level cyanide exposure and either a deficiency of the endogenous cyanide-detoxifying enzyme rhodanese or protein-calorie malnutrition with dietary sulfur deficiency. A condition resembling acute cyanide poisoning characterized by elevated blood cyanide levels that is treatable with cyanide antidotes has resulted from acute ingestion of improperly prepared cassava.[25]

Mild disorders of vitamin B_{12} and folate levels and certain thyroid function abnormalities were noted in one group of workers with chronic cyanide exposure.[2] Thyroid enlargement (goiter) and altered iodine 131 uptake have also been described in workers chronically exposed to cyanide[3] and in populations eating an iodine-deficient and monotonous diet of cassava (which contains the cyanogenic glycosides linamarin and lotaustralin).[26]

EPIDEMIOLOGY

Despite widespread cyanide and cyanogenic compound use, serious acute cyanide poisoning is rare. Of a total of 1,926,438 human poison exposures reported to the American Association of Poison Control Centers Toxic Exposure Surveillance System (TESS) during 1994, only 360 involved cyanide poisoning; of these 360, 19 were in children younger than 6 years of age, 23 were in patients 6 to 19 years of age, and 235 were in patients older than 19 years of age (the remainder were in patients of unknown age).[27] Of the 353 cases in which the reason for exposure was known, 300 were unintentional exposures, 45 were intentional exposures, and 8 were classified as other or adverse reactions.

A total of 228 (63%) of these patients were treated in a health care facility, a figure that perhaps indicates the appreciation of the potential severity of cyanide exposure.[27] Of cyanide antidotes available in the United States, amyl nitrite was not listed in the 1994 TESS database, sodium nitrite administration was recorded in 34 instances, and sodium thiosulfate administration was recorded in 50 instances. As these antidotes may be administered for other poisonings, such results do not necessarily indicate the total number of serious cyanide poisonings.

Of the 360 cyanide exposures, clinical outcome was known in only 208 cases (58%).[27] In 53 cases (15%), no signs or symptoms of cyanide poisoning developed. A total of 146 patients (41%) became symptomatic, and 13 patients (4%) developed major symptoms (life-threatening signs or symptoms; significant residual disability or disfigurement).[27] Nine patients (3%) died of cyanide poisoning during 1994.[27]

Some details of the nine fatal cyanide poisonings reported to the TESS database were available.[27] Three of these cases involved combined carbon monoxide and cyanide poisoning from smoke inhalation. Of these, two childhood fatalities demonstrated the potential synergistic effects of cyanide and carbon monoxide.

In the first pediatric case, a 2-year-old child with smoke inhalation died with an initial whole-blood cyanide level of 2.5 μg/mL and a blood carboxyhemoglobin level of 21% (neither of which alone would have been predicted to be fatal). In the second pediatric case, a 3-year-old child with smoke inhalation died with an initial whole-blood cyanide level of 3.1 μg/mL (a potentially but not always fatal concentration) and a carboxyhemoglobin level of 75% (decreased to 19% following treatment with 100% normobaric oxygen [O_2]).

Of the six "pure" fatal cyanide poisoning cases, all were in adults.[27] In these cases, ingestion of the involved cyanide compound was intentional in five; the reason for and route of exposure was unknown in the sixth. One of these adults intentionally ingested approximately 30 mL of a sodium cyanide–containing insecticide (concentration not reported).[27] The whole-blood cyanide level was 8.8 μg/mL at 1 hour after ingestion; after hyperbaric oxygenation (HBO) and specific antidote treatment, the whole blood cyanide level decreased to 1.0 μg/mL at 12 hours after ingestion; at 50 and 54 hours after ingestion, whole-blood cyanide levels were 0.3 and 0.2 μg/mL, respectively. This patient was determined to be brain dead, and organs were successfully harvested for transplantation.

An ingestion of 18.9 mg/kg of cyanide (1650 mg of potassium cyanide gold-plating solution) was survived following treatment with supportive therapy and administration of sodium nitrite and sodium thiosulfate.[28] Patients with well-documented cyanide poisoning may not always survive with supportive therapy alone.[16] Among 21 acute cyanide poisoning victims from Taiwan during the years 1984 through 1993, the following effects were noted: loss of consciousness (in 15), metabolic acidosis (in 14), cardiopulmonary failure (in 9); anoxic encephalopathy (in 6); and diabetes insipidus or conditions mimicking this condition (in 1 to 3), which may be an ominous sign.[16]

PHARMACOLOGY

Toxicokinetics

The kinetics of cyanide are not well understood. Available data are either from animal experiments or anecdotal human case reports. In dog plasma *in vitro,* cyanide is approximately 60% protein bound.[29] *In vivo,* whole-blood cyanide levels may be four or more times greater than serum levels because of the concentration of cyanide in erythrocytes.[1]

The volume of distribution (Vd) of cyanide in dogs is 0.498 L/kg.[30] A similar Vd of 0.41 L/kg was estimated in a single case of human potassium cyanide poisoning treated with sodium nitrite and sodium thiosulfate.[31] In this same case, estimates of other toxicokinetic parameters were the area under the curve (48 μg-h/mL), clearance (163 mL/min), and terminal-phase elimination half-life ($t_{1/2}$, 19 hours).[31] The last value is in contrast to the $t_{1/2}$ values of 20 to 60 minutes often quoted in the literature,[3] but it is consistent with findings in dogs showing only minimal excretion within the first 3 hours after oral administration, despite absorption of about 95%.[29] In victims of human cyanide poisoning from smoke inhalation, blood cyanide $t_{1/2}$ was approximately 60 minutes.[9]

Toxicodynamics

In a single patient not treated with specific antidotes, the average urinary cyanide excretion over nearly 40 hours was 0.64 mg/h after a probable ingestion of between 117 and 511 mg of potassium cyanide.[6] In this same patient (who was a victim of the 1982 Chicago cyanide-acetaminophen tampering incident), the mean whole-blood cyanide level 1 hour after ingestion was 8.2 μg/mL. This level increased to a mean of 19.7 μg/mL at 3 hours and to 23.4 μg/mL at 9 hours after ingestion. Despite intensive supportive treatment, this patient died about 40 hours after ingestion.

In contrast, in a patient who survived ingestion of 1 gram of potassium cyanide following treatment with sodium nitrite and sodium thiosulfate, the highest whole-blood cyanide level was 15.68 μg/mL at 1.75 hours after ingestion; this level decreased to 0.82 μg/mL at 5 hours after ingestion.[31] In another patient who survived cyanide poisoning secondary to dermal and inhalation exposure to propionitrile, treatment with the hydroxocobalamin/sodium thiosulfate antidote kit used in France caused a decrease in the whole-blood cyanide level from 5.71 μg/mL at 2 hours after exposure to 0.93 μg/mL 30 minutes later.[13] Specific antidote therapy can decrease blood cyanide levels more rapidly than is seen in patients to whom specific antidotes are not administered.

Mechanism of Action and Toxicity

Cyanide produces histotoxic hypoxia by binding with the ferric iron (Fe^{3+}) of mitochondrial cytochrome oxidase, thus inhibiting this important respiratory enzyme and disrupting the normal functioning of the electron transport chain and the ability of cells to utilize O_2 in oxidative phosphorylation.[1] The result is a shift to anaerobic metabolism, a substantial decrease in adenosine triphosphate synthesis, depletion of cellular energy stores, and greatly increased lactic acid production, which causes an elevated anion gap metabolic acidosis.[1] Numerous iron- or copper-containing enzymes may be inhibited by cyanide, but cytochrome oxidase inhibition has been considered to be the major intracellular toxic mechanism in cyanide poisoning.[3]

CLINICAL PRESENTATION

Pathophysiology

The tissue hypoxia of cyanide poisoning has several causes. Those tissues most dependent on oxidative phosphorylation—those of the heart and brain—are the most severely and rapidly affected. Central inhibition of the respiratory centers leads to hypoventilation, which in turn produces an additional hypoxic hypoxia.

Myocardial depression with decreased cardiac output produces additional stagnation hypoxia. Until the stage of respiratory depression or arrest, the blood is relatively normally oxygenated. However, the tissues are unable to extract and utilize this O_2; this leads to a greater than normal amount on the venous side and thus an increased central venous O_2 per cent saturation.

Cyanide binding to cytochrome oxidase is a reversible process. The body has a natural defense against cyanide exposure in the form of the endogenous enzyme rhodanese. This enzyme catalyzes cyanide, complexing it with sulfur and forming the much less toxic ion thiocyanate. The body's sulfur pool is small, however, and the availability of sulfur constitutes the rate-limiting factor in natural cyanide detoxification. In the absence of an exogenous source of sulfur, rhodanese activity is too slow to prevent serious toxicity or death in significant cyanide poisoning.

The mechanism by which chronic cyanide exposure might cause neurotoxicity has been poorly understood. An increase in intraneuronal calcium levels and lipid peroxidation, perhaps initiated by cyanide-induced decreased adenosine triphosphate levels, which impairs sodium and calcium extrusion processes, might be a mechanism of cyanide-induced nerve injury.[32]

Manifestations

The natural history of severe acute cyanide poisoning is a rapid progression (faster with inhalation than ingestion) to coma, convulsions, shock, respiratory failure, and death.[1] Less severely poisoned patients administered only intensive supportive care have survived,[6, 33] whereas patients also administered specific antidotes have survived with whole-blood cyanide levels as high as 40 μg/mL.[34] Most patients who recover from acute cyanide poisoning do not have permanent sequelae, although rare cases of parkinsonian-like states, with bilaterally symmetric lesions in the basal ganglia (putamen or globus pallidus) or memory deficits and personality changes, have been reported.[16, 35–37]

The clinical presentation depends on the route, dose, and time elapsed since exposure. Patients with inhalation exposure to high concentrations may experience sudden loss of consciousness after only a few breaths.[3, 38] Patients who ingest potentially fatal amounts may not develop life-threatening symptoms for up to 0.5 to 1 hour after exposure.[31] Delayed onset of symptoms (after 1 to 12 or more hours) may follow exposure to cyanogens such as laetrile, amygdalin, and nitrile compounds.[6, 15, 17, 18]

In patients who do not experience sudden collapse, the initial signs and symptoms can resemble those of anxiety or hyperventilation syndrome.[1] Early signs include those of central nervous system stimulation (giddiness, headache, anxiety), tachycardia, hyperpnea, mild hypertension, and palpitations.[6]

Late signs of poisoning are nausea, vomiting, tachycardia or bradycardia, hypotension, generalized seizures, coma, apnea, dilated pupils (either nonreactive or sluggishly reactive), and a variety of cardiac effects, including erratic supraventricular or ventricular arrhythmias, atrioventricular blocks, ischemic changes on electrocardiography, and eventual asystole.[1] Noncardiogenic pulmonary edema may occur, even following ingestion.[33]

The smell of "bitter almonds" (often described simply as "musty") may be appreciated in some cases, but the ability to detect this odor is genetically determined and thus many people cannot do so.[1] Cyanosis is a late sign that is usually only noted at the stage of apnea and circulatory collapse. The absence of cyanosis in spontaneously breathing or artificially ventilated patients who have signs compatible with severe hypoxia should suggest the diagnosis.[1]

Although some references state that systemic cyanide poisoning can occur from dermal exposure, it is difficult to find actual reported cases, other than those due to serious burns from molten cyanide salts, immersion in vats of cyanide solutions (with the potential for ingestion and vapor inhalation as well as dermal exposure), or total-body contamination in confined spaces.

DIAGNOSIS

The initial physical examination focuses on the vital signs and the respiratory, cardiovascular, and central nervous systems. Continuous vital sign and electrocardiographic monitoring should be done. Whole-blood cyanide levels are available, but generally take hours to obtain and cannot be used to guide emergent diagnosis or therapy.[1] They can, however, contribute to the documentation of the diagnosis and response to treatment.

Lactic acid, serum electrolyte, and arterial blood gas levels should be monitored as frequently as necessary to guide fluid, electrolyte, sodium bicarbonate, and respiratory therapy. If pulmonary edema develops, a chest radiograph should be obtained periodically.

Based on anecdotal case reports and animal experiments, certain screening laboratory values may help suggest the diagnosis when no history is available.[1] Cyanide produces lactic acidosis, which can be noted directly on serum lactate measurements[15, 28] or indirectly on arterial blood gas pH measurements; lactic acidosis may also be reflected by an elevated anion gap on the serum electrolyte panel (anion gap = $cNa^+ - [cCl^- + cCO_2^-]$, where c is the concentration; normal = <12 to 16 mEq/L [mmol/L]). Normal serum lactate levels are 1.0 mEq/L (mmol/L) or less; a diagnosis of lactic acidosis is usually made when serum lactate levels are greater than 2.0 mEq/L (mmol/L). In combined poisoning with carbon monoxide and cyanide from smoke inhalation, plasma lactate levels may be the best marker of the presence and severity of a cyanide poisoning component.[9, 39]

If the patient is still breathing or is receiving assisted ventilation, the arterial partial pressure of O_2 may be relatively normal. Cyanide inhibits the extraction of O_2 from the blood at the tissue level. Thus, more O_2 than normal is present on the venous side; this may be reflected by an increased (>40 mm Hg) peripheral venous partial pressure of O_2, an increased measured peripheral venous O_2 per cent saturation (>70%), or a narrowing of the normal difference between the measured arterial O_2 per cent saturation and the measured central venous or pulmonary artery O_2 per cent saturation (the normal central venous O_2 per cent saturation is about 70%).[1, 16] However, a mixed venous O_2 per cent saturation less than 90% does not, in itself, exclude acute cyanide poisoning.[15]

A smoke inhalation clinical scoring system (scale, from 1 to 10) based on the following clinical findings has been proposed: hoarseness (1 point); stridor (1 point); carbonaceous sputum (1 point); soot in the airways (1 point); singed nasal hairs (1 point); facial burns (1 point); abnormal chest auscultation findings (1 point); mental status change (1 point); and abnormal findings on chest radiography (2 points). In one case series, this clinical scoring system was predictive of a fatal outcome following smoke inhalation exposure from fire in an enclosed space; it was also the strongest predictor of assessed carboxyhemoglobin and whole-blood cyanide levels.[40]

TREATMENT

Supportive Measures

Cyanide-exposed patients with only restlessness, anxiety, or hyperventilation do not require antidote therapy, which can be dangerous as well as unnecessary. Such patients should be administered supplemental O_2 and should undergo a period of clinical monitoring. Antidotes should be administered only if more serious symptoms develop.

Rescuers must not enter areas with high airborne concentrations of cyanide without full protective clothing and proper respirators. Mouth-to-mouth breathing should be avoided if at all possible, and care must be taken by rescuers not to inhale the victim's exhaled breath. Appropriate prehospital care consists of airway management, including endotracheal intubation if required, administration of 100% supplemental O_2 by tight-fitting mask or endotracheal tube, placement of at least one large-bore intravenous line, administration of sodium bicarbonate if shock (with presumed metabolic acidosis) is present, decontamination of exposed skin or eyes, administration of standard antiarrhythmic or anticonvulsant medications if necessary, and administration of amyl nitrite by inhalation.

Amyl nitrite pearls may be broken in gauze and held close to the nose and mouth of patients who are spontaneously breathing. Alternatively, they may be placed into the lip of the face mask or inside the resuscitation bag in patients with apnea or hypoventilation. Amyl nitrite should be inhaled for 30 seconds out of each minute, and a used pearl should be replaced with a fresh one every 3 to 4 minutes. Amyl nitrite and supplemental O_2 administration alone have been efficacious in treating cyanide-poisoned patients in an occupational exposure setting.[41]

Supportive measures alone may sometimes prove to be satisfactory,[33, 38] although patients administered specific antidotes together with supportive therapy have survived with higher whole-blood cyanide levels, awakened sooner from coma, and had more rapid correction of acidosis and, thus, required less sodium bicarbonate administration.[6, 31, 34]

Standard antiarrhythmic and anticonvulsant medications are appropriate for the treatment of cyanide-induced arrhythmias and convulsions. Atropine or vasopressors may be required if symptomatic bradycardia or hypotension unresponsive to less aggressive measures are present. Metabolic acidosis should be corrected with sodium bicarbonate administration.

Decontamination and Prevention of Systemic Absorption

Exposed skin and eyes should be copiously flushed with water or normal saline. Contaminated clothing should be removed and isolated in impervious containers. Inducing emesis is contraindicated because of the potential for rapid progression to coma or seizures. Gastric lavage with a large-bore orogastric tube might be beneficial within about 60 minutes of ingestion. Older references suggest the use of various neutralizing agents in the lavage fluid, but there is no evidence for their efficacy. Although older references question the efficacy of activated charcoal administration, a single dose of approximately 1 g of activated charcoal per kilogram of body weight should be administered to patients who have ingested cyanide and related compounds.

Antidotes

In the United States and some other countries, specific therapy consists of the administration of the antidotes found in the cyanide antidote kit (Eli Lilly). Amyl nitrite has already been discussed in this chapter. Once intravenous access has been established, amyl nitrite inhalation should be discontinued and sodium nitrite administered intravenously. The usual adult dose is 300 mg (one 10-mL ampule of a 3% solution). The pediatric dose for the average child is 0.12 to 0.33 mL/kg.

Sodium nitrite has potentially significant toxicity. It is a potent vasodilator, and rapid administration may result in hypotension,[34] which can be avoided by initial slow administration, either (1) by slow intravenous push over no less than 5 minutes, or (2) by diluting the dose in 50 to 100 mL of 5% dextrose in water, initially beginning with a slow infusion rate, and then increasing to the most rapid rate possible without causing hypotension. Frequent blood pressure monitoring is mandatory during sodium nitrite administration.

Another potentially serious, although rare, adverse effect of sodium nitrite administration is induction of excessive methemoglobin levels.[34] Induction of some level of methemoglobinemia has long been thought to be the mechanism of action of sodium nitrite, as methemoglobin has a greater affinity for cyanide than cytochrome oxidase. This hypothesis has been questioned.

Excessive methemoglobin induction occurs most often in patients given excessive amounts of sodium nitrite, but it is rarely seen with therapeutic doses.[34] Methemoglobin levels should be monitored, especially when multiple doses of sodium nitrite are required. Inducing levels greater than 30% to 40% must be avoided.

Administering "enough" sodium nitrite to induce a "therapeutic methemoglobin level" of 25% has sometimes been recommended. However, patients have had excellent clinical recovery from acute cyanide poisoning with elevated whole-blood cyanide levels, even when co-oximeter–measured sodium nitrite–induced methemoglobin levels were as low as 2%.[31] The determinant of when "enough" sodium nitrite has been infused is the patient's clinical response.

Sodium nitrite should be followed by intravenous administration of sodium thiosulfate, with the adult dose being 12.5 g (one 50-mL ampule of a 25% solution). The average pediatric dose is 1.65 mL/kg. No cases of significant adverse effects from sodium thiosulfate administration have been reported in humans, despite over 50 years of clinical use of the drug. In selected patients with less severe poisoning, sodium thiosulfate and supportive measures alone may be sufficient.[15, 42] A continuous infusion of 1 g of sodium thiosulfate per hour for 24 hours was efficacious in one case of potassium cyanide ingestion poisoning.[42]

In cases of smoke inhalation with known carbon monoxide and suspected cyanide poisoning, sodium thiosulfate and 100% supplemental O_2 should be administered initially. Sodium nitrite administration should be withheld until the patient is at pressure in a hyperbaric oxygenation (HBO) chamber, where dissolved plasma O_2 can adequately compensate for induced methemoglobinemia.[8] HBO therapy itself may be beneficial, even in cases of "pure" cyanide poisoning.[28] However, when HBO was not immediately available for treatment of smoke inhalation patients, sodium nitrite has been administered successfully without complications.[43]

Second doses of sodium nitrite and sodium thiosulfate at one-half the initial amounts may be administered 30 minutes after the first doses if clinical response is inadequate. Administering further "prophylactic" doses to patients who have regained consciousness, spontaneous respirations, and stable vital signs is unnecessary and potentially dangerous. With exposure to certain nitrile compounds, however, continued metabolic release of cyanide may cause a prolonged poisoning requiring multiple antidote doses. If producing a satisfactory clinical response, sodium thiosulfate alone could be used in such cases, as its inherent toxicity is low.

Alternate antidotes in clinical use in other parts of the world such as hydroxocobalamin, dicobalt–ethylenediaminetetraacetic acid (Kelocyanor), and 4-dimethylaminophenol are not currently available in the United States.

Other Supportive Therapy

Supplemental normobaric O_2 is efficacious in treating cyanide-poisoned patients. Although not proven, HBO may be even more efficacious in patients not responsive to supportive and antidotal therapy. Reported human experience with this modality is limited, but some cyanide-poisoned patients treated with HBO have survived.[14, 28] Smoke inhalation victims with serious known carbon monoxide poisoning and suspected cyanide toxicity should be treated with HBO when available.[8]

Elimination Enhancement

Hemodialysis cannot be considered standard treatment for cyanide poisoning, but it has been efficaciously used as supportive therapy in a patient who developed renal failure secondary to rhabdomyolysis in the course of severe cyanide poisoning.[16] One patient with severe acute cyanide poisoning treated with supportive measures, antidotes, and charcoal hemoperfusion has also been reported.[4] This patient was improving following antidotal and supportive therapy at the time that hemoperfusion was begun. Hemoperfusion would presently seem to have no place in the treatment of acute cyanide poisoning.

Disposition

Asymptomatic patients with apparent minimal exposure should be observed in a controlled setting for 4 to 6 hours. If exposure was to a nitrile compound, the onset of symptoms may be delayed for 12 hours or longer; in this situation, a longer period of observation and monitoring, with probable admission, is necessary.

Patients who have serious symptoms (coma, convulsions, shock, metabolic acidosis, cardiac arrhythmias, ischemic electrocardiographic changes, and hypoventilation) and all those administered antidotes should be admitted to an intensive care unit for clinical monitoring until all symptoms have resolved, or for a minimum period of 24 hours. Outpatient followup at intervals for a period of weeks to months should be arranged in order to screen for the possible development of rare delayed central nervous system effects.

Organ Donation

Given the acute shortage of suitable organ donors, brain-dead poisoning victims should not be excluded as donors, if (1) clinical and laboratory evidence shows true brain death (*not* central nervous system depression or lack of central nervous system activity due to the continued presence of the poison); (2) the poison itself has not irretrievably damaged or destroyed the organ under consideration for transplantation; and (3) the organ being considered for transplantation is not a reservoir, such that the transplanted organ itself might secondarily poison the transplant recipient. Organs have been successfully transplanted from brain-dead acute cyanide poisoning victims without causing secondary cyanide poisoning.[7, 27, 44, 45]

References

1. Hall AH, Rumack BH: Clinical toxicology of cyanide. Ann Emerg Med *15*:1067, 1986.
2. Blanc P, Hogan M, Mallin K, et al: Cyanide intoxication among silver-reclaiming workers. JAMA *253*:367, 1985.
3. Hartung R: Cyanides and nitriles. *In* Clayton GD, Clayton FE (eds): Patty's Industrial Hygiene and Toxicology. 4th ed. Vol. II. New York, John Wiley & Sons, p 3119, 1994.
4. Krieg A, Saxena K: Cyanide poisoning from metal cleaning solutions. Ann Emerg Med *16*:582, 1987.
5. Smith RA: Controversies in toxicology: Rapid quantitative determination of cyanide in biological fluids from coyotes killed with a coyote getter. Vet Hum Toxicol *37*:580, 1995.
6. Hall AH, Rumack BH, Schaffer MI, Linden CH: Clinical toxicology of cyanide: North American clinical experiences. *In* Ballantyne B, Marrs TC (eds): Clinical and Experimental Toxicology of Cyanides. John Wright and Sons, Ltd., Bristol, England, p 312, 1987.
7. Anonymous: Cyanide poisoning associated with over-the-counter medication—Washington, State. MMWR Morb Mortal Wkly Rep *40*:161, 1991.
8. Hart GB, Strauss MB, Lennon PA, Whitcraft DD: Treatment of smoke inhalation by hyperbaric oxygen. J Emerg Med *3*:211, 1985.
9. Baud FJ, Barriot P, Toffis V, et al: Elevated blood cyanide concentrations in victims of smoke inhalation. N Engl J Med *325*:1761, 1991.
10. Norris JC, Moore SJ, Hume AS: Synergistic lethality induced by the combination of carbon monoxide and cyanide. Toxicology *40*:121, 1986.
11. Mayes RW: The toxicological examination of the British Air Tours Boeing 737 accident at Manchester in 1985. J Forensic Sci *36*:179, 1991.
12. Barr SJ: Chemical warfare agents. Top Emerg Med *7*:62, 1985.
13. Bismuth C, Baud FJ, Djeghout H, et al: Cyanide poisoning from propionitrile exposure. J Emerg Med *5*:191, 1987.
14. Scolnik B, Hamel D, Woolf AD: Successful treatment of life-threatening propionitrile exposure with sodium nitrite/sodium thiosulfate followed by hyperbaric oxygen. J Occup Med *35*:577, 1993.
15. Yeh MM, Becker CE, Arieff AI: Is measurement of venous oxygen saturation useful in the diagnosis of cyanide poisoning? Am J Med *93*:582, 1992.
16. Yen D, Tsai J, Wang L-M, et al: The clinical experience of acute cyanide poisoning. Am J Emerg Med *13*:524, 1995.

17. Kurt TH, Day LC, Reed WG: Cyanide poisoning from glue-on nail remover. Am J Emerg Med *9*:201, 1991.
18. Michaelis HC, Clemens C, Kijewski: Acetonitrile concentrations and cyanide levels in a case of suicidal oral acetonitrile ingestion. Clin Toxicol *29*:447, 1991.
19. Schulz V, Gross R, Pasch T, et al: Cyanide toxicity of sodium nitroprusside in therapeutic use with and without sodium thiosulfate. Klin Wochenschr *60*:1393, 1982.
20. Linakis JG, Lacouture PG, Woolf A: Monitoring cyanide and thiocyanate concentrations during infusion of sodium nitroprusside in children. Pediatr Cardiol *12*:214, 1991.
21. Vesey CJ, Cole PV, Linnell JC, Wilson J: Some metabolic effects of sodium nitroprusside in man. BMJ *2*:140, 1974.
22. Vesey CJ, Cole PV: Blood cyanide and thiocyanate concentrations produced by long-term therapy with sodium nitroprusside. Br J Anaesthiol *57*:148, 1985.
23. Osuntokun BO: Chronic cyanide intoxication of dietary origin and a degenerative neuropathy in Nigerians. Acta Hortic *375*:311, 1994.
24. Tylleskar T, Howlett WP, Rwiza HT, et al: Konzo: A distinct disease entity with selective upper motor neuron damage. J Neurol Neurosurg Psychiatr *56*:638, 1993.
25. Espinoza OB, Perez M, Ramirez MS: Bitter cassava poisoning in eight children: A case report. Vet Hum Toxicol *34*:65, 1992.
26. Delange F, Ekpechi LO, Rosling H: Cassava cyanogenesis and iodine deficiency disorders. Acta Hortic *375*:289, 1994.
27. Litovitz TL, Felberg L, Soloway RA, et al: 1994 Annual Report of the American Association of Poison Control Centers Toxic Exposure Surveillance System. Am J Emerg Med *13*:551, 1995.
28. Goodhart GL: Patient treated with antidote kit and hyperbaric oxygen survives cyanide poisoning. South Med J *87*:814, 1994.
29. Christel D, Eyer P, Hegemann M, et al: Pharmacokinetics of cyanide poisoning in dogs, and the effects of 4-dimethylaminophenol or thiosulfate. Arch Toxicol *38*:177, 1977.
30. Sylvester DM, Hayton WL, Morgan RL, Way JL: Effects of thiosulfate on cyanide pharmacokinetics in dogs. Toxicol Appl Pharmacol *69*:265, 1983.
31. Hall AH, Doutre WH, Ludden T, et al: Nitrite/thiosulfate treated acute cyanide poisoning: Estimated kinetics after antidote. Clin Toxicol *25*:121, 1987.
32. Bi QN, Sun PW, Gunasekar PG, Isom GE: Involvement of CA^{2+}/calmodulin-dependent protein kinase II in cyanide-induced cytotoxicity in cultured cerebellar granular cells. Abstract. Toxicologist *30*:186, 1996.
33. Graham DL, Laman D, Theodore J, Robin ED: Acute cyanide poisoning complicated by lactic acidosis and pulmonary edema. Arch Intern Med *137*:1051, 1977.
34. Feihl F, Domenighetti G, Perret C: Intoxication massive au cyanure avec évolution favorable. Schweiz Med Wschr *112*:1280, 1982.
35. Jouglard J, Fagot G, Deguigne B, Arlaud J-A: L'intoxication cyanhydrique aigüe et son traitement d'urgence. Mars Med *9*:571, 1971.
36. Rosenberg NL, Myes JA, Martin MRW: Cyanide-induced parkinsonism: Clinical, MRI, and 6-fluorodopa PET studies. Neurology *39*:142, 1989.
37. Feldman JM, Felman MD: Sequelae of attempted suicide by cyanide ingestion: A case report. Int J Psychiatr Med *20*:173, 1990.
38. Peden NR, Taha A, McSorley PD, et al: Industrial exposure to hydrogen cyanide: Implications for treatment. BMJ *293*:538, 1986.
39. Baud FJ, Imbert M, Vicaut E, et al: Time-course of lactic acidosis in acute cyanide poisonings treated with oxygen and high doses of hydroxocobalamin. Abstract. Int Toxicol *7*:38-PF-4, 1995.
40. Shusterman D, Alexeef G, Hargis C, et al: Predictors of carbon monoxide and hydrogen cyanide exposure in smoke inhalation patients. Clin Toxicol *34*:61, 1996.
41. Wurzburg H: Treatment of cyanide poisoning in an industrial setting. Vet Hum Toxicol *38*:44, 1996.
42. Heintz B, Bock TA, Kierdorf H, Sieberth HG: Cyanid Intoxikation: Behandlung mit Hyperoxigenation und Natriumthiosulfat. Dtsch Med Wochenschr *115*:1100, 1990.
43. Kirk MA, Gerace R, Kulig KW: Cyanide and methemoglobin kinetics in smoke inhalation victims treated with the cyanide antidote kit. Ann Emerg Med *22*:9, 1993.
44. Swanson-Bierman B, Krenzelok EP, Snyder JW, et al: Successful donation and transplantation of multiple organs from a victim of cyanide poisoning. Clin Toxicol *31*:95, 1993.
45. Hantson P, Mahieu P, Hassoun A, Otte J-B: Outcome following organ removal from poisoned donors in brain death status: A report of 12 cases and review of the literature. Clin Toxicol *33*:709, 1995.

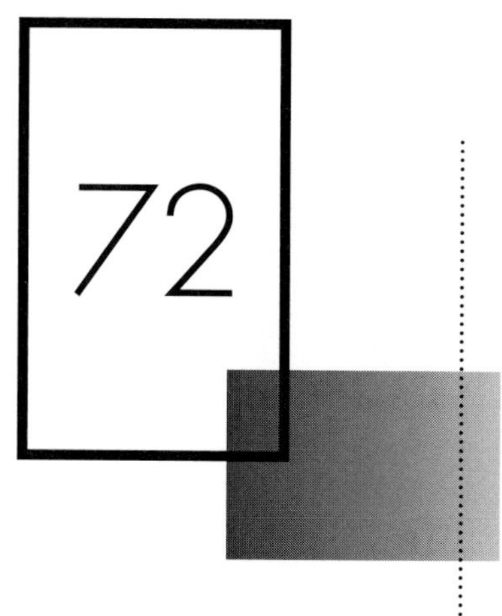

Hydrogen Sulfide

INGRID M. O. VICAS, MD

Hydrogen sulfide (H_2S) is a highly toxic, malodorous, intensely irritating gas. Poisoning with H_2S results in significant numbers of fatalities. Often, a deadly exposure affects multiple persons, as in the case of inadequately protected workers who succumb during rescue procedures.

H_2S is released from a variety of natural sources, including decaying organic material, natural gas, volcanic gases, petroleum, sulfur deposits, and sulfur springs. H_2S is routinely generated in agricultural processes and in the course of exploration for oil and natural gas. More than 70 occupational environments present some risk of H_2S toxicity, including viscose rayon manufacturing plants, paper mills, petrochemical and natural gas plants, petroleum refineries, heavy water production plants, coke oven plants, iron smelters, food processing plants, sugar beet processors, tanneries, and pesticide and sulfur production plants.[1] The petroleum industry, however, is the foremost source of H_2S exposure to workers.[2]

Because the circumstances of H_2S exposure are predominantly occupational, men tend to be more commonly affected than women.[2] However, a number of reports describe male workers' spouses[3] or children[3, 4] who have been accidentally exposed to H_2S.

MECHANISM OF ACTION

By inhibiting mitochondrial cytochrome-*c* oxidase, H_2S paralyzes the electron transport system, resulting in inhibition of cellular utilization of oxygen, metabolic acidosis secondary to anaerobic metabolism, and cytotoxic anoxia.[5] In body fluids at physiologic pH, undissociated and dissociated H_2S molecules exist in equal proportions. The undissociated acid, H_2S, is thought to be more inhibitory than its dissociated form, HS^-.[6] Although the mechanism of toxicity of H_2S resembles that of cyanide, H_2S is a more potent cytochrome-*c* oxidase inhibitor than is cyanide.[5]

PHARMACOKINETICS

Absorption

H_2S is rapidly and almost exclusively absorbed through the inhalation route. Percutaneous absorption is minimal, although toxicity and even death have been reported following cutaneous application of sulfur-containing dermatologic preparations or ammonium sulfide permanent-wave solutions.[6]

Distribution

H_2S is distributed to the brain, liver, kidney, pancreas, and small intestine.[7]

Metabolism

The metabolism of H_2S involves three different pathways: (1) oxidation to sulfate (considered to be the major metabolic pathway); (2) methylation; and (3) reaction with metallic ion– or disulfide-containing proteins. Oxidation and methylation represent detoxification routes, whereas interaction with essential proteins is responsible for the toxic action of H_2S.[8] Sulfides undergo spontaneous oxidation through both enzymatic and nonenzymatic mechanisms to nontoxic products such as thiosulfate, polysulfides, and sulfate. The major site of this conversion appears to be the liver, although other tissues such as the kidney and lung, as well as plasma, may function as secondary sites. The process of sulfide auto-oxidation consumes oxygen.[9] The reaction of H_2S with nonessential proteins containing disulfide bonds (e.g., glutathione) may represent yet another detoxification pathway with interesting therapeutic implications.[6] H_2S produced endogenously by anaerobic bacteria in the gut is detoxified through sequential methylation by intestinal tract cells.[10] The importance, if any, of this metabolic route for the detoxification of exogenously administered hydrogen sulfide remains to be determined.[8]

Excretion

Nontoxic oxidation products are excreted primarily by the kidneys.[11] Neither H_2S nor its metabolites have been shown to be excreted by the lungs.[12] Currently, H_2S is not considered a cumulative poison because it is metabolized and excreted.

Table 72–1. Physiologic Effect of Human Exposure to Hydrogen Sulfide

Concentration (ppm)	Effect
0.02	Odor threshold
100–150	Nose/eye irritation
250–500	Sore throat, cough
	Keratoconjunctivitis
	Chest tightness
	Pulmonary edema
500–1000	Headache
	Disorientation
	Loss of reasoning
	Coma, convulsions
>1000	Death

Adapted from Beauchamp RO, Bus JS, Popp JA, et al: A critical review of the literature on hydrogen sulfide toxicity. CRC Crit Rev Toxicol *13*:25–49, 1984.

CLINICAL PRESENTATION

Pathophysiology

Single sublethal doses of H_2S directly stimulate the carotid body, resulting in a brief but dramatic hyperpnea.[13] However, in persons with lethal exposures, the primary cause of death has been attributed to respiratory paralysis due to the toxic effect of sulfides on the respiratory centers of the brain.[8] Experimental evidence showing selective uptake of sulfide by the brain stem seems to support this observation.[14, 15]

Manifestations

Acute Exposure

Two major effects of H_2S on the human system can be identified: a local irritative effect, and a rapidly fatal systemic effect from the inhalation of high concentrations of H_2S.[8] The primary targets of systemic H_2S toxicity appear to be the central nervous system and the respiratory system. The mucous membranes of the eyes and the respiratory tract are the targets of local irritative and inflammatory effects. Severity of clinical effects is related to both the concentration of H_2S (Table 72–1) and the duration of exposure. Symptoms in seriously affected patients, not surprisingly, include unconsciousness, cyanosis, dilated pupils, decreased respirations or apnea, and generalized tremors or convulsions and agitation.

Neurologic Manifestations

Transient loss of consciousness, prolonged coma, lateralizing motor signs, headache, agitation, somnolence, tremulousness, convulsions, opisthotonus, and vertigo have been described as central nervous system manifestations of toxicity.[3, 17–29]

In a large series of workers exposed to H_2S, even though 75% demonstrated a period of loss of consciousness at the site of exposure, only 13% were still comatose on arrival at the hospital.[2] Table 72–2 summarizes the clinical effects observed in three series in a total of 523 patients.[2, 30, 31] Neurologic complaints consisting of altered behavior patterns, confusion, vertigo, agitation, and somnolence were common in all three series. Although headache may not necessarily occur immediately after exposure, it is usually present in 16% to 25% of patients by the time they arrive at the hospital.[2] Sudden loss of consciousness on exposure to toxic concentrations, colloquially referred to as "knockdown" by workers, is usually associated with equally sudden spontaneous recovery. Upon recovery, affected workers often continue their work without seeking medical attention until the end of the workday, when they are essentially asymptomatic. However, a knockdown may be fatal if exposure is prolonged.[32]

Pulmonary Manifestations

Minor pulmonary manifestations include cough, dyspnea, and hemoptysis (see Table 72–2). Clinical and radiologic evidence of pulmonary edema[2, 17, 20] and apnea[17–19, 21, 22] represents life-threatening pulmonary symptoms. Once respirations cease, they do not resume spontaneously, even if the patient is removed from the toxic source.[34] Apnea is often followed by convulsions, cardiovascular collapse, and death. Up to 20% of H_2S-exposed patients arriving in an emergency department demonstrated pulmonary edema.[2] This pulmonary edema can be extensive in nature, with copious frothy, bloody secretions. Experimentally, a similar massive pulmonary edema can be demonstrated after acute inhalation exposure to H_2S.[35]

Marked cyanosis is a common phenomenon described in both survivors and nonsurvivors.[17, 19–22] Although the cause of this cyanosis is unclear, several mechanisms can be considered, including (1) inadequate oxygenation due to marked pulmonary edema, (2) poor tissue perfusion due to hypotension, and (3) formation of a pigmented sulfhemoglobin. This third theoretic mechanism is controversial; some authors

Table 72–2. Clinical Features of Hydrogen Sulfide Toxicity

Symptom	No. of Patients (n = 523)	Reference		
		Kleinfeld et al (1964)[30] *(n = 52)*	*Burnett et al (1977)*[2] *(n = 221)*	*Arnold et al (1985)*[31] *(n = 250)*
Unconsciousness	309	11	163	135
Dizziness, vertigo, agitation, confusion	143	39	50	54
Headache	103	11	2?	65
Nausea or vomiting	112	12	38	62
Dyspnea	68	5	6	57
Convulsions	22	1	16	5
Pulmonary edema	50	2	34	14
Cyanosis	27	5	19	3
Conjunctivitis	67	2	19	46
Sore throat, cough	70	5	24	41
Weakness	40	13	8	19
Hemoptysis	3	—	2	1
Miscellaneous	113	34*	—	79†
Death	21	4	10	7

*Includes hoarseness, tachycardia, numbness, chest burning, tremors, and hyperreflexia.
†Includes malaise, chest pain, bradycardia, and neuropsychologic symptoms.

contend that H_2S toxicity does not induce sulfhemoglobin formation.[40]

Cardiovascular Manifestations

Myocardial infarction and electrocardiographic changes may occur.[41] However, these effects may be secondary to prolonged hypoxia rather than to a direct cardiotoxic or arrhythmogenic effect of H_2S.

Other Manifestations

Local irritating effects such as sore throat and gastrointestinal symptoms (e.g., nausea and vomiting) have been described.[2] Ocular effects include keratoconjunctivitis and subjective symptoms such as blurring of vision, "haloes" around lights ("gas eye"), photophobia, and blepharospasm. These ocular symptoms occur early in a patient with subacute exposure to H_2S, even before the manifestation of any respiratory symptoms.[8]

At concentrations of up to 30 ppm, H_2S has a rotten-egg odor, whereas at 30 ppm the odor is described as sickeningly sweet. The pungent odor of H_2S provides adequate warning at low levels of exposure. At higher concentrations, olfactory nerve fatigue and, later, paralysis of the nerve result in the inability to detect the odor. The assumption that odor warns of levels of H_2S that are life-threatening is erroneous because concentrations greater than 150 ppm may not be perceived at all.[34] Workers who recover from H_2S exposure either have no recollection of any odor or may notice a sickeningly sweet odor before loss of consciousness.

Outcome

The overall mortality in three series of H_2S victims is 4% (range, 2.8% to 6%; see Table 72–2). Ultimate survival despite complete cardiopulmonary arrest has been described.[14, 23]

In a series of 221 exposure victims, 21% of patients were seen in a physician's office and discharged. Of the 78% seen in a hospital, 65% were admitted, 6% were dead on arrival, and the remainder (29%) were discharged. Ultimately, 10% of all admitted patients required transfer to a tertiary care facility.[2] In another series of 250 workers with H_2S exposure, 22% required overnight hospitalization for observation.[31]

Permanent neurologic sequelae include prolonged coma, convulsions, increased tone with extensor muscle spasm,[37] chronic vegetative state,[4, 18] intention tremor, pseudobulbar impairment,[19] and cognitive impairment.[42–47]

The potential for increased H_2S sensitivity from repeated exposures has been considered. No good evidence supports increased or decreased sensitivity to H_2S with multiple overexposures. Although H_2S is said not to be a cumulative poison,[13] it is possible that repeated knockdown episodes result in long-term effects,[32] or that a knockdown experience renders the individual more sensitive to a lower concentration of H_2S on re-exposure.

Chronic Exposure

Whether chronic poisoning exists as an entity or whether it is a subjective response to an obnoxious agent remains unresolved.[8] Although the majority of serious exposures are acute in nature, there is continued concern about the effects of long-term exposure on an individual's general health, particularly with regard to the development of the fetus and the immature central nervous system. However, data on the teratogenic, carcinogenic, and long-term effects of chronic low-dose exposure to H_2S are incomplete.[1]

Laboratory Features

Arterial Blood Gases

Arterial partial pressure of oxygen is usually normal. However, because it binds to cytochrome-*c* oxidase, H_2S results in cellular impairment of oxygen extraction, leaving an elevated venous partial pressure of oxygen. Also, one would expect to find a decrease in the arterial-venous difference in oxygen tension in H_2S exposure, even though this has not been specifically documented.

An oxygen saturation gap (i.e., the calculated oxygen saturation minus the measured oxygen saturation) has been reported in a patient exposed to H_2S.[18] After accounting for methemoglobin and carboxyhemoglobin concentrations, it was implied that the oxygen saturation gap was due to the presence of an abnormal hemoglobin, in this case thought to be sulfhemoglobin.

Sulfhemoglobin Controversy

The presence of sulfmethemoglobin as a consequence of H_2S poisoning has been disputed. Although the formation of sulfhemoglobin has been reported or suggested after a variety of drug ingestions[38] or after H_2S exposure,[18, 21] sulfhemoglobin is thought not to occur in H_2S poisoning.[34, 39]

Radiologic Investigations

A chest radiograph may show evidence of pulmonary edema. Computed tomography of the brain has been reported to show evidence of basal ganglial lesions.[37, 40]

Sulfide Measurements

Techniques developed to measure either plasma or brain sulfide levels[14, 48] have been applied either after acute exposure to H_2S in workers[48] or in postmortem samples.[14, 49]

The brain sulfide technique involves gas dialysis and ion chromatography coupled with electrochemical detection. Endogenous brain sulfide levels have been measured experimentally in rats poisoned with H_2S or sodium sulfide,[15] in the normal human postmortem brain stem,[14] and in brain stem specimens obtained after H_2S-related death.[49] Endogenous brain sulfide levels in normal human postmortem brain stem have been measured at 0.67 ± 0.05 µg/g. This technique may be useful in confirming death due to acute H_2S poisoning by inhalation.

Brain stem selectively accumulates H_2S,[4] specifically in the myelin and mitochondrial fractions.[14] It is known that H_2S is more soluble in lipophilic solvent than in water. Because the brain stem has a higher concentration of white matter than the rest of the brain, and since white matter contains more lipid than gray matter, it is not surprising that H_2S is preferentially concentrated in the brain stem.

Treatment

Supportive Measures

Because many victims of H_2S exposure may be apneic at the scene, immediate resuscitation measures are imperative (Table 72–3). There is no evidence that performing mouth-to-mouth resuscitation on a victim of H_2S inhalation poses any danger to the rescuer. However, rescuers should first ensure that the environment is safe and should wear a self-contained breathing apparatus before they attempt to perform rescue procedures. Numerous reports[21, 24, 36, 50–55] describe rescuer exposure at the toxic environment, often with fatal outcomes.[4, 50–54]

Table 72–3. Principles of Management of Hydrogen Sulfide Exposure

Rescuer protection
Basic life support
Aggressive supportive care
Sodium nitrite (3%)
Adult: 10 mL at 2.5 to 5 mL/min
Child: 0.2 mL/kg
Hyperbaric oxygen therapy may be considered under select circumstances

In the hospital, early and aggressive management of convulsions, pulmonary edema, and acidosis may result in ultimate survival with no long-term sequelae.*

Oxygen

Experimentally, administration of oxygen alone does not affect the course of acute H_2S poisoning.[55]

Hyperbaric Oxygenation

Anecdotal evidence suggests an apparent benefit of hyperbaric oxygenation (HBO) therapy in victims of H_2S poisoning.[23, 24] In both cases, the patients did not seem to demonstrate significant improvement after standard nitrite therapy. HBO therapy, instituted even after a 10-hour delay, resulted in marked improvement in mental status as early as the administration of the first treatment.[23] In the second report, nitrite therapy administered within 30 to 60 minutes after exposure resulted in minimal improvement in mental status. Three treatments of HBO therapy at 2.5 atm for 90 minutes resulted in complete recovery.[24] Two other case reports describe patients with persistent cognitive deficits despite HBO.[42] In only one case was HBO therapy reported to be ineffective.[43]

HBO therapy is postulated to be effective by one of several mechanisms: (1) increased H_2S concentration results in increased H_2S competition for binding sites on cytochrome oxidase; (2) because oxyhemoglobin is a natural catalyst of sulfide oxidation, increased oxyhemoglobin concentration favors auto-oxidation of sulfide; (3) increased oxygen plasma diffusion results in improved oxygenation of marginally perfused tissue.[24]

Although further research is warranted, HBO therapy in H_2S exposure may be of significant benefit in

*See references 13, 17, 19, 25, 26, 28, 30, 52, and 53.

patients in whom central nervous system symptoms do not resolve either spontaneously or after prompt institution of nitrite therapy. The effect of HBO therapy in patients with marked pulmonary edema remains to be demonstrated

Antidotes

Nitrites

The similarity of the mechanisms of toxicity of H_2S and cyanide poisoning has led to the suggestion that nitrite therapy be used in H_2S poisoning.[55, 56] According to established theory, nitrites are considered effective because they induce methemoglobinemia. The resultant large available pool of ferric heme has a greater affinity for H_2S than cytochrome-*c* oxidase; thus, sulfide ions are sequestered, and cytochrome-*c* oxidase is freed. With the removal of H_2S from cytochrome-*c* oxidase, aerobic metabolism resumes. The sulfmethemoglobin complex is then detoxified through endogenous routes.[6, 57]

The application of this theory remains unclear. An understanding of the experimental and clinical evidence for and against nitrite therapy will help the clinician to make an informed and independent decision.

Experimental Evidence

A number of animal and *in vitro* studies support the use of nitrite therapy. Under experimental conditions, when cytochrome-*c* oxidase is completely inhibited by sulfide, the addition of methemoglobin results in increased oxidation of cytochrome-*c* oxidase.[6]

Pretreatment of several animal species with sodium nitrite decreased mortality and increased survival time after exposure to either parenterally administered H_2S or to H_2S gas administered by inhalation.[56, 57] However, pretreatment with sodium nitrite was ineffective with high concentrations of H_2S (1872 ppm). Pretreatment with parenteral administration of human methemoglobin protected mice from lethal doses of H_2S.[58]

In one of the few studies reported in which nitrite therapy was administered after H_2S poisoning, the nitrite treatment decreased mortality.[56] However, the dose of nitrite used was 20-fold that recommended for cyanide poisoning; it was administered 2 minutes after sulfide injection and produced up to an 82% methemoglobinemia in the animals.[59]

The effectiveness of the sulfmethemoglobin complex in sulfide detoxification is questionable in light of two observations: (1) sulfide is not bound as strongly to methemoglobin as cyanide is[58]; and (2) sulfmethemoglobin undergoes gradual auto-oxidation–reduction to ferrihemoglobin and possibly to some oxidized form of sulfur.[6] Animal experiments with cyanide poisoning have demonstrated the efficacy of nitrites even in the presence of methylene blue, which blocks methemoglobin formation.[60] Alternative explanations for the efficacy of nitrite therapy in cyanide and H_2S poisoning have been suggested, including (1) vasoactive changes in microcirculation; (2) a direct cytochrome-*c* oxidase–stimulating effect; and (3) a direct effect on H_2S–cytochrome-*c* oxidase binding that is not mediated by methemoglobin induction.[18]

Recently, this mechanism has been called into question in the case of cyanide poisoning.[60] The clinical response to nitrites occurs more rapidly than can be explained by the rate of methemoglobin formation. Some experimental evidence points to the importance of the vasodilatory effects of nitrites. α-Adrenergic blocking agents such as chlorpromazine and phenoxybenzamine in combination with thiosulfate have been shown to be as effective in treating cyanide poisoning as the nitrite-thiosulfate combination.[60] No parallel experiments questioning the traditional explanation of the effectiveness of nitrites in H_2S poisoning have been conducted.

Alternatively, it may be that nitrite-induced methemoglobinemia is a more effective oxidation catalyst for sulfide than is oxyhemoglobin.[59] *In vitro* evidence shows that both oxyhemoglobin and methemoglobin are effective catalytic agents for sulfide, with methemoglobin being somewhat more efficacious.[31] On this basis, it is not surprising that animals pretreated with nitrite show a reduced sensitivity to sulfide because the faster reaction catalyzed by the methemoglobin permits a faster turnover of sulfide. However, the oxyhemoglobin-catalyzed reaction is also rapid, resulting in elimination of more than 90% of sulfide within 20 minutes. Additionally, nitrite produces methemoglobin slowly in the presence of air or oxygen but acts more rapidly under oxygen-depleted conditions. Furthermore, nitrite inhibits H_2S detoxification catalyzed by oxyhemoglobin. From this study, the authors inferred that the time that sulfide is present in an oxygenated blood stream is on the order of minutes. Among their conclusions based on these *in vitro* data were that (1) nitrites are effective only if they are given very early in the course of management and that (2) the methemoglobinemia so produced is relatively slow in light of the rapid catalytic effect of oxyhemoglobin. Their final conclusion was that the induction of methemoglobinemia about 10 minutes after exposure confers no added benefit. These data have not been confirmed *in vivo* by either animal experimentation or human observation.

Other Antidotes

A number of alternative antidotes have been investigated experimentally. It remains to be determined whether any of these agents will prove clinically efficacious.

Thiosulfate. Experimental evidence indicates that thiosulfate confers no significant protective effect in mice.[55] Unlike cyanide poisoning, in which sodium thiosulfate is known to serve as a substrate for the enzyme rhodanese, (which catalyzes the conversion of cyanide to the nontoxic thiocyanate), no parallel rationale is known for the use of thiosulfate as an antidote to sulfide poisoning.

Pyruvate. Pretreatment with 1 g/kg of pyruvic acid offers mice approximately the same protection from the lethal effects of parenteral sodium sulfide as that afforded by nitrites.[61, 62] Additionally, pyruvic acid increases the effectiveness of sodium nitrite.[61] Pyruvic acid treatment after exposure to parenteral administration of sodium sulfide reduced the lethality *of* parenterally administered sulfide.[63]

α-Ketoglutarate. Prophylactic administration of a combination of α-ketoglutaric acid and pyruvic acid reduced the lethality of sodium sulfide when given either parenterally or orally.[63] Additionally, the protective effect of this combination was further enhanced by administration of amyl nitrite after exposure to sodium sulfide.[63]

Dithiothreitol. Dithiothreitol reduces disulfide bridges to maintain sulfhydryl groups in their reduced states. Experimental data indicate that dithiothreitol increases brain sulfide concentrations in both control and sulfide-poisoned brain homogenates.[64] This fact leads to interesting speculation about the application of such a therapeutic agent after exposure for the detoxification of sites that have been inactivated by sulfide.

Summary

Despite some uncertainty, available experimental and clinical data indicate that sodium nitrite therapy (10 mL of a 3% solution at a rate of 2.5 to 5 mL/min) may be beneficial after basic life support measures have been instituted. In the light of *in vitro* evidence, greater benefit may be realized if the nitrite therapy is instituted early in the clinical course. Further investigation of the clinical effectiveness of nitrites administered at different times after exposure may determine the usefulness of nitrite therapy beyond the first few minutes after exposure.

Clinical use of nitrite therapy in cases of H_2S poisoning is limited to a handful of anecdotal reports. Recovery after nitrite treatment may not necessarily indicate therapeutic efficacy. Victims of H_2S poisoning have survived equally well without sequelae after supportive care alone. Pulmonary edema, a cause of early death from H_2S toxicity, should be treated promptly and aggressively.

The use of hyperbaric oxygen is controversial but may be of some benefit in patients who do not respond to nitrite therapy or who demonstrate persistent neurologic abnormalities. Its role in management warrants further investigation.

A number of alternative therapeutic agents show some promise experimentally, but further research is required to determine their application in a clinical setting.

DISPOSITION

Patients who are asymptomatic at the time of presentation may be safely discharged after a thorough examination. Patients who are complaining of local irritative effects should be treated with high flow oxygen, observed for 2 to 6 hours, and then discharged. Any patient with neurologic or respiratory symptoms should be thoroughly evaluated, and hospitalization for observation should be considered. Patients should be followed up for neurologic or neuropsychiatric sequelae.

PREVENTION

A significant number of potentially preventable deaths have occurred when rescuers did not protect themselves before attempting rescue procedures. Companies and workers at risk should be aware of the dangers of exposure to H_2S and should take appropriate precautions, including the wearing of protective equipment and the development of precautionary protocols that include a "buddy system" approach. A number of symptomatic exposures have resulted from equipment failure (e.g., mask knocked off, hose pinched, or valve frozen).[31] All workers at a facility where H_2S exposure is a risk should be trained in basic life support rescue methods. An overall improvement in worker awareness as well as improvement in on-site first-aid procedures can contribute significantly to an observed decrease in overall mortality (see Table 72–2).[31]

References

1. Tabacova S: Maternal exposure to environmental chemicals. Neurotoxicology 7:421–440, 1986.
2. Burnett W, King EG, Grace M, Hall WF: Hydrogen sulfide poisoning: Review of 5 years' experience. Can Med Assoc J *117*:1277–1280, 1977.
3. Tholnan M: Sewer gas: Hydrogen sulfide intoxication. Clin Toxicol *2*:383–386, 1969.
4. Berlin CM: Death from anoxia in an abandoned cesspool. Letter. Ann Intern Med *95*:387, 1981.
5. Nicholls P: The effect of sulfide on cytochrome aa3: Isosteric and allosteric shifts of the reduced α-peak. Biochim Biophys Acta *396*:24–35, 1975.
6. Smith L, Kruszyna H, Smith RP: The effect of methemoglobin on the inhibition of cytochrome c oxidase by cyanide, sulfide or azide. Biochem Pharmacol *26*:2247–2250, 1977.
7. Voight GE, Mueller P: Versuche zum histochemischen Nachweis der Schwefelwasserstoff-Vergiftung [The histochemical effect of hydrogen sulfide poisoning]. Acta Histochem *1*:223–239, 1955.
8. Beauchamp RO Jr, Bus JS, Popp IA, et al: A critical review of the literature on hydrogen sulfide toxicity. CRC Crit Rev Toxicol *13*:25–97, 1984.
9. Evans CL: The toxicity of hydrogen sulphide and other sulphides. Q J Exp Physiol *52*:231–248, 1967.
10. Weisiger RA, Pinkus LM, Jakoby WB: Thiol *S*-methyltransferase: Suggested role in detoxification of intestinal sulfide. Biochem Pharmacol *29*:2885–2887, 1980.
11. Marcus SM: Hydrogen sulfide. Clin Toxicol Rev *5*(4), 1983.
12. Susman JL, Hornig IF, Thomae SC, Smith RP: Pulmonary excretion of hydrogen sulfide, malthanethiol, dimethyl sulfide, and dimethyl disulfide in mice. Drug Chem Toxicol *1*:327–388, 1978.
13. Amman H: A new look at physiologic respiratory: Response to H_2S poisoning. J Haz Mater *13*:369–374, 1986.
14. Warenycia MW, Goodwin LR, Benishin CG, et al: Acute hydro-

gen sulfide poisoning: Demonstration of selective uptake of sulfide by the brainstem by measurement of brain sulfide levels. Biochem Pharmacol *38*:973–981, 1989.
15. Warenycia MW, Goodwin LR, Francom DM, et al: Regional brain distribution of sulfide after H_2S poisoning. *In* Lones GR, Singer PP (eds): Proceedings of the 24th International Meeting of the International Association for Toxicology. Calgary, Alberta, University of Alberta Press, 1988.
16. Gosselin RE, Smith RP, Hodge HC: Clinical Toxicology of Commercial Products. 5th ed. Baltimore, Williams & Wilkins, 1984.
17. Kemper FD: A near-fatal case of hydrogen sulfide poisoning. Can Med Assoc J *94*:1130–1131, 1966.
18. Hoidal CR, Hall AH, Robinson MD, et al: Hydrogen sulfide poisoning from toxic inhalations of roofing asphalt fumes. Ann Emerg Med *15*:826–830, 1986.
19. Hurwitz LJ, Taylor GI: Poisoning by sewer gas. Lancet *1*:1110–1112, 1954.
20. Stine RJ, Slosberg B, Beacham BE: Hydrogen sulfide intoxication: A case report and discussion of therapy. Ann Intern Med *85*:756–758, 1976.
21. Peters JW: Hydrogen sulfide poisoning in a hospital setting. JAMA *246*:1588–1589, 1981.
22. Huang CC, Chu NS: A case of acute hydrogen sulfide (H_2S) intoxication successfully treated with nitrites. J Formos Med Assoc *86*:1018–1020, 1987.
23. Smilkstein MJ, Bronstein AC, Pickett HM, Rumack BH: Hyperbaric oxygen therapy for severe hydrogen sulfide poisoning. J Emerg Med *3*:27–30, 1985.
24. Whitcraft DD, Bailey TD, Hart GB: Hydrogen sulfide poisoning treated with hyperbaric oxygen. J Emerg Med *3*:23–25, 1985.
25. Ravizza AG, Carugo D, Cerchian EL, et al: The treatment of hydrogen sulfide intoxication: Oxygen versus nitrites. Vet Hum Toxicol *24*:4–5, 1982.
26. Milby TH: Hydrogen sulfide intoxication: Review of the literature and report of unusual accident resulting in two cases of nonfatal poisoning. J Occup Med *4*:431–437, 1962.
27. Simson RE, Simpson GR: Fatal hydrogen sulphide poisoning associated with industrial waste exposure. Med J Aust *1*:331–334, 1971.
28. Deng JF, Chang SC: Hydrogen sulfide poisonings in hot-spring reservoir cleaning: Two case reports. Am J Ind Med *11*:447–151, 1987.
29. Audeau FM, Gnanaharan C, Davey K: Hydrogen sulphide poisoning: Associated with pelt processing. N Z Med J *98*:145–147, 1985.
30. Kleinfeld M, Giel C, Rosso A: Acute hydrogen sulfide intoxication: An unusual source of exposure. Ind Med Surg *33*:656–660, 1964.
31. Arnold IMF, Dufresne RM, Alleyne BC, Stuart PIW: Health implication of occupational exposures to hydrogen sulfide. J Occup Med *27*:373–376, 1985.
32. Guidotti TL: Occupational exposure to hydrogen sulfide in the sour gas industry: Some unresolved issues. Int Arch Occup Environ Health *66*:153–160, 1994.
33. Hagley SR, South DL: Fatal inhalation of liquid manure gas. Med J Aust *2*:459–460, 1983.
34. Smith RP, Gosselin RE: Hydrogen sulfide poisoning. J Occup Med *21*:93–97, 1979.
35. Lopez A, Prior M, Reiffenstien RJ, Goodwin LR: Peracute toxic effects of inhaled hydrogen sulfide and injected sodium hydrosulfide on the lungs of rats. Fundam Appl Toxicol *12*:367–373, 1989.
36. Occupational fatality following exposure to hydrogen sulfide—Nebraska. Morb Mortal Wkly Rep *35*:533–535, 1986.
37. Matsuo M, Cummins JW, Anderson RE: Neurological sequelae of massive hydrogen sulfide inhalation. Arch Neurol *36*:451–452, 1979.
38. Park CM, Nagel RL: Sulfhemoglobinemia: Clinical and molecular aspects. N Engl J Med *310*:1579–1584, 1984.
39. Curry SC, Gerkin RD: A patient with sulfhemoglobin? Letter. Ann Emerg Med *16*:828–829, 1987.
40. Gaitonde UB, Sellar RJ, O'Hare AE: Long-term exposure to hydrogen sulphide producing subacute encephalopathy in a child. BMJ *294*:614, 1987.
41. Vathenen AS, Emberton P, Wales JM: Hydrogen sulphide poisoning in a factory worker. Letter. Lancet *1*:305, 1988.
42. Vicas IMO: Hydrogen sulfide exposure treated with hyperbaric oxygen. Vet Hum Toxicol *31*:353, 1989.
43. Kilburn KH: Case report: Profound neurobehavioral deficits in an oil field worker overcome by hydrogen sulfide. Am J Med Sci *306*:301–305, 1993.
44. Parra O, Monso E, Gallego M, Morera J: Inhalation of hydrogen sulphide: A case of subacute manifestations and long-term sequelae. Br J Ind Med *48*:286–287, 1991.
45. Tvedt B, Skyberg K, Asserud O, et al: Brain damage caused by hydrogen sulfide: A follow-up study of six patients. Am J Ind Med *20*:91–101, 1991.
46. Tvedt B, Edland A, Skyberg K, Forberg O: Delayed neuropsychiatric sequelae after acute hydrogen sulfide poisoning: Affection of motor function, memory, vision and hearing. Acta Neurol Scand *84*:348–351, 1991.
47. Snyder JK, Safir EF, Summerville GP, Middleberg RA: Occupational fatality and persistent neurological sequelae after mass exposure to hydrogen sulfide Am J Emerg Med *13*:199–203, 1995.
48. Lindell H, Jappinen P, Savolainen H: Determination of sulphide in blood with an ion selective electrode by pre-concentration of trapped sulphide in sodium hydroxide solution. Analyst *113*:839–840, 1988.
49. Goodwin LR, Francom DM, Dieken FP, et al: Determination of brain sulfide in brain tissue by gas dialysis/ion chromatography: Postmortem studies and two case reports. J Anal Toxicol *13*:105–109, 1989.
50. Deaths at a rendering plant. Morb Mortal Wkly Rep, vol 24, pp 435–436, 1975.
51. Adelson L, Sunshine I: Fatal hydrogen sulfide intoxication. Arch Pathol *81*:375–380, 1966.
52. Osbern LN, Crapo RO: Dung lung: A report of toxic exposure to liquid manure. Ann Intern Med *95*:312–319, 1981.
53. Oderda GM: Fatality produced by accidental inhalation of drain cleaner fumes. Clin Toxicol *8*:547–551, 1975.
54. Donham KJ, Knapp LW, Monson R, Gustafson K: Acute toxic exposure to gases from liquid manure. J Occup Med *24*:142–145, 1982.
55. Smith RP, Kruszyna R, Kruszyna H: Management of acute sulfide poisoning: Effects of oxygen, thiosulfate, and nitrite. Arch Environ Health *31*:166–169 1976.
56. Smith RP, Gosselin RE: Current concepts about the treatment of selected poisonings: Nitrite, sulfide, barium, and quinidine. Annu Rev Pharmacol Toxicol *16*:189–199, 1976.
57. Smith RP, Gosselin RE: The influence of methemoglobinemia on the lethality of some toxic anions: II. Sulfide. Toxicol Appl Pharmacol *6*:584–592, 1964.
58. Smith RP, Gosselin RE: On the mechanism of sulfide inactivation by methemoglobin. Toxicol Appl Pharmacol *8*:159–172, 1966.
59. Beck JF, Bradbury CM, Connors Al, Donini JC: Nitrite as an antidote for acute sulfide intoxication. Am Ind Hyg Assoc *142*:805–809, 1981.
60. Way JL, Sylvester D, Morgan RL, et al: Recent perspectives on the toxico-dynamic basis of cyanide antagonism. Fundam Appl Toxicol *4*:S231–S239, 1984.
61. Dulaney M Jr, Hume AS: Pyruvic acid protects against the lethality of sulfide. Res Commun Chem Pathol Pharmacol *59*:133, 1988.
62. Hume AS, Dulaney MD: The effectiveness of various ketocarboxylic acids in preventing sulfide-induced lethality. Toxicologist *8*:28, 1988.
63. Dulaney MD, Hume AS: The effectiveness of the combination of pyruvate (PYR) and alpha-ketoglu (AKG) as prophylactic antidotes against sulphide lethality. *In* Proceedings of the International Conference on Hydrogen Sulfide Toxicity. Banff, Alberta, 1989.
64. Warenycia MW, Reiffenstien RJ, Goodwin LR, Dieken FP: Dithiothreitol liberates additional brain sulphide. Proc West Pharmacol Soc *32*:333, 1989.
65. Finkel AJ: Hamilton and Hardy's Industrial Toxicology. 4th ed. Stoneham, MA, Butterworth, 1983.
66. Al-Mahasneh OM, Cohle SD, Haas E: Lack of response to hyperbaric oxygen in a fatal case of hydrogen sulfide poisoning. Vet Hum Toxicol *31*:353, 1989.

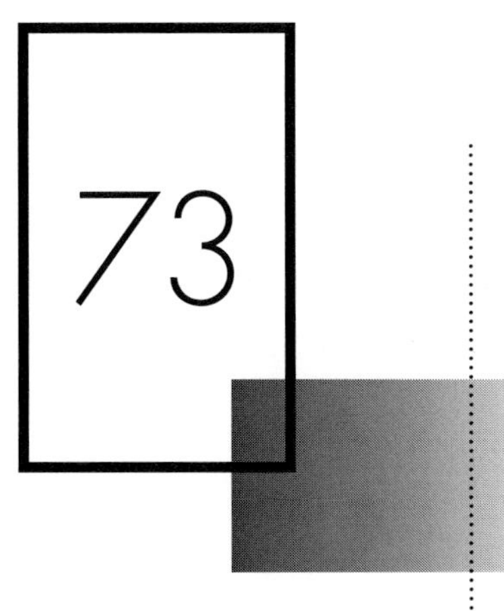

Petroleum Distillates and Turpentine

WILLIAM J. LEWANDER, MD
ALFRED ALEGUAS, JR., RPH, PHARMD

Hydrocarbons are a group of organic compounds composed entirely of hydrogen and carbon. Common hydrocarbons are derived either directly from plants (e.g., pine oil) or from petroleum distillates. Although often mixtures, petroleum distillates may be divided into three basic types: aliphatic, halogenated, and aromatic hydrocarbons. Aromatic and halogenated hydrocarbons are discussed elsewhere. Petroleum distillates are produced from the fractional distillation of crude petroleum and contain various amounts of aliphatic (straight chain) and aromatic (cyclic) hydrocarbons. Those classified predominantly as aliphatic hydrocarbons are discussed here. Some examples are kerosene, gasoline, mineral spirits, naphtha, mineral seal oil, diesel oil, and fuel oil (see Table 73–1). Turpentine is a hydrocarbon made from pine oil.

EPIDEMIOLOGY

Hydrocarbon exposures are frequent and account for an inordinate number of health care visits and hospital admissions. The American Association of Poison Control Centers reported 64,634 hydrocarbon exposures in 1994.[1] Twenty-four per cent of exposed individuals required treatment in a health care facility, and nearly 20% of these patients were considered to have suffered exposures of moderate or major severity. More than half of all exposures occur in children younger than 6 years of age, and the vast majority of exposures are accidental. Nevertheless, intentional exposures are not uncommon and frequently have greater potential for toxicity. Twenty-two deaths were reported as a result of hydrocarbon exposure in 1994.[1]

Petroleum distillates continue to be the most commonly reported cause of hydrocarbon poisoning, accounting for more than 48,000 exposures. Unmarked, poorly stored containers and an attractive aroma or color may account for the high percentage of exposures among young children. In adults, poisoning is most often by intentional ingestion, occupational exposure, or accidental aspiration when siphoning fuels. Adult ingestions generally involve larger volumes and a much greater likelihood of coingested toxins. The most common route of exposure is by ingestion, but inhalation, cutaneous, and intravenous exposures have been reported. Nearly one quarter require treatment in a health care facility. The most commonly ingested products in this group in order of frequency are (1) gasoline, (2) mineral spirits, (3) lubricating oil, (4) lighter fluid or naphtha, (5) kerosene, and (6) turpentine.[1]

PATHOPHYSIOLOGY

The major toxicity of petroleum distillates is their potential to cause a fulminant and sometimes fatal pneumonitis when aspirated. Central nervous system (CNS), gastrointestinal (GI), hepatic, renal, cardiovascular, hematologic, and cutaneous toxicity may also occur. After oral ingestion, pulmonary toxicity occurs from aspiration rather than by GI absorption. Aspiration may occur when the hydrocarbon is initially ingested or during vomiting. Although vomiting often precedes and results in aspiration, lack of vomiting does not preclude the possibility that aspiration

Table 73–1. Examples of Commercial Products Found in the Home or Garage

Brand Name	Chemical Type
Aviation Form-A-Gasket	Isopropyl alcohol
Blue Max Shield One-Step Polymer Car Coating	Petroleum distillate
Brasso	Petroleum distillate, ammonia
Bruce Cleaning Wax	Petroleum naphtha
Collinite Fleetwax	Petroleum distillate
Collinite Insulator Wax	"
Collinite Metal Wax	"
CRC Marine Formula 6-66	"
CRC Marine Lectra-Clean Motor and Equipment Cleaner	Carbon tetrachloride
CRC Marine Silicone Lubricant	Silicone, petroleum distillate
CRC Marine Zinc-Mate (Rust Preventative and Touch-up)	95% zinc
Du Pont Acrylic Enamel Reducer	Petroleum naphtha >60%
Du Pont Engine Cleaner and Degreaser	Kerosene 85%
Du Pont Good and Clean Lotion	Mineral spirits
Du Pont Imron Paint Additive	Xylene
Du Pont Plastic Cement	Toluol
Du Pont Rain Dance	Aliphatic hydrocarbons
Du Pont Windshield Washer	Methanol
Du Pont Zerex Anti-Rust Antifreeze	100% ethylene glycol
Du Pont Zerex Gas Line Antifreeze	>90% methanol
Du Pont Zerex Windshield De-Icer	90% methanol
El Pico Marine Paint and Varnish Remover	Methanol, methylene chloride, ethylene dichloride
El Pico Sandeze (Sta-Lube)	Acetone, toluene, methanol
Fixall Enamel	Mineral spirits
Fixall Varnish	"
Formby's Furniture Cleaner	Petroleum distillate
Formby's Furniture Refinisher	Methanol, toluene, methylene chloride
Formby's Furniture Treatment	Petroleum distillate
Fulton Acetone	Acetone
Fulton Lacquer Thinner	Toluol, xylol, methyl isobutyl ketone
Gulf Charcoal Lighter Fluid	Petroleum naphtha
Johnson's Paste Wax	"
Jubilee Kitchen Wax	"
Lamplight Farms Lamp Oil	Petroleum distillate
Lemon Pledge Furniture Polish (Johnson)	Petroleum naphtha
Lighting Starting Fluid	Ether, hydrocarbons
Liquid Wrench	Petroleum distillate
Mac's Brake and Electric Motor Cleaner	Trichloroethane, perchloroethylene, methylene chloride
Mac's Carburetor and Choke Cleaner	Petroleum distillate
Mac's Cleaner Wax	"
Mac's Gas Line Antifreeze	Methanol
Mac's Moisture and Rust Control	Propane, petroleum distillate
Mac's Valve Tune	Petroleum distillate
Mac's Windshield De-Icer	Methanol
Magic Pre-Wash (Armour-Dial)	Petroleum distillate
Mobil Gas Line Antifreeze	Isopropyl alcohol, methyl alcohol
Mobil Oil Cooling System Cleaner	Kerosene
Mobil Oil Fast Flush	Kerosene, orthodichloro-benzene
Mobil Oil Super Solvent	Methanol
Mobil Permazone Antifreeze	Ethylene glycol
Mobil Windshield Washer Concentrate	Methanol
Monochem T-5 Toilet Chemical	Paraformaldehyde
Napa Auto Air Conditioner Recharge Kit	Freon
Napa Balkamp Form-A-Gasket Sealant	Isopropyl alcohol
Napa Balkamp Gasket Remover	Toluene
Napa Balkamp Liquid Solder	Toluene, methyl ethyl ketone
Napa Balkamp Liquid Steel	Toluene
Napa Chain and Cable Lube	"
Napa Concrete Cleaner	Caustic soda
Napa Contact Cement	Toluene, petroleum naphtha, acetone
Napa Refrigerant 22	Monochlorodifluoromethane
Napa Spray Lube for Open Gears	Toluene
Old English Furniture Polish	Mineral seal oil
Ospho Metal Primer	Phosphoric acid
Pettit Marine Paint Old Salem Brushing Thinner	Petroleum distillate
Pine Power	Pine oil
Pinesol	Pine oil
Poco Marine Safety Clean	Hydrochloric acid
Quaker State Deluxe Motor Oil	Crude oil
Rustoleum Stops Rust	Petroleum naphtha

Table 73–1. Examples of Commercial Products Found in the Home or Garage *Continued*

Brand Name	Chemical Type
Scott's Liquid Gold	Petroleum distillate, trichloroethane
Shell Barbecue and Fireplace Lighter Fuel	Petroleum distillate
Shell Carburetor and Combustion Chamber Cleaner	Aromatic petroleum distillate
Shell Furniture Polish	Mineral spirits
Shell Lighter Fluid and Spot Remover	Petroleum naphtha
Shell Liquid Tire Chain	Methanol
Shell Parts Loosener	Petroleum naphtha
Shell Refrigerant	Freon 12
Shout Laundry Soil and Stain Remover	Petroleum naphtha
Siloo Enginkool	Sodium nitrite
Siloo Octane Treatment Gasoline Additive	Methanol, petroleum distillate
Siloo Trans Kleen Transmission Additive	Petroleum distillate, xylene
Southern Pine Denatured Alcohol	Ethyl alcohol
Southern Pine Paint Remover	Petroleum distillate
Southern Pine Pure Turpentine	Turpentine
STP Gas Treatment	Mineral spirits, xylene
3-In-1 Household Oil	Petroleum distillate
Valvoline Outboard Extreme Pressure Gear Oil	"
Valvoline Special Moly EP Grease (Ashland)	Petroleum distillate. Soap base: lithium 12-hydroxystearate, molybdenum disulfide
WD-40	Petroleum distillate

has occurred. The potential for aspiration is determined by the physical properties of viscosity, surface tension, and volatility. The risk of aspiration involving any particular petroleum distillate increases with low surface tension, low viscosity, and high volatility.[2] The most important property determining aspiration potential is viscosity, the tendency to resist flow. Low viscosity allows deeper penetration into the distal airways. Viscosity is measured in Saybolt seconds universal (SSU). Substances with a SSU value greater than 100 have a low aspiration potential (e.g., mineral and fuel oil), whereas those with a SSU value of less than 45 have a high potential for aspiration (e.g., gasoline, kerosene, mineral seal oil). Low surface tension may allow the petroleum distillate to spread from the upper GI tract to the trachea, and high volatility (i.e., tendency of a liquid to become a gas) increases the likelihood of pulmonary absorption. When aspirated, petroleum distillates inhibit surfactant, resulting in alveolar collapse, ventilation-perfusion mismatch, and subsequent hypoxemia.[2–4] Bronchospasm and direct capillary damage lead to a chemical pneumonitis and hemorrhagic bronchitis and alveolitis that peak in intensity at about 3 days.[5] A late proliferation process of alveolar thickening may occur and peak at about 10 days.[5] Upper airway injury may occur and includes hyperemia, mucosal irritation, and inflammation of the oropharynx. A case of epiglottitis has been reported after gasoline ingestion.[6]

Systemic toxicity is uncommon but may develop if a petroleum distillate contains toxic additives, if it is a vehicle for more toxic substances, or if a concomitant or massive ingestion has occurred. The specific toxin involved determines whether cardiovascular, renal, hepatic, or hematologic toxicity ensues.[7] Petroleum distillate inhalation abuse (e.g., gasoline sniffing) does not produce a chemical pneumonitis but instead leads to a complex toxicity caused by the combined effects of its many constituents (e.g., aromatic hydrocarbons, naphthenes, and tetraethyl lead).[8, 9]

CLINICAL PRESENTATION

The initial signs and symptoms following petroleum distillate ingestion usually involve three main organ systems: pulmonary, GI, and CNS. The majority of children who present to health care facilities after a petroleum distillate exposure remain asymptomatic. Patients who aspirate generally demonstrate initial symptoms (e.g., coughing, gasping, and choking) within 30 minutes, and these reach peak intensity between 24 and 48 hours after exposure.[10] During the first 24 hours, tachypnea with grunting respirations, nasal flaring, retractions, and cyanosis may develop, or these be delayed as long as 2 days.[4] The characteristic odor of the petroleum distillate may be apparent on the breath. Although auscultation may reveal rales, rhonchi, and wheezing, lower airway involvement cannot be precluded by initially normal findings on examination. Hemoptysis and pulmonary edema may be observed in severe cases. Laboratory evaluation (e.g., arterial blood gases, pulse oximetry) may reveal hypoxemia (from ventilation-perfusion mismatching) and early hypocarbia. This may progress to hypercarbia and acidosis. As many as 75% of hospitalized patients demonstrate chest film abnormalities. These abnormalities occur within 2 hours in 88% of patients and in 98% by 12 hours.[7, 11, 12] Common early changes include unilateral and bilateral basilar infiltrates, punctuate perihilar densities, and localized areas of atelectasis.[11–14] Pneumatoceles are infrequent but when they occur are delayed in onset (e.g., 3 to 15 days) and resolution (e.g., 15 days to 21 months).[15] Pleural effusion, pneumothorax, pneumomediastinum, pneumopericardium, and subcutaneous emphysema may develop.[11, 13, 16, 17] Patients' symptoms correlate poorly with radiographic findings, and both may be delayed in onset.[7, 18] It is best to treat patients and not the absence of or delayed resolution of radiographic findings. Although fever and leukocytosis may be noted during the first 48 hours, their persistence suggests bacterial superinfection.[10]

GI symptoms are common and include local irritation of the oropharynx, nausea, vomiting, and abdominal pain. Vomiting appears to increase the likelihood of aspiration.[13, 19] CNS toxicity may occur in the presence of aspiration-induced hypoxemia, large ingestions, or toxic additives (e.g., aromatic hydrocarbons). Symptoms range from lethargy (91%) or somnolence (5%) to coma (3%) and seizures (1%).[7, 20]

Cardiovascular toxicity is uncommon, but both fatal dysrhythmias and myocardial dysfunction have been reported.[21] Dysrhythmias and sudden death after siphoning gasoline may be attributed to hypoxia or absorption after aspiration resulting in myocardial sensitization to endogenous catecholamines.[7, 18] A 19-month-old girl developed severe, reversible myocardial dysfunction after ingesting paint thinner.[20] Isolated case reports of acute renal tubular necrosis,[22, 23] supraglottitis,[24] severe burns after prolonged immersion in gasoline,[25] and hemoglobinuria secondary to intravascular hemolysis have been reported.[24, 26] One case report associated turpentine ingestion with hemorrhagic cystitis.[27] Both inhalation abuse and parenteral administration of petroleum distillates have been reported to cause toxicity. CNS manifestations of inhalation abuse include confusion, dizziness, agitation, incoordination, and coma.[7, 8, 28, 29] Inhalation of leaded gasoline has also been associated with the development of organic lead poisoning.[8, 9, 28, 29] Parenteral administration has resulted in thrombophlebitis, cellulitis, and necrotizing myositis with compartment syndrome. Systemic toxicity includes seizures, hemorrhagic pneumonitis, pulmonary edema, and febrile reactions.[30–32]

DIAGNOSTIC EVALUATION

All symptomatic patients should receive medical evaluation. A thorough history should include product identification, approximate amount, concentration, time of ingestion, and symptoms before presentation. The physical examination should focus on the vital signs, respiratory system, mental status, and GI system. If significant aspiration has occurred, respiratory symptoms should develop within 6 hours and reach peak intensity 24 to 48 hours after exposure.[10] Pulse oximetry should be performed and a chest film obtained. Laboratory evaluation for symptomatic patients and for those who have ingested concomitant toxins may include arterial blood gas determination; complete blood count; determinations of electrolytes, glucose, blood urea nitrogen, and creatinine; urinalysis; and liver function tests. A directed toxic screen may help confirm the presence of toxic additives or other concomitant ingestions. Patients without symptoms for 6 hours after exposure remain asymptomatic.[10]

MANAGEMENT

Clinical and radiographic assessment of patients' respiratory status determines initial management. Patients who remain asymptomatic with normal findings on chest films (obtained 4 or more hours after exposure) may be discharged after 6 hours of observation. Patients who are symptomatic, who have abnormal findings on chest films, or who have suicidal intent should be hospitalized. Gastric decontamination is not recommended for petroleum distillate ingestions because absorption and systemic toxicity are minimal, and spontaneous or induced vomiting increases the risk of aspiration and pneumonitis.[33–35]

Patients who have ingested toxic additives or other toxins with systemic toxicity should be considered for gastric decontamination. This decision is complex, often must be individualized, and should be made after consultation with the regional poison center. The incidence of aspiration pneumonitis may be increased by either gastric lavage or ipecac-induced emesis. Either method is acceptable in an awake, alert patient.[12, 33] When GI decontamination is indicated in patients with altered mental status, the airway should first be protected by endotracheal intubation. Activated charcoal is indicated only if an adsorbable toxic additive or concomitant ingestion has occurred. Clothing that has been contaminated should be removed, and contaminated skin washed with soap and water.[7]

Patients with respiratory symptoms should be given oxygen, placed on cardiopulmonary and pulse oximetry monitors, and have intravenous access established. An arterial blood gas determination and chest film should be obtained. Findings on chest films do not always correlate with the clinical status of the patient. The need for intubation should be based on the clinical assessment of respiratory distress. Continuous positive airway pressure may be necessary to maintain oxygenation, and bronchospasm should be treated with noncardioselective bronchodilators because of potential myocardial sensitization to catecholamines.[36] Supportive care of serious petroleum distillate pneumonitis includes careful monitoring of fluid and electrolyte balance, continuous pulse oximetry, and serial chest films. Complete blood counts with differential and sputum Gram's stain and cultures help to identify bacterial superinfection. The regional poison center should be consulted. Fever and leukocytosis secondary to chemical pneumonitis are commonly noted during the first 24 to 48 hours, and prophylactic antibiotics should not be instituted.[34, 37, 38] Treatment with antibiotics should be provided only to patients with documented bacterial pneumonia (e.g., Gram's stain or culture of sputum or tracheal aspirate) or worsening of chest film findings, chest pain, leukocytosis, and fever after the first 40 hours.[7, 18] Several animal and clinical investigations have failed to demonstrate any benefit from corticosteroid treatment. Two animal studies indicate they may be harmful.[37–40] Therefore, corticosteroids should not be administered.

Several reports document the efficacy of both extracorporeal membrane oxygenation and high-frequency jet ventilation as alternative therapies when conventional treatment for respiratory failure is unsuccessful.[41–43]

Most patients with petroleum distillate poisoning recover fully with supportive care. The majority have no significant sequelae despite the report of minor pulmonary function abnormalities in as many as 82% of asymptomatic survivors of aspiration pneumonitis.[16] Long-term follow-up with pulmonary testing should be considered. When indicated, psychiatric consultation should be obtained and poison prevention education given before discharge.

TERPENES

Terpenes are aliphatic, cyclic hydrocarbons and include turpentine, pine oil, and camphor. Pine oil, a component of many household cleaners, is the product of pine trees and is composed primarily of terpene alcohols. It is normally present in concentrations of 20% to 35% and occasionally as high as 60% in products such as Pine Sol. Turpentine is a distillate from pine trees and is commonly used as a solvent for paints and varnishes. Camphor is discussed in Chapter 101.

Because of the terpenes' lower volatility and higher viscosity, the risk of aspiration is somewhat less than that with the more volatile hydrocarbons. In addition to the aspiration risk, pine oil and turpentine produce more CNS and GI symptoms than do the aliphatic hydrocarbons. Ingestions of turpentine exceeding 2 mL/kg are considered potentially toxic.[44] Although adults have survived pine oil ingestions of up to 500 g,[45] the commonly cited lethal dose is 60 to 120 g. In children, the minimum lethal dose is probably 14 g.[46]

Turpentine is readily absorbed through the GI tract and lungs[44] and distributed throughout the body. The highest concentrations are found in the liver, spleen, kidneys, and brain.[47] The details of turpentine metabolism remain unclear. Elimination of turpentine and its metabolites is primarily by the kidneys. Pine oil is also well absorbed from the GI tract and is metabolized by the epoxide pathway and excreted in the urine.[46] The volume of distribution is thought to be quite large, with the highest concentrations found in the brain, lungs, and kidneys.

Systemic toxicity of pine oil and turpentine primarily results in GI irritation and CNS depression. Signs and symptoms include nausea, vomiting, diarrhea, weakness, somnolence, or agitation. Severe cases may present as stupor or coma; seizures appear to be uncommon.[48] When systemic toxicity occurs, it usually develops within 2 to 3 hours of the exposure. GI and CNS symptoms generally resolve within 12 hours in moderately severe exposures. Dysuria and hematuria thought to be secondary to hemorrhagic cystitis have been reported in a turpentine ingestion 12 to 72 hours after exposure.[27]

The distinctive odors of pine oil and turpentine and a thorough history and physical examination are the keys to diagnosis. The examination should focus on the pulmonary, GI, and central nervous systems. No specific laboratory tests help to determine severity.[44] If aspiration is suspected, an arterial blood gas determination and appropriately timed chest radiograph should be obtained.

Treatment is largely determined by the time and amount of ingestion, evidence of aspiration, and the patient's level of consciousness. A fully alert patient who presents within 2 hours of ingesting greater than 2 mL/kg of turpentine should be considered for GI decontamination. Although not clearly defined for pine oil, lavage is generally recommended for ingestions of greater than 5 mL in adults.[49] Airway protection is recommended for all but the alert patients because of the risk of aspiration. Activated charcoal is not useful, and the apparent large volume of distribution of terpenes precludes the use of hemodialysis or hemoperfusion.

Medical disposition is based on clinical toxicity and time since ingestion. Patients who are either asymptomatic or who have only mild GI or CNS symptoms after 6 hours are unlikely to develop serious complications. All patients with evidence of significant toxicity (i.e., pulmonary or CNS) should be admitted for symptomatic and supportive care.

References

1. Litovitz TL, Felberg L, Soloway RA, et al: 1994 Annual Report of the American Association of Poison Control Centers Toxic Exposure Surveillance System. Am J Emerg Med *13*:551, 1995.
2. Gerarde HW: Toxicologic studies on hydrocarbons IX. The aspiration hazard and toxicity of hydrocarbons and hydrocarbon mixtures. Arch Environ Health *6*:329, 1963.
3. Giammona ST: Effects of furniture polish on pulmonary surfactant. Am J Dis Child *13*:658, 1967.
4. Truemper E, DeLaRocha SR, Atkinson SD: Clinical characteristics, pathophysiology, and management of hydrocarbon ingestion: Case report and review of the literature. Pediatr Emerg Care *3*:187, 1987.
5. Gross P, McNerney JM, Babyak MA: Kerosene pneumonitis: An experimental study with small doses. Am Rev Respir Dis *88*:656, 1963.
6. Grufferman S, Walker FW: Supraglottitis following gasoline ingestion. Ann Emerg Med *11*:368, 1982.
7. Ellenhorn MJ, Barceloux DG: Medical Toxicology, Diagnosis, and Treatment of Human Poisoning. New York, Elsevier, p 940, 1988.
8. Fortenberry JD: Gasoline sniffing. Am J Med *79*:740, 1985.
9. Edminster SC, Bayer MJ: Recreational gasoline sniffing: Acute gasoline intoxication and latent organolead poisoning. J Emerg Med *3*:365, 1985.
10. Anas N, Narnasonthia V, Ginsburg CM: Criteria for hospitalizing children who have ingested products containing hydrocarbons. JAMA *246*:840, 1981.

11. Eade NR, Taussig LM, Marks MI: Hydrocarbon pneumonitis. Pediatrics *54*:351, 1974.
12. Beamon RF, Siegel CJ, Landers G, et al: Hydrocarbon ingestion in children: A six year retrospective study. JACEP *5*:771, 1976.
13. Foley JC, Dreyer NB, Soule AB Jr, et al: Kerosene poisoning in young children. Radiology *62*:817, 1954.
14. Ervin ME: Petroleum distillates and turpentine. *In* Haddad LM, Winchester JF (eds): Clinical Management of Poisoning and Drug Overdose. Philadelphia, W. B. Saunders Co., p 771, 1983.
15. Bergeson PS, Hates SW, Lustgarten MD, et al: Pneumatoceles following hydrocarbon ingestion. Am J Dis Child *129*:49, 1975.
16. Gurwitz D, Kattan M, Levison H, et al: Pulmonary function abnormalities in asymptomatic children after hydrocarbon pneumonitis. Pediatrics *62*:789, 1970.
17. Brunner S, Rovsing H, Wulf H: Roentgenographic changes in the lungs of children with kerosene poisoning. Am Rev Respir Dis *89*:250, 1964.
18. Klein BL, Simon JE: Hydrocarbon poisonings. Pediatr Clin North Am *33*:411, 1986.
19. Bratton L, Haddow JE: Ingestion of charcoal lighter fluid. J Pediatr *87*:633, 1974.
20. Myocardial dysfunction after hydrocarbon ingestion. Abstract. Crit Care Med *22*:3, 1994.
21. Bass M: Death from sniffing gasoline. Letter. N Engl J Med *299*:203, 1978.
22. Barrientos A, Ortuno MT, Morales JM, et al: Acute renal failure after use of diesel fuel as shampoo. Arch Intern Med *137*:1217, 1977.
23. Crisp AJ, Bhalla AK, Hoffbrand BI: Acute tubular necrosis after exposure to diesel oil. BMJ *2*:177, 1979.
24. Adler R, Robinson RG, Binkin NJ: Intravascular hemolysis: An unusual complication of hydrocarbon ingestion. J Pediatr *89*:679, 1976.
25. Walsh WA, Scarpa FJ, Brown RS, et al: Gasoline immersion burn case report. N Engl J Med *291*:830, 1974.
26. Stockman JA: More on hydrocarbon-induced hemolysis. J Pediatr *90*:848, 1977.
27. Klein FA, Hackler RH: Hemorrhagic cystitis associated with turpentine ingestion. Urology *16*:187, 1980.
28. Poklis A, Burkett CD: Gasoline sniffing: A review. Clin Toxicol *11*:35, 1977.
29. Chessare JD, Wodarcyk K: Gasoline sniffing and lead poisoning in a child. Am Fam Physician *38*:181, 1988.
30. Wason S, Greiner PT: Intravenous hydrocarbon abuse. Am J Emerg Med *4*:543, 1986.
31. Neeld EM, Limacher MC: Chemical pneumonitis after the intravenous injection of hydrocarbons. Radiology *129*:36, 1978.
32. Tennenbein M: Hydrocarbon ingestion. Curr Probl Pediatr *16*:221, 1986.
33. Press E, Adams WC, Chittenden RF, et al: Report of the subcommittee on accidental poisoning: Co-operative kerosene poisoning study. Pediatrics *29*:648, 1962.
34. Litovitz T, Green AE: Health implications of petroleum distillate ingestion. Occup Med *3*:555, 1988.
35. Cachia EA, Fenech FF: Kerosene poisoning in children. Arch Dis Child *39*:502, 1964.
36. James FW, Kaplan S, Benzing G: Cardiac complications following hydrocarbon ingestion. Am J Dis Child *121*:431, 1971.
37. Steele RW, Conklin RH, Mark HM: Corticosteroids and antibotics for the treatment of fulminant hydrocarbon aspiration. JAMA *219*:1424, 1972.
38. Brown J, Burke B, Dajani AS: Experimental kerosene pneumonia: Evaluation of some therapeutic regimens. J Pediatr *84*:396, 1974.
39. Zieserl E: Hydrocarbon ingestion and poisoning. Compr Ther *5*:35, 1979.
40. Marks MI, Chicoine L, Legere G, et al: Adrenocorticosteroid treatment of hydrocarbon pneumonia in children. A cooperative study. J Pediatr *81*:366, 1972.
41. Scazo AJ, Weber TR, et al: Extracorporeal membrane oxyenation for hydrocarbon aspiration. Am J Dis Child *144*:867, 1990.
42. Weber TR, Tracey TF, et al: Prolonged extracorporeal support for nonneonatal respiratory failure. J Pediatr Surg *27*:1100, 1992.
43. Bysani GK, Rucoba RJ, et al: Treatment of hydrocarbon pneumonitis. Chest *106*:300, 1994.
44. McGuigan MA: Turpentine. Clin Toxicol Rev *8*:1, 1985.
45. Koppel C, Tenczer J, Tennesmarm U, et al: Acute poisoning with pine oil: Metabolism of monoterpenes. Arch Toxicol *49*:73, 1981.
46. Jill RM, Barer J, Leighton Hill L, et al: An investigation of recurrent pine oil poisoning in an infant by the use of gas chromatographic mass spectrometric methods. J Pediatr *87*:115, 1975.
47. Sperling F: *In vivo* and *in vitro* toxicology of turpentines. Clin Toxicol *2*:21, 1969.
48. Jacobziner H, Raybin HW: Turpentine poisoning. Arch Pediatr *78*:357, 1961.
49. Brook MP, McCarron MM, Mueller JA: Pine oil cleaner ingestion. Ann Emerg Med *18*:391, 1989.

74

Industrial Toxicology

MARY JO McMULLEN, MD
JEFFREY JONES, MD

A *hazardous material* is any substance that poses any threat to human life or health, either by itself or in accidents such as a fire or explosion. A material is considered hazardous if it is explosive, flammable, combustible poisonous (toxic), corrosive, or radioactive, or if it is an oxidizer. The most commonly shipped hazardous materials are gasoline, anhydrous ammonia, propane, liquefied petroleum gas, chlorine, and sulfuric acid.

More than 5 million different chemical substances are known. Chemical companies produce commercially and ship about 40,000 different dangerous chemicals to which industrial workers and others may be exposed. Toxicity data are not available for more than 80% of these agents. It is important to know about the general management of patients exposed to certain classes of chemicals and a few more common, specific compounds. It is equally important to know the sources of information that are routinely available, how to gain access to that information, and what level of help to expect in an emergency. It has been estimated that 1.6 transportation-related incidents involving hazardous materials that result in death, injury, or evacuation occur each day in the United States.

In the 17th century, Bernardo Ramazzini, often called the "father of industrial medicine," implored the physicians of Italy not only to ask patients about their symptoms but also to delve carefully into the nature of their work.[2] Today, few occupations do not involve some contact with a metal, gas, solvent, or unusual chemical that has the potential to poison, irritate, or sensitize.[3] It has been estimated that 100,000 persons in the United States die each year from industry-related disease, and about 400,000 new cases of occupational diseases are recorded each year.[4] These numbers may be significant underestimates because of the inadequacy of data collection systems and problems with recognition and diagnosis of occupational disease. Table 74–1 lists some of these problems. See Table 74–2 for a useful list of terms and Table 74–3 for abbreviations used in industrial toxicology.

Recognition of industrial poisoning is simplified when the acutely ill person is transported directly from the workplace at which an unprotected exposure to a known toxic substance has occurred. However, if there is a latent period between the time of exposure and the onset of clinical illness, if potential toxins are multiple or unknown, or if the resultant illness mimics common diseases, recognition and appropriate management of acute industrial poisoning may be delayed.[4–6] Moreover, physicians are often inadequately prepared to diagnose or treat diseases caused by exposure to industrial toxins. Formal medical school training and postgraduate programs in occupational health issues are minimal.[7]

The diagnosis of industrial poisoning is important,

Table 74–1. Obstacles to the Diagnosis of Industrial Poisoning[4, 5]

1. Most occupational illnesses are clinically and pathologically indistinguishable from common medical disorders.
2. Toxicologic data are not currently available for more than 80% of hazardous chemicals used in industry.
3. For many industrial toxins, there is a latent period (hours to days) between the toxic exposure and the onset of symptoms.
4. Nonoccupational factors (i.e., smoking) may act synergistically with occupational exposure to cause disease.
5. Many toxins occur in mixtures or may be contaminants of other products.
6. Privacy about proprietary formulations and fear of litigation limit the free flow of chemical information from employers and manufacturers.
7. Physicians often are inadequately prepared to diagnose or treat a disease caused by an industrial toxin.

not only for the care of the patient but also because accurate diagnosis makes it possible to identify potential workplace hazards and health risks to the community. *Efficient diagnosis and treatment are facilitated when emergency department personnel maintain a high index of suspicion for the possibility of industrial poisoning, familiarize themselves with industrial processes and toxic substances used locally, maintain an adequate reference library, and obtain occupational histories from their patients.*[6]

The history of work experience may provide critical information that relates the patient's symptoms and signs of exposure to a specific job hazard. Thus, Ramazzini's advice concerning the occupational history is just as relevant—if not more so—today than it was in the 17th century.

Table 74–2. Terminology in Industrial Toxicology

Absorption: the taking in of any material by direct contact with the skin.
Acid: a chemical compound of electronegative elements or groups plus one or more ionizable hydrogen(s) (H^+). Acids are very active chemically.
Alkali: a chemical compound that reacts to form the hydroxyl ion (OH^-). Also known as a base. Alkalis are very active chemically.
Asphyxiant: any chemical substance that can cause hypoxia, and potentially death, by displacing the air in a given environment.
Combustible: capable of burning; a substance with a flash point equal to or above 37.8°C (100°F). Combustion (burning) is an exothermic chemical reaction caused by light or heat, with a rapid oxidation of fuel accompanied by flames.
Corrosive: liquid or solid material that causes visible destruction or irreversible alterations in any living tissue (e.g., human skin tissue) by its chemical action. In the case of leakage from its packaging, a liquid that has a severe corrosive effect on steel.
Explosimeter: a mechanical device used to check for dangerous concentrations of gases.
Explosive: any material capable of burning or detonating suddenly and violently.
Flammable: capable of burning with a flash point below 37.8°C (100°F).
Flash point: the minimum temperature of a liquid or solid at which enough vapors are given off to form an ignitable mixture with the air.
Fumes: particulate matter floating in air; an aerosol of solid particles generated by condensation from the gaseous state.
Gas: matter that is a fluid with a vapor pressure under 40 psi at 37.8°C (100°F).
Irritant: a substance that is not classified as a poison but may produce intensely irritating fumes.
Lower explosive limit (LEL): the minimum concentration of gas or vapor in air below which the mixture will not explode.
Oxidant (oxidizer): a substance that contains oxygen and gives it up readily; supports combustion.
Poison: any substance that can cause injury, illness, or death to living tissues by chemical means. Synonymous with "toxin" or "toxic material."
Reactive: capable of reacting or tending to react chemically with other substances.
Vapor: a substance that is liquid under ordinary conditions at 25°C.
Vapor pressure: the gas pressure exerted on the sides of a closed container by the collision of molecules.
Water-reactive: describing a substance that produces hazardous vapors or that releases energy when it comes into contact with water or humid air.

Table 74–3. Abbreviations in Industrial Toxicology

LC_{50}: lethal concentration; 50% of test animals (and potentially humans) exposed to this concentration of a gas, vapor, dust, or fume in air will be killed.
LCL_0: lowest published lethal concentration.
LD 100: the dosage of an active ingredient taken by mouth that is expected to cause death.
LD_{50}: lethal dose resulting in 50% kill. This represents an experimentally derived value. This is obtained by a statistical estimate of the dosage necessary to kill 50% of an infinite population of animals. Usually expressed as weight of a substance in milligrams per kilogram of body weight.
LDL_0: lowest published toxic dose.
mg/m^3: used to measure fumes, mists, or dusts. Standards defined by the Occupational Safety and Health Act of 1970.
PPM: parts per million. This measures the parts of a gas or vapor per million parts of air. Used in environmental research more than in human studies.
TCL_0: lowest published toxic concentration of an active substance taken by mouth or absorbed by the skin that is expected to cause death in 50% of the test animals. This is reported in milligrams per kilogram of body weight.
TDL_0: lowest published toxic dose.
TLV: threshold limit value. Formerly known as the maximum allowable concentration (MAC). This term refers to airborne concentrations and represents conditions under which nearly all workers may be repeatedly exposed for 8 hours a day, 5 days a week, without harmful effects. Defined under the Toxic Substances Control Act of 1977.

CLASSIFICATION OF HAZARDOUS MATERIALS

The United States Department of Transportation requires all shipping papers to have classifications as well as identification numbers.[8] This classification and numbering system is used by many other regulatory agencies and authorities for identifying potentially hazardous substances[9] (Table 74–4).

The National Fire Protection Association (NFPA) Committee on Fire Hazards of Materials developed a hazard signal system: NFPA-704 (Fig. 74–1).[10] This includes a numeric rating scale to identify the degree of hazard in the categories of health, fire, and reactivity (Table 74–5). This system is frequently used for labeling by chemical manufacturers; however, use of

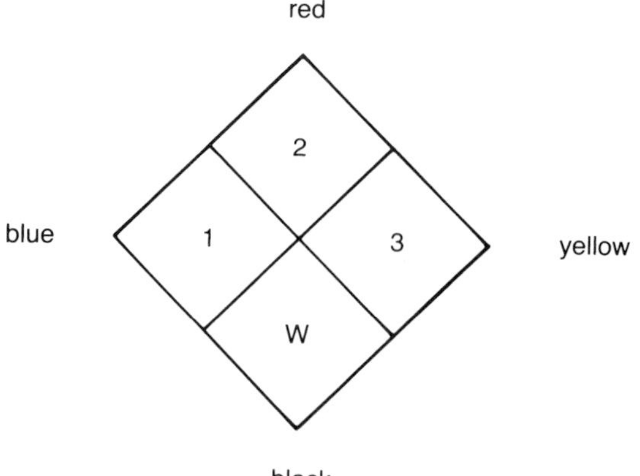

Figure 74–1. Symbol of the National Fire Protection 704 Hazard Signal System. See Table 74–5 for explanation.

this system for labeling is not required by law for chemicals transported across state lines.

The term *health hazard* refers specifically to the capacity of a material to cause personal injury from contact with or absorption into the body of a chemical. In fire fighting or other emergency conditions, the term *health hazard* refers to a single exposure, which may vary in duration from a few seconds to 1 hour. It is not applicable to the situation of an industrial worker who is exposed on as routine basis. Table 74–5 shows the NAPA-704 system's use of the five ratings of the degree of hazard of a specific chemical; the rating scale is defined as follows:

0—Materials that on exposure under fire conditions would present no hazard beyond that of ordinary combustible materials.

1—Materials that on exposure would cause irritation but only minor residual injury even if no treatment were given.

2—Materials that on intense or continued exposure could cause temporary incapacitation or possible residual injury unless prompt medical treatment were given.

3—Materials that on short exposure could cause serious temporary or residual injury even if prompt medical treatment were given.

4—Materials that on very short exposure could cause death or major residual injury even if prompt medical treatment were given.

The US Department of Labor (DOL) requires a *Material Safety Data Sheet (MSDS)* for hazardous materials with which shipbuilders work.[3] These data sheets contain detailed information about specific chemicals and their toxicity. Because of their standard format and availability, these sheets have become required by many fire department HAZMAT (*haz*ardous *mat*erials) units and in right-to-know ordinances. Since 1986, the federal Occupational Safety and Health Administration (OSHA) has required that an MSDS be available for any chemical used in the workplace. It is the responsibility of the importer or manufacturer of each chemical to prepare these forms in a standardized format. In 29CFR1910.120, OSHA defines what minimum information must be included in these sheets. The employer is required to provide an MSDS to the treating physician when an employee is involved in an acute exposure.

Table 74–4. Labeling and Classification Systems[8, 11]

US Department of Transportation

1. Class A explosives
2. Class B explosives
3. Blasting agent
4. Poison A
5. Flammable gas
6. Nonflammable gas
7. Nonflammable gas (chlorine)
8. Nonflammable gas (oxygen, pressurized liquid)
9. Flammable liquid
10. Combustible liquid
11. Flammable solid
12. Flammable solid (dangerous when wet)
13. Oxidizer
14. Organic peroxide
15. Poison B (nonflammable gas—fluorine)
16. Radioactive material
17. Corrosive material
18. Irritating material

United Nations Classification Numbers

1. Explosives
2. Gases
3. Flammable and combustible liquids
4. Flammable solids, spontaneous combustion substances
5. Oxidizers and organic peroxides
6. Poisonous materials
7. Radioactive materials
8. Corrosives
9. Miscellaneous hazardous materials

Table 74–5. NFPA Hazard Signal System "704"

Flammable (Red)

4—Extremely flammable
3—Ignites at normal temperatures below 37.8°C (100°F)
2—Ignites at temperatures below 93.3°C (200°F)
1—Must be preheated to burn
0—Will not burn

Health Hazard (Blue)

4—Too dangerous to enter vapor or liquid
3—Extreme danger
2—Hazardous
1—Slightly hazardous
0—Normal material

Reactivity (Yellow)

4—May detonate
3—Shock and heat may detonate
2—Violent chemical change
1—Unstable if heated
0—Stable

Specific Hazard (Black)

OXY—Oxidizer
ACID—Acid
ALK—Alkali
COR—Corrosive
W —Use no water
 —Radiation hazard

OCCUPATIONAL HISTORY

Obtaining a complete occupational history is too cumbersome and time-consuming for use as a screening instrument in all emergency evaluations or office visits. Goldman and Peters[5] developed a systematic approach (Fig. 74–2) for evaluating hazardous exposures. The algorithm begins with a quick survey that can be performed routinely on all patients. The clinician may then proceed to a more detailed line of questioning to follow-up any indications of toxic exposure.

Routine Survey

The first step includes asking questions about three essential topics that are easily incorporated

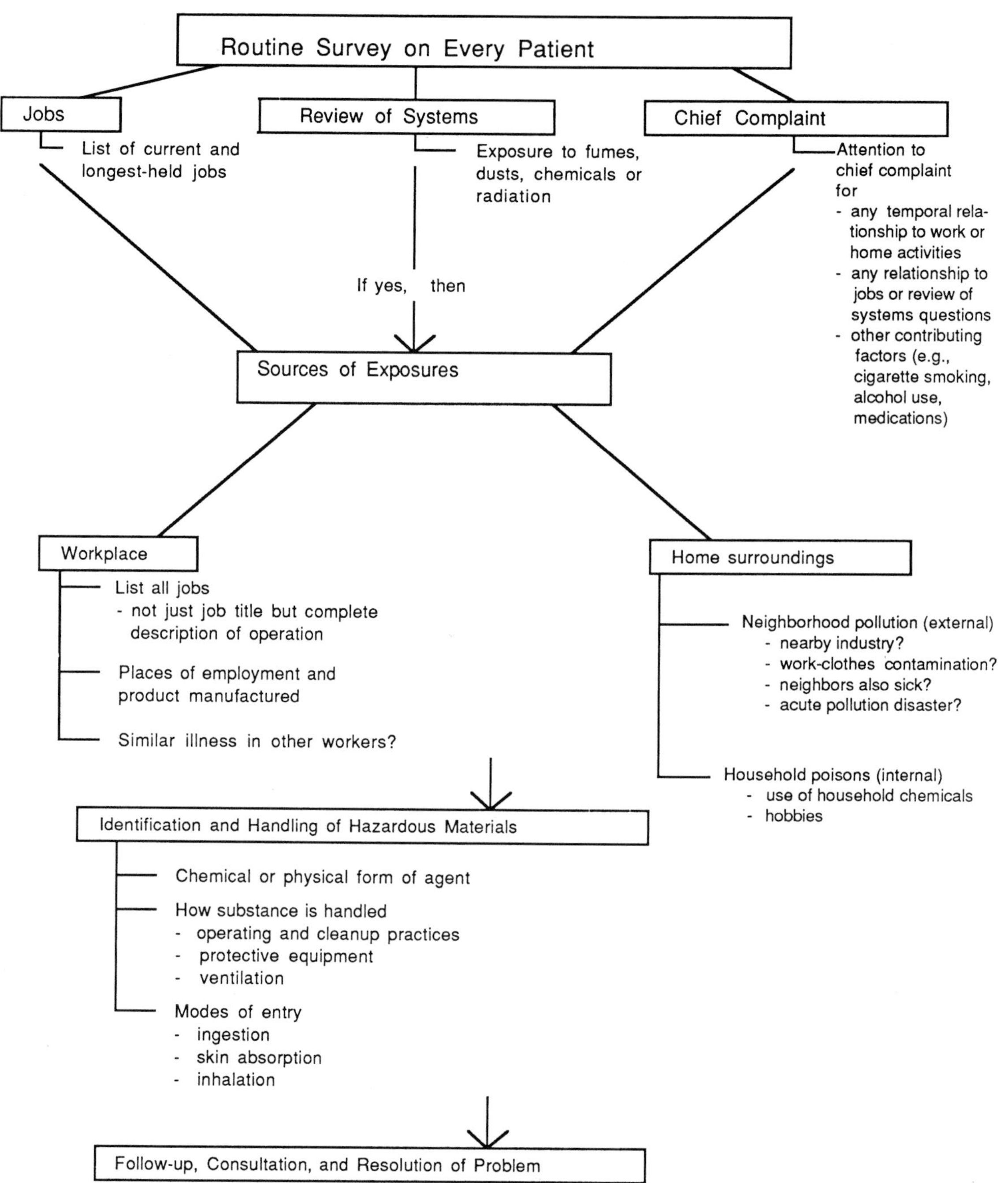

Figure 74–2. Systematic approach to history-taking and diagnosis of occupational illness. (From Goldman RH, Peters JM: The occupational and environmental health history. JAMA *246:*2831–2836, 1981. Copyright 1981, American Medical Association.)

into the routine history-taking: (1) current and past job titles; (2) known exposure to fumes, chemicals, dusts, or radiation; and (3) any temporal relationship of the chief complaint to work activities or other contributory factors. The work and exposure history acts as a broad screen to elicit potentially hazardous exposures at home or work. When conditions with short latency periods are under evaluation, such as occupational asthma, then the emphasis should be on the current job and exposures. For conditions of longer latency, such as asbestosis, the history must focus on jobs and exposures in the past. Allergic responses to agents may develop even after years of asymptomatic exposure.

A temporal relationship between the onset of symptoms and work or home activities can provide an important clue to recent sources of exposure. In general, symptoms that recede on the weekend or at vacation time and return at the start of the work week indicate some current job-related exposure.[5] For example, acute systemic solvent toxicity, which includes the symptoms of headache, gastrointestinal

TABLE 74–6. Factors That Modify Risk of Occupationally Related Illness

Modifying Factor	Known or Probable Effect
General	
Age	Youth—latency for cancer; elderly—more susceptible to toxicity
Sex	Sex differences exist for some toxicity states; reproductive effects
Smoking status	
Current smoker	Confers additive risk in some situations
Smoker at time of exposure	Confers synergistic risk in some situations
Smoking during exposure	Modifies toxic exposure in some situations, such as polymer fume fever
Family history	Hereditary conditions or predispositions may be exacerbated or triggered, such as in cancer-prone families
Exercise	
Conditioning	Fitness may reduce susceptibility in some situations
At time of exposure	Generally, increased susceptibility
Metabolic states	Activity of certain enzyme systems involved in activation, detoxification, and adaptation to toxic exposures may modify response bout within range of normal
Medical	Generally, any debilitating condition may enhance clinical susceptibility
Atopy	
Asthma	Tendency toward easy sensitization
Eczema	Increased bronchial reactivity
Chronic respiratory disease	
Respiratory insufficiency	Diminished pulmonary reserve
Bronchitis	Increased bronchial reactivity; exacerbated bronchial irritation
Chronic cardiovascular disease	
Cardiac insufficiency	Increased susceptibility
Coronary artery disease	Angina in some situations, such as carbon monoxide, methylene chloride exposure
Infection	
Acute viral illness	Increased susceptibility to bronchial irritation; possibly synergistic effect
Exposure to infectious agents	Certain exposures may depress host defenses
Immune deficiency states	Increased susceptibility to infections
Hereditary	
Immunosuppressive therapy	
Renal disease	Additive or synergistic effects may occur with exposure to nephrotoxic agents
Renal insufficiency	Increased susceptibility to toxic agents excreted via renal route
Chronic renal disease	Immunodeficiency; increased susceptibility to toxic effects
Neurologic conditions	
Diminished mental capacity	May affect judgment and response to exposure situation
Neurologic disease	Toxic effects may be additive; increased clinical susceptibility
Seizure disorder	Certain toxic exposures may alter threshold
Impaired perceptive ability (visual or hearing impairment, anosmia)	Impaired ability to avoid hazard
Dermatologic conditions	Skin rashes may increase dermal absorption; may condition response
Substance abuse	Concomitant alcohol and drug abuse may have additive or synergistic effects in some situations
Hepatic insufficiency	Increased susceptibility to toxic agents detoxified by liver; increased susceptibility to hepatotoxic agent; reduced hepatic reserve
Systemic conditions	
Malnutrition (general)	Increased susceptibility to toxic effects
Vitamin deficiency (selective)	Diminished host defenses against toxic effects
Inborn errors of metabolism	Selective susceptibility (depending on abnormality)
Genetic diseases	Certain genetic diseases associated with increased susceptibility to mutagenic effects
Mental status	Stress may increase susceptibility to some toxic exposures. Stress, affective disorders, neuroses, or psychoses may mask, mimic, or subtly modify the clinical presentation

(From Occupational and Environmental Health Committee of The American Lung Association of San Diego and Imperial Counties: Taking the occupational history. Ann Intern Med *99*:641–651, 1983.)

disturbances, and lightheadedness, usually occur within a short time of exposure and lessen within hours after removal from exposure. The expression of toxic symptoms also is influenced by the use of medications, pre-existing medical diseases, and exposure to other hazardous substances. In addition, some personal habits (e.g., the use of tobacco or alcohol) represent significant environmental exposures that may interact with or add to occupational exposures (Table 74–6).

Sources of Exposure

In assessing the likelihood of the workplace as a source of toxic exposure, the physician should obtain a complete description of all jobs that the patient has had, including the products manufactured and the processes involved. Many workers are well informed about specific exposures at the workplace, and the information that they provide is sufficient for documentation. Often, however, the taking of the exposure history requires further detective work for identification of specific components of products and for documentation of exposure levels.[4]

Patients should be asked whether fellow workers have similar complaints; the cluster of symptoms among employees may be the first clue to identifying the presence of an occupational hazard.[4] The plant's industrial hygienist, occupational medicine physician or nurse, or manager can often provide the most useful information on working conditions and chemicals in use. In addition, he or she is required to provide a copy of the MSDS.

In addition to taking the occupational history, the physician needs to be aware of possible sources of contamination in the home. The patient should be asked about neighborhood environmental exposure, such as a nearby factory or chemical waste dump. An obvious source of external pollution is dust or chemicals carried into the home on work clothes. For example, children of employees at a lead storage battery facility have shown excessive blood lead levels.[12] However, some of the most toxic industrial chemicals are readily available for home use; these include pesticides, solvents, cleaning fluids, and disinfectants. A dangerous situation may arise when two substances are mixed together in the hope of producing a more potent compound (e.g., poisonous chloramine fumes are produced when ammonia and sodium hypochlorite are mixed).

The growth and diversification of hobbies have introduced a multitude of hazardous substances into the household. Artists and craftsmen often face daily exposure to toxic substances, including solvents in paints, inks, and thinners; lead, cadmium, and other metals in pigments, pottery glazes, copper enamels, and silver solders; and dusts such as silica and asbestos in clays, talcs, and glazes.[13] Further compounding this problem is the inadequate labeling of many art materials. This brings the clinician to the next step in the algorithm: identification and description of the use of the suspected agents.

Identification

In characterizing the health effects of a chemical exposure, it is important to determine not only the generic ingredients of the compound involved, but also its physical state and concentration. For example, at high temperatures, the chlorinated hydrocarbon trichloroethylene, widely used as an industrial solvent, produces phosgene, which may cause pulmonary edema.[14] Prehospital medical care personnel or HAZMAT team members may be helpful in locating chemical labels, manifest sheets, shipping papers, or knowledgeable personnel who can identify the agent involved.

In addition to the character of an exposure, the quantity of the agent should not be overlooked in the history-taking. As in pharmacology, the effect of any substance is related to the amount that enters the body and how it is eliminated. Key elements of the quantitative exposure history include the nature and use of protective equipment and clothing, ventilation, the duration of exposure, and the general level of cleanliness of the work setting.

The final factor in the assessment of industrial poisoning is the mode of entry into the body. Industrial toxins can harm exposed workers after inhalation, skin contact, and ingestion. The most common effects are the dermatoses, consisting mainly of irritant and allergic dermatitis. Inhalation exposures to toxic fumes, vapors, and gases pose the greatest danger because they have the potential to affect many people at the same time, with immediate compromise of the respiratory system. Toxic ingestion is infrequent; however, eating, drinking, or smoking in the work area may increase exposure to the body.

Follow-Up

Despite all best efforts, the clinician is often faced with incomplete data on which to base treatment. If adequate information on the toxic agent is not available on site or from the manufacturer, then the nearest poison control center should be contacted once the chemical has been identified. Poison control centers rely on a wide variety of information sources and specialty consultants to assess toxicity and advise treatment personnel.

PATHOPHYSIOLOGY

The pathologic effects that may occur with exposure to a specific hazardous substance include direct injury, sensitization, asphyxiation, systemic toxicity, carcinogenesis, mutagenesis, and teratogenesis. The last three effects have long latency periods and thus are not considered in the category of toxicologic emergencies.

Irritant contact dermatitis is a direct injury to the *skin.* It is commonly associated with acids, alkalis (caustics), and certain metal compounds, as well as repeated exposures to detergents or solvents.[4] Strong corrosives may coagulate skin proteins or cause extensive tissue dehydration. The net effect is necrosis of the dermal cells that results in a vesicular (blistering) or ulcerative injury. Milder irritants, such as soaps and detergents, remove surface lipids and cause dryness and cracking of the skin. Generally, eyes are much more readily damaged by these actions, and ingesting the toxin can irritate mucosal surfaces on contact. Such damage leads to vomiting, diarrhea, intestinal cramping, and hemorrhage.

Irritant gases, metal dusts or fumes, and chemicals of extreme pH or reactivity may produce mucosal damage to the *respiratory tract* (Table 74–7).[17] The location of injury depends on the water solubility and particle size of the substance. The highly water-soluble gases—ammonia, hydrogen chloride, and hydrogen fluoride—dissolve readily in the moisture associated with the mucous membranes of the nose and

TABLE 74–7. Toxic Industrial Gases[4, 6, 7]

Irritant Gases	Metal Fumes	Simple Asphyxiants	Chemical Asphyxiants
Ammonia	Beryllium	Nitrogen	Carbon monoxide
Chlorine	Cadmium	Methane	Hydrogen sulfide
Nitrogen dioxide	Mercury	Carbon dioxide	Hydrogen cyanide
Ozone	Nickel	Argon	Acetonitrile
Phosgene	Vanadium	Helium	Methylene chloride
Sulfur dioxide	Zinc	Nitrous oxide	
Fluorine	Chromium	Hydrogen	
Bromine	Osmium		
Acetic acid			

upper respiratory tract. Inflammation, ulceration, edema, and necrosis may acutely obstruct the upper airway. Gases with a low solubility in water, such as ozone, nitrogen dioxide, and phosgene, reach the lower airway and produce pneumonitis and pulmonary edema. Potential late effects from the inhalation of these substances include bronchiolitis fibrosa obliterans, bronchiectasis, chronic bronchitis, and varying degrees of pulmonary fibrosis.

Most respiratory irritants are gases or vapors, but they may also exist as particulates (e.g., mist) or may be absorbed onto particulates (e.g., sulfur dioxide).[15] The particle size largely determines the extent of accessibility to small airways. Particles measuring between 1 and 5 μm can diffuse within the alveoli.[16] Pneumoconiosis is the result of chronic exposure to dusts (e.g., asbestos) and leads to the development of fibrorestrictive disease.

Hypersensitivity reactions are caused by repeated exposure to any one of a number of organic and inorganic agents. Exposure does not lead to clinical disease in every individual. The two basic immunologic reactions are the *immediate response* (type I), as is seen in bronchial asthma, and the *cell-mediated response* (type IV), as is seen in hypersensitivity pneumonitis and allergic contact dermatitis. The early appearance of hypersensitivity reactions is quite similar if not indistinguishable from that of chemical irritations.[4]

Poisonous gases need not damage the lungs directly to have adverse effects on the body. Interfering with the supply of oxygen to the tissues causes asphyxiation. When present in sufficient quantities, biologically inert gases, such as hydrogen and methane, reduce the oxygen content of inspired air. These gases are called "simple asphyxiants." Symptoms are usually evident by the time the level of these gases exceeds 20 to 30 vol% of inspired air.[18] Chemical or toxic asphyxiants include carbon monoxide and hydrogen sulfide. These gases lead to profound disruptions of cellular metabolism by blocking the delivery or utilization of oxygen. Both types of asphyxiants produce minimal direct injury to the respiratory tract but can cause marked neurologic and metabolic alterations.[19]

Many toxic agents affect other organ systems through secondary systemic spread. Under normal conditions, the skin is remarkably successful in preventing diffusion when it is exposed to toxic chemicals. The amounts of toxic chemicals absorbed are usually of little significance. Exceptions include chlorinated hydrocarbons, warfarin, organophosphates, organic mercury, tetraethyl lead, and dimethylsulfoxide.[20]

Inhalation of toxicants presents the most rapid and direct route of entry into the body because of the intimate association of air passages in the lung with the circulatory system. Once a hazardous substance has been absorbed, the clinical manifestations depend on many factors, including the inherent toxicity of the chemical, the total dose, and the duration of exposure. Exposure to other agents such as alcohol or drugs may modify the response (see Table 74–6). The clinical spectrum is accordingly very broad. When managing poisoning cases, the clinician must obtain a thorough history, perform physical examination, order appropriate laboratory studies, and be observant for injury to target organ systems, especially the *central nervous, renal, cardiac, and hepatic systems.*

Because of its strategic location, both anatomically and biochemically, the liver not only is directly exposed to cytotoxins but also is the major site in the body for biotransformation of chemical substances.[21] Hepatic enzyme systems oxidize lipid-soluble metabolites. These metabolites may then be harmlessly excreted in aqueous media such as urine or bile. However, in some instances, the oxidation system converts inactive chemicals to highly reactive toxins that can cause hepatocellular necrosis.

Table 74–8 is a guide to the clinical manifestations of acute exposure to common industrial poisons. Note that no organ system is spared. The complexity, diversity, and unpredictability of industrial poisonings require a clinical approach that concentrates on effective management of the presenting patient's problems, vital signs, symptoms complexes, and ultimately, involved major organ systems.[22, 23]

PREHOSPITAL CARE AND DECONTAMINATION

Prompt and safe removal from exposure is the first consideration in the management of industrial poisoning. If rescue of a disabled victim is required, emergency personnel should wear protective clothing and respirators appropriate for the chemical or chem-

TABLE 74–8. Clinical Signs of Industrial Poisoning[4, 16, 22, 23]

Organ System	Symptom/Sign	Exposure
Eye	Corneal burns	Caustic agents, irritant gases, solvents
	Diplopia	Carbon disulfide, CO, ethylene glycol, lead, methyl bromide, methyl chloride, methyl iodide, triethyl tin
	Miosis	Carbamates, nicotine, organophosphates
	Mydriasis	Barium, benzene, ethyl bromide, ethylene glycol, methanol, methyl chloride
	Nystagmus	Carbon disulfide, CO, ethylene glycol, mercury, methyl bromide, methyl chloride, methyl iodide
	Papilledema	Ethylene glycol, lead, methanol, phosphorus, triethyl tin
	Ptosis	Thallium
	Retinal hemorrhages	Acetylphenylhydrazine, benzene, lead, methyl bromide, triethyl tin, warfarin
	Vision disturbance	Carbon tetrachloride, dinitrobenzene, lead, methanol, naphthalene, thallium, toluene, triethyl tin
Head	Epistaxis	Acrylonitrile, benzene, bromine, chromium, phosphine, tetryl
	Gum discoloration	Arsenic, bismuth, lead, mercury
	Pharyngitis	Acetone, acrolein, antimony, formaldehyde, hydrogen sulfide, iodine, tin
	Rhinitis	Acrolein, ammonia, antimony, chlorobenzenes, epoxy resins, formaldehyde, mercury, hydrochloric acid, ozone, organic dusts, phenylenediamine, thallium
	Salivation	Arsenic, bismuth, lead, mercury, organophosphates
	Tinnitus	Carbon dioxide, heavy metals, methanol, methylbromide, nitrobenzene, toluence, xylene
Pulmonary	Asthma	Grain dusts, isocyanate, metal fumes, phenylenediamine, polyvinyl chloride, toluene
	Dyspnea	Asphyxiants, beryllium, chloramine-T, dusts, nickel carbonyl, phosphate ester insecticides
	Pulmonary edema	Hydrogen sulfide, irritant gases, metal fumes, methyl bromide, methyl chloride
Cardiovascular	Angina	Arsenic, asphyxiants, carbon disulfide, methylene chloride, nitrates
	Bradycardia	Nitrates, organophosphates
	Dysrhythmias	Arsenic, chlorinated hydrocarbons, fluorocarbons, nitrates, phenol, any agent causing ischemia
	ECG abnormalities	Antimony, arsenic, arsine
	Hypertension	Cadmium, diphenyl oxide, lead, nicotine, vanadium
	Hypotension	Arsenic, arsine, carbon tetrachloride, fluorides, iron salts, methyl bromide, nickel carbonyl, nitrities, phosphine, phosphorus
	Tachycardia	Arsenic, dinitro-*o*-cresol, dinitrophenol, iron salts, nicotine, pentachlorophenol, potassium bromate
Gastrointestinal	Abdominal colic	Arsenic, inorganic lead, organophosphates, thallium
	Constipation	Barium sulfate, lead, thallium
	Diarrhea	Arsenic, barium, carbamates, organophosphates, phosphorus, heavy metals
	Jaundice	Hepatotoxins (carbon tetrachloride), hemolytic agents (arsine, stibine)
	Melena	Corrosives, iron, thallium
	Nausea and vomiting	Chlordane, central nervous system depressants (acetone, benzene), irritants (epoxy resins, copper, tin), organophosphates, methemoglobin formers

Table continued on opposite page

icals involved. Information about such personal protective equipment is readily available from a variety of textbooks and computer programs routinely carried by fire department and industrial hazardous materials response teams.

If the chemical of exposure is unknown, attempts must be made by the initial responders to identify it. Procedures and supplies for the identification of unknown chemicals are available to most hazardous materials response teams (Hazmat). The scene of the exposure should be assessed for clues to the nature of the accident and the likelihood of associated medical or traumatic injuries. After the chemical agent has been identified, much information can be obtained to assist in rescue and evacuation.

In the past, decontamination was often the most overlooked area in the treatment of the chemically injured patient.[24] The extreme toxicity of many agents such as organophosphates and the risk of secondary contamination make thorough decontamination essential. The procedure is relatively simple unless the toxic exposure is compounded by associated injuries. Decontamination for inhaled agents, such as cyanide, generally only require removing the patient from the source of exposure and administering high-flow oxygen. The patient should be evaluated for the possibility of deposition of fumes or soot on the skin, which could pose a risk of secondary contamination.

Patients with exposure to toxic chemicals that are

TABLE 74–8. Clinical Signs of Industrial Poisoning[4, 16, 22, 23] *Continued*

Organ System	Symptom/Sign	Exposure
Renal	Anuria	Bismuth, carbon tetrachloride, chlordane, chlorohydrin, ethylene glycol, mercurials, phosphorus, trinitrotoluene, turpentine
	Hematuria	Chlorates, heavy metals, naphthalene, nitrates
	Myoglobinuria	Aniline dyes, aromatic amines, chlorate, ethylene glycol, nitrates, nitrites
	Oliguria	Lead
	Proteinuria	Arsenic, mercury, organic solvents, phosphorus
Hematopoietic	Anemia	Arsine, arsenic, benzene, copper, lead, oxidant chemicals, stibine, trinitrotoluene
	Neutropenia	Arsenic, benzene, organochlorine insecticides
	Thrombocytopenia	Benzene, organochlorine insecticides
Nervous System	Ataxia	Chlordane, heavy metals, hexane, methyl chloride, organophosphates, toluene
	Cranial neuropathy	Carbon disulfide, trichloroethylene
	Delirium	Boric acid, bromides, chlordane, DDT, lead
	Depression	Alcohols, boric acid, carbon monoxide, cationic detergents, cyanide, heavy metals, insecticides, kerosene, naphthalene, phenol, solvents
	Motor neuropathy	Lead
	Myoclonus	Benzene hexachloride, mercury
	Parkinsonism	Carbon disulfide, carbon monoxide, manganese
	Psychosis	Bromides, carbon disulfide, manganese, toluene
	Seizures	Carbon monoxide, cyanide, lead, organic mercurials, organochlorine insecticides, organotin compounds
	Sensorimotor neuropathy	Acrylamide, arsenic, carbon disulfide, carbon monoxide, DDT, hexane, mercury
	Severe headache	Carbon monoxide, carbon tetrachloride, lead, nickel, nitrates, nitrites, organophosphates, trinitrotoluene
	Tremor	Arsenic, carbon disulfide, chlordecone, DDT, manganese, mercury
Endocrine	Decreased libido	Lead, mercury, other heavy metals
	Menstrual irregularities	Bismuth, lead, mercurials
Skin	Acne	Chlorobenzene, coal tar, paraffin
	Alopecia	Arsenic, boric acid, selenium, thallium
	Bullous lesions	Carbon monoxide, caustic agents
	Burns	Acids, formaldehyde, hypochlorite, lye
	Depigmentation	Arsenic, hydroquinone, phenols
	Diaphoresis	Nicotine, organophosphates
	Eczema	Detergents, solvents, soaps
	Flushing	Boric acid, cyanide
	Hyperpigmentation	Arsenic, halogenated aromatics
	Photosensitization	Phenanthrane, tars
	Purpura	Chlorinated biphenyls, dioxins
Musculoskeletal	Arthralgias	Arsenic, dinitrotoluene, lead
	Gout	Lead
	Muscle fasciculations	Manganese, organophosphates
	Muscle weakness/paralysis	Arsenic, chlordane, lead, organophosphates, organic mercurials, thallium
	Osteomalacia	Cadmium, fluoride, phosphorus

absorbed dermally or act on the skin require aggressive cleaning for removal. Ideally, this should occur in the field, where responders trained in the use of personal protective equipment have access to the appropriate resources and equipment. In general, the first step in decontamination after removal to a safe environment is removal of the victim's clothing. This step in itself removes up to 80% of the contaminant. Following this, rinsing of the patient with a large volume of low-pressure cool water is performed. Oil-based contaminates require the addition of soap or detergent to be fully removed. The water temperature may be gradually increased as the process continues. The initial use of cool water prevents the opening of skin pores and reduces dermal absorption of the chemical.[25] Three full showers or rinsings, with special attention given to the cleansing of hair, nails, and skin folds, are considered adequate. Runoff water must be contained for proper disposal.[26, 27] Chemicals splashed into the eyes should be flushed out immediately with copious amounts of water or normal saline. In the case of exposure to an alkali or an unknown chemical, flushing of the eye should be continued until the patient reaches the hospital.

When intoxication is caused by ingestion, an attempt should be made as soon as possible to prevent further absorption by the use of activated charcoal and, in some cases, gastric lavage.[28] For a treatment overview, see the algorithm presented in Figure 74–3.

HOSPITAL MANAGEMENT

Many industrial poisoning patients have been adequately decontaminated by the time emergency phy-

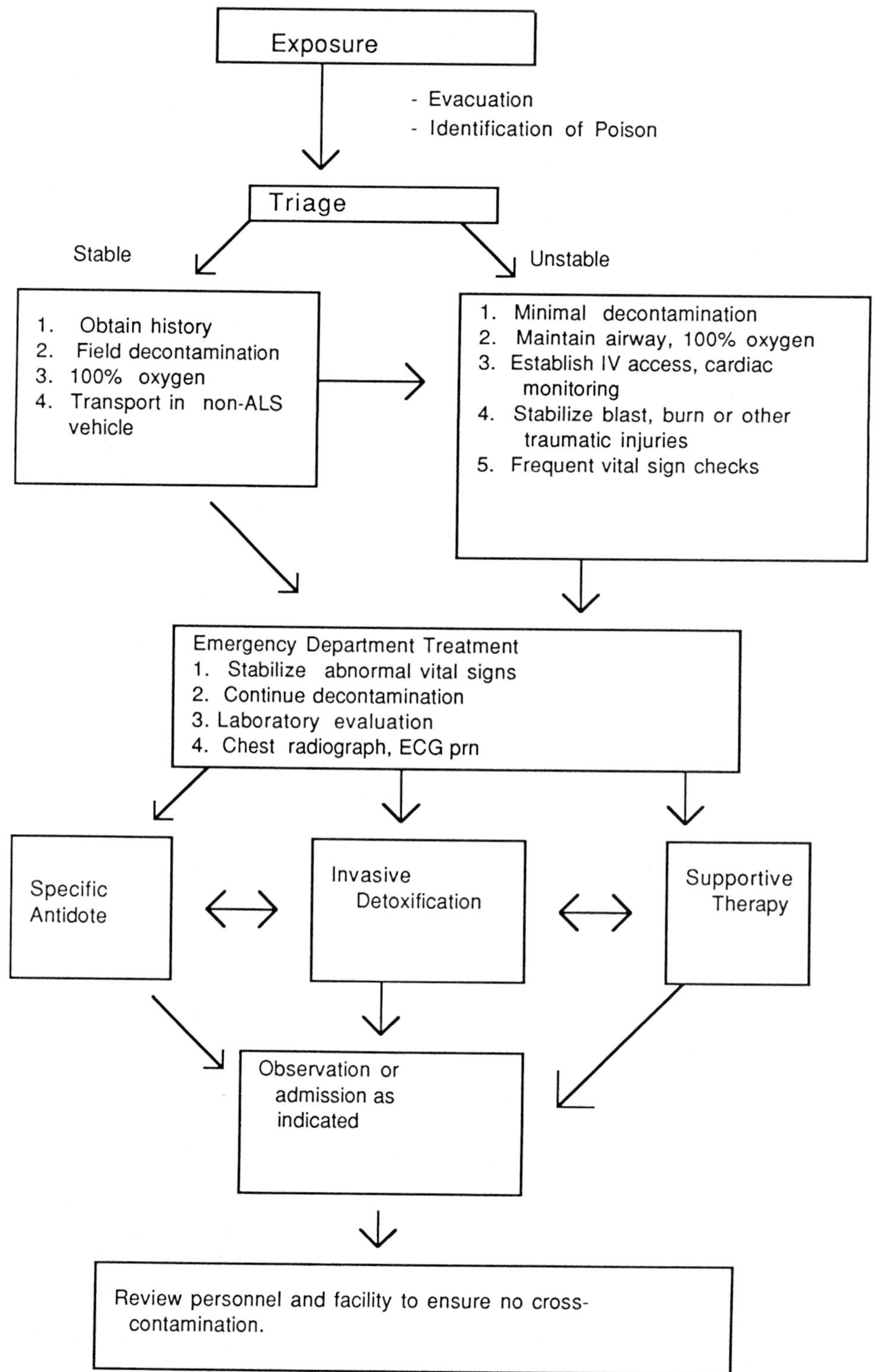

Figure 74–3. The management of industrial poisoning.

sicians become involved, but whether this is the case should always be ascertained. Specific note of the decontamination procedures should be made by physicians communicating with field personnel. If a patient arrives at the emergency department before decontamination, then the emergency department must have procedures and equipment to perform this step. Lavoie and associates reported on the success of their universal substances external decontamination procedure for hazardous chemical exposures.[29] The protection of the health care workers is essential.[30] The risk of secondary contamination depends on the toxicity of the substance and on the likelihood that quantities carried on the clothing, skin, or hair of the victims are sufficient to be a threat to the caregivers.[31] Other protocols also have been published.[1, 32–34]

Systemic absorption of ingested poisons is reduced by gastric lavage, the administration of activated charcoal, and use of cathartics.

When initial decontamination has been completed, attention is directed to aggressive airway management and supportive pulmonary therapy. Treatment may have to be concomitant with decontamination in critically ill patients. Patients exposed to noxious gases should receive humidified 100% oxygen, and a carbon monoxide level should be obtained. Transportation to a facility at which hyperbaric oxygen therapy can be given should be considered for patients who were found unconscious at the scene, have concomitant coronary artery disease, or have carbon monoxide levels over 25%. The management of inhalation injuries may require endotracheal intubation because of the presence of oropharyngeal and laryngeal edema. Occasionally, emergency cricothyroidotomy is needed. Once intubation has been accomplished, continuous positive airway pressure and positive end-expiratory pressure are useful for treating noncardiogenic pulmonary edema. Inhaled β-adrenergic agonists may be useful in patients with lower respiratory tract injury and wheezing. All patients discharged from the emergency department should be advised of the potential for late development of symptoms of respiratory distress.

As with any poisoning victim, initial management involves assessing overall severity of the illness, determining the systems affected, and preventing further absorption of the toxin. Arterial blood gas measurements are frequently helpful in evaluating both hypoxia and acidosis; also, the patient's volume status should be assessed for signs of hypovolemia. Baseline liver and renal tests should be performed. Potentially lethal arrhythmias must be identified and treated. Occasionally, central nervous system depression may be life-threatening. Patients with thermal burns and traumatic injuries need to be identified and stabilized.[17]

Treatment of minor chemical burns consists of debridement, tetanus immunization, topical application of antibiotic cream, and occlusive dressing for comfort. Because of the risk of underestimating the extent of chemical burns, close follow-up should be arranged.

Extensive burns must undergo aggressive treatment so that the patient is protected against hypovolemic shock and secondary complications such as infections.[35] Any patient with a burn that covers more than 20% of the body surface area must be transfered to a burn center. If the dermal injury is limited to superficial or localized irritation, wet dressings should be applied for comfort. A short course of systemic steroids may be necessary for extensive dermatitis. Additional treatment includes administration of oral antihistamines for sedation and relief of itching.[16]

When a chemical agent has been splashed into the eye, immediate irrigation is imperative; irrigation is generally continued during transport to a medical facility and for up to 30 minutes. Extensive irrigation is necessary in patients with alkali burns of the eyes because of the inability of the eyes to buffer pH changes of a severely basic nature and because of the capacity of alkalis to penetrate ocular tissues rapidly.[16] After irrigation, examination of the cornea with fluorescein dye and a slit lamp should be performed. A cycloplegic agent such as 0.2% scopolomine or 2% atropine may be used for associated iritis. An antibiotic ointment is generally applied. More significant injuries caused by alkalis and strong acids saponify plasma membranes, denature collagen, and cause vascular thombosis.[36] The application of collagenase inhibitors such as cysteine and calcium ethylenediaminetetraacetic acid during regeneration has greatly reduced the incidence of ulceration in patients with alkali burns; however, this therapy should be provided only with ophthalmologic consultation.[37]

Intensive supportive care is the mainstay of management of the poisoning victim. Its goal is the preservation of vital organ function until the poison has been metabolized. Care includes the early symptomatic treatment of complications such as peripheral vascular collapse, hypoxia, dysrhythmias, seizures, fluid and electrolyte disturbances, and pulmonary or cerebral edema. Hepatic, renal, and hematologic failure tend to occur somewhat later. Close expectant management of these patients has reduced the mortality in hospitalized patients to less than 1%.[38] A small group of severely poisoned patients, however, may benefit from the use of artificial organs to enhance elimination of toxins from the blood. Hemodialysis, hemoperfusion, and other modalities are considered state of the art in invasive detoxification (see Chapter 10).

LABORATORY EVALUATION

The current role of the clinical laboratory in the medical management of industrial poisoning is primarily to provide data on acid-base status, levels of hypoxia, and organ function (liver, kidney, and hematologic systems). If suspicion of a specific exposure is raised during the history-taking, additional testing such as a methemoglobin level determination may be necessary. Several types of chemical intoxication may be evaluated further with determination of the concentration of the suspected toxin or its metabolites in the blood or urine, or of the level of an affected enzyme in the blood. All patients with inhalation exposure should undergo carboxyhemoglobin level determination.

Central to the evaluation of pulmonary problems are chest radiography and pulmonary function testing. Radiography may reveal aspiration pneumonitis, noncardiogenic pulmonary edema, pleural effusions, or interstitial fibrosis. In addition to obtaining the routine posterioanterior view, one should consider obtaining oblique views if, for example, changes in the pleural surface are suspected following asbestos exposure. For diagnosis, it is helpful to be able to characterize pulmonary function abnormalities as obstructive or restrictive.[22] A xenon ventilation-perfusion lung scan may be useful in patients with suspected inhalation injury.

Abnormalities found on electrocardiography performed in the resting patient are neither very sensitive nor specific for diagnosing occupational exposure. Chemical asphyxiants or arsenic may produce an electrocardiographic picture of myocardial ischemia by interfering with cellular respiration. Both arsine and antimony have been associated with abnormalities of the T waves. Overexposure to phosphorous, organic mercury, or arsene causes QT segment prolongation and ST-T wave abnormalities.[4]

SUMMARY

Legislative measures, such as the Toxic Substances Control Act of 1976, alone may not be sufficient to reduce occupational disease significantly. Approximately 60,000 chemical substances are in common use, and several hundred new compounds are added by industrial processes each year. Unpredicted health hazards from new processes continue to emerge, and "well-known" occupational exposures still escape surveillance and control.[5] As a result, any patient presenting with an unusual symptom or group of symptoms should always prompt suspicion of an occupationally related disease. A systematic approach to recording the occupational history serves as a guide to discovering a specific toxic exposure that may be the cause of the presenting symptoms. Even when such a history is unavailable, a thorough physical examination and initial laboratory analysis often lead the clinician to an early toxicologic diagnosis.

References

1. Cox RD: Decontamination and management of hazardous materials exposure victims in the emergency department. Ann Emerg Med *23*:761–770, 1994.
2. Ramazzini B: Diseases of Workers. New York, Hafner, 1964.
3. Kunkel DB: Occupational asthma. Part II: Causes and management. Emerg Med *19*:86–94, 1987.
4. Rosenstock L, Cullen MR (eds): Clinical Occupational Medicine. Philadelphia, W.B. Saunders Co., 1986.
5. Goldman RH, Peters JM: The occupational and environmental health history. JAMA *246*:2831–2836, 1981.
6. Linz DH, Barker AF, Morton WE, et al: Occupational toxic inhalations. Top Emerg Med 7:21–33, 1985.
7. Levy B: The teaching of occupational health in American medical schools: Five year follow-up of initial study. Abstract. Am J Public Health *75*:79–80, 1985.
8. DOT Hazardous Materials Warning Placards. Washington, DC, US Department of Transportation, Research and Special Programs Administration, Materials Transportation Bureau, Office of Operations and Enforcement, 1981.
9. Stutz DR, Ricks RC, Olsen MF: Hazardous Materials Injuries: A Handbook for Prehospital Care. Greenbelt, MD, Bradford Communications Corp., 1982.
10. NFPA: Fire Protection Guide on Hazardous Materials. Boston, National Fire Protection Association, 1981.
11. Wanke LA: Toxic chemical spills. Top Emerg Med 7:9–19, 1985.
12. Increased lead absorption in children of lead workers—Vermont. MMWR Morb Mortal Wkly Rep *26*:61–62, 1977.
13. McCann M, Barazani G (eds): Health Hazards in the Arts and Crafts. Washington, DC, Society for Occupational and Environmental Health, 1980.
14. Finkl AJ: Hamilton's and Hardy's Industrial Toxicology. 4th ed. Boston, John Wright–PSG, Inc., 1983.
15. Wald PH, Balmes JR: Respiratory effects of short-term, high-intensity toxic inhalants: Smoke, gases, and fumes. J Intensive Care Med *2*:260–278, 1987.
16. Proctor NH, Hughes JP (eds): Chemical Hazards of the Workplace. 2nd ed. Philadelphia, J.B. Lippincott Co., 1988.
17. Kiser KW: Toxic inhalation. Emerg Med Clin North Am *2*:649–666, 1984.
18. Goldfrank LR, Bresnitz EA: Toxic inhalants. In Goldfrank LR, Flomenbaum NE, Lewin NA, et al (eds): Goldfrank's Toxicologic Emergencies. Norwalk, CT, Appleton-Century-Crofts, pp 651–661, 1986.
19. Hedges JR: Acute noxious gas exposure. Curr Top *2*:1–9, 1978.
20. Stokinger HE: Routes of entry and modes of action. In Key MM (ed): Occupational Diseases—A Guide to Their Recognition. Washington, DC, US Government Printing Office, pp 11–21, 1977.
21. Tolman KG: Gastrointestinal system. In Rom WN (ed): Environmental and Occupational Medicine. Boston, Little Brown & Co., pp 397–402, 1983.
22. Frank AL: The occupational history and examination. In Rom WN (ed): Environmental and Occupational Medicine. Boston, Little, Brown & Co., pp 23–32, 1983.
23. Block JB: The Signs and Symptoms of Chemical Exposure. Springfield, MA, Bannerstone House, 1980.
24. US Department of Transportation: Hazardous Materials, 1990—Emergency Response Guide. Washington, DC, US Department of Transportation, 1990.
25. Barr SJ: Chemical warfare agents. Top Emerg Med *7*:62–70, 1985.
26. US Environmental Protection Agency: Standard Operating Safety Guides. Publication 9285. 1-03 PB 963414. Washington, DC, Office of Emergency and Remedial Response, 1992.
27. Mycroft FJ, Jones JR, Olson KR: Emergency medical response to hazardous materials incidents. *In* Olson KR (ed): Poisoning and Drug Overdose. Norwalk, CT, Appleton & Lange, 1990.
28. American College of Emergency Physicians: Clinical policy for the initial approach to patients presenting with acute toxic ingestion or dermal or inhalation exposure. Ann Emerg Med *25*:570–585, 1995.
29. Lavoie FW, Coomes T, Cisek JE, Fulkenson L: Emergency department external decontamination for hazardous chemical exposures. Vet Hum Toxicol *34*:61–64, 1992.
30. Emergency Nurses Association Position Statement: Hazardous Materials Exposure. Emergency Nurses Association, Park Ridge, IL, 1994.
31. Agency for Toxic Substances and Disease Registry: Managing Hazardous Materials Incidents. Vol. III & Medical Management Guidelines for Acute Chemical Exposure. Washington, DC, US Department of Health and Human Services, Public Health Service, 1994.
32. Koehler G (ed): Hazardous Materials Medical Management Protocols. 2nd ed. Sacramento, CA, California EMS Authority, 1991.
33. Kirk MA, Cisek J, Rose SR: Emergency department response to hazardous materials incidents. Emerg Med Clin North Am *12*:461–481, 1994.
34. Borak J, Callan M, Abbott W: Hazardous Materials Exposure—Emergency Response and Patient Care. Englewood Cliffs, NJ, Prentice-Hall, 1991.
35. Klein DG, O'Malley P: A topical injury from chemical agents: Initial treatment. Heart Lung *16*:49–54, 1987.
36. Pfister RR: Chemical injuries of the eye. Ophthalmology *90*:1246–1250, 1983.
37. Slansky HH, Dohlman CH, Berman MB: Prevention of corneal ulcers. Trans Am Acad Ophthalmol Otolaryngol *75*:1208–1212, 1971.
38. Vale JA: The epidemiology of acute poisoning. Acta Pharmacol Toxicol *41*(Suppl):443–358, 1977.

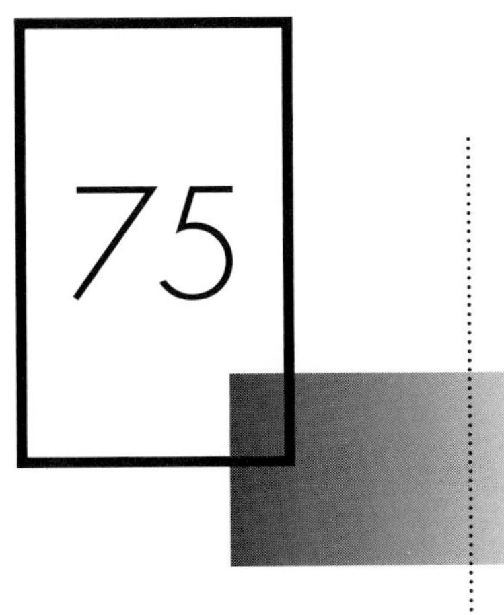

Chlorinated Hydrocarbons

KIMBERLEY C. PEARSON, MD, MPH

The chlorinated hydrocarbons are volatile chemicals that are widely encountered in industrial and commercial products. Outside of limited use as topical anesthetics or "freezing" agents, their medical applications are of primarily historic interest. Compounds of this class were among some of the earliest inhalation anesthetics; chloroform was first used in human anesthesia in 1847.[1] With the increasing use of electrical equipment in the operating room during the 1950s, trichloroethylene was an attractive nonflammable alternative to the popular anesthetic cyclopropane; however its use was limited by the induction of bradycardia and tachypnea as well as decomposition to neurotoxic byproducts on contact with hot soda lime, a component of most anesthesia breathing circuits.[2] Halothane, a chlorofluorohydrocarbon, was developed and brought into clinical use in 1956; it formed the model for most new anesthetic agents.

An evolving awareness of the toxic effects of chlorinated hydrocarbons paralleled their use in anesthesia. In the same year that chloroform was first used on humans, the first cases of jaundice and death following exposure were noted.[1]

EPIDEMIOLOGY

Chlorinated hydrocarbons are used extensively as solvents in industry due both to their excellent solvent properties and economy. However, federal regulations pertaining to the disposal of toxic wastes have significantly increased the cost of using these products such that they are being replaced in some industries by more "environmentally friendly" agents. It has been estimated that as many as 100,000 full time and 3.5 million part-time workers have been exposed to trichloroethylene at any given time.[3] These agents are also available in commercial products for home use as solvents in adhesive removers, waterproofers, and degreasers. Through industrial runoff and chlorination of public drinking water, trace and sometimes significant amounts of chlorinated hydrocarbons have been identified as contaminants in surface and ground water. The potential toxic effects of these low-level contaminants on the general population has become a topic of much debate and interest in recent years.[4]

Exposures to chlorinated hydrocarbons, therefore, may occur at the worksite or at home. Occupational exposures are generally either dermal or inhalational. The level of exposure in industry has decreased since the early 1980s due to progressive decreases in standards for exposure limits.[5] Although volitional ingestions of these agents are rare, reports of their abuse by inhalation are increasing. "Huffing," "bagging," or "sniffing" of propellants and typewriter correction fluid have led to fatalities in abusers.

PHARMACOLOGY

The agents discussed herein are short-chain aliphatic hydrocarbons. They are highly lipophilic and are therefore able to dissolve a wide variety of organic compounds. The addition of chlorine increases their stability while decreasing their flammability. Most are extremely volatile liquids at room temperature and pressure and have distinctive sweet yet slightly pungent odors. Six chlorinated aliphatic hydrocarbons are relatively commonly encountered: trichloroethylene, perchloroethylene (tetrachloroethylene), 1,1,1-trichloroethane (methyl chloroform), methylene chloride (dichloromethane), carbon tetrachloride, and chloroform. These agents are the focus of this discussion. Other more rarely encountered agents are discussed only briefly (Table 75–1). Table 75–2 provides a reference for the specific parameters of each agent.

The chlorinated hydrocarbons are volatile organic compounds, which as a group share the toxic effects of acute narcosis and dermatitis. These effects are related to their physical properties—volatility and lipophilicity—rather than to their chemical structures. The specific toxicities of the compounds are related to the manner and degree to which they are metabolized to bioactive intermediates, which varies widely among the group.

PHARMACOKINETICS

Absorption

Because these are highly volatile compounds, the most significant route of exposure is inhalation. Pulmonary uptake ranges from 50% to 80% at rest and increases during activity.[6] Dermal absorption of vapors is negligible; however, extensive contact of the skin with liquid may result in toxicity, as in the case with carbon tetrachloride.[7] Absorption through nonintact skin is more efficient. Gastrointestinal absorption is variable but usually significant.

Distribution

Because of their high lipophilicity, the chlorinated hydrocarbons distribute extensively into adipose tissue. Rate of distribution, related to the blood/air partition coefficient, tends to be rapid.

Elimination

Chlorinated hydrocarbons have two routes of elimination. They may be exhaled unchanged in the breath, or they may be enzymatically metabolized to water-soluble derivatives that can then be excreted in the urine. Individual compounds differ in the proportions of each of these routes that are utilized.

In the liver, and to a lesser extent the kidney, lung, and gastrointestinal (GI) tract, the chlorinated hydrocarbons are metabolized via the cytochrome P-450 mixed-function oxidase system. The first step in the process is to generate an intermediate that possesses a reactive group that can then be acted on in the second step to create a polar group. These reactions are shared by many compounds, both endogenous molecules and xenobiotics. In the case of the chlorinated hydrocarbons, the metabolic process may create reactive metabolites that are more toxic than the parent compounds.[8]

Figure 75–1 outlines some of these reactions in the commonly encountered chlorinated hydrocarbons. The relationship of the metabolic process to toxicity is discussed further in the following text.

Table 75–1. Uncommonly Encountered Chlorinated Hydrocarbons

Compound	Sources of Exposure	Toxic Effects
Methyl chloride	Industrial: Solvent, chemical intermediary Commercial: None Other: Local anesthetic	Gas-phase solvent at room temperature and pressure with limited use as topical anesthetic or freezing agent; primary toxicity is to CNS; few or no hepatic or renal effects
Ethyl chloride	Industrial: Chemical intermediary and solvent Other: Topical anesthetic, inhalation abuse	Volatile liquid primarily toxic to CNS producing prenarcosis symptoms; neuropsychiatric effects have been reported with chronic abuse; pre-arrhythmic effects due to myocardial sensitization
1,1-Dichloroethane 1,2-Dichloroethane	Industrial: Chemical intermediary, lead scavenger in gasoline	CNS depression accompanied by hepatic and renal dysfunction; dermal and mucous membrane irritation; 1,2-isomer is considered an animal carcinogen
1,1,2-Trichloroethane	Industrial: None Commercial: None Other: None known	Stronger anesthetic than the 1,1,1-isomer; significant hepatic toxicity; renal toxicity reported; dermal and mucous membrane irritation; suspected carcinogen
1,1,2,2-Tetrachloroethane	Excellent solvent but one of the most toxic chlorinated hydrocarbons; little or no use in United States	Similar to carbon tetrachloride but more severe
1,2-Dichloroethylene	Industrial: Extracting agent for heat-sensitive materials (perfumes, decaffeinated coffee)	Mild CNS depressant with little or no hepatic or renal toxicity
1,1-Dichloroethylene	Industrial: Reagent in the formation of copolymeric plastics	Similar to carbon tetrachloride; associated with hepatic angiosarcoma and bronchoalveolar adenoma in animals
Dichloropropane	Industrial: Soil fumigant	Irritant; significant CNS and hepatic toxicity; myocardial sensitization to catecholamines
Ethylene chlorohydrin	Industrial: Chemical intermediary, solvent	Highly toxic with pulmonary edema, vascular damage, inhibition of cardiac muscle; hepatic and renal toxicity

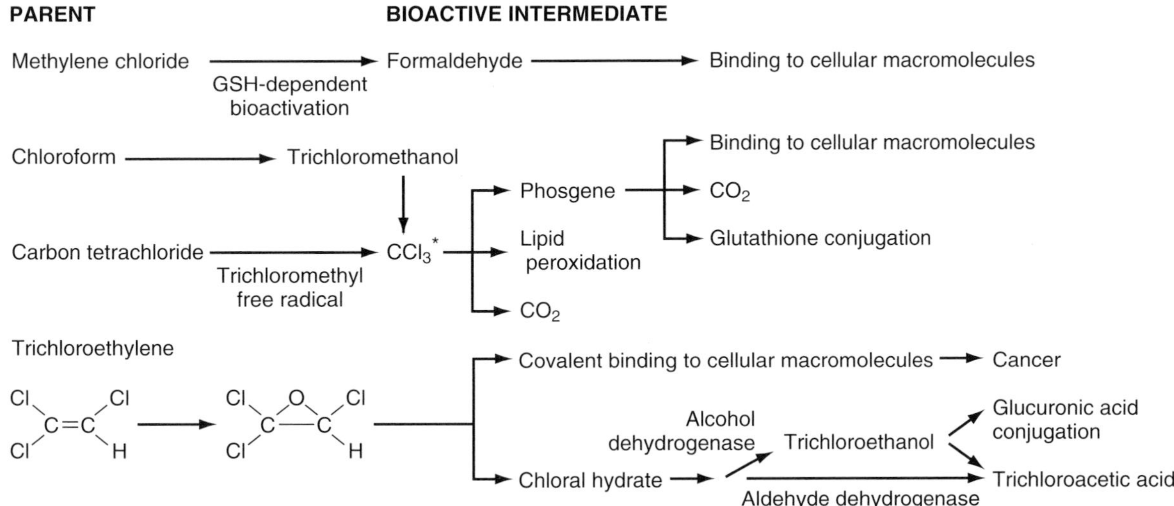

Figure 75–1. Some reactions characteristic of the commonly encountered chlorinated hydrocarbons.

Drug/Chemical Interaction

The metabolism may be affected by substances that induce or inhibit cytochrome P-450 enzymes, which may ultimately affect the toxicity. Phenobarbital and ethanol would be examples of the former. In addition, ethanol competes for alcohol dehydrogenases, which potentiates the anesthetic effect of trichloroethylene (and similarly metabolized compounds) through persistence of the active metabolite, trichloroethanol.[9] "Degreaser's flush," which is a flushing of the skin of the face and neck accompanied in some by orthostatic hypotension (similar to a disulfiram reaction) occurs in workers who consume ethanol after exposure to trichlorethylene. This may be related to an accumulation of aldehyde due to competition between trichloroethylene and ethanol for the enzyme aldehyde dehydrogenase.[10] Ketonic compounds also potentiate the toxicity of chlorinated hydrocarbons.[11]

PHARMACODYNAMICS/ MECHANISM OF ACTION AND TOXICITY

Chlorinated hydrocarbons exert their toxic effects by different mechanisms in different target end-organs. These mechanisms can be simplified into direct action of the parent compound on the target organ and bioactivation to toxic metabolites.

Direct toxicity of the parent compound is best represented by the central nervous system (CNS) toxicity, that is, narcosis or anesthesia. This effect is shared to a greater or lesser extent by all of the chlorinated hydrocarbons, in fact, by most volatile hydrocarbons. It can be considered an extension of their therapeutic actions as inhalation anesthetics. The potency of an agent to induce the anesthetic state, an absence of sensation and awareness, is directly related to their lipophilicity. The structural diversity of these implies that the site of action is not a single receptor site. Rather, interaction with a hydrophobic or amphipathic site of action is likely.[1] It is thought that these agents interact with neuronal membranes, causing reversible conformational changes and nonselective interruption of signal transmission.[12] How this leads to unconsciousness is as yet not fully described.

Chlorinated hydrocarbons exert specific end-organ toxicity through the formation of reactive intermediates that may either covalently bond to tissue or initiate destructive chain reactions (lipid peroxidation). Figure 75–1 illustrates some of these bioactivation pathways.

In the course of its oxidative metabolism, chloroform is oxidized to trichloromethanol, which breaks down to phosgene.[13] Phosgene reacts with water to produce carbon dioxide and chloride ion, and with glutathione to produce diglutathionyl dithiocarbonate. When glutathione is depleted, phosgene binds to cellular macromolecules, leading to cell necrosis.

Both covalent binding of toxic metabolites and lipid peroxidation are involved in the hepatotoxicity of carbon tetrachloride. During oxidative metabolism, the trichloromethyl free radical CCl_3* is formed by the homolytic cleavage of CCl_4. An intermediate in this metabolic pathway is a highly reactive epoxide. The free radical causes peroxidation of the polyenoic lipids, which proceeds as a chain reaction, leading to the breakdown of cellular membranes.

Epoxide formation is involved in the phase I transformation of many chlorinated hydrocarbons. Increasing chlorination of the position 1 carbon destabilizes the C-O bond and promotes binding to cellular macromolecules such as DNA, while increasing symmetry of the molecule leads to increased bond strength of the chlorinated carbon to the oxygen molecule of the epoxide and thus enhances the stability of this intermediate.[14] This may explain the toxic effects of agents such as perchloroethylene, which

Table 75–2. Commonly Encountered Chlorinated Hydrocarbons

Compound	Synonyms	Structure	Characteristics	Vapor Pressure (kPa)	Blood/Air Partition Coefficient	Oil/Air Partition Coefficient	Sources of Exposure	Absorption
Methylene chloride	Dichloromethane	CH_2Cl_2	Colorless liquid with chloroform-like odor; produces phosgene on combustion	45	9	150	Industrial: Solvent, fumigant, insecticide Commercial: paint strippers, aerosol sprays	Inhalation: Sig GI: Sig Dermal: NS
Chloroform	Trichloromethane	$CHCl_3$	Colorless liquid with a pleasant odor	21	10	400	Industrial: Production of fluorocarbons Commercial: Banned by FDA due to carcinogenicity Other: Byproduct of water chlorination	Inhalation: Sig GI: Sig Dermal: NS
Carbon tetrachloride	Tetrachloromethane	CCl_4	Colorless liquid with a characteristic ether-like odor	12	2	360	Industrial: Production of fluorocarbons, solvent in rubber and chemical industries	Inhalation: Sig GI: Sig Dermal: Sig
1,1,1-Trichloroethane	Methyl chloroform TCA	CH_3CCl_3	Colorless liquid with a mild chloroform-like odor	13	2	350	Industrial: Solvent, degreaser, insecticides Commercial: Liquid Paper, Scott's Liquid Gold, adhesive tape removal, water proofer Other: Inhalation abuse	Inhalation: Sig GI: Sig Dermal: NS
Trichloroethylene	Acetylene trichloride Trichloroethene TCE	$CHCl{=}CHCl_2$	Colorless liquid (unless dyed blue) with a chloroform-like odor	8	9	700	Industrial: Vapor degreasing Commercial: Spot removers, paint strippers, degreasers, typewriter correction fluid Other: Ground water contamination, inhalation abuse	Inhalation: Sig GI: Sig Dermal: NS
Tetrachloroethylene	Perchloroethylene PCE	$CCl_2{=}CCl_2$	Colorless liquid with a mild chloroform-like odor; decomposes in a fire to phosgene and HCl	1.9	13	1900	Industrial: Dry cleaning, degreasing Other: Ground water contamination	Inhalation: Sig GI: ?NS Dermal: NS

Sig, significant: NS, not significant; PEL, permissible exposure limit; IARC, International Agency for Research on Cancer; TCEOH, trichloroethanol; TCAA, trichloroacetic acid; CO, carbon monoxide; 2B, possibly carcinogenic to humans.

Elimination	Acute Toxicity	Chronic Toxicity	Antidote	OSHA PEL (mg/m^3)	Biologic Exposure Indices
Lung: 70% unchanged, 25–35% CO Liver: Formaldehyde	CNS: Depression; headache and lightheadedness Hepatic: Mild toxicity Renal: Rare Dermal: Significant irritant Other: Cardiac effects of COHb, pulmonary edema	None in epidemiologic study of exposed workers; IARC 2B	Hyperbaric O_2 (case series)	500	Urine: TCEOH, TCAA
Lung: 50% unchanged Liver: Phosgene	CNS: Profound depression Hepatic: Hepatitis occurs with subnarcotic dose Renal: Significant toxicity in hypoxic patients Dermal: Mucous membrane irritant, defatting dermatitis Other: Arrhythmias, cardiac arrest	IARC 2B	NAC (theoretical)	50	
Lung: 50% unchanged, 4% CO_2 Liver: 40–50% CCl_3*, phosgene, lipid peroxidation	CNS: Profound depression Hepatic: Hepatitis occurs with subnarcotic dose Renal: Significant toxicity in hypoxic patients Dermal: Mucous membrane irritant, defatting dermatitis Other: Arrhythmias, nausea, vomiting	Hepatic necrosis with prolonged or repeated exposures; IARC 2B	NAC (case series); hyperbaric O_2 (case)	10	
Lung: 90% Urine: 10% TCAA, TCE	CNS: Anesthesia Hepatic: Mild enzyme elevations Renal: Rare reports Dermal: Defatting dermatitis Other: Dysrhythmias, respiratory depression, sudden death in abusers	Reports of fatty liver in workers chronically exposed	None	350	End-exhaled air: 1,1,1-trichloroethane Urine: TCEOH, TCAA
Lung: 10% Urine: TCE 50% TCAA 40%	CNS: Anesthesia, euphoria Hepatic: Rarely reported Renal: Failure may occur Dermal: Irritant, defatting dermatitis Other: Dysrhythmias, trigeminal nerve impairment, "degreaser's flush"	? Toxic encephalopathy	None	100	
Lung: 97% Urine: TCAA 3%	CNS: Anesthesia Hepatic: moderate toxicity Renal: Rare Dermal: Significant irritant	?Neurobehavioral syndrome ?Association with liver tumors in dry cleaners; IARC 2B	None	100	End-exhaled air: PCE Blood: PCE Urine: TCAA

is associated with fatty liver development but not necrosis; however, these agents are considered to be carcinogenic. It has been postulated that their epoxides adduct to DNA molecules. This is in contrast to chloroform or carbon tetrachloride, whose highly reactive metabolite binds directly to the endoplasmic reticulum membrane and inactivates cytochrome P-450.

CLINICAL PRESENTATION

The immediate toxic effects of exposure to aliphatic chlorinated hydrocarbons are CNS depression and mucous membrane and respiratory tract irritation. These may be followed in the short term by hepatocellular injury or necrosis and/or renal dysfunction. Chronic toxic effects of exposure primarily include dermatitis, hepatic inflammation, renal tubular dysfunction, and neurobehavioral dysfunction. Effects may also be seen in the cardiovascular and peripheral nervous systems. Rare reports have been published of scleroderma associated with chlorinated hydrocarbon exposure.[14] Some agents are known to be carcinogenic or teratogenic. Individual compounds may demonstrate unique toxicities, such as methylene chloride, which is metabolized in part to carbon monoxide.[15] Acute and chronic toxic effects are discussed by system in the following text.

Central Nervous System

Acute, high-level exposure to chlorinated hydrocarbons produces signs of CNS depression or intoxication. Although the presentation may vary to some extent, depending on the narcotic potential of the compound, disorientation, euphoria, giddiness, and confusion may be followed by prenarcosis symptoms of dizziness, nausea, vomiting, incoordination, or paresthesias, progressing to unconsciousness, paralysis, convulsion, and death from respiratory or cardiovascular arrest. As discussed previously, these effects are related to the parent compound and do not depend on the bioactivation by enzyme-catalyzed reactions. Therefore, the time of onset of these effects is generally very short (i.e., minutes to hours) depending on the exposure level. Solvent-induced narcosis is the cause of death in most fatal poisonings. Recovery is usually complete in the acute setting, although long-term neurobehavioral sequelae have been reported following large exposures.

To what degree chronic exposure to low levels of solvents causes a chronic toxic encephalopathy in exposed workers has been a matter of some controversy within occupational medicine. Several studies, using batteries of psychometric tests, have sought to demonstrate changes in cognitive function and affect in workers who are exposed to either individual solvents or mixtures.[16–18] The interpretation of these studies has been hampered by a paucity of exposure data as well as poor definition of confounding variables, such as ethanol intake.

Liver

The hepatic toxicity of the aliphatic chlorinated hydrocarbons is mediated through a bioactive metabolic intermediate. Therefore, manifestation of hepatotoxicity takes a minimum of hours, if not days, after exposure. With carbon tetrachloride, centrolobular necrosis is evident by 12 hours postexposure, and hepatic necrosis by 24 hours. Recovery begins almost as soon, and may be complete by day 14.[19] Enzyme levels peak during the first 48 hours.[13] For certain compounds, particularly carbon tetrachloride, the onset of hepatic dysfunction may not be preceded by significant CNS depression. Chloroform and carbon tetrachloride induce hepatic necrosis, whereas the other agents produce only fatty liver.[20] Fatty liver may or may not be a precursor to cell death and is generally reversible. Prognosis depends on the magnitude of the exposure, the underlying state of the liver, and the presence of co-toxicants such as ethanol. Chronic exposure to solvents has been associated with elevated transaminase levels, which tend to resolve during a work absence of 2 to 4 weeks.[5]

Kidney

Nephrotoxicity occurs with some compounds in this class, such as chloroform. Acute tubular necrosis may occur with proteinuria, glucosuria, and increased blood urea nitrogen (BUN) levels. The toxicity is mediated by a reactive metabolite as in the liver. In the case of chloroform, renal tubular cytochrome P-450 enzymes catalyze the formation of trichloromethanol, which breaks down to phosgene.[21] Renal failure may also be seen secondary to massive hepatic necrosis with large exposures.

Chronic exposure to chlorinated hydrocarbons has been associated with proteinuria; however, more recent work suggests that original observations of workers may have been measuring an effect of shift work rather than of solvent toxicity.[21] An association between chronic exposure and glomerulonephritis is suggested by recent studies, although the data are not conclusive.[22, 23]

Skin

Frequent skin contact with lipid-soluble solvents can lead to a defatting of the surface of the skin and chronic irritant dermatitis. Dermatitis is the most frequent occupational disease, and exposure to solvents is thought to contribute up to 30% of the total disease burden. Chlorinated hydrocarbons are classified as mild, relative, or marginal irritants that require repeated or prolonged contact to produce inflammation.[24] Occasionally, a patient will be seen who has been using a solvent for skin cleansing. This can significantly disrupt the epidermal barrier. When a significant dermatitis is present, with disruption of the skin barrier, the solvent may be absorbed through the nonintact skin at a higher rate, leading to more significant toxicity by this route. The skin may appear thickened, scaling, and hyperkeratotic. Painful fissuring and cracking may be present. Although sensitization to solvents is rarely reported, the presence of a significant dermatitis may predispose to sensitization by other chemicals or antigens in the workplace. One agent, perchloroethylene, is a significant irritant and may cause erythema, blistering, and burns with minimal contact.

Ocular and Mucous Membrane Effects

The mucous membrane irritant effects of these substances are related to their ability to dissolve fats. They may cause pain or burning on contact. The eye may show dulling of the cornea after a significant splash. Fluorescent examination may reveal punctate staining of the epithelium. The pathophysiology appears to be scattered loss of epithelial cells due to solution of some of the fats that occur in these cells. The damage is generally reversible.[25]

Pulmonary Effects

The lungs are the primary site of exposure for most exposures to chlorinated hydrocarbons, as well as a site of excretion. Although some in situ metabolism and bioactivation takes place in the lungs, they are not a primary site of direct toxicity for most agents. Cytochrome P-450 metabolism takes place primarily in the Clara cells.[26] Although a common cause of death in fatal exposures is respiratory arrest, this is related to solvent-induced narcosis rather than to a direct pulmonary effect. Some agents, such as methylene chloride, produce pulmonary edema at high levels of exposure.[27]

Cardiovascular Effects

Chlorinated hydrocarbons can depress heart rate, contractility, and conduction.[28] The use of trichloroethylene as a general anesthetic was largely abandoned due to its effects on heart rate and blood pressure. Some of these agents sensitize the heart to the arrhythmogenic effects of β-agonists, such as endogenous epinephrine or norepinepherine. Because they are highly lipophilic, these agents readily cross the blood-brain barrier and effect cardiotoxicity through disruption of neural control of heart rate and contractility. A direct effect may also be seen on contractility due to solvent effects on membrane fluidity. Reports have been published of chronic cardiac toxicity with development of cardiomyopathy in chronic solvent exposure.[29]

Carcinogenicity and Teratogenicity

One chlorinated hydrocarbon now in very limited and controlled use is vinyl chloride. It was recognized in 1974 by an observant clinician in a vinyl chloride polymerization plant that an unusual cancer, angiosarcoma of the liver, had occurred in three workers at his plant.[30]

Most of these agents have been shown to induce tumors in one or more animal models.[31, 32] However, other than vinyl chloride, human epidemiologic studies have as yet not demonstrated a convincing association between work with these agents and cancer occurrence. Due to interspecies variations in metabolism, the animal models may not adequately predict human carcinogenicity.[33]

Transplacental transfer is generally efficient for compounds that are lipophilic, nonpolar, and have a molecular weight less than 1000 daltons. Spontaneous abortions have been associated with methylene chloride and chloroform at doses that produced maternal toxicity. Chloroprene is strongly associated with decreased sperm motility, abnormal morphology, and decreased libido in exposed males.[34]

The ubiquitous nature of low levels of these chemicals in drinking water from industrial sources as well as the generation in situ from chlorination has led to concern regarding safety of water supplies. Although several studies have suggested associations between chlorination of water and bladder or colon cancer, significant methodologic problems limit the conclusions.[35] Several epidemiologic studies have associated drinking water contamination with recalled miscarriage or fetal cardiac effects.[36] Conclusions from these studies are limited because of the recall bias and poor exposure measurements.

DIAGNOSIS

The diagnosis of chlorinated hydrocarbon toxicity relies primarily on obtaining a history of exposure. In acute exposure situations, the individual may be found with a container, or a Material Safety Data Sheet (MSDS) may be immediately available at the worksite. In making the diagnosis of chronic toxicity, the examiner may identify a clinical syndrome, suspect a causal agent in the environment, and obtain an exposure history. It is important to identify whether the exposure was to a single agent or to a mixture of agents, and to obtain some estimate of dose. The dose will depend to some degree on the conditions of use, such as temperature, work practices, environmental controls (such as ventilation), and personal protective equipment. It is important to obtain a history of non–work-related exposures, as solvents are extensively used in art, hobbies, automobile repair, home improvement, and cleaning.

Physical findings consistent with chlorinated hydrocarbon poisoning include CNS signs acutely. Later, right upper quadrant tenderness and jaundice may develop. Vital signs may show tachyarrhythmia or bradyarrhythmia. The breath may have a chloroform-like odor. Respirations may be shallow and/or slow. Temperature may be elevated. Rales may be present in the setting of aspiration. Nausea, vomiting, or generalized abdominal pain may be present. The primary survey should identify the presence of any open wounds. Telltale white smudges of titanium oxide at the nares may be found with inhalant abuse of typewriter correction fluid.

Laboratory confirmation of the exposure may be made with exhaled breath or urinary metabolite measurement if the methodology is readily available. In the workplace, biologic exposure indices are sometimes utilized as described in Table 75–1. These are generally measured at the end of a working shift. Some of these agents are radiopaque, which may be used to confirm a large ingestion.[37] Carboxyhemoglobin (COHb) measurements should be performed for methylene chloride exposures. It is important to note that COHb levels may continue to rise after cessation of exposure due to the metabolic generation of carbon monoxide.

TREATMENT

The treatment for chlorinated hydrocarbon poisoning is supportive, although an understanding of the metabolism of these agents suggests the possibility that specific interventions might be efficacious.

Immediate Supportive Measures

Standard basic and advanced life support measures should be implemented. In the case of a large ingestion, it may be prudent to protect the airway early on due to the risk of pneumonitis associated with aspiration of hydrocarbons. Hypoxemia may predispose to hepatic necrosis.[38] With ingestion in particular, CNS depression may be ongoing and attention should be paid to progressive respiratory depression. During cardiac resuscitation, avoidance of exogenous catecholamines, if feasible, should be considered, given the possibility of a lowered threshold for induced arrhythmias.

Decontamination/Prevention of Systemic Absorption

External

External decontamination is important, both to limit ongoing skin absorption of these agents and to protect the responders. The basic principles of decontamination include using the least abrasive method that is effective. Scrub brushes and hot water may cause vasodilation of the skin and enhanced absorption. The first priority should be to address mucous membranes and open wounds through which significant absorption can continue to take place. Clothing should be completely removed and bagged.

Internal

Ipecac should not be used, because of the risk of aspiration of a hydrocarbon and because of the sedative effects of these agents. Gastric lavage should be performed on any large ingestion and on any ingestion involving chloroform or carbon tetrachloride due to the risk of hepatic necrosis. A single dose of activated charcoal has been recommended in most sources; however, information as to its efficacy for most of these compounds is limited.

Antidotes

No specific antidotes for chlorinated hydrocarbons have been shown to be effective in human trials. Several case series have implicated the use of *n*-acetylcysteine (NAC) in severe poisonings with carbon tetrachloride in an attenuated course of hepatic injury.[39] The physiologic basis for this therapy is to augment the glutathione available for the detoxification of intermediates, such as phosgene, produced in the metabolism of these agents.

Case reports have been published on the use of hyperbaric oxygen for methylene chloride exposures and for carbon tetrachloride ingestions.[40, 41]

Elimination Enhancement

Hyperventilation has been used to augment respiratory elimination in a case report of perchloroethylene poisoning in which some efficacy is claimed.[42]

Dialysis is not indicated for the removal of chlorinated hydrocarbons; however, it may be necessary if renal failure occurs.

Disposition

For the majority of chlorinated hydrocarbon exposures, symptoms will abate with cessation of exposure without residual toxic effects. It is important to note, however, that the hepatic and renal toxicities are not necessarily predicted by acute CNS presentation for all agents, and observation for 24 to 36 hours may therefore be appropriate when conditions of exposure indicate the possibility of significant late hepatic toxicity.

References

1. Baden JM, Rice SA: Metabolism and toxicity of inhaled anesthetics. *In* Miller RD (ed): Anesthesia. 2nd ed. New York, Churchill Livingstone, pp 701–744, 1986.

2. Marshall BE, Wollman H: General anesthetics. *In* Gilman AG, Goodman LS, Gilman A (eds): Goodman and Gilman's The Pharmacological Basis of Therapeutics. 6th ed. New York, Macmillan, 1980.
3. National Institute for Occupational Safety and Health: Current Intelligence Bulletin No. 48: Organic Solvent Neurotoxicity. Washington, DC, NIOSH, 1987.
4. Policy Statement No. 9304: Recognizing and addressing the environmental and occupational health problems posed by chlorinated organic chemicals, American Public Health Association. Am J Public Health *84*:514, 1994.
5. Lundberg I, Hogstedt C, Liden C, Nise G: Organic solvents and related compounds. *In* Rosentock L, Cullen MR: Textbook of Clinical Occupational and Environmental Medicine. Philadelphia, WB Saunders, pp 766–785, 1994.
6. Astrand I: Effect of physical exercise on uptake, distribution, and elimination of vapors in man. *In* Fiserova-Bergerova V (ed): Modeling of Inhalation Exposure to Vapors: Uptake, Distribution, and Elimination, vol II. Boca Raton, FL, CRC Press, pp 107–130, 1983.
7. Javier Perez A, Courel M, Sobrado J, Gonzalez L: Acute renal failure after topical application of carbon tetrachloride (letter). Lancet *1*:515, 1987.
8. Anders MW: Bioactivation of halogenated hydrocarbons. J Toxicol Clin Toxicol *19*:699, 1982.
9. Larson JL, Bull RJ: Effect of ethanol on the metabolism of trichloroethylene, J Toxicol Environ Health *28*:395, 1989.
10. Muller G, Spassowski M, Henschler D: Metabolism of trichloroethylene in man: III. Interaction of trichloroethylene and ethanol. Arch Toxicol *33*:173, 1975.
11. Raymond P, Plaa GL: Ketone potentiation of haloalkane-induced hepato- and nephrotoxicity: I. Dose-response relationships. J Toxicol Environ Health *45*:465, 1995.
12. Sikkema J, de Bont JA, Poolman B: Mechanisms of membrane toxicity of hydrocarbons. Microbiol Rev *59*:201, 1995.
13. Keaton BF: Chlorinated hydrocarbons. *In* Haddad LM, Winchester JF (eds): Clinical Management of Poisoning and Drug Overdose. 2nd ed. Philadelphia, WB Saunders, pp 1216–1222, 1990.
14. Czirjak L, Pocs E, Szegedi G: Localized scleroderma after exposure to organic solvents. Dermatology *189*:399, 1994.
15. Ratney RS, Wegman DH, Elkins HB: In vivo conversion of methylene chloride to carbon monoxide. Arch Environ Health *28*:223, 1974.
16. Edling C, Edberg K, Ahlborg G Jr, et al: Long-term follow-up of workers exposed to solvents. Br J Ind Med *47*:75, 1990.
17. Gregersen P: Neurotoxic effects of organic solvents in exposed workers: Two controlled follow-up studies after 5.5 and 10.6 years. Am J Ind Med *14*:681, 1988.
18. Rasmussen K, Jeppesen HJ, Sabroe S: Solvent-induced chronic toxic encephalopathy. Am J Ind Med *23*:779, 1993.
19. Robbins SL, Cotran R, Kumar V: Pathologic Basis for Disease. Philadelphia, WB Saunders, pp 11–13, 1984.
20. Snyder R, Andrews LS: Toxic effects of solvents and vapors. *In* Klaassen CD (ed): Casarett and Doull's Toxicology: The Basic Science of Poisons. 5th ed. New York, McGraw-Hill, pp 737–771, 1995.
21. Boogaard PJ, Caubo ME: Increased albumin excretion in industrial workers due to shift work rather than to prolonged exposure to low concentrations of chlorinated hydrocarbons. Occup Environ Med *51*:638, 1994.
22. Bell GM, Gordon ACH, Lee P, et al: Proliferative glomerulonephritis and exposure to organic solvents. Nephron *40*:161, 1985.
23. Harrington JM, Whitby H, Gray CN, et al: Renal disease and occupational exposure to organic solvents: A case referent approach. Br J Ind Med *46*:643, 1989.
24. Arndt KA, Bigby M, Coopman SA: Skin disorders. *In* Levy BS, Wegman DH (eds): Occupational Health: Recognizing and Preventing Work-Related Disease. 3rd ed. Boston, Little, Brown, pp 491–506, 1995.
25. Potts AM: Toxic responses of the eye. *In* Klaassen CD (ed): Casarett and Doull's Toxicology: The Basic Science of Poisons, 5th ed. New York, McGraw-Hill, pp 583–615, 1995.
26. Nichols WK, Covington MO, Seiders CD, et al: Bioactivation of halogenated hydrocarbons by rabbit pulmonary cells. Pharmacol Toxicol *71*:335, 1992.
27. Sahu S, Lowther D, Ulsamer A: Biochemical studies on pulmonary response to inhalation of methylene chloride. Toxicol Lett *7*:41, 1980.
28. Zakhari S: Cardiovascular toxicology of halogenated hydrocarbons and other solvents. *In* Acosta D (ed): Cardiovascular Toxicology. New York, Raven Press, pp 409–454, 1992.
29. McLeod AA, Marjot R, Monaghan MJ, et al: Chronic cardiac toxicity after inhalation of 1,1,1-trichloroethane. Br Med J *294*:727, 1987.
30. Creech JL, Johnson MN: Angiosarcoma of liver in the manufacture of polyvinyl chloride. J Occup Med *16*:150, 1974.
31. International Agency for Research on Cancer: IARC Monographs on the Evaluation of Carcinogenic Risks to Humans: Overall Evaluation of Carcinogenicity: An Updating of IARC monographs vol 1 to 42, suppl 7. Lyon, France, IARC, 1987.
32. International Agency for Research on Cancer: IARC Monographs on the Evaluation of Carcinogenic Risks to Humans, vol 47. Lyon, France, IARC, 1989.
33. Green T: Species differences in carcinogenicity: The role of metabolism in human risk evaluation. Teratog Carcinog Mutagen *10*:103, 1990.
34. Welch LS: Organic solvents. *In* Paul M (ed): Occupational and Environmental Reproductive Hazards: A Guide for Clinicians. Baltimore, Williams & Wilkins, pp 267–279, 1993.
35. Lawrence CE, Taylor PR, Trock BJ, Reilly AA: Trihalomethanes in drinking water and human colorectal cancer. J Natl Cancer Inst *72*:563, 1984.
36. Bove FJ, Fulcomer MC, Klots JB, et al: Public drinking water contamination and birth outcomes. Am J Epidemiol *141*:850, 1995.
37. Dally S, Garnier R, Bismuth C: Diagnosis of chlorinated hydrocarbon poisoning by x-ray examination. Br J Ind Med *44*:424, 1987.
38. DiRenzo AB, Gandolfi AJ, Sipes IG, et al: Effect of O_2 tension on the bioactivation and metabolism of aliphatic halides by primary rat-hepatocyte cultures. Xenobiotica *14*:521, 1984.
39. Ruprah M, Mant TG, Flanagan RJ: Acute carbon tetrachloride poisoning in 19 patients: Implications for diagnosis and treatment. Lancet *1*:1027, 1985.
40. Rioux JP, Myers RA: Hyperbaric oxygen for methylene chloride poisoning: Report on two cases. Ann Emerg Med *18*:691, 1989.
41. Burkhart KK, Hall AH, Gerace R, Rumack BH: Hyperbaric oxygen treatment for carbon tetrachloride poisoning. Drug Saf *6*:332, 1991.
42. Koppel C, Arndt I, Arendt U, Koeppe P: Acute tetrachloroethylene poisoning—blood elimination kinetics during hyperventilation therapy. J Toxicol Clin Toxicol *23*:103, 1985.

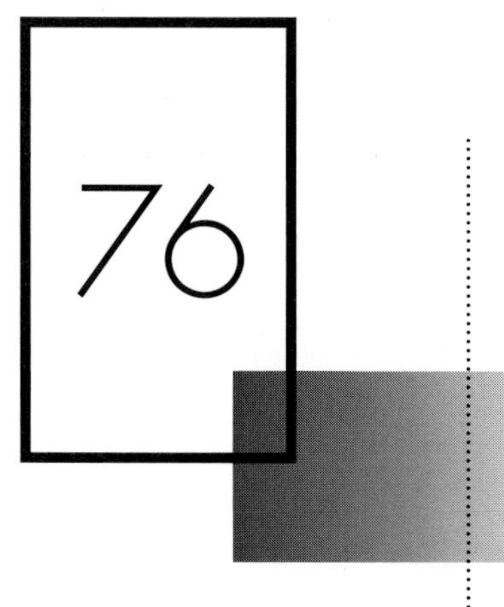

Benzene and the Aromatic Hydrocarbons

DARELL E. HEISELMAN, DO

BENZENE

Aromatic hydrocarbons are hydrocarbons that contain a benzene ring. The primary aromatic hydrocarbons are benzene, toluene, xylene, and styrene. Vinyl chloride is also included in this chapter.

The many synonyms for benzene include cyclohexatriene, benzol, coal tar naphtha, and phenyl hydride. Benzene is a clear, highly flammable liquid with a sweet, pleasant, aromatic odor. It is incompatible with chlorine, bromine, and iron. Common commercial grades contain various percentages of benzene, usually between 50% and 100%, with the remaining constituents containing other aromatic compounds such as toluene and xylene.

Benzene is often used as an industrial intermediate in the production of other chemicals such as styrene and phenol. It is involved in the distillation of coal and coal tar and is also used in the manufacturing of dyes, detergents, explosives, paints, varnishes, plastics, and rubbers.

Benzene is also a constituent in motor fuels. As the production of unleaded gasoline increases for automobiles equipped with catalytic converters, greater potential for exposure to benzene arises because the content of benzene is higher in unleaded gasoline.

Benzene's toxicity to bone marrow was recognized in the 1800s, when four fatal cases of benzene poisoning were reported in factory workers in Stockholm.[1] It was not until 1910 that Selling elucidated the important characteristic of benzene poisoning to be leukopenia with aplasia, an extreme reduction in cells produced by the bone marrow.[2]

Benzene's leukocytotoxic action was once used therapeutically in the treatment of leukemias in the early 1900s, but its toxicity limited its use, with cases of severe purpura and drastic reductions in red as well as white blood cell lines.

In the 1920s and 1930s, the Chemical and Rubber Sections of the United States National Safety Council encouraged United States industry to limit the concentration of benzene to less than 100 ppm.[3] As these safety proposals slowly became adopted, industry began to turn to safer substitutes for benzene such as toluene and liquid rubber latex.

As early as 1928, evidence that benzene might be an etiologic agent in several types of leukemias began to accumulate when Penati and Vigliani found 10 cases of leukemia in patients exposed to benzene.[4] Since that time, excessive chromosome aberrations in the nuclei of lymphocytes have been well documented, as well as a strong association between benzene exposure and leukemia.[5–8] Greenlee and colleagues have proposed a mechanism for benzene's toxicity, which may involve conversion of benzene metabolites to cytotoxic quinone and superoxide radicals.[9] These metabolites of benzene have been shown to be capable of interfering with chromosome segregation and inducing chromosomal breakage.[10]

Despite the accumulated evidence, benzene's potential for carcinogenicity has been a hotly debated issue, with strong proponents on both sides. In 1987, Rinsky and co-workers reported a large case-control study showing a strongly positive correlation between exposure to benzene and leukemia as well as multiple myeloma.[11] This was not accepted without debate, however, because 2 months later, four pages of editorial comments took issue with their findings.[12, 13] It is hard to deny a very strong if not proven association between benzene and cancer, particularly leukemia.

A similar cohort study published in the same year

involving more than 28,000 Chinese workers exposed to benzene showed similar results.[14] A follow-up study by the same group of researchers involving 100,000 Chinese workers revealed an increased incidence of acute nonlymphocytic leukemia similar to that which was treatment related after chemotherapy or radiotherapy. A greater diversity of hematologic neoplasms, including myelodysplastic syndrome, chronic granulocytic leukemia, malignant lymphoma, and aplastic anemia, was also found in this cohort.[15] Rinsky and associates estimated that the risk of cancer during 40-year period of exposure to benzene would be reduced from 154.5 to 1.7 by lowering the permissible exposure limit (PEL) from 110 ppm to 1 ppm. The National Institute for Occupational Safety and Health (NIOSH) responded by lowering the PEL from 10 ppm to 1 ppm in September of 1987, less than 6 months after the data were published.

In order to monitor benzene exposure, NIOSH recommends measuring phenol excretion in the urine by high-pressure liquid chromatography (HPLC) or gas chromatography. If more than 75 mg of phenol per liter of urine is found, monthly monitoring of complete blood counts by serial examinations should be performed for 2 to 3 months to monitor thrombocyte, leukocyte, and erythrocyte counts.[16, 17] Unfortunately, urinary phenol has been demonstrated to be a poor marker for low-level benzene exposure. A better marker for low-level benzene exposure appears to be *trans,trans*-muconic acid. *Trans,trans*-muconic acid is a minor metabolite of benzene that can be measured by using HPLC with ultraviolet detection.[18]

Pre-employment evaluation of personnel with potential benzene exposure should be comprehensive. A history should include a detailed work history to evaluate previous exposure to marrow toxins; a family and personal history of blood dyscrasias, cancer, liver, and renal function; and a history of alcohol intake and the use of medications and other drugs. Laboratory tests should include a baseline complete blood count with indices and platelet count as well as evaluation of kidney and liver function.

Treatment of Acute Exposure

The treatment of acute exposure to benzene and the other aromatic hydrocarbons is outlined in Table 76–1. The clinical signs and symptoms of acute exposure largely depend on the organ involved and the duration of contact. Benzene is a direct irritant to the eyes and skin, causing erythema and blistering, and a scaly dermatitis may develop from defatting of the subcutaneous tissues.

Lung aspiration may cause pulmonary edema and hemorrhage; therefore, emesis should not be artificially induced without adequate airway protection. Ventricular fibrillation has been reported and may be produced by aromatic hydrocarbon-produced myocardial sensitization to circulating catecholamines. This may be aggravated by the use of isoproterenol and epinephrine, so these should be reserved for patients not responding to other therapeutic maneuvers.

Table 76–1. Treatment Protocol for Acute Exposure to Aromatic Hydrocarbons

1. Remove worker from area of exposure.
2. Irrigate eyes copiously with normal saline or other irrigant if the eyes were exposed for 30 min.
3. Wash contaminated areas of the body with soap and water.
4. Perform gastric lavage if indicated, but only under experienced medical supervision. Do not induce emesis.
5. Provide oxygen for inhalation.
6. Perform cardiopulmonary resuscitation and supportive care as indicated. Be wary of isoproterenol, epinephrine, or other sympathomimetic drugs, because the myocardium may be sensitized to these medications.
7. Treat supportively any neurologic deficits or emotional lability.
8. Perform chest roentgenogram, liver profile, urinalysis, and complete blood counts as necessary. Monitor as needed.
9. Perform pregnancy testing.
10. Monitor urine for degradation products of each aromatic hydrocarbon involved.

The gastrointestinal and nervous systems may also be affected in a significant acute exposure to benzene. Nausea, vomiting, and colic are often produced by exposure, and liver damage may result. Acute exposure to benzene may also produce nervous system toxicity with severe headache. Euphoria, ataxia, dizziness, nausea, convulsions, coma, and death may also result if central nervous system (CNS) depression occurs.

Concerns related to chronic exposures to benzene at higher than permissible levels center around its potential for hematologic toxicity and myelotoxicity. Its initial effects may actually produce a nonspecific stimulation of the marrow, followed by anemia, leukopenia, thrombocytopenia, and myeloid metaplasia. Aplastic anemia may develop, and peripheral blood counts may not necessarily reflect marrow changes.

Benzene is considered by NIOSH to be leukemogenic. Evidence is substantial for benzene's induction of acute myelogenous leukemia, acute erythroleukemia, and possibly multiple myeloma; however, correlation with chronic leukemias is less substantiated.[19]

TOLUENE

Toluene is a colorless, volatile liquid with an aromatic odor. Common synonyms for toluene include toluol, methyl benzene, and phenyl methane. Although poorly soluble in water, it is rapidly absorbed, with an onset of action in minutes. Toluene is extensively metabolized via oxidation to benzyl alcohol then to benzaldehyde by alcohol dehydrogenase. Further oxidation then forms benzoic acid. Conjugation with glycine produces the major metabolite, hippuric acid, which is excreted in the urine. Benzyl glucuronide is formed in smaller amounts by conjugation with glucuronic acid. Alcohol intake during toluene exposure inhibits the metabolism of toluene by alcohol dehydrogenase and increases the internal dose of toluene. Normal therapeutic doses of propranolol and cimetidine have no measurable effect on toluene metabolism.[20]

Toluene is an organic solvent for paints and coatings. It is used in the manufacture of benzene and of products such as detergents, dyes, adhesives, lighter fluid, and explosives. Toluene is the major ingredient of model airplane glue. Unleaded gasoline may contain toluene as an additive. Printers, spray painters, shoemakers, cabinetmakers, and those involved in the manufacture or refinement of petroleum products appear to have a significant risk of constant exposure.[21–25] Commercial preparations may contain various amounts of benzene.

In comparison with other organic solvents, toluene appears to have more severe acute effects in vapor exposure than benzene. Bone marrow depression and hematologic side effects from toluene reported previously in the literature are now believed to have been secondary to contamination with benzene and not caused by toluene itself.[26] Bone marrow depression has not been described as resulting from either chronic or acute exposure to pure toluene. Toluene embryopathy can be produced by maternal toluene abuse. This syndrome produces phenotypic craniofacial abnormalities similar to those seen in fetal alcohol syndrome. Also noted is an increased incidence of premature labor, small fetal size for gestational age, postnatal growth deficiency, prenatal microcephaly, CNS dysfunction, and perinatal mortality.[27, 28]

In the early 1960s, toluene was used as an industrial solvent in place of benzene, which had known hematologic toxicity. Because of the euphoria and CNS depression caused by exposure to toluene, it has become a substance abused by "sniffers."[29] Abuse of toluene involves inhaling paint thinners, glue, fingernail polish removers, and other means. Several deaths have been reported from model airplane glue deposited in plastic bags that were then placed over an individual's head.[30] The cause of death most likely relates to narcosis and anesthesia from the toluene, followed by asphyxia in the plastic bag.

During acute exposure, toluene is an irritant to the eyes, lungs, skin, and other areas of direct exposure. Erythema, defatting dermatitis, skin paresthesias, conjunctivitis, and keratitis result from direct contact. Dilated pupils and lacrimation may be observed after exposure to toluene vapors. Arrhythmias, sudden death, respiratory arrest, and chemical pneumonitis have been reported with acute inhalation.[31–33] Nausea, vomiting, and anorexia are frequently present with acute toluene poisoning. Electrolyte and acid-base disturbances may present as type I (distal) renal tubular acidosis, hypokalemia, hypophosphatemia, and anion gap acidosis.[34] Rhabdomyolysis with elevated creatine phosphokinase levels has been described.[35] Toluene may cause headache, dizziness, mental confusion, euphoria, hallucinations, status epilepticus, incoordination, ataxia, nervousness, insomnia, muscle fatigue, and eventual narcosis.[36]

For the treatment of acute exposure to toluene, follow the recommendations given in Table 76–1. In addition, if exposure is massive, perform chest roentgenograms, hepatic and renal profiles, and urinalysis. Bicarbonate therapy should not be given until potassium and calcium are replaced adequately. Potassium replacement should be in the form of potassium phosphate, because both potassium and phosphate levels are usually low. Serial measurements of potassium, calcium, magnesium, and phosphate should be performed.

The recommendation for occupational safety and health hazards is 200 ppm at an 8-hour time-weighted average (TWA), with a 300-ppm acceptable ceiling and a 500-ppm maximum ceiling at 10 minutes.[37] Levels of exposure greater than 600 ppm cause confusion and delirium. Toluene abusers may be exposed to more than 1000 ppm for excessive periods.[38–40] The various components in abused solvent mixtures may be additive in their toxic effects.

Occupational exposure to toluene requires a comprehensive preplacement and annual medical examination, with emphasis on the liver, kidneys, and CNS. Laboratory tests should include a complete blood count, hepatic and renal profiles, and urinalysis.

Pulmonary hypertension, hemorrhagic alveolitis, sensitization of the myocardium to catecholamines, atrioventricular block, sudden death, and bradyarrhythmias have been reported during chronic exposure.[41, 42] Hypokalemic periodic paralysis may develop as a result of type I renal tubular acidosis.[43, 44] Urinalysis abnormalities include hematuria, pyuria, myoglobinuria, and proteinuria. Chronic exposure to toluene may carry the attendant risk of urinary calculi and reversible renal failure.[45, 46] Toluene exposure may produce elevated creatine phosphokinase with rhabdomyolysis.

Toluene exposure may cause dementia, cerebellar degeneration, cranial nerve abnormalities, spasticity, hyperactive tendon reflexes, corticobulbar and corticospinal damage, encephalopathy, postural tremor, and sensorineural hearing loss. In addition, peripheral and optic neuropathies, brain stem atrophy, status epilepticus, psychosis, myopathy, myoclonus, choreoathetotic movement disorders, insomnia, irritability, personality changes, and memory impairment all have been reported with toluene exposure.[47–55]

In addition to the treatment recommendations in Table 76–1, biologic monitoring of serum toxicology or urinary hippuric acid levels can be performed on all workers at risk for excessive exposure.[56] Measurement of hippuric acid levels may be inaccurate as a result of the ingestion of benzoates in food.[57]

XYLENE

Xylene is a clear, flammable liquid with an aromatic odor. Common synonyms for xylene include dimethyl benzene, xylol, and the three isomers, *o*-, *m*-, and *p*-xylene. It is produced from both petroleum and coal tar and is an organic solvent for some resins, gums, and oils. Commercial preparations usually contain 85% of the *m*- isomer and only about 5% of the *p*- isomer. Other preparations may contain benzene in various amounts. Absorption of xylene vapor is rapid via the lungs. Xylene liquid and vapor are much more slowly absorbed through the skin. Xylene is 95% metabolized to methylhippuric acid (MHA) by the liver, and 70% to 80% of the metabolites are excreted in the urine. The absorption, metabolism, and clearance of xylene can be affected by alcohol intake, exercise, cigarette smoking, gender, and hepatic and renal dysfunction.

Aromatic hydrocarbons such as xylene and benzene may be found in unleaded gasoline. Therefore, the use of unleaded gasoline increases the general population's possible exposure to these hydrocarbons. Xylene may be found in paints, lacquers, adhesives, and cements. Cleaning fluids, degreasers, dyes, inks, insect repellents, and perfumes are other sources of xylene exposure.

Temporary hepatorenal impairment and death from pulmonary edema have resulted from xylene inhalation.[58] Reports have also described reversible corneal vacuolation during xylene exposure.

Mild toxic effects on the hematopoietic system consisting of a reversible decrease in red and white blood cell counts and a concomitant increase in platelet count have been demonstrated in animal studies. Nevertheless, in humans, evidence for blood or blood-forming organ toxicity is lacking.[59–61] Rodent studies demonstrate the association of prenatal toxicity and developmental defects with mixed and individual isomers of xylene.[62, 63]

NIOSH's recommended PEL is 100 ppm (435 mg/m^3) for an 8-hour TWA.[64] After exposure, xylene can be measured in expired air and blood. The presence of MHA in the urine has been used as a diagnostic test for exposure.[65–67] The American Conference of Governmental Industrial Hygenists has recommended an upper limit of 2.0 g MHA/L urine biologic exposure index (BEI).

Xylene in liquid form is a direct irritant to the skin, causing erythema, dryness, and defatting. Vesicles may form with prolonged contact, and facial flushing has been described with acute exposure. Vapors may be irritating to the nose and throat. Ocular complications include conjunctivitis, corneal vacuolation, and keratitis.

Cardiopulmonary complications include catecholamine-induced ventricular arrhythmias, chest pain with electrocardiographic changes, dypsnea, cyanosis, acute pulmonary edema, and respiratory depression from acute exposure. Nausea, vomiting, anorexia, and abdominal pain are common; less frequently, reversible hepatic impairment occurs. High concentrations of xylene act like a narcotic and may cause dizziness, ataxia, drowsiness, excitement, incoordination, headache, confusion, vertigo, tremor, and coma.[68, 69]

Treatment of acute and chronic exposure to xylene is the same as that for exposure to other aromatic hydrocarbons (see Table 76–1). Additionally, patients suffering severe exposure should be hospitalized and observed for possible pulmonary edema, which may be delayed as much as 72 hours. A chest roentgenogram, electrocardiogram, complete blood count, determination of arterial blood gas levels, and liver and renal profiles should also be performed.

Occupational exposure to xylene requires a comprehensive preplacement medical examination. This should include special attention to symptoms of headache, dizziness, nausea, other gastrointestinal symptoms, and alcohol consumption.[70–72] Detailed examination of the eyes, lungs, mucous membranes, and skin should be performed. These medical examinations should be repeated every 2 years and should include a complete blood count, routine urinalysis, and liver function tests.[73] Biologic monitoring can be performed on all workers at risk for excessive exposure by monitoring urinary MHA levels.[74–76]

At present, no evidence indicates that xylene is toxic to blood and blood-forming organs.[77] However, xylene is often found in combination with other hydrocarbons (e.g., benzene). In these situations, the standards for any additive chemicals should be applied.

STYRENE

Commonly encountered synonyms for styrene include styrol, styrolene, vinylbenzene, cinnamene, cinnamol, and phenylethylene. Styrene is a flammable, highly lipid soluble, colorless to yellowish liquid that has an attractive sweet odor at low concentrations. This odor becomes unpleasantly penetrating at higher levels. It is a very refractive, oily liquid that boils at 145°C and polymerizes to form a plastic (polystyrene) at approximately 200°C. Styrene is a component of cigarette smoke and automobile exhaust and may occur naturally in low levels in some types of food.

Styrene is used as an industrial intermediate in combination with acrylonitrile and butadiene to form copolymer and rubber products. Styrene is also used in the synthesis of resins, as a dental filling component, as a chemical in agricultural products, in the production of insulators and polyesters, and in drug manufacturing. It is commonly used in boat and yacht manufacturing, in the reinforced plastics industry, and in photostat copying systems.

Styrene is often stabilized by the addition of terbutylcatechol or another polymerization inhibitor. Spontaneous polymerization may take place at higher temperatures or if a polymerization inhibitor is not present in sufficient levels. This may result in spontaneous rupture of containers storing this chemical. Styrene corrodes copper alloys and dissolves rubber. Contact with oxidizing agents, strong acids, or aluminum chloride should be avoided.

A fire involving styrene may release harmful byproducts, including carbon monoxide. Fumes are acrid, and the odor threshold is considerably lower than the PEL and should therefore provide adequate warning of a potential toxic exposure.

Current Occupational Safety and Health standards for styrene are 100 ppm for an 8-hour TWA, with a 200 ppm ceiling. The level defined as immediately dangerous to life or health is 5000 ppm. Workers exposed to levels exceeding 500 ppm should have a self-contained breathing apparatus with a chemical cartridge respirator with organic vapor cartridges.[78] Urinary mandelic acid and phenylglyoxylic acid have been used as markers of exposure to styrene.

Styrene in both liquid and vapor forms is irritating to the skin and mucous membranes. Humans exposed to 376 ppm experienced rapid onset of eye and nasal irritation.[79] Corneal burns have also been reported with direct contact to the eyes. Skin contact may produce acute as well as chronic dermatitis. Chest burning, wheezing, dyspnea, and angina have been reported with some acute exposures; however, objective changes in pulmonary function occurred only in workers who also smoked.[80, 81]

Styrene is a CNS depressant. After approximately 1 hour of exposure to styrene, headache, nausea, incoordination, impaired dexterity, and other signs of transient neurologic impairment develop. Studies have also shown impaired cognition, slower reaction times, and subjective feelings of tiredness after styrene exposure. Abnormal electroencephalographic findings have also been noted. These reports have been largely inconclusive observational studies, which are often subjective and difficult to interpret.[82, 83]

Studies to date have been conflicting and inconclusive regarding embryotoxicity, fetotoxicity, or teratogenicity.[84, 85] However, because birth defects have been noted, pregnant workers exposed to styrene may desire amniocentesis during pregnancy to help detect potential fetal abnormalities.

Recommendations for treating acute and chronic exposures to styrene are shown in Table 76–1. Long-term exposure to styrene may produce alterations in liver enzymes and liver function tests. Alterations in glucose metabolism have been noted, but well-defined alterations have not clearly been shown.[86]

Objective changes in pulmonary function have also been poorly documented. One study of workers exposed to styrene found that only 20% of cases showed any significant change in the forced expiratory volume in 1 second. The study was poorly controlled, and other factors may have had a primary impact on the changes observed.[80, 81]

In addition to the neurologic effects noted in acute exposure, an association with peripheral neuropathy has also been shown. Long-term exposures may result in persistent and premature dementia in some workers.[87, 88]

Reports suggest a potential for nephrotoxicity localized to the proximal tubule in rats exposed at chronic, low, nontoxic doses of styrene. Human studies are lacking.[89] Congenital defects and increases in spontaneous abortions have been reported but not supported by recent investigations.[84, 85]

Although studies to date have not conclusively shown that styrene directly causes cancer, numerous studies implicate styrene and styrene oxide as possible carcinogens. Lymphomas and leukemias have largely been associated with styrene, and Hodgson and Jones also found an increased incidence of laryngeal carcinoma.[90] A review of styrene attempted to investigate the previously reported cytogenic effects of styrene exposure. The researchers concluded that these reports were more likely attributable to the presence of other chromosome-damaging agents in the workplace or inadequate investigations.[91] To help in assessing the significance of an exposure to possible toxic quantities of styrene, biologic monitoring should be performed on all workers by monitoring urinary mandelic or hippuric acid excretion.[92, 93]

VINYL CHLORIDE

Vinyl chloride is a colorless, sweet-smelling gas that is highly explosive and flammable. Common synonyms for vinyl chloride include ethylene monochloride, monochloroethene, monochloroethylene, chloroethene, and chloroethylene.[94] It has lower and upper explosive limits of 4% and 26%, respectively. At normal temperatures, it is noncorrosive, but in contact with water and at elevated temperatures, it increases the corrosion of iron and steel. Vinyl chloride is usually handled as a liquid under pressure. The half-life in air ranges from 3 to 20 hours. Easy absorption occurs across cell membranes because of its low molecular weight, even though its low solubility impedes the process. Approximately 80% of vinyl chloride is cleared from the blood in 10 minutes after cessation of exposure.

Vinyl chloride is used as an intermediate in the production of plastics, methyl chloroform, and aerosol propellants. Vinyl chloride has been detected in small amounts in cigarette smoke (16 ng per cigarette, 27 ng per cigar).

Vinyl chloride was originally used in the early 1930s for its anesthetic action. Its use was later discontinued because of the significant cardiac arrhythmias induced during anesthesia.[95] In 1949, reports of Russian workers with liver changes consistent with hepatitis from exposure were observed. A severe neurologic disorder was described in Minamata, Japan, associated with the production of vinyl chloride in 1960.[96] Later, in 1966, acro-osteolysis was described in autoclave cleaners using vinyl chloride in Belgium.[97]

Viola and colleagues attempted to reproduce this in animal experiments, which incidentally revealed vinyl chloride–induced cancer.[98] Maltoni and Lefemine continued studies with vinyl chloride and demonstrated angiosarcoma of the liver in rodents.[99, 100]

Creech and Johnson reported two cases of hepatic angiosarcoma in employees at a chemical plant.[101] Retrospective studies of vinyl chloride workers confirmed a significant risk of 400:1 and a latency period of 12 to 30 years for liver cancer. These and other studies caused American and European industry to change acceptable exposure levels of vinyl chloride to levels of 10 ppm or less for an 8-hour TWA.

Additional evidence of the mutagenicity of vinyl chloride is demonstrated by increased chromosomal aberrations in lymphocytes of workers exposed to vinyl chloride.[102–105] Of significance is the abnormally high rate of fetal wastage found in wives of male workers with occupational exposure to vinyl chloride.[106, 107]

Exposure to vinyl chloride is usually through the lungs. Metabolic activation through a three-step process is required for vinyl chloride to become mutagenic, carcinogenic, or cytotoxic. The alcohol dehydrogenase system metabolizes vinyl chloride at low concentrations ($<$ 50 ppm) into chloroacetaldehyde and monochloroacetic acid.[108] At moderate levels ($>$ 50 ppm), oxidation by the peroxidase-catalase system produces chloroacetaldehyde. At very high levels ($>$ 250 ppm), oxidation occurs mainly via the hepatic microsomal mixed-function oxidase system (cytochrome P-450 dependent) to the end product, chloroethylene oxide. When the oxidative systems become saturated, vinyl chloride is excreted unchanged via the lungs.

Chloroethylene oxide and chloroacetaldehyde may be further oxidized or conjugated with glutathione via glutathione transferases or expoxide hydrase. The remaining nondegraded electrophilic intermediates may cause cytotoxicity by interfering with protein synthesis or forming DNA adducts (chemicals that bind to DNA). DNA adducts may cause distortion of the symmetric helical structure, resulting in mutagenic or carcinogenic interference in DNA replication.

Skin contact with vinyl chloride in liquid form can cause redness, irritation, and frostbite. Acute exposure to vapors or direct contact may cause irritation and erythema of the eyes, throat, and nose. In severe exposures, cardiac arrhythmias have been reported. Nausea, vomiting, and abdominal pain are frequent symptoms and may be associated with hepatic cell necrosis and hepatitis. Dose-related effects observed with acute vinyl chloride exposure include lightheadedness, dizziness, decreased auditory and visual responses, and disorientation.[109, 110]

Treatment of acute exposure to vinyl chloride follows the protocol given in Table 76–1. In addition, patients should have close observation for hepatic damage after significant exposure. Serial measurements of serum glutamic-oxaloacetic transaminase (SGOT), serum glutamic-pyruvic transaminase (SGPT), alkaline phosphatase, bilirubin, and albumin levels and prothrombin time should be obtained on admission and repeated every 24 hours for a 72-hour period.

Because of the long-term implications for increased incidence of tumors,[111–113] acro-osteolysis, and liver abnormalities, an extensive monitoring policy for exposed workers is recommended.[114, 115]

Occupational exposure to vinyl chloride requires a comprehensive preplacement history and physical examination, with special attention to liver and spleen enlargement. At the initial time of employment and annually thereafter, recording of alcohol intake and history of hepatitis, drugs, and chemical exposure, blood transfusions, and hospitalizations should be made. Before employment and annually thereafter, laboratory studies should be performed, including measures of SGOT, SGPT, bilirubin, γ-glutamyl transpeptidase, and alkaline phosphatase. If the person being screened has been exposed to vinyl chloride monomer production or polymerization for 10 years or more, screening should be performed every 6 months. It is recommended that no woman who is pregnant or expects to become pregnant be directly exposed to vinyl chloride monomer operations. Vinyl chloride is a demonstrated carcinogen, and NIOSH's recommended PEL is 1 ppm for an 8-hour TWA, with a 5 ppm ceiling at 15 minutes.

Although no definitive and reliable sign, symptom, or laboratory test has been found to be specific for the early diagnosis of angiosarcoma of the liver,[100] special attention should be paid to complaints of fatigue, lassitude, epigastric pain, pleuritis, chest pain, dyspnea, or gastrointestinal hemorrhage.

Chronic exposure to vinyl chloride may present with various clinical manifestations. Sclerodermatous (or scleroedema) skin changes[116] and Raynaud's phenomenon[117] may present either together with acro-osteolysis as a triad or separately. A genetic predisposition may have a role in the development of scleroderma-like skin changes with vinyl chloride exposure.[118] Acro-osteolysis has been reported in approximately 3% of workers (usually reactor cleaners) exposed to vinyl chloride.[97, 119, 120] It does not necessarily improve with removal of exposure, but radiographic improvement of phalangeal lesions has been reported. Reports suggest a possible association with malignant melanoma,[121] and a case report of vasculitic purpura has been published.[122]

Chronic exposure can cause pneumoconiosis with dyspnea and impaired pulmonary function (restrictive or obstructive insufficiency).[123–125] Biopsy abnormalities consist of desquamation of macrophages, minor interstitial and alveolar inflammatory changes, or pulmonary fibrosis.[126] An increased incidence of large cell carcinoma or adenocarcinoma of the lung has been reported in several retrospective epidemiologic studies.[127–130]

Hepatic angiosarcoma, hepatocellular carcinoma, portal hypertension, splenomegaly, and hepatic fibrosis all have been reported with exposure to vinyl chloride.[101, 131–137] A retrospective study of 1294 workers exposed to vinyl chloride revealed an increased incidence of brain cancer (glioblastoma multiforme).[138] A polyneuropathy may be associated with vinyl chloride exposure.[139] Evidence is substantial for vinyl chloride's induction of anemia, reticulocytosis, thrombocytopenia, leukopenia, and lymphatic malignancies.

References

1. Santesson CG: Chronic poisoning by benzene. Hygiea *31*:155–181, 1898.

2. Selling L: A preliminary report of some cases of purpura hemorrhagica due to benzol poisoning. Bulletin of Johns Hopkins Hospital. Johns Hopkins Hosp Rep 17:83, 1910.
3. Hamilton A: Lessening menace of benzol poisoning in American industry. J Indust Hyg *10*:227–233, 1928.
4. Penati F, Vigliani EC: Sui problema acne myelopatic aplastiche, pseudoaplastiche e leucemiche da benzelo. Rass Med Ind *9*:345–361, 1938.
5. Vigliani EC: Leukemia associated with benzene exposure. Ann N Y Acad Sci *271*:143, 1976.
6. Clare MG, Yardley JA, Maclean AC, Dean BJ: Chromosome analysis from peripheral blood lymphocytes of workers after an acute exposure to benzene. Br J Ind Med *41*:249, 1984.
7. Eikmann T, Stinner D, Prajsnar D: Haematological data relating to phenol excretion in urine with chronic benzene exposure. I: Epidemiological studies of adults (from author's translation). Zentralbl Bakteriol Mikrobiol Hyg *174*:57, 1981.
8. Mehlman MA: Carcinogenicity and Toxicity of Benzene. Princeton, NJ, Princeton Scientific Publishers, 1983.
9. Greenlee WF, Sun JD, Bus JS: A proposed mechanism of benzene toxicity; Formation of reactive intermediates from polyphenol metabolites. Toxicol Appl Pharmacol *59*:187, 1981.
10. Eastmond DA: Induction of micronuclei and aneuploidy by the quinone-forming agents benzene and *O*-phenylphenol. Toxicol Lett 67:105, 1993.
11. Rinsky RA, Smith AB, Hornung R, Filloon TG: Benzene and leukemia: An epidemiologic risk assessment. N Engl J Med *316*:1044, 1987.
12. Bader M: Benzene and leukemia. Editorial. N Engl J Med *317*:1027, 1987.
13. Hu H: Benzene associated myelofibrosis. Editorial. Ann Intern Med *106*:172, 1987.
14. Yin SN, Li GL, Tain FD, Jin C: Leukemia in benzene workers: A retrospective cohort study. Br J Ind Med *44*:124, 1987.
15. Travis LB, Li CY, Zhang ZN, Li DG, et al: Hematopoietic malignancies and related disorders among benzene-exposed workers in China. Leuk Lymphoma *14*:91–102, 1994.
16. National Institute for Occupational Safety and Health, US Department of Health, Education and Welfare: Revised Recommendation for an Occupational Exposure Standard for Benzene. (NIOSH) Publication 657–012/325. Washington, DC, US Government Printing Office, 1979.
17. National Institute for Occupational Health, US Department of Health, Education and Welfare: NIOSH Pocket Guide to Chemical Hazards. DHHS (NIOSH) Publication 85–114. Washington, DC, September 1985.
18. Ong CN, Lee BL: Determination of benzene and its metabolites: Application in biological monitoring of environmental and occupational exposure to benzene. J Chromatogr B Biomed Appl *660*:1, 1994.
19. Irons RD: Toxicology updates; benzene. J Appl Toxicol *2*:57, 1982.
20. Baelum J: Human solvent exposure. Factors influencing the pharmokinetics and acute toxicity. Pharmacol Toxicol *68*(Suppl 1):1, 1991.
21. Anshelm Olson B, Gamberale F, Gronqvist B: Reaction time among steel workers exposed to solvent vapors; a longitudinal study. Int Arch Occup Environ Health *48*:211, 1981.
22. Anshelm Olson B: Effects of organic solvents on behavior performance of workers in the paint industry. Neurobehav Toxicol Teratol *4*:703, 1982.
23. Baelum J, Anderson IB, Lundqvist GR, et al: Response of solvent-exposed printers and unexposed controls to six-hour toluene exposure. Scand J Work Environ Health *11*:271, 1985.
24. Cherry H, Hutchins H, Pace T, Waldron HA: Neurobehavioral effects of repeated occupational exposure to toluene and paint solvents. Br J Ind Med *42*:291, 1985.
25. Takeichi S, Yamade T, Shikata I: Acute toluene poisoning during painting. Forensic Sci Int *32*:109, 1986.
26. Powars D: Aplastic anemia secondary to glue sniffing. N Engl J Med *273*:700, 1965.
27. Hersh JH, Podruch PE, Rogers G, Weisskopf B: Toluene embryopathy. J Pediatr *106*:922, 1985.
28. Pearson MA, Hoyme HE, Seaver LH, Pimsza ME: Toluene embryopathy: Delineation of the phenotype and comparison with fetal alcohol syndrome. Pediatrics *93*:211, 1994.
29. Streicher HZ, Gabow PQ, Moss AH, et al: Syndromes of toluene sniffing in adults. Ann Intern Med *94*:758, 1981.
30. Paterson SC, Sarvesvaran R: Plastic bag death—a toluene fatality. Med Sci Law *23*:64, 1983.
31. Bass M: Sudden sniffing death. JAMA *212*:2075, 1970.
32. Reinhardt CF, Azar A, Maxfield ME, et al: Cardiac arrhythmias and aerosol "sniffing." Arch Environ Health *22*:265, 1971.
33. Cronk SL, Barkley DE, Farrell MF: Respiratory arrest after solvent abuse. BMJ *290*:897, 1985.
34. Fischman CM, Oster JR: Toxic effects of toluene: A new cause of high anion gap metabolic acidosis. JAMA *241*:1713, 1979.
35. Reisin E, Teicher A, Jaffe R, et al: Myoglobinuria and renal failure in toluene poisoning. Br J Ind Med *32*:163, 1975.
36. Glowa JR, DeWeese J, Natale ME, et al: Behaviorial toxicology of volatile organic solvents. I. Methods. Acute effects of toluene. J Environ Pathol Toxicol Oncol *6*:153, 1986.
37. National Institute for Occupational Safety and Health, US Department of Health, Education, and Welfare: Criteria for a Recommended Standard; Occupational Exposure to Toluene. (HSM) Publication 73-11023. Washington, DC, US Government Printing Office, pp 14–45, 1973.
38. Garriott J, Petty CS: Death from inhalant abuse: Toxicological and pathological evaluation of 34 cases. Clin Toxicol *16*:305, 1980.
39. Zee-Cheng C, Mueller CE, Gibbs HR: Toluene sniffing and severe sinus bradycardia. Ann Intern Med *103*:482, 1985.
40. Engstrand DA, England DM, Huntington RW: Pathology of paint sniffers' lung. Am J Forensic Med Pathol *7*:232, 1986.
41. Howell SR, Christian JE, Isom GE: The hepatotoxic potential of combined toluene-chronic ethanol exposure. Arch Toxicol *59*:45, 1986.
42. O'Brien ET, Yeoman WB, Hobby JA: Hepatorenal damage from toluene in a glue sniffer. BMJ *2*:29, 1971.
43. Bennet RH, Forman HR: Hypokalaemic periodic paralysis in chronic toluene exposure. Arch Neurol *37*:673, 1980.
44. Taher SM, Anderson RK, McCartney R, et al: Renal tubular acidosis associated with toluene "sniffing." N Engl J Med *290*:765, 1974.
45. Kroeger RM, Moore RJ, Lehman TH, et al: Recurrent urinary calculi associated with toluene sniffing. J Urol *123*:89, 1980.
46. Will AM, McLaren EH: Reversible renal damage due to glue sniffing. BMJ *283*:525, 1981.
47. Boor JW, Hurtig HI: Persistent cerebellar ataxia after exposure to toluene. Ann Neurol *2*:440, 1977.
48. Channer KS, Stanley S: Persistent visual hallicinations, secondary to chronic solvent encephalopathy: Case report and review of the literature. J Neurol Neurosurg Psychiatry *46*:83, 1983.
49. Ehyai A, Freemon FR: Progressive optic neuropathy and sensorineural hearing loss due to chronic glue sniffing. J Neurol Neurosurg Psychiatry *46*:349, 1983.
50. Fornazzari L, Wilkinson DA, Kapur BM, Carlen PL: Cerebellar, cortical and functional impairment in toluene abusers. Acta Neurol Scand *67*:319, 1983.
51. Hormes JT, Filley CM, Rosenberg NL: Neurologic sequelae of chronic solvent vapor abuse. Neurology *36*:698, 1986.
52. Kind MD: Neurological sequelae of toluene abuse. Hum Toxicol *1*:281, 1982.
53. Juntunen J, Matikainen E, Antti-Poika M, et al: Nervous system effects of long-term occupational exposure to toluene. Acta Neurol Scand *72*:512, 1985.
54. Prockop L: Neurotoxic volatile substances. Neurology *29*:862, 1979.
55. Lazar RB, Ho SU, Melen O, Daghestani AN: Multifocal central nervous system damage caused by toluene abuse. Neurology *33*:1337, 1983.
56. De-Rosa E, Bartolucci GB, Sigon M, et al: Hippuric acid and orthocresol as biological indicators of occupational exposure to toluene. Am J Ind Med *11*:529, 1987.
57. De-Rosa E, Brugnone F, Bartolucci GB, et al: The validity of urinary metabolites as indicators of low exposures to toluene. Int Arch Occup Environ Health *56*:135, 1985.

58. Morley R, Eccleston DW, Douglas CP, et al: Xylene poisoning: A report on one fatal case and two cases of recovery after prolonged unconsciousness. BMJ *3*:442, 1970.
59. Moszczynski P, Lisiewicz J: Enzymes of neutrophils in workers occupationally exposed to benzene, toluene, and xylene. Rev Esp Oncol *31*:435, 1984.
60. Pap M, Varga C: Sister-chromatid exchanges in peripheral lymphocytes of workers occupationally exposed to xylenes. Mutat Res *187*:223, 1987.
61. Dean BJ: Recent findings on the genetic toxicology of benzene, toluene, xylenes, and phenols. Mutat Res *254*:153, 1985.
62. Hood RD, Ottley MS: Developmental effects associated with exposure to xylene: A review. Drug Chem Toxicol *8*:281, 1985.
63. Mirkova E, Zaikov C, Antov G, et al: Prenatal toxicity of xylene. J Hyg Epidemiol Microbiol Immunol *27*:337, 1983.
64. National Institute for Occupational Safety and Health, US Department of Health, Education, and Welfare: Criteria for a Recommended Standard for Occupational Exposure to Xylene. (NIOSH) Publication 75-168. Washington, DC, US Government Printing Office, 1975.
65. Lundberg I, Sollenberg J: Correlation of xylene exposure and methyl hippuric acid excretion in urine among paint industry workers. Scand J Work Environ Health *2*:140, 1986.
66. Ogata M, Taguchi T: Quantitation of urinary metabolites of toluene, xylene, styrene, ethylbenzene, benzene, and phenol by automated high performance liquid chromatography. Int Arch Occup Environ Health *59*:263, 1987.
67. Ogata M, Taguchi T: Quantitative analysis of urinary glycine conjugates by high performance liquid chromatograph: Excretion of hippuric acid and methylhippuric acids in the urine of subjects exposed to vapours of toluene and xylenes. Int Arch Occup Environ Health *58*:121, 1986.
68. Savolainen K, Riihimaki V, Linnoila M: Effects of short-term xylene exposure on psychophysiological functions in man. Int Arch Occup Environ Health *44*:201, 1979.
69. Savolainen K, Riihimaki V, Seppalainen AM, Linnoila M: Effects of short-term xylene exposure and physical exercise on the central nervous system. Int Arch Occup Environ Health *45*:105, 1980.
70. Riihimaki V, Savolainen K, Pfaffli P, Pekari K: *m*-Xylene and ethanol. Arch Toxicol *49*:253, 1982.
71. Savolainen K, Riihimaki V, Luukkonen R, Muona D: Changes in the sense of balance correlate with concentrations of m-xylene in venous blood. Br J Ind Med *42*:765, 1985.
72. Savolainen K: Combined effects of xylene and alcohol on the central nervous system. Acta Pharmacol Toxicol *46*:366, 1980.
73. Engelmeier RL: Effective measures to reduce xylene exposure. J Prosthet Dent *53*:564, 1985.
74. Riihimaki V: Conjugation and urinary excretion of toluene and m-xylene metabolites in a man. Scand J Work Environ Health *5*:135, 1979.
75. Engstrom K, Husman K, Pfaffli P, Riihimaki V: Evaluation of occupational exposure to xylene by blood, exhaled air, and urine analysis. Scand J Work Environ Health *4*:114, 1978.
76. Sedivec V, Flek J: The absorption, metabolism and excretion of xylenes in man. Int Arch Occup Environ Health *37*:205, 1976.
77. Sollenberg J, Baldesten A: Isotachophoretic analysis of mandelic acid, phenylglyoxylic acid, hippuric acid and methylhippuric acid in urine after occupational exposure to styrene, toluene, and/or xylene. J Chromatogr *132*:469, 1979.
78. National Institutes for Occupational Safety and Health, US Department of Health, Education, and Welfare: Criteria for a Recommended Standard. Occupational Exposure to Styrene. (NIOSH) Publication 83–119. Cincinnati, OH, pp 1–250, 1983.
79. McLaughlin RS: Chemical burns of the human cornea. Am J Ophthamol *29*:1353, 1946.
80. Chmielewski J, Renke W: Clinical and experimental studies on the pathogenesis of toxic effects of styrene—Part II: The effect of styrene on the respiratory system. Bull Inst Marit Trop Med Gdynia *26*:299, 1975.
81. Stewart RD, Dodd HC, Baretta ED, Schaffer AW: Human exposure to styrene vapor. Arch Environ Health *16*:656, 1968.
82. Lorimer WV, Lillis R, Nicholson WJ, et al: Clinical studies of styrene workers—initial findings. Environ Health Perspect *17*:171, 1976.
83. Axelson O, Gustavson J: Some hygienic and clinical observations on styrene exposure. Scand J Work Environ Health *4*(Suppl 2):215, 1978.
84. Hemminki K, Franssila E, Vainto H: Spontaneous abortions among female workers in Finland. Int Arch Occup Environ Health *45*:123, 1980.
85. Harkonen H, Holmberg PCC: Obstetric histories of women occupationally exposed to styrene. Scand J Work Environ Health *8*:74, 1982.
86. Chmielewski J: Clinical and experimental research into the pathogenesis of the toxic effect of styrene—Part V: Impact of styrene on carbohydrate balance in people in the course of their work. Bull Inst Marit Trop Med Gdynia *27*:177, 1976.
87. Baker EL, Smith TJ, Landrigan PJ: The neurotoxicity of industrial solvents: A review of the literature. Am J Ind Med *8*:207, 1985.
88. Behari M, Choudhary C, Roy S, Maheshwari MC: Styrene-induced peripheral neuropathy: A case report. Eur Neurol *25*:424, 1986.
89. Chakrabarti SK, Labelle L, Tuchweber B: Studies on the subchronic nephrotoxic potential of styrene in Sprague-Dawley rats. Toxicology *44*:355, 1987.
90. Hodgson JT, Jones RD: Mortality of styrene production, polymerization and processing workers at a site in northwest England. Scand J Work Environ Health *11*:347, 1985.
91. Scott D, Preston RJ: A re-evaluation of the cytogenic effects of styrene. Mutat Res *318*:175, 1994.
92. National Institute for Occupational Safety and Health, US Department for Health and Human Services: NIOSH Recommendations for Occupational Safety and Health Standards. MMWR 35 *(Suppl 1)*: 1986.
93. National Institute for Occupational Safety and Health, US Department of Health, Education and Welfare: NIOSH Pocket Guide to Chemical Hazards. DHHS (NIOSH) Publication 85–114. Washington, DC, 1985.
94. Easter MD, Von Burg R: Vinyl chloride. J Appl Toxicol *14*:301, 1994.
95. Oster RH, Carr CJ, Krantz JC: Anesthesia: Narcosis with vinyl chloride. Anesthesiology *8*:359, 1947.
96. Kurland LT, Faro SN, Siedler H: Minamata disease. World Neurol *1*:370, 1960.
97. Cordier JM, Fievez C, Lefevre MJ, Sevrin A: Acroosteolysis and related cutaneous lesions in two workers engaged in cleaning autoclaves. Cah Med Travail *4*:14, 1966.
98. Viola PL, Bigotti A, Caputo A: Oncogenic response of rat skin, lungs, and bones to vinyl chloride. Cancer Res *31*:516, 1971.
99. Maltoni C, Lefemine GL: Carcinogenicity bioassays of vinyl chloride. 1: Research plan and early results. Environ Res *7*:387, 1974.
100. Maltoni C, Lefemine GL: Carcinogenicity bioassay of vinyl chloride: current results. Ann N Y Acad Sci *246*:195, 1975.
101. Creech JL Jr, Johnson MN: Angiosarcoma of the liver in the manufacture of polyvinyl chloride. J Occup Med *16*:150, 1974.
102. Ducatman A, Hirschhorn K, Selikoff IJ: Vinyl chloride exposure and human chromosome abberations. Mutat Res *31*:163, 1975.
103. Heath CW Jr, Dumont CR, Gamble J, Waxweiller RJ: Chromosomal damage in men occupationally exposed to vinyl chloride monomer and other chemicals. Environ Res *14*:68, 1977.
104. Leonard A, Decat G, Leonard D, et al: Cytogenetic investigations on lymphocytes from workers exposed to vinyl chloride. J Toxicol Environ Health *2*:1135, 1977.
105. Purchase IF, Richardson CR, Anderson D, et al: Chromosomal analyses in vinyl chloride–exposed workers. Mutat Res *57*:325, 1978.
106. Infante PF, Wagoner JK, Waxweiller RJ: Carcinogenic, mutagenic, and teratogenic risks associated with vinyl chloride. Mutat Res *41*:131, 1976.

107. Theriault G, Iturra H, Gingras S: Evaluation of the association between birth defects and exposure to ambient vinyl chloride. Teratology *27*:359, 1983.
108. Bolt HM, Kappus H, Buchter A, Bolt W: Metabolism of vinyl chloride. Lancet *1*:425, 1975.
109. Langauer-Lewowicka H, Kurzbauer H, Byczkowska Z, Wocka-Marek T: Vinyl chloride disease—neurological disturbances. Int Arch Occup Environ Health *52*:151, 1983.
110. Stybllova V, Lambl V, Chumcal O, et al: Neurological changes in vinyl chloride-exposed workers. J Hyg Epidemiol Microbiol Immunol *25*:233, 1981.
111. Emmerich KH, Norpoth K: Malignant tumors after chronic exposure to vinyl chlorid. J Cancer Res Clin Oncol *102*:1, 1981.
112. Nicholson WJ, Hammond EC, Seidman H, Selikoff IJ: Mortality experience of a cohort of vinyl chloride–polyvinyl chloride workers. Ann N Y Acad Sci *246*:225, 1975.
113. Tabershaw IR, Gaffey WR: Mortality study of workers in the manufacture of vinyl chloride and its polymers. J Occup Med *16*:509, 1974.
114. National Institute for Occupational Safety and Health, US Department of Health, Education, and Welfare: Criteria for a Recommended Standard for Occupational Exposure to Vinyl Chloride. (NIOSH) Publication 657–012/302. Washington, DC, US Government Printing Office, 1979.
115. National Health Council of the Netherlands, Committee on the Evaluation of Carcinogenic Substances: A scientific basis for the risk assessment of vinyl chloride. Regul Toxicol Pharmacol 7:120, 1987.
116. Ostlere LS, Harris D, Buckley C, et al: Atypical systemic sclerosis following exposure to vinyl chloride monomer. A case report and review of the cutaneous aspects of vinyl chloride disease. Clin Exp Dermatol *17*:208, 1992.
117. Falappa P, Magnavita N, Bergamaschi A, Colavita N: Angiographic study of digital arteries in workers exposed to vinyl chloride. Br J Ind Med *39*:169, 1982.
118. Black C, Periera S, McWhirter A, et al: Genetic susceptibility to scleroderma-like syndrome in symptomatic and asymptomatic workers exposed to vinyl chloride. J Rheumatol *13*:1059, 1986.
119. Cook WA, Giever PM, Dinman BD, Magnuson HJ: Occupational acro-osteolysis. Arch Environ Health *22*:74, 1986.
120. Harris DK, Adams WGF: Acro-osteolysis occurring in men engaged in the polymerization of vinyl chloride. BMJ *3*:712, 1967.
121. Storetvedt Heldass S, Andersen AA, Langard S: Incidence of cancer among vinyl chloride and polyvinyl chloride workers: Further evidence for an association with malignant melanoma. Br J Ind Med *44*:278, 1987.
122. Magnavita N, Bergamaschi A, Garcovich A, Giuliano G: Vasculitic purpura in vinyl chloride disease: A case report. Angiology *37*:382, 1986.
123. Arnaud A, Pommier de Santi P, Garbe L, et al: Polyvinyl chloride pneumoconiosis. Thorax *33*:19, 1978.
124. Lilis R: Review of pulmonary effects of poly(vinyl chloride) and vinyl chloride exposure. Environ Health Perspect *41*:167, 1981.
125. Miller A, Tierstein AS, Chuang M, et al: Changes in pulmonary function in workers exposed to vinyl chloride and polyvinyl chloride. Ann N Y Acad Sci *246*:42, 1975.
126. Cordasco EM, Demeter SL, Kerkay J, et al: Pulmonary manifestations of vinyl and polyvinyl chloride: Newer aspects. Chest *78*:828, 1980.
127. Buffler PA, Wood S, Eifler C, et al: Mortality experience of workers in a vinyl chloride monomer production plant. J Occup Med *21*:195, 1979.
128. Wagoner JK: Vinyl chloride and pulmonary cancer. J Environ Pathol Toxicol *1*:361, 1978.
129. Waxweiler RJ, Stringer W, Wagoner JK, et al: Neoplastic risk among workers exposed to vinyl chloride. Ann N Y Acad Sci *271*:40, 1976.
130. Belli S, Bertazzi PA, Comba P, et al: A cohort study on vinyl chloride manufacturers in Italy: Study design and preliminary results. Letter. Cancer *35*:253, 1987.
131. Blendis LM, Smith PM, Lawrie BW, et al: Portal hypertension in vinyl chloride monomer workers: A hemodynamic study. Gastroenterology *75*:206, 1978.
132. Block J: Angiosarcoma of the liver following vinyl chloride exposure. JAMA *229*:53, 1974.
133. Brady JS, Liberatore F, Harper P, et al: Angiosarcoma of the liver: An epidemiologic survey. J Natl Cancer Inst *59*:1383, 1977.
134. Forman D, Bennett B, Stafford J, Doll R: Exposure to vinyl chloride and angiosarcoma of the liver. A report of the register of cases. Br J Ind Med *42*:750, 1985.
135. Louagie YA, Gianello P, Kestens PJ, et al: Vinyl chloride induced hepatic angiosarcoma. Br J Surg *71*:322, 1984.
136. Sugita M, Masuda Y, Tsuchiya K: Early detection and signs of hepatoangiosarcoma among vinyl chloride workers. Am J Ind Med *10*:411, 1986.
137. Tamburro CH: Relationship of vinyl monomers and liver cancers: Angiosarcoma and hepatocellular carcinoma. Semin Liver Dis *4*:158, 1984.
138. Moss AR: Occupational exposure and brain tumors. J Toxicol Environ Health *16*:703, 1985.
139. Perticoni GF, Abbritti G, Cantisani TA, et al: Polyneuropathy in workers with long exposure to vinyl chloride: Electrophysiological study. Electromyogr Clin Neurophysiol *26*:41, 1986.

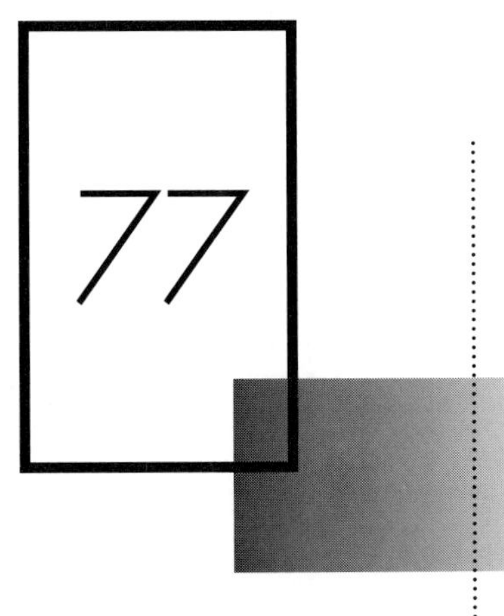

Freon and Other Inhalants

MICHELLE BLANDA, MD
JOHN V. WEIGAND, MD

FREON

Fluocarbons are a group of synthetic halogen-substituted methane and ethane derivatives containing atoms of chlorine and fluorine and are commonly known as chlorofluorocarbons (CFCs). CFCs have been used industrially since the 1930s and are generally known by commercial names such as Freon, Arcton, and Frigen. They were initially used by the armed forces in World War II and reached the civilian market in 1947. CFCs are used as refrigerants, aerosol propellants, foam-blowing agents, solvents, and polymer intermediates, as well as in fire extinguishers and anesthetics.

Common CFCs are listed in Table 77–1. Production of CFCs ceased in the United States as of December 31, 1995, because of their destructive effect on the ultraviolet radiation shield (ozone) of the atmosphere.[1] However, these compounds are still available for sale, and some areas have stockpiled supplies. Hydrogenated chlorofluorocarbons (HCFCs), which can be used instead of CFCs, are currently being manufactured with a cease production date of the year 2020, again because their effect on the ozone layer. At that time, hydrogenated fluorocarbons (HFCs) will take the place of HCFCs and CFCs.

CFCs were initially regarded as less toxic in terms of narcosis and other common solvent health effects, and thus higher levels of exposure were permitted. This led to a higher incumbent risk of problems. Many fatal cases associated with the inhalation of CFCs have been reported.[1–5] The majority of these have occurred in people in a work-related incident or in a self-induced exposure. The autopsy reports of these cases reflect generic evidence of acute cardiorespiratory failure. It is believed the toxic action of CFCs occurs through cardiac toxicity or by hypoxemic asphyxiation due to CFC saturation of the room atmosphere.[2, 6]

CFCs are known irritants to the upper airway with ambient exposure. They may also cause cryogenic effects on tissue. Liquid CFCs with low boiling points or under pressure can cause freezing of the skin if they come into contact with the body for more than 3 to 5 seconds.[7]

It should be noted that Freon does decompose into chlorine, hydrogen fluoride, phosphine, and chloride gases, all of which are extremely toxic.[8]

Pathophysiology

CFCs are absorbed rapidly by inhalation. The distribution half-life is rapid in comparison with elimination because of the slow release from fat stores. Clark and colleagues[9] reported three fatalities due to Freon exposure, and these patients had the highest concentrations in brain tissue, reflecting the high solubility of hydrocarbons. An individual who suffered a fatal exposure secondary to FC_{113} that had vaporized out of the sludge collection pit in glass lens manufacture also showed high levels in brain tissue.[5] High concentrations in heart tissue of persons suffering fatal exposures have also been found.[2, 3] Lung concentrations reported in all human cases are low, and this is probably a reflection of resuscitative efforts.

Extensive animal studies have found a relationship between CFC inhalation and cardiac arrhythmias, even without evidence of asphyxiation.[6, 9–11] Arrhythmias reported to occur in CFC exposure include ventricular arrhythmia, atrioventricular nodal block, and atrial fibrillation.[12, 13] Reinhardt and associates also reported increased sensitization to arrhythmias when epinephrine was given to dogs with exposure

Table 77–1. Common Hydrocarbons and Their Threshold Limit Values

Compound Number	Chemical Formula	Chemical Name	Threshold Limit Value (ppm)
CFC 11	CCl_3F	Trichlorofluoromethane	1000
CFC 12	CCl_2F_2	Dichlorodifluoromethane	1000
HCFC 22	$CHClF_2$	Chlorodifluoromethane	1000
CFC 13	$CClF_3$	Chlorotrifluoromethane	10
CFC 112	$Cl_2FC—CCl_2F$	1,1,2,2-Tetrachlorlo-1,2-difluoroethane	500
CFC 113	$Cl_2FC—CClF_2$	1,1,2-Trichloro-1,2,2-trifluoroethane	1000
CFC 114	$ClF_2C—CClF_2$	1,2-Dichloro-1,1,2,2-tetrafluoroethane	1000
CFC 115	$ClF_2C—CF_3$	1-Chloro-1,1,2,2,2-pentafluoroethane	1000
500		73.8% FC_{12}, 26.2% FC_{152}	
502		48.8% FC_{22}, 51.2% FC_{115}	

From Aviado DM: Fluorine-containing organic compounds. *In* Clayton GD, Clayton FE (eds): Patty's Industrial Hygiene and Toxicology. 4th ed. New York, John Wiley & Sons, pp 1177–1220, 1994 and American Conference of Governmental Industrial Hygienists, Inc.: Documentation of the Threshold Limit Values and Biological Exposure Indices. 5th ed. Cincinnati, OH, ACGIH, 1986.

to FC_{11}.[14] It has been postulated that CFCs decrease the ionic permeability of the cellular membranes, leading to transient and localized conduction blocks, altered refractory periods, and disturbance of the pacemaker ability of the heart.[15, 16] Another theory suggests that CFCs do not sensitize the myocardium to endogenous neurotransmitters but have a depressant effect on the sinus atrioventricular and ventricular conduction systems, allowing other ectopic foci to produce arrhythmias.[17]

Despite the fatal exposures and reports of arrhythmia, the documentation of arrhythmias caused by CFCs in human subjects is ambiguous. Egeland and colleagues[18] found no significant difference in atrial or ventricular premature beats, heart rate, or PR intervals in a group of 16 aerospace workers with high and low exposures. Edling and co-workers[19] studied 89 refrigerator repairmen and concluded that CFCs do not induce arrhythmias in exposed workers. However, the frequency of arrhythmia was high in these men regardless of exposure. No clear connection was found by Antti-Poika and colleagues,[4] but one subject had ectopy that may have been related to exposure. Although ectopy or other arrhythmias occurring with CFC exposure have not been associated with underlying heart disease, increased circulating concentrations of catecholamines may make patients prone to arrhythmia.[1] Caffeine intake, physical activity, and tobacco use have been suggested to have a proarrhythmic effect.[18]

Clinical Signs and Symptoms

Exposures to CFCs caused by transient low-concentration exposure result in eye, nose, and throat irritation. Frostbite of the oral cavity has been described after deliberate inhalation of a propellant.[20] Pulmonary irritation, bronchial constriction, cough, dyspnea, and chest tightness may develop after inhalation. Pulmonary edema is an autopsy finding in fatal inhalation cases.[2, 21] Edema may be secondary to aspiration or decomposition products of CFCs, which include chlorine, hydrogen fluoride, phosphine, and chloride gases.

Neurologic sequelae of CFCs involve a spectrum of symptoms that include headache, lightheadedness, dizziness, and disorientation.[22] Workers with chronic exposure to CFC 113 were found to have impaired psychomotor speed, impaired learning and memory, and emotional lability.[23] Cerebral edema has been found at autopsy.[21]

Toxic exposures to CFCs have been associated with fatal ventricular arrhythmias, atrial fibrillation, and sudden death.[6, 9–13] However, no clear connection with low-concentration exposure and cardiac arrhythmias has been documented.[4, 18, 19]

Freon exposure causing severe frostbite has been reported,[7] and a related case of compartment syndrome required amputation of the digits.[24] Direct accidental injections have also occurred, and these respond to conservative therapy with minimal tissue damage.[25, 26]

Other rare toxic effects include gastric perforation secondary to ingestion, elevation of transaminase levels, jaundice, and rhabdomyolysis.[27–30]

Specific Treatment

The first step in the management of CFC exposure is to remove the offending agent, avoiding exposure to other subjects. Attention to airway, breathing, and circulation with supplemental oxygen, symptomatic therapy, and a calming environment to avoid endogenous adrenergic stimulation are important. Use of adrenergic drugs should be avoided to prevent myocardial stimulation. Use of countershock or phenytoin may be indicated for ventricular arrhythmias.[22]

If frostbite occurs, the exposed area should be soaked in lukewarm water if possible within 20 to 30 minutes after exposure. Ice or heat should not be applied. A light coating of a bland ointment, such as petroleum jelly, should be applied and covered with a light bandage. Ocular injuries should be irrigated and assessed for injury.

ISOCYANATES

Isocyanates are polymerized with a macroglycol to produce polyurethanes. These are widely used in the manufacturing of rigid and flexible polyurethane foams, paints, adhesives, fibers, resins, and sealant. Polyurethane formation was discovered in the 1930s, and limited production was undertaken in Germany during the World War II. Large-scale production began in the United States in the 1950s.

The isocyanate-macroglycol polymer is very versatile, and demand for the product has steadily risen. This polymer is widely produced and used, and many workers are occupationally exposed to isocyanates. Persons in occupations with the potential for exposure include diisocyanate workers, polyurethane manufacturing workers, upholstery workers, spray painters, coating workers, plastic film makers, plastic molders, and rubber workers.

Methyl isocyanate was involved in one of the worst industrial disasters in history in Bhopal, India, on Dec 3, 1984 (see Chapter 22).

Chemical Structure and Properties

Isocyanates form a neutral derivative of primary mines and contain the general formula R—N=C=O. They react with compounds that contain active hydrogen atoms, which migrate to the nitrogen. Compounds containing hydroxyl groups spontaneously form esters of substituted carbon dioxide or urethanes. Combining an isocyanate with a polyol creates polyurethane. Amines are added to the volatile mixture and act as agents cross-linking hydrogen chains. Other surface-active substances or hardeners give the mixture the exact consistency desired.[31] Commonly used diisocyanates are listed in Table 77–2.

Isocyanates release cyanide when burned in fires or explosions.

Exposure hazards of isocyanates are directly proportional to volatility and molecular weight.[32] Isocyanates with low volatility and higher molecular weight are less toxic. Lower-molecular-weight and highly volatile isocyanates such as toluene diisocyanate are dermal and pulmonary irritants and in high concentrations can produce severe pulmonary damage.

Pathophysiology

The respiratory system is the main target organ for isocyanate toxicity caused by vaporization or particle formation. In humans, toxic effects of isocyanates are a result of dermal and inhalation contact.

Table 77–2. Common Isocyanates and Abbreviations

Tolulene diisocyanate (TDI)
Methylene diphenyl diisocyanate (MDI)
Hexamethylene diisocyanate (HDI)
Naphthalene diisocyanate (NDI)
Polymethylene polyphenyl isocyanate (PAPI)
Para-tolyl monoisocyanate (PTI)
Dicyclohexyl methane-4,4 diisocyanate (DMDJ)

Reasonable estimation of the respiratory exposure hazard due to isocyanates is based on molecular weight, volatility, ambient temperatures, and airborne concentration reaching a victim. The higher the dose and the longer the exposure, the quicker the symptoms develop.

Four pulmonary responses to isocyanate exposure appear to be concentration and time dependent: (1) immediate toxic bronchitis and asthma, (2) early and late bronchial asthma caused by sensitization to isocyanates, (3) accelerated decline in pulmonary function (FEV_1), and (4) extrinsic alveolitis.[33]

Immediate toxic reactions are more likely to occur when the breathing zone concentration exceeds 0.5 ppm. Symptoms may begin immediately but usually start within 4 to 8 hours. This immediate toxic reaction was noted in the Bhopal, India, disaster.

Bronchial asthma caused by hypersensitivity to isocyanates is a common problem. It affects at least 5% of workers involved with isocyanates and is one of the most frequent causes of occupationally induced asthma. The sensitization can develop within weeks of exposure or may take many years to develop. After prior sensitization, workers develop reactions at low concentrations of isocyanates. Once an individual is sensitized, asthma may be prolonged or permanent even when the worker is removed from exposure to isocyanates.

The mechanism by which isocyanates precipitate asthma is not completely understood. It appears to be multifactorial, with polygenetic susceptibility,[34] and humoral (type III) and cell-mediated (type IV) reactions resulting in inflammation and bronchospasm.[35, 36]

Isocyanate workers also suffer from an accelerated decline in pulmonary function.[37, 38] Chronic exposure appears to lead to excessive annual declines in forced expiratory volume (FEV_1) for all isocyanate-exposed workers. Hypersensitivity alveolitis is reported in some isocyanate workers.[39] Parenchymal lung involvement with infiltrates and diffusion defects are noted, as are systemic symptoms.

Clinical Signs and Symptoms

Dermal exposure can result in skin conditions ranging from localized itching to limited or widespread eczema.

Inhalation exposure to isocyanates in high vapor or aerosolized particle concentrations results in a toxic reaction. Exposed persons complain of irritation of the eyes, nose, and throat, with lacrimation and rhinitis, cough, pleuritis, wheezing, and chest tightness. If concentrations are high, pulmonary edema and hemorrhagic alveolitis may occur. This toxic reaction is what caused the thousands of deaths and injuries in the Bhopal incident.

Bronchoconstriction due to hypersensitivity to even very low atmospheric isocyanate concentrations is the most frequently reported reaction. Clinical symptoms of this reversible airway disease include cough, dyspnea, wheezing, and chest tightness. When the allergic reaction is severe, respiratory failure can result.

Hypersensitivity alveolitis presents with systemic symptoms of fever, chills, and myalgia. Cough and dyspnea may also occur. Pulmonary parenchymal infiltrates, diffusion defects, and an elevated white blood cell count may be noted.

Treatment

Acute treatment is symptomatic. Patients must first be removed from the exposure. If external exposure has occurred, patients should have the skin and mucous membranes irrigated. The airway must be maintained and suctioned as needed. High-flow oxygen should be administered. Treatment of bronchospasm with aerosolized bronchodilators and systemic steroids should be undertaken. Patients should be monitored to assess the need for intubation and mechanical ventilation. They should also be placed on a cardiac monitor to detect arrhythmias.

For workers who develop reactions from occupational exposure to isocyanates, the best treatment is to transfer them away from the exposure. Protective clothing, gloves, goggles, and respiratory equipment offer some protection to prevent the development of sensitivity to isocyanates, but once sensitivity develops, employees should avoid the environment.

Long-Term Implications

Occupational Safety and Health Administration (OSHA) recommends an exposure standard for both toluene diisocyanate and methylene bisphenyl isocyanate of 0.02 ppm. Thus, the best prevention is adequate ventilation of the work area.

The hyperactive airway disease that develops after exposure to isocyanates may be permanent. The accelerated decrease in pulmonary function may lead to permanent respiratory disability.

BORON

Boron hydrides are highly toxic chemical compounds composed of boron and hydrogen. Inhalation, ingestion, or percutaneous exposure to boranes can result primarily in pulmonary, gastrointestinal, or central nervous system (CNS) toxicity.

Boron hydrides are produced by the reaction of lithium aluminum hydride with boron fluoride to make diborane, and pyrolysis of diborane produces the remaining boranes. The three most commonly encountered in industry are diborane (B2 H6), a colorless gas with a sickly sweet, nauseating smell, like rotten eggs; pentaborane (B5 H9), a colorless volatile liquid with a sweetish, garlic-like, unpleasant odor; and decaborane (B10 H14), a white crystal with an intense bitter chocolate odor. These compounds oxidize easily, are strong reducing agents that are highly flammable, and may ignite or explode in the presence of oxygen.

Boranes are used mainly in high-energy fuels such as rocket propellants but are also used in semi-conductor manufacturing, and welding and as fungicides and bactericides. They are also used as initiators of ethylene, styrene, vinyl, and acrylic polymerization and in the vulcanization of rubber.

Pathophysiology

Boranes are highly toxic by inhalation, skin absorption, or ingestion. They may produce both acute and chronic poisoning.

Diborane gas is primarily a pulmonary irritant at 0.1 ppm. Inhalation exposure results in hydrolysis to boric acid and hydrogen.[40] Acute exposure causes pulmonary edema and hemorrhage as well as temporary damage of the liver and kidneys. Autopsies reveal rhinitis, pneumonia, and structural lung damage.[41, 42]

Pentaborane and decaborane vapor affects the nervous system and causes signs of both hyperexcitability and narcosis.[43] Pentaborane is considered to be the most toxic of the boron hydrides when inhaled, although it is also readily absorbed through intact skin. CNS norepinephrine depletion, intracranial hypertension, and cortical atrophy have been demonstrated after exposure to pentaborane and decaborane. These agents also cause gastrointestinal toxicity, with fatty necrosis of the liver and elevation of transaminase levels.

Direct myotoxic effects of the boron hydrides as well as myoclonus and seizures can result in rhabdomyolysis and myoglobinuria.

Signs and Symptoms

Acute diborane poisoning in humans results in a syndrome like that of metal fume fever, with symptoms of tightness, heaviness, and burning in the chest; cough; shortness of breath; pericardial pain; nausea; shivering; and drowsiness. Signs of intoxication may occur soon after exposure or after a latent period of up to 24 hours and may persist for 1 to 3 days or more. Long-term exposure to low concentrations results in pulmonary irritation, dizziness, headaches, weakness, and tremors.[44]

Drowsiness and nausea may occur with slight pentaborane toxicity. In moderate exposures, headaches, dizziness, nervous excitation, and hiccups may occur. Muscle pain and spasms of the muscles of the face and extremities may be noted. In more severe exposures, after 48 hours, patients may suffer loss of mental concentration, incoordination, disorientation, cramps, convulsions, and coma.

Decaborane toxicity in humans produces symptoms of restlessness, aggressiveness, depressed breathing, incoordination, general weakness, spasmodic movements, and convulsions.

Treatment

Persons exposed to boron hydrides should be immediately removed from the exposure. After contaminated clothing has been removed, victims' skin should be thoroughly washed with water. There is no known antidote for borane poisoning. Treatment is symptomatic and supportive. If high-level inhalation has occurred, hospitalization for 48 to 72 hours is recommended to monitor cardiopulmonary function, acid-base balance, and neurologic status.

Long-Term Implications

Toxic levels of some boron hydrides are below the odor threshold for humans. Exposure to others with a scent, in higher concentration, may cause loss of ability to detect an odor. Therefore, great caution must be used when working around these substances. Personal protective equipment should be used to prevent inhalation, skin, or mucous membrane exposure. Symptoms of acute toxic exposure may take several hours to develop and may persist for days. Chronic liver, kidney, and CNS impairments can result from significant exposures. Low-level exposures over time may cause CNS symptoms including poor decision making and concentration as well as apparent psychiatric symptoms of poor emotional control and personality change.

HYDRAZINES

Hydrazine is a colorless, oily fuming liquid that is used in agricultural chemicals, industry, and medicine. It is also used in photographic developing and in the manufacturing of drugs, dyes, textile treatments, explosives, and plastics.[45] Hydrazine is also a powerful explosive, used as a rocket fuel, and can self-ignite when adsorbed onto earth, cloth, wood, and asbestos. It emits toxic nitrogen compounds when heated to decomposition.

Pathophysiology

Hydrazines are a poison by ingestion, intravenous, and dermal routes. Their toxicity occurs in multiple organ systems, and they are a known carcinogen.[46] Hydrazine and its metabolite monoacylhydrazine are hepatotoxic, causing nuclear and nucleolar enlargement, mitochondrial swelling, and increased formation of antibodies and free radicals.[46, 47] Because acetylation is the pathway for metabolism, toxicity may be more common in persons who are slow acetylators.

Hydrazine is also known to produce a functional pyridoxine deficiency through inhibition of synthesis or deactivation of coenzymes.[48] Pyridoxine may be useful for treatment.

Other toxicities caused by hydrazine include a direct CNS toxicity, a negative inotropic effect on the heart leading to cardiovascular depression and hypotension, and hemolysis leading to acute tubular necrosis or nephritis.[45]

Signs and Symptoms

Hydrazines are local irritants causing ocular irritation, facial edema, salivation, and dermal irritation. Even low concentrations can cause bronchial mucous destruction and pulmonary edema. Other symptoms are nausea, vomiting, dizziness, and agitation.

Anemia due to hemolysis has been reported and can lead to renal dysfunction.[49] This blood loss can also worsen a patient's cardiovascular status and lead to progressive weakness and dyspnea.

Manifestations of the liver disease include hypoglycemia and hyperglycemia, depending on a patient's glycogen stores.

Treatment

Prompt removal of the irritant and basic life support measures are key. Dermal exposure should be treated immediately with soap and water. Ocular exposure requires copious irrigation with tepid water.

Respiratory exposure should be treated with humidified supplemental oxygen and monitoring for respiratory distress. Chest radiographs, arterial blood gas determinations, and intubation may be clinically indicated.

Oral exposures may be treated with gastric lavage and activated charcoal. Emesis must be used with caution because delayed neurologic effects, such as seizure and coma, may occur. This is dependent on the chemical ingested, the volume, and the duration of exposure.

Pyridoxine may be antidotal in hydrazine ingestions. The recommended dose is 25 mg/kg, with one third given intramuscularly and two thirds given intravenously over a 3-hour period.[45] Seizures are treated with routine medications, including diazepam, lorazepam, or phenytoin, and phenobarbital. Other routine laboratory studies include monitoring blood glucose, liver function tests, and hemoglobin measurement. If methemoglobinemia exists with a level greater than 30%, methylene blue should be used, 1 to 2 mg/kg slowly every 4 hours as needed. Treatment is otherwise supportive and symptomatic.

ACROLEIN

Acrolein, a colorless or yellowish liquid with a disagreeable odor, is ubiquitous in the environment. It is used in the manufacturing of pharmaceuticals, herbicides, food supplements, perfumes, plastics, and textiles. It is also present in cigarette smoke. Exposure occurs through inhalation and direct contact.

Pathophysiology

Most exposures to acrolein occur via inhalation. Acrolein is a severe pulmonary irritant and lacrimating agent. The strong irritant effect usually prevents serious exposures, but fatalities have been reported.[50] Studies suggest that pulmonary insult from acrolein is due to alterations of the plasma membrane–dependent transport system in the pulmonary artery endothelial cells.[51]

Skin and corneal burns may result from direct contact with the liquid. Concentrations of 0.25 ppm may cause eye irritation.

Signs and Symptoms

Splash contact may cause irritation, erythema, edema, and actual burns. Difficulty breathing, chest congestion, delayed pulmonary edema, asthma, and permanent lung damage may result from acute exposures. Nausea and vomiting are common. Ingestion may produce severe irritation of the mouth and gastrointestinal tract. Hypertension and tachycardia may result from inhalation. Inhalation can also cause loss of consciousness and coma.

Treatment

Because the primary toxic effects of acrolein involve irritation of the mucous membranes, lungs, and skin, removal of the agent is paramount. Washing with soap and water and irrigation of the eyes with tepid water are appropriate. If pain and burning persist, repeat examination is necessary.

Pulmonary support should be given as needed, including oxygen, intubation, and mechanical ventilation. Arterial blood gas measurement and chest radiograph are used to assess and monitor respiratory status. Patients with high-volume exposure may require hospitalization to be observed for delayed sequelae such as pulmonary edema.

Ingestion should be treated with gastric lavage followed by activated charcoal and cathartics. Gastric lavage should not be used in patients with neurologic deterioration without airway protection.

All other treatment is supportive and symptomatic. The use of steroids remains controversial. Antibiotic use should be aimed at treating specific infections and should not be used as a prophylactic measure.

References

1. Fitzgerald RL, Fishel CE, Bush LL: Fatality due to recreational use of chlorodifluoromethane and chloropentafluoroethane. J Forensic Sci *38:*477–483, 1993.
2. Groppi A, Polettini A, Lunetta P: A fatal case of trichlorofluoromethane (Freon 11). J Forensic Sci *39:*871–876, 1994.
3. Kaufman JD, Silverstein MA, Moure-Eraso R: Atrial fibrillation and sudden death related to occupational solvent exposure. Am J Ind Med *25:*731–735, 1994.
4. Antti-Poika M, Heikkila J, Saarinen L: Cardiac arrhythmias during occupational exposure to fluorinated hydrocarbons. Br J Ind Med *47:*138–140, 1990.
5. McGee MB, Meyer RF, Jejurikar SG: A death resulting from trichlorotrifluorethane poisoning. J Forensic Sci *35:*1453–1460, 1990.
6. Morita M, Miki A, Kazama H, et al: Case report of deaths caused by Freon gas. Forensic Sci *10:*253–260, 1977.
7. Standefer JC: Death associated with fluorocarbon inhalation: Report of a case. J Forensic Sci *20:*548–551, 1975.
8. Arena JM: Freon (dichlorodifluoromethane). *In* Kugelmass IN (ed): Poisoning. 4th ed. Springfield, IL, Charles C Thomas, Publisher, pp 624–625, 1979.
9. Clark MA, Jones JW, Robinson JJ, et al: Multiple deaths resulting from shipboard exposure to trichlorotrifluoroethane. J Forensic Sci *30:*1256–1259, 1985.
10. Flowers NC, Horan LG: Nonanoxic aerosol arrhythmias. JAMA *219:*33–37, 1972.
11. Flowers NC, Horan LG: The electrical sequelae of aerosol inhalation. Am Heart J *83:*644–651, 1972.
12. Taylor GJ, Harris WS: Cardiac toxicity of aerosol propellants. JAMA *214:*81–85, 1970.
13. Aviado DM, Belez MA: Toxicity of aerosol propellants on the respiratory and circulatory systems. I. Cardiac arrhythmia in the mouse. Toxicology *2:*31–42, 1974.
14. Reinhardt CF, Mullin LS, Maxfield ME: Epinephrine-induced cardiac arrhythmia potential of some common industrial solvents. J Occup Med *15:*953–955, 1973.
15. Lessard Y, Begue J, Paulet G: Fluorocarbons and cardiac arrhythmia: Does difluorodichloromethane (FC 12) inhibit cardiac metabolism? Acta Pharmacol Toxicol *58:*71–73, 1986.
16. Lessard Y, Paulet G: A proposed mechanism for cardiac sensitisation: Electrophysiological study of effects of difluorodichloromethane and adrenaline on different types of cardiac preparations isolated from sheep hearts. Cardiovasc Res *20:*807–815, 1986.
17. Reinhardt CV, Azar A, Maxfield ME, et al: Cardiac arrhythmias and aerosol sniffing. Arch Environ Health *22:*265–279, 1971.
18. Egeland GM, Bloom TF, Schnorr TM, et al: Fluorocarbon 113 exposure and cardiac dysrhythmias among aerospace workers. Am J Ind Med *22:*851–857, 1992.
19. Edling C, Ohlson CG, Ljungkvist G, et al: Cardiac arrhythmia in refrigerator repairmen exposed to fluorocarbon, Br J Ind Med *47:*207–212, 1990.
20. Elliott DC: Frostbite of the mouth: A case report. Mil Med *156:*18–19, 1991.
21. Lerman Y, Winkler E, Tirosh MS, et al: Fatal accidental inhalation of bromochlorodifluoromethane (Halon 1211). Hum Exp Toxicol *10:*125–128, 1991.
22. Rumack BH, Hess AJ, Gelman CR (ed): Fluorinated hydrocarbons. *In* Poisindex System. Englewood, CO, Micromedex, Inc., 1996.
23. Rasmussen K, Jeppesen HJ, Arlien-Soborg P: Psychoorganic syndrome from exposure to fluorocarbon 113—an occupational disease? Eur Neurol *28:*205–207, 1988.
24. Wegener EE, Barraza KR, Das SK: Severe frostbite caused by Freon gas. South Med J *84:*1143–1146, 1991.
25. Goetting AT, Carson J, Burton BT: Freon injection injury to the hand: A report of four cases. J Occup Med *34:*775–778, 1992.
26. Craig EV: A new high-pressure injection injury of the hand. J Hand Surg *9A:*240–242, 1984.
27. Haj M, Burstein Z, Horn E, et al: Perforation of the stomach due to trichlorofluoromethane (Freon 11) ingestion. Isr J Med Sci *16:*392–394, 1980.
28. Steadman C, Dorrington LC, Kay P, et al: Abuse of a fire-extinguishing agent and sudden death in adolescents. Med J Aust *141:*115–117, 1984.
29. Brady WJ, Stremski E, Eljaiek L, et al: Freon inhalational

abuse presenting with ventricular fibrillation. Am J Emerg Med *12:*533–536, 1994.
30. Denborough MA, Hopkkinson KC: Firefighting and malignant hyperthermia. BMJ *296:*1442–1443, 1988.
31. Hadengue P, Philbert M: Isocyanates. *In* Parmeggiani L (ed): Encyclopaedia of Occupational Health and Safety, International Labor Organisation, 1983. Geneva: International Labour Office.
32. Lewis R, Sullivan JB: Toxic hazards of plastic manufacturing. *In* Sullivan JB, Krieger GR (eds:) Hazardous Materials Toxicology. Baltimore, Williams & Wilkins, 1992.
33. Newman Taylor AJ: Occupational asthma. *In* Raffle PAB, Adams PH, Baxter PJ, Lee WR (eds): Hunter's Diseases of Occupations. 8th ed. Boston, Edward Arnold Publishers/Little, Brown & Co., 1994.
34. Bignon JS, Aron Y, Ju LY, et al: HLA Class II alleles in isocyanate-induced asthma. Am J Respir Crit Care Med *149:*71–75, 1994.
35. Fabbi LM, Piero M, Saetta M, Mapp CE: Bronchial hyperreactivity: Mechanisms and physiologic evaluation. Am Rev Respir Dis *143:*537–538, 1991.
36. Maestrelli P, Di Stefano A, Occari P, et al: Cytokines in the airway mucosa of subjects with asthma induced by toluene diisocyanate. Am J Respir Crit Care Med *151:*607–612, 1995.
37. Jones RN, Rando RJ, Glindmeyer HW, et al: Abnormal lung function in polyurethane foam products. Am Rev Respir Dis *146:*871–877, 1992
38. Parker DL, Waller K, Himrich B, et al: A cross-sectional study of pulmonary function in autobody repair workers. Am J Public Health *81:*768–771, 1991.
39. Vandenplas O, Malo J-L, Dugas M, et al: Hypersensitivity pneumonitis-like reaction among workers exposed to piphenylmethane diisocyanate (MDI). Am Rev Respir Dis *147:*338–346, 1993.
40. Carter D, Sullivan J: Intermetallic semiconductors and inorganic hydrides. *In* Sullivan J, Krieger G (eds): Hazardous Material Toxicology: Clinical Principles of Environmental Health. Baltimore, Williams & Wilkins, 1992.
41. Uemura T, Omae K, Nakashima H, et al: Acute and subacute inhalation toxicity of diborane in male ICR mice. Arch Toxicol *69:*397–404, 1995.
42. Nomiyama T, Omae K, Vemura T, et al: No-observed-effect level of diborane on the respiratory organs of male mice in acute and subacute inhalation experiments. Sangyo Eiseigaku Zasshi *37:*157–60, 1995.
43. Elinder C, Zenz C: Other metals and their compounds. *In* Zenz C, Dickerson O, Horvath E (eds): Occupational Medicine. 3rd ed. St. Louis, C.V. Mosby Co., 1994.
44. Parmeggiana L (ed): Boranes. *In* Parmeggiani L (ed): Encyclopaedia of Occupational Health and Safety. 3rd ed. International Labour Organisation, 1983. Geneva: International Labour Office.
45. Rumack BH (ed): Hydrazine. *In* Poisindex System. Englewood, CO, Micromedex Inc, 1996.
46. Albano E, Goria-Gatti L, Clot P, et al: Possible role of free radical intermediates in hepatotoxicity of hydrazine derivatives. Toxicol Ind Health *9:*529–538, 1993.
47. Ganote CE, Rosenthal AS: Characteristic lesions of methylazoxymethanol-induced liver damage. Lab Invest *19:*382–398, 1968.
48. Clark DA, Bairrington JD, Bitter HL, et al: Pharmacology and toxicology of propellant hydrazines. Aeromed Rev *11:*68, 1968.
49. Clayton GD, Clayton FE: Patty's Industrial Hygiene and Toxicology. 4th ed. New York, John Wiley & Sons, 1994.
50. American Conference of Government Industrial Hygiene: Documentation of the Threshold Limit Values. 4th ed. Cincinnati, OH, American Conference of Government Industrial Hygiene, 1980.
51. Paten JM, Block ER: Acrolein-induced injury to cultured pulmonary artery endothelial cells. Toxicol Appl Pharmacol *122:*46–53, 1993.

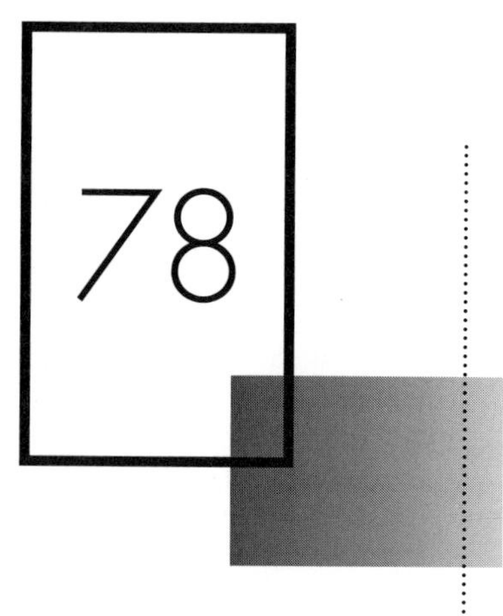

Phenol and Related Agents

CHRISTOPHER P. LANGFORD, MD
ROBERT BARTLETT, MD
LESTER M. HADDAD, MD

Case Study: While being prepared for nail bed cauterization in a podiatrist's office, a 52-year-old woman was preoperatively given what was thought to be Vistaril but in fact was 1 oz of 89% phenol.[1] On drinking the "medicine," the patient immediately clutched her throat and collapsed. Within 30 minutes she was comatose, had an unrecordable blood pressure, and sustained respiratory arrest. During endotracheal intubation, her mouth and hypopharynx were noted to be white. A lamp oil odor was detected while the patient was ventilated with bag and mask. One hour after ingestion, she experienced ventricular tachycardia, which was treated successfully with cardioversion. Supraventricular and ventricular dysrhythmias, metabolic acidosis, and a grand mal seizure occurred in the first 24 hours. Esophagitis and upper gastrointestinal bleeding occurred in the first week, and 8 days after ingestion, esophagoscopy revealed hyperkeratosis, erythema, and friable mucosa. Remarkably, she completely recovered after an eventful 15-day hospital course. At 6-month follow-up, she was asymptomatic and endoscopy revealed no evidence of stricture or impaired motility.

This chapter reviews the effects of phenol, dinitrophenol, and pentachlorophenol. All are chemically related, and exposures demonstrate some similarities in their clinical presentation; however, phenol and dinitrophenol have distinct clinical syndromes. Pentachlorophenol shares clinical effects of both phenol and dinitrophenol.

PHENOL

Phenol (also known as carbolic acid, phenic acid, phenylic acid, phenyl hydroxide, hydroxybenzene, oxybenzene) occurs naturally in animal waste and was originally produced by fractional distillation of coal tar and more recently by cumene hydroperoxidation and toluene oxidation. Lister first used phenol in the 1800s as an antiseptic to treat open fractures and reported cures of what was usually a fatal injury. Its aromatic odor masked that of pus, and its anesthetic effect decreased pain.[2] For these reasons, phenol became popular for several decades in the late 1800s. It was used as an antiseptic in the operating room in the form of soaks, ointments, sprays, and lotions for wound care (Table 78–1). During these years, symptoms of anorexia, progressive weight loss, headache, vertigo, salivation, and dark urine developed in many surgeons and operating room personnel. By 1890, the association with chronic phenol inhalation was recognized. This syndrome became known as

Table 78–1. Examples of Phenol-Related Compounds

Chemical	Use
Amyl phenol	Germicide
Creosol	Antiseptic
Creosote	Wood preservative
Guaiacol	Antiseptic
Hexachlorophene	Antiseptic
Medicinal tar	Treatment of dermatologic conditions
Phenol	Outpatient podiatric surgery
Phenylphenol	Disinfectant
Resorcinol	Bactericidal ointment
Tetrachlorophenol	Fungicide
Thymol	Fungicide and anthelmintic

Adapted from Gosselin RE, Hodge HC, Gleason MN, Smith RP: Clinical Toxicology of Commercial Products. 4th ed. Baltimore, Williams & Wilkins, 1976.

carbol (or *phenol*) *marasmus* because of its wasting effect.[2] Phenol is currently used in disinfectants and insecticides, as a reagent in chemical analysis, for nail bed cauterization by podiatrists, and in chemical peeling of skin lesions and wrinkles by facial surgeons.[3–5] It is also found in (0.1% to 4.5%) various gargles (Chloraseptic 1.4%), gels, ointments, lotions, and lozenges (Chloraseptic 32.5 mg) including Campho-Phenique (4.7%). Phenol is included in most of these as a local anesthetic for pruritus, stings, burns, bites, or sore throat, and some preparations are labeled for antiseptic use.[6] Table 78–1 lists compounds similar to phenol that produce similar clinical syndromes.

Toxicology

Phenol is rapidly absorbed into the circulation from all surfaces of the body. In concentrations of 5% or more, it rapidly denatures all proteins with which it comes into contact.[7] It is caustic and if spilled on skin or ingested causes intense pain and blanching of the area and can result in severe burns. On dermal exposure, a white layer of precipitated protein is formed. This eventually turns red and sloughs, leaving the surface stained a light brown. The keratocoagulation has been presumed to be due to disruption of the sulfur bridges of keratoprotein and aided by denaturation secondary to phenol's acidic nature.[4] Nausea, vomiting, severe abdominal pain, gastrointestinal erosion, and bleeding are commonly associated with ingestion. Stricture formation has been reported but is uncommon.[8] The extent of cutaneous absorption depends more on the total area of skin exposed than on the concentration of the solution.[4]

Lewin and Clearly[9] reported a case in which a paintbrush that had been soaking for 24 hours in an antiseptic (80% phenol) was rinsed with water before being used to apply a scabicide from the neck down to a 24-year-old inmate. He felt a stinging sensation, and 10 minutes later he became unsteady, collapsed, and began to convulse. He became cyanotic then apneic and was unable to be resuscitated. Death can occur with 64 sq in of body surface exposure, indicating the considerable toxicity of phenol.[9]

Approximately 80% of phenol is excreted through the kidneys, primarily conjugated with glucuronide but also as free phenol. A small portion is detoxified by oxidation in the liver to hydroquinone and pyrocatechol.[8] A fraction may be excreted by the lungs, imparting an aromatic odor to the breath.[1]

Systemic toxicity may include central nervous system (CNS) stimulation or depression with tremor, seizures, extremity weakness, lethargy, coma, supraventricular and ventricular dysrhythmias, circulatory collapse, respiratory stimulation, pulmonary edema, severe metabolic acidosis, and renal toxicity with darkened or black urine.[1, 10–12] Both phenol and its glucuronide conjugate have CNS effects presumed to be responsible for the excitability of the cortex and the involuntary tremors observed early in phenol poisoning.[10] Circulatory depression is thought to be due to both a central vasomotor depression and primarily to a direct toxic effect on the myocardium.[4] Rapid CNS depression with lethargy and coma was noted in Spiller and colleagues' review in 11 of 80 (14%) patients, with time of onset from 15 minutes to 1 hour.[11] Hepatic failure and renal failure with anuria have also been described with phenol poisoning.[1] Although the exact mechanism of phenol's multiorgan toxicity is unclear, Zamponi[13] reports that phenol has been shown to mimic one aspect of lidocaine's blocking effect on cardiac sodium channels. It is interesting that phenol's stimulation and depression of the CNS also resemble lidocaine's CNS toxic effects.

Occupational and environmental exposure may also occur. In 1972, Merliss[2] described a case in a laboratory technician who for 13 years had been exposed to phenol vapors inadvertently during the processing of phenol, cresol, and xylenol. His health gradually deteriorated, and he was affected by anorexia, weight loss, extremity pain, and intermittent dark urine (bilirubin negative). Examination and testing revealed hepatomegaly, right upper quadrant tenderness, and elevated liver enzymes (alanine aminotransferase greater than aspartate aminotransferase), consistent with an anicteric chemical hepatitis, presumed to be the cause of death of many physicians in the late 19th century.[2, 14–17] Phenol-contaminated drinking water resulted in an outbreak of nausea, vomiting, diarrhea, oropharyngeal burning and sores, and dark urine.[18] *These accounts underscore the importance of occupational and social histories when considering toxicologic etiologies.*

Ocular exposure results in epithelial ulceration and stromal opacity, which may lead to visual loss[19] similar to that of an acid exposure. If any symptoms persist after 30 minutes of water or saline irrigation, ophthalmologic consultation is mandatory.

Management

Management of phenol poisoning includes decontamination of the body surfaces, removal of ingested phenol, and supportive therapy. Decontamination is recommended ideally with care personnel gloved, gowned, and masked in a well-ventilated area. All clothing should be removed, and the exposed area should be wiped immediately and repeatedly with cotton-wool swabs soaked in low-molecular-weight polyethylene glycol (PEG 300 or PEG 400)[8, 20–24] (as opposed to Colyte or GoLYTELY, which is PEG 3350),[23] which may be diluted to a 50% solution with water to lessen its viscosity, decrease the heat sensation caused by the phenol/PEG mixture, and ease application without decreasing efficacy.[8] Swabbing should be continued until there is no longer an odor of phenol (aromatic or lamp oil odor). Although Pullin and colleagues' study in 1978[25] did not show a statistical benefit of PEG swabbing over copious water irrigation, other studies[8, 20, 22, 24] have determined

PEG to be the decontaminant of choice. Another alternative is glycerin solution, which is more readily available. Immediate irrigation with water as a *high-density shower* has been shown to prolong the time before which phenol exposure becomes lethal by a factor of three, whereas PEG increases it by a factor of 25 (Fig. 78–1).[8] *Lesser amounts of water irrigation only dilute the phenol and expand the area of exposure, resulting in greater morbidity.*[8] It makes no difference whether PEG is applied as an irrigation or swabbing. A second-line decontaminant is isopropyl alcohol, which has been shown to be equally efficacious in exposures of less than 5% body surface area.[21] *It is imperative that decontamination with PEG, glycerin, isopropyl alcohol, or water as a high-density shower begin as soon as possible after exposure to keep phenol absorption to a minimum.*

Removal of ingested phenol is best accomplished by careful gastric lavage. Emesis is contraindicated owing to phenol's corrosive effects and the potential for seizures and rapid CNS depression. Administration of activated charcoal, which retards phenol absorption, is indicated. Oral and esophageal burns must be evaluated endoscopically. Management of esophagitis with steroids is indicated, and long-term follow-up for strictures is appropriate. Inhalation exposure necessitates removal of the patient from the environment and supportive treatment for signs of respiratory distress.

Management of systemic toxicity is also supportive. Despite its similarities, lidocaine may be used to treat ventricular dysrhythmias. Intravenous administration of sodium bicarbonate may rapidly reverse CNS depression in the presence of metabolic acidosis.[26] Hemodialysis is not effective in removing phenol.

In all symptomatic exposures, patients must undergo cardiac monitoring and close neurologic observation. If signs of toxicity develop, patients should be admitted to an intensive care unit. If signs of toxicity have not developed within 2 to 4 hours after exposure, it is unlikely that any will develop, because of phenol's rapid absorption, and patients may be discharged.

Hexachlorophene,[27–29] a chlorinated phenolic compound, may result in gastrointestinal and CNS toxicity similar to that of phenol after oral or dermal exposure. It was used topically in the 1970s for its bacteriostatic properties in burn victims.[29] Hyperthermia, lower extremity weakness, decreased visual acuity, cerebral edema, and cardiac arrest have been reported.[29] Exposures of 160 to 250 mg/kg have resulted in death.[27] Treatment consists of lavage, activated charcoal, and support with observation for CNS effects. Emesis is contraindicated.

Also of note is propofol, a derivative of isopropyl phenol. A lipid-based, rapidly acting intravenous anesthetic, it supports rapid bacterial growth at room temperature and has been associated with bacteremia subsequent to use.[30] Recommendations therefore include wiping the outside of the ampule with alcohol immediately before opening, preparation of propofol syringes under aseptic conditions immediately before it is given, and of course use of each vial for only one patient.[31]

DINITROPHENOL

Dinitrophenol and related products are phenol derivatives that are used principally as herbicides and for control of mites and aphids. A characteristic of dinitrophenols is that they uncouple oxidative phosphorylation in cell mitochondria. The increase in oxi-

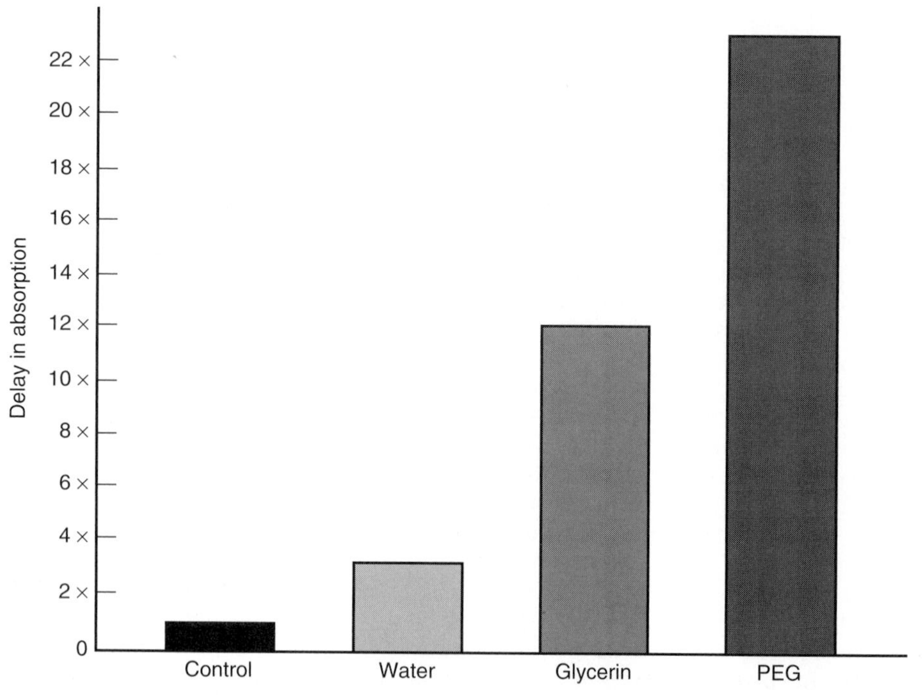

Figure 78–1. Relative efficacy of different agents in reducing absorption (and mortality) of phenol. ×, Duration of phenol exposure required for lethal absorption with no treatment. For example, polyethylene glycol (PEG 300 or 400) reduces absorption 23 times greater than no treatment and almost 8 times greater than high-density water shower. (Adapted from data in Horch R, Spilker G, Start GB: phenol burns and intoxications. Burns *20*:45, 1994.)

dative metabolism rapidly depletes body fat stores, and for this reason these compounds were once used for weight reduction.[32] Weight loss is the usual sign exhibited by patients with chronic poisoning by these agents. Dinitrophenol has recently found a role in the study of calcium metabolism and muscle physiology.[33, 34] It is absorbed by all routes, including inhalation.

Clinical Presentation

The dinitrophenols are highly toxic and can rapidly produce death. As a result of increased metabolism of body cells, patients have profuse diaphoresis, fever, thirst, tachycardia, and respiratory distress.[34] Yellow staining of the skin usually occurs after contact with dinitrophenol. Because normal cardiorespiratory function cannot keep up with metabolic demand, anoxia and metabolic acidosis rapidly ensue. Coma, convulsions, pulmonary edema, and severe hyperpyrexia usually are preterminal events. Methemoglobinemia also occurs.[32]

As with exposure to other phenols, renal and hepatic failure can occur. Delayed cataract formation and agranulocytosis have also been described.[35]

Trinitrophenol (picric acid), used in the explosives industry, has effects similar to those of dinitrophenol but can also cause intravascular hemolysis. Picric acid is also highly irritating to the eyes and skin.[35] The major differential in the diagnosis of dinitrophenol poisoning is salicylate poisoning, which also uncouples oxidative phosphorylation. Other causes of hyperpyrexia, such as anticholinergic agents, should also be included in the differential diagnosis.

Management

Management of dinitrophenol poisoning follows the general principles of management of poisoned patients. Eyes should be flushed with copious amounts of water; skin and hair should be washed with soap and water. Care must be taken to avoid contamination of hospital personnel.

Gastric lavage followed by activated charcoal and a cathartic is usually necessary to treat a patient who has ingested this substance. Salicylates and anticholinergics are contraindicated in treatment of these patients.

Supportive therapy is the mainstay of treatment. Oxygen, intravenous fluids, maintenance of acid-base and electrolyte balance, and control of hyperpyrexia with a hypothermia blanket are indicated. Diazepam may be necessary to control seizures. Significant methemoglobinemia may require treatment with methylene blue.

PENTACHLOROPHENOL

Pentachlorophenol has considerable use as an herbicide, fungicide, weed killer, molluscicide, and wood preservative. Pentachlorophenol resembles both phenol and dinitrophenol in its toxic aspects. Like phenol, it is toxic to the liver, kidneys, and CNS. It resembles dinitrophenol in that it stimulates oxidative metabolism by uncoupling oxidative phosphorylation in the mitochondria.[36]

The clinical syndromes of pentachlorophenol toxicity likewise resemble those of both phenol and dinitrophenol poisoning. Armstrong and Robson described 20 newborn infants in a small hospital who developed an unusual illness characterized by profuse generalized diaphoresis, fever, tachycardia, tachypnea, hepatomegaly, and acidosis. Two infants died. Pentachlorophenol was used in the terminal rinse of the diapers and nursery linens and was implicated as the causative agent.[36]

Treatment follows the general principles of management and is supportive. Exchange transfusion resulted in dramatic improvement and survival of six of six neonates exposed to pentachlorophenol, whereas only one of three survived with supportive therapy alone.[36] Eye exposure requires irrigation and ophthalmologic consultation for persistent symptoms.

SUMMARY

The phenols are rapidly absorbed, highly toxic compounds that require careful, immediate decontamination and supportive therapy with close monitoring and observation for all symptomatic patients. Polyethylene glycol is the decontaminant of choice for dermal phenol exposure. Less than copious amounts of water irrigation for dermal phenol exposure are contraindicated. Dinitrophenol and pentachlorophenol toxicity may resemble salicylate poisoning. Exchange transfusion may be life saving in infant exposures.

References

1. Haddad LM, Dimond KA, Schweistris JE: Case report: Phenol poisoning. J Am Coll Emerg Physicians *8*:267, 1979.
2. Merliss RR: Phenol marasmus. J Occup Med *14*:55, 1972.
3. Budavari S: The Merck Index. 11th ed. Rahway, NJ, Merck and Co., 1989.
4. Botta SA, Straith RE, Goodwin HH: Cardiac arrhythmias in phenol face peeling: A suggested protocol for prevention. Aesth Plast Surg *12*:115, 1988.
5. Byrne DS, Caldwell D: Phenol cauterization for ingrowing toenails: A review of five years experience. Br J Surg *76*:598, 1989.
6. Goodman LS, Gilman AG: The Pharmacological Basis of Therapeutics. 7th ed. New York, Macmillan Publishing Co., 1985.
7. Liao JTF, Oehme FW: Literature reviews of phenolic compounds. Vet Hum Toxicol *22*:160, 1980.
8. Horch R, Spilker G, Start GB: Phenol burns and intoxications. Burns *20*:45, 1994.
9. Lewin JF, Clearly WT: An accidental death caused by the absorption of phenol through the skin. A case report. Forensic Sci Int *19*:177, 1982.
10. Soares ER, Tift JP: Phenol poisoning: Three fatal cases. J Forensic Sci *27*:729, 1982.
11. Spiller HA, Quadrani KDA, Cleveland P: A five year evalua-

tion of acute exposures to phenol disinfectant (26%). J Toxicol Clin Toxicol *31*:307, 1993.
12. Baker EL, Landrigan PJ, Bertozzi PE, et al: Phenol poisoning due to contaminated drinking water. Arch Environ Health *33*:89, 1978.
13. Zamponi GW: Arrhythmias during phenol therapies: A specific action on cardiac sodium channels? Circulation *89*:914, 1994.
14. Kobert R: Lehrbuch der Intoxilcationen. 2nd ed. Stuttgart, Ende, 1906.
15. Devries: Therap Monatsh *4*:644, 1890.
16. Anderson W: Fatal misadventure with carbolic acid. Lancet *1*:179, 1869.
17. Deichmann WB, Gerarde HW: Toxicology of Drugs and Chemicals. New York, Academic Press, 1969.
18. Jarvis SN, Straube RC, Williams ALJ: Illness associated with contamination of drinking water supplies with phenol. BMJ *290*:1800, 1985.
19. Blanchard DL: Sting Eze keratitis. Letter. Arch Ophthalmol *107*:791, 1989.
20. Conning DM, Hayes MJ: The dermal toxicity of phenol: An investigation of the most effective first-aid measures. Br J Ind Med *27*:155, 1970.
21. Hunter DM, Timerding BL, Leonard RB, et al: Effects of isopropyl alcohol, ethanol, and polyethylene glycol/industrial methylated spirits in the treatment of acute phenol burns. Ann Emerg Med *21*:1303, 1992.
22. Brown VKH, Box VL, Simpson BJ: Decontamination procedures for skin exposed to phenolic substances. Arch Environ Health *30*:1, 1975.
23. American Medical Association: Drug Evaluations. 6th Ed. Chicago, American Medical Association, 1986.
24. Henschler D: Therapiemoglichkeiten bei akuter phenolvergiftung. Medichem *27*:211, 1972.
25. Pullin TG, Pinkerton MN, Johnston RV, Kilian DJ: Decontamination of the skin of swine following phenol exposure: A comparison of the relative efficacy of water versus polyethylene glycol/industrial methylated spirits. Toxicol Appl Pharmacol *43*:199, 1978.
26. Bennett IL, James DF, Golden A: Severe acidosis due to phenol poisoning. Ann Intern Med *32*:324, 1950.
27. Herskowitz J, Rosman NP: Acute hexachlorophenol poisoning by mouth in a neonate. J Pediatrics *94*:495, 1979.
28. Martinez AJ, Boehm V, Hadfield MG: Acute hexachlorophene encephalopathy: Clinical neuropathological correlation. Acta Neuropathol *28*:93, 1974.
29. Chilcote R, Curley A, Loughlin HH: Hexachlorophene storage in a burn patient associated with encephalopathy. Pediatrics *59*:457, 1977.
30. Bennett SN, McNeil MM, Bland LA, et al: Postop infections traced to contaminations of an intravenous anesthetic, propofol. N Engl J Med *333*:147, 1995.
31. Veber B, Gachot B, Bedos JP, Wolff M: Severe sepsis after intravenous injection of contaminated propofol. Letter. Anesthesia *80*:712, 1994.
32. Leftwich RB, Floro JF, Neal RA, Wood AJ: Dinitrophenol poisoning: A diagnosis to consider in undiagnosed fever. South Med J *75*:182, 1982.
33. Heller SL, Brooke MH, Kaiser KK, Choski R: 2,4-Dinitrophenol, muscle biopsy, and McArdle's disease. Neurology *38*:15, 1988.
34. Elz JS, Nayler WG: Calcium gain during postischemic reperfusion—the effect of 2,4-dinitrophenol. Am J Pathol *131*:137, 1988.
35. Gosselin RE, Hodge HC, Gleason MN, Smith RP: Clinical Toxicology of Commercial Products. 4th ed. Baltimore, Williams & Wilkins, 1976.
36. Armstrong RW, Robson AM: Pentachlorophenol poisoning, I and II. J Pediatr *75*:309, 1969.

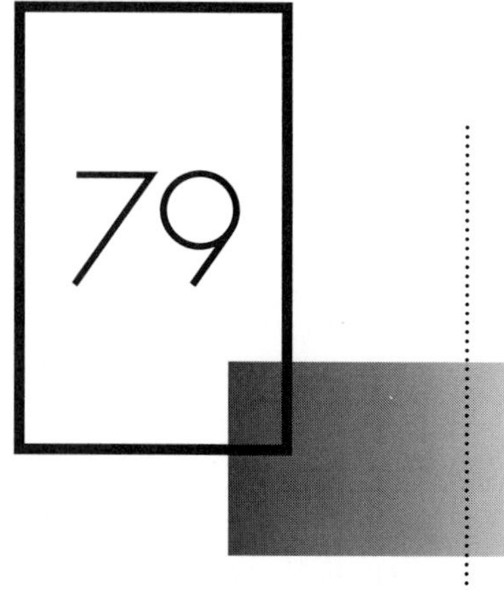

Phosgene and Phosphine

DANIEL T. SCHELBLE, MD

PHOSGENE

Phosgene is a colorless gas, heavier than air, with a musty odor resembling fresh mown hay or green corn. In high concentrations, it is reported to be pungent and mildly irritating. Smokers report a flat metallic taste when smoking in the presence of phosgene. Synonyms include carbonic dichloride, carbonyl chloride, carbon oxychloride, and chloroformyl chloride. Its chemical identification number is 1076, a potentially useful fact in identifying spills in railway or truck accidents. Phosgene is an acidic chloride with a chemical formula of $COCl_2$ and has the following structure:[1–4]

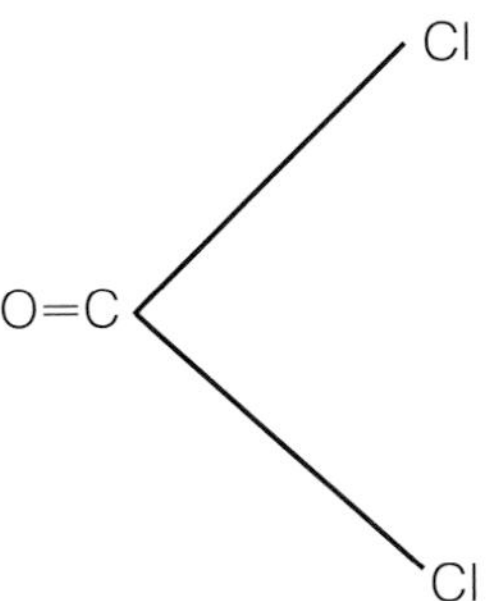

Phosgene does not occur naturally and was first synthesized by Sir Humphry Davy in 1812 by the passage of carbon monoxide and chlorine through charcoal. During the Industrial Revolution, its use in manufacturing gradually increased; however, morbidity and mortality attributable to phosgene largely went unrecognized and unreported. Because of its properties (colorless, heavier than air), phosgene was used extensively in gas warfare in World War I, and numerous writers report that it caused 80% of the deaths by gas in that conflict.[5–7]

Because of its devastating effects in World War I and follow-up studies on veterans from that war, the industrial nations recognized the need for personnel protection, and by 1940 occupational exposure standards were widely recognized in the United States and other nations. A maximum allowable concentration of 1.0 ppm (gas) or 0.4 mg/m^3 (liquid) and a threshold limit valve of 0.1 ppm continuous exposure over a 10-hour day were established and widely accepted.[3, 5] Fortunately, gas warfare was sparingly used in World War II, and exposure now is primarily industrial and relatively rare and isolated in occurrence. Public interest in gas warfare recurred during the 1991 Persian Gulf crisis (Desert Storm) owing to the stockpiling of chemical warfare agents by Iraq. Fortunately, chemical munitions were not used during that brief conflict.

Phosgene is used in synthesis of isocyanates, polyurethane, polycarbonate resins, aniline dyes, pharmaceuticals, plastics, and insecticides and in the "uranium enrichment" process. Phosgene is also a combustion or decomposition byproduct of most volatile chlorine compounds (e.g., carbon tetrachloride, chloroform, and methylene chloride). These substances are widely found in common household substances such as solvents, paint removers, and dry-cleaning fluids, which, when exposed to heat or fire, can produce phosgene gas.[8, 9] In December 1987, in Tampa, Florida, an individual was filling an air mattress with a hair dryer when the mattress exploded, burned, and released phosgene into the apartment.[10] This represents one of the many hazards to fire-fighting personnel and fire victims. Welding in a poorly ventilated, confined space in the presence of chlorinated solvents or other halides can cause phosgene to form rapidly in lethal concentrations.[11] The Occupational Safety and Health Administration placed the yearly production of phosgene in the United States at 2 million pounds and estimated that 10,000 workers are at risk of phosgene exposure.[12]

Phosgene was implicated in the Bhopal, India, tragedy in December 1984. Approximately 150,000 to 200,000 people were affected, with significant morbidity in more than 10,000 and a mortality figure of approximately 2500. This industrial accident was the worst of its kind in civilian history. In the disaster, nearly 50,000 pounds of stored methylisocyanate was released in vapor and liquid forms over 2 hours. Methylisocyanate is made from phosgene and methylamine and is used as an intermediate in the manufacture of the carbamate insecticide carbaryl (Sevin, Union Carbide Corp.). Because of the hypothesized reactions that took place within the storage tank and in the surrounding atmosphere, it is thought that methylisocyanate, phosgene, and hydrogen cyanide all had a significant role in the well-known disaster.[13]

Prevention of phosgene exposure is the key to success in the workplace and home. At work, appropriate ventilation, exhaust fans, frequent checks of tank apparatus and piping seals, respiratory protection, chemical goggles, frequent changing and washing of work clothes, regular scheduled use of phosgene dosimeters or chemically impregnated strips, and physical examinations at regular intervals all have made significant phosgene exposure a rare occurrence. Dangwal reported a spectrophotometric method for detecting phosgene in the air in concentrations as low as 0.1 μg/mL.[14] In the home, strict adherence to label precautions regarding both use and storage of chemicals and solvents should be used and encouraged.

Pathophysiology

Like most exposures, concentration, duration, and water solubility are the three key factors in the response to phosgene. Phosgene slowly hydrolyzes in mucous membrane water to produce carbon dioxide and hydrochloric acids. This reaction may take place in minutes to several hours, rarely exceeding 24 hours, depending on the concentration and the duration of exposure. Because this hydrolysis tends to occur slowly, phosgene is less irritating to the mucous membrane of the upper airway and eyes and therefore penetrates more deeply into the lungs. This initial formation of hydrochloric acid causes epithelial damage and necrosis in the bronchi and small bronchioles, with an increase in permeability and edema. In an animal model, Tobias and colleagues demonstrated the direct action of low-concentration phosgene, which caused bronchial and bronchiolar necrosis and severe pulmonary edema. The same group also demonstrated massive red blood cell hemolysis at high concentrations with resultant capillary plugging. After the epithelial damage, focal disruption of type I pneumocytes occurs, causing further alveolar and interstitital edema. This is later followed by derangements in type II pneumocytes, interstitial cell necrosis, and alveolar collapse.[15] A massive influx of neutrophils into the lungs also contributes to the worsening pulmonary edema.[16]

If the initial concentration of phosgene was high, rapid onset of direct cytoxicity and enzymatic poisoning may ensue. Because phosgene is an acidic chloride, it reacts readily with NH_2^-, OH^-, and SH^- groups. These radicals are found in essentially all living tissue as components of albumin, amino acids, intermediary metabolites, enzymes, and vitamins. For example, phosgene reacts with glutathione in renal and hepatic tissue to form diglucathionyl dithiocarbamate. As soon as the glutathione stores are depleted, the phosgene then covalently binds with proteins in cellular enzymes in macromolecules, leading to hepatic and renal necrosis.[17] Ivanhoe and Myers demonstrated in rabbits that phosgene also causes paralysis of the sympathetic system, resulting in marked pulmonary vasoconstriction, which further contributes to pulmonary edema.[18]

The end result of phosgene toxicity clinically is hypovolemia, hemoconcentration, hypotension, progressive respiratory distress with pulmonary edema and oxygenation abnormalities, and pulmonary, hepatic, and renal cellular necrosis. If unrecognized or irreversible with treatment, then full-blown adult respiratory distress syndrome develops, leading to death.

Clinical Signs and Symptoms

Eye irritation with conjunctivitis, excessive lacrimation, or corneal damage has been reported secondary to phosgene exposure in gas or liquid states. Dryness and burning of the throat, thirst, cough with thick sputum or hemoptysis, headache, nausea, vomiting, weakness, cyanosis, and chest discomfort all may be present to various degrees. Skin irritation, especially if the victim is hot and sweaty, has been reported secondary to both gas and liquid exposure. The initial constellation of signs and symptoms is proportional to the duration and concentration.[19] In terms of specific exposure levels, 3 ppm can cause immediate throat irritation, 4 ppm affects the eyes, and 5 to 10 ppm causes immediate cough. A concentration of 25 ppm for 30 minutes is very dangerous, and even brief exposure to 50 ppm or greater may be rapidly fatal. Rat studies have shown that 2 days of continuous exposure at 0.5 ppm is lethal, and 1 hour of continuous exposure at 2 ppm caused permanent lung damage.[2, 4, 5]

In most cases, a relatively asymptomatic latent period follows the initial symptoms and may last for a few minutes or as long as 72 hours. The duration of the latent period is inversely proportional to the severity of the initial exposure. Most significant exposures have a latent period of less than 24 hours, and 80% of the mortalities occur within 48 hours of the initial exposure.[7]

Other than a high index of suspicion and a very careful, detailed history evaluating for possible exposure, there are no specific diagnostic tests for phosgene. Chest x-ray findings of edema, hilar enlargement, and ill-defined central patchy infiltrates are rather late findings occurring with 6 to 8 hours of exposure. Entities that may mimic phosgene exposure include other noxious gas exposures (e.g., oxides of nitrogen, chlorine, ammonia, and sulfur dioxide) plus upper respiratory tract infections (viral or bacterial), cardiogenic pulmonary edema, pneumonia, or adult respiratory distress syndrome due to other causes.

General and Specific Treatment

Owing to the latent period, high mortality rate, and permanent morbidity, essentially all identified phosgene exposure victims should be admitted and closely observed. Obviously, victims must be immediately removed from the environment, and all contaminated clothing must be removed.

Eye and skin exposure, whether liquid or gas, should be treated with copious lavage. Treatment is aimed primarily at the pulmonary system, with supplemental oxygen delivered by the most appropriate route, pulmonary arterial catheter monitoring for fluid and oxygenation management, and administration of bronchodilators. Continuous oximeter monitoring, serial blood gas analysis, and pulmonary function testing should be used. Prophylactic use of antibiotics is recommended because autopsy studies have uniformly found pneumonia and bronchitis. Dopamine may be necessary in treatment of hypotension, bradycardia, or renal failure. The use of sedation should be weighed against the sedative effect on the respiratory center. Diuretics are contraindicated because the pulmonary edema is not hypervolemic in origin and phosgene victims tend to be hypovolemic and hypotensive.

Specific therapeutic regimens for phosgene have been controversial. Russian and German scientists during both World Wars believed that hexamethylene tetramine (HMT, methenamine; Urotropin) was a specific antidote, and both countries used the substance in their gas masks. This subject was extensively studied during and after both World Wars, and the controversy raged in the literature. Diller conducted an extensive review of the world literature plus experimentation and concluded that HMT had a limited prophylactic effect when administered *before* phosgene exposure but found no convincing proof of a therapeutic effect of HMT administered *after* phosgene exposure.[17]

Cysteine in vitro traps phosgene and converts it to a less harmful metabolite. It has therefore been suggested that the administration of *N*-acetylcysteine (Mucomyst) may afford some protection. To date, no controlled in vivo studies have been reported.[20–22] Plunkett suggests the use of aminocaproic acid (Amicar) to prevent fibrinolysis and to enhance hemostasis in the presence of a phosgene-induced bleeding diathesis.[3] Ghio and colleagues demonstrated in rats that colchicine significantly reduced the pulmonary influx of neutrophils that contributes to the pulmonary edema.[16]

Steroid administration is suggested throughout the phosgene literature and seems reasonable in light of the intense inflammation, especially in the respiratory epithelium. The Bhopal experience clearly demonstrated the efficacy of steroid use throughout the acute treatment phase.[13]

Long-Term Implications

Studies in the 1920s and 1930s on veterans implicated that phosgene exposure caused chronic and recurrent morbidity and increased mortality from bronchitis, emphysema, and reactivation of tuberculosis. However, these studies were limited by the fact that the duration and concentration of the exposure in the battlefield setting were unknown.

Polednak conducted an extensive 30-year outcome review of more than 800 uranium-processing plant workers with known levels and duration of exposure. Using standardized mortality ratios, he concluded the group of workers with low-level daily exposure (699 men) showed no evidence of excess overall mortality or mortality from diseases of the respiratory system. However, the group with known high-level exposure (106 men) did appear to have an increase in mortality and morbidity (pneumonitis, chronic bronchitis, emphysema, impaired results of pulmonary function studies), although the sample size was such that no definitive conclusions could be reached. Similarly, the same researcher concluded, with the same caveat about sample size, that no evidence showed increased lung cancer mortality after phosgene exposure.[23]

PHOSPHINE

Phosphine is colorless flammable gas with an odor of garlic or rotten, decaying fish. Synonyms include hydrogen phosphide, phosphoretted hydrogen, and phosphorous trihydride. Its chemical identification number is 2199. It has a chemical formula of PH^3 and has the following structure:

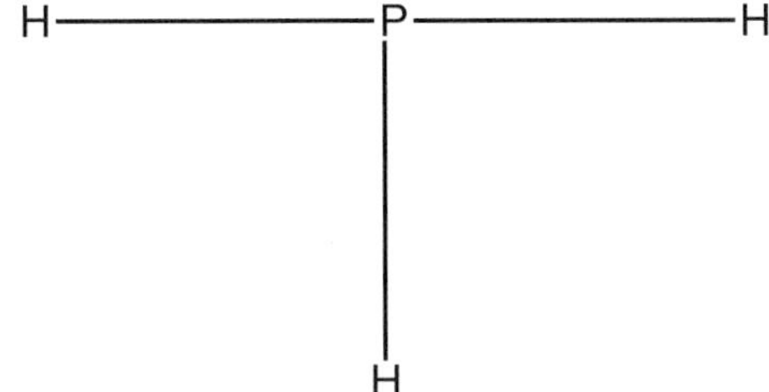

Phosphine gas is used in silicon crystal treatment in the semi-conductor industry, in the pickling of metals, and in the preparation of phosphonium halides. It is a contaminant in acetylene. Significant phosphine gas exposure is relatively rare, and from 1900 to 1958, only 59 cases of phosphine gas exposure with 26 deaths were reported in the literature.[24–27]

During the past 35 years, significant exposures with a high mortality have been reported secondary to the hydrolysis of aluminum phosphide, zinc phosphide, and calcium phosphide. When solid phosphide comes in contact with hydrochloric acid in the stomach or water in grain moisture or air humidity, it forms toxic phosphine (PH_3) gas. Aluminum phosphide, or ALP (Celphos, Phostoxin, Quick Phos), is used as a grain preservative in silos, in elevators, and aboard ships. ALP is effective against rodents and insects and is used in tablet form. Zinc phosphide, or ZNP (Field Rat Powder), is a gray crystalline powder that, like ALP, is used as a rodenticide in agricultural regions. It is often mixed with bait foods such as cornmeal and, when used indiscriminantly, represents a definite risk to pets and children. Calcium phosphide, or CAP (Polytanol), is the European form of the rodenticide. Although rare reports describe accidental exposure secondary to grain fumigation and professional exterminating, the majority of cases are intentional suicide acts. In some parts of India, ALP and ZNP became so popular as suicide agents that their production and sale were banned.[28–31] One half of a tablet (1.5 g) of ALP ingested by mouth has been reported to result in successful suicides.[32] In children, phosphide has also been reported as a homicidal agent administered by parents who themselves have taken it with suicidal intent.[33]

The threshold limit value of phosphine is 0.3 ppm (gas) or 0.4 mg/m^3 (liquid). One 3-g tablet of ALP when brought into contact with water slowly produces 1 g of phosphine gas. It is monitored in the workplace or ambient air by gas chromatographic techniques. The gas is detectable by odor at 2 ppm, and even brief exposure is fatal in the range of 400 ppm.

Pathophysiology

In general, phosphine is a protoplasmic poison that interferes with enzymes and protein synthesis and primarily attacks the cardiovascular and respiratory systems. This ultimately results in peripheral vascular collapse, cardiac arrest and failure, and pulmonary edema. Singh and colleagues have shown in animals that phosphine causes noncompetitive inhibition of cytochrome oxidase of the myocardial mitochondria.[30] Similarly, other researchers have shown that phosphine inhibits the incorporation of amino acids into myocardial protein.[32] This is consistent with autopsy studies that have demonstrated fatty degeneration with myofibril necrosis. It has been suggested that these alterations in myocardial mitochondria and protein produce permeability disturbances to Na, K, Mg, Ca, and other ions, giving rise to changes in transmembrane action potentials.[28] For yet unknown reasons, these changes are much more prevalent in the myocardium, small peripheral vessels, and pulmonary cells, sparing the large vessels and major coronary arteries.

Pulmonary edema and pneumonitis are believed to result from direct cytotoxicity to the pulmonary cells. Autopsy studies have also shown fatty infiltrates, central necrosis with hemorrhage, and lymphocytic granulomas in the liver, as well as medullary congestion and tubular epithelial degeneration in the kidneys.[34] The propensity for phosphine to attack the small peripheral vessels can cause a profound decrease in systemic vascular resistance leading to marked hypotension at times unresponsive to pressor agents.

The majority of deaths occur within the first 12 to 24 hours and are usually cardiovascular in origin. Deaths after 24 hours are usually due to liver failure.[35]

Signs and Symptoms

Symptoms are primarily related to the cardiovascular and pulmonary systems and, if oral ingestion has taken place, the gastrointestinal system. Symptoms may include restlessness, irritability, drowsiness, tremors, paresthesias, vertigo, diplopia, ataxia, cough, dyspnea, retrosternal discomfort, abdominal pain, and vomiting. Exposure of silver nitrate-impregnated filter paper to either the gastric aspirate or the breath of a patient who ingested ALP turned the filter paper black.[36]

Signs, like symptoms, are multiple and represent various stages of cardiovascular collapse. These may include hypotension, reduction in cardiac output, tachycardia, oliguria, anuria, cyanosis, pulmonary edema, tachypnea, jaundice, hepatosplenomegaly, ileus, seizures, and diminished reflexes. Electrocardiographic (ECG) findings include ST segment elevation or depression, T wave inversion, sinus tachycardia, supraventricular tachycardia, atrial fibrillation and infarction, and atrioventricular conduction problems, especially right bundle branch block and complete atrioventricular dissociation. Of interest is the fact that if a patient survives the initial 24 hours, the ECG returns to normal in 10 to 25 days, indicating that the myocardial damage is reversible. Potentially life-threatening ECG abnormalities are found in more than 50% of these patients.[35, 37]

Chest radiographs usually reveal pulmonary edema. Laboratory studies reveal abnormalities in myocardial enzymes and liver function tests. Blood urea nitrogen and creatinine levels are usually elevated. Significant hypomagnesemia and hypermagnesemia have been found to be associated with massive focal myocardial damage and cardiotoxicity.[38, 39] Blood gases demonstrate a combined respiratory and metabolic acidosis. A complete blood count may reveal leukopenia and a low red blood cell count. Chronic skin exposure to 0.6 ppm caused hyperemia and hypersensitivity to touch.[35]

Of interest, workers exposed intermittently to levels up to 35 ppm but averaging less than 10 ppm complained of mild symptoms that resolved, and no cumulative effects were noted. Chronic low-level exposure led to toothache and mandibular swelling and, ultimately, jaw necrosis, the so-called phossy jaw.[33]

Signs and symptoms may mimic, in mild form, viral upper respiratory tract infections. In more severe forms, phosphine exposure may be confused with cardiogenic pulmonary edema, viral or bacterial pneumonias, or full-blown adult respiratory distress syndrome due to any cause.

Treatment

Initially, patients must be removed as quickly and safely as possible from the environment. All clothing should be removed and the skin washed. Oxygenation, intravenous fluids, vasopressors, plasma expanders, fresh blood transfusion, bronchodilators, and digoxin or calcium channel blockers must be considered based on the clinical picture. In the setting of oral phosphide ingestion, persistent hypotension unresponsive to vasopressors (e.g., dopamine) is much more prevalent than with phosphine gas exposure. Diuretics, if the patient is not hypotensive, should be considered for pulmonary edema. Seizures are controlled by the usual therapeutic modalities.

Calcium gluconate and 25% magnesium sulfate, because of their membrane-stabilizing effects, have been advocated and used with good results. If ingestion has occurred, gastric lavage with a potassium permanganate solution (1:10,000 dilution) is recommended. Permanganate oxidizes phosphine in the stomach to form phosphate, thereby reducing the available toxic phosphine. The results from potassium permanganate lavage are much better if instituted within 60 minutes of ingestion.[40–42] Singh and colleagues reported one survival in the presence of massive renal failure by using hemodialysis.[30] The value of steroids is not proved, but their use is thought to be helpful in reducing inflammation, especially in the pulmonary system.[25]

Prevention is the ultimate treatment and consists primarily of adequate ventilation and respiratory protection from phosphine gas. Accidental ingestion of phosphide is best avoided by control of its production and distribution as well as adequate warnings and education in areas where it is used. Pediatric exposure is best prevented by continued adult vigilance. Any person with underlying cardiac, pulmonary, liver, and renal disease should be precluded from possible exposure. Annual physical examinations and chest radiographs should be conducted on potentially exposed workers. In the workplace, frequent clothing changes and appropriately located showers and eye fountains should be available and used.

Long-Term Implications

The vast majority of deaths occur with the first 24 hours and depend on the concentration and duration as well as prompt recognition and treatment. In those fortunate individuals who survived the initial 24 hours, most showed no permanent disabilities within 30 days and all had returned to normal baseline within 4 months.[37, 40, 43] All liver, pulmonary, and renal function studies as well as ECG changes were normal within this time frame. Two studies examining cytogenetic effects in rats and genotoxicity in phosphine fumigators failed to show any ill effects or mutagenicity.[44, 45] In summary, full recovery is anticipated if patients survive the initial insult.

References

1. Misra NP, Manoria PC, Sacena K: Fatal pulmonary oedema with phosgene poisoning. J Assoc Physicians India *33*:430–431, 1985.
2. Stutz DR, Ricks RC, Olsen MF: Hazardous Materials Injuries: A Handbook for Pre-Hospital Care (Protocol 12). Greenbelt, MD, Bradford Communications Corp., 1982.
3. Plunkett ER: Handbook of Industrial Toxicology. 3rd ed. New York, Chemical Publishing Co., pp 428–430, 1987.
4. Proctor NH, Hughes JP: Chemical Hazards of the Workplace. Philadelphia, J. B. Lippincott Co., pp 414–415, 1978.
5. Bradley BL, Unger KM: Phosgene inhalation: A case report. Tex Med *78*:51–53, 1982.
6. Goldfrank LR: Toxicologic Emergencies: A Comprehensive Handbook in Problem Solving. New York, Appleton-Century-Crofts, pp 213–222, 1982.
7. Haddad LM, Winchester JF: Clinical Management of Poisoning and Drug Overdose. Philadelphia, W. B. Saunders Co., pp 805–806, 1983.
8. Snyder RW, Mishel HS, Christensen GC: Pulmonary toxicity following exposure to methylene chloride and its combustion product, phosgene. Chest *101*:860–861, 1992.
9. Snyder RW, Mishel HS, Christensen GC: Pulmonary toxicity following exposure to methylene chloride and its combustion product, phosgene. Chest *102*:1921, 1992.
10. Associated Press (byline): Akron Beacon Journal. December 13, 1987.
11. Sjogren B, Plato N, Alexandersson R, et al: Pulmonary reactions caused by welding-induced decomposed trichloroethylene. Chest *99*:237–238, 1991.
12. National Institute for Occupational Safety and Health: Occupational Exposure to Phosgene: Criteria for a Recommended Standard. Washington, DC, 1976.
13. Lorin HG, Kulling PEJ: The Bhopal tragedy—what has Swedish disaster medicine planning learned from it? J Emerg Med *4*:311–316, 1986.
14. Dangwal SK: A spectrophotometric method for determination of phosgene in air. Ind Health *32*:41–47, 1994.
15. Tobias JM, Pastel S, Patt HM, et al: Localization of the site of action of a pulmonary irritant, diphosgene. Am J Physiol *158*:173–183, 1949.
16. Ghio AJ, Kennedy T, Hatch G, et al: Reduction of neutrophil influx diminishes lung injury and mortality following phosgene inhalation. J Appl Physiol *71*:657–665, 1991.
17. Diller WF: The methenamine misunderstanding in the therapy of phosgene poisoning. Arch Toxicol *46*:199–206, 1980.
18. Ivanhoe F, Meyers PH: Phosgene poisoning as an example of neuroparalytic acute pulmonary oedema. The sympathetic vasometer reflex involved. Dis Chest *46*:211–218, 1964.
19. Dreisbach RH, Robertson WO: Handbook of Poisoning: Prevention, Diagnosis, and Treatment. Norwalk, CT, Appleton & Lange, 1987, pp 162–163, 243–249.
20. Kubic VL, Anders MW: Metabolism of carbon tetrachloride to phosgene. Life Sci *26*:2151, 1980.
21. Pohl LR, Bhooshan B, Krishna G: Mechanism of activation of chloroform. Toxicol Appl Pharmacol *45*:238, 1978.
22. Sciuto AM, Strickland PT, Kennedy TP, et al: Protective effects of *N*-acetylcysteine treatment after phosgene exposure in rabbits. Am J Respir Crit Care Med *151*:768–772, 1995.
23. Polednak AP: Mortality among men occupationally exposed to phosgene in 1943–1945. Environ Res *22*:357–367, 1980.
24. Plunkett ER: Handbook of Industrial Toxicology. 3rd ed. New York, Chemical Publishing Co., pp 430–432, 1987.
25. Haddad LM, Winchester JF: Clinical Management of Poisoning and Drug Overdose. Philadelphia, W. B. Saunders Co., 1983.
26. Stotz DR, Ricks RC, Olsen MF: Hazardous Materials Injuries: A Handbook for Pre-Hospital Care (Protocol 67). Greenbelt, MD, Bradford Communications Corp., 1982.
27. Morgan DP: Recognition and Management of Pesticide Poisonings. 3rd ed. US Environmental Protection Agency. Washington, DC, US Government Printing Office, 1982, p 68.
28. Jain SM, Bharani A, Sepaha GC, et al: Electrocardiographic changes in aluminum phosphide (ALP) poisoning. J Assoc Physicians India *33*:406–409, 1985.
29. DiPalma JR: Human toxicity from rat poisons. Clin Pharm *24*:186–189, 1981.
30. Singh S, Dilawari JB, Vashist R, et al: Aluminum phosphide ingestion. BMJ *290*:1110–1111, 1985.
31. Schoonbroodt D, Guffens P, Jousten P: Acute phosphine poisoning? A case report and review. Acta Clin Belg *47*:280–284, 1992.
32. Chan LTF, Crowley RJ, Delliou D, et al: Phosphine analysis in postmortem specimens following ingestion of aluminum phosphide. J Anal Toxicol *7*:165–167, 1983.
33. Sharma A, Gathwala G: Oral aluminum phosphide poisoning in Indian children. J Trop Med Hyg *95*:221–222, 1992.
34. Dreisbach RH, Robertson WO: Handbook of Poisoning: Prevention, Diagnosis, and Treatment. Norwalk, CT, Appleton & Lange, 1987.
35. Raman R, Dubey M: The electrocardiographic changes in quick phos poisoning. Indian Heart J *37*:193–195, 1985.
36. Mital HS, Mehotra TN, Dwivedi KK: A study of aluminum phosphide poisoning with special reference to its spot diagnosis by silver nitrate test. J Assoc Physicians India *40*:473–474, 1992.
37. Chugh SN, Chugh K, Ram S, et al: Electrocardiographic abnormalities in aluminum phosphide poisoning with special reference to its incidence, pathogenesis, mortality and histopathology. J Indian Med Assoc *89*:32–35, 1991.
38. Singh RB, Singh RG, Singh U: Hypermagnesemia following aluminum phosphide poisoning. Int J Clin Pharmacol Ther Toxicol *29*:82–85, 1991.
39. Chugh SN, Jaggal KL, Sharma A: Magnesium levels in acute cardiotoxicity due to aluminum phosphide poisoning. Indian J Med Res *94*:437–439, 1991.
40. Sepaha GC, Bharani AK, Jain SM, et al: Acute aluminum phosphide poisoning. J Indian Med Assoc *83*:378–379, 1985.
41. Chugh SN: Aluminum phosphide poisoning: Present status and management. J Assoc Physicians India *40*:401–405, 1992.
42. Khosla SN, Handa R, Khosla P: Aluminum phosphide poisoning. Trop Doct *22*:155–157, 1992.
43. Shusterman D: Problem-solving techniques in occupational medicine. J Fam Pract *21*:195–199, 1985.
44. Kligerman AD, Bryant MF, Doerr CL: Cytogenetic effects of phosphine inhalation in rodents. Environ Mol Mutagen *23*:186–189, 1994.
45. Barbosa A, Bonin A: Evaluation of phosphine genotoxicity at occupational levels of exposure in New South Wales, Australia. Occup Environ Med *51*:700–705, 1994.

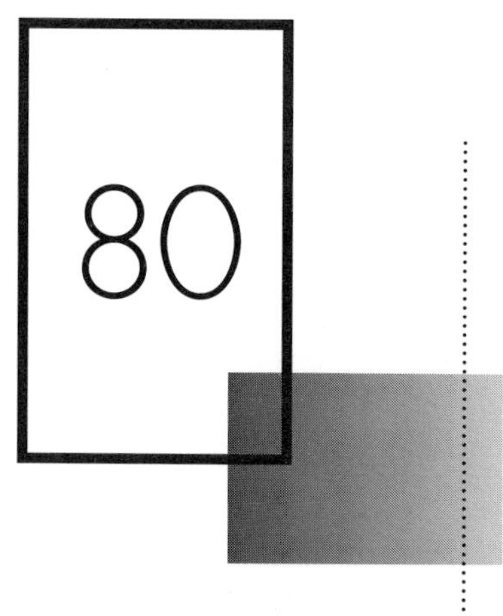

Chlorine

CHARLES A. McKAY, Jr, MD
JONATHAN BORAK, MD

Chlorine, a halogen element with atomic weight of 35.45, is a gas at standard temperature and pressure. It has a vapor pressure of 4800 mm Hg at 20°C and a relative density to air of 2.5. It is commonly used in industrial processes as a reagent in plastics manufacturing and as a bleaching agent in the paper industry.[1] Chlorine-producing compounds are also used as disinfectants and water-purifying agents. Although it was recognized in the 17th century that heating ammonium chloride and nitric acid together created an irritating gas, chlorine was first described and used as a bleaching agent in the 1770s. In 1774 chlorine was generated by oxygenation of hydrochloric acid, and it is currently produced by electrolysis of brine. More than 12 million tons was produced in the United States in 1988. The potential toxicity of this irritant gas resulted in its use as the first chemical warfare agent in World War I, although it was soon replaced by other substances such as sulfur mustard and phosgene. Of the 70,552 Americans who were victims of gassing, 1843 were reportedly exposed to chlorine.[2] Although acute mortality was infrequent, subsequent reviews demonstrated that a large number of exposed individuals had ongoing morbidity, usually noted as exertional dyspnea; as many as 52% demonstrated chronic pulmonary findings. The lack of uniform examinations and the technical limitations of studies performed 75 years ago, along with possible confounders such as smoking, tuberculosis, and other respiratory pathogens, limit the current applicability of these data. Nonetheless, the spectrum of possible acute and chronic sequelae of chlorine exposure is suggested by these early exposures.

Chlorine is the most compressible element; it is shipped as a pressurized liquid. One pound of liquid chlorine generates about 5 cu ft of gas when released. A typical rail tank car, containing more than 50 tons of liquid chlorine, would therefore be capable of releasing more than 500,000 cu ft of gas.[3] It is this potential for massive release that results in such concern about transportation and storage accidents involving chlorine.

EPIDEMIOLOGY

The 1994 summary of poisonings reported to the American Association of Poison Control Centers (AAPCC) documents 8913 exposures to chlorine-containing fumes/gases/vapors in the United States.[4] This represents 2% of all reported exposures to nonpharmaceutical agents. Table 80–1 shows the reported outcomes for some of these exposures. Clinical experience differs from the reported AAPCC data in that the most common source of chlorine exposure is the admixture of household cleaning agents. The combination of bleach (sodium hypochlorite) and acids or ammonia results in the formation of chlorine or chloramine gases, respectively.[5] Another common source of residential chlorine poisoning is from swimming pool disinfectant tablets/granules.[6–8] This is a particularly common exposure source for children. Industrial and transportation incidents account for infrequent but large-scale releases of chlorine gas.[9, 10]

MECHANISM OF TOXICITY

When chlorine comes in contact with water, hydrochloric acid and hypochlorous acid are generated (Fig. 80–1). Hypochlorous acid is thought to degenerate readily at physiologic pH to hydrochloric acid and oxygen free radicals. Hypochlorous acid is far more irritating than hydrochloric acid.[11]

As mentioned earlier, chloramine gas is generated

Table 80–1. Chlorine Exposures as Reported to the AAPCC

Substance	Exposure	Outcome				
		None	*Minor*	*Moderate*	*Major*	*Death*
Chlorine fumes:						
Acid/hypochlorite mix	749	34	378	130	1	0
Chlorine: other	5312	254	2581	783	18	2
Chloramine fumes	2852	92	1442	382	3	0

From Litovitz TL, Felberg L, Soloway RA, et al: 1994 Annual report of the American Association of Poison Control Centers toxic exposure surveillance system. Am J Emerg Med *13*:551–597, 1995.

when ammonia and bleach are mixed. Chloramine gas, when exposed to moist surfaces, also releases hypochlorous acid.[12] Chlorine itself is only moderately soluble in water, but these mixtures of household cleaning agents result in byproducts that markedly enhance its corrosive properties, resulting in coagulation necrosis and oxidative tissue damage.

CLINICAL PRESENTATION

Pathophysiology

Chlorine and chlorine-producing compounds primarily cause symptoms when inhaled in a closed space or in high concentrations. Chlorine is heavier than air (vapor density 2.5) and is recognizable in concentrated releases as a yellow-green cloud. The noxious odor does not serve as a reliable warning. The odor threshold of chlorine is less than 3 ppm, whereas the new Occupational Safety and Health Administration threshold limit value–time weighted average (TLV-TWA) for an 8-hour workday is 0.5 ppm. Extreme irritative symptoms can occur at levels as low as 1 ppm over 4 to 8 hours,[13] and levels of 30 ppm can lead to severe respiratory symptoms within minutes. Levels of 1000 ppm cause immediate death.[14]

Contact of chlorine gas with moist surfaces such as the mucous membranes of the eyes, mouth, and respiratory tract produces both upper and lower airway symptoms. Because chlorine is moderately water soluble, upper airway irritation tends to be prominent and serves as a noxious warning preventing continued voluntary exposure. For this reason, lower tract symptoms are less frequent than with other inhaled toxins having less water solubility, such as the oxides of nitrogen. However, severe lower airway damage can occur, particularly in settings of highly concentrated exposure or when victims are trapped. Persistent airways dysfunction and bronchiolitis obliterans have been described after acute exposure, although the true incidence of these chronic effects and their relation to smoking and pre-existing atopy are uncertain.[10, 15–17] Although repeated symptomatic chlorine exposures can also lead to persistent airways dysfunction, chronic exposure to controlled levels without acute symptomatic "gassing" episodes is unlikely to cause chronic pulmonary dysfunction.[18, 19]

$$Cl_2 + H_2O \longrightarrow HCl + HOCl$$

$$HOCl \longrightarrow HCl + O^-$$

Figure 80–1. Irritant products from reaction of chlorine with water.

Manifestations

The clinical spectrum following acute chlorine exposure can include mucous membrane irritation with chemical conjunctivitis, corneal burns, orofacial burns, acute tracheobronchitis, chemical pneumonitis, pulmonary edema, and hypoxemia with metabolic acidosis. Initial symptoms after exposure to chlorine fumes include cough and eye, nose, and throat irritation. Chest heaviness/burning, dyspnea, wheezing, and hemoptysis or syncope can occur with more severe exposures. Nonspecific nausea/vomiting, headache, dizziness, and chills may also be reported.

The physical findings are often unremarkable, although initial tachypnea, conjunctival injection, tearing, and wheezing may be found. Tachycardia and both mildly elevated and depressed temperature may be noted.

Various pulmonary function abnormalities have been reported in the hours after an acute exposure, including both restrictive and obstructive deficits. These changes represent the variable effects of differing concentrations of chlorine and its byproducts on the airways and parenchyma in patients with or without underlying lung diseases.[6] In one study that evaluated 18 patients after exposure to a chlorine tank leak, all subjects had evidence of moderate pulmonary obstruction, which improved over 2 weeks.[15] None developed pulmonary edema, although all were described as showing a "worsening clinical picture during the first 2 days of hospitalization, with signs of recovery noted thereafter." Despite this assessment, only one patient in that case series was treated with bronchodilators or steroids. The researchers described the presenting symptom of dyspnea as identifying individuals with a worse clinical course (slower recovery) than those with a primary complaint of paroxysmal dry cough. The former group was more likely to smoke (100% versus 25%) and to have a pre-exposure history of wheezing (50% versus 8%). This may serve as a useful triage tool in a multiple-patient encounter; however, prospective validation is lacking.

In one review of regional poison control center exposures, Mrvos and colleagues assessed symptoms in 216 individuals who were exposed to chlorine/chloramine gas from mixing household cleaners.[5] Symptoms were mild and did not require specific therapy. Most had early resolution of symptoms; only 16 had symptoms that persisted for more than 6 hours. One patient, who had underlying chronic pulmonary disease and a concurrent acute respiratory infection, was hospitalized. None developed pulmonary edema. This favorable experience can be contrasted with reports of acute pulmonary edema in two children immediately after brief exposures to vapors from containers of swimming pool chlorinator pellets.[7]

CASE SERIES

Important clinical findings from six relatively large case series of acute chlorine exposure are summarized in Table 80–2. In the poison center review mentioned earlier, Mrvos and co-workers[5] found a high prevalence of cough with little dyspnea, as well as rapid resolution of symptoms, after home exposures to mixed cleaning agents.

Fleta and associates[20] reported on 76 children (newborn to 14 years old) who were exposed to a leak of 300 L of chlorine gas from a pressurized canister used to purify municipal drinking water in Spain. Seventy of the 76 children were discharged from the hospital within 2 hours; the longest period of observation was 12 hours. No one developed pulmonary edema. Most symptoms resolved on removal from the source; those with "signs of irritation of the lower respiratory tract" were treated with oxygen and intramuscular corticosteroids.

Moulick and colleagues[17] described 82 adults (21 to 60 years old) who were within 20 yards of a chlorine storage tank leak in Bombay, India. An ambient chlorine concentration of 66 ppm was measured in the area 2 hours after the exposure. Sixty-two patients were hospitalized for 2 or more days. Two patients developed pulmonary edema within 6 to 8 hours; five had hypoxemia requiring ventilatory support. "Late" pneumonia developed in two patients. All 56 who underwent bronchoscopy had tracheobronchial mucosal congestion; 20 patients had hemorrhagic spots. Erosions or ulcerations were identified in seven patients; the presence of these correlated with more severe symptoms. All patients were treated with oxygen, aminophylline, hydrocortisone, and ampicillin. Four of 16 patients who were observed for a year or more had persistent cough for 4 to 6 weeks; no residual symptoms or chest radiographic or pulmonary function abnormalities were found at the end of the follow-up.

Hedges and Morrissey[9] summarized findings in 64 patients evaluated after a leak of approximately 4 tons of liquid chlorine from storage tanks in Philadelphia. These patients represented about 60% of the people evaluated at one medical center; after triage, the others were found to be asymptomatic and were sent home from the waiting area. All six patients admitted to the hospital with "marked tracheobronchitis" complained of dyspnea, whereas this complaint was present in only 10% of those able to be discharged. There were no deaths or cases of pulmonary edema. Symptomatic patients were treated with humidified oxygen, a combination of bronchodilators, and antitussives. Triage and treatment recommendations for management of multiple-casualty chlorine exposures were made by these researchers.

Bosse[21] reviewed 86 cases (24 adults) seen at 49 medical facilities in Kentucky with poison center recommendation of nebulized sodium bicarbonate treatment for symptomatic chlorine inhalation. Sixty-nine patients were discharged from the emergency department after one to two nebulized sodium bicarbonate treatments. Seven patients were treated with bronchodilators, and one received steroids. Seventeen patients were admitted to the hospital for 1 to 3 days. All improved; none developed pulmonary edema or required ventilatory support. Some received sodium bicarbonate; four were treated with inhaled bron-

Table 80–2. Representative Distributions of Findings in Reported Exposures to Chlorine Gas

	% Reported Occurrence					
Symptom/Sign	**Mrvos et al[5]**	**Fleta et al[20]**	**Moulick et al[17]**	**Hedges and Morrissey[9]**	**Bosse[21]**	**Weill et al[22]**
Oropharyngeal irritation	6	66	100	23	14	—
Cough	84	91	100	30	52	81
Dyspnea	19	14	100	19	51	85
Chest pain	5	14	5	17	34	—
Headache	—	9	29	9	1	—
Vomiting	3	5	24	19	8	69
Abdominal pain	<1	—	27	—	1	—
Eye complaints	2	—	—	36	—	80
Hoarseness	—	14	—	—	—	—
Loss of consciousness	—	3	—	—	—	—
Tachypnea	—	20	100	—	2	—
Shock/stupor	—	—	—	—	—	62
Rhonchi/wheezing	4	—	100	—	21	—
Rales	—	—	30	—	—	—

chodilators, and one each received inhaled steroids and intravenous aminophylline.

Weill and colleagues[22] summarized initial symptoms and results of pulmonary function follow-up in those exposed to release of up to 30 tons of liquid chlorine after a freight train derailment in Louisiana. Ambient chlorine levels in some areas 7 hours after the derailment were in excess of 400 ppm, and levels at the fringe of contamination 3 hours after the event were 10 ppm.[23] Hundreds of animals in the area died; more than 100 people developed symptoms requiring treatment. The symptoms in the 17 admitted patients of 75 who were treated at one hospital are noted in the table. One infant died shortly after severe exposure. Therapy at that time (1961) relied mainly on oxygen, postural drainage, atropine, penicillin, chymotrypsin, Alevaire (a non-ionic surfactant, sodium bicarbonate, and glycerin), and some narcotics and expectorants.

It is important to understand the circumstances of exposure when interpreting the relative prominence of findings such as those listed in Table 80–2. It should be apparent that the symptoms demonstrated by any one individual depend heavily on the circumstances of exposure and individual predisposing characteristics such as smoking history and atopy.

DIAGNOSIS

Chlorine gas toxicity is primarily a clinical diagnosis suggested by the circumstances of exposure and a cluster of symptoms and signs as described earlier. Laboratory evaluation is nonspecific, often revealing leukocytosis, metabolic acidosis, and hypoxemia or respiratory alkalosis in those who are most symptomatic. Chest radiographs may demonstrate focal areas of consolidation, central pulmonary congestion, or diffuse increased interstitial markings.[24] Pneumomediastinum has also been reported. All of these abnormalities generally correlate with more severe clinically apparent disease. Triage can be performed on a clinical basis. Laboratory studies other than pulse oximetry should have little if any role in the initial assessment and disposition of exposed individuals.

Severe exposures may cause noncardiogenic pulmonary edema. Concern about clinical deterioration after initial improvement has led to over-reliance on laboratory investigations and uncertainty about the treatment of asymptomatic patients. From available data, the following triage guidelines can be generated:

1. Mildly affected individuals improve with removal from exposure. Symptomatic treatment with humidified oxygen or bronchodilators may be beneficial. Asymptomatic individuals will not worsen.
2. Moderately affected individuals, if asymptomatic after a period of several hours after treatment, will not acutely worsen. Those with underlying pulmonary or atopic conditions may have persistence of reactive airways for weeks to months after the acute exposure. Rarely, chemical or infectious pneumonitis may develop over a few days after exposure.
3. Severely affected individuals demonstrate symptoms early and stabilize or suffer worsening of their condition; they require aggressive treatment and immediate hospitalization.

A triage algorithm is provided in Figure 80–2.

TREATMENT

After victims are removed from the source of exposure, involved skin or symptomatic eyes should be copiously irrigated with water. Attention should focus on a patient's airway and any respiratory complaints. Aggressive treatment includes high-flow humidified oxygen, inhaled bronchodilators, intravenous aminophylline, and intravenous corticosteroids. Arrhythmias are not a prominent complication of chlorine fume inhalation; once supplemental oxygen has been provided, subcutaneous epinephrine, if it is the only β-adrenergic agent available, should not be withheld for fear of provoking arrhythmias. Patients with respiratory failure secondary to pulmonary edema or the rare individual with upper airway obstruction from chlorine-induced burns may require intubation with early administration of positive end-expiratory pressure.[25] Although opiates have not been used at times because of the risks of altered mental status, respiratory depression, and cough inhibition, judicious use of parenteral opiates with close observation may be beneficial.[26]

Some investigators have advocated nebulized sodium bicarbonate for patients with persistent cough or those with evidence of severe pulmonary injury. This therapy attempts to chemically neutralize the acid products of chlorine hydration. In one animal study, 10 sheep treated with this modality after 4 minutes of exposure to 500 ppm chlorine had statistically higher PO_2 and lower PCO_2 values than animals treated with nebulized normal saline, although there was no difference in the mortality rate of 30% at 24 hours.[27] It has been recommended and used in unselected patient cohorts with anecdotal reports of improvement, but its value is unproven; no reports have described clinical worsening with this therapy.[21, 28] Although nebulized bicarbonate has been condemned because of concern about thermal injury from the heat of neutralization, this risk is theoretically minimized by the large surface area of the lungs as well as the small volumes of bicarbonate administered. Given the proposed mechanism, this therapy would seem most useful early in a patient with significant lower airway penetration of chlorine. It has been used in a dose of 3mL 8.4% sodium bicarbonate and 2mL normal saline nebulized with oxygen or air. The nebulization can be repeated if beneficial; however, there is no rationale for its continued use long after the exposure.

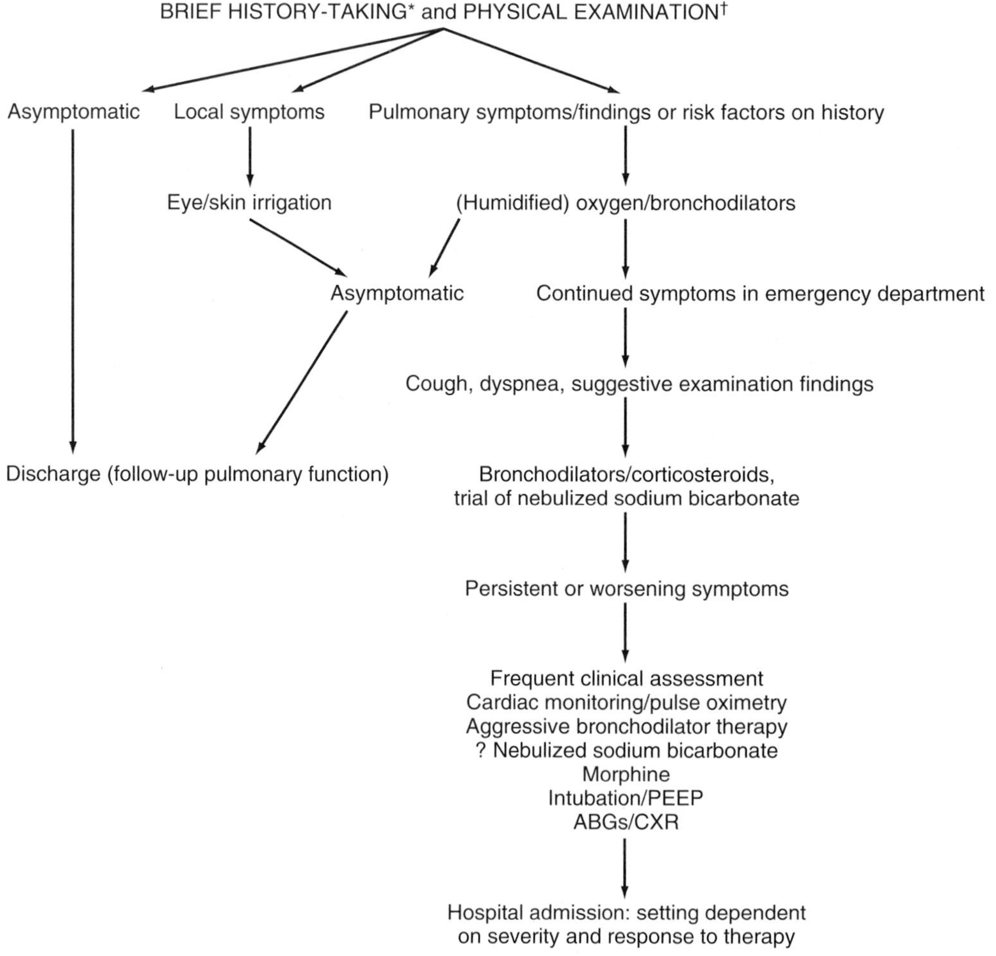

*Brief history-taking: Focus on concurrent trauma, burns, symptoms referable to mucous membrane, pulmonary signs (cough vs. dyspnea), nonspecific chest pain, nausea/vomiting, and mental status changes, as well as history of atopy, asthma, cardiopulmonary disease, or smoking.

†Physical examination: Evaluate vital signs, mucous membranes, and stridor; perform pulmonary examination.

Figure 80–2. Triage guidelines following acute chlorine exposure. PEEP, positive end-expiratory pressure; ABGs, arterial blood gases (analysis); CXR, chest radiography.

Corticosteroids have been used to treat pulmonary edema and bronchospastic symptoms. As with many proposed uses of these anti-inflammatory agents, their efficacy in the treatment of chlorine toxicity has never been subjected to a randomized trial. One report of two sisters exposed to the same chlorine release suggested that the more rapid improvement in pulmonary parameters of one patient could be attributed to the combination of hospital admission, rest, and treatment with oxygen and corticosteroids compared with the sibling who received only brief oxygen therapy.[29] To date, this anecdotal report forms the basis for any recommended use of corticosteroids after chlorine exposure.

Another potential treatment modality focuses on reducing the oxidative destruction that potentially follows chlorine-induced generation of oxygen radicals. Animal models of smoke inhalation, hydrochloric acid aspiration, and pulmonary macrophage allergic response suggest that ibuprofen can reduce pulmonary injury when administered shortly after exposure to these agents.[30, 31] Inhibition of thromboxane A_2 synthesis has been postulated to be the mechanism for these effects. No clinical reports have described the utility of this agent after chlorine inhalation.

Antibiotics, although historically used after chlorine-induced pulmonary injury, should be reserved for documented episodes of infection, which for the most part become manifested days after exposure. The initial tachypnea, sputum production, pulmonary findings, and consolidation on chest radiographs are attributable to chemical tracheobronchopneumonitis or pulmonary edema. Although this mucosal damage may provide entry for subsequent infection, prophylactic antibiotics are unlikely to contravene this process. In hospitalized individuals, the use of unnecessary antibiotics may also predispose to infection with antibiotic-resistant or other opportunistic organisms.

CHRONIC CHLORINE EXPOSURE

Other areas of potential concern about chlorine toxicity include chronic effects from low-level ambient workplace exposure and the potential carcinogenic or teratogenic effects of oral exposure to chlorinated water supplies. As described earlier, reversible obstructive airways dysfunction in workers continually exposed to chlorine has been demonstrated,[18, 19] although the effect of concurrent cigarette smoking, atopy, and the contribution of acute exposures above TLV-TWA levels ("gassing") made it difficult to sort out relative contributions. In one study, the effects of up to 2.3 ppm chlorine inhalation by rhesus monkeys for 6 hours daily for 1 year were evaluated. Conjunctival and focal tracheal irritative changes were seen only at the highest exposure levels, and not in all animals.[32] The vast majority of individuals after an acute exposure do not suffer prolonged airway dysfunction, although resolution of abnormal findings on pulmonary function tests can be prolonged, particularly in smokers and those with pre-existing pulmonary function abnormalities.[33–35]

Some halogenated compounds are known to be mutagenic. The use of chlorine, chloramine, and chlorine dioxide as disinfecting and bleaching agents in municipal water supplies and the food industry has therefore generated concern about the tradeoff between convenience, markedly improved sanitation, and the risk of increased cancer incidence. Concern has focused on the generation of trihalomethane chlorine byproducts such as chloroform. The water concentration of these byproducts is increased by the higher concentration of nitrogen waste products in surface water[36] and heat.[37] A small study demonstrated detectable chloroform in the blood of indoor competitive swimmers (mean 0.89 ng/mL), which was not found in outdoor swimmers.[38] This was associated with a "significantly elevated" β_2-microglobulin urine concentration, possibly suggesting renal damage. Patients on long-term hemodialysis are another group exposed to increased concentrations of chlorine byproducts.[39] Community-based population studies have also suggested a statistical increase in the relative risk (ranging from 1.2 to 2.2) of a number of cancers in those populations dependent on chlorinated surface water when compared with ground water users.[40, 41] The affected sites have included the bladder, kidneys, pancreas, stomach, and rectum, and malignant melanoma has also been associated. These associations obviously do not equate with causality, particularly within the individual. Various confounding variables, including socioeconomic factors or the presence of other toxic compounds, could have a role.

Similar concerns have been raised about possible reproductive toxicity of chlorine byproducts. Although severe acute exposures have resulted in fetal wastage in cows and decreased egg production in chickens,[23] low-level oral exposure to sodium hypochlorite in the drinking water of hens did not alter egg production until the chloride concentration exceeded 40 ppm.[42] Chlorine treatment of both male and female rats with up to 5 mg/kg per day resulted in no detectable reproductive or fetal changes.[43] Despite these reassurances, there have been calls to ban the use of chlorine. Caution must be exercised before abandoning the use of a substance with at most uncertain low-level toxicity in favor of other agents that have not been studied as extensively.[44] Nonetheless, given the ubiquitous nature of chlorination processes, these issues will continue to be studied.

References

1. Scone JS: Chlorine: Its Manufacture, Properties and Uses. New York, Reinhold, 1962.
2. Das R, Blanc PD: Chlorine gas exposure and the lung: A review. Toxicol Ind Health *9*:439–455, 1993.
3. Borak J: Chlorine. TEMIS 5.4. New Haven, CT, Jonathan Borak & Co., 1995.
4. Litovitz TL, Felberg L, Soloway RA, et al: 1994 Annual report of the American Association of Poison Control Centers toxic exposure surveillance system. Am J Emerg Med *13*:551–597, 1995.
5. Mrvos R, Dean BS, Krenzelok EP: Home exposure to chlorine/chloramine gas: Review of 216 cases. South Med J *86*:654–657, 1993.
6. Ploysongsang Y, Beach BC, DiLisio RE: Pulmonary function changes after acute inhalation of chlorine gas. South Med J *75*:23–26, 1982.
7. Wood BR, Colombo JL, Benson BE: Chlorine inhalation toxicity from vapors generated by swimming pool chlorinator tablets. Pediatrics *79*:427–429, 1987.
8. Martinez TT, Long C: Explosion risk from swimming pool chlorinators and review of chlorine toxicity. J Toxicol Clin Toxicol *33*:349–354, 1995.
9. Hedges JR, Morrissey WL: Acute chlorine gas exposure. JACEP *8*:59–64, 1979.
10. Jones RN, Hughes JM, Glindmeyer H, Weill H: Lung function after acute chlorine exposure. Am Rev Respir Dis *134*:1190–1195, 1986.
11. Barrow CS, Alarie Y, Warrick JC, et al: Comparison of the sensory irritation response in mice to chlorine and hydrogen chloride. Arch Environ Health *32*:68–76, 1977.
12. Krenzelok E, Mrvos R: Chlorine/chloramine. J Toxicol Clin Toxicol *33*:355–357, 1995.
13. Rotman HH, Fliegelman MJ, Moore T, et al: Effects of low concentrations of chlorine on pulmonary function in humans. J Appl Physiol *54*:1120–1124, 1983.
14. Hathaway GJ, Proctor NH, Hughes JP, et al: Chemical Hazards of the Workplace. 3rd ed. New York, Van Nostrand Reinhold, 1991.
15. Hasan FM, Gehshan A, Fuleihan FJD: Resolution of pulmonary dysfunction following acute chlorine exposure. Arch Environ Health *38*:76–80, 1983.
16. Kaufman J, Burkons D: Clinical, roentgenologic, and physiologic effects of acute chlorine exposure. Arch Environ Health *23*:29–34, 1971.
17. Moulick ND, Banavali S, Abhyankar AD, et al: Acute accidental exposure to chlorine fumes. Indian J Chest Dis Allied Sci *34*:85–89, 1992.
18. Malo JL, Cartier A, Boulet LP, et al: Bronchial hyperresponsiveness can improve while spirometry plateaus two to three years after repeated exposure to chlorine causing respiratory symptoms. Am J Res Crit Care Med *150*:1142–1145, 1994.
19. Bherer L, Cushman R, Courteau JP, et al: Survey of construc-

tion workers repeatedly exposed to chlorine over a three to six month period in a pulpmill: II. Follow up of affected workers by questionnaire, spirometry, and assessment of bronchial responsiveness 18 to 24 months after exposure ended. Occup Environ Med *51*:225–228, 1994.

20. Fleta J, Calvo C, Zuniga J, et al: Intoxication of 76 children by chlorine gas. Hum Toxicol *5*:99–100, 1986.
21. Bosse GM: Nebulized sodium bicarbonate in the treatment of chlorine gas inhalation. J Toxicol Clin Toxicol *32*:233–241, 1994.
22. Weill H, George R, Schwarz M, Ziskind M: Late evaluation of pulmonary function after acute exposure to chlorine gas. Am Rev Respir Dis *90*:374–379, 1969.
23. Joyner RE, Durel EG: Accidental liquid chlorine spill in a rural community. J Occup Med *4*:152–154, 1962.
24. Beach FXM, Jones ES, Scarrow GD: Respiratory effects of chlorine gas. Br J Ind Med *26*:231–236, 1969.
25. Heidemann SM, Goetting MG: Treatment of acute hypoxemic respiratory failure caused by chlorine exposure. Pediatr Emerg Care *7*:87–88, 1991.
26. Pino F, Puerta H, D'Apollo R, et al: Effectiveness of morphine in noncardiogenic pulmonary edema due to chlorine gas inhalation. Vet Hum Toxicol *35*:36, 1993.
27. Chisholm CD, Sigletary EM, Okerberg CV, Langinais PC: Inhaled sodium bicarbonate therapy for chlorine inhalation injuries. Abstract. Ann Emerg Med *18*:466, 1989.
28. Vinsel PJ: Treatment of acute chlorine gas inhalation with nebulized sodium bicarbonate. J Emerg Med *8*:327–329, 1990.
29. Chester EH, Kaimal PJ, Payne CB Jr, Kohn PM: Pulmonary injury following exposure to chlorine gas. Chest *72*:247–250, 1977.
30. Tamaoki J: Possible contribution of lung macrophage to airway hyperreactivity. Jpn J Thorac Dis *28*:1294–1298, 1990.
31. Shinozawa Y, Hales C, Jung W, et al: Ibuprofen prevents synthetic smoke-induced pulmonary edema. Am Rev Respir Dis *134*:1145–1148, 1986.
32. Klonne DR, Ulrich CE, Riley MG, et al: One-year inhalation toxicity study of chlorine in rhesus monkeys *(Macaca mulatta)*. Fund Appl Toxicol *9*:557–572, 1987.
33. Abhyankar A, Bhambure N, Kamath NN, et al: Six month follow-up of fourteen victims with short-term exposure to chlorine gas. J Soc Occup Med *39*:131–132, 1989.
34. Donnelly SC, FitzGerald MX: Reactive airways dysfunction syndrome (RADS) due to chlorine gas exposure. Ir J Med Sci *159*:275–276, 1990.
35. Demeter SL, Cordasco EN: Reactive airway disease after chlorine gas exposure. Letter. Chest *102*:984, 1992.
36. Rice RG, Gomez-Taylor M: Occurrence of by-products of strong oxidants reacting with drinking water contaminants—scope of the problem. Environ Health Perspec *69*:31–44, 1986.
37. Weisel CP, Chen WJ: Exposure to chlorination by-products from hot water uses. Risk Anal *14*:101–106, 1994.
38. Aiking H, van Acker MB, Scholten RJ, et al: Swimming pool chlorination: A health hazard? Toxicol Lett *72*:375–380, 1994.
39. Smith RP, Willhite CC: Chlorine dioxide and hemodialysis. Regul Toxicol Pharmacol *11*:42–62, 1990.
40. McGeehin MA, Reif JS, Becher JC, Mangione EJ: Case-control study of bladder cancer and water disinfection methods in Colorado. Am J Epidemiol *138*:492–501, 1993.
41. Morris RD, Audet AM, Angelillo IF, et al: Chlorination, chlorination by-products, and cancer: A meta-analysis. Am J Public Health *82*:955–963, 1992.
42. Damron BL, Flunker LK: Broiler chick and laying hen tolerance to sodium hypochlorite in drinking water. Poultry Sci *72*:1650–1655, 1993.
43. Carlton BD, Barlett P, Basaran A, et al: Reproductive effects of alternative disinfectants. Environ Health Persp *69*:237–241, 1986.
44. Karol MH: Toxicologic principles do not support the banning of chlorine. A society of toxicology position paper. Fund Appl Toxicol *24*:1–2, 1995.

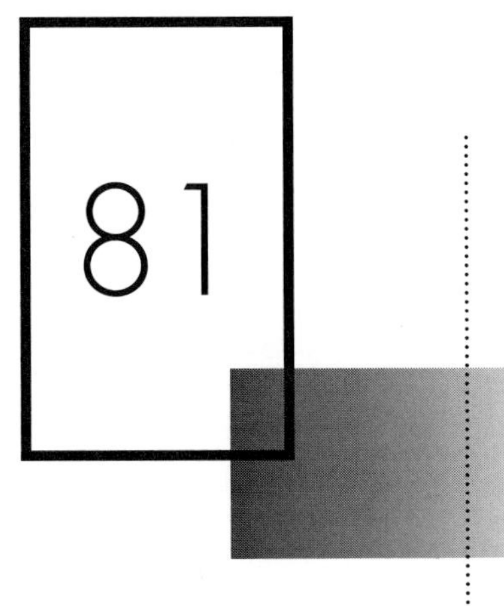

Methyl Bromide and Related Compounds

SUSAN M. POND, MBBS, MD

Methyl bromide has had a variety of industrial applications for more than a century. These have included use as an alkylating agent, fire retardant, and fumigant.[1] Its medical application as an anesthetic agent was abandoned in the early 1900s after several patients to whom it was administered died. *Methyl iodide,* a related compound, is used mainly as a methylating agent in the synthesis of pharmaceuticals and chemicals. It also has a place as an embedding material in microscopy, as a reagent for testing pyridine, as a catalyst, as a light-sensitive etching agent, and as a component of fire extinguishers.[2, 3] *Ethylene dibromide* has major roles in the fumigation of food and soil and in the scavenging of the inorganic lead compounds formed in gasoline during combustion. The use of ethylene dibromide in agriculture was banned in the United States in 1983. *Ethylene dichloride* is a chemical that is used in high volume, mostly as an intermediate in the production of vinyl chloride. It has other applications as well—as a lead scavenger in gasoline, as a solvent and dispersant, and as a component of fumigants for upholstery, carpet, and grains.[4–6]

Small amounts of methyl bromide and methyl iodide are produced by natural processes in marine algae and kelp. These processes contribute to methyl bromide's being the most abundant bromine species in the atmosphere.[7, 8] *The additional amounts of methyl bromide emitted into the atmosphere in exhaust from cars and from fumigation sites are thought to be contributing to the destruction of stratospheric ozone.*[8]

Although its use in gasoline and fire extinguishers is being curtailed, methyl bromide still fulfills a vital role as a fumigant for the control of pests not eradicated by any other means. In order to reduce the atmospheric load of this agent, microorganisms that can dehalogenate such compounds are being identified and characterized for potential environmental scavenging.[9] The approaches that have been taken to control the toxicity—particularly the neurotoxicity—of the haloalkanes are stringent industrial hygiene standards and precautions.[1, 2, 7, 10] Most cases of poisoning that have been reported involve accidental or deliberate violation of these standards.

EPIDEMIOLOGY

A comprehensive review of human poisoning by methyl bromide was published in 1983.[1] From the first case in 1899 until the publication of that review, 950 cases of death, serious systemic effects, and skin and eye injuries had been reported.[1] Many of the cases reported until 1940 involved the use of methyl bromide in fire extinguishers. This application was then abandoned except in extinguishers reserved for very specific situations. Since 1940, almost all toxic exposures have been attributed to the use of methyl bromide as a fumigant. Accounting for the relatively large number of methyl bromide poisoning cases are the absence of "warning" properties associated with the agent, such as a characteristic odor; its rapid vaporization; a density greater than that of air; its ability to penetrate many substances, including concrete, rubber, and protective clothing; slow off-gassing from fumigated material; and delayed onset of symptoms from toxicity. In an attempt to prevent exposures, many formulations with methyl bromide now contain chloropicrin, which serves as an olfactory warning agent.

Nevertheless, since 1983, a steady trickle of case

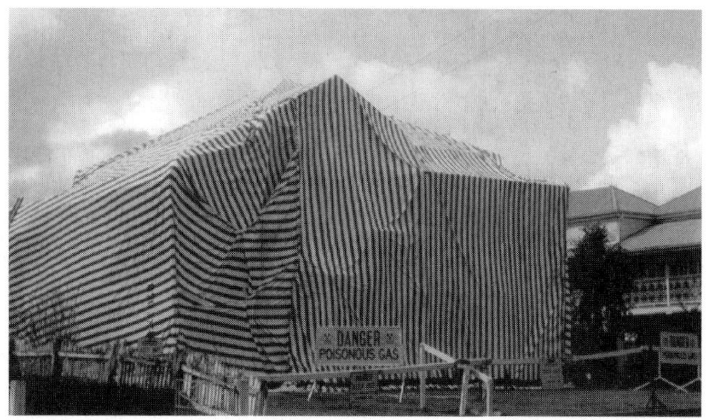

Figure 81–1. Queensland house covered with tent in preparation for fumigation with methyl bromide. (Photograph provided by the Department of Primary Industries, Queensland, Australia.)

reports has continued to appear in the literature.[7, 12–30] In one case series from Florida, six of seven poisoning cases involved burglars who entered houses that were covered with a tent, such as that shown in Figure 81–1, in preparation for fumigation with methyl bromide.[24] Despite formulation with chloropicrin, the warning agent was not sufficiently noxious nor was it retained in a concentration sufficient to prevent the illegal entry. Thus, exposure to toxic concentrations of methyl bromide retained within such a tent can lead to severe toxicity and death.

The number of reported cases of poisoning from methyl iodide[2, 3, 31–33] and the two ethyl halides, ethylene dibromide[10, 34, 35] and ethylene dichloride,[5, 6, 11] is much smaller. Methyl iodide has a chloroform-like odor, and ethylene dibromide has a powerful, disagreeable odor; these odors serve as a warning of their presence. Ethylene dichloride and ethylene dibromide have low vapor pressures which limit the concentrations that these agents reach in air. The restricted use of methyl bromide and ethylene dichloride as fumigants has reduced the number of uncontrolled and accidental exposures to them.

TOXICOLOGY

Chemical Identification and Structure

The chemical formulae and relevant chemical characteristics of the four haloalkanes are listed in Table 81–1. The three compounds that are used as fumigants are effective because of their ability to penetrate quickly and deeply into bulk materials and soil and leave an effective, long-term residue. They either leach out into the air or degrade slowly. Therefore, after reclosure of a fumigated container that has been ventilated adequately after initial fumigation, off-gassing can lead to reaccumulation of toxic concentrations of the fumigant in air.[7]

Table 81–1. Physicochemical Characteristics and Industrial Applications of the Haloalkanes

Characteristic	Methyl Bromide	Methyl Iodide	Ethylene Dibromide	Ethylene Dichloride
Chemical formula	CH_3Br	CH_3I	$C_2H_4Br_2$	$C_2H_4Cl_2$
Relative molecular mass	94.94	141.94	187.88	98.96
Chemical Abstracts Service name	Bromomethane	Iodomethane	1,2-Dibromoethane	1,2-Dichloroethane
Chemical Abstracts Service registry number	74-83-9	74-88-4	106-93-4	107-06-2
Synonym(s)	Monobromomethane	—	EDB	Dutch liquid, EDC, ethylene chloride, dichloroethylene
Boiling point at 1 atm (°C)	3.56	42.4	131.4	83.5
Vapor pressure at 20–25°C (mm Hg)	1520	400	11	64
Relative vapor density (air = 1)	3.3	4.9	6.1	3.4
Physical properties at normal temperature and pressure	Colorless gas; odorless except at high concentrations; penetrates many substances, including concrete, rubber, brick, and wood	Clear, colorless liquid; pungent odor	Heavy liquid, chloroform odor	Clear, colorless, oily liquid
Uses	Fumigation of soil, buildings, furniture, books and archived material, commodities; chemical intermediate; special purpose fire extinguishers	Chemical intermediate; microscopy, as an embedding material and reagent to test for pyridine; catalyst; etching agent; fire extinguishers	Fumigation of soil and commodities; scavenger of lead antiknock agents in gasoline	Chemical intermediate (primarily in the production of vinyl chloride); scavenger of lead antiknock agents in gasoline; solvent; fumigant

Toxicokinetics

The major route of entry of methyl bromide gas into humans is by inhalation, although concurrent dermal absorption is always possible because of the high penetrability of the toxin. Poisoning has occurred following acute, subacute, and long-term exposures. When exposure is acute, symptoms develop with a rapidity that correlates directly with the concentration. It is important to note, however, that symptoms may be delayed even with high-concentration exposures. Reported latent periods range from 1 hour to longer than 48 hours in duration.[1, 7] In general, the latent period is longer with exposures of lesser intense. Fatal poisoning has followed exposure to concentrations of methyl bromide in air of 8600 ppm or greater, and nonfatal poisoning of 390 ppm or greater.[7]

The haloalkanes are absorbed rapidly through the skin, mucous membranes, and pulmonary alveoli; they are then distributed widely throughout the body before being rapidly eliminated.[25, 36, 37] In animals, their metabolism is extensive and mediated mainly via cytosolic glutathione-*S*-transferases and microsomal cytochrome P-450.[2, 38–44] Exposure to high concentrations depletes glutathione and favors metabolism by the microsomal cytochrome P-450 system to carbon dioxide, the halide ion, and acetaldehyde and alcohol metabolites, which form conjugates with glutathione. Apart from reacting directly with the sulfhydryl group on glutathione, the haloalkanes also can undergo nucleophilic substitution with thiol and similarly reactive groups on proteins and nucleic acids. The direct glutathione conjugates are toxic and can form adducts.[41] Not surprisingly, all four compounds are mutagenic in a variety of *in vitro* tests. In animal models, their metabolites form adducts with proteins, lipids, and DNA. Adducts of hemoglobin in humans exposed to the methyl halides also have been reported.[45]

Genetic variability in the glutathione-*S*-transferase pathway has been demonstrated in humans; thus, when exposed to methyl chloride, some individuals excrete *S*-methylcysteine metabolites in urine whereas others do not.[46] Similarly, in workers exposed to methyl bromide, three of seven workers subjected to the highest exposure had high concentrations of *S*-methylcysteine hemoglobin adducts, but the four others in the same exposure group did not.[45] The implications of this genetic variability in metabolism for the susceptibility of individuals to toxicity from these agents are not known.

Mechanisms of Toxicity

The major target organs for acute toxicity of all four compounds are the central nervous system, liver, kidneys, and testes. The compounds also are severely irritating to the skin and mucous membranes.

The exact mechanisms of toxicity are not well understood because the haloalkanes produce such disastrous disruption of cellular function that it is difficult to study the sequential events after exposure. Nevertheless, the alkylation of proteins and nucleic acids by the parent compounds as well as some of their glutathione conjugates appears to be the fundamental process that produces the cellular damage. Accumulation of aldehydes also could mediate some of the toxicity via DNA-protein cross-linkages. The halide ion and alcohol metabolites are not thought to mediate the acute toxicity.

Whatever the mechanisms, the severity of toxicity is related to both the concentration and the duration of exposure, and the dose-mortality curve for these compounds is very steep.[1, 2, 5, 7, 10, 11]

On the basis of the topographic distribution of pathologic abnormalities in the brain of one patient who died 30 days after exposure to methyl bromide from a leaking fire extinguisher, Cavanagh hypothesized that the primary target of these compounds' neurotoxicity was the neuronal mitochondrion, where most cellular adenosine triphosphate is produced.[16] Classic toxins that inhibit mitochondrial respiration include cyanide, hydrogen sulfide, rotenone, and fluoroacetate. Some features of the toxicity of the haloalkanes (in particular, their targeting of the brain, which has a high requirement for adenosine triphosphate) and the metabolic acidosis that they produce are consistent with the hypothesis that these agents are mitochondrial toxins.

CLINICAL PRESENTATION

Pathophysiology

Postmortem examination of animals and patients who have died from methyl bromide intoxication reveals a range of abnormalities, the severity and extent of which correlate with the intensity (concentration and duration) of exposure.[1, 7, 13, 16, 42] Cytotoxic effects can be expected in virtually all organs and tissues. The skin and mucous membranes can be burned and blistered. The lungs can be edematous, hemorrhagic, and infiltrated with inflammatory cells. Renal tubular, hepatocellular, and myocardial necrosis develop. Neurotoxic effects can be evident throughout the central and peripheral nervous systems in the form of axonal degeneration, neuronal loss, demyelination, and hemorrhage. These findings are similar to those reported postmortem in patients who died from methyl iodide,[47] ethylene dibromide,[34, 35] and ethylene dichloride[11] toxicity.

A sural nerve biopsy in a patient who developed a peripheral neuropathy after chronic exposure to methyl bromide demonstrated loss of large axons and degenerating fibers (both myelinated and unmyelinated).[15] This patient and two others with similar exposure also had acquired color blindness, indicating the additional propensity of methyl bromide to damage the retina and cranial nerves. Optic atrophy has been observed in more severe cases.[15, 17] Electrophysiologic studies in patients with methyl bromide–

induced myoclonus implicated involvement of the sensorimotor cortex and pyramidal tracts and provide evidence for a further manifestation of its toxicity.[28]

Skin biopsies of areas of severe blistering in fumigators wearing protective breathing apparatus reveal necrotic keratinocytes, severe edema of the upper dermis, subepidermal blistering, and an inflammatory cell infiltrate, predominantly of neutrophils but with some eosinophils.[22]

Abnormal clinical chemistry and blood gas results reflect the renal tubular and hepatocellular necrosis, pneumonitis, and necrosis of other organs or tissues, including brain and muscle.

Clinical Manifestations

The clinical features of poisoning by this class of compounds have been described best for methyl bromide but are very similar in cases of poisoning by methyl iodide, ethylene dibromide, and ethylene dichloride. The chloropicrin added to methyl bromide formulations is itself an irritant, producing lacrimation as the early warning symptom.[20]

The early symptoms of acute exposure include burning and irritation of the eyes, skin, nose and throat, dizziness, headache, nausea, and vomiting. In mild cases, these may be the only manifestations. Moderate to severe intensity exposure produces respiratory manifestations ranging from cough, chest pain, and dyspnea to bronchitis, pneumonitis, pulmonary edema, and hemorrhage. In some cases, manifestations of liver failure are dominant rather than secondary clinical features.

The nervous system bears the brunt of the poisoning. It can be involved even if the exposure is insufficient to produce the premonitory symptoms from the irritative properties of the toxins. Early symptoms such as headache, vertigo, vomiting, euphoria, weakness, tremor, blurred or double vision, and dysarthria herald the development of ataxia, seizures, blindness, delirium, and coma. The peripheral nervous system does not escape injury, but severe symptoms may only become evident if the patient survives.

Deaths have followed exposure periods as short as 1 hour. Time to death has varied from 1 hour to 1 day or more after the time of exposure.[1, 7]

Extensive dermal contact—either directly with the gas or liquid, or indirectly with contaminated clothing—leads to deep burning and blistering acutely or after a time lag of 1 to 12 hours or longer, depending on the severity of exposure.[1, 22] Skin lesions are most severe in relatively moist areas of the body, such as the axilla, groin, and perineum, and in those areas subject to pressure from clothing or heavy equipment.[22] Cases of systemic poisoning due to dermal absorption have been reported.[7] When the liquid is splashed on the skin, the immediate sensation is of freezing (because the liquid evaporates quickly).

DIAGNOSIS

Clinically, the diagnosis is based on an accurate elucidation of the history of exposure to one of these toxins, the symptoms, and the findings on physical examination. Occupational use of one of these agents is the most obvious clue, but a history of inadvertant exposure to fumigated goods, to spills, or to a supposedly correctly ventilated structure after fumigation should be considered. In addition, someone working in a confined space of a structure that has been recently fumigated could become poisoned.

The area in which the patient was found should be searched for a possible source of the toxin. One patient and his dog, both of whom died from methyl bromide intoxication, had been exposed inadvertently because of a leaking fire extinguisher that contained methyl bromide. The extinguisher was found stored in the basement of the house.[27]

In the absence of a strong history or a positive search, the constellation of symptoms and signs, particularly those related to the irritative, central nervous system, and metabolic effects of the agents, brings to mind an array of possibilities that must be excluded one by one. Finding a sick or dead pet in the same area as the patient provides a clue to an environmental cause, as would noting a strong chemical odor in the case of methyl iodide, ethylene dibromide, and ethylene chloride exposures. Misdiagnosis of another illness can occur if the latent interval between exposure and the onset of symptoms is not considered.

Suspicions about the presence of one of the haloalkanes can be strengthened by measurement of the serum or urinary bromide or iodide concentrations. Bromide has a long elimination half-life of several days, so it can be detected for more than 1 week after acute poisoning.[1, 7, 34] There is some relationship between the intensity of exposure to methyl bromide and the serum bromide concentration.[1, 7] Methyl bromide can be sought as well but may not be detected because of its short half-life. In one patient, ethylene dibromide was detected at postmortem examination 64 hours after acute exposure.[34] Finally, the air in the area in which the patient is found can be sampled and analyzed for the parent compound or for bromine or iodide.

TREATMENT

Immediate Supportive Measures

Treatment of poisoning by these haloalkanes is entirely supportive. Individual problems, such as respiratory, hepatic, or renal failure, are treated as usual, as are seizures and other nervous system manifestations.

The patient should be evacuated from the area of exposure; precautions should be taken so that health care personnel are not endangered in the process of evacuation. Clothing should be stripped off quickly and sealed and stored in an isolated area. Skin and eyes should be washed thoroughly. If the toxin has been ingested, activated charcoal should be given orally or via nasogastric tube.

Specific Interventions

In animals, antidotes tested because they all contain one or more sulfhydryl groups include cysteine, glutathione, *N*-acetylcysteine, and British antilewisite. British antilewisite was only efficacious if it was administered before exposure to methyl iodide.[47] When *N*-acetylcysteine was used in individual patients, it was not thought to be harmful or beneficial.[30, 48] Any possible efficacy would become more remote the later an antidote is given after high-intensity exposure. Cavanagh suggested that glutamate receptor antagonists should be tested in animals as protectants against the neurotoxicity.[16] Follow-up work has not been reported. Various antioxidants and corticosteroids have been used sporadically but with no obvious efficacy.

Given the short half-life of the parent compounds and extensive tissue binding of the adducts, methods to enhance elimination are not practical. In one methyl bromide–poisoned patient, a reduction in serum bromide concentrations produced by hemodialysis was not accompanied by any clinical improvement.[21]

LONG-TERM OUTCOME

In patients who develop severe acute neurologic injury from any of these haloalkanes but survive, the long-term outlook is grim—both central and peripheral neurologic effects can persist indefinitely. Persistent central effects include neuropsychiatric abnormalities, such as depression and cognitive deficits, as well as classic structural deficits. Peripheral neuropathy can be a long-standing problem. For example, Moosa and associates described a patient who at 1 year after the episode was severely handicapped by neuropsychiatric disorders, incontinence, and paralysis that confined him to a wheelchair; subsequently, he was completely dependent on his caregivers.[25]

Avoiding exposure is paramount to the prevention of toxicity from this group of compounds.

References

1. Alexeeff GV, Kilgore WW: Methyl bromide. Residue Rev *88*:101, 1983.
2. Anonymous: Methyl iodide. IARC Monogr Eval Carcinog Risks Chem Hum *41*:213, 1986.
3. Appel GB, Galen R, O'Brien J, et al: Methyl iodide intoxication: A case report. Ann Intern Med *82*:534, 1975.
4. Li KM, Cheng WT: The occupational exposure level of 1,2-dichloroethane in an EM preparation laboratory. J R Soc Health *XX*:169, 1991.
5. 1,2-Dichloroethane. IARC Monogr Eval Carcinog Risks Chem Hum *20*:429, 1979.
6. National Institute for Occupational Safety and Health: Criteria for a Recommended Standard. Occupational Exposure to Ethylene Dichloride (1,2-Dichloroethane). Washington, DC: National Institute for Occupational Safety and Health; 1976. Department of Health, Education, and Welfare publication (NIOSH) 76–139.
7. World Health Organization: Environmental Health Criteria 166: Methyl Bromide. Geneva, World Health Organization, 1995.
8. Shorter JH, Kolb CE, Crill PM, et al: Rapid degradation of atmospheric methyl bromide in soils. Nature *377*:717, 1995.
9. Verschueren KHG, Seljee F, Rozeboom HJ, et al: Crystallographic analysis of the catalytic mechanism of haloalkane dehalogenase. Nature *363*:693, 1993.
10. Alexeeff GV, Kilgore WW, Li M-Y: Ethylene dibromide: Toxicology and risk assessment. Rev Contam Toxicol *112*:49, 1990.
11. Bahlman LJ, Leidel NA, Parker JC, et al: Ethylene dichloride (1,2-dichlorethane). NIOSH Curr Intell Bull *25*:A-351, 1978.
12. Anger WK, Moody L, Burg J, et al: Neurobehavioural evaluation of soil and structural fumigators using methyl bromide and sulfuryl fluoride. Neurotoxicol *7*:137, 1986.
13. Behrens RH, Dukes DCD: Fatal methyl bromide poisoning. Br J Ind Med *43*:561, 1986.
14. Bishop CM: A case of methyl bromide poisoning. Occup Med *42*:107, 1992.
15. Cavalleri F, Galassi G, Ferrari S, et al: Methyl bromide–induced neuropathy: A clinical, neurophysiological and morphological study. J Neurol Neurosurg Psychiatr *58*:383, 1995.
16. Cavanagh JB: Methyl bromide intoxication and acute energy deprivation syndromes. Neuropathol Appl Neurobiol *18*:575, 1992.
17. Chavez CT, Hepler RS, Straatsma BR: Methyl bromide optic atrophy. Am J Ophthalmol *99*:715, 1985.
18. Polkowski J, Crowley MS, Moore AM, Calder RA: Unintentional methyl bromide gas releases Florida, 1988. J Toxicol Clin Toxicol *28*:127, 1990.
19. Fuortes LJ: A case of fatal methyl bromide poisoning. Vet Hum Toxicol *34*:240, 1992.
20. Goldman LR, Mengle D, Epstein DM, et al: Acute symptoms in persons residing near a field treated with the soil fumigants methyl bromide and chloropicrin. West J Med *147*:95, 1987.
21. Herzstein J, Cullen MR: Methyl bromide intoxication in four field-workers during removal of soil fumigation sheets. Am J Ind Med *17*:321, 1990.
22. Hezemans-Boer M, Toonstra J, Meulenbelt J, et al: Skin lesions due to exposure to methyl bromide. Arch Dermatol *124*:917, 1988.
23. Hustinx WWNM, van der Laar RTH, van Huffelen AC, et al: Systemic effects of inhalational methyl bromide poisoning: A study of nine cases occupationally exposed due to inadvertent spread during fumigation. Br J Ind Med *50*:155, 1993.
24. Marraccini JV, Thomas GE, Ongley JP, et al: Death and injury caused by methyl bromide, an insecticide fumigant. J Forensic Sci *28*:601, 1983.
25. Moosa MR, Jansen J, Edelstein CL: Treatment of methyl bromide poisoning with haemodialysis. Postgrad Med J *70*:733, 1994.
26. Reidy TJ, Bolter JF, Cone JE: Neuropsychological sequelae of methyl bromide: A case study. Brain Inj *8*:83, 1994.
27. Squier MV, Thompson J, Rajgopalan B: Case report: Neuropathology of methyl bromide intoxication. Neuropathol Appl Neurobiol *18*:579, 1992.
28. Uncini A, Basciani M, Di Muzio A, et al: Methyl bromide myoclonus: An electrophysiological study. Acta Neurol Scand *81*:159, 1990.
29. Zatuchni J, Hong K: Methyl bromide poisoning seen initially as psychosis. Arch Neurol *38*:529, 1981.
30. Zwaveling JH, de Kort WLAM, Meulenbelt J, et al: Exposure of the skin to methyl bromide: A study of six cases occupationally exposed to high concentrations during fumigation. Hum Toxicol *6*:491, 1987.
31. Baselga-Mone M, Estadella-Botha S, Quer-Brossa S, et al: Occupational intoxication by methyl iodide. Med Lav *56*:592, 1965.
32. Cobb OM, Raymond LW: Methyl iodide toxicity. Ann Intern Med *85*:539, 1976.

33. Garland A, Camps FE: Methyl iodide poisoning. Br J Ind Med *2*:209, 1945.
34. Letz GA, Pond SM, Osterloh JD, et al: Two fatalities after acute exposure to ethylene dibromide. J Am Med Assoc *252*:2428, 1984.
35. Saraswat PK, Kandara M, Dhruva AK, et al: Poisoning by ethylene dibromide—Six cases: A clinicopathological and toxicological study. Ind J Med Sci *40*:121, 1986.
36. Medinsky MA, Dutcher JS, Bond RF, et al: Uptake and excretion of [^{14}C]methyl bromide as influenced by exposure concentration. Toxicol Appl Pharmacol *78*:215, 1985.
37. Morgan A, Black A, Belcher DR: Studies on the absorption of halogenated hydrocarbons and their excretion in breath using ^{38}Cl tracer techniques. Am Occup Health *15*:273, 1972.
38. Bond JA, Dutcher JS, Medinsky MA, et al: Disposition of [^{14}C]methyl bromide in rats after inhalation. Toxicol Appl Pharmacol *78*:259, 1985.
39. Bolt HM, Gansewendt B: Mechanisms and carcinogenicity of methyl halides. Crit Rev Toxicol *23*:237, 1993.
40. Davenport CJ, Ali SF, Miller FJ, et al: Effect of methyl bromide on regional brain glutathione, glutathione-*S*-transferases, monoamines, and amino acids in F344 rats. Toxicol Appl Pharmacol *112*:120, 1992.
41. Guengerich FP, Peterson LA, Cmarik JL, et al: Activation of dihaloalkanes by glutathione conjugation and formation of DNA adducts. Environ Health Perspect *76*:15, 1987.
42. Honma T, Miyagawa M, Sato M, et al: Neurotoxicity and metabolism of methyl bromide in rats. Toxicol Appl Pharmacol *81*:183, 1985.
43. Lewis SE: Inhibition of SH proteins by methyl bromide. Nature *161*:692, 1948.
44. Nachtomi E: The metabolism of ethylene dibromide in the rat: The enzymatic reaction with glutathione *in vitro* and *in vivo*. Biochem Pharmacol *19*:2853, 1970.
45. Iwasaki K, Ito I, Kagawa J: Biological exposure monitoring of methyl bromide workers by determination of hemoglobin adducts. Ind Health *27*:181, 1989.
46. van Doorn R, Borm PJA, Leijdekkers CM, et al: Detection and identification of *S*-methylcysteine in urine of workers exposed to methyl chloride. Int Arch Occup Health 46:99, 1980.
47. Buckell M: 2,3-Dimercaptopropanol (BAL) and methyl iodide intoxication. Nature *163*:330, 1949.
48. Luzhnikov EA, Lisovik ZA, Novikovskaya TV: 1,2-Dichloroethane metabolism in man after acute poisoning. Sud Med Ekspert *28*:47, 1985.

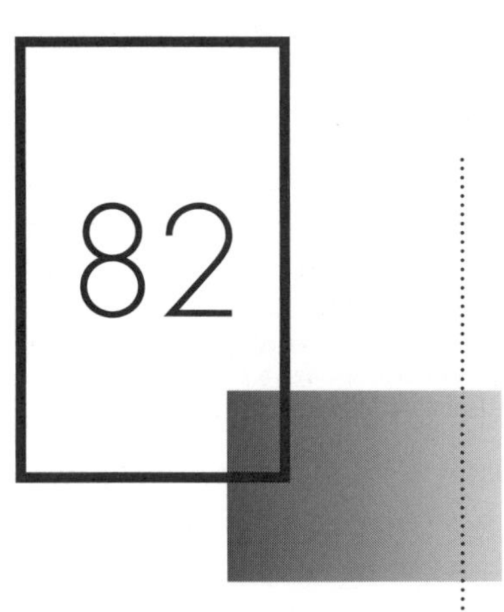

Ammonia, Nitrogen, Nitrogen Oxides, and Related Compounds

MARY JO McMULLEN, MD
THOMAS J. HETRICK, MD
LOUIS CANNON, MD

AMMONIA

The usual setting for human exposure to ammonia is an industrial accident. Industrial-strength ammonia at concentrations greater than 27% to 30% is considered an alkaline corrosive. Ammonia is most commonly used as a chemical in the manufacture of fertilizer; because ammonia has a high nitrogen content (82%), fertilizer produced with ammonia is one of the best fertilizers available commercially. Ammonia is used as a solvent in the manufacture of textiles and leather, in pulp and paper processing, and as a stabilizer in rubber manufacturing. It is used in the synthesis of nitrous oxide, plastics, pharmaceuticals, pesticides, cyanide, explosives, rocket fuels, and flame retardants. Ammonia is also used in petroleum-refining processes and in the treatment of metals. In the past, ammonia was a common refrigerant; it is still found in some food-processing installations as well as in ice production and cold storage facilities.[1–4]

When used as a household cleaner or bleaching agent, ammonia is found in a concentration of 5% to 10%, having a pH of less than 12. If an *ammonia*-containing cleaner is mixed with a *chlorine*-containing bleach, very irritating *chloramine* fumes are released. In a 5% to 10% concentration, however, ammonia is generally considered an irritant and is rarely reported to cause burns when inhaled.[5] However, three patients who attempted suicide by ingesting household ammonia were reported to have esophageal burns; among these, one fatality occurred. This patient had severe corrosive injury of the upper airway and esophagus with aspiration pneumonia. Death was attributed to adult respiratory distress syndrome and renal failure.[6] Ammonia may also be found in the home as a liniment and in spirits of ammonia.[7]

Anhydrous ammonia at atmospheric pressure is a colorless gas with an extremely pungent odor. This gas may burn but does not ignite readily; however, the pressurized container may explode in heat or fire. The explosive limit of ammonia in air is 16% to 25%. Usual shipping containers include tank cars, tank trucks, barges, and steel cylinders.[1, 3]

Pathophysiology

The extent of injury with ammonia depends on the duration of the exposure, the concentration of the gas or liquid, and, if inhaled, the depth of inhalation (Table 82–1). Ammonia vapor per se is not poisonous, but its high solubility in water is responsible for its irritant and corrosive actions. Anhydrous ammonia gas is absorbed on mucosal membranes such as the eyes, oral cavity, pharynx, and lungs, where it mixes with moisture, producing ammonium hydroxide, which is both irritating and caustic to these areas. This reaction is exothermic and produces thermal as well as chemical injury. The type of burn is a liquefaction necrosis of superficial tissues with a deeper penetration of the chemical burn and subsequent scarring. Ammonia burns feel soapy because of the saponification of the tissues. Edema of all involved tissues is common.[1–3, 7–9]

Desquamation of the epithelial layer of the upper tracheobronchial tree (tracheobronchitis) with membrane formation is the usual pathology found in the airways. There tends to be relatively little effect on the lower airways because ammonia's high solubility prevents it from reaching the distal airways. With very high concentrations of the vapors, terminal bronchiolitis and alveolar injury leading to pulmonary edema can occur. Noncardiogenic pulmonary edema is secondary to damage of the alveolocapillary membrane, with resultant increased permeability and exudation of fluid into the alveoli.[2, 4, 9–11]

Table 82–1. Effects of Ammonia at Different Concentrations

25–50 ppm	Odor threshold, tolerance may develop to the odor
25 ppm	Threshold limit value
50 ppm	Occupational Safety and Health Administration and National Institute for Occupational Safety and Health exposure limits, time-weighted average
100 ppm	Eye irritant
500 ppm	Immediate danger to life or health (IDLH)
1000 ppm	Direct caustic effects on the respiratory tract
2500 ppm	Death has been reported after 1/2 hour of exposure
30,000 ppm	Lowest concentration leading to death after 5 minutes of exposure in human references[1,3,8]

Clinical Signs and Symptoms

Facial Signs. Exposure of the head and neck region to ammonia fumes commonly causes headache, salivation, swelling around the eyes and lips, and restlessness. Concentrated ammonia fumes produce a burning sensation in the eyes, followed by lacrimation, swelling, blurred vision, and severe pain. Corneal opacification with scarring and neovascularization, iritis, lens damage, and cataract formation all are common complications of severe exposure, particularly if the patient is not treated promptly. Increased intraocular pressure produces narrow-angle closure glaucoma. Ammonia has a greater tendency to penetrate and damage the eyes than does any other alkali.[1, 3, 4, 8–9]

Lungs. Injury due to ammonia inhalation is often classified as mild, moderate, or severe, depending on the extent of pulmonary injury. Initial primary respiratory failure may result from severe local edema with acute obstruction of the airway. Patients typically present with cough, dyspnea, tightness in the chest, laryngitis, and bronchospasm with wheezing, tracheitis, and hypoxia. These patients are occasionally unable to speak. Respiratory irritation may occasionally be delayed in onset. Pulmonary edema may eventually develop, presenting with rales and rhonchi if the ammonia concentration was great enough to have penetrated the lower airways. Copious amounts of tracheal secretions are usually reported. Hemoptysis and fever are not uncommon. Consolidation and pneumonia can be seen on radiographs.[1, 3–4, 8–9]

Inhalation injury may follow a biphasic course with an initial chemical pneumonitis, edema, congestion, hemorrhage, and atelectasis. This phase is followed by some improvement during the next 48 to 72 hours. Subsequently there is the gradual onset of airway obstruction, and respiratory failure develops with sloughing of tissue; a persistent obstructive pattern may then develop. Most patients who survive the first 24 hours will recover.[3, 12]

The initial chest radiograph is usually clear but may eventually suggest tracheobronchitis and mild pulmonary edema. Xenon 133 scanning or direct examination of the airway by fiberoptic bronchoscopy helps determine the extent of injury.[4, 13]

Gastrointestinal Signs. Ingestion causes severe pain in the mouth, chest, and abdomen, accompanied by nausea and vomiting. Shock frequently occurs early owing to vomiting and third-space distribution of fluids. Severe local edema of the lips and mouth is present; burns of the soft palate may also occur. Twenty-four to 72 hours later, esophageal and gastric perforation with mediastinitis may occur. Victims with perforation have severe abdominal pain and rigidity and may have associated respiratory complications including pulmonary edema. Late complications from ulcerative esophagitis include stricture formation.[1, 8–9, 14] Alkaline corrosive ingestions are further discussed in Chapter 62.

Skin Signs. Patients initially notice sweating and a burning sensation, followed rapidly by blister or vesicle formation. Injuries may vary from mild erythema and edema after exposure to low concentrations of ammonia; severe edema with liquefaction necrosis and deep penetrating burns follows a more concentrated vapor exposure.[1, 8] Skin exposure to ammonia liquid that has a temperature of $-33°C$ produces frostbite-type injuries with first- to third-degree burns.[3, 8] Extensive systemic absorption with death has also been reported. Oral ingestion causes burns, ulcer formation, and esophageal or stomach perforation.

Laboratory Features. Laboratory results generally are nonspecific and are not helpful after an ammonia exposure. It is important to obtain serial arterial blood gas values, both to monitor the progress of respiratory failure and because these patients may develop a metabolic acidosis. The serum ammonia level does not correlate with the degree of injury.[8]

Treatment

Prehospital management must be started early and aggressively. It is necessary to evacuate patients from the exposure situation and to remove all clothing. For a skin exposure, emergency medical service personnel should wash the affected area with soap and copious amounts of water for at least 15 to 20 minutes; the area can then be covered with a dry, clean dressing. Fluid resuscitation by the standard burn protocol is recommended, but it must be remembered that noncardiogenic pulmonary edema may occur. It is important for emergency medical personnel to wash out the eyes continuously until medical care is obtained. The prehospital personnel should do nothing to induce emesis. In any case of exposure to ammonia, respiratory support with high-flow oxygen is indicated in the prehospital setting, although early intubation may be necessary.[1, 3, 5–6]

In the hospital, after skin washing, it is recommended that no ointments or burn creams be used for at least 24 hours because they are believed to promote increased penetration of the chemical into the skin.[15] Tetanus prophylaxis is indicated. Fluid resuscitation as noted earlier should be continued; central venous and pulmonary capillary wedge pressure monitoring may be required in seriously burned patients. After the eyes have been adequately irrigated to a normal pH, slit-lamp evaluation with fluorescein stain should be performed; intraocular pressure should be monitored. Use of ophthalmic antibiotics and atropine is recommended. Ophthalmic corticosteroids are frequently recommended, but no controlled trials are available to support this recommendation. For ingestions, after endoscopy, some investigators also recommend corticosteroid therapy. Although this may be beneficial in preventing stricture formation after ammonia exposure, no well-controlled trials are available to support this recommendation conclusively. Antibiotics are needed if mediastinitis develops.[3, 8] As in the prehospital setting, early aggressive control of the airway is essential. Early intubation, before edema makes it impossible, is suggested. Emergency tracheostomy may be necessary if severe upper airway obstruction develops. Humidified oxygen and bronchodilators are essential components of therapy, as is frequent suctioning. Positive end-expiratory pressure ventilation may be necessary to maintain an adequate Po_2.[2–4, 6–7, 12, 15–16]

Fiberoptic bronchoscopy can be both a diagnostic and therapeutic aid by assisting with the removal of sloughed tissue and secretions. In addition to serial arterial blood gas measurements and radiographs, serial pulmonary function testing may also be useful. Use of systemic corticosteroids for inhalation injury is controversial, although most case reports include their use. Prophylactic systemic antibiotics are not recommended.[2–4, 7–8, 12] Patients who are not having significant symptoms may be discharged from the emergency department after 2 hours' observation, with instructions to seek medical attention if late symptoms present.[17]

Long-Term Implications

Patients who survive ammonia inhalation exposures for more than 24 hours are likely to recover. Although complete pulmonary recovery is the usual outcome, residual bronchoconstriction, bronchiectasis, and small airway disease have been reported. Fibrous obliteration of the small airways, thought to be a late state of bronchiolitis obliterans, is believed to be responsible for the chronic obstructive pulmonary disease that occasionally develops.[7–8, 10, 12]

Eye damage varying in degree from mild to total blindness may be the permanent residual effect of an ocular exposure to ammonia. Cataract formation, permanent corneal ulceration, and lenticular opacification have been reported.[1, 12]

Follow-up barium swallow at 10 to 21 days is recommended for patients who have ingested ammonia because stricture formation may present at this time.

Repeated exposure to ammonia gas may cause chronic irritation of the conjunctiva and upper respiratory tract. Chronic bronchitis has been reported after repeated inhalation exposures. However, long-term exposure to low concentrations of ammonia vapor rarely causes serious injury to lung parenchyma.[1, 15]

NITROGEN OXIDES

Toxic gas inhalation involving nitrogen oxides has been reported in both single cases and mass exposures for the past 200 years. The earliest recorded case of toxic inhalation of these fumes involved a French merchant who died after breathing concentrated nitric acid fumes in 1804.[18] Nitrogen oxides were not recognized as the cause of silo filler's disease until 1956,[19] although the clinical entity had been recognized as early as 1914.[20] The mortality for silo filler's disease, based on a review of the literature, is about 30%. In one Wisconsin study, 4.2% of all farmers become symptomatic working around silos.[21] Table 82–2 lists the chemical composition of the nitrogen oxide compounds.

Sources of Exposure

The most common toxic effect of exposure to nitrogen oxide fumes is pulmonary disease, generally following exposure to silage gas (silo filler's disease).[21–25] Nitrogen oxide fumes may come from slow-burning nitrocellulose such as that found in x-ray film. Deaths in the Cleveland Clinic disaster of 1929 were largely caused by nitrogen oxides.[18] Another common occupation that involves exposure to these fumes is firefighting. Firefighters may be exposed to oxides emitted from burning materials such as bed mattresses.[22] Other common sources of exposure include acetylene welding in confined spaces, detonation of explosives (especially shot firing in coal mines and dynamite blasting), and accidents involving nitric acid. Diesel fumes or fumes from any internal combustion engine, furnace gases, and the smoke from cigarettes, cigars, and pipes can also cause low-level exposures. Nitrogen dioxide is the only measured pollutant that has actually been increasing in outdoor air.[26] Many chemical processes such as the manufacture of dyes and lacquers are associated with the release of nitrogen oxide fumes,[18, 25] as is cleaning coins.[27] Table 82–3 provides a summary of dose-response effects for nitrogen oxides.

Table 82–2. Nitrogen Oxides

Nitrogen oxide	NO (nitric oxide)
Nitrous oxide	N_2O
Nitrogen dioxide	NO_2 (red-brown or copper-colored gas)
Nitrogen peroxide	N_2O_2
Dinitrogen trioxide	N_2O_3
Dinitrogen tetroxide	N_2O_4 (nitrogen tetroxide, yellow gas)
Dinitrogen pentoxide	N_2O_5

Table 82–3. Effects of Nitrogen Oxides at Different Concentrations

1–3 ppm	NO_2	Odor detectable
3 ppm	NO_2	Maximum allowable exposure (TLV)
13 ppm	NO_2	Membrane irritation
25 ppm	NO	TLV
50–150 ppm	NO_2	Mild irritant to eyes and upper airways
174 ppm	NO_2	LD_{50} at 1 hour

TLV, threshold limit value.

Missile silos, where nitrogen tetroxide is used as a fuel oxidizer, have been the site of accidental exposures; one report described 24 workers exposed in one accident; three Apollo mission astronauts were also exposed in a chemical accident.[21, 28]

One hundred sixteen cases of nitrogen dioxide–induced respiratory illness in high school students attending hockey games in an arena in Minnesota were reported in one outbreak. Of those surveyed, 69% of students who were on or near the ice developed acute symptoms. A defective engine in the ice-resurfacing machine was blamed. No long-term sequelae were documented.[29]

Silo Filler's Disease

High concentrations of nitrogen oxides can be found when stored silage, usually corn, was grown under conditions of drought or intense sunlight or was prematurely harvested. The oxides of nitrogen are derived from nitrates in the silage, which are fermented into nitrites that combine with organic acids to form nitrous acid. This then decomposes into water and a mixture of nitrogen oxides. Nitrogen dioxide, which is reddish brown and has a pungent odor, and nitrogen tetroxide, which is yellow, are thought to be the principal agents responsible for the pulmonary injury. The decomposition process begins very shortly after putting crops into a silo (within 4 hours of filling) and continues for at least 10 days. Dangerous amounts of gas may remain in the silo for a month if the silo is not opened.[26, 30–31] One case report involved a man exposed 6 weeks after silage was stored.[32]

Pathophysiology

Because nitrogen oxides are less soluble (hydrolyze more slowly) than most irritant gases, they reach the bronchioles and alveoli, whereas more irritating gases (e.g., ammonia) do not. Within the lungs, nitrogen oxides react with water to form nitrous and nitric acids; these produce extensive local damage that results in a profound chemical pneumonitis and pulmonary edema. At lower concentrations, an inflammatory exudate and bronchoconstriction occur. Pulmonary edema occurs when high concentrations of the gases are inhaled.[21, 25, 33] Both increased airway resistance and decreased diffusion capacity occur. The acute increase in airway resistance that occurs after nitrogen dioxide exposure, even at low doses, appears to be mediated by histamine release.[18] Inhalation of as little as 0.3 ppm of nitrogen dioxide has been shown to potentiate induced bronchospasm in asthmatic individuals.[34]

Increased susceptibility to both bacterial and viral infections and interference with the ability of the lungs to remove inhaled deposited particles appear to occur after exposure to nitrogen dioxide.[22] In addition, the nitrogen oxides participate in several reactions that interfere with other biologic systems. Besides direct alveolar epithelial injury from nitrogen dioxide combined with water to form acid, nitrogen dioxide oxidizes lecithin in membranes and pulmonary surfactant, forming stable free radicals. Nitrogen dioxide is involved in direct oxidation of unsaturated fatty acids and in their *n*-nitrosation to nitrosamines; this reaction may have a significant role in gastrointestinal cancers. Poisoning of the cytochrome electron transfer reaction may also be a factor.[18]

Clinical Signs and Symptoms

Clinical presentation is generally divided into three clinical stages: acute, delayed, and subacute.[18]

Acute Phase. In this group of patients, mucosal irritation results in immediate weakness and choking, followed by dyspnea and bronchospasm, cough, nausea, vomiting, headache, conjunctivitis with eye irritation, vertigo, tachycardia, and chest pain (which may be pleuritic). Skin burns due to the mixture of nitrogen oxide fumes with sweat, producing nitric acid, may occur. Many of the effects are self-limited if exposure has been only mild and brief. Symptoms may persist for 1 to 2 weeks, usually followed by complete recovery. Leukocytosis and fever may be present at this stage.[21–22, 31, 35–37] Those with progressive disease following the acute phase have a symptom-free interval of 3 to 36 hours, occasionally lasting as long as 10 days.

Delayed Phase. This phase is characterized by the appearance of noncardiogenic pulmonary edema, which may occur even with only minimal initial symptoms. In one study, 18 of 23 patients had only a transient respiratory problem after exposure; however, 5 cases progressed to the delayed phase.[21] Symptoms and signs commonly include tachycardia, tachypnea, dyspnea, fever, cyanosis, rales, both restrictive and obstructive ventilatory defects, decreased diffusion capacity, and hypoxia. Radiographic findings generally begin with perihilar infiltrates and progress to fulminant pulmonary edema. Fibrinous bronchiectasis may be found on biopsy.[21–22, 25, 27] In one study of 34 patients, 40% of the patients who developed pulmonary edema died.[18] Those who survived either developed long-term complications, experienced a subacute phase, or recovered completely.

After delayed-phase manifestations, a further asymptomatic phase may occur during which the radiographic chest findings clear, although the patient may still have a mild cough, dyspnea, and malaise. This phase lasts from 2 to 6 weeks.[25]

Subacute Phase. This phase usually appears 2 to 4 weeks after the delayed phase. The patient again becomes acutely ill with cough, dyspnea, chest tightness, hypoxia, confusion, hypotension, fever and chills, rales, and wheezing. The chest radiographic findings at this point may again resemble those of characteristic pulmonary edema or may show multiple discrete nodules (miliary pattern). Pulmonary function testing reveals both obstructive and restrictive defects.

The pathologic picture may be that of bronchitis and bronchiolitis with persistent cough or that of bronchiolitis obliterans. Bronchiolitis obliterans appears on biopsy as a proliferation of granulation tissue with eosinophils and plasma cells in the lumen of the bronchioles and alveoli, with general preservation of the background architecture of the lung. Observed clinically is progressive deterioration with an organizing pneumonia. This stage may prove fatal.[18, 25, 28, 31]

The clinical presentation and progression of the disease depend on the concentration and duration of exposure and perhaps on a patient's predisposition to lung disease. Hypotension (direct effect of the nitrates on blood vessels), metabolic acidosis (nitrous acid and lactic acidosis), and methemoglobinemia are frequently reported.[37]

Diagnosis is based on the history of exposure to inhaled organic dusts such as occurs when entering a freshly filled silo in the summer or early fall, in exposure to a fire, or in an industrial accident. The latency period of several hours followed by the symptoms of cough, fever and chills, chest pain, dyspnea, headache, myalgias, and nausea and vomiting is very suggestive of this exposure. Differential diagnosis should include allergic lung disease due to molds (farmer's lung due to hypersensitivity reaction), pneumonia, miliary tuberculosis, viral influenza, carbon monoxide exposure, myocardial infarction, or pulmonary edema following exposure to other toxic products of combustion (see Chapter 69).

Treatment

Treatment depends on a patient's phase of clinical illness and the symptomatic presentation. High-flow oxygen and intubation with positive pressure ventilation as needed are considered the mainstays of treatment.[18, 38] Aminophylline and inhaled bronchodilators are recommended for symptomatic bronchoconstriction. Administration of albumin to raise the plasma oncotic pressure has been suggested, but its use is not well documented. Use of diuretics, digitalis, and volume reduction is not considered helpful.

Corticosteroids are thought to be beneficial in both the treatment and prevention of delayed and subacute phases of disease. High-dose corticosteroids should be continued for 8 weeks and tapered gradually to prevent relapses. Corticosteroids may assist in suppressing the diffuse alveolar damage that is induced by toxic inhalation. Many researchers report dramatic improvement in symptoms after use of corticosteroids and recurrence of the symptoms when the corticosteroids are abruptly stopped; the symptoms then respond to reinstitution of the corticosteroids.[21, 26, 28, 31, 37, 39] Corticosteroids are the treatment of choice for the phase of bronchiolitis obliterans.

Correction of acid-base abnormalities and standard therapy for methemoglobinemia are indicated. Because these patients are prone to infection, frequent sputum cultures should be obtained and antibiotics started when indicated.

In-hospital observation for 6 hours is recommended for all persons with potential nitrogen oxide exposure. If a patient is asymptomatic after that time and has relatively rapid access to medical care, he or she may be discharged for close follow-up. Repeat examinations for 6 weeks are recommended.

Long-Term Implications

In one report, 6 of 24 victims of a missile silo accident developed neurologic sequelae that have remained unexplained. In another study of 23 cases, of the 5 that progressed beyond the acute phase, all had some persistent pulmonary dysfunction on follow-up of several years.[21, 36] The ability to predict who will have long-term complications from a single acute exposure is poor, and meaningful numbers from studies are essentially nonexistent. Generally, a patient whose illness does not progress beyond the acute phase will not have subsequent problems, and patients who have pulmonary edema or whose illness evolves to bronchiolitis obliterans seem to have a high probability of developing long-term complications.

In animals, long-term exposure to nitrogen oxides has caused a pattern of emphysema, decreased body weight, and increased incidence of spontaneous tumors. The development of emphysema with continual exposure occurs in coal miners. Studies have also shown an increased incidence of bronchitis in children who have long-term low-dose exposure.[40, 41] With the release of nitrogen oxides from such sources as vehicle emissions and factories, gas stoves, water heaters, and space heaters, persistent low-level indoor and outdoor pollution from these substances is common. Several chronic health problems are postulated to occur as a result of this low-grade nitrogen oxide exposure, including increased incidence and severity of respiratory tract infections, reduced lung function, and increased symptoms in patients with asthma and chronic obstructive pulmonary disease. Multiple methodology problems and inconclusive and conflicting data leave much of this speculation.[26, 40]

LIQUID NITROGEN

Nitrogen gas accounts for 78% of the atmospheric air. It is a colorless, nonflammable elemental compound that is odorless and is liquid between −210 and 195°C. Liquid nitrogen is used in industry as a refrigerant and storage medium for nitrogen gas. It is used in cryogenic therapy in numerous medical specialities.[39]

Pathophysiology

Liquid nitrogen has two toxic mechanisms. In the gaseous phase, it can act as an asphyxiant by displacing ambient atmospheric oxygen. In the liquid or supercool gaseous phase, it acts on exposed tissues as a rapid freezing agent.

Clinical Signs and Symptoms

Inert gaseous nitrogen in sufficient quantities displaces ambient oxygen, causing asphyxia. Oxygen concentrations reduced to 15% to 16% produce symptoms. The respiratory rate and pulse initially increase and psychomotor coordination decreases. At oxygen concentrations of 10% to 12%, poor judgment, giddiness, Cheyne-Stokes respirations, and cyanosis occur; unconsciousness occurs at an oxygen concentration of 8% to 10%; rapid onset of convulsions, coma, and death occurs at oxygen levels of 6% or less.[42]

Liquid or supercooled pressurized gaseous nitrogen produces rapid freezing of exposed tissues. Mild dermal exposure causes pain on freezing and thawing, with localized erythema.[43] Transient urticarial lesions occur secondary to mast cell degranulation.[44] Bullae separating the dermal-epidermal layer generally result, with later sloughing and healing without scarring. Injury to the deeper tissues from liquid nitrogen is typical of a classic frostbite injury. The dermis can be anesthetic and pale. Bullae do not form. Red blood cell thrombi occlude the local vascular supply, with subsequent necrosis and gangrene.[44] Rockswold[39] described intraoral lesions caused by accidental inhalation of liquid nitrogen. Frank charring, inflammation, and edema of the lips were present. The patient had inspiratory stridor secondary to a pale, edematous, swollen epiglottis. Bullae of the palate subsequently developed and later sloughed, leaving an ulcerated base.

Local complications from therapeutic exposure to liquid nitrogen have included digital and ulnar nerve neuropathies,[45–46] onychodystrophy,[47] and pyogenic granulomata.[48] Patients have also suffered syncope[49] and cardiac arrest[50] during liquid nitrogen application, probably as a result of vasomotor reactions from the stress and pain of the procedure.[49]

Treatment

Asphyxiated patients should be removed from the offending environment and given 100% oxygen. Cardiac monitoring and supportive care for central nervous system complications are indicated.

For external dermal exposure, rapid rewarming in a water bath at 40 to 42°C is indicated until vascular flushing has returned. Standard frostbite management including elevation of the limb, protective dressings, and late surgical debridement of necrotic tissue should be initiated. Whether or not pharmacologic agents should be used to enhance circulation is an unresolved issue.

For intraoral injuries, acute evaluation for impending or actual upper airway obstruction is mandatory. Aggressive airway management including tracheostomy may be necessary. Use of parenteral steroids is thought to be of benefit.[39]

Long-Term Implications

Nothing is uniquely peculiar about the long-term effects of liquid nitrogen. Sequelae of tissue injury may be noted: tissue loss through gangrene, scarring, neuropathy, or changes in pigmentation. The chronic stigmata of central nervous system hypoxia may occur. As the predominant component of the atmosphere, nitrogen has no adverse environmental implications.

N-NITROSODIMETHYLAMINE

N-Nitrosodimethylamine (DMN, dimethylnitrosamine, DMNA, NDMA, *N*-methyl-*N*-nitrosomethanamine) is a yellow liquid that is soluble in water, ether, or alcohol. It is of low viscosity and has a boiling point of 152°C. It has no appreciable odor and is incompatible with strong oxidizing agents.

NDMA is used commonly as an industrial solvent in the production of dimethylhydrazine. It is used in the production of hyperbolic rocket fuels and thiocarbonyl fluoride polymers and as a cutting oil. Other potential sources of exposure include gasoline and lubricants, which use it as an additive; plasticizers for acrylonitrile polymers; and components in high-energy battery systems with active metal anode-electrolyte systems. NDMA can also be found in many cosmetic products, hand and body lotions, and shampoos. Other nitrosamines have also been patented for use in pesticides and nematocides. High levels of NDMA have been found in soil, postulated to be from the use of triazine herbicide.[51]

NDMA is classified as an occupational carcinogen by the National Institute for Occupational Safety and Health (NIOSH) and the American Conference of Governmental and Industrial Hygienists (ACGIH) and has no acceptable permissible exposure limit (PEL).

Pathophysiology

NDMA was discovered to be a powerful carcinogen more than 30 years ago, when investigators found hepatotoxicity, jaundice, and liver damage in workmen exposed to this chemical. Since that time, research has shown that NDMA is one of the most powerful carcinogenic materials recognized, its pathologic effects stemming from the alkylation of DNA. NDMA's pathologic effects appear to be both dose and time related. In rodents, a single large dose of NDMA results in renal cancer, whereas exposure to low doses for long periods causes hepatic cancer.[52–55]

It is of note that this dose- and time-related organotropism has been used in cancer chemotherapy with the drug streptozocin, an *N*-methylnitrosamine. This agent is currently being used to treat metastatic insulin-secreting tumors of the pancreas because of its high affinity and cytotoxicity to this specific cell type located in the human pancreas.[56]

Pre-employment screening of workers who may be exposed to NDMA should include attention to a family history of cancer and liver disease, smoking, the potential for pregnancy during periods of exposure, corticosteroid use, and immunocompetence.

Clinical Signs and Symptoms

Local direct exposure to NDMA produces minimal direct irritation to the skin and mucous membranes. Therefore, the warning signs of potential exposure by contact are poor. In persons with acute poisoning due to systemic exposure, headaches, a feeling of generalized malaise, fever, and weakness often occur. Gastrointestinal effects are frequent and include abdominal cramping and nausea. Vomiting and diarrhea occur within hours of absorption. Liver enlargement and jaundice may follow.[57–58]

Treatment

Workers should be removed from the area of exposure. Their eyes should be irrigated with water if the conjunctival membranes were potentially exposed. Contaminated parts of the body are washed with soap and water. It is necessary to evaluate liver function by monitoring serum albumin level, prothrombin time, conjugated bilirubin, or other indices of hepatic function. It is also necessary to monitor changes in patients' chest radiographs and renal function. Patients should be observed for other possible malignant changes as dictated by family history or other factors (i.e., breast cancer screening in female patients or sputum cytology in an employee who smokes or has a family history of lung cancer).

Chronic Poisoning or Long-Term Implications

Clinical manifestations of chronic exposure to NDMA may include severe liver damage, with acute centrolobular necrosis, jaundice, and ascites. Inhalation and ingestion of NDMA have produced malignant tumors in rodents; these have involved the liver, kidneys, and lungs. Such tumors have not been conclusively reported in humans, but in light of the potent carcinogenicity found in experimental animals, every precaution to avoid long-term exposure should be taken. Evaluation of a patient with a history of continual exposure should make optimum use of cancer screening tools such as sputum cytology, chest radiography, liver function tests, pelvic examination, and breast cancer screening in appropriate individuals as dictated by exposure and family history.[59–61]

DIETHYLAMINE AND TRIETHYLAMINE

Diethylamine (diethamine, *N*-ethylethanamine) and triethylamine (*N,N*-diethylethanamine) are alkaline, colorless liquids with a strong ammoniac or fishy odor. This odor often gives warning of their presence because the odor threshold is as low as 0.14 ppm, and the PEL is more than 100 times greater. Diethylamine and triethylamine have a PEL of 25 ppm by OSHA and of 10 ppm by ACGIH. The immediately dangerous to life or health levels are set at 2000 ppm and 1000 ppm, respectively.[62–64] Diethylamine has a boiling point of 56°C; that of triethylamine is 90°C. These compounds are incompatible with strong oxidizers and acids. Both compounds are unstable when exposed to heat, and hazardous decomposition products such as carbon monoxide and oxides of nitrogen may be released in a fire involving these compounds. Extinguishing agents should be dry chemicals, alcohol foam, or carbon dioxide.

The sources of exposure are varied. Diethylamine is often used in the petroleum and rubber industries. It is also used in manufacturing pharmaceutical products, resins, and dyes. Triethylamine is used as an antilivering agent for urea and melamine-based enamels and as a corrosion inhibitor in paint remover formulations based on methylene chloride. It is used as a rubber accelerator and propellant.

Clinical Signs and Symptoms

In the setting of an acute exposure, both of these compounds are direct irritants to the mucous membranes and the eyes. Acute dermatitis with dermal burns as well as a nonspecific irritation can result from exposure. As with all alkaline products, these compounds can significantly damage the eyes by direct contact. Exposure may result in keratitis or conjunctivitis with severe photophobia, corneal edema, coagulation necrosis of tissues, and severe eye damage.[65]

Systemic symptoms involve the respiratory tract with cough, dyspnea, chest pain, and pulmonary edema, which may be delayed until 72 hours after the initial exposure. Patients who have had significant tracheobronchial exposure should be monitored closely. A fire involving these chemicals may mean exposing victims to the breakdown products of carbon monoxide and oxides of nitrogen. Laboratory evaluation and treatment should be performed accordingly.

Treatment

Workers should be evacuated from the scene of exposure, and contaminated clothing should be removed promptly. Soap and water should be used to wash exposed areas of the body. Copious irrigation with normal saline or water should be begun as soon as possible after ocular exposure. Apply a local anesthetic and irrigate continuously, preferably with a Morgan lens, for at least 20 minutes. pH measurements should be taken to ensure satisfactory irrigation. If the pH of the eyes is still alkaline, continued irrigation must be performed to terminate liquefaction necrosis. A cycloplegic agent may be used for pain associated with ciliary spasm. An antibiotic in either drop or ointment form should be used. Ophthalmologic referral for all alkaline injuries to the eyes is recommended. Collagenase inhibitors and steroids should be used only after ophthalmologic referral.

Ingestion of either of these agents should be treated by allowing patients to take nothing by mouth and arranging endoscopy. Lavage and induced emesis are not recommended.

Oxygen should be given for all patients with inhalation exposure, and chest radiographs and arterial blood gas measurements are recommended for symptomatic patients. A high index of suspicion for delayed-onset pulmonary edema is warranted.[59]

Long-Term Implications

The condition of workers subjected to long-term exposure should be monitored with the use of liver and renal function rests, blood counts, electrocardiograms, and chest radiographs.

References

1. Occupational Health Services: Material Safety Data Sheet (MSDS), Secaucus, NJ. Occupational Health Services, 1985.
2. Flury KE, Dines DE, Roberts JR, et al: Airway obstruction due to inhalation of ammonia. Mayo Clinic Proc *58*:389–393, 1983.
3. Arwood R, Hammond J, Ward GG: Ammonia inhalation. J Trauma *25*:444–447, 1985.
4. Montague TJ, MacNeil AR: Mass ammonia inhalation. Chest *77*:496–498, 1980.

5. Blanc PD, Galbo M, Hiatt P, Olson KR: Morbidity following acute irritant inhalation in a population-based study. JAMA *266*:664–669, 1991.
6. Klein J, Olsen KR, Mckinney HE: Caustic injury from household ammonia. Am J Emerg Med *3*:320, 1985.
7. Hockberter RS: Toxic gas inhalation. Digest Emerg Med Care *3*:1–8, 1983.
8. Proctor NH, Hughes JP: Chemical Hazards of the Workplace. 2nd ed. Philadelphia, J.B. Lippincott Co., pp 373–374, 1988.
9. Kass J, Zamel N, Dobry CA, et al: Bronchiectasis following ammonia burns of the respiratory tract: A review of two cases. Chest *62*:282–285, 1972.
10. Murphy DMP, Fairman RP, Lapp NL, et al: Severe airway disease due to inhalation of fumes from cleaning agents. Chest *69*:372–376, 1976.
11. Sternbach GL: Noncardiogenic pulmonary edema. Top Emerg Med *2*:35–44, 1980.
12. Plunkett ER (ed): Handbook of Industrial Toxicology. New York, Chemical Publishing Co., 1987.
13. Chu CS: New concepts of pulmonary burn injury. J Trauma *21*:958–961, 1981.
14. Howell JM: Alkalinity of non-industrial cleaning products and the likelihood of producing significant esophageal burns. Am J Emerg Med *9*:560–562, 1991.
15. Broderick A, Schwartz DA: Halogen gases, ammonia and phosgene. *In* Sullivan JB, Kreiger GR (eds): Hazardous Materials Toxicology. Baltimore, William & Wilkins, 1992.
16. Millea TP, Kucan JO, Smoot EC: Anhydrous ammonia injuries. J Burn Care Rehabil *10*:448–453, 1989.
17. Olsen KR: Ammonia. *In* Olsen KR (ed): Poisoning and Drug Overdose. Norwalk, CT, Appleton & Lange, 1990.
18. Guidotti TL: The higher oxides of nitrogen: Inhalation toxicology. Environ Res *15*:443–472, 1978.
19. Grayson RR: Silage gas poisoning: Nitrogen dioxide pneumonia, a new disease in agricultural workers. Ann Intern Med *45*:393–396, 1956.
20. Hayhurst ER, Scott E: Four cases of sudden death in a silo. JAMA *63*:1570, 1914.
21. Horvath EP, Dopico GA, Barbee RA, et al: Nitrogen dioxide-induced pulmonary disease. J Occup Med *20*:103–110, 1978.
22. Tse RL, Bockman AA: Nitrogen dioxide toxicity—report of four cases in firemen. JAMA *212*:1341–1344, 1970.
23. Morrow PE: Toxicology data on NO_x; an overview. J Toxicol Environ Health *13*:205–227, 1984.
24. Olsen KR: Nitrogen oxides. *In* Olsen KR (ed): Poisoning and Drug Overdose. Norwalk, CT, Appleton & Lange, 1990.
25. Haggerty MA, Soto-Green M, Reichan LB: Caring for victims of toxic gas inhalation. J Crit Illness *2*:77–87, 1987.
26. Samet JM, Marbury MC, Spengler JD: Health effects and sources of indoor air polution. Part 1. Am Rev Respir Dis *136*:1486–1506, 1987.
27. Sriskandan K, Pettingale KW: Numismatist's pneumonitis: A case report of acute nitrogen dioxide poisoning. Postgrad Med J *61*:819–821, 1985.
28. Jonas DO: Case for diagnosis. Mil Med *149*:481–485, 1984.
29. Hedberg K, Hedburg CW, Iber C, et al: An outbreak of nitrogen dioxide-induced respiratory illness among ice hockey players. JAMA *262*:3012–3017, 1989.
30. Cockcroft DW, Dosman JA: Respiratory health risks in farmers. Ann Intern Med *95*:380–382, 1981.
31. Maurer WJ: Silo-filler's disease: A historical perspective and report of a case. Wisc Med J *84*:13–16, 1985.
32. Moskowitz RL, Lyons HA, Cottle HR: Silo filler's disease: Clinical, physiological and pathologic study of a patient. Am J Med *36*:457–462, 1964.
33. Fleming GM, Chester EH, Montenegro HD: Dysfunction of small airways following pulmonary injury due to nitrogen dioxide. Chest *75*:720–721, 1979.
34. Bauer MA, Utell MJ, Morrow PE, et al: Inhalation of 0.30 ppm nitrogen dioxide potentiates exercise-induced bronchospasm in asthmatics. Am Rev Respir Dis *134*:1203–1208, 1986.
35. Ramirez RJ, Dowell AC: Silo filler's disease. Nitrogen dioxide-induced lung injury. Long-term follow-up and review of the literature. Ann Intern Med *74*:569–576, 1971.
36. Yockey CC, Eden BM, Byrd RB: The McConnell missile accident. Clinical spectrum of nitrogen dioxide exposure. JAMA *244*:1221–1223, 1980.
37. Lipsett M: Oxides of nitrogen and sulfur. *In* Sullivan JB, Kreiger GR (eds): Hazardous Materials Toxicology. Baltimore, William & Wilkins, 1992.
38. Welch HW, Lull RJ, Petroff PA: The use of steroids in inhalation injury. Surg Gynecol Obstet *145*:539–544, 1977.
39. Rockswold G: Inhalation of liquid nitrogen vapor. Ann Emerg Med *11*:553–555, 1982.
40. Samet JM, Utell MJ: the risk of nitrogen dioxide: What have we learned from epidemiological and clinical studies? Toxicol Ind Health *6*:247–262, 1990.
41. Cushing AH, Samet JM: Indoor pollutants: How hazardous for children? Contemp Pediatr, Feb 1991, pp 108–127.
42. Kizer KW: Toxic inhalation. Emerg Med Clin North Am *2*:649–666, 1984.
43. Moschella SL, Heuley HJ: Dermatology. Philadelphia, W.B. Saunders Co., pp 1996–2000, 1985.
44. Fitzpatrick TB, Eisen AZ, Wolff K, et al: Dermatology in General Medicine. New York, McGraw Hill Book Co., pp 927–927, 1979.
45. Nix E: Liquid-nitrogen neuropathy. Arch Dermatol *92*:185–187, 1965.
46. Finelli PF: Ulnar neuropathy after liquid nitrogen therapy. Arch Dermatol *111*:1340–1342, 1975.
47. Caravati CM Jr, Wood BT, Richardson DR: Onychodystrophies secondary to liquid nitrogen cryotherapy. Arch Dermatol *100*:441–442, 1969.
48. Greer KE, Bishop GF: Pyogenic granuloma as a complication of cryosurgery. Arch Dermatol *111*:1536–1537, 1975.
49. Epstein AM: Syncope associated with liquid nitrogen therapy. Arch Dermatol *100*:847, 1977.
50. Goldstein N: Cardiac arrest following application of liquid nitrogen. J Dermatol Surg Oncol *5*:602, 1979.
51. Cassarett, Doull: *N*-nitrosodimethylamine. *In* The Basic Science of Poisons, New York, MacMillan, pp 668–670, 1986.
52. Magee P (ed): Nitrosamine and Human Cancer, Banbury Report 12. Cold Springs Harbor, NY, Cold Springs Harbor Laboratory, 1982.
53. O Neill IK, Borstel RC, Miller CT, et al: *N*-nitroso compounds: Occurrence, biological effects and relevance to human cancer. IARC Scientific Publication 57. Lyon, France, International Agency for Research on Cancer, 1984.
54. Searle CE (ed): Chemical carcinogens. 2nd ed. ACS Monograph 173. Washington, DC, American Chemical Society, 1984.
55. Shimkin MB: Some classics of experimental oncology. NIH Publication 80–2150. Washington, DC, US Government Printing Office, 1980.
56. American Medical Association, Department of Drugs: AMA Drug Evaluations. 5th ed. Chicago, American Medical Association, 1983.
57. US Environmental Protection Agency: Dimethylnitrosamine: Health and Environmental Effects. Publication 86. Washington, DC, Office of Solid Wastes, 1980.
58. Sax NI (ed): Dangerous properties of industrial materials, No 6 (*N*-nitrosodimethylamine). New York, Van Nostrand Reinhold, pp 65–69, 1982.
59. National Institute for Occupational Safety and Health, US Department of Health, Education and Welfare: NIOSH Pocket Guide to Chemical Hazards. Washington, DC, Department of Health and Human Services (NIOSH), pp 85–114, 1985.
60. NASA Occupational Health Office: OSHA Medical Surveillance Requirements and NIOSH Recommendations for Employees Exposed to Toxic Substances and Other Work Hazards. Washington, DC, Bio Technology, 1980.
61. National Institute for Occupational Safety and Health, US Department of Health, Education and Welfare: NIOSH recommendations for occupational safety and health standards. MMWR 35(Suppl):1s, 1986.
62. National Institute for Occupational Safety and Health, US Department of Health and Human Services and US Department of Labor: Occupational Health Guidelines for Chemical Hazards. Washington, DC, Department of Health and Human Services (NIOSH), pp 81–123, 1981.
63. American Conference of Governmental and Industrial Hygien-

ists: Diethylamine: Documentation of the Threshold Limit Values for Substances in the Workroom Air. 3rd ed. Cincinnati, OH, ACGIH, 1974.

64. American Conference of Governmental and Industrial Hygienists: Triethylamine: Documentation of the Threshold Limit Values for Substances in the Workroom Air. 3rd ed. Cincinnati, OH, ACGIH, 1974

65. Stahlbom B, Lyudh T, Floren I, et al: Visual disturbances in men as a result of experimental and occupational exposure to dimethylethylamine. Br J Indust Med *48*:26–29, 1991.

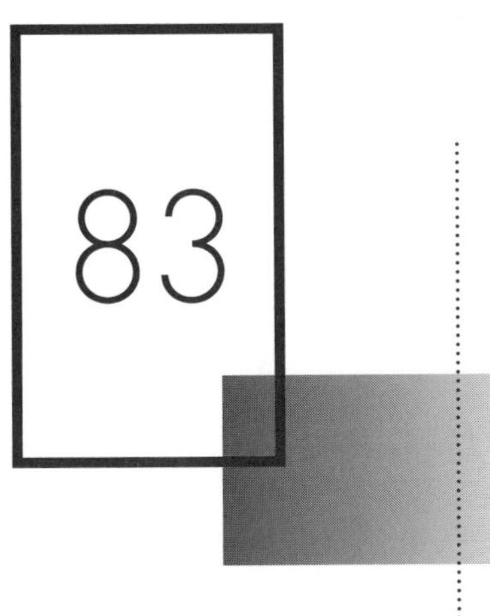

Tear Gas and Riot Control Agents

ANDIS GRAUDINS, MBBS

The term *tear gas* describes a group of chemical substances, also termed *harassing agents* or *lacrimators*, used in riot control to rapidly disable the targeted victim(s) coming into immediate contact with them. Tear gas has become widely accepted by law enforcement and military agencies as a method of controlling civilian crowds and criminal uprisings in correctional facilities. Virtually all police departments use tear gas as a nonlethal means of subduing suspected criminals. These agents are also becoming increasingly popular as nonlethal personal safety agents (in lieu of gun ownership). Large amounts of tear gas have been used worldwide. In recent times, tear gas has been released to quell demonstrations and control civil unrest in places as culturally diverse as Chile, Panama, South Korea, and the Gaza strip and West Bank in Israel. There is a paucity of literature regarding the true incidence of complications associated with the use of these agents in the field. This is primarily because of the difficulty in collecting epidemiologic information on the victims of mass exposures to tear gas agents. Consequently, the overall safety of these agents has been questioned by the medical community.[1]

Historically, various types of harassing agents have been used for centuries in the field against enemy forces. From antiquity to the Middle Ages, oxides of sulfur were combusted upwind of enemies with the aim of enveloping them in a cloud of smoke. Arsenical smoke was used sporadically from the 15th to 17th centuries. In the 20th century, the Paris police were the first to use chemical agents, in 1912. Grenades filled with ethylbromoacetate (EBA) were deployed against "lawless gangs." EBA was also used in the early phases of World War I by French ex-police conscripts.[2] Modern tear gas agents were first used in the United States during the crime waves of the 1920s to combat gangsters and as personal protection agents.[3] Subsequently, many harassing agents have been developed. Dispersal systems have also been refined in the ensuing years to improve delivery of these agents.

As many as 15 different irritants have been developed during the course of this century. Of these, only three tear gas agents and one irritant remain in common use worldwide. These are

1. 1-Chloracetophenone (CN, Mace)
2. 2-Chlorobenzylidene malonitrile (CS)
3. Dibenzoxapine (CR)
4. Capsaicin (pepper spray, "pepper Mace")

SPECIFIC IRRITANT AGENTS

Chloracetophenone

Chloracetophenone is also called simply CN. The name *Mace* originally described this agent alone. The eponym MACE was derived from a particular chemical formulation of CN: methylchloroform chloracetophenone. CN is manufactured by chlorination of acetophenone with selenium oxychloride.[4] Its chemical formula is $C_6H_5COCH_2Cl$. Chloracetophenone can be discharged as a smoke or powder but is commonly released as aerosol. Thermal grenades and artillery shells may be used to disseminate this substance. CN is heat stable, breaking down only when exposed to temperatures greater than 300°C for 15 minutes or more. When used in large amounts, CN can persist in the environment for hours to days, depending on prevailing meteorologic conditions.[5] If injected parenterally, CN can act as an alkylating agent that reacts with cellular sulfhydryl groups, with the potential for mutagenesis.[2]

The irritant effects of CN are thought to be due to the reactivity of its chloride moiety with skin and mucous membranes. Exposure results in immediate stinging and burning of the skin and mucosal surfaces, lacrimation, blepharospasm, salivation, and rhinorrhea.[4] Inhalation produces a sensation of chest constriction with dyspnea, gagging, and burning of the respiratory tract.[6] The dermal irritant effects of CN are enhanced in the presence of moisture or sweat on the skin. Hot, humid weather can produce a similar augmentation of irritant effects.[5] In most instances, the effects of CN are transient when removed from the source of exposure. A summary of the effects is listed in Table 83–1. These slowly dissipate within 20 minutes. Ocular effects are usually more prolonged. Conjunctivitis and blurred vision may persist for as long as 24 hours after exposure.[6]

CN is thought to be more toxic than CS, with a number of reports of varying toxicity abscribed to this harassing agent. Permanent corneal damage can result from CN particles embedded on the cornea, particularly when used in the aerosolized particulate form.[7] Epithelial recovery of the cornea may take months, leaving permanent corneal opacities and visual loss.[8] Direct spraying of CN and similar agents onto the face also has the potential to produce barotrauma to the eyes. Cutaneous reactions to CN have included allergic reactions and dermatitis,[9] skin burns, and bullous eruptions from prolonged exposure or direct spraying of CN onto the skin.[10] Generalized papulovesicular rashes responding to treatment with systemic steroid therapy have also been reported.[10] Death due to delayed pulmonary edema, 12 hours after exposure to CN, has occurred. The risk appears greatest in enclosed spaces, where concentrations of CN can be significantly higher than in the open.[11] Animal studies have demonstrated pulmonary exudation of protein and polymorphonuclear cells after exposure to high concentrations of CN. This is followed by suppressed phagocytic capability of immunocompetent cells. Increased susceptibility to infection is a potential consideration after large or repeated exposures to CN.[12] The actual risk of infection to humans after massive exposures to CN or other lacrimators is unknown. Additionally, little is known about the risk of chronic pulmonary toxicity, genotoxicity, or reproductive toxicologic effects associated with CN exposure.

Table 83–1. Local Effects of Riot Control Agents

Site	Effect
Eye	Discomfort or pain, blepharospasm and lacrimation
Mouth	Stinging or burning of palate and tongue, excess salivation
Nose	Rhinorrhea and discomfort
Respiratory tract	Tightness or burning sensation in the chest, coughing, sneezing, and increased tracheobronchial secretions
Skin	Stinging and burning, erythema

Modified from Balantyne B: Biomedical and health aspects of the use of chemicals in civil disturbances. *In* Scott RB, Frazer J (eds): Medical Annual. Bristol, UK, Wright & Sons, pp 7–41, 1977.

Chlorbenzylidene Malonitrile

CS was first produced in 1928 by Corson and Stoughton. CS was seen as a more potent and less toxic lacrimatory agent than CN. Large-scale production for use as a riot control agent commenced in the 1950s in the United Kingdom.[4] CS is the riot control agent most commonly used worldwide today. Its potency as an irritant is 10 times that of CN. The potential for severe toxicity with CS is reported to be much less than that of CN[1] (see comparison of effects and toxicity of agents in Table 83–2). Chemically, CS is a variant of an older, previously used irritant, bromobenzyl cyanide. It is a stable gas with a pepper-like odor.[5] CS exists as a crystalline powder and is dispersed by aerosol blowers or bursting thermal grenades. The chemical formula of CS is $ClC_6H_4CHCCN(CN)_2$. Vaporization of CS can be achieved by igniting a mixture of the powder with a fuel substance, producing clouds of white smoke containing CS vapor.[5] When detonated in the open, a CS grenade can produce a cloud of 6 to 9 m in diameter. The concentration of CS at the center of the cloud can range from 2000 to 5000 mg/m^3, rapidly declining at the periphery.[1] Detonation in an enclosed space or multiple-grenade-burst detonation has the potential for producing much higher concentrations. The lethal dose of CS for 50% of healthy adults (LD_{50}) has been estimated to be between 25,000 and 150,000 mg/m^3 per minute, based on animal studies.[2]

The clinical effects of CS appear within seconds of exposure. The threshold value for eye irritation has been determined to be 0.004 mg/m^3 (the comparable value for CN is 0.3 mg/m^3). An effective aerosol concentration of 5 mg/m^3 results in severe burning of the eyes, with lacrimation, blepharospasm, and conjunctival injection.[3] Respiratory effects include sneezing, cough, chest tightness, and rhinobronchorrhea. Tidal volume and minute ventilation have been observed to decrease with experimental exposure to CS.[13] The reasons for this are uncertain. Exposed skin stings and develops erythema. As with CN,

Table 83–2. Riot Control Agents: Comparison of Potency and Toxicity

	CN	CS	CR
Eye irritation threshold (mg/m^2)	0.3	0.004	0.002
LD_{50} (mg/kg) intraperitoneal—guinea pig	17	73	390
LD_{50} (mg/kg) oral—rabbit	118	230	1760
Estimated lethal dose (mg/min per m^3)	10×10^3	60×10^3	$>100 \times 10^3$

Modified from Beswick FW: Chemical agents used in riot control and warfare. Hum Toxicol *2*:247–256, 1983.

moist areas are more severely affected. Nausea and vomiting may result from swallowing saliva that contains CS. In most cases, with exposure to moderate concentrations of CS, symptoms should rapidly abate within 30 minutes after an exposure.[14, 15] Like CN, parenterally injected CS can act as an alkylator of cellular sulfhydryl groups. Parenteral infusion of CS is associated with its metabolism to cyanide. The metabolism of CS to cyanide is thought to be clinically insignificant after cutaneous or inhalation exposures, because systemic absorption by these routes is extremely small.[2]

Despite initial enthusiam for the use of CS as a less toxic alternative to CN, reports of significant toxicity of CS have appeared in the medical literature. Severe reactions to CS have resulted from its direct spraying onto cutaneous surfaces. Vesicular dermatitis with blistering, crusting, and marked facial swelling has developed from 12 hours to 3 days after either single or repeated exposures to CS.[16] Allergic contact dermatitis has been documented in cases of recurrent exposure to CS, with allergy subsequently confirmed by patch testing.[17] Exposure to high concentrations of CS in enclosed spaces has resulted in significant pulmonary pathology. Pulmonary edema developed 6 to 8 hours after such an exposure to CS in a previously healthy male presenting with dyspnea and wheezing.[18] Severe respiratory distress and bronchopneumonia were identified in a 4-month-old infant after exposure to CS for 2 to 3 hours in an enclosed space.[19] Persisting reactive airways dysfunction may also occur after intense exposure to CS tear gas.[20] CS powders have produced eye damage, particularly when used at close range.[7]

According to the Himsworth report, the risk of congenital anomalies, stillbirth, and spontaneous abortion was not increased in areas of heavy tear gas use in Londonderry during the late 1960s.[21] However, cytotoxic and mutagenic activity has been observed in mammalian cells in culture exposed to CS.[22] Animal studies have been unable to conclusively prove any carcinogenic or teratogenic effects after exposure to CS tear gas.[1]

Dibenzoxapine

CR is approximately 10 times more potent than CS. It is effective at concentrations of 1 mg/m^3 and higher. The lethal dose in humans has been estimated to be greater than 100,000 mg/m^3 per minute. CR is more stable than CN or CS and has a lower vapor pressure, making it much more persistent in the environment.[2] It is commonly deployed as a liquid but can also be aerosolized.

Because CR is usually delivered in solution, its effects tend to be localized to the skin and eyes. Pulmonary effects are rare owing to its low vapor pressure. On exposure to CR, skin irritation, lacrimation, eye pain, and blepharospasm develop within seconds and abate in 15 to 20 minutes after removal from exposure. Conjunctival injection and erythema of the skin develop in minutes and may persist for 1 to 2 hours. Dermal and ocular discomfort may recur up to 24 hours after exposure when exposed sites contact water.[15] CR appears to be less toxic than CN or CS in animal studies.[2] Few data exist to support or refute these observations in humans.

Capsaicin

Capsaicin (8-methyl-*N*-vanillyl-6-nonenamide) is the active ingredient largely responsible for the irritating and pungent effects of the fruits of the various species of *Capsicum*. These include the Mexican chile pepper and the Hungarian red pepper.[23] The potent topical irritant effects of capsaicin have made its use as a personal protection and immobilizing device appealing for both law enforcement agencies and the civilian population. Repeated topical capsaicin application has been used for cutaneous counter-irritant effects in chronic pain and inflammatory conditions.

The mechanism of action of capsaicin on cutaneous nerve endings has been extensively studied. Application of capsaicin to the skin or mucous membranes results in widespread excitation of cutaneous C fiber polymodal nociceptor afferent nerve terminals. Capsaicin achieves this by nonspecifically opening nerve fiber sodium, calcium, and potassium channels and releasing substance P from nerve endings.[24] This produces an intense sensation of burning pain and marked hyperalgesia to skin heating and pressure. Symptoms may be exacerbated by the presence of sweat or the application of cold water. Hyperalgesia may persist for as long as 24 hours. Cutaneous vasodilatation is also seen at the site of application and the surrounding skin via an axon flare reflex.[24] Application to the eyes results in intense pain, tearing, blepharospasm, and conjunctivitis.[25] High-pressure aerosol application to the face has the potential to produce barotrauma and mechanical injury to the eyes. Inhalation of capsaicin by asthmatic and nonasthmatic volunteers resulted in coughing and transient increases in airway resistance. This is postulated to be due to stimulation of airway sensory nerves.[26] Cutaneous application of capsaicin over days to weeks can result in habituation to its irritant effects and hypalgesia of the skin.[24]

In 1993, more than 6 million "pepper gas" spray units were sold in the United States alone.[27] When used as a harassing agent, capsaicin is used as a spray at close quarters. It is usually contained in a pressurized aerosol container in a hydrocarbon vehicle such as tetrachloroethylene, Freon, or isopropyl alcohol. When used correctly, capsaicin can result in transient, severe skin and mucous membrane irritation, incapacitating an assailant rapidly. Improper use has resulted in significant morbidity in a small number of reported cases. An 11-year-old boy developed laryngeal edema with marked stridor and pulmonary edema, requiring endotracheal intubation 4 hours after the intentional inhalation of several sprays of a capsaicin personal protection device in a hydrofluorocarbon vehicle. His clinical course improved during the next 24 hours.[28] A 4-week-old infant accidentally sprayed in the face with a 5% capsaicin aerosol developed respiratory failure and pulmonary edema, requiring extracorporeal membrane oxygenation.[27] It is difficult to ascertain the degree of influence that inhaled capsaicin had in the evolution of pulmonary injury in both cases. Exposure to high concentrations of hydrocarbon propellant may have also had a role in the development of lung injury.[27] Severe dermatitis, labeled *Hunan hand syndrome*, may result after skin exposure to capsaicin. This is particularly common in people who handle chile peppers with bare hands, resulting in severe pain and erythema of exposed surfaces.[29, 30] Relief from symptoms may be difficult to achieve. Immersion of the hands in vinegar has been successful in providing relief if applied within 30 minutes of exposure.[31] Topical lidocaine gel has also been successful in relief of irritation.[30] Prolonged immersion of hands in vegetable oil after exposure to a chile slurry has also been found to provide better long-term relief from the pain of Hunan hand than bathing in cool tap water.[32] Milk compresses have been suggested as an effective analgesic measure for the relief of capsaicin-induced dermal irritation.[33]

News reports in the lay press have raised the issue of deaths in custody temporally related to the use of capsaicin sprays. Extensive testing by the Federal Bureau of Investigation in the 1980s found no evidence of toxic problems with capsaicin use.[34] No firm scientific data currently substantiate any casual relationship between these deaths and capsaicin exposure. In these situations, victims are often in an agitated state requiring restraint, which may be implemented in a way that unintentionally produces postural asphyxia.[34] Victims are often under the influence of alcohol and drugs of abuse, which may increase aggression, mask occult trauma, and delay recognition of medical problems. In absence of any definite link between capsaicin exposure and sudden death, law enforcement agencies currently continue to use capsaicin as a harassing agent.

METHODS OF DISPERSAL OF THE HARASSING AGENTS

The way in which chemical agents are dispersed depends on the situation in which they are used. Irritant smoke can be produced by combining the agent (CN or CS) with a pyrotechnic mixture containing chlorate and lactose. The ignitor vaporizes the irritant, which then condenses into a cloud of solid or liquid particles 1 to 2 μm in diameter that can be easily inhaled.[4] This method is best used in the control of large-scale riots. CS also exists as a micropulverized powder that can be dispersed by force—blowing using a vehicle- or aircraft-mounted "smoke" generator or from a hand-held tank using carbon dioxide as a propellant.[4] This method does not require the use of a thermal agent to volatilize the irritant.

CN and CS can also be delivered by a thermal grenade or a cartridge fired from a gun. Grenades are often lauched into confined spaces by law enforcement agencies to incapacitate criminals in siege situations. Thermal grenades may produce fires.[4] There is a risk of mechanical trauma to victims hit by projectiles or in close proximity to exploding grenades.

Aerosols of irritant agents are used in small pressurized containers at close quarters to disable a would-be attacker. Capsaicin sprays (e.g., Guardian) are available commercially in some countries. CN and CS have been used with similar delivery systems in the past (e.g., Federal Streamer—CN, Paralyser—CS). The risk of persisting ocular morbidity from direct spraying of CN or CS in the eyes is significant.

In general, CS and CN used as a particulate smoke tend to affect the eyes and respiratory tract to a greater degree than the skin. Aerosols and liquid sprays are likely to produce more marked effects on the skin and eyes with less effect on the respiratory tract.

MANAGEMENT OF EXPOSURES

Most victims exposed to the tearing agents or capsaicin develop transient symptoms and signs of skin and mucosal irritation. These usually subside when victims are removed from the source of the exposure. Treatment of victims after more significant exposure begins with decontamination to reduce ongoing irritation. Prevention of contamination of emergency department staff is also extremely important. Medical and nursing staff should protect themselves with gloves, gowns, and eyewear. Victims should be treated in a well-ventilated area to prevent atmospheric accumulation of the tearing agent. Contaminated clothing should be removed and disposed of in plastic bags.[35] Exposed areas should be washed with warm water and soap. Attempted orotracheal intubation of patients exposed to CS has resulted in severe blepharospasm and lacrimation in the anesthesiologist performing the procedure owing to oropharyngeal contamination with tear gas.[36] This situation may result in difficulty or delay in airway control in a patient with otherwise normal airway anatomy.

The eyes should be irrigated for at least 30 minutes with normal saline in symptomatic patients. This should be followed by ophthalmologic assessment for ocular injury, including fluorescein examination for corneal ulceration and abrasion. Persisting symptoms and signs require formal ophthalmologic follow-up.

Contact dermatitis due to CN or CS has responded to topical or systemic corticosteroid therapy.[16, 17] Skin erythema alone does not require any treatment and usually diminishes within 24 hours.

Respiratory symptoms due to CN / CS exposure are usually transient and should disappear within 15 to 30 minutes of removal from the gas. Factors that may increase the risk of persisting pulmonary symptoms and development of pulmonary edema include prolonged exposure to CN or CS in an enclosed space, direct inhalation of capsaicin into the respiratory tract, or a history of asthma or other chronic lung disease. Bronchospasm may respond to inhaled β-adrenergic agonists and oral or parenteral corticosteroids. Patients with persisting symptoms or signs of respiratory distress may be at risk of delayed pulmonary edema and require further evaluation and admission for observation. Standard supportive measures and ventilatory support are indicated for pulmonary edema. Extracorporeal membrane oxygenation has been successfully used to support an infant with pulmonary edema after exposure to capsaicin aerosol.[27]

Finally, attention should also be paid to the potential for physical injury to victims of harassing agents. Injury may be masked by the presence of alcohol or other drugs of abuse. Trauma may be due to the violent situations in which the individuals were involved or may be a direct consequence of ballistic trauma due to the projectiles used to propel harassing agents.

SUMMARY

In most instances, exposure to harassing agents in mild to moderate concentrations in open spaces is associated with transient irritant effects. Morbidity and mortality are more likely to occur as a consequence of intense exposure to CN or CS tear gases at high concentrations, such as when used in enclosed spaces. Severe cutaneous burns and pulmonary injury are the most significant consequences of exposure. Victims of repeated exposure may develop allergic cutaneous sensitization to these agents. Capsaicin is an effective incapacitating agent when used at close quarters and appears to have minimal persisting toxicity. There is the potential for significant pulmonary injury if accidentally or intentionally inhaled in large amounts. To date, it is unclear whether any of these agents poses any significant long-term toxic risk to humans.

Management of victims exposed to the harassing agents includes decontamination of exposed surfaces and supportive care for any cutaneous or systemic sequelae. It is also important to investigate for physical injuries in patients presenting to the emergency department. In most instances, discharge after a brief period of observation is all that is required in asymptomatic patients. Persisting pulmonary symptoms or signs warrant admission and observation.

References

1. Hu H, Fine J, Epstein P, et al: Tear gas—harassing agent or toxic chemical weapon? JAMA *262*:660–663, 1989.
2. Beswick FW: Chemical agents used in riot control and warfare. Hum Toxicol *2*:247–256, 1983.
3. Sanford JP: Medical aspects of riot control (harassing) agents. Annu Rev Med *27*:421–429, 1976.
4. Compton AF: Chloracetophenone (CN). *In* Compton AF (ed): Military Chemical and Biological Agents—Chemical and Toxicological Properties. Caldwell, NJ, Telford Press, 1987.
5. Danto BL: Medical problems and criteria regarding the use of tear gas by police. Am J Forensic Med Pathol *8*:317–322, 1987.
6. Punte CL, Gutentag PJ, Owens EJ, et al: Inhalation studies with chloracetophenone, diphenylaminochlorasine and pelargonic morpholide. 11 human exposures. Am Ind Hyg Assoc J *23*:199–202, 1962.
7. Gaskins JR, Hehir RM, McCaulley DR, et al: Lacrimating agents (CS and CN) in rats and rabbits. Arch Environ Health *24*:449–454, 1972.
8. Liss G: Reaction to MACE. Letter. Am Intraocular Soc J *8*:371, 1982.
9. Frazier CA: Contact allergy to MACE. JAMA *236*:2526, 1976.
10. Thorburn KM: Injuries after use of the lacrimatory agent chloracetophenone in a confined space. Arch Environ Health *37*:182–186, 1982.
11. Stein AA, Kirwan WE: Chloracetophenone (tear gas) poisoning: A clinicopathologic report. J Forensic Sci *9*:374–382, 1964.
12. Kumar P, Kumar P, Zachariah K, et al: Effects of chloracetophenone (CN) vapor inhalation on pulmonary immune system of mice. Bull Environ Contam Toxicol *50*:69–76, 1993.
13. Cole TJ, Cotes JE, Johnson GR, et al: Ventilation, cardiac frequency and pattern of breathing during exercise in men exposed to *o*-chlorobenzylidene malonitrile (CS) and ammonia gas in low concentrations. Q J Exp Physiol *62*:341–351, 1977.
14. Holland P, White RG: The cutaneous reactions produced by chlorobenzylidene malonitrile and chloracetophenone when applied directly to the skin of human subjects. Br J Dermatol *86*:159–154, 1972.
15. Ballantyne B, Gall D, Robson DC: Effects on man of drenching with dilute solutions of *o*-chlorobenzylidene malonitrile (CS) and dibenz-1:4-oxapine (CR). Med Sci Law *16*:159–170, 1976.
16. Parneix-Spake A, Theisen A, Roujeau JC, et al: Severe cutaneous reactions to self-defense sprays. Letter. Arch Dermatol *129*:913, 1993.
17. Ro YS, Lee CW: Tear gas dermatitis. Allergic contact sensitization due to CS. Int J Dermatol *30*:576–577, 1991.
18. Krapf R, Thalman H: Akute exposition durch CS-Rauchgas und klinische beobachtungen. Schweiz Med Wochenschr *111*:2056–2060, 1981.
19. Park S, Giammona ST: Toxic effects of tear gas on an infant following prolonged exposure. Am J Dis Child *123*:245–246, 1972.
20. Hu H, Christiani D: Reactive airways dysfunction after exposure to tear gas. Letter. Lancet *339*:1535, 1992.

21. Himsworth H: Report of the enquiry into the medical and toxicological aspects of CS (orthochlorobenzylidene malonitrile), II: Enquiry into toxicological aspects of CS and its use for civil purposes. London, England, Her Majesty's Stationary Office, 1971.
22. Ziegler-Skylakakis K, Summer KH, Andrae U: Mutagenicity and cytotoxicity of 2-chlorobenzylidene malonitrile (CS) and metabolites in V79 Chinese hamster cells. Arch Toxicol *63*:314–319, 1989.
23. Virus RM, Gebhart FG: Pharmacologic actions of capsaicin: Apparent involvement of substance P and serotonin. Life Sci *25*:1273–1284, 1979.
24. Lynn B: Capsaicin: Actions on nociceptive C-fibres and therapeutic potential. Pain *41*:61–69, 1990.
25. Tominack RL, Spycker DA: Capsicum and capsaicin—a review: Case report to the use of hot peppers in child abuse. J Toxicol Clin Toxicol *25*:591–601, 1987.
26. Fuller RAW: Pharmacology of inhaled capsaicin in humans. Resp Med *85*(Suppl A):31–34, 1991.
27. Wily J, Balmier D, Farina P, et al: Severe pulmonary injury in an infant after pepper gas self defense spray exposure. Abstract. J Toxicol Clin Toxicol *33*:519, 1995.
28. Winograd HL. Acute croup in an older child: An unusual toxic origin. Clin Pediatr *16*:884–887, 1977.
29. Weinberg RB: Hunan hand. N Engl J Med *305*:1020, 1981.
30. Williams SR, Clark RF, Dunford JV: Contact dermatitis associated with capsaicin: Hunan hand syndrome. Ann Emerg Med *25*:713–715, 1995.
31. Vogl TP: Treatment of Hunan hand. N Engl J Med *306*:178, 1982.
32. Jones LA, Tandberg D, Troutman WG: Household treatment for "chile burns" of the hands. J Toxicol Clin Toxicol *25*:483–491, 1987.
33. Anderson W: Relief of capsaicin contact dermatitis. Letter. Ann Emerg Med *26*:659, 1995.
34. Krolikowski FJ: Oleo Capsicum (O.C.): The need for careful evaluation. Letter. Am J Forensic Med Pathol *15*:267, 1994.
35. Fine K, Bassin RH, Stewart MM: Emergency care for tear gas victims. J Am Coll Emerg Physicians *6*:144, 1977.
36. Bhattacharya ST, Hayward AW: CS gas—implications for the anaesthetist. Anaesthesia *48*:896–897, 1993.

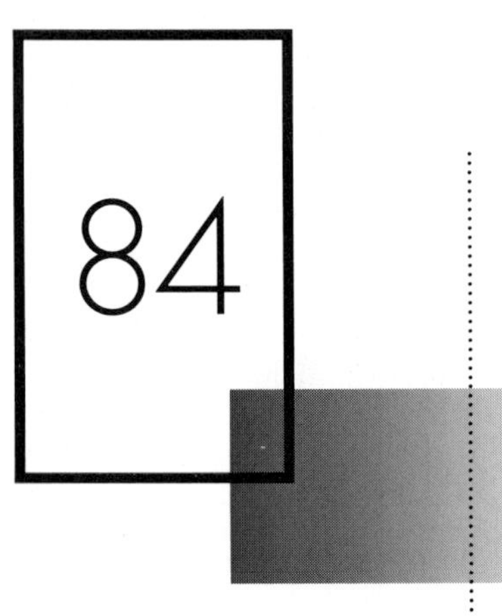

Volatile Substance Abuse

HOWARD C. MOFENSON, MD
THOMAS R. CARACCIO, PharmD
DONALD A. FEINFELD, MD

Solvent abuse is the deliberate inhalation of volatile organic compounds to produce alterations in the conscious state and perception for recreational purposes.[1] Jaffe noted that "each generation not only adds a few new substances, but seems impelled to reevaluate the old."[2] Inhalation is the primary method of administration of various volatile substances, particularly the organic solvents.

HISTORY

The inhalation of substances to produce euphoria has been traced to the ancient Greeks.[3] The modern use of inhaled substances began in the mid-1800s with the advent of halogenated hydrocarbon anesthetic agents. Trichloroethane was first used as an animal anesthetic and then in human surgery in 1847.[4] It was used consistently for nearly 100 years until less toxic drugs were developed. Another anesthetic, nitrous oxide, called "laughing gas," originated in early 1800s along with other substances such as ether; it was used as a euphoric at "frolics" by medical students.[5]

By the turn of the century, petroleum distillation yielded many new types of solvents. The early reported episodes of solvent abuse in the 20th century involved the sniffing of gasoline in the 1950s and model airplane cement in the 1960s.

EPIDEMIOLOGY

Precise epidemiologic data on inhalants are not available. Several reports have identified inhalant abuse as a problem of serious proportions.[6] Inhalant abuse is considered by many to be the gateway to abuse of other substances.[7] The pattern of inhalant abuse is exemplified by two national studies entitled the Monitoring the Future survey of 12th graders from 1975 to 1995[8] and Drug Use Among 8th Grade Students.[9] The peak age of inhalant abuse is 13 to 15 years. However, inhalant abuse may begin as early as 6 to 8 years of age and typically declines by 17 to 19 years of age. Although many young solvent abusers outgrow the habit, some inhalant abusers become chronic users and develop emotional dependendency, continuing the practice into adulthood. Others progress to use other drugs and only reduce (rather than discontinue) their inhalant use. The current use of inhalants among college students contradicts the prevailing view that inhalant abuse is largely confined to early adolescents who are poor and urban dwellers.[10, 11] Although inhalant abuse is more prevalent among the poor, it crosses all socioeconomic and ethnic barriers.[12] The National Institute on Drug Abuse monitoring of eighth graders has documented a lifetime prevalence of inhalant abuse of 21.6%, with 19.9% of eighth graders using inhalants during the previous year. A 1995 study showed that 36.4% of high school seniors surveyed admitted to having abused inhalants.[13, 14] These surveys underestimate the true prevalence because school dropouts and incarcerated youth, who have a higher rate of substance abuse, are not included. Most surveys of children and adolescents have revealed a decline in the use of mind-altering substances; however, the lifetime prevalence of inhalant abuse has increased, and inhalants have surpassed marijuana in frequency of use, according to one study.[9] In the United Kingdom, the only country that closely monitors inhalant-related mortality, use of inhalants causes approximately two deaths each week.[15] Sudden sniffing death syndrome is the most common cause of death, occasionally occurring in first-time users.[16]

Cohen identifies three groups of inhalant users. The first and largest includes the experimenters, who sample the inhalant a few times and then discontinue. The second includes social users, who use them frequently, perhaps once a month. The third group is known as the "heads," who use inhalants on a daily basis.[10] The two most important factors that contribute to continued use of inhalants are peer pressure and dysfunctional families. Chronic inhalant abuse is associated with school failure, delinquency, and social maladjustment.[17, 18]

METHODS OF INHALANT ABUSE AND IMMEDIATE EFFECTS OF INHALANTS

Abuse of volatile substances usually takes one of the following forms: "sniffing," "huffing," or "bagging." Sniffing is accomplished by direct nasal inhalation of the volatile substance, directly from the container. Huffing requires the user to thoroughly moisten a cloth with the substance and then to place the rolled cloth directly into the mouth deeply and inhale the fumes. In bagging, the user empties the volatile substance into a plastic bag and either breathes deeply through the bag's opening or places her or his head directly into the bag, inhaling deeply.

A simple but more toxic approach is to spray the substance directly into the oral cavity. Aerosol sprays can be inhaled directly, bagged, or huffed. Balloons have been used to capture the spray from the aerosol can. In all cases, the desired effects occur in seconds to minutes, beginning with euphoria, dizziness, and inhibition that rapidly progresses to central nervous system (CNS) depression.[19]

The assortment of volatile substances available for abuse is numerous and varied. Volatile agents are often complex chemical compounds that contain vehicles or excipients that may be more toxic than the active chemical for which the product was inhaled. The major categories of inhalants are hydrocarbons, anesthetics and nitrites, esters and ketones. Tables 84–1 to 84–3 list commonly abused solvents. The hydrocarbons include aliphatic hydrocarbons, aromatic hydrocarbons, and halogenated hydrocarbons. A separate category of aliphatic hydrocarbons, the nitrites, are marketed as room deodorizers or liquid incense under various names such as "Locker Room," "Rush," "Jac aroma," and "Locker Proper." Nitrites are discussed further in Chapter 13.

Nitrous oxide is still used today as a general anesthetic/analgesic (particularly in dental offices), as a propellant for whipped cream, and in rocket fuel. As a propellant, nitrous oxide is available in small metal cylinders called "whippets."[12]

MECHANISM OF ACTION OF INHALANTS

Inhalation is an effective method of administration of many physiologically active substances, varying from anesthetics to opioids. The rapid onset of action when drugs are administered by this route is due primarily to the extensive capillary network of the pulmonary alveolar system. The efficacy of drug delivery by this route of administration has been compared with intravenous injection.[20]

Inhalants are depressants that are related pharmacologically to anesthetic agents. The neurologic effects of volatile substances are a result of their lipophilic nature (especially toluene, trichloroethylene, and combinations of *n*-hexane, butanone, and methyl-*N*-butyl ketone [MnBK]) and the toxicity of these agents related to their defatting nature. Because the lipid content of myelin is the highest among all biologic membranes (75%) and the neuronal membrane contains 45% lipid, it is not surprising that such highly lipophilic substances cause

Table 84–1. Common Substances of Inhalant Abuse (by Chemical Class)

Chemical Class	Chemical Name	Product
Aliphatic hydrocarbons	*n*-Heptane	Adhesives, rubber cement, gasoline, paint thinner, solvent
	n-Hexane	Adhesives, rubber cement, model cement
	Gasoline	Gasoline, solvent
Aliphatic nitrites	Amyl nitrite	Room deodorants
	Isobutyl nitrite	
	Butyl nitrite	
Anesthetics	Carbon tetrachloride	Grain fumigant, laboratory solvent
	Enflurane	Anesthetic
	Freons	Aerosol propellant
	Chlorodifluoromethane (Halon 22)	Aerosol propellant
	Dichlorodifluoromethane (Halon 12)	Aerosol propellant, refrigerant
	Dichlorotetrafluoroethane (Halon 114)	Aerosol propellant
	Trichlorofluoromethane (Halon 11)	Aerosol propellant, refrigerant
	Halothane	Anesthetic
	Methylene chloride (dichloromethane)	Degreaser, paint thinner/stripper
	Tetrachloroethylene	Degreaser, dry cleaning
	Trichloroethylene	Degreaser, dry cleaning, gum remover
	1,1,1-Trichloroethane (methyl chloroform)	Degreaser, dry cleaning, typewriter correcting fluid
	Nitrous oxide	Foam dispensers
Aromatic hydrocarbons	Benzene	Adhesives, rubber cement, degreasers, gasoline
	Naphthalene	Adhesives, rubber cement, gasoline, paint thinner
	Styrene	Adhesives, rubber cement, model cement, airplane glue
	Toluene	Adhesives, rubber cement, aerosol sprays, degreasers, gasoline, model cement, paint thinners/stripper, spray shoe polish
	Xylene	Adhesives, rubber cement, aerosol sprays, degreasers, gasoline, model cement, paint thinner
Esters	Ethyl acetate	Adhesive, paint thinner
	N-Butyl acetate	Degreasers
	N-Proyl acetate	Paint thinner
Ketones	Acetone	Model cement, paint thinner, nail polish remover
	Methyl butyl ketone	Paint thinner
	Methyl ethyl ketone (butonone)	Degreasers, paint thinner, solvent
	Methyl isobutyl ketone	Solvent
Others	Bromochlorodifluromethane (BCF)	Fire-extinguishing agent
	n-Butane	Bottled fuel gas
	Propane	Bottled fuel gas

Data from National Institute on Drug Abuse: Inhalants: The Deliberate Inhalation of Volatile Substances, report series 30, No. 2. Rockville, MD, NIDA, 1978; and Meredith TJ, Ruprah M, Liddle A, et al: Diagnosis and treatment of acute poisoning with volatile substances. Hum Toxicol *8*:277, 1989.

Table 84–2. Common Halogenated and Aromatic Hydrocarbons

	Substance	Common Source	TLV-TWA (ppm)
Halogenated	1,2-Dichloroethane	Vinyl chloride production, solvents	1
	1,2-Dichloroethylene (acetylene chloride)	Caffeine extractant, plastics, solvents	200
	Dichloromethane (methylene chloride)	Degreasing agent, paint/varnish remover	50
	Tetrachloroethane (acetylene tetrachloride)	Solvent, paint/varnish/rust remover	1
	Tetrachloromethane	Solvent, degreaser, fire extinguisher agent	2
	Tetrachloroethylene (Tetra, Perchloroethylene, Perk)	Dry cleaning, Typewriter correction fluid, vapor degreaser	50
	Trichloroethylene	Fire retardant	
	1,1,1-Trichloroethane (methyl chloroform, Triethane, Glamorene, Scotch Guard, All Guard)	Solvent, inks, typewriter correction fluid	350
	1,1,2-Trichloroethane (vinyl trichloride)	Solvent, adhesive, insecticide	350
Aromatic	Styrene	Polystyrene plastics, latex coatings	50
	Toluene	Solvents, paints, paint/lacquer thinner	100
	Xylene	Woodworking adhesives	100

TLV-TWA, threshold limit value–time-weighted average based on the recommended limit of concentration of various substances in the air to which workers are exposed, for a 40-hour work week in parts per million (ppm). Unfortunately, it may not be useful in the evaluation of risk of concentrated inhalants, but it gives a guideline to the relative toxicity.

severe and often irreversible neurologic, neurobehavioral, and cognitive damage.

The proposed mechanism of the narcosis due to volatile substance inhalation has long been believed to be an increase in the permeability of cellular membranes of the CNS with altered neuronal function. More recent hypotheses have focused on ligand-gated ion channels, especially those associated with the glutamate and γ-aminobutyric acid-A ($GABA_A$) receptors. The anesthetic-like hydrocarbons potentiate the effects of these neurotransmitters at their receptors.[21–26]

CAUSES OF INHALANT ABUSE

The risk factors for inhalant abuse are similar to those for other types of substance abuse.[27] The reasons for choosing volatile substances for a "high" are that they are readily available, easily accessible, convenient, and inexpensive; they lack legislative control and are capable of producing a rapid, pleasurable sensory experience.[27] These same factors make inhalants more readily available to preadolescents, in contrast to other substances of abuse.

EFFECTS OF VOLATILE INHALANTS

Table 84–4 lists examples of the toxicity of various inhalants. Inhalation of these substances produces diverse effects. The effects are felt almost immediately and are similar to the early classic stages of anesthesia.

Physiologic and behavioral effects include euphoria, excitation, and disinhibition (associated with impulsive behavior). Visual and auditory hallucinations are experienced at high doses, followed by drowsiness and sleep.[28] Delusions of unusual strength or of the ability to fly may occur.

Neurologic effects include slurred speech and staggering gait. CNS depression, anesthesia, and peripheral neuropathy may occur. Coma is unusual because as the user begins to sleep, the source falls away from inhalation sites and the exposure is terminated.[29] Neurologic syndromes produced by organic solvents are listed in Table 84–4.

Gastrointestinal effects include mucous membrane irritation.

Cardiovascular effects include vasodilatation and lowering of the threshold of the myocardium to cardiac dysrhythmias.

Other systemic effects include defatting dermatitis and hepatic and renal damage.

Table 84–3. Commonly Abused Solvents

Common Products	Ingredients
Adhesives/glues	Toluene, benzene, xylene, acetone, trichloroethylene, trichloroethane
Aerosols	Fluorocarbons
Airplane glue	Toluene (polystyrene cement)
Dry cleaning	Methylene chloride, trichloroethylene, carbon tetrachloride
Dyes	Acetone, methylene chloride, petroleum distillates
Gasoline	Petroleum distillates, benzene
Lighter fluid	Butane
Liquid typewriter correction products	Trichloroethane
Nail polish remover	Acetone, amyl acetate

Table 84–4. Major Toxicity of Inhalants

Inhalant	Constituent	Major Toxicity
Acrylic paint	Toluene	Electrolyte abnormalities
Aerosols	Fluorocarbons	Dysrhythmias
	Nitrous oxide	Asphyxia
	Isobutane	Asphyxia
	Helium	Asphyxia
Gasoline	Aliphatics	Dysrhythmia
	Benzene	Aplastic anemia, dysrhythmia
	Organic lead	Lead intoxication
Glues/adhesives	Toluene	Electrolyte abnormalities
	Benzene	Central nervous system depression, dysrhythmia
	Chlorinated hydrocarbons	Cardiac dysrhythmia
Lighter refills	Butane	Asphyxia
Paints/varnishes/lacquers	Trichloroethylene	Cardiac dysrhythmia
	Methylene chloride	Carbon monoxide
Polystyrene cements	Toluene	Cardiac dysrhythmia
	n-Hexane	Polyneuropathies
	Trichloroethylene	Cardiac dysrhythmia
Rubber cement	Benzene	Aplastic anemia, dysrhythmias
	n-Hexane	Polyneuropathy
	Trichloroethylene	Cardiac arrhythmias
Shoe polish	Toluene	Electrolyte abnormalities
Chlorinated hydrocarbons		Cardiac dysrhythmia
Spot remover	Chlorinated hydrocarbons	Cardiac dysrhythmia
Typewriter correction fluid	Chlorinated hydrocarbons	Cardiac dysrhythmia
Odorizers	Nitrites	Methemoglobinemia

HC, hydrocarbons.
Modified from National Institute on Drug Abuse: Inhalants: The Deliberate Inhalation of Volatile Substances. Report series 30, No. 2. Rockville, MD, NIDA, 1978.

MORBIDITY FROM INHALANT ABUSE

Table 84–5 outlines the clinical toxicity of volatile substance abuse.

The morbidity from inhalant abuse is psychosocial as well as organic. The acute hazards of solvent abuse are loss of consciousness and control, leading to overdose and death due to respiratory arrest or irreversible damage to the brain. Acute hazards with direct aerosol spraying are laryngospasm or airway "freezing" from rapid evaporation. Evidence shows

Table 84–5. Pathology of Volatile Substance Abuse

Pathology	Specific Agent
Definite Association	
Peripheral neuropathy[41, 42, 60]	*n*-Hexane, Methyl-*N*-butyl ketone
Deafness[61, 62]	Toluene
Metabolic acidosis[48, 52, 63]	Toluene
Glomerulonephritis[48]	Toluene
Likely Association	
Embryopathy[64, 65]	Toluene
Neonatal withdrawal[66]	Multiple agents
Lung damage[67]	Paint pigments
Pulmonary[58]	Solvent
Speculative	
Trigeminal neuralgia[23, 46]	Trichloroethylene
Cardiomyopathy[34]	Glue
Heart block[68]	Glue
Ventricular dysrhythmias[48]	1,1,1-Trichloroethane
Toxic hepatitis[69, 70]	Chlorinated hydrocarbons
Decreased visual acuity[71, 72]	Toluene
Aplastic anemia[73, 74]	Benzene
Leukemia[73]	Benzene

that tolerance to the behavioral effects of volatiles occurs and may develop within 1 week with large doses.[11] Abstinence symptoms after the abrupt withdrawal of solvents have been reported.[7]

The organic morbidity resulting from chronic solvent abuse is significant. The chief site of toxicity is the lipid-rich CNS, where long-term solvent use results in dementia and cerebellar dysfunction.[22, 30, 31] Computed tomography demonstrates loss of brain mass (leukoencephalomalacia), and magnetic resonance imaging reveals white matter degeneration.[22]

Other organic effects of solvents are related to the specific categories of the abused chemicals.

MORTALITY FROM INHALANT ABUSE

The mechanisms of death from solvent abuse are varied and include asphyxia, suffocation, dangerous behavior, aspiration, or the sudden sniffing death syndrome. Fatal cardiac dysrhythmias may occur. Asphyxia is a rare theoretic effect that occurs when the partial pressure of the inhalant displaces oxygen. The British experience is that suffocation, dangerous behavior, and aspiration cause 15% of the deaths and that sudden sniffing death is responsible for 55%.[32] Suffocation occurs through nose and mouth inhalation from a plastic bag. Dangerous behavior occurs as a result of solvent-induced disinhibition. The victim may jump or fall from a height, may drown, or may cause a fire. An aspiration hazard results from vomiting and loss of airway protective reflexes and is similar to that caused by other CNS depressants.

The sudden sniffing death syndrome, originally described by Bass in 1970 as following the inhalation of fluorocarbons (trichlorofluoromethane),[16] is considered the most common cause of death associated with solvent abuse. In this circumstance, the user is suddenly startled, either by being discovered or because of a hallucination, then suddenly collapses and dies.[16] The mechanism is believed to be mediated by halogenated hydrocarbons, which are dysrhythmogenic myocardial irritants that lead to fatal dysrhythmias that are precipitated by the release of endogenous catecholamines. Sudden sniffing death can occur in first-time abusers. In one study of solvent abuse deaths, 22% of the victims had no history of prior abuse.[16, 33, 34]

In this chapter the most commonly abused solvents are briefly discussed as categoric prototypes. Further discussion may be found in the discussion of each specific agent.

AEROSOLS

Fluorinated hydrocarbons are often used as aerosol propellants.[35] They are discussed further in Chapter 77.

BENZENE

Sufficient exposure to benzene, an aromatic hydrocarbon, results in leukocytosis and anemia and eventually produces pancytopenia, myeloid leukemia, or aplastic anemia. Benzene has been shown to cause leukemia under specific exposure situations. Other toxic effects of benzene include abuse of fatty degeneration, necrosis, and ultimately yellow atrophy of the liver. Urinary phenol is a biologic marker of benzene exposure.[36, 37]

GASOLINE

Gasoline is a mixture of aliphatic hydrocarbons with a small amount of benzene and other aromatics. The vapor of gasoline contains 90% alkanes, with aromatics representing only 2% and benzene representing 0.9%. Benzene is present in amounts of about 1% in gasoline produced in the United States but can constitute as much as 5% by weight in European formulations. Directly inhaled gasoline intoxicates after 10 to 20 breaths, and the effects last 3 to 4 hours. Gasoline lowers the threshold of the myocardium for life-threatening dysrhythmias. Gasoline is a possible human carcinogen owing to the presence of benzene and 1,3-butadiene. Organic lead, usually tetraethyl, may be added to gasoline to enhance its octane activity. Gasoline that contains more than 0.05 g of lead per gram is considered leaded gasoline. Both tetraethyl and tetramethyl lead are readily absorbed by inhalation and may produce organic lead poisoning and encephalopathy.[38, 39, 40] In 1997, the use of leaded gasoline in the United States was discontinued.[40]

The major target for gasoline exposure is the CNS. Neurologic effects have been found in 95% of habitual gasoline sniffers. Gasoline sniffing has been associated with paralysis of peripheral and cranial nerves.[38, 39] Chronic perioral skin exposure can cause defatting of the skin and dermatitis. Severe gasoline intoxication can produce respiratory depression and cardiac dysrhythmia. Inadvertent gasoline aspiration can lead to fatal pneumonitis.

HEXANE AND KETONES

Continual exposure to hexane, 2-hexanone, and ketones has been associated with a profound sensorimotor polyneuropathy that consists of muscle weakness and atrophy, paresthesias, muscle atrophy, and slowed nerve conduction time.[41] Numerous reports describe neurotoxicity in abusers and in industrial workers due to *n*-hexane and MnBK.[41] The neuropathy caused by *n*-hexane and MnBK is believed to be the result of a common toxic metabolite, 2,5-hexanedione.[42] A closely related ketone, methyl ethyl ketone, does not possess such neurotoxicity.

HALOGENATED HYDROCARBONS

Table 84–2 lists commonly abused halogenated and aromatic hydrocarbons.

The toxic effects of these agents are headache, nausea, dizziness, convulsions, stupor, and coma.[43] They may also produce centrilobular necrosis of the liver and acute renal failure.[44] Sudden death attributed to cardiac dysrhythmias has been associated with inhalation of halogenated hydrocarbons, notably 1,1,1-trichloroethane, found in Liquid Paper and Wite Out.[33, 45] Trichloroethylene has been shown to cause cranial neuropathies classically involving the trigeminal nerve.[46] One 12-year-old abuser of an adhesive containing trichloroethylene suffered a left middle cerebral artery infarction, presenting with right hemiparesis.[47]

TOLUENE

Chronic effects of toluene inhalation abuse are reported to include gastrointestinal discomfort, jaundice, hepatomegaly, and one case of hepatic failure.[48]

Neurologic disturbances include tremors, emotional lability, nystagmus, cerebellar ataxia, polyneuropathies,[23, 49] and permanent encephalopathies.[23, 49] Computed tomography and magnetic resonance imaging may show abnormalities.[23] Toluene, when inhaled, can cause neurologic damage for as long as 1 year even after the abuse has ceased.[25, 26, 35] The neuropathy is usually motor or sensorimotor, ascending, progressive, and symmetric and may be irreversible.[23–26] Table 84–6 lists the major neurologic syndromes produced by organic solvents. Motor weakness and muscle atrophy have been reported in a survey of 24 chronic abusers of toluene.[30] Axonal degeneration, demyelination, and paranodal edema also occur. Magnetic resonance imaging has shown abnormalities.[23] Seizures and choreoathetosis have been reported in toluene abusers,[23] and a case of parkinsonism was reported in a 29-year-old woman who continually abused lacquer thinner containing toluene and methyl ethyl ketone.[50]

Table 84–6. Major Neurologic Syndromes Produced by Organic Solvents

Encephalopathy
Acute encephalopathy—nonspecific, high-level doses
Chronic encephalopathy—seen with repeated high-level exposures
Cerebellar ataxia
Peripheral neuropathies
Distal axonopathy
Cranial neuropathy
Primarily cranial nerves V and VII
Parkinsonism
Visual loss
Optic neuropathy
Multifocal damage
Central nervous system
Central and peripheral nervous systems

Modified from Sharp CW, Rosenberg NL: Volatile substances. *In* Lowinson J, Ruiz P, Millmen R (eds): Substance Abuse: A Comprehensive Textbook. 2nd ed. Baltimore, Williams & Wilkins, p 309, 1992.

Renal toxicity due to toluene abuse is generally one of two types: distal (type 1) renal tubular acidosis or crescentic glomerulonephritis.[48, 51] Metabolic acidosis occurs as a result of a renal dysfunction from either renal tubular acidosis with normal anion gap or with elevated anion gap due to formation of hippuric acid from toluene.[48, 50, 52–54] Nephrolithiasis is associated with renal tubular acidosis and crescentic glomerulonephritis.[48, 51]

Electrolyte abnormalities include hippuric acid acidosis, hypokalemia, and hypophosphatemia.[53, 54] The latter two disorders may account for some of the muscle weakness.

Hematologic abnormalities include reversible anemia.

A toluene embryopathy with features similar to those of ethanol embryopathy has been reported.[56]

DETECTION OF SOLVENT ABUSE

A careful physical examination is most important in recognizing solvent abuse, particularly because all organ systems may be affected. Individuals who habitually use large amounts of inhalants may be detected by their poor attention to hygiene, obvious intoxication, and the conspicuous odor of the inhalant.

The most important clue is the chemical odor on the breath because the absorbed dose is excreted in part through the lungs. Another source of odor may be from spillage or stains on the clothing. Finding intoxicating products in unusual locations, such as gasoline under the bed, is another clue.

The skin may have perioral eczema from the defat-

Table 84–7. Metabolites of Solvents

Solvent	Metabolite in Urine
Benzene	Phenol
Toluene	Hippuric acid
Trichloroethylene	Trichloroacetic acid, trichloroethanol
Xylene	Methylhippuric acid

ting action, as well as pyodermas or petechiae, and the "glue sniffer's rash" may develop.[57]

Unusual behavior may be a sign of inhalant abuse. Cognitive testing must focus on short-term memory and global function.

A routine urine drug screen is not helpful because routine screens do not detect these substances. Laboratory tests for organ dysfunction should be considered only for chronic abusers. Urinary metabolites may extend the time of detection. Of the compounds commonly abused, only toluene, xylene, and chlorinated solvents (notably trichloroethylene) have metabolites suitable for detection and measurement.[57] Urinary phenol is a biologic marker of benzene exposure and is found in non-exposed individuals at levels less than 20 mg/L.

Hippuric acid, a metabolite of toluene, may result in concentrations exceeding 200 mg/L in the urine, and creatinine concentrating levels higher than 2.5 g/g suggest toluene exposure.[53] Table 84–7 lists metabolites of solvents.

DIAGNOSIS AND MANAGEMENT

Diagnostic difficulty may arise owing to the similarity between the effects of the volatile substances and ethanol.[57] The key to successful management of volatile substance toxicity is early recognition, a high index of suspicion, and early intervention.[19]

When acute intoxication due to solvent abuse is suspected, the initial priority should be airway management, intubation and assisted ventilation if required, and supplemental warm humidified 100% oxygenation if necessary. Patients should be immediately removed from exposure.

In the event a solvent is spilled on the clothes,

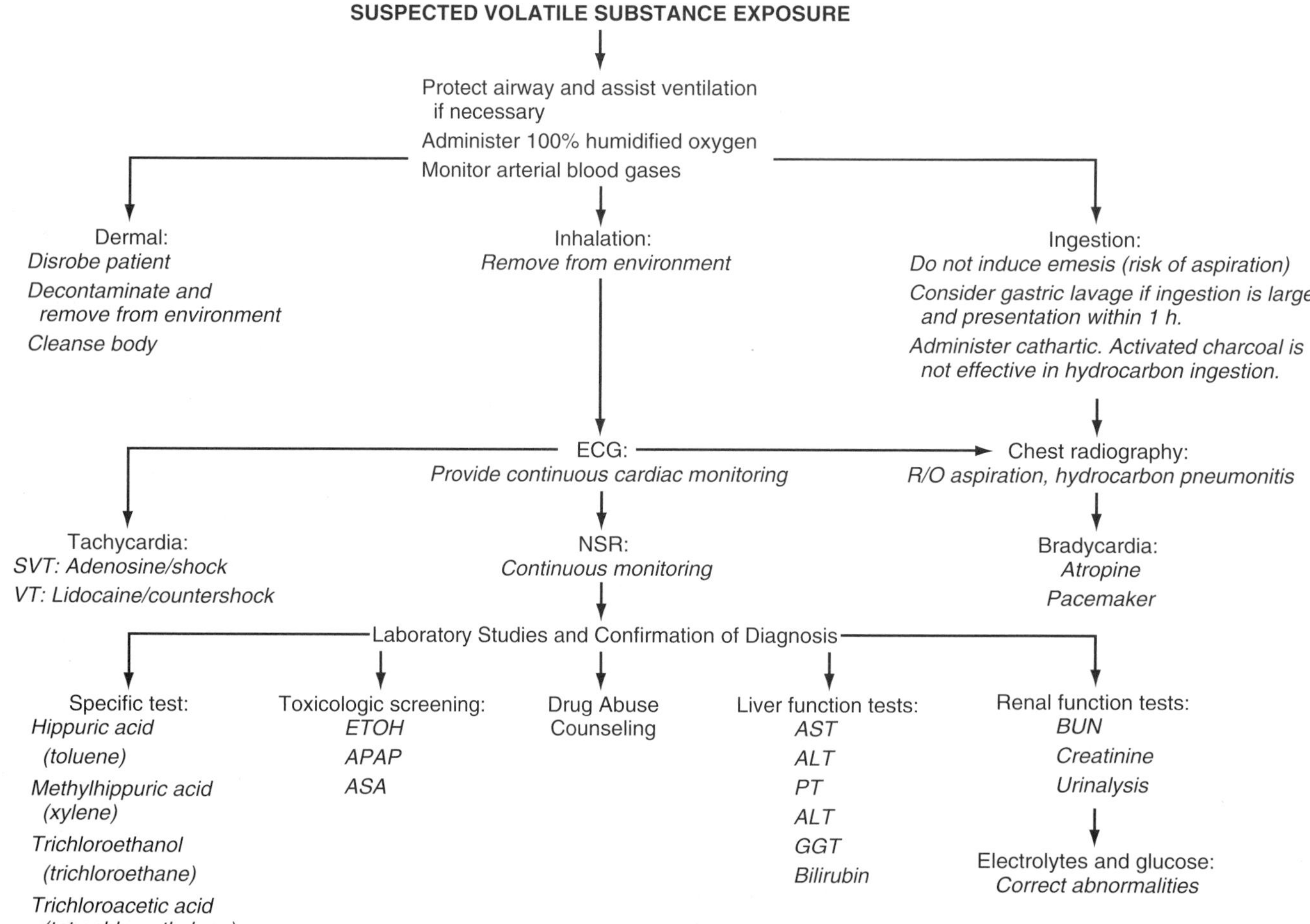

Figure 84–1. Algorithm for the clinical management of suspected volatile substance exposure. APAP, acetaminophen; ALT, alanime aminotrasferase; AST, aspartate aminotrasferase; ASA, aspirin; BUN, blood urea nitrogen; ECG, electrocardiography; ETOH, ethanol; GGT, γ-glutamyltransferase; NSR, normal sinus rhythm; PT, prothrombin time; R/O, rule out; SVT, supraventricular tachycardia; VT, ventricular tachycardia.

decontamination by disrobement should be performed, with safe disposition of the contaminated clothing. After dermal or ocular exposure to the solvent, the skin should be washed with soap and water and the eyes copiously irrigated with saline.

If solvent ingestion is suspected, consider gastric lavage in the first hour. Induction of emesis is contraindicated because of CNS depression and the risk of aspiration. Activated charcoal is ineffective in hydrocarbon ingestions.[46, 58]

In case of suspected aspiration, one may need to monitor for hydrocarbon pneumonitis with examination, pulse oximetry, and chest radiography and close observation for 24 hours (Fig. 84–1).

Monitor for and treat cardiac dysrhythmias and fluid/electrolyte disturbances. Supraventricular tachyarrhythmias may be treated first with adenosine, and ventricular tachycardias may be managed first with lidocaine or countershock as appropriate. Synchronized cardioversion or defibrillation may be necessary. Bradyarrhythmias are best treated with atropine and a pacemaker (external or transvenous) if needed. Epinephrine should be used with great caution in solvent-related exposures, because halogenated solvents lower the threshold to catecholamine-induced cardiovascular dysrhthymias. See Figure 84–1 for a recommended management algorithm.

CHRONIC INHALANT ABUSE

The most effective management is prevention, and of the potential preventive strategies, education is probably the most effective. Limiting availability of products is impractical; adding a noxious chemical to deter abuse has not proved effective.[59] Warning labeling of products identifies their abuse potential, risking increased use.

It is recommended that education before the age of experimentation with an appropriate school-based substance abuse curriculum may be the most efficient preventive strategy.[11, 21] Chronic solvent abusers must not be ignored. However, their treatment is very difficult and not highly effective.

References

1. Graham DR: Solvent abuse. *In* Haddad LM, Winchester JF (eds). Clinical Management of Poisoning and Drug Overdose. 2nd ed. Philadelphia, W.B. Saunders Co., p 1256, 1990.
2. Jaffe JH: Drug addiction and drug abuse. *In* Gilman AG, Goodman LS, Gilman A (eds). The Pharmacologic Basis of Therapeutics. 8th ed. New York, Macmillan Publishing Co., pp 522–573, 1990.
3. Carroll E: Notes on the epidemiology of inhalants. *In* Sharp CW, Bohm K (eds): Review of Inhalants: Euphoria to Dysfunction. NIDA Research Monograph 15, DHEW publication ADM 77:553. Rockville, MD, NIDA, pp 14–24, 1977.
4. Hutchens K, Kung M: Experimentation with chloroform. Am J Med *78:*715, 1984.
5. Collins VJ: Principles of Anesthesiology, 2nd ed. Philadelphia, Lea & Febiger, p 6, 1976.
6. Koblin DD, Waskell L, Watson JE, et al: Nitrous oxide inactivation of methionine synthetase in the human livers. Anesth Analg 61:75, 1982.
7. Davies B, Thorley A, O'Connor D: Progression of addiction careers in young adult solvent misusers. BMJ *290:*109, 1985.
8. Johnston LD: National survey results from the Monitoring the Future study. Drug use among the 8th, 10th and 12th graders, 1975–1995. Ann Arbor, University of Michigan, 1995.
9. Edwards RW: Drug use among 8th grade students is increasing. Int J Addict *28:*1621, 1993.
10. Cohen S: Glue sniffing. JAMA *231:*653, 1975.
11. Cohen S: *In* Beschner GM, Friedman AS (eds): Youth Drug Abuse. Lexington, MA, Lexington Books, 1979.
12. Hecht A: Inhalants: Quick route to danger. FDA Consumer *14:*10, 1980.
13. Fredlund E, Spence RT, Maxnell JC, et al: 1990 Texas school survey of substance abuse. Texas Commission on Alcohol and Drug Abuse.
14. National survey results from the Monitoring the Future study. Drug use among the 8th, 10th and 12th graders, 1975–1995. Vol. I. Ann Arbor, University of Michigan, 1995.
15. Ashton CH: Solvent abuse: Little progress after 20 years. BMJ *300:*135, 1990.
16. Bass M: Sudden sniffing death. JAMA *213:*2075, 1970.
17. Chadwick NO, Yule W, Anderson R: The examination attainments of secondary school pupils of volatile substance abuse: A review. Hum Toxicol *8:*307, 1989.
18. Evans AC, Raistrick D: Phenomenology of intoxication with toluene-based adhesives and butane gas. Br J Psychiatry *150:*769, 1987.
19. Ramsey J, Anderson HR, Bloor K, et al: An introduction to the practice, prevalence and chemical toxicology of volatile substance abuse. Hum Toxicol *8:*261, 1989.
20. Blum K: Solvent and aerosol inhalants. *In:* Blum K (ed): Handbook of Abusable Drugs. New York, Gardener Press, 1984.
21. Sharp CW, Rosenberg NL: Volatile substances. *In* Lowinson J, Ruiz P, Millmen R (eds): Substance Abuse: A Comprehensive Textbook. 2nd ed. Baltimore, Williams & Wilkins, p 309, 1992.
22. Rosenberg NL, Spitz MC, Filley CM, et al: Central nervous system effects of chronic toluene abuse—clinical, brain stem evoked response and magnetic reasonance imaging studies. Teratology *10:*489, 1988.
23. Lolin Y: Chronic neurological toxicity associated with exposure to volatile substances. Hum Toxicol *8:*293, 1989.
24. Rosenberg N: Nervous system effects of toluene and other organic solvents. West J Med *150:*571, 1989.
25. Rosenberg NL, Kleinschmidt-DeMasters BK, Davis KA, et al: Toluene abuse causes diffuse central nervous system white matter changes. Ann Neurol *23:*611, 1988.
26. Filley CM, Heston RK, Rosenberg NL: White matter dementia in chronic toluene abuse. Neurology *40:*532, 1990.
27. American Academy of Pediatrics, Committee on Substance Abuse: Role of the pediatrician in prevention and management of substance abuse. Pediatrics *91:*1010, 1993.
28. Wilford BB: Drug Abuse: A Guide For the Primary Physician. Chicago, American Medical Association, p 80, 1981.
29. Dinwiddie SH: Abuse of inhalants: A review. Addiction *89:*925, 1994.
30. Fornazzi L, Wilinson DA, Kappur BM: Cerebellar cortical and functional impairment in toluene abusers. Acta Neurol Scand *69:*319, 1983.
31. Filley CM, Heaton RK, Rosenberg NL: White matter dementia in chronic toluene abuse. Neurology *40:*532, 1990.
32. Ramsey J, Anderson HR, Bloor K, et al: An introduction to the practice, prevalence and chemical toxicology of volatile substance abuse. Hum Toxicol *8:*261, 1989.
33. Shepard R: Mechanism of sudden death associated with volatile substance abuse. Hum Toxicol *8:*287, 1989.
34. Wiseman M, Banim S: Glue sniffer's heart. BMJ *294:*739, 1987.
35. Anderson HR, MacNair RS, Ramsey JD: Deaths from abuse of volatile substances: A national epidemiologic survey. BMJ *290:*304, 1985.
36. Rinsky RA, Smith AB, Hornung R, et al: Benzene and leukemia: An epidemiologic risk assessment. N Engl J Med *316:*1044, 1987.

37. Austin H, Delzell E, Cole P: Benzene and leukemia: A review of the literature and a risk assessment. Am J Epidemiol *127:*419, 1988.
38. Coulehan JL, Hirsh W, Brillman J: Gasoline sniffing and lead toxicity of Navajo adolescents. Pediatrics *71:*113, 1983.
39. Hornfeldt CS, Ling LJ: Inhalation of gasoline fumes. Clin Pediatr *25:*114, 1986.
40. Logan D, Dart R: Gasoline Toxicity. Agency for Toxic Substances and Disease Registry: Case studies in environmental medicine, no. 31. US Department of Health and Human Services, San Rafael, CA, Delima Associates, under contract 205-90-0817, pp 1–31, 1993.
41. Yamada S: An occurrence of polyneuritis by *n*-hexane in polyethylene laminating plants. Jpn J Ind Health *6:*192, 1969.
42. Saida K, Mendell JR, Weiss HS, et al: Peripheral nerve changes induced by methyl *n*-butyl ketone and potentiation by methyl ethyl ketone. J Neuropathol *35:*207, 1976.
43. Barceloux DG, Rosenberg J: Trichloroethylene toxicity. Case studies in environmental medicine. Washington, DC, US Department of Health and Social Services, 1990.
44. Gerace RV: Near fatal intoxication by 1,1,1-trichloroethane. Ann Emerg Med *10:*533, 1981.
45. Pointer J: Typewriter correction fluid inhalation: A new substance of abuse. J Toxicol Clin Toxicol *18:*493, 1982.
46. Kimbrough R, Mitchell FL, Houk VN: Trichloroethylene: An update. J Toxicol Environ Health *15:*369, 1985.
47. Parker M, Tarlow MJ, Milne Anderson J, et al: Glue sniffing and cerebral infarction. Arch Dis Child *59:*675, 1984.
48. Marjot R, McLeod A: Chronic non-neurological toxicity from volatile substance abuse. Hum Toxicol *8:*301, 1989.
49. Press E, Done AK: Solvent sniffing. Physiologic effects and community control measures for intoxication from intentional inhalation of organic solvents I and II. Pediatrics *39:*451, 1967.
50. Uitti R, Shinotoh H, Hayward M: Parkinsonism induced by solvent abuse. Ann Neurol *35:*616, 1994.
51. Patel R, Benjamin J Jr: Renal damage associated with toluene inhalation. Clin Toxicol *24:*213, 1986.
52. Taher SM, Anderson RJ, McCartney R: Renal tubular acidosis associated with toluene "sniffing." N Engl J Med 290:765, 1974.
53. Carlisle EJF, Donnelly SM, Vasuvattakul S, et al: Glue-sniffing and distal renal tubular acidosis: Sticking to the facts. J Am Soc Nephrol *1:*1019, 1991.
54. Streicher HZ, Gabow PA, Moss AH, et al: Syndromes of toluene sniffing in adults. Ann Intern Med *94:*758, 1981.
55. Kroeger RM, Moore RJ, Lehman TH, et al: Recurrent urinary calculi associated with toluene inhalation. J Urol *123:*89, 1980.
56. Pearson MA, Hoyme HE, Seaver LH: Toluene embryopathy: Delineation of the phenotype and comparison with fetal alcohol syndrome. Pediatrics *93:*211, 1994.
57. Meredith TJ, Ruprah M, Liddle A, et al: Diagnosis and treatment of acute poisoning with volatile substances. Hum Toxicol *8:*277, 1989.
58. Cronk S, Barkley DE, Farrell MF, et al: Respiratory arrest after solvent abuse. BMJ *290:*897, 1985.
59. Kerner K: Current topics in inhalant abuse. *In* Creger RA, Rouse (eds): Epidemiology of Inhalant Abuse: An update. NIDA Research Monograph 85. Washington, DC, US Department of Health and Human Services, pp 8–12. 1988.
60. Tenenbein M, deGroot W, Ranjani KR: Peripheral neuropathy following intentional inhalation of naphtha fumes. Can Med Assoc J *131:*1077, 1984.
61. Pryor GT, Rebert CS, Dickinson J, et al: Factors affecting toluene ototoxicity in rats. Neurobehav Toxicol Tetral *6:*223, 1984.
62. Ehyai A, Freemon FR: Progressive optic and sensorineural hearing loss due to chronic glue sniffing. J Neurol Neurosurg Psychiatry *45:*349, 1983.
63. Fischman CM, Oster JR: Toxic effects of toluene. A new cause of high anion gap metabolic acidosis. JAMA *2412:*1713, 1979.
64. Pearson MA, Hoyme HE, Seaver LH, et al: Toluene embryopathy: Delineation of the phenotype and comparison with fetal alcohol syndrome. Pediatrics *93:*211, 1994.
65. Hersh JH, Podruch PF, Rogers G, et al: Toluene embryopathy. J Pediatr *106:*922, 1985.
66. Tenenbein M, Casiro OG, Seshia MMK, et al: Neonatal withdrawal from maternal inhalant abuse. Arch Dis Child *74:*F204–F207, 1996.
67. Engstand DA, England DM, Huntington RW: Pathology of paint sniffer's lung. Forensic Toxicol *7:*232, 1986.
68. Taylor G, Harris W: Glue sniffing causes heart block in mice. Science *170:*866, 1970.
69. Kaplan HG, Bakken J, Quadracci L, et al: Hepatitis caused by halothane sniffing. Ann Intern Med *90:*797, 1979.
70. Hutchens KS, Kung M: "Experimentation" with chloroform. Am J Med *78:*715, 1985.
71. Ehyai A, Freemon FR: Progressive optic and sensorineural hearing loss due to chronic glue sniffing. J Neurol Neurosurg Psychiatry *45:*349, 1983.
72. Keane JR: Toluene optic neuropathy. Ann Neurol *4:*390, 1979.
73. Aksoy M: Benzene as a leukemogenic and carcinogenic agent Am J Intern Med *8:*9, 1985.
74. Powers D: Aplastic anemia due to glue sniffing. N Engl J Med *273:*700, 1965.

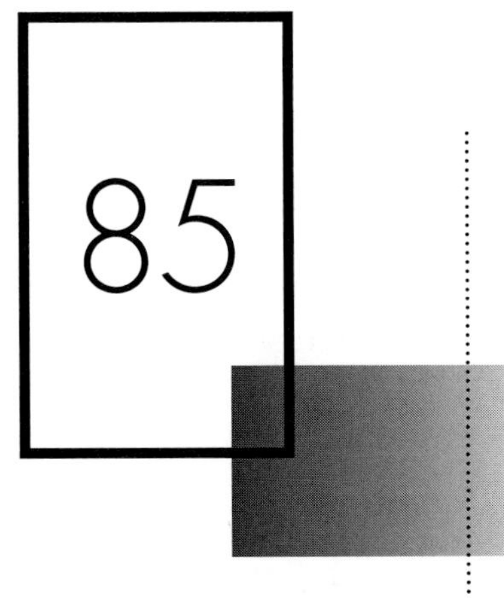

SECTION **H**

CARDIOVASCULAR AND HEMATOLOGIC AGENTS

Digitalis

LLOYD S. GOODMAN, MD

Digitalis was introduced into clinical medicine by William Withering in 1785, after his investigation of a home remedy used by herbalists in the English countryside.[1,2] He reported on 10 years of observation of 163 patients taking digitalis and recommended that

> *. . . it be continued until it acts either on the kidneys, the stomach, the pulse, or the bowel . . . let it be stopped upon the first appearance of any of these effects and I will maintain that the patient will not suffer from its exhibition, nor the practitioner be disappointed in any reasonable effects.*

He further gave a most accurate account of digitalis intoxications:

> *The Foxglove, when given in very large and repeated doses, occasions sickness, vomiting, purging, giddiness, confused vision, objects appearing green and yellow; increased secretion of urine, with frequent motions to part with it, and sometimes inability to retain it; slow pulse, even as slow as 35 in a minute, cold sweats, convulsions, syncope, death.*

SCOPE OF PROBLEM

Digitalis intoxication was once considered the most common adverse drug reaction in United States medical practice. Studies from the 1960s and 1970s showed that as many as 15% of all patients in medical admissions were taking digitalis, and 20% to 30% of these patients would have signs of toxicity. The mortality rate of toxic patients varied from 3% to 25% and was especially high in the elderly.[3,4] Prescribing habits and the incidence of toxicity have begun to change because of (1) better appreciation of digitalis pharmacodynamics and drug interactions; (2) the use of these data to determine the more appropriate maintenance dosage; (3) easy and rapid availability of serum digoxin determinations to almost every physician, thereby identifying unexpected cases; (4) better standardization of drug bioavailability; and (5) expanded drug therapy for congestive heart failure, eliminating the need to push digitalis to higher, more potentially toxic levels.[5] Nevertheless, the number of patients receiving maintenance digitalis therapy remains high, and the numerous common untoward effects still demand attention and understanding. In fact, a report by Mahdyoon and colleagues[6] showed that 56% of patients with congestive heart failure admitted to a large teaching hospital were receiving maintenance digitalis. The diagnosis of digitalis toxicity is often difficult because the margin between therapeutic and toxic doses is very small and because many abnormal rhythms can be found in patients who have advanced heart disease and are not taking digitalis. Because toxic effects are a consequence of excessive therapy, understanding the basic pharmacology of digitalis is necessary in order to treat intoxicated patients.

PHARMACOLOGY

The preparations of cardiac glycosides now used in clinical practice were initially derived from the leaves of plants from the genus *Digitalis*. Other florae that contain cardiac glycosides have occasionally led to unsuspected cardiac complications.

Several preparations of digitalis are available. However, because of their ease of oral administration and duration of action, only two preparations are used in most clinical practices today: digoxin (half-life, 33 to 34 hours) and digitoxin (half-life, 6 to 7 days). Digoxin and digitoxin are passively absorbed from the small intestine, with effective absorption of 55% to 75% for digoxin tablets, 90% to 100% for digitoxin tablets, and 90% to 100% for the liquid or encapsulated liquid form of digoxin.[7–9] Figure 85–1 illustrates the average values for absorption and half-life of digoxin and digitoxin.[10] Detailed pharmacodynamic studies have shown that the drug action depends on tissue concentration, which is relatively constant in relation to serum levels, and that the major depot in humans is skeletal muscle.[11] These findings lead to two conclusions: First, the constant relationship of myocardial digoxin concentration to serum concentration supports measuring serum levels to monitor patients' compliance; second, dosage requirements and the likelihood of toxicity can be anticipated on the basis of muscle mass and not overall body weight.

Digoxin and digitoxin are eliminated differently. Digoxin is excreted primarily via the renal route, whereas digitoxin is eliminated primarily via the metabolic change to inactive breakdown products. Because enterohepatic circulation has a role in the metabolism of both drugs, biliary production affects digitalis elimination. Bioavailability of the drug may vary because of different manufacturing processes and malabsorption syndromes and because of inactivation of gut flora, which can be altered by antibiotics.[12] Furthermore, digoxin is one of the breakdown products of digitoxin metabolism (about 8%; Figs. 85–1 and 85–2). Other important factors in patients' handling and response to digitalis include disease state, a patient's age, and drug interactions.

Basic Mechanism

Digitalis acts at the subcellular level by altering the sodium/potassium–adenosine triphosphatase (Na^+,K^+-ATPase) transport system. The net effect is intracellular loss of K^+ and gain of Na^+ and Ca^{2+}. In short, digitalis acts to increase the Ca^{2+} available to the contractile elements of the myocardium after excitation.[1] The increased Ca^{2+} augments myofibril interaction in cardiac muscle and leads to positive inotropic action.[13] Any drug affecting Na^+, K^+, or Ca^{2+} fluxes across cell membranes can exert a significant effect on conduction.

In an intact heart, the effects of digitalis can be separated into mechanical and electrophysiologic actions, with toxicity related to its excessive therapeutic effects and the status of the patient at the time of drug administration.

Normal Therapeutic Effects on Intact Heart (Summary of Actions)

A major therapeutic use for digitalis is for its inotropic effect. Digitalis augments the force of myocardial contraction by increasing the velocity of shortening and the velocity of developed tension of cardiac muscle.[13] Therefore, there is less encroachment on compensatory mechanisms, allowing greater cardiac reserve. In patients with heart failure, digitalis causes a decrease in end-diastolic pressure and volume, increasing cardiac output and stroke work. The usefulness of digoxin for congestive heart failure in patients in sinus rhythm has been the subject of some controversy. However, most conclude that digoxin is a weak inotropic agent.[13–19] (The RADIANCE study (Randomized Assessment of [the effect on] Digoxin on Inhibitors of the Angiotensin-Converting Enzyme) demonstrated that withdrawal of digoxin in patients with heart failure and abnormal systolic function could be dangerous. The Digitalis Investigators' Group trial[18] and the study by Krum and colleagues[19] demonstrated the usefulness of digoxin in congestive heart failure. In a nonfailing heart, the effects of digitalis are more controversial. Positive inotropic action may occur, but it is not manifested

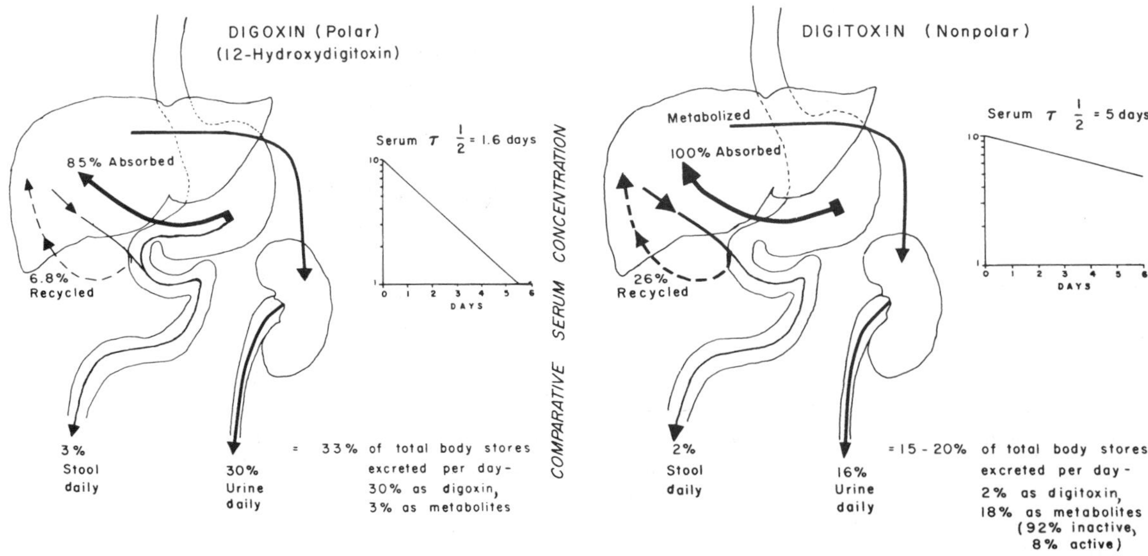

Figure 85–1. Digoxin and digitoxin pharmacokinetics, showing average values for absorption, excretion, enterohepatic circulation, and half-life. (From Doherty JE: Digitalis glycosides: Pharmacokinetics and their clinical implications. Ann Intern Med *79*:229, 1973.)

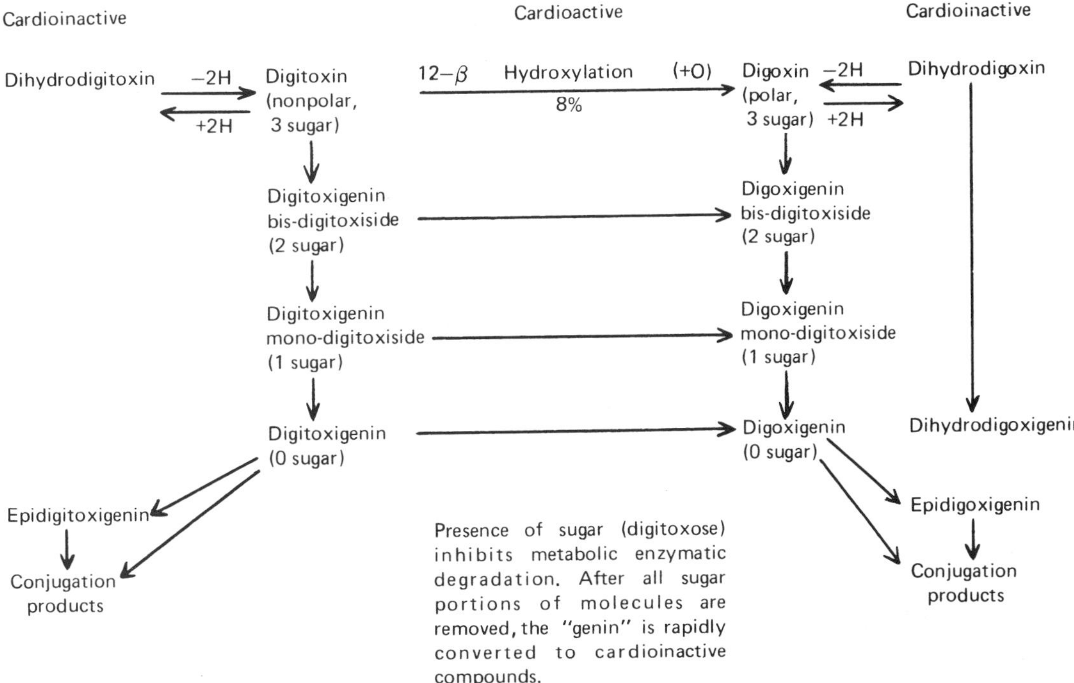

Figure 85–2. Metabolic pathways of digoxin and digitoxin. Note that digoxin is part of the metabolic pathway of digitoxin. (From Doherty JE: Digitalis glycosides: Pharmacokinetics and their clinical implications. Ann Intern Med *79*:229, 1973.)

by a measurable change in cardiac output or by a decrease in left ventricular filling pressure.[20]

The chronotropic effect of digitalis is primarily central, mediated through an increase in vagal tone, which decreases the rate of sinoatrial (SA) node depolarization. Other effects of digitalis may vary, depending on the interaction of drug concentration and autonomic tone. Digitalis decreases the refractory period of both atrial and ventricular cells and tends to increase action potential amplitude and V_{max}. These increases improve conduction within the muscle, as reflected in a shortened QT interval. The same mechanism accounts for the increased atrial rate in atrial flutter or atrial flutter-fibrillation.[21, 22]

Digitalis increases the refractory period of the atrioventricular (AV) node and the bundle of His. It prolongs phase 3 of the action potential, accounting for decreased ventricular response in atrial fibrillation. Some AV nodal effects are independent of vagal tone and affect phase 0, thus decreasing conduction velocity.[1] Most if not all effects of digitalis on the Purkinje system and ventricular muscle are direct effects and do not depend on autonomic interaction.[7–9]

Digitalis causes significant effects on myocardial automaticity (ability of tissue to undergo spontaneous depolarization) and excitability (ability of tissue to respond to a given stimulus). Inhibition of the Na^+ pump leads to an influx of Na^+ into the cell. This Na^+ influx increases phase 4 depolarization in all cardiac tissue except the SA node and leads to the appearance of new or latent pacemakers, thus increasing automaticity. This influx also lowers the resting membrane potential threshold, thus increasing excitability.[23] A number of investigators have described another and possibly more important effect of this Na^+ influx. According to Rosen, this inward current causes delayed afterpotentials (oscillations in transmembrane potentials that follow full repolarizations of the membrane), and this effect provides a more logical basis for understanding digitalis-induced arrhythmias.[24]

Digitalis possesses a relatively narrow therapeutic index; 40% to 60% of the lethal dose is required to achieve the maximal therapeutic effect. The toxic effects that occur when levels exceed the therapeutic range are almost uniformly a consequence of excessive normal physiologic responses.

Digitalis Toxicity

Digitalis toxicity can occur in any condition that increases the amount of digitalis in the body or modifies the cardiac sensitivity to digitalis. Toxicity can produce cardiac and extracardiac symptoms. Drug interactions may increase the effective level, and other factors, such as ischemia or inflammation, affect sensitivity to digitalis. The cardiac mechanism of digitalis toxicity is usually ascribed to depression of conduction and alterations of impulse formation; noncardiac symptoms are listed in Table 85–1.

Interaction with Other Drugs

The importance of drug interactions in the development of digitalis toxicity was not truly appreciated until reliable assays of digoxin levels became widespread. Several drugs, such as cholestyramine, ant-

Table 85–1. Noncardiac Symptoms of Digitalis Toxicity

	Definite Intoxication (%)	Possible Intoxication (%)	No Intoxication (%)
Vomiting	48	30	27
Anorexia	34	27	18
Dizziness	14	19	23
Fatigue	14	16	11
Visual disturbances	9	5	7
Syncope	6	3	2
Abdominal pain	6	4	0
Diarrhea	2	2	2
Headache	0	2	0
Delirium	0	1	0

Modified from Mahdyoon H, Battilana G, Rosman H, et al: The evolving pattern of digoxin intoxication: Observations at a large urban hospital from 1980 to 1988. Am Heart J *120*:1189, 1990.

acids, kaolin-pectin, and some antibiotics (such as neomycin, sulfasalazine, and *p*-aminosalicylic acid), as well as bran, alter absorption and effectively decrease the bioavailability of digoxin.[25, 26] Alteration and absorption are important, because discontinuing these drugs without changing the digoxin dose may lead to a digitoxic state. Other antibiotics (such as erythromycin and tetracycline) may significantly increase digoxin levels by altering gut flora, which is important in metabolizing digoxin.[12] This alteration is less of a problem when the capsule form is used. By far the most important drugs that cause interactions with digoxin are the antiarrhythmics. *Quinidine* causes an increase in serum digoxin in as many as 90% of patients. The magnitude of the increase varies but is often twofold. The serum digoxin level begins to increase with the onset of quinidine therapy, and the level remains elevated as long as both drugs are continued. The exact mechanism that causes this interaction is still being investigated. It is known that the half-life of digoxin is not prolonged and that total-body clearance is reduced. The findings so far are best explained by the displacement of digoxin from tissue-binding sites.[26–31] Some evidence has suggested paradoxically increased concentrations in areas of the brain and has prompted speculation that some of the toxic effects may be the result of central nervous system stimulation.[7–9] The adverse effects of elevated digoxin levels caused by quinidine are similar to those experienced with an overdose of digoxin, although the mechanism that causes this elevation is still not defined.

Another major antiarrhythmic drug that interacts with digoxin is *amiodarone*. Digoxin levels increased by 25% to 70% within 24 hours after adding amiodarone.[26] The effect is mediated via a decrease in renal and nonrenal clearance.[32] The result is more frequently bradyarrhythmias or heart block rather than tachyarrhythmias.[33]

No evidence shows that other antiarrhythmics similar to quinidine in their action (type I) interact with digoxin. Procainamide, disopyramide, lidocaine, mexiletine, and flecainide do not increase serum digoxin levels. Likewise, other antiarrhythmics, such as sotalol, aprindine, ajmaline, and moricizine do not affect digoxin levels.[26, 34]

The interaction of Ca^{2+} channel blocking drugs with digoxin varies greatly. The dihydropyridines (nifedipine, amlodipine, isradipine, nicardipine) have minimal or no effect,[26, 35] and diltiazem has such a small effect that toxicity is unlikely.[26] On the other hand, *verapamil* increases serum digoxin levels as much as 70% by altering renal and extrarenal clearance, which can lead to lethal cardiac toxicity.[26, 36, 37] Potentially toxic interaction may also occur with potassium-sparing diuretics (such as spironolactone), which inhibit tubular secretion of digoxin; with antihypertensive agents, which can significantly alter renal reperfusion and glomerular filtration rate; and with anti-inflammatory drugs, especially indomethacin, in neonates or with renal dysfunction. Some antiadrenergic agents, such as clonidine, methyldopa, reserpine, and β-blockers, in combination with digitalis, may lead to severe bradyarrhythmias, especially in patients with SA node disease.[26] Preliminary reports have shown toxicity in patients with myocarditis when cyclosporine is added to digoxin in patients who have heart failure.[27] Aside from the drug interactions discussed earlier, renal dysfunction leading to decreased renal excretion of digitalis is the major factor leading to the increased total of digitalis throughout the body. Neither dialysis nor cardiopulmonary bypass causes much body loss of digitalis.

Altering Sensitivity to Digitalis

Toxicity from digitalis is not limited to situations that increase total-body concentration of the drug but can develop with any condition that modifies the cardiac sensitivity to digitalis. Cardiac factors that increase sensitivity to digitalis and may lead to toxicity include myocardial infarction or ischemia, myocarditis, cardiomyopathy, amyloidosis, and other trauma, including surgery.[38] A healthy heart tolerates large amounts of digitalis, whereas diseased myocardium appears to develop arrhythmias at lower serum levels.[39] The myocardial disease leads to local areas of altered electrophysiology, which in turn can cause variation in digitalis uptake by cardiac tissue. The concentration differences and local ischemia lead to variation of cellular recovery times and set the stage, once again, for re-entry phenomena (Fig. 85–3). Intrinsic cardiac disease alone may produce similar rhythm disturbances, several of which are common in acute myocardial infarction. These rhythm disturbances have no specific distinguishing feature. However, digitalis toxicity can be implicated in most instances when withdrawal of the drug is followed by resolution of the arrhythmia. This increased sensitivity does not preclude careful use of digitalis when clinically indicated.[40]

Altering Metabolism

Metabolic factors are important in myocardial sensitivity to digitalis. Electrolyte abnormalities, espe-

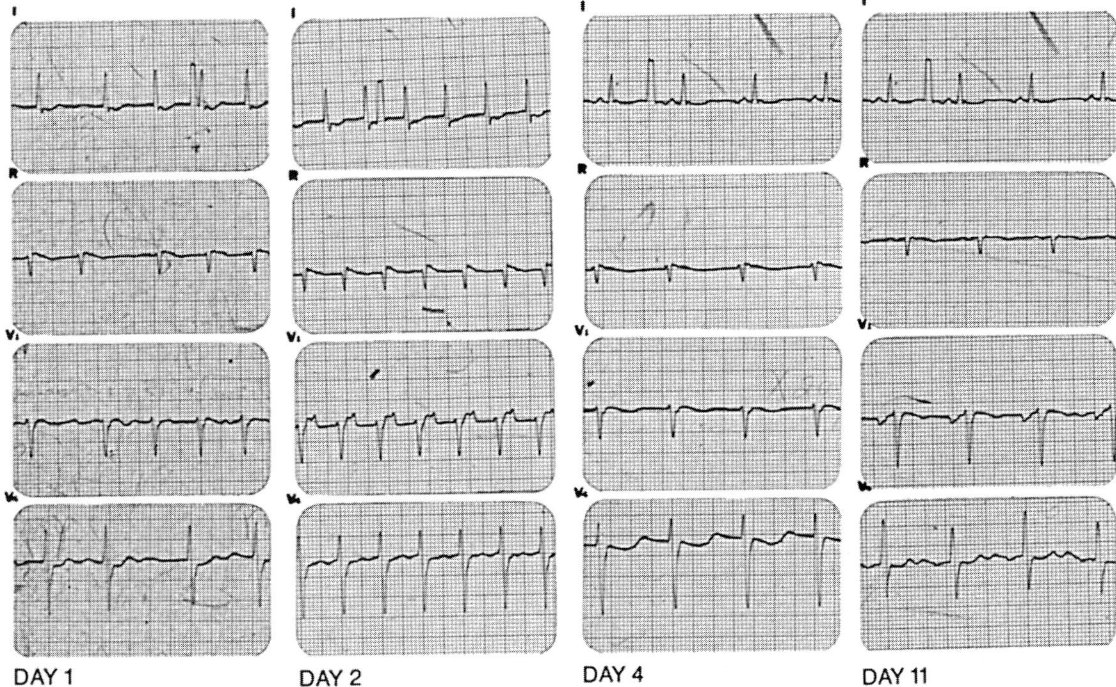

Figure 85–3. Electrocardiograms of a 67-year-old man with coronary disease and previous myocardial infarction; he was admitted to the hospital with congestive heart failure. He was receiving maintenance digoxin therapy. Day 1: The patient developed atrial fibrillation and was given an extra dose of digoxin and furosemide. Day 2: Accelerated junctional rhythm with retrograde P waves (seen clearly in V_1). Day 4: Junctional rate slowed with marked ST-T changes (K^+ level noted to be 2.3). Day 11: After fluid restriction and withholding digoxin and diuretics, sinus rhythm was re-established. This sequence demonstrates problems of digoxin toxicity worsened by ischemia.

cially hypokalemia, are well known, but aberrations of magnesium and calcium may have a role and are important to consider.[41–43] Other metabolic abnormalities, including acidosis, alkalosis, hypoxemia, and hyperthermia, may alter digitalis effect but are probably not independent risk factors. Diseases of other organ systems, especially chronic lung disease and hypothyroidism, predispose patients to digitalis toxicity. Acute cerebrovascular events may lead to toxicity by large sympathetic discharge, which may lower the arrhythmia threshold.[38] Table 85–2 contains a more complete list.

CLINICAL PRESENTATION

Pathophysiology

Digitalis toxicity represents the result of the interactions of the drug on the transmembrane potentials and ionic current flows of the cardiac cells (direct effects) and those effects related to the autonomic nervous system (indirect). These interactions have various results depending on which cells are affected; they are expressed as abnormalities of atrial, AV nodal, or ventricular pathology. Most authorities categorize the mechanism of digitalis cardiotoxic rhythms as resulting from depression of conduction or alteration of impulse formation, with increased heterogeneity of refractory periods. Fisch and Knoebel offer a somewhat more detailed classification based on probable physiologic mechanism,[44] but for simplicity, the standard mechanisms are discussed here.

Depression of Conduction

Depression of conduction is manifested as heart block at SA and AV nodes. SA nodal block is relatively common and may range from sinus pauses to the SA nodal Wenckebach phenomenon or to total SA nodal exit block (Figs. 85–4 and 85–5). AV block is usually of the type I AV nodal block. The designation of type I or II block is a relatively new approach in describing AV block based on His bundle recordings. In this scheme, block above the bundle of His is considered type I and block below the bundle

Table 85–2. Factors Predisposing to Digitalis Intoxication

Patient-related factors	Hypernatremia
Old age	Hypercalcemia
Severe heart disease	Hypomagnesemia
Myocardial infarction	Alkalosis
Myocarditis	Drugs
Recent cardiac surgery	Diuretics
Cor pulmonale	Steroids
Renal failure	Reserpine
Hemodialysis	Catecholamines
Hypothyroidism	Quinidine
Anoxia	Verapamil
Amyloidosis	Amiodarone
Electrolyte abnormalities	Cyclosporine
Hypokalemia	

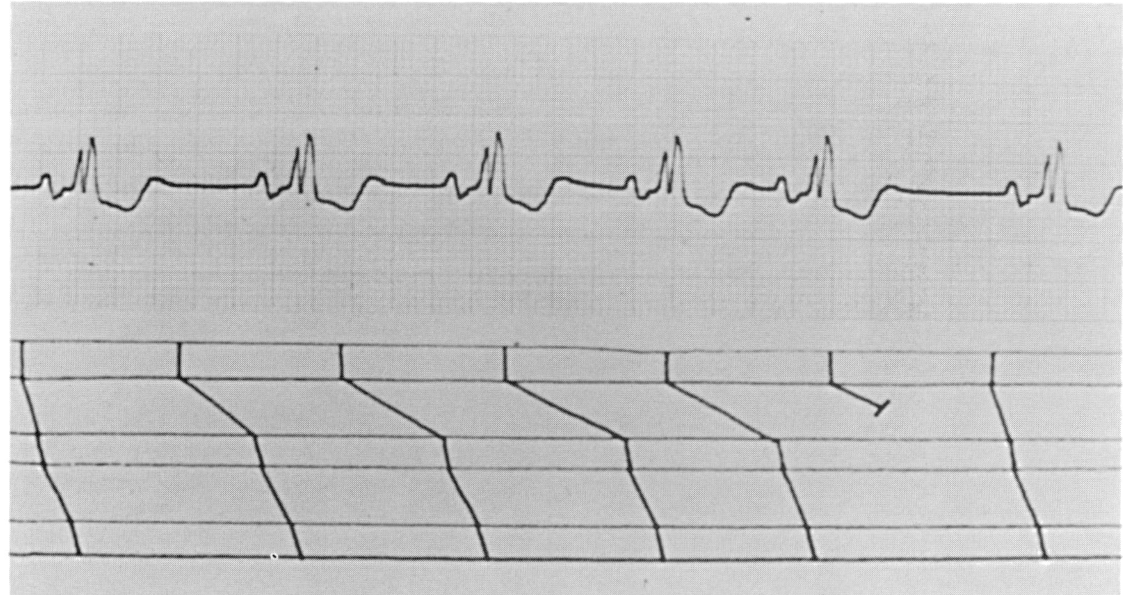

Figure 85–4. Sinus nodal Wenckebach. P-to-P interval increases by decreasing increments until P wave is dropped.

of His is type II. On an electrocardiogram, both types are consistently manifested as first-degree block (prolonged PR interval), second-degree AV block (intermittent dropped beats), or third-degree block (complete AV dissociation).[45, 46]

Digitalis is usually associated with type I block in its many forms. First-degree, second-degree, and third-degree blocks all are seen. Type II (infra-His) block and bilateral bundle branch block are rare consequences of digitalis toxicity but may be seen if underlying heart disease exists.

Alteration of Impulse Formation

Alterations of impulse formation may be divided into those that suppress higher pacemakers or those that excite lower pacemakers. Suppression of higher pacemakers is limited primarily to direct effect on the sinus node. Excitation usually takes the form of an acceleration of a lower pacer (AV node or ventricle) to every known extrasystolic mechanism. The combination of suppressant and excitant effects should be considered digitalis toxicity until proved otherwise.

Digitalis toxicity is an exacerbation of the drug's normal effects on refractory periods of the conduction system and myocardial cells. Increased heterogeneity of the refractory periods allows for the development of re-entry phenomena, which are the probable mechanisms in the development of tachyarrhythmias (Table 85–3).

Manifestations

Noncardiac

The clinical effects of digitalis intoxication are noncardiac as well as cardiac manifestations. Gastrointestinal manifestations are present in both acute and chronic intoxication. Anorexia, nausea, and vomiting are the most common. These symptoms often occur early and may be the presenting complaint. Other gastrointestinal complaints are less common but occur with both oral and intravenous forms. Neurologic and visual manifestations are also frequent and range from headache and fatigue to depression, confusion, and hallucination. The visual disturbances of blurring and alteration in color are less common. Digitalis intoxication should always be considered in older patients who are receiving the drug and present with vague gastrointestinal complaints and al-

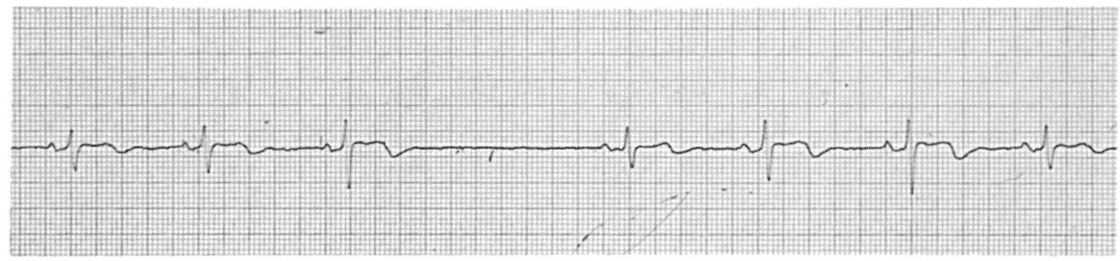

Figure 85–5. Sinus node exit block: The long pause between beat 3 and beat 4 is twice the normal sinus interval.

Table 85–3. Rhythm and Conduction Disturbances in Digitalis Intoxication

Excitant
Atrial premature beats
Atrial tachycardia
Atrial flutter (rare)
Atrial fibrillation (rare)
Junctional premature beats
Accelerated junctional rhythms
Ventricular premature beats, bigeminy and multiformed
Ventricular tachycardia
Bidirectional tachycardia
Ventricular fibrillation
Suppressant
Sinus bradycardia
Sinoatrial block
Type I second-degree AV block (Wenckebach)
Bundle branch block
Complete AV block
Type II second-degree AV block (?)
Combination excitant and suppressant
Atrial tachycardia with AV block
Sinus bradycardia with junctional tachycardia
Wenckebach with junctional premature beats
Regularization of ventricular rhythm with atrial fibrillation

AV, atrioventricular.

tered mental status. The more complete list and incidence can be found in Table 85–1. In this study, vigorous attempts were made to establish digitalis as the cause of these symptoms.[6]

Cardiac

Cardiac manifestations are the more frequent and dangerous presentations of digitalis toxicity. A healthy heart rarely has any signs of toxicity unless the amount is very high. Therefore, accidental overdoses, especially in children, rarely present any cardiac findings but may show AV conduction disturbances. On the other hand, a diseased heart presents with the more lethal arrhythmias. No arrhythmias are diagnostic of digitalis toxicity because similar rhythms may represent underlying disease. *A change in the rhythm may be the most important clue.* Nevertheless, toxicity should be suspected in any patient receiving the medication and exhibiting evidence of depressed conduction, alteration of impulse formation (automaticity), or both.

Depressed conduction is related to slowing of AV nodal conduction and prolonging nodal refractoriness from high vagal tone, but at high levels, digitalis may directly prolong AV nodal refractoriness. The result is AV block of all types.

First-degree AV block from digitalis is indistinguishable from other causes and is seen as a prolonged PR interval. Second-degree AV block is type I, often called AV nodal Wenckebach or Mobitz type I (Fig. 85–6). The resultant heart rate may be complicated because of accelerated junctional escape beats (Fig. 85–7). Third-degree block, or AV dissociation, is usually associated with a narrow QRS escape focus at adequate rates, and hemodynamic alterations are rare in the absence of other cardiac abnormalities (Figs. 85–8 to 85–10).

Impulse-forming alterations from digitalis toxicity are often manifested as suppression of atrial pacemakers, primarily the SA node. The resultant arrhythmia is frequently sinus bradycardia (Fig. 85–11) and sinus arrest or SA node exit block. The extent of the bradycardia may be quite severe, especially in elderly patients and in those with SA node disease (Fig. 85–12). Excitation is due to increased frequency of discharge of junctional or ventricular pacemakers, taking the form of accelerated junctional (Fig. 85–13) or accelerated ventricular tachycardias (Fig. 85–14). Myriad extrasystole may be seen, such as premature ventricular contractions (PVCs) (Figs. 85–15 and 85–16); ventricular parasystole, and ventricular or bidirectional tachycardia. The PVCs may be multiformed, bigeminal, paired, or in couplets. Before more current therapy, the ventricular tachycardia related to digitalis toxicity carried a 50% mortality. Bidirectional tachycardia was almost always fatal.

The combination of suppressant and excitant effects was once considered diagnostic of digitalis toxicity. However, as the number of older patients with intrinsic cardiac disease increases, these arrhythmias are less specific for digitalis toxicity. The rhythms are usually manifested by an increased sinus rate with block or second-degree AV block with accelerated lower pacer. Examples are atrial tachycardia with block or Wenckebach block with accelerated junctional escape beats (Fig. 85–17). Even though less specific, digitalis toxicity should always be considered when this type of arrhythmia is encountered.

DIAGNOSIS

Recognition of digitalis toxicity requires a high index of suspicion for any patient receiving the drug and manifesting the cardiac and noncardiac symptoms mentioned earlier. Resolution of symptoms and arrhythmias after withholding the drug was the usual method of diagnosis before the development of serum digitalis determinations.

Digitalis Levels

The concentration of digitalis in the serum is the net result of whole-body absorption, distribution, and excretion. Attempts to predict serum levels based on age, sex, and renal function have not been successful (even with computer assistance), and such attempts cannot replace actual measurement of serum levels. However, the serum level does not necessarily diagnose toxicity.[7–9, 47–50] Three major problems arise in diagnosing toxicity.

First, the accuracy and reproducibility of the tests can be a problem, but this problem has decreased with better commercial kits and longer use. Assays of different digitalis preparations often overlap, and

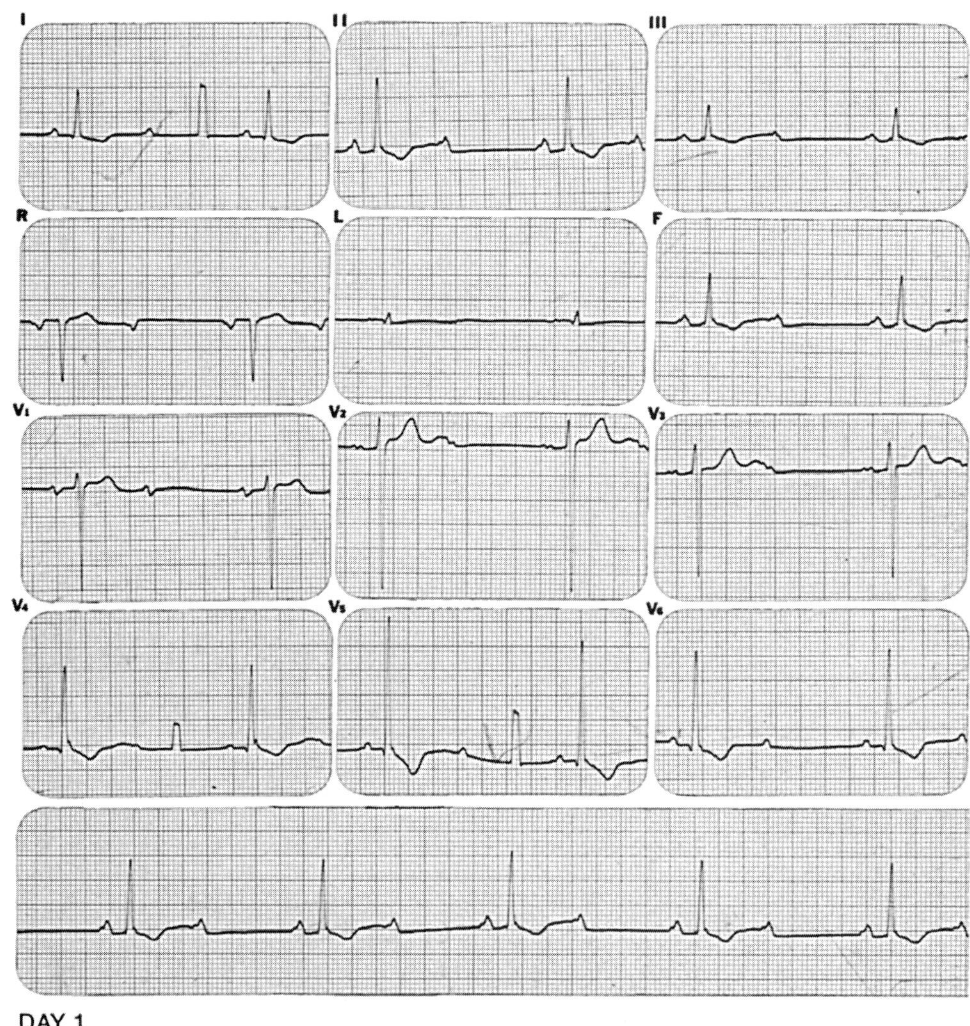

Figure 85–6. Day 1: Electrocardiograms (ECGs) of a 52-year-old woman with hypertension and congestive failure, seen in the emergency room for weakness. She was taking 0.25 mg of digoxin daily. Digoxin was withheld, and the patient was observed. Admission ECG shows 2:1 atrioventricular (AV) block, narrow QRS complex, increased voltage, and short QT and ST changes compatible with digitalis or left hypertrophy.

accurate interpretation of results is possible only if the exact preparation is known. In addition, the clinical correlations of therapeutic and toxic levels all have been made at steady-state levels. These levels are reached 6 to 8 hours after administration, and any measurements made before this time may give values two to three times greater than at steady-state levels. False-positive elevations may occur for several reasons. For example, spironolactone and hyperbilirubinemia interfere with the test. Far more frequent is a false-positive assay in patients with chronic renal failure. This elevation is thought to be caused by an endogenous circulating digoxin-like substance, which has been reported in more than 60% of patients with chronic renal insufficiency.[51]

A second problem in diagnosing toxicity arises because serum levels of patients demonstrating clinical toxicity overlap considerably. Specific and sensitive laboratory criteria are not available as alternatives to clinical assessment. The inability to define toxicity levels accurately has been a major defect in the analysis of most studies. Figure 85–18 shows the problem in an older study, but a more complete list is found in the review by Smith.[52]

A third problem is the fact that several different factors predispose patients to toxicity at levels well below the 2 ng/mL level, usually considered the upper limits of normal. Hypokalemia is the most important of these factors. Anoxia caused by chronic pulmonary disease or advanced forms of heart disease is also important. In addition, enhanced sympathetic activity for any reason seems to sensitize patients to digitalis-induced arrhythmias.[53]

Therefore, serum levels should be used only as a guide to appropriate therapeutic doses and for an indication of toxicity. Serum levels also may verify drug compliance and aid dose regulation in patients with changing renal function, those who have undergone cardiac surgery, or those with severe congestive heart failure. It must be emphasized that toxicity *cannot* be diagnosed from serum levels alone. Special consideration must be given to those patients with

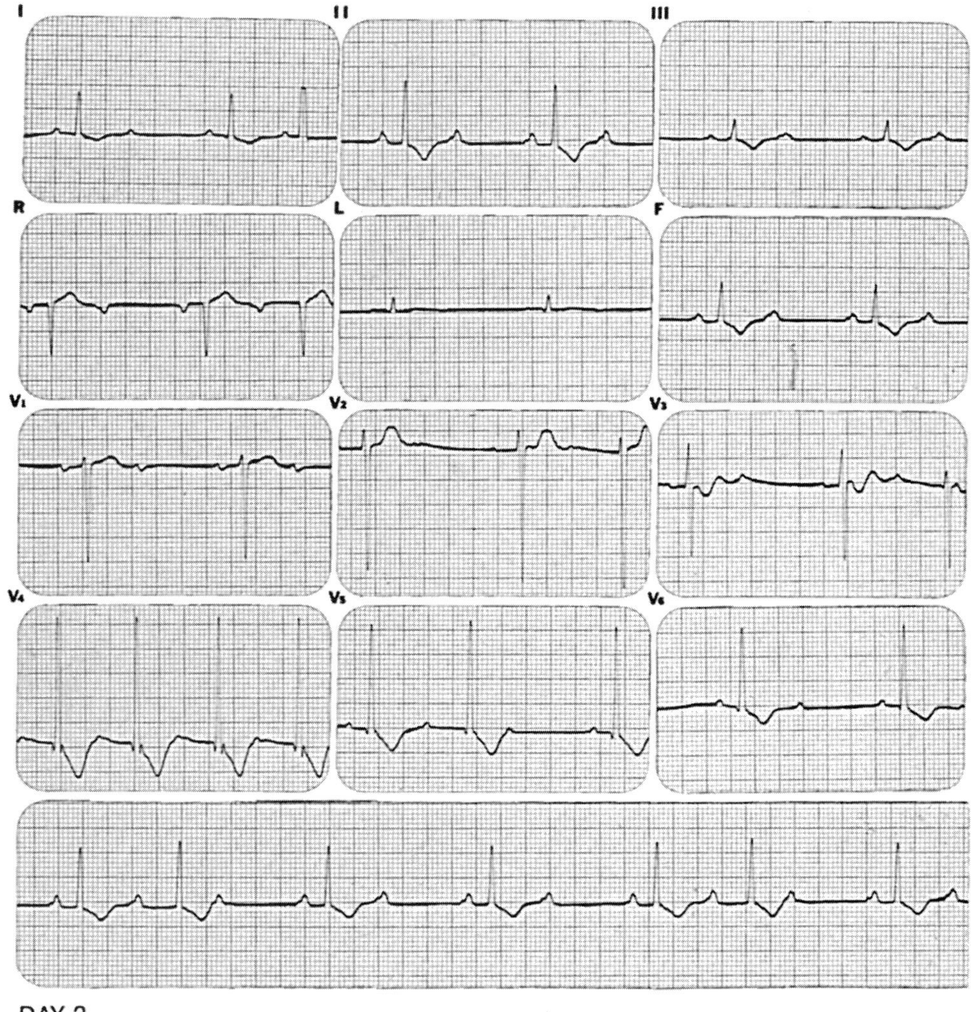

Figure 85–6 *Continued* Day 2: Day 2 ECG showed some area of 2:1 conduction but also 3:2 Wenckebach and periods of first-degree AV block (lead V_4). By day 6, the ECG showed sinus rhythm, first-degree AV block, and the typical "scooped-out" ST changes of digitalis. This sequence demonstrated first- and second-degree block associated with digitalis toxicity and 2:1 block with a narrow QRS complex (as a manifestation of type I second-degree AV block).

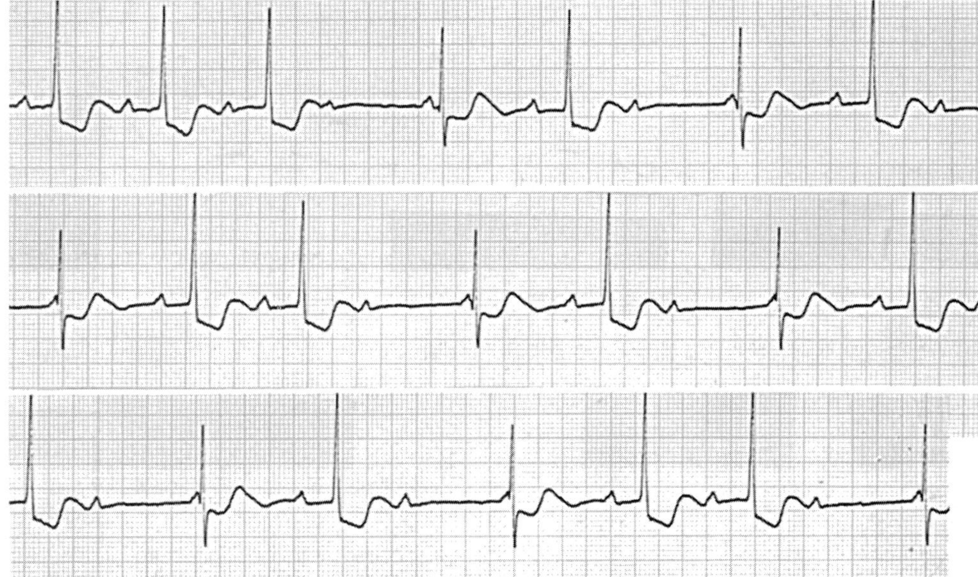

Figure 85–7. Atrioventricular nodal Wenckebach with 2:1, 3:1, and 4:1 conduction. After each dropped beat there is a junctional escape beat before re-establishment of sinus conduction. The electrocardiogram strips are continuous.

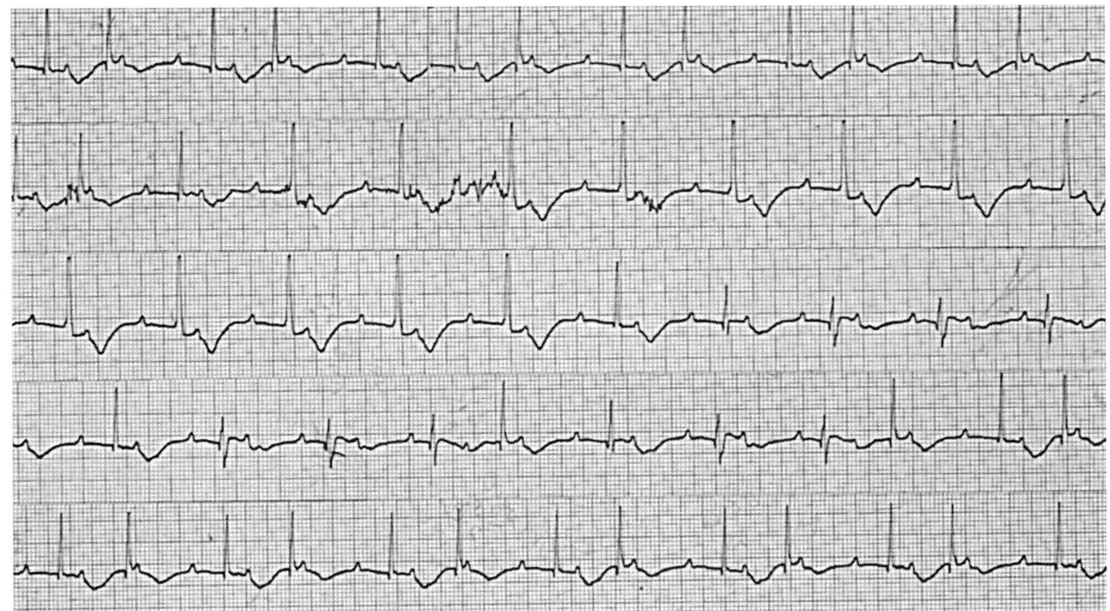

Figure 85–8. Electrocardiogram (ECG) of an elderly man receiving maintenance digoxin for congestive heart failure. He was admitted to the hospital for an irregular heartbeat and showed no other symptoms. Heart rhythm resolved to regular sinus rhythm 3 days after digoxin was discontinued. Admission ECG: Strip 1, 3:2 Wenckebach. Strip 2, 3:2 → 2:1 block. Strips 3, 4, and 5 exhibit 2:1 block changing to atrioventricular dissociation related to high-grade block. Note the slight variation in QRS configuration, the change in rate, and fusion beats (strip 3, fourth beat from right and strip 4, seventh beat). (ECG strips are continuous.)

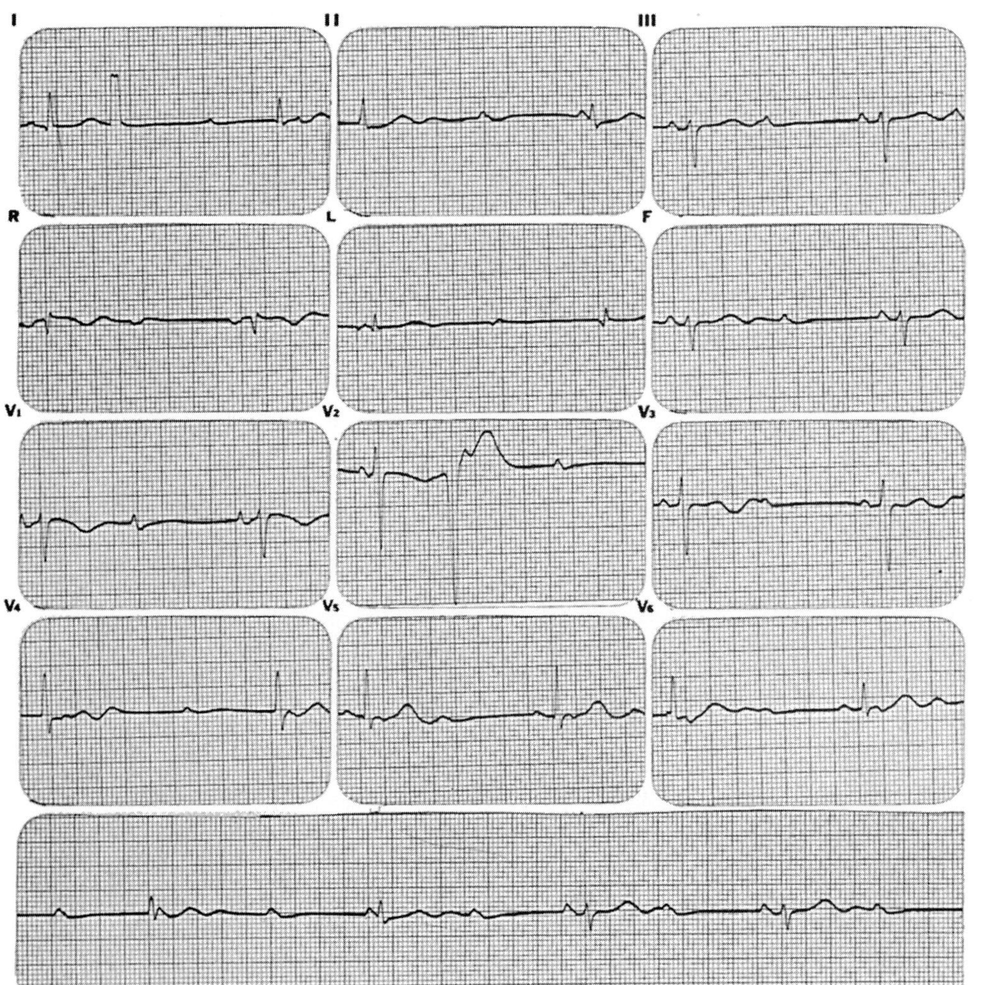

Figure 85–9. Electrocardiogram (ECG) of a 79-year-old woman admitted with shortness of breath and weight loss. She was receiving maintenance digoxin therapy. The ECG shows atrioventricular (AV) dissociation secondary to a high-grade AV block with a narrow QRS complex.

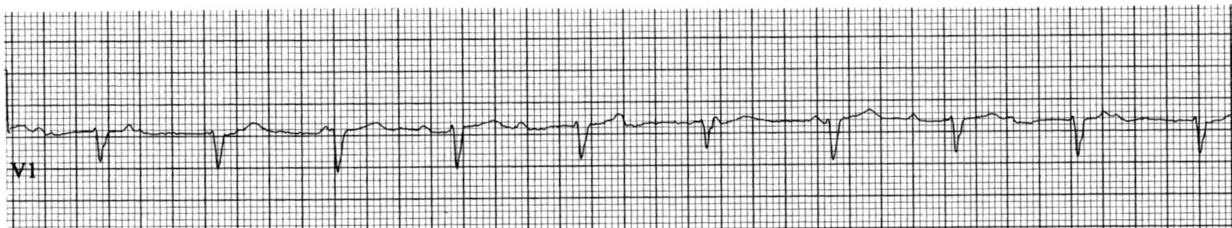

Figure 85–10. This 70-year-old was admitted to the emergency department with nausea and fever. The electrocardiogram shows sinus tachycardia with atrioventricular AV dissociation from high-grade AV block and an accelerated junctional rhythm.

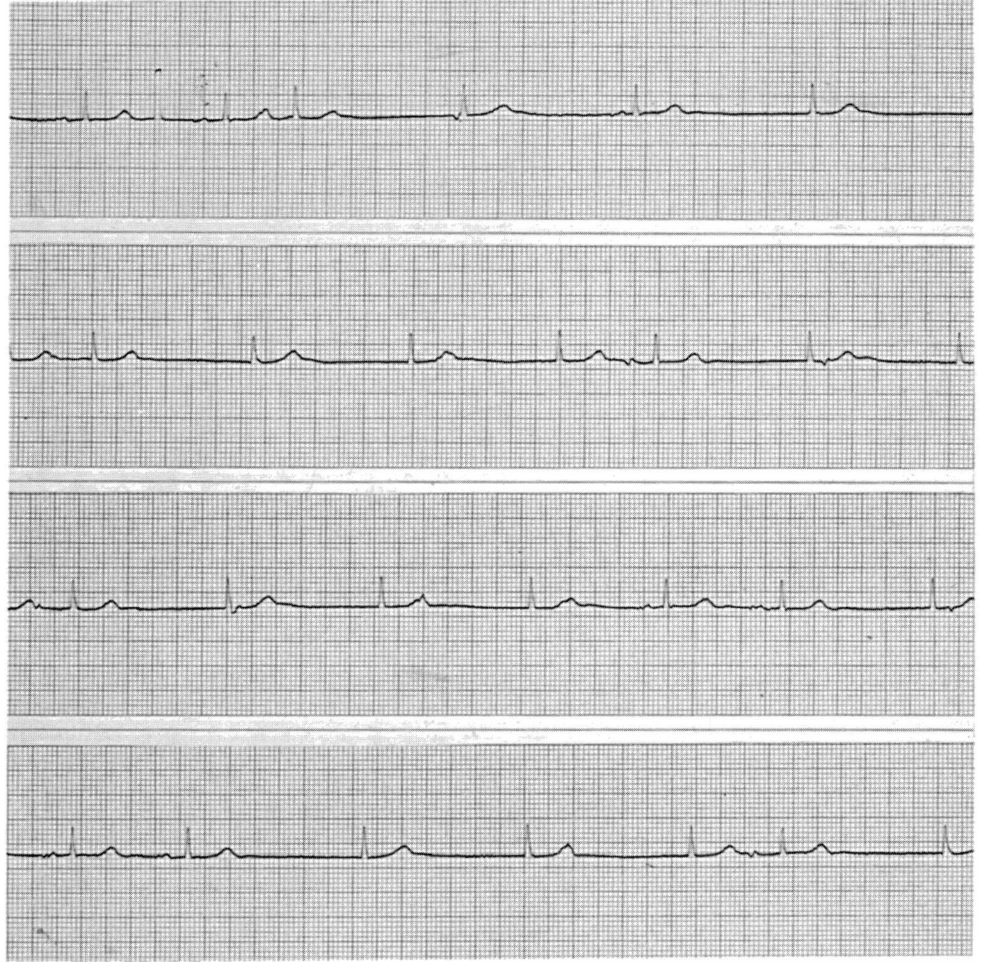

Figure 85–11. The electrocardiogram of an 82-year-old woman recently begun on digitalis shows sinus rhythm with sinus arrest and atrioventricular dissociation with slow atrial escape and faster junctional escape rhythm.

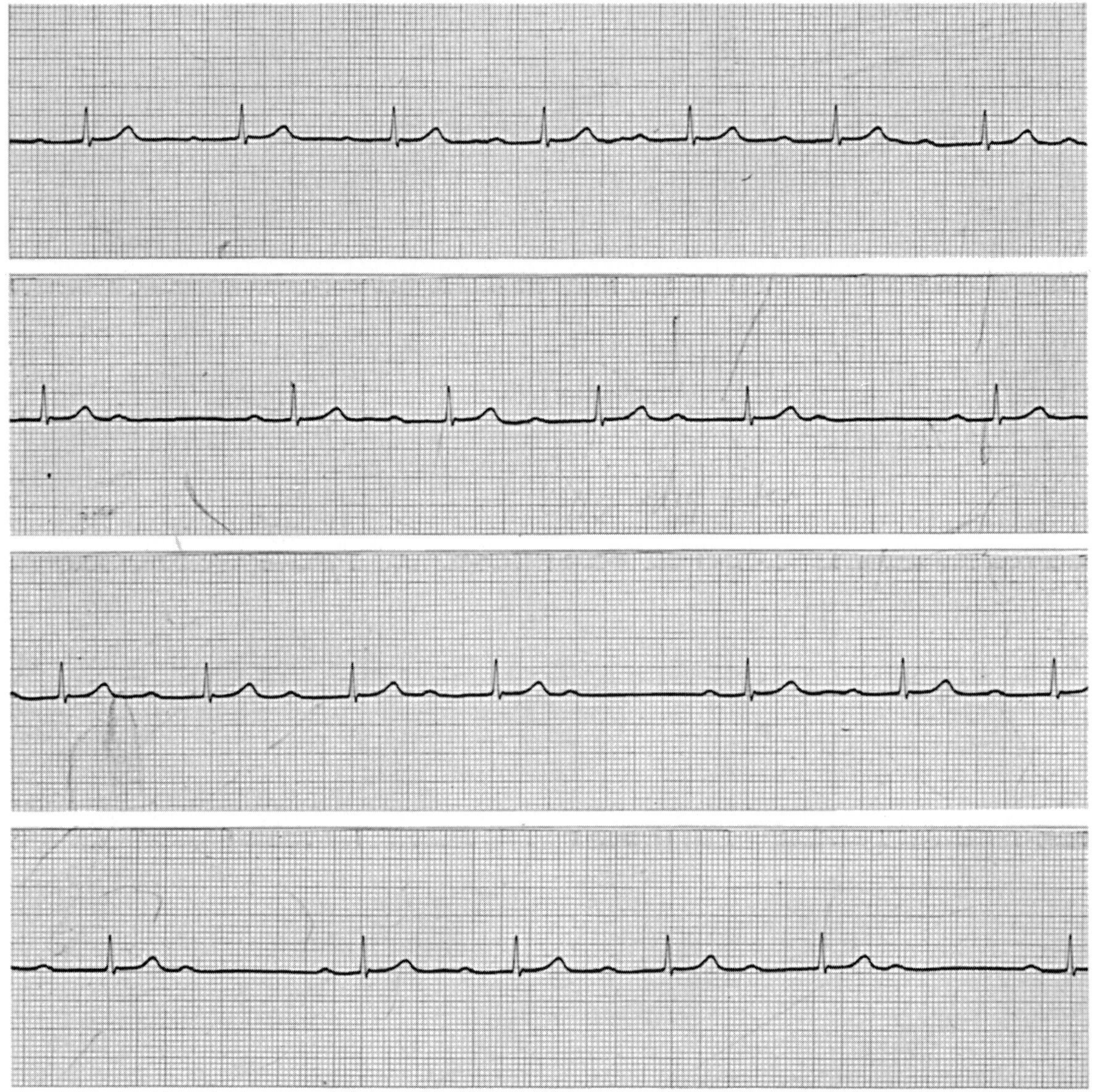

Figure 85–12. An 82-year-old man was referred for slow pulse. An electrocardiogram (ECG) 1 day before the present ECG showed 2:1 heart block. The patient was taking digoxin, 0.25 mg/day. Strips show 5:4 atrioventricular nodal block with a narrow QRS complex.

accompanying problems. These are the same problems listed in Table 85–2, as well as the type and severity of underlying heart disease. The more complete pharmacokinetic interactions are listed in Table 85–4.

THERAPY OF DIGITALIS INTOXICATION

Successful therapy of digitalis intoxication depends on early recognition. Physicians must maintain a high index of suspicion about digitalis intoxication if they are to make this diagnosis, especially in patients with predisposing factors, such as old age, renal disease, chronic lung disease, or quinidine use. Most of the patients suffer from chronic overdose as opposed to severe acute ingestion, which is usually suicidal or accidental. Three reports vividly illustrate this point. Bain reported a patient who developed digitalis toxicity from drinking herbal tea made with foxglove leaves mistaken for comfrey.[54] Wamboldt and colleagues reported three patients in whom digitalis intoxication was misdiagnosed as depression.[55] Kwan and associates reported digitalis toxicity due to a Chinese medication containing toad venom.[56]

In cases such as these, gastrointestinal manifestations, such as anorexia, nausea, or vomiting, are often the first clinical signs. The earliest electrocardiographic manifestations of digitalis effect include a prolonged PR interval and a sagging (scooped-out) ST depression with a relatively short QT interval (Fig. 85–19). However, neither ST changes nor the prolonged PR interval indicates intoxication, but it does increase suspicion.

On the other hand, arrhythmias are the hallmark of toxicity. As previously noted, the arrhythmias may take every possible form. The most common of these,

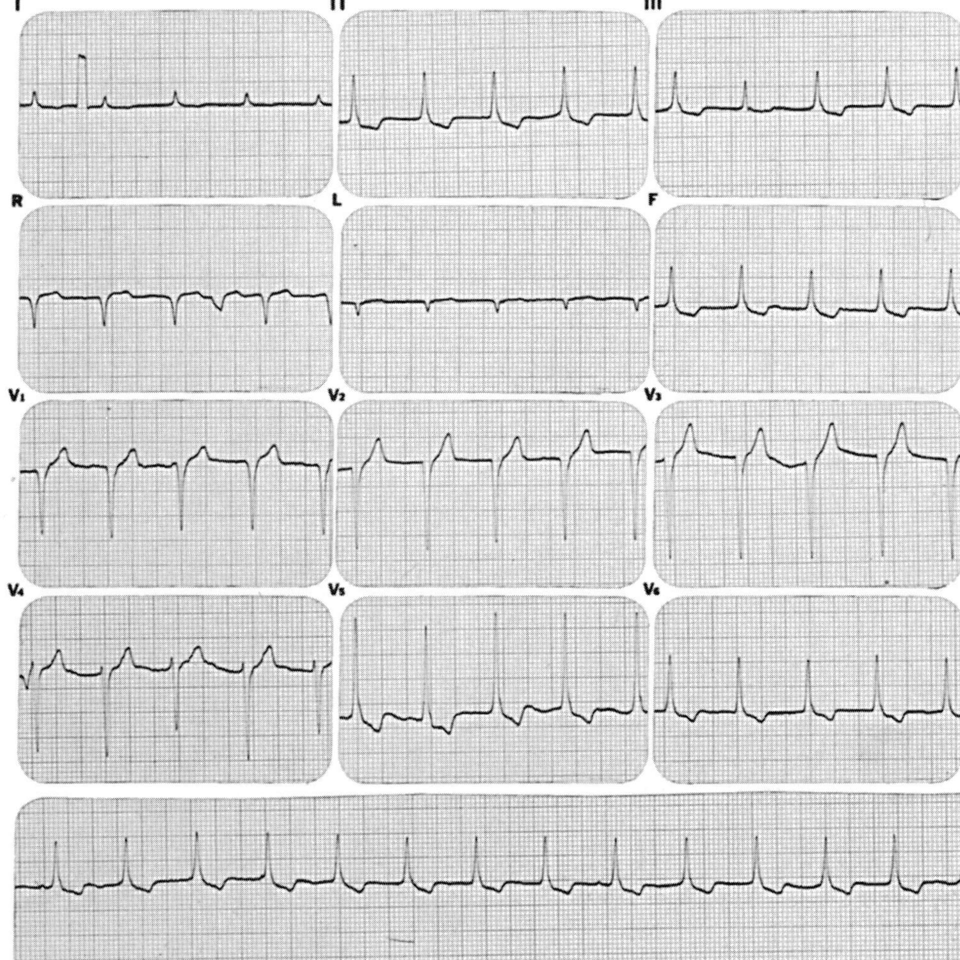

Figure 85–13. Electrocardiogram of a patient admitted to the cardiac care unit because of nausea and palpitations. Findings were an atrioventricular dissociation secondary to accelerated junctional rhythm.

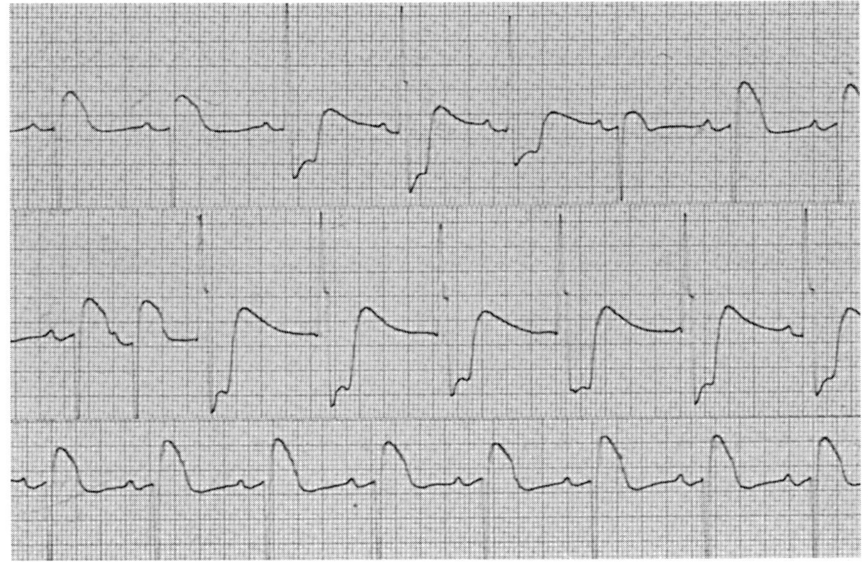

Figure 85–14. Sinus rhythm, atrioventricular dissociation related to accelerated ventricular rhythm, and occasional premature atrial contractions (second beat of middle strip) in an elderly woman admitted to the coronary care unit with a digoxin level of 9.2 ng/mL.

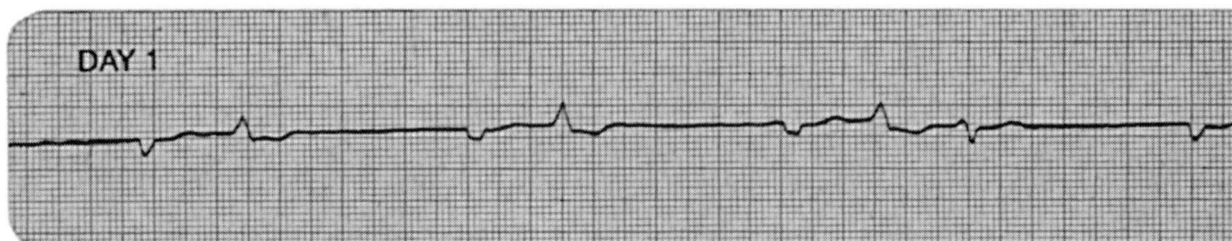

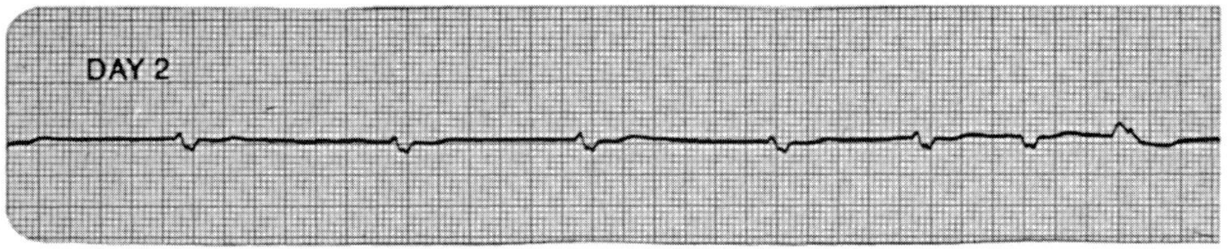

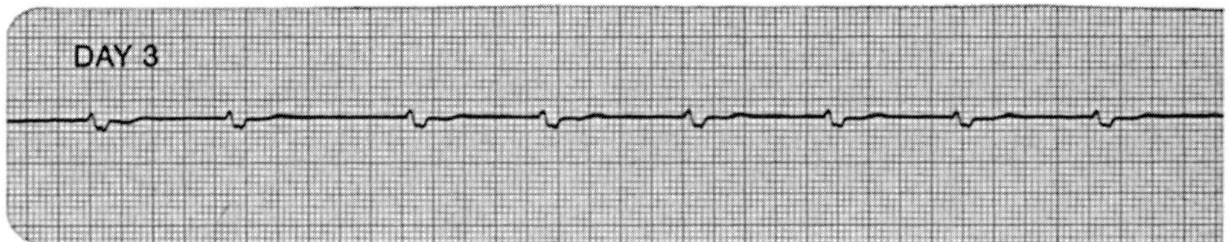

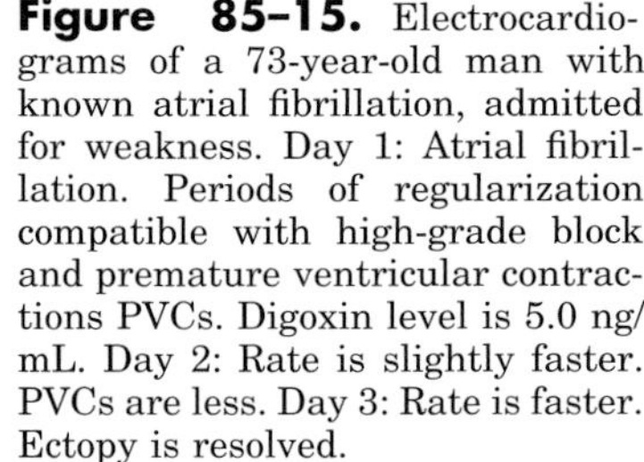
Figure 85–15. Electrocardiograms of a 73-year-old man with known atrial fibrillation, admitted for weakness. Day 1: Atrial fibrillation. Periods of regularization compatible with high-grade block and premature ventricular contractions PVCs. Digoxin level is 5.0 ng/mL. Day 2: Rate is slightly faster. PVCs are less. Day 3: Rate is faster. Ectopy is resolved.

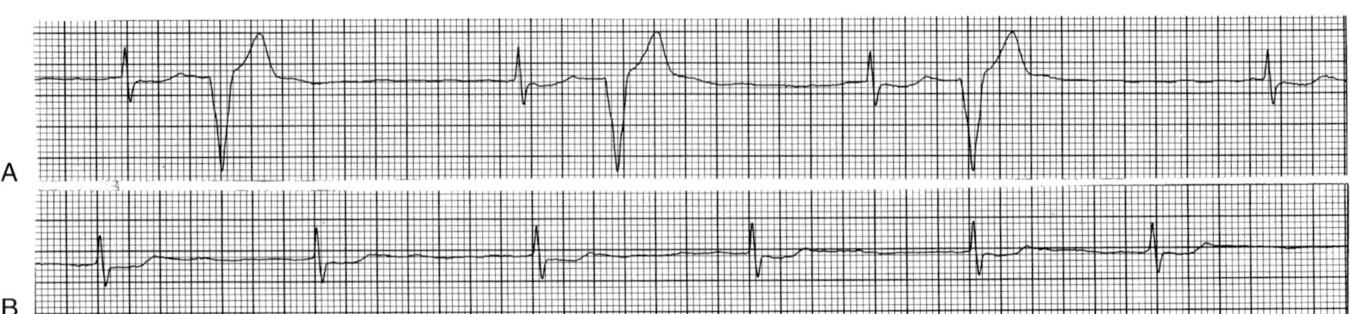

Figure 85–16. *A,* Admission electrocardiogram of an 89-year-old with a digoxin level of 2.4 ng/mL. *B,* One day later.

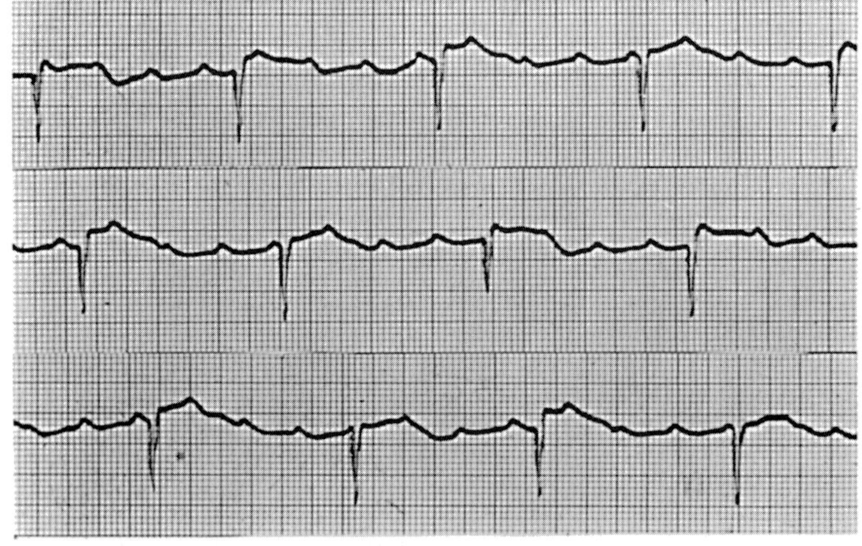

Figure 85–17. This rhythm strip shows atrial tachycardia with block. There is an atrial rate of approximately 150 per minute with a 3:1 block.

PVCs, first-degree AV block, or atrial fibrillation with a very slow rate, require no special therapy except drug withdrawal. Any disturbance that affects a patient's hemodynamic status, whether it be tachycardia or bradycardia, should be treated more aggressively (for brief overview, see Table 85–5.)

Antidotal Therapy

The most immediate decision for the physician treating suspected digitalis overdose concerns the need for antidotal therapy.

Digitalis in massive doses may be lethal, and either suicidal or accidental overdoses are not uncommon. Massive doses poison the membrane-bound Na^+,K^+-ATPase system in the heart and in all body tissues that contain this system. The poisoned membranes can no longer maintain electrolyte gradients. The abnormal membrane function leads to extremely high serum levels of potassium. In the absence of Na^+ and K^+ gradients, resting membrane potentials are reduced and the cells of the conduction system cannot function as pacemakers. The result is asystole and finally a complete loss of any cardiac electric activity.[57]

Treating massive digitalis overdose presents some difficult problems. The most immediate lethal problem is the mounting hyperkalemia. Hemodialysis, the treatment of choice for refractory hyperkalemia, may temporarily attenuate the excess serum potassium level but does not eliminate digitalis because of high tissue binding. Charcoal or resin hemoperfusion coupled with dialysis has been attempted but with minimal effect.[58]

Table 85–4. Digoxin Pharmacokinetic Interactions

Bioavailability
Decreased
Cathartics
Antacids
Cholesterol-binding agents
Malabsorption syndromes
Bowel edema
Eubacterium lentum
Gastric hyperacidity
Increased
Lanoxicaps or elixir
Antibiotics (*E. lentum*)
Omeprazole
Distribution
Decreased
Renal failure
Hyperkalemia
Aging
Hypothyroidism
Amiodarone
Increased
Hypokalemia
Hyperthyroidism
Pregnancy
Physical activity
Elimination
Decreased
Renal failure
Excessive diuretics
Aging
Indomethacin
Cyclosporine
Spironolactone
Verapamil
Quinidine
Propafenone
Increased
Diarrhea
Vasodilators

From Lewis RP: Clinical use of serum digoxin concentrations. Am J Cardiol *69*:97G, 1992.

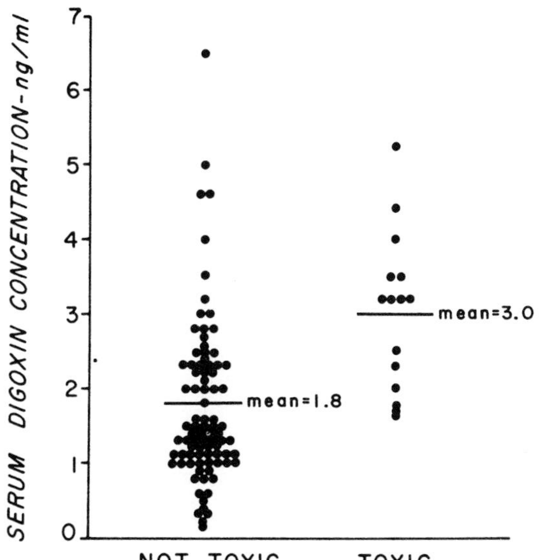

Figure 85–18. Results of 100 serum digoxin radioimmunoassay measurements. Sixteen patients were believed to be clinically toxic; their mean serum level was 3.0 ng/mL. Seven patients thought to be nontoxic also had serum levels of more than 3.0 ng/mL. Overlap of normal toxic values does occur; therefore, judgment must be used when evaluating results. (From Doherty JE: Digitalis glycosides: Pharmacokinetics and their clinical implications. Ann Intern Med *79*:229, 1973.)

The best method for treating very high levels of digitalis poisoning is the use of digoxin-specific polyclonal antibody fragments (Fab). The first report appeared in 1976[59] (Fig. 85–20.) The final report of the multicenter study was published in June 1990,[60] and the observational surveillance study in March 1991.[61] The beneficial effect in the pediatric population was reported by Woolf and colleagues.[62] As a result of these studies, the drug is now approved by the Food and Drug Administration and marketed as Digibind (Burroughs Wellcome Co., Research Triangle Park, NC).[63] The fragments (50,000 daltons) neutralize digoxin toxicity by increasing the speed of digoxin excretions and reversing tissue binding of digitalis (the affinity is higher for digoxin but can be used effectively for digitoxin). The serum concentrations reach high levels, but the small molecular size allows glomerular filtration and relatively rapid excretion.

The following protocol has been recommended by Antman and Smith[64]:

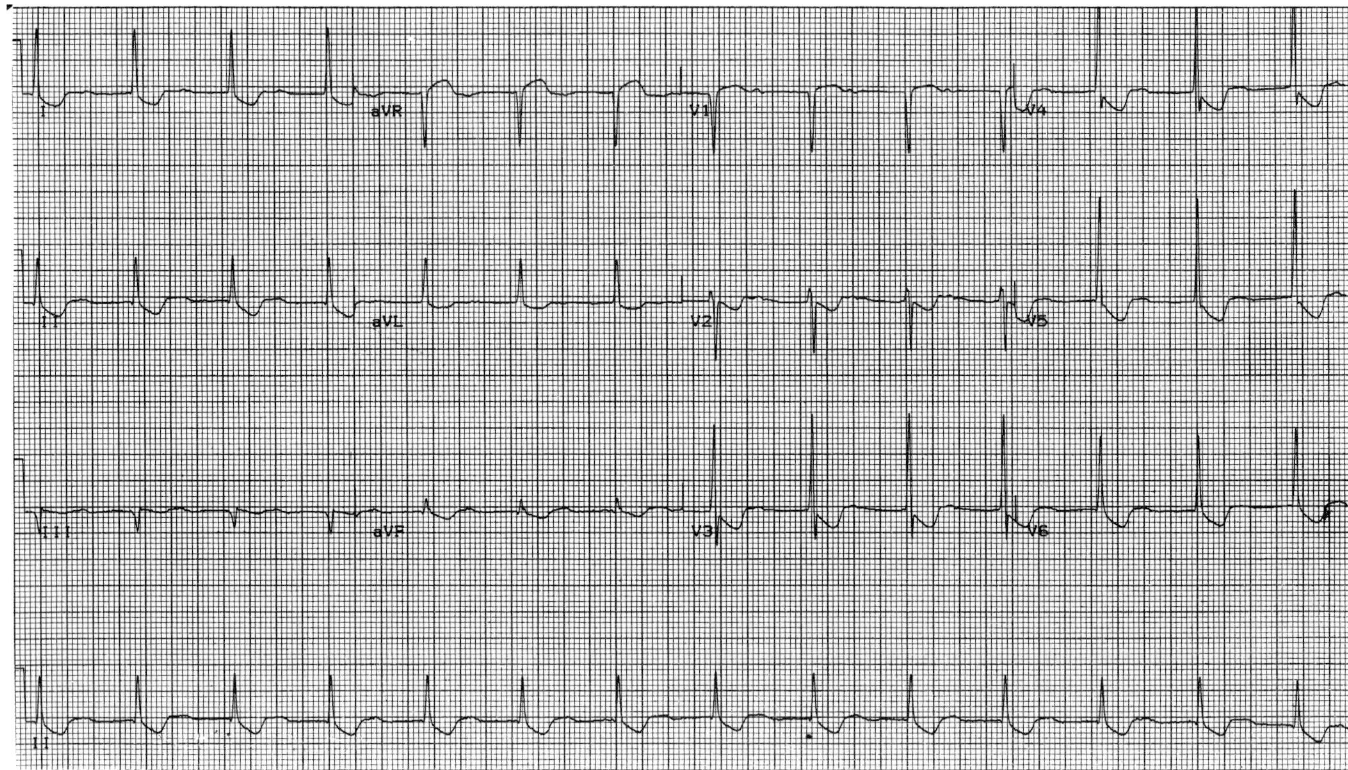

Figure 85–19. Electrocardiogram showing sinus rhythm, first-degree atrioventricular block, and marked ST changes compatible with digoxin effect. The patient was asymptomatic and had a normal digoxin level.

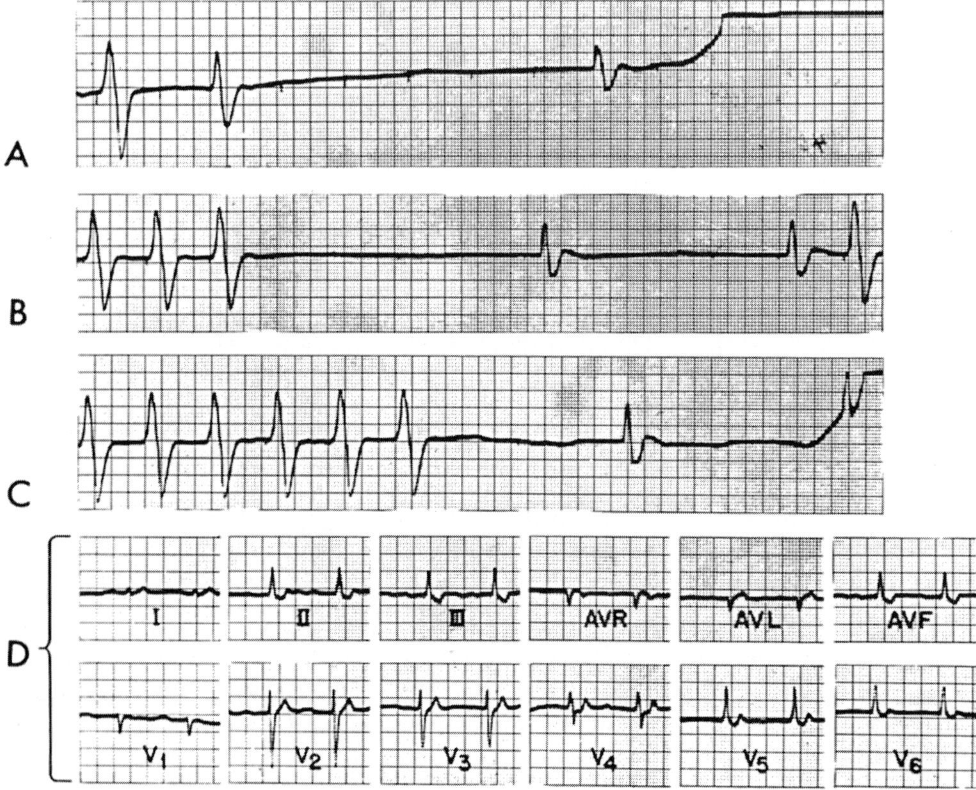

Figure 85–20. Sequential electrocardiograms recorded before, during, and after treatment with digoxin-specific Fab fragments. In *A,* the tracing recorded immediately before the start of Fab infusion, serum potassium level is 8.7 mEq/L; the escape interval when pacer stimulus is reduced below threshold is 4.60 seconds. In *B,* the tracing recorded 15 minutes after the start of Fab infusion, serum potassium level is 8.0 mEq/L; the escape interval is 3.96 seconds. In *C,* the tracing recorded 30 minutes after the start of Fab infusion, the escape interval is 2.76 seconds. In *D,* the tracing recorded 2 hours after the start of Fab infusion, the serum potassium level is 7.4 mEq/L; a sinus mechanism is present at a rate of 75 per minute, with first-degree atrioventricular block (P-R interval of 0.24 second). (From Smith TW, Haber E, Yeatman L, Butler VP Jr: Reversal of advance digoxin intoxication with Fab fragments of digoxin-specific antibodies. N Engl J Med *294:*797, 1976.)

1. Skin testing is no longer recommended. (The incidence of hypersensitivity was very small.)
2. The dose is calculated to be equimolar to the amount of digoxin estimated in the patient's body. This is derived from history and digoxin level (1 mg of digoxin for each nanogram of digoxin per milliliter of serum [Table 85–6]).
3. Administer the Fab fragments over 15 to 30 minutes. Results are usually noted within 60 minutes.
4. Monitor K^+ (potassium) level closely because reversal of Na^+,K^+-ATPase inhibition may restore transmembrane K^+ gradients, and total body K^+ is often depleted.
5. Digoxin levels may remain high, but most digoxin is bound to Fab fragments and is functionally inert. Therefore, measurement of digoxin levels is not reliable or useful. (See the articles by Antman and Smith for full explanation of the mechanism. Examples of calculations from Antman and Smith are shown in Table 85–7.)[64]

Table 85–6. Calculation of Equimolar Dose of Digoxin-Specific Fab Fragments

Calculation of body load of digoxin

Ingested amount (mg) × bioavailability of digoxin tablets = mg × 0.8

$$\frac{\text{Serum digoxin concentration (ng/mL)} \times 5.6^{*} \times \text{weight in kg}}{1000}$$

Calculation of Fab fragment dose

$$\frac{\text{MW Fab} = 50{,}000}{\text{MW digoxin} = 781} = 64 \times \text{body load (mg)} = \text{Fab dose (in mg)}$$

$$\frac{\text{Body load of digoxin (mg)}}{\text{0.7 mg neutralized/40-mg vial}} = \text{number of vials of Fab fragments}$$

MW, Molecular weight.

*Volume of distribution of digoxin in average adult (liters per kilogram). For digitoxin, use 0.56 rather than 5.6.

Modified from Antman EM, Wenger TL, Butler VP, et al: Treatment of 150 cases of life-threatening digitalis intoxication with digoxin-specific Fab antibody fragments: Final report of a multicenter study. Circulation *81*:1744, 1990.

At present, indications for this therapy are limited to severe overdoses in which actual or potential life-threatening toxicity exists. Manifestations of life-threatening toxicity include life-threatening rhythm disturbances (whether tachyarrhythmias, bradyarrhythmias, or heart block) that do not respond to conventional measures, or hyperkalemia unresponsive to the usual therapies. In addition, immunotherapy is considered appropriate in patients in whom toxic exposure is so great that satisfactory outcome with conventional therapy is unlikely. The use of Digibind should be considered when more than 10 mg of digoxin has been ingested by previously healthy adults, or 4 mg in children. In addition, a steady-state serum concentration of greater than 10 ng/mL or a serum potassium level of greater than 5 mEq/L in the setting of severe digoxin intoxication often presages cardiac arrest and satisfies the condition for use of the antidote. Continued experience has confirmed the safety of the method; its use may be extended to diagnostic testing, as well as to first-line therapy for digitalis toxicity when the diagnosis has not been confirmed.[63, 64]

Table 85–5. Summary of Treatment for Digitalis Toxicity

I. Initial approach
   A. Withdraw drug and measure serum drug level if possible.
   B. Maintain close observation in monitored setting.
   C. Reserve therapy for hemodynamically significant arrhythmias.

II. Conventional or chronic overdose
   A. Bradycardia. There is no absolute critical rate, and no therapy is needed unless the patient is symptomatic.
      1. Initiate trial of atropine first.
      2. Temporary demand pacemaker may be needed if symptomatic bradycardia persists.
      3. Avoid β-adrenergic agonists if possible. These often precipitate more serious arrhythmias.
   B. Ectopy. Reserve therapy for more complex forms.
      1. Consider normalization of K^+ unless K^+ is >5.0 mEq/L or severe renal failure exists.
      2. Lidocaine and phenytoin are antiarrhythmic drugs of first choice if K^+ replacement is unsuccessful.
      3. Other class I antiarrhythmics, such as quinidine or procainamide, are not useful as initial agents.
      4. Intravenous magnesium if K^+ level is elevated or serum magnesium is low.
      5. Verapamil is useful only if supraventricular tachycardia is present.
      6. β-Blockers have limited usefulness but may decrease automaticity.
      7. Cardioversion should be limited to patients with life-threatening arrhythmias and used at lowest effective energy level.

III. Resistant or massive overdose
   A. Digoxin-specific antibodies should be considered when:
      1. The patient has ingested >10 mg of digoxin (adult) or 4 mg (children).
      2. The serum digoxin concentration is >10 ng/mL.
      3. Serum K^+ level is >5.0 mEq/L in this setting.

Conventional Therapy

Treating Bradyarrhythmia

The majority of these expensive, time-consuming, complicated therapies for toxicity can be avoided by allocating adequate time and effort toward educating patients. Many early signs and symptoms can be easily recognized by patients. Emphasizing the potential for toxicity may help patients to avoid self-administering higher doses.

Severe bradyarrhythmias are often related to increased vagal tone. If a patient is symptomatic, a trial of atropine intravenously at a dose of 0.5 to 2.0 mg is useful. If the arrhythmia does not respond and the patient is unstable, a temporary transvenous pacemaker should be used. β-Adrenergic agonists, such as isoproterenol, should be avoided, because the risk of precipitating more severe arrhythmias is high.

Treating Ectopy

One half to three fourths of patients developing high-grade ventricular tachyarrhythmias from digi-

Table 85–7. Examples of Calculation of Equimolar Dose of Digoxin-Specific Fab Fragments

Case 1: A 75-year-old man (weight, 70 kg) with chronic coronary heart disease and atrial fibrillation receiving maintenance therapy with digoxin 0.25 mg daily. He becomes confused and takes two of his digoxin tablets daily for 2 weeks and presents with complaints of weakness and palpitations. ECG shows sustained ventricular tachycardia at 150 beats/min. SDC = 30 ng/mL.

$$\text{Body load of digoxin} = \frac{\text{SDC} \times 5.6 \times 70}{1000} = \frac{3.0 \times 5.6 \times 70}{1000} = 1.176 \text{ mg} \approx 1.2 \text{ mg}$$

$$\text{Dose of Fab fragments} = \frac{1.2 \text{ mg}}{0.6 \text{ mg neutralized/40-mg vial}} = 2 \text{ vials}$$

Case 2: A 40-year-old woman (weight, 70 kg) with no history of heart disease ingests 100 tablets of digoxin 0.25 mg in a suicide attempt. She presents 8 hours later with nausea, vomiting, hypotension, complete heart block, and an idioventricular escape rhythm at 35 beats/min. Serum digoxin concentration result not yet returned from laboratory (and not needed for Fab dose determination). Serum potassium level = 6.1 mEq/L.

$$\text{Body load} = [\text{ingested amount} \times 0.8] = 25 \text{ mg} \times 0.8 = 20 \text{ mg}$$

$$\text{Dose of Fab fragments} = \frac{20 \text{ mg}}{0.6 \text{ mg neutralized/40-mg vial}} \approx 34 \text{ vials}$$

Case 3: A 60-year-old woman (weight, 65 kg) with chronic rheumatic heart disease and mitral regurgitation maintained on digoxin 0.25 mg daily for control of the ventricular rate in atrial fibrillation. SDC = 2 ng/mL on maintenance therapy. She ingests 75 tablets of digoxin 0.25 mg during a period of depression and presents 36 hours later with fascicular tachycardia, an unusual form of ventricular tachycardia originating in or near the left anterior fascicle. Serum potassium level = 5.9 mEq/L.

$$\text{Body load} = [\text{ingested amount} \times 0.8] + \left[\frac{\text{SDC} \times 5.6 \times 65}{1000}\right] = 14.4 + 0.728 \approx 15 \text{ mg}$$

$$\text{Dose of Fab fragments} = \frac{15}{0.6 \text{ neutralized/40-mg vial}} = 25 \text{ vials}$$

SDC, serum digoxin concentration; ECG, electrocardiogram.

talis toxicity will die; aggressive therapy is essential in these situations. The following agents should be considered:

Magnesium. The use of intravenous magnesium sulfate has dramatically increased in many cardiac emergencies, and its use in digitalis toxicity has theoretic indications, especially if the magnesium level is low or, as is often the case, the potassium level is elevated.[42] Magnesium sulfate generally is packaged as 1 g of magnesium sulfate heptahydrate in 2 mL, or 50% $MgSO_4$-7 H_2O; 1 g contains 8.12 mEq of magnesium. Intravenous use for a cardiac emergency is 2 g, or 4 mL of 50% magnesium sulfate (16.24 mEq magnesium) diluted to 100 mL given over 10 minutes. This is often repeated once, followed by maintenance intravenous drips while monitoring the magnesium and potassium levels.

Lidocaine and Phenytoin. Lidocaine (and its congeners, mexiletine and tocainide) and phenytoin (Dilantin) may be useful because they have the least effect on atrial tissue and the AV node. In fact, phenytoin is more effective for digitalis-induced ectopy than for most other causes of ectopy. Lidocaine dosage regimens are well established.[54] The phenytoin dosage recommendation is 50 to 100 mg slowly intravenously, every 5 minutes, to a dose not exceeding 600 mg, while monitoring blood pressures, until toxicity is reached or arrhythmia is controlled.

Quinidine, Procainamide, and Disopyramide. These drugs are less effective for digitalis-induced ventricular ectopy. Their potential for toxicity is too high to make them initial agents. The usefulness of other type I antiarrhythmics—flecainide, moricizine, and propafenone—is unknown at this time, and these are not considered alternative therapy.

Verapamil and Cardizem. Verapamil can alter triggered automaticity and may be useful. However, experience to date has not been adequate to include this as a recommended therapy.

β-Blockers. β-Blockers may be useful by causing a decrease in automaticity. They decrease the refractory period in cardiac muscle and conduction tissue and slow conduction velocity. However, bradycardia and blood pressure reduction limit their usefulness.

Others. Intravenous potassium, once a mainstay of therapy for digitalis intoxication, is dangerous and is now used only as a last resort. Bretylium tosylate, amiodarone, sotalol, and other newer antiarrhythmics are still unproven, and their use should be reserved.[5–7, 65] Calcium should *never* be used in digitalis toxicity.

Cardioversion. Direct current countershock should be the last resort in life-threatening arrhythmias, and if used, the lowest effective energy level for cardioversion is suggested. Even at low energy levels, the highest mortality for direct current cardioversion occurs in digitalis toxicity. Safe use of cardioversion for atrial arrhythmias in patients who are taking digoxin but are *not* toxic has been reported. However, the danger remains high when the abnormal rhythm is induced by toxic digitalis levels.[66]

SUMMARY

Digitalis intoxication is one of the most common problems in medicine today. Toxicity is manifested by many systemic symptoms, the most important of which, clinically, are cardiac arrhythmias. Virtually every known arrhythmia has been reported to be caused by digitalis excess. However, each disturbance may be noted in the presence of intrinsic cardiac disease, and distinguishing one from the other is not always easy, even with measurement of serum levels. Management of arrhythmias often requires little more than drug withdrawal, but more sophisticated techniques, including the use of digoxin-specific antibodies for severe overdose, are available and should become familiar to those physicians using the drug. Hemodialysis is not useful because most of the drug has a large volume of distribution and is tissue bound. Direct current countershock either should be avoided or used at the lowest possible energy levels.

Finally, the most important aid in the successful treatment of digitalis intoxication is prevention through patient education. Patients' awareness of potential problems enables them to recognize problems early. Patient education is especially important in view of the length of digitalis use.

References

1. Schwartz A: Is the cell membrane Na^+,K^+-ATPase enzyme system the pharmacological receptor for digitalis? Circ Res *39:*1, 1976.
2. Silverman ME: William Withering and An Account of the Foxglove. Clin Cardiol *12:*415, 1989.
3. Beller GA, Smith TW, Abermann WH, et al: Digitalis intoxication: A prospective clinical study with serum level correlations. N Engl J Med *284:*989, 1971.
4. National Center for Health Statistics: Yearly Report. Washington, DC, US Government Printing Office, 1977.
5. Smith TW: Digitalis—a bicentennial progress report. West J Med *145:*92, 1986.
6. Mahdyoon H, Battilana G, Rosman H, et al: The evolving pattern of digoxin intoxication: Observations at a large urban hospital from 1980 to 1988. Am Heart J *120:*1189, 1990.
7. Smith TW, Antman EM, Friedman PL, et al: Digitalis glycosides: Mechanisms and manifestations of toxicity (in three parts): Part I. Prog Cardiovasc Dis *26:*413, 1984.
8. Smith TW, Antman EM, Friedman PL, et al: Digitalis glycosides: Mechanisms and manifestations of toxicity (in three parts): Part II. Prog Cardiovasc Dis *26:*495, 1984.
9. Smith TW, Antman EM, Friedman PL, et al: Digitalis glycosides: Mechanisms and manifestations of toxicity (in three parts): Part III. Prog Cardiovasc Dis *27:*21, 1984.
10. Doherty JE: Digitalis glycosides: Pharmacokinetics and their clinical implications. Ann Intern Med *79:*229, 1973.
11. Doherty JE, deSoyza N, Kane JJ, et al: Clinical pharmacokinetics of digitalis glycosides. Prog Cardiovasc Dis *21:*141, 1978.
12. Lindenbaum J, Rund DG, Butler VP Jr, et al: Inactivation of digoxin by the gut flora: Reversal by antibiotic therapy. N Engl J Med *305:*789, 1981.
13. Smith TW, Haber E: Digitalis. N Engl J Med *289:*945, 1973.
14. Arnold SB, Byrd RC, Meister W, et al: Long-term digitalis therapy improves left ventricular function in heart failure. N Engl J Med *303:*1443, 1980.
15. Fleg JL, Gottlieb SH, Lakatta EG: Is digoxin really important in treatment of compensated heart failure? A placebo-controlled crossover study in patients with sinus rhythm. Am J Med *73:*244, 1982.
16. Mulrow CD, Feussner JR, Velez R: Reevaluation of digitalis efficacy: New light on an old leaf. Ann Intern Med *101:*113, 1984.
17. Packer M, Gheorghiade M, Young JB, et al: Withdrawal of digoxin from patients with chronic heart failure treated with angiotensin-converting—enzyme inhibitors. N Engl J Med *329:*1, 1993.
18. Kelly RA, Smith TW: Digoxin in heart failure: Implications of recent trials. J Am Coll Cardiol *22* (suppl A):107A, 1993.
19. Krum H, Bigger TB Jr, Goldsmith RL, Packer M: Effect of long-term digoxin therapy on autonomic function in patients with chronic heart failure. J Am Coll Cardiol *25:*289, 1995.
20. Braunwald E: Effects of digitalis on the normal and the failing heart. J Am Coll Cardiol *5:*51A, 1985.
21. Smith TW: Drug therapy: Digitalis glycosides. N Engl J Med *288:*719, 1973.
22. Smith TW: Drug therapy: Digitalis glycosides. N Engl J Med *288:*942, 1973.
23. Rosen MR, Wit AL, Hoffman B: Electrophysiology and pharmacology of cardiac arrhythmias. IV. Cardiac antiarrhythmic and toxic effects of digitalis. Am Heart J *89:*391, 1975.
24. Rosen MR: Cellular electrophysiology of digitalis toxicity. J Am Coll Cardiol *5:*22A, 1985.
25. Brown DD, Juhl RP: Decreased bioavailability of digoxin due to antacids and kaolin-pectin. N Engl J Med *295:*1034, 1976.
26. Marcus FI: Pharmacokinetic interactions between digoxin and other drugs. J Am Coll Cardiol *5:*82A, 1985.
27. Robieux I, Dorian P, Klein J, et al: The effects of cardiac transplantation and cyclosporine therapy on digoxin pharmacokinetics. J Clin Pharmacol *32:*338, 1992.
28. Hager WD, Fenster P, Mayersohn M, et al: Digoxin-quinidine interaction: Pharmacokinetic evaluation. N Engl J Med *300:*1238, 1979.
29. Bigger JT Jr: The quinidine-digoxin interaction. What do we know about it? N Engl J Med *301:*779, 1979.
30. Ochs HR, Pabst J, Greenblatt DJ, Dengler HJ: Noninteraction of digitoxin and quinidine. N Engl J Med *303:*672, 1980.
31. Hirsh PD, Weiner HJ, North RL: Further insights into digoxin-quinidine interaction: Lack of correlation between serum digoxin concentration and inotropic state of the heart. J Am Coll Cardiol *46:*863, 1980.
32. Fenster PE, White NW Jr, Hanson CD: Pharmacokinetic evaluation of the digoxin-amiodarone interaction. J Am Coll Cardiol *5:*108, 1985.
33. Nademanee K, Kannan R, Hendrickson J, et al: Amiodarone-digoxin interaction: Clinical significance, time course of development, potential pharmacokinetic mechanisms and therapeutic implications. J Am Coll Cardiol *4:*111, 1984.
34. Leahey EB, Reiffel JA, Giardina E-GV, Bigger JT Jr: The effect of quinidine and other oral antiarrhythmic drugs on serum digoxin. Ann Intern Med *92:*605, 1980.
35. Schwartz JB, Raizner A, Akers S: The effect of nifedipine on serum digoxin concentrations in patients. Am Heart J *107:*669, 1984.
36. Klein HO, Land R, Di Segni E, Kaplinsky E: Verapamil-digoxin interaction. N Engl J Med *302:*160, 1980.
37. Zatuchni J: Verapamil-digoxin interaction. Am Heart J *108:*412, 1984.
38. Surawicz B: Factors affecting tolerance to digitalis. J Am Coll Cardiol *5:*69A, 1985.
39. Iesaka Y, Aonuma K, Gosselin AJ, et al: Susceptibility of infarcted canine hearts to digitalis-toxic ventricular tachycardia. J Am Coll Cardiol *2:*45, 1983.
40. Muller JE, Turi ZG, Stone PH, et al: Digoxin therapy and mortality after myocardial infarction: Experience in the MILIS study. N Engl J Med *314:*265, 1986.
41. Sonnenblick M, Abraham AS, Meshulam Z, Eylath U: Correlation between manifestations of digoxin toxicity and serum

digoxin, calcium, potassium, and magnesium concentrations and arterial pH. BMJ *286:*1089, 1983.
42. Reisdorff EJ, Clark MR, Walters BL: Acute digitalis poisoning: The role of intravenous magnesium sulfate. J Emerg Med *4:*463, 1986.
43. Tso EL, Barish RA: Magnesium: Clinical considerations. J Emerg Med *10:*735, 1992.
44. Fisch C, Knoebel SB: Digitalis cardiotoxicity. J Am Coll Cardiol *5:*91A, 1985.
45. Kastor JA: Atrioventricular block (Part 1). N Engl J Med *292:*462, 1975.
46. Kastor JA: Atrioventricular block (Part 2). N Engl J Med *292:*572, 1975.
47. Marcus FI: Current concepts of digoxin therapy. Mod Concepts Cardiovasc Dis *45:*77, 1976.
48. Ingelfinger JA, Goldman P: The serum digitalis concentration-does it diagnose digitalis toxicity? N Engl J Med *294:*867, 1976.
49. Lasagna L: How useful are serum digitalis measurements? Editorial. N Engl J Med *294:*898, 1976.
50. Lewis RP: Clinical use of serum digoxin concentrations. Am J Cardiol *69:*97G, 1992.
51. Graves SW, Brown B, Valdes RJ: An endogenous digoxin-like substance in patients with renal impairment. Ann Intern Med *99:*604, 1983.
52. Smith T: Pharmacokinetics, bioavailability and serum levels of cardiac glycosides. J Am Coll Cardiol *5:*43A, 1985.
53. Marcus FI: Use of digitalis in acute myocardial infarction. Editorial. Circulation *62:*17, 1980.
54. Bain RJI: Accidental digitalis poisoning due to drinking herbal tea. BMJ *290:*1624, 1985.
55. Wamboldt FS, Jefferson JW, Wamboldt MZ: Digitalis intoxication misdiagnosed as depression by primary care physicians. Am J Psychiatry *143:*219, 1986.
56. Kwan JE, Paiusco AD, Kohl L: Digitalis toxicity caused by toad venom. Chest *102:*949, 1992.
57. Reza MJ, Kovick RB, Shine KI, Pearce ML: Massive intravenous digoxin overdosage. N Engl J Med *291:*777, 1974.
58. Warren SE, Fanestil DD: Digoxin overdose. Limitations of hemoperfusion-hemodialysis treatment. JAMA *242:*2100, 1979.
59. Smith TW, Haber E, Yeatman L, Butler VP Jr: Reversal of advanced digoxin intoxication with Fab fragments of digoxin-specific antibodies. N Engl J Med *294:*797, 1976.
60. Antman EM, Wenger TL, Butler VP, et al: Treatment of 150 cases of life-threatening digitalis intoxication with digoxin-specific Fab antibody fragments. Circulation *81:*1744, 1990.
61. Hickey AR, Wenger TL, Carpenter VP, et al: Digoxin immune Fab therapy in the management of digitalis intoxication: Safety and efficacy results of an observational surveillance study. J Am Coll Cardiol *17:*590, 1991.
62. Woolf AD, Wenger TL, Smith TW, Lovejoy FH: Results of multicenter studies of digoxin-specific antibody fragments in managing digitalis intoxication in the pediatric population. Am J Emerg Med *9*(Suppl 1):16, 1991.
63. Burroughs-Wellcome: Digoxin-immune Fab (ovine), Digibind (package insert).
64. Antman EM, Smith TW: Digitalis toxicity. *In* Hurst JW (ed): Current Therapy of Cardiovascular Disease. 3rd ed. Philadelphia, BC Decker, pp 89–94, 1991.
65. Koch-Weser J: Drug therapy—bretylium. N Engl J Med *300:*473, 1979.
66. Ditchey RV, Karliner JS: Safety of electrical cardioversion in patients without digitalis toxicity. Ann Intern Med *95:*676, 1981.

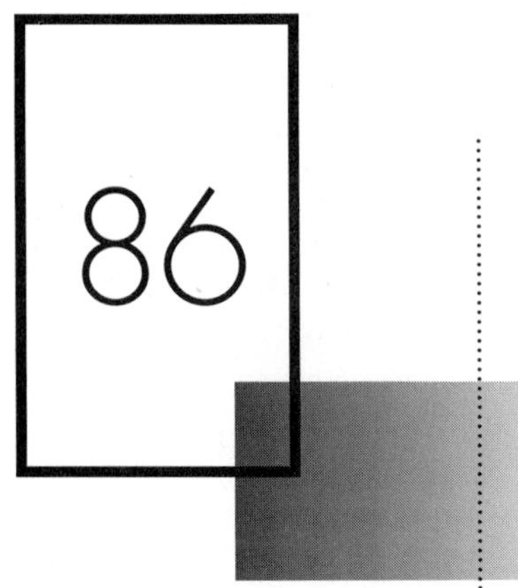

Calcium Channel Blocker Poisoning

PAUL D. PEARIGEN, MD

Calcium channel blockers have become widely used in the United States and elsewhere for the management of angina pectoris, coronary vasospasm, supraventricular arrhythmias, hypertension, hypertrophic cardiomyopathy, migraine headache, Raynaud's phenomenon, and subarachnoid hemorrhage. In addition, their use has been considered in many other disease states. Calcium channel blockers are a heterogeneous group of drugs characterized generally by three major classes: phenylalkylamine (verapamil), benzothiazapine (diltiazem), and dihydropyridine (nifedipine, amlodipine, isradipine, nicardipine, nimodipine, nisoldipine, nilvadipine, nitrendipine, felodipine). Bepridil, a newer agent used primarily for stable angina pectoris, is a diarylaminopropylamine derivative. These agents may exert profound effects on the cardiovascular system, both in therapeutic administration and in overdose.

As the calcium channel blockers have increased in therapeutic popularity and scope, so has the incidence of accidental and intentional poisoning. According to data collected by the American Association of Poison Control Centers (AAPCC), the number of exposures to and deaths from calcium channel blockers in the United States have both risen dramatically since 1985 (Fig. 86–1). These agents now account for roughly half of all deaths attributed to cardiovascular drugs. Side effects, therapeutic misadventures, and drug interactions are also frequently seen with this drug class.

PHARMACOLOGY

Chemical Identification and Structure

The clear structural differences between the phenylalkylamine, benzothiazepine, and dihydropyridine classes of calcium channel blockers appear to be associated with distinct binding sites on the "slow" calcium channel and different cardiovascular tissue affinities (Fig. 86–2 and Table 86–1). In addition, whereas the agents within the dihydropyridine class all share great similarity with the prototype nifedipine, variations in tissue affinity exist even within this group that impart selectivity profiles to these agents. Although it is an important advantage in therapeutic settings, this selectivity of the dihydropyridines generally fades in the setting of overdose. The pharmacologic profile of bepridil is even more distinctive.[1]

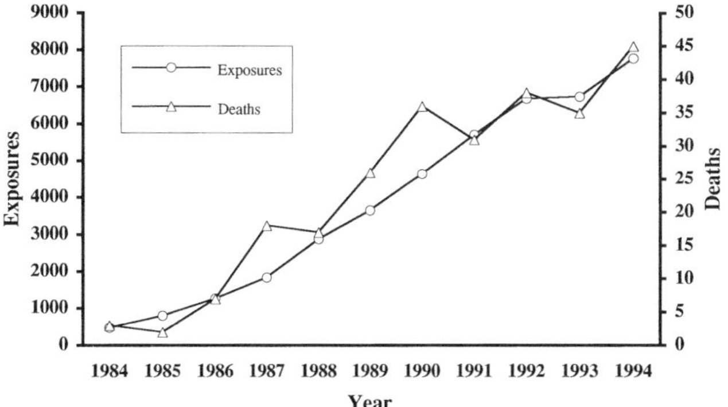

Figure 86–1. Temporal trends in exposures to and deaths from calcium-channel blocker overdose as reported by participating centers of the American Association of Poison Control Centers (AAPCC). Data extracted from reports of the AAPCC as published annually in the *American Journal of Emergency Medicine.*

Pharmacokinetics

The calcium channel blockers are rapidly and completely absorbed after oral administration, but extensive hepatic first-pass metabolism yields generally low bioavailability (Table 86–2). Exceptions to this are nifedipine and amlodipine, which may reach 60% to 70% bioavailability after an oral dose. Times to peak concentration for immediate-release formulations are 0.5 to 2 hours; however, all major classes of calcium channel blockers are now commonly administered as sustained-release preparations, with peak concentrations occurring at 3 to 7 hours. Distribution is extensive, with apparent volumes of distribution generally in the 4 to 10 L/kg range. However, nifedipine and nimodipine have the relatively small volumes of distribution of 0.8 and 0.9 L/kg, respectively. This may make these agents theoretically more amenable to enhanced elimination techniques (discussed later in the chapter). Protein binding is quite high, generally 90% to 98%. Calcium channel blockers are extensively metabolized by the liver, with limited amounts excreted unchanged in the urine. Verapamil and diltiazem possess active metabolites, norverapamil (*N*-demethylated) and desacetyldiltiazem, respectively. Terminal elimination half-lives in therapeutic trials range from 2 hours for nimodipine and 3 to 5 hours for verapamil, diltiazem, and nifedipine, to 10+ hours for felodipine, nilvadipine, nitrendipine, and amlodipine, and 42 hours for bepridil. The half-life of verapamil has been demonstrated to be prolonged in liver disease[2, 3] and in animal studies of verapamil-induced decreased hepatic blood flow.[4] Likewise, animal studies demonstrate that clearance of nifedipine is linearly related to hepatic blood flow.[5] The clearance of all the calcium channel blockers would be expected to be prolonged in disease states such as congestive heart failure, cardiomyopathy, or hypotensive overdose in which hepatic blood flow is reduced.

Pharmacokinetic Drug Interactions

Interactions between calcium channel blockers and other drugs taken therapeutically or in overdose may be due to altered pharmacokinetics and/or pharmacodynamics of the calcium channel blocker or of the other drugs.[6] Significant pharmacodynamic interactions, discussed in the following text, are most likely to occur in patients with underlying cardiac disease and in patients receiving calcium channel blockers along with other drugs that have cardiovascular activity.

A number of potentially significant pharmacokinetic drug interactions are seen with calcium channel blockers (Table 86–3). Although verapamil may elevate serum concentrations of propranolol and increase gastrointestinal absorption and decrease renal clearance of atenolol, no clinically relevant pharmacokinetic interaction has yet been demonstrated between calcium channel blockers and β-blockers.[7, 8] However, some calcium channel blockers, most nota-

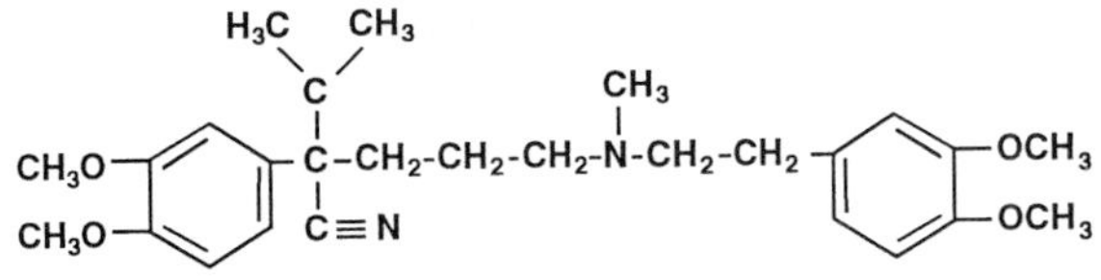

Verapamil

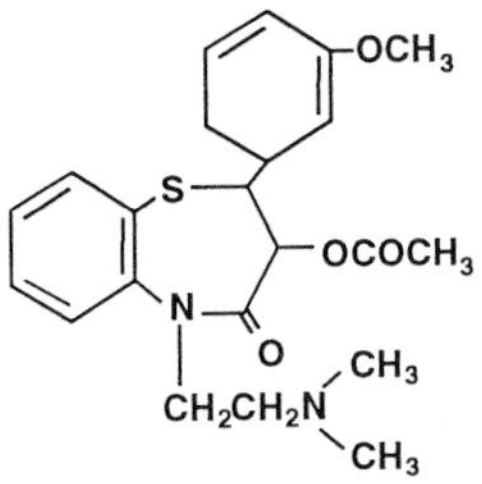

Diltiazem

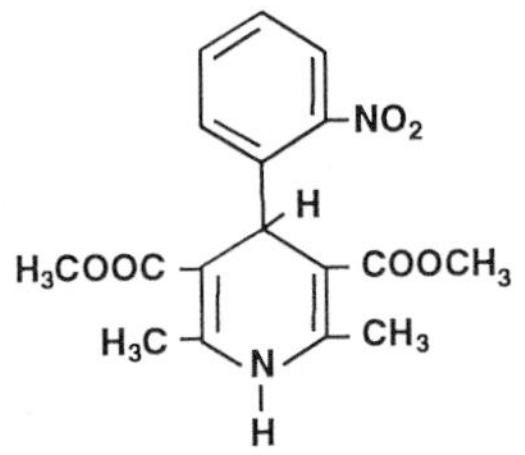

Nifedipine

Figure 86–2. *A,* Chemical structures of major calcium-channel blocker prototypes. *B,* Chemical structures of nifedipine and other dihydropyridines. *Asterisk* denotes asymmetrical center. (*B* from Abernethy DR, Schwartz JB: Pharmacokinetics of calcium antagonists under development. Clin Pharmacokinet *15*:5, 1988.)

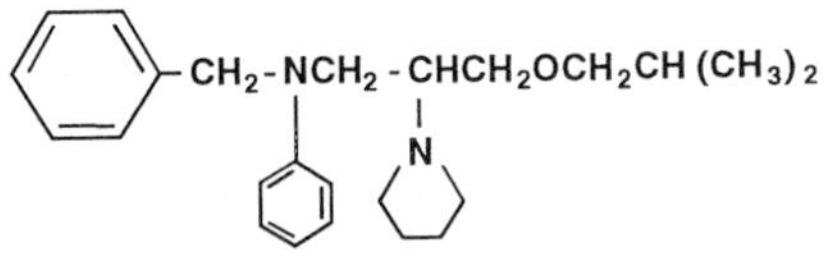

A Bepridil

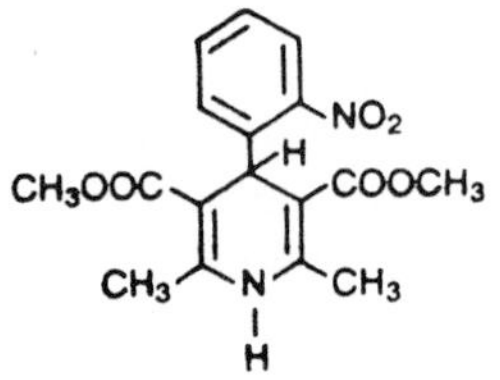

Nifedipine

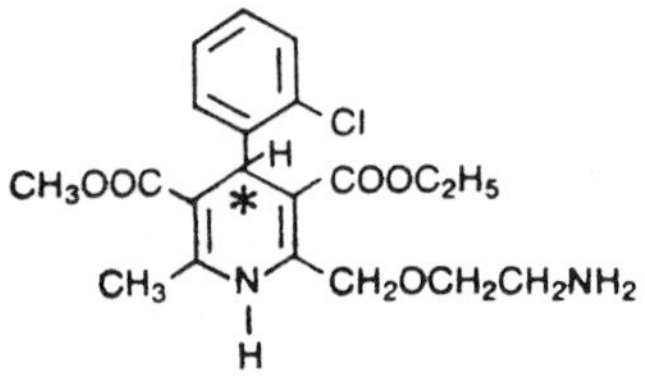

Amiodipine

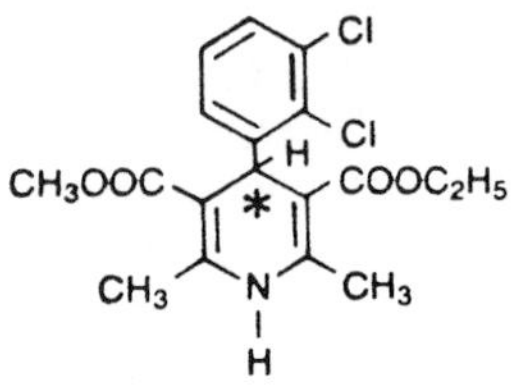

Felodipine

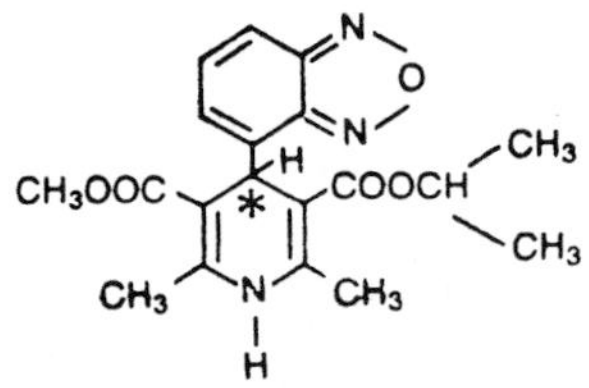

Isradipine

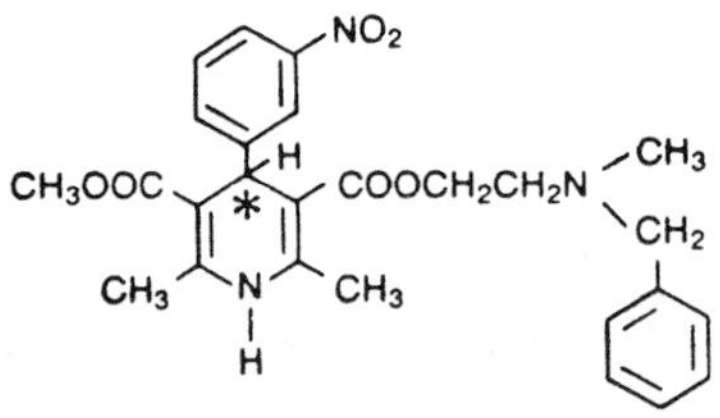

Nicardipine

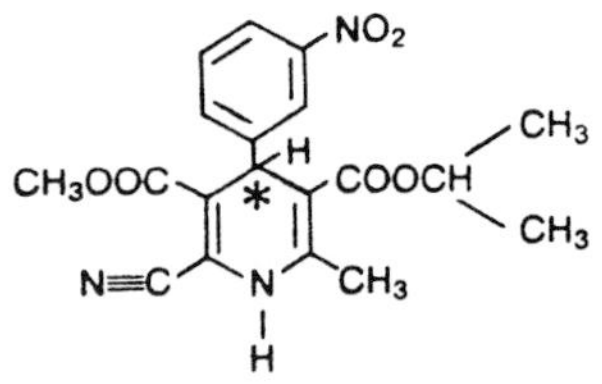

Nilvadipine

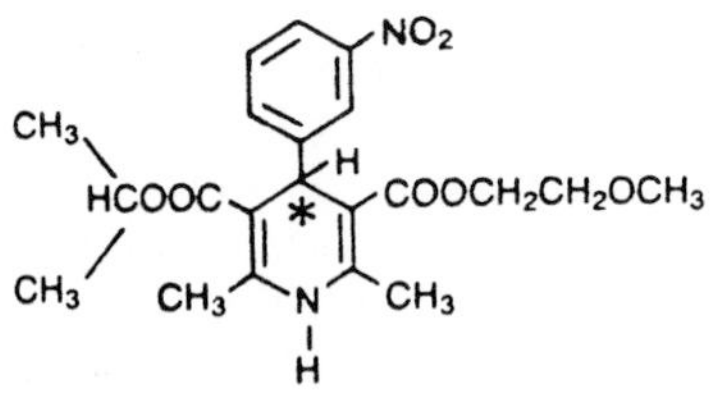

B Nimodipine

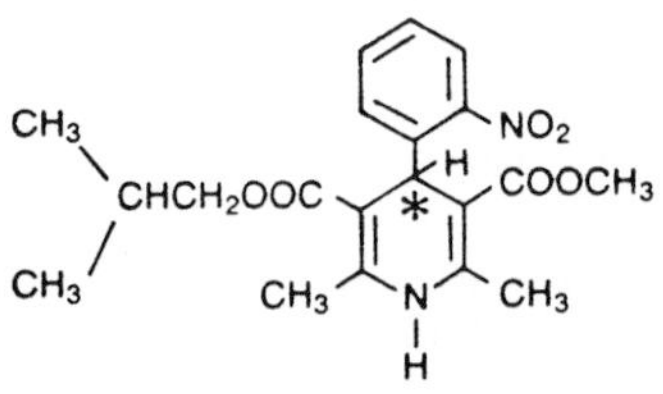

Nisoldipine

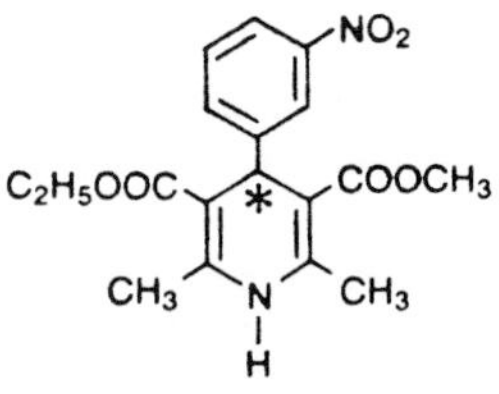

Nitrendipine

Table 86–1. Calcium Channel Blockers

Class	Agent	Trade Names
Phenylalkylamine	Verapamil	Calan*
		Isoptin*
		Verelan*
Benzothiazepine	Diltiazem	Cardizem*
		Dilacor*
		Tiazac
Dihydropyridine	Nifedipine	Procardia,* Adalat*
	Amlodipine	Norvasc
	Isradipine	DynaCirc
	Nicardipine	Cardene*
	Nimodipine	Nimotop
	Nisoldipine	Sular*
	Nilvadipine	NA†
	Nitrendipine	NA†
	Felodipine	Plendil*
Diarylaminopropylamine	Bepridil	Vascor

*Available as sustained-release preparations.
†Not available for prescription in the United States.

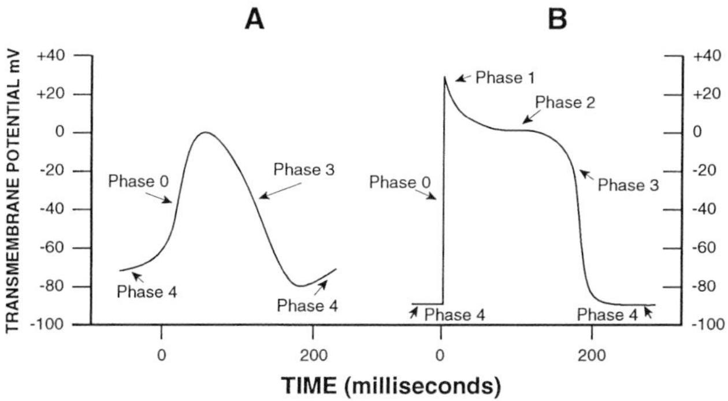

Figure 86–3. Typical action potentials recorded from cells in the sinoatrial and atrioventricular nodes *(A)* and His-Purkinje system and ventricular myocardium *(B)*. (From Antman EM, Stone PH, Muller JE, et al: Calcium-channel blocking agents in the treatment of cardiovascular disorders: I. Basic and clinical electrophysiologic effects. Ann Intern Med *93*:876, 1980.)

bly verapamil, increase serum digoxin concentrations.[8] In single- and multiple-dose verapamil studies in patients receiving digoxin, serum digoxin concentrations increased by 70% as a result of reduced digoxin clearance, both renal and nonrenal.[9, 10] Considering the frequency of concomitant use of verapamil and digoxin, the narrow therapeutic window of digoxin and the propensity of both drugs to cause high-degree heart block in excess, this interaction could certainly lead to toxic effects. Diltiazem and the dihydropyridines have less pronounced and more variable effects on serum digoxin concentrations, leading to no apparent clinical pharmacokinetic significance.[8, 11] Bepridil also increases serum digoxin concentrations, but the clinical significance is unclear thus far.[12]

Some calcium channel blockers, especially verapamil and diltiazem, are potent inhibitors of hepatic microsomal enzymes.[8] This has led to toxicity with carbamazepine, phenytoin, and theophylline during combined therapy.[8, 13, 14] Although the potential exists for drug interactions with highly protein-bound drugs as a result of competition for binding sites, no clinically significant interactions have yet been demonstrated to be on this basis.

Drugs that inhibit hepatic enzymes (e.g., cimetidine, ranitidine) may slow elimination of calcium channel blockers, potentially increasing their cardiovascular effects and producing toxicity. Conversely, liver enzyme inducers, such as rifampin and sulfinpyrazone, may significantly lower bioavailability of verapamil as a result of increased first-pass metabolism.[6, 15]

Pharmacodynamics

Calcium channel blockers inhibit movement of calcium from extracellular sites through cell membrane–based voltage-sensitive L-type calcium channels. This pharmacodynamic action affects cardiac electrophysiology, myocardial contractility, and vascular smooth muscle tone and accounts for the most significant manifestations of toxicity.[6] In the action potential of sinoatrial (SA) and atrioventricular (AV) nodal pacemaker cells, phase 0 depolarization is primarily controlled by calcium influx through “channels” (Fig. 86–3*A*).[16] The calcium channel blockers

Table 86–2. Pharmacokinetics of Calcium Channel Blockers

	Absorption (%)	Bioavailability (%)	Volume of Distribution (L/kg)	Protein Binding (%)	Terminal Half-Life (h)
Verapamil	>90	10–22	4.7	90	3–7
Diltiazem	>90	30–60	5.3	80–90	4
Nifedipine	>90	65–70	0.8–1.4	90	5
Amlodipine	100	60–65	21.4	>95	35
Felodipine	—	10–25	9.7	>99	10.2
Isradipine	—	15–20	69–161 L	>95	8
Nicardipine	—	15–43	—	98	5
Nilvadipine	—	14	—	—	11
Nimodipine	—	6.6	0.94	—	1–2
Nisoldipine	—	8.4	2.3	—	4
Nitrendipine	>80	10–30	6.6	98	12
Bepridil	100	60	8.0	>99	33–48

Adapted from Pearigen PD, Benowitz NL: Poisoning due to calcium antagonists: Experience with verapamil, diltiazem and nifedipine. Drug Saf *6*:418, 1991.

Table 86–3. Drug Interactions Involving Calcium Channel Blockers

Drug	Interacting Drug	Effect	Probable Mechanism	Comments
Verapamil Bepridil (other calcium channel blockers possible, but less likely)	β-Blockers	Heart block, cardiac failure, asystole (after IV verapamil)	Additive depression of AV conduction, myocardial contractility	Primarily seen with verapamil; should be used with caution in patients on β-blockers
	Digitalis	Aggravates heart block; asystole	Additive depression of cardiac conduction	Avoid use of calcium channel blockers in patients with digitalis toxicity
Verapamil Diltiazem	Propranolol	Reduced oral clearance with increased levels of propranolol	Inhibition of first pass metabolism	Propranolol dose may need to be reduced
Verapamil Diltiazem Bepridil (possibly)	Digoxin	Reduced digoxin clearance, increased digoxin levels	Inhibition of metabolism and renal excretion of digoxin	Reduce digoxin dose after starting verapamil or diltiazem; monitor serum digoxin concentration
Verapamil Diltiazem	Cyclosporine	Increased cyclosporine levels	Uncertain	Reduce cyclosporine dose after starting verapamil or diltiazem; monitor cyclosporine level
Verapamil	Quinidine	Hypotension (after IV verapamil)	Additive α-adrenergic blockade	Use IV verapamil cautiously in patients taking quinidine or other drugs with α-blocking activity
Verapamil	Prazosin	Increased prazosin levels; greater hypotensive effect	Reduced clearance; additive α-blocking effect	Use combination cautiously; may need to decrease prazosin dose
Verapamil	Halothane	Bradycardia Hypotension	Additive depression of sinus node function and myocardial contractility	Avoid co-administration
Verapamil Diltiazem	Disopyramide Flecainide	Cardiac failure	Additive depression of myocardial contractility	Avoid use if possible, particularly in patients with impaired myocardial function
Bepridil	Quinidine Disopyramide Procainamide Sotalol	Ventricular arrhythmias Torsades de pointes	Additive prolongation of QT interval	Avoid co-administration
Verapamil Diltiazem	Amiodarone Flecainide	Sinus arrest Heart block	Additive depression of sinus node function and AV nodal conduction	Use combination with extreme caution
All calcium channel blockers	Oral hypoglycemic agents	Hyperglycemia	Inhibition of insulin release usually stimulated by sulfonylurea drugs	May need to increase oral hypoglycemic doses or use insulin to maintain glucose control; beware of hypoglycemia when calcium channel blockers are discontinued
All calcium channel blockers	Cimetidine	Increased oral bioavailability of calcium channel blockers	Inhibition of metabolism; reduced presystemic metabolism	Reduce calcium channel blocker dose 30–40%
Verapamil	Rifampin Sulfinpyrazone	Reduced oral bioavailability of verapamil	Accelerated metabolism; increased presystemic metabolism	Increase verapamil dose; use alternative calcium channel blocker with less presystemic metabolism

are able to block this calcium influx, slowing conduction time through the AV node (negative dromotropic effect) and depressing the sinus node discharge rate (negative chronotropic effect).[6] Verapamil may also depress phase 4 depolarization, leading to sinus bradycardia and even sinus arrest. These electrophysiologic effects are most prominent for verapamil, diltiazem, and bepridil and are seldom encountered with the dihydropyridines, even in overdose.

Rapid depolarization during phase 0 of the action potential of His-Purkinje cells and atrial and ventricular myocytes is a function of fast inward sodium channels. In these cells, calcium entry through slow channels during phase 2 plateau (see Fig. 86–3*B*) triggers release of calcium from intracellular stores as well as further influx of extracellular calcium.[6] This intracellular calcium release, essential for muscle contraction, is inhibited when calcium channel blockers impede influx of calcium through the slow membrane channels. The resultant depression of myocardial contractility is most pronounced in overdose or in therapeutic doses in patients who already have depressed myocardial function from underlying disease or from additional drugs.[6] In contrast to verapamil and diltiazem, the dihydropyridines, such as nifedipine, have minimal effect on contractility.

As with cardiac muscle, contraction of vascular smooth muscle is mediated by calcium influx, which is inhibited by calcium channel blockers.[17] Sensitivity to calcium channel blockers is much greater in arterial vascular smooth muscle, yielding significant reduction in arterial resistance and blood pressure. All classes of calcium channel blockers are vasoactive and effective in treating hypertension. Particularly early in the course of therapy, the effect of vasodilatation on systemic blood pressure may be lessened by a reflex sympathetic increase in heart rate and cardiac output, especially seen with nifedipine and other dihydropyridines.

The particular similarities and differences in pharmacodynamic profiles among the calcium channel blockers are demonstrated in Table 86–4. In summary, all calcium channel blockers decrease arterial vascular resistance and lower blood pressure, although bepridil appears to have the least effect on systemic blood pressure while still producing notable coronary vasodilation. Verapamil and diltiazem decrease resting heart rate, atrioventricular (AV) nodal conduction, and contractility to similar degrees, whereas nifedipine and other dihydropyridines generally have little to no effect on AV nodal conduction or contractility and may even produce an increase in resting heart rate. Bepridil mildly decreases heart rate and slows AV nodal conduction, but it has a much less negative inotropic effect than conventional calcium antagonists, perhaps due in part to its inhibition of sodium-calcium exchange and its impediment of calmodulin's role in intracellular calcium availability.[18]

The most serious consequences of calcium channel blocker toxicity are essentially extensions of this cardiovascular profile. As is discussed later in the section on clinical presentation of overdose, these effects vary somewhat depending on the presence of underlying cardiac disease, the concomitant administration or co-ingestion of other cardiovascular agents, and whether the ingested agent is verapamil, diltiazem, or a dihydropyridine. No reported cases of overdose from bepridil have yet appeared in the literature.

Pharmacodynamic Drug Interactions

Due to combined depressant effects on cardiac conduction, heart rate, and myocardial contractility, significant pharmacodynamic effects are common during combination therapy with calcium channel blockers and β-blockers, digoxin, nitrates, or other antihypertensives or antiarrhythmics that affect the cardiovascular system (Table 86–3 and Fig. 86–4). These combined effects may be used to therapeutic advantage, but caution and careful monitoring in combining these agents is advised. This is especially true in patients with underlying sinus node disease, conduction abnormalities, or congestive heart failure. Verapamil in particular has been associated with bradycardia, advanced heart block, asystole, cardiac failure, and hypotension when given in combination with β-blockers or digoxin.[19–22] Nifedipine and other dihydropyridines are relatively safe when combined with β-blockers in therapeutic doses, particularly in patients with normal left ventricular function, but hypotension-induced worsening of angina pectoris has been reported in patients in whom nifedipine was added to regimens of β-blockers, nitrates, or diuretics.[23, 24]

Enhanced blood pressure lowering has also been demonstrated in combination therapy of calcium channel blockers with nitrates, diuretics, and angiotensin-converting enzyme (ACE) inhibitors.[8] Because it possesses some α-adrenergic blocking properties (especially when administered intravenously), verapamil may produce a greater hypotensive effect when combined with quinidine or prazosin.[25] The combined use of drugs that depress myocardial contractility, especially antiarrhythmics such as disopyramide and flecainide, with the calcium channel blockers verapamil and diltiazem may result in additive depression of myocardial function. In addition, flecainide and amiodarone may exhibit additive depression of the sinus node and AV conduction when combined with calcium antagonists.[6, 26]

CLINICAL PRESENTATION

Pathophysiology

As noted previously, the most serious toxic effects of calcium channel blockers result from their alteration of transmembrane flow of calcium throughout

Table 86–4. Cardiovascular Profile of Calcium Channel Blockers

	Resting Heart Rate	Blood Pressure	Systemic Vascular Resistance	Cardiac Contractility	AV Nodal Conduction
Verapamil	↓	↓	↓	↓↓	↓↓↓
Diltiazem	↓	↓	↓↓	↓	↓↓
Nifedipine	↔ or ↑	↓↓	↓↓↓	±	±
Bepridil	↓	↓	↓	±	↓↓

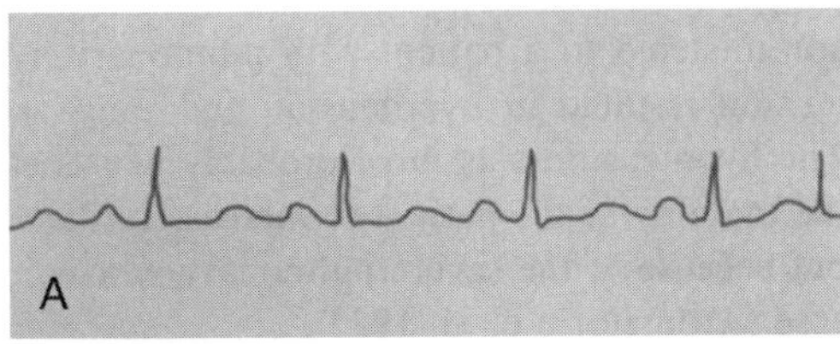

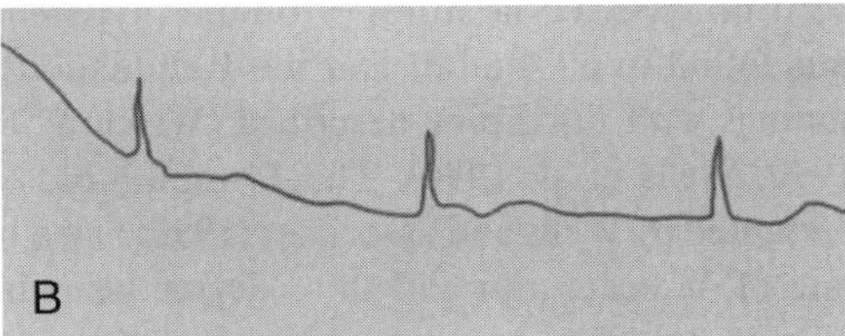

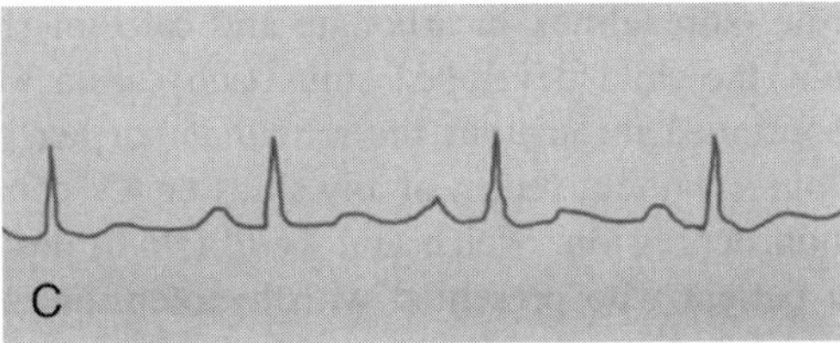

Figure 86–4. An elderly woman was in normal sinus rhythm with a PR interval of 152 ms when she was admitted for elective surgery *(A)*. Postoperatively, rapid atrial fibrillation developed and was controlled by digoxin and verapamil (not shown). After 1 week, the verapamil was discontinued and atenolol, 25 mg each morning, was substituted. When return to surgery was required 1 week later, postoperative orders inadvertently resulted in concomitant administration of digoxin, 0.125 mg, verapamil SR, 240 mg, and atenolol, 25 mg. Eight hours later, hypotension to a systolic blood pressure of 60 mm Hg accompanied a junctional rhythm that was accelerated to 70 beats/min with atropine *(B)*. Twelve hours later, with all medications withheld, sinus rhythm was present, but the PR interval was still prolonged from baseline at 196 ms *(C)*. (From Pearigen PD, Benowitz NL: Poisoning due to calcium antagonists: Experience with verapamil, diltiazem and nifedipine. Drug Safety *6*:413, 1991.)

the cardiovascular system and elsewhere, and are generally an extension of their therapeutic effects on heart rate, conduction, myocardial contractility, and systemic vascular resistance (Fig. 86–5). Although there is some variability—depending on the specific agent involved, the presence of co-ingestants, and the presence or absence of underlying heart disease—the general pathophysiology of calcium channel blocker overdose is the same. Slowing of the heart rate resulting from decreased automaticity or diminished AV nodal conduction and a decrease in myocardial contractility combine to produce a drop in cardiac output. With associated decreased systemic vascular resistance due to vascular smooth muscle dilation, progressive hypotension and even shock ensue.

Manifestations

Cardiovascular

Bradycardia and conduction defects are among the most frequent findings in overdose with verapamil or diltiazem, and hypotension is present in most significant exposures to any calcium antagonist (Table 86–5).[6, 27] Varying degrees of AV block and dissociation, junctional or idioventricular rhythms, and even bundle-branch blocks and asystole have been reported.[28, 29] Ventricular tachyarrhythmias are not typical of calcium channel blocker overdose, and their presence suggests underlying cardiac disease or toxic effects of drugs other than calcium channel blockers. Examples of electrocardiographic (ECG) abnormalities typical of calcium channel blocker poisoning are shown in Figures 86–4 and 86–6. Signs and symptoms of calcium channel blocker poisoning generally begin within 1 to 2 hours of ingestion, but the onset of moderate to severe cardiovascular manifestations may be delayed as much as 24 hours when a sustained-release preparation has been ingested.[30, 31]

Verapamil may dangerously accelerate conduction through an accessory pathway when given intravenously to patients with anomalous or accessory AV conduction (e.g., Wolff-Parkinson-White syndrome).[32] It should not be given to patients with atrial fibrillation and evidence of preexcitation on ECG. Intravenous verapamil has also been associated with cardiovascular collapse when given to patients in combination with β-blockers and to neonates with supraventricular tachycardia and heart failure.[33] Oral verapamil or diltiazem in therapeutic doses may depress the sinus node and AV conduction, particularly in patients with underlying conduction system disease or during combination therapy with β-blockers or digoxin. Diltiazem commonly produces hypotension from diminished cardiac output and/or systemic vasodilatation as well as AV conduction disturbances.[34] Nifedipine and other dihydropyridines produce the greatest vasodilatory effects of the calcium channel blockers, both therapeutically and

Table 86–5. Clinical Manifestations of Calcium Channel Blocker Poisoning

Cardiovascular
- Hypotension, shock
- Bradycardia and other arrhythmias
- Sinus bradycardia
- Accelerated AV nodal rhythm
- Secondary and tertiary AV block with nodal or ventricular escape rhythm
- Sinus arrest with AV nodal escape rhythm
- Asystole

Central Nervous System
- Lethargy, slurred speech, confusion
- Coma
- Respiratory arrest
- Seizures

Gastrointestinal
- Nausea, vomiting
- Ileus, obstruction
- Bowel ischemia, infarction

Metabolic
- Hyperglycemia
- Lactic acidosis

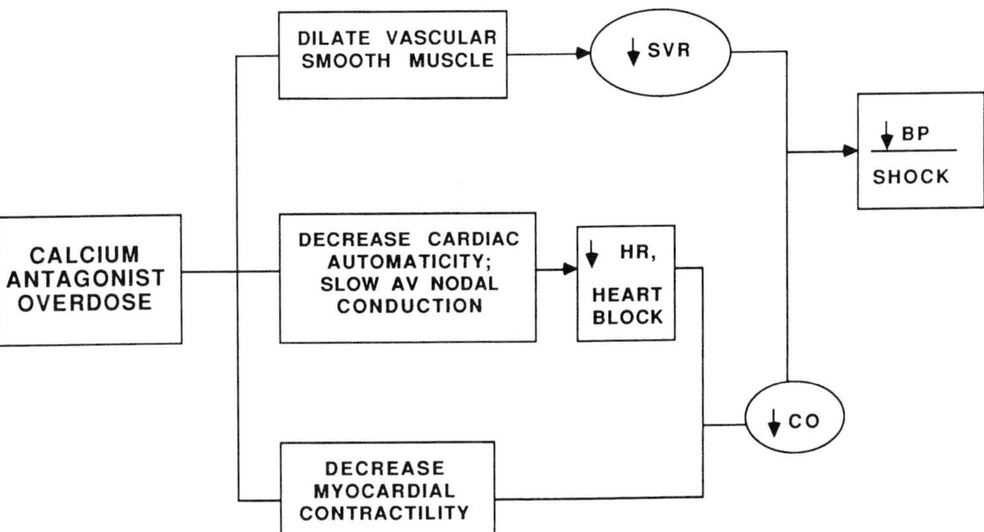

Figure 86–5. Pathophysiology of cardiovascular consequences of calcium-channel blocker overdose.

in overdose. Profound hypotension, often associated with reflex tachycardia, is therefore common in nifedipine overdose.[35–37] Conduction defects are rarely seen with nifedipine toxicity unless a very large dose is ingested.

Therapeutic use of any calcium channel blocker in patients with severe myocardial dysfunction, hypertrophic outflow obstruction, obstructive valvular disease, or concomitant therapy with other myocardial depressants may aggravate cardiac failure and precipitate pulmonary edema.

Central Nervous System

Confusion, agitation, dizziness, lethargy, and slurred speech may be present in the patient with overdose of a calcium channel blocker. Coma most commonly occurs in the setting of cardiovascular collapse with profound hypotension. Seizures are rare, but have been described in case reports of overdose due to verapamil, diltiazem, and nifedipine.[28, 36, 38] Stroke from hypotension-induced cerebral hypoperfusion has also been reported.[39]

Gastrointestinal

Nausea and vomiting frequently develop in the patient with overdose of calcium channel blockers. Verapamil has been associated with paralytic ileus and small bowel obstruction, with and without mechanical obstruction, as well as with fecal impaction.[40, 41] Mesenteric ischemia and colonic infarction have also been described and are likely related to the systemic hypotensive effects of calcium channel blocker overdose.[42, 43] Concretion formation with associated mechanical obstruction and prolonged release of drug may complicate overdose with sustained-release preparations.

Metabolic/Endocrine

The effect of therapeutic doses of calcium channel blockers on glucose tolerance and insulin release is controversial, as studies in animals and humans have shown conflicting results. However, hyperglycemia is a common finding in overdose from calcium channel blockers. It is reversible and usually resolves within 24 hours, but it may necessitate insulin therapy.[44, 45] Metabolic acidosis is a common finding in severe poisonings and is likely a result of tissue hypoperfusion.

Other

Adverse cutaneous reactions to calcium channel blockers are rare, but they have included Stevens-Johnson syndrome, erythema multiforme, exfoliative dermatitis, toxic epidermal necrolysis, cutaneous vasculitis, angioedema, and urticaria.[46]

Nifedipine has been associated with acute, reversible deterioration in renal function in several patients despite the absence of any documented episodes of systemic hypotension. Altered renal hemodynamics and possible worsening of left ventricular failure as a result of negative inotropism were implicated as possible explanations.[47]

DIAGNOSIS

Recognizing conduction disturbances and hypotension as hallmarks of calcium channel blocker poisoning aid in making the diagnosis, particularly when a history of access to such agents is not available. Although other agents, most notably β-adrenergic blockers, produce a similar syndrome in overdose, considering the possibility of calcium channel blocker poisoning is essential in such cases because of the potential severity of the overdose. These agents are not identified on routine qualitative urine drug screening. Further, specific quantitative measurement of calcium channel blockers in body fluids is not routinely available in acute care settings and correlates poorly with clinical toxicity and outcome.[6] Therefore, laboratory methods are not generally use-

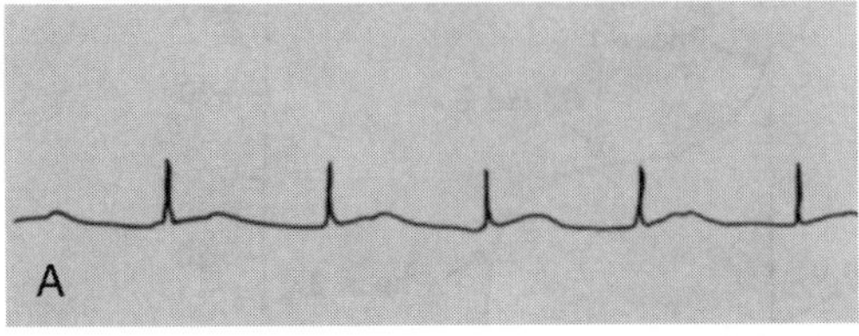

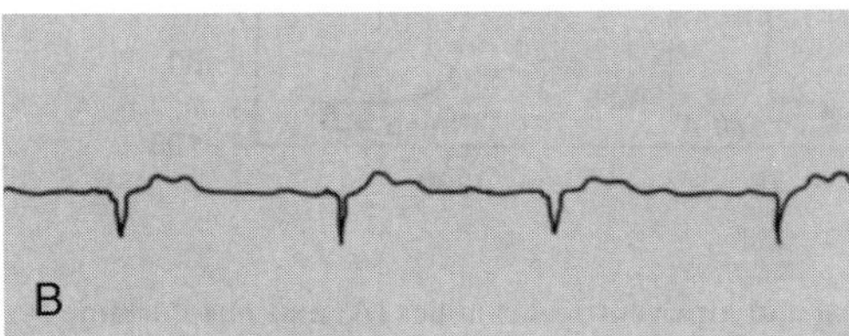

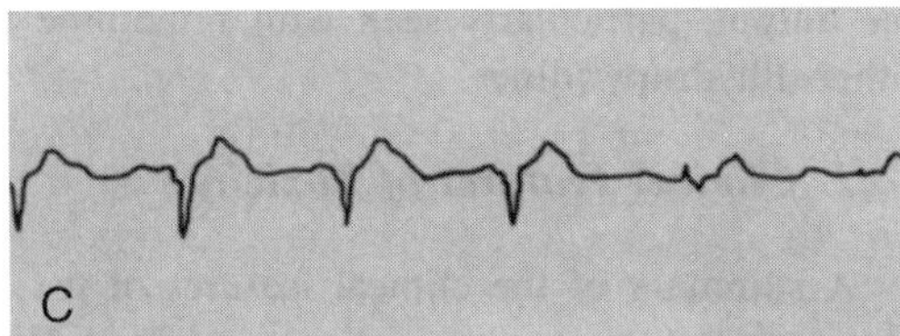

Figure 86–6. A 24-year-old woman ingested 10 to 15 sustained-release verapamil tablets, 240 mg, 2 hours prior to presentation with lethargy, a systolic blood pressure of 50 mm Hg, and a heart rate of 40 beats/min. This series of lead II rhythm strips shows accelerated junctional rhythm (rate, 62/min) at 3 hours postingestion *(A)*; type I (Wenckebach) AV nodal block with wide QRS complex at 5 hours *(B)*; and accelerated wide QRS rhythm (rate, 65/min) with AV dissociation followed by primary AV block with narrow QRS at 5½ hours *(C)*. Treatment with calcium chloride had resulted in a serum calcium level of 19.0 mg/dL measured at approximately 6 hours after ingestion. (From Pearigen PD, Benowitz NL: Poisoning due to calcium antagonists: Experience with verapamil, diltiazem and nifedipine. Drug Safety *6*:412, 1991.)

ful in making the diagnosis of poisoning due to calcium channel blockers. Twelve-lead ECG and continuous ECG monitoring may reveal early signs of conduction disturbance before more overt cardiovascular symptoms develop. Again, delays in manifestations may occur in patients who have ingested a sustained-release preparation.

TREATMENT

Immediate Supportive Measures

Initial management of poisoning due to calcium channel blockers is similar to that for other toxic drug exposures with support of the airway, adequate ventilation and oxygenation, and attention to circulatory status (Table 86–6). If the calcium channel blocker is being administered therapeutically, it should be discontinued immediately. Intravenous calcium chloride as an emergency antidote should first be administered in a patient whose condition is critical. Seizures, when present, should be treated initially with intravenous benzodiazepines, followed by phenytoin or phenobarbital.

Arrhythmias

Specific therapy of sinus node depression and/or AV nodal conduction disturbances from calcium channel blocker toxicity is only necessary when they contribute to hemodynamic compromise. However, preparations for drug therapy and for transcutaneous or transvenous cardiac pacing are recommended, as these disturbances of automaticity or of conduction may worsen in patients who present with such findings. Calcium salts may be administered, but they are usually ineffective at improving conduction. Bradyarrhythmias that contribute to hypotension may be treated initially with atropine or isoproterenol.[48] In patients unresponsive to drug therapy, or in the patient in whom more definitive management of conduction is necessary, transvenous pacing may be required. Due to the effects of calcium channel blockers on the myocardium and on the peripheral vasculature, it is not uncommon for hypotension to persist despite correction of electrical activity and conduction.

Hypotension

Hypotension should be addressed based on the mechanisms of pathophysiology discussed previously

Table 86–6. Management of Calcium Channel Blocker Poisoning

General Management
Airway, ventilatory, circulatory support
Activated charcoal (with or without gastric lavage)
Whole-bowel irrigation in sustained-release ingestion
Intravenous calcium chloride in critical patients
Admit to ICU and initiate continuous ECG monitoring
Seizures: Lorazepam, 1–2 mg/dose IV; phenytoin, 15 mg/kg IV, or phenobarbital, 15 mg/kg IV, each loaded over 20–30 min
Arrhythmias
Asymptomatic: Supportive measures and continued ECG monitoring
Symptomatic: Atropine, isoproterenol, or cardiac pacing
Hypotension
Treat significant bradyarrhythmias as above
Calcium salts: Calcium chloride, 1 g (10 mL of 10% solution), *or* calcium gluconate, 3 g (30 mL of 10% solution) IV over 5 min; repeat as needed if favorable response
0.9% Sodium chloride, 200 mL IV every 10 min up to 1–2 L or evidence of pulmonary edema
Glucagon, 2–5 mg IV over 5 min; repeat or initiate continuous infusion
If patient remains hypotensive, place pulmonary artery catheter and consider administration of the following: Norepinephrine, neosynephrine, dopamine, dobutamine, amrinone
Investigational Therapies
4-Aminopyridine
Calcium entry promoters (Bay k 8644)
Cardiac glycosides (digoxin)
Hyperinsulinemic euglycemia

(see Fig. 86–5). It may result from depressed myocardial contractility, bradycardia, or decreased systemic vascular resistance. Calcium salts are often quite effective in treating hypotension due to depressed myocardial contractility, although in many cases patients have failed to respond to calcium, necessitating the use of other pharmacologic or artificial devices to assist pump function.[28, 35, 49] If cardiac output is impaired because of significant bradycardia, measures to increase ventricular rate, as described previously, are indicated. Finally, intravenous fluids and vasoconstrictors such as norepinephrine, neosynephrine, or dopamine (often in high doses) may be successful in treating hypotension that is primarily due to peripheral vasodilation.

Decontamination

Gastrointestinal decontamination is appropriate in an attempt to limit systemic absorption of ingested calcium channel antagonists. If accidental or intentional oral ingestion has occurred, gastrointestinal lavage (if within 1 hour of exposure) and administration of activated charcoal orally or via nasogastric tube is indicated. Syrup of ipecac–induced emesis should be avoided, as rapid deterioration of mental status and vital signs is possible, and increased vagal tone due to vomiting may worsen bradycardia and hypotension. Repeated doses of activated charcoal and the early use of whole-bowel irrigation should be considered in cases involving the ingestion of sustained-release preparations.

Antidotes

Calcium

In humans, calcium reverses the myocardial depression induced by calcium channel blockers, occasionally increases sinus rate, and improves AV nodal conduction. As noted previously, enough reports of benefit from administration of calcium salts to patients with adverse cardiovascular effects from any of the calcium channel blockers have appeared in the literature to justify the early administration of calcium to such patients. However, it is important to recognize that only some effects of the overdose may be reversed and that in severe cases of poisoning, patients may fail to respond to calcium.[6]

Administration of calcium chloride, 1 g (27% calcium) in a 10% solution, given intravenously over 5 minutes, is typically used. This may be repeated every 10 to 20 minutes for three to four additional doses or more, depending on the response. Calcium gluconate is only 9% calcium; thus, 3 g must be administered to deliver the same amount of calcium as is found in 1 g of calcium chloride. The dose of calcium chloride required for optimal effect in human poisoning is unclear. Reports have been published of large total amounts of calcium being given to patients with calcium channel blocker poisoning.[27, 49–51] The concern about hypercalcemia appears to be a theoretical one.

Glucagon

Glucagon is a polypeptide hormone with positive inotropic and chronotropic actions that are unaffected by adrenergic depletion or blockade. It increases cyclic adenosine monophosphate (cAMP) levels by stimulating adenyl cyclase, and it thereby appears to promote calcium ion influx via calcium channels. By this mechanism, glucagon circumvents the β-receptors and has therefore become quite useful in treating toxicity from β-blockers. Glucagon has been shown to reverse myocardial depression and increase heart rate and blood pressure in animal models of calcium channel blocker poisoning, and it has been the basis for some anecdotal reports of success in human cases of calcium channel blocker overdose.[52–55] Although clearly not all cases will respond to glucagon, this intervention appears to hold promise and may be given to the patient whose symptoms do not respond to other measures. An initial intravenous dose of 2 to 5 mg, followed by a maintenance infusion, is recommended.

Others

Additional modalities that may play a role in calcium channel blocker poisoning include phosphodiesterase inhibitors, 4-aminopyridine, calcium agonists, cardiac glycosides, and hyperinsulinemic euglycemia. By inhibiting the breakdown of cAMP, phosphodiesterase inhibitors, such as amrinone, may promote calcium flux and improve cardiac function. Animal studies and case reports suggest that amrinone may be useful in calcium channel blocker poisoning that is refractory to other measures.[48] 4-Aminopyridine is an antagonist of nondepolarizing neuromuscular blocking agents that has been used by electrophysiologists to block outward potassium channels, indirectly facilitating inward calcium movement. It has been shown to reverse verapamil cardiotoxic effects in feline and canine models, and it showed equivocal benefit in conjunction with other measures in one human poisoning.[56–58] Bay k 8644, a dihydropyridine analog that acts as a calcium entry promoter, reverses all conduction and hemodynamic effects of verapamil in animal models of intoxication, but its severe coronary vasoconstrictive effects may preclude its use in humans.[6, 59] Some researchers have suggested that cardiac glycosides, such as digoxin, may have a beneficial effect on conduction and contractility in the setting of calcium channel blockade as demonstrated in animal studies.[60] Finally, the use of hyperinsulinemic euglycemia in animal models of verapamil toxicity has been shown to improve myocardial metabolic parameters, perhaps promoting improved myocardial contractility.[61] The clinical role of these investigational modalities remains uncertain.

Enhanced Elimination

Calcium channel blockers are generally both highly protein-bound and extensively distributed in tissues. They are also rapidly metabolized, primarily to inactive metabolites. Therefore, enhanced elimination techniques such as hemodialysis and hemoperfusion would not be expected to be of benefit. Indeed, clinical reports have failed to support a role for accelerated drug removal in therapeutic or overdose settings.[58, 62–64]

Disposition

Symptomatic patients and those who may have ingested sustained-release preparations of calcium channel blockers should be admitted to an intensive care unit for continuous ECG monitoring for at least 24 hours.

References

1. Hollingshead LM, Faulds D, Fitton A: Bepridil: A review of its pharmacological properties and therapeutic use in stable angina pectoris. Drugs *44*:835, 1992.
2. Somgyi A, Albrecht M, Kliems G, et al: Pharmacokinetics, bioavailability and ECG response of verapamil in patients with liver cirrhosis. Br J Clin Pharmacol *12*:51, 1981.
3. Woodcock BG, Rietbrock I, Vohringer HF, et al: Verapamil disposition in liver disease and intensive-care patients: Kinetics, clearance, and apparent blood flow relationships. Clin Pharmacol Ther *29*:27, 1981.
4. Hamann SR, Blouin RA, Chang SL, et al: Effects of hemodynamic changes on the elimination kinetics of verapamil and nifedipine. J Pharmacol Exp Ther *231*:301, 1984.
5. McAllister RG, Hamann SR, Blonin RA: Pharmacokinetics of calcium-entry blockers. Am J Cardiol *55*:30B, 1985.
6. Pearigen PD, Benowitz NL: Poisoning due to calcium antagonists: Experience with verapamil, diltiazem and nifedipine. Drug Saf *6*:408, 1991.
7. McGourty JC, Silas JH, Tucker GT, et al: The effect of combined therapy on the pharmacokinetics and pharmacodynamics of verapamil and propranolol in patients with angina pectoris. Br J Clin Pharmacol *25*:349, 1988.
8. Kirch W, Kleinbloesem CH, Belz GG: Drug interactions with calcium antagonists. Pharmacol Ther *45*:109, 1990.
9. Klein HO, Lang R, Weiss E, et al: The influence of verapamil on serum digoxin concentration. Circulation *65*:998, 1982.
10. Pedersen KE, Dorph-Pedersen A, Hvidt S, et al: Digoxin-verapamil interaction. Clin Pharmacol Ther *30*:311, 1981.
11. Schwartz JB: Digoxin and nifedipine. Am J Cardiol *55*:31E, 1985.
12. Belz GG, Wistuba S, Matthews JH: Digoxin and bepridil: Pharmacokinetic and pharmacodynamic interactions. Clin Pharmacol Ther *39*:65, 1986.
13. Beattie B, Biller J, Mehlhaus B, et al: Verapamil-induced carbamazepine neurotoxicity. Eur Neurol *28*:104, 1988.
14. Hunt BA, Self TH, Lalonde RL, et al: Calcium channel blockers as inhibitors of drug metabolism. Chest *96*:393, 1989.
15. Mooy J, Bohm R, van Baak M, et al: The influence of antituberculous drugs on the plasma level of verapamil. Eur J Clin Pharmacol *32*:107, 1987.
16. Antman EM, Stone PH, Muller JE, et al: Calcium channel blocking agents in the treatment of cardiovascular disorders: I. Basic and clinical electrophysiologic effects. Ann Intern Med *93*:875, 1980.
17. Frohlich ED: Clinical pharmacology of calcium antagonists. Hypertension *11*(Suppl I):I222, 1988.
18. Gill A, Flaim SF, Damiano BP, et al: Pharmacology of bepridil. Am J Cardiol *69*:11D, 1992.
19. Wayne VS: Interaction of calcium channel and beta-blocking drugs. J Am Coll Cardiol *2*:594, 1983.
20. Packer M, Meller J, Medina N, et al: Hemodynamic consequences of combined beta-adrenergic and slow calcium channel blockade in man. Circulation *65*:660, 1982.
21. Carruthers SG, Freeman DJ, Bailey DG: Synergistic adverse hemodynamic interaction between oral verapamil and propranolol. Clin Pharmacol Ther *46*:469, 1989.
22. Zatuchni J: Verapamil-digoxin interaction. Am Heart J *108*:412, 1984.
23. Vetrovec GW, Parker VE: Acute electrophysiologic, hemodynamic and ventricular effects of nifedipine and beta-blocker interactions. Am J Cardiol *55*:21E, 1985.
24. Boden WE, Korr KS, Bough EW: Nifedipine-induced hypotension and myocardial ischemia in refractory angina pectoris. JAMA *253*:1131, 1985.
25. Maisel AS, Motulsky HJ, Insel PA: Hypotension after quinidine plus verapamil. N Engl J Med *312*:167, 1985.
26. Lee TH, Friedman PL, Goldman L, et al: Sinus arrest and hypotension with combined amiodarone-diltiazem therapy. Am Heart J *109*:163, 1985.
27. Howarth DM, Dawson AH, Smith AJ, et al: Calcium channel blocking drug overdose: An Australian series. Hum Exp Toxicol *13*:161, 1994.
28. Horowitz BZ, Rhee KJ: Massive verapamil ingestion. Am J Emerg Med *7*:624, 1989.
29. Zoghbi W, Schwartz JB: Verapamil overdose: Report of a case and review of the literature. Cardiovasc Rev Rep *5*:356, 1984.
30. Rankin RJ, Edwards IR: Overdose of sustained-release verapamil. N Z Med J *103*:165, 1990.
31. Tom PA, Morrow CT, Kelen GD: Delayed hypotension after overdose of sustained release verapamil. J Emerg Med *12*:621, 1994.
32. McGovern B, Garan H, Ruskin JN: Precipitation of cardiac arrest in patients with Wolff-Parkinson-White syndrome. Ann Intern Med *104*:791, 1986.
33. Epstein ML, Kiel EA, Victorica BE: Cardiac decompensation following verapamil therapy in infants with supraventricular tachycardia. Pediatrics *75*:737, 1985.
34. Ferner RE, Odemuyima O, Field AB, et al: Pharmacokinetics and toxic effects of diltiazem in massive overdose. Hum Toxicol *8*:497, 1989.
35. Welch RD, Todd K: Nifedipine overdose accompanied by ethanol intoxication in a patient with congenital heart disease. Int J Cardiol *4*:275, 1990.
36. Wells TG, Graham CJ, Moss MM, et al: Nifedipine poisoning in a child. Pediatrics *86*:91, 1990.
37. Ramoska EA, Spiller HA, Winter M, et al: A one-year evaluation of calcium channel blocker overdoses: Toxicity and treatment. Ann Emerg Med *22*:196, 1993.
38. Malcolm N, Callegari P, Goldberg J, et al: Massive diltiazem overdosage: Clinical and pharmacokinetic observations. Drug Intell Clin Pharm *20*:888, 1986.
39. Shah AR, Passalacqua BR: Case report: Sustained-release verapamil overdose causing stroke: An unusual complication. Am J Med Sci *304*:357, 1992.
40. Ward DJ, Ward JW, Griffo W, et al: Intravenous calcium for fecal impaction secondary to verapamil. N Engl J Med *307*:1709, 1982.
41. Fauville J-P, Hantson P, Honore P, et al: Severe diltiazem poisoning with intestinal pseudo-obstruction: Case report and toxicological data. Clin Toxicol *33*:273, 1995.
42. Sporer KA, Manning JJ: Massive ingestion of sustained-release verapamil with a concretion and bowel infarction. Ann Emerg Med *22*:603, 1993.
43. Gutierrez H, Jorgensen M: Colonic ischemia after verapamil overdose. Ann Intern Med *124*:535, 1996.
44. Enyeart JJ, Price WA, Hoffman DA, et al: Profound hyperglycemia and metabolic acidosis after verapamil overdose. J Am Coll Cardiol *2*:1228, 1983.
45. Heyman SN: Verapamil intoxication and hyperglycemia. J Emerg Med *7*:407, 1989.
46. Stern R, Khalsa JH: Cutaneous adverse reactions associated

with calcium channel blockers. Arch Intern Med *149*:829, 1989.
47. Diamond JR, Cheung JY, Fang LST: Nifedipine-induced renal dysfunction: Alterations in renal hemodynamics. Am J Med *77*:905, 1984.
48. Goenen M, Col J, Compere A, et al: Treatment of severe verapamil poisoning with combined amrinone-isoproterenol therapy. Am J Cardiol *58*:1142, 1986.
49. Haddad LM: Case report: Resuscitation of nifedipine (Procardia) overdose exclusively with intravenous calcium chloride. Am J Emerg Med *14*:602–603, 1996.
50. Buckley N, Dawson AH, Howarth D, et al: Slow-release verapamil poisoning: Use of polyethylene glycol whole-bowel lavage and high-dose calcium. Med J Aust *158*:202–204, 1993.
51. Luscher TF, Noll G, Sturmer T, et al: Calcium gluconate in severe verapamil intoxication (letter). N Engl J Med *330*:718–720, 1994.
52. Jolly SR, Kipnis JN, Lucchesi BR: Cardiovascular depression by verapamil: Reversal by glucagon and interactions with propranolol. Pharmacology *35*:249, 1987.
53. Zaritsky AL, Horowitz M, Chernow B: Glucagon antagonism of calcium channel blocker-induced myocardial dysfunction. Crit Care Med *16*:246, 1988.
54. Doyon S, Roberts JR: The use of glucagon in a case of calcium channel blocker overdose. Ann Emerg Med *22*:1229, 1993.
55. Walter FG, Frye G, Mullen JT, et al: Amelioration of nifedipine poisoning associated with glucagon therapy. Ann Emerg Med *22*:1234, 1993.
56. Agoston S, Maestrone E, van Hezik EJ, et al: Effective treatment of verapamil intoxication with 4-aminopyridine in the cat. J Clin Invest *73*:1291, 1984.
57. Gay R, Algeo S, Lee R, et al: Treatment of verapamil toxicity in intact dogs. J Clin Invest *77*:1805, 1986.
58. ter Wee PM, Hovinga TKK, Uges DRA, et al: 4-Aminopyridine and haemodialysis in the treatment of verapamil intoxication. Hum Toxicol *4*:327, 1985.
59. Korstanje C, Jonkman FAM, Van Kemenade JE, et al: Bay k 8644, a calcium entry promoter, as an antidote in verapamil intoxication in rabbits. Arch Int Pharmacodyn Ther *287*:109, 1987.
60. Ramo MP, Grupp I, Pesola MK, et al: Cardiac glycosides in the treatment of experimental overdose with calcium-blocking agents. Res Exp Med *192*:335, 1992.
61. Kline JA, Leonova E, Raymond RM: Beneficial myocardial metabolic effects of insulin during verapamil toxicity in the anesthetized canine. Crit Care Med *23*:1251, 1995.
62. Hanyok JJ, Chow MSS, Kluger J, et al: An evaluation of the pharmacokinetics, pharmacodynamics, and dialyzability of verapamil in chronic hemodialysis patients. J Clin Pharmacol *28*:831, 1988.
63. Roberts D, Honcharik N, Sitar DS, et al: Diltiazem overdose: Pharmacokinetics of diltiazem and its metabolites and effect of multiple dose charcoal therapy. Clin Toxicol *29*:45, 1991.
64. Rosansky SJ: Verapamil toxicity—treatment with hemoperfusion. Ann Intern Med *114*:340, 1991.

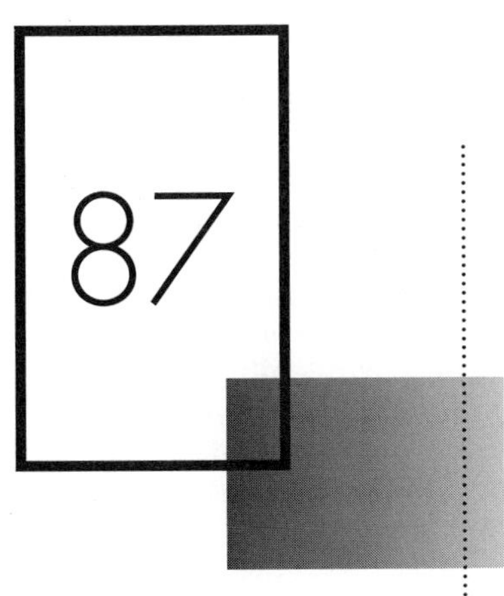

β-Adrenergic Blocker Toxicity

LESLIE RAE WOLF, MD

β-Adrenergic blocking agents (β-blockers) were initially developed for the treatment of angina pectoris and dysrhythmias. In 1964, while treating patients with β-blockers, Prichard discovered the hypotensive effect of these agents.[1] This discovery led to an increase in the use of β-blockers for the treatment of hypertension. Since that time, the therapeutic indications for the use of these agents continue to increase in number and include dysrhythmias, angina, hypertension, dissecting aneurysm, status post myocardial infarction, mitral valve prolapse, idiopathic hypertrophic subaortic stenosis, thyroid storm, essential tremors, glaucoma, migraine prophylaxis, anxiety, withdrawal states, and pheochromocytoma.[2]

As the use of β-blockers increases, the incidence of β-blocker toxicity also increases, with an average of

4700 cases of overdose occurring annually.[3] The first review of cases of β-blocker toxicity was published by Frishman and colleagues in 1979.[4] From 1988 to 1992, there was a 5% annual increase in deaths from β-blockers reported to the American Association of Poison Control Centers (AAPCC).[3, 5–7] In 1994, nine deaths attributable β-blocker were reported.[8]

By the year 2030, an estimated 21% of the population in the United States will be older than 60 years of age.[9, 10] As the use of β-blockers in the elderly increases, the incidence of toxicity will probably also continue to increase. Because of the refractory nature of the cardiovascular compromise often seen with β-blocker toxicity, treatment can be challenging. An understanding of the pharmacology and clinical presentation of β-blocker toxicity aids in the early diagnosis and effective management of this increasingly frequent problem.

PHYSIOLOGY

β-Adrenergic Receptors

In 1948, Ahlquist initially distinguished α- and β-adrenergic receptors.[11] The understanding of β-blocker toxicity requires a review of β-adrenergic receptor activity. The binding of catecholamines to β-receptors results in phosphorylation of the G protein complex in the cell membrane. This allows adenylate cyclase to catalyze cyclic adenosine monophosphate (cAMP) formation in the cell. In the myocyte, the cAMP then stimulates protein kinases within the sarcoplasmic reticulum; this results in calcium release. In the presence of calcium, excitation-contraction coupling of the cell occurs.[12]

In 1967, Lands and associates characterized β_1 and β_2-adrenergic receptors.[13] β_1-Adrenergic receptors are located in the myocardium, kidney, and the eye, and they have equal affinities for epinephrine and norepinephrine.[13] β_1-Adrenergic stimulation increases the inotropy and chronotropy of the heart as a result of increases in sinoatrial node rate, myocardial contractility, atrial conduction velocity, atrioventricular node and ventricular tissue conduction velocity, and non–sinus node pacemaker automaticity. Renin secretion and aqueous humor production in the anterior chamber also are increased by β_1-adrenergic stimulation. β_2-Adrenergic receptors are located in adipose tissue, pancreas, liver, and smooth and skeletal muscle, and they have a greater affinity for epinephrine than for norepinephrine. β_2-Adrenergic stimulation dilates bronchial smooth muscle and arterioles in skeletal muscle, relaxes the gravid uterus, stimulates insulin secretion, increases lactic acid production, lipolysis, and glycogenolysis.[2] β_2-Adrenergic stimulation also affects the distribution of potassium, resulting in the movement of this electrolyte into the cells[14] (Table 87–1).

Table 87–1. β-Receptor Effects

β_1 Adrenergic Effects	β_2 Adrenergic Effects
Eye: increased acqueous humor production *Kidney:* increased renin production *Heart:* increased chronotropy and inotropy	*Lung:* bronchial dilation *Vascular:* arteriolar dilation *Metabolic:* increased insulin release, lipolysis, glycogenolysis, increased lactic acid production *Other:* movement of potassium into cells

Pathophysiology

In patients with normal hearts, myocardial performance is not dependent on sympathetic tone. The toxic effects associated with β-blockers may be the result of several factors, including decreases in cAMP levels, unopposed α-adrenergic receptor stimulation, membrane stabilization, and class III antiarrhythmic action. Most reports of serious adverse effects occur in overdoses with β-blockers with significant membrane stabilizing activity.[15]

The decrease in cellular cAMP concentrations results in decreased myocardial contractility, decreased automaticity in pacemaker cells, and decreased conduction velocity through the atrioventricular node.[16] Cardiac contraction is altered by the reduction of the capacity of the sarcoplasmic reticulum and plasma membrane sites to accumulate calcium for subsequent release.[17] Serum calcium may also be affected by β-blocker inhibition of parathyroid hormone release.[18] Unopposed α-adrenergic receptor stimulation can result in vasoconstriction and tachycardia. The membrane-stabilizing (local anesthetic) effects result in a reduction of membrane permeability to the fast inward current of sodium ions.[2] Central nervous system (CNS) effects are due to lipid solubility and membrane stabilization.[2, 4] Respiratory depression probably is the result of a central action,[19, 20] and centrally-mediated hypotension also may occur.[20] Sotalol, with its unique electrophysiologic action, increases the time of repolarization and lengthens the effective refractory period and duration of the action potential in Purkinje fibers as well as in atrial and ventricular muscles.[21]

PHARMACOLOGY

Classification of β-Blockers

Although selectivity is often lost in large-dose administrations, β-blockers can be classified on the basis of their cardioselectivity (β_1-adrenergic selectivity), membrane stabilizing activity, partial agonist activity, and class III antiarrhythmic action (Table 87–2). β_1-Selective agents include acebutolol, atenolol, metoprolol, and esmolol.[4, 22] Because of these agents' cardioselectivity at therapeutic doses, the risk of bronchospasm, peripheral vasoconstriction,

Table 87–2. Classification of β-Blockers

Agent	β_1-Selective	Partial Agonist	Membrane Stabilization	Lipid Solubility
Acebutolol	Yes	Yes	Yes	Moderate
Atenolol	Yes	No	No	Weak
Esmolol	Yes	No	No	Weak
Labetalol	No	Yes	No	Weak
Metoprolol	Yes	No	No	Moderate
Nadolol	No	No	No	Weak
Oxprenolol	No	Yes	Yes	Moderate
Pindolol	No	Yes	Yes	Moderate
Propranolol	No	No	Yes	High
Sotalol	No	No	No	Weak
Timolol	No	No	No	Weak

Adapted from Frishman W, Jacob H, Eisenberg E, et al: Appraisal and reappraisal of cardiac therapy: Clinical pharmacology of the new β-adrenergic blocking drugs: VIII. Self-poisoning with β-adrenoreceptor blocking agents: Recognition and management. Am Heart J *98*:798, 1979.

and alteration in serum glucose is decreased. Agents with membrane stabilizing effects include propranolol, acebutolol, labetalol, oxprenolol, pindolol, and alprenolol. Overdose with these agents is more likely to result in CNS effects, including sedation, coma, and seizures. Depression of myocardial contractility and decreased intraventricular conduction velocity also are more common with these agents, resulting in hypotension and heart block.[2]

Nonselective β-blockers produce both negative chronotropic and inotropic effects, but they also can cause bronchospasm and predispose to hypoglycemia.[2] *Partial agonist agents* (pindolol, practolol, alprenolol, acebutolol, oxprenolol) produce a low-grade stimulation of the β-receptor. This intrinsic sympathomimetic activity often results in a less severe presentation in overdose. Sotalol is a nonselective β-blocker with a unique type III antiarrhythmic effect: dose-dependent QT segment prolongation.[23] Labetolol causes blockade of β- and α-adrenergic receptors at a ratio of 3:1, resulting in a hypotensive effect at therapeutic doses without depression of cardiac output or heart rate.[24]

Pharmacokinetics and Toxicokinetics

In general, absorption of β-blockers after ingestion is rapid, with non–sustained-release agents producing peak effects in 1 to 4 hours.[24] Propranolol and metoprolol are available as sustained-release products. All β-blockers have a volume of distribution greater than 1 L/kg. Half-lives range from 10 minutes (esmolol) to 24 hours (nadolol). Lipophilic agents include propranolol, pindolol, metoprolol, labetalol, and alprenolol. Lipid solubility is greatest with propranolol.[24] Increased lipid solubility results in increased ability to cross the blood-brain barrier, which in turn leads to greater CNS toxicity. CNS propranolol levels are 10- to 20-fold those in the plasma.[25] Highly lipid soluble agents also have greater membrane-stabilizing activity.

Highly lipid-soluble agents, like propranolol and metoprolol, are extensively metabolized in the liver, with little unchanged drug being excreted in the urine.[26] Elimination is prolonged in the presence of liver disease, decreased hepatic blood flow, or hepatic enzyme inhibition.[24] Among those β-blockers metabolized by the liver, propranolol has an active metabolite (4-hydoxy-propranolol) that extends its biologic half-life.[2] Hydrophilic agents (nadolol, sotalol, and atenolol) are eliminated unchanged in the urine[26]; thus, abnormalities of renal function result in an increase in the half-lives of these agents.

Drug Interactions

Drugs that induce hepatic enzymes (e.g., phenytoin, phenobarbital, rifampin) accelerate the metabolism of propranolol and metoprolol. Conversely, the bioavailability of these two agents is increased by drugs that inhibit hepatic enzymes (e.g., cimetidine and erythromycin). Nonsteroidal anti-inflammatory agents may alter the elimination of renally excreted β-blockers.

Adverse drug interactions are most common in patients taking other myocardial depressant agents, such as calcium channel blockers or antiarrhythmics. In patients with depressed cardiac function, hypotension and congestive heart failure may result if β-blockers are combined with calcium channel blockers.[27–30] The sympathetic blocking activity of amiodarone may have an additive myocardial depressant effect. The combination of β-blockers and vasodilators may be useful in the treatment of hypertension because of the ability of β-blockers to inhibit reflex tachycardia. But profound hypotension can occur if intravenous hydralazine or diazoxide is given to patients taking β-blockers. Postural hypotension may result from the coadministration of β-blockers and prazosin. The combination of nonselective β-blockers with exogenous or endogenous epinephrine can result in unopposed α-adrenergic effects, causing severe hypertension with subsequent myocardial infarction or cerebrovascular accident.[22]

CLINICAL EFFECTS

A summary of the clinical effects of β-blocker toxicity is presented in Table 87–3.

Adverse Effects from Therapeutic Doses

Serious adverse effects from therapeutic doses of β-blockers usually occur in patients with underlying medical disease or after the coadmininstration of other drugs[4] (Table 87–4). In patients with poor ventricular function who rely on sympathetic tone for maintenance of cardiac output, the administration of β-blockers may result in hypotension or pulmonary edema. Bronchospasm usually occurs in patients with a history of asthma or chronic obstructive pulmonary disease.[22] In patients with underlying intraventricular conduction delays or sinus node disease, bradyarrhythmias may occur. After therapeutic doses, prolongation of the PR interval and slowing of the sinus rate are often noted on electrocardiography.[22] Patients taking sotalol often have QT prolongation. Antagonism of β_2-adrenergic arteriolar dilation with persistent α-mediated constriction can result in cold extremities in the absence of underlying peripheral vascular disease. In children taking therapeutic doses of β-blockers, hypoglycemia has been reported after decreased oral intake.[22] Hypoglycemia can also occur in diabetic patients taking hypoglycemic drugs and in uremic patients. In therapeutic doses, lipid-soluble β-blockers can cause various CNS effects, such as depression, insomnia, or vivid dreaming.

Table 87–3. Clinical Effects of β-Blocker Toxicity

Cardiovascular
Blood pressure
Hypotension
Hypertension (partial agonists)
Cardiac rhythm
Bradycardia, atrioventricular block, asystole
Tachycardia (partial agonists)
Prolonged QT interval (sotalol)
Prolonged QRS complex (membrane-stabilizing agents)
Ventricular dysrhythmias (membrane-stabilizing agents, sotalol)
CNS (Lipid-soluble and Membrane-stabilizing Agents)
Depressed level of consciousness
Seizures
Respiratory
Respiratory depression, apnea, cyanosis
Bronchospasm
Gastrointestinal
Esophageal spasm
Mesenteric ischemia
Metabolic
Hypoglycemia
Other
Renal failure

CNS, central nervous system.

Table 87–4. Adverse Effects from Therapeutic Doses of β-Blockers

Cardiac
Hypotension, pulmonary edema (in patients with underlying ventricular dysfunction)
Electrocardiographic changes
Bradycardia
Prolonged PR interval
Prolonged QT interval (sotalol)
Respiratory
Bronchospasm (in patients with underlying airway disease)
Vascular
Cold extremities
CNS (Lipid-soluble Agents)
Depression
Insomnia
Vivid dreams
Metabolic
Hypoglycemia

Predisposing Factors for Toxicity

The elderly are at higher risk for adverse effects owing to changes in metabolism and to changes in the action of pharmaceutical agents that occur with aging. Also, the risk of unintentional overdose in the elderly is greater because of the increase in polypharmacy and failing eyesight.[10] Patients with underlying cardiovascular disease usually present with a more severe clinical picture after overdose than those who do not have such disease. Renal failure or hepatic disease also increase the risk for toxicity.

Timing

In acute ingestions of non–sustained-release β-blockers, symptoms usually occur within 1 to 3 hours, but the onset of symptoms may occur from 15 minutes to 10 hours after ingestion.[4, 23, 31–36] Sudden deterioration with cardiovascular collapse is a common presentation.[4] A delay in the onset of symptoms may occur with sustained-release preparations or with coingestion. In one review of β-blocker overdoses, all patients with propranolol toxicity presented with symptoms in less than 2 hours.[36] If sotalol is excluded, all adult patients who require treatment for cardiovascular toxicity from non–sustained-release β-blocker overdose present with symptoms within 6 hours, and 97% have symptoms within 4 hours.[37] Owing to the long elimination half-life of sotalol after overdose, signs of cardiotoxicity have been reported to occur for as long as 2 days after ingestion.[23, 38] In most cases of β-blocker toxicity, symptoms resolve within 72 hours of ingestion.[26]

Cardiovascular Effects

Hypotension, bradycardia, low-output cardiac failure, and cardiogenic shock due to conduction delays

and decreased contractility are the most common features of severe β-blocker intoxication. In one review of 90 β-blocker overdoses, 64 patients had a systolic blood pressure less than 80 mm Hg, and 65 had a heart rate less than 60 beats per minute.[39] The most serious toxicity generally occurs after ingestion of agents with membrane-stabilizing activity. Patients can present with sinus bradycardia, atrioventricular block, junctional rhythm, loss of atrial activity, widening of the QRS complex, intraventricular rhythm, right bundle branch block, or asystole.[40] QRS complex prolongation occurs with membrane-stabilizing agents.[4, 31, 33, 41] QT prolongation occurs in all patients with toxic ingestions of sotalol and may occur after ingestion of therapeutic doses, resulting in an increased incidence of ventricular arrhythmias.[23] The occurrence of ventricular arrhythmias parallels the degree of prolongation of the QT interval and the serum sotalol concentration.[23] After sotalol ingestion, premature ventricular contractions, bigeminy, ventricular tachycardia, ventricular fibrillation, and torsades de pointes have all been reported.[23, 38, 42–44]

In most serious cases of β-blocker intoxication, patients develop profound hypotension, and this hypotension can occur despite a normal heart rate.[2, 34, 35, 45] Hypotension is secondary to a decrease in cardiac output, which is most often due to a reduction in myocardial contractility. Bradydysrhythmias commonly occur and may potentiate the hypotension. However, the magnitude of bradycardia alone is not a useful indicator of the severity of poisoning. Because partial agonist agents cause less slowing of the heart rate and can cause vasoconstriction, patients with overdoses of these agents may present with tachycardia and hypertension.

Central Nervous System Effects

Effects of β-blocker intoxication on the CNS can range from alterations in level of consciousness to seizures or coma. These effects are more commonly seen with lipid-soluble agents and those with membrane-stabilizing effects. Generally, coma is preceded by evidence of cardiovascular toxicity. Although it should always be considered, hypoglycemia has rarely been documented in patients with seizures after β-blocker overdose.[36] Coingestion must also be considered in patients with altered mental status. Low output–induced hypoxia may also result in CNS effects, but these effects often persist despite maintenance of an adequate hemodynamic status[36]; also, cerebral impairment can be out of proportion to cardiovascular toxicity. Primary CNS effects probably occur as a result of the blockade of fast sodium channels in the brain.[2, 4] Seizures are seen in over 58% of patients with propranolol overdose and are usually generalized and brief and have no sequelae.[36, 46] Propranolol-induced seizures usually occur after ingestions of greater than 1600 mg.[36] CNS recovery is usually rapid and complete, even after prolonged resuscitation efforts in patients with massive overdose.

Respiratory Effects

Central respiratory depression, apnea, and cyanosis can occur after β-blocker overdose. In one review of 90 cases, respiratory insufficiency was documented in 34 patients and was unrelated to the type of β-blocker ingested or to the presence of hypotension.[39] A study in rats demonstrated the occurrence of respiratory arrest before cardiac failure as the severity of the intoxication progressed,[20] suggesting that circulatory failure may be in part due to respiratory failure. In rats who were artificially ventilated, larger doses of β-blockers were tolerated before death. Although uncommon,[15] bronchospasm may also occur and has been reported in patients both with and without a history of previous airway disease.

Gastrointestinal Effects

Esophageal spasm that obstructs the insertion or withdrawal of an orogastric or nasogastric tube has been reported with propranolol overdose.[47] Esophageal spasm could be due to mechanical irritation by the tube or by pill fragments, or as a consequence of β-blockade. Inhibition of β-mediated smooth muscle relaxation with unopposed α-mediated contraction results in increased esophageal and lower esophageal sphincter contraction.[47, 48] Mesenteric ischemia has also been reported after massive propranolol overdose.[49]

Metabolic Effects

Because β_2-adrenergic stimulation results in the movement of potassium into cells,[14] β-blockade could theoretically result in an elevated serum potassium level. Both hyper- and hypoglycemia have been reported after β-blocker overdose.[36, 50] Hypoglycemia should be considered in any patient with coma or seizures, although it has rarely been documented after β-blocker overdose.

Other Effects

Acute renal failure after labetalol overdose has been reported and, on the basis of biopsy results, was compatible with vasomotor nephropathy.[35]

LABORATORY AND ANCILLARY STUDIES

Drug Levels

Drug levels can be determined with the use of high-pressure liquid chromatography or gas chromotography/mass spectrometry, but there appears to be no relationship between blood and plasma levels of β-blockers and outcome after poisoning. Determination of levels may confirm toxicity but does not aid in initial management.

Ancillary Studies

All patients with suspected β-blocker toxicity should undergo electrocardiography. In patients with respiratory symptoms or in those with severe toxicity, chest radiography should also be performed. Serum electrolytes, arterial blood gases, and serum glucose levels should also be evaluated in patients with evidence of toxicity. In cases of altered mental status or seizure, performance of computed tomography of the head or lumbar puncture should be considered to rule out other causes. A digoxin level is the only drug level that may be of some value in patients who present with bradycardia and altered mental status of unknown cause.

DIFFERENTIAL DIAGNOSIS

Patients with β-blocker poisoning most commonly present with sudden development of hypotension and bradycardia. In patients who present with bradycardia, hypotension, and altered mental status, the differential diagnosis should include toxicity from calcium channel blockers, clonidine, cardiac glycosides, antiarrhythmics, opiates, organophosphates, cyanide, hydrogen sulfide, barbiturates, chloroquine, or end-stage sympathomimetic or cyclic antidepressant toxicity. The broader differential diagnosis of nontoxicologic causes of altered mental status should also be considered.

MANAGEMENT

General

The first priority in treatment is evaluation of the "ABC's" (*a*irway, *b*reathing, and *c*irculation; Fig. 87–1). In patients with altered mental status or seizures, rapid assessment of serum glucose levels should be performed, with correction of hypoglycemia. Because hypoxia and acidosis potentiate cardiotoxicity, and because artificial ventilation reduces the toxicity of β-blockers in an animal model,[51] early ventilatory control is essential.

Gastrointestinal Decontamination

Gastrointestinal decontamination should be performed after initial supportive care has been provided. Due to the risk of rapid deterioration, altered mental status, and seizures after β-blocker ingestion, the use of ipecac is contraindicated. Gastric lavage, after adequate airway protection, should be performed in patients who present within 1 to 2 hours after ingestion. Activated charcoal (1 g/kg) should be administered to all patients; multiple doses may be of benefit in interrupting enterohepatic circulation. Whole-bowel irrigation with a polyethylene glycol solution (2 L/h in adults and 0.5 L/h in children) should be considered in patients who ingest sustained-release preparations.

Specific Therapeutic Agents for Cardiovascular Toxicity

Glucagon

Glucagon is a single-chain pancreatic polypeptide whose positive inotropic and chronotropic effects were first discovered in animals who were treated with insulin that was contaminated with glucagon.[52] Glucagon activates myocardial adenylate cyclase. This results in an increase in cAMP synthesis and a subsequent increase in myocardial contractility and heart rate.[53, 54] This increase in cAMP is similar to that seen after administration of catecholamine agents, but glucagon acts at a distinct glucagon re-

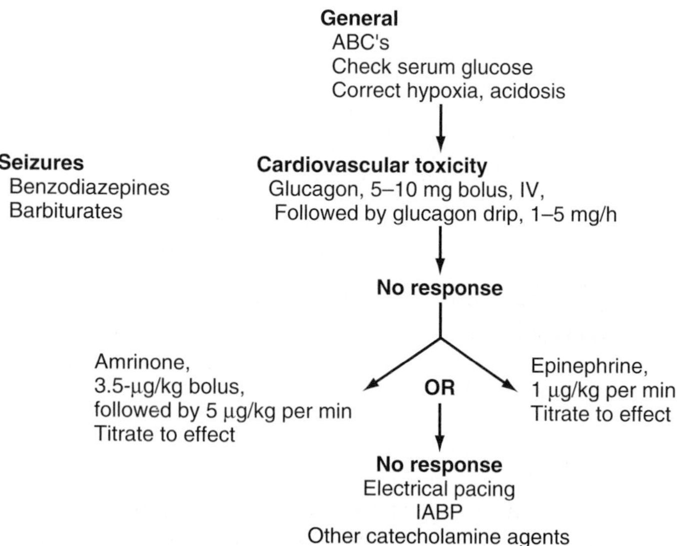

Figure 87–1. Treatment of β-blocker overdose. ABC's, airway, breathing, and circulation; IABP, intra-aortic balloon pump; IV, intravenous.

ceptor that is not affected by β-blockade.[55–58] Glucagon augments the movement of calcium into the myocardial cell and produces significant increases in cardiac index, arterial pressure, and contractility, as well as a slight decrease in systemic vascular resistance and no change in left ventricular end-diastolic pressure.[54, 58–60] Although it may not be able to reduce the effects of membrane stabilization, glucagon is the most consistently effective agent used in β-blocker toxicity[15, 36] and is considered the drug of choice.

Glucagon can be given intravenously, intramuscularly, or subcutaneously, but the intravenous route is preferred. The recommended initial dose is 50 to 150 μg/kg (3.5 to 5 mg in an adult), but up to 10 mg may be required.[36, 53] Hemodynamic actions begin 1 to 3 minutes after administration of the bolus dose and become maximal at 5 to 7 minutes.[54] Because its duration of action is only 15 to 20 minutes, a continuous infusion should be initiated at 1 to 5 mg/h (0.07 mg/kg per hour) after the bolus has been administered.[36] A continuous intravenous infusion of glucagon has been shown to produce a more sustained stabilization of blood pressure than repeated intermittent bolus doses.[61] The normal diluent supplied with glucagon contains phenol (2 mg of phenol per 1 mg of glucagon), which can cause toxicity in doses of 50 mg or greater.[62] Therefore, the continuous infusion should be mixed with normal saline or 5% dextrose solutions.

The most common side effects from glucagon therapy are gastrointestinal, with nausea and vomiting occurring in one third of patients.[54, 60, 63–65] Hyperglycemia can occur, but the stimulation of insulin release by glucagon can also result in hypoglycemia. Decreased serum potassium levels may result from cellular shifts of potassium induced by insulin release. Although very uncommon, erythema multiforme,[66] Stevens-Johnson syndrome, and allergic reactions have all been reported after glucagon administration.[67] No increased risk of arrhythmias has been associated with glucagon use. Contraindications to glucagon therapy include insulinoma, pheochromocytoma, and glucagon sensitivity. The major limitation to the use of glucagon is the institutional availability of sufficient quantities to manage a severely intoxicated patient.[68, 69]

Catecholamine Agents

Because binding to the β-receptor is reversible and surmountable, the addition of high doses of exogenous β-agonists would be expected to reverse β-blockade. However, the response of β-blocker intoxication to different catecholamine agents has been variable and frequently ineffective. In Weinstein's review of the treatment of 39 cases of overdose, epinephrine had the greatest effect of all catecholamine agents used, resulting in improvement of heart rate in 4 patients (67%) and in blood pressure in 3 patients (50%). Dopamine improved blood pressure in 50% but had no effect on heart rate, and isoproterenol improved heart rate in 11% and blood pressure in 22%.[36] The doses of catecholamines needed after β-blocker overdose are much greater than those required for other indications. In human volunteers given labetalol, 26-fold the control dose of isoproterenol was required.[70] In dogs poisoned with propranolol, 15 times the normal dose of isoproterenol and 5 times the normal dose of dopamine were needed.[71] Isoproterenol increases myocardial oxygen demand and predisposes to arrhythmias; in addition, its β_2-agonism can result in vasodilation and cardiovascular collapse. However, in one case report, a patient intoxicated with propranolol and ethanol responded to high-dose administration of isoproterenol (200 μg/min) in combination with other therapies.[50]

Phosphodiesterase Inhibitors

Prior to the introduction of amrinone, the only positive inotropic drugs available in the United States to treat congestive heart failure were cardiac glycosides and catecholamine agents.[72] Amrinone, milrinone, and theophylline all inhibit phosphodiesterase, thus inhibiting the breakdown of cAMP. Milrinone is 30 to 50 times more potent than amrinone.[73] Although it has relatively low inotropic potency with associated neurologic, gastrointestinal, and arrhythmogenic side effects, aminophylline use has been reported in two cases of β-blocker toxicity.[50, 74] Amrinone has been shown to be effective in the canine model of β-blocker poisoning, resulting in a positive inotropic effect without a concomitant increase in myocardial oxygen demand.[75] However, when amrinone and glucagon are combined to treat β-blocker intoxication in dogs, there appears to be no advantage over glucagon treatment alone.[76] Amrinone should be administered in a bolus dose of 0.5 to 3.5 μg/kg, followed by a continuous infusion starting at 5 μg/kg per minute and titrated to desired hemodynamic effect.[77] The dose of amrinone required for a positive inotropic effect may be as great as 40 μg/kg per minute.[77]

Atropine

Although atropine is the most frequently used agent in the treatment of β-blocker toxicity, it is the least effective.[36, 39] Atropine improves heart rate in 25% of cases but has no effect on blood pressure.[36] Because the cardiovascular effects of β-blockade are not due to a vagal effect, atropine would not be expected to have a significant effect. Atropine may have some effect because of the slight inhibition of the parasympathetic component of the baroreflex, which may explain the transient acceleration of heart rate with no effect on blood pressure. The absence of effect of a 1-mg dose of atropine on blood pressure and heart rate may be diagnostic for β-blocker poisoning.

Pacing

Transvenous or external cardiac pacing is often attempted to treat β-blocker–induced bradycardia, but it may be ineffective. In Weinstein's study, pacing restored heart rate in 8 patients but had no effect on blood pressure.[36] Overdrive pacing may be necessary in cases of torsades de pointes associated with sotalol intoxication.[44]

Intra-Aortic Balloon Pump

Insertion of an intra-aortic balloon pump may restore perfusion, particularly if other measures fail. Successful use of an intra-aortic balloon pump was reported in a 17-year-old patient who experienced cardiac arrest after an ingestion of 8 g of propranolol.[78]

Experimental Therapies

Prenalterol—a new, cardioselective β-agonist not yet available in the United States—has been successfully used to treat metoprolol toxicity in dogs.[79] It appears to be less arrhythmogenic than other β-agonists and has also been used effectively to treat human poisonings from atenolol, propranolol, and metoprolol.[31, 80]

The root of an Indian coleus plant contains a diterpene, forskolin, which has positive inotropic and vasodilatory properties. The mechanism of action of this substance is stimulation of adenylate cyclase at a site distinct from the β-adrenergic receptor, with marked increases in cAMP being observed *in vitro*.[81] Although it is insoluble in water, forskolin is effective when administered orally or intravenously. Its use for the treatment of congestive heart failure may be limited by its prominent positive chronotropic effects,[82] but these effects may be advantageous in the treatment of β-blocker toxicity.

Sotalol Intoxication

Sotalol-induced ventricular arrhythmias have been treated successfully with lidocaine, magnesium, overdrive pacing, and defibrillation.[23, 25] Because of sotalol's low protein binding and volume of distribution, its removal with hemodialysis may be effective.

Treatment of Seizures

Initial therapy for seizures should include prompt reversal of hypoxia and hypoglycemia. Conventional treatment of seizures should be employed, with initial administration of benzodiazepines. If benzodiazepines are ineffective, barbiturates should be used. Phenytoin should be avoided because of its ability to block sodium ion channels in the CNS.

Treatment of Bronchospasm

Although rare, bronchospasm should be treated with aerosolized β-agonists. Parenteral β-agonist therapy with epinephrine may be required in severe cases.

Extracorporeal Removal

Hemodialysis and hemoperfusion are usually not effective in the treatment of toxicity from β-blockers owing to their large volumes of distribution and high lipid solubility. Extracorporeal removal can be considered for those agents with volumes of distribution less than 2 L/kg, low endogenous clearance, and long half-lives (acebutolol, atenolol, nadolol, sotalol). Although extracorporeal removal has not been well-studied, it has been used in cases of toxicity from propranolol,[33] atenolol,[83] and a combination of metoprolol and diltiazem.[84]

DISPOSITION

All patients with symptomatic β-blocker toxicity and patients with a history of sotalol overdose should be admitted to a hospital. Those with significant signs and symptoms, including altered mental status, bradycardia, or hypotension, should be managed in the intensive care unit. With the exception of those with toxicity from sustained-release preparations, patients with suspected β-blocker overdose who are initially asymptomatic and who have a normal electrocardiogram and normal vital signs should receive activated charcoal and be medically observed for at least 8 to 10 hours. Patients who ingest sustained-release products require observation for a minimum of 24 hours.

PROGNOSIS

Thirty per cent to 40% of β-blocker overdose patients remain asymptomatic,[26] but the mortality rate in severe cases can be as great as 26%.[39] In one literature survey, 75% of deaths from propranolol toxicity occurred at home[26]; thus, if a patient arrives alive and if appropriate treatment is initiated early, the prognosis is good. Prolonged resuscitation is indicated after β-blocker overdose because survival without neurologic sequelae has been reported even after massive β-blocker ingestion.

References

1. Prichard BNC: Hypotensive action of pronethalol. BMJ *1*:1227, 1964.
2. Hoffman BB, Lefkowitz RJ: Adrenergic receptor antagonists. *In* Gilman AG, Rall TW, Nies AS, et al (eds): Goodman and Gilman's The Pharmacologic Basis of Therapeutics. 8th ed. New York, Pergamon Press, pp 229–243, 1990.
3. Litovitz TL, Schmitz BF, Bailey KM: 1989 Annual report of the American Association of Poison Control Centers national data collection system. Am J Emerg Med *8*:394, 1990.
4. Frishman W, Jacob H, Eisenberg E, et al: Appraisal and reap-

praisal of cardiac therapy: Clinical pharmacology of the new β-adrenergic blocking drugs: VIII. Self-poisoning with β-adrenoreceptor blocking agents: Recognition and management. Am Heart J *98*:798, 1979.

5. Litovitz TL, Bailey KM, Schmitz BF, et al: 1990 Annual report of the American Association of Poison Control Centers national data collection system. Am J Emerg Med *9*:461, 1991.
6. Litovitz TL, Holm KC, Bailey KM: 1991 Annual report of the American Association of Poison Control Centers national data collection system. Am J Emerg Med *10*:452, 1992.
7. Litovitz TL, Holm KC, Clancy C, et al: 1992 Annual report of the American Association of Poison Control Centers national data collection system. Am J Emerg Med *11*:494, 1993.
8. Litovitz TL, Felberg L, Soloway RA, et al: 1994 Annual report of the American Association of Poison Control Centers toxic exposure surveillance system. Am J Emerg Med *13*:551, 1995.
9. Hecker MM: Health promotion for older Americans. Public Health Rep *100*:225, 1985.
10. Dean BS, Krenzelok EP: Poisoning in the elderly: An increasing problem for health care providers. Clin Toxicol *25*:411, 1987.
11. Ahlquist RP: Study of adrenotropic receptors. Am J Physiol *153*:586, 1948.
12. Colucci WS, Wright RF, Braunwald E: New positive inotropic agents in the treatment of congestive heart failure: Mechanisms of action and recent clinical developments. N Engl J Med *314*(Part I):290, 1986.
13. Lands AM, Arnold A, McAuliff, et al: Differentiation of receptor systems activated by sympathomimetic amines. Nature *214*:597, 1967.
14. Brown MJ, Brown DC, Murphy MB: Hypokalemia from β_2-receptor stimulation by circulating epinephrine. N Engl J Med 309:1414, 1983.
15. Critchley JA, Ungar A: The management of acute poisoning due to β-adrenoreceptor antagonists. Med Toxicol 4:32, 1989.
16. Whitsitt LS, Lucchesi BR: Effects of β-receptor blockade and glucagon on the atrio-ventricular transmission system in the dog. Circ Res *23*:585, 1968.
17. Nayler WG, Chang A: Cellular pharmacology of β-blocking drugs. *In* Barrett AM (ed): New Perspectives in Beta-Blockade: Ciba Symposium. Aarhus, Denmark, Scanticon, pp 41–71, 1972.
18. Amundson DE, Brodine SK: A fatal case of propranolol poisoning. Drug Intell Clin Pharmacol *22*:781, 1988.
19. Campbell SC, Lauver GL, Cobb RB: Central ventilatory depression by oral propranolol. Clin Pharmacol Ther *30*:758, 1981.
20. Langemeijer J, de Wildt D, de Groot G, et al: Central origin of respiratory arrest in β-blocker intoxication in rats. Toxicol Appl Pharmacol *89*:399, 1987.
21. Strauss HC, Bigger JT, Jun T, et al: Electrophysiological and β-receptor blocking effects of MJ 1999 on dog and rabbit cardiac tissue. Circ Res *26*:661, 1970.
22. Benowitz NL: Beta-adrenoreceptor blocker poisoning. *In* Haddad LM, Winchester JF (eds): Clinical Management of Poisoning and Drug Overdose. 2nd ed. Philadelphia, W.B. Saunders Co., pp 1315–1326, 1990.
23. Neuvonen PJ, Elonen E, Vuorenmaa T, et al: Prolonged Q-T interval and severe tachyarrhythmias, common features of sotalol intoxication. Eur J Clin Pharmacol *20*:85, 1981.
24. Hoffman BB: Adrenoreceptor-blocking drugs. *In* Katzung BG (ed): Basic and Clinical Pharmacology. 6th ed. Norwalk, CT, Appleton & Lange, pp 137–146, 1995.
25. Cruickshank JM: The clinical importance of cardioselectivity and lipophilicity in β-blockers. Am Heart J *100*:160, 1980.
26. Taboulet P, Cariou A, Berdeaux A, et al: Pathophysiology and management of self-poisoning with β-blockers. Clin Toxicol *31*:531, 1993.
27. Benaim ME: Asystole after verapamil. BMJ *15*:169, 1972.
28. Wayne VS, Harper RW, Laufer E, et al: Adverse interaction between β-adrenergic blocking drugs and verapamil: Report of three cases. Aust N Z J Med *12*:285, 1982.
29. Anastassiades CJ: Nifedipine and β-blocker drugs. BMJ *281*:1251, 1980.
30. Opie LH, White DA: Adverse interaction between nifedipine and β-blockade. BMJ *281*:1462, 1980.
31. Brimacombe JR, Scully M, Swainston R: Propranolol overdose: A dramatic response to calcium chloride. Med J Aust *155*:267, 1991.
32. Lindvall K, Personne M, Sjögren A: High-dose prenalterol in β-blockade intoxication. Acta Med Scand *218*:525, 1985.
33. McVey FK, Corke CF: Extracorporeal circulation in the management of massive propranolol overdose. Anaesthesia *46*:744, 1991.
34. O'Mahony D, O'Leary P, Molloy MG: Severe oxprenolol poisoning: The importance of glucagon infusion. Hum Exp Toxicol *9*:101, 1990.
35. Smit AJ, Mulder PO, de Jong PE, et al: Acute renal failure after overdose of labetalol. BMJ *293*:1142, 1986.
36. Weinstein RS: Recognition and management of poisoning with β-adrenergic blocking agents. Ann Emerg Med *13*:1123, 1984.
37. Love JN: β-Blocker toxicity after overdose: When do symptoms develop in adults? J Emerg Med *12*:799, 1994.
38. Adlerfliegel F, Leeman M, Demaeyer Ph, et al: Sotalol poisoning associated with asystole. Intensive Care Med *19*:57, 1993.
39. Langemeijer JJ, de Wildt DJ, de Groot G, et al: Intoxication with β-sympathicolytics. Neth J Med *40*:308, 1992.
40. Kerns W, Kline J, Ford MD: β-Blocker and calcium channel blocker toxicity. Emerg Med Clin North Am *12*:365, 1994.
41. Nicolas F, Villers D, Rozo L, et al: Severe self-poisoning with acebutolol in association with alcohol. Crit Care Med 15:173, 1987.
42. Edvardsson N, Varnauskas E: Clinical course, serum concentrations and elimination rate in a case of massive sotalol intoxication. Eur Heart J *8*:544, 1987.
43. Gupta K: Hazards of β-blockers in the elderly: Severe bradycardia due to Sotacor overdose. Br J Clin Pract *39*:116,1985.
44. Tötterman KJ, Turto H, Pellinen T: Overdrive pacing as treatment of sotalol-induced ventricular tachyarrhythmias (torsades de pointes). Acta Med Scand *668*(Suppl):28, 1982.
45. Chen TW, Huang TP, Yang WC, et al: Propranolol intoxication: Three cases' experience. Vet Hum Toxicol *27*:528, 1985.
46. Weinstein RS, Cole S, Knaster HB, et al: β-Blocker overdose with propranolol and with atenolol. Ann Emerg Med *14*:161, 1985.
47. Panos RJ, Tso E, Barish RA, et al: Esophageal spasm following propranolol overdose relieved by glucagon. Am J Emerg Med *4*:227, 1986.
48. Christensen J: Pharmacology of the esophageal motor function. Annu Rev Pharmacol *15*:243, 1975.
49. Pettei MJ, Levy J, Abramson S: Nonocclusive mesenteric ischemia associated with propranolol overdose: Implications regarding splanchnic circulation. J Pediatr Gastroenterol Nutr *10*:544, 1990.
50. Agura ED, Wexler LF, Witzburg RA: Massive propranolol overdose: Successful treatment with high-dose isoproterenol and glucagon. Am J Med *80*:755, 1986.
51. Langemeijer J, de Wildt D, de Groot, et al: Respiratory arrest as main determinant of toxicity due to overdose with different β-blockers in rats. Acta Pharmacol Toxicol *57*:352, 1985.
52. Farah A, Tuttle R: Studies on the pharmacology of glucagon. J Pharmacol Exp Ther 129:49, 1960.
53. Lewin NA: Antihypertensive agents. *In* Goldfrank LR, Flomenbaum NE, Lewin NA, et al (eds): Goldfrank's Toxicologic Emergencies, 5th ed. East Norwalk, CT, Appleton & Lange, pp 701–704, 1994.
54. Parmley WW, Glick G, Sonnenblick EH: Cardiovascular effects of glucagon in man. N Engl J Med *279*:12, 1968.
55. Murad F, Vaughan M: Effect of glucagon on rat heart adenyl cyclase. Biochem Pharmacol *18*:1053, 1969.
56. Jolly SR, Kipnis JN, Lucchesi BR: Cardiovascular depression by verapamil: Reversal by glucagon and interactions with propranolol. Pharmacology *35*:249, 1987.
57. Levey GS, Epstein SE: Activation of adenyl cyclase by glucagon in cat and human heart. Circ Res *24*:151, 1969.
58. Abel FL: Action of glucagon on canine left ventricular performance and coronary hemodynamics. Circ Shock *11*:45, 1983.
59. Manchester JH, Parmley WW, Matloff JM, et al: Effects of glucagon on myocardial oxygen consumption and coronary blood flow in man and in dog. Circulation *41*:579, 1970.
60. Diamond G, Forrester J, Danzig R, et al: Acute myocardial

infarction in man: Comparative hemodynamic effects of norepinephrine and glucagon. Am J Cardiol *27*:612, 1971.
61. Illingworth R: Glucagon for β-blocker poisoning. Practitioner *223*:683, 1979.
62. Brancato DJ: Recognizing potential toxicity of phenol. Vet Hum Toxicol *24*:29, 1982.
63. Parmley WW, Matloff JM, Sonnenblick EH: Hemodynamic effects of glucagon in patients following prosthetic valve replacement. Circulation *39*(Suppl):163, 1969.
64. Vander Ark CR, Reynolds EW: Clinical evaluation of glucagon by continuous infusion in the treatment of low cardiac output states. Am Heart J *79*:481, 1970.
65. Williams JF, Childress Rh, Chip JN, et al: Hemodynamic effects of glucagon in patients with heart disease. Circulation *39*:38, 1969.
66. Edell SL: Erythema multiforme secondary to intravenous glucagon. Am J Roentgenol *134*:385, 1980.
67. Zavras GM, Kounis NG, Dimopoulos JA: Glucagon-induced severe anaphylactic reaction. ROFO *152*:110, 1990.
68. Smith RC, Wilkinson J, Hull RL: Glucagon for propranolol overdose. JAMA *254*:2412, 1985.
69. Love JN, Tandy TK: β-Adrenoreceptor antagonist toxicity: A survey of glucagon availability. Ann Emerg Med *22*:267, 1993.
70. Richards DA, Prichard BNC, Boakes AJ, et al: Pharmacological basis for antihypertensive effects of intravenous labetalol. Br Heart J *39*:99, 1977.
71. Avery GJ, Spotnitz HM, Rose EA, et al: Pharmacologic antagonism of β-adrenergic blockade in dogs: I. Hemodynamic effects of isoproterenol, dopamine, and epinephrine in acute propranolol administration. J Thorac Cardiovasc Surg *77*:267, 1979.
72. Colucci WS, Wright RF, Braunwald E: New positive inotropic agents in the treatment of congestive heart failure. N Engl J Med *314*(Part II):349, 1986.
73. Sys S, Goenen MJ, Chanlant CH, et al: Inotropic effects of amrinone and milrinone on contraction and relaxation of isolated cardiac muscle. Circulation 73(Suppl):25, 1986.
74. Perrot D, Bui-Xuan B, Lang J, et al: A case of sotalol poisoning with fatal outcome. Clin Toxicol *26*:389, 1988.
75. Alousi AA, Canter JM, Fort DJ: The beneficial effect of amrinone on acute drug-induced heart failure in the anaesthetised dog. Cardiovasc Res *19*:483, 1985.
76. Love JN, Leasure JA, Mundt DJ: A comparison of combined amrinone and glucagon therapy to glucagon alone for cardiovascular depression associated with propranolol toxicity in a canine model. Am J Emerg Med *11*:360, 1993.
77. DiBianco R: Acute positive inotropic intervention: The phosphodiesterase inhibitors. Am Heart J *121*:1871, 1991.
78. Lane AS, Woodward AC, Goldman MR: Massive propranolol overdose poorly responsive to pharmacologic therapy: Use of the intra-aortic balloon pump. Ann Emerg Med 16:1381, 1987.
79. Andersson T, Heath A, Mattsson H: Prenalterol as antidote to massive doses of metoprolol: A cardiovascular study in the dog. Acta Med Scand Suppl *659*:71, 1982.
80. Freestone S, Thomas HM, Bhamra RK, et al: Severe atenolol poisoning: Treatment with prenalterol. Hum Toxicol *5*:343, 1986.
81. Daly JW: Forskolin, adenylate cyclase, and cell physiology: An overview. Adv Cycl Nucl Protein Phosphoryl Res *17*:81, 1984.
82. Linderer T, Biamino G, Brhggeman T, et al: Hemodynamic effects of forskolin: A new drug with combined positive inotropic and vasodilating properties. J Am Coll Cardiol *3*:562, 1984.
83. Saitz R, Williams BW, Farber HW: Atenolol-induced cardiovascular collapse treated with hemodialysis. Crit Care Med *19*:116, 1991.
84. Anthony T, Jastremski M, Elliott W, et al: Charcoal hemoperfusion for the treatment of a combined diltiazem and metoprolol overdose. Ann Emerg Med *15*:1344, 1986.

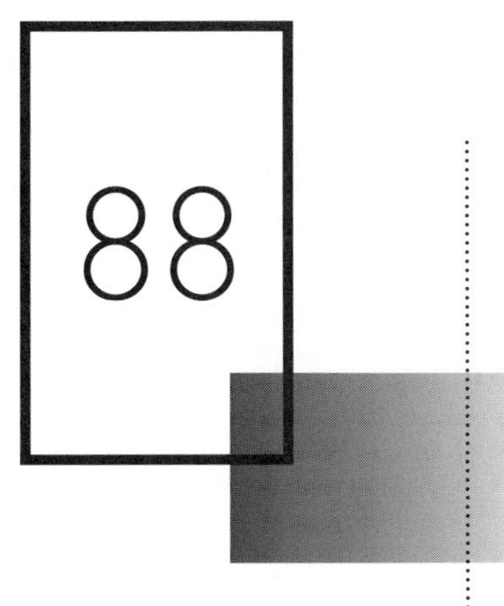

Nitroprusside, ACE Inhibitors, and Selected Antihypertensive Agents

DAVID A. FLOCKHART, MD, PHD
MILOU-DANIEL DRICI, MD, PHD

USAGE PATTERNS OF ANTIHYPERTENSIVE DRUGS

The pattern of toxicity among drugs used to treat hypertension is diverse and unpredictable. Drugs that most commonly present in poisonings are not necessarily the most frequently recommended for the treatment of hypertension. The recommendations by the Joint National Committee for the treatment of hypertension reflect the most recently gathered expert opinion on how physicians should treat hypertension.[1] These guidelines recommend that therapy be initiated with diuretics or β-blockers. Despite this, it remains the case that if drug therapy is necessary for the treatment of hypertension, the initial agent used may simply reflect the biases of the prescribing physician rather than any generalizable interpretation of the literature.[2] The number of antihypertensive drugs implicated in poisoning and overdose therefore are more likely to reflect the influence of pharmaceutical marketing and individual drug toxicity. Table 88–1 presents the most current data available: national data on the incidence of overdoses of antihypertensive agents and the outcomes reported to the American Association of Poison Control Centers in 1994. These data show that calcium antagonists were involved in more episodes of poisoning with more morbidity than the other antihypertensives recorded, including 45 deaths. β-Blockers were also involved in 12 reported poisoning deaths and thiazides in 1 death. It is of note that few poisonings due to α-blockers were recorded and that no separate reporting for ACE inhibitors was conducted. The only exclusively inpatient medication listed is nitroprusside, and few episodes are listed, a finding that may reflect the fact that this therapy is usually administered by trained personnel in highly monitored settings.

NITROPRUSSIDE TOXICITY

Intravenous nitroprusside has been used for more than 30 years as a rapid hypotensive agent in critical care settings, where it has been recognized since 1955 that *short* infusions can be used with great effect, and toxicity can be closely monitored.[3] The approved indications for its use are severe hypertension and blood pressure management during surgery. The mechanisms of nitroprusside's actions are directly related to its spontaneous breakdown products, nitric oxide and cyanide. Although the mechanism of nitroprusside's hypotensive action is almost certainly via the release of nitric oxide[4] and the vasodilatory properties of that molecule,[5] its toxicity is principally although not exclusively due to the release of cyanide that occurs.[6–8] The risks of cyanide toxicity that attend the routine clinical use of nitroprusside are an important part of the knowledge base required to use the drug safely. Effective and available management strategies are essential.

Routine use of nitroprusside at doses greater than 2 μg/kg per minute or at any dose for more than 24

Table 88–1. Poisonings and Overdoses of Antihypertensive Agents Reported to the American Association of Poison Control Centers in 1994

Antihypertensive Agent	Number of Exposures	Number Treated in a Health Care Facility	No Morbidity	Minor Morbidity	Moderate Morbidity	Major Morbidity	Death
α-Blockers	231	123	103	39	20	2	0
β-Blockers	5788	3337	2421	699	654	114	12
Calcium antagonists	7787	4400	3248	922	735	215	45
Hydralazine	201	89	80	42	12	2	0
Long-acting nitrates	728	237	349	66	21	4	0
Nitroprusside	35	35	8	6	5	2	0
Furosemide	1273	466	436	234	61	5	0
Thiazides	1277	477	517	164	48	2	1

hours has been questioned for several years.[9] Specifically, Robin and McCauley at the Tsurai Indian Health Care Clinic[8] have estimated that the use of nitroprusside may be as high as 480,000 patient-days per year. They calculated that if the excess mortality associated with its use were as high as 1.0%, then the number of deaths attributable to nitroprusside toxicity would be more than 1000 per year.

These risks were emphasized by a change in the labeling of nitroprusside by the United States Food and Drug Administration in 1991 "to highlight the risk of potentially lethal cyanide toxicity."[10] In announcing the new labeling, the Food and Drug Administration emphasized that cyanide toxicity is increasingly likely with prolonged administration at infusion rates faster than 2 μg/kg per minute and recommended that "infusion should be started at a very low rate (0.3 μg/kg/min) with upward titration until the desired effect is reached or the maximum recommended dosage is reached."

Pharmacology of Nitroprusside Toxicity Due to Cyanide

Nitroprusside is composed of a ferrous ion center complexed with five cyanide moieties (44% of the total molecular weight) and a nitrosyl group. The breakdown and metabolism of nitroprusside is depicted in Figure 88–1. Nitroprusside is spontaneously soluble in blood and can interact rapidly with oxyhemoglobin to form methemoglobin with the spontaneous release of cyanide and nitric oxide.[7] Cyanide may then react immediately with methemoglobin to form cyanomethemoglobin.[7] Normal adult total methemoglobin concentration in blood is able to bind the cyanide released from approximately 18 mg of sodium nitroprusside.[11] Cyanide that exceeds this binding capacity is available for transport into tissues, particularly the liver and kidneys, where the mitochondrial enzyme rhodanase interacts with thiosulfate stores to catalyze conversion to thiocyanate. Thiocyanate is then removed slowly by renal filtration; its half-life is approximately 4 days but is prolonged in renal failure.[11] Endogenous thiosulfate stores are sufficient to detoxify approximately 50 mg of sodium nitroprusside in healthy subjects.[12, 13] Patients with low thiosulfate stores due to malnutrition or diuretics are not only theoretically but actually vulnerable to greater toxicity.[13] Toxicity is presumably due to free cyanide radical binding to mitochondrial cytochrome oxidase, with resultant cessation of transport along the electron transport chain, and of oxidative phosphorylation. An inevitable cellular reliance on anaerobic metabolism for the synthesis of ATP follows, with eventual accumulation of lactate generated by glycolysis. Although cyanide concentrations exceeding 40 μM are clearly associated with toxicity,[13] the clinical utility of measured levels is limited because of the difficulty of protecting samples from light[14] and the inevitable time delay (at least several hours) before concentrations can be reported.

Clinical Presentation and Management of Nitroprusside Toxicity

Severe nitroprusside toxicity due to cyanide presents with mental status changes, seizures, and

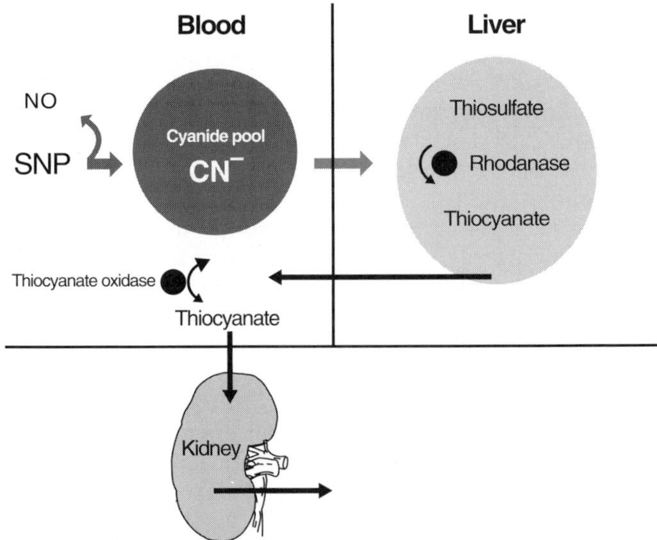

Figure 88–1. Human metabolism of nitroprusside. Nitroprusside delivered intravenously is metabolized primarily in the liver and kidneys by the enzyme rhodanase, which catalyzes the production of thiocyanate from thiosulfate and cyanide ion. Thiocyanate is subsequently removed from the body by renal filtration. SNP, sodium nitroprusside; CN, cyanide ion.

eventual coma; as cardiovascular instability in the form of arrhythmias and ST-T changes on the electrocardiogram (ECG); and with lactic acidosis. Although these symptoms occur late and neural toxicity (in the form of neuropathic symptoms, with nausea, weakness, tinnitus, muscle spasms, disorientation, and psychosis) may occur with low-level exposure, lactic acidosis as represented by an increasing anion gap is an important harbinger that many believe can serve as a surrogate for the intensity of cyanide exposure.[12, 15] Baud and colleagues[15] have shown that plasma lactate concentrations greater than 10 mM can serve as a sensitive indicator of cyanide intoxication, as defined by a coincident cyanide concentration exceeding 40 μM.

A reasoned clinical approach that incorporates the importance of acidosis, short-term infusion rate, and total drug infused has been proposed by Vesey and Cole,[16] who recommend bolus infusions of 25 mL of a 50% solution of sodium thiosulfate over 10 minutes for patients with acidosis, more than 1.5 mg/kg of nitroprusside in the short term, or an infusion rate of 4 μg/kg/min for more than 12 hours.[17] Although concurrent infusions of thiosulfate, in a 10:1 ratio with nitroprusside, effectively reduce serum and red blood cell concentrations of cyanide,[18] physicians should bear in mind that thiocyanate itself can produce toxic effects in high concentration[12, 19, 20]; therefore, this strategy may result in accumulation of toxic thiocyanate at high infusion rates and in patients with renal insufficiency. The use of prophylactic sodium thiosulfate has not been tested formally in clinical trials, but numerous case reports of its efficacy in treatment have been presented.[8] Administration of thiosulfate has been reported to be effective, even after complications occur.[18, 19]

If clinically important cyanide toxicity appears, the Cyanide Antidote Kit (Eli Lilly, Indianapolis, IN) is useful. It contains amyl nitrite and sodium nitrite designed to promote the conversion of hemoglobin to methemoglobin. Health care providers should be aware that rapid infusions of sodium nitrite can cause clinically important hypotension. *The use of intravenous methylene blue to treat cyanide-induced methemoglobinemia is contraindicated, because large quantities of cyanide may be liberated after the conversion of methemoglobin to hemoglobin.*

Hydroxocobalamin, an analogue of vitamin B_{12} (vitamin B_{12a}) has also been suggested as a safe and effective treatment for cyanide toxicity associated with the use of nitroprusside in animals and humans.[21] The mechanism used involves the replacement of the hydroxyl group of hydroxocobalamin by cyanide liberated from nitroprusside to form cyanocobalamin, which is vitamin B_{12}, which is then excreted in the urine.[22] Cottrell and colleagues[23] investigated the ability of nitroprusside infusions alone and in combination with a 25-mg/h concurrent infusion of hydroxocobalamin (100 mg in 100 mL of 5% dextrose in water) to produce cyanide toxicity in surgical patients. They observed a 60% reduction in erythrocyte cyanide concentrations in patients receiving combined nitroprusside/hydroxocobalamin therapy. These researchers recommend that hydroxocobalamin infusions be continued for 10 hours after the discontinuation of nitroprusside infusions, because the half-life of cyanide within erythrocytes is approximately 10 hours.[23]

During the use of nitroprusside, a high level of clinical suspicion for cyanide and thiosulfate toxicity is clearly warranted. Monitoring of the anion gap should be conducted particularly carefully if anemia, malnutrition, decreased renal function, or decreased hepatic function is identified. If the clinical suspicion for cyanide toxicity becomes high, anticyanide therapy in the form of amyl nitrite, thiosulfate, or hydroxocobalamin therapy should be considered. Simultaneously with the introduction of anticyanide therapy, use of various other agents, including labetalol and diazoxide, should be considered.

HYDRALAZINE

Although hydralazine is a commonly prescribed antihypertensive agent, reports of acute human poisoning are uncommon. Hydralazine is removed from the body primarily by hepatic acetylation.[24] Most of the literature focuses on chronic toxicity, most notably the drug-induced systemic lupus erythematosus syndrome, which occurs more commonly in slow acetylators.[25–27] Of note, a genetic test for the specific enzyme involved, *N*-acetyltransferase-2, has been developed[28, 29] to allow the prediction of whether a patient is a slower acetylator with a higher risk for hydralazine-induced lupus.

A case of acute hydralazine overdose associated with marked ST segment depression in the ECG of a young adult was reported.[30] Although the patient also had mild hypotension, acidemia, and ethanol intoxication, the ECG abnormality was alarming and suggestive of myocardial ischemia. The patient was treated conservatively in an intensive care unit setting, and the metabolic and ECG abnormalities resolved. Clinical and experimental data on acute hydralazine exposure suggest that the possibility of direct drug effects, including positive inotropic and chronotropic effects and myocardial cell injury, should be considered.

Acute hydralazine overdose usually results in profound hypotension. Treatment should be directed toward maintaining cerebral perfusion by placing patients in the Trendelenburg position and by aggressive use of intravenous fluids and of dopamine as a pressor. Because of the possibility that direct cardiac effects of hydralazine may result in arrhythmias, telemetry should be used and drugs with arrhythmogenic potential avoided.

MINOXIDIL

Minoxidil is useful as a systemic antihypertensive agent because it is a potent and relatively pure arterial vasodilator. It use in hypertension is confined to refractory cases, and its toxicity in overdose is primarily due to profound vasodilation and resultant hypotension. The most noticeable side effect of minoxidil therapy is hirsutism. In 1988, a 2% topical solution of minoxidil was approved for use in male pattern baldness and is now used by a large number of men and women. This preparation is currently among the top 200 drugs used in the United States, with annual sales of more than $100 million.

Toxic ingestions of the topical preparation have been reported. A 52-year-old man ingested 60 mL of 2% topical minoxidil solution, resulting in severe hypotension and tachycardia.[31] He was resuscitated with intravenously administered crystalloid solution and treated with intravenously administered dopamine, and this therapy resulted in a partial hemodynamic improvement. Further treatment with intravenously administered phenylephrine infusion resulted in resolution of hypotension. The patient suffered a non–Q wave myocardial infarction as a result of the ingestion. The toxicity of this increasingly common preparation is profound[32] and cannot be underestimated. Treatment in overdose should be directed toward maintaining cerebral perfusion by placing patients in the Trendelenburg position, with aggressive use of intravenous fluids and of dopamine as a pressor.

Toxicity of minoxidil tablets ingested in overdose appears similar. In 1992, a 20-year-old woman ingested an unknown quantity of minoxidil tablets as a suicide gesture.[33] She presented to the emergency department about 90 minutes later with tachycardia, diffuse T wave inversion, and ST segment depression on the ECG; labile hypotension; and a substantially elevated total serum minoxidil concentration of 3140 ng/mL. She responded to supportive therapy with intravenous fluids and was discharged 32 hours later with stable blood pressure and mild residual tachycardia. Slower resolution of symptoms might be expected in subjects with hepatic compromise, because minoxidil is cleared primarily by hepatic elimination.[34]

A particular toxicity associated with minoxidil has been fluid retention that presents more commonly in patients with renal failure and has been associated with pericardial effusion.[35] Alternative antihypertensive therapy seems appropriate in this context, with slow diuresis if necessary.

ANGIOTENSIN-CONVERTING ENZYME INHIBITORS

ACE inhibitors are widely used in therapeutics, and many nonpeptide angiotensin II receptor antagonists are being developed. The eight available ACE inhibitors are captopril (Capoten), enalapril (Vasotec) and its active metabolite enalaprilat (Vasotec injection), lisinopril (Prinivil, Zestril), benazepril (Lotensin), fosinopril (Monopril), quinapril (Accupril), ramipril (Altace), spirapril (Renormax), and moexipril (Univasc). Among these ACE inhibitors, only captopril and lisinopril are active compounds that require no metabolic conversion for their activity.[36] The other compounds require the cleavage of their ester moiety by hepatic esterases to produce the active form of the drug: enalaprilat, benazeprilat, or fosinoprilat. Poisoning and overdosage have been reported with captopril and enalapril in adults, children, and neonates.

The first reported case of captopril toxicity was an intentional ingestion by a 33-year-old woman who ingested an estimated oral dose of 500 to 750 mg of captopril together with 10 mg of alprazolam, leading to a plasma drug concentration of 5.9 mg/L of captopril 6 hours after ingestion.[37] When she was admitted to the hospital 5 hours later, her systolic blood pressure was 80 mm Hg, and this responded to intravenous fluids and dopamine at 10 μg/kg per minute within 30 minutes. Further episodes of hypotension occurred 18.5 and 24.5 hours after admission, but all responded to use of dopamine. Her blood pressure remained stable afterward throughout hospitalization, and no other symptoms developed.

Four cases of enalapril overdosage in adults are published. The first[38] was a deliberate oral ingestion of 300 mg of enalapril (between 8 and 30 times the usual dose range) and 225 mg of oxazepam by a 46-year-old hypertensive woman. She was found to have a peak enalaprilat serum concentration of 1.45 mg/L 10 hours after the ingestion. This was followed by hypotensive episodes (with a systolic blood pressure in the 80 to 100 mm Hg range and a diastolic blood pressure between 50 and 80 mm Hg) that improved with the infusion of intravenous plasma (250 mL) and saline (2 L over 24 hours). No further complications were observed, but although plasma ACE activity and angiotensin II returned to normal after 7 days, it took 3 weeks for the blood pressure to reach hypertensive values.

A subsequent report involved a 56-year-old woman who had congestive heart failure and who ingested 440 mg of enalapril with 42 mg of warfarin.[39] She presented with severe hypotension (blood pressure of 50/30 mm Hg) and became stuporous. She responded well to intravenous infusion of plasma and saline (6.8 L over 2 days), but renal dysfunction ensued. Serum enalaprilat concentration was 2.85 mg/L 15 hours after ingestion and remained above the normal range for about a week. Renal function gradually improved during the following week. The patient recovered from the overdose but died 40 days later of heart failure.

A third case was reported in a 66-year-old man who ingested 100 mg of enalapril. In this case, the outcome was uneventful apart from a moderate decrease in blood pressure that did not necessitate intravenous fluids. At 56 hours after the emergency, enalaprilat plasma levels were 5.7 ng/mL with a half-life of 7 hours. The terminal elimination half-life in this patient was approximately 36 hours,[40] as compared with 11 hours in normal patients.[41]

Jackson and colleagues reported a fourth case involving an overdose of 600 mg of enalapril together with 7200 mg of sustained-release verapamil and 100 mg of temazepam in a 46-year-old hypertensive man.[42] The patient presented alert and oriented but with a blood pressure of 75/40 mm Hg and a pulse of 40, in sinus rhythm. Central venous monitoring, infusion of dopamine (3 μg/kg per minute), and epinephrine (0.02 μg/kg per minute) were started. His blood pressure was then 80/50 mm Hg, his pulse was 40, and he had a junctional rhythm and oliguria. Electrolytes were unremarkable, with a blood urea nitrogen value of 9.1 mmol/L and creatinine level of 231 μmol/L. It was conjectured that oliguria was due to a profound lack of glomerular arterial tone, and infusion of angiotensin was started at 3 μg/min and increased to 18 μg/min for the first 3 hours, then to 5 μg/min for 2 hours. His urine output increased dramatically, his blood pressure improved, and his cardiac rhythm returned to normal. These variables remained stable despite enalaprilat concentrations of 0.26 mg/L 12 hours after discontinuation of the infusion.

A retrospective case study of ACE inhibitor ingestion in children age 5 years or younger did not show any important clinical effect.[43] Forty-eight cases were identified, involving doses up to 300 mg of captopril or 30 mg of enalapril. Twenty cases were treated in the hospital with ipecac syrup, 7 were treated similarly by parents at home, 16 were only observed by parents at home, and 5 were unavailable for follow-up. Apart from treatment-induced vomiting, all patients remained asymptomatic.

The use of dialysis has been proposed for reversal of acute renal failure that developed in a neonate whose mother received enalapril for pregnancy-induced hypertension. Because the neonate developed anuria, peritoneal dialysis was started 60 hours after birth and discontinued after 10 days when diuresis exceeded 1 mL/kg per hour. Enalapril levels decreased from 28 ng/mL before dialysis to less than 0.16 ng/mL after dialysis. However, serum creatinine and plasma renin levels remained elevated until the age of 3 months.[44]

In conclusion, ACE inhibitor overdosage seems to induce episodes of hypotension that are remarkably responsive to the infusion of fluids, as well as dopamine when necessary. The usually favorable evolution of the overdosage, independently of the underlying condition, renders the need for dialysis unlikely. It is important to note that both captopril and enalaprilat are dialysable, should the need arise.

α-ADRENERGIC BLOCKERS

Although the most clinically relevant effects of α-adrenergic stimulation are observed in the cardiovascular system, actions on both the central nervous system and the periphery are also important. The stimulation of α-adrenergic receptors in vascular smooth muscle cells is responsible for maintaining peripheral vascular resistances and is critical to the maintenance of blood pressure during postural changes. Agents that block the α_1-adrenergic receptor are widely used in the treatment of essential hypertension and include prazosin, doxazosin, and terazosin. Yohimbine is the only selective α_2-antagonist available, whereas phentolamine is an α-blocker that has similar affinity for both α_1- and α_2-adrenergic receptors. The use of phentolamine is confined to the management of pheochromocytoma.

Prazosin

Prazosin is an arterial dilator that operates via blockade of postsynaptic α-adrenergic receptors in vascular smooth muscle cells. The major toxicity with prazosin is related to severe sudden hypotension, often referred to as *first-dose phenomenon,* at the initiation of treatment. Fluid retention is also common. More than 90% of an administered dose of prazosin is metabolized in the liver, and the mean elimination half-life is approximately 3 hours in healthy volunteers.[45] It follows that inadvertent hypotension is more likely to occur in individuals with poor liver function, advanced age, or congestive heart failure.

Four cases reports of overdose related to prazosin are published in the literature. They include a 19-year-old man who ingested 200 mg of prazosin[46] and experienced tachycardia of 140 bpm with hypotension of 95/60 mm Hg (resting in bed for 36 hours permitted recovery); a 25-year old man who took 150 mg of prazosin[47] and had priapism that led to a cavernospongiosum shunt with a late recovery; a 75-year-old man who ingested 80 mg of drug and recovered from drowsiness and hypotension 18 hours after gastric lavage, charcoal administration, and intravenous fluids;[48] and a 72-year-old man who ingested 120 mg of prazosin and experienced severe hypotension, coma with Cheyne-Stokes respiration, respiratory failure with pulmonary edema, and acidosis. He was treated with dopamine, angiotensin, atropine, intravenous fluids, and ventilation in an intensive care unit, and he recovered after 48 hours.[49]

Headache, vertigo, paresthesia, and weakness have been reported with α_1-antagonist overdose.[50] Other neuropsychiatric effects have been described in patients with chronic renal failure, such as confusion, visual hallucinations, paranoia, or uninhibited behavior.[50] Dyspnea, nasal congestion, gastrointestinal symptoms, and sweating could also be noted in cases of prazosin overdose. Of note, physicians should be particularly careful in situations in which an α_1-antagonist is coadministered with verapamil, because the effect on blood pressure appears synergistic.[51]

Terazosin and Doxazosin

Experience with these two drugs is limited, and no report of overdosage has been published. Hypotension usually follows overdosage and can be severe enough to induce collapse, but postural hypotension can also occur during standard treatment and may be sudden and unexpected, leading to syncope.

In general, the hypotensive effects of α-blockers are exacerbated by coadministration of other drugs that cause hypotension.[50] Monitoring of blood pressure, cardiac rhythm, and urine output is indicated for at least 48 hours, after use of gastric lavage or activated charcoal or both if necessary. Hypotension should be corrected by supine position with leg raising; intravenous fluids, plasma expanders, and atropine may be required. Epinephrine should be avoided because of a possible β-adrenergic–mediated vasodilation. Because α-blockers are highly bound to plasma protein, hemodialysis or hemoperfusion is of little help. Decreasing gastrointestinal absorption and correction of hypotension with intravenous fluids usually enable a full recovery within 48 hours.

DIURETICS

Diazoxide

The early clinical development of oral diazoxide preparations was complicated by its most common side effects: hyperglycemia and hypertrichosis. Pancreatitis and hypertrophic cardiomyopathy[52] with prolonged use have also been reported.

The drug has been used succesfully in parenteral formulations in the treatment of hypertensive emergencies, but prolonged use clearly can result in hyperglycemia with hyperosmolar coma[53] or acute ketoacidosis.[54] Although diazoxide remains a rational therapeutic alternative, because of difficulty with blood pressure monitoring, its use has largely been replaced by use of sodium nitoprusside and labetalol. This is largely because of the greater control over blood pressure that is possible with the latter two drugs. One study conducted between 1975 and 1985 documented the care of 454 children who presented with severely raised blood pressures deemed to require emergency management in a pediatric renal unit.[55] At presentation, 84 of 110 had symptoms and signs of long-standing hypertension with neurologic involvement. Between 1975 and 1980, bolus intravenous injections of diazoxide or hydralazine or both were used with the aim of reducing the blood pressure to within the normal range for age in the first 12 to 24 hours after admission. Of 57 patients treated in this way, 13 developed hypotensive complications, and 4, whose blood pressures returned to normal within 24 hours of admission, suffered irreversible neurologic damage. After 1980, the management changed to the use of intravenous infusions of labetalol (1 to 3 mg/kg per hour) or sodium nitroprusside (0.5 to 8 μg/kg per minute) or both to enable a more gradual controlled reduction of blood pressure during the first 96 hours of admission. Between 1980 and 1985, 53 patients were treated using this regimen. In all cases, blood pressure reduction was achieved in a more controlled manner without further neurologic impairment or serious irreversible side effects.

Uremic patients are vulnerable to enhanced hypotensive effects of diazoxide, because concentrations of free drug are greater when a significant proportion of diazoxide is displaced from serum albumin by nonspecific factors present in uremic blood. Diazoxide overdose is generally managed with positional preservation of cerebral perfusion, administration of half-normal saline, and careful attention to glucose concentrations, with the use of insulin if necessary. Because diazoxide in the oral form has a serum half-life of between 24 and 36 hours and this may be prolonged after overdosage or in patients with impaired renal function, lengthy monitoring may be necessary.

Thiazides

Acute intoxication as a result of thiazide diuretics is extremely rare. The most frequent adverse effect by far is hypokalemia, which is usually treated by potassium supplementation or by the addition of a potassium-sparing agent such as triamterene. Drug-induced acute pancreatitis has been associated with thiazide therapy,[56] as has choroidal effusion, transient myopia,[57] and a single case of acute angle-closure glaucoma.[58]

Potassium-Retaining Compounds

These drugs include amiloride, spironolactone, and triamterene. Their most important toxicity is potassium retention itself, with hyperkalemia and its attendant cardiac risks. Renal dysfunction predisposes to this form of hyperkalemia, as does diabetes. Hyperkalemia should be managed with saline hydration and loop diuretics, with orally administered cation exchange resins (e.g., sodium polystyrene sulfate, or Kayexelate) if necessary. Exchange resins should be administered as soon as possible, because their onset of action is 1 to 2 hours after administration.

Triamterene has for some time been associated with nephrolithiasis,[59] but a review of urinary stone analyses performed during the past decade by a single laboratory revealed an increasing incidence of triamterene stones. This study group recommend that awareness of the calculogenic potential of triamterene-containing medications be re-emphasized. Spironolactone has well-documented endocrine effects that result in gynecomastia, as well as occasional amenorrhea with prolonged use.

Loop Diuretics

Loop diuretics include furosemide, bumetanide, and ethacrynic acid. The major toxicities of these drugs are arrhythmogenic hypokalemia[60] and ototoxicity.[61] Loop diuretics may induce hypokalemia, hypocalcemia, and hypomagnesemia. Although severe hypokalemia may cause muscle weakness, severe hypomagnesemia is associated with muscle spasms and tetany, which cannot be corrected by potassium and calcium supplementation alone. These electrolyte changes can be managed by careful replacement during cardiac telemetry monitoring in situations in which the serum potassium concentration declines below 3.5 mM or when other risks for cardiac arrythmia are a factor.

Transient or permanent loss of hearing due to these drugs is well described. Animal experiments show that these drugs act on the stria vascularis, producing edema of these tissues and loss of function, resulting in a decrease of the endocochlear potential. Animal data indicate that the risk of ototoxicity may be increased in hypoalbuminemia, when the access of unbound furosemide to its site of ototoxic action in the cochlea may be improved.[62] Short of discontinuation of the drug, no current therapy is available.[61]

In addition to these toxicities, thiamine deficiency as a result of prolonged furosemide use has been well described in patients with congestive heart failure. These patients have been shown to benefit from thiamine replacement.[63] Chronic furosemide use has also been associated with a 3.9-fold increase in adjusted risk for hip fracture in elderly patients.[64]

References

1. Joint National Committee on Detection: The Fifth Report of the Joint National Committee on Detection, Evaluation and Treatment of High Blood Pressure (JNCV). Arch Intern Med *153:*154–183, 1993.
2. Avorn J, Soumerai SB: Improving drug therapy decisions through educational outreach. A randomized, controlled trial of academically-based "detailing". N Engl J Med *308:*1457–1461, 1983.
3. Page IH, Corcoran AC, Dustan HP, Koppanyi T: Cardiovascular actions of sodium nitroprusside in animals and hypertensive patients. Circulation *11:*188–198, 1955.
4. Kowaluk EA, Seth P, Fung HL: Metabolic activation of sodium nitroprusside to nitric oxide in vascular smooth muscle. J Pharmacol Exp Ther *262:*916–922, 1992.
5. Ignarro LJ: Biologic actions and properties of endothelium-derived nitric oxide formed and released from artery and vein. Circ Res *65:*1–21, 1989.
6. Johnson CC: Mechanisms of actions and toxicity of nitroprusside. Proc Soc Exp Biol Med *26:*102–103, 1928.
7. Smith RP, Kruszyna H: Nitroprusside produces cyanide poisoning via reaction with hemoglobin. J Pharmacol Exp Ther *191:*557–563, 1974.
8. Robin ED, McCauley R: Nitroprusside-related cyanide poisoning. Time (long past due) for urgent, effective interventions. Chest *102:*1842–1845, 1992.
9. Sarvotham SS: Nitroprusside therapy in post-open heart hypertensives. A ritual tryst with cyanide death? Letter. Chest *91:*796, 1987.
10. Food and Drug Administration: New labelling for sodium nitroprusside emphasised risk of cyanide toxicity. JAMA *265:*847, 1991.
11. Hall VA, Guest JM: Sodium nitroprusside-induced cyanide intoxication and prevention with sodium thiosulfate prophylaxis. Am J Crit Care *1:*19–27, 1992.
12. Friedrich JA, Butterworth JF: Sodium nitroprusside: Twenty years and counting. Anesth Analg *81:*152–162, 1995.
13. Curry SC, Arnold-Capell P: Toxic effects of drugs used in the ICU: Nitroprusside, nitroglycerin and angiotensin converting enzyme inhibitors. Crit Care Clin *7:*555–581, 1991.
14. Bisset WI, Butler AR, Glidewell C, Reglinski J: Sodium nitroprusside and cyanide release: Reasons for re-appraisal. Br J Anaesth *53:*1015–1018, 1981.
15. Baud FJ, Barriot P, Toffis V, et al: Elevated blood cyanide concentrations in victims of smoke inhalation. N Engl J Med *325:*1761–1766, 1991.
16. Vesey PV, Cole CJ: Sodium thiosulphate decreases blood cyanide concentrations after the infusion of sodium nitroprusside. Br J Anaesth *59:*531–537, 1987.
17. Vesey CJ, Cole PV: Blood cyanide and thiocyanate concentrations produced by long-term therapy with sodium nitroprusside. Br J Anaesth *57:*148–155, 1985.
18. Schulz V, Gross R, Russe J, Loescheke G: Cyanide toxicity of sodium nitroprusside in therapeutic use with and without sodium thiosulfate. Klin Wochenschr *60:*1393–1400, 1982.
19. Schulz V: Clinical pharmacokinetics of nitroprusside, cyanide, thiosulfate and thiocyanate. Clin Pharmacokinet *9:*239–251, 1984.
20. Wald MH, Lindberg HA, Barker MH: The toxic manifestations of the thiocyanates. JAMA *112:*1120–1126, 1939.
21. Zerbe NF, Wagner BK: Use of vitamin B_{12} in the treatment and prevention of nitroprusside-induced cyanide toxicity. Crit Care Med *21:*465–467, 1993.
22. Posner MA, Tobey RE, McElroy H: Hydroxocobalamin therapy of cyanide intoxication in guinea pigs. Anesthesiology *44:*157–160, 1976.
23. Cottrell JE, Casthely P, Brodie JD: Prevention of nitroprusside-induced cyanide toxicity with hydroxocobalamin. N Engl J Med *298:*809–811, 1978.
24. Reidenberg MM, Drayer D, Demarco A, Bello CT: Hydralazine elimination in man. Clin Pharmacol Ther *14:*970–976, 1973.
25. Timbrell JA, Faccini V, Harland SJ, Mansilla-Tinoco R: Hydralazine-induced lupus: Is there a toxic, metabolic pathway? Eur J Clin Pharmacol *27:*555–559, 1984.
26. Russel GI, Bing RF, Jones JA, et al: Hydralazine sensitivity: Clinical features, autoantibody changes and HLA-DR phenotype. Q J Med *65:*845–852, 1987.
27. Sturman SG, Kumararatne D, Deevers DG: Fatal hydralazine-induced systemic lupus erythematosus. Lancet *2:*1304, 1988.
28. Blum M, Grant DM, McBride W, et al: Human arylamine *N*-acetyltransferase genes: Isolation, chromosomal localization, and functional expression. DNA Cell Biol *9:*193–203, 1990.
29. Hickman D, Sim E: *N*-acetyltransferase polymorphism: Comparison of genotype and phenotype in humans. Biochem Pharmacol *42:*1007–1014, 1991.
30. Smith BA, Ferguson DB: Acute hydralazine overdose: Marked ECG abnormalities in a young adult. Ann Emerg Med *21:*326–330, 1992.
31. McCormick MA, Forman MH, Manoguerra AS: Severe toxicity from ingestion of a topical minoxidil preparation. Am J Emerg Med *7:*419–421, 1989.
32. MacMillan AR, Warshawski FJ, Steinberg RA: Minoxidil overdose. Chest *103:*1290–1291, 1993.
33. Poff SW, Rose SR: Minoxidil overdose with ECG changes: Case report and review. J Emerg Med *10:*53–57, 1992.
34. Gottlieb TB, Thomas RC, Chindsey CA: Pharmacokinetic studies of minoxidil. Clin Pharmacol Ther *13:*436–440, 1972.
35. Zarate A, Gelfand MC, Horton JD, et al: Pericardial effusion associated with minoxidil therapy in dialyzed patients. Int J Artif Organs *3:*15, 1980.
36. Jackson EK, Garrison JC: Renin and angiotensin. *In* Hardman JG, Limbird LE, Molinoff RW, et al (eds): Goodman and Gilman's The Pharmacologic Basis of Therapeutics. New York, McGraw Hill Book Co., pp 733–758, 1996.
37. Augenstein WL, Kulig KW, Rumack BH: Captopril overdose resulting in hypotension. JAMA *259:*3302–3305, 1988.
38. Waeber B, Nussberger J, Brunner HR: Self poisoning with enalapril. BMJ *288:*287–288, 1984.
39. Lau CP: Attempted suicide with enalapril. N Engl J Med *315:*197, 1986.
40. Varughese A, Taylor AA: Consequences of angiotensin-converting enzyme imhibitor overdose. Am J Hypertens *2:*355–357, 1989.

41. Todd PA, Heel RC: Enalapril: A review of its pharmacodynamic and pharmacokinetic properties, and therapeutic use in hypertension and congestive heart failure. Drugs *31:*198–248, 1986.
42. Jackson T, Corke C, Agar J: Enalapril overdose treated with angiotensin infusion. Lancet *341:*703–705, 1993.
43. Spiller HA, Udicious TM, Muir S: Angiotensin converting enzyme inhibitor ingestion in children. J Toxicol *27:*345–353, 1989.
44. Schubiger G, Flury G, Nussberger J: Enalaphil for pregnancy-induced hypertension: Acute renal failure in a neonate. Ann Intern Med *108:*215–216, 1988.
45. Bateman DN, Hobbs DC, Twomey TM, et al: Prazosin pharmacokinetics and concentration effect. Eur J Clin Pharmacol *16:*177–181, 1979.
46. McLean WJ: Prazosin overdose. Med J Aust *1:*592, 1976.
47. Robbins DN, Crawford D, Lackner LH: Priapism secondary to prazosin overdose. J Urol *130:*957, 1983.
48. Rygnestad TK, Dale O: Self-poisoning with prazosin. Acta Med Scand *213:*157–158, 1983.
49. Lenz K, Druml W, Kleinberger G, et al: Acute intoxication with prazosin: Case report. Hum Toxicol *4:*53–56, 1985.
50. Gyh L, Re F: Poisoning with anti-hypertensive drugs: Alpha-adrenoceptor antagonists. J Hum Hypertens *9:*523–526, 1995.
51. Meredith PA, Elliot HL: An additive or synergistic drug interaction: Application of concentration-effect modeling. Clin Pharmacol Ther *51:*708–714, 1992.
52. Parker JJ, Allen DB: Hypertrophic cardiomyopathy after prolonged diazoxide therapy for hyperinsulinemic hypoglycemia. J Pediatr *118:*906–909, 1991.
53. Harrison BDW, Rutter TW, Taylor RT: Severe non-ketotic hyperglycaemic pre-coma in a hypertensive patient receiving diazoxide. Lancet *2:*599–561, 1972.
54. Updike ST, Harrington AR: Acute diabetic ketoacidosis—a complication of intravenous diazoxide treatment for refractory hypertension. N Engl J Med *280:*768–771, 1969.
55. Deal JE, Barrat TM, Dillon MJ: Management of hypertensive emergencies. Arch Dis Child *67:*1089–1092, 1992.
56. Lankisch PG, Droge M, Gottesleben F: Drug induced acute pancreatitis: Incidence and severity. Gut *37:*565–567, 1995.
57. Soylev MF, Green RL, Feldon SE: Choroidal effusion as a mechanism for transient myopia induced by hydrochlorothiazide and triamterene. Arch Opthalmol *120:*395–397, 1995.
58. Geanon JD, Perkins TW: Bilateral acute angle closure glaucoma associated with drug sensitivity to hydrochlorothiazide. Arch Opthalmol *113:*1231–1232, 1995.
59. Carr MC, Prien ELJ, Babayan RK: Triamterene nephrolithiasis: Renewed attention is warranted. J Urol *144:*1339–1340, 1990.
60. Chvilicek JP, Hurlbert BJ, Hill GE: Diuretic-induced hypokalemia inducing torsades de pointes. Can J Anaesth *42:*1137–1139, 1995.
61. Rybak LP: Ototoxicity of loop diuretics. Otolaryngol Clin North Am *26:*829–844, 1993.
62. Whitworth C, Morris C, Scott V, Rybak LP: Dose-response relationships for furosemide ototoxicity in rat. Heart Res *71:*202–207, 1993.
63. Shimon I, Almog S, Vered Z, et al: Improved left ventricular function after thiamine supplementation in patients with congestive heart failure receiving long-term furosemide therapy. Am J Med *98:*485–490, 1995.
64. Heidrich FE, Stergachis A, Gross KM: Diuretic use and the risk for hip fracture. Ann Intern Med *115:*1–6, 1991.

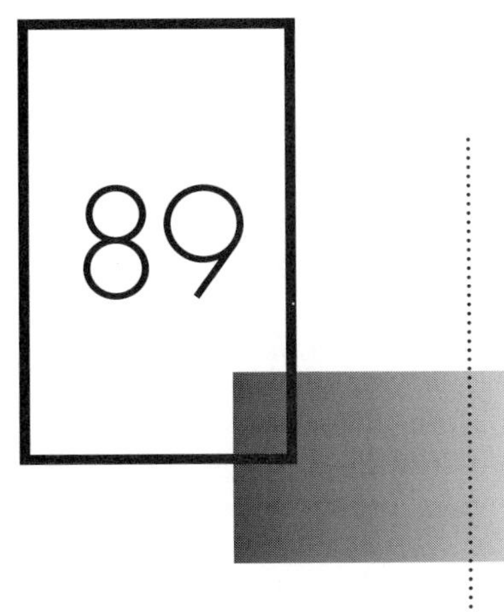

Clonidine and Related Imidazoline Derivatives

JAMES F. WILEY II, MD

Clonidine and the related drugs, guanabenz, guanfacine, methyldopa, oxymetazoline, naphazoline, xylometazoline, and tetrahydrozoline, share similar toxicity. Clonidine, guanabenz, guanfacine, and methyldopa have been used primarily as antihypertensive medications, although new indications have recently been developed for clonidine and guanfacine. Oxymetazoline, tetrahydrozoline, naphazoline, and xylometazoline are topical vasoconstrictors for application to the nasal mucous membranes and are found in many over-the-counter nasal drops and sprays. Tetrahydrozoline is also found in over-the-counter eye drops. Most of the severe toxicity reactions attributable to this class of drugs have occurred with clonidine.

Clonidine was initially developed as a topical nasal decongestant in 1962. It was subsequently found to be a potent antihypertensive agent, with sympatholytic effects not attributable to ganglionic blocking.[1] Clonidine is synergistic in antihypertensive effect with diuretics and has been employed as a second or third agent in the treatment of essential hypertension. Recently, the introduction of converting enzyme inhibitors has resulted in decreased use of clonidine as an antihypertensive agent. Alternative indications in adults include the induction of spinal anesthesia, the ultra-short detoxification of opiate dependence, alcohol withdrawal, smoking cessation, and alleviation of postmenopausal hot flashes.[2–5] In children, clonidine is being used for the treatment of refractory attention deficit disorder with hyperactivity, conduct disorder, and Gilles de la Tourette syndrome and as a provocative agent for the diagnosis of growth hormone deficiency.[6–8] Recently, guanfacine has been evaluated for the treatment of children with both attention deficit disorder with hyperactivity and Tourette syndrome[9] and has been shown to induce growth hormone secretion without the concomitant hypotension or sedation common with clonidine.[10]

Clonidine exposure is responsible for approximately 1 in 1000 poisonings and is notable for serious signs and symptoms following many ingestions.[11, 12] Children are especially susceptible to the toxic effects of clonidine, with as little as one 0.1-mg tablet causing major signs and symptoms.[13] Exposure to over-the-counter nose drops and eye drops containing other imidazolines is more frequent than exposure to clonidine but tends to be uneventful.[14] Guanabenz, guanfacine, and methyldopa are rarely prescribed or ingested and appear to cause similar but lesser effects than clonidine.[15–17]

PHARMACOLOGY

Chemical Identification and Structure

Clonidine, guanabenz, guanfacine, oxymetazoline, tetrahydrozoline, naphazoline, and xylometazoline are related imidazolines with central and peripheral α_2-adrenergic agonist effects. In addition, some of the central antihypertensive effects may be attributable to binding of specific imidazoline receptors. As sympathomimetic agents, imidazolines have little or no β-adrenergic effect and have peripheral vasoconstrictive properties similar to those of specific α_1-adrenergic agonists. However, imidazolines differ markedly from most sympathomimetics in their central inhibition of sympathetic outflow.[18] Methyldopa, which was developed as an analogue of 3,4-dihydroxyphenylalanine (DOPA), is chemically unrelated to the imidazolines but stimulates α_2-adrenergic receptors centrally through its metabolite, α-methyl norepinephrine.[19]

Pharmacokinetics

Clonidine is available in 0.025- (Dixarit, United Kingdom), 0.1-, 0.2-, and 0.3-mg tablets (Catapres) and in combination with chlorthalidone (Combipres). Rapid absorption follows oral administration of clonidine, with drug bioavailability of 75% to 96% after a single oral dose.[20] Bioavailability falls with chronic administration to 65%.[21] Maximal hypotensive effect coincides with peak plasma concentration 1 to 3 hours after ingestion. Therapeutic clonidine levels range from 0.5 to 2 ng/ml, with a close relationship between plasma concentration and clinical effects.[19] Clonidine is 20% to 40% protein bound and has a volume of distribution of 2.9 to 5.3 L/k.[19, 20] It undergoes hepatic metabolism to inactive compounds, but approximately half of a single oral dose is excreted unchanged in the urine. The elimination half-life is 12 to 16 hours and is prolonged in patients with renal insufficiency, often necessitating decreased dosing.[22] In preoperative patients, clonidine may be given sublingually or rectally, with pharmacokinetics similar to oral administration.[23, 24]

A patch formulation of clonidine is available in dosages of 2.5 mg, 5.0 mg, and 7.5 mg. These systems provide a constant rate of transdermal clonidine administration over 7 days. Maximum plasma concentration occurs 2 to 3 days after application and peaks at 0.1 to 0.5 ng/ml. Elimination half-life ranges from 26 to 55 hours while the patch is applied. Drug delivery varies by application site, with the highest absorption from the left arm and the lowest from the thigh.[25] From 20% to 75% of residual clonidine may remain in the patch after 7 days of use.[26]

The pharmacology of guanfacine and guanabenz relative to clonidine is shown in Table 89–1. Naphazoline, tetrahydrozoline, oxymetazoline, and xylometazoline are approved and intended only for topical use, so pharmacokinetic data based on ingestion are not available.

Significant drug interactions are rare with imidazolines. Three sudden deaths were reported in children taking the combination of clonidine and methylphenidate for attention deficit disorder with hyperactivity. However, circumstances in each case led the United States Food and Drug Administration to conclude that both clonidine and methylphenidate have potential cardiotoxicity, but no convincing evidence exists for a lethal drug interaction involving these two medications.[27, 28] Cyclic antidepressants potentially interfere with the antihypertensive effect of clonidine. Klonopin (clonazepam) and clonidine sound alike and one may be inadvertently mistaken for the other.

A withdrawal syndrome can occur after sudden cessation of clonidine. This state is characterized by hypertension, tachycardia, sweating, anxiety, insomnia, abdominal pain, nausea, and palpitations. Rarely, clonidine withdrawal can cause malignant hypertension and cardiac dysrhythmias in patients with heart disease. Withdrawal occurs 1 to 3 days after the abrupt termination of chronic clonidine therapy and coincides with elevated urine and plasma catecholamine levels.[29, 30] Patients on concomitant β-blocker therapy at the time clonidine is stopped are at higher risk of serious effects. Reinstitution of clonidine therapy usually suffices to treat clonidine withdrawal, but occasionally patients may require nitroprusside infusion for control of hypertension.[31] Use of β-blockers should be avoided since they could produce unopposed α-adrenergic effects that may worsen hypertension in the setting of withdrawal. Abrupt cessation of guanabenz and guanfacine therapy may also cause mild withdrawal symptoms but to a lesser degree than clonidine.[32]

Pharmacodynamics, Mechanism of Action, and Toxicity

The imidazolines produce effects by a complex interaction with central α_2-adrenoceptors, peripheral α_2-adrenoceptors, and central imidazoline receptors. Elucidation of the receptor-binding properties for the drugs under discussion have involved radioligand studies using [^{3}H]clonidine. Clonidine strongly binds to central α_2-adrenergic receptors located in the brain stem (nucleus tractus solitarii). This binding has a central inhibitory effect on norepinephrine release, resulting in decreased sympathetic outflow.[33–35] Therapeutically, this action causes bradycardia, sedation, and reduced blood pressure. The hypotensive changes are not seen in quadriplegic patients who receive clonidine.[33] Clonidine also inhibits acetylcholine release. Clinically, this effect is manifest as dry mouth in therapeutic doses. In the hypothalamus,

Table 89–1. Pharmacokinetics of Clonidine, Guanfacine, and Guanabenz

Drug	Bioavailability (%)	T_{max} (hr)	$T_{1/2}$ (hr)	Vd (L/kg)	Protein Binding (%)	Elimination
Clonidine	75–96	1–3	12–16	3–5	20–40	Renal
Clonidine patch	25–80*	40–80	26–55	3–5	20–40	Renal
Guanfacine[54, 55]	95–100	1–3	17–24	4–6	20–30	Renal
Guanabenz[14, 56]	75	2–5	7–14	7–17	90	Hepatic

*After 7 days 20% to 75% of drug remains in the patch.[23]

clonidine stimulates the release of growth hormone and has varying effects on sympathetic tone and blood pressure. In the spinal cord, clonidine decreases sympathetic tone and blood pressure and has analgesic properties that are similar to narcotic medications.[33, 36]

The similarity in effects found on stimulation of central α_2-adrenergic receptors and opiate receptors has prompted much investigation into a possible molecular link between these sites. Clinical evidence supporting such a link include the use of clonidine for ultra-short detoxification of opiate dependence,[3] the successful use of clonidine for spinal analgesia,[36] the similarity of toxicity found after overdose with narcotics and clonidine, the reversal of clonidine toxicity with naloxone in some patients,[12] and the decreased density of central α_2-adrenergic receptors in heroin addicts.[37] Both opiate and central α_2-adrenergic receptors act through G proteins. The possibility of "cross-talk" between these receptors through the G protein complex has been raised, although initial studies in a neuroblastoma–glioma cell line were not supportive.[38] Another unproved theory suggests that clonidine may incompletely bind to opiate receptors. Improved understanding concerning the relationship of central α_2-adrenergic and opiate receptors must await further study.

Peripheral imidazoline effects are varied, relate to agonist effects at α_2-adrenergic receptors, and are usually overshadowed by central α_2-adrenergic receptor effects. Agonist activity at postsynaptic peripheral α_2-adrenergic receptors located in some blood vessels causes vasoconstriction. This action explains why intravenous administration of clonidine and supratherapeutic levels of clonidine are associated with hypertension and pallor in some patients. Stimulation of presynaptic peripheral α_2-adrenergic receptors, however, reduces vasomotor tone in other blood vessel sites and inhibits renin release, which would lead to synergism with central effects.[33] The net effect is a reduction of blood pressure and sympathetic outflow in both hypertensive and normotensive patients who receive clonidine.

Specific imidazoline (I) receptors of multiple types have been identified in a variety of tissues and animal species. Current nomenclature delineates I1 and I2 receptors, with a further breakdown of I2 receptors into I2a (amiloride-sensitive) and I2b (amiloride-insensitive).[39] These receptors do not act through G proteins.[40] Clonidine has strong affinity at I1 receptors, which are located in the ventrolateral medulla in humans. Binding at these sites leads to decrease in blood pressure independent of central α_2-adrenergic effects.[41] An endogenous substance with imidazoline receptor affinity, called clonidine displacing substance, has also been discovered, but its physiologic role has yet to be elucidated. Guanabenz is an agonist at I2 imidazoline receptors, which are strongly linked to MAO-A and MAO-B expression, but the mechanism of action and function of I2 receptors are uncertain and require further study.[42]

CLINICAL PRESENTATION

Pathophysiology

In overdose, the sympatholytic effects of imidazolines predominate. The organs most commonly affected are the brain and the heart. Decreased norepinephrine release in the central nervous system causes lethargy, coma, miosis, hypotonia, respiratory depression, apnea, and hypothermia.[11, 12] Cardiac consequences of imidazoline toxicity include bradycardia (sinus or first-degree atrioventricular [AV] block) and hypotension related to central α_2-adrenergic and imidazoline receptor stimulation.[11, 12] Peripheral α_2-adrenergic effects may cause vasoconstriction with hypertension. Rarely, malignant hypertension and seizures occur, particularly in patients with renal insufficiency who ingest large doses of clonidine.[43] Children are particularly sensitive to the toxic effects of the imidazolines. As little as 0.1 mg of clonidine or 2.5 mL (1/2 teaspoon) of 0.05% tetrahydrozoline eye drops has caused significant toxicity.[13, 44]

Manifestations

Clinical findings of clonidine and other imidazoline poisoning appear soon after ingestion. In one series of clonidine poisoning in children, 75% of patients had signs of toxicity within 1 hour of ingestion, and no new findings occurred in any patients more than four hours after poisoning.[12] Topical imidazoline exposure by unintentional oral ingestion or nasal administration in infants and young children can cause lethargy and coma within 1 hour.[45] Close observation of patients who ingest imidazolines is imperative because of the potential for rapid decompensation.

The relative frequencies of clinical findings in children and adults with clonidine poisoning are shown in Table 89–2. Lethargy and coma universally accompany serious clonidine toxicity and occur soon after ingestion. Miosis, hyporeflexia, and hypotonia are common associated findings, particularly in children. This constellation of neurologic findings closely mimics opiate toxicity. Frequently, pediatric patients with clonidine intoxication and coma have transient responsiveness to painful stimuli, such as intravenous line placement or phlebotomy, but quickly revert back to profound central nervous system depression. Irritability, dilated pupils, and the presence of a Babinski sign occur less frequently in children and are rarely seen in adults.

Bradycardia and hypotension follow clonidine ingestion in approximately one third of children and one half of adults. Sinus bradycardia is the most common rhythm in these patients, with first-degree AV block seen occasionally. Though complete AV block and supraventricular tachycardia complicated clonidine ingestion in a 22-year-old woman with systemic lupus erythematosus and renal insufficiency,[46] second-degree block or complete AV dissociation should prompt the consideration of toxicity from

Table 89–2. Frequency of Clinical Findings in Children and Adults after Clonidine Poisoning*

Finding	Children (<10 ys)	Adults (>18 ys)
No. of patients	180	37
Central Nervous System		
Lethargy/coma	87%	78%
Miosis	16%	3%
Hypotonia	12%	2%
Irritability	11%	1%
Hyporeflexia	10%	1%
Unreactive pupils	6%	—
Babinski sign present	4%	—
Mydriasis	4% (2/47)	—
Cardiovascular System		
Bradycardia	32%	49%
Hypotension	25%	32%
Arrhythmia	11%	—
Hypertension	7%	11%
Cardiac arrest	0%	3%
Respiratory System		
Respiratory depression	16%	5%
Apnea	7%	—
Other Findings		
Pallor	22%	16%
Hypothermia	17% (8/47)	—
Dry mouth	2%	11%

*Data from Stein B, Volans GM: Dixarit overdose: The problem of attractive tablets. BMJ *2*:667–668, 1978; and Wiley JF II, Wiley CC, Torrey SB, Henretig FM: Clonidine poisoning in young children. J Pediatr *116*:654–658, 1990. Age-specific definitions of bradycardia, hypotension, and hypertension were used for pediatric findings.

other drugs, such as digoxin, calcium channel blockers, or β-adrenergic blockers. Hypotension may be quite profound but usually responds readily to rapid intravenous fluid administration.[12] Hypertension is associated with a large ingested dose of clonidine and is usually transient.[47] Severe hypertension with encephalopathy or seizures attributed to clonidine exposure has been described in a patient with renal insufficiency.[43] Hypertension may also be precipitated by naloxone administration.[12, 48] Cardiac arrests have been described in adults with clonidine poisoning, but not in children.[11]

Apnea and respiratory depression occur more commonly after clonidine exposure in children but also complicate clonidine poisoning in adults. In many patients, the degree of respiratory compromise necessitates endotracheal intubation. Stimulation of the pediatric patient often increases respiratory rate and effort transiently. This finding may be useful in differentiating apnea caused by clonidine poisoning from the apnea associated with opiate intoxication. Occasional findings with clonidine intoxication include dry mouth, hypothermia, and pallor. The duration of symptoms following ingestion of clonidine tablets is less than 24 hours, with an averaged reported duration of 9 to 16 hours.[11, 12] To date, no deaths have been reported in children or adults who have ingested clonidine, despite the severity of clinical findings they may manifest.

Other imidazolines could potentially cause any of the clinical findings seen with clonidine poisoning. Most topical imidazoline exposures result in no symptoms. Guanabenz, guanfacine, and methyldopa are rarely used or ingested. The most commonly reported adverse findings in symptomatic patients who have been exposed to an imidazoline other than clonidine, however, are coma, miosis, bradycardia, and respiratory depression.[14–17, 44, 45]

DIAGNOSIS

History and physical findings are strongly relied on to make the diagnosis of imidazoline poisoning. In general, imidazoline exposure should be suspected in any patient who has the signs of opiate intoxication without responsiveness to high doses of naloxone or who improves with naloxone administration but has no identifiable opiate ingestion. Improvement in coma, apnea, and bradycardia with stimulation or hypertension after naloxone administration also suggest imidazoline poisoning, especially clonidine. No specific routine laboratory findings exist for imidazoline toxicity. Furthermore, imidazolines are not found on comprehensive toxicology screening evaluations. Specific drug levels have been established for clonidine, guanabenz, and methyldopa toxicity to confirm the diagnosis, but determination of blood levels usually takes several days, limiting the usefulness of specific levels for patient management.

TREATMENT

Immediate Supportive Measures

Careful attention to stabilization procedures supersedes all other treatment modalities in importance when managing serious imidazoline overdose. These patients frequently require immediate interventions targeted at airway control and reversal of hemodynamic compromise. In one series, 12% of children who ingested clonidine required endotracheal intubation because of apnea, deep coma, or respiratory depression.[12] Although naloxone administration may reverse symptoms of respiratory depression, it has not prevented the need for endotracheal intubation in the majority of reported patients.[12, 49] When performing endotracheal intubation in these patients, atropine and muscle relaxant administration should precede laryngoscopy to avoid bradycardia and difficulty due to patient agitation, respectively.

All patients suspected of a significant imidazoline overdose should have an intravenous line placed. Bradycardia typically responds well to administration of a routine dose of atropine (0.02 mg/kg, up to 1 mg). Hypotension should be treated with rapid infusion of 20 to 40 mL/kg of isotonic crystalloid, either normal saline or Ringer's lactate. Dopamine infusion has been used successfully in the minority of patients who do not improve after fluid administration.[12] Hypertension after clonidine ingestion is usually transient and frequently requires no treatment. If treatment is instituted, a short-acting agent such as sodium nitroprusside or hydralazine is recommended. β-adrenergic blockers should be avoided for imidazoline-induced hypertension to prevent unopposed α effects and worsening of hypertension. A search for an adherent clonidine patch should occur during skin exposure and examination of patients suspected of imidazoline poisoning.[50]

Decontamination and Prevention of Systemic Absorption

The most useful method of decontamination following imidazoline overdose varies based on the type of exposure and the drug formulation. A single dose of activated charcoal is indicated following the oral ingestion of clonidine pills or imidazoline topical preparations. Gastric emptying with syrup of ipecac is contraindicated because of the potential for rapid onset of central nervous system depression. Gastric lavage prior to administration of activated charcoal may be useful in patients who have recently ingested a large amount of pills or liquid. Toxicity following nasal or ocular administration of imidazoline drops in young children is unlikely to be significantly altered by any means of gastric decontamination.

Ingestion of a clonidine patch preparation presents a special challenge. Two reports highlight the beneficial use of cathartics in this situation. In one case, a 29-month-old girl had persistent findings of clonidine intoxication 26 hours after presumed ingestion of a patch. Administration of magnesium citrate led to passage of the patch 30 hours later.[51] Another patient had spontaneous passage of a clonidine patch after 4 hours of whole bowel irrigation with polyethylene glycol at 500 mL/hour.[52] Based on this experience, administration of a single dose of activated charcoal followed by whole bowel irrigation may be an effective method for the prevention of clonidine absorption after transdermal patch ingestion.

Antidotes

There is no true antidote for imidazoline poisoning. Naloxone has reversed signs of imidazoline toxicity in some patients, however. The mechanism by which naloxone works in imidazoline poisoning is unknown. The response rate is approximately 15% to 40% in patients receiving up to 0.1 mg/kg of naloxone.[12] A total dose of 10 mg of naloxone may need to be administered before determining that naloxone is ineffective.[51] Naloxone infusion after an initial response is rarely needed in patients who ingest clonidine. Given the low risk of naloxone administration in the emergency setting, it should be given to patients with significant central nervous system, cardiovascular, or respiratory compromise. Patients with severe imidazoline poisoning often need immediate supportive care, such as endotracheal intubation, atropine administration, and rapid crystalloid infusion, despite having received naloxone.[12]

Tolazoline, an α-adrenergic antagonist, was initially used in the treatment of clonidine poisoning but was frequently ineffective.[53] In addition, it has adverse effects of tachycardia, hypertension, and dysrhythmias. Given the excellent outcome in patients poisoned with imidazolines who receive supportive care alone, the risk of giving tolazoline outweighs the potential benefit.

Elimination Enhancement

The imidazolines are not amenable to any form of elimination enhancement.

Disposition

Patients who ingest imidazolines but remain asymptomatic may be watched for 4 to 6 hours from the time of ingestion and medically cleared if no physical findings of imidazoline poisoning occur. Symptomatic patients who respond to naloxone should be admitted and monitored to ensure no recrudescence of toxicity. These patients often can receive adequate treatment on a regular inpatient ward. Symptomatic patients who do not respond to naloxone require immediate supportive care and admission to an intensive care unit. In most instances, patients fully recover from imidazoline poisoning within 1 to 2 days.

References

1. Lowenstein J: Clonidine. Ann Intern Med *92:*74–77, 1980.
2. Gold MS, Redmond DE Jr, Kleber HD: Clonidine blocks acute opiate-withdrawal symptoms. Lancet *2:*599–602, 1978.
3. Riordan CED, Kleber HD: Rapid opiate detoxification with clonidine and naloxone. Lancet *1:*1079–1080, 1980.
4. Glassman AH, Stetner F, Walsh T, et al: Heavy smokers, smoking cessation, and clonidine: Results of a double-blind, randomized trial. JAMA *259:*2863–2866, 1988.
5. Clayden JR, Bell JW, Pellard P: Menopausal flushing: Double-blind trial of a non-hormonal medication. BMJ *9:*490, 1974.
6. Hunt RD, Minderaa RB, Cohen DJ: Clonidine benefits children with attention deficit disorder and hyperactivity: Report of a double-blind placebo-crossover therapeutic trial. J Am Acad Child Psychiatry *24:*617–629, 1985.
7. Cohen DJ, Young JG, Nathanson JA, Shaywitz BA: Clonidine in Tourette's syndrome. Lancet *2:*551–553, 1979.
8. Gil-Ad I, Topper E, Laron Z: Oral clonidine as a growth hormone stimulation test. Lancet *2:*278–280, 1979.
9. Chappell PB, Riddle MA, Seahill L, et al: Guanfacine treatment of comorbid attention-deficit hyperactivity disorder and Tourette's syndrome: Preliminary clinical experience. J Am Acad Child Adolsc Psychiatry *34:*1140–1146, 1995.
10. Balldin J, Berggren U, Briksson E, et al: Guanfacine as an alpha-2-agonist inducer of growth hormone secretion—a comparison with clonidine. Psychoneuroendocrinology *18:*45–55, 1993.
11. Stein B, Volans GN: Dixarit overdose: The problem of attractive tablets. BMJ *2:*667–668, 1978.

12. Wiley JF II, Wiley CC, Torrey SB, Henretig FM: Clonidine poisoning in young children. J Pediatr *116:*654–658, 1990.
13. Bamshad MJ, Wasserman GS: Pediatric clonidine intoxications. Vet Hum Toxicol *32:*220–223, 1990.
14. Lewis S, Giffen SL: Pediatric imidazoline exposures: Incidence of serious effects. Vet Hum Toxicol *34:*333, 1992.
15. Hall AH, Smolinske SC, Kulig KW, Rumack BH: Guanabenz overdose. Ann Intern Med *102:*787–788, 1985.
16. Rogers SJ: Guanabenz overdose (letter). Ann Intern Med *104:*445, 1986.
17. Shnaps Y, Almog S, Halkin H, et al: Methyldopa poisoning. J Toxicol Clin Toxicol *19:*501–503, 1982.
18. Langer SZ, Cavero I, Massingham R: Recent developments in noradrenergic neurotransmission and its relevance to the mechanism of action of certain antihypertensive agents. Hypertension *2:*372–382, 1980.
19. Bobik A, Jennings G, Jackman G, et al: Evidence for a predominantly central hypotensive effect of alpha-methyldopa in humans. Hypertension *8:*16–23, 1986.
20. Dollery CT, Davies DS, Draffan GH, et al: Clinical pharmacology and pharmacokinetics of clonidine. Clin Pharmacol Ther *19:*11–17, 1976.
21. Frisk-Holmberg M, Paalzow L, Edlund PO: Clonidine kinetics in man—evidence for dose dependency and changed pharmacokinetics during chronic therapy. Br J Clin Pharmacol *12:*653–658, 1981.
22. Pettinger WA: Pharmacology of clonidine. J Cardiovasc Pharmacol *1*(Suppl):S21–S28, 1980.
23. Cunningham FE, Baughman VL, Peters J, Laurito CE: Comparative pharmacokinetics of oral versus sublingual clonidine. J Clin Anesth *6:*430–433, 1994.
24. Lonnqvist PA, Bergendahl HT, Eksborg S: Pharmacokinetics of clonidine after rectal administration in children. Anesthesiology *81:*1097–1101, 1994.
25. Ebihara A, Fujimura A, Ohashi K, et al: Influence of application site of a new transdermal clonidine, M-5041T, on its pharmacokinetics and pharmacodynamics in healthy subjects. J Clin Pharmacol *33:*1188–1191, 1993.
26. MacGregor TR, Matzed KM, Keirns JJ, et al: Pharmacokinetics of transdermally delivered clonidine. Clin Pharmacol Ther *38:*278–284, 1985.
27. Fenichel RR: Post-marketing surveillance identifies three cases of sudden death in children during treatment with clonidine and methylphenidate. J Child Adolesc Psychopharmacol *5:*157–166, 1995.
28. Popper CW: Combined methylphenidate and clonidine: News reports about sudden death. J Child Adolesc Psychopharmacol *5:*155–156, 1995.
29. Ram CVS, Engelman K: Abrupt discontinuation of clonidine therapy. JAMA *242:*2104–2105, 1979.
30. Planz G, Beckenbauer U, Bundschu HD: Response of plasma catecholamines and blood pressure to clonidine and to sudden withdrawal of the drug in subjects with essential hypertension. Int J Clin Pharmacol Ther Toxicol *29:*474–478, 1982.
31. Campbell BC, Reid JL: Regimen for the control of blood pressure and symptoms during clonidine withdrawal. Int J Clin Pharm Res *5:*215–222, 1985.
32. Zamboulis C, Reid JL: Withdrawal of guanfacine after long-term treatment in essential hypertension. Observations on blood pressure and plasma and urinary noradrenaline. Eur J Clin Pharmacol *19:*19–24, 1981.
33. Reid JL: Alpha-adrenergic receptors and blood pressure control. Am J Cardiol *57:*6E–12E, 1986.
34. Van Zwieten PA: Overview of alpha$_2$-adrenoceptor agonists with a central action. Am J Cardiol *57:*3E–5E, 1986.
35. Hoffman BB, Lefkowitz RJ: Alpha-adrenergic receptor subtypes. N Engl J Med *302:*1390–1396, 1980.
36. Niemi L: Effects of intrathecal clonidine on duration of bupivacaine spinal anaesthesia, haemodynamics, and postoperative analgesia in patients undergoing knee arthroscopy. Acta Anaesth Scand *38:*724–728, 1994.
37. Gabilondo AM, Meana JJ, Barturen F, et al: Mu-opioid receptor and alpha 2-adrenoceptor agonist binding sites in the postmortem brain of heroin addicts. Psychopharmacology *115:*135–140, 1994.
38. Gracsor D, Neubig RR: Compartmentation of receptors and guanine nucleotide-binding proteins in NG108-15 cells: Lack of cross-talk in agonist binding among the alpha 2-adrenergic, muscarinic, and opiate receptors. Mol Pharmacol *43:*434–443, 1993.
39. Ernsberger PR, Westbrooks KL, Christen MO, et al: A second generation of centrally acting antihypertensive agents act on putative I1-imidazoline receptors. J Cardiovasc Pharmacol *20:*S1–S10, 1992.
40. Bricca G, Greney H, Zhang J, et al: Human brain imidazoline receptors: Further characterization with [3H]clonidine. Eur J Pharmacol *266:*25–33, 1994.
41. Bousquet P, Feldman J, Tibirica E, et al: Imidazoline receptors: A new concept in central regulation of the arterial blood pressure. Am J Hypertension *5*(4):47S–50S, 1992.
42. Hudson A: Imidazoline receptors. Tocris Cookson Monograph, January 1996.
43. Hunyor SN, Bradstock K, Somerville PJ, Lucas N: Clonidine overdose. Letter. BMJ *4:*23, 1975.
44. Higgins GL, Campbell B, Wallace K, Talbot S: Pediatric poisoning from over-the-counter imidazoline-containing products. Ann Emerg Med 20:655–658, 1991.
45. Mack RB: "Pack up the moon and dismantle the sun"—imidazoline overdose. Contemp Pediatr *13:*67–79, 1996.
46. Williams PL, Krafcik JM, Potter BB, et al: Cardiac toxicity of clonidine. Chest *72:*784–785, 1977.
47. Yagupsky P, Gorodischer R: Massive clonidine ingestion with hypertension in a 9-month-old infant. Pediatrics *72:*500–502, 1983.
48. Gremse DA, Artman M, Boerth RC: Hypertension associated with naloxone treatment for clonidine poisoning. J Pediatr *108:*776–778, 1986.
49. Banner W, Lund ME, Clawson L: Failure of naloxone to reverse clonidine toxic effect. Am J Dis Child *137:*1170–1171, 1983.
50. Reed MT, Hamburg EL: Person-to-person transfer of transdermal drug delivery systems: A case report. Letter. N Engl J Med *314:*1120, 1986.
51. Knapp JF, Fowler MA, Wheeler CA, Wasserman GS: Case 01-1995: A two-year-old female with alteration of consciousness. Pediatr Emerg Care *11:*62–65, 1995.
52. Henretig FM, Wiley JF II, Brown L: Clonidine patch toxicity: The proof's in the poop! Abstract. J Toxicol Clin Toxicol *33:*520, 1995.
53. Olsson JM, Pruitt AW: Management of clonidine ingestion in children. J Pediatr *103:*646–650, 1983.
54. Sorkin BM, Heel RC: Guanfacine: A review of its pharmacodynamic and pharmacokinetic properties and therapeutic efficacy in the treatment of hypertension. Drugs *31:*301–306, 1986.
55. Kiechel JR: Pharmacokinetics of guanfacine in patients with impaired renal function and in some elderly patients. Am J Cardiol *57:*18E–21E, 1986.
56. Guanabenz (Wytensin): A new antihypertensive drug. Med Lett Drugs Ther *25:*11–12, 1983.

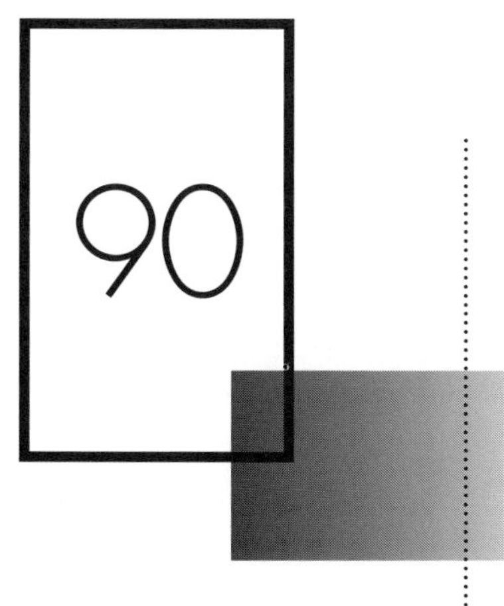

Class IA Antiarrhythmics: Quinidine, Procainamide, and Disopyramide

JANE K. WITMAN, MD
R. BRENT FURBEE, MD

The class IA antiarrhythmics include quinidine, procainamide, and disopyramide. Although dissimilar in structure (Fig. 90–1), all three drugs suppress cardiac dysrhythmias via the same mechanisms and produce adverse effects typical of the group. In the past, these drugs were widely used for the control of both atrial and ventricular arrhythmias, but because of the high incidence of adverse effects with therapeutic use and overdose, they have been largely replaced by newer, safer agents.

HISTORY

Quinidine and its optical isomer, quinine, are extracted from the South American cinchona tree. Centuries ago, it was noted that patients with both malaria and atrial fibrillation, when treated with cinchona for malaria, were sometimes also cured of their arrhythmia. Jean-Baptiste de Senac, of Paris, recorded using cinchona in the treatment of atrial fibrillation in 1749. In 1936, Mautz demonstrated procaine to be effective in decreasing ventricular irritability, but this compound was rapidly metabolized and was too neurotoxic to be of clinical value. Procainamide, a congener of procaine, was introduced in 1955. Disopyramide was introduced in 1978.[1]

PHARMACOKINETICS

Quinidine is well absorbed after ingestion, with a bioavailability of between 70% and 80%. Quinidine sulfate levels peak at 1.5 hours. The gluconate and bisulfate or polygalacturonate salts are sustained-release preparations, and blood levels of these may not peak until 4 hours after ingestion. Peak levels may be significantly prolonged in overdose.[2, 3] Quinidine is 75% to 95% protein bound and is metabolized by the liver via hydroxylation, with a half-life of approximately 6 hours.[4] Quinidine has two metabolites with antiarrhythmic properties: 2′-quinidinone and 3-hydroxyquinidine. Its apparent volume of distribution is 3 L/kg. Approximately 20% of quinidine is excreted unchanged in the urine.[2]

Oral procainamide is absorbed well from the small intestine; levels peak 1 to 2 hours after ingestion. After intravenous administration, the drug distributes to the tissue within 30 minutes. Procainamide diffuses well into tissue and has a volume of distribution of 2 L/kg. Protein binding is approximately 15% to 20%.[5] Procainamide is hydrolyzed by the liver into several active metabolites, the most significant being 1,4,2,-*N*-acetylprocainamide (NAPA).[6] Procainamide has a half-life of 3 hours, and NAPA of 6 hours. Fifty per cent of procainamide is excreted in the urine unchanged.[7]

Disopyramide is well absorbed orally, with peak levels occurring 2 to 3 hours after ingestion.[8] Protein binding is 30%, and the volume of distribution is 0.8 L/kg. Disopyramide is partially metabolized by the liver, with 55% being excreted unchanged in the urine. The half-life of disopyramide is approximately 8 hours.[9]

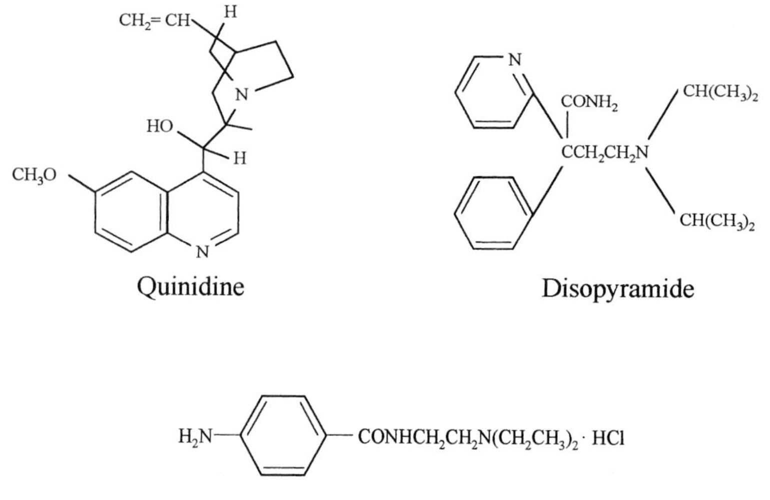

Quinidine

Disopyramide

Procainamide

Figure 90–1. Although dissimilar in structure all class IA antiarrhythmic agents share therapeutic and toxic effects.

PATHOPHYSIOLOGY

Anticholinergic Effects

Many of the symptoms associated with class IA antiarrhythmics are related to the anticholinergic activity of these compounds. Disopyramide is the most anticholinergic, followed by procainamide and then quinidine. Confusion, hallucinations, tachycardia, decreased gastrointestinal motility, urinary retention, and dry mucous membranes all may occur with their use. Because some patients may suffer from cinchonism, the clinical presentation may be a confusing combination of the two syndromes. A summary of reported adverse effects of these agents is found in Table 90–1.

Immune System

Hypersensitivity reactions most commonly occur with quinidine but may also occur with procainamide and disopyramide. Hypersensitivity may be manifested as fever, rashes, thrombocytopenia, neutropenia, agranulocytosis, hepatitis, hemolytic anemia, or lymphadenopathy.[3, 10–12] These reactions are frequently unrelated to dose.

Procainamide is the most common cause of drug-induced lupus. Antinuclear antibodies occur in 50% to 75% of patients treated with procainamide, and 20% to 30% of those patients develop components of drug-induced lupus.[13] Patients suffer from arthralgias, myalgias, malar rash, fever, pleuritis, pleural effusion, and pericarditis. Renal involvement is rare with drug-induced lupus.[14] The mechanism responsible for the development of drug-induced lupus remains under investigation. Metabolic products of procainamide have been found to inhibit the covalent binding of C4 to C2 in the complement cascade, which is thought to decrease the clearance of immune complexes.[15, 16]

Thrombocytopenia has been reported to occur with therapeutic use of quinidine and procainamide.[17, 18] Drug-induced thrombocytopenia is an immune-mediated reaction. The sensitizing drug induces antiplatelet antibodies, which cause the rapid destruction of platelets. Recovery is usually complete within 5 days of removal of the drug.[18]

Table 90–1. Noncardiac Effects of Class IA Antiarrhythmics at Therapeutic Doses

Central nervous system	Giddiness, depression, hallucinations,† blurred vision, sedation‡
Pulmonary	Pleural fibrosis,† pneumonitis
Gastrointestinal	Nausea, vomiting, diarrhea, hepatitis*
Genitourinary	Urinary retention
Musculoskeletal	Myopathy with muscle weakness†
Skin	Rashes, lichen planus*
Hematologic	IgG-mediated agranulocytosis,† thrombocytopenia,† IgM-mediated hemolysis (most often in patients with glucose-6-phosphate dehydrogenase deficiency)
Rheumatologic	Systemic lupus erythematosus†
Other	Hypoglycemia‡

*Primarily quinidine.
†Primarily procainamide.
‡Primarily disopyramide.
Data from references 58 to 62.

Metabolic

Symptomatic hypoglycemia has been reported to occur after therapeutic doses of disopyramide. Goldberg and colleagues demonstrated hypoglycemia with administration of disopyramide. This could be reproduced on readministration of the drug.[19] One suggested mechanism is that quinidine, like the sulfonylureas, has the ability to block potassium efflux from pancreatic β cells, thus leading to increased insulin secretion resulting in hyperinsulinemia (Fig. 90–2). Hyperinsulinemia is well documented with use of quinine, a stereoisomer of quinidine, and with

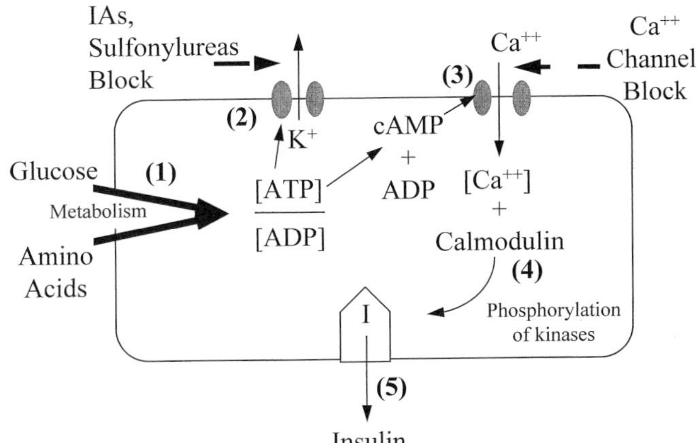

Figure 90–2. The presence of glucose or amino acids triggers the conversion of adenosine triphosphate (ATP) to cyclic adenosine monophosphate (cAMP) (1). cAMP is needed to open calcium channels in the β-cell. Calcium ions then enter the cell (3) and bind with calmodulin to activate kinases such as myosin–light chain kinase or protein kinase C (4) to stimulate the release of insulin (5). The initial depolarization of the β-cell triggers potassium efflux (2). The IA antiarrythmics (IAs) are thought to block the potassium efflux out of β-cells in the pancreas. This would prolong the "depolarization" of the cell and increase secretion of insulin. (Adapted from Gerich JE: Oral hypoglycemic agents. N Engl J Med *321*:18, 1990.)

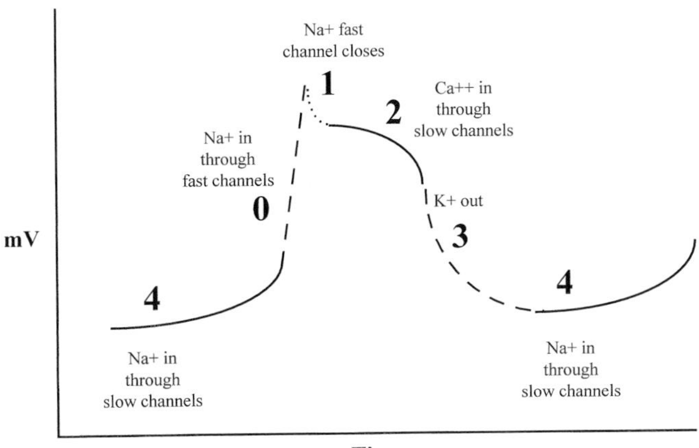

Figure 90–3. Ion flow during Purkinje's cell action potential.

disopyramide, but its occurrence in the presence of other class IA antiarrhythmics has not been supported by the work of other researchers.[14, 19, 20]

Cardiac

The class IA antiarrhythmics, although structurally dissimilar, produce similar effects on the heart. Dysrhythmias can occur at therapeutic as well as toxic serum concentrations of these drugs. The cardiac effects of quinidine are the most studied, but all the agents in this class act in a similar manner. Procainamide has less cardiotoxicity at therapeutic doses than quinidine and disopyramide. Disopyramide exhibits the greatest negative inotropic effect of the three and has been reported to cause congestive heart failure with therapeutic use.[3, 21] Class IA antiarrhythmics cause numerous cardiac arrhythmias, including heart block, atrial tachycardia, premature ventricular contractions, torsades de pointes, ventricular tachycardia, and ventricular fibrillation. The drug actions responsible for these arrhythmias are sodium channel blockade, potassium efflux blockade, sodium/potassium–adenosine triphosphatase and inhibition of the (Na^+, K^+ ATpase) pump.

In a normal Purkinje cell, the rapid influx of sodium ions in phase 0 causes the interior of the cell to become more positive (Figs. 90–3 and 90–4). Phase 1 is associated with slow leakage of sodium out of the cell, causing a decrease in positive charge within the cell. During phase 2, voltage-dependent calcium channels open, allowing calcium ions to enter. This calcium influx, which sustains the positive charge within the cell, is reflected as the plateau of phase 2. The slow leak of potassium from the cell during phase 2 has little impact on the overall charge within. In phase 3, however, further leakage of potassium out of the cell (potassium efflux) occurs in order to repolarize the cell. In phase 4, the charge within the cell has returned to its resting potential and sodium begins to leak into the cell. This moves the cell membrane potential toward threshold again, and the next action potential can occur. Late phase 4 and phase 0 represent *depolarization* of the cardiac cell, whereas phases 1, 2, and 3 represent *depolarization*. Phases 0 to 3 correspond to systole, and phase 4 corresponds to diastole.

Afterdepolarizations and Triggered Activity

Afterdepolarization is essentially electric oscillations of the conductive cell membrane that occur late in phase 2, throughout phase 3, or early in phase 4. This activity appears to occur primarily in Purkinje's cells or deep subendocardial regions of the ventricular wall.[22] Afterdepolarizations that occur in phase 2 or 3 are known as *early afterdepolarizations*. Afterdepolarizations occurring in phase 4 are termed *de-*

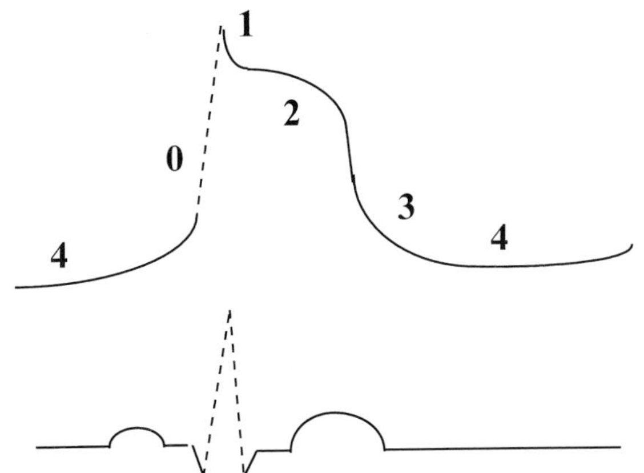

Figure 90–4. Normal Purkinje's action potential and corresponding electrocardiogram pattern.

layed afterdepolarizations. The IA antiarrhythmics are capable of producing both.

Not all afterdepolarizations lead to dysrhythmias. Because they occur during the relative refractory period of cellular repolarization, some of these membrane oscillations do not cause the cell to fire again. If the cell has sufficiently repolarized, some afterdepolarizations are capable of reaching threshold and can cause abnormal firing and dysrhythmias. Dysrhythmias produced by afterdepolarizations that reach threshold are referred to as *triggered activity.* They are distinguished from arrhythmias that are due to increased automaticity. The latter do not require an initial depolarization to occur. They may be caused by catecholamines, infarction, or electrolyte abnormalities. Triggered activity is responsible for the tachyarrhythmias that occur at therapeutic levels of the IA antiarrhythmics.[23] Early afterdepolarization triggered activity from the IA antiarrhythmics tends to result in torsades de pointes. Delayed afterdepolarization activity tends to be more closely associated with premature ventricular contractions.

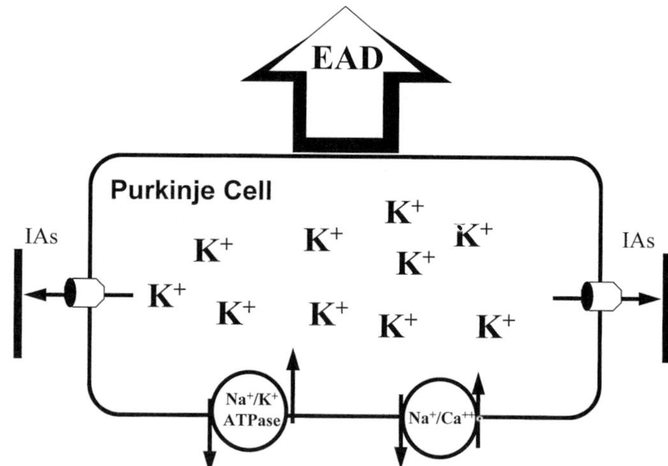

Figure 90–6. IA antiarrhythmics and other toxins may block the efflux of K^+ from the cardiac cell, driving the charge on the interior of the cell membrane in a less negative direction, toward threshold. This change in charge leads to early afterdepolarization (EAD) formation.

Arrhythmias at Therapeutic Levels

Quinidine syncope, which occurs at therapeutic and subtherapeutic levels, was initially thought to be caused by hypotension, secondary to the vasodilatory effect of this drug. Ventricular tachyarrhythmias were then determined to be responsible. Fifty per cent of patients who develop torsades de pointes do so within the first 5 days of therapy; the remainder of the cases occur weeks to years later, often after a dosage change.[24] Disopyramide and procainamide, although less frequently than quinidine, have also been reported to cause fatal arrhythmias in the therapeutic range.[25–27] The arrhythmias are usually nonsustained but have occasionally been fatal. Sudden death while on quinidine therapy has been estimated at 0.5%.[10] Both polymorphic ventricular tachycardia and torsades de pointes have been reported. Both rhythms produce a rotating axis on an electrocardiogram but respond differently to various therapeutic interventions.[28] Torsades de pointes may be distinguished from polymorphic ventricular tachycardia by the following criteria: The initial complex follows a pause or sudden rate deceleration, which produces a long preceding RR interval. The initiating complex also has an accentuated U wave (Fig. 90–5). Torsades de pointes is associated with a prolonged QT interval and is caused by early afterdepolarization activity. Drugs such as quinidine, procainamide, and disopyramide block the efflux of potassium from the Purkinje cell during phase 2 or phase 3 of cardiac depolarization. When this occurs, the interior of the cell becomes more positive, making it more likely to reach threshold and depolarize again.[23, 29] (Figs. 90–6 and 90–7). When a multitude of cells become hypopo-

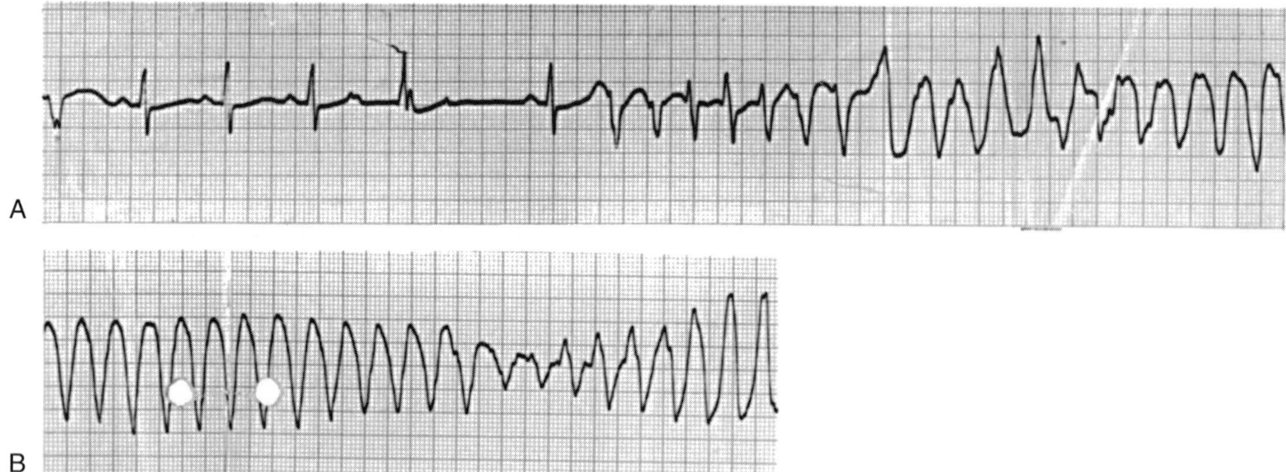

Figure 90–5. Rhythm strip of a patient with torsades de pointes suffering from chronic procainamide toxicity. Procaine level was 27.5 μg/mL; *N*-acetylprocainamide level was 62.4 μg/mL. *A,* Note prolonged R-R interval and accentuated U wave prior to onset of torsades de pointes. *B,* Torsades de pointes is characterized by a rotating axis on the ECG.

larized, the action potential is effectively lengthened. This change in the action potential corresponds to prolongation of the QT interval. Salata and Wasserstrom demonstrated that quinidine's K^+ efflux blockade predominates at lower heart rates. Therefore, early afterdepolarization is more likely at slower heart rates.[30] As the heart rate increases, quinidine's blockade of slow Ca^{2+} and Na^+ channels is greater. Blockade of the movement of these positive ions into the interior of the cell keeps it hyperpolarized, and thus the potassium efflux is counterbalanced.[30] The inside of the cell remains relatively more negative, making early afterdepolarization activity less likely and decreasing the risk of developing torsades de pointes.

Arrhythmias Occurring in Toxicity

Arrhythmias occurring in class IA toxicity include ventricular tachycardia, bradycardia, sinus pause or arrest, junctional or ventricular block, ventricular fibrillation, and asystole.[3, 10, 31]

Sodium Channel Blockade

The IA antiarrythmic agents can produce widening of the QRS, ventricular tachycardia, and decreased inotropy by blocking fast sodium channels in cardiac cells. Electric conductance in the Purkinje fibers is dependent on the rapid influx of sodium through fast sodium channels (phase 0). A number of toxins are capable of blocking the fast sodium channels and slowing the influx of sodium ions in phase 0. In terms of the action potential, this slows the rate of rise of phase 0 (V_{max}). Because phase 0 corresponds to the QRS complex, any toxin that slows the influx of sodium ions through the fast channels produces a widened QRS complex (Fig. 90–8). The class IA antiarrhythmics' ability to block Na^+ channels is dose dependent and is clinically significant only with high drug levels.[31] At toxic serum concentrations, QRS widening, bundle branch block, and sinoatrial or atrioventricular block may be present. Villemaire and colleagues found that dogs overdosed with procainamide had more severe conduction delays when hyperkalemic. The exact mechanism remains unclear, but hyperkalemia may reduce the membrane potential of the cardiac cell, which favors Na^+ channel inactivation.[32] Lee and associates reported that intravenous procainamide, given in therapeutic doses, increased the effective refractory period of the cardiac cycle, with a greater relative increase at shorter cell cycles than would be expected from rate alone.[33] Normally, as the heart rate increases, both action potential duration and effective refractory period shorten. This occurs because of an accumulation of extracellular K^+ and intracellular Ca^{2+} that hastens repolarization. Fast heart rates shorten diastole and impede complete recovery of inward currents that compose phase 4, or repolarization of the action potential. The increase in refractory period caused by procainamide reflects a voltage-independent but time-dependent suppression of excitability. More simply stated, procainamide may cause rate-dependent Na^+ channel blockade, which becomes more pronounced as the heart rate increases. Therefore, patients experiencing ventricular tachycardia secondary to procainamide toxicity, and possibly toxicity due to disopyramide and quinidine, should not be treated with overdrive pacing because of possible worsening of the Na^+ channel blockade.

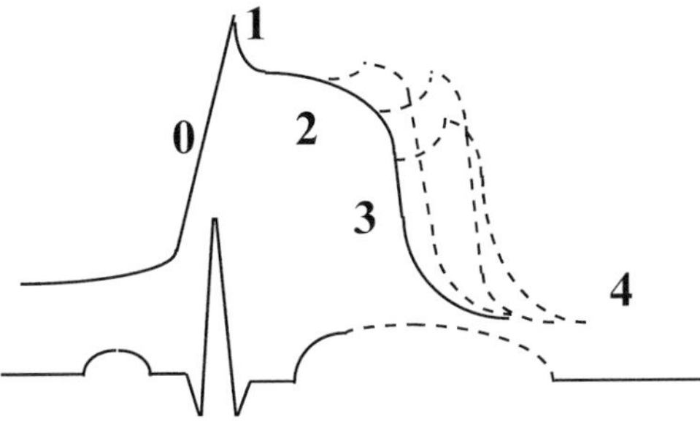

Figure 90–7. Blockade of potassium in the cells leads to membrane oscillations or early afterdepolarizations. If they attain threshold voltage, triggered activity will occur.

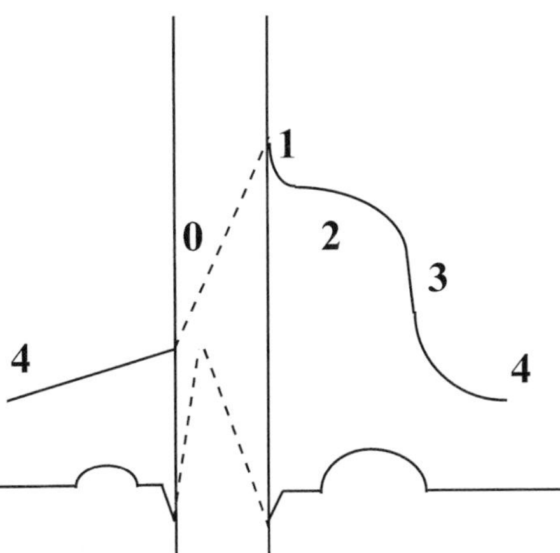

Figure 90–8. When sodium channels are blocked, the rate or rise of phase 0 (V_{max}) is decreased. This corresponds to a widening of the QRS complex.

The premature ventricular contractions observed in overdose may be caused by inhibition of the Na^+, K^+-ATPase pump in cardiac cells. The Na^+, K^+-ATPase pump functions to repolarize the cell after contraction by transporting three intracellular Na^+ ions out of the cell in exchange for two K^+ ions. Class IA agents, in a fashion similar to digoxin, inhibit the Na^+, K^+-ATPase pump, resulting in intracellular Na^+ accumulation.[34] The Na^+ is exchanged for Ca^{2+} by the Na^+-Ca^{2+} pump, causing an increase in intracellular Ca^{2+} (Fig. 90–9). Normally, the sarcoplasmic reticulum takes up cytoplasmic Ca^{2+} and stores it; however, excessive intracellular Ca^{2+} is thought to overload the sequestration mechanism of the sarcoplasmic reticulum. The increased intracellular Ca^{2+} then activates the Na^+-Ca^{2+} pump, which increases the exchange of intracellular Ca^{2+} for extracellular Na^+. This creates an inward current of Na^+ ions

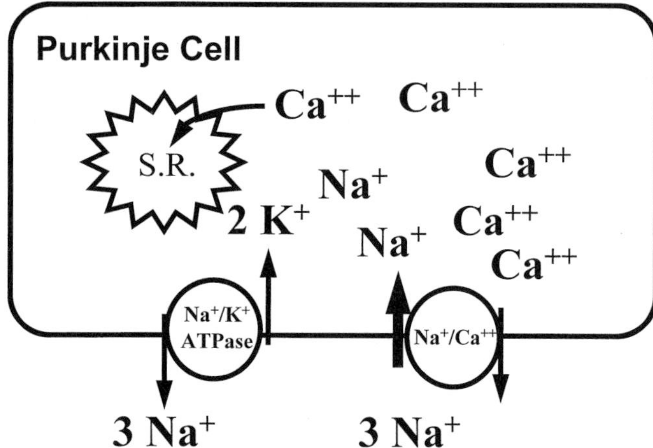

Figure 90–9. Ordinarily, the inhibition of the Na^+, K^+-ATPase pump leads to an increase of intracellular Na^+. This in turn leads to an exchange of Na^+ for Ca^{2+} via the Na^+/Ca^{2+} pump. The excess Ca^{2+} is sequestered in the sarcoplasmic reticulum (SR).

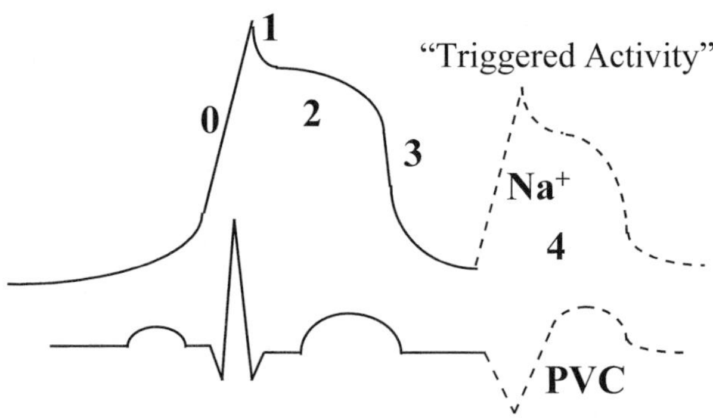

Figure 90–11. If the delayed afterdepolarization reaches threshold, triggered activity occurs, leading to dysrythmias. PVC, premature ventricular contraction.

that is carried by the Na^+ channels and results in a delayed afterdepolarization[23] (Figs. 90–10 and 90–11). The frequency of delayed afterdepolarizations' reaching threshold increases as the heart rate accelerates.[34] Dzimiri and Almotrefi demonstrated increasing inhibition of the Na^+, K^+-ATPase pump with decreasing serum potassium levels, which may explain the exacerbation of arrhythmias caused by class IA antiarrhythmics by hypokalemia.[34] Low serum potassium levels further inhibit the Na^+, K^+-ATPase pump, worsening intracellular Ca^{2+} overload and resulting in increased activity of delayed afterdepolarization with resultant arrhythmias. Conditions associated with this increased activity all result in intracellular Ca^{2+} overload. Other conditions responsible for such increased activity include digitalis toxicity, hypernatremia, hypokalemia, and catecholamines.

CLINICAL PRESENTATION

Significant ingestions of these drugs produce primarily neurologic and cardiovascular consequences.[10, 35] Ingestion of more than 1 g of quinidine by an adult has been reported to produce symptoms. As little as 7 g of procainamide and 1.5 g of disopyramide is potentially toxic. In assessing the severity of a toxic ingestion, it is important to remember that the reported history of the amount of a drug ingested is very unreliable and individual responses to these drugs vary greatly. Underlying cardiac disease may make some patients symptomatic at lower than expected doses.

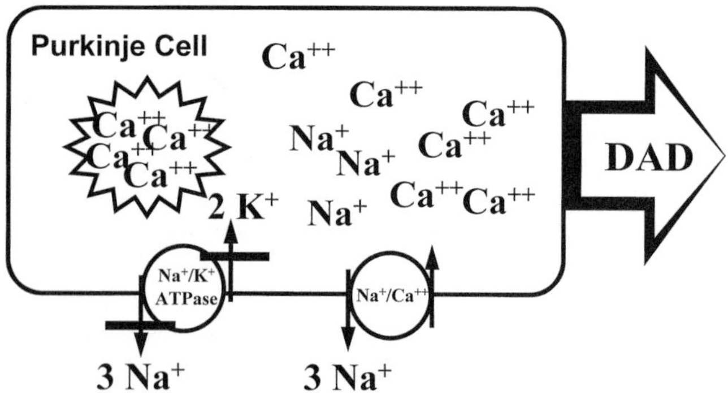

Figure 90–10. If inhibition of the Na^+, K^+-ATPase pump leads to Ca^{2+} overload of the cell, the sarcoplasmic reticulum is unable to compensate by sequestration and the internal charge begins to increase, leading to delayed afterdepolarization (DAD) formation.

Central Nervous System

Poisoning with a class IA antiarrhythmics may cause mydriasis and blurred vision. A patient's mental status may range from lethargy and confusion to coma. Convulsions independent of hypotension secondary to quinidine have been reported.[35] Summers and colleagues reported on a 69-year-old man who developed confusion and hallucinations while receiving quinidine during hospitalization for myocardial infarction.[36] The patient's mental status cleared after the administration of physostigmine, leading the investigators to conclude that mental status changes were due to anticholinergic toxicity.

Cardiovascular

The cardiotoxic effects of this class of drugs are the most threatening to patients. Although tachycardia may be present early in a serious poisoning, bradycardia secondary to conduction delays and blocks is most common. Other arrhythmias reported in overdose include atrial tachyarrhythmias, ventricular tachycardia, and fibrillation. QT prolongation and widening of the QRS duration serve as reliable markers of cardiac toxicity. Prolongation of the QT interval by greater than 50% is considered a marker for severe poisoning.[35] Hypotension and shock associated with class IA antiarrhythmics are primarily related to depressive actions on the heart rather than to direct effects on the peripheral vasculature.[37, 38]

Gastrointestinal

Dry mouth is a frequent complaint of patients exposed to class IA antiarrhythmics. Nausea, vomiting, and diarrhea are also common, although decreased bowel sounds, constipation, and ileus may occur secondary to the anticholinergic effects of these drugs.

Cinchonism

First described in association with quinine, the complex of symptoms called *cinchonism* may occur in chronic overuse or acute overdose of quinidine, although it is more common with quinine. This syndrome is characterized by abdominal pain, diarrhea, nausea, vomiting, hearing loss, tinnitus, visual disturbances, encephalopathy, coma, and seizures.[10] Symptoms typically resolve after removal of the causative agent.

Genitourinary

Urinary retention and anuria have been reported. They are thought to be associated with the anticholinergic effects of these drugs.

Musculoskeletal

Myositis, muscle weakness, and myopathy have been associated with therapeutic use. One patient has been described with diaphragmatic paralysis while taking 750 mg of procainamide twice daily.[39]

Pregnancy

The class IA antiarrhythmic agents clearly cross the placenta. No evidence shows that they are teratogenic. Disopyramide has been associated with premature uterine contractions, which resolved on discontinuance of the drug.[40]

DRUG INTERACTIONS

A particular form of cytochrome P-450 inhibition has been described with quinidine use. Debrisoquin, which is an antihypertensive agent used in Europe, is metabolized by the cytochrome P-450 isozyme CYP2D6 (debrisoquin hydroxylase). A number of other drugs are metabolized by the same isozyme. Ten per cent of the western population are genetically deficient in this enzyme and are slow metabolizers of debrisoquin. Quinidine, although not metabolized by this isozyme, binds to CYP2D6, interfering with its function. Commonly prescribed medications metabolized by this pathway, when taken with quinidine, are metabolized more slowly, causing higher than expected serum concentrations.[41] Drugs metabolized by the CYP2D6 and potentially affected by quinidine are listed in Table 90–2.

Quinidine and Digitalis

Quinidine is thought to decrease the volume of distribution of some cardiac glycosides. This seems particularly true in the presence of digoxin. When these drugs are given concomitantly, the usual digoxin dose should be reduced by 50%.[42]

LABORATORY STUDIES

Serum quinidine levels of 1 to 4 μg/mL are considered therapeutic. Toxic symptoms are expected at levels greater than 5 μg/mL. Combined serum levels of both procainamide and its active metabolite, NAPA, must be measured for evaluation of procainamide toxicity. A combined level of greater than 30 μg/mL is potentially cardiotoxic. Combined levels of greater than 60 μg/mL are likely to cause lethargy and hypotension. Disopyramide levels of greater than 5 μg/mL are considered toxic.

TREATMENT

General Management

Treatment of an overdose of a class IA antiarrhythmic should include early and aggressive management of the airway. The possibility of rapid decline in mental status and the onset of cardiac arrhythmias places these patients at very high risk of aspiration and pulmonary compromise. Once the airway is controlled, gastrointestinal decontamination should be a priority. Gastric lavage may be helpful in recent

Table 90–2. Drugs Metabolized by CYP2D6

β-Blockers	Timolol Propranolol Metoprolol Propafenone
Tricyclic antidepressants	Nortriptyline Amitriptyline Desipramine Imipramine Clomipramine
Neuroleptics	Thioridazine Fluphenazine Perphenazine Trifluperidol
Monoamine oxidase inhibitors	Amiflamine Methoxyphenamine
Antiarrhythmics	Flecainide Encainide
Other	Codeine Dextromethorphan Phenformin Methamphetamine

ingestions, and oral activated charcoal should be administered. Repeat doses of charcoal are of minimal clinical benefit and may be harmful to patients with decreased gastrointestinal motility. Admission to an intensive care setting for cardiac monitoring is appropriate for all symptomatic patients.

Seizures secondary to use of class IA antiarrhythmics respond readily to administration of benzodiazepines. Loading with other anticonvulsants is not indicated unless the seizures are recurrent or prolonged. Phenobarbital, 15 mg/kg intravenously, should be used for persistent seizure activity. Monitoring of creatine phosphokinase levels for evidence of rhabdomyolysis should be carried out for any patient "found down" (obtunded) for an unknown period.

Cardiac Toxicity

Class IA antiarrhythmics' strong cardiac sodium channel blocker activity is responsible for the intraventricular conduction delays in overdose.[36] *Wide complex rhythms may respond to intravenous administration of a sodium bicarbonate bolus.*[43, 44] The exact mechanism of action of sodium bicarbonate in the treatment of ventricular tachycardia secondary to Na^+ blockade may be related to either the physical displacement of the drug from the Na^+ channel by increased serum Na^+ concentration[43] or decreased binding to the channel by increasing the serum pH.[44, 45] Bradycardia unresponsive to atropine may require transcutaneous or transvenous pacing.[35] Hypotension should initially be treated with intravenous fluids. Patients with a history of cardiac dysfunction should be closely monitored for signs of fluid overload and may need placement of a Swan-Ganz catheter for continued evaluation of fluid status. Both epinephrine and dopamine have been reported to be effective in treating associated hypotension.[46, 47]

Torsades de pointes, an arrhythymia occurring at subtherapeutic and therapeutic levels of class IA antiarrhythmics, is usually preceded by a relatively slow heart rate and a prolonged QT interval.[48, 49] Antiarrhythmics routinely used for ventricular tachycardia are often ineffective in its treatment. *Patients presenting with torsades de pointes of any origin should be given 2 g of intravenous magnesium sulfate followed by a 1- to 2-g/h infusion.*[50, 51] Although the exact mechanism by which magnesium sulfate terminates torsades de pointes is not understood, research suggests it suppresses early afterdepolarization activity by shortening the plateau phase of cardiac depolarization.[52] Hypokalemia should also be corrected. If these measures are ineffective, transvenous overdrive pacing may convert torsades de pointes.[24, 49, 53] Isoproterenol may be considered but must be used with caution in patients with underlying cardiac disease.

Extracorporeal Drug Removal

Hemodialysis and hemoperfusion are ineffective in the treatment of acute quinidine poisoning because of this drug's large volume of distribution and extensive protein binding.[2] The half-life of disopyramide has been shown to be significantly reduced in patients undergoing hemodialysis and should be considered in patients not responding to supportive therapy.[54] Hemodialysis has been shown to double the clearance of procainamide and to provide a fourfold increase of elimination of NAPA, the active metabolite of procainamide.[55] Braden and colleagues demonstrated that hemoperfusion is superior to hemodialysis in the clearance of procainamide and NAPA.[56] Douglass and co-workers demonstrated continuous arteriovenous hemofiltration to provide even higher clearance than episodic hemoperfusion.[57] Dialysis equipment now capable of high flow rates may provide drug clearance that is equal if not superior to that of both hemofiltration and continuous arteriovenous hemofiltration.

References

1. Bigger JT, Hoffman B: Antiarrhythmic drugs. *In* Gilman AG, Roll TW, Nies AS, et al (eds): Goodman and Gilman's the Pharmacological Basis of Therapeutics. 8th ed. New York, Pergamon Press, pp 848–850, 1990.
2. Ochs HR, Greenblatt DJ, Wood E: Clinical pharmacokinetics of quinidine. Clin Pharmacokinet *5:*150, 1980.
3. Kim S, Benowitz N: Poisoning due to class IA antiarrhythmic drugs. Drug Saf *5:*393, 1990.
4. Palmer K, Martin B, Baggett B, et al: The metabolic fate of orally administered quinidine gluconate in humans. Biochem Pharmacol *18:*1845, 1969.
5. Karlsson E: Clinical pharmacokinetics of procainamide. Clin Pharmacokinet *3:*97, 1978.
6. Giardina E-GV, Bigger JT, Shaw JM, Schreiber EC: Metabolism of procainamide in normal and cardiac subjects. Clin Pharmacol Ther *19:*339, 1976.
7. Galeazzi RI, Sheiner LB, Lockwood T, Benet LZ: The renal elimination of procainamide. Clin Pharmacokinet *19:*55, 1976.
8. Bryson SM, Whiting B, Lawrence JR: Disopyramide serum and pharmacologic effect kinetics applied to the assessment of bioavailability. Br J Clin Pharmacol *6:*409, 1978.
9. Hinderling PH, Garrett ER: Pharmacokinetics of the antiarrhythmic disopyramide in healthy humans. J Pharmacokinet Biopharm *4:*199, 1976.
10. Tiliakos N, Waites T: Multiform quinidine toxicity. South Med J *74:*1267, 1981.
11. Cohen I, Jick H, Cohen S: Adverse reactions to quinidine in hospitalized patients: Findings based on data from the Boston Collaborative Drug Surveillance Program. Prog Cardiovasc Dis *20:*151, 1977.
12. Danielly J, DeJong R, Radke-Mitchell CC, Uprichard ACG: Procainamide-associated blood dyscrasias. Am J Cardiol *74:*1179, 1994.
13. Heyman M, Flores RH, Edelman BB, Carliner NH: Procainamide-induced lupus anticoagulant. South Med J *81:*934, 1988.
14. Strathman I, Cohen A, Nitzberg DM: Hypoglycemia in patients receiving disopyramide phosphate. Drug Intell Clin Pharm *17:*635, 1983.
15. Yung R, Richardson F: Drug-induced lupus. Rheum Dis Clin North Am *20:*61, 1994.
16. Yung R, Quddus J, Chrisp CE, Johnson KJ, et al: Mechanism of drug-induced lupus. J Immunol *154:*3025, 1995.
17. Chong B, Berndt MC, Koutts J, Castaldi PA: Quinidine-induced thrombocytopenia and leukopenia: Demonstration and characterization of distinct antiplatelet and antileukocyte antibodies. Blood *62:*1218, 1983.
18. Landrum E, Siegert EA, Hanlon JT, Currie MS: Prolonged

thrombocytopenia associated with procainamide in an elderly patient. Ann Pharmacother *28:*1172, 1994.
19. Goldberg I, Brown LK, Rayfield EJ: Disopyramide (Norpace)-induced hypoglycemia. Am J Med *69:*463, 1980.
20. Croxson M, Shaw DW, Hemley PG, Gabriel HDLL: Disopyramide-induced hypoglycaemia and increased serum insulin. N Z Med J *100:*407, 1987.
21. Podrid P, Schoeneberger A, Lown B: Congestive heart failure caused by oral disopyramide. N Engl J Med *302:*614–617, 1980.
22. Sicouri S, Antzelevitch C: Drug-induced afterdepolarizations and triggered activity occur in a discrete subpopulation of ventricular muscle cells (M cells) in the canine heart: Quinidine and digitalis. J Cardiovasc Electrophysiol *4:*48, 1993.
23. Binah O, Rosen M: Mechanisms of ventricular arrhythmias. Circulation *85:*1, 1992.
24. Jackman W, Friday KS, Anderson JL, Aliot EM, et al: The long QT syndromes: A critical review, new clinical observations and a unifying hypothesis. Prog Cardiovasc Dis *31:*115, 1988.
25. Riccioni N, Castiglioni M, Bartolomei C: Disopyramide-induced QT prolongation and ventricular tachyarrhythmias. Am Heart J *105:*870, 1983.
26. Olshansky B, Martins J, Hunt S: *N*-Acetyl procainamide causing torsade de pointes. Am J Cardiol *50:*1439, 1982.
27. Starasberg B, Scarovsky S, Erdberg A, et al: Procainaide-induced polymorphous ventricular tachycardia. Am J Cardiol *47:*1309, 1981.
28. Tzivoni D, Banai S, Schuger C, et al: Treatment of torsade de pointes with magnesium sulfate. Circulation *77:*392, 1988.
29. Waldo A, Wit A: Mechanisms of cardiac arrhythmias. Lancet *341:*1189, 1993.
30. Salata J, Wasserstrom A: Effects of quinidine on action potentials and ionic currents in isolated canine ventricular myocytes. Circ Res *62:*324, 1988.
31. Hoffman BF, Rosen MR, Wit AL: Electrophysiology and pharmacology of cardiac arrhythmias: VII. Cardiac effect of quinidine and procaine amide B. Am Heart J *90:*117, 1975.
32. Villemaire C, Nattel S: Modulation of procainamide's effect on cardiac conduction in dogs by extracellular potassium concentration. Circulation *89:*2870, 1994.
33. Lee R, Cohen TJ, Franz MR: Relation between repolarization and refractoriness in the human ventricle: Cycle length dependence and effect of procainamide. J Am Coll Cardiol *19:*614, 1992.
34. Dzimiri N, Almotrefi A: Interaction between potassium concentration and inhibition of myocardial Na^+-K^+-ATPase by two class IA antiarrhythmic drugs: Quinidine and procainamide. Arch Int Pharmacodyn *314:*34, 1991.
35. Kerr F, Kenoyer G, Bilitch M: Quinidine overdose: Neurological and cardiovascular toxicity in a normal person. Br Heart J *33:*629, 1971.
36. Summers WK, Allen RE, Pitts FN: Does physostigmine reverse quinidine delirium? West J Med *135:*411–412, 1981.
37. Grant A, Starmer F, Strauss H: Antiarrhythmic drug action: Blockade of the inward sodium current. Circ Res *55:*427, 1984.
38. Li G, Ferrier G: Effects of quinidine on arrhythmias and conduction in an isolated tissue model of ischemia and reperfusion. J Cardiovasc Pharmacol *17:*239, 1991.
39. Javaheri S, Logemann TN, Corser BC, et al: Diphragmatic paralysis. Am J Med *86:*623, 1989.
40. Leonard RF, Braun TE, Levy AM: Initiation of uterine contractions by disopyramide during pregnancy. N Engl J Med *299:*84, 1978.
41. Caporaso N, Shaw G: Clinical implications of the competitive inhibition of the debrisoquin-metabolizing isozyme by quinidine. Arch Intern Med *151:*1985, 1991.
42. Thatcher SK, Lemberg L: Digitalis-quinidine interaction. Heart Lung *9:*352, 1980.
43. Ranger S, Sheldon R, Fermini B, Nattel S: Modulation of flecainide's cardiac sodium channel blocking actions by extracellular sodium: A possible cellular mechanism for the action of sodium salts in flecainide cardiotoxicity. J Pharmacol Exp Ther *264:*1160, 1993.
44. Wasserman F, Brodsky L, Kathe JH, et al: The effect of molar sodium lactate in quinidine intoxication. Am J Cardiol: *4:*294, 1959.
45. Bellet S, Hamdan G, Somlyo A, Lara R, et al: The reversal of cardiotoxic effects of quinidine by molar sodium lactate: An experimental study. Am J Med Sci *237:*165, 1959.
46. Nolan M, Prichard J: Non-fatal overdose with disopyramide. Ir Med J *77:*209, 1984.
47. Villalba-Pimentel L, Epstein LM, Sellers EM, et al: Survival after massive procainamide ingestion. Am J Cardiol *32:*727, 1973.
48. El-Sherif N, Bekheit SS, Henkin R, et al: Quinidine-induced long QTC interval and torsade de pointes: Role of bradycardia-dependent early afterdepolarizations. J Am Coll Cardiol *14:*252, 1989.
49. Bauman J, Bauerafeind RA, Hoff JV, Strasberg B, Swiryn S, Rosen KM: Torsade de pointes due to quinidine: Observations in 31 patients. Am Heart J *107:*425, 1984.
50. Tzivoni D, Banai S, Schuger C, et al: Treatment of torsade de pointes with magnesium sulfate. Circulation *77:*392, 1988.
51. Vukmir R: Torsade de pointes. Am J Emerg Med *9:*250, 1991.
52. Kaseda S, Gilmour R, Zipes D: Depressant effect of magnesium on early afterdepolarization and triggered activity induced by cesium, quinidine, and 4-aminopyridine in canine cardiac Purkinje fibers. Am Heart J *118:*458, 1989.
53. Swiryn S, Kim S: Quinidine-induced syncope. Arch Intern Med *143:*314, 1983.
54. Horn J, Hughes M: Disopyramide dialysability. Letter. Lancet *2:*214, 1978.
55. Atkinson A, Krumlovsky FA, Huang CM, del Greco F, et al: Hemodialysis for severe procainamide toxicity: Clinical pharmacokinetic Observations. Clin Pharmacol Ther *20:*585, 1976.
56. Braden G, Fitzgibbons JP, Germain MS, Ledewitz HM, et al: Hemoperfusion for treatment of *N*-acetylprocainamide intoxication. Ann Intern Med *105:*64, 1986.
57. Douglass T, Dornoto DT, Broun MW, Bruggensmith P, et al: Removal of toxic levels of *N*-acetylprocainamide with continuous arteriovenous hemofiltration or continuous arteriovenous hemodiafiltration. Ann Intern Med *106:*550, 1987.
58. Mc Crum ID, Guidry JR: Procainamide-induced psychosis. JAMA *12:*1265, 1978.
59. Sheikh S, Seggev J: Procainamide-induced pleural fibrosis. Am J Med *91:*313, 1990.
60. Poukkula A, Paakko P: Quinidine-induced reversible pneumonities. Chest *106:*304, 1994.
61. Worman HJ, Ip JH, Winters SL, et al: Hypersensitivity reaction associated with acute hepatic dysfunction following a single intravenous dose of procainamide. J Intern Med *232:*361, 1992.
62. Thompson D, Skaehill P: Drug-induced lichen planus. Pharmacotherapy *14:*561, 1994.

91

Lidocaine

PHILIP D. WALSON, MD
MARCEL CASAVANT, MD

Since its discovery as a local anesthetic about 50 years ago, lidocaine has gained widespread use, first as an anesthetic and then as a parenteral antiarrhythmic agent. Less established indications for its use include headache,[1] seizures,[2, 3] tinnitus,[4] intubation-induced responses,[5] pain,[6] and even prevention of deep venous thrombosis.[7] Lidocaine also is used as a cocaine substitute; this is not surprising because procaine and then lidocaine were originally developed to replace cocaine. Mexiletine and tocainide are oral antiarrhythmic drugs with similar mechanisms, structures (Fig. 91–1), and toxicity; however, these two agents are not covered in this chapter because they are safer than lidocaine when taken orally and are much less commonly used.[8] Toxicity from lidocaine—as a result of therapeutic or illicit use, or after accidental or intentional overdose—is relatively common.[8] The diverse causes of lidocaine toxicity include the mistaken use of undiluted 20% lidocaine formulations,[9, 10] therapeutic use,[10–13] direct intravenous injection in suicide[14] or homicide attempts,[15] use as a cocaine substitute,[16] inadvertent intravenous or intra-arterial administration during local anesthesia,[17, 18] aspiration,[19] or ingestion (oral lidocaine).[20–22] Regardless of its cause, it is important for physicians to be aware of the presentation and treatment of lidocaine toxicity.

PHARMACOLOGY AND PHYSIOLOGY OF OVERDOSE

Lidocaine stabilizes the membranes of excitable cells, probably through inhibition of the tetrodotoxin-sensitive sodium channel but not the slow channel, to prevent the transmembrane sodium shifts that cause depolarization. In peripheral nerves, this results in conduction blockade and anesthesia. In the heart, depolarization of excitable cells is blocked, especially in ischemic cells and at rapid heart rates. At least part of lidocaine's effects may be the result of sympathetic inhibition. The end result of these actions depends on unbound drug concentrations, as well as on the type of cell and its physiologic state. The effect on cardiac activity depends on the ability of low lidocaine concentrations to slow conduction and increase refractoriness in diseased cardiac muscle while not altering nondiseased specialized atrial fibers, atrial muscle cells, and the sinoatrial or atrioventricular nodes. At usual concentrations, lidocaine has little effect on normal automaticity or conduction. However, at higher concentrations, lidocaine can decrease both automaticity and conduction by shortening the action potential and the refractory period of both His-Purkinje cells and healthy ventricular muscle. This can also occur at therapeutic concentrations in the presence of pre-existing sinus nodal dysfunction, abnormal His-Purkinje conduction, ischemia, or catecholamine-induced junctional escape arrhythmias. The specificity of lidocaine for His-Purkinje cells explains its effectiveness for ventricular rather than atrial arrhythmias. Lidocaine's widespread use in coronary care units is the result of its ability to increase the fibrillation threshold and decrease re-entry arrhythmias during or soon after acute coronary occlusion.[23–25]

Lidocaine is a type Ib antiarrhythmic drug. Unlike many other antiarrhythmic drugs, at usual therapeutic concentrations it has little if any effect on the QRS complex or QT interval, pulse, blood pressure, or cardiac contractility. However, at toxic concentrations (5 to 10 μg/mL; Table 91–1), lidocaine can directly decrease cardiac contractility and cause conduction abnormalities and life-threatening arrhythmias. After overdose, sodium conduction can be decreased even in normal tissue and can produce quinidine-like, wide QRS-complex arrhythmias, depressed contractility, vasodilation, low-output shock,

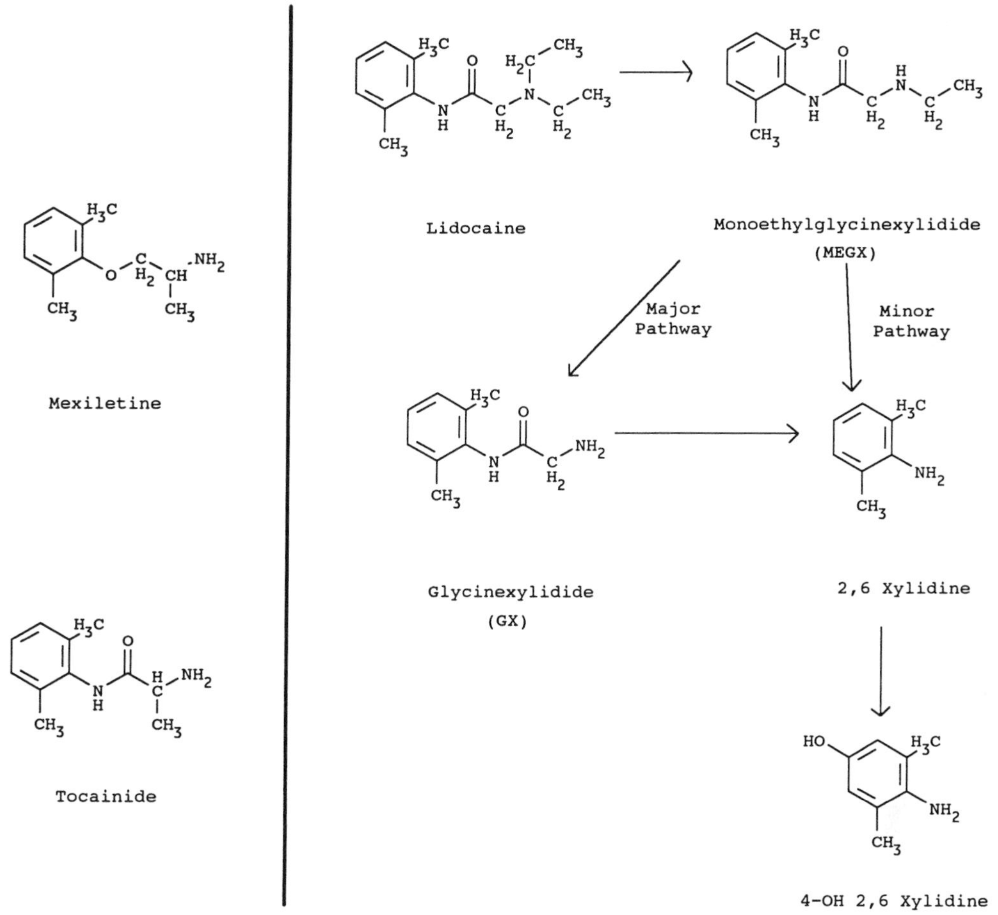

Mexiletine

Tocainide

Lidocaine

Monoethylglycinexylidide (MEGX)

Major Pathway

Minor Pathway

Glycinexylidide (GX)

2,6 Xylidine

4-OH 2,6 Xylidine

Figure 91–1. Chemical structure of mexiletine, tocainide, and lidocaine, as well as the metabolic pathway for lidocaine.

and decreased automaticity with slow ventricular rhythm or even asystole.[23–25]

The duration of action of lidocaine is dependent on many factors, including the dose, rate, and site of drug administration; the disease being treated; the lidocaine concentration before and after administration of the dose; the patient's clearance of the drug; the percentage of protein-bound lidocaine; the patient's physiologic state; the presence of other drugs; and the concentration of lidocaine metabolites.[23]

CLINICAL PRESENTATION OF OVERDOSE AND OTHER EFFECTS

Toxic signs and symptoms are largely the result of the cocaine-like effects (see Chapter 39) of lidocaine and its metabolites on the central nervous and cardiovascular systems. Gastrointestinal, hematologic, pulmonary, and immunologic signs are indirect or less common.

Central nervous system toxicity with seizures and respiratory arrest is also seen in severe intoxication. Inhibitory neurons are blocked first, followed by excitatory neurons; this leads to initial stimulation and convulsions followed by central nervous system depression. Nonsystemic toxicity (e.g., neuritis or aseptic meningitis) may result from high concentrations at the site of administration.

Toxic signs are age and dose dependent. Early symptoms consist of light-headedness, visual disturbances, paresthesias (especially perioral), feelings of intoxication, euphoria, gastrointestinal upset, and blurred vision. These symptoms may proceed to dysarthria, ataxia, memory loss, tinnitus, hearing loss, confusion, and disorientation; these are followed by seizures or coma and muscle fasciculations, then by paralysis, cardiac arrhythmias, and decreased cardiac contractility or congestive heart failure. Anaphylaxis and methemoglobinemia have also been reported; the latter is especially important in glucose-6-phosphate dehydrogenase–deficient patients and in children taking other methemoglobin-producing compounds. In neonates, apnea, dilated pupils, hypotonia, loss of oculocephalic reflexes, and seizures have also been seen,[8] especially after direct injection into the fetus during delivery. True allergic reactions occur but are rare and may be the result of reactions to preservatives rather than to lidocaine itself.

Rapid, sensitive assays are available for measuring concentrations of lidocaine and its monoethylglycylxylidide (MEGX) metabolite. When properly interpreted, the results of these assays can be used to increase lidocaine's clinical efficacy and decrease its toxicity, as well as to identify lidocaine toxicity in the nontherapeutic setting.

Table 91–1. Clinical Features of Lidocaine Intoxication

Central Nervous System

Lightheadedness, anxiety, visual disturbances, dilated pupils
Paresthesias, dysarthria, feelings of intoxication
Ataxia, memory loss, tinnitus, hearing loss
Euphoria, agitation, drowsiness
Confusion, disorientation, psychosis, coma
Shivering, muscle fasciculations, tremor, paralysis
Hypotonia (in neonates)
Seizures
Respiratory arrest

Cardiovascular

Arrhythmias

Sinus arrest
Sinus bradycardia
Atrioventricular junctional or ventricular bradycardia
Second- or third-degree heart block
Asystole
QRS complex prolongation*
Ventricular tachycardia or fibrillation*

Hypotension

Vasodilation
Depressed myocardial contractility and low cardiac output, congestive heart failure

Gastrointestinal

Nausea, vomiting

Hematologic

Methemoglobinemia

Local

Necrosis
Neuritis
Aseptic meningitis
Loss of vision (common with retrobulbar use)

Immunologic

Rash
Anaphylaxis

*In massive poisoning.

PHARMACOKINETICS (Table 91–2)

Absorption

Lidocaine is usually administered intravenously, subcutaneously, or topically. The oral absorption of lidocaine is rapid and almost complete; however, there is rapid and extensive (50% to 75%) first-pass metabolism to metabolites (especially MEGX) that are more toxic than lidocaine itself.[25] The failure to appreciate this factor is responsible for numerous cases of iatrogenic toxicity from the oral use of oral lidocaine. However, patients with hepatic cirrhosis or portacaval shunts may absorb 90% or more of a lidocaine dose unchanged into their circulation. Rectal doses can deliver up to 70% of a lidocaine dose unmetabolized in most patients. However, in most patients, oral administration is too toxic and rectal administration too erratic for either to be advised. In all patients, lidocaine is well absorbed from mucous membranes of the nose, mouth, esophagus, intestine, respiratory tract, vagina, and bladder.[26] There have been many cases of significant toxicity reported from use of nasal lidocaine, ingestion of lidocaine by a "body packer" unwittingly carrying the drug instead of cocaine, use of topical lidocaine sprays for invasive procedures such as bronchoscopy or endoscopy,[27] and oral or vaginal use of lidocaine. To decrease the chances of iatrogenic toxicity, it is important to be aware of the difference between low percentage concentrations and low dosages. As an example, a 10-kg child who ingests only 10 mL of a 2% lidocaine solution receives 200 mg of lidocaine. This dose (20 mg/kg) is more than twice the milligram-per-kilogram dose that produced mild central nervous system toxicity in 5 of 12 adult patients given a 750-mg dose.[28] The confusion about low concentrations and amounts is also responsible for cases of systemic toxicity after local use, such as for cardiac catheterization.[29, 30] Lidocaine is also well absorbed after intramuscular injections. The rate of absorption depends on the muscle group and on individual differences in muscle blood flow; for example, injections are more rapidly absorbed from the deltoid muscle than the gluteal muscle. The absorption of lidocaine after perivascular use also depends on the site of injection and whether epinephrine is added as a vasoconstrictor to slow absorption. Absorption rate increases progressively, from subcutaneous to brachial plexus to epidural to intercostal sites.[23]

Distribution

Intravenous lidocaine is distributed throughout the body. It is first rapidly (distribution half-life, 4 to 12 minutes) distributed to well-perfused tissues (e.g., brain and heart), with subsequent slower redistribution to less well–perfused tissues and much slower metabolism (half-life, 1 to 8 hours). It readily crosses the placenta, and it distributes into red blood cells with a red blood cell–to–plasma ratio of 1.1:1.5. Distribution is much less important with nonintravenous routes of administration. Because the volume of distribution of lidocaine is about 1.5 ± 0.3 L/kg (less in patients with congestive heart failure), each 1-mg/kg intravenous dose raises the lidocaine concen-

Table 91–2. Average Pharmacokinetic Values of Lidocaine in Healthy Adults

Parameter	Value
Oral availability (%)	35
Usual dose	1–4 mg/min IV
Per cent urinary excretion* (unchanged)	2
Plasma protein binding (%)	50†
Volume of distribution (L/kg)	1.1
Clearance (mL/min per kg)	10–15
Half-life (h)	1–8
"Therapeutic" serum concentration (mg/L)	1.5–5.5‡
Minimally effective concentration for premature ventricular contractions	0.6–2.0§

*Renal excretion is pH dependent; excretion is greater in acid urine.
†Protein binding is concentration dependent; 30% bound at 20 mg/L.
‡Total concentrations given; may be altered by protein binding and metabolite concentrations.
§Toxicity can occur at <5 μg/mL, and concentrations as high as 8 μg/mL have been required and tolerated.

tration by about 1 μg/mL. Thus, when given 100 mg, a 50-kg patient with a lidocaine level of 4 μg/mL may attain a level of 6 μg/mL; in contrast, a 100-kg patient with no lidocaine may only attain a level of 0.5 μg/mL. After a single intravenous dose, the lidocaine concentration in a "normal" patient decreases by one half within 15 to 20 minutes, primarily as a result of distribution. This is why patients may experience seizures after rapid intravenous administration of a dose yet have therapeutic lidocaine concentrations minutes later. In patients with poor perfusion, previous lidocaine accumulation, or slow metabolism, the decrease is much slower. After the initial distribution, plasma concentrations decrease much more slowly (elimination half-life, 110 ± 24 minutes). Adults of normal size with normal clearance require an infusion rate of 1 to 3 mg/min for maintenance of therapeutic concentrations, but patients with slow clearance accumulate lidocaine if they are given this much. Failure to properly determine and interpret lidocaine concentrations, as well as an incomplete appreciation of lidocaine pharmacokinetics, can result in iatrogenic lidocaine toxicity.

Protein binding of lidocaine is concentration dependent; it is 80% bound at 3 μg/mL, 60% bound at 10 μg/mL, and only 30% bound at 20 μg/mL. Protein binding is largely to α_1-acid glycoprotein (70%); a smaller amount (about 30%) binds to albumin. However, this ratio is dependent on the concentrations of albumin, lidocaine, and α_1-acid glycoprotein. Although not routinely measured, unbound concentrations are more indicative of drug effects than are total concentrations. Unbound concentrations can be as much as twofold greater in newborns and in patients with hepatitis than in normal patients because of decreased α_1-acid glycoprotein concentrations. In contrast, patients with uremia or cancer, those who have had myocardial infarction, and those who have undergone cardiac surgery or anticonvulsant treatment may have lower unbound concentrations due to increased concentrations of α_1-acid glycoprotein[23] (an acute phase reactant).

Elimination

Lidocaine elimination is best described by a two-compartment open model: elimination is from the central compartment, primarily by hepatic de-ethylation (see Fig. 91–1) to two active metabolites, MEGX and glycine xylidide (GX), both of which are renally excreted to a greater degree than is lidocaine. The initial, rapid lidocaine distribution phase is followed by a slower, metabolic β phase. The rate of metabolism varies widely among patients and disease states. MEGX and GX can accumulate because they are cleared more slowly than is lidocaine (terminal half-lives, about 2 and 10 hours for MEGX and GX, respectively). It appears that the significant gastrointestinal and central nervous system toxicity caused by these metabolites—and not poor absorption—limits the oral use of lidocaine.[8] In most patients, lidocaine has a high hepatic extraction ratio (about 0.7); therefore, lidocaine clearance (mean, 13 mL/min per kilogram)[23] is primarily determined by hepatic blood flow. Lidocaine clearance is generally unaffected by the concentrations of hepatic drug–metabolizing enzymes. However, this extraction ratio may be much lower in patients with cirrhosis, congestive heart failure, active hepatitis, or cardiogenic shock, as well as in patients taking drugs that interfere with hepatic metabolism (e.g., cimetidine) or decrease cardiac output and hepatic flow (e.g., β-blockers or norepinephrine) in whom use of usual lidocaine infusion rates can cause accumulation and life-threatening toxicity. The hypotensive, low-output state induced by severe lidocaine toxicity also can cause delayed lidocaine elimination.

Renal elimination of lidocaine is minor (about 10% of total clearance), but it may be more important in patients with severe hepatic dysfunction and for lidocaine metabolites (especially GX).

TREATMENT OF LIDOCAINE POISONING

As for any patient with toxicity, treatment consists of correct diagnosis, supportive care, minimization of further exposure, and if possible, hastening of toxin elimination and administration of antidotal or physiologic antagonists.

A high level of suspicion is sometimes necessary to diagnose lidocaine toxicity. This is especially important in patients who are not known to be receiving lidocaine. Even in patients being treated with lidocaine, toxicity can be missed. The diagnosis should be considered in any symptomatic patient who is given, is taking, or has access to a lidocaine-containing preparation. This includes infants whose mothers received lidocaine for local anesthesia during delivery (i.e., infant toxicity is either secondary to maternal toxicity or the result of accidental fetal injection). Young infants in whom topical lidocaine or Emla (2.5% each of lidocaine and prilocaine) has been applied—especially on or near mucous membranes or skin that can be put in the mouth—also are at risk, as are children, adolescents, and adults who have access to nonmedical "cocaine" or in whom any formulation of lidocaine was used therapeutically.

Toxic symptoms may occur at concentrations just above the therapeutic range, and plasma lidocaine concentrations correlate fairly well with effects (Table 91–3). Once toxicity is suspected, blood should be sent for lidocaine therapeutic drug monitoring. MEGX concentrations should also be determined in selected cases. If a urine toxicologic screen is ordered, the finding of lidocaine or its metabolites should not be ignored because it may be significant, even in a patient treated with topical or intravenous lidocaine. Treatment (Table 91–4) should not be delayed even for the brief time needed for therapeutic drug monitoring results to be reported (1 to 2 hours). False-positive results can occur if venous samples are

Table 91–3. Relationship Between Concentration and Toxic Effect

Concentration (µg/mL)		
1.5–6	*6–8*	*>8*
Anxiety Dizziness Drowsiness Feeling of cold, heat, numbness	Nausea/vomiting Visual changes Tinnitus Tremors Twitching	Troubled breathing Severe dizziness or fainting Bradycardia Seizures

From Drug Information for the Health Care Professional, US Pharmacopeial Convention: US Pharmacopeia Dispensing Information (USP DI). 15th ed. Taunton, MA, Rand McNally & Co., 1995.

drawn from extremities where the drug has been given or through lines used to administer the drug. Skin puncture samples can be contaminated with drug used topically or by fingers put into the mouth after oral lidocaine administration. Any delay in obtaining blood also should be taken into consideration when the results are interpreted. Even short delays between the onset of symptoms and blood collection can lead to significant decreases in concentration, and as a result the diagnosis of lidocaine toxicity may not be made. Failure to measure metabolite concentrations also can obscure the diagnosis of toxicity.

Primary treatment (see Table 91–4) involves discontinuing further lidocaine administration and observation until absorption is complete. This may involve turning off the intravenous infusion and discarding any lidocaine-containing fluid in the tubing, decreasing venous drainage from injection sites, removing ruptured body packing condoms, or washing off contaminated mucous membranes. Lavage should be performed and activated charcoal administered for intestinal exposures. Induction of emesis is contraindicated even after oral administration because of the risk of seizures and aspiration. The remainder of treatment is supportive and involves therapy for heart block, convulsions, respiratory compromise, or cardiac arrest. It is especially important not to use lidocaine to treat cardiac arrhythmias caused by unsuspected lidocaine toxicity. Examples include bronchoscopy or endoscopy patients with overdoses of topically applied lidocaine, cardiac patients inadvertently given overdoses of undiluted 20% lidocaine, and drug abusers who unknowingly have overdoses of lidocaine substituted for cocaine. It is also prudent to avoid the use of drugs which, like lidocaine, block sodium transport (e.g., phenytoin). The presence of severe bradyarrhythmias or asystole may require pacing.

The therapy provided also depends on the original indication, if any, for use of the drug. In selected cardiac patients (e.g., patients with ventricular arrhythmias deliberately given high doses in preparation for cardioversion), lidocaine use may even be continued and pacing added. In most patients, high-dose sodium administration (sodium bicarbonate) may be useful for arrhythmias and high-dose barbiturates or benzodiazepines for seizures. Anesthesia should be considered for patients with unresponsive status. Except in patients with continued absorption (e.g., after oral ingestion) or delayed clearance (e.g., in patients with liver dysfunction or congestive heart failure) the symptoms are usually short lived. Although oral activated charcoal administration has not been proved to be effective, its use should be considered because little else can be done immediately to hasten elimination and block further absorption. Hemodialysis is probably not useful. Urine acidification increases renal clearance, but the increase is unlikely to be clinically useful because so little lidocaine is cleared renally. Also, acidification has significant risks, especially in the presence of acidemia and myoglobinemia. Therefore, acidification is not recommended. Hemoperfusion might be useful for toxicity with lidocaine or its metabolites. However, hemoperfusion would be extremely difficult to perform without cardiac bypass in the presence of the cardiac decompensation, which is likely to be present in patients sufficiently poisoned for its use to be considered. Clinically significant methemoglobinemia should be treated and attempts should be made to correct hypotension and poor hepatic perfusion with administration of fluids or pressor agents,

Table 91–4. Treatment of Lidocaine Overdose

General Management

Discontinue further administration
Oral ingestion: Administer charcoal and possibly lavage
Seizures: Administer diazepam, up to 5–10 mg IV

Impaired Myocardial Conduction

Sodium bicarbonate: Administer 0.5–1 mEq/kg IV; repeat every 5–10 min to maintain arterial pH of 7.4–7.5

Arrhythmias

Bradyarrhythmias

Isoproterenol
Cardiac pacemaker

Ventricular Tachycardia

Overdrive pacing
(Avoid using other type Ib antiarrhythmic drugs)

Hypotension

Administer normal saline, 2–3 mL/kg every 10 min until response, 15–30 mL/kg has been given, or evidence of pulmonary edema demonstrated
If patient is still hypotensive, consider pulmonary arterial catheter insertion:
If low systemic vascular resistance, administer dopamine or norepinephrine
If low cardiac output, administer isoproterenol, dobutamine, or epinephrine
If patient has intractable cardiogenic shock, consider intra-aortic balloon pump assistance or cardiopulmonary bypass
Methemoglobinemia: Consider administering 1–2 mg/kg of 1% methylene blue if the patient is cyanotic or symptomatic, or has a methemoglobin level >30%

Accelerated Drug Removal

Consider hemoperfusion in patients with massive poisonings with circulatory and/or liver failure (possibly combined with cardiopulmonary bypass)

IV, intravenously.

the use of pump-assist devices or cardiac bypass, or, in selected cases, extracorporeal membrane oxygenation.[31]

ACKNOWLEDGMENT

Supported by NICHD Pediatric Pharmacology Research Unit HD31316 and by grant 5F32 ES 05651–02 from the National Institute of Environmental Health Sciences, National Institutes of Health.

References

1. Kaube H, Hoskin KL, Goadsby PJ: Lignocaine and headache: An electrophysiological study in the cat with supporting clinical observations in man. J Neurol *241*:415–420, 1994.
2. Lemmen LJ, Klassen M, Duiser B: Intravenous lidocaine in the treatment of convulsions. JAMA *239*:2025, 1978.
3. Morris HH: Lidocaine: A neglected anticonvulsant? South Med J *72*:1564, 1978.
4. Lyttkens L, Larsson B, Wasterstrom SA: Local anesthetics and tinnitus: Proposed peripheral mechanism of action of lidocaine. ORL J Otorhinolaryngol Relat Spec *46*:17–23, 1984.
5. Brown RH, Robbins W, Staats P, Hirshman C: Prevention of bronchoconstriction by an orally active local anesthetic. Am J Respir Crit Care Med *151*:1239–1243, 1995.
6. Rowlingson JC, DiFazio CA, Foster J, et al: Lidocaine as an analgesic for experimental pain. Anesthesiology *52*:20–22, 1980.
7. Cooke ED, Lloyd MJ, Bowcock SA, et al: Intravenous lidocaine in prevention of deep venous thrombosis after elective hip surgery. Lancet *2*:797–799, 1977.
8. Benowitz N: Lidocaine, mexiletine, and tocainide. *In* Haddad LM, Winchester JF (eds): Clinical Management of Poisoning and Drug Overdose. 2nd ed. Philadelphia, W.B. Saunders Co., pp 1371–1379, 1990.
9. Kempen PM: Lethal/toxic injection of 20% lidocaine: A well-known complication of an unnecessary preparation? Anesthesiology *65*:564–565, 1986.
10. Pfeifer HJ, Greenblatt DJ, Koch-Weser J: Clinical use and toxicity of intravenous lidocaine: A report from the Boston Collaborative Drug Surveillance Program. Am Heart J *92*:168–173, 1976.
11. Boston Collaborative Drug Surveillance Program: Drug-induced convulsions. Lancet *2*:677–679, 1972.
12. Davison R, Parker M, Atkinson AJ Jr: Excessive serum lidocaine levels during maintenance infusions: Mechanisms and prevention. Am Heart J *104*:203–208, 1982.
13. Tjon a Ten WE: Lidocaine poisoning in a newborn infant following perineal infiltration for episiotomy. Review. Tijdschr Kindergeneeskunde *60*:49–52, 1992.
14. Dawling S, Flanagan RJ, Widdop B: Fatal lignocaine poisoning: Report of two cases and review of the literature. Hum Toxicol *8*:389–392, 1989.
15. Peat MA, Deyman ME, Crouch DJ, et al: Concentrations of lidocaine and monoethylglycylxylidide (MEGX) in lidocaine-associated deaths. J Forensic Sci *30*:1048–1057, 1985.
16. Nichols GR II, Davis GJ: Body packing with a twist: Death of a salesman. Am J Forensic Med Pathol *13*:142–145, 1992.
17. Alfano SN, Leicht MJ, Skiendzielewski JJ: Lidocaine toxicity following subcutaneous administration. Ann Emerg Med *13*:465–467, 1984.
18. Grimes DA, Cates W Jr: Deaths from paracervical anesthesia used for first trimester abortion. N Engl J Med *295*:1397–1399, 1976.
19. Garrettson LK, McGee EB: Rapid onset of seizures following aspiration of viscous lidocaine. J Toxicol Clin Toxicol *30*:413–422, 1992.
20. Hess GP, Walson PD: Seizures secondary to oral viscous lidocaine. Ann Emerg Med *17*:725–727, 1988.
21. Smith M, Wolfram W, Rose R: Toxicity: Seizures in an infant caused by (or related to) oral viscous lidocaine use. J Emerg Med *10*:587–590, 1992.
22. Geraets DR, Scott SD, Ballew KA: Toxicity potential of oral lidocaine in a patient receiving mexiletine. Ann Pharmacother *26*:1380–1381, 1992.
23. Stargel WW: Lidocaine. *In* Taylor WJ, Diers-Caviness MH (eds): A Textbook for the Clinical Application of Therapeutic Drug Monitoring. Irving, TX, Abbott Laboratories, pp 109–123, 1986.
24. Drug Information for the Health Care Professional, US Pharmacopeial Convention: US Pharmacopeia Dispensing Information (USP DI). 15th ed. Taunton, MA, Rand McNally & Co., pp 1720–1728, 1995.
25. Ritchie JM, Greene NM: Local anesthetics. *In* Gilman AG, Rall TW, Nies AS, Taylor P (eds): Goodman & Gilman's The Pharmacological Basis of Therapeutics. 8th ed. New York, Permagon Press, pp 311–331, 1990.
26. Watson WA, Sands MF, Barlow JC, et al: Lidocaine absorption and metabolism after oropharyngeal application in young and young-elderly adults. DICP *25*:463–465, 1991.
27. Lin SY, Wang SJ, Tso HS, et al: A case report of possible lidocaine intoxication due to sprays of 8% lidocaine. Acta Anaesthesiol Sin *32*:219–222, 1994.
28. Perucca E, Richens A: Reduction of oral bioavailability of lidocaine by induction of first-pass metabolism in epileptic patients. Br J Clin Pharmacol *8*:21–31, 1979.
29. Palmisano JM, Meliones JN, Crowley DC, et al: Lidocaine toxicity after subcutaneous infiltration in children undergoing cardiac catheterization. Am J Cardiol *67*:647–648, 1991.
30. Ryan CA, Robertson M, Coe JY: Seizures due to lidocaine toxicity in a child during cardiac catheterization. Pediatr Cardiol *14*:116–118, 1993.
31. Ellenhorn MJ, Barceloux D: Medical Toxicology: Diagnosis and Treatment of Human Poisoning. New York, Elsevier Science Publishing Co., pp 183–186, 1988.

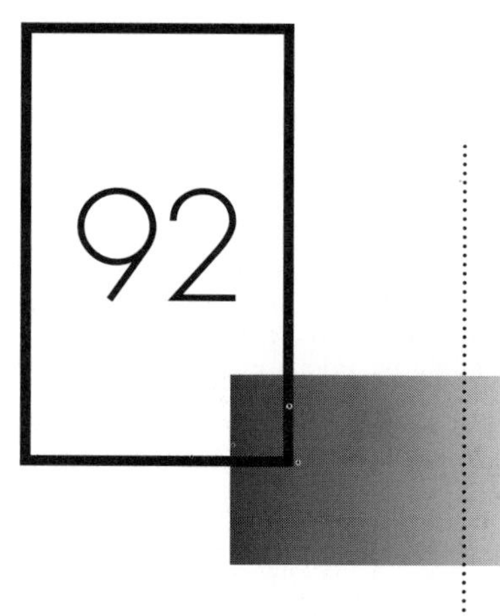

The New Cardiac Antiarrhythmic Agents

GRADY H. HENDRIX, MD

Pharmacologic therapy of cardiac arrhythmias is now an established principle. Antiarrhythmic drugs are widely disseminated, and many patients are using them for treatment of cardiac arrhythmias. The opportunity for chronic overdosage when used in a therapeutic manner, acute overdosage when inadvertently ingested, and acute overdosage when these drugs are intentionally ingested in excessive amounts are widespread. Emergency physicians encounter many patients taking these drugs and must be prepared to treat acute and chronic toxicity whether intentional or unintentional. The potential benefits of antiarrhythmic therapy are that they may decrease arrhythmia-related symptoms and decrease mortality. Although many patients do benefit from reduced symptoms of their underlying rhythm disorder, the evidence that these drugs reduce mortality has been proved only in the case of β-adrenergic blockers. Some of them clearly increase mortality, but adequate data are not available for the majority of them as far as their effect on mortality is concerned (Table 92–1).[1] The risks of antiarrhythmic therapy in general in addition to the prorhythmic effects are those associated with depressing ventricular function. Except in the case of amiodarone, most of the known noncardiac risks are those of nuisance-type symptoms rather than anything that could be life threatening. Information is desperately needed and clinical trials are now under way to help to identify the relative risks and benefits of many drugs as well as devices such as implantable cardioverter defibrillators that prevent death due to cardiac arrhythmias.

Life-threatening ventricular arrhythmias may be treated by administering the maximum tolerated dose of an antiarrhythmic agent to ensure suppression of a life-threatening electric disturbance. For safety reasons, starting doses of antiarrhythmic drugs under these circumstances are best established in a hospital. One must guide their therapy and incremental dose increases by careful monitoring and in some cases repeated electrophysiologic studies.

GENERAL MECHANISMS OF ACTION AND CLASSIFICATION

The normal Purkinje fiber action potential of the myocardial cell remains the basic landmark in understanding electrophysiology at the cellular level and the mechanism of action of antiarrhythmic drugs. Figure 92–1 illustrates the normal Purkinje fiber action potential of the myocardial cell. Depolarization of the Purkinje cell occurs in phase 0, and at that

Table 92–1. Effects of Long-Term Antiarrhythmic Therapy on Mortality in Placebo-Controlled, Randomized Trials

Effect	Therapy
Increases mortality	Encainide
	Flecainide
	Moricizine (short-term)
Reduces mortality	β-Adrenergic blockers
Adequate data not available	Amiodarone
	Disopyramide
	Mexiletine
	Moricizine (long-term)
	Procainamide
	Propafenone
	Quinidine
	Tocainide
	Sotalol
	Implanted cardioverter-defibrillators

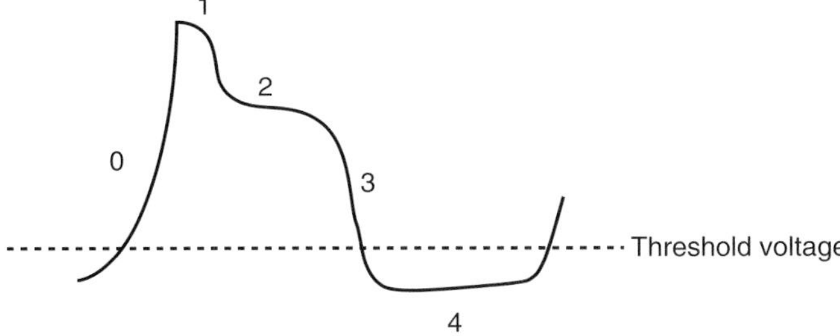

Figure 92–1. The normal Purkinje fiber action potential of the myocardial cell. Depolarization occurs in phase 0; phase 1 is overshoot, phase 2 is plateau, phase 3 leads repolarization, and phase 4 is spontaneous depolarization back to the threshold voltage, where the process will repeat itself. During phase 0 the fast sodium inward channel is activated, sodium and slow calcium inward currents occur during phase 1 and 2, and in phase 3, potassium moves out of the cell and the sodium and calcium channels cease to move inward.

point the fast sodium inward channel is activated. In phases 1 and 2, which are the plateau and repolarization phases, sodium and slow calcium channel inward currents occur, and in phase 3, potassium moves out of the cell during repolarization. After depolarization has ended, diastole occurs and the resting voltage slowly rises to the threshold level again, at which point the process repeats. All antiarrhythmic drugs have a mechanism of action that involves some of these electrophysiologic characteristics of the Purkinje cell.

The Vaughan Williams classification of antiarrhythmic drugs (Table 92–2) is the present electrophysiologic concept.[2] The class I drugs act principally by decreasing the fast inward sodium current in a dose-dependent manner. This slows the rate of phase 0 depolarization (V_{max}) and the rate of conduction of the cardiac impulse. Class I drugs are divided into three classifications because of otherwise different electrophysiologic activity.

Class IA drugs, which include quinidine, procainamide, and disopyramide, slow conduction only slightly at therapeutic doses. With excessive doses, this action is exaggerated and the QRS interval is prolonged. Class IA drugs also prolong action potential duration, and this results in increasing the effective refractory period. The most dangerous effect of class IA drugs is prolongation of the QT interval, which can lead to a torsades de pointes type of polymorphic ventricular tachycardia and fibrillation.

Class IB drugs, which include lidocaine, mexiletine, tocainide, and moricizine, slow phase 0 markedly in abnormal tissue but not in normal tissue. These drugs shorten the action potential duration very slightly and have no effect on the QT interval.

Class IC drugs, which include flecainide and propafenone, markedly depress phase 0 with slowing of conduction and prolongation of the QRS even at therapeutic doses. They have little effect on the action potential duration and do not prolong the QT interval.

The class II drugs are the β-adrenergic blockers. Sotalol is included in this group as well as in class III. Both the conventional β-blockers and the unusual β-blocker sotalol lengthen the action potential in all cardiac tissues. Sotalol does prolong the QT interval and has been known to produce torsades de pointes.

The class III antiarrhythmic drugs prolong the action potential duration and the effective refractory period. The QT interval is prolonged, and this can lead to torsades de pointes. Drugs in this group are amiodarone and bretylium; sotalol is considered primarily in this group but also in class II.

Class IV antiarrhythmic drugs are the calcium channel blockers.

Many of the modern antiarrhythmic agents have effects that straddle the four major categories of the Vaughan Williams classification. This serves to make things more complicated and is an unpleasant fact of life but must be recognized. A new classification scheme that categorizes antiarrhythmic drugs individually based on 11 different parameters has been proposed. This is known as the Sicilian gambit (Table 92–3).[3]

One should keep in mind some basic principles when dealing with patients using antiarrhythmic drugs:

1. For safety reasons, therapy with an antiarrhythmic drug for serious arrhythmias should be initiated with the patient in the hospital. This is dictated for most of the newer drugs by the package insert and by the Food and Drug Administration (FDA).
2. Adequate arrhythmia control must be assessed in follow-up by some form of continuous long-term recording rather than observation of the patient for a few minutes on electrocardiograms.
3. Any risk of developing torsades de pointes during therapy with drugs that prolong the QT interval is exaggerated at slow heart rates. Therefore, patients who have or who develop sinus bradycardia of 50 beats per minute or less should not receive such drugs.
4. The QRS duration should not be allowed to rise more than 50% above baseline in those patients receiving drugs that prolong the QRS interval.
5. The rate-corrected QT interval should not be allowed to exceed 550 ms in those patients taking drugs that prolong the QT interval.
6. Any degree of heart block other than first degree should be taken as evidence of toxicity in patients receiving those drugs that prolong atrioventricu-

Table 92–2. Vaughan Williams Classification of Antiarrhythmic Drugs

I	A Quinidine, procainamide, disopyramide
	B Tocainide, mexiletine, moricizine, lidocaine
	C Flecainide, propafenone
II	β-Adrenergic blockers, sotalol
III	Amiodarone, bretylium, sotalol
IV	Calcium channel blocker

Table 92–3. Characteristics of Selected Antiarrhythmic Drugs Using the Criteria of the Sicilian Gambit

	Channels				Receptors				Pumps
	Na⁺								
Drug	Fast	Medium	Slow	CA^{2+} K^+ I_F	α	β	M_2	*P*	Na^+, K^+-*ATPase*
Propafenone		◇				xx			
Flecainide			◇	x					
Sotalol				xxx		xxx			
Amiodarone	x			x xxx	xx	xx			

Relative blocking potency: x, low; xx, medium; xxx, high; ◇, high activated-state blocker.

lar (AV) conduction. The drugs should be discontinued.

7. Serum potassium and magnesium levels must be closely monitored in patients taking drugs that have a possibility of inducing torsades de pointes.
8. One should always be alert for signs of declining systolic ventricular function. Many antiarrhythmic drugs can precipitate congestive heart failure.
9. Drug interactions must be carefully watched for at all times. These are numerous, and one is frequently surprised by what may interact with the antiarrhythmic drug that one is prescribing. Some of the more common interactions involving drugs that are frequently used are listed in Table 92–4.

Table 92–5 summarizes the pharmacologic effects, electrophysiologic properties, and side effects of the new antiarrhythmic drugs.

INDIVIDUAL ANTIARRHYTHMIC DRUGS

This section discusses new antiarrhythmic drugs such as sotalol, propafenone, and moricizine and older established antiarrhythmic drugs that have new uses such as flecainide and amiodarone. Their use in atrial fibrillation and other supraventricular arrhythmias is addressed.

The remainder of this chapter is devoted to a discussion of individual antiarrhythmic drugs listed earlier, including their mechanism of action, indications, contraindications, drug interaction characteristics, and toxicology. Recognition and treatment of toxicity and overdoses are outlined in Table 92–6.

Sotalol

Sotalol is now recognized as a major therapeutic agent in the treatment of cardiovascular disorders including arrhythmias. It was introduced in 1965 as a β-adrenergic blocking agent, but its unique electrophysiologic properties have been recognized for about the past decade.[4, 5] Sotalol is now regarded as an important class III antiarrhythmic agent as well as a β-adrenoreceptor blocking agent. It selectively lengthens the cardiac action potential and competitively antagonizes β-adrenoreceptors. It is a nonse-

Table 92–4. Drugs Interacting with Antiarrhythmics and Their Effects

	Moricizine	**Amiodarone**	**Sotalol**	**Propafenone**
Antiarrhythmics				
Amiodarone			Hypotension	↓ HR
Flecainide		↑ [Flecainide]	Cardiac arrest	
Procainamide		↑ [Procainamide]		
Propafenone		Bradycardia, ↓ HR	↓ HR, CHF	
Propranolol		Bradycardia, ↓ HR	↓ HR, CHF	
Quinidine		↑ [Q], torsades de pointes	Torsades de pointes	↑ [Propafenone]
Antibiotics				
Cyclosporine		↑ [Cyclosporine]		↑ [Cyclosporine]
Rifampicin				↓ [Propafenone]
Anticoagulants				
Coumadin	↑ PT	↑ PT		
Bronchodilators				
Theophylline	↑ [Theophylline]			↑ [Theophylline]
Calcium Blockers				
Diltiazem		Bradycardia	Bradycardia	
Verapamil		Bradycardia	Bradycardia, ↓ BP	
Digoxin		↑ [Digoxin]		↑ [Digoxin]

[], Concentrations; ↑, increase; ↓, decrease; HR, heart rate; BP, blood pressure; PT, prothrombin time; CHF, congestive heart failure.

Table 92–5. Pharmacologic Effects, Electrophysiologic Properties, and Side Effects of Antiarrhythmics

Drug	Relative Potency of Receptor Blockade		Electrophysiologic Properties	Electrocardiographic Effects	Important Side Effects
Amiodarone	K^+ channel	+ + +	Prolongs action potential, slows AV nodal conduction velocity (increases AH interval)	Prolongs QT interval, prolongs PR interval, ↓ HR	CNS, hepatic, gastrointestinal, thyroid, pulmonary, cutaneous
	Na^+ channel	+			
	α-Adrenergic	+			
	β-Adrenergic	+			
	Ca^{2+} channel	+			
Sotalol	β-Adrenergic	+ + +	Prolongs action potential, prolongs AH interval, mild β-blocker effects	Prolongs QT interval, prolongs PR interval, ↓ HR	Torsades de pointes at low heart rates, thyroid, pulmonary bronchospasm
	K^+ channel	+ +			
Propafenone	Na^+ channel	+ + +	Prolongs AH interval, prolongs HV interval, mild β-blocker effects	Prolongs PR interval, prolongs QRS duration, minimal ↓ HR	Proarrhythmia at high heart rates, heart failure, bronchospasm
	β-Adrenergic	+			
	Ca^{2+} channel	+			
	K^+ channel	+			
Moricizine			Shortens action potential and ERP. Prolongs AV, AH, and HV intervals	Prolongs PR interval, prolongs QRS duration	Proarrhythmia, sinus bradycardia, arrest

AV, atrioventricular; CNS, central nervous system; HR, heart rate; ERP, effective refractory period.

lective β-adrenoreceptor antagonist; it depresses sinus node function and slows AV nodal conduction. It does not possess membrane-stabilizing properties. It prolongs the action potential and lengthens the atrial, AV nodal, and ventricular refractory period and is consistent with potassium channel blockade.[6] The toxicity and potential for overdose of this drug should be considered in light of the fact that it is both a class II and class III drug in the Vaughan Williams classification.

Sotalol is marketed as Betapace, manufactured by Berlex Laboratories in 80-, 160-, and 240-mg tablets. Patients normally do not take more than 320 mg daily except in unusual cases, when doses have been pushed as high as 480 to 640 mg daily.

The drug is approved by the FDA for use in ventricular arrhythmias. However, a major off-label use at present is for rate control for patients in atrial fibrillation as well as for prophylaxis to keep patients in normal sinus rhythm after being converted from atrial fibrillation.

The major drug interactions are detailed in Table 92–4. The side effects of sotalol are related to both its β-blocking and potassium-blocking properties. The β-blocker activity includes *hypotension, dyspnea, fatigue, bradycardia,* signs of *congestive heart failure,* and any sign that might be an aggravation of preexisting congestive heart failure.[6, 7] Sotalol potassium channel blocking activity prolongs the action potential, thus lengthening the QT interval. Therefore, torsades de pointes is a possibility in such patients, and other drugs that may be likely to cause prolongation of the QT interval, such as quinidine, and electrolyte imbalance, such as hypokalemia, should be carefully avoided. Patients with a significant bradycardia of 50 beats per minute or less should not receive sotalol. Fortunately, the torsades de pointes occurring during sotalol therapy is dose dependent, unlike that during quinidine therapy, which is idiosyncratic.

Overdose of the drug would be expected to produce the previously mentioned signs as well as usually marked hypotension. Hypoglycemia is common. *The immediate antidote for sotalol overdose is glucagon* (see Chapter 87 for further discussion). Adjunctive agents that have β-adrenergic properties, which have positive inotropic activity, and which may be administered intravenously and rapidly include epinephrine, isoproterenol, dopamine, and dobutamine. Supportive therapy such as cardiac pacing for AV block and extreme bradycardia, aminophylline for bronchospasm, direct current cardioversion for ventricular tachycardia or fibrillation, magnesium and potassium replacement, and intravenous furosemide for pulmonary edema may be in order. If the ingestion is excessive, gastric lavage is advised. Fortunately, because of the lack of protein binding, hemodialysis is useful for reducing sotalol plasma concentrations. The elimination half-life of sotalol is 12 hours.

Flecainide

Flecainide is a class IC drug whose most important action is blockade of the sodium channel, resulting in prolongation of the QRS interval to a modest degree. It has a somewhat variable effect on action potential duration, decreasing it in Purkinje fibers and increasing it in ventricular muscle.[8] Flecainide was originally approved and available as a ventricular antiarrhythmic drug; however, the Cardiac Arrhythmia Suppression Trial (CAST) demonstrated that it increased mortality. Although the drug is still available for that purpose, it is not used for such, and its sister drug, encainide, has now been removed from the market completely.[9] Flecainide is now approved by the FDA for the treatment of atrial fibrillation, however, and is considered an excellent drug for prophylaxis to keep patients prone to atrial fibrillation in normal sinus rhythm. It is the only drug, other than quinidine, that is approved by the FDA

Table 92–6. Toxicology and Treatment: Acute Effects Due to Intentional or Unintentional Excessive Levels

Drug	Symptoms	Antidote	Lavage	Dialyzable	Supportive Therapy	Elimination Half-Life	Manufacturer
Sotalol	AV block, bradycardia, CHF, hypotension, bronchospasm, hypoglycemia, QT prolongation, torsades de pointes, PVCs, VT, VF	Glucagon, β-adrenergic (epinephrine), dopamine (dobutamine), isoproterenol	Yes	Yes	Cardiac pacing, aminophylline, DC cardioversion, atropine, IV furosemide	12 h	Berlex Laboratories 300 Fairfield Rd. Wayne, NJ 07470 1-800-888-2407
Flecainide	PVCs, VT, bradycardia, AV block, congestive heart failure, QRS prolongation, hypotension	Hypertonic Na lactate or bicarbonate	Yes	No	Cardiac pacing, DC cardioversion, IV furosemide, vasopressors, atropine	14–19 h	3M Pharmaceuticals P.O. Box 33275 Minneapolis, MN 55343 1-800-328-0255
Propafenone	Hypotension, somnolence, bradycardia, AV block, convulsions, QRS prolongation, VT and VF, CHF	None	Yes	No	Cardiac pacing, defibrillation, atropine, vasopressors, Na bicarbonate	2–10 h	Knoll Pharmaceuticals 301 Jefferson Rd. Whippany, NJ 07981 1-800-526-0221
Moricizine	Emesis, lethargy, coma, syncope, hypotension, CHF, VT, VF, AV block, sinus arrest	None	Yes	No	Cardiac pacing, defibrillation, atropine, vasopressors	1.5–3.5 h	Roberts Pharmaceuticals 4 Industrial Way West Eatontown, NJ 07724 1-800-992-9306
Amiodarone (oral)	Pneumonitis, sinus bradycardia, VT, VF, torsades de pointes, hypotension	None	Yes, carefully because drug is very toxic to lungs	No	Vasopressors, cardiac pacing, atropine, β-adrenergic blockers	19–52 d	Wyeth Laboratories P.O. Box 8299 Philadelphia, PA 19101 1-610-688-4400
Amiodarone (IV)	Hypotension, shock, bradycardia, AV block, hepatotoxia	Discontinue IV infusion	NA	No	Vasopressors, inotropic agents, volume expansion, cardiac pacing	20–47 d	Wyeth Laboratories P.O. Box 8299 Philadelphia, PA 19101 1-610-688-4400

AV, atrioventricular; CHF, congestive heart failure; PVCs, premature ventricular contractions; VT, ventricular tachycardia; VF, ventricular fibrillation; IV, intravenous; DC, direct current.

for converting atrial fibrillation to normal sinus rhythm and for maintaining a normal sinus rhythm.

Flecainide does increase the QT interval with therapeutic use by prolonging the QRS complex. It produces no prolongation of the JT interval, however, and therefore, torsades de pointes is rare with the use of this drug. It is well absorbed orally, and its elimination half-life is 14 to 19 hours.

Toxicity is as outlined in Table 92–6. The primary toxic effects are conduction delays with bradycardia and a negative inotropic effect, which reduce cardiac output. Prorhythmic effects rarely occur in the presence of normal ventricular function and normal potassium and magnesium levels. Previously noted was the fact that this drug is rarely used for patients with severe left ventricular dysfunction. Toxic effects are premature ventricular contractions with ventricular tachycardia, which may progress to ventricular fibrillation, sinus bradycardia, AV block, precipitation or exacerbation of congestive heart failure, and usually QRS prolongation. Patients may be hypotensive. A fatality has been reported in a patient who ingested a large amount of oral flecainide in conjunction with a large dose of propranolol.[10] A few reports have noted that hypertonic sodium lactate or bicarbonate may be beneficial in flecainide overdose.[11] The drug is not dialyzable. Early after ingestion, gastric lavage would be helpful, and the drug does not cause pulmonary toxicity if aspirated (other than what would normally be expected). Supportive therapy would be the method of approach, including cardiac pacing, cardioversion, intravenous furosemide for congestive heart failure, atropine, and vasopressors.

The drug is manufactured by 3M and is marketed as Tambocor in tablets of 50 mg, 100 mg, and 150 mg.

Propafenone

Propafenone is a class IC drug with some structural resemblance to β-adrenergic blockers, but its most conspicuous action is in the first inward sodium current.[12] It prolongs the PR and QRS intervals. It weakly antagonizes calcium channels. It does have weak β-blocking activity and can slow the heart rate slightly. It has little effect on sinus node function and does not cause sinus bradycardia.

This agent is approved by the FDA for the treatment of premature ventricular contractions and for suppressing recurrence of ventricular tachycardia. However, a major off-label use is for patients with atrial fibrillation, as a prophylaxis in attempts to keep them in a normal sinus rhythm once they have been converted from atrial fibrillation. Obviously, any bradyarrhythmia would be a contraindication for the use of this drug. It does have a negative inotropic effect on left ventricular function, and congestive heart failure is considered a contraindication to its use. Prorhythmic effects range from an increase in frequency of premature ventricular contractions to the development of more severe ventricular arrhythmias. Torsades de pointes has occurred. This drug is highly metabolized by the liver and should be administered cautiously to patients with impaired hepatic function.

In terms of important drug interactions, propafenone used concurrently with digitalis increases the digoxin level. Used with quinidine, propafenone has an increased effect. Propafenone also causes cyclosporine levels to be increased, and this is an important factor in transplant recipients.

Toxic manifestations of this drug are detailed in Table 92–6.

Premature ventricular contractions, ventricular tachycardia, ventricular fibrillation, hypotension, sinus bradycardia, AV block, QRS prolongation, and congestive heart failure all occur with overdose of propafenone. Because of the intraventricular conduction delays, bundle branch block may occur as a manifestation of overdoses of this drug. Acute propafenone overdose has been reported in a child. It was manifested by seizures, marked prolongation of the QRS, first-degree AV block, hypotension, and progressive bradycardia resulting in cardiac arrest. Atropine, dopamine, and sodium bicarbonate were successful in reversing this outcome.[13] The usual supportive therapy for such patients *in extremis* would be as detailed in Table 92–6.

Propafenone is marketed as Rhythmol by Knoll Pharmaceutical, in tablets of 150, 225, and 300 mg. Patients normally do not take more than 900 mg/d.

Moricizine

Moricizine is a class IB antiarrhythmic agent with potent local anesthetic activity and myocardial membrane-stabilizing effects. It reduces the fast inward currents carried by sodium ions. It prolongs AV conduction by prolonging both the AV nodal conduction time and the His-Purkinje conduction time. The PR interval is also prolonged. Moricizine has very little effect on sinus node recovery time.

This drug is used for the treatment of ventricular arrhythmias that are believed to be life threatening, such as sustained ventricular tachycardia. It is not considered a first-line drug. It is rarely used for any off-label purposes such as control of atrial fibrillation.

Drug interactions are not very prominent with this agent, but two very important ones are prolongation of the prothrombin time in patients taking oral anticoagulants and increase of the theophylline level in patients taking theophylline as a bronchodilator.

Moricizine does have a prorhythmic effect. This is usually in the form of increasing frequency of premature ventricular contractions or leading to more severe ventricular arrhythmias such as ventricular tachycardia. The usual guidelines should be used in recommending this agent in that it should not be used with other drugs that have similar toxic effects or in patients with significant bradycardia.

Toxic effects of the drug are emesis, lethargy, coma, syncope, hypotension, congestive heart failure, ventricular tachycardia, ventricular fibrillation, AV block, and sinus arrest. There is no immediate antidote. Lavage should be used if appropriate. The agent is not dialyzable. Survival after toxic overdoses depends primarily on supportive therapy such as use of vasopressors and positive inotropic agents, cardiac pacing, defibrillation, and support of the patient until the toxic effects dissipate.

This drug is marketed as Ethmozine in doses of 200, 250, and 300 mg. Patients are unlikely to be taking more than 900 mg/d. It is fortunate from the standpoint of toxicity that the elimination half-life is 1.5 to 3.5 hours.

Amiodarone

Oral

Amiodarone is a highly lipid-soluble benzofuran derivative that primarily decreases potassium ion conductants and thus lengthens the action potential and refractoriness.[14] It is a Vaughan Williams class III drug, but it possesses other properties that contribute to its antiarrhythmic action such as inhibition of α- and β-adrenergic receptors. Some calcium channel blocking activity has also been demonstrated.[15] It prolongs the refractory period of all cardiac tissues and decreases AV nodal conduction velocity.

This drug is primarily used to treat serious ventricular arrhythmias. It has life-threatening side effects and is recommended primarily for patients with hemodynamically unstable ventricular tachycardia or recurrent ventricular fibrillation. However, its use is being liberalized, and it is believed to be particularly effective for patients who have left ventricular systolic dysfunction and congestive heart failure because it has no significant negative inotropic activity. A major off-label use has developed for control of atrial fibrillation and as prophylaxis for recurrence of atrial fibrillation in patients who have been converted to a normal sinus rhythm.

There has been great interest in this drug and its use after myocardial infarction, particularly in lower doses than those previously recommended. The only significant reductions in mortality that have been observed have been in small numbers of patients, although studies involving larger groups of patients have shown some evidence to this effect. However, at this point it is difficult to make a case for routine use of amiodarone in postinfarct patients who have ventricular arrhythmias.[16, 17]

Drug interactions with amiodarone are diverse (see Table 92–4). One should particularly note that amiodarone and digoxin used concurrently elevate the digoxin level, and patients taking anticoagulants have a greater degree of anticoagulation than expected. The drug interactions associated with cardiac antiarrhythmic drugs are quite complex and are listed. It should be noted that transplant recipients have an elevated level of cyclosporine if they are concurrently receiving amiodarone.

The pharmacokinetics of amiodarone contribute to its many and well-known toxicities because it absorbs slowly and concentrates extensively into adipose, hepatic, pulmonary, and cardiac tissue.[14, 15, 18] A steady state may not be reached for more than a month, and the elimination half-life may vary from 1 week to 6 months. Absorption in the intestinal tract is poor and highly variable. It is very difficult to predict appropriate doses because of individual variability and peak plasma concentration, elimination half-life, and partition coefficients in the drug between plasma and tissue.[19] This drug induces side effects of some type in approximately 75% of patients treated with at least 400 mg daily, but only about 10% to 15% have to discontinue use because of side effects. The incidence of side effects correlates with both dose and duration of therapy.[20] Side effects of therapy include ataxia, tremors, dizziness, hepatic and gastrointestinal effects, and ocular effects. Amiodarone causes inhibition of thyroxine deiodination in the thyroid gland and results in hypothyroidism.[21] Thyrotoxicosis also may occur.[21] Pulmonary toxicity is a grave side effect of amiodarone use, and the instance of clinically significant toxic pneumonitis is from 2% to as much as 17%.[22] Pulmonary toxicity increases greatly at doses exceeding 400 mg/d but occurs even at lower doses. Approximately 30% of patients who develop major pulmonary toxicity do not survive.

The daunting side effects of amiodarone make dosage very critical. The usual dose is 400 mg/d for suppression of ventricular arrhythmias after the loading is complete. After 1 year of therapy, in most instances this is reduced to 200 mg/d. Serum concentrations do not give an indication of the risks involved because so much drug is deposited in tissues.[23]

The steady-state serum concentrations of amiodarone are achieved slowly with therapeutic dosing, and the onset of toxicity may be delayed for several weeks. The long elimination half-life of amiodarone, 19 to 52 days, results in a prolonged duration of toxicity when it is encountered.[24] Amiodarone can cause torsades de pointes and increased ventricular arrhythmias in the absence of a prolonged QT interval. The toxic effects, which may be acute, are primarily those associated with the cardiovascular system as the daunting side effects require cumulative doses. Bradycardia, torsades de pointes, ventricular tachycardia, ventricular fibrillation, and hypotension would be expected. There is no specific antidote. Lavage must be performed very carefully, because aspiration of amiodarone into the lungs causes a far greater problem than the gastric contents would otherwise. Supportive therapy such as vasopressors, cardiac pacing, and atropine is important. Patients who have ventricular arrhythmias have been reported anecdotally to respond quite well to β-adrenergic blockers. One patient survived the ingestion of 8 g without any clinical toxicity.[25]

The maximum dose of oral amiodarone that a patient would likely be taking therapeutically is 600 mg/d on a long-term basis. Amiodarone is marketed

Table 92–7. Effects of Intravenous and Oral Amiodarone on Electrophysiologic Parameters

Formulation	SCL	QRS	QTc	AH	HV	ERP RA	ERP RV	ERP AVN
Intravenous	↔	↔	↔	↑	↔	↔	↔	↑
Oral	↑	↔	↑	↑	↔	↑	↑	↑

ERP, effective refractory period; RA, right atrium; RV, right ventricle; AVN, atrioventricular node; ↔, no change.

by Wyeth Laboratories as Cordarone in 200-mg tablets.

Intravenous

Intravenous amiodarone has now been approved by the FDA for use in intractable ventricular arrhythmias. It is marketed as Cordarone intravenous by Wyeth Laboratories. As noted previously, amiodarone is a class III antiarrhythmic drug. It prolongs intranodal conduction and refractoriness of the atrioventricular node but has little or no effect on sinus cycle length, refractoriness of the atrium, repolarization, and infranodal conduction. It does not prolong the QT interval. Its properties differ somewhat from oral amiodarone (Table 92–7).

Intravenous amiodarone is indicated for initiation of treatment and prophylaxis of frequently recurring ventricular fibrillation and hemodynamically unstable ventricular tachycardia. A popular off-label use is for intravenous conversion of atrial fibrillation to normal sinus rhythm.

Hypotension is the most common adverse effect of intravenous amiodarone. Sinus bradycardia also is not an unusual occurrence. Patients with a known previous history of bradycardia and AV block should be treated cautiously with intravenous amiodarone. Torsades de pointes has occurred, although rarely, with this agent. The usual complications of long-term oral administration of amiodarone do not occur with short-term intravenous use of the drug. The acute toxic effects, in addition to the ones noted earlier, are hepatotoxicity and AV block. Obviously, discontinuing the intravenous infusion reverses most toxicity. There is no other specific antidote, and it is not dialyzable. Vasopressors, inotropic agents, volume expansion, and cardiac pacing all are supportive therapy that may be necessary.

The recommended dosage schedule is 150 mg during the first 10 minutes followed by an infusion of 360 mg during the next 6 hours with a maintenance infusion of 540 mg over the remaining 18 hours. The maintenance infusion rate may be continued past 24 hours. It is believed that this can be continued for 2 to 3 weeks. It should be administered through a central venous catheter with an in-line filter.

References

1. Roden DM: Risks and benefits of antiarrhythmic therapy. N Engl J Med *331*:785, 1994.
2. Vaughan Williams EM: Classification of anti-arrhythmic drugs. *In* Sandoe E, Flenstod-Jensen E, Olesen K (eds): Cardiac Arrhythmias. Sodertalje, Sweden, Ad Astra, pp 449–473, 1970.
3. Task Force of the Working Group on Cardiac Arrhythmias of the European Society of Cardiology: The Sicilian gambit: A new approach to the classification of antiarrhythmic drugs based on their action on arrhythmogenic mechanisms. Eur Heart J *84*:1831, 1991.
4. Lisk PM, Weikel JH, Dungan KW: Pharmacological and toxicological properties of two new beta-adrenergic receptor antagonists. J Pharmacol Exp Ther *149*:161, 1965.
5. Singh BN, Vaughan Williams EM: A third class of antiarrhythmic action: Effects on atrial and ventricular intracellular potentials, and other pharmacological actions on cardiac Muscle of MJ 1999 and AH 3676. Br J Pharmacol *39*:675, 1970.
6. Hohnloser SH, Woosley RL: Sotalol. N Engl J Med *331*:31, 1994.
7. Kirschenbaum HL, Rosenberg JM: Clinical experience with sotalol in the treatment of cardiac arrhythmias. Clin Ther *16*:346, 1994.
8. Ikeda N, Singh BN, Davis LD, et al: Effects of flecainide on the electrophysiologic properties of isolated canine and rabbit myocardial fibers. J Am Coll Cardiol *5*:303, 1985.
9. Echt DS, Lieberson LB: Mortality and morbidity in patients receiving encainide, flecainide, or placebo. The Cardiac Arrhythmia Suppression Trial. N Engl J Med *324*:781, 1991.
10. Brown CR, Buchanan JF: Combined flecainide and propranolol over dosage. Clin Toxicol Update *8*:9, 1986.
11. Pentel PR, Dunbar DN: New cardiac antiarrhythmic agents. *In* Haddad LM, Winchester JF, Shannon MW (eds): Clinical Management of Poisoning and Drug Overdose. 2nd ed. Philadelphia, W.B. Saunders Co., pp 1380–1390, 1990.
12. Shen EN: Propafenone, a promising new antiarrhythmic agent. Chest *98*:434, 1990.
13. McHugh TP: Propafenone ingestion. Ann Emerg Med *16*:437, 1987.
14. Mason JW: Amiodarone. N Engl J Med *316*:455, 1987.
15. Gill J, Heel RC, Fitton A: Amiodarone, An overview of its pharmacological properties, and review of its therapeutic use in cardiac arrhythmias. Drugs *43*:69, 1992.
16. Ceremzynski L, Kleizar E, Krzeminska-Pakula M, et al: Effect of amiodarone on mortality after myocardial infarction: A double-blind, placebo controlled, pilot study. J Am Coll Cardiol *20*:1056, 1992.
17. Burkart F, Pfisterer M, Kiowski W, et al: Effect of antiarrhythmic therapy on mortality in survivors of myocardial infarction with asymptomatic complex ventricular arrhythmias: Basel Antiarrhythmic Study of Infarct Survival (BASIS). J Am Coll Cardiol *16*:1711, 1990.
18. Puech P: Practical aspects of the use of amiodarone. Drugs *41*(Suppl 2):67, 1991.
19. Brennan FJ, Brien JF, Armstrong PW: Plasma concentration, time course and pharmacological effects of a standardized oral amiodarone dosing regimen in humans. Can J Cardiol *7*:117, 1991.
20. Shetty HGM, Woodhouse KW: Use of amiodarone for elderly patients. Age Aging *21*:223, 1992.
21. Trip MD, Wierienga W, Plomp TA: Incidence, predictability and pathogenesis of amiodarone-induced thyrotoxicosis and hypothyroidism. Am J Med *91*:507, 1991.
22. Roca J, Heras M, Rodriguez-Raisin R, et al: Pulmonary com-

plications after long term amiodarone treatment. Thorax *47*:372, 1992.
23. Follath F: The utility of serum drug level monitoring during therapy with class III antiarrhythmic agents. J Cardiovasc Pharmacol *20*(Suppl 2):41, 1993.
24. McGovern B, Garan H, Kelly E, et al: Adverse reaction during treatment with amiodarone hydrochloride. BMJ *287*:175, 1983.
25. Bonati M, D'Aranno V, Galletti F, et al: Acute overdose of amiodarone in a suicide attempt. J Clin Toxicol *20*:181, 1983.

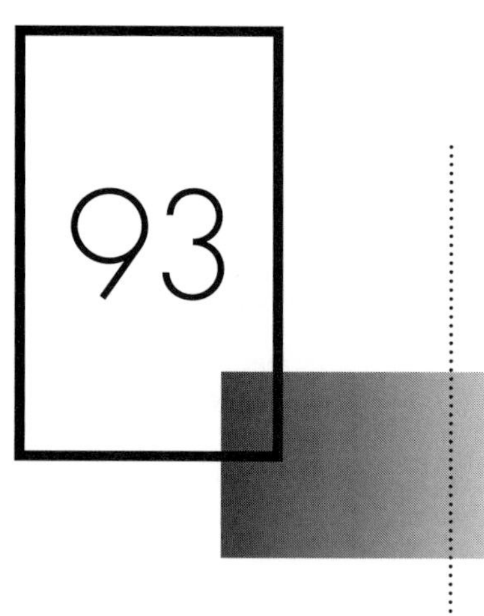

Sympathomimetics

MICHAEL T. KELLEY, MD

A large portion of the medications used in modern therapeutics accomplish their desired effects by altering autonomic nervous system functions. Cardiac output and vascular resistance are altered to control blood pressure. Bronchioles are dilated to control asthma. Nasal vessels are constricted to control the symptoms of the common cold. The autonomic nervous system is divided into parasympathetic and sympathetic divisions. This chapter focuses on the toxicology of drugs that stimulate the sympathetic division. All sympathomimetics are variations of a basic structure of a benzene ring and an ethylamine side chain (Fig. 93–1).[1] Norepinephrine (the neurotransmitter) and epinephrine (the hormone) are the major sympathomimetics in the body. All of the stimulants discussed in this chapter are analogues of these two natural substances.

Drugs that stimulate the sympathetic division of the autonomic nervous system are called *sympathomimetics*. The sympathomimetics exert their effects by interacting with α- and β-adrenergic receptors. The α-adrenergic receptors are subdivided into α_1- and α_2-adrenergic receptors. Only a few times in this chapter are the subclassifications of the α-adrenergic receptors considered, as the physiologic effects of the stimulation of both the α_1- and α_2-adrenergic receptors are similar, particularly in overdose situations.

The β-adrenergic receptors are also subdivided into β_1- and β_2-adrenergic receptors. Selective stimulation of the β-adrenergic receptors produces different physiologic effects. Table 93–1 lists the physiologic effects of the stimulation of α-adrenergic and β-adrenergic receptors.

Unless multiple drugs have been ingested, the diagnosis of an overdose of a sympathomimetic medication can often be based on the recognition of patterns of specific physiologic responses. These responses have been termed "autonomic clinical syndromes."[2] By noting the effects on blood pressure, pulse, pupil size, skin and mucous membrane moisture, lung sounds, and bowel sounds, an overdose of a particular drug can be classified into a particular syndrome. Proper treatment can then proceed in a logical manner. Table 93–2 summarizes the sympathetic clinical syndromes.

SYMPATHETIC SYNDROMES

The α-adrenergic syndrome is caused by relatively pure α-agonists. The blood pressure is increased owing to constriction of the peripheral arteriolar beds. Reflex bradycardia often accompanies this elevation in blood pressure. The pupils are dilated. The mucous membranes are dry because of decreased blood flow to the capillary beds, but sweating is frequently present. Bowel sounds are decreased due to decreased gut motility.

Some of the β-adrenergic agents are selective therapeutically; however, in overdose, both β_1- and β_2-

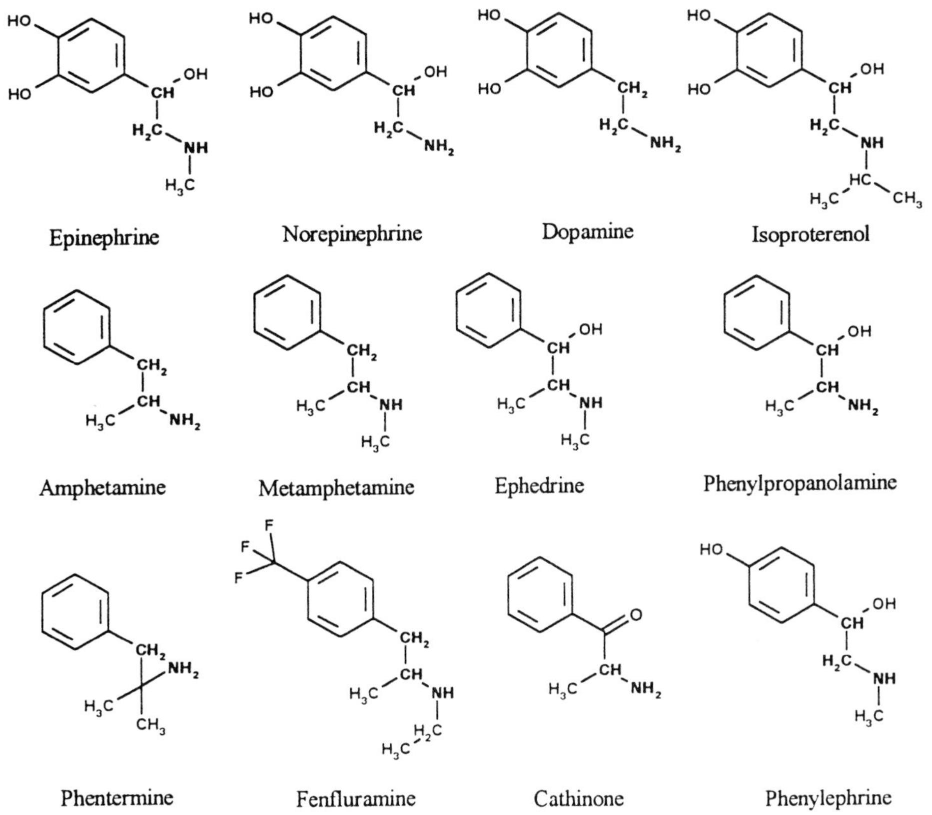

Figure 93–1. Structures of various sympathomimetics.

adrenergic receptors usually are stimulated,[3] and the β-adrenergic syndrome results. Heart rate is increased because of β_1-adrenergic receptor stimulation. β_2-Adrenergic stimulation causes vasodilatation and hypotension. Gut motility may be decreased. The pupils are relatively unaffected by β-adrenergic stimulation.

The *mixed α- and β-adrenergic syndrome* is seen with the use of both agents, which increase central sympathetic output, as well as with the use of those that stimulate both α- and β-adrenergic receptors. Blood pressure is increased because of vasoconstriction as well as β_1-adrenergic stimulation of the heart (positive inotropic effect). Because of the β_1-adrenergic stimulation, tachycardia also is seen (positive chronotropic effect). The combination of hypertension with tachycardia differentiates this syndrome from the pure α-adrenergic syndrome, in which hypertension occurs with reflex bradycardia. The pupils are dilated in the mixed adrenergic syndrome. Mucous membranes are dry, but sweating often is present. Bowel sounds are diminished because of decreased gut motility.

SPECIFIC AGENTS

Phenylpropanolamine

Many of the sympathomimetics are available over-the-counter as well as by prescription. It is intriguing that a 75-mg dose of phenylpropanolamine (PPA),

Table 93–1. Sympathomimetic Effects

α-Stimulation	β_1-Stimulation	β_2-Stimulation
Pupillary dilatation	Increased heart rate	Skeletal muscle, pulmonary, visceral, and renal arterial
Arterial vasoconstriction: skin, mucosal, skeletal, cerebral, pulmonary, visceral, renal, salivary	Increased cardiac contraction	Dilatation
Systemic venoconstriction	Increased cardiac automaticity	Relaxation of bronchial smooth muscle
Decreased bowel motility		Decreased gastrointestinal motility
Increased gastrointestinal sphincter tone		Relaxation of urinary bladder
Increased trigone and urinary bladder sphincter tone		Increased glycogenolysis and gluconeogenesis
Pilomotor contraction		Increased lipolysis
Increased sweating in palms		Increased pancreatic and glandular secretions
Decreased pancreatic secretions		Hypokalemia
Platelet aggregation		

Table 93–2. Sympathetic Clinical Syndromes

	Blood Pressure	Pulse	Pupil Size	Sweating	Peristalsis
α-Adrenergic	+ +	−/0	+ +	+	0/−
β-Adrenergic	+/−	+ +	0	0	0
Mixed adrenergic	+ +	+ +	+ +	+ +	0/−

+, increased; −, decreased; 0, variable or no effect.
Modified from Olsen KR, Pentel PR, Kelley MT: Physical assessment and differential diagnosis of the poisoned patient. Med Toxicol 2:52–81, 1987.

when used as a nasal decongestant, is a prescription medication (Entex LA), but the same 75-mg dose of PPA can be purchased without a prescription in the form of an appetite suppressant (Dexatrim). There are hundreds of other over-the-counter and prescription medications that contain PPA, and the list of them grows each year.

PPA is an almost pure α-agonist. It has some β-agonist activity, but in overdose situations the α effects predominate. PPA is used clinically as a decongestant and an appetite suppressant. On the street, it may be sold illegally in "speed" look-alikes. The speed look-alikes may contain up to 50 mg of PPA as well as ephedrine and caffeine. Some of the slang names for these drugs are "pink ladies," "black beauties," and "speckled pups."

Pharmacology

PPA (D,L-norephedrine) is structurally similar to amphetamine, differing only by the addition of a hydroxyl group on the β carbon (see Fig. 93–1).[1] The addition of a hydroxyl group on the side chain β carbon inhibits the action of catechol *O*-methyltransferase, which decreases the clearance and increases the duration of action of the drug. A hydroxyl group on the β carbon also makes the drug less lipid soluble and less likely to cross the blood-brain barrier.[1] Small amounts of PPA do cross the blood-brain barrier and produce some limited central nervous system (CNS) activity. Amphetamine is more lipophilic than PPA and readily crosses the blood-brain barrier because it has no hydroxyl groups on the β carbon or benzene ring. Ironically, the lower CNS activity of PPA often leads to more severe overdose than occurs with amphetamine because the abuser does not experience the expected amphetamine high and thus takes more of the drug. This results in more dangerous peripheral effects.

PPA stimulates adrenergic receptors and acts indirectly by stimulating the release of norepinephrine at the nerve terminals.[1–7] PPA is a weak base and is rapidly absorbed in the small intestine. The average time to maximal concentration after a normal dose is 1.5 hours. The volume of distribution is 3.0 to 4.5 L/kg, making the patient with PPA toxicity a poor candidate for hemodialysis. The half-life after administration of a therapeutic dose is 4 to 6 hours. The duration of action ranges from 3 hours for the regular capsules to 12 to 16 hours for the extended-release tablets. Ninety per cent of administered PPA is eliminated unchanged by the kidneys.[8]

PPA is a relatively safe drug when it is taken as directed. However, it has a low therapeutic index—that is, adverse symptoms can occur at doses two- to threefold of normal.[9] The recommended dose daily dose is 75 to 150 mg.

Methyldopa, monoamine oxidase inhibitors, and β-blockers can potentiate the hypertensive effects of PPA. Caffeine can potentiate the effects of PPA, and PPA increases blood levels of both caffeine and theophylline. The Food and Drug Administration banned the sale of combination drugs containing PPA and caffeine in 1983. However, illicit street preparations may still contain this combination.

Clinical Presentation

Hypertension is a common presenting problem in patients with PPA overdose.[10–13] Hypertension is a result of increased cardiac output, increased peripheral vascular resistance, increased stroke volume, and increased ejection fraction. The increase in blood pressure induces a reflex decrease in heart rate. Hypertensive crisis manifested by severe headache and encephalopathy,[14] as well as intracerebral hemorrhage, subarachnoid hemorrhage, and CNS vasculitis have been reported after PPA overdose.[8, 9]

PPA overdose has caused cardiac arrhythmias.[10, 11, 13, 15] Bradycardia is the most common arrhythmia, but supraventricular tachycardia, premature ventricular and atrial tachycardia, and ventricular tachycardia have been reported.[16]

Seizures have also been reported in patients with PPA toxicity,[14] but it is questioned whether these seizures were due to PPA or to another ingredient in the combination drug. Anxiety, agitation, and psychotic behavior, which are often seen with amphetamine abuse, can occur with PPA overdose.[10, 11]

Treatment

The treatment for sympathomimetics overdose is primarily stabilization of the vital signs. All of the sympathomimetics fall into one of three categories: α-agonists, β-agonists, or mixed α- and β-agonists. PPA management is a prototype for α-agonist management.

Decontamination and removal of the drug is the most important therapeutic measure in any drug overdose. However, if a patient has severe hypertension, the blood pressure should be reduced before emesis is induced or lavage is performed because both therapies may further increase intracranial pressure. Activated charcoal decreases the absorption of PPA and should be administered as soon as possible.

Although acidification of the urine enhances the elimination of PPA, this therapy is not warranted and may be dangerous. PPA excretion usually is fairly rapid, and the toxicity often lasts less than 6 hours. In PPA overdoses, increased muscular activity is often seen. The increased muscular activity or vasoconstriction, or both, that accompany PPA overdose may cause myoglobinemia. Acidification of the urine may cause precipitation of myoglobin in the kidney and thus cause acute renal failure. Furthermore, the use of specific antagonists to PPA avoids the risks of acidification, and thus its benefits probably outweigh those of this formerly recommended practice.

Hypertension should be treated on the basis of the symptoms and not the absolute blood pressure. For example, it is not uncommon for an adolescent or small adult with a PPA overdose to present with a blood pressure of 190/110. Although some elderly adults with long-standing hypertension can tolerate this pressure, most adolescents or small adults have baseline pressures of about 100/60. For children, treatment should be considered if the blood pressure is above the 95th percentile for age. Treatment is recommended if the blood pressure is above the 95 percentile and the child is symptomatic. Before the hypertension is treated, an intracerebral hemorrhage has to be ruled out by a good physical examination. Lowering the blood pressure too much or too quickly in patients with an intracerebral hemorrhage can increase brain destruction.

Initial therapy for hypertension can begin with placing the patient in an upright position to take advantage of orthostatic effects. Many antihypertensive agents can be used to lower blood pressure emergently (Table 93–3). If there are indications of intracranial hemorrhage, sodium nitroprusside is the drug of choice. Slow, precise regulation of the blood pressure can be obtained by titrating this drug. In the less emergent setting, phentolamine, a short-acting α-antagonist, a calcium channel blocker, nitroglycerin paste, or sublingual nitroglycerin are effective. In an overdose patient, the duration of the toxic effects may be longer than the duration of the effects of these agents. Therefore, frequent blood pressure monitoring is required for determining the need for repeated doses.

Tachycardia is uncommon in pure α-agonist overdose, but if it is present and compromising cardiac function, esmolol or another β-blocker can be used.[12] However, a β-blocker should not be used to treat the tachycardia without the administration of an agent to treat the hypertension, such as an α-blocker, calcium channel blocker, or a nitrate. Blocking the β-adrenergic receptors in the periphery may cause unopposed α vasoconstriction, which leads to a further increase in blood pressure.

It is neither necessary nor advisable to treat bradycardia unless the patient has symptomatic hypotension or cardiac compromise. Hypotension is rare in a PPA overdose, and the bradycardia is normally a physiologic reflex to hypertension caused by PPA. Therefore, increasing the heart rate with an anticholinergic drug like atropine works against the corrective mechanism of the body and may worsen hypertension.

Should seizures occur, administration of a benzodiazepine like lorazepam or diazepam is an appropriate treatment. Barbiturates also are effective and should be considered if the seizures are recurrent. The occurrence of seizures should increase the index of suspicion for cerebral hemorrhage. If computed tomography of the head cannot be performed, then the blood pressure should be lowered slowly and carefully.

Pre-existing medical conditions that increase toxicity and complicate treatment include coronary artery disease, hypertension, arrhythmias, glaucoma, hyperthyroidism, and prosthetic hypertrophy. Patients with these conditions require close observation, and symptoms should be treated accordingly.

Phenylephrine

Phenylephrine is used as a topical nasal decongestant and as an ophthalmic mydriatic in 2.5% and 10% solutions. Phenylephrine, like PPA, is primarily an α-agonist. Even though phenylephrine is a topical agent, it is readily absorbed orally. However, only 38% of the drug reaches the systemic circulation owing to first-pass metabolism by monoamine oxi-

Table 93–3. Therapeutic Drugs

Drug	Indication	Dose (Adult)	Dose (Pediatric)
Nitroprusside	Hypertension	0.5–10 μg/kg per min†	Same
Phentolamine	Hypertension	2.5–5 mg IV*	0.05–0.1 mg/kg*
	Extravasation	5–10 mg in 10 mL saline locally	Same
Propranolol	Tachycardia	0.5–1.0 mg IV slow	10–20 μg/kg IV
Labetalol	Hypertension	20 mg IV q 10 min to a maximum of 300 mg	Unknown
Esmolol	Tachycardia	50–200 μg/kg per min after 500-μg/kg bolus	
Diazepam	Seizures	5–10 mg	0.1–0.3 mg/kg
Lorazepam	Seizures	0.05 mg/kg	0.05 mg/kg

*Dose can be repeated in 5–10 minutes until the desired effects are obtained.
†Titrate as needed.

dase in the gut wall.[8] This decrease in bioavailability greatly decreases the oral toxicity of phenylephrine. The half-life of elimination is 2 to 3 hours; thus, any toxicity that occurs is short. Cardiovascular reactions have been reported after the use of topical phenylephrine in infants, in geriatric patients, and in patients with underlying cardiovascular disease or hypertension.[17, 18] Myocardial infarction[18] and subarachnoid hemorrhage secondary to hypertension[19] have been reported as adverse effects of phenylephrine use. Psychosis after chronic use of phenylephrine also has been reported.[16]

Duration of action of phenylephrine is short, being about 30 to 60 minutes. However if symptoms persist, therapy should follow the guidelines for treating PPA toxicity.

Ephedrine and Pseudoephedrine

Ephedrine and its optical isomer pseudoephedrine are structurally very similar to methamphetamine (see Fig. 93–1). In illicit drug laboratories, simple dehydrogenation is used to make methamphetamine from ephedrine. Ephedrine and pseudoephedrine are common over-the-counter medications. However, in many states, ephedrine is being reclassified as a schedule V drug. This classification makes it available directly from the pharmacist only, not freely over the counter.

In areas where its sale is not regulated, ephedrine is purchased in gas stations and truck stops by long-distance truckers who use the drug for its arousal properties. It also can be purchased in health food stores as a diet aid or energy booster. Also, mail-order distribution of the drug is large. Illegal entrepreneurs distribute the drug without recommendations on amount or frequency of dosing. This practice is common on campuses and in gyms, where ephedrine has been touted to enhance performance and muscle development. Neither claim has any merit or been substantiated by scientific proof. The common street name for ephedrine is "white crosses."

Many health food stores products contain ephedrine, even if it is not listed as one of the ingredients. In 1993, a Swedish athlete was tested positive for ephedrine after taking a ginseng product. Analysis of the product revealed that it contained no ginsenoisides, only high quantities of ephedrine.[20] Ma huang, or Ephedra, is a Chinese herb found in many products sold in health food stores as diet aids or energy boosters. A 1995 Drug Enforcement Agency report examined these products and found that they contained, in addition to ephedrine, norephedrine, methylephedrine, pseudoephedrine, norpseudoephedrine, and methylpseudoephedrine. In many of the products, synthetic ephedrine was found in addition to the natural ephedrine in ma huang. Also, ephedrine-containing products are sold in pyramid schemes as energy boosters and are marketed to the geriatric population.

Ephedrine is relatively safe when it is used in recommended doses. The toxicity and abuse potential is related to dose. In a study of incarcerated males, a high dose of ephedrine was found to have an effect equal to that of amphetamine, methamphetamine, phenmetrazine, and methylphenidate on ratings of drug liking and measures of addiction.[21] Using a similar model and smaller doses of ephedrine, Chait found no increased abuse liability in college students and university staff.[22]

Pseudoephedrine's major use is in oral preparations as a nasal decongestant. Ephedrine also has β_2-adrenergic effects and can produce bronchodilation. It was first used in the treatment of asthma by Chen and Schmidt in 1930. It is combined with theophylline in some preparations because of this effect. Unfortunately, this combination has been shown to potentiate the toxic effects of theophylline without improving the therapeutic response.

Pharmacology

Both ephedrine and pseudoephedrine have α- and β-adrenergic agonist effects. The pharmacologic effects of the drugs are a result of direct stimulation of the adrenergic receptors and the release of norepinephrine. Pseudoephedrine is readily absorbed, with peak concentrations being reached about 1.5 to 2 hours after administration. However, when combined with antihistamines, as many of these preparations are, the absorption and the attainment of peak levels can be delayed. The volume of distribution is about 3 L/kg; thus, patients with toxicity are not good candidates for hemodialysis. Pseudoephedrine is a less potent bronchodilator than ephedrine and has 25% of ephedrine's vasopressor effects. Ephedrine results in less CNS stimulation than methamphetamine because of the β carbon hydroxylation, but it is more potent than methamphetamine in raising blood pressure and heart rate. This combination of effects is particularly dangerous if the drug is abused for its CNS activity.

Clinical Presentation

Typical signs and symptoms in overdose are headache, dilated pupils, nausea, vomiting, diaphoresis, hypertension, ventricular ectopy, tachycardia, myocardial ischemia, agitation, psychosis, and seizures.[10, 23] Intracerebral hemorrhage, presumably due to a direct cerebrovascular effect, has also been reported.[24] Chronic ephedrine use can produce delusional disorders, manic conditions, insomnia, restlessness, anxiety, and toxic psychosis that may be more likely to occur in predisposed individuals.[25]

Treatment

The treatment of overdoses of the mixed α- and β-agonist sympathomimetic drugs like ephedrine and pseudoephedrine is somewhat different than that for toxicity from the relatively pure α-agonists. However, decontamination and support of vital signs are the mainstays of therapy.

The majority of overdoses with pseudoephedrine are mild, and no therapy except decontamination and administration of activated charcoal is necessary. Ipecac is not indicated because of the possibility of seizure activity and increased intracranial pressure. Lavage can also increase intracranial pressure; when present, severe hypertension should be treated first (see Table 93–3).

Unlike the α-agonists, which produce hypertension and bradycardia, mixed α- and β-agonists taken in overdose commonly produce hypertension and tachycardia. These overdoses also can be treated with a variety of medications. As in cases of α-agonist overdose, severe hypertension or hypertension with signs of intracranial hemorrhage should be treated with sodium nitroprusside to titrate the drug to lower blood pressure. In addition, emergent tachycardia can be treated with the short-acting β-blocker esmolol. In other cases, a combination of an α- and a β-antagonist can be used.[26] Labetalol has mixed α- and β-antagonistic effects. However, the β effects are sevenfold the α effects, and persistent elevations in blood pressure may necessitate treatment with additional agents. β-Blockers have good membrane stabilizing effects and are beneficial for tachyarrhythmias which can occur with overdoses of these drugs. Calcium channel blockers and nitrates can also be used to control the hypertension.

Acidification of the urine enhances elimination of these drugs, but the risk of this procedure in this setting exceeds any potential benefits.

Agitation and psychosis should be treated with a benzodiazepine. The antipsychotics should be avoided because their anticholinergic effects can worsen cardiovascular toxicity. Agitation and psychosis can also cause increases in temperature. Care should be taken to evaluate the core body temperature and to provide necessary treatment.

Epinephrine

Epinephrine, a natural sympathomimetic hormone, has many therapeutic uses and can be found in over-the-counter inhalers. Asthma, anaphylaxis, cardiac arrest, hemostasis, nasal congestion, and glaucoma are examples of the many conditions treated with epinephrine preparations.

Pharmacology

Epinephrine is a potent stimulator of both α- and β-adrenergic receptors. The duration of action of epinephrine is relative short. It is metabolized in the blood by the catechol *O*-methyltransferase and monoamine oxidase systems.

Clinical Presentation

Adverse effects and symptoms of overdose have been seen after administration of conventional doses.[27] Most problems occur after the inadvertent intravenous administration of concentrations intended for subcutaneous delivery. In general, epinephrine should not be administered intravenously to anyone who has a normal blood pressure. It is the drug of choice for treating anaphylaxis; however, for bronchospasm secondary to asthma, the β_2-agonist inhalers are safer.

After administration of epinephrine, constriction of the vascular beds in the skin, mucosa, and kidney cause a rapid dose-dependent increase in blood pressure. Usually, the increase in systolic pressure is greater than the increase in diastolic pressure. This large increase in blood pressure may lead to a reflex bradycardia, but tachycardia is more common. The rapid increase in blood pressure may produce headache, encephalopathy, and cerebral hemorrhage.

Myocardial infarction can occur secondary to the increased cardiac work and oxygen consumption. Infarction is not a result of coronary artery constriction. Epinephrine dilates coronary arteries.[27]

Epinephrine can also produce cardiac arrhythmias.[28] The arrhythmias probably result from a combination of factors. The increased oxygen demand creates an ischemic myocardial state. Stimulation of the β-adrenergic receptors causes direct myocardial irritation. Further, epinephrine administration produces a hypokalemia secondary to stimulation of β_2-adrenergic receptors.[29]

Diaphoresis and mydriasis also occur in overdose settings.

Treatment

Because the duration of action of epinephrine is short, treatment may not be necessary. If indicated, treatment should follow the guidelines for the treatment of toxicity with other mixed agonists, ephedrine, and pseudoephedrine (see Table 93–3).

Cases of the accidental injection of epinephrine into the digits have been reported. These cases usually involve the automatic injection devices used in the treatment of anaphylaxis. Epinephrine can also extravasate into the local subcutaneous tissues during intravenous infusions. The α-antagonist phentolamine can be infused into the area to reverse the vasoconstriction, returning blood flow to the area.

Imidazolines

The imidazolines have α-adrenergic stimulation properties.[30] Clonidine, rilmenidine, guanfacine, and guanabenz are α_2-agonists that act centrally to decrease the sympathetic output from the brain. As such they are used in the treatment of hypertension. Because they act as sympatholytic agents, they are not discussed in this chapter. Clonidine was initially developed for use as a nasal decongestant. Other imidazolines are used clinically because of their ability to produce vasoconstriction; thus, they are categorized as sympathomimetics.

Oxymetazoline, Xylometazoline, Tetrahydrozoline, and Naphazoline

The imidazoline derivatives oxymetazoline, xylometazoline, tetrahydrozoline, and naphazoline are common ingredients in topical ophthalmic and nasal decongestant products. Many formulations are available for over-the-counter purchase. Abuse and overuse of these produces is common. They are generally used as topical vasoconstrictors in the nose and eye, but systemic absorption and adverse effects can occur.

The clinical effects and, consequently, the adverse effects are mediated through stimulation of the α_2-adrenergic receptor. As a group, the imidazolines are potent vasoconstrictors. However, like their antihypertensive cousins, they can have central effects. Penetration into the CNS is dependent on their lipophilicity and chemical substitution of the derivative.[31] Chronic psychosis and hallucinosis has occurred with chronic nasal use.[32] Central stimulation of α_2-adrenergic receptors increases vagal tone and may cause bradycardia. Glazener and associates reported a case of a patient who was about to undergo pacemaker placement because of syncope secondary to bradycardia and hypotension.[33] Surgery was canceled when it was noted that the patient frequently used an oxymetazoline-containing nasal spray. When use of the nasal spray was discontinued, the bradycardia resolved. In children, oxymetazoline can cause sedation, seizures, agitation, insomnia, and hallucinations.[34]

Retinal artery occlusion has been reported after topical ophthalmic use. The occlusion was thought to be secondary to the α-adrenergic receptor–stimulated increase in platelet aggregation.[35] Constriction of uterine vessels and decreased perfusion led to uteroplacental insufficiency in a nearly full-term woman who used nasal spray.[36]

Sometimes, these agents are used as fillers in illicit cocaine. Nine cases of intravenous injection of what was thought to be cocaine but was actually 97% naphazoline were reported by van Montfrans and associates.[37] After intravenous injection, diaphoresis, nausea, drowsiness, headaches, syncope, and seizures occurred. In addition, sinus bradycardia with normal blood pressure was present. One of the patients was treated with atropine because of bradycardia and ectopic beats. She subsequently experienced an abnormal increase in blood pressure and an intracerebral hemorrhage.

Treatment

Generally, for mildly symptomatic patients, all that is necessary is observation. Intravenous administration of phentolamine is effective treatment for the adverse α effects of the drug (see Table 93–3). Seizures should be treated with a benzodiazepine.

β-Agonists

The β-adrenergic receptor stimulators are primarily used clinically for the treatment of bronchospasm. Isoproterenol has the added therapeutic role of increasing heart rate in symptomatic bradycardia unresponsive to atropine.

Isoproterenol

Isoproterenol stimulates β_1- and β_2-adrenergic receptors but has almost no α-agonist effects. It has also been used as a bronchodilator; however, it is no longer the drug of choice since more selective β_2-agonists have become available.

Headache, flushing of skin, cardiac arrhythmias, and myocardial ischemia from increased oxygen demand are some of the major untoward effects of isoproterenol therapy. Hypotension can also occur secondary to the stimulation of β_2-adrenergic receptors in the peripheral vasculature and subsequent vasodilatation.

β_2-Agonists

The selective β_2-agonists are used in the therapy of bronchospasm. They can be administered via inhalation, by mouth, or subcutaneously. The toxicity is much less when the drug is administered via inhalation. The amount of drug in an entire albuterol inhaler canister is only slightly greater than the 24-hour oral dose of the drug.[38]

Metaproterenol actually stimulates both β_1- and β_2-adrenergic receptors. However, when used in its inhaled form, the β_1 effects are minimized.

Terbutaline is also relatively selective in stimulation of β_2-adrenergic receptors. However, when it is given parenterally, it loses its selectivity. A reflex tachycardia can occur due to β_2-induced vasodilatation. Skeletal muscle tremors also are more frequent after oral or subcutaneous administration.

Albuterol has relatively selective β_2 stimulation. Fine tremor, hypotension, and reflex tachycardia are side effects of albuterol use.

The β_2-agonist compounds are relatively nontoxic. A review of albuterol overdoses revealed that up to 20-fold the oral daily dose produced no deaths.[39] In overdose tremor, hypotension and tachycardia can occur. Arrhythmias caused by the β stimulation of the heart or the β_2-induced hypokalemia may be seen.[40]

A case of myocardial infarction that occurred after the intravenous use of albuterol has been reported.[41] After the infusion of albuterol, the patient became hypotensive. Electrocardiography showed ST segment depression and multiple premature ventricular beats. Symptoms resolved in 30 minutes; however, significant elevation of cardiac enzyme levels was noted.

A 7-year-old girl had seizures following a dose of

terbutaline that was threefold normal.[42] She responded to treatment with diazepam.

Usually, intravenous fluid administration is adequate for the treatment of hypotension caused by these drugs. Tachycardia, if compromising cardiac function, can be treated with propranolol or esmolol.

Treatment

The treatment of β-agonist overdose is similar to that of overdose with other sympathomimetics—namely, control of the vital signs and decontamination (see Table 93–3).

Lavage and emesis are not contraindicated because the β-agonists do not aggravate hypertension or induce seizures. However, because the effects of β-agonists are relatively mild in overdose, these measures may not be necessary, and use of activated charcoal only may be sufficient for oral ingestions.

Support of blood pressure and control of tachycardia are the major therapeutic interventions. β-Agonist–induced hypotension usually responds to fluid therapy, and vasopressors are rarely needed. Tachycardia that produces cardiac compromise can be treated with a short-acting β-blocker like esmolol. β-Blockers may worsen asthmatic symptoms; thus, if overdose occurs in an asthmatic patient, these agents must be used with extreme caution.

Overdoses of these drugs can cause decreases in potassium level, and small doses of potassium can be added to intravenous fluids to support the heart when electrocardiographic changes are noted. The decrease in potassium is not a loss of body potassium but rather a shift of potassium into the cells induced by stimulation of the β-adrenergic receptor. Therefore, small doses of potassium—and not replacement doses—are indicated. When the β-agonist drug is cleared from the system, potassium will leave the cells and the potassium level will normalize.

Other Sympathomimetic Agents

Fenfluramine and Phentermine

The sympathomimetics fenfluramine and phentermine are among the newest agents used in appetite control. These drugs have actually been used for the treatment of obesity for many years, and both are schedule IV controlled substances. As is the case with many other diet aids, there are no acceptable studies demonstrating these drugs' effectiveness for long-term weight loss.

Fenfluramine does not produce CNS stimulation but can produce decreased levels of consciousness in overdose. It can potentiate the hypotensive effects of antihypertensive drugs. Pulmonary hypertension and increased muscular activity can occur, but no cardiac effects or seizures have been reported.[43]

Phentermine has a long half-life (19 to 24 hours). Its abuse potential is apparently low despite the fact that it does have central catecholamine effects.[43]

Overdoses of these two drugs are likely to occur together because of their combination use in appetite control. Treatment of hypertension or tachycardia should follow the guidelines established for ephedrine overdose.

Cathine

Cathine (*S,S*-(+)-phenylpropanolamine or (+)-norpseudoephedrine) is a diastereomer of PPA. Cathine is derived from the major alkaloid of the *Catha edulis* or khat plant. This plant is widely used as a stimulant in countries of East Africa and the Arabian Peninsula.[44] The leaves are chewed to achieve the stimulant effect. In Yemen, khat is used during social gatherings and other cultural events. Cathinone is a keto-analogue of cathine. It is more lipophilic than cathine; thus, it readily crosses the blood-brain barrier and is a highly potent CNS stimulant. This natural amphetamine produces marked euphoria and psychostimulant effects. In Europe, it is used as an appetite suppressant. The United Nations Convention of Psychotropic Substances has determined this substance to be a schedule I drug.

SUMMARY

Overdoses with sympathomimetic preparations are not uncommon. Treatment requires a good understanding of both autonomic physiology and autonomic pharmacology.

Many of the drugs listed in this chapter are used in combination with other drugs. These other drugs may have their own toxicity and symptomatology. For instance, antihistamines are commonly combined with the decongestants PPA, ephedrine, and pseudoephedrine. The antihistamines have anticholinergic effects and can alter expected symptoms.

Decontamination is usually the appropriate initial therapy. However, lavage can cause vagal stimulation or increased intracranial pressure. In some cases, specific therapies are needed first.

In general, vital signs should be normalized. However, abnormal vital signs do not always indicate a need for treatment. Treatment of bradycardia in the hypertensive patient may worsen the bradycardia.

Finally, the underlying medical conditions of the patient should be considered. Consultation with the local poison center and a toxicologist is often necessary for appropriate management.

References

1. Hoffman BB, Lefkowitz RJ: Catecholamines, sympathomimetic drugs, and adrenergic receptor antagonists. *In* Hardman JG, Limbird LE, Molinoff PB, et al (eds): Goodman and Gilman's The Pharmacological Basis of Therapeutics. 9th ed. New York, McGraw-Hill Book Co., pp 199–248, 1996.
2. Olson KR, Pentel PR, Kelley MT: Physical assessment and differential diagnosis of the poisoned patient. Med Toxicol *2*:52–81, 1987.

3. Benowitz NL, Goldschlager N: Cardiac disturbances in the toxicologic patient. *In* Haddad LM, Winchester JF (eds): Clinical Management of Poisoning and Drug Overdose. Philadelphia, W.B. Saunders Co., pp 65–9998, 1983.
4. Bravo EL: Phenylpropanolamine and other over-the-counter vasoactive compounds. Hypertension *11*(Suppl II):II7–II10, 1988.
5. Nickerson M, Nomaguchi GM: Response to sympathomimetic amines after Dibenamine blockade. J Pharmacol Exp Ther *107*:284–299, 1953.
6. Greiner TH, Garb S: The influence of drugs on the irritability and automaticity of heart muscle. J Pharmacol Exp Ther *98*:215–233, 1950.
7. Trendelenburg U, de La Sierra BGA, Muskus A: Modification by reserpine of the response of the atrial pacemaker to sympathomimetic amines. J Pharmacol Exp Ther *141*:301–309, 1963.
8. Kanfer I, Dowse R, Vuma V: Pharmacokinetics of oral decongestants. Pharmacotherapy *13*:116S–128S, 1993.
9. Horowitz JD, Lang WJ, Howes LG et al: Hypertensive responses induced by phenylpropanolamine in anorectic and decongestant preparations. Lancet *1*:60–61, 1980.
10. Pentel P: Toxicity of over-the-counter stimulants. JAMA *252*:1898–1903, 1984.
11. Bernstein E, Diskant BM: Phenylpropanolamine: a potentially hazardous drug. Ann Emerg Med *11*:311–315, 1982.
12. Pentel PR, Asinger RW, Benowitz NL: Propranolol antagonism of phenylpropanolamine-induced hypertension. Clin Pharmacol Ther *37*:488–494, 1985.
13. Pentel PR, Mikell FL, Zavoral JH: Myocardial injury after phenylpropanolamine ingestion. Br Heart J *47*:51–54, 1982.
14. Mueller SM, Solow EB: Seizures associated with a new combination "pick-me-up" pill. Ann Neurol *11*:322, 1982.
15. Woo OF, Benowitz NL, Bialy FW, et al: Atrioventricular conduction block caused by phenylpropanolamine. JAMA *253*: 2646–2647, 1985.
16. Cetaruk EW, Aaron CK: Hazards of nonprescription medications. Emerg Clin North Am *12*:483–510, 1994.
17. Fraunfelder FT, Meyer SM: Possible cardiovascular effects secondary to topical ophthalmic 2.5% phenylephrine. Am J Ophthalmol *99*:362–363, 1985.
18. Fraunfelder FT, Scafidi AF: Possible adverse effects from topical ocular 10% phenylephrine. Am J Ophthalmol *85*:447–453, 1978.
19. Solosko D, Smith RB: Hypertension following 10% phenylephrine ophthalmic. Anesthesiology *36*:187–189, 1972.
20. Cui J, Garle M, Eneroth P, et al: What do commercial ginseng preparations contain? Lancet *334*:134, 1994.
21. Martin WR, Sloan JW, Sapira JD, et al: Physiologic, subjective and behavioral effects of amphetamine, methamphetamine, ephedrine, phenmetrazine and methylphenidate in man. Clin Pharmacol Ther *12*:245–258, 1971.
22. Chait LD: Factors influencing the reinforcing and subjective effects of ephedrine in humans. Psychopharmacology *113*:381–387, 1994.
23. Hughes DTD, Empey DW, Land M: Effects of pseudoephedrine in man. J Clin Hosp Pharm *8*:315–321, 1983.
24. Loizou LA, Hamilton JG, Tsementzis SA: Intracranial haemorrhage in association with pseudoephedrine overdose. J Neurol Neurosurg Psychiatry *45*:471, 1982.
25. Capwell RR: Ephedrine-induced mania from an herbal diet supplement. Letter. Am J Psychiatry *152*:647, 1995.
26. Mariani PJ: Pseudoephedrine-induced hypertensive emergency: treatment with labetalol. Am J Emerg Med *4*:141–142, 1986.
27. Barach EM, Nowak RM, Lee TG, et al: Epinephrine for treatment of anaphylactic shock. JAMA *251*:2118–2122, 1984.
28. Sullivan TJ: Cardiac disorders in penicillin-induced anaphylaxis: association with intravenous epinephrine therapy. JAMA *248*:2161–2162, 1982.
29. Brown MJ: Hypokalemia from beta$_2$-receptor stimulation by circulating epinephrine. Am J Cardiol *56*:3D–9D, 1985.
30. Timmermans PB, deJonge A, van Zwieten PA: Comparative quantitative studies on central and peripheral alpha adrenoceptors. Chest *83*:354–357, 1983.
31. Fornai F, Blandizzi C, del Tacca M: Central alpha-2 adrenoceptors regulate central and peripheral functions. Pharmacol Res *22*:541–554, 1990.
32. Escobar JI, Karno M: Chronic hallucinosis from nasal drops. JAMA *247*:1859–1860, 1982.
33. Glazener F, Blake K, Gradman M: Bradycardia, hypotension, and near-syncope associated with Afrin (oxymetazoline) nasal spray. N Engl J Med *309*:731, 1983.
34. Söderman P, Sahlberg D, Wiholm BE: CNS reactions to nose drops in small children. Letter. Lancet *1*:573, 1984.
35. Magargal LE, Sanborn GE, Donoso LA, et al: Branch retinal artery occlusion after excessive use of nasal spray. Ann Ophthalmol *17*:500–501, 1985.
36. Baxi LV, Gindoff PR, Pregenzer GJ, et al: Fetal heart rate changes following maternal administration of a nasal decongestant. Am J Obstet Gynecol *153*:799–800, 1985.
37. van Montfrans GA, van Steenwijk RP, Vyth A, et al: Intravenous naphazoline intoxication. Acta Med Scand *209*:429–430, 1981.
38. Spangler DL: Review of side effects associated with beta agonists. Ann Allergy *62*:59–62, 1989.
39. Prior JG, Cochrane GM, Raper SM, et al: Self-poisoning with oral salbutamol. BMJ *282*:1932, 1981.
40. Higgins RM, Cookson WO, Lane DJ, et al: Cardiac arrhythmias caused by nebulized beta-agonist therapy. Letter. Lancet *2*:863–864, 1987.
41. Santo M, Sidi Y, Pinkhas Y: Acute myocardial infarction following intravenous salbutamol. S Afr Med J *58*:394, 1980.
42. Friedman R, Zitelli B, Jardine D, et al: Seizures in a patient receiving terbutaline. Am J Dis Child *136*:1091–1092, 1982.
43. US Pharmacopoeia Dispensing Information (USP DI): Drug Information for the Health Care Professional. 15th ed. Taunton, Mass., Rand McNally & Co., pp 381–383, 1995.
44. Kalix P: The pharmacology of psychoactive alkaloids from Ephedra and catha. J Ethnopharmacol *32*:201–208, 1991.

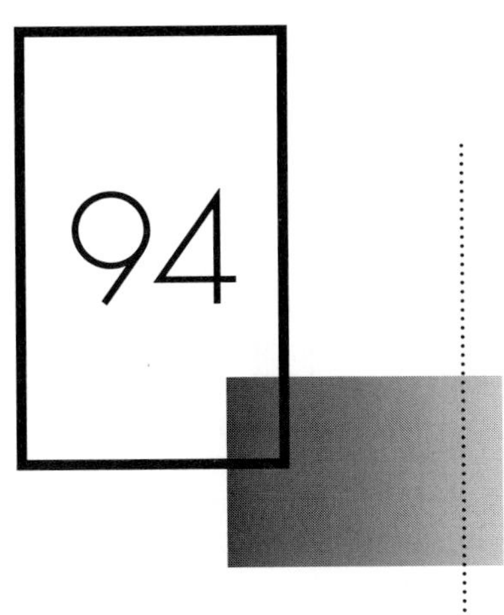

Ergot

DONALD B. KUNKEL, MD
MICHAEL W. CARLTON, MD

Ergot has a long and rich history. Medicinal use of ergot can be traced back over 3000 years to ancient China, where it was used as an obstetric agent.[1] Two thousand years ago, an ancient Assyrian tablet referred to ergotized grain as "a noxious pustule in the ear of grain." Several hundred years later, the first known reference to disease caused by ergot was made in one of the *Sacred Books of Parsees,* in which the author referred to ergotized grain as "noxious grasses that cause pregnant women to drop the womb and die in childbed."

Physicians, including Hippocrates and Galen, knew of the effects of ergotized grain. The first century naturalist Carus Plinius wrote that ergotized grains should be fed to cattle rather than humans. However, mass outbreaks of ergot-related disease (ergotism) were not reported in Europe until 857 AD. In that year, the *Annals of Xanthes* tell how "a great plague of swollen blisters consumed the people by a loathsome rot so that their limbs were loosened and fell off before death."[2] During the next 1000 years, over 100 outbreaks of ergotism would be recorded. As many as 40,000 people died in a single epidemic.

Many of ergot's victims turned to the saints for aid. The most famous patron of the disease, St. Anthony of Egypt, is enshrined in Dauphine, France. In 1090, a wealthy nobleman vowed before Anthony's tomb that if his son, Gerin, would be cured of the disease, he would use his fortune to aid victims of ergot's *ignis sacer* ("holy fire"). Gerin was cured, and together he and his father founded the Order of St. Anthony, a brotherhood of monks dedicated to the care of ergot victims. Since that time, the disease has been known as "St. Anthony's fire." Many ergotism victims reported healing following a pilgrimage to the Shrine of St. Anthony. However, many became sick again when they returned home owing to re-exposure to infected grain.

In 1676, Dodart reported to the French Academy of Sciences that the gangrenous form of the disease was associated with ergotized grains.[3] The same association was made with the convulsive form by Brunner in 1695. After this knowledge had been gained, ergot epidemics became increasingly less frequent. However, outbreaks have continued into the 20th century in the Soviet Union (1926), Ireland (1929), France (1951), and Ethiopia (1978).

Ergots were used by midwives as early as the 16th century, and they became popular with American physicians after John Sterns published his experience in 1808. The worldwide presence of ergotized grain has led some to suggest that these agents may have had a role in the witch trials of Salem, Massachusetts,[4] and in many Christian religious revivals of the American frontier.[5] Ergots and their adverse effects continue to be a source of concern to the modern medical community. The authors have hospitalized a woman with peripheral vasospasm secondary to the use of dihydroergotamine for migraine headaches.

BOTANY

The term *ergot* is generally used to describe species of the fungal genus *Claviceps,* the sclerotia formed by the fungi (especially *C. purpurea*), and the wide range of unique alkaloids produced by the fungi following the infestation of grain.

Three species of *Claviceps (C. purpurea, C. paspali,* and *C. cinerea)* have been known to parasitize the grains of various cultivated and wild grasses in the United States, with resultant animal disease.[6] Historically, however, *C. purpurea* infection of rye grain has been closely associated with human illness worldwide, and the sclerotium of this fungal species has become the source of many pharmacologically active principles.

Infection of grains occurs at the time of flowering of the grass. A parasitic spore of *Claviceps* germinates within the ovary of grass, and penetrating hyphae form a dense mass of tissue, the *mycelium,* which supplants the ovary. This mass gradually hardens into a dark, purplish resting body known as a *sclerotium.* The small, club-shaped (whence the name *Claviceps*) sclerotium may superficially resemble the host grain and may be processed and consumed with the grain itself. In the past, some grain harvests have consisted of over 30% ergot sclerotia; today, strict controls over maximal concentration of sclerotia account for the decreased incidence of natural ergotism.

Sclerotia of *C. purpurea* contain, in addition to certain pharmacologically active alkaloids (discussed later in this chapter), alkaloids of unproven pharmacologic use. Also isolated from sclerotia have been such diverse compounds as tyramine, tyrosine, tryptophan, histamine, histidine, choline, acetylcholine, and ergosterol.[7]

PHARMACODYNAMICS

All ergots are derivatives of the tetracyclic compound 6-methylergoline and have a common lysergic acid base. The ergot alkaloids may be divided into three classes: (1) the amine alkaloids; (2) the amino acid alkaloids; and (3) the synthetically derived dihydrogenated amino acid derivatives (Table 94–1). The structural similarity between the lysergic acid base and the endogenous catecholamines dopamine, norepinephrine, epinephrine, and serotonin account for most of the effects of the ergot alkaloids.

No other pharmacologic class of drugs has such a varied and diverse spectrum of activity (Table 94–2). The effects can be broadly divided into central and peripheral effects. *Central effects* are secondary to their dopaminergic properties and include hallucinations, delirium, emetogenicity, diarrhea, bradycardia, inhibition of the baroreceptor arc, tremors, and decrease in lactation. *Peripheral effects* include vasoconstriction, uterotonic activity, bradycardia, and hypercoagulable state, and they are mediated through α-adrenergic and serotonergic receptors. The precise distribution of effects depends on the substitutions made to the lysergic acid base.

Table 94–1. Clinically Significant Ergot Alkaloids

Amine Alkaloids	Amino Acid Alkaloids	Dihydrogenated Alkaloids
Ergonovine	Ergotamine	Dihydroergotamine
Methylergonovine	Bromocriptine	Dihydrogenated ergot alkaloids
Methysergide		
Lysergic acid diethylamide		
Lisuride		
Lergotrile		
Methergoline		

Absorption and Distribution

Most of the ergot alkaloids are poorly absorbed when they are taken by enteral or rectal routes. Absorption by both routes is increased when these agents are taken with caffeine, which increases the dissolution rate. Bioavailability is inconsistent following intramuscular use owing to varied absorption. Ergots are rapidly and widely distributed into tissues. The distribution half-life of ergotamine is 3 minutes.

Metabolism and Elimination

Ergot alkaloids are extensively metabolized by hepatic enzyme systems. Bioavailability is greatly diminished following oral administration due to first-pass metabolism. Bioavailability following rectal administration may be 20-fold that after oral administration. The elimination half-lives range from 1.4 hours for ergotamine to 6.2 hours for bromocriptine and to 10 hours for methysergide. Eighty per cent to 90% of the metabolites are eliminated in the bile, with the remaining portion excreted in the urine.

Ergotamine and Dihydroergotamine

Ergotamine and dihydroergotamine share many pharmacologic properties and differ only in degree of activity. Their actions are mediated through their activity on 5-HT_{1B}, 5-HT_{1C}, 5-HT_{1D}, and α-adrenergic receptors.[8–10] Ergotamine is the most potent vasoconstrictor of the ergots. Both of these drugs possess veno- and arterioconstrictive activity owing to their action on α-adrenergic and serotonergic receptors.[11, 12] Focal lesions of the central and peripheral nervous systems have been caused by arterioconstriction. Both drugs possess agonist and antagonist activity with respect to α-adrenergic and serotonergic receptors. Although dihydroergotamine's vasoconstrictive action is markedly less than that of ergotamine, its action may be more pronounced in the capacitance vessels, accounting for its utility in treating orthostatic hypotension. Ergotamine has little dopaminergic effect, with the exception of its high emetogenic potential, whereas dihydroergotamine is a nonselective antagonist of sympathetic ganglia. Ergotamine is highly uterotonic, whereas dihydroergotamine is active only on the pregnant uterus.

Methysergide

Peripherally, methysergide is a potent serotonergic antagonist; centrally, it is a partial agonist, particu-

Table 94–2. Pharmacologic Activity of Ergot Alkaloids*

	Ergotamine	Dihydroergotamine	Methylergonovine	Bromocriptine	Methysergide	Dihydroergotoxine
Pressor activity	1000	120	<10	<10	30	30
α-Adrenergic blockade	50	350	<0.4	230	<0.4	1000
Emetic activity	1000	85	210	410	<1	540
Serotonin blockade	10	40	250	3	1000	10
Uterotonic activity	500	Inhibition of methylergonovine	1000	Inhibition of methylergonovine	40	Inhibition of methylergonovine

*Based on an arbitrary potency of 1000 for the most active compound.

Adapted from Berde B, Sturmer E: The ergot alkaloids. *In* Berde B, Schild HO (eds): Handbook of Experimental Pharmacology. Vol. 49. Berlin, Springer-Verlag, p 4, 1978.

larly in the brain stem. It has a high affinity for 5-HT_2 receptors in the central nervous system, but it also is active at the 5-HT_{1C} receptor.[13] Methysergide also prevents mast cell–induced histamine release and serotonin-induced platelet aggregation, and it decreases the release of prostaglandin and kinins. Unlike most of the ergots, methysergide has a low first-pass effect and a bioavailability that approaches 100%. It has weak uterotonic and vasoconstrictor ability and is slightly emetic. Retroperitoneal, pleural, and pericardial fibrosis is the most severe complication of methysergide; however, it occurs after prolonged use and is not a complication of acute toxicity or overdose. A 1-month drug holiday has been suggested to prevent this complication.

TOXICITY AND CLINICAL PRESENTATION

In the past, ergotism was observed to have two forms: (1) gangrenous and (2) convulsive.[14] In epidemics, one form or the other usually predominated, although mixed outbreaks did occur. It is not clear why a particular geographic region tended to have repeated episodes of the same disease form. It has been suggested that nutritional deficiencies or variations in toxic contents of sclerotia had a role. Although most of the symptoms of the two forms were different, hallucinations were common in both.

Ergotismus gangraenosis, common in France, presented with lassitude, vomiting, and pain in the lower limbs. A severe feeling of inner heat lead many to plunge their afflicted extremity into ice water, and this led to frostbite. Limbs turned charcoal black and eventually became numb. Autoamputation of extremities at joints frequently occurred, usually without blood loss.

Ergotismus convulsivus primarily presented in Germany's Rhine valley. Symptoms began as soon as 6 hours after ingestion and could last from hours to months. Symptoms started with formication, diaphoresis, nausea, vomiting, and diarrhea, followed by pressure and pain in the chest and a heaviness of the head, arms, and legs. Convulsive muscular spasms and twitching began in the toes and progressed proximally. The convulsive symptoms could be limited to the extremities, face, vocal cords, or even the esophagus, or they could become generalized. The patient could lie for hours with paralytic spasms of the extremities. Repeated episodes could be expected, often with complete symptom resolution between incidents.

Today, acute toxicity presents either following administration of a large ergot dose or after longer exposure to a more moderate dosing. There is, however, a single case report of a 32-year-old woman who developed ergotism after a single dose of ergotamine tartrate.[15] Acute toxicity begins with formication, nausea, and vomiting within 4 hours of exposure. A feeling of severe thirst, diarrhea, and evidence of dermatologic hypoperfusion (pallor, coldness of the extremities, cyanosis, and pain) follow. Cardiovascular toxicity includes tachycardia or bradycardia, hypertension or hypotension, chest pain, and myocardial ischemia or infarct. Central nervous system features consist of restlessness, agitation, confusion, seizures, and coma. A 75-year-old man with temporal arteritis developed necrosis of the tongue while taking ergotamine tartrate.[16]

Toxic and fatal doses have not been strictly determined. Pediatric exposures are especially noteworthy because of their association with high mortality rates.[17, 18] One neonate developed respiratory failure and convulsions following administration of 0.5 mg of ergometrine.[19] A 29-year-old man suffered a myocardial infarction followed by a series of cardiac arrests after ingestion of 120 mg of ergotamine and 6 mg of caffeine.[20] Cardiac arrest and death have been reported after small doses of ergonovine during evaluation for variant angina pectoris.[21] Patients with underlying hepatic, renal, or vascular disease or with sepsis or toxemia may be predisposed to acute toxicity due to impaired ability to metabolize the drug or secondary to underlying disease.

Subacute and chronic toxic exposure often result from the misuse of headache preparations. It is noteworthy that ergotamine administration can cause headache and that headache may be precipitated by drug withdrawal following chronic use. Smokers may be at increased risk for ergot-induced vascular injury. Patient presentation depends on which vascular bed is affected by the drug. The usual effect is vasoconstriction. Extremities are most frequently affected. Symptoms may be unilateral or symmetric. The authors have admitted a 41-year-old woman for dihydroergotamine-induced vasospasm. She initially complained of burning pain in the left foot; this pain became bilateral and eventually involved all four extremities. Her extremities became cool, pale, and pulseless and, subsequently, cyanotic. She later developed chest pain, shortness of breath, and arrhythmias secondary to myocardial ischemia. Some authors have reported that residual sensory loss or paresthesia may persist. Blindness, myocardial infarction, and ischemic bowel and renal failure have all been reported as result of vascular impairment.

Central nervous system effects include nausea, vomiting, headache, fatigue, insomnia, restlessness, excitement, delirium, dementia, seizures, and respiratory depression. Hallucinogenic effects of lysergic acid diethylamide, bromocriptine, ergonovine, methylergonovine, and methysergide have all been well documented. In the French epidemic in 1951, which was caused by the ingestion of ergotized grain used by a local baker, hallucinations were common.[22]

Drugs that interact with ergots are rare, but one notable exception is macrolide antibiotics. Both troleandomycin[23, 24] and erythromycin[25] have been associated with an increased incidence of vasospastic disease when used in combination with ergotamine. Propranolol has also been claimed to interact with ergotamine.[26] However, this interaction was reported before propranolol was commonly used to prevent migraine, and given the large number of patients using prophylactic propranolol therapy who concomitantly use ergotamine, it is likely that the reported case represented toxicity from the ergotamine alone.

LABORATORY EVALUATION AND ANCILLARY TESTS

No specific ancillary tests for ergot-induced disease are available. While adverse reactions occur more frequently when blood levels of ergotamine exceed 1.8 ng/mL,[27] blood levels are generally neither available nor useful. Serum creatinine measurement, blood urea nitrogen determination, and urinalysis are used for assessing renal damage. Hepatic transaminase levels reflect the degree of liver injury. Metabolic acidosis with elevated lactate levels may occur. Serial serum creatinine phosphokinase determinations are necessary to confirm myocardial infarct and may be useful in assessing the degree of ischemic peripheral muscle injury.

Electrocardiography is useful when myocardial ischemia or infarction are suspected. Continuous cardiac monitoring is important for arrhythmia detection. Arteriography is an effective means of documenting arteriospasm and thrombosis. Computed tomography or magnetic resonance imaging can be used for assessing cerebral and cerebellar insult.

TREATMENT

Because intestinal absorption of ergots is incomplete, gastric decontamination should prove useful following acute ingestion of toxic quantities of ergots. Administration of syrup of ipecac may lead to prolonged vomiting and a delay in the administration of activated charcoal. Altered mental status and respiratory depression predispose the patient to aspiration of vomitus. Therefore, emetogenic measures should be avoided. Nasogastric and orogastric lavage with the use of small-bore tubes is unlikely to retrieve significant quantities of medication. Orogastric tubes with calibers sufficiently large for retrieval of intact pills and pill fragments should be used if gastric lavage is to be initiated, but large diameter limits the utility of gastric lavage in the pediatric population. Activated charcoal should be administered to bind any remaining medication left in the intestinal tract. No specific antidotes are available.

In mild cases of toxicity, withdrawal of the offending agent, hydration, and the use of minor analgesics (acetaminophen) may be sufficient. Oral administration of vasodilators may be necessary in more severe cases. In one case, ergotamine-induced vasospasm was reduced within 24 hours with prazosin, 1 mg three times per day.[28] In another report, ergotamine-induced peripheral vasospasm was relieved within 6 hours with the use of captopril, 50 mg three times per day.[29] Nifedipine has also been reported to be useful in a dosage of 10 mg by mouth three times per day.[30]

Nitroprusside has been the treatment of choice to combat severe vasospasm. Therapy is usually initiated intravenously or intra-arterially at a 0.3 μg/kg per minute, and dosage is titrated to effect. The usual therapeutic range is 2 to 10 μg/kg per minute. To avoid cyanide toxicity, thiosulfate should be added in a 10-to-1 ratio for each milligram of nitroprusside used. Various other intra-arterial vasodilators such as tolazoline, ethanol, niacin, and papaverine have been used with mixed results. Administration of intravenous heparin or low-molecular-weight dextran has been recommended to minimize thrombosis caused by stasis and endothelial damage.

The arterial and venous spasm induced by ergots is likely secondary to the combined effects of adrenergic and serotonergic receptor agonism.[8–10] The degree of the effect may vary from species to species and from one vascular bed to another.[11, 12] In isolated human femoral veins, vasospasm is a function of both adrenergic and serotonergic effects, but serotonin has more potent effects on veins than on arteries. Cyproheptadine, a serotonin antagonist, inhibited the vasoconstrictive effects of dihydroergotamine in isolated rat aorta.[31] A single case of dihydroergotamine-induced vasospasm in a 41-year-old woman treated with cyproheptadine is reported in the literature.[32] She improved dramatically following administration of cyproheptadine, 4 mg three times per day. These data suggest that cyproheptadine should be considered in other cases of dihydroergotamine-induced vasospasm.

Coronary artery vasospasm should be treated with nitroglycerin. Sublingual, intravenous, and intracoronary routes of administration have been reported to be efficacious.[33–35] Verapamil has also been used to reduce the coronary artery spasm induced by ergonovine testing.[36]

ACUTE BROMOCRIPTINE TOXICITY

Bromocriptine deserves special attention because of recent changes in its approved labeling. In the United States, bromocriptine's approved indications are for hyperprolactinemia-associated dysfunctions, acromegaly, and Parkinson's disease. It has also been used in the treatment of neuroleptic malignant syndrome and cocaine withdrawal. In 1980, the Food and Drug Administration approved the use of bromocriptine for prevention of physiologic lactation. However, following reports of serious adverse reactions (seizures, strokes), the manufacturer agreed to withdrawing this as an approved indication.

Through its structural relationship to dopamine, bromocriptine is an agonist of the dopamine D_2 receptor and an antagonist of the D_1 receptor. Nausea, vomiting, dizziness, lethargy, pupillary dilation, hypertension, and tachycardia are common presenting symptoms.[37] Both sympathomimetic signs (tachycardia, hypertension, hallucinations, paranoid behavior) and anticholinergic findings (mydriasis, flushed skin, tachycardia, fever, hallucinations, confusion, mania) may be noted in overdose.

Recovery is usually rapid with adequate gut decontamination and supportive care, with particular attention to the airway, hypo- and hypertensive crises, and management of delirium. No human deaths have been reported. Use of the drug generally seems to have a broad margin of safety.[38]

References

1. Bove FJ: The Story of Ergot. New York, S. Karger AG, p 136, 1970.
2. Merhoff CG, Porter JM: Ergot intoxication. Ann Surg *180*:773–779, 1974.
3. Barger G: Ergot and Ergotism. London, Gurney Jackson, p 59, 1931.
4. Caporael LR: Ergotism: The Satan loosed in Salem? Science *192*:21–26, 1976.
5. Massey JM, Massey EW: Ergot, the "jerks," and revivals. Clin Neuropharmacol *7*:99–105, 1984.
6. Kingsbury JM: Poisonous Plants of the United States and Canada. Englewood Cliffs, NJ, Prentice-Hall, pp 80, 86, 1964.
7. Morton JF: Major Medicinal Plants. Springfield, IL, Charles C Thomas, p 6, 1977.
8. Roquebert J, Grenie B: Alpha 2-adrenergic agonist and alpha 1-adrenergic antagonist activity of ergotamine and dihydroergotamine in rats. Arch Int Pharmacodyn Ther *284*:30–37, 1986.
9. Buzzi MG, Moskowitz MA: Evidence for 5-HT1B/1D receptors mediating the antimigraine effect of sumatriptan and dihydroergotamine. Cephalalgia *11*:165–168, 1991.
10. Brown AM, Patch TL, Kaumann AJ: The antimigraine drugs ergotamine and dihydroergotamine are potent 5-HT1C receptor agonists in pig choroid plexus. Br J Pharmacol *104*:45–48, 1991.
11. Glusa E, Markwardt F: Studies on 5-hydroxytryptamine receptors on isolated human femoral veins and arteries and the influence of dihydroergotamine. Pharmacology *29*:336–342, 1984.
12. Muller-Schweinitzer E, Rosenthaler J: *Ex vivo* studies after oral treatment of the beagle with dihydroergotamine. Eur J Pharmacol *89*:1–8, 1983.
13. Vhora S, Chiba S: Functional 5-HT receptor subtypes in the isolated canine common carotid artery. Heart Vessels *9*:235–240, 1994.
14. Haller JS: Smut's dark poison: Ergot in history and medicine. Trans Stud Coll Physicians Phila *3*:2–79, 1981.
15. Harrison TE: Ergotaminism after a single dose of ergotamine tartrate. J Emerg Med *2*:23–25, 1984.
16. Bondeson J, Ericsson UB, Falke P, et al: Tongue necrosis in temporal arteritis provoked by ergotamine. J Intern Med *232*:541–544, 1992.
17. Edwards WM: Accidental poisoning of newborn infants with ergotamine maleate. Clin Pediatr *10*:257–260, 1971.
18. Jones WM, Williams B: Two cases of ergotamine poisoning in infants. BMJ *1*:466, 1966.
19. Kenna AP: Accidental administration of syntometrine to a newborn infant. J Obstet Gynecol Br Common *79*:764–766, 1972.
20. Carr P: Self-induced myocardial infarction. Postgrad Med J *57*:654–655, 1981.
21. Buxton A, Goldberg S, Hirschfeld JW, et al: Refractory ergonovine-induced coronary vasospasm: Importance of intracoronary nitroglycerine. Am J Cardiol *46*:329–334, 1980.
22. Fuller JG: The Day of St. Anthony's Fire. New York, Macmillan Publishing Co., p 51, 1968.
23. Hayton AC: Precipitation of acute ergotism by triacetyloleandomycin. N Z J Med *69*:42, 1969.
24. Matthews MB, Havill JH: Ergotism with therapeutic doses of ergotamine tartrate. N Z J Med *89*:476–477, 1979.
25. Ghali R, De Léan J, Douville Y, et al: Erythromycin-associated ergotamine intoxication: Arteriographic and electrophysiologic analysis of a rare cause of severe ischemia of the lower extremities and associated ischemic neuropathy. Ann Vasc Surg *7*:291–296, 1993.
26. Baumrucker JF: Drug interaction—propranolol and cafergot. N Engl J Med *288*:916–917, 1973.
27. Orton DA, Richardson RJ: Ergotamine absorption and toxicity. Postgrad Med J *58*:6–11, 1982.
28. Cobaugh BS: Prazosin treatment of ergotamine-induced peripheral ischemia. JAMA *244*:1360, 1980.
29. Zimran A, Ofek B, Hershko C, et al: Treatment with captopril for peripheral ischemia induced by ergotamine. BMJ *288*:364, 1984.
30. Dagher FJ, Pais SO, Richards W, Queral LA: Severe unilateral ischemia of the lower extremity caused by ergotamine: Treatment with nifedipine. Surgery *97*:369–373, 1988.
31. Glusa E, Markwardt F: Influence of endothelium on the vasoconstrictor effect of dihydroergotamine in the isolated rat aorta. Arch Int Pharmacodyn Ther *296*:66–75, 1988.
32. Carlton MC, Kunkel DB, Curry SC: Ergotism treated with cyproheptadine. Clin Toxicol *33*:552, 1995.
33. Eurin B, Samii K, Rouby JJ, Glaser P: Ergot and sodium nitroprusside. N Engl J Med *298*:632–633, 1978.
34. O'Dell CW, Davis GB, Johnson AD, et al: Sodium nitroprusside in the treatment of ergotism. Radiology *124*:73–74, 1977.
35. Heupler FA Jr, Proudfit WL, Razavi M, et al: Ergonovine maleate: Provocative tests for coronary artery vasospasm. Am J Cardiol *41*:631–640, 1978.
36. Waters DD, Szlachcic J, Theroux P, et al: Ergonovine testing to detect spontaneous remissions of variant angina during long-term treatment with calcium antagonist drugs. Am J Cardiol *47*:179–183, 1981.
37. Vermund SH, Goldstein RG, Romano AA, Atwood SJ: Accidental bromocriptine ingestion in childhood. J Pediatr *105*:838–840, 1984.
38. Mack RB: Mairzy doats and dozy doats and a kiddle eat almost anything: Bromocriptine (Parlodel) overdose. N C Med J *49*:17–18, 1988.

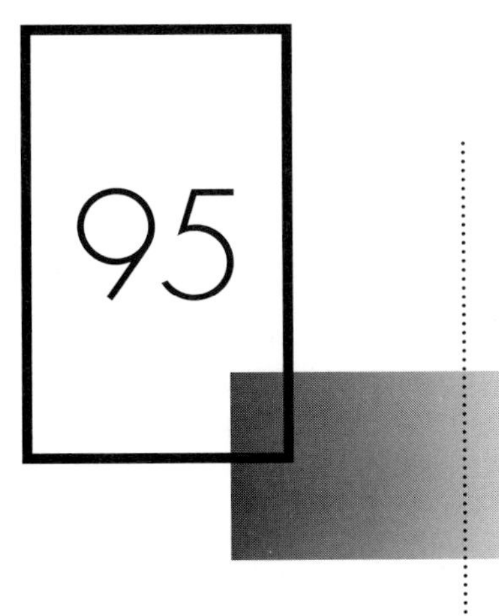

Theophylline and Caffeine

MICHAEL W. SHANNON, MD, MPH

Theophylline, caffeine, and theobromine are the major members of a group of pharmacologic agents known as *methylxanthines*. These drugs have obtained a ubiquitous position in society: Caffeine is used around the world for the pleasure that its mild stimulation provides. For almost a century, theophylline has been used for the treatment of respiratory ailments.

THEOPHYLLINE

Theophylline is currently used to treat various illnesses. At one time it was the primary therapy for asthma, considered valuable both for acute treatment and for long-term prophylactic therapy.[1] Through the years, β-adrenergic agonists have largely replaced theophylline for this indication, having greater safety and efficacy. However, theophylline is still used as a primary agent in areas where β-adrenergic agonists are less available and for individuals who have asthma that is resistant to β-adrenergic agonist and corticosteroid therapy. Moreover, data suggesting that theophylline has anti-inflammatory properties have led to a slight increase in its use.[2, 3] Besides asthma, theophylline is used for other syndromes of airway obstruction including chronic obstructive pulmonary disease in adults and bronchiolitis in infants.[4, 5] Finally, theophylline is prescribed for neonates, particularly premature neonates, who have apnea and bradycardia.[6]

Individuals develop theophylline intoxication by two general mechanisms. First, its general availability makes theophylline an agent that can be ingested by curious toddlers or suicidal adolescents or adults. Second, because of its highly variable pharmacokinetics, theophylline is often responsible for unintentional chronic intoxication. By whatever mechanism, theophylline poisoning leads to a host of clinical and metabolic complications that often result in disastrous consequences, including death. A thorough understanding of theophylline intoxication, including rational and effective treatment algorithms, is therefore necessary for management of this overdose.

Structure and Structural Relationships

As illustrated in Figure 95–1, the methylxanthines are purines that are structurally related to the nucleotides adenine and guanine. Theophylline is 1,3-dimethylxanthine. It is closely related to caffeine (1,3,7-trimethylxanthine) and theobromine (3,7-dimethylxanthine). Caffeine is found in high concentration in coffee and certain teas. Theobromine is primarily found in cocoa. A related drug, pentoxifylline, is prescribed for peripheral vascular disease. Adenosine, which is an adenine-ribose nucleoside, is closely related to theophylline in structure and appears to have an important role in theophylline's pharmacologic actions and toxic effects.

More than 100 theophylline products are available as solutions, tablets, sustained-release capsules, and intravenous preparations. Many of these products include additional agents to increase theophylline's solubility, including bromide ion, choline, and salicylate. For example, because of theophylline's poor solubility in water, the intravenous form, aminophylline, contains an ethylenediamine salt; aminophylline is approximately 80% theophylline.[7]

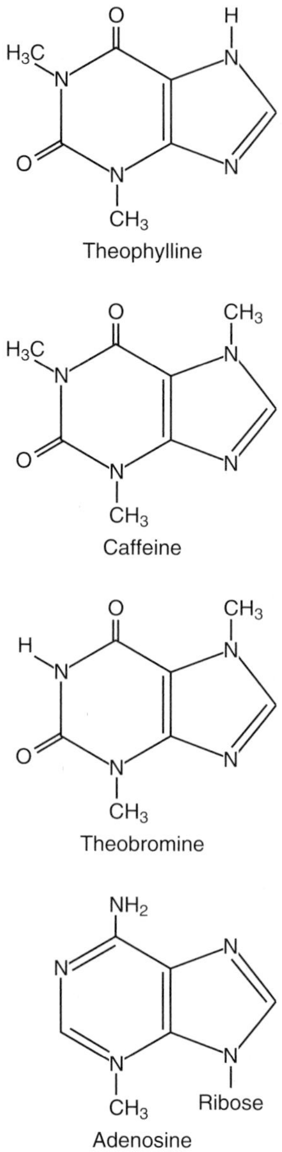

Theophylline

Caffeine

Theobromine

Adenosine

Figure 95–1. Theophylline and related compounds.

Pharmacology

Pharmacokinetics

In its oral form, theophylline is most commonly prescribed as a sustained-release capsule; although liquid preparations and standard-release formulations are still available, they are used in a minority of circumstances. The type of preparation influences absorption pattern. Sustained-release theophylline is designed to provide stable serum concentrations by having a gastrointestinal (GI) absorption rate that approximates that of drug elimination. These agents are not completely absorbed until 6 to 8 hours after ingestion. Overdoses of sustained-release theophylline can be associated with 15 to 24-hour delays to peak absorption. However, absorption of theophylline is complete; there is no significant presystemic clearance (first-pass effect) of the drug.

Once absorbed, theophylline is distributed in the body with a relatively small volume of distribution (average 0.45 L/kg, with a range of 0.3 to 0.7 L/kg).[7] Young infants and the elderly tend to have larger volumes of distribution. Plasma protein binding is 40% to 65%. The therapeutic serum concentration of theophylline is generally considered to be 10 to 20 μg/mL, although lower serum concentrations can produce the desired therapeutic effect. As a general rule, 1 mg/kg of administered theophylline raises serum theophylline concentration by 2 μg/mL. Theophylline freely crosses the placenta and enters breast milk.[7]

The metabolism of theophylline occurs through its biotransformation by the cytochrome P-450 system. The specific enzymes of this superfamily that have been associated with theophylline metabolism are CYP1A2, CYP2E1, and CYP3A3. The primary metabolic step is *N*-demethylation by the enzyme CYP1A2, producing the pharmacologically active agent 3-methylxanthine. The secondary metabolic pathway is hydroxylation, forming inactive 1,3-dimethyluric acid. Neonates also have the ability to metabolize theophylline by its methylation, producing caffeine. Moreover, neonates excrete approximately 50% of theophylline in urine unchanged (versus only 10% in children and adults).[7]

The rate of theophylline metabolism is variable. Age is an important influence on metabolism (Table 95–1). Neonates and the elderly eliminate the drug relatively slowly. Theophylline clearance is maximal between the ages of 1 and 9 years before decreasing by approximately 50% to adult rates.[7] The reason for such age-dependent elimination rates is unclear but may be related to the relative activity of cytochrome P-450 enzymes.

Theophylline also exhibits Michaelis-Menten (saturable) kinetics. As a result, across a narrow range, increments in dose are associated with corresponding increments in serum theophylline concentration. At high doses, however, increments lead to dispropor-

Table 95–1. Theophylline Elimination Patterns by Age

Population	Age	Half-Life (h)	Clearance (mL/kg/ per min)
Neonates and Infants			
Premature neonates	1 wk	30	0.29
Premature neonates	41 d	20	0.64
Term infants	18 wk	6.9	0.80
Term infants	34 wk	3.7	2.0
Children and Adolescents	4–15 y	3.0	1.55
Adults			
Asthmatic nonsmokers	31 y	9.4	0.65
Healthy nonsmokers	22–35 y	8.1	0.86
Healthy elderly nonsmokers	67 y	7.4	0.59
Healthy elderly nonsmokers	>70 y	9.8	NA

NA, not available.
Data from references 7, 67, and 88.

tionate elevations in serum concentration.[8] Conversely, with severe theophylline intoxication, initial drug elimination rates are extremely slow, following zero-order (dose-dependent) kinetics. With decreasing serum theophylline concentration, first-order (dose-independent) kinetics eventually appear, leading to abrupt increases in elimination rate. It is these kinetics that are often responsible for inadvertent theophylline intoxication.

Drug-Drug Interactions

Theophylline is a drug whose metabolism is highly subject to alteration by concomitant drug use. A growing list of drugs, when prescribed with theophylline, can result in either increased or decreased clearance. Chronic theophylline intoxication is often a result of unrecognized drug interactions.

The drugs that have been associated with increased clearance of theophylline are relatively few; all are known to be inducers of cytochrome P-450 enzymes. These agents include phenobarbital, phenytoin, carbamazepine, and tobacco smoke. Patients who are taking these drugs often have difficulty maintaining therapeutic serum theophylline concentrations and require inordinately high doses. If these patients discontinue their medications or quit smoking because they feel unwell, elimination rates can quickly revert. For example, theophylline clearance falls by approximately 40% within 1 week of abstinence from cigarette smoking).[7]

The list of agents that decrease theophylline clearance is extensive (Table 95–2). It is also notable that among drug classes, one member may inhibit clearance but the others do not; cimetidine, a histamine$_2$ (H_2)-antagonist, is a potent inhibitor of theophylline metabolism. However, the H_2-antagonists ranitidine and famotidine do not appear to have this action (although case reports have suggested that ranitidine occasionally reduces theophylline clearance). Common drugs that diminish theophylline clearance include the macrolide antibiotics (e.g., erythromycin/clarithromycin) and the quinolone antibiotics (e.g., ciprofloxacin/norfloxacin). The erythromycin-theophylline interaction has been characterized as appearing between days 3 and 7 of their concomitant use, with serum theophylline concentrations rising by an average of 30% to 35% if dosing adjustments are not made.

Table 95–2. Drugs Reported to Reduce Theophylline Metabolism

Allopurinol	Nifedipine
Cimetidine	Norfloxacin
Ciprofloxacin	Ofloxacin
Clarithromycin	Pefloxacin
Diltiazem	Pentoxifylline
Disulfiram	Pipemidic acid
Enoxacin	Propafenone
Erythromycin	Propranolol
Estrogen	Roxithromycin
Ethanol	Tacrine
Fluvoxamine	Thiabendazole
Furosemide	Ticlopidine
Idrocilamide	Troleandomycin
Interferon (recombinant α)	Verapamil
Methotrexate	Viloxazine
Mexiletine	

Adapted from American Academy of Pediatrics Committee on Drugs: Precautions concerning the use of theophylline. Pediatrics *89*:781, 1992; and Hendeles L, Jenkins J, Temple R: Revised FDA labeling guidelines for theophylline oral dosage forms. Pharmacotherapy *15*:409, 1995.

Drug-Disease Interactions

Several medical conditions have significant impact on theophylline pharmacokinetics. In young children, febrile illness can markedly reduce theophylline elimination; it is recommended that the dose of theophylline be reduced by one half in children who are febrile for more than 24 hours.[6] Influenza and respiratory syncytial virus have also been reported as infectious agents that can reduce theophylline elimination.[6] Cardiac disease, particularly congestive heart failure, can reduce theophylline clearance by as much as 50%, presumably through secondary hepatic dysfunction.[7] Primary hepatic disease can also reduce theophylline clearance by as much as 50%. Both cystic fibrosis and hyperthyroidism have been associated with increased clearance, resulting in larger dosing requirements. Renal disease has no important effect on theophylline pharmacokinetics.

Pharmacologic Actions

Methylxanthines have a number of pharmacologic actions that give them therapeutic value. They relax smooth muscle, including that of the bronchi, esophagus, and gastroesophageal sphincter. They are central nervous system (CNS) stimulants that can reduce fatigue and increase concentration. Physiologic dependence may occur with this action: Acute abstinence from caffeine is associated with malaise, headaches, emotional lability, and depression. Other CNS actions include stimulation of the CNS respiratory center, increasing minute volume. Cardiovascular effects include reduced peripheral vascular resistance with increased cardiac chronotropy and inotropy.[9] Improved muscle function can result in improved racing performance and improved pulmonary dynamics. Evidence indicates that theophylline is a potent inhibitor of renal erythropoietin production.[10] Methylxanthines are also diuretics.

Mechanism of Action

Four major theories have been proposed to explain theophylline's pharmacologic effects. First is the theory that theophylline acts as an inhibitor of phosphodiesterase, the enzyme that breaks down intracellular cyclic adenosine monophosphate (cAMP). According to current theories, cAMP is created by the membrane-bound enzyme adenylate cyclase, in response to a number of receptor-linked stimuli. cAMP next effects a number of actions, including regulation of gated potassium channels. These actions are terminated when cAMP is metabolized by phosphodiesterase. Theophylline was historically thought to be an inhibitor of phosphodiesterase. However, data now suggest that phosphodiesterase inhibition is negligible at therapeutic serum concentrations of theophylline, indicating that this mechanism alone cannot account for theophylline's actions.[11, 12] Phosphodiesterase inhibition has not been studied in victims of theophylline intoxication.

A second theory proposed for theophylline's actions is that of sympathetic nervous system stimulation. In therapeutic doses, theophylline produces marked increases in the level of circulating catecholamines, particularly epinephrine and norepinephrine.[13–16] Theophylline's actions of bronchodilation, cardiorespiratory stimulation, and even metabolic changes such as depression in serum potassium may result from augmented plasma catecholamine activity. In a canine model of theophylline poisoning, hypokalemia, increased oxygen consumption, metabolic acidosis, and cardiac disturbances have been directly related to plasma catecholamine activity.[13, 14]

The third potential mechanism of theophylline's action is competitive antagonism of endogenous adenosine. Adenosine, which is recognized as a bronchoconstrictor, anticonvulsant, and regulator of cardiac rhythm, interacts closely with theophylline through its competition for adenosine receptors.[10] The structural similarity between these chemicals and their opposite physiologic functions supports this theory of adenosine receptor antagonism.

Finally, theophylline's actions may result directly from changes in intracellular calcium transport. For example, caffeine has been shown to inhibit the uptake and storage of calcium by the sarcoplasmic reticulum of striated muscle, thereby producing increased strength in skeletal muscle.[9]

Clinical Toxicity

Having a narrow therapeutic index, theophylline is associated with a high rate of adverse effects. For example, as many as 15% of patients complain of adverse effects when their serum theophylline concentration is in the therapeutic range. Once serum theophylline concentrations exceed the therapeutic range (> 20 μg/mL), the prevalence of adverse effects exceeds 65% to 70%. More than 90% of patients with serum theophylline concentrations greater than 30 μg/mL demonstrate signs of toxicity.[7] It is also notable that theophylline intoxication has a high rate of iatrogenic origin; Schiff and colleagues found that in 68% of patients hospitalized with theophylline intoxication, inpatient or emergency department drug administration was responsible or contributed to toxicity.[17]

Clinical Manifestations

The signs and symptoms of theophylline intoxication can be placed into five categories: GI, musculoskeletal, cardiovascular, neurologic, and metabolic.[7, 18–21]

Gastrointestinal. The GI tract seems most sensitive to theophylline's toxicity. The most common complaints associated with theophylline use are abdominal pain, heartburn, and vomiting.[22] In some cases, hemorrhagic gastritis can occur. These effects result from GI actions that include increased production of gastric acid and pepsin as well as relaxation of the lower esophageal sphincter. With moderate to severe theophylline intoxication, vomiting can be difficult to control despite antiemetic therapy.[23]

Musculoskeletal. Victims of theophylline intoxication often complain of generalized muscle aches. With moderate toxicity, muscular hypertonicity with frank myoclonus may develop. Coarse tremor has also been reported as a manifestation of toxicity.[22] These effects have been attributed to the potassium disturbances that accompany theophylline intoxication or disturbances in intracellular calcium transport. Elevations in serum creatine phosphokinase levels have been reported with severe intoxication.[24]

Cardiovascular. Theophylline has several cardiovascular effects, some of which can be life threatening. Even when serum theophylline concentrations are in the therapeutic range, sinus tachycardia is often present. Greater toxicity has effects on vascular tone and cardiac rhythm.

Peripheral vasodilation is invariable with significant theophylline intoxication. This results in a widened pulse pressure and a decline in systemic vascular resistance.[25] Hypotension is generally present rather than hypertension.[13, 14] The mechanism of vascular disturbances is thought to be stimulation of peripheral vascular β-adrenergic receptors, produced by circulating plasma catecholamines.

Theophylline is arrhythmogenic.[26] Myocardial irritability appears with mild to moderate theophylline intoxication; electrocardiograms most often reveal ventricular premature beats. These are usually of no consequence. However, more severe myocardial irritability occurs with serious intoxication, producing bigeminy and other potentially unstable rhythms. These dysrhythmias may be a prelude to life-threatening cardiac arrhythmias such as ventricular tachycardia.

Although sinus tachycardia is one of the most common of manifestations of toxicity, appearing in as many as 82% of cases,[22] rhythm disturbances are a sign of severe theophylline intoxication and the most common cause of theophylline-induced fatalities. Sinus tachycardia can quickly progress to life-threatening rhythms, which can be either ventricular or supraventricular in origin.[27] Supraventricular disturbances reported after theophylline intoxication include supraventricular tachycardia, atrial fibrillation, atrial flutter, and multifocal atrial tachycardia.[28] Many of these rhythms, such as multifocal atrial tachycardia, are characteristic of theophylline intoxication.[29] Supraventricular tachyarrhythmias result in increased myocardial oxygen demand, compromised cardiac output, shock, metabolic acidosis, and myocardial ischemia or infarction. Life-threatening arrhythmias of ventricular origin consist of ventricular tachycardia and ventricular fibrillation.

The mechanism of cardiac rhythm disturbances is unclear. Rhythm disturbances may also be secondary to elevated plasma catecholamine activity. Data now suggest that the mechanism of rhythm disturbances is theophylline inhibition of cardiac adenosine receptors.

Neurologic. Neurologic manifestations of theophylline intoxication appear at relatively low serum concentration; users of theophylline may complain of anxiety and insomnia. In children, theophylline may produce important behavioral disturbances that interfere with school function.[30, 31] Although results of clinical investigations have been mixed, most data have failed to demonstrate a consistent effect on learning, although some children are likely to have a detrimental neurobehavioral response to the medication.[32]

With moderate theophylline intoxication, more striking signs of neurologic disturbance appear. An early sign of intoxication is tachypnea, representing stimulation of CNS respiratory centers and often resulting in respiratory alkalosis. Worsening clinical toxicity is attended by anxiety, agitation, and delirium or hallucinosis.[22]

The single most serious consequence of theophylline intoxication is the appearance of seizures. Theophylline-induced seizures can present in many patterns. These seizures are usually generalized, although focal seizures have been described.[33] In young infants, seizures may be subtle, consisting of generalized hypertonicity, eye deviation, and lip smacking without a clonic component. Theophylline-induced seizures can be single or repeated. They can appear without warning, although irritability, vomiting, and headache may be premonitory signs.[6] Seizures may occur at serum theophylline concentrations less than 20 μg/mL.[6] Once they appear, those seizures can be extremely difficult to treat, being resistant to standard anticonvulsant therapy. Seizures due to theophylline use often predict a poor outcome; earlier case series reported a mortality of 50% to 100% among those who developed seizures.[34, 35] Numerous case reports and case series have reported disabling, permanent neurologic sequelae in those who develop theophylline-induced seizures.[6, 36–41] Neurologic complications can include amnesia, personality changes, quadriplegia, and intractable seizure disorder. In young infants, associated intracerebral hemorrhage has been reported.[37] Neurologic sequelae are more common after long-term theophylline overmedication rather than acute single overdose.

The mechanism of theophylline-induced seizures is not completely understood and is likely multifactorial. However, as many as 34% of children and 12% of adults develop abnormalities on electroencephalogram while taking the medication.[36, 42] Theophylline-induced seizures have been linked to dysfunction of GABAergic inhibitory neurons; in an animal model, pyridoxine, which promotes γ-aminobutyric acid (GABA) synthesis, was found to ameliorate theophylline-induced seizures.[43]

Theophylline's relationship to CNS adenosine receptors has received considerable attention in recent years. The CNS has a dense population of adenosine receptors. These modulate the activity of various populations of neurons (e.g., cholinergic and glutaminergic). *In vitro* and *in vivo* studies have proved the importance of endogenous adenosine in regulating neuronal depolarization. For example, adenosine antagonists lead to marked alterations in seizure pattern after experimental administration of proconvulsant agents, producing uninterrupted electric discharge. Studies with radiolabeled theophylline have also shown it can displace adenosine from its receptor sites. In an animal model of theophylline-induced seizures, Shannon and Maher demonstrated that direct CNS administration of adenosine could forestall theophylline-induced seizures.[44]

In addition to its direct neuroexcitatory effects, theophylline has marked effects on cerebral vascular tone, an action that is also related to adenosine activity.[45] Adenosine is a potent stimulator of cerebral vasodilation; marked increases in CNS adenosine activity occur in response to cerebral ischemia, representing another cerebroprotective effect.[9] Theophylline antagonizes this action, producing sustained cerebrovasoconstriction, which compromises CNS delivery of oxygen and nutrients as well as removal of toxic metabolic wastes.

Metabolic. Metabolic complications of theophylline intoxication are many.[46, 47] Even in therapeutic doses, theophylline can produce depressions in serum potassium and elevations in blood glucose levels. With more severe intoxication, profound hypokalemia can result. Serum potassium concentrations as low as 1.7 mEq/L have been reported after theophylline poisoning.[25, 48]

The mechanism of theophylline-induced hypokalemia is well defined. Although early theories attributed it to potassium losses as a result of vomiting or diuresis, this is unlikely to be the cause.[49] For example, Amitai and Lovejoy demonstrated that the hypokalemia often precedes vomiting.[50] The current belief is that hypokalemia results from intracellular transport of potassium ion, produced by increased activity of sodium/potassium adenosine triphosphatase (Na^+, K^+-ATPase) or opening of calcium-linked potassium channels. This effect occurs secondary to catecholamine-induced β_2-adrenergic stimulation.[49, 51–53] As a result, total-body potassium is preserved. Theophylline-induced hypokalemia promptly reverses as serum theophylline concentration declines, without potassium supplementation. The clinical consequences of theophylline-induced hypokalemia are unclear. Although hypokalemia has been implicated in the genesis of theophylline-induced cardiac arrhythmias, this is only speculative and is not supported by available data. Blood glucose elevations also appear to be a result of circulating plasma catecholamines. Serum blood glucose can rise to levels greater than 400 mg/dL.[25]

Metabolic acidosis with depression of serum bicarbonate levels is usually modest but can be severe, resulting in a high anion gap. Serum bicarbonate concentrations as low as 5 mEq/L have been reported after serum theophylline poisoning. Acidosis appears to result from the combination of increased lactate production and lipolysis with increased free fatty acid circulation.[54]

Other metabolic disturbances associated with theophylline intoxication include hypercalcemia, which has been reported in as many as 15% of patients.[55] Hypomagnesemia, hypophosphatemia, and respiratory alkalosis have also been reported.[46, 48]

Theophylline has not been proved to have significant human genotoxicity or fetotoxicity.[7, 56] However, it is listed as a pregnancy category C drug by the Food and Drug Administration.

Acute Versus Chronic Intoxication

The clinical course of patients with theophylline poisoning is highly variable and often unpredictable. The reasons for such wide variations in reaction to a drug whose toxic manifestations are so clearly recognized have been an enigma that continues to challenge clinicians who must provide appropriate care to theophylline-poisoned patients in order to prevent disastrous outcomes. During the past 15 years, a series of important modulators of theophylline poisoning have been identified.

Early descriptions of the clinical course of theophylline intoxication suggested that serum theophylline concentrations were highly predictive of outcome. For example, in a study of 28 children with acute theophylline intoxication, Gaudrealt and colleagues demonstrated that life-threatening toxicity did not appear with serum theophylline concentrations less than 70 μg/mL and that the lower the serum theophylline concentration, the less likely the risk of major toxicity.[57] Bertino, Aitken, and others subsequently published case series indicating that serum theophylline concentration was not always predictive of outcome and that patients with relatively low serum theophylline concentrations often had fatal outcomes.[36, 58–60]

In 1985, Olson and colleagues were the first to clearly demonstrate that the clinical course of patients with theophylline intoxication was largely influenced by the mechanism of their poisoning. This study found that victims of acute theophylline intoxication, although they were more likely to have metabolic consequences such as hypokalemia and hyperglycemia, seemed to tolerate elevated serum theophylline concentrations better than those with chronic overmedication. Those in the latter category had a lower incidence of metabolic disturbances but were more likely to have life-threatening seizures or cardiac disturbances. Moreover, these life-threatening events occurred at lower serum theophylline concentrations than in those with acute intoxication who developed life-threatening events.[61]

Subsequent studies have attempted to clarify differences in outcome as influenced by method of intoxication. Consequently, three types of patients with theophylline intoxication have been identified: those with acute overdose, those with chronic overmedication, and those with acute-on-therapeutic intoxication. According to current definitions, the victim of acute theophylline overdose is one who has not been taking or receiving theophylline but is then exposed to a single dose exceeding 10 mg/kg. A patient who suffers an acute toxic overdose and who has been taking theophylline for only 1 or 2 days, not having reached steady-state concentrations (which require 4 to 5 half-lives), is considered a victim of acute overdose. Common causes of acute overdose include ingestion by children, attempted suicide by young adults, and inadvertent administration of an excess dose. Tenfold errors in drug administration are a common cause of acute intoxication in children.

The findings of Gaudreault and colleagues have been borne out by larger, subsequent clinical investigations: Patients with acute theophylline overdose generally exhibit signs of minor toxicity at serum theophylline concentrations of 20 to 40 μg/mL, moderate toxicity with concentrations of 40 to 80 μg/mL, and severe toxicity with concentrations of greater than 70 to 80 μg/mL. In the absence of prompt, aggressive care, serum theophylline concentrations of greater than 100 μg/mL are often fatal (although survival with only supportive care has been reported with serum theophylline concentrations of 203 and 300 μg/mL[62, 63]).

Victims of chronic theophylline overmedication differ from those with acute poisoning in several respects. First, epidemiologically, these patients are more likely to be very young (i.e., neonates) or elderly. They invariably have pre-existing cardiorespiratory disease, which is the reason why they are taking the medication. Unintentional overmedication can result from a number of causes, most commonly inappropriate dosing by the patient or health care provider (Table 95–3). Those with chronic overmedication have a substantially higher risk of major toxicity than those with acute intoxication (49% versus 10% in one study[28]). This higher incidence occurs despite lower serum theophylline concentrations in those with chronic overmedication.[64]

Table 95–3. Common Causes of Chronic Theophylline Overmedication

Cause	%
Increased dosing by patient or parent	31%
Physician dosing error	14%
Drug interaction	7%
Cardiac disease	10%
Viral illness	3%
Hepatic disease	1%
Unknown	35%

Adapted from Shannon M, Lovejoy F: The influence of age vs. peak serum concentration of life-threatening events after chronic theophylline intoxication. Arch Intern Med *150*:2045, 1990.

The most distinctive feature of chronic theophylline overmedication is the complete loss of predictive value provided by serum theophylline concentration. Victims of chronic overmedication may have seizures, arrhythmias, and fatalities at serum theophylline concentrations as low as 20 to 30 μg/mL.[39] Conversely, patients may survive serum concentrations as high as 100 μg/mL. Olson and co-workers suggested that among those with chronic overmedication, serum theophylline concentrations have some predictive value; however, others have not found this. Studies now indicate that age rather than peak serum theophylline concentration is most predictive of major toxicity after chronic theophylline overmedication; proportional increases in the risk of a life-threatening event occur with advancing age.[28, 65] In the pediatric age group, the opposite is true; the younger the patient, the greater the risk of major toxicity.[19, 64] Age does not have an important role in the risk of major toxicity for those with acute theophylline overdose.

Acute-on-therapeutic theophylline intoxication acts in an intermediate fashion, with metabolic disturbances and clinical consequences occurring in a pattern that lies between the other two populations.[28, 64, 66]

Differences between those with acute versus chronic theophylline intoxication are also evident in patients' metabolic profile. For example, in those with acute intoxication, 85% to 95% develop hypokalemia, in contrast to 25% to 32% of those with chronic overmedication.[61, 66] Serum glucose level is typically higher and serum bicarbonate level lower in those with acute theophylline overdose.

Diagnosis of Theophylline Poisoning

The diagnosis of theophylline poisoning is made in various ways. With acute overdose, patients, friends, or caretakers offer a history of recent use. In those with chronic overmedication, the diagnosis may be more elusive, with vague and nonspecific presenting complaints. Complaints of nausea, vomiting, and diarrhea may be erroneously diagnosed as gastroenteritis. In the elderly, the presenting complaint is often respiratory decompensation; in such cases, the development of chronic theophylline overmedication has likely resulted from improper self-medication (i.e., taking extra doses). In many cases of theophylline intoxication, seizures may be the presenting feature. Various presenting signs require a high index of suspicion as well as a detailed review of medications that the patient is taking. Because increasing numbers of drugs are being found to inhibit cytochrome P-450 activity, close attention should be paid to those patients taking theophylline in combination with another drug.

In those who receive inadvertent intravenous theophylline overdoses, representing either acute or acute-on-therapeutic poisoning, the error is often discovered when the clinical status deteriorates and tachycardia, agitation, or frank seizures appear.

Serum theophylline concentrations are readily measured. However, theophylline may not be a part of a general toxic screen, and thus the test must be specifically requested. Because serum theophylline concentrations may be of limited value in patients with chronic theophylline overmedication, it is essential that a thorough clinical assessment be performed. After an acute toxic ingestion, theophylline concentrations should be measured every 2 to 4 hours until a plateau is documented because of the risk of delayed peak absorption after ingestion of sustained-release theophylline preparations.[7, 67]

Ancillary laboratory tests that are important in the treatment of patients with theophylline intoxication include an electrocardiogram; chest radiograph; measurement of arterial blood gas, serum electrolytes, calcium, and blood sugar; and occasionally liver function tests. Because seizures may be associated with a cerebrovascular accident, cranial tomography should be considered for those who develop convulsions.

Management of Theophylline Poisoning

Supportive Measures

General management principles are key in the care of patients with theophylline poisoning. For those with respiratory compromise, cardiac disturbances, or seizures, initial interventions must be airway control, assisted ventilation, and vascular access. Patients who present with respiratory failure as a result of exacerbation of their pulmonary disease or seizure require immediate endotracheal intubation. Hypotension may reflect theophylline-induced vasodilatation, dehydration, or myocardial infarction. In such cases, based on clinical assessment and, ideally, central venous pressure monitoring, modest fluid boluses should be administered. If vasopressor therapy is needed, there are theoretic advantages to using phenylephrine, a potent peripheral vasoconstrictor. However, more conventional vasopressors, including dopamine, dobutamine, and norepinephrine, are also effective for blood pressure support.

Cardiac arrhythmias also require immediate intervention and can be treated according to advanced cardiac life support algorithms. Isolated ventricular premature beats without hemodynamic compromise require no treatment. More significant signs of myocardial irritability should be treated with appropriate doses of lidocaine. Although the proconvulsant actions of lidocaine pose theoretic risks, no evidence shows that lidocaine is detrimental when used in appropriate doses. Supraventricular arrhythmias can be treated with agents including β-blockers, verapamil, or adenosine. Propranolol has been shown to reverse peripheral vasodilatation, hypotension, tachycardia, hypokalemia, and hypercalcemia after theophylline poisoning.[25, 53, 55, 68] It may, however, produce bronchoconstriction in susceptible individuals. Esmolol, a very short-acting β_1-specific antagonist, has been used successfully for reversal of tachycardia.[69, 70] The calcium channel blocker verapamil, although effective in the treatment of supraventricular tachycardia, carries the risk of exacerbating hypotension.[71]

The intimate relationship between theophylline and adenosine justifies the use of adenosine (Adenocard) as first-line treatment for theophylline-induced tachyarrhythmias. Supraventricular tachycardia is very responsive to adenosine therapy. If the basis of theophylline-induced tachyarrhythmias is cardiac adenosine receptor antagonism, exogenous adenosine can be considered an "antidote" in reversing this action. The dose of adenosine is 6 to 20 mg for adults and 0.1 mg/kg for children. Adenosine is effective only if delivered into the central circulation by rapid bolus. Having an elimination half-life of approximately 10 seconds, adenosine may not produce sustained control of arrhythmias. Like propranolol, adenosine has been associated with the occurrence of bronchoconstriction.

Seizures are an ominous occurrence with theophylline intoxication because they are often multiple, are highly resistant to anticonvulsant therapy, and are associated with permanent neurologic disability. This recognition has led some physicians to recommend prophylactic anticonvulsant therapy to those patients who present with severe theophylline intoxication.[7] In many victims, however, particularly those with chronic theophylline overmedication (who have the greatest likelihood of seizures), status high-risk patients is difficult to identify, making it unclear who should receive preventive anticonvulsant therapy. Certainly, once they appear, seizures should be treated aggressively. The initial anticonvulsant should be a benzodiazepine (diazepam or lorazepam). Benzodiazepines are considered agents of choice because benzodiazepine receptor is linked to GABAergic neurons. Large doses of benzodiazepines may be necessary to control seizures. The second anticonvulsant choice is a barbiturate such as phenobarbital.[72] Like the benzodiazepines, barbiturates have actions at the GABA receptor; they are effective at terminating theophylline-induced seizures. Barbiturates do, however, have two disadvantages. First, they have a delayed onset of action. Also, being CNS depressants, they may produce severe respiratory depression if administered in conjunction with benzodiazepines. Phenytoin is relatively contraindicated in the treatment of theophylline-induced seizures, based on both empirical observation that it is ineffective in terminating theophylline-induced seizures as well as animal data that suggest that phenytoin increases the risk of theophylline-induced seizures.[72] If anticonvulsants are ineffective in terminating seizures, skeletal muscle paralysis may be necessary to prevent the complications of prolonged tonic-clonic activity. However, with theophylline intoxication, paralysis carries the risk of masking continued seizure activity. Because experimental data suggest that continued electric discharge and resulting metabolic disturbances are pivotal in theophylline-induced neurologic injury, every effort should be made to provide electroencephalographic monitoring.

GI disturbances, although generally not considered life threatening, have a critical role in the management of theophylline intoxication because they prevent both successful GI decontamination and elimination enhancement with multiple-dose activated charcoal. Therefore, a treatment priority is control of vomiting. Vast clinical experience indicates that conventional interventions including antiemetic suppositories and low-dose metoclopramide are ineffective therapies. Phenothiazines are also disappointing as antiemetics; they also may precipitate seizures because of their ability to lower seizure threshold.

Several agents are effective in control of theophylline-induced emesis. Parenteral histamine$_2$ antagonists, particularly ranitidine, control gastric acid secretion and reduce the mucosal irritation that contributes to vomiting (Fig. 95–2).[73] Metoclopramide is an effective antiemetic if given in adequate doses. For control of theophylline-induced vomiting, the recommended dose is 0.5 to 1 mg/kg; lower doses are unlikely to be effective. Because metoclopramide doses of this magnitude have been associated with the development of acute dystonic reaction, diphenhydramine should be made readily available or administered prophylactically. Ondansetron, a nonsedating antiemetic that acts as an inhibitor of CNS

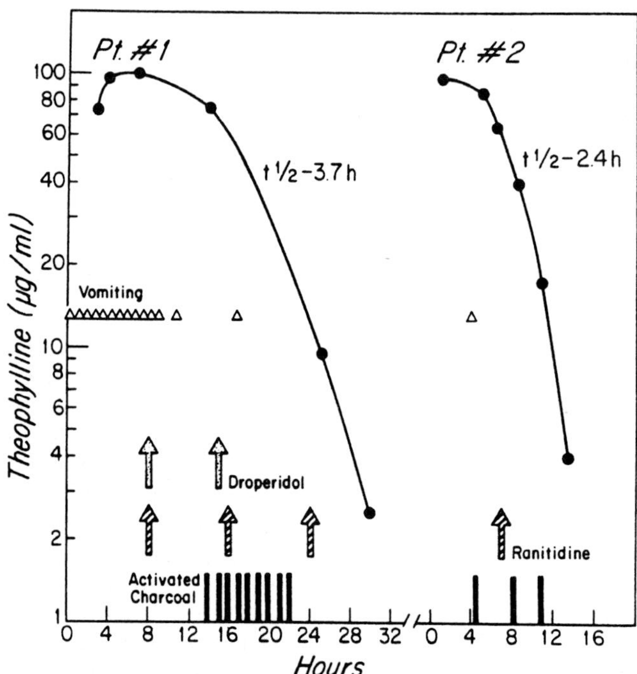

Figure 95–2. Serum theophylline concentrations and frequency of vomiting in two patients before and during treatment with ranitidine, droperidol, and repetitive activated charcoal. $t_{1/2}$, elimination half-life of theophylline. (From Amitai Y, Yeung AC, Moye J, Lovejoy FH: Repetitive oral activated charcoal and control of emesis in severe theophylline toxicity. Ann Intern Med *105*:386, 1986.)

serotonergic neurons, has also been successfully used to control theophylline-induced vomiting.[74] Another agent that may be effective is droperidol.[73]

Aggressive GI decontamination is important because sustained-release theophylline tablets can coalesce, forming bezoars.[75] Activated charcoal should be administered as soon as possible. A cathartic can be added to enhance elimination of the activated charcoal-theophylline complex. Whole-bowel irrigation has been advocated for the treatment of sustained-release theophylline ingestion; however, whole-bowel irrigation fluids may promote theophylline desorption from activated charcoal. One study has suggested that whole-bowel irrigation offers no additional benefit over activated charcoal.[76] If confirmed by additional studies, these data would support omission of whole-bowel irrigation as an adjunct to use of activated charcoal after theophylline ingestion.

Metabolic disturbances generally do not require aggressive management. Insulin therapy is not recommended for hyperglycemia because blood glucose elevations are transient and inconsequential.[25] Significant metabolic acidosis should be treated with administration of sodium bicarbonate.

The most significant metabolic abnormality is hypokalemia, which can be profound. Because total-body potassium is unchanged, exogenous potassium theoretically is not needed. However, because hypokalemia may be a risk factor for cardiac disturbances, it is appropriate to treat severe depressions of serum potassium concentration. Potassium supplementation should be provided cautiously and with close monitoring of serum potassium values to prevent iatrogenic hyperkalemia. D'Angio and Sabatelli described a patient with theophylline intoxication who was treated with aggressive potassium replacement. As the patient's serum theophylline concentration fell, however, serum potassium level rose, resulting in a hyperkalemic cardiac disturbance.[77]

Elimination Enhancement

Having a favorable pharmacokinetic profile, theophylline can be removed by a number of methods; because of its life-threatening toxicity, the drug should be removed as quickly as possible.

Multiple-dose activated charcoal is very effective at enhancing the elimination of theophylline from the body, even if toxic doses have been administered intravenously.[73, 78] Theophylline has the unusual property of diffusibility across the gut mucosa, such that if activated charcoal is present in the GI lumen, theophylline adsorbs to charcoal, and is eliminated in the stool. This action is referred to as *GI dialysis* or *enterocapillary exsorption* (see Chapter 1). Animal models and case reports have demonstrated the efficiency with which repeat oral charcoal doses can eliminate theophylline that has been administered intravenously. Theophylline clearance rates as high as 100 mL/min, corresponding to serum elimination half-lives as low as 1 to 2 hours, have been reported with use of multiple-dose activated charcoal.[7, 67, 73] Because it is so effective yet noninvasive, multiple-dose activated charcoal is the cornerstone of elimination enhancement procedures in patients with theophylline intoxication.

For treatment of theophylline intoxication, activated charcoal should be administered in a dose of 1 g/kg (maximum 50 g) every 4 hours. If vomited, the dose should be repeated. Cathartics, if used, should not be administered with every charcoal dose because of the risk of fluid and electrolyte disturbances. Alternative administration strategies include 20 g every 2 hours or continuous nasogastric infusion of activated charcoal.[79, 80] Aggressive antiemetic therapy is usually necessary to permit retention of charcoal. Continuous assessment of bowel motility is important because of the risk of intestinal pseudo-obstruction, which has been associated with use of multiple-dose activated charcoal in theophylline intoxication.[81] Repeat doses of charcoal can be safely administered to young infants.[82]

In 1979, Russo demonstrated that theophylline could be rapidly removed from the body by hemoperfusion.[83] Theophylline clearance rates that were four to six times greater than endogenous clearance could be produced by hemoperfusion, making this procedure extremely valuable in treating theophylline intoxication.[38] With hemoperfusion, theophylline extraction ratios as high as 0.75, corresponding to elimination half-lives of 1 to 2 hours, were initially reported. Three hours of hemoperfusion removed more than 65% of a theophylline dose in early experiences.[84] In contrast, hemodialysis, an alternative to hemoperfusion, could only double theophylline clearance rates.[67]

Hemoperfusion has become widely considered to be the definitive treatment for theophylline intoxication. Because newer high-flux hemodialysis machines are capable of increasing theophylline clearance rates to greater than 200 mL/min, perhaps identical to rates associated with hemoperfusion,[67] *hemodialysis is now becoming considered to be an equal option to charcoal hemoperfusion for serious theophylline intoxication.*

The criteria for hemodialysis (or hemoperfusion[HD/HP]) after theophylline intoxication are controversial. Park and colleagues proposed the criteria of peak serum theophylline concentration greater than 60 μg/mL or a concentration of greater than 30 μg/mL in patients older than 60 years.[40] Olson and co-workers have recommended hemoperfusion in those with acute intoxication and serum theophylline concentrations of greater than 100 μg/mL and in those with chronic overmedication and peak concentrations greater than 40 to 60 μg/mL.[61] Greenberg and associates recommended that hemoperfusion be performed only in those with intractable hypotension, ventricular ectopy, or resistant seizures.[71] Notably, all investigators have emphasized that a criterion for HD/HP is the appearance of seizures or arrhythmias, suggesting that HD/HP is also effective in reducing morbidity and mortality once major toxicity is manifested. However, data now suggest that

Table 95–4. Recommendations for Elimination Enhancement After Theophylline Intoxication

Acute Intoxication

1. Multiple-dose activated charcoal for all patients
2. HD/HP for patients with peak serum [theo] >80–100 μg/mL*
3. HD/HP for patients with peak serum [theo] >60–80 μg/mL and intractable vomiting
4. HD/HP for those with seizures or cardiac arrhythmias and serum [theo] >100 μg/mL

Chronic Overmedication

1. Multiple-dose activated charcoal for all patients
2. HD/HP for all patients younger than 6 mo or older than 65 y with serum [theo] >30–40 μg/mL

HD/HP, hemodialysis or hemoperfusion.
*Exchange transfusion may be used as an alternative therapy for neonates.

the majority of patients who received HD/HP *after* they had a seizure or cardiac arrhythmia continued to have these life-threatening events. In contrast, as few as 5% of patients who receive HD/HP before major toxicity eventually develop a life-threatening event.[28] Therefore, HD/HP is best considered a preventive intervention rather than a procedure that offers great benefit after major toxicity has developed.

Based on the growing data that have analyzed major toxicity and its predictors as a function of method of intoxication, the following recommendations are rational (Table 95–4): For all patients with theophylline intoxication (serum theophylline concentration > 20 to 30 μg/mL), treatment should be initiated with multiple-dose oral charcoal. For those with acute theophylline intoxication, HD/HP should be performed in patients with a serum theophylline concentration of greater than 80 to 100 μg/mL. If uncontrolled vomiting prevents successful charcoal administration, HD/HP should be performed for all those with serum theophylline concentrations that exceed 60 to 80 μg/mL.

The decision to perform HD/HP after chronic theophylline intoxication is more difficult for several reasons. First, the patients at greatest risk for seizures and cardiac arrhythmias cannot be identified on the basis of peak serum theophylline concentration. Second, these victims are usually very young or very old, ages at which HD/HP is technically more difficult. Finally, patients with chronic theophylline intoxication often have seizures and cardiac arrhythmias as their presenting manifestations, making the value of HD/HP less clear. Nonetheless, because of the evidence that high-risk patients are those at extremes of age, hemodialysis should be considered in all patients with a serum theophylline concentration of greater than 30 μg/mL, particularly those younger than 6 months or older than 65 years.

Because of the technical difficulty in performing HD/HP in neonates, alternative methods of extracorporeal drug removal have been evaluated. Among these, exchange transfusion is the procedure with the greatest promise. Although an early case report found no benefit from exchange transfusion in infants with severe acute theophylline intoxication,[63] two recent case reports have demonstrated that significant amounts of theophylline can be removed with exchange transfusion, making this therapy a viable option in acutely poisoned neonates.[85, 86]

Plasmapheresis has also been successfully used in the treatment of theophylline intoxication, reducing elimination half-life to 1.7 hours.[87, 88]

CAFFEINE

Caffeine is a plant alkaloid found in a wide variety of foods and beverages. Coffee, tea, and chocolate have the largest natural concentrations of caffeine. Caffeine is also added to carbonated beverages and a large number of over-the-counter medications including weight control aids, "alertness" tablets, pain relievers, diuretics, and cold remedies (Table 95–5). Finally, caffeine is prescribed for the treatment of apnea/bradycardia in newborns and as adjunctive therapy for cerebrovascular (migraine) headache.

Clinical Pharmacology

Caffeine can be administered by a number of routes, including oral, intravenous, subcutaneous, and rectal. After ingestion, it is well absorbed, with an absorption pattern relatively unaffected by the presence of food. Peak plasma concentrations are achieved 30 to 60 hours after ingestion.[89] Absorption after rectal and subcutaneous administration is equally rapid. It has an apparent volume of distribution of 1 L/kg. As with theophylline, caffeine metabolism occurs via biotransformation in the cytochrome P-450 system. The primary metabolic pathway for caffeine is its demethylation. 1-Demethylation pro-

Table 95–5. Average Caffeine Content of Beverages, Foods, and Pharmaceuticals

	Dose Range (mg)
Beverages	
Coffee (5 oz)	
Brewed	40–200
Instant	30–150
Decaffeinated	1–5
Tea (5 oz)	
Brewed	20–100
Instant	25–50
Iced (12-oz glass)	65–80
Carbonated beverages, 12 oz	25–200
Chocolate milk	2–10
Food	
Dark chocolate, 1 oz	5–30
Nonprescription Pharmaceuticals	
Weight control aids	100–200
Alertness agents	100–200
Analgesics	30–65
Diuretics	100–200
Cold remedies	15–30

duces theobromine (3,7-dimethylxanthine), a pharmacologically active methylxanthine found widely in chocolate. 7-Demethylation of caffeine produces theophylline; as a result, caffeine ingestion produces measurable serum theophylline concentrations. The elimination half-life of caffeine is variable and highly age dependent; the average half-life in a nonsmoking adult is 3 to 6 hours. In contrast, premature neonates can have elimination half-lives that range from 1.5 to 6 days.[89] Agents associated with induction of cytochrome P-450 enzymes (e.g., smoking) produce shorter half-lives. Approximately 5% of caffeine is excreted unchanged in the urine. Significant amounts of caffeine are excreted into breast milk.

Caffeine has a number of pharmacologic actions. Its most important property, mild CNS stimulation, is the basis for the worldwide enjoyment of caffeinated beverages, particularly coffee. This CNS stimulation is associated with increased alertness and concentration as well as mood elevation. In excessive doses, undesirable effects including hyperactivity (particularly in children), anxiety, and insomnia appear.

Caffeine has become extremely valuable therapy in the treatment of the neonatal apnea/bradycardia syndrome. Newborns with this syndrome have recurrent hypoventilation, often accompanied by bradycardia. Both theophylline and caffeine are effective in treating this syndrome; stimulation of central respiratory centers by methylxanthines results in decreased apnea, increased minute ventilation, normalization of breathing pattern, increased ventilatory response to carbon dioxide, and reduction in both the need for and duration of mechanical ventilation. Another beneficial effect in newborns is increased cardiac output.[90] Caffeine offers the advantages of excellent absorption after ingestion and a longer elimination half-life; these provide more sustained serum concentrations and more predictable pharmacokinetics. The therapeutic serum concentration of caffeine is 8 to 20 μg/mL.

Caffeine is also a cardiotonic agent, producing positive inotropy and chronotropy. However, it does not consistently produce significant increases in pulse or blood pressure.[91] In susceptible individuals, caffeine occasionally leads to the development of premature ventricular contractions, which are usually of no clinical consequence. Important vascular effects of caffeine include cerebral vasoconstriction and renal vasculature relaxation. Because cerebral vasodilation often contributes to the pathophysiology of headache, constriction of cerebral blood vessels by caffeine can be therapeutic. Enhanced renal blood flow is associated with a modest diuretic effect.

Caffeine has two important GI effects: smooth muscle relaxation and stimulation of gastric secretion. Smooth muscle relaxation is most pronounced at the lower esophageal sphincter, where gastroesophageal reflux can result from caffeine use. In concert with increased secretion of both gastric acid and digestive enzymes, reflux can result in esophagitis (heartburn). These GI effects are also noted after ingestion of decaffeinated coffee, suggesting they are mediated by alkaloids other than caffeine. Metabolic effects of caffeine include increased fatty acid oxidation and glycogenolysis. According to one study, typical doses of caffeine, unlike theophylline, do not usually produce marked increases in circulating plasma catecholamines.[92] However, catecholamine elevations have been reported in victims of caffeine intoxication.[93]

Caffeine exhibits all the properties of an addictive drug (tolerance, dependence, and an abstinence syndrome on immediate withdrawal). Tolerance to all its pharmacologic effects develops after repeated use.

Clinical Toxicology

Undesirable effects of caffeine can appear after ingestion of as little as 50 mg; at these doses, anxiety, GI upset, and insomnia may occur. More significant toxicity appears after ingestion of 15 to 30 mg/kg. At this range, moderate toxicity marked by vomiting, myoclonus, and myocardial irritability appear. Vomiting may be severe; frank hematemesis may occur.[94] Fatal oral doses of caffeine have ranged from 5 to 50 g, with a mean of 10 g; the lethal dose is estimated to be 100 to 200 mg/kg. Clinical toxicity correlates with serum caffeine concentrations. Several cups of coffee yield a serum caffeine level of 5 to 10 μg/mL. Agitation and myoclonus occur at levels of 15 to 30 μg/mL; cardiac arrhythmias and seizures develop at 50 to 100 μg/mL. Fatalities have been associated with serum caffeine concentrations as low as 80 μg/mL to as high as 1560 μg/mL,[95] although concentrations as high as 200 μg/mL have been associated with survival. Deaths have also been reported from the use of coffee enemas as a naturopathic therapy.[96]

Many but not all of the consequences of caffeine poisoning are identical to those of theophylline, although they are associated with comparably higher serum caffeine concentrations. Seizures can appear without warning and are often repeated. Opisthotonos, decerebrate posturing, and generalized muscular hypertonicity are also common.[97] Cardiac arrhythmias can be supraventricular or ventricular (ventricular tachycardia or fibrillation). Other manifestations of severe intoxication are rhabdomyolysis with resultant acute renal failure and pulmonary edema.[98] Rhabdomyolysis has been attributed to increased muscular activity. Pulmonary edema is a frequent occurrence with severe poisoning and is thought to result, in part, from pulmonary vasculature dilation.[89, 97] Victims of caffeine intoxication develop the metabolic disturbances of hyperglycemia, hypokalemia, leukocytosis, ketosis, and metabolic acidosis.

Chronic caffeine intoxication (caffeinism) is manifested by irritability, insomnia, anxiety, emotional lability, and chronic abdominal pain. Cardiovascular disease, myocardial irritability, and fibrocystic disease of the breast all have been associated with long-term caffeine consumption.[92, 99, 100] However, for all these diseases, the association with caffeine has been controversial and inconsistent in clinical investigations.

Caffeine is both mutagenic and teratogenic in laboratory animal species.[89] A study of women suggested that more than 600 mg of caffeine daily could result in an increased incidence of spontaneous abortion and premature birth.[89] The Food and Drug Administration has advised pregnant women to avoid or limit caffeine intake.

Caffeine has now been proved to produce a physiologic abstinence syndrome (withdrawal). Although it has been well recognized that abrupt termination of caffeine consumption could produce insomnia, malaise, and headache, little scientific investigation has addressed these phenomena. Silverman[101] and Strain[102] and their colleagues have shown that withdrawal from caffeine can produce an increase in depressive symptoms, anxiety, fatigue, headache, and decreased performance. Abstinence was also associated with a marked increase in the use of medications (e.g., headache relievers).

Management

In patients with an acute caffeine overdose, initial attention should be directed to airway, breathing, and circulation. The sudden appearance of airway compromise and hypoxia as a result of seizures, cardiac disturbances, or pulmonary edema should be anticipated, particularly in patients who ingest more than 30 to 50 mg/kg of caffeine.

Management of seizures and cardiac disturbances parallels their treatment in patients with theophylline intoxication. Therefore, seizures are preferably treated with a benzodiazepine (e.g., diazepam) or phenobarbital. No evidence shows that phenytoin is ineffective in the treatment of caffeine-induced seizures; however, because all methylxanthines are presumed to have similar mechanism of toxicity, phenytoin's lack of efficacy in theophylline-induced seizures argues against its use. Cardiac disturbances should be treated according to standard management strategies. Adenosine, verapamil, and β-blocking agents all are effective treatments for supraventricular arrhythmias.[94, 103] Ventricular arrhythmias should be treated initially with intravenous lidocaine.

GI decontamination measures should include administration of activated charcoal with a cathartic. Vomiting is likely in those with significant ingestion. Although this provides gastric evacuation, it thwarts efforts at activated charcoal administration. Aggressive antiemetic therapy should therefore be provided. Antiemetic therapy should include the administration of histamine$_2$ antagonists, which reduce gastric hypersecretion. Other beneficial agents include metoclopramide, 10 to 50 mg intravenously, and ondansetron, 0.6 mg/kg intravenously.

Laboratory evaluation should include electrolytes, blood glucose, creatine phosphokinase, arterial blood gas, and an electrocardiogram. Hypokalemia should be treated with modest potassium supplementation (because total-body potassium is preserved). Insulin is not recommended for treatment of hyperglycemia, although it has been suggested by others.[104]

Enhanced elimination is the final component of managing caffeine poisoning. A number of measures have been shown to be effective, including multiple-dose activated charcoal, peritoneal dialysis,[94, 98] and HD/HP.[97] Although a proportion of caffeine is excreted from the urine unchanged, forced diuresis has no role in management. Diuresis should be provided only if patients have clinical evidence of severe rhabdomyolysis.

Multiple-dose activated charcoal has not been clearly shown to enhance caffeine elimination but does eliminate any theophylline that is generated; it is therefore considered an integral component of treatment. Use of several antiemetic agents may be necessary to end vomiting. Peritoneal dialysis has been used but is unlikely to be more helpful than multiple-dose activated charcoal. Hemodialysis is the procedure that provides greatest efficacy with the lowest complication rate. Indications for hemodialysis are not clearly established but should include a serum caffeine concentration of greater than 100 μg/mL and life-threatening seizures or cardiac arrhythmias, regardless of serum caffeine concentration. Because it is both invasive and unlikely to be more effective than hemodialysis, hemoperfusion has little to no role in the management of caffeine intoxication.

References

1. Szefler SJ, Bender BG, Jusko WJ, et al: Evolving role of theophylline for treatment of chronic childhood asthma. J Pediatr *127*:176, 1995.
2. Epstein PE: Hemlock or healer? The mercurial reputation of theophylline. Ann Intern Med *119*:1216, 1993.
3. McFadden ER: Methylxanthines in the treatment of asthma: The rise, the fall, and the possible rise again. Ann Intern Med *115*:241, 1991.
4. Murciano D, Auclair M-H, Pariente R, Aubier M: A randomized, controlled trial of theophylline in patients with severe chronic obstructive pulmonary disease. N Engl J Med *320*:1521, 1989.
5. Drazen JM, Gerard C: Reversing the irreversible. N Engl J Med *320*:1555, 1989.
6. American Academy of Pediatrics Committee on Drugs: Precautions concerning the use of theophylline. Pediatrics *89*:781, 1992.
7. Hendeles L, Jenkins J, Temple R: Revised FDA labeling guidelines for theophylline oral dosage forms. Pharmacotherapy *15*:409, 1995.
8. Weinberger M, Ginchansky E: Dose-dependent kinetics of theophylline disposition in asthmatic children. J Pediatric *91*:820, 1977.
9. Rall TW: Drugs used in the treatment of asthma: The methylxanthines, cromolyn sodium, and other agents. *In* Gilman AG, Rall TW, Nies AS, Taylor P (eds): Goodman and Gilman's The Pharmacological Basis of Therapeutics. New York, Pergamon Press, pp 619–630, 1990.
10. Bakris GL, Sauter ER, Hussey JL, et al: Effects of theophylline on erythropoetin production in normal subjects and in patients with erythrocytosis after renal transplantation. N Engl J Med *323*:86, 1990.
11. Fredholm BB: On the mechanism of action of theophylline and caffeine. Acta Med Scand *217*:149, 1985.

12. Polson JB, Krzanowski JJ, Goldman AL, Szentivanyi A: Inhibition of human pulmonary phosphodiesterase activity by therapeutic levels of theophylline. Clin Exp Pharmacol Physiol *5*:535, 1978.
13. Curry SC, Vance MV, Requa R, Armstead R: Cardiovascular effects of toxic concentrations of theophylline in the dog. Ann Emerg Med *14*:547, 1985.
14. Curry SC, Vance MV, Requa R, Armstead R: The effects of toxic concentrations of theophylline on oxygen consumption, ventricular work, acid base balance and plasma catecholamine levels in the dog. Ann Emerg Med *14*:554, 1985.
15. Higbee MD, Kumar M, Galant SP: Stimulation of endogenous catecholamine release by theophylline: A proposed additional mechanism of action for theophylline effects. J Allergy Clin Immunol *70*:377, 1982.
16. Vestal RE, Eiriksson CE, Musser B, et al: Effect of intravenous aminophylline on plasma levels of catecholamines and related cardiovascular and metabolic responses in man. Circulation *67*:162, 1983.
17. Schiff GD, Hegde HK, LaCloche L, Hryhorczuk DO: Inpatient theophylline toxicity: Preventable factors. Ann Intern Med *114*:748, 1991.
18. Paloucek FP, Rodvold KA: Evaluation of theophylline overdoses and toxicities. Ann Emerg Med *17*:135, 1988.
19. Shannon MW, Lovejoy FH, Woolf A: Prediction of serum theophylline concentration after acute theophylline intoxication. Abstract. Ann Emerg Med *19*:627, 1990.
20. Skinner MH: Adverse reactions and interactions with theophylline. Drug Saf *5*:275, 1990.
21. Stavric B: Methylxanthines: Toxicity to humans. Food Chem Toxicol *26*:541, 1988.
22. Baker MD: Theophylline toxicity in children. J Pediatr *109*:538, 1986.
23. Amitai Y, Lovejoy FH: Characteristics of vomiting associated with acute sustained release theophylline poisoning: Implications for management with oral activated charcoal. Clin Toxicol *25*:539, 1987.
24. Ng R, Roe C, Funt D, Statland B: Increased activity of creatine kinase isoenzyme MB in a theophylline-intoxicated patient. Clin Chem *31*:1741, 1985.
25. Biberstein MP, Ziegler MG, Ward DM: Use of beta-blockade and hemoperfusion for acute theophylline poisoning. West J Med *141*:485, 1984.
26. Lin C-K, Chuand I-N, Cheng K-K, Chiang BN: Arrhythmogenic effects of theophylline in human atrial tissue. Int J Cardiol *17*:289, 1987.
27. Sessler CN, Cohen MD: Cardiac arrhythmias during theophylline toxicity—a prospective continuous electrocardiographic study. Chest *98*:672, 1990.
28. Shannon M: Predictors of major toxicity after theophylline overdose. Ann Intern Med *119*:1161, 1993.
29. Bittar G, Friedman HS: The arrhythmogeneicity of theophylline—a multivariate analysis of clinical determinants. Chest *99*:1415, 1991.
30. Rachelefsky GS, Wo J, Adelson J, et al: Behavior abnormalities and poor school performance due to oral theophylline use. Pediatrics *78*:1133, 1986.
31. Rappaport L, Coffman H, Guare R, et al: Effects of theophylline on behavior and learning in children with asthma. Am J Dis Child *143*:368, 1989.
32. Schlieper A, Alcock D, Beaudry P, et al: Effect of therapeutic plasma concentrations of theophylline on behavior, cognitive processing and affect in children with asthma. J Pediatr *118*:449, 1991.
33. Nakada T, Keww IL, Lerner AM, Remler MP: Theophylline-induced seizures: Clinical and pathophysiologic aspects. West J Med *138*:371, 1983.
34. Zwillich CW, Sutton FD, Neff TA, et al: Theophylline-induced seizures in adults. Ann Intern Med *82*:784, 1975.
35. Phung ND: Theophylline toxicity in ambulatory elderly patients. Immunol Allergy Pract *8*:17, 1986.
36. Richards W, Church JA, Brent DK: Theophylline-associated seizures in children. Ann Allergy *54*:276, 1985.
37. Woody RC, Laney M: A second case of infantile intracranial hemorrhage and severe neurological sequelae following theophylline overdose. Dev Med Child Neurol *28*:120, 1986.
38. Sahney S, Abarzua J, Sessums L: Hemoperfusion in theophylline neurotoxicity. Pediatrics *71*:615, 1983.
39. Bahls F, Ma KK, Bird TD: Theophylline-associated seizures with "therapeutic" or low toxic serum concentrations: Risk factors for serious outcome in adults. Neurology *41*:1309, 1991.
40. Park GD, Spector R, Roberts RJ, et al: Use of hemoperfusion for treatment of theophylline intoxication. Am J Med *74*:961, 1983.
41. Parish RA, Haulman NJ, Burns RM: Interaction of theophylline with erythromycin base in a patient with seizure activity. Pediatrics *72*:828, 1983.
42. Shucard DW, Spector SL, Euwer RL, et al: Central nervous system effects of anti-asthma medication: An EEG study. Annals Allergy *54*:177, 1985.
43. Glenn GM, Krober MS, Kelly P, et al: Pyridoxine as therapy in theophylline-induced seizures. Vet Hum Toxicol *37*:342, 1995.
44. Shannon M, Maher T: Anticonvulsant effects of intracerebroventricular Adenocard in theophylline-induced seizures. Ann Emerg Med *26*:65, 1995.
45. Pinard E, Riche D, Puiroud S, Seylaz J: Theophylline reduces cerebral hyperaemia and enhances brain damage induced by seizures. Brain Res *511*:303, 1990.
46. Hall KW, Dobson KE, Dalton JG, et al: Metabolic abnormalities associated with intentional theophylline overdose. Ann Intern Med *101*:457, 1984.
47. Sawyer WT, Caravati EM, Ellison MJ, Krueger KA: Hypokalemia, hyperglycemia, and acidosis after intentional theophylline overdose. Am J Emerg Med *3*:408, 1985.
48. Robertson NJ: Fatal overdose from a sustained-release theophylline preparation. Ann Emerg Med *14*:154, 1985.
49. Buckley BM, Braithwaite RA, Vale JA: Theophylline poisoning. Lancet *2*:618, 1983.
50. Amitai Y, Lovejoy FH: Hypokalemia in acute theophylline poisoning. Am J Emerg Med *6*:214, 1988.
51. Clausen T, Flatman JA: Beta-2 adrenoceptors mediate the stimulating effect of adrenaline on active electrogenic Na-K-transport in rat soleus muscle. Br J Pharmacol *68*:749, 1980.
52. Clausen T: Adrenergic control of Na-K-homeostasis. Acta Med Scand *672*(Suppl):111, 1983.
53. Kearney TE, Manoguerra AS, Curtis GP, Ziegler MG: Theophylline toxicity and the beta-adrenergic system. Ann Intern Med *102*:766, 1985.
54. Ryan T, Coughlan G, McGing P, Phelan D: Ketosis, a complication of theophylline toxicity. J Intern Med *226*:277, 1989.
55. McPherson ML, Prince SR, Atamer ER, et al: Theophylline-induced hypercalcemia. Ann Intern Med *105*:52, 1986.
56. Neff RD, Leviton A: Maternal theophylline consumption and the risk of stillbirth. Chest *97*:1266, 1990.
57. Gaudrealt P, Wason S, Lovejoy F: Acute pediatric theophylline overdose: A summary of 28 cases. J Pediatr *102*:474, 1983.
58. Aitken ML, Martin TR: Life-threatening theophylline toxicity is not predictable by serum levels. Chest *91*:10, 1987.
59. Bertino JS, Walker JW: Reassessment of theophylline toxicity—serum concentrations, clinical course, and treatment. Arch Intern Med *147*:757, 1987.
60. Covelli HD, Knodel AR, Heppner BT: Predisposing factors to apparent theophylline-induced seizures. Ann Allergy *54*:411, 1985.
61. Olson KR, Benowitz NL, Woo OF, Pond SM: Theophylline overdose: Acute single ingestion versus chronic repeated overmedication. Am J Emerg Med *3*:386, 1985.
62. Dean LS, Brown JW: Massive theophylline overdose—survival without hemoperfusion. JAMA *248*:1742, 1982.
63. Wells DH, Ferlauto JJ: Survival after massive aminophyline overdose in a premature infant. Pediatrics *64*:252, 1979.
64. Shannon M, Lovejoy F: Effect of acute versus chronic intoxication on clinical features of theophylline poisoning in children. J Pediatr *121*:125, 1992.
65. Shannon M, Lovejoy F: The influence of age vs. peak serum concentration of life-threatening events after chronic theophylline intoxication. Arch Intern Med *150*:2045, 1990.
66. Shannon M, Lovejoy FH: Hypokalemia after theophylline

intoxication—the effects of acute vs. chronic poisoning. Arch Intern Med *149*:2725, 1989.
67. Heath A, Knudsen K: Role of extracorporeal drug removal in acute theophylline poisoning —a review. Med Toxicol *2*:294, 1987.
68. Amin DN, Henry JA: Propranolol administration in theophylline overdose. Lancet *1*:520, 1985.
69. Gaar GG, Banner W, Laddu AR: The effects of esmolol on the hemodynamics of acute theophylline toxicity. Ann Emerg Med *16*:1334, 1987.
70. Seneff M, Scott J, Friedman B, Smith M: Acute theophylline toxicity and the use of esmolol to reverse cardiovascular instability. Ann Emerg Med *19*:671, 1990.
71. Greenberg A, Piraino BH, Kroboth PD, Weiss J: Severe theophylline toxicity—role of conservative measures, antiarrhythmic agents and charcoal hemoperfusion. Am J Med *76*:854, 1984.
72. Blake KV, Massey KL, Hendeles L, et al: Relative efficacy of phenytoin and phenobarbital for the prevention of theophylline-induced seizures in mice. Ann Emerg Med *17*:1024, 1988.
73. Amitai Y, Yeung AC, Moye J, Lovejoy FH: Repetitive oral activated charcoal and control of emesis in severe theophylline toxicity. Ann Intern Med *105*:386, 1986.
74. Roberts JR, Carney S, Boyle SM, Lee D: Ondansetron quells drug-resistant emesis in theophylline poisoning. Am J Emerg Med *11*:609, 1993.
75. Bernstein G, Jehle D, Bernaski E, Braen GR: Failure of gastric emptying and charcoal administration in fatal sustained-release theophylline overdose: Pharmacobezoar formation. Ann Emerg Med *21*:1388, 1992.
76. Burkhart KK, Wuerz RC, Donovan JW: Whole-bowel irrigation as adjunctive treatment for sustained-release theophylline overdose. Ann Emerg Med *21*:1316, 1992.
77. D'Angio R, Sabatelli F: Management considerations in treating metabolic abnormalities associated with theophylline overdose. Arch Intern Med *147*:1837, 1987.
78. Kulig KW, Bar-Or D, Rumack BH: Intravenous theophylline poisoning and multiple-dose charcoal in an animal model. Ann Emerg Med *16*:842, 1987.
79. Ohning BL, Reed MD, Blumer JL: Continuous nasogastric administration of activated charcoal for the treatment of theophylline intoxication. Pediatr Pharmacol *5*:241–245, 1986.
80. Park GD, Radomski L, Goldberg MJ, et al: Effect of size and frequency of oral doses of charcoal on theophylline clearance. Clin Pharmacol Ther *34*:664, 1983.
81. Longdon P, Henderson A: Intestinal pseudo-obstruction following the use of enteral charcoal and sorbitol and mechanical ventilation with papaveretum sedation for theophylline poisoning. Drug Saf *7*:74, 1992.
82. Shannon M, Amitai Y, Lovejoy FH: Multiple-dose activated charcoal for theophylline poisoning in young infants. Pediatrics *80*:368, 1987.
83. Russo ME: Management of theophylline intoxication with charcoal-column hemoperfusion. N Engl J Med *300*:24, 1979.
84. Goldberg MJ, Park GD, Berlinger WG: Treatment of theophylline intoxication. J Allergy Clin Immunol *78*:811, 1986.
85. Osborn H, Henry G, Wax P, et al: Theophylline toxicity in a premature neonate — elimination kinetics of exchange transfusion. Clin Toxicol *31*:639, 1993.
86. Shannon M, Wernovsky G, Morris C: Exchange transfusion in the treatment of severe theophylline poisoning. Pediatrics *89*:145, 1992.
87. Laussen P, Shann F, Butt W, Tibballs J: Use of plasmapheresis in acute theophylline toxicity. Crit Care Med *19*:288, 1991.
88. Gaudrealt P, Guay J: Theophylline poisoning—pharmacological considerations and clinical management. Med Toxicol *1*:169, 1986.
89. Dalvi R: Acute and chronic toxicity of caffeine: A review. Vet Hum Toxicol *28*:144, 1986.
90. Walther FJ, Erickson R, Sims M: Cardiovascular effects of caffeine therapy in preterm infants. Am J Dischild *144*:1164, 1990.
91. Myers M: Effects of caffeine on blood pressure. Arch Intern Med *148*:1189, 1988.
92. Chelsky L, Cutler J, Griffith K, et al: Caffeine and ventricular arrhythmias—an electrophysiological approach. JAMA *264*:2236, 1990.
93. Benowitz N, Osterloh J, Goldschlager N: Massive catecholamine release from caffeine poisoning. JAMA *248*:1097, 1982.
94. Walsh I, Wasserman G, Mestad P, Lanman R: Near fatal caffeine intoxication treated with perioneal dialysis. Pediatr Emerg Care *3*:244, 1987.
95. Mrvos R, Reilly P, Dean B, Krenzelok E: Massive caffeine ingestion resulting in death. Vet Hum Toxicol *31*:571, 1989.
96. Eisele J: Deaths related to coffee enemas. JAMA *244*:1608, 1980.
97. Dietrich AM, Mortensen M: Presentation and management of an acute caffeine overdose. Pediatr Emerg Care *6*:296, 1990.
98. Wrenn K, Oschner I. Rhabdomyolysis induced by a caffeine overdose. Ann Emerg Med *18*:94, 1989.
99. Minton NA, Glucksman E, Henry JA. Prevention of drug absorption in a simulated theophylline overdose. Hum Exp Toxicol *14*:170, 1995.
100. Lubin F, Ron E, Wax Y, et al: A case-control study of caffeine and methylxanthines in benign breast disease. JAMA *253*:2388, 1985.
101. Silverman K, Evans SM, Strain E, Griffiths R: Withdrawal syndrome after the double-blind cessation of caffeine consumption. N Engl J Med *327*:1109, 1992.
102. Strain E, Mumford G, Silverman K, Griffiths R: Caffeine dependence syndrome—evidence form case histories and experimental evaluations. JAMA *272*:1043, 1994.
103. Price K, Fligner D: Treatment of caffeine toxicity with esmolol. Ann Emerg Med *19*:44, 1990.
104. Sullivan J: Caffeine poisoning in an infant. J Pediatr *90*:1022, 1977.

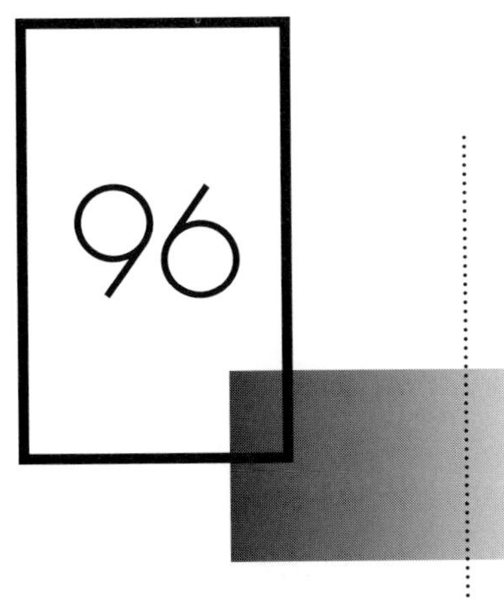

Thrombolytic Agents and Anticoagulants

WILLIAM E. DAVIS, MD
DARLENA M. MONET, MD

BACKGROUND

Thrombosis is a complex process that involves multiple elements of the blood and vascular system and is essential to maintaining the integrity of the vascular system. Platelets, vascular endothelium, hemostatically active components of blood vessel walls, and the plasma coagulation system play primary roles in clot formation. Normally, the coagulation and fibrinolytic systems maintain a dynamic equilibrium. When this homeostatic balance is disrupted, pathologic thrombosis or bleeding may result. Spontaneous venous thrombosis and pulmonary thromboembolism are major sources of postoperative morbidity and mortality. Spontaneous arterial thrombosis, usually at the site of atheromatous plaque, is the primary pathogenesis of myocardial infarction and stroke. Numerous antithrombotic agents, such as heparin, warfarin, and aspirin, act at specific points in the coagulation system to inhibit thrombus production. Other agents, in particular the thrombolytic agents streptokinase (SK), urokinase (UK), and tissue-type plasminogen activator (t-PA), act to accelerate thrombus destruction. These potent agents have shown great potential in the rescue of ischemic tissue and have become widely used in the management of acute pathologic thrombosis. However, they have also demonstrated that their use carries a substantial risk of serious complication. This chapter reviews the mechanisms and control of thrombogenesis, the principal thrombolytic and antithrombotic agents, the complications of thrombolytic therapy, and the basic management of the patient suffering these complications.

PHARMACOLOGY AND MOLECULAR BIOLOGY

Overall three major processes are active in the natural history of thrombosis. These are platelet aggregation, fibrin production through the coagulation system, and fibrinolysis. These processes are the same in both physiologic hemostasis and pathologic thrombosis.

Platelet Aggregation and Thrombosis

The adhesion, activation, and aggregation of platelets is the pivotal first step in thrombosis. A thrombus begins with the adherence of platelets by means of specific membrane glycoprotein receptors, GpIb, to specific adhesion molecules on the activating surface. These adherent platelets expose their glycoprotein receptor GpIIb/IIIa, to which fibrinogen and von Willebrand's factor bind. Fibrinogen and von Willebrand's factor are the major adhesion molecules in platelet aggregation. As these activated platelets coalesce, they synthesize thromboxane A_2 and degranulate releasing platelet activators and more adhesion molecules. These released factors in turn recruit and activate additional platelets.

Contact with the activated platelet surface initiates the coagulation cascade quickly and directly (see subsequent discussion). Soluble fibrinogen adheres to the GpIIb/IIIa receptors of the activated platelet surfaces to form a bridging web of fibrinogen. Additional platelets then adhere to the fibrinogen mesh to form further platelet aggregate layers. This process of platelet adhesion, platelet aggregation, and fibrinogen deposition proceeds through successive layers, forming the primary hemostatic plug. The thrombin generated by the activated coagulation system then converts the fibrinogen within the thrombus to the fibrin monomers. The later "stabilized" fibrin polymers thereby form a structural skeleton around the platelets, producing the platelet-fibrin thrombus, or secondary hemostatic plug.[1]

Coagulation and Fibrin Production

Blood coagulation is the result of the sequential activation of circulating coagulation factors from their proenzyme (zymogen) forms into their active forms. This coagulation cascade occurs primarily on cellular or molecular surfaces. The circulating clotting factors concentrate selectively, or "assemble," through specific receptor binding on molecular "surfaces" such as activated platelet membranes, endothelial cell membranes, collagen, or complex glycoproteins to accelerate the rate of these enzymatic reactions drastically. This surface catalysis is essential for the rapid explosive propagation of the coagulation cascade. Thrombin is the principal product of this catalytic sequence, and thrombin generation is a pivotal step in thrombogenesis. Thrombin promotes platelet activation and aggregation and plays a positive feedback role by further activating factors V, X, VII, VIII, XIII, and protein C. When thrombin reaches sufficient concentration to overcome circulating antithrombins and other protease inhibitors, this enzyme converts soluble fibrinogen into an insoluble fibrin gel.

Classically, the coagulation system is divided into an intrinsic pathway and an extrinsic pathway that converge to produce thrombin. The intrinsic pathway is activated by contact of the blood with negatively charged surfaces, primarily activated platelets and collagen, or with a foreign material, for example, a prosthetic heart valve. All intrinsic pathway factors (high molecular weight kininogen; prekallikrein; factors XII, XI, IX, VIII, and X; as well as phospholipid and calcium cofactors) are contained in circulating blood. The extrinsic pathway (factors VII and X with phospholipid and calcium) is activated by tissue thromboplastin, which leaks into the blood from damaged tissue cells following injury. The systems themselves are interconnected so that activating one pathway can activate the other pathway. Both systems are necessary to provide normal hemostasis. The extrinsic and intrinsic pathways meet in the "common" pathway generating the factor Xa complex (the suffix "a" denotes the activated form of the clotting factor). This complex of factor Xa, factor V, Ca^{2+}, and phospholipid is the thrombin generator that converts prothrombin to thrombin.

Thrombin cleaves fibrinogen to produce the insoluble gel of fibrin monomers. Following conversion of fibrinogen into a fibrin gel, thrombin-activated factor XIIIa stabilizes the fibrin monomers by linking them end to end with covalent bonds to create fibrin polymers, which in turn cross-link with peptide bonds. This process of polymerization and cross-linking proceeds to create an increasingly stable degradation-resistant clot.[2]

Control of Coagulation, Thrombosis and Fibrinolysis

Four major and several less important endogenous systems control coagulation and regulate the formation or accumulation of fibrin. All of these systems function to inhibit thrombin production primarily by inhibiting factor Xa complex, thrombin activity, or fibrin deposition. The major systems are the tissue factor pathway inhibitor system, the protein C–thrombin–thrombomodulin system, the antithrombin III–heparin system, and the plasminogen–plasminogen activator assembly system. All of these systems are intimately related to endothelial cell surface and function.

1. Tissue factor pathway inhibitor, also referred to as lipoprotein-associated inhibitor, is a member of a superfamily of proteins (known as kunins) homologous to aprotinin. It is secreted by endothelial cells, monocytes, and macrophages in response to the presence of cytokines and anoxia. Tissue factor pathway inhibitor complexes with factor VIIa to directly inhibit factor Xa. This inhibition of factor Xa appears to in part regulate extrinsic pathway activation and is under study as a pharmacologic agent.
2. Protein C is a circulating proenzyme whose synthesis is vitamin K dependent. When activated, it becomes a serine protease. Protein C is produced in response to inflammatory mediators. It is activated by thrombin when the thrombin is complexed with thrombomodulin, an endothelial cell surface protein, and Ca^{2+}. Activated protein C inhibits coagulation by inactivating clotting factors Va and VIIIa and prolongs the activated partial thromboplastin time. Because factor Va is an essential component of the factor Xa complex, activated protein C inhibits the rate of thrombin generation.[2] The activity of protein C is greatly enhanced when it combines with protein S, another vitamin K–dependent plasma protein. In addition, activated protein C complex increases fibrinolytic activity by neutralizing plasminogen activator inhibitor types 1 and 3.[3] Recombinant protein C has been studied as an anticoagulant, using direct infusion in animals.[4] Protein C is vitamin K dependent and has a short half-life compared with those of most other vitamin K–dependent coagulation factors. Inhibition of vitamin K–dependent activation of coagulation factors by warfarin-related compounds also inhibits protein C activity, resulting in a relative hypercoagulable state. This state persists until the remaining

vitamin K–dependent cofactor activity decreases to the point that the loss of protein C inhibition of coagulation is counterbalanced.

3. Antithrombin III (AT-III) is a member of a class of proteins known as serpins, a family that includes most of the inhibitors that regulate the proteases of the coagulation and fibrinolytic pathways. Serpin is a contracted form of serine protease inhibitors. AT-III is the principal circulating anticoagulant and directly inhibits numerous activated clotting factors including thrombin and factor Xa. Heparin acts by allosterically catalyzing the tight binding of AT-III and thrombin. AT-III–thrombin complexes are removed by the reticuloendothelial system. Hirudin and its analogues effectively mimic the role of AT-III as direct antithrombins but produce an irreversible inhibition of thrombin rather than a competitive inhibition such as that of AT-III.
4. Plasmin, the active form of plasminogen, is the central component of the fibrinolytic system. Plasminogen is a single-chain glycoprotein with a molecular weight of approximately 90,000 daltons that is produced by the liver and normally circulates in concentrations of approximately 20 mg/dL. Plasminogen also binds to multiple substrates throughout the circulatory system, including fibrin, fibrinogen, platelet membrane surfaces, and endothelial cell surfaces. Plasminogen activators cleave the inactive plasminogen into a two-chain plasmin molecule. Plasmin is a nonspecific serine protease that acts to degrade multiple substrates. Most important, plasmin degrades fibrin and fibrinogen. However, plasmin is generated wherever plasminogen is bound, resulting in the nonspecific degradation of several other important sites. Plasmin degrades von Willebrand's factor, degrades the platelet glycoprotein receptors GpIb and GpIIb/IIIa,[5] converts single-chain tissue plasminogen activators to double-chain molecules, and degrades other factors important to maintaining a stable thrombus.[6] Plasmin production by plasminogen activators is primarily regulated by plasminogen activator inhibitors. The plasminogen activator inhibitors rapidly bind circulating active forms of plasminogen activators. When bound to the endothelial cell surface, both UK and t-PA are significantly protected from inactivation by plasminogen activator inhibitor type 1. The process of plasminogen activation by t-PA on endothelial cell surfaces is thereby greatly enhanced. In addition to the inhibition of platelet aggregation noted earlier, plasmin directly inhibits factors Va and VIIIa of the coagulation cascade.[7] Unbound plasmin is rapidly inhibited directly by circulating α_2-antiplasmin and more slowly bound by α_2-macroglobulin. Plasmin not only clips apart the fibrin skeleton that supports a thrombus but also inhibits the production of new fibrin and degrades the adhesion and aggregation ability of platelets.[8] This lytic process allows the clot to break apart under the stress of vascular flow.

Of lesser importance in the physiologic control of coagulation and thrombosis is α_2-macroglobulin, a serpin that partially neutralizes thrombin. Other circulating inhibitors are heparin cofactor II, C_1-inhibitor, and α_2-antitrypsin. Protease nexin-1 is a similar but noncirculating inhibitor of thrombin that is secreted directly by the cells, acts locally, and then is rapidly reabsorbed. Though individually not as important as the major regulatory systems noted previously, the nonspecific depletion of these lesser coagulation inhibitors contributes to the procoagulant thrombin-activating effect of tissue plasminogen activator.

Plasminogen Activators and the Regulation of Fibrinolysis

Plasminogen activators are generally grouped into three distinct classes based on their naturally occurring homologues: UK-type plasminogen activator (u-PA), t-PA, and SK. Although t-PA is the primary physiologic plasmin generator, both SK and UK were identified and studied earlier. SK was discovered in the 1930s and named streptococcal fibrinolysin.[9] Fibrinolytic activity was first identified in human urine in 1947[10] and subsequently named UK.[11] In 1947, t-PA was also described[12] but could not be characterized fully until it was successfully isolated from melanoma cell line cultures in 1981.[13] Currently, there are five commercially available plasminogen activators: recombinant t-PA (rt-PA), UK, pro-urokinase (scu-PA or single-chain urokinase), SK, and anistreplase (anisoylated plasminogen activator complex, APSAC). Numerous other agents are under development or investigation, including mutant recombinant forms of t-PA such as reteplase and the long-known but recently rejuvenated staphylokinase. Each of these hopes to improve on the basic characteristics of native t-PA, which is the primary fibrinolytic activator *in vivo*.

All of the plasminogen activators act by cleaving plasminogen to plasmin. The broad range of therapeutic and adverse effects of the plasminogen activators on the hemostatic mechanism derive almost exclusively from the actions and effects of plasmin described earlier. The plasminogen activators vary in several basic characteristics that influence the rate, site, and duration of plasmin generation.

The first characteristic is relative fibrin specificity. The first-generation agents, SK and UK, act equally on both "fibrin bound" and "circulating unbound" plasminogen. Unlike SK or UK, t-PA manifests the relative propensity to cleave only the plasminogen bound to fibrin. Theoretically, this higher fibrin specificity should confer relative "clot selectivity" so that the majority of plasmin generation and consequent fibrinolysis would occur within a thrombus rather than in the general circulation. Similarly, the lower levels of circulating plasmin would spare the circulating fibrinogen and thus avoid hypofibrinogenemia. This fibrin-binding "clot selectivity" of t-PA accelerates thrombolysis and should, at least relatively, preserve the systemic coagulation system. At pharmacologic doses, rt-PA loses much of this clot selectivity. When given at therapeutic doses, none of the currently available agents can distinguish between the pathologic thrombus and the physiologic hemostatic plug that maintains the integrity of the vascular system. Although the accelerating effects of fibrin selectivity remain, the systemic benefits remain largely theoretic.

The second characteristic is the propensity to generate a systemic lytic state. This lytic state is characterized by fibrinogen depletion, plasminogen depletion, depletion of clotting factors V and VIII, alterations in platelet function, elevated plasmin levels, and accumulation of fibrin degradation products and D-dimers. As noted earlier, the ability to induce this systemic plasma proteolytic state is in part influenced by fibrin specificity of the plasminogen activator. The activity of the agent as infused also influences the induction of the systemic lytic state. An inactive proenzyme form of a plasminogen activator would not lyse the circulating plasminogen and could avoid inactivation by the circulating plasminogen activator inhibitor. One theoretic benefit of infusing a proenzyme form of a fibrin-specific plasminogen activator is that the circulating drug would not induce a systemic lytic state because it is not active until bound to the thrombus. This was part of the rationale behind the development of both APSAC and scu-UK. Both agents are activated only after binding to fibrin, whereas rt-PA is active when infused. Despite this theoretic advantage, APSAC induces a marked systemic lytic state at currently used clinical doses.[14] Two other related characteristics are the plasma half-life and duration of the lytic effects. Activation time, plasma clearance, and relative resistance to binding by inhibitors are major determinants of the duration of effect of an agent. For example, circulating t-PA is rapidly bound by plasminogen activator inhibitor and deactivated by the liver. The circulating half-lives for t-PA and rt-PA are approximately 4 and 6 minutes, respectively, so that the drug must be administered as a continuous infusion to sustain a fibrinolytic effect. The *systemic* lytic state, as a result of this very short half-life, resolves rapidly after stopping t-PA infusion to reveal a procoagulant effect noticeable within 2 hours in the absence of heparin or other anticoagulant therapy. Owing to the high affinity of t-PA for fibrin and the marked protection of bound t-PA from inactivation by plasminogen activator inhibitor, increased fibrinolytic activity may persist *in thrombi* for several more hours. Anistreplase, which has a 70-minute activation half-life, possesses a 90 to 120 minute circulating half-life, and is relatively protected from plasminogen activator inhibitor, produces a systemic lytic lasting more than 24 hours. Agents vary considerably in lytic potency *in vivo* and *in vitro*, with t-PA having the greatest lytic potency of any currently available agent.

In general, there is little correlation between the serum levels of plasminogen activators and the effectiveness of thrombolysis, in large part because of the circulating inhibitors. In addition, numerous other factors influence the ability of plasminogen activators to dissolve a thrombus. Of particular importance are clot-dependent factors. The effectiveness of plasminogen activators depends on the amount of plasminogen bound in the clot, the surface area of clot exposed to activators, the plasminogen activator accessibility to the clot, and the age of the clot. Thrombus resistance to plasmin degradation increases rapidly. With time, the fibrin becomes more cross-linked and the fibrin polymers grow longer, making the clot more resistant to degradation.

Finally, all of the plasminogen activators induce a paradoxical procoagulant effect that contributes significantly to the rethrombosis phenomenon. This effect is largely mediated by the activator-induced plasminemia. Elevated thrombin activity, the depletion of heparin cofactor and antithrombin III, and the positive feedback of thrombin clotting factor activation are characteristic effects of plasminogen activators.[15] This is one of the reasons that antithrombotic agents such as aspirin or heparin are important adjuncts to thrombolytic therapy.

Currently, plasminogen activators are used for the treatment of acute myocardial infarction (AMI), deep venous thrombosis, acute thrombotic stroke, pulmonary embolism, peripheral arterial thrombosis, and catheter occlusion. A clear benefit has been demonstrated for all but pulmonary embolism; current series have not been large enough to demonstrate a significant benefit over that provided by heparin alone.

The principal plasminogen activators currently in clinical use are discussed below.

PRINCIPAL THROMBOLYTIC AGENTS

Streptokinase

SK is a single-chain protein secreted by β-hemolytic streptococci that has 415 amino acid residues and a molecular weight of 45,000 to 50,000 daltons.[16] It is produced by chemical purification of bacterial culture filtrates.

Unbound SK is not an active enzyme. Plasminogen activation by SK requires two steps. SK must first bind to plasminogen or plasmin, which unmasks the catalytic center of the SK to form the enzymatically active complex. The SK-plasminogen and SK-plasmin complexes are potent plasminogen activators. These active complexes must then bind to plasminogen and act to cleave plasminogen to plasmin. Neither fibrin nor fibrinogen has specific SK binding sites, so SK acts equally on both fibrin-bound and circulating plasminogen. SK and the active SK complexes have a plasma half-life of approximately 23 minutes. The duration of thrombolytic effect lasts for approximately 6 hours.

Table 96–1. Indications and Standard Dosage Regimens for Streptokinase

Indication	Route	Total Dose	Bolus	Infusion Rate	Infusion Time
Acute MI	Peripheral IV	1.5 million units	None	1.5 million units	1 h
Acute MI	Intra-arterial	140,000 units	20,000 units	2,000 units/min	1 h
Pulmonary embolism	Peripheral IV	2.65 million units	250,000 units over 30 min	100,000 units/h	24 h
Deep venous thrombosis	Peripheral IV	7.45 million units	250,000 units over 30 min	100,000 units/h	72 h
Peripheral arterial occlusion	Peripheral IV	2.65–7.45 million units	250,000 units	100,000 units/h	24–72 h
Peripheral arterial occlusion	Intra-arterial	Up to 8.6 million units	20,000 units over 30 min	2,000 units/min	Up to 72 h
Acute CVA	Not recommended				
Catheter occlusion	Intracatheter	500,000 units	250,000 units over 60 min	250,000 units	60 min

MI, myocardial infarction; CVA, cerebrovascular accident; IV, intravenous.

Because SK is a foreign antigenic protein, it is significantly allergenic and produces the full spectrum of pulmonary, gastrointestinal, cutaneous, and cardiovascular side effects. These include fever, anaphylaxis, angioedema, bronchospasm, serum sickness, interstitial nephritis, and many less significant complaints. The likelihood of allergic side effects increases dramatically with recent prior exposure either from treatment with SK and APSAC or from streptococcal infection.

SK is also associated with a significant incidence of profound hypotension at the time of administration that is not of apparent allergic etiology. This effect is related to the dose and the rate of infusion. Table 96–1 summarizes the usual indications and the standard clinical dosages for SK.

Anistreplase

Anistreplase is a *p*-anisoylated derivative of human lys-plasmino-streptokinase complex and has a molecular weight of 131,000 daltons. It is prepared by the binding of SK to human lys-plasminogen in the presence of a specific acylating agent. The lys-plasminogen is the plasminogen moiety with a high affinity for fibrin and fibrinogen.

APSAC is not an active enzyme until it undergoes deacylation through ester hydrolysis. The inactive acyl form is relatively stable and resistant to degradation or inhibition by circulating inhibitors. Thus, the fibrin-binding sites on the plasminogen component of the acylated complex are immediately available for binding. This provides time for fibrin binding before unmasking the enzymatic site. The deacylation half-life is approximately 105 minutes in human blood at body temperature.[17] Deacylation produces a free activator complex with greater lytic potency than that of SK.

The clearance half-life of APSAC parallels the deacylation half-life of 90 to 120 minutes. Degradation occurs enzymatically in the plasma so that renal and hepatic function have little direct impact on APSAC metabolism. The duration of the thrombolytic effect continues, however, for more than 20 hours.

Because APSAC contains SK, the likelihood of allergic side effects is comparable to that of SK. APSAC is also associated with usually mild hypotensive effects comparable to those produced by a similar dose of SK administered over 1 hour. The usual dose used in clinical practice is listed in Table 96–2.

Urokinase

UK is a human naturally occurring double-chain polypeptide with a molecular weight of approximately 54,000 daltons, although it may exist in lower molecular weight forms. It is one of two endogenous circulating plasminogen activators that are prevalent in the intercellular matrix and it is concentrated in the urine. Its physiologic role is probably to decrease intercellular adhesion and thereby facilitate cell migration through the interstitium. UK is manufactured by purification of human urine, made by cell cultures, and manufactured using recombinant DNA technology.

UK cleaves plasminogen to form plasmin with only a slight preference for fibrin-bound plasminogen; hence it has a low level of fibrin specificity. It is cleared rapidly by the liver with only 3% to 5% of clearance by the kidney.[18] The circulating half-life is approximately 16 minutes with normal hepatic function. The duration of the thrombolytic activity is probably less than 4 hours.

UK, although a naturally occurring human protein, has been rarely associated with allergic side effects in clinical trials. Table 96–3 summarizes the current clinical indications and dosages for UK.

Table 96–2. Indications and Standard Dosage Regimen for Anistreplase (APSAC)

Indication	Route	Total Dose	Bolus	Infusion Rate	Infusion Time
Acute myocardial infarction	Peripheral intravenous	30 units	30 units	None	3–5 min

Table 96–3. Indications and Standard Dosage Regimens for Urokinase

Indication	Route	Total Dose	Bolus	Infusion Rate	Infusion Time
Acute MI	Intra-arterial	Up to 500,000 units	None	6,000 units/min	Up to 120 min
Pulmonary embolism	Peripheral IV	3.9 million units	300,000 units	300,000 units/h	Up to 12 h
Peripheral arterial occlusion	Intra-arterial	Up to 2.64 million units	4000 units/min for 120 min	1000–2000 units/min	Up to 48 h
Acute CVA	Not recommended	Not recommended	Not recommended	Not recommended	Not recommended
Catheter occlusion	Intracatheter	500,000 units	250,000 units for 60 min	250,000 units for 60 min	2 h

MI, myocardial infarction; CVA, cerebrovascular accident; IV, intravenous.

Pro-Urokinase

Pro-urokinase is a naturally occurring single-chain proenzyme form of urokinase that when infused possesses a high degree of fibrin affinity, thrombolytic efficacy, and pharmacodynamics similar to those of t-PA. The scu-PA is very stable in plasma and has a high affinity for fibrin despite the apparent lack of specific receptors or direct binding to the fibrin molecule. This high-affinity fibrin-dependent activity of scu-PA is distinctly different from the mechanism of action of t-PA. The scu-PA itself possesses significant thrombolytic potency at the fibrin surface. Plasmin further "activates" scu-PA on the fibrin surface by proteolytic cleavage of several sites, creating several active molecular forms of u-PA. The dominant and most thrombolytically potent product of this activation is the two-chain form.

Like other plasminogen activators, clearance of scu-PA follows a two compartment model. It has an initial phase half-life of approximately 4 to 8 minutes.[19] Once activated, it is susceptible to binding by plasminogen activator inhibitor, and, like u-PA, is predominantly cleared by the liver.

A recombinant form of scu-PA, saruplase, which as a result of its bacterial source of production differs from the native scu-PA in the lack of a carbohydrate side chain, has a slightly longer half-life than wild-type.[20]

Tissue-Type Plasminogen Activator

Human t-PA is a single-chain polypeptide with a molecular weight of approximately 64,000 daltons. This single-chain form can be cleaved to a two-chain form. On the surface of clots the single-chain form is usually converted by plasmin into the double-chain form. Though initially produced from melanoma cell cultures, it is primarily manufactured using recombinant DNA technology (rt-PA).

Both the single-chain and the double-chain forms are equivalent in their ability to activate plasminogen and in their high degree of fibrin specificity.[21] The single-chain form is less reactive with low molecular weight substrates and inhibitors than the double-chain form. The single-chain rt-PA has a shorter initial half-life in humans of 4.3 minutes compared with 5.2 minutes for the double-chain form. As a result of a shorter half-life, the concentration of t-PA achieved with a 1-hour infusion of single-chain rt-PA achieves only around 70% of the plasma concentration of a similar infusion of the double-chain form. Early rt-PA production was of the two-chain variety. Now the majority (80%) of rt-PA in the lots produced is of the single-chain variety.

Circulating t-PA is rapidly bound by plasma activator inhibitor and is rapidly cleared by the liver with no significant contribution by the kidneys. The clearance of both forms of rt-PA is best understood using a two-compartment model in which the initial α-phase half-life is approximately 5 minutes and the β-phase half-life is approximately 40 minutes. The volume of distribution is approximately 7.3 liters.[22, 23] There are no known active metabolites of t-PA. Despite the short half-life, the duration of fibrinolytic activity may be prolonged in the areas of clot formation owing to the avid fibrin binding.

As a human protein naturally present throughout the circulatory system, t-PA is nonallergenic. However, rt-PA has been associated with a low but definite incidence of allergic-type reactions.

Use of the accelerated regimen for t-PA has shown a slight survival advantage over that for SK for AMI, but there has been no advantage shown over SK with use of the standard t-PA regimen. Table 96–4 illustrates the current indication and standard dosage regimens of t-PA currently used in clinical practice.

Intra-Arterial Thrombolytic Therapy

The intra-arterial "local" delivery of plasminogen activator directly to the clot was the method of choice in the early clinical experience with thrombolytic therapy. The appeal of this technique was based largely on its theoretic ability to avoid systemic toxicity. This technique fell into relative disfavor for the treatment of AMI when clinical trials demonstrated the equivalent efficacy of peripheral venous administration without the delay to initiation of therapy and the bleeding complications associated with an invasive intra-arterial procedure. However, intra-arterial treatment has remained the mainstay of therapy for peripheral arterial occlusion.

The clinical effect and complications of intra-arte-

Table 96–4. Indications and Standard Dosage Regimens for Tissue-Type Plasminogen Activator (t-PA)

Indication	Route	Total Dose	Bolus	Infusion Rate	Infusion Time
Acute MI, "standard"[24]	Peripheral IV	100 mg	10 mg	50 mg over 1 h	Then 20 mg/h for 2 h
Acute MI, weight adjusted, "accelerated"[25]	Peripheral IV	1.25 mg/kg up to 100 mg	15 mg	0.75 mg/kg up to 50 mg over first 30 min	0.5 mg/kg up to 35 mg over next 1 h
Pulmonary embolism[26]	Peripheral IV	100 mg	None	50 mg/h	2 h
Acute CVA[27]	Peripheral IV	0.9 mg/kg up to 90 mg	10% of the dose		1 h
Proximal DVT	Peripheral IV	Up to 150 mg	None	0.05 mg/kg/h	24 h
Proximal DVT	Peripheral IV	Up to 150 mg	None	0.5 mg/kg	4 h

MI, myocardial infarction; CVA, cerebrovascular accident; DVT, deep venous thrombosis; IV, intravenous.

rial thrombolytic therapy are essentially the same as those for peripheral therapy and relate similarly to the duration of the thrombosis, the risk factors of the patient, the dose of agent used, and the duration of the infusion. Even the lowest doses of intra-arterial SK overwhelm the local vascular system to induce a systemic lytic state similar to that with peripheral therapy, resulting in the same rate of hemorrhagic complications.

The current interest in thrombolytic therapy for acute thrombotic cerebrovascular (CVA) accidents and the substantial advancement in techniques of selective arterial catheterization have combined to rekindle the interest in direct intra-arterial therapy.

The principal antithrombotic agents are discussed at the end of the chapter.

COMPLICATIONS AND ADVERSE REACTIONS TO THERAPY

Thrombolytics and antithrombotic agents are examples of the proverbial double-edged sword that promises dramatic saves as well as the possibility of disastrous consequences. Currently, thrombolytic therapy has six major clinical indications: AMI, acute nonhemorrhagic cardiovascular accident, acute pulmonary embolism, acute peripheral arterial thrombosis, proximal deep venous thrombosis, and thrombotic occlusion of parenteral catheters or grafts. The overwhelming majority of our information on the frequency and spectrum of complications is derived from two sources: primarily from the numerous trials of thrombolytic therapy for AMI and to a much lesser degree from the trials of thrombolytic therapy for pulmonary embolism. The risk factors for complications of thrombolytic treatment as well as the nature and spectrum of the complications are the same in all clinical settings. The prevalence of risks of therapy, the thrombolytic regimen used, and the resultant absolute rates of adverse reactions are the aspects that vary. This discussion focuses primarily on the clinical experience from thrombolytic therapy for AMI to review the risks, spectrum, and mechanisms of toxicity.

The major complications of thrombolytic therapy regardless of agent employed are hemorrhage, stroke, and thromboembolism. In the case of SK or APSAC, allergic reaction and anaphylaxis must be added to this list.

Hemorrhage

Thrombolytic and anticoagulant therapy impair the ability of the body to form hemostatic plugs through numerous mechanisms. Current thrombolytic therapy induces this hemostatic defect by alterations in the function of the blood components, the vessel wall, and the hemostatic plug itself.[28] The actions of these thrombolytic agents induce a systemic hypocoagulable lytic state that both dissolves preexisting hemostatic plugs and severely impairs the body's ability to repair any new insults to the integrity of the blood vessel. In the setting of an uninjured vascular system, anticoagulation alone does not induce bleeding.[29] Vascular injury or disease causes the bleeding; the thrombolytic or antithrombotic agents only intensify and prolong it. This fact is supported by and explains the observation that the incidence of major noncerebral and intracerebral hemorrhage cannot be predicted from laboratory measures of the severity (e.g., fibrinogen levels) or the duration of the lytic state (as detected by elevated fibrin degradation products). The overall incidence of hemorrhagic complications does not vary substantially among patients who use SK, APSAC, UK, and t-PA despite marked variation in the intensity and duration of the induced lytic states associated with each agent.[30] The majority of bleeding occurs at sites of vascular invasion or injury as in hemorrhagic cardiovascular accident, active peptic ulcer disease, or cardiac catheterization. In general, it is useful for the purpose of discussion to classify hemorrhage associated with anticoagulant and thrombolytic treatment as one of the following:

- Intracranial bleed (ICB), including hemorrhagic strokes, intraparenchymal hemorrhage, and subdural or epidural hematomas
- Major noncerebral bleed (MNCB), if it requires transfusion or is life threatening
- Minor, if none of the above

The absolute incidence of major noncerebral and intracranial hemorrhage in these clinical trials is dependent largely on the prevalence of factors known to increase the risks of bleeding in the population under study and, to a lesser degree, on the thrombolytic regimen employed.

Major Noncerebral Bleeding

Thrombolytic therapy itself results in an overall two- to threefold increase in the incidence of MNCB and ICB when compared with that resulting from the use of heparin or aspirin alone as evidenced by the early controlled trials of thrombolytic therapy in the treatment of both deep venous thrombosis and AMI.[31] The overall incidence of MNCB associated with fibrinolytic therapy in an overview of the nine largest randomized trials was 1.1% compared with 0.4% for controls.[32] This degree of increased incidence of MNCB was consistent among all subgroups by age, history of hypertension, and smoking.

In the ISIS-3 study,[33] the overall incidence of other bleeding, MNCB, and all bleeding complications was essentially the same when comparing the use of t-PA, APSAC, and SK: 0.8%, 1.0%, and 0.9% for MNCB and 5.2%, 5.4%, and 4.5% for all bleeding, respectively.[33]

Experience from trials in the management of pulmonary embolism and peripheral arterial thrombosis provides evidence that the incidence of MNCB and ICB increases significantly with the duration of the thrombolytic treatment.[34]

Adjunctive therapy with aspirin, aspirin plus heparin, heparin, or hirudin increases the likelihood of both major bleeding and intracerebral hemorrhage. The use of heparin in ISIS-3 resulted in an increase in the rate of MNCB from 0.75% to 1.2%.[33] In the TIMI 9a trial of heparin versus hirudin in conjunction with t-PA or SK, major bleeding was much more frequent than expected, occurring in 3% of heparin-treated and 7% of hirudin-treated patients.[35]

Invasive procedures are a significant risk factor for MNCB. Cardiac catheterization when performed within 48 hours of thrombolytic therapy can produce a significant increase in major bleeding complications predominantly related to access site bleeding.[36] The absolute transfusion rates range from 2% to 19% higher than those for comparable controls in the TAMI-1, TIMI IIa, TIMI IIb, SWIFT,[37] and TAMI-5 trials. This increased risk of MNCB associated with cardiac catheterization, however, does not extend to an increase in the risk of ICB.

Advancing age, especially an age older than 70 years, is a significant risk factor for all bleeding complications of thrombolytic administration, including both MNCB and ICB. Age alone though is no longer a contraindication to thrombolytic therapy for AMI owing to the high mortality without treatment.[38] In the ISIS-3 patient population of suspected AMI, the risk of ICB and noncerebral bleeding associated with adjuvant aspirin and heparin therapy increased with age. The rate of all MNCB for persons younger than 70 using aspirin plus heparin was 5.0% and using aspirin alone was 3.4%. The rate for persons 70 years or older using aspirin plus heparin was 9.8% and using aspirin alone was 5.3%. The mechanism of this association of bleeding complications with advancing age is uncertain. It may be that the frequency of other risk factors associated with advancing years accounts for this higher complication rate. Following SK therapy for massive pulmonary embolism the rate of complication did not increase in the elderly when other suspected risk factors were excluded from the trial.[39]

Diabetes with diabetic retinopathy has traditionally been cited as a risk factor for complication of thrombolytic therapy and a relative contraindication to its use. Although vitreous hemorrhage is a reported bleeding complication,[40] diabetic retinopathy does not appear to present a substantial increase in risk for this rare event. A review of clinical experience in the United Kingdom using thrombolytic therapy for AMI in patients with varying degrees of diabetic retinopathy failed to identify any instance of intraocular hemorrhage.[41]

Active menstruation has historically been a criteria for exclusion from thrombolytic therapy owing to the perceived risk of major hemorrhage. The limited published clinical experience to date suggests that although there may be a minor increase in uterine bleeding, it is well tolerated and should not preclude treatment with thrombolytics.[42]

Cardiopulmonary resuscitation has also been considered a contraindication to thrombolytic therapy owing to perceived hemorrhagic risk. The experience reported to date suggests that even prolonged cardiopulmonary resuscitation does not itself significantly increase the risk of fatal bleeding. Although there may be some bleeding associated with chest compression, there is only one reported case of fatal intrapulmonary hemorrhage. The majority of major bleeding complications in patients undergoing cardiopulmonary resuscitation with thrombolysis are related to vascular access sites, and the overall rate of serious bleeding in resuscitated patients is the same as that in patients not requiring resuscitation.[43]

Clinical Outcome of Major Noncerebral Bleeding

The overwhelming majority of instances of MNCB are nonfatal and can be managed by standard measures, including transfusion. The location of the bleed is the major determinant of outcome. The majority of hemorrhages in clinical trials occur at vascular access sites and can be treated with compression. Occasionally, however, the location is more occult and life or limb threatening. Some of these cases include retroperitoneal bleeding,[44] spontaneous splenic ruptures,[45] esophageal dissection,[46] and bilateral forearm and hand compartment syndromes following radial artery puncture.[47]

Cardiac rupture represents the most lethal of the MNCB and generally is not reported separately owing to the associated mortality. An accelerated incidence of cardiac rupture is proposed to account for the increased first-day mortality of patients treated with plasminogen activators compared with that of controls. Although there is a higher incidence of early cardiac rupture, the overall rate of cardiac rupture appears to be the same as that in the nonthrombolytic groups.[48]

Stroke and Intracranial Bleeding

Stroke of all varieties has always been a major source of morbidity and mortality in patients with AMI. Historically, the absolute incidence of acute stroke is about 0.4% among AMI patients. The use of t-PA or APSAC is associated with an approximately twofold increase in the incidence of ICB and total stroke rate when compared with the use of SK for the treatment of AMI. In the ISIS-3 study, of 41,299 patients, the overall incidence of stroke was significantly higher in patients receiving t-PA (1.39%) than in patients treated with SK (1.04%). Most of these strokes occurred within the first day and were attributable to ICB; the rates were 0.66%, 0.55% and 0.24% for the use of t-PA, APSAC, and SK, respectively. This increased rate of both ICB and nonhemorrhagic cardiovascular accident is more pronounced with increasing age. For those younger than 70, overall stroke rate was 0.23% with SK use and 0.48% with t-PA use. For those older than 70, the rate of stroke with SK use was still 0.25%, whereas with t-PA use the rate increased to 1.16%. Some criticize the ISIS-3 data because the t-PA form used was the higher potency two-chain form of rt-PA (duteplase), resulting in the equivalent of 150 mg or more of the more commonly used predominantly single-chain rt-PA (alteplase). Despite that reservation, other studies have also shown an increase in the incidence of overall stroke and ICB when t-PA rather than SK was used.

The total dose and rate of administration also influence the incidence of severe hemorrhagic complications. Early studies revealed that using 150 mg of t-PA instead of 100 mg of t-PA resulted in a higher rate of stroke (1.6% versus 0.6%) and ICB (1.3 versus 0.4%).[49] The rate of stroke and ICB associated with the accelerated rt-PA plus intravenous heparin protocol of GUSTO-1 was 1.55% and 0.70%, whereas for SK plus intravenous heparin the rates were 1.39% and 0.64%, respectively.[50]

On analysis of strokes in the GISSI-2 trial,[51] older age, higher Killip class, and anterior infarction significantly increased the overall risk of stroke, whereas previous hypertension, diabetes, higher body-mass index, and smoking did not. After adjusting for other risks, age was no longer a risk for ICB but Killip class and anterior infarction remained. Diastolic hypertension on admission was strongly associated with overall incidence of stroke and ICB but systolic hypertension alone was not. The incidences of all strokes and ICB for diastolic blood pressure lower than 100 were 1.1% and 0.3%; for diastolic blood pressure of 100 to 110 they were 1.2% and 0.5%; and for diastolic blood pressure higher than 110 they were 3.2% and 1.9%, respectively. Also of interest in this study was that aspirin reduced the incidence of all strokes and ICB.[52]

Multiple logistic regression analysis of the GUSTO-1 data identified age, low body weight, prior cerebrovascular disease, diastolic hypertension, history of hypertension, accelerated t-PA, and systolic hypertension as major independent risk factors for stroke and ICB in that order.[50] Increasing age, lower body weight, and elevated presenting blood pressures were continuously variable risks without clear cutoff points. These data did not confirm the findings of other investigators that pulse pressure was predictive of intracranial hemorrhage.[53] Of particular importance is that a history of prior cerebrovascular disease was associated with a marked increased rate of stroke. The overall rate of stroke with thrombolytic therapy was 1.4%. The rate of stroke in patients with a prior history of transient ischemic attack or CVA was 5.5% and 6.9% respectively. Approximately 45% of these strokes were ICB.

The use of adjunctive antithrombotic therapy strongly influences the incidence of ICB. The use of heparin in the ISIS-3 study resulted in an increase in the rate of ICB from 0.40% without heparin use to 0.56% with heparin use.

The intensity of adjunctive anticoagulation appears to correlate with the risk of ICB. In both the original GUSTO-I trial and the GUSTO-IIa trials there was a significant correlation between marked prolongation of the activated partial thromboplastin time and rate of ICB.[25, 54] Several more recent multicenter studies evaluating the use of hirudin or heparin, or both, as adjunctive anticoagulant therapy were stopped prematurely owing to an excessive rate of intracerebral hemorrhage. In GUSTO IIa the incidence of ICB among the patients treated with heparin alone was 1.3% and with hirudin alone was 0.7%. However, in patients receiving either t-PA or SK, ICB rates were 1.8% compared with 0.3% in the nonlytic therapy group. Among the group treated with thrombolysis, heparin therapy was associated with a 1.5% rate of hemorrhagic stroke, whereas hirudin-treated patients had a 2.2% incidence of hemorrhagic stroke.[54] The TIMI 9a trial of heparin versus hirudin in conjunction with t-PA or SK also reported an ICB rate of 1.9% with heparin treatment and 1.7% with hirudin.[35] Even with a 25% to 30% reduction in hirudin dosage from that used in the TAMI 9a and the GUSTO IIA trials, the HIT-III study found the incidence of excessive ICB and major hemorrhage in the hirudin group sufficient for the termination of the trial.[55] The reason for the high complication rates in all of these trials is not well understood at this time. However, these studies illustrate the risks associated with more potent antithrombotic therapy in conjunction with plasminogen activator therapy.

Clinical Presentation and Outcome of Intracranial Bleeding

The most detailed information on the natural history of ICB associated with rt-PA and heparin therapy is provided by the TIMI II trial,[56] in which the study carefully tracked the onset and evolution of ICB in 23 patients. The t-PA was administered over a 4-hour period with 60 mg the first hour, 20 mg the second, and 5 mg each of the next 2 hours. The time in hours from initiation of t-PA infusion to onset of symptoms was as follows:

Hours	Patients
<1	0
1–4	7
4–8	5
8–12	3
12–16	2
16–20	2
20–24	0
24–28	2
>28	2

The presenting signs or symptoms were decreased level of consciousness in 15 patients (65%), focal neurologic deficit in 8 (35%), vomiting in 6 (26%), seizure in 5 (22%), headache in 3 (13%), and coma in 2 (9%). Fourteen of the 23 patients reached maximal deficit within 6 hours and another four in the next 6 hours.

The overall outcome in this analysis of ICB in TIMI II was a 48% 1-month mortality. Those who presented with a decreased level of consciousness had a 65% mortality. Of interest is that in those patients whose brains were examined for pathologic conditions following the ICB, amyloid angiopathy was present in the majority of bleeding sites.[56] This has led to speculation that the majority of all ICB complicating fibrinolytic therapy is due to underlying significant vascular disease and raised the question of whether plasmin directly lyses the amyloid proteins deposited in the vessel walls.

This is consistent with the ISIS-3 experience, in which the respective percentages for 176 t-PA-treated and 141 SK-treated patients with strokes were that 49% and 47% died in-hospital, 32% and 34% had significant disability, and 18% and 19% had no disability.

Thrombolytic Therapy for Acute Cerebral Artery Thrombosis

Interest in the use of thrombolytic therapy for acute thrombotic stroke has developed as well as that for treatment of AMI. The devastating impact and high incidence of ICB in patients with cerebrovascular disease has slowed the growth of clinical experience. The growing availability of emergency CT scanning to exclude the highest risk patients has allowed the completion of several larger clinical trials leading to clinical use of thrombolytics in acute nonhemorrhagic cardiovascular accident.[27, 57] These studies of t-PA report a significant therapeutic benefit in functional outcome with therapy but at a substantial risk with the current regimens.

As expected from the experience in AMI, even with restrictive exclusion criteria the incidence of major ICB is much higher in treatment of acute cerebrovascular accident than in treatment of AMI. The ECASS study,[57] using a 1.1 mg/kg dose of t-PA, reported a 20% incidence of ICB and an 18% 30-day mortality compared with 7% and 12% in the placebo group, respectively. The NINDS study[27] used a slightly lower dose of t-PA (0.9 mg/kg up to 90 mg) and reported an incidence of ICB within 36 hours of treatment of 6.4% compared with 0.6% in the control group. The overall mortality between the groups was not statistically significant, however.

Allergic Reaction and Hypotension

Allergic reactions including flushing, urticaria, bronchospasm, and anaphylaxis occur with plasminogen activator injection. This is expected with the injection of bacterial protein–derived SK analogue. Surprisingly, allergic reactions are also observed after treatment with native t-PA. However, APSAC and SK use are associated with a significantly higher incidence of allergic reactions than the pharmaceutical preparations of t-PA, with rates of 5.1% (APSAC), 3.6% (SK), and 0.8% (t-PA) given. Of these, approximately 10% were reported to cause persistent symptoms, and the rest were minor transient reactions.[33]

A decline in blood pressure with thrombolytic infusion is common. The mechanism for the hypotension is not known, but it is neither a hypersensitivity reaction nor an occult hemorrhage. The prevalent theories are that the hypotensive effect is secondary to (1) plasmin-mediated generation of bradykinin through proteolysis of kallikrein and (2) plasmin-induced complement activation and endothelial prostacyclin secretion. Clinically significant hypotension occurs with surprising frequency with all plasminogen activators. In ISIS-3, hypotension was more frequent with the use of APSAC and SK than t-PA, with rates reported of 12.5%, 11.8%, and 7.1%, respectively. About half of these instances of hypotension required drug therapy. This compared with a 1.5% rate of hypotension in patients who did not receive fibrinolytic therapy. In earlier studies of streptokinase infusion, blood pressure lower than systolic 90 mm Hg has been noted in up to 38% of the patients.[58] A later evaluation of this side effect also noted a 34% incidence of systolic blood pressure lower than 90 and a 20% incidence of systolic blood pressure lower than 80 mm Hg. when using a 1.5 million–unit SK infusion over 1 hour. The average decline in systolic blood pressure was 35 mm Hg. There was a definite association between lowest systolic blood pressure and both early and 1-year mortality. The 2-week mortality was 22% in the group with hypotension versus 11% in the group without hypotension. On multivariate analysis, the hypotensive effect was independently related only to initial systolic blood pressure before infusion, age, and a history of diabetes mellitus. Infarct location, mortality, gender, history of heart disease, Q wave development, and administration of metoprolol were not independently associated. This suggests that the mortality difference between the groups is due to age and preinfusion systolic blood pressure.[59]

Emboli

Thromboembolism associated with fibrinolytic therapy is a well-recognized but infrequent complication of treatment. It is not surprising that as the plasmin clips apart the thrombus a clinically significant piece of the clot may break loose and migrate downstream. When this occurs on the venous side, it is rarely a serious clinical problem. Arterial embolization, however, can be devastating. Nonlethal and lethal strokes have been reported due to cerebral embolization from cardiac mural thrombi[60] and from prosthetic cardiac valve thrombosis.[61] Unlike distal embolization from peripheral arterial emboli, the acute cerebral embolus cannot be treated with continued thrombolytic infusion.

TREATMENT OF COMPLICATIONS OF THROMBOLYTIC THERAPY

The most important considerations in the management of complications of thrombolytic therapy are initial patient selection for thrombolytic therapy and avoidance of invasive procedures, especially at noncompressible sites. It is essential to screen for prior exposure to SK or recent streptococcal infections when planning to use SK or APSAC. Although there are numerous factors that may increase the risks of therapy, the final decision to use plasminogen activators or antithrombotic therapy must be based on relative risk-benefit considerations. The high mortality associated with ICB places those risks at the top of our list of relative contraindications. Hemorrhagic cerebrovascular accident, recent head injury or intracranial surgery, intracranial neoplasm, or severe uncontrolled hypertension on admission virtually preclude any therapeutic benefit to thrombolysis. Similarly, active bleeding from noncompressible sites outweighs the potential benefits of thrombolytic therapy, which essentially excludes patients with active gastrointestinal bleeding or recent thoracoabdominal surgery. In consideration of both ICB and MNCB risk, "recent" is not clearly defined, but most sources agree that less than 10 days is "too recent" for comfort.

Nonhemorrhagic Complications

Allergic reactions should be managed in the usual fashion using parenteral antihistamines, bronchodilators, and epinephrine if needed for severe reactions. Though not specifically studied, most researchers suggest initial treatment with intravenous benadryl and hydrocortisone.

The optimal management of plasminogen activator infusion-related hypotension is not well defined. Because it is not an allergic reaction, antihistamines are not effective. The initial treatment is to slow or temporarily stop the infusion, and this should be done in all cases of serious hypotension. Approximately 50% of the hypotensive episodes require additional therapy. Of those who require additional treatment, 50% will respond to a combination of atropine and fluids, 15% will require intravenous pressors, and the remainder will require further intervention.[59]

Hemorrhagic Complications

Minor bleeding or localized hematomas in compressible sites, even when large, do not warrant cessation of lytic therapy or reversal of the lytic state. Careful monitoring of the patient and compression of the bleeding sites is generally sufficient even though limited transfusion may occasionally be necessary.

Reversal of the Lytic State

The first step in the treatment of the serious hemorrhagic complications of thrombolytic therapy is to stop the infusion of the plasminogen activator and any antithrombotic therapy. Pharmacologic treatment must then focus on reversal of the "lytic state." Four major attributes of the lytic state must be addressed.

Increased Plasminogen Activator Activity

Laboratory assessment of residual plasminogen activator activity utilizes the euglobulin lysis time, chromogenic substrate assays for tissue plasminogen activator, or similar assays of plasmin activity. Unfortunately, in the setting of an acute severe hemorrhagic complication such assays are generally not available in a timely fashion. Consequently, initial management should be based on the half-lives of the plasminogen activator used. Assuming that increased plasminogen activator activity will persist for up to 24 hours after infusion is reasonable. Laboratory assays can then be used to monitor ongoing therapy.

Plasminogen activator inhibitor infusions are not available for human use at this time. Exogenous plasminogen activator inhibitor would be the obvious agent of choice to correct this aspect of the lytic state. Because plasmin is the mediator of the fibrinolytic effect of plasminogen activator therapy, therapeutic interventions now focus on inhibition of plasmin effects.

Increased Plasmin Levels and Activity

Plasmin is a serine protease that acts in two steps. It first binds fibrinogen and fibrin and then cleaves the molecule producing the characteristic fibrin degradation products. Current pharmacologic treatment to reduce fibrinolysis focuses on inhibiting the binding of plasmin to fibrin or fibrinogen and inhibiting the enzymatic activity of plasmin.

Lysine Analogues.[6] Agents of this class are synthetic lysine analogues that bind and activate plasminogen but then allosterically block the enzymatically active site, rendering it unable to bind fibrin or fibrinogen. EACA (6-amino-hexanoic acid or ϵ-aminocaproic acid) and AMCA (trans-*p*-aminomethyl-cyclohexanecarboxylic acid or tranexamic acid) are available for clinical usage. Other than mild differences in potency and pharmacokinetics, these drugs are essentially equivalent.

EACA (ϵ-aminocaproic acid, brand name Amicar) is well absorbed from the gastrointestinal tract and rapidly cleared by the kidneys with approximately 80% excretion within 3 hours after an intravenous dose. The drug is widely distributed in the extravascular space and may be detectable in the urine up to 36 hours later. EACA is usually given as an initial intravenous infusion of 0.1 gm/kg over 30 minutes, followed by a maintenance dose of 0.5 to 1.0 g/h by continuous intravenous infusion. The EACA maintenance dose may also be given in an equivalent dose by an intermittent regimen every 1 to 4 hours, either orally or intravenously. The plasmin inhibitory effect of a single dose of EACA lasts approximately 3 hours.

AMCA (tranexamic acid) is also excreted rapidly in the urine and has a serum half-life similar to that of EACA of 1 to 2 hours. Because AMCA is a much more potent inhibitor than EACA, the inhibitory effect of a single dose lasts 7 to 8 hours. As a result, the dose of AMCA can be lower or the dosing interval longer than that for EACA. The recommended intravenous dose of AMCA is 10 mg/kg of body weight given three to four times daily. The recommended oral regimen is 25 mg/kg body weight taken three to four times daily.

These agents occasionally produce serious side effects, including cerebral thrombosis, venous thrombosis, myonecrosis, disseminated intravascular coagulation, and allergic reactions. Rhabdomyolysis, as suggested by myoglobinuria and muscle weakness, requires cessation of therapy. AMCA and EACA should not be used in pregnant patients.

Aprotinin. Aprotinin (Trasylol) is a low molecular weight polypeptide serine protease inhibitor derived from bovine lung, parotid, and pancreas extract. It is a potent inhibitor of plasmin and other serine proteases, including kallikrein and trypsin.

The standard dose is 2 million kallikrein inhibitory units given intravenously over 10 minutes followed by 70,000 units per hour infusion until hemostasis is obtained. The drug is generally well tolerated but may induce sensitization with a risk of anaphylaxis on repeated exposure.[34]

Most of the clinical experience is derived from its use in cardiac and liver transplantation. There are some reports of the successful use of aprotinin after thrombolysis.[62] The relative efficacy of this agent in the treatment of hemorrhagic complications of thrombolytic therapy compared with that of AMCA is not certain. Table 96–5 gives standard dosages and regimens of antifibrinolytic agents.

Fibrinogen Depletion

Fibrinogen depletion is characteristic of the lytic state and is often profound after standard plasminogen activator therapy. Although fibrinogen levels are not useful in predicting which patient will suffer serious hemorrhage, repletion of fibrinogen is essential in reversal of the hypocoagulable state.

Administration of fresh frozen plasma or cryoprecipitate will replete fibrinogen. Replacement should continue to maintain a minimum of 50% of the normal level of fibrinogen.

Severe Platelet Dysfunction and Thrombocytopenia

Plasmin and plasminogen activator disruption of platelet function plays a significant role in the lytic state. This effect is compounded by the standard use of direct antiplatelet agents in conjunction with plasminogen activator therapy. Although some of the effects are reversible, the time course is uncertain.

Administration of platelets is an essential component of the treatment of the acute hemorrhage. All of the hematologic parameters noted earlier should be followed and maintained for 36 hours following the hemorrhagic events. Serial monitoring of the platelet count, fibrinogen level, activated partial thromboplastin time, bleeding time, and plasmin activity or euglobulin lysis time (if available) should be considered.

In summary, the specific treatment of an acute serious hemorrhagic complication of thrombolytic therapy is to (1) stop the infusion of the lytic agent and any antithrombotic agents (reversal of heparin may be indicated), (2) initiate EACA 0.1 g/kg intravenously over 30 minutes to begin reversal of the fibrinolytic state, (3) immediately infuse fresh frozen plasma to begin to replete the fibrinogen levels, and (4) promptly transfuse the patient with platelets. These interventions should continue through the complete reversal of the lytic state in conjunction with appropriate measures specific for the patient's clinical condition and complications.

PRINCIPAL ANTITHROMBOTIC AGENTS

The prevention and treatment of thrombosis includes use of the just-discussed thrombolytic agents; the antiplatelet drugs such as aspirin, ticlopidine, and the new agent abciximab (ReoPro); and the anticoagulants, heparin, hirudin, and warfarin.

Table 96–5. Antifibrinolygic Agents: Standard Dosage and Regimen

Agent	Initial Dose	Maintenance Dose	Route and Interval
ε-Aminocaproic acid (EACA)	0.1 g/kg IV over 30 min	0.5–1.0 g/h	IV continuous infusion or IV intermittent q1–q4 h or orally q1–q4 h
Tranexamic acid (AMCA)	10 mg/kg IV	10 mg/kg IV or 25 mg/kg orally	q6–q8 h
Aprotinin	2 million kallikrein units IV over 10 min	70,000 units/h IV	IV continuous infusion

Heparin

Intravenous heparin is primarily indicated in the in-hospital management of deep venous thrombosis and pulmonary embolism and has a major role in the emergency management of AMI. Heparin is also useful while performing vascular procedures and inserting prosthetic heart valves. Heparin has limited use as an outpatient drug in patients resistant to oral anticoagulants, in pregnant patients, and in nursing mothers.[63–65] The use of low molecular weight heparin in patients with a recent myocardial infarction treated with SK and heparin and in long-term outpatient management of deep venous thrombosis is presently undergoing evaluation.[66, 67]

Heparin is a naturally occurring glycosaminoglycan. Heparin inhibits coagulation by enhancing the effect of antithrombin III in the inhibition of activated clotting factors IX, X, XI, XII, and thrombin. By definition, 1 unit of heparin renders 1 mL of sheep blood incoagulable.

The dosage of heparin is variable and is presently in evolution. *A standard therapeutic dose of intravenous heparin for acute pulmonary embolus, acute myocardial infarction, and deep venous thrombosis is a 5000 unit (IU) intravenous bolus initially, or 80 IU/kg as an initial loading dose, followed by heparin as a continuous intravenous infusion at 1000 units (IU)/hour, or a maintenance dose of 10 to 25 IU/kg per hour.* The use of weight-adjusted intravenous heparin protocols is gaining favor at many institutions. Careful monitoring of the activated partial thromboplastin time is necessary; it should be maintained at 1.5 to 2.5 times the normal range, or a general therapeutic range of 50 to 85 seconds. Intravenous heparin has a half-life of 60 to 90 minutes. Heparin-induced thrombocytopenia occurs in 1% to 3% of patients.

Bleeding is the most common complication of intravenous heparin use, and because of its short half-life, stopping the infusion may be all that is necessary. For critical cases, intravenous protamine is the antidote. Protamine sulfate is a strongly basic drug that combines with heparin and neutralizes it. One mg of protamine neutralizes 100 units of heparin. Generally up to 50 mg of protamine should be given intravenously over 10 minutes to reverse the effects of heparin. Because the half-life of heparin is only 60 to 90 minutes, the dose of protamine should be halved for every 60 minutes from the time of heparin administration. Protamine has an even shorter half-life than heparin, so "rebound" hemorrhage may occur, requiring the administration of additional protamine.

Hirudin

Hirudin is the specific inhibitor of thrombin originally extracted from the salivary gland of the leech. Hirudin is a 65-amino acid compound that is an irreversible inhibitor of thrombin. Recombinant hirudin is presently being evaluated as an intravenous agent to prevent restenosis after coronary angioplasty and to manage unstable angina.[68–70] Intravenous hirudin is given as an initial bolus injection of 40 mg followed by a continuous intravenous infusion of 0.2 mg/kg per hour for 24 hours, followed by subcutaneous hirudin 40 mg twice daily for 3 days.[69] Although hirudin was impressive compared with heparin in the reduction of major cardiac events in the first 96 hours following coronary angioplasty in one study, it demonstrated no long-term advantage over heparin.[69] Furthermore, bleeding complications are difficult to manage, as there is no specific antidote.

Abciximab (ReoPro)

Abciximab is the fragment antigen binding (Fab) fragment of the chimeric human-murine monoclonal antibody 7E3 (c7E3 Fab). It has been approved for use as an adjunct to percutaneous transluminal coronary angioplasty to prevent abrupt closure of the coronary vessel after angioplasty.[71–74]

Abciximab prevents platelet aggregation by binding to the platelet GpIIb/IIIa receptor and prevents the binding of adhesive glycoproteins to the surface of activated platelets.[71]

Intravenous abciximab is given at a bolus dose of

0.25 mg/kg, followed by continuous infusion of 10 μg/min for 12 hours. Bleeding time exceeds 30 minutes during infusion and returns to normal in 12 to 24 hours.

Evaluation of abciximab in the EPIC trial indicated favorable results, showing a reduction of acute ischemic complications and of clinically evident restenosis following percutaneous transluminal coronary angioplasty.[74] However, bleeding episodes are increased significantly (from 13% for placebo to 24% for abciximab in one study), and there is no specific means of reversing the effects of abciximab.[74] Fresh frozen plasma may be given in the hopes of stopping hemorrhage.

Warfarin

Warfarin (Coumadin) is the most widely used anticoagulant today. Coumadin is indicated for the outpatient management of atrial fibrillation, pulmonary embolism, deep venous thrombosis, and after coronary stent and prosthetic valve placement.[75] The prothrombin time should be maintained at an international normalized ratio of 2.0 to 3.0 in all situations except for mechanical prosthetic valves, in which the ratio is maintained at 2.5 to 3.5.

Warfarin is also a commonly used rodenticide. The anticoagulant rodenticides were discussed in Chapter 68.

Warfarin is an antagonist of the fat-soluble vitamin K and inhibits vitamin K–dependent coagulation factors II (prothrombin), VII (Stable factor), IX (Christmas factor), and X (Stuart factor).

Warfarin is almost completely absorbed and reaches maximal concentration in plasma within 1 hour. It is 99% bound to albumin, with only the free fraction being metabolically active. Metabolism of warfarin is by hepatic microsomal enzymes. The mean half-life of warfarin is 35 hours, and the duration of action may be up to 5 days, although this is highly variable, depending on the patient's diet and other medications.[76] Green vegetables such as spinach, Brussels sprouts, broccoli, cabbage, and lettuce are high in vitamin K content. Drugs such as erythromycin, metronidazole, cimetidine, anabolic steroids, thyroxine, isoniazid, and trimethoprim-sulfamethoxazole enhance anticoagulant effects and prolong the prothrombin time, whereas barbiturates, penicillin, rifampin, griseofulvin, and carbamazepine impair anticoagulant effects and shorten the prothrombin time.[63, 75, 76]

Bleeding is the most common complication, and if the bleeding is minor, such as microscopic hematuria, stopping the drug is all that is necessary. However, with significant hemorrhage, 10 mg of intravenous vitamin K_1 (Aquamephyton) may be administered slowly, diluted in physiologic normal saline at no more than 0.5 mg/min. If given rapidly, intravenous vitamin K_1 has caused ventricular fibrillation.[76–78] In less emergent circumstances vitamin K_1 may be administered as 10 mg subcutaneously. Because the half-life of vitamin K_1 is only 1.7 hours, repeat doses every 4 to 6 hours may be required over a 24-hour period until the prothrombin time returns to normal.[76] If more than 25 mg of vitamin K_1 is administered, the patient will be refractory to further anticoagulation for several days. Because the half-life of warfarin is 35 hours, fresh frozen plasma may be necessary to treat critically bleeding patients.

References

1. Hawiger J: Blood-vascular wall interface in thrombosis and rethrombosis. *In* Haber E, Braunwald E (eds): Thombolysis: Basic Contributions and Clinical Progress. St. Louis, Mosby, 1991.
2. Verstraete M: Biology and chemistry of thrombosis. *In* Haber E, Braunwald E (eds): Thombolysis: Basic Contributions and Clinical Progress. St. Louis, Mosby, 1991.
3. Comp PC, Esmon CT: Generation of fibrinolytic activity by infusion of activated protein C into dogs. J Clin Invest *68:*1221, 1981.
4. Gruber A, Hanson SR, Kelly AB, et al: Inhibition of thrombus formation by activated recombinant protein C in a primate model of arterial thrombosis. Circulation *82:*578, 1990.
5. Kamat SG, Michelson AD, Benoit SE, et al: Fibrinolysis inhibits shear stress-induced platelet aggregation. Circulation *92:*1399, 1995.
6. Sherry S, Marder VJ: Therapy with antifibrinolytic agents. *In* Colman RW, Hirsch J, Marder VJ, et al (eds): Hemostasis and Thrombosis: Basic Principles and Clinical Practice. 3rd ed. Philadelphia, J.B. Lippincott, 1994.
7. Hajjar KA, Nachman RL: The human endothelial cell plasmin-generating system. *In* Colman RW, Hirsch J, Marder VJ, et al (eds): Hemostasis and Thrombosis: Basic Principles and Clinical Practice. 3rd ed. Philadelphia, J.B. Lippincott, 1994.
8. Coller BS: Platelets and thrombolytic therapy. N Engl J Med *322:*33, 1990.
9. Tillett WS, Garner RL: The fibrinolytic activity of hemolytic streptococci. J Exp Med *58:*485, 1933.
10. McFarlane RG, Pilling J: Fibrinolytic activity of normal urine. Nature *159:*779, 1947.
11. Sobel GW, Mohler SR, Jones NW, et al: Urokinase: An activator of plasma profibrinolysin extracted from urine. Am J Physiol *171:*768, 1952.
12. Astrup T, Permin PM: Fibrinolysis in animal organism. Nature *159:*681, 1947.
13. Rijken DC, Collen D: Purification and characterization of the plasminogen activator secreted by human melanoma cells in culture. J Biol Chem *256:*7035, 1981.
14. Hoffman JJML, van Rey FJW, Bonnier JJRM, et al: Systemic effects of BRL 26921 during thrombolytic treatment of acute myocardial infarction. Thromb Res *37:*567, 1985.
15. Kornowski R, Battler A: Activated protein C and antithrombin-III activity during arterial thrombolysis with recombinant tissue-type plasminogen activator in rabbits. Coron Artery Dis *4:*1115, 1993.
16. Jackson KW, Tang J: Complete amino acid sequence of streptokinase and its homology with serine proteases. Biochemistry *21:*6220, 1982.
17. Monk JP, Heel RC: Anisoylated plasminogen streptokinase activator complex (APSAC): A review of its mechanism of action, clinical pharmacology and therapeutic use in acute myocardial infarction. Drugs *34:*25, 1987.
18. Rutherford RB, Comerota AJ: Urokinase. *In* Messerli FH (ed): Cardiovascular Drug Therapy. 2nd ed. Philadelphia, W.B. Saunders Co., 1996.
19. Van de Werf F, Nobuhara M, Collen D: Coronary thrombolysis with human single-chain urokinase-type plasminogen activator (scu-UK) in patients with acute myocardial infarction. Ann Intern Med *104:*345, 1986.

20. Van de Werf F, Vanhecke J, De Geest H, et al: Coronary thrombolysis with recombinant single-chain urokinase-type plasminogen activator (rscu-UK) in patients with acute myocardial infarction. Circulation *74:*1066, 1986.
21. Rijken DC, Hoylaerts M, Collen D: Fibrinolytic properties of one-chain and two-chain human extrinsic (tissue-type) plasminogen activator. J Biol Chem *257:*2920, 1982.
22. Verstraete M, Bounameauz H, deCock F, et al: Pharmacokinetics and systemic fibrinolytic effects of recombinant human tissue-type plasminogen activator (rt-PA) in humans. J Pharmacol Exp Ther *235:*506, 1985.
23. Garabedian HD, Gold HK, Leinbach RC, et al: Comparative properties of two clinical preparations of recombinant human tissue-type plasminogen activator in patients with acute myocardial infarction. J Am Coll Cardiol *9:*599, 1987.
24. TIMI Research Group: Comparison of invasive and conservative strategies after treatment with intravenous tissue plasminogen activator in acute myocardial infarction: Results of the thrombolysis in myocardial infarction (TIMI) phase II trial. N Engl J Med *320:*618, 1989.
25. GUSTO Investigators: An international randomized trial comparing four thrombolytic strategies for acute myocardial infarction. N Engl J Med *329:*673, 1993.
26. Goldhaber SZ, Haire WD, Feldstein ML, et al: Alteplase versus heparin in acute pulmonary embolism: Randomized trial assessing right ventricular function and pulmonary perfusion. Lancet *341:*507, 1993.
27. The NINDS rt-PA Stroke Study Group: Tissue plasminogen activator for acute ischemic stroke. N Engl J Med *333:*1581, 1995.
28. Marder VJ, Sherry S: Thrombolytic therapy: Current status. N Engl J Med *318:*1512, 1988.
29. Pitney WR, Pettit JE, Armstrong L: Control of heparin therapy. BMJ *4:*139, 1980.
30. Levine MN, Goldhaber SZ, Gore JM, et al: Hemorrhagic complications of thrombolytic therapy in the treatment of myocardial infarction and venous thromboembolism. Chest *108:*291S, 1995.
31. Marder VJ, Hirsch J, Bell WR: Rationale and practical basis of thrombolytic therapy. *In* Colman RW, Hirsch J, Marder VJ, et al (eds): Hemostasis and Thrombosis: Basic Principles and Clinical Practice. 3rd ed. Philadelphia, J.B. Lippincott, 1994.
32. Fibrinolytic Therapy Trialists' (FTT) Collaborative Group: Indications for fibrinolytic therapy in suspected acute myocardial infarction: Collaborative overview of early mortality and major morbidity results from all randomized trials of more than 1000 patients. Lancet *343:*311, 1994.
33. Third International Study of Infarct Survival Collaborative Group: ISIS-3: A randomised comparison of streptokinase vs tissue plasminogen activator vs anistreplase and of aspirin plus heparin vs aspirin alone among 41,299 cases of suspected acute myocardial infarction. Lancet *1:*753, 1992.
34. de Bono DP, More RS: Prevention and management of bleeding complications after thrombolysis. Int J Cardiol *38:*1, 1993.
35. TIMI-9A Investigators: Hirudin in acute myocardial infarction. Circulation *90:*1624, 1994
36. TIMI Research Group: Immediate vs delayed catheterization and angioplasty following thrombolytic therapy for acute myocardial infarction. JAMA *260:*2849, 1988.
37. SWIFT (Should We Intervene Following Thrombolysis?) Trial Study Group: SWIFT trial of delayed elective intervention vs consecutive treatment after thrombolysis with anistreplase in acute myocardial infarction. BMJ *302:*555, 1991.
38. Topol E, Califf R: Thrombolytic therapy for elderly patients. N Engl J Med *327:*45, 1992.
39. Meneveau N, Bassand J, Schiele F, et al: Safety of thrombolytic therapy in elderly patients with massive pulmonary embolism: A comparison with nonelderly patients. J Am Coll Cardiol *22:*1075, 1993.
40. Greckos ZG, Schocken DD: Bilateral vitreous hemorrhages as a consequence of thrombolytic therapy successfully treated with vitrectomy in a patient without diabetes. Am Heart J *130:*611, 1995.
41. Higgs ER, Parditt VJ, Harney BA, et al: Use of thrombolysis for acute myocardial infarction in the presence of diabetic retinopathy in the UK, and associated ocular haemorrhagic complications. Diabet Med *12:*426, 1994.
42. Sekyema YF, Baltazar RF: Is thrombolytic therapy safe during active menstruation? J Emerg Med *13:*345, 1995.
43. Scholz KH, Tebbe U, Herrmann C, et al: Frequency of complications of cardiopulmonary resuscitation after thrombolysis during acute myocardial infarction. Am J Cardiol *69:*724, 1992.
44. Ellis SG: Interventions in acute myocardial infarction. Circulation *81*(S4):43, 1990.
45. Blankenship JC, Indeck M: Spontaneous splenic rupture complicating anticoagulant or thrombolytic therapy. Am J Med *94:*433, 1993.
46. Jishi F, Sissons CE, Silverstone EJ, et al: Oesophageal dissection after thrombolytic treatment for myocardial infarction. Thorax *47:*835, 1992.
47. Thomas WO, Harris CN, D'Amore TF, et al: Bilateral forearm and hand compartment syndrome following thrombolysis for acute myocardial infarction: A case report. J Emerg Med *12:*467, 1994.
48. Becker RC, Charlesworth A, Wilcox RG, et al: Cardiac rupture associated with thrombolytic therapy: Impact of time to treatment in the late assessment of thrombolytic efficacy (LATE) study. JACC *25:*1063, 1995.
49. Gore JM, Sloan M, Price TR, et al: Intracerebral hemorrhage, cerebral infarction, and subdural hematoma after acute myocardial infarction and thrombolytic therapy in the thrombolysis in myocardial infarction study. Thrombolysis in myocardial infarction, phase II, pilot and clinical trial. Circulation *83:*448, 1991.
50. Gore JM, Granger CB, Simoons ML, et al: Stroke after thrombolysis: Mortality and functional outcomes in the GUSTO-1 trial. Circulation *92:*2811, 1995.
51. Grupo Italiano per lo Studio della Sopravivenza Nell'infarto Miocardico—GISSI 2: A factorial randomized trial of alteplase versus streptokinase and heparin versus no heparin among 12,490 patients with acute myocardial infarction. Lancet *336:*65, 1990.
52. Maggioni AP, Franzosi MG, Santor E, et al: The risk of stroke in patients with acute myocardial infarction after thrombolytic and antithrombotic treatment. N Engl J Med *327:*1, 1992.
53. Selker HP, Beshansky JR, Schmid CH, et al: Presenting pulse pressure predicts thrombolytic therapy-related intracranial hemorrhage: Thrombolytic predictive instrument (TPI) project results. Circulation *90:*1657, 1994.
54. GUSTO IIa Investigators: Randomized trial of intravenous heparin versus recombinant hirudin for acute coronary syndromes. Circulation *90:*1631, 1994.
55. Neuhaus KL, Essen R, Tebbe U, et al: Safety observations from the pilot phase of the randomized r-hirudin for improvement of thrombolysis (HIT-III) study. Circulation *90:*1638, 1994.
56. Sloan MA, Price TR, Petito CK, et al: Clinical features and pathogenesis of intracerebral hemorrhage after rt-PA and heparin therapy for acute myocardial infarction: The thrombolysis in myocardial infarction, phase II, pilot and randomized clinical trial combined experience. Neurology *45:*649, 1995.
57. Hacke W, Kaste M, Fieschi C, for the ECASS Study Group: Intravenous thrombolysis with recombinant tissue plasminogen activator for acute hemispheric stroke. JAMA *274:*1017, 1995.
58. Lew AS, Laramee P, Cercek B, et al: The hypotensive effect of intravenous streptokinase in patients with acute myocardial infarction. Circulation *72:*1321, 1985.
59. Herlitz J, Hartford M, Solveigh A, et al: Occurrence of hypotension during streptokinase infusion in suspected acute myocardial infarction, and its relation to metoprolol therapy. Am J Cardiol *71:*1021, 1993.
60. Bautista RE: Embolic stroke following thrombolytic therapy for myocardial infarction in a patient with preexisting ventricular thrombi. Stroke *26:*324, 1995.
61. Pape LA, Love DG, Gore JM: Massive thromboembolic stroke and death after fibrinolytic therapy of St. Jude prosthetic

mitral valve thrombosis: Documentation by transthoracic Doppler echocardiography. Am Heart J *128:*406, 1994.
62. Akhtar TM, Goodchild CS, Boylan MKG: Reversal of streptokinase-induced bleeding with aprotinin for emergency cardiac surgery. Anaesthesia *47:*226, 1992.
63. Harker LA: Antithrombotic therapy. *In* Bennett JC, Plum F (eds): Cecil Textbook of Medicine. 20th ed. Philadelphia, W.B. Saunders, pp 115–122, 1996.
64. Mahaffey KW, Granger CB, Collins R, et al: Overview of randomized trials of intravenous heparin in patients with acute myocardial infarction treated with thrombolytic therapy. Am J Cardiol *77:*551, 1996.
65. Hirsh J: Heparin. New Engl J Med *324:*1565, 1991.
66. Glick A, Kornowski R, Michowich Y, et al: Reduction of reinfarction and angina with use of low-molecular-weight heparin therapy after streptokinase (and heparin) in acute myocardial infarction. Am J Cardiol *77:*1145, 1996.
67. Levine M, Gent M, Hirsh J, et al: A comparison of low-molecular-weight heparin administered primarily at home with unfractionated heparin administered in the hospital for deep vein thrombosis. N Engl J Med *334:*677, 1996.
68. Fuchs J, Cannon CP, and the TIMI 7 Investigators: Hirulog in the treatment of unstable angina. Circulation *92:*727, 1995.
69. Serruys PW, Herrman JPR, Simon R, and others for the Helvetica Investigators. A comparison of hirudin with heparin in the prevention of restenosis after coronary angioplasty. N Engl J Med *333:*757, 1995.
70. Mruk JS, Zoldhely P, Webster MWJ, et al: Does antithrombotic therapy influence residual thrombus after thrombolysis of platelet-rich thrombus? Circulation *93:*792, 1996.
71. Abciximab to prevent vessel closure after angioplasty. Med Lett *37:*52, 1995.
72. Coller BS, Anderson K, Weisman HF: New antiplatelet agents. Thromb Haemost *74:*302, 1995.
73. The EPIC Investigators: Use of a monoclonal antibody directed against the platelet glycoprotein IIb/IIIa receptor in high-risk coronary angioplasty. New Engl J Med *330:*956, 1994.
74. Lefkovits J, Ivanhoe RJ, Califf RM, et al: Effects of abciximab on acute and six-month outcomes after PTCA for acute myocardial infarction. Am J Cardiol *77:*1045, 1996.
75. Spandorfer JM, Merli GJ: Outpatient anticoagulation issues for the primary care physician. Med Clin North Am *80:*475, 1996.
76. Schuh A, Keating A: Anticoagulants. *In* Haddad LM, Winchester JF (eds): Clinical Management of Poisoning and Drug Overdose. 2nd ed. Philadelphia, W.B. Saunders Co., pp 308–320, 1990.
77. Lefrere JJ, Girot R: Acute cardiovascular collapse during intravenous vitamin K_1 injection. Thromb Haemost *58:*790, 1987.
78. Pelletier G, Attali P, Ink O: Arrest cardiorespiratoire après injection intraveineuse de vitamine K_1. Gastro Clin Biol *10:*615, 1986.

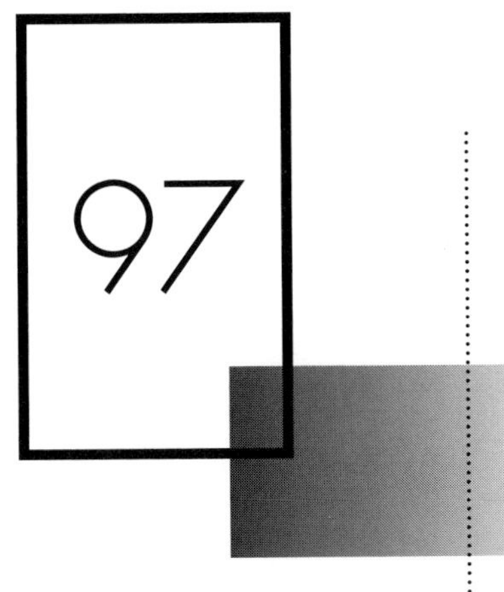

SECTION I

HERBAL MEDICINE AND MISCELLANEOUS AGENTS

Herbal, Traditional, and Alternative Medicine

MICHAEL W. SHANNON, MD, MPH

Despite the continued development of medical and pharmacologic therapies for the treatment of illness, as many as 50% of people worldwide use alternative treatments, including herbal and traditional medicines.[1] Even in industrial nations, where there is no dearth of pharmaceutical agents, many seek "natural" products for their ailments. In one of the few studies of its kind, Eisenberg and colleagues, investigating the prevalence of use of unconventional medicine in the United States, found that one third of a sample population had used at least one unconventional therapy in the prior year.[2] Highest use was found among those with relatively more education and higher incomes. Annual prevalence was 3% for herbal medicines, 1% for homeopathy, and almost 1% for folk remedies. Reasons for using these therapies were extensive, including treatment of back pain, anxiety, headaches, cancer, and insomnia. In a similar pediatric study, 11% of children were found to have received one or more forms of alternative therapy since their birth.[3] Parents stated that they chose alternative medicines after hearing about them from a friend, because of a fear of drug side effects, because they were dissatisfied with conventional medicine, or because they received more personal attention from alternative medicine practitioners. In a study conducted in a New York emergency department near the Chinatown district, Pearl and associates found that 43% of patients had used a traditional Chinese therapy within a week of their emergency department visit.[4] Fifty-eight per cent of these had used at least one oral herbal preparation. Eleven patients admitted using therapies that included unidentified tablets, nose drops, or topical preparations and animal preparations such as deer antler. Finally, it is of epidemiologic importance that psychoactive plant materials such as jimsonweed, nutmeg, and morning glory seeds are often ingested as substances of abuse.

The increasing interest in alternative medicines as well as their proven therapeutic value[5–8] led in 1992 to the establishment of the Office of Alternative Medicine at the National Institutes of Health. Through this organization, investigators can obtain support for research designed to determine the range of benefit that alternative medicines offer, with the goal of "integrating validated alternative medical practice with current conventional medical procedures."[9] Additional evidence of the public's interest in alternative medicine was shown in a survey that found that 10% of American pharmacies carry herbal remedies.[10] The potential routes of administration of alternative medicines include topical, rectal, and vaginal application as well as ingestion, injection, and inhalation.[11]

Nonetheless, alternative medicines, including herbs and "nutritional supplements," are repeatedly associated with episodes of poisoning. In some cases, mass poisonings have occurred because these substances are widely used before their toxicity is realized. The Food and Drug Administration (FDA) is given responsibility for protecting the public from dietary, nutritional, and medical hazards. Unfortunaly, the FDA has been given limited power to regulate herbal, homeopathic, and nutritional agents because they fall into an ambiguous category.[12] When Congress passed the Dietary Supplement Health and Education Act, the FDA's ability to regulate alternative medicines was further weakened.[9, 10] As a result of this new law, alternative medicines are placed in a category that is virtually immune from FDA regulation. Six major features of this law are as follows:

1. Alternative medicines can be marketed with no testing of efficacy.
2. Companies do not have to prove that their product is safe before marketing. Instead, the FDA must prove that the product is unsafe.
3. Supplements need not be manufactured according to any standards (quality control standards will be introduced eventually).
4. Certain product claims are permitted. For example, products cannot be claimed to cure a disease, but the label can discuss how a supplement affects the body's function.
5. Label statements do not require extensive supportive evidence.
6. FDA approval is not needed for marketing claims.

As a result of this law, intoxication by alternative medications of all types poses an even greater threat. In an attempt to identify adverse effects of these medicines, the FDA has implemented MEDWATCH. Adverse reactions from alternative medications can and should be reported immediately (telephone number 1-800-332-1088).[12]

HERBAL MEDICINES

An herbal medicine can be defined as a plant extract that is used in relatively unrefined form to achieve a therapeutic effect. Mushrooms and other fungi are also considered to be herbal medicines. There is no controversy that many of these medicines have potent pharmacologic actions.[13, 14] It is this same potency that often makes them responsible for inadvertent poisoning.

The use of herbs and medicinal plants spans history and has been universal, occurring in every culture on earth. For example, Egyptian writings chronicled the use of medicinal herbs more than 4000 years ago; at that time, for example, poppy extracts were used to quiet crying children. Ayurvedic medicine (literally, "knowledge of how to live") emphasized the value of herbal medicines in texts dating back to 2500 BC. The Chinese Materia Medica lists about 5800 medicinal plants; approximately 2500 medicinal herbs are listed in Indian medical texts, and at least 800 are used in tropical Africa. As a general rule, herbalists regularly use a repertoire of 150 to 200 plants. Herbalists uncommonly prescribe animal parts, metals, and minerals.

One of the most widely practiced and enduring herbal traditions has been that of Chinese herbal medicine. This form of herbal medicine has been traced back to about 2500 BC. In Chinese culture, herbs are considered basic to the treatment of all illness, in conjunction with aids such as acupuncture or acupressure. Generally speaking, among all alternative medical practices, Chinese herbal medicine has become the form most familiar to practitioners.

Herbs are prescribed in standard formulas created by a trained herbalist or an individual with limited knowledge of herbal medicine. Typical prescriptions consist of 10 to 15 herbs.[15] When herbs are used to make herbal remedies, any or all parts of the plant can be used. These include flowers, leaves, seeds, roots, sap/resins, fruit, bark, or bulbs. These herbs can be administered in a number of forms (decoctions and so on); they can be eaten in isolation or with food. Common terminology for herbal remedies includes the following:[14]

Infusion—Herbs that are steeped in hot water, similar to tea.
Decoction—A technique that extracts more of the plant's ingredients by soaking then boiling the plant in water.
Tincture—An herb extract prepared by steeping the herb in a 25% mixture of water and alcohol.
Syrup—An herb extract prepared in honey or sugar in order to make it less unpleasant.
Compress—A cloth pad soaked in a hot herbal extract and applied to a painful area.
Poultice—Similar to a compress, except that the entire herb is applied rather than an extract.
Emmenagogue—An herb that induces or increases menstrual flow.
Carminative—An herb that reduces or prevents flatulence.

Systematic studies of poisoning due to herbal remedies are few. In a study conducted in China, 0.2% of all hospital admissions were the result of adverse reactions to Chinese herbal medicines.[15] Another Chinese study reviewed 33 hospitalizations resulting from toxicity related to herbal medicine.[15, 16] The most common herb leading to toxic reactions was aconitine (accounting for 61%). In nine patients, adverse effects were life threatening; one fatality was reported.

A number of factors magnify the toxicity of herbal preparations that should otherwise be beneficial:

Dose. Unlike the pharmaceutical industry, in which the quantity of active agent is consistent from pill to pill, quantities of active drug in a plant are highly variable. Also, the content of active drug is influenced by the particular species of plant, the growing conditions, the part of the plant, and its form when used (wet versus dry).

Route of Exposure. Many herbs are applied topically, particularly those used to treat skin and musculoskeletal conditions. Although topical herbs occasionally produce systemic toxicity, their adverse effects are usually confined to development of contact dermatitis or phytodermatitis.[17] Many herbs are smoked as substitutes for tobacco. Because of the richness of the pulmonary blood supply and the lipophilicity of the active principles in these herbs, effects can be immediate. Herbs that are commonly smoked include yohimbine, California poppy, catnip, cinnamon, hops, hydrangea, juniper, kavakava, lobelia, passion flower, periwinkle, prickly poppy, snakeroot, thorn apple, wild lettuce, and wormwood.[18]

Duration of Use. Many herbs with little to no toxicity after short-term use can produce adverse effects if they are ingested for a considerable time.

For example, chronic use of pyrrolizidine alkaloids produces hepatic veno-occlusive disease, whereas short-term ingestion has no apparent hazards. Chronicity is also an important factor in the development of malignancies after use of carcinogenic teas such as sassafras and comfrey.[19, 20]

Pre-existing Disease. As the study by Eisenberg and colleagues illustrates,[2] herbal remedies are often sought as alternative treatments for illness or disease. Therefore, those using them may have pre-existing disease that modulates the effect of that agent. For example, in those who are taking coumarin anticoagulant and begin to ingest herbs such as tonka bean or melilot, a bleeding diathesis can occur. Similarly, in those with an allergy to ragweed, ingestion of chamomile tea could lead to severe allergic reaction.

Improper Identification. Although trained herbalists can confidently prescribe herbs, an untrained or poorly trained herbalist sometimes misidentifies an herb and prescribes it, with disastrous consequences. For example, comfrey is similar to foxglove in appearance. Ingestion of foxglove, from which digitalis is derived, could lead to severe cardiac disturbances. The same risk of misidentification can occur when names are confused. Cohosh, a common herb used as a sedative and anti-inflammatory agent, generally refers to *Cimicifuga racemosa* (black cohosh) or *Caulophyllum thalictroides* (blue cohosh). However, in other regions, cohosh refers to the toxic baneberry.[19]

Herb Preparation. How an herb is prepared has the most important influence on both the pharmacologic and toxicologic actions of the herb. Again, an untrained herbalist may prescribe all parts of a plant when only the leaf or flower should be used. The bark of the elder has considerable therapeutic value, but its stem is extremely toxic, containing cyanogenic alkaloids.[19] Equally important, an herb may be administered according to its dry weight rather than wet weight. Because the dried product almost always has a higher concentration of active agent than the fresh form, inadvertent overdose can occur.

Contamination. Herbs can become contaminated by toxins by a number of means. The herbs sold by herbalists as well as those that are picked in the wild can be contaminated by agents including metals if they are grown in regions with contaminated soil, particularly if the plant is capable of incorporating the toxin. Teas prepared from herbs have been reported to contain lead, cadmium, mercury, copper, zinc, fluoride, and arsenic.[20] Another means by which contamination can occur is by using plant products from improper sources. For example, commercial plant seeds may be used to prepare an herbal remedy. However, these seeds often contain pesticides or fungicides designed to lengthen their shelf life. If these seeds are ingested, serious toxicity can result. Finally, because herbs are often processed into tablets, capsules, and other pharmaceutical forms (commonly referred to as Chinese proprietary medicine), accidental or intentional adulteration by pharmaceutical agents can occur. Table 97–1 summarizes the clinical toxicity of popular herbs.

Herbal Teas

The preparation of teas is the most common use of herbal medicines. The illnesses associated with the use of herb teas can be placed into system categories of gastrointestinal (GI) (including hepatic), hematologic, autonomic, neurologic, cardiac, allergic, and carcinogenic.

Gastrointestinal. GI upset is the most common adverse effect associated with the use of herb teas. Although this is generally mild, severe vomiting and diarrhea can be produced by ingestion of poke root (*Phytolacca americana*), buckthorn (*Hipthothae rhamnoides*), and senna (*Cassia angustifolia*).

The term *herbal hepatitis* has been coined to describe the relatively frequent occurrence of herb-associated liver injury.[21] For example, fatal hepatitis has been associated with ingestion of wild germander (*Teucrium chamaedrys*).[22] Use of "chaparral" teas was associated with development of hepatitis (leading to the need for liver transplantation in one patient). This tea, which is derived from the ground leaves of the creosote bush (*Larrea tridentata*), has been promoted as an antioxidant, a blood purifier, and an inhibitor of aging.[23, 24] Another reported outbreak of hepatitis was associated with the use of Chinese herbs[25]; in this case, the responsible toxin was not identified.

Hematologic. Herbs may contain alkaloids that are toxic to red blood cells. Among these are salicylate-containing agents such as willow bark; these can lead to hemolysis if ingested by an individual with glucose-6-phosphate dehydrogenase (G-6-PD) deficiency. Other herbs contain coumadin-like agents, including tonka beans (*Coumarouna oppositifolia*), melilot (*Melilotus officinalis*), and woodruff (*Galium odoratum*); excess consumption can produce a coagulopathy.[20]

Autonomic. Herbs that affect the autonomic nervous system include those containing the anticholinergic drugs atropine, scopolamine, and hyoscyamine.[20] These include mandrake (*Mandragon officinarum*), thorn apple (*Datura* spp.), lobelia (*Lobelia inflata*), burdock root (*Arctium lappa*), and jimson root (*Datura stramonium*).[26] Other agents acting on the autonomic nervous system include sympathomimetics, e.g., mormon tea (*Ephedra nevadensis*), which contains ephedrine; snakeroot tea (*Rauwolfia serpentina*), which contains reserpine; and yohimbe bark (*Corynanthe yohimbe*), which contains yohimbine, a central nervous system α_2-adrenergic antagonist.

Neurologic. A large number of herbal teas contain psychoactive substances that are the basis of their use (e.g., those containing caffeine). Teas associated with central nervous system toxicity include the kavakava (*Piper methysticum*), jimson root (*Datura* spp.), and nutmeg.[27, 20]

Table 97–1. Clinical Toxicity of Selected Herbs

Common Name	Botanic Name	Therapeutic Uses	Potential Toxicity
Aconite (monkshood, wolfsbane)	*Aconitum* spp.	Sedative, analgesic, antihypertensive	Cardiac arrhythmias
Aloe	*Aloe* spp.	Burns, skin diseases	Nephritis, GI upset
Betel nut	*Areca catechu*	Mood elevation	Bronchoconstriction, oral cancers
Bloodroot	*Sanguinaria canadensis*	Emetic, cathartic, eczema	GI upset, vertigo, visual disturbances
Chaparral (greasewood)	*Larrea tridentata*	Aging, free radical scavenging	Hepatitis
Compound Q	*Trichosanthes kirilowi*	Antihelminthis, cathartic	Diarrhea, hypoglycemia, CNS toxicity
Dandelion	*Taraxacum officinale*	Diuretic, heartburn remedy	Anaphylaxis
Figwort (xuan shen)	*Scrophularia* spp.	Anti-inflammatory, antibacterial	Cardiac stimulation
Ginseng	*Panax quinquefolium*	Antihypertensive, aphrodisiac, stimulant, mood elevation, digestive aid	Ginseng abuse syndrome
Goldenseal	*Hydrastis canadensis*	Digestive aid, mucolytic, anti-infective	Uterine, cardiac stimulation; GI upset, leukopenia
Hellebore	*Vertrum* spp.	Antihypertensive	Vomiting, bradycardia, hypotension
Hyssop	*Hyssopus officinalis*	Asthma, mucolytic	Seizures
Juniper	*Juniperus communis*	Hallucinogen	GI upset, seizures, renal injury, hypotension, bradycardia
Kavakava	*Piper methysticum*	Sedative	Inebriation
Kombucha		Stimulant	Metabolic acidosis, hepatotoxicity, death
Licorice	*Glycyrrhiza* spp.	Indigestion	Mineralocorticoid effects
Lily of the valley	*Convallaria* spp.	Cardiotonic	GI (nausea, vomiting), cardiac arrhythmias
Linn	*Salix caprea*	Purgative	Hemolysis with glucose-6-phosphate dehydrogenase deficiency
Lobelia (Indian tobacco)	*Lobelia* spp.	Stimulant	Nicotine intoxication
Ma Huang	*Ephedra sinica*	Stimulant	Sympathetic crisis, especially with monoamine oxidase inhibitors
Mandrake	*Mandragora officinarum*	Hallucinogen	Anticholinergic syndrome
Mormon tea	*Ephedra nevadensis*	Stimulant, asthma, antipyretic	Hypertension, sympathomimetic
Nutmeg	*Myristica fragrans*	Hallucinogen, abortifacient	Hallucinations, GI upset
Oleander	*Nerium oleander*	Cardiac stimulant	Cardiac arrhythmias
Passion flower	*Passiflora caerulea*	Hallucinogen	Hallucinations, seizures, hypotension
Periwinkle	*Vinca* spp.	Anti-inflammatory, diabetes	Alopecia, seizures, hepatotoxicity
Pokeweed	*Phytolacca* spp.	Arthritis, chronic pain	GI upset, seizures, death
Sabah	*Sauropus androgynus*	Weight loss, vision	Pulmonary injury
Sage	*Salvia* spp.	CNS stimulant	Seizures
Snakeroot	*Rauwolfia serpentina*	Sedative, antihypertensive	Bradycardia, coma
Squill	*Urginea maritima*	Arthritis, cardiac stimulant	Seizures, arrhythmias, death
Thorn apple	*Datura stramonium*	Hallucinations	Anticholinergic
Tonka bean	*Dipteryx odoratum*	Anticoagulant	Bleeding diathesis
Valerian root	*Valeriana* spp.	Sedative	Sedation, obtundation
Wild (squirting) cucumber	*Ecbalium elaterium*	Constipation, anti-inflammatory, rheumatic disease	Airway obstruction
Wormwood (mugwort)	*Artemisia* spp.	Stimulant, hallucinogen	Hallucinations, seizures, uterine stimulation
Yohimbine	*Coryanthe yohimbe*	Aphrodisiac, stimulant	Hypertension, sympathetic crisis

GI, gastrointestinal; CNS, central nervous system.

Cardiac. Herbal teas associated with cardiotoxicity include those prepared from squill (*Urginea maritima*), lily-of-the-valley (*Convallaria majalis*), and oleander (*Thevetia* spp.). Some cardiac glycosides (e.g., those in oleander) produce toxic manifestations that resemble digitalis poisoning and that, like digitalis, respond to the administration of digoxin antibody fragments (Digibind).

Allergic. Chamomile (from *Chamomilla* spp.) is a popular sedative. However, it is closely related to the ragweed and chrysanthemum families. Exposure to this tea can therefore produce a mild allergic reaction or frank anaphylaxis.

Carcinogenic. Sassafras is a popular tea that was once prescribed for a number of therapeutic effects. However, its active principle, safrole, is a recognized hepatic carcinogen. As a result, safrole has been banned from use by the FDA.[28] However, sassafras can still occasionally be found in health food or herbal stores.

Pyrrolizidine Toxicity

Many herbal teas contain pyrrolizidine alkaloids. These are a group of approximately 200 distinct substances found widely among plants.[29] The teas, such as comfrey, are prescribed as sedatives and as treatment for amenorrhea. However, since the first description of *Senecio* disease (hepatic veno-occlusive syndrome) in 1920, epidemics of pyrrolizidine-associated hepatic disease have repeatedly occurred. These alkaloids are highly hepatotoxic and, in some cases, carcinogenic.[30]

The hallmark of pyrrolizidine intoxication is the development of veno-occlusive disease, a hepatic disorder that is similar but not identical to the Budd-Chiari syndrome. The mechanism of pyrrolizidine toxicity appears to be formation of toxic pyrroles by P-450 enzymes; these pyrroles alkylate nucleophilic groups on cell macromolecules.[31] Pyrrolizidine alkaloids can be transmitted across the placenta; in one case in which a woman ingested an herbal tea during her pregnancy, her newborn developed fatal hepatic veno-occlusive disease.[32] Despite their well-characterized toxicity, which can occur after ingestion of as little as 85 mg of pyrrolizidine alkaloid, pyrrolizidine-containing teas are widely available in herbal and health food stores.[30] The herbs most commonly associated with hepatic veno-occlusive disease are *Heliatropim, Crotolaria, Senecio,* and *Symphytum.* Other herbs containing pyrrolizidine are listed in Table 97–2. Plant roots can contain 10 times more alkaloid than the leaf. Other toxicities associated with pyrrolizidine alkaloids include disturbances of GI, pancreatic, and renal function. Interestingly, inadvertent exposure to pyrrolizidine agents can also occur through their contamination of dietary staples. For example, as a result of contaminated grain, epidemics of hepatic veno-occlusive disease occurred in both Afghanistan and India in 1976, affecting more than 2000 persons and causing more than 30 deaths.[29, 31] Epidemiologically, consumption of pyrrolizidine-containing plants is widespread in Africa, South and Central America, and Jamaica.[31] Jamaican bush tea, a popular drink, is largely prepared with *Crotolaria* species, making veno-occlusive disease endemic on this island.[31] Pyrrolizidine poisoning has also been blamed for major cases of livestock loss in the Pacific Northwest.[29, 31]

Table 97–2. Pyrrolizidine-Containing Teas

Common Name	Botanic Name
Coltsfoot	*Tussilago farfara*
Comfrey	*Symphytum officinale*
Gordolobo	*Senecio longilobus*
Groundsel	*Senecio vulgaris*
Mate	*Ilex paraguayensis*
Tansy ragwort	*Senecio jacobea*
T'u-san-chi	*Gynura segetum*

The clinical presentation of hepatic veno-occlusive disease begins with severe abdominal pain and vomiting. Physical examination reveals hepatomegaly, abdominal distention, and ascites. In children, the clinical picture can mimic Reye's syndrome.[31] On biopsy, characteristic histopathology consists of perivenular congestion, sinusoidal dilatation, and occlusion of terminal venules by connective tissue. This is also the pattern seen in the Budd-Chiari syndrome.

The diagnosis of pyrrolizidine hepatotoxicity is made on the basis of history, clinical evidence of veno-occlusive disease, and pathognomonic histopathology. Treatment is supportive.

Clinical Toxicity of Specific Herbs

Ginseng. *Ginseng* is a Chinese word meaning "the essence of man."[33] This herb has been used for centuries to treat a broad range of illnesses.[19] From the botanic genus *Panax,* ginseng is promoted as a respiratory, digestive, and central nervous system stimulant; a cure for fatigue; a treatment for ulcers; and a cholesterol-lowering agent. Ginseng's most active principles are alkaloids known as *saponins* (also referred to as *panaxosides* or *ginsenoisides*). Scientific investigations have shown that these agents can release histamine; block calcium mobilization in smooth muscle, producing hypotension; stimulate α_2-adrenergic receptors; stimulate erythropoiesis; increase adrenocorticotropic hormone, antidiuretic hormone, and cortisol secretion; raise sperm count; increase glucose utilization; increase levels of circulating immunoglobulins; and inhibit the cells of tumor cells cultivated *in vitro.*[33] Therapeutically, ginseng has been prescribed for the treatment of shock, hypertension, hyperlipidemia, diabetes mellitus, depression, cough, headaches, and fever.

Excessive use of ginseng (more than 3 g daily) is associated with a ginseng abuse syndrome consisting of diarrhea, anxiety, insomnia, nonspecific dermatitis, depression, amenorrhea, and hypertension.[19] Treatment of this transient, self-limited condition is supportive.

Aconite. Aconites are among the most popular yet toxic herbs. At one time, execution of criminals was performed by the administration of aconite decoctions. The *Aconitum* genus includes many species, the most common being *A. napellus,* popularly referred to as monkshood, wolfsbane, or friar's cap. Aconite is found in Chinese decoctions or soups including Fu Zi, Wu Tao, Cao Wu, Chuan Wu, Ts'ao Wu, Futxu, Xue Shang Yi Zhi Gao, Shi-I, Fu Zi, and Sen Fu. Herbalists generally prescribe aconite for treatment of musculoskeletal complaints, angina, and congestive heart failure and as a sedative. The active principles of aconite have been shown to have pharmacologic properties that include stimulation of adrenocorticotropic hormone secretion.[34]

With the GI tract, nervous system, and heart as target organs, aconites, when taken in overdose, produce a distinctive clinical picture. GI effects occur initially, consisting of nausea, vomiting, and hypersalivation. These are followed by neurologic effects including paresthesias, blurred vision, skeletal muscle weakness or frank paralysis,[35] coma, and seizures. Cardiac disturbances, which can be fatal,[36, 37] include bradycardia, hypotension, ectopy, cardiac conduction disturbances (prolonged QRS or QT interval), and intractable ventricular tachyarrhythmias.

Treatment of aconite poisoning consists of stabilization of the airway, aggressive treatment of cardiac disturbances, and early GI decontamination. Subsequent treatment is supportive because there are no known antidotes and no identified mechanism for enhanced elimination of the toxin.

Nutmeg. The mood-elevating, aphrodisiac, narcotic, and hallucinogenic effects of nutmeg have been exploited for centuries. This spice remains popular, particularly as a hallucinogen. Prepared from the fruit of the evergreen tree *Myristica fragrans,* nutmeg is an easily obtained spice. The nutmeg seed contains a number of alkaloids including myristicin, eugenol, isoeugenol, methyleugenol, methylisoeugenol, safrole, geraniol, borneal, and elemicin. Among these, myristicin is the most psychoactive compound. Myristicin is metabolized to the hallucinogen 3-methoxy-4,5-methylenedioxyamphetamine (MMDA), a substance closely related to methylenedioxymethamphetamine (MDMA, "ecstasy"). Another alkaloid in nutmeg, elemicin is metabolized to a hallucinogen.

Ingestion of 5 to 30 g of nutmeg produces symptoms promptly, with GI upset predominating. Within 3 hours, hallucinogenic effects appear, consisting of vivid visual hallucinations. The duration of this action can be as long as 2 to 3 days. Chronic abuse of this potent hallucinogen is limited by the GI disturbances it produces. Treatment of acute nutmeg intoxication consists of reducing environmental stimuli and attempting to calm the patient. Benzodiazepines may be valuable as adjunctive therapy.

Kombucha mushroom. Kombucha is a plant that has recently gained popularity as a "fountain of youth." It has been promoted as a treatment for cancer, hypertension, fatigue, declining T cell counts, arthritis, wrinkles, constipation, and gray hair. Prescribed and marketed by naturopathic healers in the United States, kombucha is often cultivated at home and passed on to friends.[38] Not a true mushroom, the plant is a yeast-bacterial aggregate surrounded by a membrane. Use of this mushroom has been blamed for sporadic cases of hepatotoxicity and severe metabolic acidosis, which was fatal in one case.[38, 39] The toxic principles have not been identified; toxicity may result from kombucha contamination by other yeasts or bacteria.

Sabah. Marketed in the United States under the name "Defat," this vegetable has been associated with an epidemic of pulmonary disease in Taiwan. One report described 44 individuals, primarily women, who developed respiratory distress, insomnia, and obstructive pulmonary disease after consumption of the Sabah vegetable (*Sauropus androgynus*).[40] This vegetable, which is a regular part of the diet in many parts of the world, was being ingested in large daily quantities as a means of improving vision, reducing lipids, treating constipation, and hemorrhoids, or as a weight loss measure. An epidemiologic investigation was undertaken after repeated reports to the Taiwan Poison Center of illness related to ingestion of this vegetable. Victims were primarily females who had been taking the vegetable whole or in juice form. The average duration of consumption before the appearance of disease was 35 days. Initial symptoms consisted of insomnia and excitation, followed by difficulty in breathing, cough, and chest tightness. In many cases, illness developed after consumption of the vegetable had ceased. In a patient who underwent a lung biopsy, histopathology suggested bronchiolitis obliterans with organizing pneumonia. Four fatalities occurred. By Dec 1, 1995, 169 cases of Sabah-associated illness had been reported. An exact cause has yet to be determined.[41]

Chinese Patent (Proprietary) Medicines

In addition to herbs being prescribed and sold in their unadulterated form, herbs are often combined to form Chinese patent medicines. Chinese patent medicines, unlike Chinese herbal medicines, are mass produced in a fashion similar to pharmaceutical manufacture.

The potential problems with these medicines are several. First, Chinese proprietary medicines are often sold in unlabeled or poorly labeled packages. Second, they typically contain a combination of products such that a distinctive clinical syndrome may not be present after an intoxication. Jin Bu Huan tablets, prescribed for muscle spasm, pain, and insomnia, were associated with the poisoning of three children when they were discovered to contain an herb not usually a part of them.[42] In a later report, hepatitis was also associated with Jin Bu Huan.[12] Third, combining herbs from various sources poses a greater probability of product contamination. Fourth, because of sometimes relatively poor quality control in production, proprietary medicines can be entirely mislabeled, containing a product completely different from what is stated. Finally, these products can be adulterated with pharmaceutical agents. Several cases of intoxication have been attributed to these preparations.[43] For example, Gan Mao Tong Pian, a remedy prescribed for viral illness, produced aplastic anemia in a child as a result of its adulteration by phenylbutazone.[43] One Chinese proprietary product, *Chuei-Fong-Tou-Gen-Wan,* has been found to contain agents including phenacetin, phenylbutazone, mercuric sulfide, lead, cadmium, and arsenic.[15, 16, 43, 44] In one study, eight of nine Chinese patent medicines tested were found to be contaminated with arsenic and mercury.[44] In a 5-year study of hospital admissions resulting from use of Chinese proprietary medicines, Chan and colleagues identified 71 patients, of whom 42 were found to have elevated serum concentrations of aspirin or acetaminophen.[45] Products containing acetaminophen included *Superior Yinchiao, Chieh, Tu Pien, Yinchiao Chieh Tu Pien, Ganyanquing Pian, and Suxiaao Shangfeng.*

TRADITIONAL ("FOLK") MEDICINE

A folk remedy can be defined as an unrefined product that is taken for medicinal purposes. Unlike herbal medicines, folk remedies are regularly derived from animals, plants, or minerals. The use of folk medicines has a strong component of religious ritual (e.g., shamanism). Folk treatments may consist of physical modalities (e.g., "coining" or "cupping"), widely practiced in Asian cultures, as well as religious practices.[46] The use of so-called ethnomedical therapies is most prevalent among minority groups, especially among families who have either recently emigrated or who have a family member who has inherited knowledge about folk remedies. In many cases, the basis of therapies is a nonorthodox belief about disease processes (e.g., the humoral [hot-cold] theory).[47] However, folk medicines are also used to treat well-defined western diseases. These diseases may be referred to by archaic names such as rheumatism (musculoskeletal inflammation), dropsy (congestive heart failure), or consumption (tuberculosis). Folk medicines are also sought by those under the care of physicians because of frustration with the ability of western medicine to cure a disease or because of a desire to use natural remedies rather than pharmaceutical agents. With increasing frequency, these traditional medicines can be purchased in the United States. For example, in Hispanic populations, local *botanicas* usually provide religious objects as well as folk remedies.[47]

A list of folk medicines associated with clinical toxicity is found in Table 97–3. For example, the remedy alcanfor contains 20% camphor, sufficient to produce toxic manifestations.[47] Several folk remedies used in the treatment of GI disturbances contain lead. In some cases, use of these agents can produce lead-induced abdominal pain (lead colic), resulting in further use and more severe lead poisoning.

Identifying the ingredients in fok remedies is often assisted by knowledge of the cultural origins of the disease being treated. For example, empacho, one of the most common illnesses among Hispanic cultures, is treated by various means including massages with olive oil (or other type of oil/grease), laxatives, conventional stomach remedies (e.g., bismuth subsalicylate [Pepto-Bismol]), chamomile tea, and antacids, as well as the folk remedies *greta* or *azarcon* (both of which contain up to 90% lead).[48] Other lead-containing folk medicines are listed in Table 97–3.

Pachter and associates described other potential toxicities from traditional medicines.[47] For example, azogue, which contains elemental mercury, is generally used as a talisman. However, if it is dispersed about the room to ward off evil spirits, inhalation of toxic mercury vapors could occur.

Ayurvedic Medicine

Ayurveda is a traditional system of medicine practiced primarily in Asian countries (Tibet, Burma,

Table 97–3. Common Folk Medicines by Cultural Origin

Name	Contents	Potential Toxicity
Hispanic		
Siete jarabes	Almond, castor oil, tolu, wild cherry licorice, cocillana, honey	GI upset, catharsis, electrolyte disturbances
Agua maravilla	Witch hazel, ethanol	Ethanol toxicity
Jarabe maguey	Maguey (*Agave* spp.)	GI upset
Alcanfor	Camphor	Camphor toxicity
Azarcon	Lead	Lead intoxication
Greta	Lead	Lead intoxication
Azogue	Elemental mercury	Mercury intoxication
Ipecacuanha	Ipecac	Vomiting, myopathy
Southeast Asian		
Paylooah	Lead	Lead intoxication
India and Ayurvedic		
Surma	Lead	Lead intoxication
Deshi Dawa	Lead	Lead intoxication

GI, gastrointestinal.

Pakistan, Sri Lanka, India, Bangladesh). Practitioners of Ayurvedic medicine not only rely on herbal remedies but often prescribe animal products, metals, and minerals as well. Increasingly, Ayurvedic remedies are being used in western areas, including Europe and North America. Also, in becoming a commercial industry, Ayurvedic medicine has begun to include large-scale distribution of these drugs.

Because Ayurvedic medicine includes therapy with metals and minerals, inadvertent metal intoxication is the most significant potential occurrence. Ayurvedic medicines are typically sold in an "ash" powder form, packaged in capsules and produced by the repeated pyrolysis of the metal. Zinc, iron, lead, tin, mercury, and silver are among the metals that may be contained in an Ayurvedic "tonic." As such, both consumers and manufacturers of these products are at risk for metal intoxication. Lead intoxication has been reported with the use of these medicines.[49, 50]

ALTERNATIVE MEDICINES

Although herbal and traditional medicines, such as chiropractic medicine and acupuncture, all can be placed under the broad classification of alternative medicines, they are therapies that are neither herbal nor traditional. Practices that can be placed in this category include homeopathy, naturopathy (a method of treating disorders that involves the use of diet, herbal medicine, and environmental modifications), nutritional supplementation, and novel therapies, such as hyperoxygenation and oligotherapy (the administration of trace elements to improve health).[3]

Homeopathy

Homeopathy is a popular alternative therapy that advocates the use of toxic substances in small amounts. It is extremely popular in Europe, Latin America, and Asia and has been used by an estimated 1% of the American population.[8] The principle was introduced by Samuel Hahnemann in the late 18th century. Treatments in homeopathic medicine are based on three principles: "like cures like," "efficacy improves with increasing dilution," and "treatments need to be individualized."[51] Under this principle, a toxin when administered in small doses can have therapeutic value. Such a theory is not a great departure from western medicine, as it is the basis of desensitization therapy for allergies. However, the theory that the smaller the dose of medicine, the more effective, has not been well documented in scientific study. Homeopathy also requires that therapy be individualized; therefore, in principle, homeopathic medications should not be shared with another person.

Homeopathic medicines are generally toxins derived from plants, animals, or minerals.[8] Common agents include strychnine, ipecac, arsenic, mercury, podophyllin, and sulfur.[8] Preparations of accepted therapeutic value are recorded in the United States Homeopathic Pharmacopoeia, published by the American Institute of Homeopathy.[51] Homeopathic products often are packages of capsules or tablets with the ingredients listed by their Latin names. Scientifically rigorous studies have suggested efficacy of some of these medicines.[5, 7, 8]

Homeopatic tinctures are generally made by adding 1 part of a toxin to 20 parts of alcohol. This tincture is diluted as needed to 1:1000, 1:10,000, and even further dilutions. A homeopathic product may therefore contain on its label a symbol of 1× (1:10 dilution), 2× (1:100 dilution), 3×, and so forth. Another dilution technique is the centidecimal ("c" or "cH"), in which 1 part of active substance is diluted in 99 parts of an alcohol mixture.[51] Therefore, a substance labeled 30C has had the active substance diluted 1:100 in a water/alcohol solution 30 times, yielding a final concentration of 1×10^{-60}.[8]

Because of the minute quantities of toxin, ingestion of homeopathic medications should rarely produce toxicity, even if as many as 100 tablets are ingested. Important exceptions to this rule would be if the product were homemade, thereby potentially having dilutions lesser than planned, or in the potential case of an allergic reaction, which could occur after exposure to small quantities of the active agent. Reports have described homeopathic products adulterated with active agents.[5]

Nutrition Supplements

In addition to using herbal and alternative medications, the public commonly takes substances that are promoted as nutrition supplements, designed to improve health. The use of these is widespread: an examination of advertisements in 12 health and bodybuilding magazines disclosed 311 supplements, containing 235 unique ingredients. Most common among these were amino acids, followed by herbs, vitamins, minerals, and steroids.[52] The toxicity of vitamins is discussed in Chapter 99. Specific nutrition supplements that have been reported to have clinical toxicity are discussed next.

γ-Hydroxybutyrate. γ-Hydroxybutyrate (GHB) is a health food supplement that became popular in 1990 after its promotion as a bodybuilding and diet aid. Shortly after widespread use began, cases of a toxic syndrome related to its ingestion were reported. Dyer described a series of 16 cases of GHB toxicity reported to the San Francisco Regional Poison Center; manifestations included coma and seizures.[53] Other signs of toxicity were confusion, agitation, hallucinations, and bradycardia. These effects occurred after ingestions of as little as ¼ tsp of GHB (sold as a white powder). Shortly after similar reports throughout the country, individual states banned the product.[53]

L-Tryptophan. L-Tryptophan is an essential amino acid. As a precursor to the neurotransmitter serotonin, it has been touted as an effective treatment for ailments including insomnia, depression, and premenstrual syndrome. Its use, however, has been associated with at least two syndromes of intoxication.

An epidemic of multisystem disease occurred in the fall of 1989 when patients who had been ingesting L-tryptophan developed eosinophilia and severe myalgia. During the course of 6 to 9 months, an estimated 5000 to 10,000 developed this syndrome; more than 36 fatalities occurred. Eighty-four per cent of victims were female. Prominent symptoms were peripheral eosinophilia (with eosinophil counts of >1000/mm^3), severe diffuse myalgias, and dermatologic changes resembling scleroderma. Termed the eosinophilia-myalgia syndrome (EMS), this disease had other features that included pulmonary disturbances (dyspnea, cough, pulmonary infiltrates, and pulmonary hypertension, which occurred in approximately 60%), peripheral neuropathy, alopecia, edema, coronary artery spasm, and cardiac arrhythmias.[41, 54] The illness bore a striking resemblance to the unexplained "toxic oil" epidemic that occurred in Spain in 1981.[41, 55] When it was found that all cases of EMS could be traced to L-tryptophan synthesized by a single manufacturer, analysis revealed that owing to changes in the manufuacturing method, the tryptophan was contaminated with an impurity, 1,1′-ethylidenebis (tryptophan).[41] There is still controversy about whether the true cause of EMS was discovered. Nonetheless, after the FDA's ban of tryptophan-containing products, the disease quickly and almost completely disappeared. This important mass poisoning has been extensively reviewed by others.[56–62]

Adverse effects have also occurred with the simultaneous use of tryptophan and antidepressants of the monoamine oxidase (MAO) inhibitor or serotonin reuptake inhibitor classes. In the case of MAO inhibitors, tryptophan was once recommended as adjunctive therapy for those who had a poor response to MAO therapy.[63] However, after this combination began being used more consistently, reports began to describe hypertensive crises, myoclonus, and delirium after their combined use.[64] This syndrome, now referred to as a *serotoninergic syndrome,* appears to result from excess stimulation of central nervous system serotonin receptors and can include other features such as myoclonus, hyperreflexia, diaphoresis, priapism, and tremor. At its extreme, the serotoninergic syndrome can produce seizures, coma, and death. In addition to MAO inhibitors, the newer serotonin reuptake inhibitors (e.g., fluoxetine, paroxetine, and sertraline) have the potential to produce this syndrome after ingestion of tryptophan.

Calcium Supplements. Use of calcium supplements has increased considerably during the past decade as the diminishing calcium intake of Americans is documented and the relationship between deficient calcium intake and osteoporosis, particularly in women, is recognized. Some calcium supplements that are derived from bone meal are reported to contain lead.

Hyperoxygenation Therapy

Hyperoxygen therapy is being increasingly promoted as a health aid. It has become particularly popular as an alternative treatment for AIDS. Acting in a fashion similar to white blood cells in their destruction of microbial agents, ingestion of oxygen-liberating agents is thought to augment host defense mechanisms. Hydrogen peroxide is the most common agent used for hyperoxygenation therapy. Hydrogen peroxide used for this purpose is generally sold in a 25% to 50% concentration, in contrast to the 5% concentration of household hydrogen peroxide. The user is directed to ingest several drops daily. Because the agent is refrigerated, the potential for inadvertent ingestion is increased.[65]

Toxicity from hyperoxygen therapy has been reported after ingestion of excess amounts. The two major consequences of this ingestion are corrosive injury of the GI tract and excess liberation of oxygen, resulting in the formation of gas emboli. One milliliter of a concentrated hydrogen peroxide solution can liberate approximately 115 mL of oxygen; ingestion of two ounces of 35% hydrogen peroxide could release 6.9 L of oxygen in the stomach.[65, 66] Several researchers have described life-threatening or fatal gas emboli after ingestion of concentrated hydrogen peroxide.[65–67]

Treatment of concentrated hydrogen peroxide therapy includes supportive care, assessment of the esophagus and stomach for corrosive injury, and anticipation of air emboli. Diluting agents should not be administered because of their potential to enhance oxygen liberation.

Other Therapies

The promotion of tonics, extracts, and elixirs has a consistent ability to entice consumers. Their list is constantly changing. In rare circumstances, these alternative medicines prove to have therapeutic value. In most cases, they have no beneficial action but also no toxicity. These agents can occasionally be highly toxic. For example, Laetrile was promoted in the early 1980s as an alternative treatment for cancer. Prepared from crushed apricot pits, this agent contained high concentrations of amygdalin, a cyanogenic alkaoid. Although it was not proved to have therapeutic value, Laetrile did result in cases of cyanide intoxication after overdose.[68]

Other therapies, including ingestion of shark cartilage, boiled urchin, and algae, continue to be promoted without clear, scientifically proven benefit.

References

1. Verhoef MJ, Sutherland LR, Brkich L: Use of alternative medicine by patients attending a gastroenterology clinic. Can Med Assoc J *142:*121–125, 1990.
2. Eisenberg DM, Kessler RC, Foster C, et al: Unconventional

medicine in the United States—prevalence, cost, and patterns of use. N Engl J Med *328:*246–252, 1993.
3. Spigelblatt L, Laine-Ammara G, Pless IB, Guyver A: The use of alternative medicine by children. Pediatrics *94:*811–814, 1994.
4. Pearl WS, Leo P, Tsang WO: Use of Chinese therapies among Chinese patients seeking emergency department care. Ann Emerg Med *26:*735–738, 1995.
5. Sampson W, London W: Analysis of homeopathic treatment of childhood diarrhea. Pediatrics *96:*961–964, 1995.
6. Weizman Z, Alkrinawi S, Goldfarb D, Bitran C: Efficacy of herbal tea preparation in infantile colic. J Pediatr *122:*650–652, 1993.
7. Kleijnen J, Knipschild P, terRiet G: Clinical trials of homeopathy. BMJ *302:*316–323, 1991.
8. Jacobs J, Jimenez LM, Gloyd SS, et al: Treatment of acute childhood diarrhea with homeopathic medicine: A randomized clinical trial in Nicaragua. Pediatrics *93:*719–725, 1994.
9. Delbanco TL. Bitter herbs; mainstream, magic and menace. Ann Intern Med *121:*803–804, 1994.
10. Reports C: Herbal roulette. Consumer Reports, pp 698–705, Nov 1995.
11. Pereira CAL, Nishioka SDA: Poisoning by the use of Datura leaves in a homemade toothpaste. Clin Toxicol *32:*329–332, 1994.
12. Woolf GM, Petrovic L, Rojter SE, et al: Acute hepatitis associated with the Chinese herbal product Jin Bu Huan. Ann Intern Med *121:*729–735, 1994.
13. Bakhiet AO, Adam SEI: Therapeutic utility, constituents and toxicity of some medicinal plants: A review. Vet Hum Toxicol *37:*255, 1995.
14. Ody P: The Complete Medicinal Herbal. London, Dorling Kindersley Limited, p 192, 1993.
15. Chan TY, Chan JC, Tomlinson B, Critchley JA: Poisoning by Chinese herbal medicines in Hong Kong: A hospital-based study. Vet Hum Toxicol *36:*546–547, 1994.
16. Chan TYK, Critchley JA: The spectrum of poisonings in Hong Kong: An overview. Vet Hum Toxicol *36:*135–137, 1994.
17. Lee T, Lam T: Allergic contact dermatitis to Yunnan Paiyao. Contact Dermatitis *17:*59–60, 1987.
18. Siegel RK: Herbal intoxication—psychoactive effects from herbal cigarettes, tea and capsules. JAMA *236:*473–476, 1976.
19. Saxe T: Toxicity of medicinal herbal preparations. Am Fam Physician *35:*135–142, 1987.
20. Ridker PM: Toxic effects of herbal teas. Arch Environ Health *42:*133–136, 1987.
21. Katz M, Saibil F: Herbal hepatitis: Subacute hepatic necrosis secondary to chaparral leaf. J Clin Gastroenterol *12:*203–206, 1990.
22. Mostefa-Kara N, Pauwels A, Pines E, et al: Fatal hepatitis after herbal tea. Lancet *340:*674–675, 1992.
23. Gordon DW, Rosenthal G, Hart J, et al: Chaparral ingestion—the broadening spectrum of liver injury caused by herbal medications. JAMA *273:*489–490, 1995.
24. Centers for Disease Control (CDC): Chaparral-induced toxic hepatitis—California and Texas, 1992. MMWR *41:*812–814, 1992.
25. Perharic L, Shaw D, Leon C, et al: Possible liver damage with the use of Chinese herbal medicine for skin disease. Vet Hum Toxicol *27:*563–566, 1995.
26. Chan TY: Anticholinergic poisoning due to Chinese herbal medicines. Vet Hum Toxicol *37:*156, 1995.
27. Coremans P, Lambrecht G, Schepens P, et al: Anticholinergic intoxication with commercially available thorn apple tea. Clin Toxicol *32:*589–592, 1994.
28. Segelman AB, Segelman FP, Karliner J, Sofia D: Sassafras and herb tea—potential health hazards. JAMA *236:*477, 1976.
29. Ridker PM, Ohkuma S, McDermott WV, et al: Hepatic venocclusive disease associated with the consumption of pyrrolizidine-containing dietray supplements. Gastroenterology *88:* 1050–1054, 1985.
30. Huxtable RJ, Luthhyy J, Zweifel U: Toxicity of comfrey-pepsin preparations. N Engl J Med *315:*1095, 1986.
31. Huxtable RJ: Herbal teas and toxins: Novel aspects of pyrrolizidine poisoning in The United States. Perspect Biol Med *24:*1–14, 1980.
32. Roulet M, Laurini R, Rivier L, Calame A: Hepatic veno-occlusive disease in newborn infant of a woman drinking herbal tea. J Pediatr *112:*433–4436, 1988.
33. Huang KC: The Pharmacology of Chinese Herbs. Boca Raton, FL, CRC Press, p 388, 1993.
34. Bisset NG: Arrow poisons in China. Part II. Aconitum—botany, chemistry, and pharmacology. J Ethnopharmacol *4:*247–336, 1981.
35. Chan TY, Tomlinson B, Critchley JA, Cockram CS: Herb-induced aconitine poisoning presenting as tetraplegia. Vet Hum Toxicol *36:*133–134, 1994.
36. Fatovich DM: Aconite: A lethal Chinese herb. Ann Emerg Med *21:*309–311, 1992.
37. Tai Y-T, But PP-H, Young K, Lau C-P: Cardiotoxicity after accidental herb-induced aconite poisoning. Lancet *340:*1254–1256, 1992.
38. Perron AD, Patterson JA, Yanofsky NN: Kombucha “mushroom” hepatotoxicity. Ann Emerg Med *26:*660–661, 1995.
39. CDC: Unexplained severe illness possibly associated with consumption of Kombucha Tea—Iowa, 1995. MMWR *44:*892–900, 1995.
40. Lin T-J, Lu C-C, Chen K-W, Deng J-F: Outbreak of obstructive ventilatory impairment associated with consumption of sauopus androgynus vegetable. Clin Toxicol *34:*1–8, 1996.
41. Spyker D, Love LA, Brooks SM: An outbreak of pulmonary poisoning. Clin Toxicol *34:*15–20, 1996.
42. CDC: Jin Bu Huan toxicity in children—Colorado, 1993. MMWR *42:*633–636, 1993.
43. Nelson L, Shih R, Hoffman R: Aplastic anemia induced by an adulterated herbal medication. Clin Toxicol *33:*467–470, 1995.
44. Espinoza EO, Mann M-J, Bleasdell B: Arsenic and mercury in traditional Chinese herbal balls. N Engl J Med *333:*803–804, 1995.
45. Chan TYK, Lee KKG, Chan AYW, Critchley JAJH: Poisoning due to Chinese proprietary medicines. Hum Exp Toxicol *14:*434–436, 1995.
46. Pachter LM: Culture and clinical care—folk illness beliefs and behaviors and their implications for health care delivery. JAMA *271:*690–694, 1994.
47. Pachter LM, Cloutier MM, Bernstein BA: Ethnomedical (folk) remedies for childhood asthma in a mainland Puerto Rican community. Arch Pediatr Adolesc Med *149:*982–988, 1995.
48. Risser AL, Mazur L: Use of folk remedies in a Hispanic population. Arch Pediatr Adolesc Med *149:*978–981, 1995.
49. McElvaine MD, Harder EM, Johnson L, et al: Lead poisoning from the use of Indian folk medicines. JAMA *264:*2212–2213, 1990.
50. Kulshrestha MK: Lead poisoning diagnosed by abdominal x-rays. Clin Toxicol *34:*107–108, 1996.
51. Spoerke DG: Toxicity of homeopathic products. Vet Hum Toxicol *31:*259, 1989.
52. Philen RM, Ortiz DI, Auerbach SB, Falk H: Survey of advertising for nutritional supplements in health and body building magazines. JAMA *268:*1008–1011, 1992.
53. Dyer JE: Gamma-hydroxybutyrate—a health-food product producing coma and seizurelike activity. Am J Emerg Med *9:*321–324, 1991.
54. Swygert LA, Maes EF, Sewell LE, et al: Eosinophilia-myalgia syndrome—results of national surveillance. JAMA *264:*1698–1703, 1990.
55. Hertzman PA, Falk H, Kilbourne EM, et al: The eosinophilia-myalgia syndrome: The Los Alamos conference. J Rheumatol *18:*867–873, 1991.
56. Hertzman PA, Blevins WL, Mayer J, et al: Association of the eosinophilia-myalgia syndrome with the ingestion of tryptophan. N Engl J Med *322:*868–873, 1990.
57. Belongia EA, Hedberg CW, Gleich GH, et al. An investigation of the cause of the eosinophilia-myalgia syndrome associated with tryptophan use. N Engl J Med *323:*357–365, 1990.
58. Kamb ML, Murphy JJ, Jones JL, et al: Eosinophilia-myalgia syndrome in L-tryptophan–exposed patients. JAMA *267:*77–82, 1992.
59. CDC: Analysis of L-tryptophan for etiology of eosinophilia-myalgia syndrome. MMWR *39:*789–790, 1990.

60. CDC: Eosinophilia-myalgia syndrome: Follow-up survey of patients—New York, 1990–1991. MMWR *40*:401–403, 1991.
61. Slutsker L, Hoesly FC, Miller L, et al: Eosinophilia-myalgia syndrome associated with exposure to tryptophan from a single manufacturer. JAMA *264*:1213–1217, 1990.
62. Swygert LA, Maes EF, Sewell LE, et al: Eosinophilia-myalgia syndrome—results of national surveillance. JAMA *264*:1698–1703, 1990.
63. Pope HG, Jonas JM, Hudson JI, Kafka MP: Toxic reactions to the combination of monoamine oxidase inhibitors and tryptophan. Am J Psychiatry *142*:491–492, 1985.
64. Blackwell B: Monoamine oxidase inhibitor interactions with other drugs. J Clin Psychopharmacol *11*:55–59, 1991.
65. Luu TA, Kelley MT, Strauch JA, Avradopoulos K: Portal vein gas embolism from hydrogen peroxide ingestion. Am J Emerg Med *21*:1391–1393, 1992.
66. Giberson TP, Kern JD, Pettigrew DW, et al: Near-fatal hydrogen peroxide ingestion. Ann Emerg Med *18*:778–779, 1989.
67. Rackoff WR, Merton DF: Gas embolism after ingestion of hydrogen peroxide. Pediatrics *85*:593–594, 1990.
68. Hall AH, Linden CH, Kulig KW, et al: Cyanide poisoning from Laetrile ingestion: Role of nitrite therapy. Pediatrics *78*:269–272, 1986.

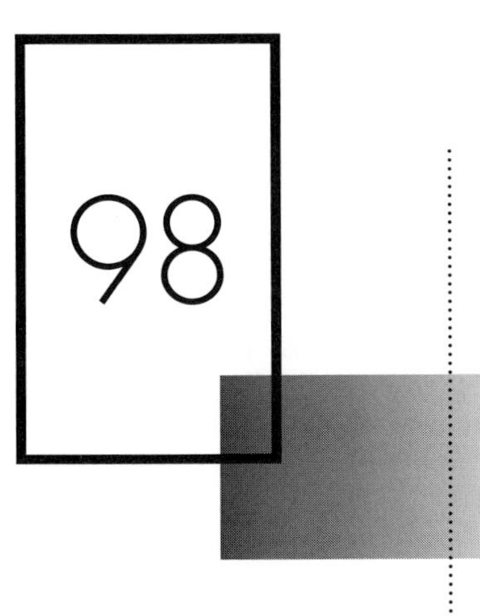

Thyroid

K. M. MOHAMED SHAKIR, MD
PAUL W. LADENSON, MD

Thyroid hormone–containing tablets are commonly prescribed drugs. Despite the fact that large numbers of thyroid hormone–containing drugs are prescribed each year in the United States to an estimated 4% of the adult population, only a small proportion of patients suffer accidental or intentional poisoning.[1, 2] For example, only 4917 thyroid hormone overdoses (based on extrapolation from the National Capital Poison Control Center statistics) were documented in the United States in 1994.[2] It is probable that many cases may be unreported because children and young adults may tolerate relatively large doses of thyroid preparations without any untoward effects.

THYROID PHYSIOLOGY

Hypothalamic-Pituitary-Thyroid Axis

The hypothalamic-pituitary-thyroid system, an integrated organ complex, regulates the control of thyroid hormone secretion from the thyroid gland. This organ complex begins in the cells of the supraoptic nucleus of the hypothalamus. These cells secrete a tripeptide, thyrotropin-releasing hormone, which is carried via the pituitary portal circulation to the anterior pituitary gland. Thyrotropin-releasing hormone stimulates the pituitary gland to secrete thyroid-stimulating hormone (TSH) into the general circulation. TSH in turn causes the thyroid gland to secrete thyroxine (T_4) and triiodothyronine (T_3).

Thyroid Hormone Synthesis

Iodine is a major constituent of thyroid hormones. T_4 has four iodine atoms per molecule, and iodine makes up 66% of T_4 by weight. In contrast, T_3 has three iodine atoms per molecule and is 58% iodine by weight (Fig. 98–1).

Dietary iodine is reduced to iodide and is absorbed in the small intestine within 1 hour after ingestion. Thyroid follicular cells actively transport plasma iodide into their cytoplasm. Iodine is stored in the

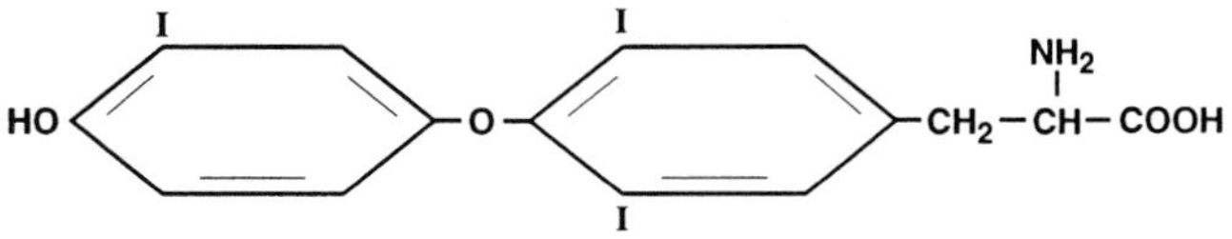

3′, 5, 3 - Triiodothyronine (T_3)

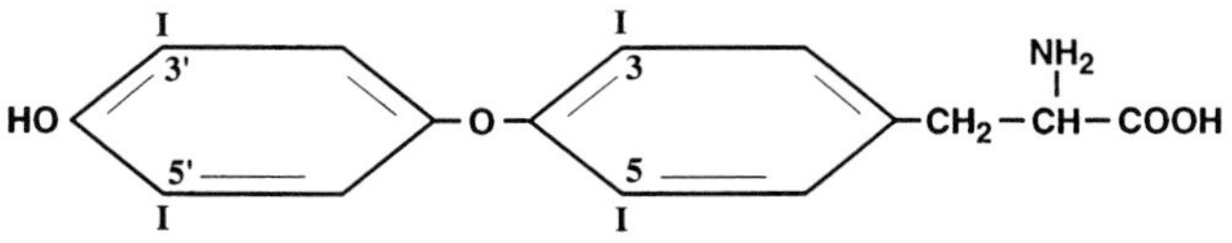

3, 5, 3′, 5′ - Thyroxine (Tetraiodothyronine, T_4)

Figure 98–1. Chemical structure of thyroxine (T_4) and triiodothyronine (T_3).

thyroid gland in thyroglobulin, a large glycoprotein that has a pivotal role in the synthesis and storage of thyroid hormones. Iodide ions transported into the thyroid follicular cells are oxidized to a higher valence state before binding to tyrosyl residues present in the thyroglobulin molecules. Iodination of the tyrosyl residues within thyroglobulin, a process called *organification of the iodine*, is catalyzed by thyroid peroxidase. If one iodine atom replaces a hydrogen atom, then monoiodotyrosine is formed; if two iodine atoms are joined in the tyrosyl ring, diiodotyrosine is the resultant product. Monoiodotyrosine and diiodotyrosine then undergo oxidative condensation to yield various iodothyronines. These include 3,5,3′-triiodothyronine (T_3) and 3,5,3′,5′-tetraiodothyronine (thyroxine, T_4) (see Fig. 98–1). During this process, other iodine-containing compounds, such as iodinated proteins and iodotyronines, are deiodinated and their iodine is recycled within the thyroid gland. Thyroglobulin is secreted into the follicular lumen, where it is stored as colloid. Under normal circumstances, only a small fraction of stored hormones, about 1%, turns over each day. The colloid in the follicular lumen is reabsorbed by pinocytosis into follicular cells. Normally, thyroglobulin undergoes digestion by proteolytic enzymes to release T_4 and T_3 into circulation. All the steps in the biosynthesis of thyroid hormone are stimulated by TSH.

Approximately 120 nmol of T_4 and 47 nmol of T_3 are secreted into circulation per day. The serum concentrations of these hormones are determined by the balance between production and degradation. Nutrition, nonthyroidal illness, exercise, medication use, and age affect this balance.[3–6] The total body hormone store or pool for T_4 is around 850 nmol • 70 kg^{-1} whereas the value for T_3 is 76 nmol • 70 kg^{-1}.[7]

The thyroid hormones T_4 and T_3 are reversibly bound to plasma proteins synthesized by the liver. Transthyretin (TTR), previously known as *thyroid-binding prealbumin*, has a low affinity and rapid dissociation constant; therefore, it has a greater role in delivering iodothyronines to various tissues. In contrast, thyroxine-binding globulin (TBG), with its relatively high binding affinity and slower dissociation constant serves as a stable hormone reservoir in the circulation. Albumin has low binding affinity and thus may act similarly to TTR to provide tissue delivery of the hormone.[7]

Circulating T_4 is almost entirely bound (99.97%) to these plasma proteins. T_4 is predominantly bound to T_4-binding globulin (75% to 80%). TTR binds approximately 15% to 20% and albumin binds 5% to 10%. Compared with T_4, plasma T_3 is bound to a lesser extent (99.7%). Throughout a wide range of binding protein concentrations, production rate and steady-state free hormone levels remain nearly constant. Thus, measurement of the free fractions of T_3 or T_4 in the plasma is critical, especially when changes occur in the transport proteins. Furthermore, target tissue responses are related principally if not exclusively to these free fractions of circulating T_4 and T_3. With overdoses of thyroid hormones, the concentration of TBG is changed little, and the levels of free hormone increase directly or even disproportionately with the total serum thyroid hormone concentrations.

Generation of T_3 from T_4 by removing either iodine atom from the outer ring (at 3′ or 5′ position) of the T_4 molecule results in a metabolically more active hormone. Peripheral deiodination contributes 80% to 85% of the daily T_3 production. Thus, most total daily T_3 production results from extrathyroidal deiodination in such tissues as the liver and kidneys.

Thyroid Hormone Metabolism and Actions

Medications containing thyroid hormones are generally administered by the oral route. T_4 absorption generally varies from 50% to 80%, depending on its formulation. Studies have demonstrated the fractional gastrointestinal (GI) absorption of a levothyroxine preparation (Synthroid) of 81%, a value considerably higher than the earlier estimate of 48%.[8] T_3 is almost completely absorbed. Absorption can also be affected by food intake or drugs, such as cholestyramine, ferrous sulfate, aluminum hydroxide–containing antacids, or sucralfate.[9–12]

T_4, after entering the circulation and equilibrating with body pools, is distributed in a plasma equivalent volume of 10 L and normally disappears, with a half-life of 6 to 7 days. In contrast, T_3 is distributed in 38 L and has a half-life of 1 to 2 days. T_4 has a metabolic clearance rate of 0.8 to 1.4 L/d and a fractional turnover rate of 10% to 14% per day. The metabolic clearance of both T_4 and T_3 is altered by several factors, such as age, underlying thyroid status, and coadministered drugs. The T_4 half-life may be halved in children, whereas in the elderly the half-life may be prolonged. Hormone turnover is slowed in hypothyroid and increased in hyperthyroid states. Although most studies of thyroid hormone metabolism in hyperthyroidism have evaluated patients with Graves' disease, the findings have been corroborated by observations of factitious hyperthyroidism from ingested thyroid hormone preparations.[6, 7]

Approximately 35% of T_4 entering the circulation is converted to T_3 in the peripheral tissues such as the liver and kidneys by type I and II deiodinases, which act on the phenolic ring. T_3 is also generated intracellularly as an intermediate in T_4 action, especially in the central nervous system and pituitary.[7] The large pool of T_4 and its slow metabolism provide for the steady generation of T_3. The three main pathways of thyroid hormone degradation are (1) deiodination, (2) side chain metabolism, and (3) conjugation with glucuronic acid and sulfate. The first pathway accounts for 80% of T_3 and T_4 disposal. The deiodination process probably occurs in all tissues, but deiodinases are distributed in the highest concentrations in the liver, kidneys, muscle, brain, and heart.[7] The iodothyronines eventually are totally deiodinated, but the diphenyl-ether link of the thyronine nucleus remains intact. The alanine side chain of T_3 and T_4 undergoes metabolism by enzyme systems in peripheral tissues, yielding acetic, lactic, and pyruvic acids. Additionally, a pathway involving conjugation of the hydroxyl group and biliary excretion accounts for a significant proportion (20%) of thyroid hormone degradation.[7]

Conjugates of T_3 and T_4 undergo different metabolic fates.[7] Sulfoconjugation is most important for T_3, whereas T_4 undergoes glucuronidation.[4] Hydrolysis of the conjugates probably occurs in the GI tract, as evidenced by the absence of conjugates in the stool. Thyroid hormone released from conjugates in the gut is available for reabsorption, and interruption of this enterohepatic circulation by cholestyramine has been used as an adjunct in the management of thyroid hormone intoxication.[11]

T_4, when administered intravenously, usually takes 6 to 8 hours to exert initial effect, and peak effect may not occur until the following day. With massive oral doses of T_4 administration, however, clinical effects may be seen in 3 to 16 hours. Approximately a third of extrathyroidal hormone is stored in the liver, and circulating thyroid hormone slowly saturates other tissues to reach equilibrium in several days.

The principal actions of thyroid hormones in target tissues are initiated by the binding to specific nuclear receptors, termed *T_3 receptors*, which were first identified as cellular homologues of the avian erythroblastosis virus oncogene (c-*erb*A). These receptors have properties of (1) binding T_3 with high affinity; (2) binding specific oligonucleotide sequences, called T_3 regulatory elements, which are present in the the regulatory regions of thyroid hormone–responsive genes; and (3) binding one another to form dimers, a property that has been shown to be an important aspect of T_3 action. Within hours of thyroid hormone administration, T_3 binding to these receptors stimulates transcription of certain messenger RNAs that are then translated into proteins (e.g., β-myosin heavy chain in myocardium), which are ultimately responsible for effecting thyroid hormone actions in various tissues. Those actions include increases in metabolic rate, body temperature, heart rate, and myocardial contractility.[13]

Laboratory Tests of Thyroid Function

Determination of serum levels of thyroid hormones is necessary for an accurate assessment of patients. Serum total T_4 and T_3 concentrations are readily determined by a number of specific, sensitive, and widely available immunoassay techniques.

Alterations in serum T_4 binding proteins may result in hyperthyroxinemia or hypothyroxinemia. Therefore, it is important to define the levels of free thyroid hormone in blood.[7, 14] Two techniques are available for clinical use, the calculated free T_4 index (FTI) and direct free immunoassays. The FTI is calculated by multiplying the serum total T_4 by the percentage of T_3 resin uptake. The calculated FTI is useful in distinguishing altered TBG binding from states of true hyperthyroxinemia or hypothyroxinemia. The FTI generally correlates well with the results of both the free T_4 immunoassay and the more complex determination of free T_4 concentration by equilibrium dialysis. However, numerous conditions may alter the protein binding to produce a spurious free T_4 index value. A free T_3 index, calculated by multiplying the serum total T_3 and the T_3 uptake ratio, provides a reasonable estimate of serum free T_3. It may be used in the diagnosis of T_3 toxicosis.

Various commercial immunoassay kits are available for measuring free T_4. Assays using a two-step analogue procedure for free T_4 have demonstrated values comparable to equilibrium dialysis, in many clinical disorders. However, the analogue method may not yield accurate results in certain situations in which there may be an aberrant increase in TTR or T_4 binding to albumin.

Serum thyrotropin (TSH) is a reliable indicator of primary hypothyroidism. Second- and third-generation assays of TSH with greater sensitivity show undetectable levels of TSH in hyperthyroid patients. Thus, a suppressed basal serum TSH level determination diagnoses thyrotoxicosis, iatrogenic or endogenous, in more than 95% of cases.

Thyroglobulin is normally secreted in small amounts and can be assayed in serum by commercially available radioimmunoassays. When thyroid hormone, in the form of T_4 or T_3, is taken orally, no thyroglobulin or very low levels of thyroglobulin are detectable in serum. Although desiccated thyroid or purified thyroglobulin preparations contain thyroglobulin, the protein is degraded in the GI tract by proteolytic enzymes before absorption; therefore, no significant amount is detectable in the serum. Measurement of serum thyroglobulin thus allows differentiation of excessive thyroid hormone ingestion from other forms of thyrotoxicosis.[14] Serum thyroglobulin antibodies can, when present, interfere with the assay of serum thyroglobulin. A study has shown that measurement of fecal thyroxine levels may also help to confirm factitious thyrotoxicosis.[15]

COMMERCIAL THYROID HORMONE PREPARATIONS

Thyroid hormone preparations fall into three groups: biologic products containing T_4 and T_3, synthetic T_3, and synthetic T_4 (Table 98–1).

Biologic Products Containing T_4 and T_3. These preparations include desiccated forms of thyroid gland obtained from hogs, cattle, and sheep. This yellow insoluble powder, containing both T_4 and T_3, has a characteristic metallic odor and a saline taste. The recommended maintenance doses are 60 to 120 mg/d. Although the preferred therapy is synthetic T_4 (levothyroxine), patients who have used desiccated thyroid extract preparation in the past may be continued on these drugs. These thyroid tablets are now required by the U.S. Pharmacopeia to contain specified amounts of T_4 and T_3. This is a more reliable index of potency than the previous standardization by the total iodine content.

Liothyronine Sodium. The sodium salt of the L-isomer of T_3 is prepared as a tan crystalline powder, slightly soluble in water and alcohol. It is available as a parenteral preparation in addition to the previously available oral preparation. Liothyronine is occasionally indicated when a quicker response or faster disappearance of thyroid hormone effect is preferred. However, the resulting wide fluctuations in serum levels may result in cardiovascular side effects, especially in those with underlying coronary artery disease.

Levothyroxine Sodium. Synthetically prepared T_4 is a hygroscopic, cream-colored, odorless, tasteless powder slightly soluble in alcohol and water. The sodium salt is better absorbed from the GI tract than is the free acid. It may be given orally or intravenously when reconstituted with saline. An aqueous preparation for parenteral use is also currently available. Currently, 1.6 μg/kg is considered the average replacement dose. Thus, the daily maintenance dose is 88 to 125 μg for most adults of average body weight.

Generally, T_4 is the preferred thyroid hormone preparation in most clinical circumstances. Thyroid hormone is used clinically as a replacement therapy in the treatment of primary and secondary hypothyroidism. Additionally, thyroid hormone is used for suppression of benign thyroid nodules, nontoxic nodular and diffuse goiters, chronic autoimmune thyroiditis, and thyroid carcinoma. Concurrent administration of T_3 and tricyclic antidepressants has been recommended for treatment of refractory depression.[16] Other indiscriminate uses of thyroid hormones are unjustified. Thyroid hormones should not be used for menstrual, dietary, somatic, or fertility disorders not specifically related to thyroid disease.

THYROID HORMONE TOXICITY

Clinical Features

Thyroid hormone intoxication typically occurs in several settings: childhood ingestions, overdose in adults, suicidal overdoses, and subacute or chronic iatrogenic or factitious thyrotoxicosis. Most of the reported cases of acute T_4 ingestions have been in children. Acute overdose in adults is rare, although mild overdoses can result from medication errors by physicians, pharmacists, nurses, or patients. In 1994, 69% of reported thyroid hormone overdoses were in children younger than 6 years. Individuals between 6 and 19 years of age accounted for 9% of reported overdoses, and the remaining 22% occurred in adults.[2]

Factitious thyrotoxicosis is a well-documented clinical entity that is self-induced by long-term ingestion of excessive amounts of T_4. Some patients may become iatrogenically thyrotoxic on thyroid hormone doses that were previously considered appropriate or that become excessive as hormone metabolism declines with advancing age.[3] "Hamburger thyrotoxicosis" is a syndrome that follows the ingestion of ground beef contaminated with thyroid tissues.[17] Cooking the contaminated meat does not inactivate iodothyronines. Serum levels of T_3 and T_4 in such cases are elevated in association with low radioactive iodine uptake, suggesting a pattern similar to factitious thyrotoxicosis. Although inclusion of the thyroid gland in meat product preparations is now banned in most states in the United States, this

Table 98–1. Thyroid Preparations

Generic Name	Brand Name	Substrate	Available Doses
Pork thyroid "liquid" capsule USA	S-P-T	Pork thyroid with T_4 and T_3 in a ratio of 2.5:1	1 grain, 2 grain, 3 grain, 5 grain
Liothyronine sodium	Cytomel	3,3,5′-triiodo-L-thyronine sodium T_3 (synthetic)	5 μg and 25 μg
Levothyroxine	Synthroid Levoxyl Levothroid Eltroxin	3,5,3′,5′-tetraiodothyronine, T_4 (thyroxine sodium)	25 μg, 50 μg, 75 μg, 88 μg, 112 μg, 125 μg, 137 μg, 150 μg, 175 μg, 200 μg, 300 μg

Only the preparations available in the United States are listed. However, preparations other than the ones mentioned in this table may be available in other countries. The tablets are colored coded. Levothyroxine and liothyronine are also available commercially as parenteral preparation.

entity still should be considered in the differential diagnoses of thyrotoxicosis presenting with elevated serum T_3 and T_4 and low radioactive iodine uptake, especially occurring in a cluster pattern.

Effects of thyroid hormone overdose are observed primarily in the cardiovascular, neurologic, and GI systems. Typical cardiovascular responses include tachycardia, shortness of breath, palpitations, vasodilatation, systolic hypertension, and increased force of myocardial contraction.[18–20] Hypotension, congestive heart failure, and cardiovascular collapse can occur if the cardiovascular system is stressed beyond its capacity. Typical associated tachyarrhythmias are sinus tachycardia, atrial fibrillation, paroxysmal atrial tachycardia, and atrial flutter.[19] Electrocardiographic changes are nonspecific.[20] Common neurologic symptoms include sympathetic nervous system overactivity, including anxiety, mydriasis, diaphoresis, and agitation. Patients have been reported to develop periodic paralysis in subacute overdoses, a phenomenon most often affecting Asian men.[21] Intense muscle weakness with elevated serum creatinine kinase and aldolase levels may occur.[22] Patients may develop slurred speech.[21] Rare central nervous system manifestations of hormone overdose include extreme agitation, acute psychosis, seizures, and coma.[22, 23] GI manifestations include diarrhea and vomiting, but acute abdominal pain and peptic ulceration have been reported.[24] Constitutional features of thyroid hormone intoxication may include fever and malaise. In one report, patients developed intense laminar desquamation of the palms and soles late in the course of the illness.[22] Laboratory evaluation may reveal glucose intolerance; elevations in levels of blood urea nitrogen, creatinine, creatinine kinase, and aldolase; and abnormal results of liver function tests.

Thyroid hormone overdoses are generally well tolerated by pediatric patients. In this population, the clinical features include irritability, hyperactivity, vomiting, insomnia, diarrhea, fever, diaphoresis, flushing, abdominal pain, tachycardia, and leukocytosis.[25–27] Furthermore there may be little apparent relationship between the severity and type of symptoms and the ingested amount or serum T_4 levels.[25–31] Some children tolerate relatively large doses of thyroid hormone without symptoms of overdose. Funderburk and Spaulding[27] have reported an overdose of 13.2 mg of levothyroxine in a 3-year-old child with only modest symptoms. A retrospective study by Tunget and colleagues[25] showed no significant symptoms of toxicity with acute ingestions of less than or equal to 2 mg (0.13 mg/kg) T_4 equivalent in a pediatric age group. These researchers concluded that ingestion of less than 5 mg T_4 equivalent of thyroid hormone is not associated with significant toxicity. Of six adult patients with acute thyroxine ingestion, none developed thyroid storm despite serum T_4 levels ranging from 3 to 16 times the average level.[32] However, a rapid downhill course following massive ingestion of the thyroid hormone in adults has been reported.[22] It is important to note that these features may develop as late as 3 days after ingestion.[22]

Acute thyroid hormone overdose alone has only rarely been reported to cause fatality in pediatric or adult populations in the United States. Of 36,796 cases of thyroid hormone overdoses collected by the United States Poison Control Center from 1983 to 1993, only three fatalities were reported.[2, 25] Other ingested medications were believed to be the principal cause of death in each of these cases. Severe toxicity including sepsis, pneumonia, acute renal failure, myopathy, and left ventricular failure occurred in five adults in Spain who were erroneously administered between 70 and 1200 mg of levothyroxine for 2 to 12 days.[22] In this series, the only reported fatality due to thyroid hormone poisoning occurred in an adult patient who ingested 125 mg/d for 2 days.

Euthyroid persons appear to tolerate the effects of acute or chronic overdose relatively well. It has been reported that patients without underlying cardiovascular diseases tolerate intravenous T_4 doses of 750 μg.[33] However, patients of advanced age and with associated cardiovascular diseases can be quite vulnerable to even modest overdoses. Some investigators have suggested that women may tolerate excess thyroid hormone less well than men.[34]

The nature of the thyroid hormone preparation influences the clinical course of patients with thyroid hormone overdose. Because T_4 has a relatively long half-life, the clinical course may be prolonged.[35] In contrast, T_3, with its shorter half-life, may be better tolerated.[36] Patients ingesting large doses of desiccated thyroid extract may present with both acute and prolonged clinical manifestations.

Differential Diagnosis of Thyroid Hormone Intoxication (Table 98–2)

Patients presenting with full-blown clinical features of thyroid storm or crisis are rare. A history of drug ingestion can be difficult to obtain.[31] A thorough history should be obtained not only from the patient

Table 98–2. Differential Diagnosis of Thyroid Hormone Overdose

Hyperthyroidism
- Endogenous hyperthyroidism due to Graves' disease, multinodular goiter, solitary functioning adenoma, thyroiditis
- Hyperthyroidism associated with drug use such as thyroid hormone preparations, amiodarone, iodide-containing compounds, interferon, lithium
- Hyperthyroid state and ingestion of sympathomimetic drugs

Acute disorders associated with sympathetic nervous system activation: infection, heatstroke, hemorrhage, trauma, conditions associated with severe pain

Toxic drug ingestion
- Amphetamine
- Cocaine
- Tricyclic antidepressants
- Salicylates
- Dinitrophenol and pentachlorophenol
- Nicotine overdose

but from family members and friends. Questions should be asked about the possible availability of thyroid hormones (e.g., a personal history or family history of thyroid disorders, previous neck surgery, "weight problems" treated with medications, or history of depression being treated with a T_3-tricyclic combination).[16, 37] Because T_4 tablets are color coded, a specific description of the drugs ingested provides valuable dose information. Most cases of factitious hyperthyroidism occur in paramedical personnel[38] or in patients eager to lose weight.

Although physical findings may be nonspecific, attention should be focused on vital signs and cardiovascular and neurologic system manifestations. Accurate body temperature monitoring and early detection of hyperthermia are vital. Systolic hypertension and tachycardia may be noted. In addition, a hyperdynamic point of maximal cardiac impulse, systolic flow murmur, and atrial flutter or atrial fibrillation may be observed. Sympathetic nervous system overactivity may be manifested as diaphoresis, tremor, or eyelid lag. Neurologic findings such as restlessness, brisk deep tendon reflexes, delirium, and rarely psychosis or coma may be encountered.

Other acute conditions occasionally presenting with prominent sympathetic nervous system activation may mimic thyroid overdoses. These disorders include infection, heatstroke, hemorrhage, trauma, and profound pain. Acute psychosis due to other causes may at times be difficult to distinguish from thyroid hormone poisoning, especially in a patient with a history of drug overdose. The clinical history and a complete physical examination can usually distinguish these disorders from thyroid hormone overdose. Thyroid hormone poisoning should be considered in any patient presenting with hyperthermia.

It is critical to differentiate between endogenous thyrotoxicosis and overdose. The relatively short duration of symptoms and the absence of exophthalmos, pretibial myxedema, onycholysis of fingernails, thyroid bruit, and goiter are helpful in ruling out endogenous hyperthyroidism. Thyrotoxicosis occurring in association with the use of certain drugs should also be considered in the differential diagnosis. These drugs include amiodarone and other compounds containing iodides, thyroid hormones used to treat depression and obesity, and lithium carbonate. Sympathomimetic drugs taken alone with large doses of thyroid hormones may result in an acute clinical presentation or may even precipitate thyroid storm.[39, 40] In children presenting with symptoms and signs of thyrotoxicosis, especially in those younger than 5 years, overdose is a more likely diagnosis, because endogenous hyperthyroidism is unusual in this age group.

Compounds stimulating cellular metabolism, if ingested, may result in a clinical picture similar to that of thyroid overdose. These substances include amphetamine, cocaine, tricyclic antidepressants, salicylates, and phenol derivatives. A toxicologic analysis is helpful in confirming the diagnosis. Salicylates (aspirin, oil of wintergreen) poisoning may be difficult to distinguish from thyroid overdose; however, acid-base disturbance, glucose and coagulation abnormalities of salicylism, and positive results of a urine ferric chloride test are helpful. Serum salicylate levels further confirm the diagnosis. Phenol derivatives (dinitrophenol, pentachlorophenol) uncouple oxidative phosphorylation. These compounds are used in small doses for treating obesity in some countries and can produce an increase in pulse rate, respiratory rate, body temperature, and oxygen consumption, as well as diaphoresis. Ingestion of these caustic agents may result in mucous membrane and GI toxicity. Anoxia, acidosis, and delayed renal and hepatic toxicity may be apparent. The clinical course in these patients runs a significantly downhill course, compared with the course of thyroid hormone overdose. Nicotine toxicity may be ruled out by the absence of salivation and the presence of miosis. Absence of diaphoresis helps to rule out anticholinergic overdose.

Laboratory Diagnosis

In the hours after thyroid hormone ingestion, the serum T_4 and T_3 levels may not accurately reflect the severity of the clinical thyrotoxicosis. Furthermore, the early laboratory values are of limited use in defining the prognosis for patients with an overdose or in mandating the aggressiveness of therapy. Patients often may not have significant thyrotoxic symptoms on admission despite the high serum concentrations of T_3 and T_4.[32] Sudden death has been reported with only modest serum thyroid hormone level elevations and during periods when levels are decreasing. Furthermore, accurate laboratory assessment may be elusive in severely ill patients.[41] Hepatic, renal, and infectious diseases among others (euthyroid sick syndrome) can lower serum T_3 and to a lesser extent serum T_4 levels. With acute thyroid hormone overdose, the initial serum TSH level may not be suppressed until pituitary thyrotrophs respond to thyroid hormone excess and circulating TSH is metabolically cleared.

Despite these shortcomings, it is critical to monitor thyroid functions at least daily to correlate with the patient's clinical course. Useful testing may include serum free T_4 and total T_3 levels. Measurement of serum thyroglobulin may be helpful in differentiating endogenous from exogenous thyrotoxicosis. Very low or undetectable levels of thyroglobulin in the serum allow differentiation of other rare forms of endogenous hyperthyroidism with a low thyroidal radioactive iodine uptake, such as silent thyroiditis, functioning metastatic thyroid carcinoma, and struma ovarii. In contrast to patients with thyroid hormone overdose, these patients have normal or increased serum levels of thyroglobulin. Endogenous hyperthyroidism due to Graves' disease or nodular thyroid disease can also be differentiated from thyroid hormone overdose by measuring thyroidal uptake of iodine[123] or technetium 99m. The uptake is increased in hyperthyroidism due to Graves' disease or nodular thyroid disease, whereas it is suppressed with overdose. However, it should be kept in mind that the uptake is also suppressed in hyperthyroidism associated with thyroiditis, metastatic thyroid cancer, and struma ovarii. Measurement of fecal thyroxine levels may also be used to diagnose thyroid hormone overdose.[15]

In addition, these patients should also be monitored for electrolyte imbalance and liver dysfunction.

MANAGEMENT OF THYROID HORMONE OVERDOSE

Several factors should determine the aggressiveness with which a patient who has ingested excessive amounts of thyroid hormone should be treated. These include (1) the type of thyroid hormone preparations (i.e., T_4 or T_3 or both); (2) estimated dose of medication; (3) time since ingestion; (4) associated ingestion of other compounds; and (5) perhaps most important, the patient's age and underlying cardiac status and other associated disorders.[22, 34] As noted earlier, some healthy adults and children may tolerate even relatively large doses of thyroid hormone without serious consequences.[25–32, 35] On the other hand, life-threatening toxicity can occur in elderly patients with underlying cardiac disease and even occasionally in children.[26–34]

Special considerations apply to management of intoxication, depending on the type of thyroid hormone preparation ingested. T_3 ingestion may cause symptoms and signs to appear sooner, and the acute manifestation tends to be more serious. In contrast, T_4 overdose tends to be initially milder, and signs and symptoms may not appear until several days after ingestion.[22] Overdose with desiccated thyroid extract or thyroglobulin preparations may result in a combination of both acute and delayed symptoms.

The initial clinical evaluation should include the most precise possible history regarding the type of thyroid hormone preparation, the dose and time of thyroid hormone ingestion, current symptoms and signs of thyrotoxicosis, and any past history or signs of cardiac or other significant underlying disease. In the pediatric age group, the risks of overdose must be weighed against the risks of decontamination. Significant morbidity and mortality attributable to the use of syrup of ipecac, activated charcoal gastric lavage, and cathartic have been reported in this age group.[25] A report by Tunget and colleagues[25] recommended that GI decontamination not be performed with ingestions of less than or equal to 5 mg T_4 equivalent of thyroid hormone. Administration of activated charcoal is indicated in conscious adults. Serum measurements of electrolytes, glucose, urea nitrogen, creatinine, creatinine kinase, aldolase, calcium, T_3, T_4, and TSH should be ordered, as well as liver function tests.[22, 27–32] However, the previously noted limitations of serum thyroid function testing in assessing the severity and prognosis of thyroid hormone intoxication should be kept in mind.

The following generally are indications potentially justifying inpatient treatment: (1) severe symptoms or signs (e.g., tachycardia >120 beats per minute); (2) underlying cardiopulmonary disease; (3) elderly age; (4) ingestion of more than 100 μg/kg of T_4 or 30 μg/kg of T_3; and (5) serum T_4 concentrations greater than 50 μg/dL and/or T_3 levels greater than 350 ng/dL.

Supportive measures should include correction of hyperpyrexia, maintenance of fluid and electrolyte balance, and monitoring of cardiac rhythm and respiratory status. Acetaminophen should be used as an antipyretic because aspirin can increase the serum free T_4 fraction. Fulminant hyperthermia, although more common in thyroid storm due to endogenous hyperthyroidism, may present as a therapeutic challenge. The traditional treatment includes acetaminophen, sedation, neuromuscular blockade, and active cooling. Dantrolene sodium has been used in treating hyperpyrexia associated with thyroid crisis, improving clinical status without significant side effects.[42, 43]

In T_3 ingestion, hospital observation should continue until the patient is only mildly symptomatic and the serum T_3 has declined to less than 350 to 400 ng/dL. For T_4 ingestion in vulnerable adults, hospitalization generally should be continued for several days after the peak serum T_4 concentration. A briefer period of hospital observation may be reasonable for children, whereas more prolonged inpatient care may be appropriate for individuals with known cardiac disease or other complications. In pure T_3 ingestions, these criteria may be satisfied within 12 to 24 hours, whereas hospitalization for 1 week or longer can be anticipated for some T_4 ingestions in adults not treated with extracorporeal detoxification. Asymptomatic or mildly symptomatic and otherwise healthy patients may be monitored at home for approximately 1 week, particularly if T_4 was the major thyroid hormone ingested.

Propranolol is useful to ameliorate tachycardia, systolic hypertension, diaphoresis, and tremulousness accompanying hyperthyroidism. Propranolol, 10 to 80 mg orally every 6 hours or 1 to 3 mg intravenously every 4 hours, may be used in patients with no contraindication (e.g., pulmonary edema, bronchospasm, heart block). Children should receive a lower oral dose, no more than 0.2 mg/min intravenously. The propranolol dose should be titrated to the patient's response; a heart rate less than 120 beats per minute is a reasonable goal. A completely normal heart rate is not easily restored; an attempt to achieve it may cause hypotension. Esmolol, an ultrashort-acting β-blocking drug, has been used in cases of severe thyrotoxicosis and thyroid storm. A loading dose of 250 to 500 μg/kg over one minute followed by continuous infusion rates of 50 to 100 μg/kg per minute may be given. These drugs are relatively contraindicated in the presence of cardiovascular collapse or shock. In patients with a history of bronchial asthma, diltiazem, 30 to 60 mg orally four times daily with a maximum dose of 360 mg/d, may be administered. Diltiazem can also be given intravenously as a bolus injection (0.25 mg/kg); 20 mg is a reasonable initial dose for the average patient. This is then followed by a continuous infusion of 5 to 10 mg/h.

Cardiac glycosides such as digoxin may facilitate control of atrial fibrillation but should be expected to be less effective in controlling heart rate in patients with thyroid hormone overdose. Although the metabolic clearance rate for digoxin is increased in hyperthyroidism, toxicity nevertheless results if the dosage is titrated on the basis of heart rate. The phenothiazine group of drugs such as chlorpromazine has been suggested as a useful therapeutic adjunct as an adrenergic and cholinergic antagonist and antiemetic with sedative properties. However, these drugs may exacerberate hyperthermia and cause depression of cardiac and ventilatory functions.[27] Phenobarbital has been used for sedation, especially in the pediatric population.[25]

Administration of glucocorticoids may be useful in diminishing T_4 to T_3 conversion. However, actual adrenal insufficiency is exceedingly rare in these patients. Propylthiouracil (PTU), iopanoic acid, other radiocontrast dyes, and amiodarone all inhibit extrathyroidal T_4 to T_3 conversion but have no clearly demonstrated utility in the management of thyroid hormone ingestions. Because the thionamides, such as propylthiouracil and methimazole (Tapazole), do not block the action of ingested thyroid hormones, they have little role in treating exogenous thyroid hormone intoxication.

Bile acid sequestrants may serve as useful adjunctive therapy for these patients. Interruption of the enterohepatic circulation of thyroid hormones with a bile acid sequestrant such as cholestyramine has been shown to be useful in treating iatrogenic thyrotoxicosis[11] (Fig. 98–2). Similarly, cholestyramine has been used in treating patients with Graves' disease.[44] It has been shown that 50 mg of cholestyramine can bind at least 3000 μg of thyroxine[11] and thus enhance the clearance of thyroid hormone. This resin may be administered in a dosage of 4 g four times daily after the initial diagnosis. The drug may be continued until the patient recovers clinically and the serum thyroid hormone level becomes completely normal.

Diuresis and hemodialysis are not usually used in accelerating clearance of thyroid hormones because of their binding to plasma proteins too large to pass through glomerular capillary and dialysis membranes, respectively. Peritoneal dialysis, the first effective method for speeding thyroid hormone removal, reduces the T_4 half-life to less than 24 hours.[45] Exchange transfusion with donor blood effectively provides unsaturated serum proteins but has the usual risks associated with blood transfusion.[46]

Two extractive techniques, plasmapheresis and hemoperfusion, are now available for use in the treatment of thyroid hormone overdose[22, 46–48] (Fig. 98–3). Because thyroid hormones are firmly bound to plasma proteins, plasmapheresis, at least on a theoretic basis, should reduce the pool of thyroid hor-

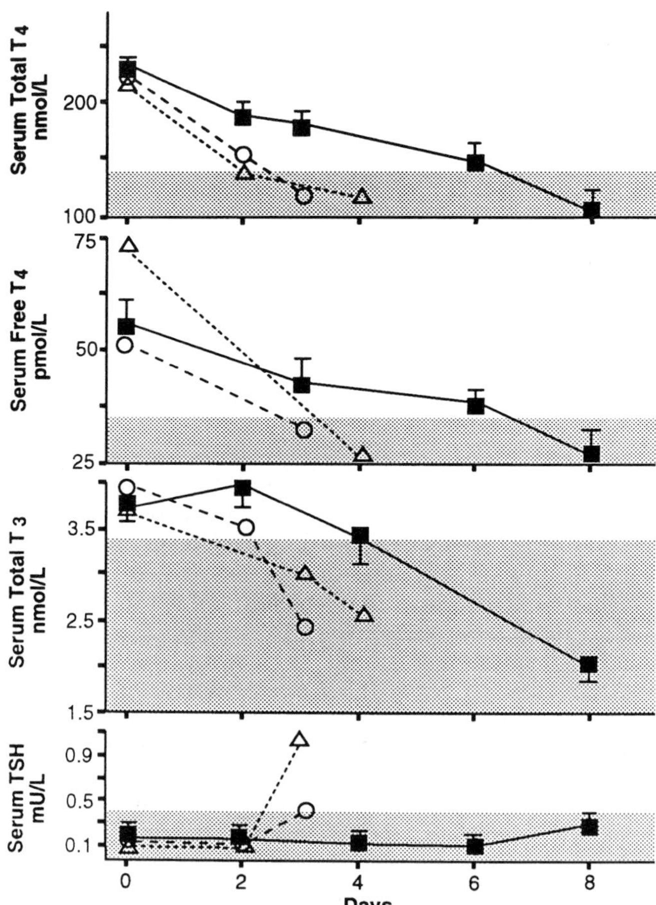

Figure 98–2. The use of the bile acid sequestrant cholestyramine to lower serum thyroid hormones in iatrogenic hyperthyroidism. Two patients with iatrogenic hyperthyroidism were treated with 4 g of cholestyramine four times a day. The alterations in serum total T_4, free T_4, total T_3, and thyroid-stimulating hormone (TSH) levels in patient 1 (O---O), patient 2 (△---△), and control patients (■---■) (n = 3, values = mean ± SE) are shown. The normal serum values are as follows: total T_4, 51 to 142 nmol/L; free T_4, 10 to 36 pmol/L; total T_3, 1.2 to 3.4 nmol/L; and TSH, 0.4 to 3.5 mU/L. The *shaded areas* show the upper normal range values for T_4 and T_3 and the lower normal range values for TSH. (From Shakir KMM, Michaels RD, Hays JH, et al: The use of bile acid sequestrants to lower serum thyroid hormones in iatrogenic hyperthyroidism. Ann Intern Med *118*:113, 1993.)

mones in circulation. Thus, plasmapheresis with reinfusion of hormone-free proteins to the patient may be more efficient than hemoperfusion. However, hemoperfusion has been shown to remove bound as well as free hormones. Hemoperfusion with activated charcoal has emerged as an effective approach to remove circulating thyroid hormone quickly. Charcoal hemoperfusion for 8 hours or less has produced clinical improvement and normalization of serum T_3 and T_4 levels within 36 hours. Both protein-bound and free hormones are absorbed, the hazards of transfusion are avoided, and the procedure can be accomplished quickly and safely in experienced hands. Charcoal or XAD-4 resin hemoperfusion may be indicated for patients with severe existing or potential cardiac toxicity or after failure of conventional supportive and β-adrenergic antagonist therapy after

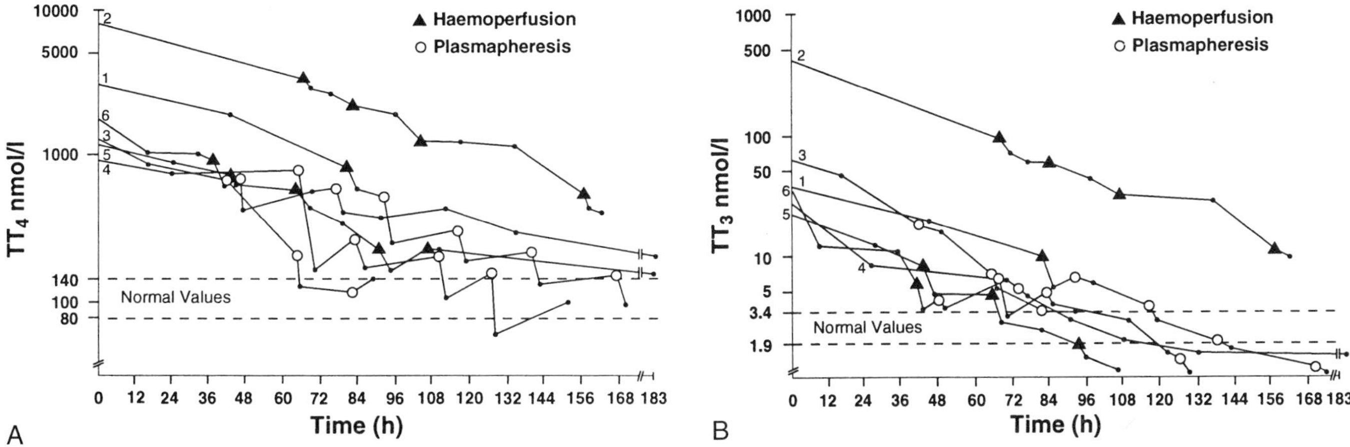

Figure 98–3. *A*, The changes in serum total T_4 (TT_4) in response to hemoperfusion or plasmapheresis in six patients. These patients ingested between 70 and 1200 mg of L-thyroxine for 2 to 12 consecutive days. Extraction techniques were started 8 to 14 days after the first dose of L-thyroxine. The plasma disappearance rate of TT_4 with plasmapheresis was 30 times higher than with standard medical treatment. With hemoperfusion, the plasma disappearance rate was five times higher than with medical treatment. *B*, The changes in serum total T_3 (TT_3) in response to hemoperfusion or plasmapheresis. The clinical details are mentioned in *A*. The plasma disappearance rates for TT_3 were higher under hemoperfusion than under plasmapheresis. (From Binimelis J, Bassas L, Marruecos L, et al: Massive thyroxine intoxication: Evaluation of plasma extractions. Intensive Care Med *13*:36, 1987.)

24 hours.[48] Binimelis and colleagues[22] have demonstrated that both plasmapheresis and hemoperfusion are effective in decreasing the duration of thyrotoxicosis. These investigators found that plasmapheresis is more effective than hemoperfusion in the extraction of T_4 (see Fig. 98–3). However, other investigations have shown that plasmapheresis may not be as effective in thyroid hormone overdose.[49–50]

INTOXICATIONS WITH THYROID ANTAGONISTS

Antithyroid drugs are drugs that interfere with one or more steps in iodine metabolism, hormone formation, or hormone release by the thyroid gland. Perchlorate and thiocyanate, rarely used in clinical practice, inhibit the transport of iodide ion across the basal membrane of the thyroid follicular epithelium. Thionamides, such as propylthiouracil and methimazole, inhibit iodide organification. Finally, drugs that prevent the secretion of thyroid hormones include iodide and lithium. In this section, only the thionamides are addressed. The toxicity of iodine (see Chapter 60) and lithium (see Chapter 33) is discussed elsewhere.

The thionamides inhibit organification of iodide and the coupling of iodotyrosines to form hormonally active iodothyronines. Both are readily absorbed from the GI tract within an hour, and inhibition of thyroid iodine organification begins within 20 to 30 minutes. The volume of distribution for PTU is approximately 0.3 L/kg, and 80% is protein bound. The plasma half-lives of PTU and methimazole are 1 to 2 hours and 6 to 13 hours, respectively. Intrathyroidal accumulation of drug occurs. Both PTU and methimazole cross the placental barrier and appear in human milk.

Most toxic reactions to thionamides occur within a few weeks or months of beginning therapy. Mild side effects include skin rash, urticaria, loss of hair, and itching in 2% to 5% of patients. Serious side effects include agranulocytosis, which has a rapid onset and is usually heralded by fever and a sore throat. The reported incidence of agranulocytosis is approximately two to three per 1000 patients. A mild dose-dependent leukopenia also may occur in as many as 10% of patients. Management of agranulocytosis and other toxicities includes early recognition and prompt withdrawal of the drug. Methimazole-induced agranulocytosis has been treated with recombinant human granulocyte colony-stimulating factor.[51] Other side effects may include GI distress, hepatitis, arthritis, and rarely headache, drowsiness, vertigo, visual and hearing disturbances, ageusia, allergic vasculitis, aplastic anemia, coagulopathy, and hypoglycemia. Hepatic injury is generally mild but rarely may be life threatening.

In one case report of overdose with PTU, a 12-year-old girl took between 5000 and 13,000 mg of the drug.[52] No symptoms were noticed, and laboratory evaluation revealed normal blood counts, renal functions, and prothrombin time. Her serum alkaline phosphatase level was slightly elevated. Urinary levels of PTU were 90 mg/dL 17 hours after ingestion. Serum levels of thyroid hormones declined for several days. This patient completely recovered because of ideal conditions for rapid clearance of PTU (i.e., short drug plasma half-life, normal renal and hepatic function, and thyroidal accumulation). However, PTU overdose could run a more complicated course in patients with previously impaired liver or renal functions.

In the event of thionamide overdose, complete blood count and liver function test results should be monitored daily for at least 3 to 5 days. Renal function should be assessed initially. The mild hypothyroid state should not require treatment in previously euthyroid individuals. Hydration and other supportive measures should be instituted. No experience with extracorporeal detoxification for PTU has been reported; in view of its serum protein binding, only hemoperfusion techniques would seem promising.

References

1. Nyström E, Lindstedt G, Lundberg PA: Minor signs and symptoms of toxicity in a young woman in spite of massive thyroxine ingestion. Acta Med Scand *207*:135, 1980.
2. Litovitz TL, Felberg L, Soloway RN, et al: 1994 Annual Report of the American Association of Poison Control Centers Toxic Exposure Surveillance System. Am J Emerg Med *13*:551, 1995.
3. Green WL: Werner and Ingbar's The Thyroid: A Fundamental and Clinical Text. 6th ed. Philadelphia, J.B. Lippincott Co., pp 322–402, 1991.
4. Sterling K, Chodos RB: Radiothyroxine turnover studies in myxedema, thyrotoxicosis and hypermetabolism without endocrine disease. J Clin Invest *35*:806, 1956.
5. Haddad HM: Rates of I^{131}-labelled thyroxine metabolism in euthyroid children. J Clin Invest *39*:1590, 1960.
6. Rose E, Sanders TP, Webb WL: Occult factitial thyrotoxicosis. Ann Intern Med *71*:309, 1969.
7. Reed L, Pangaro LN: Principles and Practice of Endocrinology and Metabolism. 2nd ed. Philadelphia, J.B. Lippincott Co., pp 285–291, 1995.
8. Fish LH, Schwartz HL, Cavanaugh J, et al: Replacement dose, metabolism, and bioavailability of levothyroxine in the treatment of hypothyroidism. Role of triiodothyronine in pituitary feed back in humans. N Engl J Med *316*:764, 1987.
9. Campbell NRC, Hasinoff BB, Stalts H, et al: Ferrous sulfate reduces thyroxine efficacy in patients with hypothyroidism. Ann Intern Med *117*:1010, 1992.
10. Sherman SI, Tielens ET, Ladenson PW: Sucralfate causes malabsorption of L-thyroxine. Am J Med *96*:531, 1994.
11. Shakir KMM, Michaels RD, Hays JH, Potter BB: The use of bile acid sequestrants to lower serum thyroid hormones in iatrogenic hyperthyroidism. Ann Intern Med *118*:112, 1993.
12. Liel Y, Sperber AD, Shany S: Nonspecific intestinal adsorption of levothyroxine by aluminum hydroxide. Am J Med *97*:363, 1994.
13. Brent GA: The molecular basis of thyroid hormone action. N Engl J Med *331*:847, 1994.
14. Smallridge RC: Principles and Practice of Endocrinology and Metabolism. 2nd ed. Philadelphia, J.B. Lippincott Co., pp 299–306, 1995.
15. Bouillon R, Verresen L, Staels F, et al: The measurement of fecal thyroxine in the diagnosis of thyrotoxicosis factitia. Thyroid *3*:101, 1993.
16. Cole PA, Bostwick JM, Fajtova VT: Thyrotoxicosis in a depressed patient on L-triiodothyronine. Psychosomatics *34*:539, 1993.
17. Hedberg CW, Fishbein DB, Janssen RS, et al: An outbreak of thyrotoxicosis caused by the consumption of bovine thyroid gland in ground beef. N Engl J Med *316*:993, 1987.
18. Bhasin S, Wallace W, Lawrence JB, et al: Sudden death associated with thyroid hormone abuse. Am J Med *71*:887, 1981.
19. Rogers HM: Cardiovascular manifestations of induced thyrotoxicosis. Ann Intern Med *26*:914, 1947.
20. Sandler G: Effect of thyrotoxicosis on the electrocardiogram. Br Heart J *21*:111, 1959.
21. Layzer RB, Goldfield E: Periodic paralysis caused by the abuse of thyroid hormone. Neurology *24*:949, 1974.
22. Binimelis J, Bassas L, Marruecos L, et al: Massive thyroxine intoxication: Evaluation of plasma extraction. Intensive Care Med *13*:33, 1987.
23. Roberts JA: Correct use of thyroxine. Med J Aust *2*:650, 1975.
24. Garbart AC: Simultaneous occurrence of active peptic ulcer and active hyperthyroidism. J Mt Sinai Hosp *17*:787, 1951.
25. Tunget CL, Clark RF, Turchen SG, et al: Raising the decontamination level for thyroid hormone ingestions. Am J Emerg Med *13*:9, 1995.
26. Dahl IL: Thyroid crisis in a three year old. Acta Paediatr Scand *57*:55, 1968.
27. Funderburk SJ, Spaulding JS: Sodium levothyroxine intoxication in a child. Pediatrics *45*:298, 1970.
28. Lehrner LM, Weir MR: Acute ingestions of thyroid hormones. Pediatrics *73*:313, 1984.
29. Tennebein M, Dean HJ: Benign course after massive levothyroxine ingestion. Pediatr Emerg Care *2*:5, 1986.
30. Golightly LK, Smolinske SC, Kulig KW, et al: Clinical effects of accidental levothyroxine ingestion in children. Am J Dis Child *141*:1025, 1987.
31. Lewander WJ, Lacouture PG, Silva JE, et al: Acute thyroxine ingestion in pediatric patients. Pediatrics *84*:262, 1989.
32. Matthews SJ: Acute thyroxine overdosage: Two cases of parasuicide. Ulster Med J *63*:170, 1993.
33. Ridgway EC, McCammon JA, Benotti J, et al: Acute metabolic responses in myxedema to large doses of intravenous L-thyroxine. Ann Intern Med *77*:549, 1972.
34. Likoff WB, Levine SA: Thyrotoxicosis as the sole cause of heart failure. Am J Med Sci *206*:425, 1943.
35. Von Hofe SE, Young RL: Thyrotoxicosis after a single ingestion of levothyroxine. JAMA *237*:1361, 1977.
36. Dahlberg PA, Karlsson FA, Wide L: Triiodothyronine intoxication. Lancet *2*:700, 1979.
37. Cooper N, Palmer B: Thyroid hormone in a health food capsule. N Z Med J *107*:231, 1994.
38. Gorman CA, Wahner HW, Tauxe WN: Metabolic malingerers. Am J Med *48*:708, 1970.
39. Jacobson T, Steckler T, Wilson BE: Sympathomimetic drug abuse masking an endogenous hyperadrenergic state, Graves' disease. Behav Med *20*:91, 1994.
40. Wilson BE, Hobbs WN: Case report: Pseudoephredrine-associated thyroid storm: Thyroid hormone catecholamine interactions. Am J Med Sci *306*:317, 1993.
41. Vos RA, De Jong M, Bernard BF, et al: Impaired thyroxine and 3,5,3′-triiodothyronine handling by rat hepatocytes in the presence of serum of patients with nonthyroidal illness. J Clin Endocrinol Metab *80*:2364, 1995.
42. Christensen PA, Nissen LR: Treatment of thyroid storm in a child with dantrolene. Br J Anaesth *59*:523, 1987.
43. Bennett MH, Wainwright AP: Acute thyroid crisis on induction of anesthesia. Anaesthesia *44*:28, 1989.
44. Solomon BL, Wartofsky L, Burman KD: Adjunctive cholestyramine therapy for thyrotoxicosis. Clin Endocrinol (Oxf) *38*:39, 1993.
45. Herrmann J, Schmidt HJ, Krüskemper HL: Thyroxine elimination by peritoneal dialysis in experimental thyrotoxicosis. Horm Metab Res *5*:180, 1973.
46. Ashkar FS, Katims RB, Smoak III WM, et al: Thyroid storm treatment with blood exchange and plasmapheresis. JAMA *214*:1275, 1970.
47. Van Heukelom LHS, der Kinderen PJ, Vingerhoeds ACM: Plasmapheresis in L-thyroxine intoxication. Vet Hum Toxicol *21*:33, 1979.
48. Seyffart G: Dialysis and Hemoperfusion in Poisonings. Bad Homburg, Fresenius Foundation, 1977.
49. Henderson A, Hickman P, Ward G, et al: Lack of efficacy of plasmapheresis in a patient overdosed with thyroxine. Anaesth Intensive Care *22*:463, 1994.
50. May ME, Mintz PD, Lowry P, et al: Plasmapheresis in thyroxine overdose: A case report. J Toxicol Clin Toxicol *20*:517, 1983.
51. Tamai H, Mukuta T, Matsubayashi S, et al: Treatment of methimazole-induced agranulocytosis using recombinant human granulocyte colony-stimulating factor (rhG-CSF). J Clin Endocrinol Metab *77*:1356, 1993.
52. Jackson GL, Flickinger FW, Wells LW: Massive overdose of propylthiouracil. Ann Intern Med *91*:418, 1979.

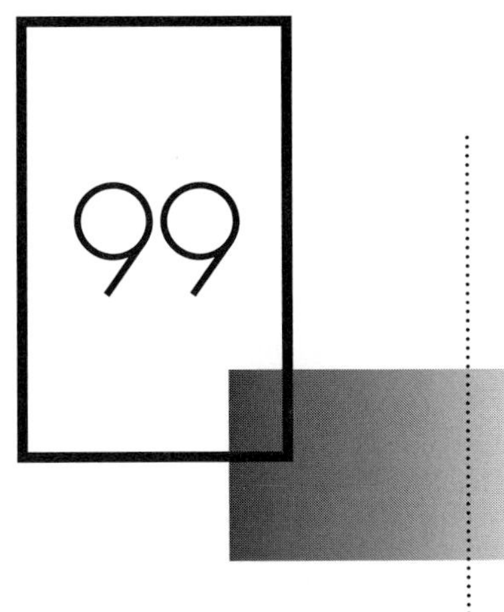

The Vitamins

FRED M. HENRETIG, M.D.

The vitamins are a defined group of essential organic micronutrients that are required in the human diet for optimal nutrition and to prevent a specific deficiency syndrome.[1, 2] This requirement is due to either a complete inability to synthesize these nutrients *de novo* or an inadequate rate of synthesis to maintain optimal health. Medical uses for the vitamins include the prevention or treatment of deficiency states and the treatment of rare vitamin-responsive inborn errors of metabolism.

A less accepted current usage of vitamins has been routine high-dose consumption by healthy adults. This practice has gained popularity with the lay public and some health care workers in an effort to enhance appearance, longevity, athletic performance, or to prevent or ameliorate nondeficiency-specific disease states. The clinically significant vitamin exposures occur most often under these circumstances of intentional chronic overdose. The water-soluble vitamins are typically excreted renally when ingested in excess, although very large doses taken chronically have resulted in adverse effects. The fat-soluble vitamins are stored in tissues, and excessive consumption is thus more likely to result in toxicity. Accidental overdose of pediatric multivitamin preparations by children also occurs frequently, although this is rarely a cause for significant concern aside from coingested iron in combination products. (Even serious iron toxicity is rare in this context.) Occasionally, vitamins are chosen as an intentional acute overdose agent. An unfortunately not uncommon scenario is the acute overdose by a young pregnant woman of her prescribed prenatal vitamin and mineral supplement. In this context, with a typical elemental iron content of 62.5 mg per tablet, serious iron poisoning may occur, although toxicity related to coingested vitamins is again rarely of significance (see also Chapter 56 on Iron).

The medical use of vitamins can be traced to the 1753 discovery by British naval surgeon James Lind of the protection from scurvy afforded to sailors by the addition of fresh citrus fruits to their diets during long voyages.[1] Ascorbic acid (vitamin C) was, of course, subsequently identified as the antiscorbutic factor and became the first of the 13 named vitamins. Vitamins are currently divided into nine that are water soluble (ascorbate, thiamine, riboflavin, niacin, pyridoxine, biotin, pantothenic acid, folate, and B_{12}) and four that are fat soluble (vitamins A, D, E, and K). Several of the vitamins exist in nature or *in vivo* as different but closely related chemical compounds referred to as *vitamers.* The water-soluble vitamins or their derivatives function primarily as coenzymes for apoenzymes. An example is pyridoxine (when converted to pyridoxal phosphate) as coenzyme to the glutamic acid decarboxylase apoenzyme, forming a holoenzyme that synthesizes γ-aminobutyric acid from glutamic acid. The mechanism of action of the fat-soluble vitamins is less well understood, except for the role of vitamin K in promoting prothrombin and factors VII, IX, and X synthesis. However, recent work has found hormonal or prohormonal effects, with the discovery of a "superfamily" of specific intracellular receptors, for vitamins A and D.[2]

Amounts of vitamins necessary daily to protect normal, healthy persons from vitamin deficiency states range from micrograms to milligrams and are designated the *minimum daily requirements* (MDRs). In the United States, the Food and Nutrition Board, Institute of Medicine of the National Academy of Sciences, periodically reviews the scientific evidence and sets recommended dietary allowances (RDAs), which in general are set two to six times higher than MDRs in order to provide an ample but safe intake for the overall population.[1] The most recent RDAs were published in 1989[3] and are summarized in Table 99–1. These RDAs vary considerably, ranging from 2 μg (B_{12}) to 60 mg (C) a day for the water-

Table 99–1. Recommended Dietary Allowances

Fat-Soluble Vitamins	A (μg)	D (μg)	E (μg)	K (μg)
Infants	375	7.5–10	3–4	5–10
Children	400–700	10	6–7	15–30
Males (>11 y)	1000	5–10	10	45–80
Females (>11 y)	800	5–10	8	45–65
Pregnant	800	10	10	65
Lactating	1200–1300	10	11–12	65

Water-Soluble Vitamins	C (mg)	Thiamine (mg)	Riboflavin (mg)	Niacin (mg)	B_6 (mg)	Folate (μg)	B_{12} (μg)
Infants	30–35	0.3–0.4	0.4–0.5	5–6	0.3–0.6	25–35	0.3–0.5
Children	40–45	0.7–1.0	0.8–1.2	9–13	1.0–1.4	50–100	0.7–1.4
Males (>15 y)	50–60	1.2–1.5	1.4–1.8	15–20	1.7–2.0	150–200	2.0
Females (>15 y)	50–60	1.0–1.1	1.2–1.3	13–15	1.4–1.6	150–180	2.0
Pregnant	70	1.5	1.6	17	2.2	400	2.2
Lactating	90–95	1.6	1.7–1.8	20	2.1	260–280	2.6

Adapted from Marcus R, Coulston AM: The vitamins: Introduction. *In* Hardman JG, Gilman AG, Limbard LE (eds): Goodman and Gilman's The Pharmacologic Basis of Therapeutics. 9th ed. New York, McGraw-Hill, pp 1547–1553, 1996.

soluble vitamins and from 5 to 10 μg (D) to approximately 10 mg (E) for the fat-soluble vitamins. Megadose usage typically involves self-administration of doses 20 to 600 times in excess of these RDAs.[1]

In the United States, efforts to regulate vitamin usage have had a complex and politically charged history. Currently, the U.S. Food and Drug Administration (FDA) has the authority to regulate the labeling of vitamin and mineral supplements. The FDA proposed in 1973 to classify all vitamin/mineral supplements that contained more than 150% of RDAs as drugs, but the regulation was reversed by court order. Similar attempts to specifically limit the total dosage of vitamin A and D supplements sold without prescription were also blocked.[2] Currently, the FDA does not regulate the nutrient content of vitamin supplements, except those intended for use by children less than 12 years of age and by pregnant or lactating women, despite the well-recognized hazards of megadose vitamin usage.

A number of vitamin-responsive metabolic disorders have been described, involving at least eight of the nine water-soluble vitamins and vitamin D.[1, 4, 5] Classic examples include pyridoxine-dependent infantile convulsions, pernicious anemia, and vitamin D–sensitive rickets. Pyridoxine dependency was first described in the early 1950s,[1] and the same era witnessed the observation that the dementia associated with pellegra (niacin deficiency) was similar in some ways to that of schizophrenia.[4, 5] Early studies in the psychiatric literature suggested beneficial results in treating schizophrenia with massive doses of niacin, prompting further extension of this concept to other vitamins and to other illnesses.[4, 6]

Pauling's 1970 monograph *Vitamin C and the Common Cold*[7] helped popularize the use of megadoses of vitamins for prevention and treatment of a number of illnesses ranging from the viral infections to cancer. The increased interest in personal fitness and preventive health of the 1970s provided fertile ground for the expansion of this concept of vitamin megadosing. By the 1980s, more than 70% of Americans believed that vitamins could prevent fatigue, and 21% believed that diseases such as cancer and arthritis were caused by vitamin deficiency.[4, 8] A 1987 survey found that one half of adult Americans took occasional vitamin supplements, and more than 20% took vitamins daily.[9] The popularity of megavitamins is currently often reinforced by broad media coverage of findings from studies of the positive effects of "antioxidant" vitamins (A, C, and E) on the prevention of cancer and atherosclerotic heart disease.[10, 11] In general, although many nutritional surveys have demonstrated a protective effect from dietary consumption of foods rich in these nutrients, clinical trials of supplementation with high doses of exogenous vitamins have thus far tended to show negative or equivocal results.[12, 13] Most recognized nutritional authorities continue to counsel that healthy adults, other than women who are pregnant or breast feeding, satisfy their vitamin needs with a normal, varied diet[14] and recommend only increasing the amount of fresh fruits, vegetables, and cereal fiber that are unfortunately often omitted in the modern "fast-food" diets many Americans consume.[15, 16]

FAT-SOLUBLE VITAMINS

In general, toxic effects of vitamins are most often related to overdosing of the fat-soluble vitamins and have been observed particularly with excessive ingestion of vitamin A as well as with vitamin D (Table 99–2). Adverse effects ascribed to vitamins E and K have been uncommon and noted primarily with parenteral use. In view of the prominent place afforded to vitamin A toxicity in reported medical literature, this vitamin is here reviewed in some detail relative to the other vitamins covered in this chapter.

Vitamin A

Vitamin A has a long and fascinating history. As early as 1500 BC, night blindness that could be reme-

Table 99–2. Vitamin Toxicity Overview

Vitamin	Toxic Dose	Principal Toxic Effects
A	Acute: 75,000–100,000 IU (P) >1,000,000 IU (A) Chronic: 18,000 IU/d (P) 20,000–50,000 IU/d (A) Teratogenic: >10,000 IU/d	Initial: CNS; increased ICP with headache, irritability, lethargy, ophthalmoplegia, papilledema Later: hair loss, peeling skin, hepatomegaly CNS: increased ICP, pseudotumor cerebri Mucocutaneous: dry, scaly, peeling skin; hair loss, brittle nails; cheilitis, stomatitis, gingivitis Hepatic: early–hepatomegaly, anorexia, vomiting, +/− abnormal LFTs late–hepatic fibrosis, ascites, cirrhosis, esophageal varices Skeletal: bone pain, cortical hyperostoses; premature epiphyseal closure (P) Reproductive: teratogenic effects on face, ears; occasional CNS, cardiac (less so than with isotretinoin)
D	1600–2000 IU/d (P) 60,000 IU/d (A) Teratogenic: (?) 2000–4000 IU/d Probably variable, with idiosyncratic hypersensitivity	Metabolic: hypercalcemia Renal: hypercalciuria, nephrocalcinosis CV: metastatic calcifications in heart, vessels CV: infantile hypercalcemia, supravalvular aortic stenosis syndrome
E	(?) 400–3000 IU/d	CNS: headache, weakness GI: Nausea, cramps, diarrhea Heme: increased effect of anticogulants
K	(?) (Occurs with therapeutic IV dose)	Anaphylactoid reaction Heme: hemolysis, jaundice in newborns (esp with G6PD deficiency)
Pyridoxine	117–500 mg/d	Peripheral sensory neuropathy
Niacin	3.0–4.5 g/d	Cutaneous: flushing, pruritus GI: cholestatic jaundice, hepatitis Heme: thrombocytopenia CV: atrial fibrillation Misc: gout, myopathy
Thiamine	Acute: (?) (rare, occurs with therapeutic IV dose) Chronic: 5 mg/d	Anaphylactic reaction Misc: headache, irritability, tachycardia
C	(?), probably > 4 g/d	GI: nausea, cramping, diarrhea Renal: nephrolithiasis (esp in predisposed patients) Heme: hemolysis with G6PD deficiency Misc: rebound scurvy after withdrawal

A, adult; CNS, central nervous system; CV, cardiovascular; esp, especially; GI, gastrointestinal; G6PD, glucose-6-phosphate dehydrogenase; Heme, hematologic; ICP, intracranial pressure; LFTs, liver function tests; Misc, miscellaneous; P, pediatric.

died by the topical application of roasted liver was described in Egypt, and Hippocrates later recommended the ingestion of cow liver as a cure.[17] In 1865, ophthalmia brasiliana, an eye disorder of poorly nourished slaves, was described. Further linkage of keratomalacia to nutritional deficiency was provided in the 1880s with descriptions of night blindness among Russian Orthodox Catholics who fasted during Lent and particularly with the description of corneal sloughing in breast-fed infants of fasting mothers.[17] Perhaps the oldest and largest recorded experience with vitamin toxicity is associated with both acute and chronic exposure to excess vitamin A. The 19th century Arctic explorer Elisha Kane described a syndrome of severe headache, vomiting, drowsiness, and irritability occurring a few hours after the ingestion of polar bear liver.[18] This syndrome is recognized today as being quite likely due to acute hypervitaminosis A–induced pseudotumor cerebri. Modern authors continue to describe similar phenomena, e.g., the 1984 report of a 25-year-old Sri Lankan woman who developed pseudotumor and markedly elevated serum vitamin A levels one week after consuming a meal of shark liver (discussed later).[19]

Physiology and Pharmacology

The vitamin A family consists of several related compounds, with their respective stereoisomers, which exhibit the vitamin's biologic effects. Retinol, also referred to as vitamin A_1, is the alcohol form, which is found primarily as an ester in the liver of many animals and saltwater fish (Fig. 99–1). Retinal, which is the vitamin A aldehyde, functions as the chromophore of the retina when it combines with the protein opsin to form rhodopsin. β-Carotene, or provitamin A, is a dimer of retinal that occurs in many pigmented plants. Retinoic acid, the carboxylic acid of retinol, is believed to be the relevant vitamer at the cellular level for most functions of vitamin A other than in the visual cycle.

Vitamin A is classically quantified by bioassay in rats, although purified preparations may also be

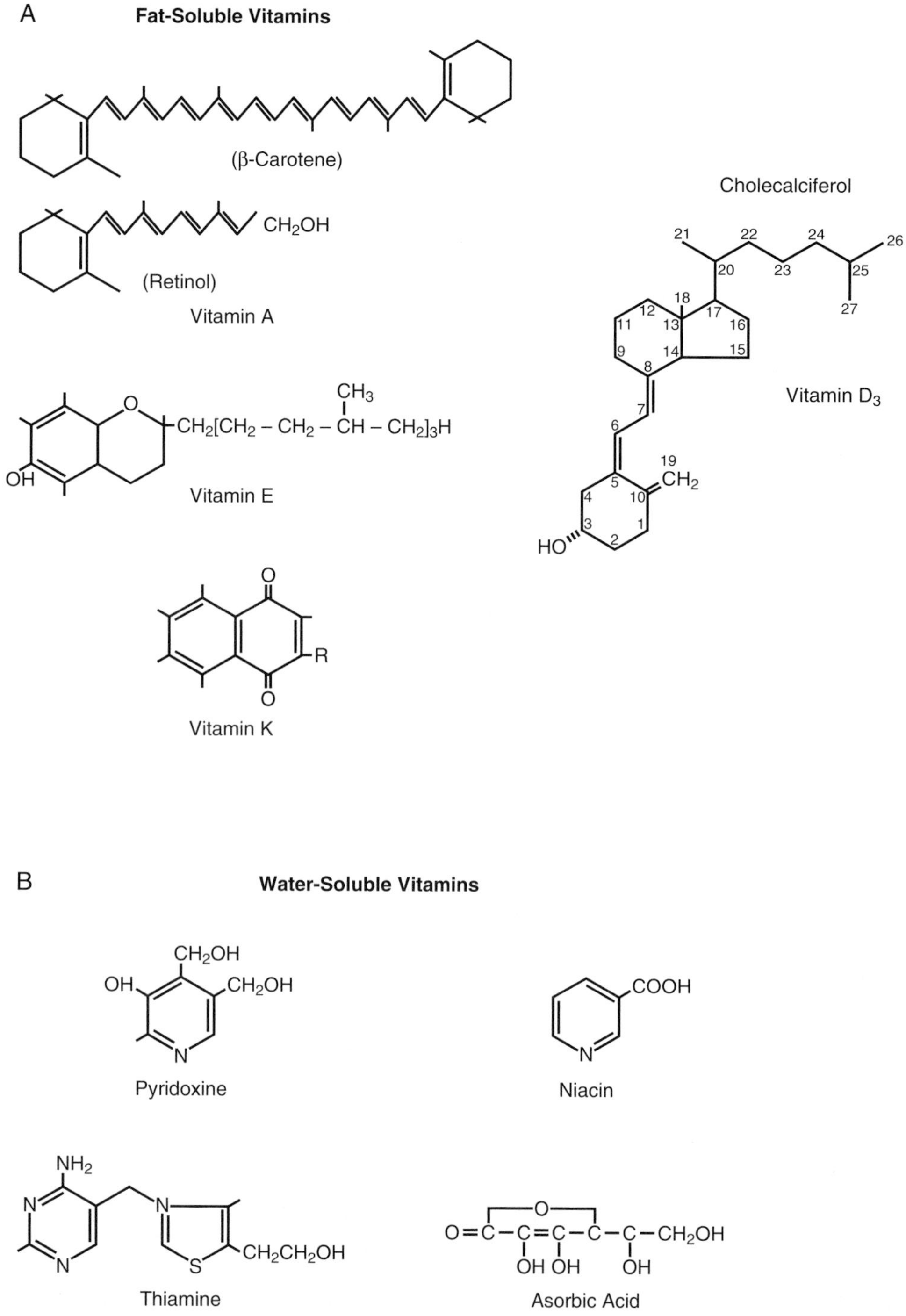

A **Fat-Soluble Vitamins**

(β-Carotene)

CH_2OH

(Retinol)

Vitamin A

CH_3

$CH_2[CH_2 - CH_2 - CH - CH_2]_3H$

OH

Vitamin E

O

R

O

Vitamin K

Cholecalciferol

Vitamin D_3

CH_2

HO

B **Water-Soluble Vitamins**

CH_2OH

OH

CH_2OH

N

Pyridoxine

COOH

N

Niacin

NH_2

CH_2CH_2OH

Thiamine

$O=C-C=C-C-C-CH_2OH$

OH OH OH

Asorbic Acid

Figure 99–1. Fat- *(A)* and water-soluble *(B)* vitamins reported to have toxic effects in humans.

determined spectrophotometrically.[17] The "retinol equivalent" is equal to 1 μg of all-*trans*-retinol (3.3 IU) or 6 μg of dietary β-carotene (10 IU).

Vitamin A is believed to act through hormone-like activity on intracellular receptors, in addition to the well-understood specific effect of one of its vitamers, retinal, as the chromophore in the visual light-sensing cells. Vitamin A is essential in the visual cycle, in the maintenance of the functional and structural integrity of epithelium in mucus-secreting or keratinizing tissues, in bone growth, and in reproduction and embryologic development. It has an important role in enhancing immune function and reducing sequelae of some infections, e.g., measles in young children,[20] and may play a significant role in anticarcinogenesis. Several synthetic analogues of vitamin A have been developed as pharmaceutical agents for dermatologic applications.

In the visual system, both rods and cones utilize 11-*cis*-retinal as the chromophore. In the photoreceptor cells of the rods, especially sensitive to low-intensity light, this vitamer combines with the membrane protein opsin to form rhodopsin, which is the light-absorbing holoreceptor. The cones, which are the color-sensitive photoreceptor cells, are of three types, each having a separate protein that when combined with 11-*cis*-retinal responds optimally to red, green, or blue wavelengths of light. The visual cycle involves an interaction of the photon-activated rhodopsin with a G protein and interconversions of 11-*cis*-retinal to several stereoisomers.[21]

The basal mucus-secreting cells of many epithelia depend on vitamin A for normal structure and mucus secretion. These influences appear to be mediated primarily by retinoic acid, via changes in nuclear transcription. Retinoic acid receptors have been described that belong to a receptor "superfamily" that includes receptors for calcitriol as well as thyroid and steroid hormones.[17]

Possible anticarcinogenic effects of vitamin A have been attributed to its ability to induce differentiation of malignant cells and to function in the synthesis of cell-surface glycoproteins and glycolipids that may play an important role in cell adherence and communication. Splenic lymphocyte proliferation and killer cell cytotoxic activity is impaired in vitamin A deficiency. Therefore, differentiation of these immune cells may play a role in the vitamin's beneficial effect on immunity and resistance to infection.[22]

The primary food sources for vitamin A are liver, dairy products, egg yolk, and fish (providing retinol or retinol esters) and yellow and green vegetables (providing β-carotene).[17] In the average American diet, about 50% of the vitamin intake comes from animal-based products and 50% from vegetable sources. Absorption and utilization of the vitamin is complex, and varies with the source. Most animal-derived vitamin A is consumed in the form of retinol esters, typically retinyl palmitate, and, when vitamin A is ingested in usual dietary amounts, absorption is virtually complete. These esters are hydrolyzed in the intestinal lumen and brush border and then taken up by the intestinal cells bound to a cellular retinol-binding protein (CRBP). There they are re-esterified and incorporated into chylomicrons for transport to the liver, in which they are stored. Hepatic vitamin A storage capacity is considerable (average content of retinyl esters is 100 to 300 μg/g), with reserves sufficient to withstand several months of a vitamin A–free diet before the plasma concentration decreases markedly or deficiency symptoms appear. The liver normally releases vitamin A after hydrolysis to retinol, 95% of which is bound to an α-1-globulin, the retinol-binding protein (RBP). When the liver becomes saturated with vitamin A due to excessive ingestion or hepatic disease or both, retinyl esters may appear in the blood, eventually accounting for as much as 65% of the total circulating retinoids. Circulating retinol is carried to cells of various target organs, where it is taken up by a membrane-bound protein very similar to CRBP, re-esterified, then hydrolyzed and delivered to the appropriate intracellular sites by a cytosolic CRBP. The fate of ingested carotenoids is slightly different.[17, 23] Only about one third of the carotene content of a meal is absorbed. Some β-carotene is cleaved in the intestinal mucosa and esterified and transported to the liver via the lymphatics, while some is absorbed intact. When carotenoids are present in large amounts in the diet, they may cause an elevated blood carotene level (normal range 50 to 200 μg/dL), associated with a benign and reversible yellowish (or "golden suntan") discoloration of the skin (but not the sclera, as occurs in jaundice). Excessive consumption of carotene does not lead to hypervitaminosis A, presumably because only limited conversion to retinol occurs.

In addition to hepatic storage and tissue uptake, some retinol is glucuronidated. Other water-soluble metabolites are also excreted, with no retinol normally found unchanged in the urine.[17]

Deficiency

In adults, vitamin A deficiency is usually related to chronic illnesses associated with fat malabsorption such as inflammatory bowel disease, biliary or pancreatic insufficiency, and cirrhosis. Children suffering from general malnutrition are especially susceptible, and it is believed that vitamin A deficiency is responsible for more than 250,000 cases per year worldwide of irreversible pediatric blindness, in addition to greatly enhanced mortality from infectious diseases, especially measles.[17, 20] Features characteristic of vitamin A deficiency include night blindness and keratomalacia progressing to permanent blindness, keratinization and drying of the skin with follicular hyperkeratosis, increased incidence of respiratory infections, urinary calculi due to associated changes in the urinary tract epithelium, diarrhea, and occasional impairment of hearing, taste, and smell.[17]

Toxicity

With excessive vitamin A intake, hepatic storage capacity is exceeded, and the previously noted normal pattern of almost all circulating vitamin A existing as retinol bound to RBP is altered, with an increasing proportion of plasma retinoids being present as retinyl esters loosely associated with lipoproteins. Clinical case reports of vitamin A toxicity typically involve normal or only slight elevation of retinol (normal range 30 to 70 μg/dL), with markedly elevated retinyl esters (normal less than 7 μg/dL, or 5% to 8% of plasma retinol).[24, 25] In more advanced cases of hypervitaminosis A, one may find an elevation of retinol to more than 100 μg/dL, and some authors suggest that excess circulating free retinol, e.g., a molar ratio of retinol to RBP of greater than 1, is important to clinical toxicity.[26] However, most recent reviews suggest that retinyl esters, which exhibit surfactant properties, are more likely responsible for toxic effects.[17, 25] Retinyl esters—and perhaps free retinol—probably cause cellular toxicity via altered membrane lipoprotein phenomena. The precise mechanism of the increased intracranial pressure that is so characteristic of vitamin A toxicity is unclear, but it may relate to such altered membrane function in the choroid plexus.[27] As hepatic stores of vitamin A become saturated, another characteristic feature, hepatotoxicity, is observed when marked accumulation of retinyl esters and lipid develops in the perisinusoidal fat storage cells (Ito cells in the space of Disse). This process may stimulate transformation of these cells to fibroblasts[25]; clinically, progression is observed to sinusoidal fibrosis, portal fibrosis, central vein sclerosis, and eventually cirrhosis.

Toxicity may occur as the result of either acute or chronic overdose.[25] In children, single doses of 75,000 to 100,000 IU are necessary to produce toxicity, while in adults the range is usually in excess of 1,000,000 IU. Chronic exposures of 18,000 to 60,000 IU/day in infants and children, and 50,000 to 100,000 IU/day in adults will result in toxicity. One adult patient has been reported recently with hepatotoxicity resulting from habitual daily ingestion of 20,000 IU.[28] Clinical manifestations of chronic toxicity may vary in terms of total dosage and duration of exposure; most case reports observe periods of excessive intake of months to years, although infants treated with 18,000 IU/day became symptomatic within 6 weeks.[29] Persons with underlying liver disease, or who develop acute hepatitis, are at increased risk. For acute intoxication, most reported cases are due to the ingestion of liver with high vitamin A content, e.g., bear, seal, or fish livers, with iatrogenic cases representing another sizable group. With chronic exposures, the most common cause is excessive intake via self-medication or food faddism in adults, or overzealous vitamin treatment of children by their parents.[17, 25, 29, 30]

Clinical Manifestations

Classically, vitamin A intoxication is stratified by age of patient and chronicity of exposure, although there is considerable overlap of symptomatology. The target body areas most typically affected are the central nervous system, liver, bone, and skin and mucous membranes.

Accounts of acute vitamin A toxicity are relatively uncommon, but typical early features are primarily neurologic. These include irritability, tiredness with intense sleep desire progressing to somnolence, increased intracranial pressure that may manifest as a bulging fontanelle in infants or signs of acute pseudotumor cerebri in older children and adults, anorexia, and vomiting.[25] Within a few days, cheilitis, hair loss and skin peeling, hepatomegaly, and epistaxis or miscellaneous hemorrhages may ensue. Laboratory abnormalities may include increased serum retinyl esters (and retinol in severe cases), hypercalcemia, and slight changes in liver function tests. An illustrative case report was provided by Misbah et al.[19] A 25-year-old Sri Lankan woman ingested a meal of cooked shark liver and presented after several days of headache, vomiting, and diplopia. The examination was notable for bilateral florid papilledema, enlarged blind spots, and bilateral partial abducens palsies. Routine serum chemistry, liver function, and hematology values were normal, but total serum vitamin A level (retinol versus retinyl esters not specified) was elevated at 177 μg/dL. She recovered over an 8-week period, becoming asymptomatic with only residual but receding papilledema.

Far more common is the occurrence of chronic vitamin A toxicity, which tends to involve all four of the major target organ systems. The central nervous system and ophthalmologic effects include headache, fatigue but difficulty sleeping, visual disturbances, anorexia and weight loss, and signs of increased intracranial pressure with bulging fontanelles in infancy and pseudotumor cerebri in older children and adults. Changes of the integument and mucous membranes, including dry, pruritic, scaly, and peeling skin; hair loss; brittle nails; and cheilitis, stomatitis, and gingivitis are regular and often early signs. Involvement of the liver is manifested as hepatosplenomegaly, nausea, abdominal pain, ascites, esophageal varices, and cirrhosis. Liver function tests may be abnormal, but patients with severe hepatic involvement and ascites and without jaundice have been reported, as have patients with minimally altered or normal liver function tests, although prothrombin time may be increased owing to hypoprothrombinemia.[24, 26, 29, 30] A vicious circle may be conceptualized wherein early vitamin A hepatotoxicity results in decreased liver storage capacity or RBP synthesis or both; continued chronic excessive ingestion results in escalating release of retinyl esters, and in some cases unbound retinol, with resultant systemic toxicity. The skeletal system is also frequently affected, particularly in children with growing long bones. Bone pain and tenderness is often noted, and children may manifest painful swelling of overlying soft tissues.[30] Radiographic findings may include areas of osteoporosis or hypermineralization, periosteal calcifications and cortical hyperostosis of the cranium, clavicles, long bones, and metatarsals, as well as cup-shaped deformity of the metaphyses.[31, 32] Permanent deformity and growth retardation may occur in children due to partial or complete premature epiphyseal closure. Associated laboratory abnormalities of hypercalcemia and increased alkaline phosphatase are noted on occasion; these may represent effects of stimulation of osteoclastic resorption or inhibition of osteoblastic activity or both.[32]

Another area of concern related to vitamin A and its derivatives involves potential *teratogenic* effects. Isotretinoin, 13-*cis*-retinoic acid, has been used widely in the United States and Europe as a systemic agent for the treatment of nodulocystic acne vulgaris. A specific embryopathy has been well characterized for this agent, with a calculated relative risk of 26.5%.[33] Typical malformations include those related to four main structural areas: the brain, head and face, heart and great vessels, and thymus. These include hydrocephalus and/or areas of cerebral agenesis or hypoplasia; micrognathia, cleft palate, microtia and/or anotia; transposition of the great vessels, Fallot's tetralogy, or truncus arteriosus; and thymic hypoplasia or aplasia. Further studies have found that the crucial exposure period occurs during the first trimester (especially the second to fifth postconceptional weeks), and that the prevalence of malformations averages 85% for involvement of the brain, 70% for the ears, and 50% for the cardiovascular system.[34] Congenital malformations noted after high-dose maternal vitamin A therapy have also been reported; these tend to primarily involve facial and otic defects, with less frequent neurologic and cardiac involvement.[25, 34] An attempt to calculate relative risks for vitamin A prenatal exposure has been recently reported from data collected on more than 20,000 pregnant women in the United States as part of a large prospective cohort study of congenital malformations.[35] These researchers compared outcomes in women taking supplements of more than 10,000 IU/day with those taking less than 5,000 IU/day and found a relative risk for cranial–neural crest defects of 4.8 (95% CI 2.2 to 10.5). They concluded that doses of supplemental vitamin A in excess of 10,000 IU/day pose a significant risk of teratogenicity.

Diagnosis

The recognition of the characteristic clinical syndromes of acute or chronic hypervitaminosis A, along with finding a history of exposure, are the most important steps in diagnosis. As noted previously, routine serum chemistries and liver function tests may be normal or only minimally elevated. Some patients manifest hypercalcemia or hypoprothrombinemia. Characteristic radiographic findings have been described and may be present in patients with chronic toxicity. Patients may be symptomatic at a time when serum vitamin A levels are normal. However, a retinol serum level exceeding 100 μg/dL is highly suggestive of toxicity, as is an elevated proportion of retinyl esters (more than 5% to 8% of total, or over 7 μg/dL), if specific tests are available. Characteristic liver pathology and an elevated liver vitamin A content may be found on biopsy in occult cases.

Treatment

The most crucial specific intervention is immediate discontinuation of vitamin A; this measure alone suffices in most cases. Most symptoms resolve over several weeks to months. Routine principles of gastrointestinal decontamination are probably appropriate in the uncommon situation of a patient seen soon after an acute overdose exceeding 75,000 to 100,000 IU in children or 1,000,000 IU in adults. Patients with severe hepatotoxicity obviously require significant supportive care. Vitamin K may be of value for patients with hypoprothrombinemia. Associated increased intracranial pressure may occasionally require intervention depending on duration and severity. Neurologic consultation is probably advised prior to instituting a regimen that might include repeated lumbar punctures; diuretics (e.g., furosemide, initial IV dose 0.5 to 1 mg/kg up to 40 mg); mannitol (initial IV dose 0.25 to 0.5 mg/kg up to 1 g); acetazolamide (adult PO dose of 250 mg QID); and/or steroids (e.g., prednisone 0.5 to 1.0 mg/kg up to 40 mg PO per day) as necessary. Hypercalcemia may also require specific treatment, although initial management with intravenous normal saline to enhance hydration usually suffices.[32] If hypercalcemia is severe or persistent, additional treatment may be warranted. Adjuvant therapy has included diuretics such as furosemide to enhance renal calcium excretion. Corticosteroids (e.g., prednisone in adult doses of 20 mg/d[36]) may also lower serum calcium by increasing renal excretion, as well as decreasing intestinal calcium absorption and bone resorption.

Vitamin D

Vitamin D is another of the fat-soluble vitamins that produces a classic toxic syndrome following excessive ingestion. Vitamin D shares with vitamin A the properties of a hormone. However, in some respects it is not truly a vitamin because, for most persons living in tropical or temperate geographic zones, cutaneous photobiosynthesis of the nutrient is sufficient to supply optimal nutritional needs.[37, 38]

Physiology and Pharmacology

Vitamin D congeners are secosterol (split sterol) derivatives of the cholesterol precursor 7-dehydrocholesterol.[37] Vitamin D_3 (cholecalciferol) is formed when this precursor absorbs ultraviolet light in the skin and splits the C9-C10 bond in the B ring of the sterol skeleton. Preformed vitamin D congeners with biologic equivalency to endogenous skin-derived vitamin D_3 may be absorbed from the diet, especially fish liver oils. Vitamin D_3 from all sources enters the circulation bound to a specific α-1-globulin, the vitamin D–binding protein, and is transported to the liver where it undergoes hydroxylation to 25-hydroxyvitamin D [25(OH)D]. The production of 25(OH)D is influenced by feedback inhibition but is not tightly controlled, and levels of this congener rise dramatically in states of excess vitamin D exposure (normal range 5 to 80 ng/ml). At physiologic levels, 25(OH)D is not thought to exhibit significant biologic activity, but it appears to be active at very elevated concentrations and may be responsible for much of the toxicity associated with hypervitaminosis D. The 25(OH)D is transported to the kidneys bound to the vitamin D–binding protein, where under the influence of parathyroid hormone, it is further hydroxylated to 1,25-dihydroxyvitamin D, also known as *calcitriol.*

The synthesis of calcitriol is closely regulated by fluctuations in serum calcium. Hypocalcemia stimulates parathyroid hormone secretion and thus the synthesis of calcitriol, which is believed to be the significant biologically active congener at physiologic levels. Calcitriol is carried to target organs—particularly the intestine and bone—by the vitamin D–binding protein. (Normal serum concentration of total calcitriol ranges from 16 to 65 pg/ml.) Free calcitriol is taken up by cells and exhibits its hormone-like effect by complexing with a specific nuclear receptor, a member of the same receptor superfamily that includes receptors for retinol, steroids, and thyroid hormone. The calcitriol-receptor complex activates transcription of genes for the synthesis of an intestinal calcium-binding protein and bone osteocalcin, which increase intestinal calcium absorption and bone resorption, respectively, and result in increased serum calcium. Thus, vitamin D plays a central role in calcium homeostasis. Receptors for calcitriol have been identified in several other tissues, but their function is less well understood.

Daily requirements for vitamin D range from 200 to 400 IU (5 to 10 μg) per day.[37] In latitudes where and during seasons when sunlight intensity is limited, this MDR must be met by dietary intake, which was difficult to achieve in the era before widespread fortification of milk and bread products. The classic nutritional vitamin D deficiency state manifests as rickets in infants and growing children and as osteomalacia in adults. Several disorders in synthesis or response to calcitriol may require treatment with supraphysiologic doses of vitamin D analogues, e.g., vitamin D–resistant and vitamin D–dependent rickets and renal osteodystrophy. Today, most persons in the United States receive adequate vitamin D through their diet, unless they suffer from a primary intestinal malabsorption syndrome, or hepatic or biliary dysfunction. Rickets and osteomalacia have also been observed in patients on chronic anticonvulsant therapy with phenobarbital or phenytoin, although the mechanism for this is not well understood.

Toxicity

Hypervitaminosis D has been recognized for decades,[27] principally in persons treated with pharmacologic doses for diseases unrelated to vitamin D deficiency but thought likely to benefit from such treatment, such as rheumatoid arthritis. Occasional acute vitamin D exposures may occur from ingestion of vitamin D–containing rodenticides or massive ingestions of multivitamins. Chronic vitamin D consumption in excess of even four times the RDA may be hazardous to young infants; adults may experience toxicity at doses of 60,000 IU/d for weeks to months. Large numbers of infants were oversupplemented in England during World War II, typically with daily intakes of 2000 to 4000 IU/d. A number of such children developed hypercalcemia; a nonfamilial congenital syndrome related to maternal hypervitaminosis D, and/or abnormal fetal or infantile vitamin D sensitivity was also described with cerebral, cardiovascular, and renal anomalies, particularly supravalvular aortic stenosis.[39] The toxicity of excess vitamin D is thought to be due primarily to its exaggerated physiologic effects, resulting in hypercalcemia, hypercalciuria, and metastatic soft tissue calcification.

Clinical Manifestations

Classically described clinical effects include initial symptoms of systemic hypercalcemia, including weakness, headache, fatigue, nausea, and vomiting. Subsequently, manifestations of soft tissue calcification may occur, including hypertension, polyuria, and polydipsia related to nephrocalcinosis, which may progress to uremia, as well as signs referable to calcifications in myocardium, vessels, muscle, lung, and skin; death may result. An outbreak of hypervitaminosis D due to overfortification of milk (up to 200,000 IU per quart) by a dairy in Massachusetts in 1988 to 1991 has allowed for case-control studies that have reinforced the association of these effects with excess vitamin D exposure.[40, 41]

Diagnosis and Treatment

The clinical findings and exposure history may be characteristic. Observed laboratory abnormalities include hypercalcemia with variable phosphate levels, decreased renal function with albuminuria and anemia, and elevated levels of 25(OH)D and free calcitriol. (Total calcitriol is usually normal or only slightly elevated.[42]) Radiographic findings may include ectopic calcifications in kidneys, heart, and vessels as well as skeletal changes of periosteal thickening.

Prompt withdrawal of vitamin D supplements and implementation of a diet low in calcium and vitamin D are sufficient therapy for mild to moderate cases. In the acute overdose situation, as of a vitamin D–based rodenticide, appropriate gastrointestinal decontamination is warranted. Patients with persistent hypercalcemia may benefit from further measures as detailed previously for vitamin A toxicity. Renal failure may require dialysis for a period of time. The induction of hepatic enzymes with glutethimide to facilitate degradative metabolism of vitamin D has been reported successful in one case.[43] Other case series have suggested a benefit in treating hypercalcemia and hypercalciuria with the biphosphonates, clodronate[44] and pamidronate.[45]

Vitamin E

Although vitamin E was isolated in 1936, its role in human nutrition is still controversial, and there is currently little unequivocal evidence that a specific deficiency state exists for it in otherwise normal term infants, in children, or in adults.[17] In premature babies, in persons with severe fat malabsorption, and in those with the rare genetic disease abetalipoproteinemia, vitamin E seems to protect against a hemolytic anemia, although other nutrients may play a role. In animals, particularly rodents, vitamin E appears vital for normal reproduction and neuromuscular function. α-Tocopherol (see Fig. 99–1) is believed to be the most important vitamer and displays the most biologic activity in most bioassays. The vitamin has come under intense scrutiny in recent years because of its known antioxidant properties and the publicity surrounding studies evaluating its possibly protective effect from atherosclerosis and carcinogenesis.[10–12]

Toxicity

Case series of persons taking large doses of vitamin E (400 IU to more than 3000 IU) have reported a variety of symptoms, including fatigue, headache, muscle weakness, nausea, intestinal cramps, and diarrhea.[46] In addition, vitamin E may antagonize vitamin K, with resulting increased clotting time and effect of oral anticoagulants.[46, 47] However, most large controlled studies (typical dose 400 to 800 IU) have failed to find significant differences in the incidence of adverse effects between treated cases and controls.[11, 48] Of historical interest was the tragic epidemic of morbidity (pulmonary deterioration, hepatic and renal failure, and thrombocytopenia) and 38 deaths in premature infants treated in the winter of 1983–1984 with an intravenous preparation of vitamin E (E-Ferol). This syndrome was subsequently determined to be due to the carrier, a mixture of polysorbate 80 and polysorbate 20 (oleate and laurate esters of sorbitol condensed with ethylene oxide).[49]

Vitamin K

Vitamin K activity is found in two natural sources, a plant-derived form (phytonadione, vitamin K_1) and the form synthesized by intestinal bacteria (menaquinone, vitamin K_2).[17] Both are utilized as essential cofactors in the hepatic biosynthesis of blood coagulation factors II, VII, IX, and X. Other vitamin K–dependent proteins include the anticoagulant proteins C and S, as well as bone osteocalcin. Deficiency of vitamin K results in a hemorrhagic diathesis. A coumarin embryopathy has been described with skeletal abnormalities that may represent the effects of fetal vitamin K deficiency on osteocalcin synthesis.

Chronic ingestion of excess vitamin K is unusual because it is not available in the typical multivitamin supplements subject to abuse.[27] Large amounts may inhibit the desired effects of anticoagulant medications.[46] Water-soluble congeners (menadiones) given to newborns for hemorrhagic disease prophylaxis, particularly if there is glucose-6-phosphate dehydrogenase (G6PD) deficiency, may cause hemolysis and jaundice; phytonadione is rarely associated with this effect.[27, 46] Intravenous administration of phytonadione may result in an anaphylactoid reaction of flushing, chest pain, hypotension, and death; it is unclear if this is due to the vitamin itself or the vehicle.[17] Recently some concern has been raised about a potential association of the routine use of prophylactic vitamin K in healthy newborns and increased risk of subsequent childhood cancer; however, careful controlled studies have failed to substantiate this association, and authorities continue to recommend this use of vitamin K.[50]

WATER-SOLUBLE VITAMINS

Significant toxicity is well established for chronic excessive consumption of pyridoxine and niacin (see Table 99–2). Adverse effects have also been ascribed to thiamine and ascorbate, and are briefly reviewed.

Pyridoxine

The pyridoxidine congeners are utilized by mammals after hepatic conversion to the active form, pyridoxal phosphate, which in turn is an important coenzyme in numerous metabolic reactions of amino acids.[51] Pyridoxine is supplied by meats, whole grains, soybeans, and various vegetables. A deficiency state has been observed with mucocutaneous manifestations (seborrhea-like lesions and stomatitis), and seizures due to diminished γ-aminobutyrate (GABA) production. This role of pyridoxine as a cofactor in GABA synthesis underlies its use as an antidote in the treatment of isoniazid overdose and hydrazine-mushroom poisoning (see Chapter 25), as well as its previously noted use in pyridoxine dependency, an inherited disorder of pyridoxine metabolism resulting in neonatal seizures. Pyridoxine has found similar usage in the treatment of xanthurenic aciduria and homocystinuria.

Pyridoxine toxicity is most likely to occur with chronic ingestion in excess of 500 mg/day, often taken for self-treatment of premenstrual syndrome or as a body-building adjunct. Symptoms suggestive of a dependency state have been noted in patients taking 200 mg/day.[51] Toxic effects have been reported with consumption of average total doses as low as 117 mg/day for 3 years.[52] The toxic syndrome manifests as a striking sensory axonal neuropathy, typically without weakness or central nervous system involvement.[53] Patients present with unsteady gait and difficulty in handling small objects. Neurologic findings include ataxia, severely impaired position and vibration sense, and less dramatic effects on light touch, pain sensation, and temperature. Diminished deep tendon reflexes and Lhermitte's sign (neck pain and tingling that shoots down the spine to the legs and feet after neck flexion) are also present. Dose response characteristics were studied in five healthy volunteers administered 1 g or 3 g/day and closely followed for clinical symptoms and sural nerve electrophysiology.[54] Subjects receiving higher doses became symptomatic earlier, and symptoms persisted for 2 to 3 weeks after discontinuation of pyridoxine, a phenomenon termed "coasting" by the authors. An infant exposed *in utero* to pyridoxine (maternal dose 50 mg/d) was born with amelia of one leg.[55] At least one patient has been reported who developed motor weakness after 5 years of 10 g/day consumption.[56] An unusual episode of acute toxicity occurred in two patients who received an iatrogenic parenteral, massive (exceeding 100 g) pyridoxine overdose during treatment of *Gyromitra* mushroom poisoning.[57] These patients manifested weakness, lethargy, nystagmus, and respiratory depression in addition to severe sensory neuropathy. At follow-up 4 years after exposure, one of these patients had persistent profound sensory loss, although the motor abnormalities had disappeared.[58] Chronic pyridoxine intake at doses as low as 25 mg/day have been reported to antagonize the antiparkinsonian effect of L-dopa, and similar antagonisms have been observed for barbiturates and phenytoin.[46] The treatment of pyridoxine toxicity consists of its withdrawal, which usually results in gradual recovery,[52] although some patients may have long-term or permanent sequelae.

Niacin

Niacin has been long recognized as the antipellegra factor missing in diets based largely on corn.[51] The vitamin exists as nicotinic acid (niacin) and nicotinamide (niacinamide) (see Fig. 99–1), with equivalent biologic vitamin activity but different pharmacologic effects. In both forms, niacin is converted to either nicotinamide-adenine dinucleotide (NAD) or its phosphate (NADP), which are vital coenzymes for a variety of enzymes involved in oxidation-reduction reactions necessary for tissue aerobic metabolism. Tryptophan may also be utilized in the biosynthesis of NAD, and diets rich in tryptophan will offset low niacin intake in preventing deficiency. Pellegra is rare in the United States today, where dietary intake of animal protein tends to be high, but is classically manifested with cutaneous, gastrointestinal, and neurologic abnormalities. This clinical syndrome is often recalled with a mnemonic, the "three Ds": dermatitis, diarrhea, and dementia.[51] Typical clinical findings include desquamating skin rash; sialorrhea, stomatitis, and diarrhea; and headache, depression, memory loss, hallucinations and dementia, and motor and sensory changes.

Niacin toxicity has been primarily associated with the chronic therapeutic use of large doses of nicotinic acid as a lipid-lowering agent, although an epidemic has been reported in 17 persons after an acute "overdose" of pumpernickel bagels.[46, 59–63] Clinical effects predominate in the skin and gastrointestinal tract. Cutaneous manifestations of flushing and pruritus are very common and have classically been attributed to histamine release,[46] although more recent work suggests that prostaglandin E_2 is responible and that pretreatment with prostaglandin inhibitors such as aspirin ameliorate this effect.[61] Hyperkeratosis and acanthosis nigricans have also been described in chronic users. Gastrointestinal effects include those that are likely mediated by prostaglandin, such as exacerbation of peptic ulcer disease, and hepatotoxicity, which may range from mild cholestatic jaundice to severe hepatitis with fulminant hepatic failure.[61–63] Hepatitis is typically associated with dosages ranging from 3 to 4.5 g/day for 1 to 18 months, although a patient has been reported to have developed hepatic dysfunction after 10 years of treatment without apparent prior side effects.[62] Recent studies suggest that time-release forms of niacin are more hepatotoxic.[61, 62] Occasional additional findings include thrombocytopenia,[62] increased serum uric acid and gouty arthritis, glucose intolerance,[59] skeletal muscle myopathy,[60] and increased cidence of atrial fibrillation and other arrhythmias.[27, 59] In most cases, all these effects have regressed with discontinuation of the niacin.

Thiamine

Thiamine was the first of the B-complex vitamins to be identified. Its history is traced back to the 19th century Japanese navy; it was shown that adding fish, meat, and vegetables to the sailors' poor diet of polished rice reduced the incidence of beriberi.[51] Today thiamine deficiency is still common in western societies among chronic alcoholics, and is observed in patients with other malnourished states including AIDS, cancer, hyperemesis gravidarum, and eating disorders. It is also endemic among breast-fed infants in Third World countries where rice consumption is high. Thiamine deficiency is classically associated with neurologic and cardiovascular abnormalities and includes the neurologic syndromes of alcoholic neuritis, Wernicke's encephalopathy, and Korsakoff's psychosis[51, 64, 65] and the cardiovascular effects of peripheral vasodilation, biventricular heart failure, and peripheral edema. Thiamine pyrophosphate, the biologically active form of the vitamin, is a vital coenzyme in numerous metabolic pathways involving carbohydrate metabolism. It has been observed that rapid infusion of hypertonic glucose solutions to treat endogenous hypoglycemia may precipitate both neurologic and cardiac deterioration in thiamine-deficient patients, and concomitant thiamine administration is recommended.[65]

Thiamine's oral absorption is relatively limited, and large doses (e.g., 100 mg, or almost 100 times the RDA) are usually administered intravenously for the emergency treatment of suspected thiamine deficiency. In this context, a few severe anaphylactic reactions have been described,[66] while in a series of more than 1000 thiamine treatments given IV to 989 consecutive patients over a 6-month period only one patient with generalized pruritus was considered to have a possible precursor of anaphylaxis (less than 0.1%), and 11 patients with localized burning at the infusion site.[67] Of note, any patient with prior history of thiamine reaction (number not stated) was excluded. The incidence of local reactions may be decreased if thiamine is administered slowly via relatively larger veins.[64, 67] While thiamine is no longer used commonly in chronic therapeutic regimens, there are reports from the 1940s of headache, irritability, insomnia, tachycardia, and weakness said to resemble hyperthyroidism with doses as low as 5 mg/day for 4 to 5 weeks.[59, 67]

Vitamin C (Ascorbic Acid)

Scurvy, the vitamin C deficiency state, has been recognized as a disease since the Middle Ages, and its relation to diets lacking fresh fruit and vegetables has been understood since the 16th to 18th centuries.[51] The human (along with other primates, guinea pigs, and Indian fruit bats) is one of the few mammals unable to synthesize vitamin C from glucose. This vitamin functions as an important cofactor for numerous hydroxylation and amidation reactions and has antioxidant properties. It is vital to normal synthesis of collagen, proteoglycans, and other components of the intercellular matrix, and therefore the structural integrity of tooth, bone, and capillary endothelium.[51] Scurvy is rarely encountered today, but occasional cases are still reported in malnourished persons, especially shut-ins and those espousing exaggerated food faddism.[68] Cutaneous findings include perifollicular hemorrhages, hyperkeratotic papules, petechiae, ecchymoses, and poor wound healing.[51, 68] Additional effects include bone pain with subperiosteal hemorrhage, gingivitis and loosening of the teeth, and anemia.

Vitamin C's antioxidant (or free radical scavenger) effects have prompted widespread and largely unsupervised experimentation with megadose treatment (e.g., in excess of 1 g/day).[46, 48, 59] Numerous adverse effects have been ascribed to such usage, although with little controlled study.[69] These effects may include gastrointestinal disturbances of nausea, cramping, and diarrhea; urinary calculi, primarily from oxalates but also with urates and cystine; and hemolysis in G6PD-deficient patients.[70] Rebound scurvy has been seen in persons abruptly discontinuing long-term high-dose therapy and also occurs in infants of mothers taking such doses.[46, 51] Concern has been raised about increased blood estradiol levels noted in women taking oral contraceptive pills and high-dose vitamin C, as well as about this vitamin's potential to increase iron absorption in patients with iron overload states such as hemolytic anemia and hemochromatosis.[46, 69] In contrast, most recent reviews have found that dosages of up to 4 g/day are actually unlikely to result in significant toxicity in otherwise healthy persons.[47, 48, 71] In particular, a prospective cohort study on over 45,000 men aged 40 to 75 years compared those taking 1500 mg/day or more to those taking less than 250 mg/day, and found no increased incidence of kidney stones in the high-dose patients.[72] Withdrawal of vitamin C (with surveillance for rebound scorbutic effects) and supportive care should suffice for treatment of presumed toxicity. It is probably prudent to caution against the use of high-dose vitamin C therapy for patients with known nephrolithiasis, G6PD deficiency, iron overload conditions, pregnancy, and perhaps for women taking oral contraceptives.

References

1. Rudman D, Williams PJ: Megadose vitamins—use and misuse. N Engl J Med *309:*488, 1983.
2. Marcus R, Coulston AM: The Vitamins: Introduction. *In* Hardman JG, Gilman AG, Limbard LE (eds): Goodman and Gilman's The Pharmacologic Basis of Therapeutics. 9th ed. New York, McGraw-Hill, pp 1547–1553, 1996.
3. Food and Nutrition Board, National Research Council: Recommended Dietary Allowances. 10th ed. Washington, D.C., National Academy of Sciences, 1989.
4. Davidson RA: Complications of megavitamin therapy. Southern Med J *77:*200, 1984.
5. Evans CDH, Lacey JH: Toxicity of vitamins: Complications of a health movement. BMJ *292:*509, 1986.
6. Hoffer A, Osmond H: Treatment of schizophrenia with nicotinic acid: A ten-year follow-up. Acta Psychiatr Scand *40:*171, 1964.
7. Pauling L: Vitamin C and the Common Cold. San Francisco, W H Freeman Co., 1970.
8. Jukes TH: Revolution and counterrevolution in nutrition. Ann Nutr Health *28:*8, 1973.
9. Subar AF, Block G: Use of vitamin and mineral supplements: Demographics and amounts of nutrients consumed. The 1987 Health Interview Survey. Am J Epidemiol *132:*1091, 1990.
10. Rapola JM, Virtamo J, Haukka JK, et al: Effect of vitamin E and beta-carotene on the incidence of angina pectoris: A randomized, double-blind, controlled trial. JAMA *275:*693, 1996.
11. Stephens NG, Parsons A, Schofield PM, et al: Randomised controlled trial of vitamin E in patients with coronary disease: Cambridge Heart Antioxidant Study (CHAOS). Lancet *347:*781, 1996.
12. α-Tocopherol, β-Carotene Cancer Prevention Study Group. The effect of vitamin E and β-carotene on the incidence of lung cancer and other cancers in male smokers. N Engl J Med *330:*1029, 1994.
13. Greenberg ER, Baron JA, Karagas MR, et al: Mortality associated with low plasma concentration of β-carotene and the effect of oral supplementation. JAMA *275:*699, 1996.
14. Council on Scientific Affairs: Vitamin preparations as dietary supplements and as therapeutic agents. JAMA *257:*1929, 1987.
15. Rimm EB, Ascherio A, Giovannucci E, et al: Vegetable, fruit, and cereal fiber intake and risk of coronary heart disease among men. JAMA *275:*447, 1996.
16. Wynder EL, Stellman SD, Zang EA: High fiber intake: Indicator of a healthy lifestyle. JAMA *275:*486, 1996.
17. Marcus R, Coulston AM: Fat-soluble vitamins. *In* Hardman JG, Gilman AG, Limbard LE (eds): Goodman & Gilman's The Pharmacologic Basis of Therapeutics. 9th ed. New York, McGraw-Hill, pp 1573–1590, 1996.
18. Kane EK: Arctic Explorations in the Years 1853, 1854, 1855. Philadelphia, Childs & Peterson Pub., Vol. 1:392, 1856.
19. Misbah SA, Peiris JB, Atukorala TMS: Ingestion of shark liver associated with pseudotumor cerebri due to acute hypervitaminosis A. J Neurol Neurosurg Psych *47:*216, 1984.
20. Hussey GD, Klein M: A randomized, controlled trial of vitamin A in children with severe measles. N Engl J Med *323:*160, 1990.
21. Stryer L: Visual excitation and recovery. J Biol Chem *266:*10711, 1991.
22. Ross AC: Vitamin A status: Relationship to immunity and the antibody response. Minireview. Proc Soc Exp Biol Med *200:*303, 1992.
23. Olson JA: The irresistible fascination of carotenoids and vitamin A: The 1992 Atwater lecture. Am J Clin Nutr *57:*833, 1993.
24. Carpenter TO, Pettifor JM, Russell RM, et al: Severe hypervitaminosis A in siblings: Evidence of variable tolerance to retinol intake. J Pediatr *111:*507, 1987.
25. Biesalski HK: Comparative assessment of the toxicology of vitamin A and retinoids in man. Toxicology *57:*117, 1989.
26. Mendoza FS, Johnson F, Kerner JA, et al: Vitamin A intoxica-

tion presenting with ascites and a normal vitamin A level. West J Med *148:*88, 1988.

27. Dipalma JR, Ritchie DM: Vitamin toxicity. Ann Rev Pharmacol Toxicol *17:*133, 1977.
28. Kowalski TE, Falestiny M, Furth E, Malet PF: Vitamin A hepatotoxicity: A cautionary note regarding 25,000 IU supplements. Am J Med *97:*523, 1994.
29. Persson B, Tunell R, Ekengran K: Chronic vitamin A intoxication during the first half year of life: Description of 5 cases. Acta Pediatr Scand *54:*49, 1965.
30. James MB, Leonard JC, Fraser JJ, Stuemky JH: Hypervitaminosis A: A case report. Pediatrics *69:*112, 1982.
31. Rosenberg HK, Berezin S, Heyman S, et al: Pleural effusion and ascites: Unusual presenting features in a pediatric patient with vitamin A intoxication. Clin Pediatr *21:*435, 1982.
32. Baxi SC, Dailey GE: Hypervitaminosis A: A cause of hypercalcemia. West J Med *137:*429, 1982.
33. Lammer EJ, Chen DT, Hoar RM, et al: Retinoic acid embryopathy. N Engl J Med *313:*837, 1985.
34. Rosa FW, Wilk AL, Kelsey FO: Teratogen update: Vitamin A congeners. Teratology *33:*355, 1986.
35. Rothman KJ, Moore LL, Singer MR, et al: Teratogenicity of high vitamin A intake. N Engl J Med *333:*1369, 1995.
36. Bergman SM, O'Malia J, Krane NK, Wallin JD: Vitamin A induced hypercalcemia: response to corticosteroids. Nephron *50:*362, 1988.
37. Marcus R: Agents affecting calcification and bone turnover: Calcium, phosphate, parathyroid hormone, vitamin D, calcitonin, and other compounds. *In* Hardman JG, Gilman AG, Limbard LE (eds): Goodman & Gilman's The Pharmacologic Basis of Therapeutics. 9th ed. New York, McGraw-Hill, pp 1529–1536, 1996.
38. Haddad JG: Vitamin D: Solar rays, Milky Way or both? N Engl J Med *326:*1213, 1192.
39. British Paediatric Association: Hypercalcemia in infants and vitamin D. BMJ *2:*149, 1956.
40. Jacobus CH, Holick MF, Shao Q, et al: Hypervitaminosis D associated with drinking milk. N Engl J Med *326:*1173, 1992.
41. Blank S, Scanlon KS, Sinks TH, et al: An outbreak of hypervitaminosis D associated with the overfortification of milk from a home-delivery dairy. Am J Public Health *85:*656, 1995.
42. Pettifor JM, Bikle DD, Caveleros M, et al: Serum levels of free 1,25-dihydroxyvitamin D in vitamin D toxicity. Ann Intern Med *122:*511, 1995.
43. Iqbal SJ, Taylor WH: Treatment of vitamin D_2 poisoning by induction of hepatic enzymes. Br Med J *285:*541, 1982.
44. Rizzoli R, Stoermann C, Ammann P, Bonjour JP: Hypercalcemia and hyperosteolysis in vitamin D intoxication: Effects of clodronate therapy. Bone *15:*193, 1994.
45. Selby PL, Davies M, Marks JS, Mawer EB: Vitamin D intoxication causes hypercalcaemia by increased bone resorption which responds to pamidronate. Clin Endocrinol *43:*531, 1995.
46. Toxic effects of vitamin overdosage. Med Letter Drug Ther *26:*73, 1984.
47. Garewal HS, Diplock AT: How safe are antioxidant vitamins? Drug Safety *13:*8, 1995.
48. Diplock AT: Safety of antioxidant vitamins and β-carotene. Am J Clin Nutr *62:*1510S, 1995.
49. Alade SL, Brown RE, Paquet A: Polysorbate 80 and E-Ferol toxicity. Pediatrics *77:*593, 1986.
50. Brousson MA, Klein MC: Controversies surrounding the administration of vitamin K to newborns: A review. Can Med SSOC J *154:*307, 1996.
51. Marcus R, Coulston AM: Water-soluble vitamins: The vitamin B complex and ascorbic acid. *In* Hardman JG, Gilman AG, Limbard LE (eds): Goodman & Gilman's The Pharmacologic Basis of Therapeutics. 9th ed. New York, McGraw-Hill, pp 1555–1572, 1996.
52. Dalton K, Dalton MJ: Characteristics of pyridoxine overdose neuropathy syndrome. Acta Neurol Scand *76:*8, 1987.
53. Schaumberg H, Kaplan J, Windebank A, et al: Sensory neuropathy from pyridoxine abuse: A new megavitamin syndrome. N Engl J Med *309:*445, 1983.
54. Berger AR, Schaumberg HH, Schroeder C, et al: Dose response, coasting and differential fiber vulnerability in human toxic neuropathy: A prospective study of pyridoxine neurotoxicity. Neurology *42:*1367, 1992.
55. Gardner LI, Welsh-Sloan J, Cady RB: Phocomelia in infant whose mother took large doses of pyridoxine during pregnancy. Lancet *1:*636, 1985.
56. Morra M, Philipszoon HD, D'Andrea G, et al: Sensory and motor neuropathy caused by excessive ingestion of vitamin B6: a case report. Functional Neurology *8:*429, 1993.
57. Albin RL, Alpers JW, Greenberg HS, et al: Acute sensory-neuropathy-neuronopathy from pyridoxine overdose. Neurology *37:*1729, 1987.
58. Albin RL, Albers JW: Long-term follow-up of pyridoxine-induced acute sensory neuropathy-neuronopathy. Neurology *40:*1319, 1990.
59. Alhadeff L, Gualtieri T, Lipton M: Toxic effects of water-soluble vitamins. Nutrition Reviews *42:*33, 1984.
60. Litin SC, Anderson CF: Nicotinic acid-associated myopathy: A report of three cases. Am J Med *86:*481, 1989.
61. Rader JI, Calvert RJ, Hathcock JN: Hepatic toxicity of unmodified and time-release preparations of niacin. Am J Med *92:*77, 1992.
62. Reimund E, Ramos A: Niacin-induced hepatitis and thrombocytopenia after 10 years of niacin use. J Clin Gastroenterol *18:*270, 1994.
63. Gibbons LW, Gonzalez V, Gordon N, Grundy S: The prevalence of side effects with regular and sustained-release nicotinic acid. Am J Med *99:*378, 1995.
64. Doyon S, Roberts JR: Reappraisal of the "coma cocktail": Dextrose, flumazenil, naloxone, and thiamine. Emerg Med Clin N Am *12:*301, 1994.
65. Wrenn KD, Slovis CM: Neurologic complications of alcoholism. Emerg Med Clin N Am *8:*835, 1990.
66. Stephen JM, Grant R, Yeh CS: Anaphylaxis from administration of intravenous thiamine. Am J Emerg Med *10:*61, 1992.
67. Wrenn KD, Murphy F, Slovis CM: A toxicity study of parenteral thiamine hydrochloride. Ann Emerg Med *18:*867, 1989.
68. Kronauer CM, Buhler H: Skin findings in a patient with scurvy. N Engl J Med *332:*1611, 1995.
69. Sestili MA: Possible adverse health effects of vitamin C and ascorbic acid. Seminars Oncol *10:*299, 1983.
70. Goldfrank LR: Vitamins. *In* Goldfrank LR, Flomenbaum NE, Lewin NE, et al (eds): Toxicologic Emergencies, 5th ed. Norwalk, Conn, Appleton and Lange, pp 535–544, 1994.
71. Meyers DG, Maloney PA, Weeks D: Safety of antioxidant vitamins. Arch Intern Med *156:*925, 1996.
72. Curhan GC, Willett WC, Rimm EB, Stampfer MJ: A prospective study of the intake of vitamins C and B_6, and the risk of kidney stones in men. J Urol *155:*1847, 1996.

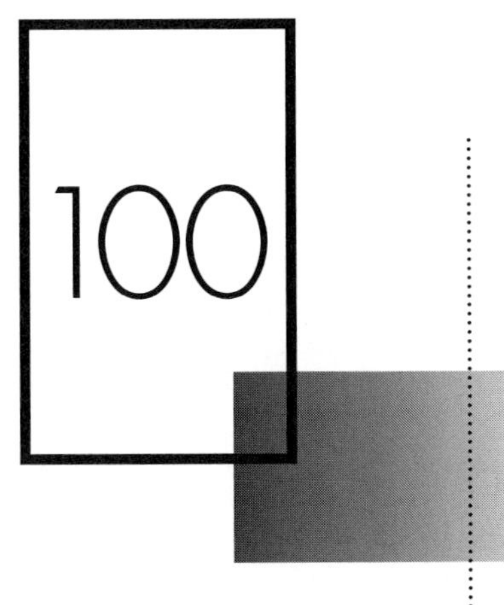

Pharmaceutical Excipients

THOMAS W. McKEE, MD
KATHERINE JONES, PharmD

In addition to their active or therapeutic ingredients, most pharmaceutical products contain presumably inert ingredients known as *excipients*. These additives are usually designed to provide stability and to increase the bioavailability of drug products. Excipients are generally considered to be inert, but past experiences have proved this not always to be true. The goal of this chapter is to acquaint practitioners with the importance of excipients and their potential adverse effects. The incidence of adverse reactions to excipients is not known, because many problems undoubtedly are unrecognized. A detailed account of all excipients and their adverse effects is beyond the scope of this chapter. Those readers seeking a comprehensive listing are referred to more detailed reviews.[1, 2]

HISTORICAL BACKGROUND[3]

In 1937, 5 years after the discovery of the antibacterial properties of sulfa products, a liquid preparation of sulfanilamide, known as Elixir Sulfanilamide, was produced and distributed by a small pharmaceutical firm in Tennessee. Within weeks of initial distribution, unexpected deaths due to acute renal failure related to ingestion of this product were recognized. The drug was recalled, and the majority retrieved before distribution. Nevertheless, 105 individuals died during a 4-week period as a result of ingesting this product. Subsequent study of Elixir Sulfanilamide demonstrated that the toxic ingredient was diethylene glycol, the solvent used to dissolve the sulfanilamide. Safety or efficacy testing had not been performed.

In response to this tragedy, Congress passed the 1938 Federal Food, Drug, and Cosmetic (FD&C) Act, which required pharmaceutical companies to demonstrate product safety of new drugs and to list all active ingredients. Before this time, the Food and Drug Administration (FDA) functioned primarily as a policing agency, responding to violations after they occurred. Safety or efficacy of new drugs had not been addressed. In 1962, companies were also required to demonstrate both safety and efficacy of new drugs. Subsequently the FDA has required listing of additives known to cause adverse reactions. A current listing of approved excipients is maintained in the FDA inactive ingredient guide.[4]

The Elixir Sulfanilamide tragedy is perhaps the most dramatic example of excipient toxicity in modern medicine in the United States. Despite current safety testing, adverse effects from presumed inert drug excipients continue to be recognized. The following discussion of examples of excipients that have been shown to cause adverse reactions is organized according to their function.

BULK AGENTS

Bulk agents are used to provide mixing, homogeneity, and stability to medications. Solid enteral excipients are generally thought to be safe. Commonly used solids include starch, lactose, dextrose, cellulose, talc, gluten, povidone, calcium salts, citric acid, and bicarbonate salts. Of these, lactose has the potential to cause cramping and diarrhea in lactase-deficient individuals. Although the amount of lactose ingested in drugs is quite small, even these amounts can cause symptoms in highly sensitive individuals. Gluten, or wheat protein, causes epithelial damage to the small bowel in sensitive individuals and can lead to malabsorption, although significant clinical problems are rarely caused by these excipients.

SOLVENTS

Solvents used in pharmaceuticals include water, ethanol, glycerin, and glycols. They are used in both enteral and parenteral preparations.

Polyethylene glycols are added to nonabsorbed electrolyte solutions that are used for bowel preparations. Mallory-Weiss tears,[5] esophageal perforation,[6] pulmonary edema,[7] urticaria,[8] and possibly anaphylaxis[9] have been associated with polyethylene glycols used in this fashion. Absorption of polyethylene glycols in burn creams is believed to have been responsible for renal injury, metabolic acidosis, and death in patients with large body surface area burns.[10] Urticaria[11] and delayed contact allergic reactions[12] are also well documented as resulting from topical preparations using polyethylene glycol.

Ethanol, commonly used in elixirs, can cause symptoms if ingested in large enough quantities. It represents a particular problem for infants, who may ingest toxic amounts of many commonly used pharmaceuticals[13] (see Chapter 34). Ethanol intoxication has also been reported in elderly patients receiving intravenous nitroglycerin.[14] Disulfiram-like reactions have occurred in patients taking ethanol-containing medications.[15]

Propylene glycol is a widely used pharmaceutical solvent that also has antimicrobial activity. It has been associated with a wide variety of adverse effects. Hyperosmolality has occurred in small infants receiving propylene glycol in multivitamin preparations,[16] in burned patients treated with a propylene glycol–containing antibiotic cream,[17] and in elderly patients who have renal insufficiency and who receive propylene glycol in intravenous nitroglycerin solution.[18] Central nervous system toxicity has been reported in children receiving propylene glycol as a vehicle for liquid enteral medication.[19] Lactic acid is also produced from propylene glycol, resulting in metabolic acidosis.[20] Life-threatening arrhythymias have been reported in patients receiving intravenous injections of phenytoin with propylene glycol used as the solvent, although a definite cause-effect relationship has not been established.[21] It also has been implicated as causing seizures in low-birth-weight infants,[22] stupor,[23] heparin resistance,[24] contact dermatitis,[25] and phlebitis.[26]

Glycerol is used as a solvent, sweetener, and preservative. The combination of glycerol and ethanol used as a vehicle for oral medication has been reported to cause hyperosmolality in neonates.[27] Although complications are reported to result from its use as a therapeutic agent, adverse effects from glycerol used as an excipient are rare.

COATINGS

Coatings for medicinal products are varied and include gelatins, silicones, shellac, gluten, various polymers, paraffins, and waxes. As excipients, they are ingested in small amounts and are generally believed to be safe.

FLAVORING AGENTS

Flavoring agents are commonly added to oral medications. As an example, a recent review found that 89 of 91 surveyed pediatric oral antibiotic preparations contained added flavorings.[28] These additives have been subjected to limited study. Often provided by the food industry, they are considered trade secrets, and listing is not required by the FDA. New substances may be manufactured from any of the GRAS chemicals. In 1985, the flavor and extract manufacturer's association of the United States listed 1750 GRAS chemicals.[29] Flavoring agents may be derived from a number of sources, including natural flavors from fruits and vegetables, aromatic oils from plants, and chemically synthesized flavors. Often a mixture of many different chemicals, flavorings are generally used in small amounts in pharmaceuticals. Although adverse effects appear to be rare, documentation is difficult owing to the many different ingredients potentially involved.

SWEETENERS

Commonly used sweeteners include sucrose, glucose, fructose, sorbitol, saccharin, aspartame, and cyclamate. All have the potential to alter bioavailability of active ingredients. Sugars, especially sorbitol, sucrose, and fructose, can cause osmotic diarrhea if ingested in large enough amounts.[30] Sucrose in liquid medications has been associated with increased dental disease in children.[31] Long-term use of saccharin and cyclamate has been associated with an increased incidence of cancer in laboratory animals.[32] Interestingly, saccharin is widely used in the United States; in one study, it was found in a third of oral antibiotics.[33] The amounts of these agents ingested as excipients in pharmaceuticals are much less than current dietary ingestion in our society, and their roles as drug excipients are believed to be minimal.

COLORING AGENTS

Coloring agents are commonly used to provide an identifiable or distinctive appearance to pharmaceutical products. The FDA has 129 permanently listed color additives for pharmaceutical, food, and cosmetic use.[34] Of these, the azo dye tartrazine is the only one for which labeling is required. It has been associated with a number of adverse reactions, especially in aspirin-sensitive individuals, including bronchospasm,[35] urticaria,[36] and rarely anaphylaxis.[37] Confirmation of tartrazine's role in causing the allergic reactions is not consistent, however, and its role has been questioned.[38] Other dyes have also occasionally been associated with bronchoconstriction, urticaria, and contact dermatitis. Adverse effects of dyes are listed in Table 100–1. Concerns about hyperkinesis and behavioral changes in children as a result of ingestion of artificial dyes have not been supported by scientific investigation.[39]

BUFFERING AGENTS

Many drugs contain buffering agents that adjust pH and thus improve bioavailability. They are not generally thought to be likely causes of untoward effects in pharmaceuticals.

SUSPENDING AND EMULSIFYING AGENTS

Suspending and emulsifying agents are used to alter the physical properties of pharmaceuticals and provide uniformity in dosing and delivery. These agents are used in many topical, enteral, parenteral, and aerosolized products. Polysorbate emulsifiers have been implicated as a possible contributing cause of renal and hepatic injury and death in newborns receiving a parenteral vitamin E formulation.[40] Similar symptoms have been reported in patients receiving intravenous amiodarone with the same polysorbate excipient.[41]

Polyethoxylated castor oil is associated with histamine-like reactions when used as an emulsifier with certain anesthetic agents.[42] It has also been associated with various immediate reactions when used as a vehicle with intravenous cyclosporine.[43]

PRESERVATIVES

Preservatives are added to prevent degradation and contamination of pharmaceuticals. They include antioxidants, antimicrobials, and chelating agents.

Sulfiting agents are a well-recognized cause of hypersensitivity reactions in sensitized individuals.[44]

Table 100–1. Various Dyes and Their Adverse Effects

Dye	Adverse Effects
Azo Dyes	
Tartrazine (FD&C yellow No. 5)	Anaphylactoid reactions; angioedema; asthma; urticaria; contact dermatitis; rhinitis; hyperkinesis in hyperactive patients; eosinophilia; cross-reactivity with aspirin, sodium benzoate, and indomethacin
Sunset yellow (FD&C yellow No. 6)	Anaphylactoid reactions; angioedema; anaphylactic shock; vasculitis; retching; abdominal pain; purpura; vomiting; belching; cross-reactivity with aspirin, acetaminophen, sodium benzoate, and other azo dyes
FD&C No. 4 (Ponceau Sx)	Bronchoconstriction
FD&C red No. 36	Contact dermatitis
FD&C No. 17	Contact dermatitis
Quinoline Dyes	
Quinoline yellow (FD&C yellow No. 10)	Contact sensitization
Quinoline yellow SS (FD&C No. 11)	Contact sensitization
Triphenylmethane Dyes	
FD&C blue No. 1	Bronchoconstriction in asthmatic patients
FD&C blue No. 2 (brilliant blue)	Weak sensitizer
FD&C green No. 3 (fast green)	Erythema multiforme–like skin rash
	In general, photosensitizer, anaphylactoid and asthmatic reactions
Xanthene Dyes (Fluran Dyes)	
FD&C No. 3 (erythrosin)	Potent photosensitizer, elevation of protein-bound iodine
FD&C orange No. 5	None reported
FD&C yellow No. 7 (fluorescein)	Urticaria, angioedema, syncope, shock, anaphylaxis
FD&C orange No. 10	None reported
FD&C red No. 19 (rhodamine)	None reported
FD&C red No. 21 (tetrabromofluorescein)	None reported
FD&C red No. 22 (eosin)	Potent photosensitizer
FD&C red No. 27 (tetrabromotetraclorofluorescein)	None reported
Others	
Carmine	Allergic cheilitis, asthma

From Kumar A, Rawlings RD, Beaman DC: The mystery ingredients: Sweeteners, flavorings, dyes and preservatives in analgesic/antipyretic, antihistamine/decongestant, cough and cold, antidiarrheal, and liquid theophylline preparations. Pediatrics *91*:932, 1993.

Their use in fresh fruits and vegetables has been banned. They are, however, found in many preserved foods and are used as antioxidants in a number of parenteral and inhaled medications. Paradoxically, use of sulfite-containing nebulized bronchodilators can precipitate bronchospasm in asthmatic patients.[45]

The antioxidant propyl gallate in infant formula has been linked to methemoglobinemia in infants with gastroenteritis.[46] Benzyl alcohol was found to cause metabolic acidosis, encephalopathy, renal failure, shock, and death in low-birth-weight infants when used as a preservative in bacteriostatic saline flush.[47] Chlorbutol as a preservative in heparin has been associated with hypotension in adult patients undergoing cardiac surgery.[48] Benzalkonium chloride–preserved inhalation agents have been implicated as causing bronchospasms in asthmatic patients,[49] as well as dermal and ocular hypersensitivity reactions. Other antimicrobial preservatives recognized as causing adverse reactions include chlorocresol, phenyl mercurial salts, thimerosal, parabens, benzoates, and sorbic acid.[50]

EVALUATION OF POSSIBLE ADVERSE REACTION TO AN EXCIPIENT

I. Determining the excipient components in a medication
   A. Inactive ingredients are required to be listed on the label of all parenteral medications. Despite recommendations from physicians' organizations,[51] the labeling of excipients is not required for oral or over-the-counter drugs. Some inactive ingredients, such as flavorings and dyes, may be considered trade secrets. The only coloring agent for which labeling is required is tartrazine (FD&C Yellow No. 5). The manufacturer, if requested, may disclose the inactive ingredients of an oral medication, although the concentrations may also be considered trade secrets. Manufacturers may also change excipients as long as FDA-approved agents are used.

II. Determining the excipient role in adverse drug reactions
   A. The patient's risk for an adverse reaction to an excipient must be assessed. Most adverse reactions from additives appear to be the result of direct toxicity, hypersensitivity, or allergy, although intolerance idiosyncrasy, immunotoxicity, and pseudoallergic reactions are also described.[52] Not surprisingly, those patients at greatest risk are those who are prone to hypersensitivity reactions (i.e., asthmatic patients) and those with altered kinetics (i.e., the elderly, premature infants, and patients with organ system dysfunction). These are the same patient groups at greatest risk for adverse reactions to active ingredients in medications.
   B. The risk of the excipient as the causal agent must be assessed. This can be done if the excipient in question has a track record of causing the recognized adverse effect. Unfortunately, standard references such as the *Physicians' Desk Reference*[53] do not differentiate adverse effects caused by excipients from those caused by active ingredients.

III. Defining the excipient as the causal agent
   A. For suspected allergic reactions, skin testing may be performed. This method may be of benefit if future exposure is likely and avoidance of the offending ingredients is necessary.
   B. Alleviation of an adverse effect on removal of a medication is strong evidence of causation. However, the reaction cannot definitively be attributed to the medication without a repeat challenge. This may not be feasible owing to the severity of the reaction. Neither technique differentiates which component of the drug is causative. Repeat challenge with a different preparation of the active ingredient without the offending excipient, if available, may provide presumptive evidence of causation.
   C. Adverse reactions to excipients should be reported to the FDA. All inactive ingredients are regulated by the FDA, and labeling, if not already in place, may be required for excipients recognized to cause adverse effects.

References

1. Golightly LK, Smolinske SS, Bennett ML, et al: Pharmaceutical excipients: Adverse effects associated with "inactive" ingredients in drug products (parts I and II). Concepts Toxicol Rev *3*:128–165, 209–240, 1988.
2. Weiner M, Bernstein IL: Adverse Reactions to Drug Formulation Agents: A Handbook of Excipients. New York, Marcel Dekker, 1989.
3. Wax PM: Elixirs, diluents, and the passage of the 1938 Federal Food Drug and Cosmetic Act. Ann Intern Med *122*:456–461, 1995.
4. Food and Drug Administration: Inactive Ingredient Guide, Washington, D.C. Division of Drug Information Resources, Center for Drug Evaluation and Research Office of Management, Washington, D.C., October 1993.
5. Santoro MJ, Chen YK, Collen MJ: Polyethylene glycol electrolyte solution–induced Mallory-Weiss tears. Am J Gastroenterol *88*:1292–1293, 1993.
6. McBride MA, Vanagunas A: Esophageal perforation associated with polyethylene glycol electrolyte lavage solution. Gastrointest Endosc *39*:856–857, 1993.
7. Papp CM, Erlich R: Acute pulmonary edema after polyethylene glycol intestinal lavage in a child. Ann Pharmacother *27*:1044–1047, 1993.
8. Brullet E, Moron A, Calvert X, et al: Urticarial reaction to oral polyethylene glycol electrolyte lavage solution. Gastrointest Endosc *38*:400–401, 1992.
9. Schuman E, Balsam P: Probable anaphylactic reaction to polyethylene glycol electrolyte lavage solution. Gastrointest Endosc *39*:411, 1991.

10. Bruns DE, Herold DA, Rodenheaver GT, Edlich RF: Polyethylene glycol intoxication in burn patients. Burns *9*:49–52, 1982.
11. Fisher AA: Contract urticaria due to polyethylene glycol. Cutis *19*:409–412, 1977.
12. Fisher AA: Immediate and delayed allergic contact reactions to polyethylene glycol. Contact Dermatitis *4*:135–138, 1978.
13. Pruitt AW, Anyan WR, Hill RM, et al: American Academy of Pediatrics Committee on Drugs: Ethanol in liquid preparations intended for children. Pediatrics *73*:405–407, 1984.
14. Brown SH, Comer JB: Intravenous nitroglycerin and ethanol intoxication. Ann Intern Med *102*:274, 1985.
15. Korn SH, Comer JB: Intravenous nitroglycerin and ethanol intoxication. Ann Intern Med *97*:621–622, 1982.
16. Glscow AM, Boeckx RL, Miller MK, et al: Hyperosmolality in small infants due to propylene glycol. Pediatrics *72*:353–355, 1983.
17. Berkeris L, Baker C, Fenton J, et al: Propylene glycol as a cause of an elevated serum osmolality. Am J Clin Pathol *72*:633–636, 1979.
18. Demey H, Daelemans R, De Broe ME, Bossaert L: Propylene glycol intoxication due to intravenous nitroglycerin. Lancet *1*:1360, 1984.
19. Arulanantham K, Genel M: Central nervous system toxicity associated with ingestion of propylene glycol. J Pediatr *93*:515–516, 1978.
20. Cate JC, Hendrick R: Propylene glycol intoxication and lactic acidosis. N Engl J Med *303*:1237, 1980.
21. Golightly LK, Smotinke SS, Bennett ML, et al: Pharmaceutical excipients: Adverse effects associated with "inactive" ingredients in drug products (Part I). Concepts Toxicol Rev *3*:162, 1988.
22. MacDonald MG, Getson PR, Glasgow AM, et al: Propylene glycol: Increased incidence of seizures in low birth weight infants. Pediatrics *79*:622–625, 1987.
23. Martin G, Finberg L: Propylene glycol: A potentially toxic vehicle in liquid dosage form. J Pediatr *77*:877, 1970.
24. Col J, Col-Debeys C, Lavenne-Pardonge E, et al: Propylene glycol-induced heparin resistance during nitroglycerin infusion. Am Heart J *110*:171–173, 1985.
25. Angelini G, Meneghini CL. Contact allergy from propylene glycol. Contact Dermatitis *7*:197–198, 1981.
26. Mattila MAK, Ruoppi M, Korhonen M, et al: Prevention of diazepam-induced thrombophlebitis with cremaphor as a solvent. Br J Anaesth *51*:891–894, 1979.
27. Vander Westuyzen JH, Berger GMB, Beyers N, Moosa A: Iatrogenic hyperosmolality in a neonate. S Afr Med J *60*:996–998, 1981.
28. Kumar A, Weatherly MR, Beaman DC: Sweeteners, flavorings, and dyes in antibiotic preparations. Pediatrics *87*:352–360, 1991.
29. Osler BL, Weil CS, Woods LA, Bernard BK: GRAS substances. Food Technol *39*:108–117, 1985.
30. Johnson KR, Govel LA, Andritz MH: Gastrointestinal effects of sorbitol as an additive in liquid medications. Am J Med *97*:185–191, 1994.
31. Feigal RJ, Jensen ME, Mensing CA: Dental caries potential of liquid medications. Pediatrics *68*:416–419, 1981.
32. Council on Scientific Affairs: Saccharin, review of safety issues. JAMA *254*:2622–2624, 1985.
33. Kumar A, Weatherly MR, Beaman DC: Sweeteners, flavorings, and dyes in antibiotic preparations. Pediatrics *87*:352–360, 1991.
34. Food and Drug Administration: Permanently listed color additives. Inactive Ingredient Guide. Washington, DC, Division of Drug Information Resources, Center for Drug, Evaluation and Research Office of Management, October 1993, Appendix.
35. Samter M, Beers RF: Intolerance to aspirin: Clinical studies and considerations of its pathogenesis. Ann Intern Med *68*:975, 1968.
36. Stevenson DD, Simon RA, Lumry WR, Mathison DA: Adverse reactions to tartrazine. J Allergy Clin Immol *78*:182–191, 1986.
37. Desmund RE, Trautlein JJ: Tartrazine (FD&C Yellow #5) anaphylaxis: A case report. Ann Allergy *46*:81–82, 1981.
38. Simon RA, Stevenson DD: Adverse Reactions to Food and Drug Additives. *In* Allergy, Principles and Practice. St. Louis, Mosby–Year Book, p 1700, 1993.
39. David TJ: Reactions to dietary tartrazine. Arch Dis Child *62*:119–122, 1987.
40. Alade SL, Brown RE, Paquet A: Polysorbate 80 and E-ferol toxicity. Pediatrics *77*:593–597, 1986.
41. Rhodes A, Eastwood JB, Smith SA: Early acute hepatitis with parenteral amiodarone: A toxic effect for the vehicle? Gut *34*:565–566, 1993.
42. Watkins J: The allergic reactions to intravenous induction agents. Br J Hosp Med *36*:45–48, 1986.
43. Kahn BD, Wideman CA, Flechner S, van Buren CT: Anaphylactic reaction—intravenous cyclosporin. Lancet *1*:52, 1984.
44. Jamieson DM, Guill MF, Wray BB, May JR: Metabisulfite sensitivity: Case report and literature review. Ann Allergy *54*:115–121, 1985.
45. Koepke JW, Christopher KL, Chai H, et al: Dose-dependent bronchospasm from sulfites in isoetharine. JAMA *251*:2982–2983, 1984.
46. Nitzan M, Volovitz B, Topper E: Infantile methemoglobinemia caused by food additives. Clin Toxicol *15*:273–280, 1974.
47. Brown WJ, Buist NRM, Gipson HTC, et al: Fatal benzyl alcohol poisoning in a neonatal intensive care unit. Lancet *1*:250, 1982.
48. Bowler GMR, Galloway DW, Meiklejohn BH: Sharp fall in blood pressure after injection of heparin containing Chlorbutol. Lancet *1*:848–849, 1986.
49. Beasley CRW, Rafferty P, Holgate S: Benzalkonium chloride and bronchoconstriction. Lancet *2*:1227, 1986.
50. Golighly LK, Smolinske SS, Bennett ML, et al: Pharmaceutical excipients: Adverse effects associated with inactive ingredients in drug products (Part I). Med Toxicol *3*:132–145, 1988.
51. American Academy of Pediatric Committee on Drugs: "Inactive" ingredients in pharmaceutical products. Pediatrics *76*:635–643, 1985.
52. Weiner M, Berstein IL: Adverse Reactions to Drug Formulation Agents: A Handbook of Excipients. New York, Marcek Dekker, pp 17–22, 1989.
53. Physicians' Desk Reference. Muntrale, NJ, Medical Economics, 1995.

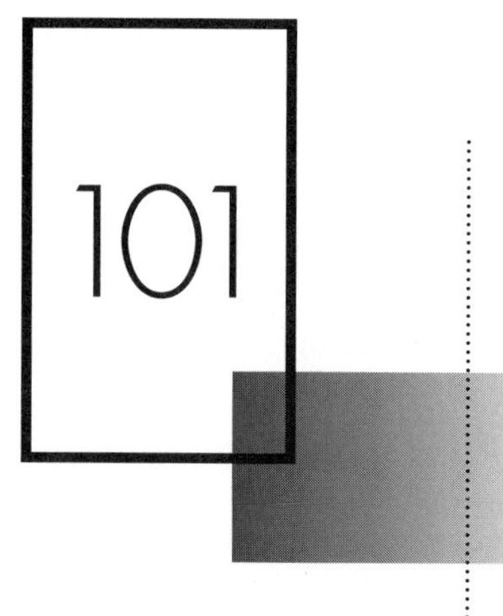

Baby Powder, Borates, and Camphor

YOUNG-JIN SUE, MD
HEIDI PINKERT, MD

BABY POWDER

Of the 80 baby powder preparations in the United States, the major component of 70 is talc,[1] a hydrous magnesium silicate.[2] Because it is obtained through commercial mining, it may be contaminated by minerals that occur in natural juxtaposition,[3] and industrial talc may contain asbestos.[4] Manufacturers of cosmetic-grade talc set forth purity guidelines in 1976; contamination from asbestos is therefore not a concern in today's baby powders.[5] Those powders that do not contain talc utilize cornstarch as the major ingredient.[1] Literature with regard to toxic effects from such powders is lacking.

Means of exposure to baby powder generally occur either via its routine use by women as a dusting powder in the perineal area[6] or via accidental inhalation by infants and children. Workers are variably exposed to talc in the course of mining it.[7] Oral ingestion of talc is not likely to be toxic; it is contained in some pills, but there is no evidence to suggest adverse effects from moderate intake.[4]

Range of Toxic Effects

A number of studies have attempted to ascertain whether perineal exposure to talc in women increases the risk of ovarian cancer.[8] Frequency and duration of use have also been examined.[5] To date, a clear-cut relationship between perineal talc exposure and ovarian cancer has not been clearly established.

Data on the toxic effects of talc inhalation originally came from a few case reports of accidental massive exposures in infants and children.[9–15] Many of the individuals died as a result of the exposure. More recent literature has reported on milder cases of baby powder inhalation, with the majority of children doing well.[2]

Clinical Presentation

A frequent scenario for significant inhalation involves a child grabbing the baby powder container during diaper changing,[16] with resultant spilling of contents into the mouth from a loose or opened top. Another common event involves the child playing with the powder container (whose shape is similar to that of a bottle used for feeding) and placing it in the mouth.[16] An older sibling may also "powder" the baby, covering the face and causing inhalation.[13] Regardless of the inciting event, the child is usually found coughing, often with dyspnea, sneezing, and vomiting.[2] The airway may be completely obstructed in some instances.[17] In many cases, the initial symptoms resolve, and an asymptomatic period ensues.[12] This, in turn, gives way to respiratory distress, usually after a few hours. The degree of respiratory distress is variable, but it may easily progress to respiratory failure when significant amounts of powder are inhaled.

Toxicokinetics/Pathophysiology

The physical properties of talc account for its toxicity when inhaled. It is insoluble in water and not biodegradable; it thus may obstruct the airways to variable degrees.[14] The size of talc particles, which averages less than 5 μm,[18] would allow them to reach the alveoli; this has indeed been confirmed on pathologic specimens.[10] Other pathologic findings after talc inhalation consist of inflammatory changes in the airway and interstitium, bronchiolitis with bronchiolar obstruction, atelectasis, emphysema, and fibrosis.[10, 11, 14] These pathologic findings are in accord with the observation that the clinical picture may resemble severe bronchiolitis.[13]

Management

Management of baby powder inhalation consists first of recognizing the potential for respiratory distress and failure, despite several hours of an asymptomatic period.[9, 11, 12, 19] Even if the patient appears to have made initial clinical improvement, follow-up is necessary, and the caretaker should be advised of the potential for subsequent development of symptoms.

Management of respiratory distress is essentially supportive; intubation and mechanical ventilation may be necessary as in any child with severe respiratory distress and/or failure. The use of corticosteroids has been reported to result in clinical improvement in some cases,[11, 13, 20, 21] presumably by decreasing the inflammatory response noted on pathologic examination of the lung.[9] Bronchoalveolar lavage is another therapeutic modality that has been instituted in some cases,[12] but its use may be limited by the insolubility of baby powder in aqueous solution.[14] The use of lavage in combination with steroid therapy has produced favorable results in one series of 13 patients.[22] No evidence exists to suggest that antibiotics play a beneficial role.[12, 13]

As with many ingestions, prevention of initial exposure is the best way to avoid problems. Indeed, many physicians have advocated strongly against the use of baby powder as being unnecessary and a potential hazard.[2, 17, 23, 24]

BORATES

Borates and borate-mineral concentrates such as borax ($Na_2B_4O_7 \cdot 10H_2O$) are salts or esters of boric acid, H_3PO_3. Postulated original uses for borax include its use as a flux for working gold by the Babylonians more than 4000 years ago, and references have been found to the use of boron by the Egyptians for mummifying, medicinal, and metallurgic purposes. Today's uses for borate-mineral concentrates include as micronutrients in fertilizer, in fire retardants, in laundry bleaches, and in glass and related vitreous applications.[25] Boric acid is an odorless, colorless compound that can occur in crystalline, granular, or white powder form. Its introduction as a medication in the 18th century is credited to Wilhelm Homberg; its original uses were as a sedative, antispasmodic, and analgesic. In the mid-19th century, Lister began using boric acid as an antiseptic, and it was subsequently used as a bowel irrigant in dysentery and typhoid. Other uses included irrigation of surgical wounds and abscesses, as a wash for the urinary bladder and prostatic bed, and as a wash for eyes, nose, and throat, as well as treatment for oral thrush. Dermatologic uses for boric acid have also existed (e.g., for treatment of burns and skin eruptions). Boric acid acts as a buffer against alkali, and it allows powders with which it is mixed to flow more freely. Because of these properties and its mild antiseptic and antifungal properties, boric acid has been used in talcum powders;[26] indeed many of the reported cases of serious poisonings and fatalities have been linked to use of "medicated" talcum powders in babies.[27] Boric acid suppositories have been used to treat vulvovaginal candidiasis in adult women.[28] Current nonmedical applications for boric acid include use as a pesticide and for cockroach control.[25]

Although boron is a ubiquitous element, borates and borax are found only in areas where the geography is conducive to formation of borates from boric acid and steam. Tibetan lakes are thought to have been the earliest source,[25] with Italy being an important source for Europe in the 19th and early 20th centuries. Today, Turkey is the largest producer of borate products worldwide.[29] The only source of borax in the United States is from large deposits in southern California.

Range of Toxic Effects

Most data regarding the range of toxic effects from boric acid ingestion come from case reports and case series.[27, 30–32] Due in part to the fact that more than one route of exposure may result in toxic responses, estimating the quantity ingested can be difficult. A case series review by Goldbloom and Goldbloom[27] noted a general trend of increased mortality in the very young, specifically newborns and infants younger than 1 year. Dermal exposure in this group was a significant cause of toxic effects and death. Wong and colleagues[30] reported a case series of oral boric acid intoxications in a newborn nursery. Their data revealed that between 4.5 and 15.0 g of boric acid had been ingested by those infants who died. Deaths occurred as a result of drinking formula accidentally prepared with a 2.5% boric acid solution. Serum borate levels in these infants ranged from 40 to 160 mg/dL. Infants who survived the poisoning but were symptomatic ingested amounts ranging from 2.0 to 4.5 g and had serum borate levels of 2 to 15 mg/dL. A report has been published, however, of two children (a 2- and a 3-year-old) with serum borate levels of 7.9 and 7.4 mg/dL, respectively, who were completely asymptomatic.[33] In general, a dose of 2 to 3 g in newborns and infants and 5 g in children is regarded as lethal. Because boric acid solutions usually range in concentration from 2.5% to 5.0%, a significant amount must be ingested for toxicity to occur. Of greater concern is the ingestion of boric acid powder, crystals, or granules; 1 teaspoonful of 100% boric acid in these forms contains 2.9 to 4.4 g.[34] The literature regarding adults describes four deaths due to acute boric acid or sodium borate ingestion since 1921.[35] Based on these data and other case series, it has been estimated that the adult human median lethal dose (LD_{50}) is likely to be greater than 30 g. Although case series reveal a wide range for toxicity,[27, 32] ingestion of 15 to 20 g of boric acid is generally cited as the lethal dose for adults.[61]

Clinical Presentation

The potential routes of exposure to borate compounds are several. Workers exposed to borax dust, boron oxide, and boric acid powder were studied to determine the effects of inhalation exposure.[37, 38] Symptoms that correlated with chronic exposure to these compounds included eye irritation; sore throat; mouth, nose, or throat dryness; and productive cough.[37] Radiographic abnormalities on chest x-ray were not found commonly in workers exposed to borax dust. Smokers exposed to borax dust were noted, however, to have small decreases in forced expiratory volume (FEV_1) following exposure. These compounds are classified as simple respiratory irritants when inhalation is the route of exposure.

Irrigation of body cavities and wounds with boric acid solution was responsible for a number of deaths in the late 19th and early 20th centuries.[26] Other routes of exposure include dermal contact or oral ingestion. A number of reports of infant poisonings cite application of boric acid powder or "medicated" baby powder containing boric acid to an excoriated diaper area.[27, 39, 40] The clinical picture typically associated with toxicity from dermal application of boric acid consists of vomiting and diarrhea. A blue-green color has inconsistently been noted in vomitus and stool. Significant dehydration may occur as a result of gastrointestinal symptoms. The central nervous system (CNS) is involved, with seizures and/or irritability noted, as well as lethargy. A bright erythematous rash often becomes generalized (the so-called boiled-lobster appearance), with significant desquamation occurring 1 to 2 days after the rash is first noted. In infants, the rash is very similar in appearance to toxic epidermal necrolysis (Staphylococcal scalded-skin syndrome).[42] Vomiting and diarrhea are accompanied by nausea and abdominal cramps. The neurologic manifestations in adults are more likely to be those of CNS depression rather than excitation. Erythema of the skin is followed by exfoliation. Fatalities from dermal application have been noted in this population as well.[41]

Oral ingestion of boric acid has occurred in adults, both with intention to do harm and accidentally.[35, 43] Many oral infant poisonings resulted from accidental preparation of formula with boric acid solution instead of water.[30, 44, 45] Clinical manifestations from oral intoxication are strikingly similar to those seen with cutaneous application of boric acid, that is, vomiting and diarrhea (often with a blue-green color), neurologic abnormalities, and a diffuse erythematous eruption that desquamates 1 to 2 days after appearance. Oliguria and proteinuria have been reported, usually preceding acute tubular necrosis, but this is uncommon. Abnormalities of liver function have rarely been noted as well.[32] The American Academy of Pediatrics recommends that boric acid be eliminated from pediatric sections and newborn nurseries of hospitals for two reasons: (1) because of the potentially serious consequences of boric acid ingestion in infants, and (2) because it is thought that boric acid is unnecessary for the care of infants.[46]

Toxic response to borates may also occur with chronic exposure. The limited literature on this topic suggests a clinical picture different from that noted with acute exposures: infants given pacifiers dipped in a borax and honey compound came to medical attention with the onset of generalized seizures.[31, 47] All had been exposed in this manner for greater than 4 weeks. Two of the infants lacked any gastrointestinal symptoms, despite blood boric acid levels of 14.5 and 9.44 mg/dL, respectively, at the time of presentation.[47] All infants had cessation of seizures with withdrawal of the borax and honey compound, and follow-up several years later showed them to be seizure-free and otherwise doing well. Case reports in adults suggest that alopecia may result from chronic exposure to boric acid, either orally or via inhalation.[48, 49] In one case, a young woman presented with diffuse alopecia after utilization of several bottles of mouthwash daily for at least a year. She had been swallowing the boric acid-containing mouthwash after use and was noted to have in increased serum boron level on presentation. The alopecia resolved after discontinuation of this practice.[48] A storekeeper whose job included filling a soap dispenser with a borax washing powder similarly complained of alopecia. He had been working in an unventilated storeroom with the washing compound for more than 6 years. A few months after limiting the patient's contact with borax, hair growth returned to normal.[49]

Toxicokinetics

Absorption of boric acid occurs easily through abraded or excoriated skin,[40, 41, 50] but absorption through intact skin is negligible.[33, 51] Oral ingestion results in rapid and complete absorption of boric acid from the gastrointestinal tract. Distribution then occurs throughout body water, but with highest concentrations in certain organs, specifically brain, liver, and kidneys.[44, 52, 53] The overwhelming majority of ingested boric acid is excreted unchanged by the kidneys; greater than 50% of the oral dose is gone within 24 hours, and greater than 90% is excreted within 96 hours of ingestion.[32, 54] Various numbers for the half-life of boric acid have been reported, ranging from 5 to 21 hours.[32, 44]

Pathophysiology

Autopsy findings in patients who die as a result of boric acid poisoning note significant involvement of several organ systems: skin, gastrointestinal tract, kidneys, brain, and liver all appear to be affected.[27, 40, 50] In those individuals with skin eruptions, pathologic specimens are consistent with an exfoliative dermatitis. The gastrointestinal tract demonstrates inflammatory changes, with congestion, edema, and mucosal exfoliation. Boric acid is not caustic, however, so stricture formation should not be a concern in oral intoxication. Renal changes are somewhat variable, ranging from gross pallor to cloudy swelling and tubular degeneration. The CNS as a target organ demonstrates congestion and edema of the brain and has in some studies been noted to be the organ with the highest concentration of boric acid in intoxicated individuals.[27] The liver, despite being the organ with the second highest concentration of boric acid, rarely demonstrates clinical manifestations of boric acid toxicity.[27, 53, 54] Pathologic findings consist of fatty change and congestion. Rare findings include intracytoplasmic inclusion bodies in pancreatic acinar cells.[26]

Animal studies have demonstrated that borax and boric acid at very high levels may lead to growth suppression and decreased efficiency of food utilization in rats. Testicular degeneration has been noted in both rats and dogs at very high boron levels, and rats were sterile.[55] Similar reproductive effects have recently been demonstrated in mice.[56] A study by Whorton and others[57] concluded that no such reproductive effects existed among male employees at a borate mining and production facility, where average length of employment was 18 years.

In trying to elucidate a specific mechanism of action whereby borates exert their toxic effects, it has been noted that boric acid acts as a teratogen in chick embryos. The resulting malformations resemble those characteristic of riboflavin deficiency.[58, 59] It was further demonstrated by Roe and associates[60] that toxicity from boric acid was markedly reduced in animals fed supplemental riboflavin. Greatly increased urinary riboflavin excretion has been documented in humans after boric acid ingestion;[61] this naturally raises the question of the possible utility of riboflavin supplementation in the treatment of borate toxicity. No data on the efficacy of such treatment currently exist.

Diagnosis

The diagnosis of boric acid poisoning requires careful history-taking with the appropriate clinical picture. At one time, the turmeric paper test was used as an assay for the presence of boric acid. The urine of the patient to be tested was acidified with concentrated hydrochloric acid. Turmeric paper was dipped into this solution, then air dried. With drying, the turmeric paper turns a pink to red color in the presence of borate. A confirmatory test is performed by placing a drop of ammonia water on the test paper and observing a transient blue-black color.[27, 30] The major difficulty with this test is that it is overly sensitive and may be positive even in the presence of normal borate levels. Because boron is ubiquitous, small amounts of boric acid are normally present in the body due to dietary intake of fruits, vegetables, cereals, and breads. Data from a study by Fisher and Freimuth[33] indicated an average blood boron level of 0.25 μm/mL (range, 0.00 to 1.25 μm/mL) in infants exposed only to dietary sources. The average normal serum boric acid level for an adult is reported as 1.4 μm/mL.[26] Because most hospital laboratories do not have the capability to quickly determine serum borate levels, this information cannot be relied on to make the diagnosis of borate toxicity. However, because individual susceptibility varies greatly, and no correlation is noted between serum borate levels and the clinical picture, such levels are chiefly of academic interest. Two commercial laboratories are able to quantitate serum borate levels: National Medical Services, Inc., 2300 Stratford Ave., P.O. Box 433A, Willow Grove, PA, 19090, telephone (215) 657–4900; and West Coast Analytical Services, Inc., 9840 Albgurtis Ave., Sante Fe Springs, CA 90670, telephone (310) 948–2225. The U.S. Borax and Chemical Co. provides a 24-hour telephone number for medical emergencies related to borates: (800) 228–5635, extension 144 (Strong P: oral communication, 1996).

Management

As no antidote exists for boric acid poisoning, supportive care is the backbone of treatment. Gastric emptying should be performed in cases of acute oral ingestion, regardless of the time relative to ingestion; recovery of large concentrations of boric acid has been reported even 24 hours after ingestion.[30] Charcoal should not be given in cases in which borates alone have been ingested, as it is ineffective.[62] If toxicity is due to any form of borate administration, it should be discontinued. Intravenous fluid administration may be necessary in the patient who has experienced significant vomiting and/or diarrhea. In the presence of dermatologic manifestations of poisoning, with skin desquamation, local skin care should be initiated, but antibiotics are useful only if secondary bacterial infection becomes evident.

Other modes of treatment have been suggested, including hemodialysis, peritoneal dialysis, and exchange transfusion.[32, 39, 45] The last treatment is generally not considered effective and is no longer used. No specific recommendations have been made regarding when dialysis should be instituted. Baker and Bogema[44] suggest its use in patients whose serum levels exceed 200 μm/mL or in those who are severely symptomatic. Others suggest that it be used early on in almost any patient, even in the absence of clinical symptoms.[63] Certainly, renal failure is an indication for dialysis.

Given the awareness of the medical community regarding the potential for toxicity from boric acid, and recognition of its limited utility in this field, significant poisonings secondary to medicinal use are rare in adults. It appears that at present, the greatest risk may be from ingestion of highly pure boric acid crystals utilized as insecticides and for cockroach control.

CAMPHOR

Camphor, the pungent distillate of the tree by the same name, has been used historically as an aphrodisiac, anti-aphrodisiac, lactation suppressant, abortifacient, contraceptive, and "circulatory stimulant."[64] In the 1930s, Ladislav Meduna induced seizures with intramuscular injections of camphor to treat catatonia, a therapeutic predecessor to electroconvulsive therapy.[65] The use of parenteral camphor as an analeptic to rouse patients with cardiac or respiratory "collapse," syncope, or sedation following anesthesia persisted into the 1940s.[66] Although no longer available in sterile parenteral solutions, camphor continues to be ubiquitous in over-the-counter preparations such as local anesthetics, antipruritics, rubefacients, antitussives, and "chest cold" inhalants. Despite its lack of therapeutic value and the availability of safer alternatives for all of its purported uses, the placebo effect associated with its intense odor and local warmth contributes to its continued popularity in over-the-counter preparations.

Most accidental overdoses of camphor have occurred when it has been mistakenly administered for castor oil or cough syrup. Often produced in similar packaging and stocked on adjacent shelves in pharmacies, the confusion of camphorated oil, a 20% mixture of camphor and cottonseed oil, for castor oil was predictable. In 1983, the FDA ruled that over-the-counter products cannot contain camphor in excess of 11%. However, the older products containing higher concentrations of camphor continue to surface in childhood poisonings.[67] For 1993, the American Association of Poison Control Centers Toxic Exposure Surveillance System reported 7635 cases of toxic exposures to camphor.[68] Of these, the vast majority (7380) were unintentional, and most (6055) occurred in children younger than 6 years. Seventy-four were judged to have had a moderately severe outcome, and 15 suffered major morbidity. No fatalities ensued.

Pharmacology

Camphor is a crystalline ketone, related to the terpenes, that was originally steam-distilled from the bark of the camphor tree *Cinnamomum camphora*. Now it is synthetically produced from alpha-pinene ($C_{10}H_{10}$), a hydrocarbon extracted from turpentine oil.[66] Chemically, it is described as a bicyclo-monoterpenoid or 1,7,7-trimethyl-bicyclo (2.1.1)-2-heptanone.[69, 70]

The mechanism of toxicity of camphor is unclear. Topically, camphor is a rubefacient, producing local hyperemia and warmth. It is felt to generate its perceived therapeutic benefits via the "counterirritant analgesic effect" in which moderate visceral pain is masked by a milder skin irritation.[71] Camphor's intense odor and sensation of warmth on application contributes to the feeling of relief from pain or congestion that may be greater than that actually physiologically present. Although the biochemical basis by which camphor leads to central nervous system excitation and seizures is not well understood, it is felt to act directly to stimulate nervous tissue. Smith and Margolis, in 1954, attempted to describe the pathologic findings associated with camphor poisoning. In a 19-month-old child who died 5 days after the ingestion of an estimated 1 tsp of camphorated oil, they found "extensive degenerative changes" selectively involving the neurons of the cerebral cortex, basal ganglia, and hippocampus. The same investigators found no neurologic pathologic lesions in mice when seizures were prevented by the concomitant administration of pentobarbital with camphor. These findings suggest that the neuronal damage found in camphor fatalities may result from seizures and anoxia rather than from a direct action of camphor on neurons.[64]

Camphor is readily absorbed from the gastrointestinal tract, although the presence of food may delay the rate of absorption. In a 2-year-old child who ingested an estimated 1 to 2 tsp of Campho-Phenique (11% camphor), gas-liquid chromatography detected camphor in serum drawn as early as 20 minutes following ingestion.[72] Although most poisonings result from ingestion, toxicity has been reported from absorption via other routes. Skoglund and colleagues reported the case of a 15-month-old boy who developed prolonged seizures after crawling through a quantity of spirits-of-camphor that had been spilled on the floor. The child recovered and was well until a year later when he developed a brief generalized seizure coincident with exposure to a nebulized camphor solution for an upper respiratory infection. The child was reported to be well prior to the camphor exposures. Nevertheless, reports of toxicity following inhalational and dermal exposure are not common, and one wonders whether this patient had a pre-existing CNS focus that predisposed him to seizures.[73] In another case, a 48-year-old woman developed seizures after self-administration of several milliliters of a camphor-containing nose-drop solution for nasal congestion. Although some absorption may have taken place from the nasal mucosa, swallowed camphor solution was probably more important in the resulting toxicity.[74]

In liver microsomes, camphor undergoes metabolism to several compounds. Koppel and associates analyzed the serum and urine of two young men who had ingested camphor. Using gas chromatography/mass spectrophotometry, they detected, in addition to the parent compound, 3-, 5-, 8- and 9-hydroxycamphor, 5-ketocamphor, 8- or 9-camphor carbonic acid trimethylsilylester and isoborneole.[69] Glucuronide conjugation renders certain of these metabolites water-soluble, allowing for renal excretion. Others, distributing to fatty tissues, may have prolonged retention times. The rapid onset of symptoms following ingestion implies that the parent compound is largely responsible for the toxicity of camphor. It is not clear to what extent, if any, the metabolites are responsible for the clinical findings.

Camphor has been reported to distribute across the placental barrier. In one case, a pregnancy ended with fetal death, and camphor was measured in fetal tissues and amniotic fluid.[75] In another case, the odor of camphor was apparent on the otherwise uncomplicated delivery of the infant.[76] Camphor was just detectable in the serum of this infant.

Clinical Presentation

On ingestion, local symptoms are immediate, whereas systemic complaints may develop within minutes to hours. Immediately, individuals tend to complain of burning of lips, oral mucosa, and throat; thirst; epigastric pain; and nausea and vomiting.[77] In more serious ingestions, local symptoms may be followed by twitching, confusion, irritability, coma, and seizures.[78] Although most significant toxicity occurs early, there have been reports of cases in which severe symptoms were delayed for several hours. A 61-year-old man ingested 2 oz of camphorated oil and presented 6 hours later to a hospital in status epilepticus.[79] Although he required treatment with anticonvulsants, he recovered fully. More typically, in 1919, Benz described 20 children, ages 4 to 10 years, who had accidentally received from 1 to 1½ tbsp of camphorated oil instead of castor oil. Symptoms developed in the first child within 45 minutes. All of the children's symptoms progressed to seizure activity. Although no child died, one suffered prolonged symptoms and coma before recovering 29 hours after ingestion.[80]

Rated a class 4 or "very toxic" compound, the lethal dose range of camphor has been reported to be 50 to 500 mg/kg.[81] Most patients recover fully with supportive care, and fatalities are usually due to respiratory arrest following prolonged seizure activity. In fact, one would expect that death from accidental poisoning with camphor should become vanishingly rare given the availability of contemporary medical intensive care capabilities. Historically, as little as 1 g has been reported to be fatal in a child. A 19-month-old child, reported to be previously healthy, ingested approximately 1 tsp of camphorated oil (1 g of camphor).[64] Other than vomiting within a few minutes of ingestion, he remained relatively symptom free for 3 hours. At that point, he developed "salivation and rigidity," most certainly seizure activity, and was brought to medical attention. The child was febrile (41.5°C) and had tachycardia. Peripheral blood count revealed a leukocytosis with left shift at 40,000/mm^3, with 93% segmented neutrophils. The care at the time (1954) included administration of meperidine, caffeine, sodium benzoate, phenobarbital, oxygen, and fluids by hypodermoclysis as well as sponge baths. Although seizures may account for the vital sign and hematologic abnormalities, it is apparent that an infectious etiology was considered, as penicillin was also administered. The premorbid course was characterized by coma and intermittent tonic seizures. Signs of increased intracranial pressure developed and the child died on the fifth day following admission. At the other extreme, an adult was reported to have survived an ingestion of 30 g.[82] An adult male, in a suicide attempt, ingested 150 mL of camphorated oil. He developed severe vomiting, shock, and generalized seizures. Treated with gastric lavage, endotracheal intubation, and diazepam, he recovered within 36 hours of ingestion.

A few cases of the use of camphor in pregnancy have been described. In at least one, no apparent adverse effect resulted. A young pregnant woman at term accidentally ingested 2 oz of camphorated oil in orange juice and shortly thereafter developed seizure activity.[76] The woman was treated with diazepam and supportive care. The following day, she delivered an infant who, although redolent of camphor, was well and without any signs of camphor toxicity. Riggs and associates describe another case in which a young pregnant woman, admitted to the hospital at term for symptoms of preeclampsia, inadvertently ingested 12 g of camphor instead of castor oil. Confusion and seizures developed within several minutes, and the patient was treated with gastric lavage, amobarbital, and phenobarbital. Labor, which began 17 hours following ingestion, was complicated by abruptio placentae, vaginal bleeding with grossly bloody amniotic fluid, and fetal bradycardia. The mother did well, but the infant was never successfully resuscitated and died at 30 minutes following delivery. Although the authors reported the case as camphorated oil intoxication in pregnancy, the preeclampsia and placental abruption probably were the dominant contributors to the neonatal death.[75]

Although most reports of camphor poisoning result from acute exposure, there have been a few reports of toxicity following chronic ingestion. Jiminez and co-workers described a 6-month-old male infant in whom coma and hepatomegaly developed following a 2-day upper respiratory febrile illness. Liver function abnormalities, hypoglycemia, and the neurologic findings following a viral syndrome led to a suspicion of Reye's syndrome. Eventually, the parent admitted to the chronic administration of a home remedy containing camphor for "fretfulness and cold." Beginning at the age of 1 month, the infant had received daily dropperfuls of a solution containing 3% camphor and 33% ethanol. Hepatic histologic examination supported neither the diagnosis of Reye's syndrome nor that of chronic ethanolism, consisting of irregularly sized and located fat deposits within the hepatocytes. Although the infant's hepatitis improved, his neurologic status continued to deteriorate, and he died on the fifth hospital day.[83] In another case of chronic camphor exposure, McCollam and others reported the case of a 72-year-old woman who presented to a hospital complaining of weakness, fever, pruritus, anorexia, and weight loss.[84] Liver biopsy, prompted by the finding of hepatomegaly, revealed a granulomatous picture with necrosis and eosinophilia. When the patient returned 4 months later with the same complaints, extensive questioning uncovered a history of chronic self-medication with Vicks VapoRub (5% camphor) for the "relief of mild bronchospasm." Total consumption was estimated at 5 small bottles over the period of 5 years. On discontinuation of this practice, the patient recovered without sequelae.

Diagnosis

As most instances of camphor intoxication occur following accidental ingestion, patients usually promptly seek medical attention and willingly offer historical information relevant to the poisoning. Even in the absence of such historical information, however, the presence of camphor is readily apparent due to its intense and characteristic odor, which may be detected on the breath, vomitus, clothes, and hair. This is further aided by the typical clinical picture of gastrointestinal distress, agitation, somnolence, and seizures. Hyperthermia and tachycardia usually accompany prolonged agitation and seizures. No laboratory derangements are specifically characteristic of camphor poisoning, though transient liver function abnormalities have been reported in some cases.[76, 79] Camphor may be quantitatively determined in serum by gas chromatography/mass spectrophotometry, but this assay is not generally available in most clinical laboratories nor does it contribute significantly to the acute management of camphor poisoning. When it has been measured, camphor levels have varied widely and have not been predictive of serious toxicity. For example, a level of 0.0015 mg/dL (0.015 mg/L) was detected in a 2-year-old girl with vomiting only.[72] Two young men with agitation but no seizures had levels of 300 and 400 ng/mL (or 0.3 and 0.4 mg/L).[69]

Patients who experienced seizures had levels ranging from 0.0017 to 3.1 mg/L.[85–87] Due to the frequency of emesis, accurate quantitation of absorbed camphor is difficult, and dose-concentration relationships are not available for camphor. As the clinical consequences of camphor intoxication are played out long before plasma concentrations are available, assay of camphor levels does not contribute to the management of camphor poisoning.

Management

Supportive care, the mainstay of treatment for any intoxication, is generally sufficient for most camphor poisonings. Appropriate attention to airway integrity, judicious use of anticonvulsants, and precautions to avoid trauma supersede all other immediate considerations in the actively seizing patient. Because of the potential for rapid onset of lethargy and seizures, emesis induction by syrup of ipecac is contraindicated. Gastric lavage may be considered, but only if the patient comes to medical attention very early in the course of intoxication. Nevertheless, gastric lavage may pose a threat to the airway in the obtunded or actively convulsing patient while accomplishing little to remove the rapidly absorbed camphor from the gut. Cutaneous exposures merit prompt removal of contaminated clothing and washing of affected skin and mucous membranes, whereas removal to fresh air suffices for inhalational exposures. Activated charcoal is currently recommended as a sorbent to prevent camphor absorption from the gut, but its efficacy has been questioned. Though they do not offer data to support their claim, Holt and Holz listed camphor in a discussion of substances demonstrated to be moderately adsorbed *in vitro* to charcoal.[88] More recently, an *in vivo* study failed to show statistically significant differences in mean serum camphor concentrations and area-under-the-absorption curves in rats who received activated charcoal with camphor versus control rats who received camphor alone. A limitation of the study, as the authors concede, was that activated charcoal was administered in a charcoal-to-toxin ratio of only 2:1 instead of the conventionally recommended ratio of 10:1. The authors cite camphor's molecular weight, nonpolar nature, and high lipid solubility as characteristics that lend a rationale for its adsorption to activated charcoal.[89]

Due to the relative undesirability of gastric emptying interventions, and the lukewarm support for the efficacy of activated charcoal, a number of extracorporeal methods for postabsorptive removal of camphor have been explored. Hemodialysis using a soybean oil dialysate was performed in a 56-year-old camphor-intoxicated woman.[79] The patient recovered, and the authors noted an increasingly noticeable odor of camphor in the dialysate coil compartment during the 4-hour procedure. A 37-year-old man underwent hemoperfusion with Amberlite resin, another hydrophobic compound, and hemodialysis with vegetable oil.[85] Post-hemoperfusion sampling (Amberlite) revealed complete extraction, whereas post-hemodialysis sampling (vegetable oil) yielded about 60% extraction. The patient clinically improved within 2.5 hours of therapy and recovered within 1 day. In a second report of Amberlite hemoperfusion, seizures ceased in a 53-year-old woman during therapy, but there was no perceptible improvement of coma grade.[86] Furthermore, the investigators demonstrated that while Amberlite hemoperfusion produced nearly complete clearance of camphor (89% to 95%) following ingestion of 200 mg of camphor by a volunteer, only a total of 35 mg was ultimately removed by the procedure, most likely as a consequence of camphor's large volume of distribution (estimated at 2 to 4 L/kg). Mascie-Taylor and associates investigated charcoal hemoperfusion and lipid hemodialysis in a 60-year-old woman who had accidentally ingested camphor. Again, although the charcoal column produced nearly complete clearance of camphor from the blood, less than 1% of the total estimated ingested dose was removed. While the efficacy of the lipid dialysis could not be assessed due to the previous high clearance by the charcoal column, the procedure itself was limited in this case by a small degree of hemolysis.[87]

Although many factors contribute to the ultimate decision regarding disposition of patients following camphor intoxication, it is probably safe to discharge to home the patient who has accidentally ingested a small amount and has been observed for several hours with mild or no gastrointestinal symptoms. Any patient who has been poisoned with intent to do self-harm or with greater than minimal symptoms should be admitted to the hospital for observation and treatment.

References

1. Computerized clinical information. Denver, Micromedex, Inc., 1974–1988,.
2. Mofenson HC, Greensher J, DiTomasso A, et al: Baby powder—a hazard. Pediatrics *68*:265, 1981.
3. Cosmetic talc powder (editorial). Lancet *1*:1348, 1977.
4. Wehner AP: Biological effects of cosmetic talc. Food Chem Toxicol *32*:1173, 1994.
5. Harlow BL, Cramer DW, Bell DA, et al: Perineal exposure to talc and ovarian cancer risk. Obstet Gynecol *80*:19, 1992.
6. Rohl AN, Langer AM, Selikoff IJ, et al: Consumer talcums and powders: Mineral and chemical characterization. J Toxicol Environ Health *2*:255, 1976.
7. Gamble JF: A nested case control study of lung cancer among New York talc workers. Int Arch Occup Environ Health *64*:449, 1993.
8. Hartge P, Stewart P: Occupation and ovarian cancer: A case-control study in the Washington D.C. metropolitan area, 1978–1981. J Occup Med *36*:924, 1994.
9. Hughes WT, Kalmer T: Massive talc aspiration: Successful treatment with dexamethasone. AJDC *111*:653, 1966.
10. Molnar JT, Nathenson G, Edberg S: Fatal aspiration of talcum powder by a child: Report of a case. N Engl J Med *266*:36, 1962.
11. Gould SR, Bernardo ED: Respiratory distress after talc inhalation. Br J Dis Chest *66*:230, 1972.
12. Pfenniger J, D'Apuzzo V: Powder aspiration in children: Report of two cases. Arch Dis Child *52*:157, 1977.
13. Brouillette F, Weber, ML: Massive aspiration of talcum powder by an infant. Can Med Assoc J *119*:354, 1978.
14. Motomatsu K, Adachi H, Uno T: Two infant deaths after inhaling baby powder. Chest *75*:448, 1979.
15. Cruthrids TP, Cole FH, Paul RN: Pulmonary talcosis as a result of massive aspiration of baby powder. South Med J *70*:626, 1977.
16. McCormack MA, Lacouture PG, Gaudreault P, et al: Hazards associated with diaper changing. JAMA *248*:2159, 1982.
17. Cotton WH, Davidson PJ: Aspiration of baby powder (letter). N Engl J Med *313*:1662, 1985.
18. Abraham JL, Brambilla C: Particle size for differentiation between inhalation and injection pulmonary talcosis. Environ Res *21*:94, 1980.
19. Jenkins MQ: Dusting powder inhalation. J S C Med Assoc *59*:62, 1963.
20. Reyes de la Rocha S, Brown MA: Normal pulmonary function after baby powder inhalation causing adult respiratory distress syndrome. Pediatr Emerg Care *5*:43, 1989.
21. Pairaudeau PW, Wilson RG, Hall MA, et al: Inhalation of baby powder: An unappreciated hazard. Br Med J *302*:1200, 1991.
22. Gouveau FP, Gonsalves PE, Lebrun E, et al: Aspiracao aguda de talco e outrous pos: Terapeutica per lavagem bronquica. Rev Hosp Clin Fac Med Sao Paulo *21*:49, 1966.
23. Rumack BH: Diapers and poisons (editorial). JAMA *248*:2164, 1982.
24. Moss MH: Dangers from talcum powder (letter). Pediatrics *43*:1058, 1969.
25. Woods WG: An introduction to boron: History, sources, uses, and chemistry. Environ Health Perspect *102S*:5, 1994.
26. Valdes-Dapena MA, Arey JB: Boric acid poisoning: Three fatal cases with pancreatic inclusions and a review of the literature. J Pediatr *61*:531, 1962.
27. Goldbloom RB, Goldbloom A: Boric acid poisoning: Report of four cases and a review of 109 cases from the world literature. J Pediatr *43*:631, 1953.
28. Swate TE, Weed JC: Boric acid treatment of vulvovaginal candidiasis. Obstet Gynecol *43*:893, 1974.
29. Sprague RW: Boron. Metals and Minerals Annual Review, 1992.
30. Wong LC, Heimbach MD, Truscott DR, et al: Boric acid poisoning: Report of 11 cases. Can Med Assoc J *90*:1018, 1964.
31. O'Sullivan K, Taylor M: Chronic boric acid poisoning in infants. Arch Dis Child *58*:737, 1983.
32. Litovitz TL, Klein-Schwartz W, Oderda GM, et al: Clinical manifestations of toxicity in a series of 784 boric acid ingestions. Am J Emerg Med *6*:209, 1988.
33. Fisher RS, Freimuth HC: Blood boron levels in human infants. J Invest Dermatol *50*:85, 1958.
34. Toxicology update: Boron, boric acid, borates, and boron oxide. J Appl Toxicol *12*:149, 1992.
35. Ishii Y, Fujizuka N, Takahashi T, et al: A fatal case of acute boric acid poisoning. Clin Toxicol *31*:345, 1993.
36. Seyffart G: Poison Index: Dialysis and Haemoperfusion in Poisoning. Munich, Fresenius Foundation, ed. 1977.
37. Garabrant DH, Bernstein L, Peters JM, et al: Respiratory and eye irritation from boron oxide and boric acid dusts. J Occup Med *26*:584, 1984.
38. Garabrant DH, Berstein L, Peters JM, et al: Respiratory effects of borax dust. Br J Ind Med *42*:831, 1985.
39. Baliah T, MacLeish H, Drummond KN: Acute boric acid poisoning: Report of an infant successfully treated by peritoneal dialysis. Can Med Assoc J *101*:166, 1969.
40. Skipworth GB, Goldstein N, McBride WP: Boric acid intoxication from "medicated talcum powder." Arch Dermatol *95*:83, 1967.
41. Jordon JW, Crissey JT: Boric acid poisoning: A report of a fatal adult case from cutaneous use: A critical evaluation of the use of this drug in dermatologic practice. Arch Dermatol *75*:720, 1957.
42. Rubenstein AD, Musher DM: Epidemic boric acid poisoning simulating staphylococcal toxic epidermal necrolysis of the newborn infant: Ritter's disease. Pediatr Pharmacol Ther *77*:884, 1970
43. Restuccio A, Mortensen ME, Kelley MT: Fatal ingestion of boric acid in an adult. Am J Emerg Med *10*:545, 1992.
44. Baker MD, Bogema SC: Ingestion of boric acid by infants. Am J Emerg Med *4*:358, 1986.
45. Connelly JP, Crawford JD, Soloway AH: Boric acid poisoning in an infant. N Engl J Med *259*:1123, 1958.
46. American Academy of Pediatrics, Subcommittee on Accidental Poisonings: Statement on hazards of boric acid. Pediatrics *26*:884, 1960.
47. Gordon AS, Prichard JS, Freedman MH: Seizure disorders and anemia associated with chronic borax intoxication. Can Med Assoc J *108*:719, 1973.
48. Stein KM, Odum RB, Justice GR, Martin GC: Toxic alopecia from ingestion of boric acid. Arch Dermatol *108*:95, 1973.
49. Tan TG: Occupational toxic alopecia due to borax. Acta Derm Venereol *50*:55, 1970.
50. Ducey J, Williams DB: Transcutaneous absorption of boric acid. J Pediatr *43*:644, 1953.
51. Friis-Hansen B, Aggerbeck B, Aas Jansen J: Unaffected blood boron levels in newborn infants treated with a boric acid ointment. Food Chem Toxicol *20*:451, 1982.
52. McNally WD, Rust CA: The distribution of boric acid in hu-

man organs in six deaths due to boric acid poisoning. JAMA *90*:382, 1928.
53. Brooke C, Boggs T: Boric acid poisoning: Report of a case and review of the literature. AJDC *82*:465, 1951.
54. Schillinger BM, Berstein M, Goldberg LA, Shalita AR: Boric acid poisoning. J Am Acad Dermatol *7*:667, 1982.
55. Weir RJ, Fisher RS: Toxicologic studies on borax and boric acid. Toxicol Appl Pharmacol *23*:351, 1972.
56. Chapin RE, Ku WW: The reproductive toxicity of boric acid. Environ Health Perspect *1025*:87, 1994.
57. Whorton MD, Haas JL, Trent L, et al: Reproductive effects of sodium borates on male employees: Birth rate assessment. Occup Environ Med *51*:761, 1994.
58. Landauer W: Malformations of chicken embryos produced by boric acid and the probable role of riboflavin in their origin. J Exp Zool *120*:469, 1952.
59. Landauer W: Genetic and environmental factors in the teratogenic effects of boric acid on chicken embryos. Genetics *38*:216, 1953.
60. Roe DA, McCormick DB, Lin R: Effects of riboflavin on boric acid toxicity. J Pharmacol Sci *61*:1081, 1972.
61. Pinto J, Huang YP, McConnell RJ, et al: Increased urinary riboflavin excretion resulting from boric acid ingestion. J Lab Clin Med *92*:126, 1978.
62. Decker WJ, Combs HF, Corby DG: Adsorption of drugs and poisons by activated charcoal. Toxicol Appl Pharmacol *13*:454, 1968.
63. Martin GI: Asymptomatic boric acid intoxication: Value of peritoneal dialysis. NY State J Med *71*:1842, 1971.
64. Smith AG, Margolis G: Camphor poisoning. Am J Pathol *30*:857, 1954.
65. Fink M: Meduna and the origins of convulsive therapy. Am J Psychiatry *141*:1034, 1984.
66. Aronow R, Spigiel RW: Implications of camphor poisoning. Drug Int Clin Pharmacol *10*:631, 1976.
67. Kauffman RE, Banner W, Berlin CM, et al: Camphor revisited: Focus on toxicity. Pediatrics *94*:127, 1994.
68. Litovitz TL, Clark LR, Soloway RA: 1993 Annual report of the American Association of Poison Control Centers Toxic Exposure Surveillance System. Am J Emerg Med *12*:546, 1994.
69. Koppel C, Tenczer J, Scirop T, et al: Camphor poisoning. Arch Toxicol *51*:101, 1982.
70. Trestrail JH, Spartz ME: Camphorated and castor oil confusion and its toxic results. Clin Toxicol *11*:151, 1977.
71. Skoutakis VA, Koumbourlis TC: Camphor intoxication: Diagnosis and management. Clin Toxicol Consultant *3*:131, 1981.
72. Phelan WJ III: Camphor poisoning: Over-the-counter dangers. Pediatrics *57*:428, 1976.
73. Skoglund RR, Ware LL, Schanberger JE: Prolonged seizures due to contact and inhalation exposure to camphor. Clin Pediatr *16*:901, 1977.
74. Seife M, Leon JL: Camphor poisoning following ingestion of nose drops. JAMA *155*:1059, 1954.
75. Riggs J, Hamilton R, Homel S, et al: Camphorated oil intoxication in pregnancy. Obstet Gynecol *25*:255, 1965.
76. Weiss J, Catalano P: Camphorated oil. Pediatrics *52*:713, 1973.
77. Jacobziner H, Raybin HW: Camphor poisoning. Arch Pediatr *79*:28, 1962.
78. Craig JO: Poisoning by the volatile oils in childhood. Arch Dis Child *28*:475, 1953.
79. Antman E, Jacob G, Volpe B, et al: Camphor overdosage. N Y S J Med *78*:896, 1978.
80. Benz RW: Camphorated oil poisoning with no mortality. JAMA *72*:1217, 1919.
81. Gleason MN, Gosselin RE, Hodge HC, Smith RP: Clinical Toxicology of Commercial Products, 3rd ed. Baltimore, Williams & Wilkins, p 56, 1969.
82. Vasey RH, Karayannopoulos SJ: Camphorated oil. Br Med J *8*:112, 1972.
83. Jiminez JF, Brown AL, Arnold WC, Byrne WJ: Chronic camphor ingestion mimicking Reye's syndrome. Gastroenterology *84*:394, 1983.
84. McCollam A, Block R, Lipscomb JW, et al: Chronic camphor ingestion: A case report of granulomatous hepatitis. Vet Hum Toxicol *31*:337, 1989.
85. Kopelman R, Miller S, Kelly R, et al: Camphor intoxication treated by resin hemoperfusion. JAMA *241*:727, 1979.
86. Koppel C, Martens F, Schirop T, et al: Hemoperfusion in acute camphor poisoning. Intensive Care Med *14*:431, 1988.
87. Mascie-Taylor BH, Widdop B, Davison AM: Camphor intoxication treated by charcoal hemoperfusion. Postgrad Med J *57*:725, 1981.
88. Holt LE, Holz PH: The black bottle. J Pediatr *63*:306, 1963.
89. Dean BS, Burdick JD, Geotz CM, et al: In vivo evaluation of the adsorptive capacity of activated charcoal for camphor. Vet Hum Toxicol *34*:297, 1992.

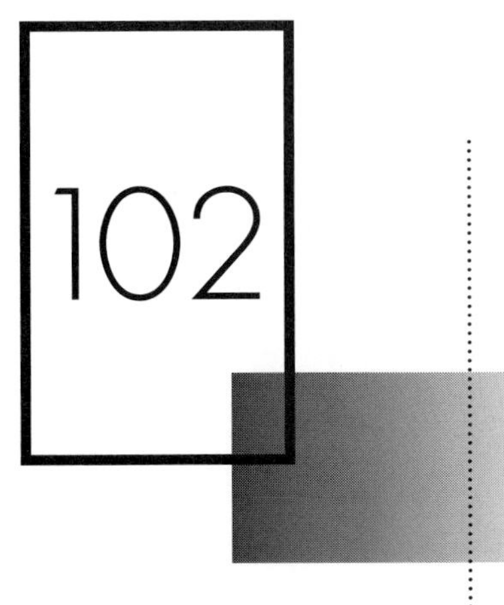

Cosmetics and Toilet Articles

JUDITH K. LUCAS, MD

Human self-decoration is and has always been an integral part of all cultures, spanning both time and geography. Decorations have consisted of beads, feathers, body tattoos, and facial and body paints. Decorative applications may be to skin or hair, they may be permanent or temporary, and they may be purely esthetic or offer health advantages. Regulation of any substance applied to the hair or body for the purpose of altering or enhancing appearance falls under the auspices of the Food and Drug Administration (FDA), specifically the Food, Drug, and Cosmetic Act, USFDCA, which defines *cosmetics* as follows:

"1. Articles intended to be rubbed, poured, sprinkled, or sprayed on, introduced into, or otherwise applied to the human body or any part thereof for cleansing, beautifying, promoting attractiveness, or altering the appearance, and

"2. articles intended for use as a component of any such article; except that such term shall not include soap."[1]

Basic to an agent's classification as a cosmetic is that it not be poisonous when used according to labeling information. In fact, information in this chapter deals with responses to the emergency situation only; unless grossly misused, cosmetics generally present a limited threat to health.

The approach to the adversely exposed patient begins with identifying the ingredients in the cosmetic product. Today, ingredients are listed either directly on the product container or on the cosmetic package. If the chemical is unfamiliar, the agent can be identified in the *CTFA Cosmetic Ingredient Dictionary* (available through the Cosmetic, Toiletry, and Fragrance Association, Inc., 1110 Vermont Ave NW, Washington, DC 20005; 202/331–1770),[2] which provides significant information about each chemical. Unfortunately, no 800 number is available for customer or emergency services at the CTFA; therefore, for gross ingestions or severe exposures, one should refer to the regional poison center.

In addition to regulation by the FDA, cosmetics must also abide by the requirements of the 1970 US Poison Prevention Packaging Act and of the Fair Packaging and Label Act. Under these regulations, cosmetics must be packaged in child-resistant containers and labeling must be accurate to the product.

Colors, shadings, and dyes used in cosmetics are also scrutinized by the FDA. However, some hair color preparations are permitted to use dyes that are *not* on the FDA safety list. Such preparations should be clearly labeled: "*Caution*—this preparation contains ingredients that may cause skin irritation in certain individuals, and a preliminary test according to accompanying directions should first be made. This product must not be used for dyeing eyelashes or eyebrows; to do so may cause blindness." The package must provide the directions for performing a patch test 24 hours prior to application.

The remainder of the chapter provides general information on the basic composition of cosmetic groups, such as hair products, soaps, and facial paints. Toxic exposures may occur via three routes: ingestion, skin exposure, and ocular exposure.

There are two major classes of serious poisonings that may occur with certain cosmetics: alcohol (isopropyl or ethanol) ingestions and ingestions of caustic agents. For detailed management of these poisonings, refer to respective chapters.

HAIR PRODUCTS

Hair Colors

Hair colors are either permanent or semi-permanent. The permanent agents contain oxidizing agents that interact with the dye intermediate to cause the color molecule to fix onto the hair shaft. The most common oxidizing agent is hydrogen peroxide, usually in a 6% by volume solution. Occasionally the concentration of hydrogen peroxide is 12%. Common dye intermediates, used in a 1:1 concentration with the hydrogen peroxide, are paraphenylenediamine, resorcinol, or aminophenols. The remaining ingredients are soaps, largely synthetic detergents, and other components that allow viscosity, spreadability, and penetration.

The major difference between semi-permanent and permanent hair colors is that the semi-permanent hair colors do not contain oxidizing agents. As a result, the chemical reaction does not fix the color onto the hair shaft. Rather, the dye is deposited along the hair cuticle. These agents are used mostly for "touch-ups" to cover gray hair as opposed to lightening or changing natural hair pigment. They are washed out after five or six washings.

Temporary hair colors, or colors whose effects last only a washing or two, are rarely used today, largely because of the profound "rub-off" effect (e.g., on clothing, skin, bed linens), due to the superficial deposit of the color onto the hair shaft.

If ingested, the oxidizing agents (permanent hair colors) can be fairly toxic; however, it is unlikely that one could ingest a quantity sufficient to induce toxicity, as the free ammonia or ethanolamine present in these products is highly emetogenic, and vomiting results before injury can occur.[3] Should ingestion occur, rinsing the mouth with water and drinking milk should alleviate any gastric symptoms. It should be noted that some formulations (Grecian Formula, for example) may contain lead, and ingestion may warrant measurement of blood lead levels.

Skin exposure rarely results in irritation except in the hypersensitive or allergic individual. Should irritation occur, conventional measures, such as washing the area with soap and water and possibly administering antihistamines is all that is necessary.

Thorough and immediate rinsing of the eyes is mandatory in the case of ocular exposure. Injury is generally limited to conjunctival irritation or burning and itching with the 6% hydrogen peroxide–containing products, and there are no long-term adverse effects. However, should the product contain higher concentrations, such as 12% hydrogen peroxide, immediate flushing with saline solution and thorough ocular assessment is required, with possible referral to an ophthalmologist.

Hair Lighteners

Hair lightening agents contain oxidizers in addition to the hydrogen peroxide, such as ammonia, potassium, or sodium persulfate. Other agents are also added to affect thickening, stabilizing, or dispersing. The pH of these solutions usually ranges between 9.5 and 11.5, and they are therefore considered gastrointestinal (GI) irritants.

The foul odor and taste generally prevent significant accidental ingestion. However, intentional ingestion of a large amount can produce clinical toxicity, which is characterized by vomiting, hematemesis, and diarrhea. Management should be as with any highly irritating corrosive ingestion, as detailed in Chapter 62.

Hair Waving Agents

Hair waving involves "softening" the hair by altering its molecular structure, followed by reshaping or curling and then rehardening. The softeners are thioglycolic acid salts, sodium sulfite or ammonium sulfite. Once the agents are applied, the hair is wrapped around curlers and the solution is left in place for a period of time. Continued alteration of the hair structure is halted by the rinsing out of the softening agent and addition of the "neutralizing agent," which generally is a solution of hydrogen peroxide or sodium bromate in a dilute acidic solution.

Waving products that contain thioglycolic acids are moderately toxic because of the corrosive nature of the chemical. If ingested, irritation of the mouth and throat occur, followed by nausea, vomiting, and possibly diarrhea. The mouth should be rinsed thoroughly.

The softeners with ammonium or sodium sulfite are only mildly alkaline, with pH levels ranging from 7.0 to 8.5. Although these agents are nontoxic, water or milk may still have a soothing effect on the irritated gastric mucosa.

The neutralizers contain bromates that are highly toxic. Very concentrated preparations (2% solution) produce serious poisoning in children between ages 1 and 3 years at doses of 1 to 2 tsp (1.5 to 3.0 g). An adult lethal dose is 10 g. GI symptoms begin within 30 minutes of ingestion. The otic and renal systems are most sensitive, and damage may be permanent. Renal failure is the primary cause of death.[4, 5] For detailed management of bromate toxicity, see Chapter 60.

Typically, in sensitive individuals, contact with neutralizers may result in erythema, burning, and edema. Thorough, gentle washing with copious amounts of water is the treatment for excessive contact.

Because of their alkalinity, the hair waving products can be highly irritating to the eyes. Ocular exposure should be treated by immediate irrigation.

Hair Straighteners

Hair straightening products are extremely toxic. These products are caustics, and ingestion or ocular exposure constitute medical emergencies. Hair straighteners are composed of sodium hydroxide at a concentration of 1% to 3%, with a pH of 13. Precise instructions for application must be followed, as accidental contact with skin or eyes, or even prolonged contact with hair and scalp, can produce serious injury. If these products are ingested, immediate attention at an emergency health care facility is required. At this time, there is controversy regarding the benefits versus risks of immediate dilution. The rate of injury to esophageal and gastric mucosa is extremely rapid, rendering questionable the benefit of dilution and raising the risk of vomiting, thus worsening the situation. Likewise, unless a substantial amount of fluid is administered, an exothermic reaction is initiated, resulting in thermal injury that worsens the already serious caustic injury. For specific recommendations on alkaline corrosives (see Chapter 62).

Should prolonged contact with scalp or inadvertent skin contact occur, wash immediately with copious amounts of lukewarm water. Ocular contact with hair straightening agents warrants evaluation at an emergency health care facility with irrigation with saline, monitoring of ocular pH, and examination by an ophthalmologist.

Hair Sprays

Hair sprays are applied to hair after it is combed into place. There are two formulations of hair spray, a liquid pump form and an aerosolized propellant form containing butane, isobutane, or propane.[6] They maintain a hairdo through the application of a resin that, when dry, forms a film on the hair. The resins are numerous and are typically polymers, such as vinyl acetate, methyl vinyl ether, and acrylamides. Toxicity from these chemicals is very rare, as their concentrations are small enough to be insignificant if ingested. The resin, however, is delivered in a solvent; ethyl alcohol is the most common solvent, constituting up to 95% of the product formulation. Should ingestion of a large enough volume occur, management as for ethyl alcohol toxic ingestion should be undertaken.

Skin contact, unless it occurs in a hypersensitive or allergic individual, does not result in untoward effects. If hair spray is inadvertently sprayed into the eyes, flushing with water is generally all that is necessary. If persistent stinging or burning occurs, further evaluation and treatment are warranted.

Shampoos and Conditioners

Shampoos and conditioners are of such tremendous variety that it is impossible to list all of the ingredients. These products are made up of a variety of nonanionic and anionic surfactants, fragrances, artificial coloring agents, and preservatives. They may contain small amounts of ethyl alcohol, but not enough to be considered toxic. These hair care products are nontoxic if ingested, with the most likely manifestation being mild nausea and GI distress. Milk may be given to soothe the stomach upset and to dilute the product. The only adverse skin effects are in persons with a hypersensitivity to the product. A mild, temporary conjunctivitis may result if shampoo or conditioner gets into the eyes. Rinsing the eyes with lukewarm water is the only intervention necessary.

BATH PREPARATIONS

Soaps, Bubble Baths, and Bath Oils

Soaps and bubble baths are similar to shampoos in that they are composed largely of non-anionic and anion surfactants and are essentially nontoxic or mildly toxic if ingested, resulting in mild GI distress. The bath oils are essentially mineral oils and vegetable oils, although occasionally a product may contain an essential oil (e.g., sage, eucalyptus, or pennyroyal). If large enough quantities are ingested, GI distress with nausea, vomiting, and cramping may occur as well as central nervous system (CNS) depression. Chemical lipoid pneumonia results from aspiration of these oils. The remainder of the constituents are emulsifiers, preservatives, and surfactants.

Bath Salts

Bath salts are generally inorganic salts, such as sodium chloride, and are nontoxic; however, if large enough quantities are ingested, electrolyte disturbances may ensue.

COLOGNES, PERFUMES, AND TOILET WATER

The toxicity of colognes, perfumes, and toilet waters depends on the ethanol concentration, which can be as high as 95%. There are no adverse effects from skin contact, except in hypersensitive persons. If these products get into the eyes, they can be irritating; this is best managed by rinsing the eyes. Ingestions should be managed as toxic ethanol ingestions, using the product label and the volume missing from the bottle to determine the dose of ethanol ingested.

FACIAL AND BODY PAINTS

Body Paints and Makeup

Body paints are also largely ethanol-containing products, with small amounts of color additives, emulsifiers, and preservatives. The management of a toxic ingestion of these products is identical to that for colognes, perfumes, and toilet waters.

Lipsticks and facial makeups are virtually nontoxic. The ingredients are, for the most part, waxes, oils, fats, and water. Blushers mostly consist of talcs that have been blended to a semi-solid state with vegetable oils. The risk of aspiration of these talc-containing products is negligible. Besides the innocuous ingredients, the small volume in each package further ensures these products' safety.

Nail Polish

Nail polishes are primarily hydrocarbon solvents, such as xylenes and toluenes, in addition to alcohol solvents, ethanol and methanol. Colors and plasticizers are added. Because of the small bottle volume, the potential injury from ingestion is low, with stomach upset being the primary manifestation of toxicity. Likewise, skin irritation or adverse effects are rare, and thorough rinsing of the eyes is all that is indicated in the case of ocular contact.

Nail Polish Removers

Nail polish removers consist primarily of acetone and/or ethanol. Weight for weight, nail polishes and removers are equally toxic, but the larger-volume bottle of nail polish remover lends itself to a greater potential for toxicity. For management of acetone toxicity, refer to the chapter on toxic alcohols (Chapter 35).

False nails are removed with a highly toxic compound, *acetonitrile.* Acetonitrile is metabolized via the P-450 system to several compounds, one of which is cyanohydrin, which is further metabolized to aldehyde and cyanide. Clinical manifestations of acetonitrile toxicity are identical to those of cyanide but are delayed by anywhere from 3 to 24 hours. Thus, although the patient initially appears stable, serious effects may still occur.[7] Management is the same as for cyanide poisoning (Chapter 71).

POWDERS

Body, dusting, and baby powders are scented talcs, starches, or both, with smaller amounts of various inorganic carbonates, stearates, and fragrances. Their only significant toxicity is inhalational, resulting in severe pneumonitis. Their management is specifically addressed in Chapter 101.

DENTIFRICES

Toothpastes

Toothpastes and gels as well as powders for cleaning teeth are generally nontoxic. They contain varying amounts of abradants, such silica or calcium carbonate, humectants (gels or pastes), flavoring, and coloring. Fluorinated products generally contain stannous fluoride or sodium monofluorophosphate. Both of these are fluoride formulations of low solubility and are therefore considered relatively nontoxic.[8] Should large amounts of any of the dentifrices be ingested, GI discomfort could occur, which can be managed by the administration of milk. Significant fluoride intoxication is unlikely to result from these ingestions.

Denture Cleaners

Likewise, *non–bleach-containing* denture cleaners are considered nontoxic; they contain little more than water, surfactants, polishing agents, and buffering agents, along with flavoring and coloring. The bleach-containing denture cleaners, however, contain potassium persulfate and/or sodium perborate as well as trisodium phosphate and sodium carbonate. Ingestion of these agents is moderately irritating, producing a burning sensation in the mouth and throat, epigastric pain, and vomiting. Of greater concern is the toxicity associated with ingestion of a large volume of sodium perborate–containing denture cleaner. Sodium perborate is broken down into sodium borate and peroxide, resulting in borate poisoning ("boiled lobster" appearance, CNS irritability or lethargy, and acute tubular necrosis). The peroxide may induce severe GI distress with vomiting, diarrhea, and hematochezia. Management is supportive and is directed at symptomatic relief.

Mouthwashes

Mouthwashes are only toxic based on their ethanol concentration, and management appropriate to alcohol toxicity is indicated. Other components of mouthwashes include flavoring, sweeteners, essential oils, preservatives, and, occasionally, astringents. The volume of these components is insignificant and not problematic.

TOILETRIES OF HYGIENE

Soaps

Soaps, whether in bar or liquid form, are invariably anionic and cationic surfactants with vegetable or mineral oils and fragrances; they occasionally contain added antibacterial agents. All of these are nontoxic and at most cause a mild stomach upset if swallowed. Ocular contact, likewise, results in little more than irritation, which responds to rinsing with lukewarm water.

Creams and Lotions

Creams and lotions are similar to soaps in that they are composed of various combinations of water, fats, and waxes in surfactants. Alcohol, if present, is in a concentration less than 10%. The remainder of the ingredients are colors, perfumes, and preservatives. Ingestion of creams and lotions results in similar GI discomfort as from soap ingestion. The consequences of ocular exposure are also limited to minor irritation.

Deodorants

Deodorants mask body odor and are generally considered nontoxic. They contain alcohol, water, and a deodorizing compound (less than 5% concentration by weight). Antiperspirants are similar to deodorizers, but they contain aluminum hydroxychloride, which inhibits eccrine sweat glands. Antiperspirants are also nontoxic if ingested. These products are nonirritating to the skin in most persons, although some persons are sensitive. Ocular exposure requires thorough rinsing. The remaining ingredients, e.g., soaps and skin lotions, are essentially waxes, surfactants, humectants, and preservatives.

Depilatories

Hair removers, or depilatories, are considered moderately toxic because they are caustic agents. Application of these products allows hair removal or hair dissolution by either sodium hydroxide (1% to 10% solution) or calcium hydroxides. They also contain thioglycolates, which are also alkaline and produce injury similar to that produced by sodium hydroxide, although not as severe. The remaining ingredients are not dissimilar from lotions, creams, or soaps. Symptom severity is dependent on the volume ingested; management, likewise is also volume dependent. The reader is referred to Chapter 62 for details of management. Depilatories can also be quite irritating to skin due to their alkaline nature. Should erythema or burning sensation begin, the affected areas should be washed thoroughly with large volumes of lukewarm water. The eyes, if contact occurs, should be flushed with at least a liter of fluid in each eye, and arrangements for immediate follow-up with an ophthalmologist should be made.

SKIN LIGHTENERS

Skin lighteners or spot removers achieve their results through the use of hydroquinones in concentrations of up to 5%. The remaining ingredients, water, glyceryl stearate, glycerin, and fragrance, are inert. If large enough volumes are ingested, the hydroquinones are very toxic, producing dyspnea, cyanosis, GI distress, and convulsions. Gastric decontamination in a health care facility is indicated; supportive care is given as needed. Contact with the eyes can

Table 102–1. Toxic Components of Cosmetics and Toiletries

Toxicity	Toxic Ingredient	Clinical Manifestations
Nontoxic		
Shampoos		
Conditioners		
Soaps		
Bubble bath		
Bath oil		
Body paints		
Lipstick		
Facial makeup		
Nail polish		
Toothpastes/gels		
Body creams and lotions		
Deodorants/antiperspirants		
Fairly toxic		
Hair coloring agents	Oxidizers	GI
Hair lightening agents	Oxidizers/sodium persulfate	GI
Hair spray	Ethyl alcohol	GI/CNS
Bath salts	Sodium chloride	Electrolyte
Powders	Talc/starch	Pulmonary
Moderately or severely toxic		
Hair straightening	Sodium hydroxide	GI (corrosive)
Hair waving (neutralizers)	Thioglycolic salts	GI (irritant)
	Sodium bromate	Otic/renal
Colognes, perfumes, aftershaves	Ethanol	GI/CNS
Nail polish remover	Acetone/ethanol	GI/CNS
False nail remover	Acetonitrile	CV (cyanide)
Bleach-containing denture cleaner	Sodium perborate	Skin/CNS/renal
Mouthwash	Ethanol	GI/CNS
Depilatories	Sodium hydroxide	GI (corrosive)
	Thioglycolic salts	GI (irritant)
Skin lighteners	Hydroquinones	Pulmonary/GI/CNS

GI, gastrointestinal; CNS, central nervous system; CV, cardiovascular.

cause corneal injury and ophthalmologic referral is therefore indicated.

SUMMARY

Table 102–1 divides cosmetics or ingredients into those that are nontoxic or mildly so, fairly toxic, and moderately to severely toxic. Essentially, most are nontoxic unless ingested in very large volumes. The *CTFA Cosmetic Ingredient Dictionary* is the standard compendium for cosmetic ingredients and can describe the physical properties and toxicities for the various chemicals used in toiletries. No detailed management for any specific ingestion has been described in this chapter; rather, the reader is referred to the appropriate chapter for the type of anticipated injury.

References

1. Federal Food, Drug, and Cosmetic Act, current, as amended. Superintendent of Documents, US Government Printing Office, Washington DC, 1990.
2. CTFA Cosmetic Ingredient Dictionary. 2nd ed. The Cosmetic, Toiletry, and Fragrance Association, Washington, DC, 1976.
3. Gosselin RE, Hodge HD, Smith RP, et al: Clinical Toxicology of Commercial Products. 4th ed. Baltimore, Williams & Wilkins, 1976.
4. Hymes LC, Bruner BS, Rauber AP: Bromate poisoning from hair permanent preparations. Pediatrics *76*:975–977, 1985.
5. Quick CA, Chole RA, Mauer SM: Deafness and renal failure due to potassium bromate poisoning. Arch Otolaryngol *101*:494–495, 1975.
6. Sullivan JB, Krieger GR: Hazardous Materials Toxicology: Clinical Principles of Environmental Health (part 5). Baltimore, Williams & Wilkins, 1992.
7. Geller RJ, Ekins BR, Iknoian RC: Cyanide toxicity from acetonitrile-containing false nail remover. Am J Emerg Med *9*:271–272, 1991.
8. Shannon M: Fluoride. Clin Toxicol Rev *8*:91, 1985.

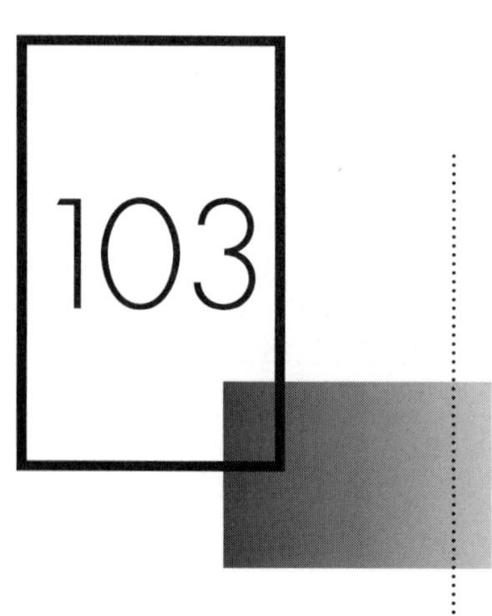

The Volatile Oils

T. J. RITTENBERRY, MD
RICHARD FELDMAN, MD

The volatile oils are a group of complex mixtures of hydrocarbons derived from plant sources that share the characteristic of readily evaporating at room temperature. Also known as *ethereal* or *essential oils*, these compounds generally impart agreeable odors or pleasant tastes at extremely low concentrations when combined with other materials. Since antiquity, such spice extracts have been valued as perfumes, flavorings, and medicaments, making them prominent and influential factors in the commercial intercourse of nations.[1] Today, their medical role is extremely limited; medical interest is almost entirely confined to the treatment of accidental ingestion or topical exposure to these oils.

Renewed interest in herbal medicines and self-treatment as well as the ready availability of a number of concentrated volatile oils from health food stores, mail-order establishments, and pharmacies has increased the likelihood of a toxic incident. As food additives, use of these oils is regulated by the Food and Drug Administration (FDA) at concentrations limited to less than 300 ppm, making toxicity through ingestion of flavored foodstuffs a trivial risk. However, for herbal or nondrug preparations there is no such regulation, and the threat of serious toxicity exists.[2, 3] The more common volatile oils include chenopodium, clove, cinnamon, pennyroyal, peppermint, lemon grass, eucalyptus, pine, sandalwood, and sassafras oils (Table 103–1).[4]

VOLATILE OILS

Chenopodium Oil

Chenopodium oil, also known as American wormseed oil, is a pale yellow liquid with an unpleasant odor and bitter taste distilled from the American wormseed or Jerusalem oak plant. The weed is common in the southeastern United States. Once a standard part of the physician's armamentarium for the treatment of ascariasis and other intestinal parasitic infestations, chenopodium is now of largely historical interest, having been abandoned in favor of other less toxic anthelmintics. Its principal component is ascaridole, with lesser amounts of cymene, camphor, and limonene.[5] Oil of chenopodium is a strong local irritant, causing inflammation of mucous membranes.[5, 6] Minor toxic reactions following ingestions include nausea, vomiting, abdominal pain, dizziness, headache, and paresthesias, whereas in fatal ingestions, central nervous system (CNS) symptoms such as seizures, paralysis, or coma predominate.[7] Acute ingestions have also been associated with mydriasis, temporary impairment of vision, and postingestion optic atrophy.[8] Salant approximated the fatal oral dose of chenopodium in rabbits at 250 mg/kg, noting that lesser ingestions repeated after 1 or 2 days caused increased toxicity.[9] Autopsy findings in man give evidence for acute cerebral edema, enteritis, nephritis, and hepatitis as well as interstitial pulmonary edema.[5, 10]

Pennyroyal Oil

Pennyroyal oil or tea (made from the leaves of the immature *Mentha pulegium* or *Hedeoma pulegioides* plant) have been used since the days of the Roman Empire as a stimulus for menses and as an abortifacient. Its actions are believed by herbalists to involve irritation of the uterus and bladder, triggering contractions.[11] Ingestion of as little as 3.5 mL in an adult has been associated with protracted emesis, abdominal pain, erythematous rash, delirium, and seizures.[12–15] Sullivan and associates reported one fatality from the ingestion of 1 oz of pennyroyal oil.[15] The patient, an 18-year-old woman who was attempting to abort a suspected pregnancy, presented with generalized rash and persistent emesis, which was positive for blood. Her steadily downward course over the next 7 days was significant for metabolic acidosis, disseminated intravascular coagulation (DIC), hepatocellular dysfunction with markedly elevated liver enzyme levels, pneumonia, and subsequent renal failure. Postmortem findings demonstrated congestion and consolidation of the lung parenchyma as well as massive centrilobular hepatic necrosis. Vallance[16] reported a similar case in which a 24-year-old woman presented with fever and generalized rash after ingesting an unknown amount of pennyroyal oil. Nausea, vomiting, abdominal pain, and diarrhea progressed to anuric renal failure, spontaneous abortion of an approximately 12-week pregnancy, hemolysis, and pneumonia over a 10-day course. Necropsy revealed renal tubular degeneration with pigmented casts consistent with acute hemolysis and "transfusion kidney," cerebral edema, and consolidated pulmonary parenchyma. Acute hepatic and pulmonary necrosis has been caused in mice at doses of 400 mg/kg, with the major constituent of pennyroyal oil, R(+)-pulegone, being primarily responsible.[17] There is suggestive evidence that pulegone may cause tissue necrosis via a toxic intermediate in a fashion similar to acetaminophen.

Peppermint Oil

Peppermint oil has long been used medically as a carminative, augmenting relaxation of gastrointestinal smooth muscle both *in vivo* and *in vitro.* More recently it has been helpful in controlling spasm and hypermotility in the large colon.[18] Doses of 0.2 mL

Table 103–1. The Volatile Oils

Oil	Plant Source	Principal Component	Plant Part
Chamomile	*Anthemias flores*	Tiglic oil	Flowers
Chenopodium	*Chenopodium ambrosioides* (American wormseed)	Ascaridole	Plant tops
Cinnamon	*Cinnamonum loureirii* or *zeylanieum*	Cinnamon aldehyde	Bark, leaves
Clove	*Eugenia carophyllus*	Eugenol	Flower buds
Eucalyptus	*Eucalyptus dives* or *radiata*	Eucalyptol	Leaves
Juniper	*Juniperus communis*	Pinene	Fruit
Lemon grass		Citral	Leaves
Pennyroyal	*Mentha pulegium* *Hedeoma pulegioides*	Pulegone	Leaves
Peppermint	*Mentha piperita*	Menthol	Leaves
Sandalwood	*Santalum album*	Santalol	Leaves
Sassafras	*Sassafras albidum*	Safrole	Root

have provided some improvement in symptoms of irritable bowel syndrome, and enteric-coated preparations of peppermint oil (Mintec and Colepermin), which are available in the United Kingdom, have been used to this end.[19, 20] The toxicity of peppermint oil is generally considered to be minimal, yet its two major constituents (up to 90% menthol and up to 30% menthone) have been implicated in toxic reactions. Menthol is a ubiquitous constituent of over-the-counter medications, toothpastes, mouthwashes, shaving creams, and analgesic balms as well as foods and candies. It has been found to cause hypersensitivity reactions when used topically, causing hot flashes, dermatitis, and urticaria.[21] Menthol has also been implicated in the development of chemical pneumonitis in an infant after exposure to a medicated aerosol, and in jaundice in neonates with glucose-6-phosphate dehydrogenase (G6PD) deficiency treated with menthol-containing powders.[22, 23] The menthone component of peppermint oil is considered a strong topical irritant. Parys reported a case of chemical burn secondary to peppermint oil exposure proceeding to frank skin necrosis, which was ascribed to the menthone component.[24] Oral exposure to peppermint oil has caused acute allergic reactions in the mouth with massive edema of oral and pharyngeal tissues.[25] Large ingestions of peppermint oil have resulted in the development of cataracts in rabbits, whereas topical exposure has caused temporary corneal clouding. Accidental rubbing of the eyes with menthol or peppermint oil in humans, however, has caused only a transient burning sensation.[8] The oral median lethal dose (LD_{50}) of menthol at 48 hours in rats was found to be approximately 2.5 g/kg, consistently producing CNS symptoms of seizures, ataxia, limb paralysis, and respiratory depression.[26] Subchronic toxicity occurred in rats given much smaller daily doses of 40 mg/kg to 100 mg/kg over a 3-month period, resulting in cystic white matter lesions of the cerebellum and chronic progressive nephropathy with hyaline deposition in the proximal renal tubules.[27]

Eucalyptus Oil

Eucalyptus oil is a clear to pale yellow liquid with a distinctive camphoraceous aroma and pungent, cooling taste. Since first described by John White, an Australian physician, in 1790, it has been used as a traditional remedy for a variety of common ailments, particularly of the respiratory tract. It is among the most toxic of the volatile oils. The predominant constituent is 8-cineole, or eucalyptol, which constitutes up to 70% of the oil. Hydrocyanic acid (prussic acid) is present in lesser amounts but may be the constituent most responsible for the oil's specific toxicologic profile.[28] The safe oral adult dosage is quoted as 0.06 to 0.2 mL.[29] There is no recommended pediatric oral dose.

A review of 31 fatalities due to eucalyptus oil ingestion from the British and Australian literature by Gurr notes that burning of the oral mucosa, abdominal pain, and vomiting are common early findings. Pulmonary involvement includes acute bronchospasm, bronchorrhea, tachypnea, and the development of chemical pneumonitis.[30] Dizziness, slurred speech, giddiness, ataxia, headache, and drowsiness are common neurologic symptoms. Serious ingestion may rapidly progress to coma with loss of deep tendon reflexes and respiratory depression.[30–32] Seizures have occurred in children but have not been common in adults.[29] Death in adults has followed ingestion of as little as 4 mL.[34] Convalescing patients may have the odor of eucalyptus on their breath for days, and work by Boyd and Pearson suggests that the respiratory excretion of eucalyptol may be responsible for pulmonary irritation.[35]

Clove Oil

Clove oil contains eugenol, a phenolic compound, in concentrations up to 92%, with lesser amounts of caryophillin and vanillin. It is ubiquitous as a flavoring and fragrance added to candies, medications, toothpastes, and soaps. It is often applied to the gingiva as a traditional treatment for odontalgia. The principal compound, eugenol, is an effective disinfectant and a rapid-acting anodyne, making it useful in dentistry for root canal procedures as well as in the treatment of hyperemic and inflamed pulp.[36] Topical exposure to clove oil causes irritation to the skin and oral mucosa. Prolonged contact with eugenol in dental packs has caused inflammation and frank necrosis.[37, 38] As with many of the other volatile oils, clove oil is capable of eliciting allergic reactions when mucosal or skin surfaces have been previously sensitized. It has been responsible for cases of contact dermatitis and stomatitis.[39, 40] The initial stinging and irritation after topical exposure may progress to permanent local anesthesia and anhidrosis if contact is prolonged.[41] This is supported by Kozam, whose studies with eugenol on frog sciatic nerve indicate a direct, progressive, dose-related neurotoxic effect.[42] Clove oil splashed into the eye may cause acute pain, blepharospasm, lacrimation, and conjunctival edema, with loss of corneal epithelium.[43] When injected into the cornea, an acute inflammatory reaction with hypopyon of the anterior chamber results.[8]

Reported cases of clove oil ingestion in humans have been infrequent; therefore toxic effects can only be inferred from animal studies. Dogs given oral doses of 0.25 g/kg of eugenol demonstrated vomiting, weakness, lethargy, and ataxia.[44] At 0.5 g/kg, eugenol is capable of causing coma and death within 24 hours. The LD_{50} of eugenol in rats has been determined to be 1.8 mL/kg (1.93 g), with postmortem findings being consistent with sudden cardiovascular collapse.

Clove cigarettes (approximately 40% dried clove and 60% tobacco) may also cause toxicity. They are imported from Indonesia and are readily available throughout the United States. Nausea, vomiting, dyspnea, bronchospasm, pulmonary edema, hemoptysis, and epistaxis have been reported and may be due to the direct effects of eugenol or as a result of eugenol-induced anesthesia of the mucous membranes, allowing more vigorous inhalation of the tobacco constituent.[45, 46] When instilled directly into the trachea of rats, eugenol causes interstitial hemorrhage, acute emphysema, and acute pulmonary edema.[46] Moreover, the low LD_{50} of 11 mg/kg in these rats emphasizes the potential toxicity of clove oil if aspirated during ingestion or gastric removal.

Cinnamon Oil

Cinnamon oil is also readily available in food stores and pharmacies and is commonly used as a flavoring agent and as a carminative. Through the years it has also found use as a germicide, a mild astringent, and as a treatment for colic.[47] Cinnamon oil is predominantly composed of cinnamic aldehyde (60% to 80%) with lesser amounts of other volatile components, including eugenol. Cinnamon aldehyde is oxidized *in vivo* to cinnamic acid and excreted renally as benzoic and hippuric acids.[48] Most cases of cinnamon oil toxicity have been related to hypersensitivity reactions or to direct irritation from contact to skin or mucous membranes. In addition to allergic contact dermatitis and stomatitis, perioral leukoderma due to exposure to cinnamon-flavored toothpastes has been reported.[49, 50] Prolonged topical exposure has been noted to cause a chemical burn.[45] Cinnamon oil has been used by herbalists as a carminative and an antidiarrheal in adults at doses of 0.06 to 0.2 mL, whereas larger doses have been associated with gastrointestinal irritation. Cases involving severe toxicity or death from ingestion have been rarely published, yet similarities to the other volatile oils, as well as limited experience in animal models, suggest that 5 to 10 mL taken orally may be capable of inducing seizures, respiratory depression, and altered mentation.[52, 53] A case of cinnamon oil toxicity in a 7-year-old child who ingested 2.5 mL/kg on a dare has been reported, which resulted in diplopia, lightheadedness, lethargy, nausea, vomiting, diarrhea, abdominal cramping, and rectal burning, which resolved after 5 hours when treated with diluent, ipecac, and activated charcoal.[54] There have also been recent reports of cinnamon oil abuse by adolescents seeking the sudden onset of the sensations associated with rapid heartbeat, facial flushing, lightheadedness, or shortness of breath. Dipping hard candy, fingers, or toothpicks in the oil, which are then sucked, is the common method of delivery. Thirty-two cases of such abuse were reported by the Pittsburgh Poison Center, which noted facial erythema, abdominal pain, and oral burning from oral ingestion, erythema and blistering from dermal exposure, and immediate burning on accidental ocular exposure in their review. No serious toxic effects resulted from any of the exposures.[48]

Lemon Grass Oil

The predominant constituent of lemon grass oil is citral, a diolefinic aldehyde, which may constitute up to 80% of the oil. It is often used in fragrances, cosmetics, and flavorings as well as in disinfectants and pet repellents. As with several of the other volatile oils, it, too, may be a primary irritant or sensitizing agent, giving rise to contact dermatitis with topical exposure.[55, 56] In animal studies using rabbits and monkeys, vascular endothelial damage has been caused with single oral doses as small as 5 μg/kg.[57] Humans seem less sensitive to citral. Two grams of orange peel contains approximately 50 μg of citral, yet such toxic effects have not been reported in humans who have ingested orange peel.

Sassafras Oil

Oil of sassafras was once used as a treatment for pediculosis capitis, as an abortifacient, and as a flavoring and fragrance. Containing 80% safrole with small amounts of pinene and camphor, its use dropped dramatically in 1960 when the FDA prohibited its use in foods, citing evidence that safrole was a proven carcinogen in rats and mice. Today, its availability is limited to products in health food stores, such as sassafras tea or small quantities of the oil. The acute toxicity profile of sassafras oil is similar to that of eucalyptus oil. Craig reviewed five cases of sassafras oil ingestion in young children, which rapidly caused vomiting, vertigo, aphasia, stupor, and shock. An adult male died after taking 1 tsp of the oil.[32] Chronic use of sassafras teas, with as much as 200 mg/kg of safrole available in one tea bag,[58, 59] may increase the risk for hepatocarcinoma.

TREATMENT OF POISONING

Clinical experience with volatile oil poisoning is extremely limited. Treatment is therefore *symptomatic* and *supportive*. Owing to their common irritant and allergenic sensitizing qualities, skin and eye exposures should be handled with rapid removal and copious irrigation. Following eye exposure, a complete ophthalmologic examination with appropriate referral is necessary, especially with oil of cloves. Ingestion of seemingly small amounts of oils should be aggressively treated with rapid gastric removal of the substance. Because of the danger of aspiration pneumonitis and the altered mental status often seen with the volatile oils, emesis with ipecac is potentially hazardous. A case of a 60-mL ingestion of cinnamon oil in a child previously mentioned was, however, successfully treated with diluent and ipecac with no adverse outcome.[54] Finally, ingestion of these oils must be considered, at least in theory, to be similar to hydrocarbon ingestion (eugenol has a viscosity similar to that of turpentine), and their possible aspiration with emesis or gastric lavage may cause pneumonitis.[60] Prudent care would probably dictate protection of the airway with endotracheal intubation when gastric removal is performed. Dialysis has been used in one case in which ethanol and eucalyptus oil were coingested, with dubious improvement.[30] Presently, dialysis is only indicated in the presence of progressing renal failure. Although no clear evidence exists that any chemotherapeutic agent may act as an antidote in volatile oil ingestion, further investigation may be fruitful. Work to date suggests that the toxicity of lemon grass and pennyroyal oils may be mechanistically similar to the hepatotoxicity of acetaminophen.[15] Pretreating mice prior to pennyroyal challenge with diethyl maleate has been noted to decrease hepatic gluthathione levels by 30%, with an associated increase in hepatic injury.[17] That the toxic effects of citral can be reversed in animals by administration of antioxidant sulfhydryl compounds such as cysteine supports this assumption.[57]

References

1. Gildemeister E: The Volatile Oils. 2nd ed. Vol 1 and 2. New York, John Wiley & Sons, 1913.
2. Lewin NA, Howland MA, Goldfrank LR, et al: Herbal preparations, *In* Toxicologic Emergencies. 3rd ed. Norwalk, CT, Appleton-Century-Crofts, p 560, 1986.
3. Doull J (ed): Casarett and Doull's Toxicology: The Basic Science of Poisons. 2nd ed. New York, Macmillan, p 600, 1980.
4. Morton JF: Major Medicinal Plants. Springfield, IL, Charles C Thomas, pp 359–381, 1977.
5. Gayton WL: Poisoning due to oil of chenopodium. JAMA *132*:330, 1946.
6. Salant W, Nelson ER: The toxicity of oil of chenopodium. Am J Physiol *36*:440, 1915.
7. Birnberg TL, Steinberg CL: Case of oil of chenopodium poisoning: Treatment with forced perivascular (spinal) drainage. Arch Pediatr *56*:304, 1939.
8. Grant WM: Toxicology of the Eye. 3rd ed. Springfield, IL, Charles C. Thomas, pp 199, 576, 1986.
9. Salant W: The pharmacology of the oil of chenopodium. JAMA *69*:2016, 1917.
10. Ingham SD, Courville CB: Diffuse cerebral changes in poisoning with oil of chenopodium. Bull L A Neurol Soc *1*:152, 1936.
11. Gunby P: Plant known for centuries still causes problems today. JAMA *241*:2246, 1979.
12. Early DF: Pennyroyal poisoning: A rare case of epilepsy. Lancet *2*:580, 1961.
13. Holland GW: A case of poisoning from pennyroyal. Va Med Semimonthly *7*:319, 1902.
14. Kimball HW: Poisoning by pennyroyal. Atlanta Med Weekly *9*:397, 1898.
15. Sullivan JB, Rumack BH, Thomas H, et al: Pennyroyal poisoning and hepatotoxicity. JAMA *242*:2873, 1979.
16. Vallance WB: Pennyroyal poisoning: A fatal case. Lancet *2*:850, 1955.
17. Gordon WB, Forte AJ, McMurtry RJ, et al: Hepatotoxicity and pulmonary toxicity of pennyroyal oil and its constituent terpenes in the mouse. Toxicol Appl Pharmacol *65*:413, 1982.
18. Nolen HW, Friend DR: Menthol-β-D-glucuronide: A potential prodrug for treatment of irritable bowel. Pharm Res *11*:1707, 1994.
19. Rees WDE: Treating irritable bowel syndrome with peppermint oil. Br Med J *2*:835, 1979.
20. Friedman G: Treatment of irritable syndrome. Gastroenterol Clin North Am *20*:325, 1991.
21. Papa CM, Shelly WB: Menthol hypersensitivity. JAMA *189*:546, 1964.
22. Krueger RP: Chemical pneumonitis from medicated vapor aerosol spraying. Clin Pediatr *6*:465, 1967.
23. Olowe SA, Ransome-Kuti O: The risk of jaundice in glucose-6-phosphate dehydrogenase deficient babies exposed to menthol. Acta Pediatr Scand *69*:341, 1980.
24. Parys BT: Chemical burns resulting from contact with peppermint oil mar: A case report. Burns *9*:374, 1983.
25. Smith ILF: Acute allergic reaction following the use of toothpaste. Br Dent J *125*:304, 1968.
26. Eickholt TH, Box RH: Toxicities of peppermint and *Pyncnanthemun albescens* oils, Fam. Labiateae. J Pharm Sci *547*:1071 1965.
27. Spindler P, Madison C: Subchronic toxicity study of peppermint oil in rats. Toxicol Lett *62*:21, 1992.
28. Whitman BW, Ghazizadeh H: Eucalpytus oil: Therapeutic and toxic aspects of pharmacology in humans and animals. J Paediatr Child Health *30*:190, 1994.
29. Martindale W: The Extra Pharmacopoeia. 27th ed. London, Pharmaceutical Press, 1977.
30. Gurr FW: Eucalyptus oil poisoning treated by dialysis and mannitol infusion. Aust Ann Med *4*:238, 1965.
31. Foggie WE: Eucalyptus oil poisoning. Br Med J *1*:359, 1911.
32. Craig JO: Poisoning by the volatile oils in childhood. Arch Dis Child *28*:475, 1953.
33. Patel S, Wiggins J: Eucalyptus oil poisoning. Arch Child Dis *55*:405, 1980.
34. MacPherson J: The toxicology of eucalyptus oil. Med J Aust *1*:313, 1925.
35. Boyd EM, Pearson GL: On the expectorant action of volatile oils. Am J Med Sci *211*:602, 1946.
36. Gurney B: Eugenol utility versus toxicity. Oral Hygiene *55*:74, 1965.
37. Waerhaug J, Loe H: Tissue reaction to gingivectomy pack. Surgery *10*:923, 1957.
38. Guglani LM, Allen F: Connective tissue reaction to implants and periodontal packs. J Peridontol *36*:279, 1965.
39. Sternberg L: Contact dermatitis: Cases caused by oil of cloves and by oil of camomile tea. J Allergy *8*:185, 1937.
40. Silvers SH: Stomatitis and dermatitis venenate with purpura resulting from oil of cloves and oil of cassia. Dent Items Interest *61*:649, 1939.
41. Isaacs G: Permanent local anaesthesia and anhidrosis after clove oil spillage. Lancet *1*:882, 1983.
42. Kozam G: The effect of eugenol on nerve transmission. Oral Surg *44*:799, 1977.
43. Libby GF: Ocular injury from oil of cloves. Ophthalmic Rec *21*:189, 1912.
44. Lauber FU, Hollander F: Toxicity of the mucigogue, eugenol, administered by stomach tube to dogs. Gastroenterology *15*:481, 1950.
45. Centers for Disease Control: Illnesses possibly associated with smoking clove cigarettes. MMWR *34*:297, 1985.
46. LaVoie EJ, Adams JD, Reinhardt J, et al: Toxicity studies on clove cigarette smoke and constituents of clove: Determination of the LD50 of eugenol by intratracheal instillation in rats and hamsters. Arch Toxicol *59*:78, 1986.
47. Hoover J: Remington's Pharmaceutical Sciences. Easton, PA, Mack Publishing Co., 1975, p 1229.
48. Perry P, Dean B, Krenzelok E: Cinnamon oil abuse by adolescents. Vet Hum Toxicol *32*:162, 1990.
49. Drake TE, Maibach HI: Allergic contact dermatitis and stomatitis caused by a cinnamic aldehyde-flavored toothpaste. Arch Dermatol *112*:202, 1976.
50. Mathias CGT, Maibach MI, Conant MA: Perioral leukoderma simulating vitiligo from use of a toothpaste containing cinnamic aldehyde. Arch Dermatol *116*:1172, 1980.
51. Sparks TS: Cinnamon oil burn. West J Med *142*:835, 1985.
52. Osal A: The Dispensatory of the United States of America. 25th ed. Philadelphia, J.B. Lippincott, 1955.
53. Rumack BH: Poisindex. Denver, Micromedex, Inc., 1989.
54. Pilapil V: Toxic manifestations of cinnamon oil ingestion in a child. Clin Pediatr *28*:276, 1989.
55. Rothenborg HW, Menné T, Sjolin KE: Temperature dependent

primary irritant dermatitis from lemon perfume. Contact Dermatitis *3*:37, 1977.
56. Mendelsohn HV: Lemon grass oil: A primary irritant and sensitizing agent. Arch Dermatol Syph *53*:94, 1946.
57. Leach EH, Lloyd JPF: Citral poisoning. Proc Nutr Soc *15*:15, 1956.
58. Segelman AB, Segelman FB, Karlinger J, et al: Sassafras and herb tea: Potential health hazards. JAMA *236*:477, 1976.
59. Hagan EC, Jenner PM, Jones WI, et al: Toxic properties of compounds related to safrole. Toxicol Appl Pharmacol 7:18, 1965.
60. Weast RC (ed): CRC Handbook of Chemistry and Physics. 68th ed. Boca Raton, FL, CRC Press, Inc., 1987.

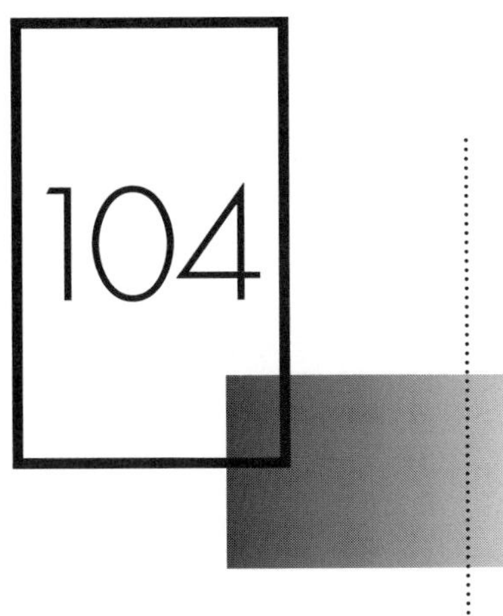

Cyanoacrylates

ANDREW R. DONATO, MD

Cyanoacrylates undergo rapid and spontaneous polymerization to cured resins and have excellent adhesive properties. The ability of these compounds to bind a whole range of materials almost instantly has made them very popular for both commercial and home use. The focus of this chapter is the treatment of patients with both accidental and occupational exposure to cyanoacrylates, because these groups include the vast majority of patients seeking medical care in relation to these compounds.

SOURCES

Cyanoacrylates were first synthesized by Ardis in 1949.[1] This original work involved a thermal polymerization, and it was not until the early 1950s that scientists at Eastman Kodak discovered the rapid room temperature cure and excellent adhesion of these materials, essentially by accident.[2] The unique properties of these substances have led to their widespread use in industry, as well as a smaller yet significant use in the medical field.[1, 3–5] Today, some of the main manufacturers and their trademarks include Loctite (Duro SuperGlue, SuperGonder), Toagosei (Krazy Glue, Aron Alpha), National Starch (Permabond), Three Bond (Super Three), and Henkel (Sicomet).

The standard monomer for a cyanoacrylate adhesive is ethyl 2-cyanoacrylate, which readily undergoes anionic polymerization when brought into contact with any weakly basic surface. The presence of adsorbed surface moisture is adequate to initiate the curing reaction. The resultant polymers are hard, clear thermoplastic resins with high tensile strength and excellent adhesion to a wide variety of surfaces. Apparently, few materials do not bond to some extent with the cyanoacrylate adhesives.[6]

CLINICAL PRESENTATION

Dermal

Cyanoacrylate adhesives form an almost instantaneous bond when applied to the skin. Adherent body surfaces should be treated by flushing the affected area with warm water. This serves to weaken and release the bond gradually because these substances do not possess good heat resistance and begin losing their bond strength at about 70°C.[6] Although the tensile strength of the cyanoacrylates across adherent planes is high, the peel or rolling strength is poor.[7] Therefore, the recommended management after irrigation is to peel gently or roll the surfaces apart using a blunt object. In the event that these measures are unsuccessful, manufacturers recommend soaking the affected area in acetone for several minutes, followed by repeat attempts at separation. A nonsurgical approach to these patients should be emphasized to avoid unnecessary iatrogenic complications. Similarly, previously recommended solvents such as nitromethane, xylene, methylene chloride, and toluene, which are toxic and irritate the skin, should be avoided in lieu of safer alternatives mentioned earlier.[7]

Adhesive cured on the skin without bonding to an opposing surface and residual solidified adhesive after separation of bonded skin can be conservatively approached by soaking in warm water. Dry glue in contact with a skin surface separates over a period of 1 to 2 days as desquamation occurs.[8]

In rare cases, a thermal burn may result from these substances as they cure. Highly exothermic polymerization can result from direct addition of catalytic substances such as water, alcohols, and bases (amines, ammonia, or caustics) or from contamination with any of the commercially available surface activator solutions. Thermal injuries should be managed as any other thermal burns.[2]

Oral

Inadvertent bonding of the lips can be managed in much the same way as dermal exposure. Irrigate the area with applied moisture externally and with saliva internally. Apply a gentle peeling/rolling force to separate.

Ingested cyanoacrylate becomes adherent to the oral or buccal mucosa. The material generally separates in 1 to 2 days. Patients should be made aware of this fact to minimize the risk of aspiration when separation does occur. Although no specific reports in the literature document ingested cyanoacrylate polymers, these materials are generally accepted to be nontoxic. Oral doses of 6400 mg/kg failed to produce lethal toxicity in laboratory rats.[2] Also, no reports in the literature describe airway compromise secondary to accidental cyanoacrylate exposure.

Ophthalmic

Inadvertent instillation of cyanoacrylate into the eye generally results in adherence of the lids, either with or without involvement of the conjunctival and corneal surfaces. Conservative management in such cases is vital. The involved area should be copiously irrigated with warm water. Forced separation of the lids should never be attempted, because damage to the lid margins may result. After irrigation, the eye should be patched and these patients referred to an ophthalmologist who will monitor them for spontaneous separation of the lids, which should occur in 1 to 4 days. Mineral oil may be applied judiciously to the glue surface to help weaken the bond. Acetone should be avoided in these cases to prevent excessive drying of the corneal epithelium.[9]

Cyanoacrylates adhere rapidly to the protein substance of the cornea and conjunctiva, resulting in significant lacrimation and double vision. Direct irritation induced by the rough glue surface can generate sufficient trauma to the ocular surface to produce a mechanical keratoconjunctivitis leading to epithelial breakdown and infectious keratitis. Abrasions of the corneal and conjunctival epithelium are common as solid flakes of polymerized adhesive are released into the conjunctival sac.[5] Temporary binding of cyanoacrylate to the cornea and conjunctiva spontaneously resolves in several hours. Examination of the eye at that time may reveal areas of fluorescein dye uptake, indicating an abrasion. Management should include local application of ophthalmic antibiotic drops with subsequent patching of the eye. A cycloplegic may be used in cases associated with significant discomfort.[7]

Occupational

Several case reports in the literature describe adverse dermatologic and respiratory effects from prolonged contact with cyanoacrylates. Allergic contact dermatitis had been considered to be very unlikely in response to these adhesives, mainly because of their immediate bonding to surface keratin, which means that molecules do not reach immunocompetent cells deeper in the skin. Despite this mechanism, several reports document occupational allergic contact dermatitis from cyanoacrylates, as confirmed by patch testing.[10–12] Treatment with topical or oral corticosteroids has been shown to be of therapeutic benefit in these patients, as has avoidance of the specific allergen.

Exposure to cyanoacrylate in poorly ventilated work areas has been reported to cause symptoms of ocular and bronchial irritation. In addition, asthma and rhinitis have been associated with prolonged exposure to cyanoacrylates. Although the exact mechanism of this association is not known, evidence suggests that immunologic sensitization is an important etiologic factor.[13, 14] Standard asthma therapeutics are used in such cases, along with avoidance as described earlier.

References

1. Ronis ML, Harwick JD, Funy R, Dellavecchia M: Review of cyanoacrylate tissue glues with emphasis on their otorhinolaryngological applications. Laryngoscope *94*:210–213, 1984.
2. Kroschwitz JI: Encyclopedia of Chemical Technology. 4th ed. New York, John Wiley & Sons, pp 344–351, 455, 1991.
3. John LC, Awad WI, Anderson DI: Retrograde pulmonary embolectomy by flushing of the pulmonary veins. Ann Thorac Surg *60*:1404–1406, 1995.
4. Sheta SM, Hida T, McCuen BW: Cyanoacrylate tissue adhesive in the management of recurrent retinal detachment caused by macular hole. Am J Ophthalmol *109*:28–32, 1990.
5. Cavanaugh TB, Gottsch JD: Infectious keratitis and cyanoacrylate adhesive. Am J Ophthamol *111*:466–472, 1991.
6. Sherst I: Handbook of Adhesives. 2nd ed. New York, Van Nostrand Reinhold Co., pp 569–578, 1977.

7. Maitra AK: Management of complications of cyanoacrylate adhesives. Br J Clin Pract *38*:284–286, 1984.
8. Wight RG, Bull PD: Clinical records "Superglue ear." J Laryngol Otol *101*:706–707, 1987.
9. Dean BS, Krenzelok EP: Cyanoacrylates and corneal abrasion. J Toxicol Clin Toxicol *27*:169, 1989.
10. Bruze M, Bjorkner B, Lepoittevin JP: Occupational allergic contact dermatitis from ethyl cyanoacrylate. Contact Dermatitis *32*:156–159, 1995.
11. Fitzgerald DA, Bhaggoe R, English JS: Contact sensitivity to cyanoacrylate nail adhesive with dermatitis at remote sites. Contact Dermatitis *32*:175–176, 1995.
12. Jacobs MC, Rycroft RJ: Allergic contact dermatitis from cyanoacrylate. Contact Dermatitis *33*:71, 1995.
13. Chan CC, Cheong TH, Lee HS, et al: Case of occupational asthma due to glue containing cyanoacrylate. Ann Acad Med Singapore *23*:731–733, 1994.
14. Kopp SK, McKay RT, Miller DR, et al: Asthma and rhinitis due to ethylcyanoacrylate instant glue. Ann Intern Med *102*:613–615, 1985.

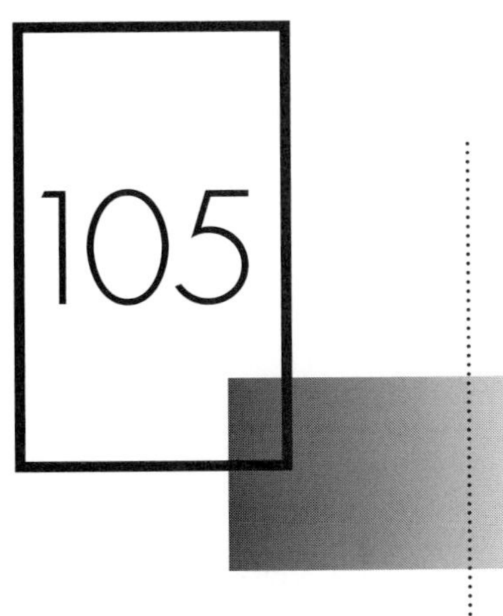

Muscle Relaxants

MICHAEL W. SHANNON, MD, MPH

The skeletal muscle relaxants are a relatively heterogeneous group of drugs, which makes them difficult to describe in general terms. Instead, their disparate origins make them responsible for a wide range of toxic reactions when ingested and requires their description as distinct drugs.

What muscle relaxants have in common is an ability to reduce skeletal muscle tension. This effect may occur at the level of the central nervous system (CNS), the spinal cord, or directly within the muscle. Having this effect, they are generally prescribed to two types of patients: (1) those with a chronic disease associated with muscle spasm (e.g., multiple sclerosis or cerebral palsy) and (2) those with acute post-traumatic muscle spasm (e.g., torticollis or low back pain). The efficacy of many of these drugs in muscle relaxation can be strongly questioned; indeed, many of these agents are relatively useless in conditions of muscle spasm, offering little more benefit that local heat, anti-inflammatory drugs, and massage therapy. It is also recognized that many skeletal muscle relaxants have significant abuse potential.[1, 2]

One of the most common classes of skeletal muscle relaxants, the benzodiazepines, is discussed in Chapter 44. Outside of the benzodiazepine class, there are 10 skeletal muscle relaxants of clinical and toxicologic importance: baclofen, carisoprodol, cyclobenzaprine, chlorzoxazone, chlormezanone, dantrolene, methocarbamol (and related chlorphenesin), metaxalone, and orphenadrine. The indications for these drugs and their major toxic effects are summarized in Table 105–1.

BACLOFEN

Baclofen (Lioresal) is unique among skeletal muscle relaxants in many respects. Chemically, baclofen is para-chlorophenyl-γ-aminobutyric acid; it differs from γ-aminobutyric acid (GABA) only by an additional phenylchloride group. Baclofen is also closely related to an increasingly popular street drug, γ-hydroxybutyrate (GHB). Because GABA is an inhibitory neuron, baclofen is thought to act as a GABA agonist at the spinal cord level; the relative absence of CNS effects after baclofen use in therapeutic doses supports this isolated mechanism of action. Because of its potent effects at the spinal cord level and its relatively poor penetration across the blood-brain barrier, baclofen is also unique in being occasionally administered as an intrathecal drug.

Table 105–1. Summary of Muscle Relaxants and Their Toxicities

Generic Name	Trade Name	Chronic Exposure	Acute Toxicity
Baclofen	Lioresal	Neuropsychiatric disturbances, urinary retention, GI upset, physical dependence	Coma, seizures, hypothermia, apnea
Carisoprodol	Soma	Sedation, abdominal upset, orthostatic hypotension, allergic reactions, physical dependence	Coma, hypotension, seizures, shock, nystagmus
Chlorphenesin	Maolate	Sedation, confusion, headache, allergic reactions	Sedation
Chlorzoxazone	Parafon Forte	Sedation, amnesia, paresthesias, allergic reactions, abdominal pain, hepatotoxicity	CNS depression, abdominal pain, hypotonia, areflexia, hypotension
Cyclobenzaprine	Flexeril	Anticholinergic syndrome, orthostatic hypotension, headache, syncope	Coma, tachycardia
Chlormezanone	Trancopal	Sedation, hypersensitivity reaction, hepatotoxicity, physical dependence	Sedation, hypotension, cyclic coma, hepatotoxicity
Dantrolene	Dantrium	Hepatic injury (dose-dependent and idiosyncratic), sedation, confusion	Hypotonia, sedation
Metaxalone	Skelaxin	Syncope, neurobehavioral changes, hypersensitivity reactions	Sedation, GI upset, hepatotoxicity, nephrotoxicity
Methocarbamol	Robaxin	Syncope, neurobehavioral changes, abdominal upset, hypotension, hypersensitivity reactions	Sedation, rarely seizures
Orphenadrine	Norflex	Anticholinergic syndrome	CNS excitation or coma, seizures, wide-complex arrhythmias, apnea

The pharmacokinetics of baclofen include rapid and complete absorption, although absorption decreases as dose is increased.[3] Its volume of distribution is approximately 1.3 L/kg. Therapeutic serum concentrations range from 80 to 395 ng/mL. Baclofen crosses the placenta and, at therapeutic concentrations, has approximately 30% protein binding. Elimination half-life has been reported at 2.5 to 4.0 hours. However, Gerkin and associates performed a kinetic analysis in a woman who ingested 2 g of baclofen, calculating an elimination half-life of 8.6 hours.[4] Although one case report has described a half-life as long as 34.5 hours in a case of overdose, the possibility of continued absorption from the gut and/or drug redistribution were not adequately evaluated.[5] Seventy per cent to 80% of drug is eliminated in the urine unchanged; only an estimated 15% is metabolized in the liver.[3]

Adverse effects associated with the use of baclofen are numerous and include CNS depression, nausea, muscle weakness, and headache. Among those with a history of psychiatric illness, behavioral disturbances (e.g., hallucinations, excitation, depression, confusion, or anxiety) may be unveiled by the use of baclofen. Other CNS toxic effects include insomnia, paresthesias, tremor, dystonia, nystagmus, diplopia, dysarthria, and incoordination. In patients with epilepsy, seizure control can deteriorate. Adverse effects to other organ systems include genitourinary dysfunction (e.g., urinary retention or enuresis, bladder spasm, sexual dysfunction), cardiovascular symptoms (e.g., hypotension or hypertension, palpitations, bradycardia, flushing, diaphoresis), gastrointestinal (GI) disturbances (e.g., constipation, vomiting, dry mouth, abdominal pain, diarrhea, fecal incontinence), and dermatologic problems (e.g., rash, pruritus). Chronic use of baclofen can result in physical dependence. Once dependence occurs, abrupt withdrawal of the drug can lead to profound dysautonomia, auditory and visual hallucinations, piloerection, paranoia, or seizures.

Acute overdoses of baclofen can produce life-threatening toxicity. Death has been associated with ingestion of 2 g or more. In fatal cases, victims have died of apnea or intractable arrhythmias. Ingestion of 1 g of baclofen may result in areflexia, vomiting, hypotonia, salivation, coma, respiratory depression, and seizures. Coma may occur after ingestion of as little as 100 mg.[6] Respiratory failure results from the combined effect of diminished CNS respiratory drive and weakness of the diaphragm. The mechanism of seizures is unclear; however, they are potentially explained by the greater affinity of baclofen for the GABA-β site, which is a presynaptic inhibitory receptor that, when stimulated, would cause diminished GABA release from the presynaptic neuron. Seizures may not appear for as long as 12 hours after ingestion.[6] Persistent CNS symptoms in baclofen overdose, long after return of serum levels to the normal level, are explained by the drug's delayed clearance from the CNS.[4, 7] Hypotonia can continue for several days after an overdose, also explained by the drug's slow elimination from the CNS.[3]

Other toxic effects associated with acute baclofen overdose include cardiac rate disturbances (either tachycardia or bradycardia),[8] blood pressure changes (hypotension or hypertension), pupillary changes (either mydriasis or miosis), and hypersalivation.

On Feb 28, 1997, in a bizarre mass exposure, 14 adolescents ingested large amounts of baclofen (as much as 600 mg) during a party. All developed weakness, nausea, vomiting, and lethargy. Ten children developed respiratory failure necessitating intubation and ventilatory support. The onset of symptoms was delayed as long as 2 hours after ingestion and was heralded by sudden onset of coma, hypotonia, and respiratory depression. Other toxic manifestations were seizures, areflexia, premature ventricular beats, hypothermia, hypertension requiring nifedipine therapy, and hypotension. All were extubated 24 to 48 hours postingestion; there were no obvious sequelae. Serum baclofen concentrations were as high as 6000 ng/mL and did not correlate with clinical symptoms (Shannon M: Unpublished data, 1997).

Treatment of acute baclofen overdose requires attention to airway, breathing, and circulation. Victims of severe baclofen intoxication are at high risk for respiratory failure; emergency intubation and assisted ventilation may be necessary. Cardiac disturbances are uncommon but, if present, should be treated with standard supportive measures. Seizures should be treated with benzodiazepines. A theoretical argument against the use of flumazenil is that it may be proconvulsant when combined with a potential GABA antagonist, such as baclofen. The coma of baclofen overdose has been reversed by the administration of physostigmine.[9] However, with its known inherent toxic effects (cardiac and CNS), physostigmine should be used cautiously, if ever. Atropine has been shown to be beneficial in the treatment of baclofen-associated hypotension and bradycardia.[10] Gastrointestinal decontamination should be performed by administration of activated charcoal. No role has been established for repeated doses of oral charcoal. Because a large fraction of baclofen is excreted in the urine unchanged, a brisk diuresis may facilitate its elimination.

With aggressive supportive care, the general outcome of baclofen overdose is one of survival without sequelae. Both serum and urine baclofen levels can be measured, but they are of little to no importance in guiding clinical management.

CARISOPRODOL

Carisoprodol is a popular muscle relaxant sold under the trade name Soma. Carisoprodol-containing medication may include aspirin (Soma compound) or aspirin and codeine (Soma compound with codeine). Each tablet contains 200 or 350 mg of carisoprodol.

Carisoprodol is structurally related to the sedative-hypnotic meprobamate. Like meprobamate, it is a potent CNS depressant. As with other muscle relaxants, evidence of a direct effect on skeletal muscle is lacking, and the drug's action can be attributed to a sedative effect (although in animal models carisoprodol can depress polysynaptic spinal reflexes). Unlike baclofen, carisoprodol is ineffective for diseases of muscle spasticity (e.g., cerebral palsy).

Carisoprodol is quickly absorbed after ingestion, with the onset of its actions appearing within 30 minutes. Its volume of distribution is approximately 1 L/kg. Therapeutic serum levels are 4 to 7 mg/L.[11] Carisoprodol crosses the placenta and is distributed into breast milk. Its distribution into breast milk is high (carisoprodol concentrations in milk are 2 to 4 times higher than those in plasma).[12] The drug is metabolized in the liver, having an elimination half-life of approximately 8 hours. Meprobamate is the major metabolite of carisoprodol; within 6 hours of ingestion, 92% of carisoprodol is measured as meprobamate[12]; very little carisoprodol is excreted in urine unchanged. Chronic ingestion of carisoprodol induces hepatic microsomal activity. Like meprobamate, carisoprodol can produce tolerance, dependence, and with- drawal (manifested by nausea, abdominal cramps, dysautonomia, and headache). Carisoprodol has significant abuse potential; victims are referred to as "Soma addicts."[13, 14]

Adverse effects associated with the use of carisoprodol include drowsiness, agitation, irritability, and other neurobehavioral disturbances. GI effects include stomach upset with nausea and vomiting. Cardiovascular effects, such as orthostatic hypotension and facial flushing, may occur. The excipient sodium metabisulfite is often used in carisoprodol medications and may lead to severe allergic-type reactions or anaphylaxis in susceptible individuals.[11] Carisoprodol may precipitate symptomatic acute intermittent porphyria.

Overdose of carisoprodol produces a clinical picture similar to that seen with meprobamate overdose (Chapter 43). Coma, seizures, hypotension, and shock can appear abruptly and lead to death.[12] Nystagmus is another prominent feature of acute intoxication. Coma can be long-lasting (up to 2 days). Fatalities have occurred after ingestions of as little as 1 g; ingestions as large as 14.7 g have been associated with survival.

Treatment of carisoprodol intoxication includes cardiorespiratory support and GI decontamination. Severe respiratory depression and/or hypotension should be anticipated. After careful assessment of airway, breathing, and circulation, gastrointestinal decontamination should be performed by administration of activated charcoal. Neither hemodialysis nor peritoneal dialysis has a proven role in enhancing carisoprodol elimination. However, because meprobamate is effectively removed by hemoperfusion, this procedure should be effective as an adjunct to supportive care. Supportive care is adequate treatment in the vast majority of circumstances. Carisoprodol withdrawal is treated with comfort measures or with reinitiation of drug followed by a controlled taper.

CHLORZOXAZONE

Chlorzoxazone is popularly sold under the trade name Parafon Forte. Although its mechanism of action is not clearly established, this drug also seems to act as a CNS depressant. Chlorzoxazone has rapid GI absorption after ingestion, a relatively small volume of distribution (<1 L/kg), and an elimination half-life of approximately 1 hour.[15] Chlorzoxazone metabolites are excreted in the urine; there is little renal elimination of unchanged drug.

In therapeutic doses, chlorzoxazone leads to a number of important adverse effects. In addition to expected CNS effects of sedation and lightheadedness, paresthesias and amnesia may occur. Dermatologic effects include urticaria and other hypersensitivity reactions. GI effects include anorexia, nausea, vomiting, and abdominal pain. However, the most important adverse effect associated with chlorzoxazone is hepatotoxicity. This idiopathic effect is associated with increases in levels of transaminases and bilirubin. Onset of hepatotoxicity is variable, occurring within 1 month or, occasionally, after more than 5 months of use. Histopathologically, variable types of hepatic injury are seen, the most common being centrilobular necrosis.[15] Hepatic injury is usually reversible; however, fatal hepatotoxicity has been reported.[15] Fulminant hepatic necrosis is idiosyncratic and may be related to formation of a toxic metabolite.

Chlorzoxazone overdose is associated with CNS depression, GI upset, and hypotonia. The degree of muscle relaxation can be profound, resulting in flaccidity, areflexia, and respiratory failure. Hypotonia may occur with maintenance of a relatively intact sensorium. Cardiac toxic effects are rare and are generally confined to hypotension.

Treatment consists of supportive care and GI decontamination. There are no established means of elimination enhancement.

CYCLOBENZAPRINE

Cyclobenzaprine (Flexeril) is a central muscle relaxant that is structurally related to the tricyclic antidepressant amitriptyline. Direct muscle actions have not been identified in humans.[16]

After ingestion, cyclobenzaprine is slowly but completely absorbed; peak concentrations may not be achieved for 4 to 6 hours after ingestion. Volume of distribution is approximately 6 L/kg; plasma protein binding is 90% to 95%. The drug undergoes extensive hepatic biotransformation with the creation of metabolites that may be pharmacologically active. Cyclobenzaprine and its metabolites undergo enterohepatic cycling.[16] Elimination half-life is substantially longer than that of other muscle relaxants (1 to 3 days).

General adverse effects of cyclobenzaprine are those that would be expected of a drug with anticholinergic properties (e.g., drowsiness, blurred vision, dry mouth, and urinary retention).[17, 18] Severe headache is another common adverse effect.[17] Cardiovascular effects include sinus tachycardia, hypotension, and palpitations. Severe orthostatic hypotension can result in lightheadedness or frank syncope.

Cyclobenzaprine overdose produces a picture resembling that of a mild tricyclic antidepressant overdose.[19] Severe ingestions may produce CNS depression (including coma) and tachycardia.[20] These manifestations may not appear for as long as 12 hours after ingestion. However, in contradistinction to tricyclic antidepressant overdose, seizures and cardiac conduction disturbances are uncommon with cyclobenzaprine overdose, and fatalities after cyclobenzaprine overdose are extremely rare. The absence of classic tricyclic antidepressant toxicity has been attributed to the relatively low doses of cyclobenzaprine ingested (as it is provided in 10 mg tablets, the drug is rarely ingested in quantities greater than 250 to 500 mg) or to a low degree of potency.

Cyclobenzaprine use (or overdose) produces a positive urine or serum assay for amitriptyline.[21]

Treatment of cyclobenzaprine intoxication begins with the provision of general supportive measures. The need for airway protection and blood pressure support should be anticipated. An electrocardiogram should be obtained in all patients. In the rare event that conduction disturbances appear (e.g., widening of the QRS interval), sodium bicarbonate should be administered. It is unknown whether conduction disturbances after cyclobenzaprine ingestion carry the same prognosis as that after tricyclic antidepressant overdose. Although it is theoretically efficacious because it can reverse anticholinergic manifestations, physostigmine has no proven benefit when used for cyclobenzaprine overdose[20]; its use is not recommended. Because cyclobenzaprine absorption may be delayed after overdose, GI decontamination should be performed in all patients, even those who present many hours after a cyclobenzaprine overdose. Activated charcoal with a cathartic should be administered. There is no established role for repeated dosing of activated charcoal, although it may be beneficial.

CHLORMEZANONE

Chlormezanone (Trancopal) is a muscle relaxant with central actions. Like carisoprodol, it is structurally related to meprobamate. It is commonly prescribed as adjunctive therapy for acute muscle injuries, acting primarily as an anxiolytic and a sedative.[22] Adverse effects to chlormezanone are primarily neurologic. However, severe hypersensitivity reactions (e.g., erythema multiforme, Stevens-Johnson syndrome) have also been reported. Hepatitis or cholestatic jaundice can also result after prolonged use. In an action similar to meprobamate and carisoprodol, abrupt discontinuation of chlormezanone can result in an acute abstinence (withdrawal) syndrome.[22]

Overdoses of chlormezanone produce severe CNS depression and hypotension or shock. There may be an unusual profile of cyclic coma after chlormezanone overdose, resulting either from erratic GI absorption or enterohepatic recycling of active metabolites. Acute hepatic injury has been reported after acute single overdose.[23] Treatment consists of supportive care and administration of activated charcoal.

DANTROLENE

Dantrolene (Dantrium) is unique in having a direct action; the mechanism of its relaxant effects is not neuronal. The agent is a structural analogue of phenytoin and acts by inhibiting the release of calcium by the sarcoplasmic reticulum of skeletal muscle; decreased force of muscle contraction occurs promptly after use of dantrolene. The drug has no effect on cardiac or smooth muscle.[24] Because of its potent muscle-relaxing actions, dantrolene has had utility in the treatment of malignant hyperthermia, neuromuscular malignant syndrome, and monoamine oxidase inhibitor overdose, all of which may be associated with severe muscle hypertonia.

Dantrolene has the following pharmacokinetic profile: GI absorption is poor with only about 35% of an oral dose being absorbed.[24] Peak absorption may not be attained for 4 to 6 hours after ingestion. Metabolism is hepatic, with an elimination half-life of 6 to 8 hours.[24]

Regular use of oral dantrolene is associated with a host of adverse effects. A reversible chemical hepatitis can result in elevations of transaminases and bilirubin. Hepatosplenomegaly may be present. Idiopathic fulminant hepatic necrosis can occur after chronic use.[25, 26] GI upset, nausea, and vomiting usually precede the onset of hepatotoxicity.[24] CNS toxic effects are less common, but visual disturbances, confusion, and hallucinations may occur.

Acute overdoses of dantrolene can be expected to produce severe muscle weakness and, occasionally, CNS depression. Hypotension may also occur. Nonetheless, acute single overdose is associated with a low mortality.[27] Treatment is supportive.

METAXALONE

Metaxalone (Skelaxin) is a centrally acting skeletal muscle relaxant that also bears structural similarities to phenytoin. Adverse effects after overdose include CNS manifestations (e.g., drowsiness, dizziness, headache, confusion, and, rarely, seizures), GI disturbances, hypersensitivity phenomena, and liver function abnormalities, and nephrotoxicity may occur.[28] Treatment consists of supportive care and GI decontamination.

METHOCARBAMOL

Methocarbamol (Robaxin) is structurally related to chlorphenesin. It is rapidly and almost completely absorbed after ingestion.[29] Its onset of action appears within 30 minutes of ingestion. The volume of distribution of methocarbamol is 1 to 2 L/kg; serum elimination half-life is approximately 1 hour. Adverse effects in therapeutic doses include neurobehavioral disturbances, GI upset, hypotension, syncope, and bradycardia. Hypersensitivity phenomena may also occur.[28]

Acute methocarbamol overdose can result in CNS depression and, rarely, seizures. However, there is a near-complete absence of important cardiac disturbances. The drug therefore carries a low risk of life-threatening toxicity. Methocarbamol has been ingested in quantities as large as 50 g without fatality. Treatment of this overdose consists of appropriate supportive care, GI decontamination, and observation.

Chlorphenesin (Maolate) is a muscle relaxant chemically related to methocarbamol. It is also a CNS depressant whose relaxant effects are attributed to sedation. Chlorphenesin has similar pharmacokinetics with rapid absorption after ingestion. Its metabolism is hepatic, with a half-life of 2 to 5 hours.[29]

Adverse effects from chlorphenesin use are primarily CNS and include drowsiness, dizziness, confusion, and headache. GI effects include nausea and abdominal pain. Chlorphenesin preparations may contain tartrazinc, a potent allergen. Therefore, allergic-type reactions may also occur. Overdose of this agent can be expected to result in sedation. Treatment consists of supportive care and GI decontamination.

ORPHENADRINE

Orphenadrine (Norflex) is a unique drug in several respects. Structurally related to diphenhydramine,[30] its muscle-relaxing effects are attributed to CNS actions. Orphenadrine also has analgesic effects that contribute to relief from muscle spasm.

In therapeutic doses, orphenadrine is readily absorbed after ingestion; however, absorption may be delayed in overdose due to anticholinergic effects. Its volume of distribution has not been fully characterized but appears to be large.[30] Protein binding is approximately 20%. Orphenadrine has significant enterohepatic cycling. The drug's elimination half-life is approximately 14 hours. In addition to antimuscarinic and antihistaminic properties, orphenadrine has a direct, quinidine-like action, which can result in significant myocardial depression and conduction disturbances.[31]

Orphenadrine overdose typically presents as a classic antimuscarinic toxidrome, with dry mouth, agitated delirium, blurred vision, urinary retention, mydriasis, and tachycardia. With more severe intoxication, life-threatening symptoms can appear rapidly (within 2 hours of ingestion), consisting of coma, seizures, tachycardia, or cardiac arrest. Death can result from apnea, complications of status epilepticus, or intractable ventricular arrhythmias. Wide-complex tachyarrhythmias are common; torsades de pointes has also been described.[32] Unlike diphenhydramine, orphenadrine generally produces CNS excitation rather than depression; victims often present with agitation, hallucinations, and delirium. Without prompt, aggressive intervention, orphenadrine overdose can be lethal.[33–35] In one series, death after orphenadrine overdose was associated with ingestion of greater than 20 to 25 mg/kg in adults and 70 to 75 mg/kg in children.[31, 36] Other manifestations of severe toxicity include hypoglycemia, hypothermia, disseminated intravascular coagulation, and pulmonary hemorrhage.[31]

Treatment consists of airway and circulatory support followed by GI decontamination. Activated charcoal should be administered as quickly as possible. Physostigmine has been used with success in reversing both central and peripheral manifestations of toxicity after orphenadrine overdose and has been recommended as an effective antidote.[37, 38] However, as with other intoxications in which physostigmine has potential benefits, its hazards will generally outweigh them.

Multiple-dose activated charcoal is recommended for the management of orphenadrine overdose, based on pharmacokinetic data obtained in an overdose patient that demonstrated accelerated drug clearance using this intervention (Shannon M, Linakis J: Unpublished data, 1989). There are no other known means of enhancing the elimination of orphenadrine.

References

1. Elder N: Abuse of skeletal muscle relaxants. Am Fam Physician 44:1223–1227, 1991.
2. Schifano F, Marra R, Magni G: Orphenadrine abuse. South Med J 8:546–547, 1988.
3. American Hospital Formulary Service: Baclofen. *In* McEvoy GK (ed): Drug Information. Bethesda, MD, American Society of Health-System Pharmacists, pp 951–954, 1996.
4. Gerkin R, Curry SC, Vance MV, et al: First-order elimination kinetics following baclofen overdose. Ann Emerg Med 15:843–846, 1986.
5. Ghose K, Holmes K: Complications of baclofen overdosage. Postgrad Med J 56:865–867, 1980.
6. Lee T-H, Chen S-S, Su S-L, Yang S-S: Baclofen intoxication: Report of four cases and review of the literature. Clin Neuropharmacol 15:56–62, 1992.
7. Cook D, Glasstone M: Baclofen poisoning in children. Vet Hum Toxicol 36:448–450, 1994.
8. Nugent S, Katz MD, Little TE: Baclofen overdose with cardiac conduction abnormalities: Case report and review of the literature. Clin Toxicol 24:321–328, 1986.
9. Muller-Schwartz G, Penn R: Physostigmine in the treatment of intrathecal baclofen overdose. J Neurosurg 71:273–275, 1989.
10. Cohen MB, Gailey R, McCoy GC: Atropine in the treatment of baclofen overdose. Am J Emerg Med 4:552–553, 1986.
11. American Hospital Formulary Service: Carisoprodol. *In* McEvoy GK (ed): Drug Information. Bethesda, MD, American Society of Health-Systems Pharmacists, pp 968–971, 1996.
12. Adams H, Kerzee T, Morehead C: Carisoprodol related death in a child. J Forensic Sci 20:200–202, 1975.
13. Good PJ: Soma (carisoprodol): A challenge to a DRE evaluation. The DRE (Drug Recognition Expert) 7:14–15, 1995.
14. Luehr J, Meyerle K, Larson E: Mail order drug dependence. JAMA 263:657, 1990.
15. American Hospital Formulary Service: Chlorzoxazone. *In* McEvoy GK (ed): Drug Information. Bethesda, MD, American Society of Health-Systems Pharmacists, 1996, pp 957–958.
16. American Hospital Formulary Service: Cyclobenzaprine. *In* McEvoy GK (ed): Drug Information. Bethesda, MD, American Society of Health-Systems Pharmacists, pp 958–959, 1996.
17. Azoury F: Double-blind comparison of Parafon Forte and Flexeril in the treatment of acute musculoskeletal disorders. Curr Ther Res 26:189–197, 1979.
18. Nibbelink D, Strickland S: Cyclobenzaprine (Flexeril): Report of postmarketing surveillance program. Curr Ther Res 28:894–903, 1980.
19. O'Riordan W, Gillette P, Calderon J, Stennes RL: Overdose of cyclobenzaprine, a tricyclic muscle relaxant. Ann Emerg Med 15:592–593, 1986.
20. Linden C, Mitchiner J, Lindzon R, Rumack B: Cyclobenzaprine overdose. J Toxicol Clin Toxicol 20:281–288, 1983.
21. Tasset J, Schroeder T, Pesce A: Cyclobenzaprine overdose: The importance of a clinical history in analytical toxicology. J Anal Toxicol 10:258, 1985.
22. American Hospital Formulary Service: Chlormezanone. *In* McEvoy GK (ed): Drug Information. Bethesda, MD, American Society of Health-Systems Pharmacists, 1996, pp 1727–1728.
23. Sheu B-S, Lin C-Y, Chen K-W, Chi C-Hea: Severe hepatocellular damage induced by chlormezanone overdose. Am J Gastroenterol 90:833–835, 1995.
24. American Hospital Formulary Service: Dantrolene sodium. *In* McEvoy GK (ed): Drug Information. Bethesda, MD, American Society of Health-Systems Pharmacists, 1996, pp 959–962.
25. Chan C: Dantrolene sodium and hepatic injury. Neurology 40:1427–1432, 1990.
26. Wilkinson S, Portmann B, Williams R: Hepatitis from dantrolene sodium. Gut 20:33–36, 1979.
27. Robillart A, Bopp P, Vailly B, Dupeyron J: Cardiac failure due to dantrolene overdose. Ann Fr Anesth Reanim 5:617–619, 1986.
28. American Hospital Formulary Service: Metaxalone. *In* McEvoy GK (ed): Drug Information. Bethesda, MD, American Society of Health-Systems Pharmacists, 1996, pp 962–963.
29. American Hospital Formulary Service: Methocarbamol. *In* McEvoy GK (ed): Drug Information. Bethesda, MD, American Society of Health-Systems Pharmacists, 1996, pp 963–964.
30. American Hospital Formulary Service: Orphenadrine citrate. *In* McEvoy GK (ed): Drug Information. Bethesda, MD, American Society of Health-Systems Pharmacists, 1996, pp 965–966.
31. Bozza-Marrubini M, Frigerio A, Ghezze R: Two cases of severe orphenadrine poisoning with atypical features. Acta Pharmacol Toxicol 41(suppl 2):137–152, 1977.
32. Henderson R, Lane S, Henry J: Life-threatening ventricular arrhythmia (torsades de pointes) after haloperidol overdose. Hum Exp Toxicol 10:59–62, 1991.
33. Sangster B, Van Heijst A, Zimmerman A: Intoxication by orphenadrine HCl: Mechanism and therapy. Acta Pharmacol Toxicol 41(suppl 2):129–136, 1977.
34. Robinson A, Holder A, McDowall R: Forensic toxicology of some orphenadrine-related deaths. Forensic Sci 9:53–62, 1977.
35. Millar W: Deaths after overdoses of orphenadrine. Lancet 2:566, 1977.
36. Clarke B, Mair J, Rudolf M: Acute poisoning with orphenadrine. Lancet 1:1386, 1985.
37. Danze L, Langdorf M: Reversal of orphenadrine induced ventricular tachycardia with physostigmine. J Emerg Med 9:453–457, 1991.
38. Snyder B, Kane MK, Plocher D: Orphenadrine overdose treatment with physostigmine. N Engl J Med 295:1435, 1976.

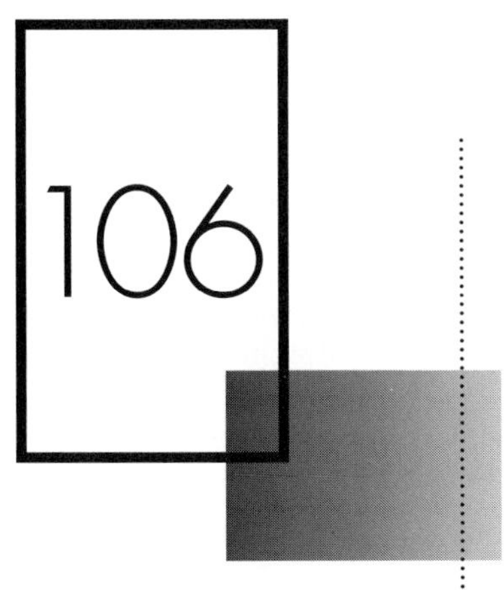

LSD, Natural Hallucinogens, and Miscellany

LESTER M. HADDAD, MD

LSD AND NATURAL HALLUCINOGENS

Man has forever tried to expand the limits of his reality, whether by religious experiences, near-death experiences, or the use of hallucinogens and mind-altering drugs. The history of hallucinogens dates to antiquity and has often been central to tribal religious ceremonies. Hallucinogen abuse first appeared with the emergence of the drug culture in the 1960s and it is experiencing a resurgence,[1] especially in adolescents, on college campuses, at rock concerts, and at "rave" parties.

Hallucinations are psychedelic experiences that exist only within the mind. It is characteristic of drug-induced hallucinations that the user usually remains aware that the experienced visual images are drug-induced. In addition to the hallucinogens, which are taken primarily for their hallucinogenic properties, medical conditions (e.g., hypoglycemia, impending delirium tremens, thyrotoxicosis) and several therapeutic medications (e.g., tricyclic antidepressants, methylphenidate, and carbamazepine) may produce hallucinations.

This chapter discusses LSD and the natural hallucinogens psilocybin, peyote and mescaline, dimethyltryptamine, the morning glory plant, and nutmeg. Δ^9-Tetrahydrocannabinol (THC) is discussed in Chapter 38; phencyclidine is reviewed in Chapter 40; "ecstasy" (MDMA) and "eve" (MDEA)[2] and the psychotomimetic amphetamines are discussed in Chapter 41; the hallucinogenic designer drugs are discussed in Chapter 42; and *Datura stramomium,* the jimson weed, and the anticholinergic agents are discussed in Chapter 46.

LSD

LSD, or D-lysergic acid diethylamide, was discovered by Dr. Albert Hofmann, a Swiss chemist, who was doing research on synthesis of ergot as found in *Claviceps purpurea*. On April 16, 1943, he discovered that the ergot derivative LSD-25 caused an "intense kaleidoscopic play of colors and fantasies." Further experiments by Dr. Hofmann and psychiatrists at the University of Zurich established that as little as 50 to 100 μg could produce a full-scale LSD "trip."

LSD has been intensely studied in the scientific community for possible legitimate use. LSD is a remarkable drug in that it makes cats afraid of mice, causes fish to swim backward, and produces fever in rabbits but hypothermia in pigeons.[3] LSD was experimentally tried by the psychiatric community for treatment of medical conditions and was given to patients to bring to consciousness repressed thoughts and memories, but this practice has obviously fallen into disfavor. Reports[4,5] of chromosomal damage from LSD in the late 1960s received sensational media attention, and the LSD "chromosome scare" dramatically curtailed the casual use of LSD.

Structurally, LSD is an indole derivative and chemically resembles serotonin. It has recently been observed that treatment of LSD psychosis with selective serotonin reuptake inhibitors severely aggravates the patient's condition, and this should be avoided.[6] LSD is a racemic mixture of four stereoisomers: D-LSD, L-LSD, D-iso-LSD, and L-iso-LSD, the only hallucinogen being D-LSD. LSD is colorless, tasteless, odorless, and water soluble, which accounts for its ease of illicit distribution. Street names often reflect the form in which it is marketed. LSD is available as capsules, tablets, powder, or, as is primarily the case today, as drops of solution on blotting paper ("blotter acid").[7] LSD on thin squares of gelatin ("windowpanes") or as purple-colored drops of solution on an aspirin tablet ("purple micro-dots") or a sugar cube are most uncommon. Colorful transferable decals of cartoon characters have been impregnated with LSD, raising the fear that children may inadvertently become exposed to LSD. Case reports of childhood exposure are primarily from inadvertent exposure to the parent's illicit possession of LSD.[8, 9] LSD is well absorbed and has a volume of distribution of 0.27 L/kg, with more than 80% being protein bound. LSD has a half-life of 3 hours; most of the drug accumulates in the bile within 3 hours, with subsequent fecal excretion of the inactive hepatic metabolites.[10]

An LSD "trip" usually begins 15 to 45 minutes after oral ingestion, and its hallucinogenic effect generally lasts 2 to 6 hours, depending on dosage. LSD produces markedly dilated pupils, often resulting in photophobia, but its physiological effects are generally minor, except in overdose. It is of course the psychic effects of LSD that are noteworthy, and feelings of depersonalization, derealization, and loss of body image often ensue. Visual illusions appear with a magnified sense of color. Shape and distance are altered, and time sense is lost. *Synesthesias and "trails" are characteristic of LSD.* Synesthesias are a translation of one sensory modality into another, such as seeing colored vibrations of music, or smelling purple.[10] Trails are formed positive afterimages that remain immediately behind an object as it moves across the subject's visual field.[11]

Adverse reactions to LSD are common. Acutely, LSD can produce a "bad trip." Frightening thoughts overwhelm the user, with a loss of insight that this is a drug experience; the resulting acute panic reaction generally necessitates a visit to the emergency department. Acute mania,[12] schizophrenia,[13] depression, and permanent psychoses have resulted from LSD abuse, particularly in someone of borderline stability. Tolerance occurs, but there is no withdrawal state.

LSD *flashbacks* are another interesting phenomenon, in which the LSD experience is triggered without the use of the drug.[14, 15] The first such case ever treated by this author was of a sailor who experienced a flashback while watching a radar screen at sea; he had not used the drug since he had been home months before. Flashbacks may be perceived as flashes of light; geometric figures that come and go; objects that move in the peripheral field of vision (such as a flowerpot moving across the windowsill); halos around objects; intensification of colors; objects growing large (macropsia) or small (micropsia); images that appear within an image; double exposures of an image; and trails.[11] Persistent palinopsia, or prolonged afterimages, has been described in three patients who have continued to be symptomatic up to 3 years after they ceased to ingest the drug.[15]

Massive overdose of LSD was once described in eight patients who variably experienced coagulopathy (8), coma (5), bleeding (4), hyperthermia (4), and hypertension (3) after inadvertently snorting milligram dosages of pure LSD when intending to abuse cocaine.[16]

Peyote and Mescaline

The legal use of peyote and mescaline in the United States today is limited to Indian tribes in the Native American Church who use the peyote as part of their religious ceremony. Peyote is the common name for the North American cactus *Lophophora williamsii,* found in the deserts of the Southwestern United States and Mexico.[17] Peyote is a spineless cactus, which forms buttons with 7 to 10 ribs. Mescaline is the major active alkaloid of peyote. The cactus contains about 6% mescaline when dried. Peyote buttons are the round fleshy tubercles from the cactus, which maintain their hallucinogenic potency while in storage for later use.

Mescaline, the active phenylethylamine alkaloid, was first isolated from peyote in 1896; the average hallucinogenic dose of synthetic mescaline is 5 mg/kg. One peyote button contains about 40 to 50 mg of mescaline, which explains the tradition of consuming 4 to 12 peyote buttons during each Indian ceremony.[10] Mescaline sold on the street is usually LSD, PCP, or a designer drug.

The clinical effects usually occur approximately one hour following ingestion, and begin with a gastrointestinal phase, predominantly nausea and vomiting, and may be accompanied by diaphoresis, hypertension, mydriasis, and ataxia. This is followed by the psychoactive phase, which generally peaks at 4 to 6 hours and resembles LSD intoxication. This temporal pattern of transition from the gastrointestinal phase to the psychoactive phase is markedly uniform and is characteristic of mescaline intoxication.[10]

Symptoms usually resolve within 12 hours of ingestion. Deaths are rare, and are usually associated with accidents due to the user's altered perception.

Psilocybin

Psilocybe cubensis mushrooms are usually found in moist tropical climates, such as the coasts of Georgia, South Carolina, and the Gulf coast. Other species of *Psilocybe* are found primarily in the Pacific Northwest. *Psilocybe caerulipes* is found on the Northeastern Atlantic coast. *Psilocybe coprophila* is weakly hallucinogenic, and is widely distributed in North America. Some *Panaeolus* and *Gymnopilus* mushrooms also are reported to contain psilocybin or psilocin and are considered to be hallucinogenic, and they are widely distributed in North America (Table 106–1).[17–21]

Psilocybin mushrooms have an ancient history; they have been discovered to be part of a mushroom cult more than 3000 years ago in Central America. The magic mushrooms known as "Teonanacatl" ("flesh of the gods") in Aztec rituals were taken from Mexico and identified as *Psilocybe mexicana* in Europe. The two psychoactive components of the mushrooms are derivatives of dimethyltryptamine, psilocybin, and psilocin.[9, 22] Psilocybin, which is 1.5 times more potent than psilocin, bears a striking resemblance to serotonin.

Psilocybin mushrooms grow overnight in cow pastures after a rainfall. Quite scarce, they are treasured among the young as producing the most vivid colors and images during hallucinosis. One high school student presented to our emergency department one late afternoon, "flying high." He had eaten several mushrooms from the grounds of the local orphanage. He was aware of his condition and said he could control his hallucinations. He then proceeded to point in my direction and exclaimed, "Wow, I'm making you melt to the ground."

Characteristically, the stalks of some psilocybin mushrooms turn blue in handling. Psilocybin is quite stable, and both dried mushrooms and boiled extract retain their potency. Psilocybin mushrooms, although eaten directly, usually are boiled for sanitary reasons, as they usually grow on or near dung. The quantity ingested is variable, as concentrations of psilocybin vary greatly from mushroom to mushroom. Intravenous use has been described in a case report from Phoenix, Arizona.[23] Psilocybin sold on the street is hardly ever psilocybin, but is usually mushrooms adulterated with LSD or other substances. The effects are similar to those of LSD and have an onset of roughly 1 hour; the hallucinatory effects last from 4 to 6 hours. The intoxication is usually self-limiting. Although fever or convulsions have been reported in children,[17, 24] they must be quite rare, as are other complications. Should complications occur, the physician should consider other sources of intoxication or illness (see Chapter 25 and accompanying color plates for more information).

DMT

Dimethyltryptamine (DMT) is known as Yurema in Brazil and is basic to the Brazilian Indian Kariri religion. DMT is prepared as snuff from the seeds, leaves, and pods of *Piptadenia peregrina, Prestonia amazenicum,* and *Mimosa hostilis.* DMT intoxication closely resembles that of LSD, except that its effects last only 30 to 60 minutes.

Morning Glory

Morning glory is the common name for plants of the *Convolvulaceae* family, many of which have been used for their hallucinogenic properties. A garden morning glory is a beautiful funnel-shaped flower with heart-shaped leaves. The seed, which is toxic, was ground into flour by American Indians, then soaked in cold water and strained with a cloth. The filtrate was then consumed during a religious ceremony. Mexican ololiuqui was the derivative of the morning glory *Rivea corymbosa. Ipomoea violaceae* is one of the common morning glory plants sold in garden catalogues in the United States; those with blue flowers are called Heavenly Blue, those with crimson flowers Scarlett O'Hara, and those with white flowers Pearly Gates.[25] The Hawaiian baby woodrose *(Argyreia nervosa)* and Hawaiian woodrose *(Merremia tuberosa)* also have hallucinogenic properties, but these are considerably more potent.

Ingram[26] was one of the first to report a case of morning glory intoxication in a 20-year-old college student who ingested 5 packets (250 seeds) of *Ipomoea violaceae,* and experienced an LSD-type reaction. Indeed, analysis of the alkaloid content of these seeds reveals D-lysergic acid amide, D-isolysergic acid amide, and related compounds.

Table 106–1. Some Hallucinogenic Mushrooms of North America[17–21]

Scientific Name	Common Name (Variable by Region)	Geographic Location
Psilocybe baeocystis	Potent *Psilocybe*	Pacific Northwest
Psilocybe caerulipes	Blue-foot *Psilocybe*	Eastern United States to the Midwest
Psilocybe coprophila		North America
Psilocybe cubensis	Bluestain smoothcap	Georgia, South Carolina, Gulf Coast
Psilocybe cyanescens	Bluing *Psilocybe*	Canada and Pacific Northwest
Psilocybe montana	Mountain moss *Psilocybe*	Western United States and Canada
Psilocybe pelliculosa	Conifer *Psilocybe*	Western United States and Canada
Psilocybe semilanceata	Liberty cap	North America
Psilocybe stuntzii	Blue legs	Pacific Northwest
Gymnopilus spectabilis	Showy flamecap	North America
Panaeolus campanulatus	Bell mottlegill	North America
Panaeolus foenisecii		Eastern North America
Panaeolus subbalteatus	Girdled *Panaeolus*	North America

Table 106–2. Clinical Effects of Hallucinogen Abuse

	LSD-25	MDMA	PCP
Street name	Acid	Ecstasy	Angel dust
Pharmacologic effect	Hallucinogenic	Sympathomimetic	Hallucinogenic
Preparation	Blotter paper	Gelatin capsule	Cigarette
Half-life (hr)	3	7–34	24
Pupils	Dilated	Dilated	Pinpoint, may be dilated
Nystagmus	No	No	Yes
Anesthesia and analgesia	No	No	Yes
Hypertension	No	Yes	Yes
Social behavior	Contemplative or bizarre	Outgoing and energetic	Violent, agitated

Nutmeg

Nutmeg is the dried seed kernel of the fruit of a tall evergreen tree, *Myristica fragrans,* native to the Molucca Islands of the South Pacific and now cultivated on Grenada and Trinidad. Tried unsuccessfully for many medical conditions, nutmeg is found in every home as a spice, particularly at Christmas. The toxic dose of nutmeg is one to three whole nutmegs, or 5 to 15 g of the ground spice. Scattered case reports of ingestion appear in the literature,[27, 28] and symptoms usually appear 3 to 6 hours after ingestion, and may persist up to 60 hours! Patients are miserable and often have a sense of impending doom. They experience nausea, epigastric pain, facial flushing, decreased salivation, and hypothermia (which distinguishes the syndrome from anticholinergic poisoning). Pinpoint pupils may be seen initially, which may also help to distinguish the clinical picture from that of atropine poisoning, which is accompanied by dilated pupils.

MANAGEMENT OF HALLUCINOGEN ABUSE

Emergency management of a hallucinating patient can be a major challenge. The emergency physician must first distinguish whether the patient has truly ingested a hallucinogen, is truly psychotic, or has an organic psychosis from a medical condition, such as hypoglycemia, hyperthermia, impending delirium tremens, or salicylate, anticholinergic, or tricyclic antidepressant poisoning. Thyrotoxicosis may also present in a similar fashion.[29]

A thorough history from friends or family or EMS personnel is most helpful, as is a physical examination. For example, if the patient experienced gastrointestinal symptoms before the onset of hallucinations, the patient may have ingested mescaline. The physical examination and clinical course may offer valuable clues as to the etiologic agent of the acute hallucinosis (Table 106–2). Nystagmus, pinpoint pupils, and sensory anesthesia suggest phencyclidine ingestion. The physical examination is also critical in ruling out signs of trauma and sexual mutilation, as these patients may act out their distorted perceptions. Laboratory studies for blood glucose and serum electrolyte levels, and hematologic and other studies such as thyroid profile and ethanol and salicylate levels, may be indicated in ruling out other medical conditions or toxic effects. An electrocardiogram may be helpful if tricyclic antidepressant overdose is suspected.

In general, if the patient has ingested LSD or one of the plant hallucinogens and is experiencing an acute panic reaction, he or she is best treated in a calm, quiet, and reassuring manner. "Talking the patient down" with compassionate support will suffice in the majority of cases.[10, 29, 30] Gastric lavage is to be avoided, as are restraints or an abusive, judgmental approach. Although activated charcoal is indicated for multiple drug ingestion, it may or may not be necessary. Benzodiazepines such as diazepam provide excellent relief for the patient, who is often in psychic torment. Phenothiazines should be avoided, as should selective serotonin reuptake inhibitors, as these will often aggravate the toxic effects. Physostigmine is indicated *only* if one is sure that the toxic etiology is anticholinergic poisoning. The majority of patients with hallucinosis from LSD and the plant hallucinogens will respond to these supportive measures. Haloperidol may be indicated in the event of prolonged psychosis.

Patients with prolonged coma or hallucinosis, seizures, hypertensive crisis, hyperpyrexia, bleeding, or other diverse complications require admission to an intensive care unit, and further evaluation and treatment may be indicated, as one may be faced with hallucinations from ingestion of phencyclidine or one of the psychotomimetic amphetamines or designer drugs, with all of their attendant complications. Further evaluation and treatment measures are outlined in Chapters 40 through 42.

Once the patient becomes coherent and stable, psychiatric evaluation and follow-up are indicated. Fortunately, one "bad trip" is usually enough to dissuade the casual user from repeating his or her experience.

MISCELLANY

The purpose of this section is to present vignettes on a variety of subjects that the physician may either face or be queried about from time to time.

Aquarium Products

A common phone call to emergency departments and poison control centers concerns home aquarium products. Aquarium products include antimicrobials used to control algae, fungi, bacteria, and parasites; antichlorine products, such as sodium thiosulfate; pH indicators, such as bromothymol blue; and miscellaneous substances, including vitamins, aquarium salts, and copper sulfate.

With the exception of copper sulfate, these products generally are of low toxicity, although some pH test kits do contain sodium hydroxide. Should one be consulted about any of these substances, the physician should inquire about the particular ingredient on the label, in case the product contains any potentially toxic ingredients.

Birth Control Pills (Oral Contraceptives)

Pediatric ingestion of birth control pills is quite common. They generally contain estrogen or progesterone or their derivatives, either in combination or in sequence. Oral contraceptives presently are not considered to be harmful in a single acute ingestion.

Calamine Lotion

Calamine lotion or cream is an 8% solution of calamine and is often used either alone, as calamine lotion, or as Caladryl, which now contains 1% pramoxine (in contrast to the old formulation, which contained diphenhydramine) for the relief of itching caused by poison ivy or oak and insect bites, and for soothing relief of mild sunburn. Calamine itself is a pink powder composed of roughly 99% zinc oxide and 0.5% ferric oxide. Ingestion of large quantities of either calamine lotion or Caladryl has caused gastritis and vomiting. Supportive care may be indicated.

Diet Medications

This group includes fenfluramine (Pondimin), phentermine (Fastin), and dexfenfluramine (Redux). Redux has been available in Great Britain since 1989 but has just been released in the United States in 1996. All are derivatives of amphetamine and are marketed for appetite suppression. All three medications are sympathomimetic amines.

Fenfluramine differs from amphetamine in that it produces more central nervous system depression than stimulation. It is indicated in the management of infantile autism. Phentermine has a long half-life of 19 to 24 hours and is often used in combination with fenfluramine.

Both fenfluramine and dexfenfluramine have been implicated in the etiology of primary pulmonary hypertension.[31–35] In a study from France,[31] 15 of 73 patients (20%) with primary pulmonary hypertension had used fenfluramine or dexfenfluramine and presented with exertional dyspnea. Pulmonary hypertension was confirmed by right heart catheterization. Only 3 of 15 patients improved after withdrawal of the drug; 3 patients died.

Dexfenfluramine was associated with a non Q-wave acute myocardial infarction in a 31-year-old woman,[36] who had taken 15 mg of dexfenfluramine three times daily (instead of the recommended dose of 30 mg daily) for 8 days prior to admission.

Several reports of fenfluramine overdose have been noted in the literature. One fatal case[37] involved a 17-year-old girl who ingested 1600 mg of fenfluramine and presented within 3 hours of ingestion with agitation and sinus tachycardia. She subsequently developed seizures, cardiac arrhythmia, and cardiac arrest, which was unresponsive to resuscitative measures. Hyperthermia has also been noted.

In the event of ingestion of fenfluramine, dexfenfluramine, or phentermine, gastric decontamination, careful monitoring of vital signs, and observation are clearly indicated. Severe hypertension may require management with nitroprusside, although intravenous (IV) nitroglycerin or a β-blocker such as esmolol or labetalol may be sufficient. Hospitalization is necessary in significant cases, particularly in patients who develop hypertension that is severe enough to require therapy, seizures, hyperthermia, or cardiac arrhythmia. Patients with minor ingestions who manifest only sinus tachycardia that resolves after extended observation in the emergency department may be considered for discharge (see Chapter 93 for further discussion of management).

Fertilizers

Fertilizers are plant foods that contain one of more of the three chemical elements necessary for plant growth: nitrogen, phosphorus, and potassium. Most commercial fertilizers bear a series of three numbers indicating the content of these three elements. For example, Southern States Ferty Care 12-4-8 fertilizer contains 12% by weight of total nitrogen, 4% of phosphorus as phosphoric acid (P_2O_5), and 8% of potassium as soluble potash (K_2O). The total nitrogen is further divided into nitrate nitrogen, ammoniacal nitrogen, water-soluble organic nitrogen, and water-insoluble nitrogen. Nitrogen is usually supplied as ammonium nitrate, sodium nitrate, or ammonium sulfate or ammonium phosphate, urea, urea formaldehyde, or sewage sludge. Phosphorus is usually present in the form of animal bone meal, superphosphate, or potassium phosphate. Potassium is usually provided in the form of potash.

Nitrogen is vital to the plant for color and leaf development. Phosphate improves root growth and plant food storage capability, whereas potash is important for growth, improves the hardiness of the plant, and promotes resistance to drought.

Fertilizers generally contain trace elements as micronutrients, including iron as iron oxide, chlorine, zinc as zinc oxide, manganese, magnesium, boron as sodium borate, copper as copper oxide, and molybdenum. Table 106–3 lists some common fertilizers.

Pediatric ingestion of fertilizers that contain *only* the three main elements usually causes no symptoms other than vomiting or diarrhea. It is possible that the nitrate present in these compounds may produce methemoglobinemia, particularly in children younger than 1 year. The first report[38] of methemoglobinemia from contamination of well-water with nitrate fertilizers appeared in 1945; since that time, numerous reports of similar cases have been published, particularly in farm families.[39, 40] The Environmental Protection Agency (EPA) estimates that up to 20% of private wells exceed advisory water nitrogen-nitrate levels.[41, 42] Levels should not exceed 10 ppm for nitrate-nitrogen or 45 ppm for nitrate.[43, 44]

A few fertilizer products may also contain herbicides, insecticides, or other additives that may in themselves be toxic, and which, in the event of exposure, may require specific attention. The explosive potential of fertilizers containing ammonium nitrate was painfully dramatized in the April 19, 1995 Oklahoma City bombing of the U.S. Government Murrah Federal Office Building.

In the event of ingestion, it is important to determine the specific chemical mix of the involved fertilizer, if at all possible. Management of fertilizer ingestion is primarily supportive.

Hydrogen Peroxide

Hydrogen peroxide is commercially available as a 3% solution. It is a popular home antiseptic. Pediatric ingestions are common but are generally of low toxicity, as hydrogen peroxide rapidly decomposes to water and oxygen in the gastrointestinal tract prior to absorption. Since 1 mL of 3% hydrogen peroxide liberates 10 mL of oxygen, ingestion of large quantities of hydrogen peroxide may cause gastric distention. A case has been reported[45] of portal venous gas embolism following ingestion of 3% hydrogen peroxide in a 2-year-old boy who was managed as an outpatient and discharged without sequelae.

Oral ingestion of industrial strength hydrogen peroxide (30% to 40%) has been implicated in four fatalities.[46, 47] Further reports include a patient[46] who suffered seizures, metabolic acidosis, diffuse hemorrhage and edema of the stomach, and respiratory arrest, but survived with aggressive airway and ventilatory management and general supportive care; a case[48] of portal vein gas embolism that necessitated hospitalization, but in which no long-term sequelae were seen; and an 84-year-old man who ingested 35% hydrogen peroxide obtained from a health food store and suffered multiple cerebral infarctions with residual neurologic deficits.[49] Treatment is supportive.

Licorice

Natural licorice is an extract of the root of the plant *Glycyrrhiza glabra,* and contains glycyrrhizic acid, a compound with well-documented mineralocorticoid activity. The syndrome of pseudoprimary hyperaldosteronism is a known complication of excessive licorice ingestion.[50, 51] This syndrome is rarely reported in the United States, because commercial products usually contain artificial licorice flavoring, nor is it observed in the Middle East, where anise (which has a similar flavor but a different chemical structure) is used for flavoring. Patients demonstrate the classic features of exogenous mineralocorticoid excess: sodium retention (hypertension, dyspnea, and peripheral edema) and hypokalemia (lethargy, muscle cramps, paresthesia, and tetany); serum studies confirm depressed serum renin and aldosterone levels. Treatment involves withdrawal of licorice and potassium supplementation, which usually suffices to correct the problem.

Nicotine*

Nicotine was once one of the leading causes of toxic death in the United States. Before World War II

*For this section of the chapter we are indebted to the contributions of Kenneth V. Iserson, M.D., to earlier editions of this book.

Table 106–3. Some Common Fertilizer Products

Trade Name	Total Nitrogen* (%)	Phosphorus as Available Phosphoric Acid (P_2O_5)(%)	Potassium as Potash (K_2O)(%)
Scotts Super Bonus S 30–3–10	30	3	10
MMSD Milorgamite 6–2–0	6	2	0
Pennington Penngreen 14–7–7	14	7	7
True Value Green Thumb 26–3–3	26	3	3
Nitram ammonium nitrate	34	0	0
Ferti-Lome Centipede lawn fertilizer	15	0	15
Ferti-Lome Classic lawn food	16	4	8
Kmart Kgro 10–14–14	10	14	14
Kmart Kgro 5–10–10	5	10	10
Kmart ammonium nitrate	34	0	0

*Total nitrogen is further classified in one or more of the following types: nitrate nitrogen, ammoniacal nitrogen, water-soluble organic nitrogen, and water-insoluble nitrogen. For example, Kmart ammonium nitrate contains 34% total nitrogen, of which 17% is nitrate nitrogen and 17% is ammoniacal nitrogen.

and the development of DDT, nicotine was the most commonly used insecticide and thus accounted for a major number of exposures.

Today, even with the prevalence of the nicotine "patch," the most common cause of nicotine exposures are chewing and swallowing of cigarettes by children.[52] In fact, an unexpected finding in one report[52] of childhood poisoning found that 15% of cases were due to cigarette ingestion. Fortunately, this has not amounted to serious toxicity, as the children generally stop ingestion because of the bad taste; the uncommon child who manages to ingest 2 entire cigarettes may require charcoal and emergency department observation.[53]

Death from nicotine poisoning is rare today, there being only one recent report of cardiac arrest and death from ingestion of concentrated nicotine alkaloid solution.[54] A recent report of nicotine toxicity from the "patch" did not result in fatality.[55]

Nicotine is now most commonly used as tobacco, as a transdermal "patch" for smoking cessation, and as an animal-tranquilizing dart. The use of smokeless tobacco products, such as chewing tobacco, dip, and snuff, has dramatically increased on college campuses. One insecticide that is available on the market still contains nicotine. Table 106–4 lists some common nicotine products.

Common blends of tobacco vary in their nicotine content. The average cigarette contains 15 to 25 mg of nicotine. Cigarette smoke contains less than 3 mg; nonfiltered cigarettes, 1.5 to 2.5 mg; and filtered cigarettes, 0.2 to 1.0 mg. Up to 90% of the nicotine in the smoke is absorbed by the smoker. Nicotine gum contains 2 or 4 mg per piece.

Animal tranquilizing darts contain nicotine sulfate at a concentration of 240 mg/mL. Nicotine transdermal systems ("the nicotine patch") variably contain from 5 to 22 mg of nicotine released over a 16- to 24-hour period.

Nicotine is an alkaloid obtained from the dry leaves and stems of the *Nicotiana* species. These include *N. tabacum* (cultivated tobacco), *N. attenuata* (wild tobacco), *N. glauca* (tree tobacco), and *N. trigonophylla* (desert tobacco). Lobeline, the chief constituent of Indian tobacco, is obtained from the leaves and tops of *Lobelia inflata*.[56]

Nicotine is 1-methyl-2-(3-pyridyl) pyrrolidine. It is a colorless, strongly alkaline, volatile liquid and is responsible for the brown color and classic odor of tobacco. Nicotine is water-soluble and is readily absorbed from the oral mucosa, skin, gastrointestinal tract, and respiratory system. It is primarily metabolized in the liver to cotinine, its major metabolic product.[57] Elimination via the kidney is generally complete in 16 hours; acidification of the urine increases urinary excretion approximately fourfold. Nicotine is also excreted in the milk of breast-feeding mothers and may be a cause of pediatric colic.

Cigarette smoking[58] is the number one cause of preventable death in the United States. Cigarette smoking is a major cause of cancer,[59] heart attacks, cardiovascular disease,[60] lung disease,[61] cardiac arrest, burns, and death by fire. A recent study[62] by the Canadian Coronary Atherosclerosis Intervention Trial documents that smoking accelerates coronary progression and new lesion formation by serial quantitative coronary arteriography. Because this is such an important health issue, the reader is referred to selected treatises on the impact of cigarette smoking, nicotine dependence, and smoking cessation.[63–70]

The risk of "passive smoking," or environmental exposure to tobacco smoke, has just begun to be assessed.[71] Several epidemiologic studies[71–75] indicate that nonsmokers exposed to environmental tobacco smoke show a 20% increase in coronary heart disease, but this association remains controversial.

The physiologic response to nicotine includes stimulation of the central nervous system and cardiovascular systems. Nicotine stimulates the sympathetic ganglia, the adrenal medulla, and the aortic and carotid bodies, producing an increase in heart rate and blood pressure.[76]

Nicotine poisoning occurs by an initial, direct stimulation of the nicotinic receptors of the autonomic ganglia, followed by a subsequent depression of autonomic ganglia.[76] Classic findings of cholinergic excess are initially seen, followed by neuromuscular blockade from persistent membrane depolarization in severe cases. Profuse salivation, vomiting, abdominal pain, and diarrhea often follow significant oral ingestion. Coma, seizures, hypotension, and cardiopulmonary arrest may be seen with severe exposure. The adult lethal dose is estimated to be 60 mg.

A milder form of nicotine toxicity is "green tobacco sickness," a condition that occurs in young, often inexperienced, tobacco workers who handle uncured tobacco when it is wet.[77–79] Symptoms are described as being similar to being "seasick," characterized by nausea, vomiting, dizziness, and fluctuations in vital signs. Twelve of 47 patients in a Kentucky study[78] required hospitalization for up to 48 hours; of these, two required intensive care management for hypotension and bradycardia. As the source of nicotine toxicity is by dermal absorption, this syndrome is generally prevented by using rubber gloves and protective (waterproof) clothing while harvesting tobacco.

Emergency department resuscitation may be necessary for cases of critical nicotine poisoning. Rapid-

Table 106–4. Some Common Nicotine Products

- Black Leaf–40 (40% nicotine)
- Black Leaf–40 garden spray (40% nicotine)
- Cigarettes and cigars
- Smokeless tobacco products
  - Red Man chewing tobacco
  - Kensington snuff
  - Kodiak dip
- Nicorette and Nicorette DS (nicotine 2 and 4 mg)
- Nicotine transdermal systems
  - Habitrol (24-h release) (nicotine 21, 14, and 7 mg)
  - Nicoderm (24-h release) (nicotine 21, 14, and 7 mg)
  - Nicotrol (16-h release) (nicotine 15, 10, and 5 mg)
  - Prostep (24-h release) (nicotine 22 and 11 mg)

sequence intubation[80] may be indicated with an agent such as thiopental to prevent seizures. Treatment of the mild to moderate exposure includes supportive care, the use of activated charcoal for ingestions, or extensive irrigation of the skin for dermal exposures, as nicotine is absorbed through intact skin. Atropine may be indicated for the patient who manifests mild cholinergic symptoms. Seizures are managed with diazepam or barbiturates. Intravenous fluids and supportive care are indicated for patients with "green tobacco sickness."

References

LSD and Natural Hallucinogens

1. Johnston LD, O'Malley PM, Bachman JG: National Survey Results on Drug Use from the Monitoring of the Future Study, 1975–1992. Washington, DC, National Institute of Drug Abuse, 1993.
2. Box SA, Prescott LF, Freestone S: Hyponatraemia at a rave. Postgrad Med J *73*:53–54, 1997.
3. Louria DB: Lysergic acid diethylamide. N Engl J Med *278*:435–438, 1968.
4. Cohen MM, Marinello M, Bark N: Chromosomal damage in human leukocytes induced by lysergic acid diethylamide (LSD-25). Science *155:*1417–1419, 1967.
5. Corey MJ, Andrews JC, McLeod MJ, et al: Chromosome studies on patients (in vivo) and cells (in vitro) treated with LSD-25. N Engl J Med *282:*939–942, 1970.
6. Markel H, Lee A, Holmes RD, et al: LSD flashback syndrome exacerbated by selective serotonin reuptake inhibitor antidepressants in adolescents. J Pediatr *125:*817–819, 1994.
7. Schwartz RH: LSD. Pediatr Clin North Am *42:*403–413, 1995.
8. Ianzito BM, Liskow B, Stewart MA: Reaction to LSD in a two-year-old child. J Pediatr *80:*643–645, 1972.
9. Brown RT, Braden NJ: Hallucinogens. Pediatr Clin North Am *34:*341–347, 1987.
10. Litovitz TL: Hallucinogens. *In* Haddad LM, Winchester JF (eds): Clinical Management of Poisoning and Drug Overdose. Philadelphia, WB Saunders Co., pp 455–466, 1983.
11. Abraham HD: Visual phenomenology of the LSD flashback. Arch Gen Psychiatry *40:*884–889, 1983.
12. Lake CR, Licitra-Stirba A, Kinneman RE, et al: Mania associated with LSD ingestion. Am J Psychiatry *138:*1508–1509, 1982.
13. Roy A: LSD and the onset of schizophrenia. Can J Psychiatry *26:*64–65, 1961.
14. Kaminer Y, Hrecznyj B: Lysergic acid diethylamide-induced chronic visual disturbances in an adolescent. J Nerv Ment Dis *179:*173–174, 1991.
15. Kawasaki A, Purvin V: Persistent palinopsia following ingestion of lysergic acid diethylamide (LSD). Arch Ophthalmol *114:*47–50, 1996.
16. Klock J, Boermer V, Berher C: Coma, hyperthermia and bleeding associated with massive LSD overdose: A report of 8 cases. Clin Toxicol *8:*191–203, 1975.
17. Foster S, Caras R: Peterson Field Guides: Venomous Animals and Poisonous Plants. Boston, Houghton Mifflin Co., pp 116–117, 1994.
18. Lincoff GH: National Audobon Society Field Guide to North American Mushrooms. New York, Knopf, 1995.
19. Pacioni G: Simon and Schuster's Guide to Mushrooms. New York, Fireside, pp 198–209, 1981.
20. Scates K: Poisonous Mushroom Chart of North America. Post Falls, ID, Kit-Scate Myco-Charts, 1996.
21. Jordan P: The New Guide to Mushrooms. New York, Smith Mark Publishers, 1996.
22. Schneider SM: Mushroom Toxicity. *In* Auerbach PS (ed): Wilderness Medicine. pp 891–907, 1995.
23. Curry SC, Rose MG: Intravenous mushroom poisoning. Ann Emerg Med *14:*900–902, 1985.
24. McPartland JM, Vilgalys RJ, Cubeta MA: Mushroom poisoning. Am Fam Phys *55:*1797–1812, 1997.
25. Thomas DS: Time-Life Books' Complete Guide to Gardening and Landscaping. New York, Simon & Schuster, pp 210–211, 1991.
26. Ingram AL: Morning glory seed reaction. JAMA *190:*107–108, 1964.
27. Green RC: Nutmeg poisoning. JAMA *171:*1342–1344, 1959.
28. Payne RB: Nutmeg intoxication. N Engl J Med *269:*36–38, 1963.
29. Haddad LM: Management of hallucinogen abuse. Am Fam Phys *14:*82–87, 1976.
30. Haddad LM: Acute poisoning. *In* Bennett JC, Plum F (eds): Cecil Textbook of Medicine, 20th ed. Philadelphia, WB Saunders, pp 503–510, 1996.

Diet Medications

31. Brenot F, Herve P, Petitpretz, et al: Primary pulmonary hypertension and fenfluramine use. Br Heart J *70:*537–541, 1993.
32. Thomas SHL, Butt AY, Corris PA, et al: Appetite suppressants and primary pulmonary hypertension in the United Kingdom. Br Heart J *74:*660–663, 1995.
33. Douglas JG, Munro JF, Kitchin AH, et al: Pulmonary hypertension and fenfluramine. Br Med J *283:*881–883, 1981.
34. Abenhaim L, Moride Y, Brenot F, et al for the International Primary Pulmonary Hypertension Study Group: Appetite-suppressant drugs and the risk of primary pulmonary hypertension. N Engl J Med *335:*609–616, 1996.
35. Atanassoff PG, Weiss BM, Schmid ER, et al: Primary hypertension and dexfenfluramine (letter). Lancet *339:*436, 1992.
36. Evrard P, Allaz AF, Urban P: Myocardial infarction associated with the use of dexfenfluramine (letter). Br Med J *301:*345, 1990.
37. Veltri JC, Temple AR: Fenfluramine poisoning. J Pediatr *87:*119–121, 1975.

Fertilizers

38. Comly HH: Cyanosis in infants caused by nitrates in well water. JAMA *129:*112–116, 1945.
39. Lukens JN: The legacy of well-water methemoglobinemia. JAMA *257:*2793–2795, 1987.
40. Johnson CJ, Bonrud PA, Dosch TL, et al: Fatal outcome of methemoglobinemia in an infant. JAMA *257:*2796, 1987.
41. Johnson CA: Methemoglobinemia: Is it coming back to haunt us? Environ Digest *1:*3–4, 1988.
42. National Pesticide Survey: Project Summary. Environmental Protection Agency, Washington, DC, 1990.
43. National Pesticide Survey: Another Look. Phase II Report. Environmental Protection Agency, Washington, DC, 1992.
44. Kross BC, Ayebo AD, Fuortes LJ: Methemoglobinemia: Nitrate toxicity in rural America. Am Fam Physician *46:*183–187, 1992.

Hydrogen Peroxide

45. Rackoff WR, Merton DF: Gas embolism after ingestion of hydrogen peroxide. Pediatrics *85:*593–594, 1990.
46. Giberson TP, Kern JD, Pettigrew DW, et al: Near-fatal hydrogen peroxide ingestion. Ann Emerg Med *18:*778, 1989.
47. Christensen DW, Faught WE, Black RE, et al: Fatal oxygen embolization after hydrogen peroxide ingestion. Crit Care Med *20:*543–544, 1992.
48. Luu TA, Kelley MT, Strauch JA, et al: Portal vein gas embolism from hydrogen peroxide ingestion. Ann Emerg Med *21:*1391–1393, 1992.
49. Sherman SJ, Boyer LV, Sibley WA: Cerebral infarction immediately after ingestion of hydrogen peroxide solution. Stroke *25:*1065–1067, 1994.

Licorice

50. Blachley JD, Knochel JP: Tobacco chewer's hypokalemia: Licorice revisited. N Engl J Med *302:*784, 1980.

51. Walker BR, Edwards CRW: Licorice-induced hypertension and syndromes of apparent mineralocorticoid excess. Endocrinol Metab Clin North Am *23*:359–377, 1994.

Nicotine

52. Petridou E, Polychronopoulou A, Kouri N, et al: Childhood poisonings from ingestion of cigarettes (letter). Lancet *346*:1296, 1995.
53. Sisselman SG, Mofenson HC, Caraccio TR: Childhood poisonings from ingestion of cigarettes (letter). Lancet *347*:200, 1996.
54. Lavoie FW, Harris TM: Fatal nicotine ingestion. J Emerg Med *9*:133–136, 1991.
55. Montaldo N, Brackett CC, Sobol T: Use of transdermal nicotine systems in a possible suicide attempt. J Am Board Fam Pract *7*:417–420, 1994.
56. Lampe KF, McCann MA: AMA Handbook of Poisonous and Injurious Plants. Chicago, Chicago Review Press, 1985.
57. Benowitz NL, Jacob P III, Denaro C, et al: Stable isotope studies of nicotine kinetics and bioavailability. Clin Pharmacol Ther *49*:270–277, 1991.
58. Fiore MC: Cigarette smoking: A clinical guide to assessment and treatment. Trends in cigarette smoking in the United States: The epidemiology of tobacco use. Med Clin North Am *76*:289–304, 1992.
59. Newcomb PA, Carbone PP: The health consequences of smoking: Cancer. Med Clin North Am *76*:305–332, 1992.
60. McBride PE: The health consequences of smoking: Cardiovascular diseases. Med Clin North Am *76*:333–354, 1992.
61. Sherman CB: The health consequences of smoking: Pulmonary disease. Med Clin North Am *76*:355–376, 1992.
62. Waters D, Lesperance J, Gladstone P, et al: Effects of cigarette smoking on the angiographic evolution of coronary arteriosclerosis. Circulation *94*:614–621, 1996.
63. Benowitz NL: Nicotine replacement therapy: What has been accomplished—can we do better? Drugs *45*:157–170, 1993.
64. Department of Health and Human Services: The Health Consequences of Smoking: Nicotine Addiction: A Report of the Surgeon General, 1988. DHHS publ No. CDC 88-8406, Government Printing Office, Washington, DC, 1988.
65. Department of Health and Human Services: Preventing Tobacco Use Among Young People: A Report of the Surgeon General. Government Printing Office, Washington, DC, 1994.
66. Benowitz NL, Henningfield JE: Establishing a nicotine threshold for addiction. N Engl J Med *331*:123–125, 1994.
67. Henningfield JE: Nicotine medications for smoking cessation. N Engl J Med *333*:1196–1203, 1995.
68. Benowitz NL, Porcher H, Sheiner L, et al: Nicotine absorption and cardiovascular effects with smokeless tobacco use: Comparison with cigarettes and nicotine gum. Clin Pharmacol Ther *44*:23–8, 1988.
69. Russell MAH: The future of nicotine replacement. Br J Addiction *86*:653–658, 1991.
70. Henningfield JE, Kozlowski LT, Benowitz NL: A proposal to develop meaningful labeling for cigarettes. JAMA *272*:312–314, 1994.
71. Taylor AE, Johnson DC, Kazemia H: Environmental tobacco smoke and cardiovascular disease. Circulation *86*:1–4, 1992.
72. Dobson AJ, Alexander HM, Heller RF, et al: Passive smoking and the risk of heart attack or coronary death. Med J Aust *154*:793–797, 1991.
73. Humble C, Croft J, Gerber A, et al: Passive smoking and 20-year cardiovascular disease mortality among non-smoking wives in Evans County, Georgia. Am J Public Health *80*:599–601, 1990.
74. Steenland K, Thun M, Lally C, et al: Environmental tobacco smoke and coronary heart disease in the American Cancer Society Cancer Prevention Study II. Circulation *94*:622–628, 1996.
75. Pirkle JL, Flegal KM, Bernert JT, et al: Exposure of the U.S. population to environmental tobacco smoke. JAMA *275*:1233–1240, 1996.
76. Hardman JG, Limbird LE, Molinoff PB, et al (eds): Goodman and Gilman's The Pharmacological Basis of Therapeutics, 9th ed. New York, McGraw-Hill, pp 191–193, 1996.
77. Gehlbach SH, Williams WA, Pery LD, et al: Green tobacco sickness: An illness of tobacco harvesters. JAMA *229*:1880–1883, 1974.
78. Green tobacco sickness in tobacco harvesters—Kentucky, 1992. MMWR *42*:237–240, 1993.
79. Ballard T, Ehlers J, Freund E, et al: Green tobacco sickness: Occupational nicotine poisoning in tobacco workers. Arch Environ Health *50*:384–389, 1995.
80. Walls RM: Rapid sequence intubation. Ann Emerg Med *22*:1008–1013, 1993.

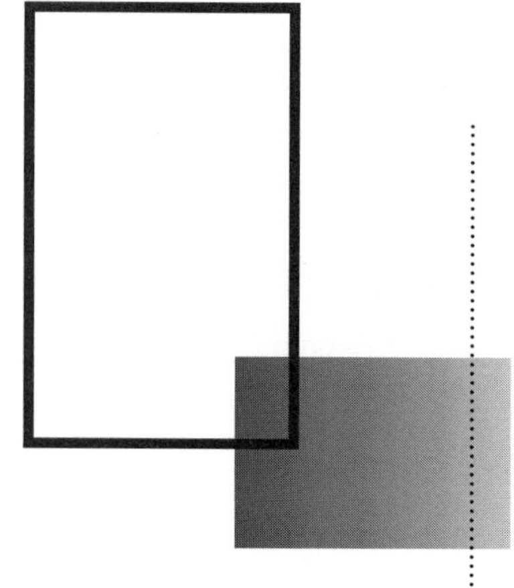

APPENDIX

Chemical Conversions of Toxicologic Laboratory Values

THOMAS S. HERMAN, PhD

THE METRIC SYSTEM

1 kilogram (kg) = 1000 grams (g)
1 gram (g) = 1000 milligrams (mg)
1 milligram (mg) = 1000 micrograms (mcg or μg)
1 microgram (μg or mcg) = 1000 nanograms (ng)
1 nanogram (ng) = 0.001 *or* 1×10^{-3} *or* $\frac{1}{1000}$ microgram
= 0.000001 *or* 1×10^{-6} *or* $\frac{1}{1,000,000}$ milligram
= 0.000000001 *or* 1×10^{-9} *or* $\frac{1}{1,000,000,000}$ gram

1 milliliter (mL) = 1 cc = 1 g = 15 drops or minims
5 mL ≅ 1 teaspoon
15 mL ≅ 1 tablespoon
30 mL ≅ 1 ounce
100 mL = 1 deciliter (dL)
1000 mL = 1 liter (L) = 1 kilogram (kg)
1 mg % (milligram per cent) = 1 milligram per 100 mL = 1 mg/dL = 1000 mcg/dL or μg/dL = 1,000,000 ng/dL
1 nanogram/mL = 0.001 μg/mL

CALCULATION OF MILLIEQUIVALENTS

1 milliequivalent (mEq) =

$$\frac{\text{the relative atomic mass of a substance in grams}}{\text{valence} \times 1000}$$

Example: How many mEq of sodium are in a 3-gram sodium diet?

1. Determine the atomic mass from the periodic table of the elements. Na = 23
2. Thus, 1 mEq of Na = $\frac{23}{1 \times 1000}$ = 0.023 g or 23 mg.
3. Thus, 1 mEq of Na = 23 mg of sodium.
4. Per 3 grams of sodium, there are $\frac{3000 \text{ mg}}{23 \text{ mg}}$ = 130.4 mEq of sodium.

OTHER CONVERSIONS

1 grain = 60 mg (occasionally rounded off to 65 mg)
ppm = parts per million = mg/liter
ppb = parts per billion = μg(mcg)/liter

Percentage Expressions

As 0.1% ethanol = 100 mg/100 cc = 0.1 g/dL = 1 g/L = 100 mg/dL = 1 mg/mL
As 10% Mucomyst = 10 grams/100 cc = 10 g/dL = 100 g/L = 10,000 mg/dL = 100 mg/mL

Example: Calculation of the Dose of Mucomyst for Acetaminophen Overdose

The initial dose of *N*-acetylcysteine (Mucomyst) for acetaminophen overdose is 140 mg/kg; subsequent doses are 70 mg/kg.

Suppose the patient weighs 132 pounds and your pharmacy has 10% Mucomyst. How much Mucomyst do you give your patient?

1. 1 kilogram = 2.2 pounds 132/2.2 = 60 kilograms
2. 10% Mucomyst means that there is 1 gram of Mucomyst in 10 mL of Mucomyst. The initial dose is 140 mg/kg. Thus, the patient should receive 60 × 140 or 8400 mg or 8.4 grams of Mucomyst (*N*-acetylcysteine).

Answer: The patient should receive 84 mL of 10% Mucomyst or 42 mL of 20% Mucomyst.

THE INTERNATIONAL SYSTEM OF UNITS

Laboratory values today are expressed in the United States in traditional units—for example, mg/dL.

In 1960, the Eleventh General Conference on Weights and Measures established the International System of Units (SI, or Systême Internationale)[1–4] as a practical system of units of measurement. SI units are laboratory standard in Europe, the Commonwealth countries, and others. An example of international units is moles per liter.

In the United States, the National Committee for Clinical Laboratory Standards has recommended phasing in most SI units in reporting clinical laboratory data.[4] Many American medical and scientific journals require that both traditional and SI units be reported. Thus, until SI units are universally accepted, practitioners should be conversant with two measurement systems.

Several aids for the interconversion of traditional and SI units commmonly encountered in toxicology are given here. The conversion aids are designed for traditional units reported as or converted to metric mass per volume and require the relative molecular or atomic mass (M_r) of the compound/element of interest. The M_r of many toxicologic compounds is listed in Table 2.

To Convert American (Traditional) Units to SI Units

1. Determine the factor from Table 1 by matching the desired SI unit column with the traditional unit row.
2. Determine the relative molecular or atomic mass (M_r) of the particular compound/element in Table 2.
3. SI unit = traditional unit ÷ (M_r × factor)
   Example: Convert 1.5 μg/L of digoxin to nmol/L:
   SI unit = 1.5 μg/L ÷ (781 × 10^{-3}) = 1.92 nmol/L

To Convert SI Units to Traditional Units

1. Determine the factor from Table 1 by matching the desired traditional unit row and SI unit column.
2. Determine the relative molecular or atomic mass (M_r) of the compound/element in Table 2.
3. Traditional unit = SI unit × (M_r × factor)
   Example: Convert 80 μmol/L of phenytoin to mg/dL:
   Traditional unit = 80 μmol/L × (252 × 10^{-4}) = 2 mg/dL

Table 1. Factors for Interconversion of SI Units and Traditional Units

Traditional Units	SI Units			
	nmol/L	μmol/L	mmol/L	mol/L
pg/mL	1	10^3	10^6	10^9
pg/dL	10^2	10^5	10^8	10^{11}
pg/L	10^3	10^6	10^9	10^{12}
ng/mL	10^{-3}	1	10^3	10^6
ng/dL	10^{-1}	10^2	10^5	10^8
ng/L	1	10^3	10^6	10^9
μg/mL	10^{-6}	10^{-3}	1	10^3
μg/dL	10^{-4}	10^{-1}	10^2	10^5
μg/L	10^{-3}	1	10^3	10^6
mg/mL	10^{-9}	10^{-6}	10^{-3}	1
mg/dL	10^{-7}	10^{-4}	10^{-1}	10^2
mg/L	10^{-6}	10^{-3}	1	10^3
g/mL	10^{-12}	10^{-9}	10^{-6}	10^{-3}
g/dL	10^{-10}	10^{-7}	10^{-4}	10^{-1}
g/L	10^{-9}	10^{-6}	10^{-3}	1

[1]Doumas BT: IFCC documents and interpretation of SI units—a solution looking for a problem. Clin Chem *25*:655, 1979.

[2]Lines JG: SI units: Another view. Clin Chem *25*:1331, 1979.

[3]Page CH, Vigouraux P (eds): The International System of Units (SI). NBS Special Publication 330. Washington, DC, US Government Printing Office, 1974.

[4]Quantities and Units: SI. NCCLS Proposed Position Paper: PCP-11. Villanova, PA, National Committee for Clinical Laboratory Standards, 1979.

Table 2. Relative Molecular Mass (M_r) of Selected Products[1–6]

Product	Trade Name	M_r	Product	Trade Name	M_r
acetaminophen	Tylenol	151.16	haloperidol	Haldol	375.87
acetone		58.08	halothane		197.38
aluminum		26.98	heroin		369.42
amitriptyline	Elavil	277.41	hydrogen sulfide		34.08
ammonia		17.03	hydromorphone	Dilaudid	285.33
amphetamine	Benzedrine	135.21	imipramine	Tofranil	280.40
amyl nitrate		117.15	lidocaine	Xylocaine	234.33
aniline		93.12	lindane		290.83
arsenic		74.92	lithium		6.94
borate		58.83	LSD		323.44
bromide		79.90	meperidine	Demerol	247.35
butabarbital	Butisol	211.25	meprobamate	Miltown	218.25
butalbital	Fiorinal	224.26	methadone	Dolophine	309.45
caffeine		194.19	methanol		32.04
carbamazepine	Tegretol	236.26	methaqualone	Quaalude	250.29
carbaryl	Sevin	201.22	methocarbamol	Robaxin	241.25
carbon monoxide		28.01	methotrexate		454.44
carbromal	Carbrital	237.11	methsuximide	Celontin	203.24
carisoprodol	Soma	260.33	methyl bromide		94.95
chloral hydrate	Noctec	165.40	methyprylon	Noludar	183.25
chloramphenicol		323.14	morphine		285.33
chlordiazepoxide	Librium	299.76	nicotine		162.23
chlorpromazine	Thorazine	318.86	nortriptyline	Aventyl	263.37
chlorpropamide	Diabinese	276.74	oxazepam	Serax	286.72
chlorazepate	Tranxene	313.72	oxycodone	Percodan	315.38
cocaine		303.35	parathion		291.27
codeine		299.36	phencyclidine	(PCP)	243.38
cyanide		26.03	phenobarbital		232.23
desipramine	Norpramin	266.39	phenytoin	Dilantin	252.26
diazepam	Valium	284.75	procainamide	Pronestyl	235.33
diazinon		304.36	promethazine	Phenergan	284.42
digitoxin		764.96	propoxyphene	Darvon	339.49
digoxin		780.95	propranolol	Inderal	259.34
diphenhydramine	Benadryl	255.37	protriptyline	Vivactil	263.38
disopyramide	Norpace	339.47	salicylate		180.15
doxepin	Sinequan	279.39	secobarbital	Seconal	238.29
ethanol		46.07	theophylline		180.17
ethchlorvynol	Placidyl	144.60	thioridazine	Mellaril	370.56
ethinamate	Valmid	167.21	tobramycin	Nebcin	467.52
ethosuximide	Zarontin	141.17	tolbutamide	Orinase	270.35
ethylene glycol		62.07	toluene		92.13
fluoride		18.99	valproic acid	Depakene	144.21
flurazepam	Dalmane	387.88	warfarin	Coumadin	308.32
formaldehyde		30.03	xylene		106.16
glutethimide	Doriden	217.27	zinc		65.37

NOTE: The molecular mass (M_r) reflects the weight of the principal base, anhydrous compound *only*. Cations such as sodium or anions such as chloride are *not* included. For example, 308.32 is the M_r for warfarin, *not* for warfarin sodium.

[1]The United States Pharmacopeia. 20th rev. Rockville, MD, US Pharmacopeia Convention, Publishers, 1980.

[2]Osol A, Pratt R (eds): The United States Dispensatory. 27th ed. Philadelphia, J.B. Lippincott Co., 1973.

[3]Physicians' Desk Reference. 34th ed. Oradell, NJ, Medical Economics Co., 1980.

[4]The Merck Index. 9th ed. Rahway, NJ, Merck and Company, 1976.

[5]Baselt RC: Analytical Procedures for Therapeutic Drug Monitoring and Emergency Toxicology. Davis, CA, Biomedical Publications, 1980.

[6]Baselt RC: Biological Monitoring Methods for Industrial Chemicals. Davis, CA, Biomedical Publications, 1980.

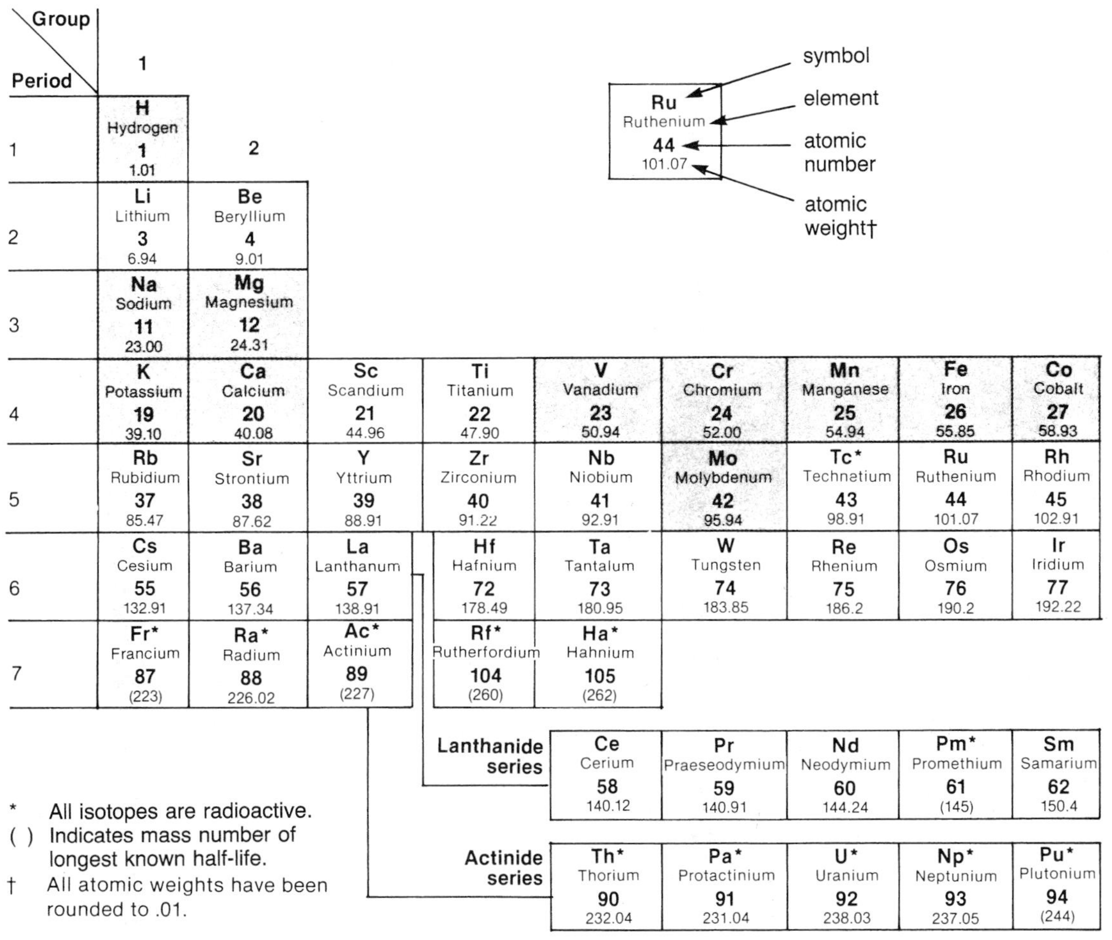

THE PERIODIC TABLE OF THE ELEMENTS

Period \ Group	1	2							
1	H Hydrogen 1 1.01								
2	Li Lithium 3 6.94	Be Beryllium 4 9.01							
3	Na Sodium 11 23.00	Mg Magnesium 12 24.31							
4	K Potassium 19 39.10	Ca Calcium 20 40.08	Sc Scandium 21 44.96	Ti Titanium 22 47.90	V Vanadium 23 50.94	Cr Chromium 24 52.00	Mn Manganese 25 54.94	Fe Iron 26 55.85	Co Cobalt 27 58.93
5	Rb Rubidium 37 85.47	Sr Strontium 38 87.62	Y Yttrium 39 88.91	Zr Zirconium 40 91.22	Nb Niobium 41 92.91	Mo Molybdenum 42 95.94	Tc* Technetium 43 98.91	Ru Ruthenium 44 101.07	Rh Rhodium 45 102.91
6	Cs Cesium 55 132.91	Ba Barium 56 137.34	La Lanthanum 57 138.91	Hf Hafnium 72 178.49	Ta Tantalum 73 180.95	W Tungsten 74 183.85	Re Rhenium 75 186.2	Os Osmium 76 190.2	Ir Iridium 77 192.22
7	Fr* Francium 87 (223)	Ra* Radium 88 226.02	Ac* Actinium 89 (227)	Rf* Rutherfordium 104 (260)	Ha* Hahnium 105 (262)				

Lanthanide series	Ce Cerium 58 140.12	Pr Praeseodymium 59 140.91	Nd Neodymium 60 144.24	Pm* Promethium 61 (145)	Sm Samarium 62 150.4
Actinide series	Th* Thorium 90 232.04	Pa* Protactinium 91 231.04	U* Uranium 92 238.03	Np* Neptunium 93 237.05	Pu* Plutonium 94 (244)

* All isotopes are radioactive.

( ) Indicates mass number of longest known half-life.

† All atomic weights have been rounded to .01.

THE PERIODIC TABLE OF THE ELEMENTS *(Continued)*

In each A group, the number of electrons (#e⁻) in the outer shell of each element is the same.

In each period, the identifying number (*n*) for the outer shell of each element is the same.

			3	4	5	6	7	8
								He Helium 2 4.00
			B Boron 5 10.81	C Carbon 6 12.01	N Nitrogen 7 14.01	O Oxygen 8 16.00	F Fluorine 9 19.00	Ne Neon 10 20.18
			Al Aluminium 13 26.98	Si Silicon 14 28.09	P Phosphorus 15 30.97	S Sulfur 16 32.06	Cl Chlorine 17 35.45	Ar Argon 18 39.95
Ni Nickel 28 58.71	Cu Copper 29 63.55	Zn Zinc 30 65.37	Ga Gallium 31 69.72	Ge Germanium 32 72.59	As Arsenic 33 74.92	Se Selenium 34 78.96	Br Bromine 35 79.90	Kr Krypton 36 83.8
Pd Palladium 46 106.4	Ag Silver 47 107.87	Cd Cadmium 48 112.40	In Indium 49 114.82	Sn Tin 50 118.69	Sb Antimony 51 121.75	Te Tellurium 52 127.60	I Iodine 53 126.90	Xe Xenon 54 131.30
Pt Platinum 78 195.09	Au Gold 79 196.97	Hg Mercury 80 200.59	Tl Thallium 81 204.37	Pb Lead 82 207.2	Bi Bismuth 83 208.98	Po* Polonium 84 (210)	At* Astatine 85 (210)	Rn* Radon 86 (222)

Eu Europium 63 151.96	Gd Gadolinium 64 157.25	Tb Terbium 65 158.93	Dy Dysprosium 66 162.50	Ho Holmium 67 164.93	Er Erbium 68 167.26	Tm Thulium 69 168.93	Yb Ytterbium 70 173.04	Lu Lutetium 71 174.97

Am* Americium 95 (243)	Cm* Curium 96 (247)	Bk* Berkelium 97 (247)	Cf* Californium 98 (251)	Es* Einsteinium 99 (254)	Fm* Fermium 100 (257)	Md* Mendelevium 101 (257)	No* Nobelium 102 (255)	Lr* Lawrencium 103 (256)

(From Berlow PB, Burton DJ, Routh JI: Introduction to the Chemistry of Life. Saunders College Publishing, Philadelphia, 1982.)

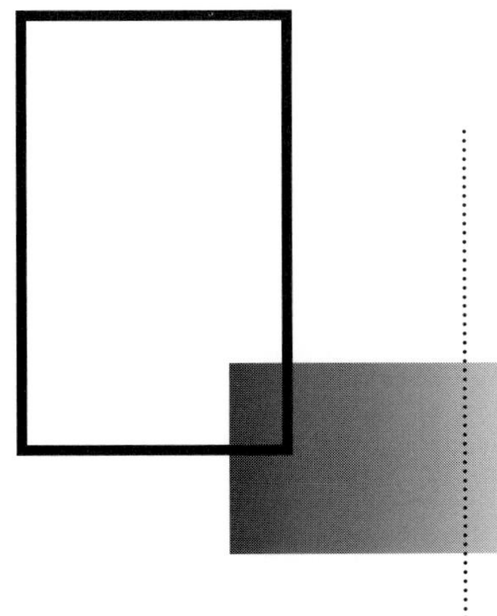

Index

Note: Page numbers in *italics* refer to illustrations; page numbers followed by t refer to tables.

ISBN 0-7216-6409-1